GEORGIAN COLLEGE
BARRIE
College & Career
Preparation Program

Nursing Foundations

A Canadian Perspective

NURSING

FOUNDATIONS

A Canadian Perspective

BEVERLY WITTER DU GAS, RN, BA, MN, EdD, LLD
President, Witter-DuGas Consultants Limited

EMILY R. KNOR, RN, BScN, MA
Langara College

Appleton & Lange Canada
Scarborough, Ontario

Canadian Cataloguing in Publication Data

Du Gas, Beverly Witter
Nursing foundations

Includes bibliographical references and index.
ISBN 0–8385–7064–X

1. Nursing. 2. Nursing — Canada. I. Knor, Emily R.
II. Title

RT41.D84 1994   610.73   C94–931522–2

© 1995   Appleton & Lange Canada
A Division of the Simon & Schuster Higher Education
Publishing Group
1870 Birchmount Road, Scarborough,
Ontario, M1P 2J7

ISBN 0–8385–7064–X

Acquisitions: Cliff Newman
Managing Editor: Marta Tomins
Production Editor: Imogen Brian
Assistant Editor: Emily Meetsma
Cover and Interior Design: Carole Giguère
Cover Image: Alex Murchison
Page Layout & Technical Illustrations: Zofia Moczulak
Medical Illustrations: Dave Mazierski, Stephen Mader

    4 5 CW 99 98 97

Printed and bound in the United States of America

Photo credits

Augustine Medical, Inc.: 759.

CanadaWide: 1173, 1237.

Canadian Nurses Association: 71, 90 , 188, 195.

Courtesy of the Canadian Red Cross Society: 692 (right).

Lyle Morrison Creelmann: 205.

Beverly Du Gas/Emily Knor: 14, 15, 18, 66, 164, 167, 174, 175, 178 (top and bottom), 180, 182, 183, 185, 186 (top and bottom), 192, 193, 196, 201, 222, 223, 226, 227, 230, 263, 279, 293, 462, 463, 464, 573, 762, 863, 880, 882, 887, 895, 935, 968, 1044, 1171, 1172, 1198, 1208, 1209, 1214, 1215, 1224.

City of Toronto Archives: 118.

Cindy Goodman, North Shore News, Courtesy of Lion's Gate Hospital, North Vancouver, BC: 162, 697.

Grey Nuns of Montreal, Sister Cécile Castonguay: 23, 225.

Langara College, Nursing Department, Vancouver, BC.: 461, 669.

Courtesy of Lion's Gate Hospital, North Vancouver, BC: 2, 112, 136, 255, 306, 308, 330, 334, 505, 572, 758, 764, 789, 794, 795, 797, 811, 824, 825, 838, 839, 851, 865, 875 (right), 921, 964, 965, 974, 981, 990, 991, 1012, 1013 (bottom right), 1014, 1022, 1040, 1041, 1052, 1054, 1146 (left), 1170, 1236, 1249.

Lauchlin McKenzie: 214, 309, 357, 364 (all), 377 (left and right), 387, 415, 421, 516, 520, 530, 540, 555, 559 (left and right), 587, 609, 654 (left and right), 655 (all), 656 (Figure 22.9 A, B, E, F, G, H), 658 (Figure 22.11), 659, 660 (all), 662, 664 (A, B), 665 (left and right), 667, 671, 688, 692 (left), 709, 738 (left and right), 742, 748 (all), 787, 808 (all), 809 (all), 861, 871, 909 (left and right), 910, 911, 912 (top and bottom), 914 (top and bottom), 915 (top and bottom), 916, 917 (top and bottom), 918, 919, 920, 923 (all), 931, 1013 (top, Figure 31.2), 1017 (top and bottom), 1018 (top and bottom), 1019 (all), 1020 (all), 1021 (all), 1026 (Figure 31.3), 1027 (all), 1028 (all), 1029 (all), 1030 (all), 1031 (all), 1032 (all), 1033, 1055, 1067 (all), 1075, 1080, 1090, 1111, 1113, 1123 (all), 1124 (all), 1125, 1126 (all), 1127 (all), 1133 (all), 1134 (all), 1139, 1140 (all), 1144, 1145, 1146 (right), 1150, 1187.

Memorial Nurse Portrait Collection of the BC History of Nursing Groups. Dolls designed by Sheila Rankin Zerr: 89.

Multicultural Health Education Program of the Vancouver Health Department: 9, 50, 61, 76, 81, 100, 145, 163, 165, 181, 254, 266, 278, 280, 356, 401, 420, 460, 477, 928, 949, 1213.

National Archives of Canada: 6.

Courtesy of the National Archives of Canada, Henri Beau (artist): 7.

North Shore News, Courtesy of Lion's Gate Hospital, North Vancouver, BC: 307, 875 (left).

Courtesy of the Registered Nurses Association of British Columbia: 3, 39, 86, 87, 113, 210 (top and bottom), 331, 350, 417, 430, 447, 449, 720, 929, 1091, 1114, 1143.

Courtesy of Respiratory Services, St. Paul's Hospital, Vancouver, BC: 60, 446, 703, 713, 728.

Alice Katherine Smith: 299.

Marta Tomins: 862.

University of Alberta, Office of Public Affairs: 269.

University of British Columbia Library, Special Collections and University Archives Division: 149.

Courtesy of the Vancouver General Hospital Nurses Alumnae Association Archives: 4, 44.

The Vancouver Health Department: 137, 426.

Courtesy of Vancouver Hospital and Health Sciences Centre: 608, 656 (C and D), 658 (Figure 22.10), 663 (top and bottom), 664 (C, D, E, F).

Victoria General Hospital, Winnipeg, MN: 786.

Victorian Order of Nurses for Canada: 43.

Kate Williams, Courtesy of The Richmond Hospital, Richmond, BC: 5, 38, 390, 400, 860, 876, 922, 924, 930, 940.

Figure credits

Figure 2.1: copyright by American Public Health Association

Figures 2.7, 2.10, 2.11, 12.1, 12.2, 12.3, 12.4, 12.5, 12.6, 12.7, 29.1. Tables 12.1 and 12.2: Reproduced by authority of the Minister of Industry, 1994. Readers wishing further information on data provided through the cooperation of Statistics Canada may obtain copies of related publications by mail from: Publication Sales, Statistics Canada, Ottawa, Ontario, K1A 0T6, by calling 1-613-951-7277 or toll-free 1-800-267-6677. Readers may also facsimile their order by dialling 1-613-951-1584.

Figures 2.13, 2.14, 2.15, 4.2, 4.3: Reproduced with the permission of the Minister of Supply and Services Canada 1994.

Figure 3.3: From *Preliminary Estimates of Health Expenditures in Canada: Provincial/Territorial Summary Report 1987-1991*, Health Canada, 1994. Reproduced with permission of the Minister of Supply and Services Canada 1994.

Figure 4.1: Special thanks to The Danish Nurses' Organization, The Association of Registered Nurses of Newfoundland and Dr. Dorothy Hall.

Figures 5.1, 5.2, 5.4, 5.6, 5.7, 5.9: Reproduced with permission from *The Canadian Nurse/L'infirmière canadienne*.

Figure 9.2: Reprinted with permission of Aspen Publishers, Inc.

CONTRIBUTORS

CHRISTINA M. BECKETT, RN, Dip. Critical Care,
Dip. Business Management Administration
Manager, Client Services
Health Vision Corporation
Richmond, B.C.
Chapter 18

E. GAIL BREMER, RN, BSN
Faculty, Nursing Department, Langara College
IV Therapist, Vancouver Hospital and Health
Sciences Centre
Vancouver, B.C.
Chapter 22, 23

RHODA L. BROOKE, RN, BSN, MEd
Faculty, Nursing Department
Langara College
Vancouver, B.C.
Chapter 33

LYNN CHASE, RN, BScN
Instructor, Education Department
Vancouver Hospital and Health Sciences Centre
Chapter 22

HEATHER CLARKE, RN, PhD
Nursing Research Consultant
Registered Nurses Association of British Columbia
and Adjunct Professor
School of Nursing
University of British Columbia
Vancouver, B.C.
Chapter 7

BETTY DAVIES, RN, PhD
Professor, School of Nursing, University of British
Columbia and Investigator, Research Division
B.C.'s Children's Hospital
Vancouver, B.C.
Chapter 36

KAREN E. DEIGHTON, RN, BSN, MEd
Faculty, Nursing Department
Langara College
Vancouver, B.C.
Chapter 19, 20

KATIE DE LEON-DEMARE, RN, BN, MN
Lecturer, Faculty of Nursing
University of Manitoba
Winnipeg, Manitoba
Chapter 24

LENORE DU GAS, RN, BScN
Enterostomy Therapist,
Prince George Regional Hospital
Prince George, B.C.
Nurses at Work, Chapter 17

JANET ERICKSEN, RN, MA
Assistant Professor, School of Nursing
University of British Columbia
Vancouver, B.C.
Chapter 6

WENDY FALLIS, RN, BScN, MN
Director of Research and Special Projects
Victoria General Hospital, Winnipeg, Manitoba
Chapter 24

HEATHER D. FRASER-DAVEY, RN, PhD
Associate Professor
School of Nursing
Dalhousie University
Halifax, Nova Scotia
Chapter 8

SUSAN C. GALLOWAY, RN, MScN
Clinical Nurse Specialist — General Surgery
Sunnybrook Health Science Centre
North York, Ontario
Chapter 32

ANN GASSON, RN, BA
Staff Nurse
Children's Hospital of British Columbia
Vancouver, B.C.
Nurses at Work, Chapter 10

LINDA D. GOMEZ, RN, MSN
Faculty, Nursing Department
Langara College
Vancouver, B.C.
Chapter 33

J. KIRSTINE GRIFFITH, BASc (Nursing), MA
(Adult Education)
Freelance research assistant
Looking Back vignettes

DORIS GRINSPUN, RN, MSN, CRRN
Program Director, Nursing
Mount Sinai Hospital
Toronto, Ontario
Chapter 13

BARBARA HESTRIN, RN
Nursing Clinician
B.C.'s Women's Hospital and Health Centre
Vancouver, B.C.
Chapter 34

PAULA L. HUSBAND, RN, BSN
Instructor, Nursing Department
Camosun College, Victoria, B.C.
Chapter 23

PATRICIA L. JESSELSON, RN, BScN
Manager, Patient Care Information Department
Greater Victoria Hospital Society
Chapter 18

NANCY JOHNSTON, RN, MHSc
Chief Executive Officer, Nursing
The Clarke Institute of Psychiatry
Toronto, Ontario
Chapter 16

ANN S. KARL, RN, MScN
Assistant Director of Care
and Clinical Coordinator
Amherst Private Hospital
Vancouver, B.C.
Chapter 18

YVES LAFORTUNE, BEd, MEd
Manager, Business Development and Test
Administration
Canadian Nurses Association, Testing Division
Ottawa, Ontario
CNA *Nurse-Registration/Licensure Examination*

VANESSA LAM, BScN, RN
Community Health Nurse
Vancouver Health Department, West Main Unit
Vancouver, B.C.
Nurses at Work, Chapter 9

CHRISTINE M. MACDONALD-CLARKSON, RN, MSN
Faculty, Nursing Department
Langara College
Vancouver, B.C.
Chapter 21

SUE MAVINIC, RN, BScN
Clinical Supply and Equipment Coordinator
Lions Gate Hospital
North Vancouver, B.C.
Chapter 15

CHERRY NETTLETON, RN, BScN
Case Manager
Boundary Health Unit
Surrey, B.C.
Nurses at Work, Chapter 11

DIANNE L. Noel, RN, CCOHN
Occupational Health Nurse
Surrey Memorial Hospital
Surrey, B.C.
Chapter 29

PATRICIA A. PICKETTS, RN, MEd
Instructor, Grant MacEwan Community College,
Edmonton, Alberta
Instructor, Athabasca University
Athabasca, Alberta
Chapter 15, Health History Guides

WANDA PIERSON, RN, MSN
Faculty, Nursing Department
Langara College
Vancouver, B.C.
Chapter 25, 26

BARBARA J. STODDARD, BSR
Acting Chief, Rehabilitation
The Richmond Hospital
Richmond, B.C.
Chapter 28

D. ROBERTA SWANSON, RN, MSN
Faculty, Nursing Department
Langara College
Vancouver, B.C.
Chapter 7

AUDREY J. TOLHURST, RN, BN, MEd
Faculty, Nursing Department
Langara College
Vancouver, B.C.
Chapter 28

CHRISTINE WASYLISHYN, RN, BScN
Faculty, Nursing Department
Langara College
Vancouver, B.C.
Chapter 30

MOIRA M. WALKER, RN, CIC
Senior Infection Control Nurse
Vancouver Hospital and Health Sciences Centre
Vancouver, B.C.
Chapter 31

SUSAN WARD, BSc, MHA
Acting Manager, Test Development and
Consultation
Canadian Nurses Association, Testing Division
Ottawa, Ontario
CNA *Nurse-Registration/Licensure Examination*

ANN WESTWOOD, RN, BScN, MSN
Faculty, Nursing Department
Langara College
Vancouver, B.C.
Chapter 10

CAROLINE WIEBE, RN, BScN,
Community Health Nurse
Inuvik Regional Health Services
North West Territories
Nurses at Work, Chapter 12

GLENNIS N. ZILM, RN, BSN, BJ, MA
Writer and editor in the nursing field
Surrey, B.C.
Looking Back vignettes

CELESTE BARRETT, RN, MScN
Assistant Professor
School of Nursing
Dalhousie University
Halifax, Nova Scotia

P. LYNN BUHLER, BScN, RN
Manager, Prevention Program
Vancouver Health Department, West Main Unit
Vancouver, B.C.
Chapter 11

PAMELA NOVAK CAWLEY, RN, BSN, MEd
Faculty, Nursing Department
Langara College
Vancouver, B.C.
Chapter 22

MARGARET CHAD, BSN
Instructor
Diploma Nursing Program
SIAST, Kelsey Institute
Saskatoon, Saskatchewan

WANDA CHERNOMAS, PhD, RN
Lecturer
Faculty of Nursing
University of Manitoba
Winnipeg, Manitoba

BARBARA DAVIES, RN, MScN
Assistant Professor
School of Nursing
University of Ottawa
Ottawa, Ontario
Chapter 7

MARILYN E. DEWIS, RN, MEd
Assistant Professor
Faculty of Nursing
University of British Columbia
Vancouver, B.C.

GAYE GREAVES, RN, BNSc, MEd, EdD
Assistant Professor
Faculty of Nursing
Queen's University
Kingston, Ontario

NORA J. HAMMELL, RN, MEd.,MScN
Nursing Policy Consultant
Canadian Nurses Association
Ottawa, Ontario
Chapter 5

SYLVIA M. HINZ, RN, BSN
Instructor
Diploma Nursing Program
SIAST, Kelsey Institute
Saskatoon, Saskatchewan

SYLVIE LE MAY, RN, MScN
Assistant Professor
Faculty of Nursing
University of Montreal
Montreal, Quebec

JUDY RISEBROUGH, RN, MA(Ed)
Director of Nursing
Al-Salma Hospital
Jeddah, Saudi Arabia
Chapter 2, 22

ANNIE J. STARR, PhD, RN
Assistant Professor
Faculty of Nursing
University of Western Ontario
London, Ontario

DANA WERTENBERGER, PhD, RN
Director, University of Alberta Hospitals
and Professor
School of Nursing
University of Alberta
Edmonton, Alberta

CATHERINE WINTERHALDT, RN, BScN, DipPH
Regional Nursing Officer, Pacific Region
Medical Services Branch, Health Canada
Chapter 12

SHEILA J. RANKIN ZERR, RN, MEd
Visiting Assistant Professor
School of Nursing
University of Victoria
Victoria, B.C.
Chapter 13

CONSULTANTS

HELEN E. ARMSTRONG, RDN
    Chairman
    Nutrition & Food Services Management
        Department
    Langara College,
    Vancouver, B.C.
        Chapter 19

RUTH A. BROMLEY, BHE, MEd, RDN
    Faculty
    Nutrition & Food Services Management
        Department
    Langara College,
    Vancouver, B.C.
        Chapter 19

BUD DU GAS, Dip Mgmt Admin
    Director, Assessments
    Workers' Compensation Board of British Columbia
        Chapter 29

SHARON HELIN (MPH) and Associates
    Community Health Consultants
    Richmond, B.C.
        Chapter 12

SUSAN E. HICKS, RN, MScN
    Nursing Policy Consultant
    Canadian Nurses Association
    Ottawa, Ontario
        Chapter 5, 6

INA JUSUFOVIC, RT
    Teaching Technologist
    The Canadian Red Cross Society
    Vancouver, B.C.
        Chapter 22

A. P. (AIME) LEHOUILLIER, Captain
    Fire Prevention Officer, Fire Department
    West Vancouver, B.C.
        Chapter 29

SHARON E. LIVERSIDGE, RN, BSN
    Faculty, Nursing Department
    Langara College
    Vancouver, B.C.
        Chapter 33

SHARON L. NIELD, RN, BN, MA
    Nursing Policy Consultant
    Canadian Nurses Association
    Ottawa, Ontario
        Chapter 5

FOCUS GROUP PARTICIPANTS

LINDA BARRETT, RN, BA, MA
    Instructor
    Faculty of Nursing
    British Columbia Institute of Technology

MARILYN DEWIS, RN, MED
    Assistant Professor
    Faculty of Nursing
    University of British Columbia
    Vancouver, B.C.

KATHERINE DOYLE, RN, BN, MA
    Instructor
    Faculty of Nursing
    British Columbia Institute of Technology

CHERYL ENTWHISTLE, MSN, RN
    Program Director
    Nursing Outreach Program
    University of British Columbia
    Vancouver, B.C.

FRANCES JOHNSON, BScN, MEd
    Instructor
    General Nursing Program
    Douglas College

MARY KRUGER, RN, MScN, EdD
    Faculty, Nursing Department
    Langara College
    Vancouver, B.C.

SHEILA J. RANKIN ZERR, RN, MEd
    Visiting Assistant Professor
    Department of Nursing
    University of Victoria
    Victoria, B.C.

SUPPLEMENTAL TEACHING AND LEARNING AIDS

Instructor's Manual

This valuable teaching aid includes:
- Chapter overviews
- A list of the diagrams, tables, and boxed material found in the text
- Key terms with page numbers
- Central questions referenced in detail to the relevant sections of the text
- Ideas for classroom teaching
- Ideas for laboratory/clinical experience
- Suggested resources

Test Item File

The TIF has more than 1500 multiple-choice questions with page number references and answers.

Computerized Test Item File

This best-selling state-of-the-art test generation software program is available free to adopters.

Application Problem Test Bank

This second test bank contains in-depth application questions to test students' understanding of the principles covered in the text.

Transparencies/Transparency Masters

These transparencies and black-line transparency masters contain a selection of key diagrams, tables and boxes from the text for classroom use.

Study Guide

An invaluable supplement for students, the Study Guide helps to review the theories, concepts and techniques presented in the text. It contains:
- Learning objectives
- Key terms
- Detailed chapter outlines
- 800 self-test questions with answers at the back
- 400 review questions

ACKNOWLEDGEMENTS

In the preparation of this book we have had the help of a great many nursing colleagues and other individuals whom we would like to acknowledge here. First of all, we would like to thank the numerous nursing teachers who contributed ideas and made suggestions in focus groups or through written input which helped to shape the direction this book has taken. Then, there are the colleagues who contributed content for various chapters and the people we consulted on specific topics, each of whom enriched the subject matter with their specialized expertise. Their names are listed on the preceding pages. In addition, because we were covering new ground with much of the content of this book, we enlisted the help of some of our colleagues to review various chapters and these individuals we would also like to thank for their helpful suggestions on content and organization. Their names are also listed.

We would also like to thank Lauchlin McKenzie for his patience and his skill in taking photographs for most of the clinical chapters in the book and Jean Blake, Betty Ross and Denise Sharron of the Lion's Gate Hospital for their excellent photos of nurses at work in their clinical setting. We are also grateful to the Vancouver Health Department, the Registered Nurses Association of British Columbia, the Richmond Hospital, the Canadian Red Cross Society, the Vancouver Hospital and Health Sciences Centre and the Respiratory Services of St. Paul's Hospital who gave us permission to use some of their photographs in this book.

The assistance of Kirstine Griffith with research for this book and supportive help through the various stages of its preparation is gratefully acknowledged. We would also like to give a special thank-you to Frank Knor for his invaluable assistance with the technological aspects that are so important in this day of electronic writing, as well as his help in researching material for the text. Nor should we forget the assistance of Martha Ippersiel and staff of the Helen K. Mussallem Library at the Canadian Nurses Association and Joan Andrews and Carol MacFarlane and staff at the Helen Randal Library of the Registered Nurses Association of British Columbia.

We would also like to express our appreciation to the Victorian Order of Nurses for permission to use material from the unpublished history of that organization.

Special thanks are due to Walter Bailey who believed in the need for a basic nursing text with a Canadian perspective and started us on our joint writing endeavours.

We must also give thanks to the editors, artists and production staff of Appleton & Lange Canada and Allyn & Bacon Canada who provided helpful advice and supportive encouragement throughout the lengthy process of preparing this text and readying it for publication.

This book was written to provide a basic nursing text for students and their teachers that is in line with current trends in health care in Canada and around the world. *Nursing Foundations* has a health-promotion orientation based on health rather than illness, with emphasis on the socioeconomic and environmental determinants of health and well-being that go beyond the lifestyle model. As so beautifully and succinctly stated by Sister Simone Roach, nursing is the professionalization of caring, a philosophy that is evidenced in a holistic approach to the care of individuals, families and communities.

The authors believe that beginning nursing students should have an understanding of the health care system in which they will practise as graduates, the philosophy on which the system is based and their role in providing nursing services to individuals, families and communities. We also believe that, in their introductory courses in nursing, students should gain a solid foundation of knowledge and skills in basic nursing on which to build in more senior courses.

The book has been divided into seven units. Unit 1 introduces students to the role of the nurse in today's health services in both hospitals and the community. Writing from a Canadian perspective, the authors discuss first of all, changing views on health and its determinants as these have evolved over the years. This is followed by a description of the development and present structure of Canada's health care system and the services provided for people under our national health insurance program—services that are increasingly based on a primary health care philosophy that emphasizes health promotion throughout the life cycle. The remaining chapters in this unit outline nursing practice and nursing education in Canada, the legal and ethical basis of practice and the role of research in nursing practice.

The focus of Unit 2 is on health as it relates to basic human needs of the individual, the family and the community, with a chapter on the health needs of people of different cultural and ethnic backgrounds. Included in this chapter is a discussion on meeting the health needs of the people of our First Nations.

The third unit introduces students to the theoretical basis of nursing and to the methodology of nursing practice, giving them both a conceptual framework and the tools needed to begin their clinical practice. Included are chapters on nursing theories and conceptual frameworks, on nursing process and on clinical assessment, on communication and teaching and learning skills and on the documentation of nursing care.

In Units 4–7, the student is introduced to the care of people who need help in meeting their basic needs regardless of their medical diagnosis. Starting with basic physiological needs, this half of the book looks at needs throughout the life cycle. Emphasis is placed on the nurse's role in promoting optimal health through helping people make decisions and take control of their own health and in providing supportive assistance as needed. The nursing process serves as an organizing framework for these chapters which cover assessment, diagnostic reasoning, planning, implementation and evaluation of nursing care related to each of the basic needs. Nursing interventions for health promotion and health protection, for health restoration and supportive care are included for each basic human need. Strategies for promoting health in everyday living are highlighted.

Features which enrich this book include historical and modern vignettes of Canadian nurses and selected research reviews. The historical vignettes of "first ladies" in Canadian nursing which appear in each chapter in Units 1 and 2 introduce students to the rich heritage of nursing in this country, while the vignettes in Unit 3 of Canadian nurses at their daily work paint a vivid picture of the diversity of current nursing practice. The selected research reviews in clinical chapters in the final units bring to life for students the concept of research-based practice through examples of the use of nursing research in clinical practice.

Except for the first chapter, which serves as an introduction to the text, each chapter begins with an outline of content and a set of central questions as guides to learning. Each contains an introduction and a review, a list of key terms, a set of learning activities and a list of references and selected readings to aid students. In addition, inset boxes emphasize principles of care and highlight other important material in each chapter.

In this text, the authors have opted to use the term "patient," rather than "client" to refer to the recipient of nursing care. Our rationale for doing so is our belief that "client" is a generic term, referring to anyone who seeks help from a professional practitioner, regardless of the nature of that person's practice. That is to say, a person becomes a "client" when seeking the services of a lawyer, an engineer, an accountant or any other individual who has special qualifications for practice in his or her field. On the other hand, the term "patient" refers specifically to an individual who has sought the help of a health professional. In this sense, both "client" and "patient" can be considered correct, with "patient" the more specific term.

Common Abbreviations

Note: Abbreviations in common use can vary widely from place to place. Each institution's list of acceptable abbreviations is the best authority for its records.

°C	degrees Centigrade
@	at
ABG	arterial blood gas
a.c.	before meals
ad lib	freely as desired
ADL	activities of daily living
AIDS	acquired immunodeficiency syndrome
AM	morning
Ba	barium
b.i.d.	two times a day
BM, bm	bowel movement
BMR	basal metabolic rate
BP	blood pressure
BRP	bathroom privileges
BSA	body surface area
BUN	blood urea nitrogen
č	with
Ca	calcium, cancer, carcinoma
CAD	coronary artery disease
cap	capsule
CAT	computed axial tomography
CBC	complete blood count
CBR	complete bed rest
cc	cubic centimetre
CCU	coronary care unit, critical care unit
CDC	Centres for Disease Control
CHF	congestive heart failure
CHO	carbohydrate
Cl	chlorine
cm	centimetre
CNS	central nervous system
CO	carbon monoxide
CO_2	carbon dioxide
COPD	chronic obstructive pulmonary disease
CPR	cardiopulmonary resuscitation
CSF	cerebrospinal fluid
CT	computed tomography
CVA	cerebrovascular accident, costovertebral angle
CVP	central venous pressure
D&C	dilation and curettage
DC	discontinue
DOE	dyspnea on exertion
dx, DX	diagnosis
ECF	extracellular fluid
ECG (EKG)	electrocardiogram
EEG	electroencephalogram
elix	elixer
ER	emergency room
ESR	erythrocyte sedimentation rate
EST	electroshock therapy
Fe	iron
FEV	forced expiratory volume
FHR	fetal heart rate
FRC	functional residual capacity
FUO	fever of unknown origin
g, gm, Gm	gram
GI	gastrointestinal
gtt	drops
GU	genitourinary
GYN, Gyn	gynecological
H_2O	water
h (hr)	hour
H^+	hydrogen ion
Hb (Hgb)	hemoglobin
Hct	hematocrit
Hg	mercury
HIV	human immunodeficiency (AIDS) virus
hs (h.s.)	at bedtime
I&O	intake and output
IC	inspiratory capacity
ICP	intracranial pressure
ICU	intensive care unit
IDDM	insulin-dependent diabetes mellitus
Ig	immunoglobulin
IgA, etc	immunoglobulin A, etc
IM	intramuscular
IOP	intraocular pressure
IPPB	intermittent positive pressure breathing
IV	intravenous
K	potassium
kg	kilogram
KVO	keep vein open
L	litre
LLE	left lower extremity
LLQ	left lower quadrant
LUE	left upper extremity
LUQ	left upper quadrant
m	metre
MAP	mean arterial pressure
mcg	microgram
mg	milligram
Mg	magnesium
MI	myocardial infarction
ml	millilitre
mm	millimetre
mm^3	cubic millimetre
mm Hg	millimetres of mercury
MRI	magnetic resonance imaging
N	nitrogen
Na	sodium
nm	nanometre
NMR	nuclear magnetic resonance
NPO	nothing by mouth
NS	normal saline
O_2	oxygen
OD	right eye; optical density; overdose
OL	left eye
OOB	out of bed
OS	left eye
OT	occupational therapy
OTC	over-the-counter
p.c.	after meals
PCP	pulmonary capillary pressure
PCWP	pulmonary capillary wedge pressure
PE	physical examination
PEEP	positive end expiratory pressure
PEG	pneumoencephalography
per	through, by way of
PERRLA	pupils equal, round, and reactive to light and accommodation
pH	hydrogen ion concentration (acidity and alkalinity)
PKU	phenylketonuria
PM	evening
p.o.	orally
ppm	parts per million

p.r.n. (prn)	when required, as often as necessary
PT	physical therapy; prothrombin time
PTT	partial thromboplastin time
q.	every
q.2.h.	every 2 hours
q.3.h.	every 3 hours
q.4.h.	every 4 hours
q.d.	every day
q.h.	every hour
q.i.d.	four times a day
qs	quantity sufficient
R/O	rule out
RDA	recommended daily (dietary) allowance
Rh+	positive Rh factor
Rh−	negative Rh factor
RLE	right lower extremity
RLQ	right lower quadrant
ROM	range of motion
RUE	right upper extremity
RUQ	right upper quadrant
Rx	take; treatment
š	without
SC	subcutaneous
Sig	write on label
sol	solution, dissolved
SR	sedimentation rate
ss	half
stat	immediately
susp	suspension
t.i.d.	three times a day
TKO	to keep open
TLC	total lung capacity
TPN	total parenteral nutrition
TPR	temperature, pulse and respirations
tr	tincture
URI	upper respiratory infection
UTI	urinary tract infection
via	by way of
VC	vital capacity
VDA	visual discriminatory acuity
VS	vital signs
V$_T$	tidal volume
WBC	white blood cell, white blood count

Prefixes

adeno-	gland
ante-	before, forward
arthro-	joint
bi-	double
bili-	bile
brachio-	arm
brady-	slow
broncho-	bronchus (pl. bronchi)
cardio-	heart
cervico-	neck
chole-	gall or bile
chondro-	cartilage
colpo-	vagina
contra-	against, opposite
costo-	ribs
cranio-	skull
cysto-	bladder
cyto-	cell
derma-	skin
dorso-	back
encephal-	brain
entero-	intestine
eryth-	red
gastro-	stomach
glosso-	tongue
glyco-	sugar
hemo-	blood
hepato-	liver
hyper-	too much, high
hypo-	not enough, low
hystero-	uterus
laparo-	loin, flank, abdomen
laryngo-	larynx
leuk-	white
litho-	stone
mast-	breast
medio-	middle
myelo-	bone marrow, spinal cord
myo-	muscle
nephro-	kidney
neuro-	nerve
oculo-	eye
os-	mouth, bone
osteo-	bone
oto-	ear
ped-	child, foot
pharyngo-	pharynx
phleb-	vein
pneumo-	air, lungs
post-	after
pre-	before
pyelo-	pelvis of kidney
rhin-	nose
salpingo-	tube
sclero-	hard, hardening
skeleto-	skeleton
sub-	under, below
super-	above, excess
supra-	above
tachy-	fast
teno-	tendon
thoraco-	chest
thyro-	thyroid, gland
trache-	trachea
trachel-	neck
vaso-	vessel

Suffixes

-cele	tumour, swelling
-centesis	surgical puncture to remove fluid
-ectomy	a cutting out or excision
-emia	blood
-itis	inflammation
-lithiasis	presence of stones
-lysis	disintegration
-oma	tumour
-opathy	disease of
-orrhaphy	surgical repair
-oscopy	examination by means of a lighted instrument
-ostomy	formation of a fistula or opening
-otomy	a cutting or incision
-pexy	fixation
-plasty	plastic surgery
-plegia	paralysis
-rhage	to burst forth
-rhea	excessive discharge

Special Features Boxes and Procedures

ℬRIEF ℐABLE OF ℭONTENTS

Detailed Table of Contents

UNIT 2 DIMENSIONS OF HEALTH   162

UNIT 6 PROTECTION AND SAFETY NEEDS   928

UNIT 7 PSYCHOSOCIAL NEEDS   1170

NURSING
FOUNDATIONS

A Canadian Perspective

U N I T 1

Health Care
and the Practice of Nursing

Introduction to Health Care

OUTLINE

INTRODUCTION

Caring is the most common criterion of humanness. . . . No discipline is seen to be so directly and intimately involved in caring needs and behaviours as nursing. . . . Nursing is (in essence) the professionalization of caring.

Sister Simone Roach, 1992

The mission of nursing is to serve humanity by assisting people in the promotion, protection and restoration of health or to comfort and support them in the event of incurable illness. In carrying out this mission, nursing responds to the needs of the people it serves, constantly modifying its practice to meet the challenges brought about by ever-changing societal forces. As beginning students in nursing, you are entering the profession at a time when nursing is poised to take a major role in the restructuring of health services in this country. In this chapter we will introduce some of the changes that are taking place in our society and examine the effects these changes are having on nursing.

THE CHANGING IMAGE OF NURSING

Nursing in Canada has a long and honourable history — it has played an integral role in Canadian society from the time the first colonists arrived on the shores of New France. Long before Florence Nightingale ushered in the era of modern nursing in Britain, French nursing sisters were practising a comprehensive type of nursing care in the precarious environment of the New World.

Nursing still remains at the forefront of health care in Canada. Nurses constitute the largest single group of health care providers in the country. At the present time, most nurses work in hospitals where their expertise is considered the key determinant of excellence in hospital care, according to the Chief Executive Officers of hospitals (Banning, 1992). In Canada, nursing has always been held in high regard; today, nursing is a career with growing opportunities and attractive financial rewards.

FROM SCIENCE TO HUMANISM

The latter half of this century has been characterized by a tremendous explosion of knowledge in all the sciences. The amount of knowledge in the biomedical field alone was said to have more than doubled in the 25 years between 1950 and 1975 — and the field has continued to expand. During the 1950s and 1960s and well into the following decade, we were enamoured with science and all the technological wonders that were becoming part of our everyday lives. In the biomedical field, increasingly complex surgery, such

Arrival of Ursuline Nuns at Quebec, 1639

as organ transplants and micro-optic and laser surgery, became possible. From the end of the 1970s, however, we have been witnessing a growing disenchantment with science. The technological age has had a tendency to depersonalize many aspects of our lives, as machines have taken over so many tasks that people used to do. Patients tell us they feel dehumanized and alienated as they are hooked up to various bottles and machines and surrounded by faceless people in masks and gowns. They long for a human touch and some recognition of their existence as people — not just appendages at the end of a machine. At the same time, nurses often feel as if they are spending their time caring for machines rather than people and they feel frustrated that they cannot give patients the personal type of care they know they should give.

While science has provided answers to many questions in the health field, it has, in many cases, ignored the human component of care. This has brought about a return to *humanism* — an approach that puts the human being back at the centre of care. We see this shift to a more human approach in the workplace in general as well as in the health field. In factories, assembly lines are being replaced with small teams of workers who share in company policy-making and participate in management of the organization. Employees in a number of companies buy into the organization, in many instances to save it from bankruptcy, and they develop a keen sense of identity with the company. Job-sharing is another recent innovation that helps to better meet the needs of parents by enabling them to maintain their professional careers while fulfilling family commitments.

This shift towards humanism has been particularly evident in health care. The traditional values on which nursing is based — those of caring and nurturing — are becoming universally recognized as essential ingredients in the process of healing. Until fairly recently, caring and nurturing were looked upon as strictly women's work and, as such, of not

JEANNE MANCE 1606–1673

Jeanne Mance, nurse and extraordinary hospital administrator, was the first woman to earn an important place in the history of New France. She was founder of the Hôtel-Dieu de Ville-Marie (hospital) and is considered, along with Paul de Chomedey de Maisonneuve, cofounder of Montreal.

Jeanne Mance was born in 1606, the tenth child in a distinguished and well-to-do family in Langares, France. She was educated in an Ursuline convent, where she learned the basics of nursing, as befitted a woman destined to head a household, although she soon announced she would devote her life to the Church. During her young adult years, France was at war and, as her home was in a battle area, she assisted with nursing care of the sick and wounded. Then, in 1640, she heard of a proposal to found a second colony in New France, and resolved to establish a hospital there. She immediately began to raise funds for the enterprise and obtained sufficient capital from Madame Angelique Faure de Bullion to enable her to join the expedition.

After a gruelling voyage, Jeanne and the other members of the expedition were forced to remain the winter in Quebec City, where she learned more nursing skills by working with the trained Augustinian sisters who had established the first hospital in Canada. In the Spring of 1642, the colonists journeyed on to Ville Marie, now Montreal, and Jeanne Mance built her hospital. Although the first year she did not have many patients, she soon was required to use all her nursing skills and by 1645 needed a larger building. During the next 28 years, she made three voyages to France to raise funds and to bring out trained nuns for her growing hospital. She died in 1673, in Montreal, respected and revered throughout the Colony she had helped to found.

Glennis Zilm

---

much value in the "real world." Psychologists tell us that the distinction between what are considered male and female attributes is rapidly blurring, however, and personality traits like sensitivity and compassion are being recognized as legitimate for men as well as women. Fathers are encouraged in many cultures to express their nurturing instincts more openly; they help with child care as well as cooking meals and sharing household tasks in most two-parent households. An increasing number of men are entering nursing schools; even in our North American "pioneer" society, nursing has become a socially acceptable profession for men.

These are exciting times for nurses — and for all who work in the health field. In Canada, we are in the process of undergoing major health reforms as we redefine health and reconsider what constitutes health care, how it should be managed and where and how it should be delivered. Our ponderous health care system is finally shifting from one that was disease-oriented and hospital-based to one that is focussed on health and is based primarily in the home and the community. Patients and families are regarded as important and active participants in health and in healing. Nurses at all levels must be able to function as effectively in the home and in the community as they do in the hospital.

The reforms in health care that are currently taking place have accelerated changes in nursing. The nurse's role as a member of the health team has undergone rapid change in the past two decades. Gone are the days when the nurse was "handmaiden" to the physician. Instead, we see the nurse as someone who participates as an equal member of the health team and shares a collegial relationship with other health professionals. Graduates of today's nursing schools are prepared with the knowledge and skills to identify health needs, to articulate these to other members of the health team and to participate fully in decisions regarding care. Furthermore, nurses are demanding — and receiving — a share in the governance of health services. Authority is being decentralized in health care agencies as supervisory positions are eliminated and head nurses assume more direct control of all aspects of care on their units, including hiring staff and writing policies. Staff nurses now sit on senior management committees in many hospitals and nurses participate in health policy-making decisions at all levels of government — local, provincial and federal.

The education of nurses is also changing and, again, the momentum has picked up in recent years. The Canadian Nurses Association in 1982 recommended the baccalaureate as the entry level requirement for professional nursing practice and in all parts of the country this transition is now in process. In a number of provinces, colleges and universities have formed collaborative partnerships for developing and offering baccalaureate programs in nursing. Some of the programs are designed with exit points midway through the course of studies, permitting students to enter the workforce earlier, if they so wish. A common curriculum, shared by a number of institutions, facilitates re-entry into the program at a later date. The curricula for nursing education are also shifting to reflect a health rather than illness orientation. For example, the new baccalaureate program at the University of Prince Edward Island has developed a curriculum that is based on principles of health promotion.

The number of graduate programs in nursing has increased at universities across Canada. Doctoral programs in nursing are offered at several Canadian universities. At the time of writing, there are doctoral programs at the Universities of Alberta, British Columbia and Toronto, and a conjoint program offered by McGill University and the University of Montreal.

The establishment of master's and doctoral level programs in nursing has spurred the development of research in the field. Nurses now sit on the esteemed Medical Research Council of Canada and, in some universities, nursing scholars are attracting more research funding than the members of many other faculties. Research-based nursing practice is becoming a fact of life, as we will discuss more fully in Chapter 7, Research and Nursing Practice.

OUR CHANGING POPULATION

The face of Canada has changed dramatically during this century. We have become a nation with a rapidly growing older segment and an increasing diversity of ethnic origins among our people. Family patterns have altered. While the nuclear family, composed of a mother, a father and two or more children, is still the standard in Canadian households, the traditional situation in which the father was bread-winner and the mother was homemaker has changed. The new family structure is one in which both parents pursue careers and share equal responsibility in the home. Many other family patterns have also emerged, including single-parent, blended, cohabiting, and gay and lesbian families.

We no longer live in the small, close-knit communities that once characterized most of this country. The majority of the population now live in increasingly large cities. Our economic base has also shifted. From one that was built on logging, fishing, farming and mining, it moved first to manufacturing as we developed a strong industrial base in Central Canada and now it is shifting again. A major restructuring of our economy is currently going on as we move from the industrial to the information age.

AGING

The aging of populations is a world-wide phenomenon. Much of it is expected to occur in the developing world over the next 20 years, as life expectancy is lengthened in many countries due to improvements in health. But, we are also seeing a rapid growth in the number of older persons in the population of Canada. From approximately 10 percent of the population in 1986, the number of persons over the age of 65 is expected to grow to 20 percent by the year 2021, with the biggest increase coming after 2011 when members of the baby boom generation begin to reach retirement age. The increasing number of older adults is already posing a challenge to our health service. The impact will be even greater in the years to come. Particularly important in this regard is the fact that the fastest growing segment of the older population is the group over the age of 85 whose numbers are expected to increase to 11 percent by the year 2031. This is the group who consume the most hospital days of all age groups in the country and almost all of the long-term care facilities (Beckingham, 1993).

FAMILY PATTERNS

The aging of the Canadian population is occurring at a time when there has been increasing fragmentation of the family unit. Grownup children now often live thousands of miles away from their parents. With more women working outside the home there is often no one at home to look after an aging mother or father. As people are living longer, many women in their middle years are being caught caring for children at home and having to look after aging parents who also need care. Alternative services have had to be developed to assist older people to remain independent as long as possible and facilities have had to be built to care for them when they are no longer able to care for themselves.

The number of single-parent families represented 13 percent of all families in Canada in 1991. This situation, combined with the increased numbers of women in the workforce, has meant that social institutions such as day care centres, schools, churches and community centres must provide many services that once were provided by parents in the home. The day-to-day management of many transient and chronic problems of children's illnesses may be delegated to the day care worker, the teacher or the school nurse. For example, the school nurse or the teacher may be asked to give a child medication at specified times after the acute phase of an illness is past and the parent must return to work.

URBANIZATION

We have also had to cope with the need for rapid expansion of health services in our cities, as new immigrants came into the country and more people migrated to urban centres in search of employment opportunities. All too often, the number of people moving into the city far outstrips the capacity of its health services. This is particularly true in inner-city neighbourhoods where overcrowding and poverty frequently compound the situation. It is the inner-city neighbourhoods, too, that usually have the most new immigrants. This situation results in a rich cultural mix among inhabitants, but often poses problems for health workers both in terms of overcoming language barriers and in understanding different beliefs and customs about health and illness.

The trend towards increasing urbanization is beginning to change, however. As the cities become more crowded, and the pace of life more hectic, many people are seeking an alternative lifestyle and moving to the suburbs or to smaller communities. We are seeing this shift among the older population as retirement villages and other housing options for elders are developed in small communities. But, we are also seeing the trend among young people who can afford houses in small towns that they could never hope to afford in a big city.

A health educator discusses health issues with community residents

CHANGES IN THE ECONOMY

The current restructuring of our economy is wreaking havoc among the working population. As we move from the industrial age into the information age, and into a global economy, thousands of people have found themselves suddenly unemployed and having to learn new skills in order to compete in the labour market. There is more poverty in Canada than ever before. And along with poverty have come all its resultant social problems, not the least of which is the effect on people's health. People cannot eat well-balanced diets if they do not have enough money to buy food and pay the rent. Despite Canada's universal health care system, surveys have shown that ill health is more common among the poor, and that access to needed health services is more difficult for them.

Poverty also breeds crime, and we have seen a distressing increase in violent crime in our cities in recent years. Our health services have had to learn to cope with gunshot wounds and stabbings in increasing numbers. There is a growing need for mental health and social services to help victims deal with the trauma of violent acts.

Given these troubling changes, it is no wonder that stress is considered the most common illness of our times.

ETHNICITY

Canada has been called the world's first international nation (*Royal Bank Reporter*, Spring 1992). Diversity has characterized the Canadian people ever since the French and then the British settlers joined the country's long-

established North American Indians and Inuit to form the fledgling nation that was to become Canada. As wave after wave of immigration has populated our country, the ethnic diversity of our peoples has become more pronounced. Today, there are more than 100 distinct ethnic groups among our population. Most of us (82 percent, according to a 1991 Angus Reid survey) live in neighbourhoods with persons of different ethnic or racial backgrounds and nearly three quarters of us can name people of different ethnic or cultural backgrounds among our close friends. Intermarriage between different racial and ethnic groups — once a social taboo — has become common, with 40 percent of Canadians stating that they have family members of different ethnic or racial backgrounds.

Immigration continues to swell our numbers as people from every corner of the globe come in the hope of a better life. We are seen as a growing nation with great economic potential where people can be free to worship as they choose and where political diversity is tolerated. Along with Sweden, the United States and Australia, we are among the world's leaders in refugee resettlement. We will discuss the topic of transcultural nursing in Chapter 12. The remarkable ethnic diversity of our population is one of the most interesting challenges faced by workers in the health field as they try to tailor care to meet the needs of patients.

CHANGING PATTERNS OF DISEASE

The nature of the illnesses that affect us has changed dramatically over the years and this too has had an impact on health services. The tremendous advances in medical science in the twentieth century have radically altered disease patterns in Western societies and have revolutionized our health care. Most of the communicable diseases that necessitated lengthy hospitalization and took such a toll on human lives at the beginning of the century, such as smallpox, diphtheria, typhoid and scarlet fever, have been virtually eliminated by improvements in public health measures coupled with the discovery and widespread use of specific immunity-producing agents. However, other diseases, such as the world-wide epidemic of Acquired Immunodeficiency Syndrome (AIDS), continue to come forward to plague us.

The massive migration of refugees, the global nature of travel these days and, in our country especially, the influx of immigrants from all over the world have also brought different patterns of disease. Even in our northern part of the globe, we need to be aware that our patients may recently have come from a country where malaria, dengue, yellow fever and the like are common. The care of people with tropical diseases is no longer something for study only by missionaries going off to foreign lands. All Canadian health workers need to know how to identify the symptoms of these diseases and how to care for people suffering from them.

The miracle drugs of the 1940s and 1950s, the sulfonamides and the antibiotics, radically changed methods of patient care by hastening recovery and lowering fatality rates from infections. The rapid advances in surgical techniques in the latter half of the century have made procedures simpler and safer with day surgery and home recovery possible for many operations that used to require lengthy hospital stays. The advances in medical and surgical techniques have also contributed to increasing the life span of people in our society. The longer people live, however, the more likely they are to suffer from chronic and degenerative diseases — heart conditions, cerebrovascular accidents (strokes) and cancer are among the leading causes of death in Canada today. These diseases also figure prominently on the list of chronic conditions from which people suffer.

Many of our present-day health problems are directly attributable to the way we live. Faster cars, driven at high speeds, have contributed to making the care and treatment of accident victims a major portion of the workload in hospitals. External causes of death, including accidents, violence and poisonings, are the third leading cause of death for men in Canada, and the fourth for women. Many hospitals have Trauma Units staffed with physicians and nurses who have taken specialist courses in the field. Rehabilitation services are needed to help restore people who have had accidents to an active, functioning role in society. The number of people permanently handicapped as a result of accidents and other acts of violence adds to the demand for long-term care services.

The heightened tempo of life in today's world has led to many stress-related health problems. There has been a marked increase in the incidence of mental illness, for example, especially among young people, and we are also see-

ing much evidence of the tragic effects of alcohol and drug abuse. Suicide, homicide and other acts of violence are on the increase, as we noted above.

CHANGING PERSPECTIVES OF HEALTH AND HEALTH CARE

Our ideas about health and the factors affecting health have undergone considerable change over the past century. We have moved from looking at health and illness from a purely biological viewpoint to a perspective which includes the effects of individual behaviours and more recently, social, economic and environmental factors as major contributors to health (Health and Welfare Canada, 1987).

Today's view portrays health as a part of everyday living and as an essential dimension of the quality of life. "Quality of life" in this context implies the opportunity to make choices and to gain satisfaction from living. Health is envisaged as a resource which permits people to manage and even change their surroundings. Today's view of health recognizes freedom of choice and emphasizes the role of individuals, families, groups and communities in defining the meaning of and in making decisions about their health (Epp, 1986). With this view comes a change in health care from a focus on the cure of disease to an emphasis on the promotion and protection of health. "Armed with the knowledge that health goes beyond lifestyle and medical care, we can insist that policies in housing, education, justice, taxation and other areas take health into account" (Government of Ontario, 1993). Nurses, therefore, work collaboratively with people from other sectors of the community such as business, education and community organizations to better the health of Canadians.

In keeping with the changing perspectives on health, there is a shift in the relationship between the nurse (and other health care professionals) and the individual, family, group or community for whom health services were established. No longer is it one in which the nurse or health care professional is provider of care and the individual, family, group or community are passive recipients. The relationship is viewed as an equal partnership — where the nurse or health care professional and the recipients collaborate to achieve the best level of health possible for them.

WHAT DOES ALL THIS MEAN FOR NURSING?

The redefinition of health to include socioenvironmental determinants as well as biological factors and lifestyle has changed the direction of health care policy and the nature of health care services in Canada. Nurses are playing a key role in helping to determine health policy and to restructure the health care system. In addition to their traditional caring functions, nurses' roles now encompass those of facilitator, advocate, community organizer, political activist and lobbyist. These roles involve collaboration with other health professionals as well as professionals from other sectors of society, such as economists, urban planners and environmentalists (RNABC, 1990). In order to undertake these new roles, nurses need highly developed skills in the caring aspects of nursing. Additionally, nurses need to be able to work with individuals and groups to enable them to determine their own needs and take control of their own health. A nurse, for example, may now be asked to assist a group working to improve housing for low-income families in the community.

The realignment of our health care system, with the shift towards more ambulatory and home-care services, has increased the number of nurses working in the community. Here, nurses are playing an increasingly large role in identifying patient needs, coordinating the various services available, and providing care. Community health nurses require skills in assessing the health status of individuals and families, enabling them to promote their health and to cope with the effects of illness or disability. Nurses' practice takes them into homes, schools, industry and clinics in the community. It is anticipated that in the future an even greater number of nurses will be needed in these settings.

People coming into acute-care hospitals are usually very ill. Many, such as the accident victim with multiple injuries or the person who has just suffered a heart attack or a stroke, require intensive nursing care. The complexity of care and the highly sophisticated machinery used require specialized skills. Many nurses are taking advanced training to become clinical specialists in various fields.

As so many of the diseases prevalent in our society today are attributable to high-pressure urban living, it is important for nurses to have a good understanding of the nature of stress and ways of coping with it. Nurses are as vulnerable to the effects of stress as their patients are. Nurses must examine their own health practices carefully to make sure that their daily activities include sufficient rest, exercise and recreation in order to offset stress encountered in the work environment.

An increasingly large number of nurses are involved in working with older people, who now constitute such a large part of our society. Many nurses are providing health services for people in senior citizen housing units, helping them to keep well and as active and independent as possible, for as long as possible. Nurses are also the principal providers of care in nursing homes and extended-care facilities, where so many of the sick elderly are in residence.

WHAT DOES ALL THIS MEAN FOR NURSING STUDENTS?

The only constant in the emerging world is change — and the accelerating rate of that change.

Burton, 1992

As nursing responds to the changes occurring in society, it is important to remember that the traditional values on which nursing was founded — those of caring, nurturing, compassion and commitment — have withstood the test of time. Nursing in Canada has a long and honourable history. It has played an integral role in Canadian society from the time the first colonists arrived on the shores of New France. As beginning students, you should have a sense of the rich history of nursing in this country and in this context we introduce some of the illustrious "first ladies" of Canadian nursing. We start in this chapter with Jeanne Mance, who is honoured as the first nurse in Canada. You should also know something about the profession you have chosen, its mandate in society and how this mandate is carried out in practice.

The rapid and extensive changes in health care will inevitably have an impact on you, the nursing student. First, you need a good grounding in the scientific basis of nursing. The underlying foundation for nursing lies in its theoretical underpinnings — the theories that have been articulated about the phenomenon of nursing and the processes by which nursing is carried out in practice. Second, you will need a broad base of knowledge in the social sciences, as well as in the biological sciences. Third, you will have to develop intellectual skills in problem-solving, critical thinking and decision-making as part of the process of giving care. And finally, you will need to gain skills in communication, human interaction and group process. These requirements are, of course, in addition to the basic techniques and procedures that are the traditional foundation of nursing practice.

The provision of expert nursing care is a highly developed skill acquired over time with experience and continued learning. As first-year students you will be introduced to the problem-solving process and you will develop the beginning skills necessary for nursing practice. You will learn to give care to people in their homes, in community clinics, in long-term care facilities as well as in acute-care hospitals. The basic knowledge and skills you gain from your introductory course in nursing will provide you with a solid foundation on which to build.

But you need more than just the basic skills. You will also need an understanding of health, the factors that affect the health of individuals, families, groups and communities and the perceptions people have of health in general and their own health in particular. Not everyone views health in the same way. As new people have come to settle in Canada, they have brought customs and traditions from their native lands, and sometimes "healers" or traditional practitioners of the healing arts have emigrated as well. It is often a challenge for health workers to practise culturally sensitive care and adapt interventions to meet the needs of people with different backgrounds from their own. It is helpful, then, to know something about the health beliefs and practices of some of the major ethnic groups who have made Canada their home. A particular case in point for Canadian nurses is health care for people of the First Nations. This field of nursing, and particularly the challenges of nursing in Canada's North, has not only attracted Canadian nurses but has also lured nurses from around the globe.

As well as understanding health, you, as future health practitioners in Canada, need to know something about the health care system in which you will be working. We mentioned the shift to community-based care that is occurring. It makes sense, then, to learn something about the direction community-based care is taking and how nurses can work effectively with people in the community, both on an individual and a group basis. With the focus on health rather than illness, nurses need skills in health promotion and health protection — skills that depend to a large extent on communication and teaching abilities. The interpersonal skills that enable nurses to collaborate with other health care professionals and with people from other sectors of the community are invaluable in making our communities healthy places in which to live.

REFERENCES AND READINGS

BANNING, J. (1992). New perspectives in nursing. *Canadian Nurse*, 88.

BECKINGHAM, A. (1993). Aging in Canada. In A.C. Beckingham and B.W. Du Gas. *Promoting healthy aging: A nursing and community perspective*. St. Louis: Mosby.

DEVELOPING RESOURCEFUL HUMANS (1992). L.E. Burton (Ed.). New York: Routledge.

EPP, J. (1986). *Achieving health for all: A framework for health promotion*. Ottawa: Ministry of Supply and Services. (Catalogue No. H39 – 102/1986E)

GOVERNMENT OF ONTARIO. (1993). *Nurturing health*. Report of the Premier's Council on Health, Well-being and Social Justice (1987 – 1991). Toronto: Queen's Printer. (Catalogue No. 01 – 93 – 20M)

HEALTH AND WELFARE CANADA. (1987). *The active health report: A framework for health promotion*. Ottawa: Ministry of Supply and Services. (Catalogue No. H39 – 106/1987E)

LALONDE, M. (1974). *A new perspective on the health of Canadians: A working document*. Ottawa: Information Canada.

A NATION WITH A DIFFERENCE. (1992). *Royal Bank Reporter*. Spring Edition.

REGISTERED NURSES ASSOCIATION OF BRITISH COLUMBIA (RNABC). (1990). *Health promotion: A discussion paper*. Vancouver: Author.

ROACH, S.M. (1992). *The human act of caring: A blueprint for the health professions*. Ottawa: Canadian Hospital Association Press.

STATISTICS CANADA. (1992). Families: Number, type and structure. *The Nation*. Ottawa: Ministry of Industry, Science and Technology. (Statistics Canada Catalogue No. 93 – 312)

WORLD HEALTH ORGANIZATION (WHO). (1984). *A discussion document on the concept and principles of health promotion*. Geneva: Author.

CHAPTER 2

Health and Wellness

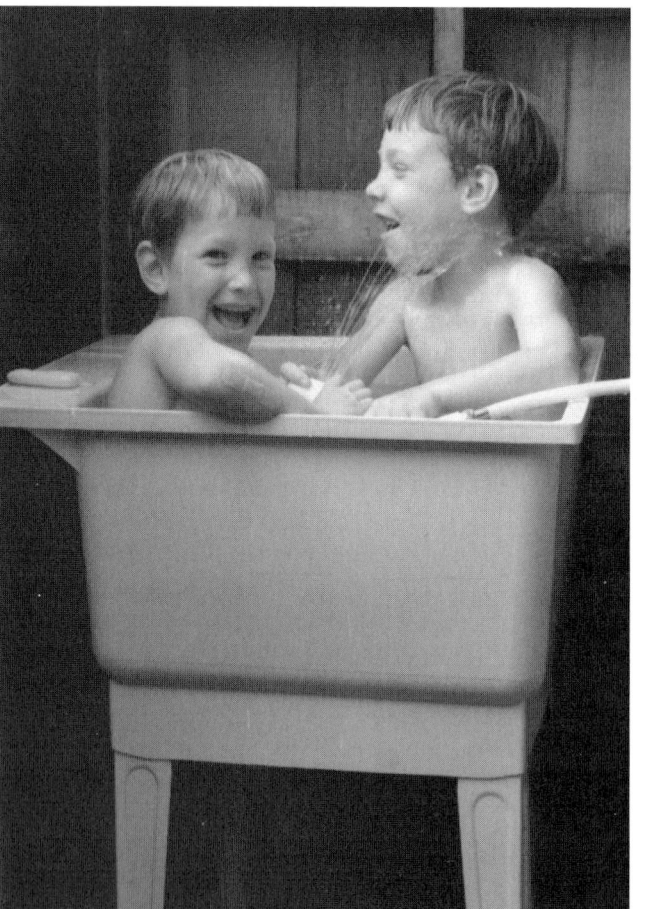

CENTRAL QUESTIONS

1. What are the meanings of health, well-being, wellness, illness and disease?

2. What do the terms holistic health and health within illness mean?

3. How have ideas of health changed over the past century?

4. How does the socioeconomic model of health differ from its predecessors — the biomedical and behavioural models?

5. What are the major factors that determine a person's health?

6. How does the World Health Organization define health?

7. What are the main indicators of health status used by most countries?

8. How does the health status of Canadians compare with that of people in other countries?

9. What are the leading causes of death in Canada?

10. What are the most common illnesses experienced by Canadians?

11. What are the most common disabilities?

12. What are the main causes of hospitalization?

13. How do Canadians feel about their health?

INTRODUCTION

Good health is the bedrock on which social progress is built. A nation of healthy people can do those things which make life worthwhile and, as the level of health increases, so does the potential for happiness.

Lalonde, 1974

Canadians today are a highly health-conscious people. And it is health, rather than illness, that is becoming the focus of our health care system. Over the past two decades, there has been a major change, a "paradigm shift," in the philosophy of health care in Canada, in the United States and, indeed, in most countries of the world. We appear at long last to have swung towards a more positive approach. It is an approach that stresses the promotion of health and the prevention of illness as matters of primary concern, and one that focusses on restoration to optimum health (or a peaceful death), not merely on the curing of disease, as the goal of therapeutic care.

As knowledgeable professionals to whom other people turn for advice on health matters, nurses need a good understanding of what health and illness are all about. They also need to be aware of current thinking in regard to the factors that contribute to good health and those that predispose a person to illness — what are referred to in today's terminology as the determinants of health.

THE MEANINGS OF HEALTH, WELLNESS, ILLNESS AND DISEASE

Health is a complex phenomenon which cannot be simply defined. There is a wide variation in definitions of health and in personal meanings and perceptions of health. Older people might accept a few aches and pains as a normal part of the aging process, whereas runners may feel that they are not in good health unless they can cover 25 kilometres easily. The concept of health has been viewed from a variety of perspectives and has been interpreted in many ways. Broadly defined, **health** is a positive state of being that includes physical fitness, mental (or emotional) stability and social and spiritual ease. It is not a constant or absolute entity but rather an ever-changing and evolving state in which people actively strive to achieve the highest level of functioning that is possible for them. In order to describe the concept of health more fully, we must first define the terms *disease* and *illness*, as well as *wellness* and *well-being*.

The word *health* conveys a positive meaning, whereas *disease* and *illness* have negative connotations. We prefer to talk of a person as having a "health problem" or a "health deficit," rather than to say that he or she is ill. **Disease** is

seen from this perspective as an interruption in the continuous process of health, manifested by abnormalities or disturbances in the structure and function of body parts, organs or systems. When these abnormalities appear clustered together, they become recognizable as the signs and symptoms of a particular disease, for example, the high temperature, cough and chest pain commonly seen in people with pneumonia. Pneumonia is a medical label or diagnosis the physician assigns to the complex of symptoms manifesting the disease process.

Illness is the personal experience of feeling unhealthy. A person may feel ill because of a disease, or may just not feel well. However, a person may also not feel ill even though disease is present. For instance, a man may have a serious illness, according to his physician, and yet feel very healthy because he is able to carry out his normal activities for daily living. On the other hand, another man may wake up in the morning with a headache and may feel so ill that he decides he is not well enough to go to work. In either case, illness involves changes in the person's state of being and in social function (Clark 1990). What is important in the experience is how people feel and what they do because of those feelings (Leddy and Pepper, 1993).

A term associated with disease and illness is sickness. **Sickness** is a status, defined as the social actions or roles assumed by individuals who experience illness or are diagnosed with a disease (Clark, 1990). When a person is considered to be sick, certain behaviours are sanctioned that otherwise might not be acceptable. For instance, someone who is sick with the flu is expected to stay at home in bed. But staying at home in bed is not socially acceptable for someone who stayed out late the night before and is simply tired.

Well-being is defined as "a subjective perception of ability, harmony and vitality" (Leddy and Pepper, 1993). Like illness, well-being is a relative, changing state experienced in the course of everyday living. When it is experienced at the lowest levels, people perceive themselves as ill, but when it is experienced at the highest levels, they feel maximum satisfaction, understanding and a sense of contribution in life (Leddy and Pepper, 1993). Often, physical symptoms of illness (headache, tiredness, etc.) may be negated — or reinforced — by environmental conditions. Well-being fluctuates towards illness or towards health depending on various factors that influence the individual at a particular time.

Well-being may be viewed on a continuum that ranges from extreme illness when death is imminent to peak or high-level wellness (Dunn, 1959). Dunn describes a health (well-being) grid which analyzes the possible interaction of environment with health and the resulting degrees of well-being and illness (see Figure 2.1). The grid consists of a health axis and an environmental axis, which intersect to make the health and wellness quadrants. The quadrants are labelled as follows: poor health in an unfavourable en-

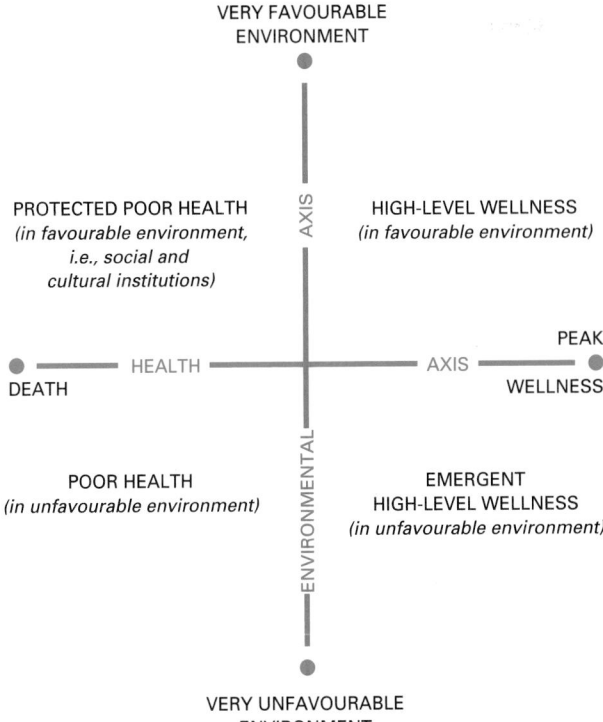

FIGURE 2.1 Dunn's health (well-being) grid, its axes and quadrants

SOURCE: From Dunn, H.L. High-level Wellness for Man and Society. *American Journal of Public Health*, 1959, 49:788. Reproduced with permission.

vironment; protected poor health in a favourable environment; emergent high-level wellness in an unfavourable environment; and high-level wellness in a favourable environment. The environmental axis includes the physical and biological aspects of the environment as well as the socioeconomic conditions affecting an individual's health. The health grid ranges from death at the extreme left through serious illness, minor illness, and good health to peak wellness at the right. According to Dunn, high-level wellness can only occur in a favourable environment because people are never isolated from the effects of the world in which they live (Dunn, 1959).

Wellness is a basic concept that underlies the framework for modern-day health care. Simply defined as a state of optimal health or optimal functioning, this concept is based on the assumption that individuals possess their own optimal level of functioning, which represents the best state of well-being that is possible for them. This definition allows for the fact that most people have some type of minor health deficit. They may have a minor physical problem, such as an allergy to certain foods, or a small speech impediment, or they may be "shy" and have a problem meeting people. Some people have an unreasonable fear of heights or of cats — problems in the psychological realm of functioning. People rarely attain perfection in all aspects of their health — phys-

ical, mental and social — and certainly do not achieve it all of the time, but each individual has a unique optimal level of functioning that is attainable for him or her.

Wellness is described by Dunn as "an integrated method of functioning which is oriented toward maximizing the potential of which the individual is capable. It requires that the individual maintain a continuum of balance and purposeful direction within the environment where he [or she] is functioning" (1959, 447). Dunn viewed high-level wellness not as an optimum state but rather as a progression or growth towards an ever-higher potential of functioning and an open-ended and ever-expanding challenge to live at a fuller potential. *Potential* in this sense means the best a person is capable of doing within the confines of his or her physical or mental limitations. High-level wellness involves a progressive integration (or maturation) of the whole being of the individual — one's body, mind and spirit — at increasingly higher levels throughout the life cycle. In optimum health, individuals function at a high level within a dynamic and ever-changing environment (Dunn, 1959, 1973; Pender, 1987).

Leddy and Pepper conceptualize wellness as "an actively continuing process that involves initiative, ability to assume responsibility for health, value judgements and integration of the total person" (1993, 222). While wellness is difficult to evaluate objectively, there are a number of indicators that can be used. These include:

- the capacity of people to perform to the best of their ability
- the ability to adjust and adapt to varying situations
- a reported feeling of well-being
- a feeling that "everything is together" and "harmonious."

TWO BASIC CONCEPTS: HEALTH WITHIN ILLNESS AND HOLISTIC HEALTH

HEALTH WITHIN ILLNESS

In the concept of **health within illness**, illness is regarded as "an event that can expand human potential" (Moch, 1989, 23). It is seen not as an enemy the patient is expected to fight against but as an opportunity for personal growth and transformation. Many people in our society have serious chronic health problems, yet they are able to live normal, healthy lives, often of a better quality than before they became ill. It is not unusual to hear people with conditions such as diabetes, for example, say that they have "never felt better" or "more alive" once their diabetic state was regulated and they have learned to live with the limitations of the disease. To use another example, a young woman afflicted with multiple sclerosis who has lost the function of one side of her body may never regain total functioning of her affected arm and leg, but may nonetheless be able to achieve independence in daily activities and maintain an active role in society. In the course of daily living, such a person would not see herself as being ill, unless she had a cold or a case of the flu. For people like her, health means living with and mastering the handicaps imposed by the disease process, while focussing on activities that increase the quality of life and maximize the physical, mental, emotional and social potential of which they are capable.

There is an expanding body of evidence indicating that people grow and become stronger as human beings, particularly in the psychological, social and spiritual dimensions, during the experience of illness (Jones and Meleis, 1993; Jaffe, 1980; Siegel, 1986). They may develop a heightened sense of self and of their personal potential, feel a greater spiritual inner peace and discover new meaning and purpose in life. They may also experience changes in themselves, their personal goals, their values and their relationships with others. As well, the experience of illness may bring an increased awareness of nature and the environment in which they live. Through the experience of illness, people "may emerge healthy rather than vulnerable" (Jones and Meleis, 1993, 3). A wonderful example of a person who made life a healthy, positive experience in the face of terminal illness was Terry Fox, of Coquitlam, British Columbia. His 1980 "Marathon of Hope," in which he ran across Canada, despite having bone cancer, to increase awareness of cancer and raise funds for research into this life-threatening disease, has been immortalized in statues, plaques and public edifices throughout the world. And, more importantly, it has inspired annual fund-raising marathons around the country.

HOLISTIC HEALTH

Holistic health is an approach to wellness that recognizes the interaction between the whole person and his or her environment, and emphasizes harmony with oneself, with nature and with the world (Flynn, 1980). This approach is based on the premise that "things and events cannot be analyzed by reducing them to component parts without destroying or distorting the integrity of the whole" (Flynn, 1980, 9). That is to say, an individual's health must be considered in terms of his or her total functioning. One cannot separate the physical, social and emotional components of health; nor can one separate the whole person from his or her environment. This interaction works in both directions — an illness, even a minor one, such as influenza or a short-lived gastrointestinal upset, can affect

This woman is able to live a normal, healthy life and to maintain an active, fulfilling role in society.

a person's mental outlook and interactions with other people; and an emotional problem, such as anxiety over examinations or an argument with someone, can affect appetite, digestion and other aspects of physical functioning.

Flynn (1980) considers holistic health to be synonymous with Dunn's "high-level wellness" and sees wellness as "an ever-changing growth toward fulfilling an individual's potential considering individual needs, abilities and disabilities" (p.12). Holistic health care focusses on the individual rather than on the disease. Learning about the person who has the disease is considered more important than finding out about the disease itself. The ill person is viewed as having a "dynamic disturbance in the equilibrium of the body–mind–spirit environment. Health requires a harmonious integration of the body, mind, spirit and the environment, while illness indicates a degree of imbalance among them" (p.12). Illness, while often painful and frightening, is regarded as having a positive potential, providing an opportunity "to further clarify values, affirm individual priorities and direction and deepen a sense of the meaning and value of life" (p 28).

Returning to the example of the young woman with multiple sclerosis, it is easy to see that her physical disability will interfere with both her emotional and social well-being. She will undoubtedly feel grief over the loss of physical functioning. She may feel that she is no longer the person she used to be, or that she is a burden to her husband. Her illness may require lengthy hospitalization from time to time when she will be cut off from normal social activities with family and friends. Holistic care for this woman will extend beyond the therapeutic intervention needed for the physical problems caused by the disease itself. Her feelings and her relationships with her husband and others will have to be explored and she will need help to restore harmony, balance and a sense of meaning and direction in her life.

CHANGING PERSPECTIVES ON HEALTH

Over the years, our ideas about health and illness have changed considerably. At one time, health was defined simply as the absence of illness; people were considered healthy as long as they were not sick. Health care focussed on determining the causes of disease and on developing new and better ways to treat it. We subsequently went through a period when we put considerable emphasis on people's own behaviour — smoking, overeating, lack of exercise — as a cause of many illnesses. Health care began to focus on encouraging people to change lifestyles in order to promote their health. Today, we recognize that health is affected not only by physiological and lifestyle factors, but also by the social and economic conditions in which people live. The World Health Organization states that "health begins at home, in schools and factories. It is there where people live and work, that health is made or broken" (WHO, 1981).

In order to improve health, then, it is necessary not only to treat disease and encourage healthy habits, but also to improve living and working conditions, for as these conditions improve, so does health (Epp, 1986). In this section of the chapter, we explore the evolution of our current definition of health as exemplified in the biomedical, behavioural and socioeconomic models of health. We will discuss the models chronologically, in the order in which they successively dominated the health field in Canada.

THE BIOMEDICAL MODEL

As we noted in Chapter 1, tremendous advances have been made in the biomedical and physical sciences over the past 100 years. The application of these sciences in medicine and medical technology has dominated health care in Western cultures for the better part of this century. This purely empirical approach to health, based on scientific research and teaching, is known as the *biomedical model*. It focussed on the physiological determinants of health and disease. The body was likened to an intricate machine, with disease considered to be the result of a breakdown somewhere in the mechanism. Restoration to health required first, a diagnosis to determine the cause, and second, intervention to remedy the condition. Medications and phys-

ical or surgical measures were the common treatments. Efforts to prevent illness concentrated on measures to control or eradicate the physical causes of disease, by such means as mosquito control to prevent malaria or immunizations for communicable diseases such as typhoid, tetanus, diphtheria, smallpox and polio. Considerable progress was made in the areas of diagnosis and therapeutic treatments for disease during the time the biomedical model dominated the health field. Gradually, it was realized, however, that all ills could not be solved through the use of diagnostic and therapeutic measures alone.

The first challenge to the biomedical model came in 1948 when the World Health Organization defined health as "a state of complete physical, mental and social well-being and not merely the absence of disease or infirmity" (WHO, 1948). This definition set the stage for a new perspective on health which moved beyond looking only at the physiological basis of illness. As with all new ideas, the more holistic approach to health, which incorporated an individual's social and mental attributes as well as physical well-being, took time to be accepted. The WHO definition was criticized for being too vague and all-inclusive — critics claimed that it would be difficult to measure a person's health by quantitative scientific means using this definition.

THE BEHAVIOURAL MODEL

In Canada, the next major challenge to the biomedical model of health came with publication in 1974 of a working document prepared by the Research and Planning Division of the Department of Health and Welfare (Lalonde, 1974). The document was aptly titled *A New Perspective on the Health of Canadians* (also referred to as the Lalonde Report). It suggested that health should be looked at in terms of a *health fields* approach. The basic premise of this concept was that there were four principal factors affecting both individual and group health, namely, heredity, environment, lifestyles and health care organization. Because of this emphasis, it became known as the *behavioural model*. See Figure 2.2.

The *New Perspective* document also suggested that the goal of health care should be to increase freedom from disability, as well as to promote a state of well-being sufficient to perform at adequate levels of physical, mental and social activity, taking age into consideration (Lalonde, 1974).

While acknowledging the contribution of medical science and technology to improvements in the health of Canadians since the turn of the century, the Lalonde Report pointed out that further improvements would come about, not from further advances in medical science, but from strategies such as improving our environment, moderating self-imposed risks and adding to our knowledge of human biology.

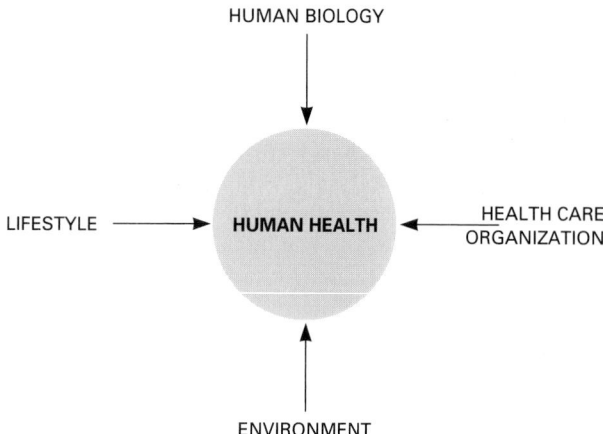

FIGURE 2.2 Behavioural model of health

SOURCE: *Introduction to Patient Care*, 4th edition, 34

The *New Perspective* document was a landmark in Canadian health care. It not only extended the boundaries of the health field, but also suggested that the *outcomes of care* were more important than *accessibility to care*, which was seen as a variable that might or might not improve one's health (Crichton, Hsu & Tsang, 1993).

The *New Perspective* document put considerable emphasis on the importance of lifestyle as a contributing factor in most of the five leading causes of death in Canada — heart disease, cancer, strokes, chronic obstructive lung disease and accidents. Following this report, a Health Promotion Directorate was established in the Federal Department of Health and Welfare. Programs were subsequently initiated by federal, provincial and municipal governments and by voluntary agencies, including the Canadian Heart Association and others, to encourage us to improve our lifestyles. And, there is no doubt that the programs have achieved a certain amount of success. The *Active Health Report* on the findings of a 1985 study on the health and health behaviour of Canadians indicated that many of us had improved our health habits — we were exercising more, we were more conscious of the benefits of eating a healthy diet, and a great many people had stopped smoking. There has been a considerable reduction, too, in the number of accidents due to the deadly combination of drinking and driving (Health and Welfare Canada, 1987).

Although the Health Fields concept (Behavioural Model) was seen to be an improvement over the biomedical model, its usefulness was limited by the fact that it failed to take into consideration the impact of the socioeconomic environment on health.

THE SOCIOECONOMIC MODEL

Addressing these limitations and looking back at several earlier reports on the effect of social and economic conditions

on health, the World Health Organization expanded the *Health Fields* concept to include socioeconomic factors. In 1977, the Thirtieth World Health Assembly stated that "the main social target of governments and WHO in the coming decades should be the attainment by all citizens of the world by the year 2000 of a level of health that will permit them to lead a socially and economically productive life (WHO, 1981). And at the 1978 International Conference on Primary Health Care in Alma-Ata, USSR, the importance of the relationship between health and the economic and social dimensions of a community was once again emphasized. The WHO publication *Health for All by the Year 2000* (1981) outlined strategies to implement the socioeconomic, or "healthy people," vision of health espoused at the Alma-Ata conference. The deliberations of the Alma-Ata Conference also led WHO to propose the following definition of health:

> Health is defined as the extent to which an individual or group is able, on one hand, to realize aspirations and satisfy needs; and, on the other hand, to change or cope with the environment. Health is, therefore, seen as a resource for everyday life, a dimension of our "quality of life," and not the object of living; it is a positive concept emphasizing social and personal resources, as well as physical capabilities (World Health Organization, 1984).

All countries belonging to the World Health Organization were urged to work towards the goal of "*Health for All by the Year 2000*" using ways and means best suited to their particular situation to implement the new vision of health. In Canada, the strategies to implement the new vision emerged from the findings of two studies, a *National Health Survey* which was undertaken from 1977 to 1979 and the *Health Promotion Survey* of 1985. The findings from both studies clearly showed the role of poverty, unemployment and pollution in health. These findings led to the development of Health and Welfare Canada's discussion paper entitled *Achieving Health for All: A Framework for Health Promotion* (Epp, 1986). The paper was presented at an international conference on health promotion, held in Toronto in 1986, which was sponsored jointly by the World Health Organization, Health and Welfare Canada, and the Canadian Public Health Association. From this conference came the *Ottawa Charter for Health Promotion* (see Figure 2.3).

The Epp Report and the Ottawa charter recommended the reduction of health inequities caused by socioeconomic and environmental factors. They identified the prerequisites of health as "peace, shelter, food, income, a stable ecosystem, sustainable resources, social justice and equity." These documents were another landmark in Canadian health care, signifying a major shift in thinking about both health and health care. We have moved to a socioeconomic model in which our ideas about health have broadened to include social and economic factors, as the list of prerequisites for health cited above indicates. The emphasis has shifted away from therapeutic care to health promotion and

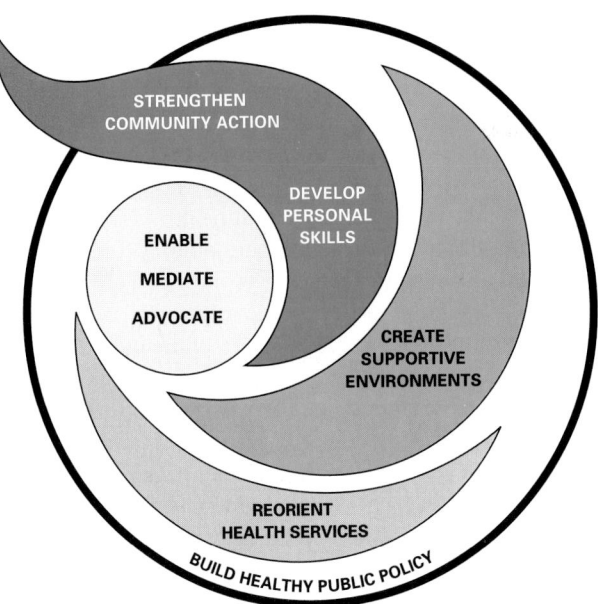

FIGURE 2.3 Ottawa Charter for Health Promotion

SOURCE: Canadian Public Health Association, 1986. Ottawa

health protection, aimed at getting at the causes of ill health, rather than only at its cure. Actions to improve health are community-based and **multisectoral**; involving collaboration between the health care sector and the business, education, justice and law enforcement sectors. The pivotal concepts in the socioeconomic model of health are *empowerment* and *community*. Use of the term "empowering" indicates a shift in the power base in public health from bureaucracies to the community (Green and Raeburn, 1988). It also implies that individuals should take an active role in making decisions as well as in creating and using resources to achieve their health potential. We will discuss these concepts further in subsequent chapters throughout the book.

The primary responsibility for administration and management of our National Health Insurance program is vested

A *Vision of Health for Ontario*

We see an Ontario in which people live longer in good health, and people are empowered to realize their full health potential through a safe, non-violent environment, adequate income, housing, food and education, and a valued role to play in family, work and the community.

We see people having equitable access to affordable health care regardless of geography, income, age, gender or cultural background. Finally, we see everyone working together to achieve better health for all.

SOURCE: Government of Ontario (1993). *Nurturing Health*. Report of the Premier's Council on Health, Well-being and Social Justice (1987–1991). Toronto: Queen's Printer.

in the provinces. Following the Epp Report, studies have been undertaken in all provinces to look at ways and means of implementing its recommendations and, at the time of writing, the provinces are at various stages of implementing the findings of these studies. A province-by-province comparison is made in Chapter 3.

In Ontario, the Premier's Council on Health, Well-being and Social Justice (1987–1991) published a summary of their research on the factors which determine our health. The summary was entitled *Nurturing Health* (1993) and it embodies many of the precepts of the socioeconomic model of health.

DETERMINANTS OF HEALTH

The Ontario Nurturing Health Model (see Figure 2.4) identifies four key factors, or *determinants*, of health:

1. living and working conditions
2. social support
3. genetic makeup
4. individual behaviours.

You will notice that two of these factors — individual behaviours and genetic makeup — are essentially the same as the lifestyles and heredity factors of the behavioural model. The other two factors, which have the most influence on health, according to the Ontario report, relate to two aspects of the environment — living and working conditions, and the social support available to people. You will notice, too, that the fourth factor identified in the behavioural model — health care organization — is missing from the Ontario Nurturing Health Model. In the approach outlined in this version of the socioeconomic model, health care is viewed as a part of both living and working conditions (community and occupational health) and as a component of social support (emergency services, and therapeutic, rehabilitative and palliative care). The integration of health care organization into living and working conditions and social support is not intended to devalue the importance of health care. Nor does it mean that there will be less need for doctors and nurses. Rather, it underscores the need for the coordination of efforts by all sectors to improve the health of people in our society. Let us take a look at each of the elements in the Nurturing Health model.

LIVING AND WORKING CONDITIONS

The *Nurturing Health* Report suggests that the factors with the greatest influence on people's health are their living and working conditions and the social support available to

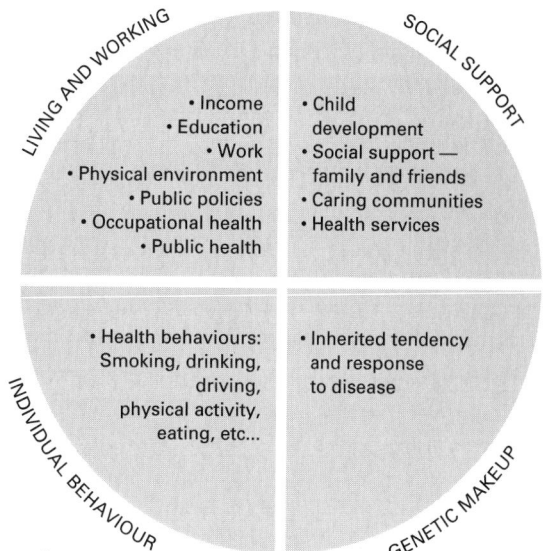

FIGURE 2.4 Beyond Lifestyle: The Ontario Nurturing Health Model

SOURCE: Government of Ontario (1993). *Nurturing Health*. Premier's Council on Health, Well-being and Social Justice (1987–1991). Toronto: Queen's Printer, 4. Adapted with permission.

them. Lifestyle is determined as much by circumstance as by the decisions made, consciously or unconsciously, by people about the way they choose to live. Single parents on welfare, for example, may be at a disadvantage in terms of their health if they cannot afford to join a health club or a local community centre. They also need considerable social support from family, from friends, and from health and social services in order to maintain their family. A good income, on the other hand, can make life more comfortable and go a long way towards enhancing one's "quality of life," even for people with health problems.

In looking at living and working conditions, we will consider such elements as income, education, work (including occupational health), the physical environment (including public health) and public policies.

Income

Recent studies on health have shown some very interesting findings about the relationship between income and general health. The *Active Health Survey* showed that people's health is directly related to income. Men in the upper income groups can expect to live six years longer than men with lower incomes; slightly less difference (three years) was found for women. People with higher incomes can also look forward to more disability-free years — fourteen more for men and eight for women.

In much of the developing world, many health problems are directly attributable to a lack of the basic essentials of life (such as adequate nutrition and housing), resulting from widespread poverty among large segments of the pop-

ulation. In countries with a small gap between the rich and the poor, such as Japan, the Netherlands and Norway, people have a greater overall life expectancy than in countries such as the United States and France where there is a large gap between rich and poor (Government of Ontario, 1993).

Poor people are more likely to have poor health. They have a higher incidence of mental health disorders, high blood pressure and disorders of the joints and limbs than do people with higher incomes. They are also more likely to die from accidental falls, chronic respiratory conditions, pneumonia, tuberculosis and cirrhosis of the liver. And unfortunately, Canada, despite its wealth, is not entirely exempt from the influence of poverty on the health of its people. Particularly vulnerable are certain groups within the low-income bracket, namely, older people, the unemployed, welfare recipients, single women supporting families, people of the First Nations and immigrants. Among people of the First Nations, where the rate of poverty is more than twice the national average, the infant mortality rate is also more than double the average Canadian rate (Government of Ontario, 1993; Epp, 1986).

Although Canada is considered a rich country by international standards, it is estimated that a million Canadian children live in poverty, that is, in families with incomes below the poverty line. Given the established connection between poverty and ill health, this situation is of great significance to all health care workers.

Education

The more highly educated people are, the better equipped they are to look after their health. WHO, for example, has found that teaching mothers to read is one of the most effective ways to improve the health of families (UNICEF and WHO, 1993). In Canada, more people with post-secondary education rate their health as good or excellent (70 percent) than those with less than secondary education (46 percent).

Education contributes to good health in many ways. The *Nurturing Health* document lists the following health benefits:

- Education increases job and income security and job satisfaction

- Education equips people with the skills they need to identify and solve individual and collective problems

- Education can unlock the innate creativity in people, thereby adding to our collective ability to generate wealth

- Education improves "health literacy" — the ability to gain access to information and services that keep you and your family healthy.*

---

* Government of Ontario (1993). *Nurturing Health*. Premier's Council on Health, Well-being and Social Justice (1987–1991). Toronto: Queen's Printer, 10.

Work

Most adults spend about one-quarter of their lives at work, so a healthy workplace is an important component of conditions for healthy living. A healthy and safe physical environment is essential and, in our country, provincial Workers' Compensation Boards are very concerned with this aspect of working conditions (see Chapter 3 for a full discussion). Also, it is increasingly being recognized that stress is one of the major contributors to decreased productivity and absenteeism. This topic is discussed further in Chapter 29 on Safety Needs, where we talk about the role of the occupational health nurse.

Employers are coming to recognize that they can positively influence the health of their employees by improving working conditions — many are offering ongoing education and training programs, incentives for work well done, job security, employee involvement in decision-making, working as a member of a team and adjustments to accommodate employees with both home and workplace responsibilities. And many firms now offer health promotion and wellness programs in the workplace. The need for occupational health nurses can be expected to increase over the next few years.

The Physical Environment

The physical environment includes both the natural and the artificial aspects of the physical world that surrounds us. Considerable research is currently being done on the effects of weather (an important part of our natural environment) on people's health. We know that many people, particularly those with rheumatism, arthritis or asthma, are sensitive to atmospheric changes. With impending changes in the weather, some individuals experience a variety of symptoms including severe pain, breathing difficulties, fatigue and depression. It has been observed that the rate of suicide is considerably

LOOKING BACK

MARGUERITE D'YOUVILLE 1701–1771

Marie-Marguerite Dufrost de Lajemmerais d'Youville was the founder of the Order of the Sisters of Charity of Montreal, commonly known as the Grey Nuns. This Order became one of the pioneering nursing orders, mainly involved as visiting nurses in the community; its members introduced both hospitals and district nursing throughout Canada, especially on the frontiers of the west and the north.

Marguerite de Lajemmerais was born in 1701 into one of the great and wealthy families of New France, but the death of her father when she was seven left the family financially insecure. Her marriage to François d'Youville in 1722 was not a happy one and was marked by the death, in early infancy, of four of her six children. Her husband died in 1730, leaving a debt-burdened estate. Following his death, Madame d'Youville, who had turned increasingly to her religion during the latter years of her marriage, worked actively with the established sisterhoods and soon was applying herself to service of the poor and the ill.

In 1737, with two other women, she established a lay order both to care for the sick poor and to raise money for their care, drawing on her own needlework skills as a means of raising money. The women chose a simple grey habit and, because it was not a cloistered order, did mainly visiting nursing. However, they also took into their house many abandoned children and ill elderly. Their reputation as district nurses grew rapidly. In 1747, the Governor asked Marguerite d'Youville and her Sisters of Charity to take over the running of the bankrupt and filthy general hospital of Montreal, which she soon had running smoothly and well. This became the main headquarters for their care, although the Grey Nuns continued their community nursing. The hospital was all but destroyed in a fire a few years later, but despite that and despite epidemics, war (during which they nursed both French and English soldiers), poor harvests and government interference, Madame d'Youville managed to establish a firm foundation for the growing and increasingly respected nursing sisterhood. In 1755, the Order of the Sisters of Charity was accepted as a religious order by the Roman Catholic Church.

Despite increasing ill health, Mother Marguerite d'Youville was a tireless worker and remained a remarkable administrator until her death in 1771. The Order she founded continued to grow and, in the 1800s and 1900s, established branches throughout Canada, the United States and other parts of the world. Marguerite d'Youville was personally credited with several miraculous cures and in December 1990 she was canonized by the Roman Catholic Church. Saint Marguerite became Canada's first Canadian-born saint.

Glennis Zilm

greater in the Northern coastal areas of British Columbia, where the rainfall is highest, than in other parts of Canada.

Many other aspects of the physical environment have been created by human beings, and are now beginning to be controlled by us as well, in order to make our surroundings more conducive to healthy living. One of the major factors in the improvement of health in the Western world during the past century and a half has been the reduction of known environmental hazards through the application of public health measures. These have included such basic measures as establishing standards for housing; provisions to ensure safe water, food and milk supplies; safety standards for places where people work; and the control of communicable disease.

Although we have greatly reduced the effect of environmental factors on health in Canada, there is still much lack of uniformity in the application of basic public health measures across the country. Housing for many people is still inadequate or even unsafe. Access to a safe water supply is not guaranteed to all. In some homes, there is still no running water or indoor plumbing. Raw sewage still pours into many of our lakes and rivers, and insects, rats and other disease-carrying pests infest many poverty-stricken neighbourhoods.

Then, too, other environmental problems have emerged in recent years, many as a result of industrialization and increasing urbanization. The contamination of our waterways by industrial pollutants is a matter of major concern. There is growing alarm about the threat to health of air pollution, particularly in large urban centres. Many cities have installed monitoring devices and have instituted controls to curb industrial activity when air pollution reaches a level considered harmful to health.

The effect of increasing urbanization on both the physical and social environment is also causing considerable concern to people in the health field. In many instances, cities and new communities have grown too rapidly to cope with the housing, sewage and other basic services needed by the population. Overcrowding, lack of recreational facilities, excessive noise, violence and solitude are among the social factors resulting from urbanization that contribute to the health problems of city-dwellers.

Public Policy

At every level of government — national, provincial and municipal — health programs are based on policies that the prevailing government either initiated or endorsed from a previous government.

"Public policy has the power to provide people with opportunities for health, as well as to deny them such opportunities. All policies, and hence all sectors, have a bearing on health" (Epp, 1986, 10). Many policies outside the health sector have a direct bearing on health; examples of these include regulations for safe housing, the control of agricultural pesticides, high taxation on alcohol and tobacco and regulations for a smoke-free environment. Politicians are becoming more aware and are accepting greater accountability for the effect policies in their sectors have on health. The role of public policy on health is explored in more detail in Chapter 3.

SOCIAL SUPPORT

In looking at the determinants of health, we must remember that human beings are social animals. Their relationships with other people are very important to the satisfaction of many of their basic needs. Relationships with other people in the home, in the work or school setting and in the numerous other activities in which people engage contribute positively or negatively to their health. A number of studies have shown the influence of a supportive social environment on good health and a long life. (Epp, 1986; *Nurturing Health*, 1993). Social support is a lifelong need. Essential to this social support is the positive interaction with others that gives a person a sense of belonging and fosters his or her self-esteem (Muhlenkamp & Sayles, 1986). We will be talking about the importance to health of supportive social relationships when we discuss health and the individual, health and the family and health and the community in subsequent chapters.

Under the rubric of social support, the Nurturing Health model includes: child development, the support given by family and friends and that provided in caring communities. In our consideration of social support, we also include the emergency, restorative and palliative care services which provide a network of health support for people in our society. These were included in the original Nurturing Health model.

Social support, in the form of health and social programs administered by different levels of government, also provides a buffer to help people cope with stresses faced in everyday living. Canada is called a "welfare state" because of the network of social and economic supports built into our governmental system. These include the National Health Insurance Program, Old Age Pension, the Social Assistance (Welfare) Program, the Canada Assistance Program (which supplements the OAP and other social assistance programs), Unemployment Insurance, Family Allowance, Workers' Compensation and the Canada and Quebec Pension Plans. While these resources are available to all Canadians, not everyone makes the best use of them. In fact, it is often those who are most in need of social assistance who do not use the services, either because they do not know that they are there or they do not know how to access them. Furthermore, a lack of self-esteem or low self-image all too frequently prevents people from taking the initiative to mobilize these resources for their own needs (Grant, 1988).

GENETIC MAKEUP

Biological factors that influence human health include an individual's genetic inheritance, the processes of maturation and aging and the complex network of structures and systems that compose the human body. The role of genetics, in particular, is the subject of much recent health research.

A number of specific diseases are now known to be passed down through families. One example is Huntington's chorea, a progressive degenerative disorder of the nervous system that is transmitted through a single dominant gene and may affect both males and females in a family. Another is hemophilia, the so-called bleeder's disease, which has afflicted several generations of males in the Hapsburg family and other royal families. The more common disease, diabetes, is also believed to have an inherited component, although its exact mode of transmission is still not well understood. Down's syndrome (mongolism) is thought to be caused by a defective chromosome, which may or may not be inherited.

Although many disorders present at birth may have a genetic component, others may result from problems encountered by the unborn infant *in utero*. These are called **congenital** problems and include such things as heart malformations, cleft palate (a division in the roof of the mouth) and spina bifida (a defect in the spinal canal). Other disorders present at birth are caused by difficulties during delivery; cerebral palsy (an involuntary muscular disorder) is an example.

In many other disorders that affect human beings, the effect of genetic inheritance is suspected but the relationship has not yet been fully established. We do not know for certain at this point in time, for example, the extent of the role of heredity as a causative factor in heart trouble, or in hypertension, or in a number of other health problems. Nor do we yet know why some diseases seem to afflict people of one ethnic group more than another, as, for example, the high prevalence of diabetes among Jewish women, or of glaucoma (increased tension within the eyeball) among people in many of the West Indian ethnic groups.

INDIVIDUAL BEHAVIOUR

The ways of life of people in a community, and their individual lifestyles, also have a significant impact on health. Lifestyle is determined in part by circumstance and in part by the decisions made, consciously or unconsciously, by people about the way they choose to live. Lifestyle depends to a large extent on the occupation of the head of the household, the income level of the family, and the things that income can purchase.

In addition to circumstantial factors, the element of personal decision-making that enters into an individual or family lifestyle plays an important role in determining health.

One of the by-products of affluence in the developed world has been obesity, which is considered a major health problem in North American society. Although other factors contribute to obesity — many of which are not yet fully understood — individual choice of diet has a great deal to do with it. Obesity has been linked to many of the diseases that afflict large numbers of North Americans today, such as heart conditions, hypertension, diabetes and the like. At the other end of the spectrum, malnutrition can occur even in the midst of a plentiful food supply, as indicated by the eating patterns of some adolescent females who starve themselves because they think that being thin is beautiful. Malnutrition in wealthy nations may also result from poor food choices, such as the eating of too many snack foods and sweets instead of regular, well-balanced meals.

The sedentary way of life among many people in Canada (and among people in higher socioeconomic groups in other parts of the world) must also be considered as a lifestyle factor affecting health. It too is a by-product of the affluent society, in which most people rely on cars for transportation and television sets for entertainment. A lack of exercise contributes to a generally lowered state of physical fitness. When the body is deprived of physical activity, the accompanying physical decline includes decreased muscle strength, stiffened joints, increased brittleness of the bones, impairment of digestion and a general decline in endurance, strength and physical skills. This "atrophy through disuse" may occur at any age. It is encouraging to see so many of our young — and older — people today engaging in programs of regular exercise.

Another example of individual behaviour that has an enormous impact on health is the terrible toll on human lives caused by excessive speed and careless driving on the highways. A very heavy burden is put on our health care

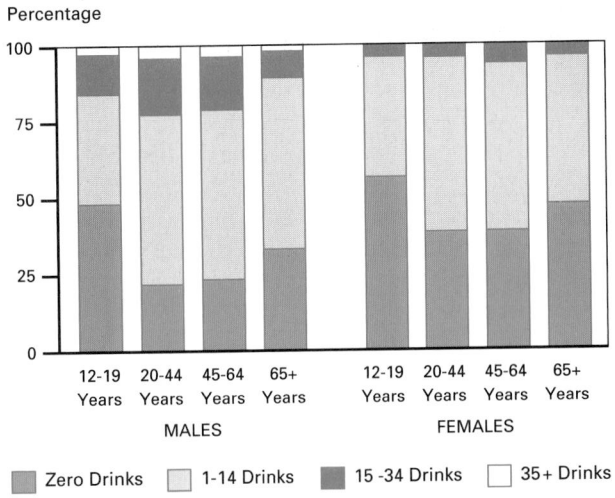

Percentage

FIGURE 2.5 Alcohol consumed in last seven days

SOURCE: Ontario Ministry of Health (1992) *Ontario Health Survey 1990: A Working Document*. Toronto: Government of Ontario.

system for the care, treatment and rehabilitation of count-less victims of automobile accidents.

Numerous other major problems of increasing concern in the health field today can also be attributed to individual lifestyle factors. These include tobacco use, alcoholism, drug addiction, sexually transmitted diseases and suicide. It is especially troubling that these are affecting increasing numbers of young people (see Figure 2.5 on page 25).

THE HEALTH OF CANADIANS

In this section, we are going to discuss the health of Canadians as measured by objective standards using statistical data that has been collected over the years. Then, we will look briefly at how Canadians perceive their own health, as documented in recent studies undertaken by the federal government and by the Government of Ontario. The objective standards we will examine include commonly used health status indicators; the perceptions of health status come from the findings of two surveys.

HEALTH STATUS INDICATORS

In this chapter we have discussed comparisons between the health status of different groups of people within Canada and between that of people in different countries. We said, for example, that the poor are at a disadvantage health-wise, and that certain low-income groups are especially vulnerable to illness. We also said that the health status of people in some developed countries, for example, Japan, Norway and the Netherlands, is better than that in other countries. The basis for these statements is found in the statistical data that governments collect about the health of people in the country. In Canada, Statistics Canada (an arm of the federal government) regularly undertakes surveys, collects data and compiles information about the health status of Canadians. The governments of most countries in the world routinely collect data about illness and death among the people living in their countries. The kinds of statistical information usually compiled on an annual basis by national governments include:

1. the average life span of people (*life expectancy*)
2. the number of deaths relative to the population (*mortality rates*)
3. the reasons for these deaths (*causes of death*)
4. the incidence of illness (*morbidity data*).

These statistical measures are considered four of the main health status indicators for a given population. They provide a base for identifying major health problems, that is, those problems responsible for the most deaths and those

causing the greatest amount of disability to people. They also help to give some insight into the principal factors affecting the health of the population. Because virtually every country in the world collects information on these four indicators, it is possible to look at differences between countries, and where statistical information has accumulated over a number of years, to look at trends over time.

In Canada, health care for people of the First Nations has been a responsibility of the federal government, which has kept separate statistical information on the health status of this segment of Canadian society. There are many differences in the health status of people of the First Nations vis-à-vis that of other Canadians as measured by the various indicators listed above. In this chapter, we will simply note differences. In Chapter 12, Health and Ethnicity, we discuss some of the causes of these discrepancies and look at health services for people of the First Nations.

LIFE EXPECTANCY

The average life span of people in a given country reflects, among other things, the total effect of its economic development and its health care programs. In the developed countries of the world, such as Canada, life expectancy has increased dramatically since the turn of the century — from a little under 50 years in 1900 to 77 years in 1991. The biggest changes in life expectancy occurred during the first half of the century, with smaller but still significant gains made since 1950 (see Figure 2.6).

FIGURE 2.6 Gains in expectation of life at birth, for five-year periods, Canada, 1931-1991

SOURCE: Statistics Canada Longevity and Historical Life Tables. Cat. 89-506 and author calculations for recent periods. In Duman, J., Lavoie, Y. (1992). *Statistics Canada 1992 Report on the Demographic Situation in Canada*. Ottawa: Ministry of Supply and Services, 61.

The remarkable extension of the life span in Canada — and in most countries of the developed world — during this century can be attributed to a constellation of factors. These include the general overall raising of standards of living, improved sanitation, the development and widespread use of immunity-producing agents to protect people from communicable disease, improvements in health care services and advances in medical science and technology.

One interesting trend in the statistics on life expectancy in Canada is the widening gap between men and women (see Figure 2.7). In 1900, women outlived men by an average of approximately two years. By 1991, this figure had increased to approximately 6.9. The average life span for men is now 73.7 years and for women it is 80.6 years (Statistics Canada, 1992). Comparable figures from the United States are 71.6 years for men and 78.6 years for women. A major factor in the lengthening of the life span for women has been the reduction in maternal death rates.

Among the reasons women live longer than men do is the fact that they have not until fairly recently smoked as much as men have. Additionally, it is only in the past two decades that women have participated in such great numbers in the labour force, where stress is thought to contribute to ill health. The increased stress created for women by having to balance career and family demands may reduce the life expectancy gap between men and women in the future.

At present, however, the existing imbalance between the sexes, particularly in the older age group, has brought about changes in the structure of our society. One of the unfortunate results of this trend is that widowhood and loneliness all too often contribute to the health problems of many of our senior citizens. It can be difficult to maintain a well-balanced, nutritious diet when cooking for one. Many older women find it difficult to find the initiative to go out with friends. Depression is common, affecting a sizable minority of older adults (Ross and Casey, 1993; Du Gas, 1993).

There is a considerable gap between the life expectancy of people in developed countries and that of people in many developing countries. The average life expectancy for people in Mauritania, at the extreme low end of the scale, is still only 47 years, while that in Canada is 77 years. One cannot group all developing countries into the same bracket, however, as great strides have been made in improving health conditions in many countries over the past 40 years.

Equally important in both developed and developing countries is the difference that exists between various groups within the population. The figures quoted above for Canada represent average life expectancies at birth for Canadians. Through data collected by Statistics Canada, it is possible to compare differences in life expectancies for various groups within the population. The findings of such comparisons show, as was noted in the Epp report, that there is considerable difference in life expectancy between rich and poor, and among certain groups within the low-income category. The same discrepancy holds true for people in developing countries where the rich, who enjoy a much higher standard of living, better educational opportunities and easier access to health care, are much healthier than the poor. According to Statistics Canada reports, the differences in all-cause mortality among different income groups in Canada have diminished between 1971 and 1986 — perhaps as a result of the introduction of our national health insurance program, which provided easier access to health care for all citizens.

Life expectancy at birth is a standard measurement used internationally that serves as a convenient means of comparison between countries. However, you will also see in statistical reports the term *Potential years of life lost* (or PYLL), which is now being used in Canada and some other countries to look at the potential wastage of life due to premature death from preventable causes. This measure is based on the assumption that everyone has the potential to live to old age. The ages of 65, 70 and 75 years have been used in different studies to calculate the PYLL due to different causes. To calculate this measure, the deceased's age at death is subtracted from 75 (if this is the figure selected) to estimate the potential years of life lost. For example, if a young man were killed in a car accident at the age of 21, the potential years of life lost would be 75–21 = 54 years. Individual PYLLs are added together to obtain the total PYLLs for each preventable cause of death. The Potential Years of Life Lost for major causes of death in Canada in 1990 are shown in Figure 2.8.

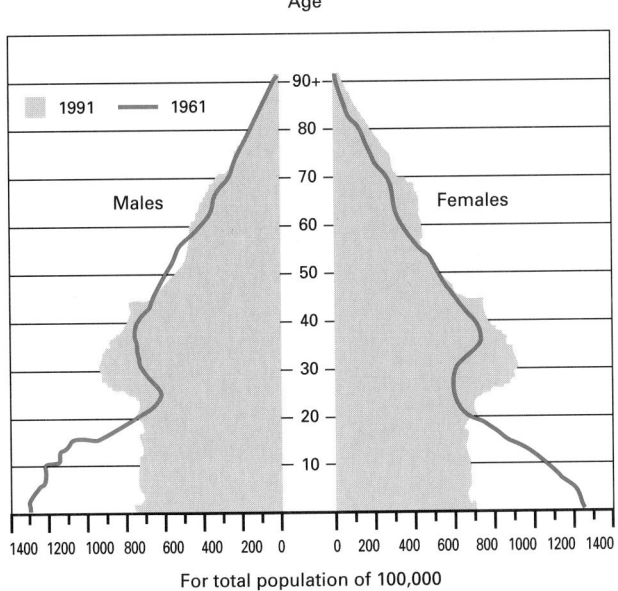

Age

FIGURE 2.7 Population distribution, by age and sex, 1961 and 1991

SOURCE: Statistics Canada Demographic Division. In McKie, C. (1993). *Population aging: Baby boomers into the 21st century. Canadian Social Trends.* Ottawa: Minister of Supply and Services. Cat. No. 11-008E. *29*, 6.

MORTALITY RATES

People in Canada today have a much better chance of living to old age than did the early immigrants to this country whose estimated life span in the eighteenth century was only 35 years (Charbonneau, 1970). Although life became a little less perilous during the nineteenth century, it was not until the twentieth century that we began to see the remarkable extension in the life span that we discussed above. This increased longevity is reflected not only in the statistics on average life span, but also in the annual figures compiled on death rates in the country. The proportion of deaths to the population (**mortality rate**) is now a minimal 7.26 per 1000 population — in the United States, the figure is 8.20, and in Latin America the current level of overall mortality is equivalent to the level that existed in Canada and the United States 50 years ago (1989 figures as quoted in Statistics Canada *Health Reports*, 1992, *4*(2); Pan American Health Organization, 1990).

Among Canada's First Nations, death rates have declined in recent years, although they still remain higher than the national level. These rates were 9 per 1000 population in 1986 — about one and a half times that of the general population. Young people of the First Nations, under 35 years of age, appear to be more at risk; the death rate for this group was three times that of other Canadians. In contrast, the rate for older adults, between 70 and 74 years of age, was lower than the general rate for older adults the same age in Canada (Bobet, 1989).

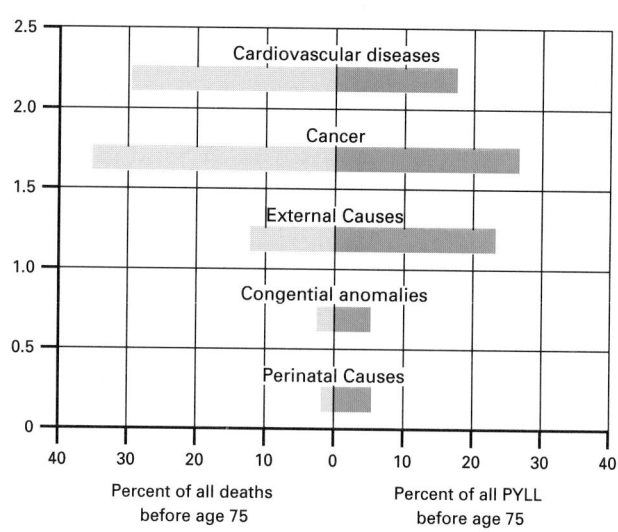

FIGURE 2.8 Deaths and potential years of life lost (PYLL) before age 75 for major causes of death, Canada, 1990 (as a percent of deaths, or PYLL from all causes)

SOURCE: From Brancker, A. (1992). Highlights: causes of death 1990. *Health Reports*. Statistics Canada catalogue 82-003, Ottawa: Minister of Supply and Services Canada, *4*, 189.

A major factor in the lengthening of the average life span in Canada among the general population and among the people of the First Nations has been the dramatic reduction in the number of maternal and infant deaths.

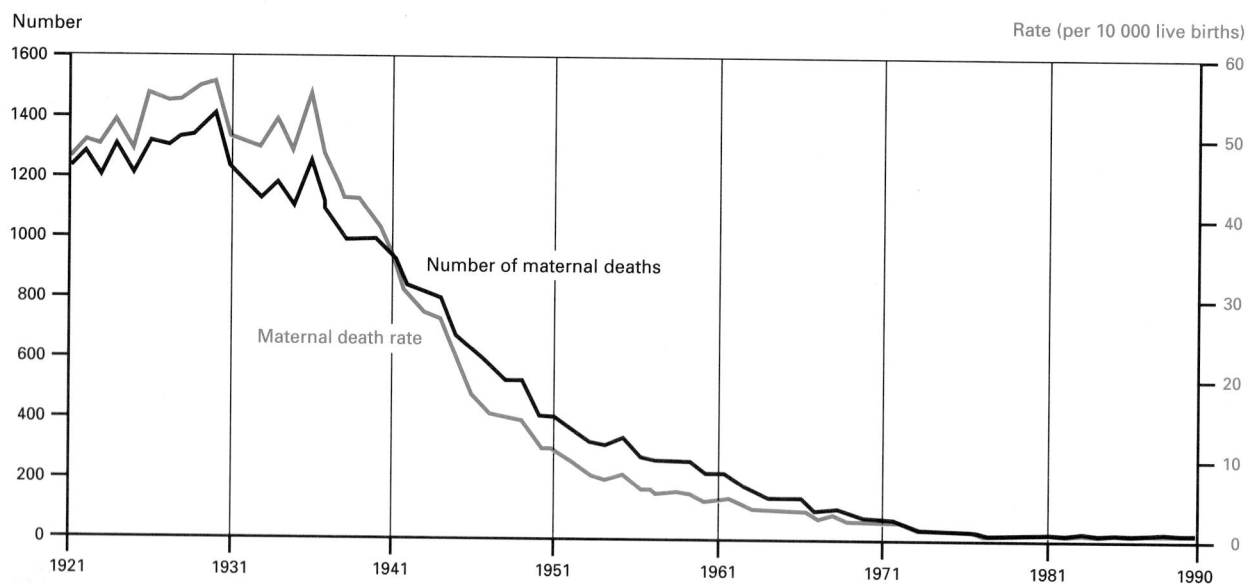

FIGURE 2.9 Number of maternal deaths and maternal death rate, Canada, 1921–1990

SOURCE: From Wadhera, S. and Strachan, J. (1992). Selected infant mortality and related statistics, Canada, 1921–1990. *Health Reports*. Statistics Canada catalogue 82-003, Ottawa: Minister of Supply and Services Canada, *4(4)* 434.

Maternal Mortality

Maternal mortality has shown a remarkable decline in Canada during this century, particularly since 1921, as shown in Figure 2.9 on the preceding page.

Not many women in Canada die as a result of childbirth these days; the maternal mortality rate was 2 per 100 000 live births in 1990. This is down from the 1988 figure of 7 per 100 000 in Canada, which was considerably lower than the rate of 13 per 100 000 in the US for the same year (Statistics Canada figures as reported in Nair, Karim and Nyers, 1992).

Maternal deaths are considered to be largely preventable. The importance of early and adequate prenatal care cannot be overstressed. The reduction in maternal death rates in Canada is attributed mainly to improved prenatal care for pregnant women and to improved care during and after delivery. Although Canada's record is very good, there are still differences in the extent of care received by women in different socioeconomic groups. Unfortunately, it is often the women at highest risk who delay prenatal care until late in pregnancy. These include women from First Nations, recent immigrants, adolescents and those with low incomes.

In many developing countries, maternal mortality rates are considerably higher, sometimes as much as ten times higher than in developed countries. The high maternal mortality rates in developing countries is felt in part to be the result of discrimination against women in predominantly male-dominated societies. The International Conference on Maternity without Risk (Nairobi, 1987) issued a "Call for Action," stating that "high maternal death rates (particularly in developing countries) are a reflection of underlying disadvantages for and discrimination against women. This is particularly true in regard to their legal status, and their access to education, adequate nutrition, dignified employment, financial resources and satisfactory health care, including family planning services" (PAHO, 1992, 121-122).

Infant Mortality

Infant mortality is considered one of the most sensitive indicators of a nation's health status. In Canada, major accomplishments in this area are reflected in the significant drop in infant mortality rates, from 102 deaths per 1000 live births reported in 1921 to 6.8 per 1000 in 1991. However, as with most of the other health status indicators we have discussed, there is much room for improvement in the differences between segments of the population divided on socioeconomic and geographic lines. Infant mortality rates are considerably higher among the lowest income groups in Canada — 9.9 per 1000 live births in 1986, as compared to 6.0 per 1000 in the highest income group

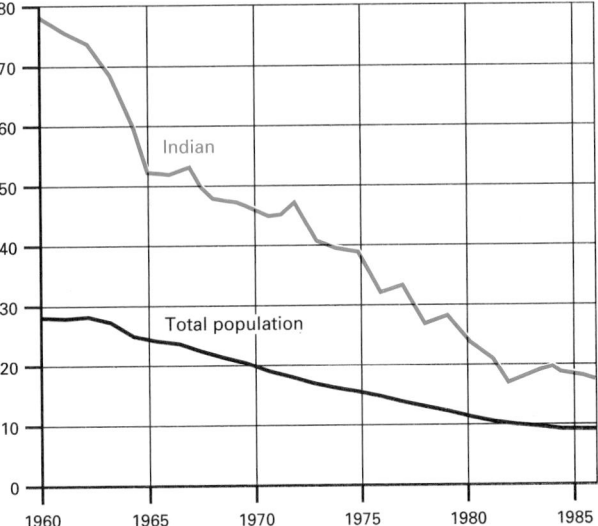

Deaths per 1000 live births

FIGURE 2.10 Infant mortality rates for First Nations people (Indians) and total population (Canada), 1960-1986

SOURCES: Statistics Canada, Catalogue 84-206, and Health and Welfare Canada, Medical Services Branch. In Bobet, E. (1989). Indian Mortality. *Canadian Social Trends*. Ottawa: Minister of Supply and Services. Cat. No. 11-008E. *15,* Winter. 14.

(King, Gartrell & Trovalto, 1991). Despite considerable improvement in the infant mortality rate among people of the First Nations (see Figure 2.10), which has helped to lower the overall rate for Canada from approximately 25 per 1000 live births during the late 1950s and 1960s to 6.8 per 1000 today, the infant mortality rate for First Nations' people is still more than double the average Canadian rate (Government of Ontario, 1993, 9, 17).

The majority of early infant deaths (neonatal) are associated with the status of the infant at birth. Later infant deaths (postnatal), with the exception of those caused by congenital anomalies, are more likely to be associated with environmental factors. In Canada, the decrease in infant mortality has shown a continuous decline in both neonatal and postnatal deaths. In other words, babies are both getting a better start in life (an important factor here is better prenatal care for mothers) and are having greater chances of survival through the first year, owing to improved environmental factors including improved nutrition and better infant health care.

In many developing countries, infant deaths remain excessively high, although considerable improvement has been made in many countries in recent years. There is no doubt that a large number of infant deaths could be prevented by further improvements in disease prevention and environmental sanitation and by better programs of maternal–child health care. The startling difference in infant mortality rates in various developed and developing countries is evident in Table 2.1.

TABLE 2.1 Infant mortality rates for recent years. Selected countries.

Japan	4.4	(1991)
Netherlands	6.5	(1991)
Canada	6.8	(1991)
Germany	7.0	(1990)
United Kingdom	7.3	(1991)
Denmark	7.5	(1991)
Australia	8.2	(1990)
New Zealand	8.3	(1991)
United States	8.9	(1991)
Barbados	15.1	(1991)
Republic of Korea	25.0	(1988)
Argentina	25.1	(1990)
China	32.0	(1988)
Brazil	63.0	(1988)
South Africa	72.0	(Year Not Given)
Mauritania	124.0	(1991)
Sierra Leon	154.0	(1988)

SOURCE: United Nations (1992). *Demographic Yearbook 1991*. New York: The United Nations Secretariat. Department of International Economic and Social Affairs.

NOTE: Over the years, the differences between Canadian and US infant mortality rates have been slight. In the late 1950s and early 1960s, the infant mortality rate in both countries was relatively constant at approximately 25 per 1000 live births, declining by 1977 to 14.1 per 1000 in the US and to 14.3 per 1000 in Canada. Today, the situation is reversed, with Canada's rate at 6.8 per 1000 live births and the US at 8.9 per 1000 live births.

Early Childhood Deaths

The mortality rate for children under the age of five years is another indicator that is frequently used to assess the relative health status of people in different countries. It is considered to reflect the overall socioeconomic and environmental conditions in a country. Here, again, there is a wide gap between developed and developing countries. In Canada, deaths among young children have declined dramatically since the beginning of the century, particularly for the age group one to five years. As the infectious diseases which caused so many deaths among young children in the early 1900s have been brought under control (primarily by immunization), non-infectious diseases and conditions have taken over as the leading cause of death among young children. Accidents are the most common cause of early childhood deaths in Canada today, with congenital anomalies and neoplasms next highest on the list. The change in the primary causes of early childhood deaths in Canada from 1926, when infectious diseases were still rampant, to the mid-1980s is shown in Table 2.2.

In Canada, the United States, and most other industrialized countries, early childhood death rates are now very low. Infectious diseases continue to take their toll in many developing countries, however, and the number of early childhood deaths remains high. The mortality rate for children under age five is 8 per 100 000 in Canada, and 13 per 100 000 in the US (Nair, Kari, Nyers, 1992), whereas in Mauritania it is 217 per 100 000 (UNICEF, 1991). Most early childhood deaths in developing countries are the result of infectious diarrheal diseases, with poverty and resultant malnutrition, poor sanitation and inadequate access to health services combining to make life tenuous for small children.

PRINCIPAL CAUSES OF DEATH

Statistical data on the leading causes of death help to identify the major health problems in a country. The pattern in leading causes of death in Canada has changed considerably since the turn of the century. In 1900, deaths from infectious diseases headed the list. These included pneumonia/influenza, tuberculosis and diarrhea/enteritis. Also on the list of major killers at that time were nephritis (for the most part, postinfectious) and diphtheria. By 1940, the noninfectious disorders of heart disease, cancer and cerebrovascular accidents had become the three leading causes of death, although tuberculosis, pneumonia and nephritis were still among the major causes. By the early 1970s, influenza/pneumonia was the only infectious disease still a major cause of death in Canada.

TABLE 2.2 Percentage of deaths among children aged 1-4 due to selected causes, 1926-1985.

	INFECTIOUS DISEASES	NONINFECTIOUS		
		ACCIDENTS	CONGENITAL ANOMALIES	NEOPLASMS
1926–1930	72.6	8.4	1.3	0.8
1931–1935	66.8	11.1	1.7	1.6
1936–1940	64.8	12.0	2.3	2.0
1941–1945	58.5	17.1	4.0	3.1
1946–1950	49.6	23.2	5.8	5.0
1951–1955	41.2	29.2	7.1	7.3
1956–1960	33.3	32.6	10.4	9.5
1961–1965	26.9	37.3	11.2	10.6
1966–1970	22.0	41.1	13.2	11.1
1971–1975	15.6	44.4	14.7	10.4
1976–1980	12.5	45.0	14.8	10.3
1981–1985	10.2	41.5	16.3	11.0

SOURCE: Statistics Canada, Vital Statistics and Causes of Death as published from 1926-1985. In King, M., Gartrell, J., & Trovalto, F. (1991) Early childhood mortality, 1926-1986. *Canadian Social Trends*. Ottawa: Minister of Supply and Services. Cat. No. 11-008E. *21*, Summer, 9.

Deaths per 100 000 population

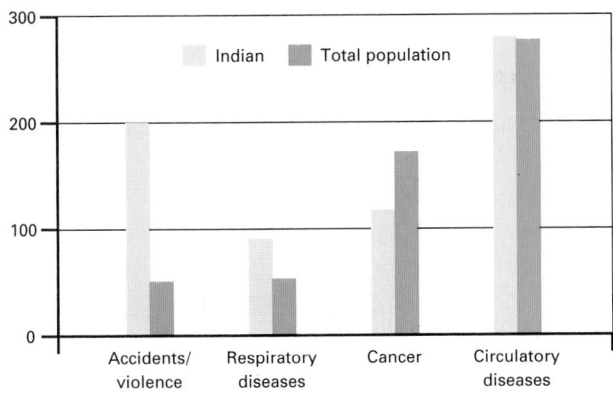

FIGURE 2.11 Age-standardized death rates for First Nations people (Indians) and total population, by cause, 1983–1986 average (Canada)

SOURCE: Health and Welfare Canada, Medical Services Branch. In Bobet, E. (1989). Indian Mortality. *Canadian Social Trends.* Ottawa: Minister of Supply and Services. Cat. No. 11-008E. *15,* Winter, 14.

The leading causes of death in Canada are now cardiovascular diseases (including heart disease and stroke) and cancer, which between them cause more than two thirds of all the deaths each year. These are followed by respiratory diseases, accidents and violence, diseases of the digestive system and endocrine, nutritional and metabolic diseases, of which diabetes mellitus is the most frequent contributor (Brancker, 1987).

Among our First Nations population, the major causes of death are similar to those in the overall population, but the proportion of deaths due to various causes is different. As shown in Figure 2.11, Native (North American) Indians are much more likely to die as a result of accidents or violence than are the rest of the population. There has been a decline in recent years in the number of deaths due to accidents/violence, but it is still much higher than for the general population. Motor vehicle accidents account for almost one third of these deaths, shootings and drownings account for another ten percent each. Respiratory diseases also continue to be a major cause of death, particularly among Indian infants and native people over 55 years of age (Bobet, 1989).

Cardiovascular diseases Cardiovascular diseases, which include both heart disease and stroke, accounted for 39 percent of all deaths in Canada in 1990. The number of deaths from cardiovascular disease declined considerably during the 1970s and continued to decline during the 1980s — in fact, the decline accelerated during these years. A number of factors are felt to have contributed to this. Fewer people are smoking, and our dietary habits have improved; we no longer eat as much saturated fat as we used to and we include more fibre in our diet. More of us are exercising regularly. Emergency medical services have improved in

their ability to respond quickly. There are better methods for the treatment of people with hypertension and we have a greater number of coronary care units better equipped to handle acute cases. Still, heart disease and strokes continue to account for the greatest source of acute illness and major disability among the total population (Brancker, 1992).

Cancer Cancer is the second leading cause of death in Canada, accounting for a little more than one quarter of all deaths in 1987. Cancer strikes people of all ages and becomes a principal cause of death and disability among people from the latter half of the young adult years onward. Lung cancer was responsible for one third of deaths in men in 1987. While the number of deaths from lung cancer has levelled off in the past few years, the number of deaths in women from lung cancer has increased by an average of eight percent each year for the past decade (Brancker, 1989). At the same time, there has been a decline in the number of men smoking. Among young people, aged 15–24, approximately one in three people (both sexes) are smokers (Health and Welfare Canada, 1992).

The figures for breast cancer have remained fairly constant over the past few decades. Breast cancer accounted for the largest proportion (one fifth) of all deaths among women (Brancker, 1992). There is, however, a reduced incidence of breast cancer among younger women. But, it is now showing up in older women much more than it did a few years ago.

There have been improvements in the methods of treating various types of cancer, such as Hodgkin's disease (a malignant disease of the lymph glands and nodes) and childhood leukemia. These advances have also helped to cut the incidence of cancer mortality among young people.

Respiratory diseases Despite our progress in the control of infectious diseases, influenza/pneumonia continues to show up among the leading causes of death in Canada. It is a principal cause of death in infants under one year of age and remains an important cause of death and a major cause of acute illness throughout the life span. Together with chronic obstructive lung problems, influenza/pneumonia is listed as the third leading cause of death in Canada for women, and the fourth for men. The primary respiratory diseases are pneumonia and influenza, chronic bronchitis, emphysema and asthma and other chronic obstructions of the airway (Brancker, 1989). These diseases are also a major cause of illness throughout the life span.

Accidental and violent deaths Accidental and violent deaths are the third leading cause of death for men in Canada, and the fourth for women. Of these deaths, more than half are the result of motor vehicle accidents, while suicides make up the largest portion of remaining deaths in this category (Brancker, 1992). Accidents are the leading cause of death for the male population from one to

44 years of age and for women from one to 34 years. Motor vehicle accidents and suicides are the leading causes of death in young adults from age 15 upwards (Brancker, 1989). They are also a major cause of acute hospitalization. The residual effects of accidents in the form of long-term disability constitute a very major health problem.

Diseases of the digestive system Among the disorders included under this category are chronic liver disease and cirrhosis of the liver, noninfectious enteritis and colitis, peptic ulcer (with and without hemorrhage) and gastrointestinal hemorrhage. The proportion of deaths from digestive disorders in Canada is relatively small (3.5 percent for men and 4 percent for women), although they are listed as the fifth leading cause of death and are among the ten leading causes of acute-care hospitalization (Brancker, 1989; Statistics Canada, 1993).

Endocrine, nutritional and metabolic diseases These accounted for 2.7 percent of all deaths in 1987. The largest portion of deaths in this category (almost 75 percent) was caused by diabetes mellitus. The rate of deaths attributed to this cause has declined slightly over the past decade (Brancker, 1989).

All other causes All other causes accounted for 9.7 percent of all recorded deaths in 1987. Although AIDS (Acquired Immune Deficiency Syndrome) is not showing up, as yet, on the lists as a major cause of death in Canada, it has been causing increasing concern since the early 1980s. The total number of deaths in Canada in 1990 was under 1000, most of them (937) in men, particularly in those over 30 years, with relatively few deaths from AIDS (45) reported in women (Duman and Lavoie, 1992).

MORBIDITY DATA

The list of leading causes of death alone does not give us a full picture of all the major health problems in Canada today. A large amount of data is collected on the prevalence of illness (**morbidity**) which helps to enlarge our perspective on the health of Canadians. Three major sources of information on morbidity data are: the data collected on hospitalization, on communicable diseases and on people with disabilities. Data on communicable diseases is discussed in Chapter 31, so we will not go into that aspect further here.

Hospitalization We have mentioned, in the sections on mortality data and on causes of death above, some of the major causes of acute illness and hospitalization. To recapitulate, the major causes of acute-care hospitalization in Canada (as measured by total number of days spent in hospital by all persons in 1990–1991) are as follows:

1. Diseases of the circulatory system (7 958 000 days)
2. Mental disorders (5 374 000 days)
3. Diseases of the respiratory system (3 901 000 days)
4. Neoplasms (3 576 000 days)
5. Diseases of the nervous system and sensory organs (3 272 000 days)
6. Injury and poisoning (3 173 000 days)
7. Diseases of the digestive system (2 921 000 days)
8. Complications of pregnancy (2 134 000 days)
9. Diseases of the musculoskeletal system and connective tissue (2 043 000 days)
10. Symptoms, signs and ill-defined conditions (1 489 000 days).*

People with disabilities A *Health and Activity Limitation Survey* conducted by Statistics Canada in households in the fall of 1986 and in health-related institutions in the spring of 1987 yielded some interesting data on persons with disabilities. To begin with total numbers, there are an estimated 3.3 million persons in Canada with disabilities. There is a greater amount of disability among older people than among other segments of the population, and more men than women up to the age of 55 years who are disabled. After that age, more women than men have disabilities, and the difference becomes greater as age increases.

Only an approximate 7.5 percent of people with disabilities reside in long-term care facilities and homes for older people. The remainder live in households in the community. Of the disabled persons living in households, there are approximately 275 000 children under the age of 14. Among people residing in institutions, most are over 65 years of age (78.9 percent) and are severely disabled (72.9 percent). Women with disabilities are more likely to reside in an institution than men with disabilities: 9.1 percent of women with disabilities are institutionalized, whereas only 5.6 percent of men are.

The most frequently reported types of disability are agility and mobility disabilities. Less common but still disabling for many people are vision, hearing and speaking problems. Other types of disabilities such as mental handicaps and emotional, psychiatric and learning disabilities are much more prevalent in people living in institutions than those living in the community (see Figure 2.12).

Three out of four severely disabled adults are living in the community, where it appears clear that they receive a high degree of social support. Approximately 40 percent receive help with meal preparation and with personal finances and approximately 60 percent receive help with shopping and housework, as shown in Figure 2.13. The

---

* Statistics Canada (1993). *Hospital Morbidity, 1990-1991*. Ottawa: Minister of Industry, Science and Technology. Catalogue No. 82-217. Table 1. Separations and Days, Rates per 100 000 population and Average Days per separation, pages 2,4,6,8.

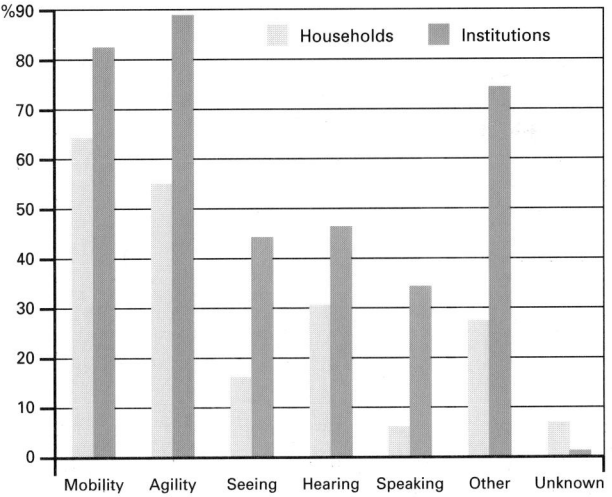

FIGURE 2.12 Adults with disabilities by nature of disability by type of living arrangement (Canada), 1986-87

SOURCE: Adams, O., Dowler, J., Lafleur, L., Jordan-Simpson, D.A., & Wilkins, R.(1991). *Profile of persons with disabilities residing in health care institutions in Canada.* Prepared for Statistics Canada. Special Topic Series from the Health and Activity Limitation Survey. Ottawa: Minister of Supply and Services Canada. Catalogue 82-615, vol. 6.

availability of social support to help people with these activities is quite likely an important factor in making it possible for severely disabled adults to stay in the own homes.

Among severely disabled adults, those who are in long-term care facilities are more likely to be more severely disabled than those living at home. There is, in these cases, a resultant higher degree of dependence on others for help with personal care and with moving about within the residence (Adams, Dowler, Lafleur, Jordan-Simpson, and Wilkins, 1991).

PERCEIVED HEALTH STATUS

As the data discussed throughout the chapter indicates, the health of Canadians (measured by objective standards) has improved considerably during this century. Although there are still areas for improvement, particularly with respect to certain segments of the population, Canada's record in increasing life expectancy and in reducing maternal and infant mortality and the number of deaths in early childhood is highly commendable. According to international comparisons, the health of people in this country is good.

Most studies on the health of Canadians, such as those discussed above, have focussed on illness and recognizable health problems. But, we have come to realize that health is not merely the presence or absence of disease, but, rather, "a resource for everyday living" (WHO, 1986).

As such, it is a concept that health professionals have found difficult to define and to measure. Canada's Health Promotion Survey of 1985 and the Ontario Health Survey of 1990 both reflect the new orientation to health. Both attempted to obtain a portrait of the health of the people as they live it and see it. Therefore, they asked people how they rated their own health (Health and Welfare Canada, 1987; Government of Ontario, 1992).

The findings of the Health Promotion Survey undertaken in 1985 by the Health Promotion Directorate of Health and Welfare Canada and conducted on its behalf by Statistics Canada indicated that most Canadians perceive their health as excellent or very good (61 percent), while only 12 percent consider it to be fair or poor (see Figure 2.14).

The findings in this survey were similar through all age groups and for both sexes and showed that even people with various serious health problems rated their health as good to excellent, as shown in Figure 2.15.

According to the report of the 1990 Ontario Health Survey, numerous studies indicate that the way people assess their own health status is very similar to the physical and social well-being assessments made by objective measures. "People who rate their health as poor tend to have poor physical health and to engage in fewer health maintenance and promotion practices. They are also more likely to experience higher rates of social isolation, depression and unhappiness" (Government of Ontario, 1992, 9). Findings from the Ontario Survey were much like those of the national Health Promotion Study in finding that most people rate their health as good, very good or excellent.

FIGURE 2.13 Severely disabled adults residing in households[1] showing proportion receiving help with selected activities because of their condition by type of activity, Canada, 1986

[1] Excluding the disabled population residing in northern areas.

SOURCE: Adams, O., Dowler, J., Lafleur, L., Jordan-Simpson, D.A., & Wilkins, R.(1991). *Profile of persons with disabilities residing in health care institutions in Canada.* Prepared for Statistics Canada. Special Topic Series from the Health and Activity Limitation Survey. Ottawa: Minister of Supply and Services Canada. Catalogue 82-615, vol. 6.

Excellent 25% Very Good 36% Good 27%

Fair 9% Poor 3%

FIGURE 2.14 How Canadians rate their health

SOURCE: Health and Welfare Canada (1987). *The Active Health Report: Perspectives on Canada's Health Promotion Survey 1985*. Ottawa: Minister of Supply and Services Canada, 8.

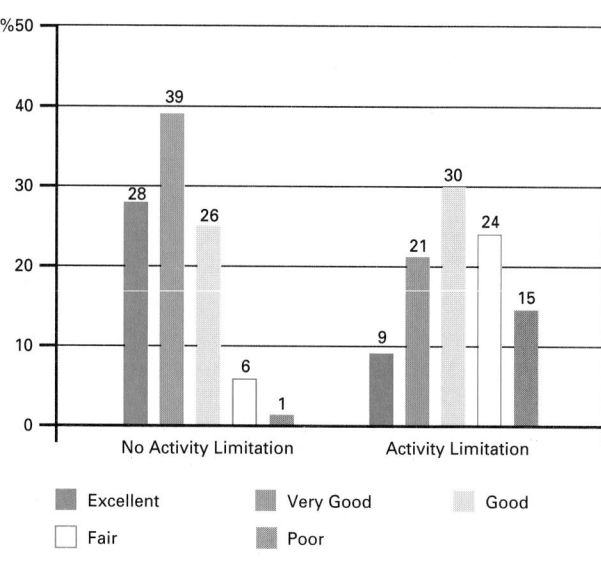

Excellent Very Good Good

Fair Poor

FIGURE 2.15 Self-rated health and activity limitation

SOURCE: Health and Welfare Canada (1987). *The Active Health Report: Perspectives on Canada's Health Promotion Survey 1985*. Ottawa: Minister of Supply and Services Canada, 9.

The Ontario Health Survey found that, although there was not much difference in perceived health status between the sexes, the ratings of this indicator did vary with age, with older people (over 65 years) reporting more frequently (almost one in four) that their health was only fair or poor and less than half reporting it as good or excellent. The number of health problems reported by respondents also increased with age. Almost three in four people over the age of 65 reported two, three or more health problems. It should be noted, however, that 13 percent of people over 65 reported that they were free of even minor health problems (Government of Ontario, 1992).

The Ontario survey also found that two out of every three people in the province had had one or more health problems in the twelve months preceding the survey. The most common problems reported were musculoskeletal (25 percent), respiratory (23 percent), injuries and poisonings (12 percent) and circulatory (12 percent) (Government of Ontario, 1992, 5).

The Active Health Survey looked at health behaviours in addition to self-rated health reports. The Ontario Health Survey looked at both of these, as well as several other aspects of health, including perception of pain, suffering, social support and family functioning. Their findings provided valuable information about the role of social and psychological factors on health. We will discuss some of the findings of both surveys in later chapters.

KEY TERMS

health p. 16	well-being p. 16	biomedical model p. 19	congenital p. 25
disease p. 16	wellness p. 17	behavioural model p. 19	mortality rate p. 28
illness p. 16	health within illnes p. 17	multisectoral p. 21	morbidity p. 32
sickness p. 16	holistic health p. 18	empowerment p. 21	

IN REVIEW

Health is an ever-changing and evolving state of being in which people strive to achieve the highest level of functioning that is possible for them. Well-being, which is a person's subjective perception of ability, harmony and vitality, may be viewed on a continuum that ranges from extreme illness when death is imminent to high-level wellness. High-level wellness involves a progressive integration (or maturation) of the whole being — one's body, mind and spirit — at increasingly higher levels throughout the life cycle. Individuals may achieve wellness during the experience of illness. The concept of health within illness views illness as an opportunity for growth and transformation, particularly in the psychological, social and spiritual dimensions. Holistic health considers an individual's health in terms of his or her total functioning. The physical, social and emotional components of a person's health cannot be separated, nor can the person be separated from his or her environment. Illness is viewed as a disturbance in the dynamic equilibrium of the body–mind–spirit–environment. Holistic health care extends beyond therapeutic interventions and focusses on restoring harmony, balance and a sense of meaning and direction in life.

During the past century, we have modified our beliefs about health, moving from a biomedical model which emphasized the physiological causes of disease, to a behavioural model which included lifestyle as a major causative factor in illness, and then to a socioeconomic model that acknowledges the role of social and economic factors in health. The major determinants of health are now considered to be living and working conditions, social support, genetic makeup and individual behaviours.

The Epp Framework for Health Promotion set the stage for major reforms in health care in this country in keeping with the broadened view of health. The Ontario Nurturing Health Model provides an example of a guide for new directions in health care as provincial governments look at ways to implement the socioeconomic model of health in their jurisdictions. Health promotion and health protection are being emphasized through community and personal empowerment, shifting the focus away from the disease and hospital orientation that has long dominated our health care system.

According to international standards, the health of people in this country is good and most Canadians rate their health as good by their personal standards. During the past century, life expectancy has greatly increased and Canadian infant, maternal and early childhood mortality rates have declined to the point where they are among the best in the world. Most communicable diseases have been brought under control through a combination of public health measures and widespread immunization. Still, new diseases such as AIDS have become serious concerns, and tuberculosis has started to be a problem again. There are also some segments of the population for whom there is room for improvement in health status. These groups include people who are economically disadvantaged, older adults on low incomes, single mothers, immigrants and people of the First Nations.

The five leading causes of death in Canada are cardiovascular diseases, cancer, respiratory diseases, accidents and violence and diseases of the digestive system. These conditions are also responsible for a large proportion of acute-care hospitalization, although mental disorders are now the second leading cause of hospitalization.

Over three million people in Canada suffer from some form of disability. Most are living in their own homes — only seven percent reside in institutions. Those who live at home need (and appear to receive) a considerable amount of social support.

LEARNING ACTIVITIES

1. Explore personal meanings of health. Ask a number of people of different ages what health means to them. How are personal meanings of health similar? How are they different? How do people's views of health change as they grow older?

2. Explore how people with a chronic health condition perceive their state of health. Talk with two or three people who have a chronic health condition (for example, arthritis, emphysema, diabetes, Parkinson's disease or hypertension). Do they consider themselves to be healthy or ill? How do they maintain their optimal level of functioning?

3. Go to the library and find out the main health status indicators in your province and community. Determine the infant and maternal mortality rates and causes of death, morbidity and disability. How do these compare to the rest of Canada?

4. From a hospital in your area, find out the major reasons for hospital admissions for infants, children, adults and older adults.

5. Talk to a community health nurse about the number of people on the nurse's case load who have chronic conditions and disabilities. What is the nature of these conditions or disabilities?

REFERENCES AND READINGS

ADAMS, O., DOWLER, J., LAFLEUR, L., JORDAN-SIMPSON, D.A. and WILKINS, R. (1991). *Profile of persons with disabilities residing in health care institutions in Canada.* (Vol. 6). Prepared for Statistics Canada. Special topics from the Health and Services Canada Catalogue 82-615. Ottawa: Canadian Centre for Health Information.

BOBET, E. (1989). Indian mortality. *Canadian Social Trends*, *15*, 11–14. (Supply and Services Canada Catalogue No. 11–008E)

BRANCKER, A. (1989). Causes of death 1987. *Health Reports*. (Statistics Canada Catalogue 82-003) Ottawa: Minister of Supply and Services, 1(1) 97-105.

BRANCKER, A. (1992). Highlights: causes of death 1990. *Health Reports*, *4*, 185–189. (Statistics Canada Catalogue No. 82–003)

CANADA'S FIRST NATIVE-BORN SAINT. (1990). *The Montreal Gazette*, Dec. 9, 1990, A 10.

CANADIAN PUBLIC HEALTH ASSOCIATION. (1986). Ottawa Charter for Health Promotion. *Report of the International Conference on Health Promotion*. Ottawa: Author.

CHARBONNEAU, H. (1970). *Tourouvre-au-perche aux XVII et XVIII siècles: Etude de démographie historique*. Paris: Presses universitaires de France, 424 pages (Travaux et documents, published by l'Institut national d'études démographiques, cahier 55). As cited in Duman and Lavoie (1992), 111.

CLARKE, J.N. (1990). *Health, illness, and medicine in Canada*. Toronto: McClelland and Stewart.

COMMUNITY HEALTH PROMOTION STRATEGIES. (1987, Spring). *Health Promotion*, *32*, 5–10.

CRICHTON, A., HSU, D, and TSANG, S. (1993). *Canada's health care system: Its funding and organization*. Ottawa: The Canadian Health Association.

DU GAS, B.W. (1993). Healthy lifestyles. In A. Beckingham and B.W. Du Gas. *Promoting healthy aging*. St. Louis: Mosby, 129–160.

DUMAN, J. and LAVOIE, Y. (1992). *Statistics Canada 1992 report on the demographic situation in Canada*. Ottawa: Minister of Supply and Services.

DUNN, H.L. (1959a). High-level wellness for man and society. *American Journal of Public Health*, *49*(6), 786–792.

DUNN, H.L. (1959b). What high-level wellness means. *Canadian Journal of Public Health*, *50*(11), 447 –457.

DUNN, H.L. (1973). *High-level wellness*. Arlington: R.W. Beatty, Ltd.

EPP, J. (1986). *Achieving health for all: A framework for health promotion*. Ottawa: Minister of Supply and Services. (Catalogue No. H39–102/1986E)

FLYNN, P.A.R. (1980). *Holistic health*. Bowie, MD: Robert J. Brady.

GIBBON, J.M., and MATHEWSON, M. (1947). *Three centuries of Canadian nursing*. Toronto: Macmillan.

GOVERNMENT OF BRITISH COLUMBIA. (1992). Selected vital statistics and health status indicators. *One hundred year report. Annual report 1991*. Victoria, BC: Division of Vital Statistics, BC Minister of Health and Minister Responsible for Senior Citizens.

GOVERNMENT OF BRITISH COLUMBIA. (1992). *Health indicator workbook* (1st ed.). Victoria, BC: Office of Health Promotion. BC Minister of Health and Minister Responsible for Senior Citizens.

GOVERNMENT OF CANADA. (1981). *Fitness for the older Canadian. Don't take it easy*. Ottawa: Minister of State for Fitness and Amateur Sport.

GOVERNMENT OF ONTARIO. (1992). *Ontario health survey 1990*. Toronto: Ontario Minister of Health.

GOVERNMENT OF ONTARIO. (1993). *Nurturing health*. Report of the Premier's Council on Health, Well-being and Social Justice (1987–1991). Toronto: Queen's Printer. (Catalogue No. 01–93–20M)

GRANT, K.R. (1988). The inverse care law in Canada: Differential access under universal free health insurance. In Bolaria, B. Singh and H.D. Dickinson. (1988). *Sociology of health care in Canada*. Toronto: Harcourt, Brace Jovanovich, 118–134.

GREEN, L.W. and RAEBURN, J.M. (1988). Health promotion: What is it? What will it become? *Health Promotion*, (Oxford), *3*(2), 151.

HEALTH AND WELFARE CANADA. (1981). *The health of Canadians: Report of the Canada health survey 1978–79*. Ottawa: Minister of Supply and Services.

HEALTH AND WELFARE CANADA. (1987). *The active health report: Perspectives on Canada's health promotion survey 1985*. Ottawa: Minister of Supply and Services. (Catalogue No. H39–106/1987E)

HEALTH AND WELFARE CANADA. (1992). *Alcohol and other drug use by Canadian youth*. Ottawa: Minister of Supply and Services.

JAFFE, D.T. (1980). *Healing from within*. New York: Knopf.

JONES, P.S. and MELEIS, A.I. (1993). Health is empowerment. *Adv Nurs Sci*, *15*(3), 1–14.

KING, D. (1980). *The Grey Nuns and the Red River settlement*. Agincourt, ON: Book Society of Canada.

KING, M., GARTRELL, J., and TROVALTO, F. (1991). Early childhood mortality, 1926–1986. *Canadian Social Trends*, *21*(9), 6–11. (Supply and Services Canada Catalogue No. 11–008E)

LABONTE, R. (1987). Community health promotion strategies. *Health Promotion*. Spring 1987, 5–10, 32.

LACELLE, C. (1979). Dufrost de Lajemmerais, Marie-Marguerite (Youville). In F. Halpenny (Ed.), *Dictionary of Canadian biography 1771 to 1800* . Toronto: University of Toronto Press, 234–239

LALONDE, M. (1974) *A new perspective on the health of Canadians*. Ottawa: Information Canada.

LEDDY, S. and PEPPER, J.M. (1993). *Conceptual bases of professional nursing* (3rd ed.) Philadelphia: Lippincott.

MCKIE, C. (1993). Population aging: baby boomers into the 21st century. In *Canadian Social Trends*, *29*, 6. (Supply and Services Canada Catalogue No. 11–008E)

MOCH, S.D. (1989). Health within illness: Conceptual evolution and practice possibilities. *Adv Nurs Sci*, *11*(4), 23–31.

NAIR, C., KARIM, R. and NYERS, C. (1992). Health care and Health status: A Canada – United States statistical comparison. *Health Reports 1992*, *4*(2), 175–183.

PAN AMERICAN HEALTH ORGANIZATION. (1990). *Health Conditions in the Americas 1990 (Vols 1 and 2)*. Washington, DC: Pan American Sanitary Bureau, World Health Organization.

PENDER, N.J. (1987). *Health promotion is nursing practice* (2nd ed.). Norwalk, CT: Appleton & Lange.

REGISTERED NURSES ASSOCIATION OF BRITISH COLUMBIA (RNABC). (1992). *Determinants of health: Empowering strategies for nursing practice*. (RNABC Publication No. 24). Vancouver, BC: Author.

ROSS, M. and CASEY, A. (1993). Health concerns associated with aging. In A. Beckingham and B.W. Du Gas. *Promoting healthy aging*. St. Louis: Mosby.

SIEGEL, B. (1986). *Love, medicine and miracles*. New York: Harper and Row.

SISTERS OF CHARITY OF MONTREAL. (1987). *Marguerite d'Youville: Mother of universal charity, Foundress of the Sisters of Charity of Montreal "Grey Nuns."* Montreal: Sadifa Media.

STATISTICS CANADA. (1992). *Health Reports*, *4*(2). (Statistics Canada Catalogue No. 82–003)

STATISTICS CANADA. (1993). *Hospital Morbidity, 1990–1991*. Ottawa: Minister of Science and Technology. (Catalogue No. 82–217)

SUTHERLAND, R. and FULTON, J. (1988). *Health care in Canada*. Ottawa: The Health Group.

TWADDLE, A.C. and HESSLER, R.M. (1987). *A sociology of health* (2nd ed.). New York: Macmillan.

UNICEF. (1992). *The state of the world's children*. New York: Oxford University Press for UNICEF.

UNITED NATIONS. (1992). *Demographic Yearbook 1991*. New York: The United Nations Secretariat. Department of International, Economic, and Social Affairs, Statistics Section.

WADHERA, S. and STRACHAN, J. (1992). Selected infant mortality and related statistics, Canada, 1921–1990. *Health Reports*, *4*(4), 429–433. (Statistics Canada Catalogue No. 82–003)

WILKINS, R., ADAMS, O. and BRANKER, A. (1989). Changes in mortality by income in urban Canada from 1979–1986. *Health Reports*, *1*(2), 137–167. (Catalogue No. 82-003)

WORLD HEALTH ORGANIZATION. (1948). *Constitution of the World Health Organization.*

WORLD HEALTH ORGANIZATION. (1978). *Alma Ata 1978: primary health care*. Geneva: Author.

WORLD HEALTH ORGANIZATION. (1980). *Health for all by the year 2000*. Pan-American Health Organization, Regional Office of the Pan-American Sanitary Bureau. Washington, DC: Author.

WORLD HEALTH ORGANIZATION. (1981). *Global strategy for health for all for the year 2000*. (Health for All series No. 3) Geneva: Author.

WORLD HEALTH ORGANIZATION. (1984a). *Health promotion glossary*. Copenhagen: WHO Regional Office for Europe.

WORLD HEALTH ORGANIZATION. (1984b). *Concepts and principles of health promotion* (Report on a WHO meeting, Copenhagen, 1984). Copenhagen: WHO Regional Office for Europe.

WORLD HEALTH ORGANIZATION. (1985). *Health manpower requirements for the achievement of health for all by the year 2000 through primary health care* (Report of a WHO Expert Committee). (Technical Report Series 717). Geneva: Author.

CHAPTER 3

Health Care
in Canada

CENTRAL QUESTIONS

1. What do the terms *welfare state*, *welfare society*, *healthy public policy* and *social safety net* mean?

2. What were some of the major events leading to the national health insurance program Canada has today?

3. How does Canada's national health care model differ from those of Great Britain and the United States?

4. What are the five principles on which the Canadian model was founded? How are these principles carried out in practice?

5. Why is each provincial and territorial health insurance program different from those of other provinces?

6. What specific hospital, outpatient, extended care and medical services are included in all provincial and territorial health care insurance programs?

7. What other services are included in each of the provinces and territories?

8. Why is everyone concerned about health care costs?

9. Why has every province and territory in Canada embarked on major health care reforms?

10. What are some of the commonalities of these reforms across provinces?

11. What are some of the specific changes taking place in the various provinces and the territories that are of particular interest to nurses?

INTRODUCTION

Health is said to be a human right, that is, a condition to which everyone has a just claim. The very acceptance of the notion of human right implies that society assumes a responsibility and will give high priority to carrying it out.

Lalonde, 1974

The provision of adequate health services is an essential component of a country's overall social policies. The impact of all public policies on health is powerful. Indeed, the Epp Report (1986) identified healthy public policy as one of the principal strategies for reforming the health care system in Canada.

Today we view health as encompassing social, economic and environmental factors, as well as biological and lifestyle factors. This enlarged understanding of health has led us to broaden our concept of what is involved in the "right to health." A statement of philosophy developed by the B.C. South Fraser Valley Health Council (1992) provides an example of this broader view. The statement reads, "We believe everyone has the right to those things that contribute to healthy living, including a safe physical environment, an effective social support system, a broad base of health services, and the information needed to make informed decisions about their own [health] behaviour" (South Fraser Valley Health Council, 1992).

Canada is seen as a **welfare state** because of its **social safety net** that provides a wide range of health and social support services to its citizens. Crichton, Hsu and Tsang (1994) suggest that the welfare state is becoming a **welfare society** characterized by:

1. a multisectoral approach to promoting health
2. the participation of consumers in the formulation of health and social policies
3. partnerships between business, government, educational institutions and health agencies in research and training.

They claim that we have moved beyond the basic health policy goals of equal access to care and promotion of income security for those most in need to the recognition of the importance of human rights (or equality of condition) in health care issues (Crichton, Hsu and Tsang, 1994).

In this chapter, we will discuss the concept of *healthy public policy*, as well as the development of the Canadian social safety net that has emerged as a result of our social policies. We will also look at our National Health Insurance Program as it has evolved and at its administration in the different provinces and territories. We will also discuss the health care reforms that are currently being initiated in every province and territory.

Because of our close social and economic ties to both Great Britain and the United States, we will also include a brief comparison of the health care systems in our country and in theirs.

POLICY-MAKING

A **policy** is a decision or action taken in an organization by which other specific proposals are judged for their acceptability. It provides guidelines for the actions of people within that organization. As a student, you were probably introduced to school policies in your orientation classes, for example, in regard to the "dress code" for class and for clinical experiences.

According to Blum, **public policy** is "an established and legislatively enacted proposal by a public body duly constituted to make policy in the area of concern. It stipulates ends and it may provide resources. It may spell out specific means to reach these ends" (1981, cited in Pederson, Edwards, Marshall, Allison and Kelner, 1989, 11). For example, the Royal Commission on Health Services (Government of Canada, 1964), in examining health and health services in Canada, found that there was an acute shortage of qualified health personnel across the country — doctors, nurses, dentists, pharmacists, physiotherapists and occupational therapists, laboratory and X-ray technicians were in short supply. Indeed, in virtually all categories of health personnel, we were highly dependent on people from other countries to fulfill our needs. Each year we were bringing into the country more doctors than we were graduating from our Canadian medical schools. In response to recommendations of the Royal Commission, a policy decision was made by the prevailing government, in consultation with the provinces, to increase the Canadian supply of health workers so that Canada could become self sufficient in the production of qualified health personnel. To this end, the federal government passed the Health Resources Act (1966), allocating resources totalling $500 million to be expended over a 15-year period to help the provinces develop the educational facilities and clinical practice areas to prepare the needed health workers. The money was to be distributed to the provinces by means of matching grants (whereby the federal government and the provincial government share equally in the cost). A Health Manpower Directorate was established within the Department of National Health and Welfare to administer the fund. A Manpower Planning Division was incorporated to develop strategies for planning for the country's future needs.

The enactment of policy decisions in legislation is a complex and lengthy process. In our democratic Canadian society, we believe that everyone should be given the opportunity to voice opinions on the issue through public forums, written briefs in reaction to "White Papers" or other means. A formal policy statement of the government's intent, such as the Nova Scotia Ministry of Health's *Health Care for the Nineties: Managing Better Health* (1990) or

Saskatchewan's *Vision of Health* (1992), is then set out. Consensus needs to be built, through another round of public forums or meetings with all stakeholders. With federal legislation, this may be done through federal–provincial meetings. Then, proposals must go through the parliamentary (or legislative) committee process. Following these steps, during which many changes may be made, proposed legislation is drafted and debated in Parliament or Legislative Assembly. If this is passed, the Senate then takes a "second look" at the bill in the case of federal legislation. This step is followed by official signing of the bill by the Governor-General, or the Lieutenant-Governor of the province, at which stage the bill becomes law.

HEALTHY PUBLIC POLICY

A relatively new term that has come into use in recent years is **healthy public policy**. This has been defined as "policy enacted by the various levels of government that is characterized by explicit concern for health and equity, and by accountability for health impact" (B.C. Government, 1991b, 1). According to Pederson et al. (1989), the goal of this concept is "to suggest a new way of thinking about health and government policy that is participatory, multisectoral, and ecological" in order to make health a higher priority on the political agenda.

An example of a healthy public policy that has been enacted at the national level of government is the Tobacco Control Act (1987), which included strengthening of the government's smoking prevention program by adding efforts to achieve cessation and a regulatory strategy (Pederson et al., 1989). The enactment of this legislation required collaboration between the Ministers of Health, Justice, Labour and the Secretary of the Treasury. An example of a provincially enacted healthy public policy is the mandatory seat belt legislation that almost all provinces have now passed (which has required the cooperation of health, justice and transport ministries). Healthy public policies can be enacted at municipal levels as well. In January, 1991, the Richmond (B.C.) City Council passed a by-law (subsequently approved by the Ministry of Health) requiring licensed bars and restaurants to post signs warning that drinking alcoholic beverages during pregnancy can cause birth defects (see Figure 3.1).

Sometimes, governments do not explicitly espouse certain policies, but may demonstrate support for them through the allocation of funds or other resources such as space. Many interested groups try to influence both policy decisions and the form and substance of proposed legislation by lobbying members of the law-making body through the use of advertisements on radio, in the newspapers and on television, or by staging demonstrations and other means to gain public support and the attention of politicians. Nursing or-

FIGURE 3.1 Fetal Alcohol Syndrome Warning Sign.

SOURCE: In B.C. Ministry of Health. (1991a). *A Guide for communities to enact health-promoting policies.* Victoria, B.C.: Queen's Printer, 23.

ganizations in Canada have only in recent years become aware of the tremendous impact they can have on the political process by virtue of the sheer size of the nursing community. (We are the largest group of health workers, numbering over 200 000 at the latest count.) Nursing's involvement in the political process has increased greatly in recent years (Larsen and Baumgart, 1992; Lefort, S.M., 1993). We will discuss the topic of nurses and politics further in Chapter 5, Nursing in Canada. Meanwhile, it should be noted that everyone can participate in bringing about healthy policy changes. At the community and neighbourhood level, local residents can often introduce changes such as getting the city to install a light at a busy intersection for the safety of children and older adults. People can also attend public forums, express their opinions through "Letters to the Editor" in their local paper or write letters to their Member of the Legislative Assembly (MLA) or Member of Parliament (MP).

THE CANADIAN SOCIAL SAFETY NET

As pointed out in the Epp Report, health cannot be separated from the social conditions in which people live (Epp, 1986). In discussing the Canadian health care system, then, we will also consider the role of Canada's social welfare programs, which ensure income security for those in need. These programs include unemployment insurance, old age pension, Canada and Quebec contributory pension programs for working people, family allowance and social assistance programs for those in financial need. The combination of our national health plan, which includes both hospital and medical care, and our social welfare programs is frequently referred to as the Canadian social safety net. Canadians today view these social programs as a right to which all are naturally entitled, but they came about through a long, slow process of policy development, consensus building, policy finalization, endorsement by the provinces, drafting and debating of legislation and the final step of enactment into law.

HISTORICAL PERSPECTIVE

EARLY HEALTH CARE IN CANADA

The early immigrants who settled in this land, although fiercely independent in most things, accepted the reality of having to band together for mutual aid when someone was ill or in need. Until late in the nineteenth century, health and welfare were seen as primarily the responsibility of individuals and their families — with help from church and community in times of need. In French Canada, the tradition of church involvement in health and social welfare was established by the early settlers who sent back to France for members of the religious orders to care for the sick. In the English-speaking colonies, municipalities passed legislation similar to the English Poor Law of 1598 in which municipalities accepted responsibility for the care of those unable to care for themselves.

During these early years, sisters of the Roman Catholic Church set up hospitals and provided nursing services, following the settlers westward as the country was opened up. After the British conquest of Canada in 1767, the French nursing sisterhoods continued their work in the parishes of the Roman Catholic church. The British, on their part, set up military hospitals, with male nurses. Some secular hospitals developed in the larger towns but, for the most part, these were dirty and poorly managed. In those times, it was considered part of a woman's role to look after anyone who was ill in the household, with only the homeless having to seek refuge in a hospital.

Secular hospitals in Canada remained very primitive for a number of years. The massive wave of immigrants into the country in the early 1800s brought an increased number of health problems, however, and stimulated the development of health personnel. A number of both French and English-speaking nursing sisterhoods were established. In addition to the Roman Catholic Church, other religious groups became involved in the provision of health services, including the Eastern Orthodox and Anglican churches as well as the Home Mission Boards of the Methodist, Presbyterian and United Churches. English-speaking hospitals began to emerge, operated by these religious groups,

as, for example, the Anglican and United Church Mission hospitals that dotted the coasts of Labrador, Newfoundland and British Columbia, as well as the Far North (Victorian Order of Nurses, 1983).

"Poorhouses," which sheltered the indigent sick, the mentally ill and older people without families to care for them, were under municipal jurisdiction. Maternity care was generally undertaken by lay midwives, except in rare cases where the few physicians who had settled in the new land were available.

With the passage of the British North America Act in 1867, Canada became a federated state. The Act carefully laid out the respective powers of the federal and provincial governments, assigning the responsibility for health and welfare matters to the provinces. Jurisdiction over the collection of the revenue necessary to pay for these services, however, was invested primarily with the federal government — a situation which has been a major source of federal–provincial conflict ever since.

Increasing urbanization and industrialization marked the post-Confederation years. Towns were often unable to cope with the floods of farm labourers seeking work in the new factories and immigrants coming from other lands to seek a better life in the "New World." Crowded conditions, poor housing, a lack of health services and inadequate sewage and garbage disposal combined to make disease rampant and mortality rates high. The poor health conditions brought about the passage of a Public Health Act in each of the provinces, modelled after a British act passed in 1875. These acts established provincial and local boards of health and provided for the appointment of medical health officers and sanitary inspectors.

Hospitals and care of the needy were, however, still mainly the responsibility of the church and charitable organizations. The secular hospitals were, regrettably, "generally distinguished by a prevalence of rats, dirt, stale air and lack of order and good management" (Victorian Order of Nurses, 1983, 8, 9). Nursing in the secular hospitals was carried out by poorly educated girls who were paid a miserable wage. Nursing was not something that girls from good families did.

Florence Nightingale can be given credit for changing the image of nursing and for improving hospital conditions in Great Britain, North America and throughout the western world. Her work in saving the lives of hundreds of soldiers through the good management of military hospitals in the Crimean War during the mid-1850s brought her acclaim from a grateful British nation. In return they raised funds to enable her to establish a training school for nurses (VON, 1983; Canadian Nurses Association, 1968).

We will discuss the Nightingale school further in Chapter 5 when we talk about the development of nursing education. In addition to her work in hospitals, Florence Nightingale was concerned about the unsanitary conditions and ignorance of health matters of people living in the crowded slums of London and other towns and in the

1600 1700 1800 1900

1650 1750 1850 1950

LOOKING BACK

LADY ABERDEEN 1857–1939

The founding of the Victorian Order of Nurses of Canada, like many historical firsts in nursing, was the work of a "woman of influence" — one of those women of earlier centuries who were denied access to the political and employment arenas but who applied their energies and positions to the promotion of better health care. Countess Ishbel Aberdeen was the wife of the Governor General of Canada during the years 1894 to 1898 and used her position during those years to bring into being a visiting nursing order that continues to the present day. The Victorian Order of Nurses of Canada is a voluntary charitable organization that has initiated many major advances in public health care for almost a century.

The third daughter in the wealthy Marjoribanks family, Ishbel Maria married John Gordon, seventh Earl of Aberdeen, in 1877. He was politically active, and the young couple soon had a brief viceregal appointment in Ireland. On their return to England, she began to take an active role in current events and accepted the presidency of the newly formed International Council of Women. When her husband was appointed Governor General of Canada, she immediately began to work for a Canadian National Council of Women. During a tour of Canada, members of western branches of the Council stressed the hardships of sick women and children in isolated settlements, where there was no medical assistance and no hospitals. Lady Aberdeen was familiar with the Jubilee Institute of District Nurses, formed in Britain for such work, and believed a project of home helpers would be ideal for Canada.

Nora E. Livingston, Lady Superintendent of the Montreal General Hospital, proposed to Lady Aberdeen that the Order should consist of qualified nurses, with extra preparation in district nursing. Once convinced, Lady Aberdeen set out to raise the funds for such an undertaking and to lay the political groundwork for it to be a success. Her proposal was at first strongly opposed by the medical profession, especially the powerful Ontario Medical Association, who were concerned that the nurses would practice midwifery and thus cut into their incomes. Through some well-placed lobbying efforts, aided by Dr. Alfred Worcester, founder of the Waltham Training School for District Nurses in the United States, she managed to gain medical endorsements and the support of the Canadian government. She also managed to convince Charlotte Macleod, a Canadian who was superintendent at Waltham, to return to Canada to become the national director. Lady Aberdeen herself became the first president of the VON Canada national board.

Four VON branches were established in 1897, in Halifax, Montreal, Ottawa and Toronto. These were, as they are now, run by local, voluntary, charitable, not-for-profit boards in each community. The boards raised money and then recruited nurses through the VON national director. Communities decided on the services to be offered, but these generally included district nursing care for those with infectious diseases, care of women and their newborns, and care for the elderly and poor who could not afford medical or hospital care. Education was a vital part of the role.

Lady Aberdeen continued her mentorship of the project, taking care that the VON received favourable publicity whenever possible. She was responsible for arranging for four VON nurses to travel to the Yukon to provide care during the Klondike Gold Rush of 1898 as one means of making the service known throughout Canada. The Victorian Order of Nurses of Canada is a tribute to her political acumen, hard work, and influential support.

— Glennis Zilm and Kirstine Griffith

rural villages of England. She was emphatic that "the nurse must combat in the home, 'dirt, drink, diet, damp, draughts, drains' " (VON, 1983, 12). Her influence was felt in the development of the Queen's Own Visiting Nurse service in Great Britain and, subsequently, the Victorian Order of Nurses in Canada.

By the turn of the century, hospitals were beginning to flourish. People who could not afford to pay for the services of a hospital were, however, still dependent on charity if they fell ill. To provide an alternative to charity, fraternal societies like the Masons, the Foresters and the Knights of Columbus began to emerge. Each member contributed to a common fund which was used to help members and their families who were sick, unemployed or otherwise in need. Because government scholarships and bursaries were offered to only a select few, many students received financial assistance from one of the fraternal societies to go through normal school (teacher training) or nurses' training, or to complete a university education.

By the end of the nineteenth century, medical and nursing schools were well established, standards had been raised for the qualifications of health practitioners, and hospital conditions had improved considerably. Institutions were built for the mentally ill, people with tuberculosis, the blind and the deaf. In addition, a number of voluntary organizations had been established, among them the Children's Aid Societies, the Red Cross Society and the Victorian Order of Nurses (Health and Welfare Canada, 1989; VON 1983).

Industrialization in the latter part of the nineteenth century also brought about the development of unions. Like the fraternal societies, they were interested in the welfare of their members. In addition to being concerned with raising living standards, they also wanted to protect workers from losing their income if they were ill, unemployed or had been injured on the job. The Ontario Workmen's Compensation Act, passed in 1914, and those subsequently passed in other provinces, were the first modern social security programs in Canada (see Chapter 4 for a discussion of services provided by Workers' Compensation Boards).

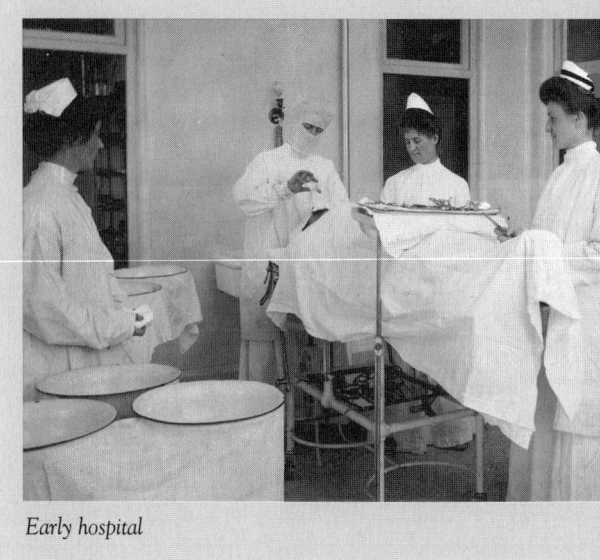

Early hospital

THE WAR YEARS

Canada's entry into World War I, in 1914, accelerated the trend towards industrialization and urbanization. There was a demand for assistance to widows and children, as well as to older family members who had lost sons who would have supported them in their old age. Manitoba responded to this demand by passing a Mothers' Pension Act in 1916 which was followed soon after by similar legislation in other provinces. The Mothers' Pension was not available to everyone, however, but only to those in financial need. The demeaning philosophy of the Poor Law still prevailed. Receiving charity of any kind was considered a sign of personal failure. To have to admit that you were in need of assistance (whether from government, church or other charitable organization) by undergoing a means test in order to qualify for the Mothers' Pension was demeaning.

During the war years, people in rural towns and villages in Saskatchewan had a problem enticing doctors to set up practice because so many people could not pay for the doctor's services. They began to pool their resources to employ a physician for the community. Passage of the Rural Municipality Act in 1916 legitimized this practice, giving towns and villages the power to raise taxes by local levy to pay for a physician's services.

Between World War I and World War II, provincial and municipal governments began to get more involved in providing medical care for the needy and in financing hospitals for the sick. Agitation for social legislation by veterans looking for work as they returned to their homes across the country stimulated the first policy proposals for national health insurance, unemployment insurance and old age pensions. These proposals were incorporated as components of the Liberal election platform in 1919 — but the Liberals did not win. The federal government did get together with the provinces, though, in sharing half the costs for an old age pension program in 1927. The program paid twenty dollars a month, again only to those determined to be in need by a means test.

During the Depression of the 1930s, British Columbia and Alberta both made unsuccessful attempts to bring in health insurance legislation to ease the bleak situation. Saskatchewan, however, always the pioneer, passed a Municipal Medical and Hospital Services Act in 1939 which extended the rights of municipalities to allow them to collect a levy for both hospital and physicians' services (Taylor, 1978, 1990; Guest, 1985).

In 1941, the federal government brought in an unemployment insurance program to forestall some of the social unrest anticipated when the soldiers came home after the war. They also commissioned an extensive study on the feasibility of national health insurance, but the recommendations of the Heagerty Commission were not implemented, because of disputes over money during federal–provincial consultations. Parliament did, however, pass a **Family Allowance** Act in 1945, which was the first universal social program in Canada. There was no means test — every family with children received a certain allowance, according to the number of children. The National Health Grants Act, passed in 1948, helped the provinces through matching grants to improve hospitals and community health services.

THE BEGINNINGS OF MEDICARE

Saskatchewan introduced the first province-wide universal hospital insurance in 1948, followed by British Columbia and Alberta in 1949. After several rounds of federal–provincial negotiation, Parliament finally passed a Hospital Insurance and Diagnostic Services Act in 1957 based on a fifty–fifty sharing of costs with provinces who met the criteria for entry into the program. All provinces had qualified and were enrolled by 1961.

During the 1950s, the federal government expanded its social service network to include cost-sharing programs with the provinces, such as universal **Old Age Security** (OAS), established in 1951, and programs for the disabled and the blind. Revisions were also made to the Unemployment Insurance Act.

The 1960s saw the birth of **Medicare** after a lengthy battle with physicians who objected to the idea of "socialized medicine" and would have preferred privately sponsored medical insurance. Saskatchewan took the lead once again, introducing a provincial Medical Care Act in 1962. A mass exodus of doctors from the province followed, their numbers being quickly replaced by physicians from Great Britain who were unhappy with the even more socialized system there. To explore the feasibility of going ahead with plans to implement a national program, the federal government had appointed a Royal Commission on Health Services. The Report of the Commission recommended that, although the country was short of the needed health personnel, the government should proceed with its plans (Government of Canada, 1964). To overcome the shortage of human resources in the health field, the government enacted the Health Resources Act (mentioned earlier in the chapter) in 1966. Also in 1966, Parliament passed the Medical Care Act, in which the federal government agreed to share the cost of the programs with the provinces (it was implemented in 1968). By 1972, all provinces and territories had joined the plan.

The 1960s also saw great strides in the development of other social programs. In the Vocational Rehabilitation of Disabled Persons Act of 1961, the federal government shared with the provinces the cost of comprehensive vocational rehabilitation services for physically and mentally disabled persons. The **Canada Pension Plan** (CPP) was introduced in 1966. Contribution to this plan is compulsory for all employed persons in Canada, with the exception of Quebec which has its own pension plan. The plan was intended to augment income in the event of retirement, disability or the loss of a spouse. In 1966, Parliament passed the Canada Assistance Plan Act to provide subsidies to provinces and municipalities for social assistance and other welfare services.

Many of our older adults were in the labour force before generous retirement pension programs were made an integral component of most employee benefit packages. Those who weren't able to save enough money when they were working are now having a hard time living on the government old age pension. Women who stayed at home to look after their families are in a particularly vulnerable position because it was only those who worked outside the home who contributed to, and can benefit from, pension programs. Additionally, a man's pension often died with him, leaving a widow in dire circumstances. Older people receiving the OAS who are on a low income benefit from the Guaranteed Income Supplement introduced in 1967. In 1975, a Spouse's Allowance was added to the OAS for spouses aged 60–64 to augment the income of low-income families. By the end of the 1960s, a fairly comprehensive social safety net for Canadians was in place. All citizens had access to required medical and hospital services, regardless of their income, and a minimum income was guaranteed to those in need (Taylor, 1990; Guest, 1985).

RESTRUCTURING THE SAFETY NET

The 1970s was a time for refining systems. The rapid rise of hospital costs prompted reconsideration of the national health program by both federal and provincial governments. It became evident that, under the National Health Grants program, too many hospitals had been built (Rachlis and Kushner, 1989; Sutherland and Fulton, 1988). By the end of the decade, it was also acknowledged that the capacity of medical schools had perhaps been increased too much and we were heading for a surplus of doctors. The Lalonde Report of 1974 set the tone for a new direction in health care in Canada, pointing out that further gains in the health of Canadians were not likely to come from a sickness-oriented system, but rather from measures such as improving people's lifestyles and physical environment. The provinces began to agitate for more control of the health care dollar, demanding relaxation of federal control over spending so that they could experiment with innovative ways of delivering health care, such as community health centres, home care programs and the utilization of nurse practitioners.

Negotiations which went on for several years resulted in the passage of the Established Programs Financing Act in 1977. Provincial governments traded the fifty–fifty open-ended cost-sharing of programs with the federal government for a significant number of personal income and corporate tax benefits. The federal government's contribution was to be in the form of block grants, with an equalization formula for provinces designated as low-income provinces — all but British Columbia, Alberta and Ontario have been so designated. Also introduced in 1977 was the federal Extended Health Care Services program, providing funds of twenty dollars per person so that the provinces could experiment with lower-cost alternative services, such as community health centres and home care.

By the end of the decade, health care services were taking an increasingly large share of provincial budgets. There was also concern about the erosion of the system by practices such as extra billing by doctors and the levy of premiums by provincial governments, such as a daily charge for hospital care. Another Royal Commission on Health Services, chaired once again by Justice Emmott Hall, was appointed to study the system. The 1980 Report pointed out that the principles on which the National Health Care

Program had been based were indeed being eroded and recommended a return to the original intent of the program. A new Canada Health Act was passed in 1984 which placed controls on extra billing and additional provincial levies for basic services. This act replaced the Hospital and Diagnostic Services Act of 1957 and the Medical Care Insurance Act of 1968, and remains the basis of health care in this country. As costs of maintaining the system continue to increase, many Canadians are questioning whether we can keep our national health care system intact. We will discuss this topic further in a later section of this chapter.

Canada's Social Safety Net Time-Line

1867	British Parliament	British North America Act
1882	Ontario	First provincial Bureau of Health
1890s	Private sector	VON, Red Cross, Children's Aid societies established
1914	Ontario	First provincial Workmen's Compensation Act
1916	Saskatchewan	Rural Municipality Act
1916	Manitoba	Mothers' Pension Act
1927	Federal Government	Old Age Pension Act
1939	Saskatchewan	Municipal Medical and Hospital Services Act
1941	Federal Government	Unemployment Insurance Act
1945	Federal Government	Family Allowance Act
1946	Saskatchewan	Universal hospital insurance introduced
1948	Federal Government	National Health Grants
1951	Federal Government	Old Age Security Act (OAS)
		Programs for the disabled and blind
1957	Federal Government	National Hospital Insurance and Diagnostic Services Act
1961	Federal Government	National Fitness and Amateur Sport Act
1962	Saskatchewan	Medical Care Insurance Act
1962	Federal Government	National Welfare Grants
1964	Federal Government	Hall Commission Report Youth Allowances program
1966	Federal Government and Quebec	Canada/Quebec Pension Plans (CPP/QPP)
	Federal Government	Canada Assistance Plan (CAP)
	Federal Government	Health Resources Act
1966	Federal Government	Medical Care Act
1974	Federal Government	Lalonde Report
1975	Federal Government	Spouse's Allowance
		National Health Research and Development Program (NHRDP)
1977	Federal Government	Established Programs Financing Act
1980	Federal Government	Hall Commission Report on Canada's national health insurance program
1984	Federal Government	Canada Health Act

SOURCES: (1) Du Gas, B. and Beckingham, A. The emergence of gerontological nursing. In A. Beckingham and B. Du Gas (1993). *Promoting Healthy Aging*. St. Louis: Mosby, 50–79. (2) Health and Welfare Canada (1989). *Health and Welfare in Canada*. Ottawa: Ministry of Supply and Services Canada; Gibbon, J.M. and Mathewson, M.S. (1947). *Three Centuries of Canadian Nursing*. Toronto: The Macmillan Company of Canada Limited. Adapted from Canada's Social Security Network Time-line, in Beckingham and Du Gas.

NOTE FOR STUDENTS: You will sometimes find different dates for the passage of legislation in different sources. Acts of Parliament are sometimes passed in one year but not promulgated until the next. We have chosen to use the dates given in an official publication by Health and Welfare Canada (Health and Welfare Canada, 1989).

NATIONAL HEALTH CARE

MAJOR NATIONAL HEALTH CARE MODELS

Sutherland and Fulton (1988) describe three basic models for the organization of health care services in a country:

1. the national health services model, in which services are provided and organized by a national government
2. the national (public) insurance model, in which the government is the insuring agency. People pay the government (or a **quasi-governmental agency***) a predictable sum, either through a premium or through taxes, to cover health care costs.
3. the entrepreneurial model, in which health services are provided by private agencies and paid for by the consumer of these services.

Canada's health care system is basically a public insurance model, although it contains elements of the other two.

The system in Great Britain is a **national health services model** and you will often hear British people refer to it as "the NHS." In this model, health services are organized and delivered by the government, most often through a Ministry of Health. In Britain, all services are under the direct control of the national Ministry of Health; the service is therefore considered a centralized system. In some countries — Sweden and Finland are examples — the services are decentralized. Most Canadian health services are not operated by government agencies, although some are. Government operated services in Canada include community health services in most provinces, provincial hospitals and services for the mentally ill, provincial laboratory services and provincial ambulance systems. The federal government also provides direct services to certain groups within the Canadian population. We will discuss the services provided by different levels of government in Canada in Chapter 4.

In Canada, we have opted for a **national insurance model** in which the government funds most services. This model is sometimes referred to as a "one payer system." National health insurance operates on the same principle as any other type of insurance. That is to say, people pay a predictable sum on a regular basis to cover unpredictable expenses for health care. Payments are made directly by individuals to the insuring agency, through payroll deductions (usually on a cost-sharing basis with employers), or

they may be included in the provincial tax system, where payment is correlated with income. The insuring agency in some cases is the government. In others it is an agency closely associated with and accountable to the government, such as a Crown Corporation (sometimes spoken of as quasi-governmental). In some provinces the Ministry of Health is the insuring agency; in others a Crown Corporation has been established to administer the plans.

Although funded primarily by provincial governments, with contributions from the federal government, most health services in Canada are administered and delivered by agencies other than government. Most hospitals, for example, are called "public general hospitals" but are run by a private "hospital society." In national health insurance systems, the government may fund, regulate and plan health services but these services may be carried out by employees of non-governmental "non-profit" agencies or by non-governmental agencies for profit. The Ontario and Nova Scotia governments contract out home nursing services to the Victorian Order of Nurses (a non-profit voluntary agency). The B.C. Ministry of Health hires private agencies such as Comcare (a private agency) to provide home care services to people, in addition to those provided by employees of the Ministry's own community health agencies. Ninety-five percent of the physicians in Canada are in private practice and people are free to choose their own physicians. Government is the sole payer for all insured services, including those provided by physicians. The physicians are paid for carrying out these services on a fee-for-service basis, according to a schedule for different services negotiated between the provincial medical association and the government (Sutherland and Fulton, 1988).

In the **entrepreneurial model**, services are provided by private agencies and paid for by the consumer so that market forces control the supply and demand aspects of health care. The government does not play a role in either the funding or provision of services. The health care system in the United States is closer to this model, although it has elements of each of the other two (Sutherland and Fulton, 1988). The US federal government does fund services for older people through its Medicare program and services for the poor through **Medicaid**. State Departments of Health also fund and deliver some health services; for example, community health programs and municipal governments usually plan, fund and deliver school health programs. In the United States, private health insurance is the principal method of health care financing for people under the age of 65. Much of the insurance is employer-paid as a fringe benefit of employment.

THE CANADIAN MODEL

Although the federal government contributes funding, the health care system in Canada is administered by provincial

---

* A quasi-governmental agency is one that is closely related to government and is responsible to it, but operates autonomously. Crown Corporations are quasi-governmental agencies.

and territorial governments. The National Health Insurance program was founded on the following five principles:

1. public administration
2. comprehensiveness
   a. hospital services
   b. outpatient services
   c. extended care services
   d. medical services
3. universality
4. portability
5. accessibility.

These five principles provided the basis for both the Hospital Insurance and Diagnostic Services Act of 1957 and the Medical Care Act of 1966. These principles were reaffirmed in the Canada Health Act of 1984. The criteria which provincial health insurance plans must meet in order to receive full cash contributions for their plans from the federal government were derived from these principles, and are set out in the Canada Health Act.

Conditions Certain conditions were spelled out in the Canada Health Act which the provinces and territories must meet in order to be eligible for full cash payments for insured health services, as well as extended care services. These include keeping Health Canada informed regarding operation of the provincial and territorial plans and appropriate recognition for Federal contributions. Provisions were also built into the 1984 Act to ban extra billing and user charges for insured services. The federal minister of health is empowered to withhold cash payments to the provinces if the criteria and conditions are not met. Indeed, until some provinces succeeded in banning extra billing or discontinued the practice of user fees for some insured services, cash payments were withheld. At the time of writing, all provinces have complied, although from time to time, these practices tend to recur.

Services The insured health services covered by the Canada Health Act include all necessary hospital services, physician services and surgical-dental services carried out in a hospital. The Act also includes provisions for extended care services. These include nursing homes, intermediate care, adult residential care, home care and ambulatory care. Within this broad framework, provincial and territorial governments are free to develop their own health care plans and, as we will discuss in the next section, each is different.

Criteria required to obtain federal funding

1. PUBLIC ADMINISTRATION The plan must be administered and operated on a non-profit basis by a public authority, responsible to the provincial government and subject to audits of its accounts and financing transactions.

2. COMPREHENSIVENESS The plan must insure all insured health services provided by hospitals, medical practitioners or dentists, and, where permitted, services rendered by other health care practitioners.

3. UNIVERSALITY One hundred percent of the insured persons of a province must be entitled to the insured health services provided for by the plan on uniform terms and conditions.

4. PORTABILITY Residents moving to another province must continue to be covered for health services by the home province during any minimum waiting period imposed by the new province of residence, not to exceed three months. For persons temporarily absent from their home provinces:
   a. Out-of-province (but within Canada) insured services are to be paid for by the home province at the rate of the host province unless other fiscal arrangements have been made between the provinces. Prior approval may be required for elective services.
   b. Out-of-country services are to be paid, as a minimum, on the basis of the amount that would have been paid by the home province for similar services rendered in-province. Prior approval may also be required for elective services.

5. ACCESSIBILITY The health care plan of a province must provide for:
   a. insured health services on uniform terms and conditions and reasonable access by insured persons to insured health services unprecluded or unimpeded, either directly or indirectly, by charges or other means;
   b. reasonable compensation to physicians and dentists for all insured health services rendered;
   c. payments to hospitals in respect of the cost of insured health services.

SOURCE: Canada Health Act Overview (1992). In Health and Welfare Canada. *Canada Health Act Annual Report 1991–1992.* Ottawa: Ministry of Supply and Services. Cat. HI-4/1992.

PROVINCIAL AND TERRITORIAL HEALTH CARE PLANS

All provinces and territories must conform to the guidelines set out in the Canada Health Act. However, the guidelines are broad and allow for considerable flexibility. The result of this flexibility is that we essentially have ten health care plans, each one slightly different from the other. Each province or territory has the responsibility for financing its program (with contributions from the federal government). Provinces and territories can, almost as much they wish, set their own priorities, select the policies they want to follow and plan their own health services. In looking at provincial plans, we will discuss similarities and differences under each of the principles on which the National Health Insurance Program was founded.

Public administration   In all provinces and territories, hospital and medical insurance are operated by the Ministry of Health and/or a public body that is responsible to it, for example a quasi-governmental insurance agency.

Comprehensiveness   Bearing in mind the conditions of the Canada Health Act regarding compulsory payments for insured services, provinces are free to allocate resources, to set standards for services, to administer the services and to evaluate them. They may also deliver services. These services include physician's and dental services, ambulance services, hospital and other inpatient services such as nursing homes, as well as community health services (Sutherland and Fulton, 1988). The specific services covered by all provinces are as follows:

- HOSPITAL SERVICES
  - accommodation and meals at standard ward level

  - necessary nursing services, including private duty if required

  - radiological and other diagnostic services (laboratory, x-ray or other)

  - drugs, biologicals (medicinal compounds prepared from living organisms) and related procedures performed in hospitals

  - routine surgical supplies

  - use of Operating Room, Case Room and anesthetic facilities

  - use of radiotherapy and physiotherapy services where available

- OUTPATIENT SERVICES
  - laboratory, diagnostic and radiology procedures where available

  - radiotherapy and physiotherapy

  - the hospital component of other outpatient services, for example, plaster room and Operating Room services

- EXTENDED CARE SERVICES
  - nursing home intermediate care (care requiring some nursing service) — daily room service charge may be levied for this service

  - assistive devices, such as wheelchairs, prostheses and hearing aids for people with disabilities or long-term incapacitating illness (in Alberta and Saskatchewan assistive devices come under a separate plan, called the Aids for Independent Living).

- MEDICAL SERVICES

  All provinces provide the basic services outlined in the Canada Health Act. Some provide payment for the services of other practitioners, such as optometrists and podiatrists or chiropodists,* either on the same basis as for physicians or with a "user fee." For example, one may have to pay a five-dollar user fee per visit for physiotherapy treatment (in the physiotherapist's office), over and above the fee the practitioner receives from the government plan for the service. The number of visits per year permitted under the plan may also be limited. Some provincial plans have a Seniors' Drug Plan under which older people do not have to pay for prescription drugs or may be charged only for the pharmacist's dispensing fee. Drug plans may be extended to other specific groups, for example, to people with diabetes. Ambulance services must be provided by all provinces. All charge a small "user fee" except Ontario, the Yukon and the Northwest Territories. Emergency transportation by ambulance may be exempted from the user fee. For any or all of the medical, dental and hospital services not covered by the provincial plan, insurance may be obtained from a third party. Many employee health benefit plans, for example, contain options for semi-private or private room hospital coverage, for dental plans and for other services.

Universality   All insured persons of each province are entitled to coverage. Not eligible for coverage are people who are looked after under other health programs. For example, the federal government provides direct service for members of the armed services and members of the Royal Canadian Mounted Police, and also has special programs for First Nations people and the population of prisons. Some provinces collect a premium for health insurance but, in most provinces, money comes from general tax revenues.

---

*   Podiatrists and chiropodists are both foot care specialists — the difference between them is that podiatry is taught in university degree programs, and chiropody in college programs.

Portability   Most provinces entitle a person to become a beneficiary on the first day of the third month following their arrival in the province. First day (immediate) coverage is extended to certain specific groups, such as landed immigrants, in some provinces.

Accessibility   Additional charges (user fees) may be levied on services not performed in hospital, such as physiotherapy in a therapist's office, and on services provided by practitioners other than physicians or dentists — podiatrists, for example. No person is denied access to services because they cannot pay for them. A distinguishing number on an individual's health care identification card enables agency receptionists to identify that person as eligible for additional benefits, such as no "user fees" for services for people on social welfare, low-income seniors or people with certain chronic diseases.

Table 3.1 provides a comparison of the differing aspects of the various provincial health insurance plans.

HEALTH CARE AND THE MONEY IT COSTS

Canada's health care plan is basically "a publicly funded program which pays private providers" (Rachlis and Kushner, 1989). When the national hospital and medical in-

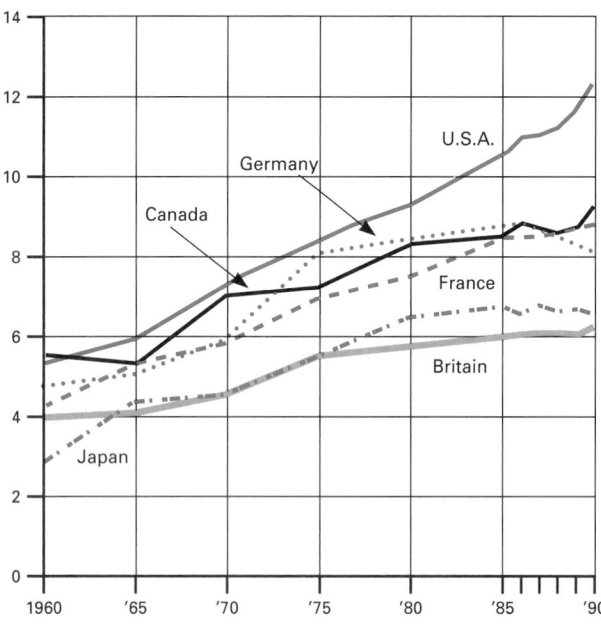

FIGURE 3.2 Total health care spending as a percentage of GDP, Canada and selected other countries

SOURCE: OECD Health Systems: Facts and Trends, 1992. In C. Nair, R. Karim and C. Nyers. *Health Care and Health Status: A Canada–United States Comparison. Health Reports 1992.* 4 (2) Statistics Canada, Cat. 82–003.

A dental hygienist teaches a boy proper use of a toothbrush.

surance programs were introduced, the federal government agreed to sharing costs with the provinces on a fifty–fifty "open-ended" basis. In other words, there were no limits on the amount the federal government was required to contribute. Under the Established Programs Financing Act of 1977, these arrangements were changed, as the provinces negotiated successfully for a transfer of some tax credits (that is, the right to impose certain taxes on personal and/or corporate income) together with a cash grant. This grant was to be given as a block of money for health, welfare and education services. Provinces were free to allocate these funds as they wished. Quebec opted for a larger share of tax credits and smaller cash grant than the other provinces — a choice which later developments have shown to have been a wise one.

THE EXPENDITURES

In 1960, Canada was spending 5.5 percent of its gross domestic product (GDP) on health care. By 1991, this figure had increased to 9.9 percent of the GDP, an increase of 67 percent. Figures for the United States show that their increase in health expenditures was 135 percent from 1960 to 1990 (from 5.2 percent of GDP to 12.2 percent). Figure 3.2 shows that the rise in Canada's spending on health as a proportion of GDP is close to the average for most of the countries in the Organization for Economic Cooperation and Development (OECD).

The health care systems of Canada and the United States share some similarities, although the structure of

TABLE 3.1 A Comparison of Provincial and Territorial Health Insurance Plans, Selected Points

CRITERIA	NFL	PEI	NS	NB	PQ	ONT	MAN	SASK	ALTA	BC	YUK	NWT
Public Administration												
Hospital Plan												
MOH	x	–	x	x	x	x	–	x	x	x	–	x
Other public body	–	x	–	–	–	–	x	–	–	–	x	–
Medical Plan												
MOH	–	–	–	x	–	x	–	x	x	–	–	x
Other public body	x	x	x	–	x	–	x	–	–	x	x	–
Comprehensiveness												
Additional services:												
Children's Dental Plan	x	x	x	–	x	–	–	x	–	–	–	–
Prescription Drugs												
• Senior's Plan	x	x	x	x	x	x	x	x	x	x	x	–
• For other groups	–	x	x	x	x	x	x	x	x	x	x	x
Other practitioners												
• chiropractors	–	–	–	–	–	x	–	x	x	x	–	–
• podiatrists/chiropodists	–	–	–	–	–	x	–	x	x	x	–	–
• naturopaths	–	–	–	–	–	–	–	–	–	x	–	–
• physiotherapists*	–	–	–	–	–	x	–	–	x	x	–	–
• massage therapists	–	–	–	–	–	–	–	–	–	x	–	–
• osteopaths	–	–	–	–	–	x	–	–	–	–	–	–
Universality												
Premiums	–	–	–	–	–	–	–	–	x	x	–	–
Portability												
Day 1, Third month	x	x	x	x	x	x	x	x	x**	x	x**	x**
First-day coverage for landed immigrants	x	x	x	–	–	–	x	x	x	–	x	x
Extended Care Services												
Home care	x	x	x	x	x	x	x	x	x	x	x	x
Extramural hospitals	–	–	–	x	–	–	–	–	–	–	–	–

* For services performed outside of hospital or home care services.
** Not to exceed 3 months. Day not specified in report.

x = Yes
– = No

SOURCE: Health and Welfare Canada (1992). *Canada Health Act Annual Report 1991–1992*. Ottawa: Minister of Supply and Services. Cat. H1-4/1992.

services differs to meet the respective needs of the two countries. As noted, Canada spends less per capita on health than does the United States. Canadian hospitals operate with proportionately less staff than American hospitals which helps to account for the fact that hospital expenditures are also lower in Canada, despite higher admission rates and longer average length of stay. The health status of Canadians and Americans also varies on a number of health status indicators. We noted some of these in Chapter 2; for example, life expectancy is greater in Canada and infant and maternal mortality rates are lower (Nair, Karim and Nyers, 1992).

In 1990, Canadians spent roughly $2100 per capita on health care, approximately one third less than Americans, but more than the people in either Great Britain or Japan. And where, you may ask, does the money go? The largest share of the health care dollar goes to hospital care. In 1991, expenditures for hospitals and other institutional services took almost one half of the total national expenditures on health care. Physician services took over 15 percent and professional services by dentists and other health professionals a little over six percent. Drugs, including both prescribed and non-prescribed, took almost 14 percent, a considerable increase from the 1987 figure of approximately 12 percent. Other health expenses, including administration, public health, capital expenses, research and miscellaneous items accounted for the rest. See Figure 3.3.

CONCERNS ABOUT HEALTH SPENDING

Economists tell us that our health care costs have been controlled reasonably well (Rachlis and Kushner, 1989). But this contradicts the media and general public's perception that there is a crisis in Medicare. The concern over health care costs started almost as soon as our social programs were established at the end of the 1960s. The federal government began to go into deficit spending, in order to finance its health programs, during the 1970s. The Lalonde Report (1974) was developed primarily as a result of the government's desire to curb health expenditures in general, and hospital spending in particular. The Report advocated less emphasis on the "sickness" side of health care and more on community health measures and public education.

As you can see from the pie chart on health care expenditures shown in Figure 3.3, community services continue to consume a very small portion of the health care dollar, being relegated to the category "other expenditures" along with other items that consume relatively small proportions of the total expenditure on health. Hospitals and physicians are still responsible for the largest part of expenditures. The national deficit continued to grow during the 1970s but it was not until the middle of the 1980s that the federal government began to take action to reduce it — in large part by cutting transfer payments to the provinces for health and welfare programs, which resulted in increased financial burdens on the

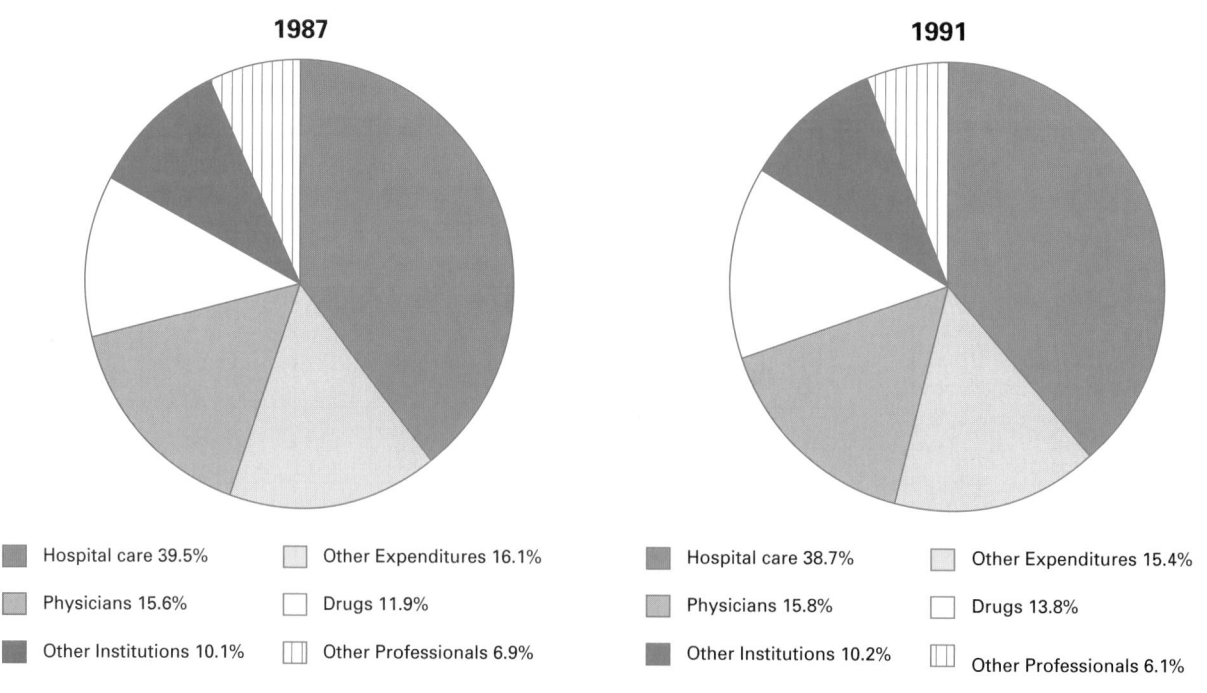

FIGURE 3.3 Distribution of National Health Expenditures by Category, Canada, 1987 and 1991

SOURCE: Health Information Division, Policy and Consultation Branch, Health Canada, February 1994, 16.

provinces (Boothe and Johnston, 1993; Rachlis and Kushner, 1989; Crichton, Hsu and Tsang, 1994).

The provinces are justifiably concerned about the spiralling cost of health care to them for three reasons:

1. Health care services are taking an increasingly large share of the total provincial budget each year; expenditures went up an average of approximately 42 percent for all provinces in the four-year period between 1988–89 and 1991–92. During the period from 1985 to 1990 hospital expenditures rose by 12 percent in Canada (37 percent in the United States). In British Columbia and Ontario they increased by 50 percent over the period (Nair et al, 1992). Meanwhile, the federal share of the costs declined from almost 20 percent in the 1988–89 year to less than 15 percent in 1991–92 as the federal government tried to lower the deficit (Boothe and Johnston, 1993).

2. The provinces' ability to pay for the services has lessened because of the slow state of the economy. Some provinces suffered more than others during the recession of the early 1990s, although equalization grants have helped to cushion the blow somewhat for the "have-not" provinces.

3. The provinces have little control over the amount to be spent on health care, although they have to pay for services. Hospitals, for example, are given funds from the provincial coffers but, if they overrun their budget, the province has always had to pay the deficit. Physicians are "gatekeepers" to most services and have so far had a free rein in ordering services for their clients (Rachlis and Kushner,1989).

HEALTH CARE REFORM ACROSS THE COUNTRY

The need for changes in the health care system in Canada was acknowledged in the early 1970s, both because the system was beginning to cost more than we could afford to pay and, as the Lalonde Report pointed out, we could not expect much more improvement in health status from pouring more money into the system. The need for trimming costs became more urgent during the 1980s, but provincial enquiries into health care reform at the time tended to focus on cost containment, rather than on severe cost cutting.

As we began to change our ideas about the determinants of health (we discussed these in Chapter 2), the federal government and the provinces realized that radical changes were needed in the system — simply tinkering with it to lower costs was not enough. It was realized that further improvements in the health of Canadians required "not so much . . . attempts to diagnose and cure diseases

and remedy disabilities as . . . non-medical efforts to improve social and economic ills" (*Health Promotion Matters in Ontario*, 1987a, 127). In other words, it was time to spend less money on the detection and treatment of disease and more on remedying some of the social and economic ills that were major contributors to health problems.

Publication of the Epp Report (1986), which outlined strategies for promoting health, set the stage for provincial enquiries into ways of reforming the system to both promote better health and, at the same time, lower costs. The result has been an unprecedented number of reports and papers on health care reform in each province. Some provinces have moved more quickly than others and are busy implementing the changes recommended in the reports. We talked earlier in this chapter about public participation in the process of policy formulation. In all provinces, people have had the opportunity to voice their opinions. The Canadian Nurses Association and its provincial counterparts have been active in presenting briefs, speaking at public forums and developing position papers. Each province has come up with different reform packages but the following common trends have emerged:

1. a strong movement to home- and community-based care
2. a reduction in the number of hospital beds
3. regionalization or decentralization of services
4. increasing public participation in policy-making, planning and management of care
5. increased intersectoral collaboration (that is, collaboration between health and other sectors of the community, such as business, justice, etc.)
6. attempts to reduce inequities existing between regions within a province as well as between specific groups within the population
7. more effective utilization of health personnel
8. attempts to control hospital costs
9. efforts to decrease the rapid rise in the number of physicians in the country
10. a cap on expenditures for medical care.

We will now attempt to give you a brief outline of the changes in health care reform planned or being implemented in all the provinces at the time of writing. This summary is based on the following sources: Crichton et al, 1994, Government of Canada, 1992; *CNA Today*, 1992, 1993 and 1994.

NEWFOUNDLAND

In attempts to improve management and to control costs, three commissions were set up:

1. the Royal Commission on Hospital and Nursing Home Costs, 1983–84

2.   an Advisory Committee on Nursing Workforce
3.   the Green Paper entitled Our Health Care System Expenditures and Funding, 1986.

In response to the reports of these commissions, the Newfoundland government initiated a plan in 1991–92 to regionalize community health services, and had four regional boards in place by 1993. The government has also moved to decrease the number of acute care beds and to increase the number of long-term care beds. The role of small community hospitals has also been changed — they have become integrated health care centres, combining community health care services with traditional hospital services. A precedent-setting primary health care project, planned and initiated by nurses in 1990, was the first complete nurse-run PHC pilot project in Canada and proved the cost-effectiveness and capability of nurses as primary health care providers (Hall, 1989; *CNA Today*, 1994).

PRINCE EDWARD ISLAND

Prince Edward Island did not set up any commissions or public enquiries. The government did, however, establish a health care task force which reported during 1991–92 on directions and approaches to addressing current trends and pressures in health care in the province. A review of women's health was sponsored by consumers. A 1990 needs assessment study of people in the west central part of the island resulted in a community-initiated Farm Heart Health project. An Active Living Program is also underway to encourage healthier lifestyles. As we mentioned in Chapter 1, the new baccalaureate program in nursing at the University of Prince Edward Island was developed using the concept of primary health care. The curriculum focusses on health promotion and illness prevention as they relate to this concept (*CNA Today*, Nov/Dec 1992).

NEW BRUNSWICK

A Commission on Selected Health Care Programs proposed 64 recommendations (1989). A Statement of Vision was subsequently prepared, followed by plans to implement changes, based on the notion of a continuum of care from wellness to illness. During the 1991–92 year, the Minister of Health and Community Services tabled a number of hospital system reforms in the provincial legislature and these are now in effect. They encompass a strong shift away from hospitals and towards community services. The role of many hospitals is being changed, and the "extramural hospital" (hospital care given in the home) is receiving wide publicity as an increasing number of hospitals in the province move in this direction (*CNA Today*, May 1993). There has also been an expansion of long-term care assessment to make nursing home care a last resort (Stewart, 1993).

NOVA SCOTIA

A Royal Commission on Health Care was established in 1987 to examine the financing and delivery of health care in the province (The Nova Scotia Royal Commission on Health Care, 1989). In responding to the 103 recommendations of the Commission, the Health Ministry contracted advisory services to prepare intersectoral communication and comprehensive health planning guidelines. The Nova Scotia Ministry of Health subsequently published a policy paper entitled *Health Care for the Nineties: Managing Better Health* (1990). Action has been taken to start the process of **regionalization** — decentralizing the health care system by giving local authorities the power to make decisions about health care (Crichton et al, 1994). During the 1991–92 year, the Minister of Health announced a commitment to reduce the number of hospital beds to five per thousand by 1993–94 and to control expenditures with tight budgetary restrictions. Ministerial task forces were appointed to look into physician policy development, nursing and primary health care. A community-based care pilot project was initiated in late 1992, operated out of the Sacred Heart Hospital in Cape Breton. A nurse coordinator was appointed to head up the project (*CNA Today*, Nov/Dec 1992).

QUEBEC

The Quebec (Castonguay) model developed in the early 1970s was based on the principles of universal access, preventive medicine and community development. It set a health-outcome model that has influenced the rest of Canada. A province-wide system of community clinics with community advisory boards was established. The CLSCs, as they are known, provided health and social services and had a mandate for community development. During the 1980s the Quebec government appointed the Rochon Committee to review the progress made in implementing the Castonguay model and to assess its current appropriateness.

The Commission made a number of recommendations on better ways to promote health and prevent social and health problems. Strategies were also recommended to improve the participation of community members in care for one another and to encourage consumer involvement in policy-making and in participative management of health and social services. It also recommended that the CLSCs should become more streamlined to deal with the medical and social problems of their locality. Subsequent enquiries have been conducted on mental health policy (Boudreau, 1987), on the work of nurses and on the new technologies of human reproduction. Responding to the recommendations of these committees, the Ministry published a document entitled *Improving Health and Well-Being in Quebec: Orientations* (1989). Another paper, published in 1990, suggested reforms for primary care services (Gouvernement du

Québec, 1990). During 1992, a broad public consultation was held on the major stakes involved in financing health and social services. The discussion identified objectives to be pursued and suggested ways of containing increases in health and social services expenditures. In June 1992, the Quebec Legislative Assembly passed legislation about social services and about amending previous legislation. The Bill is considered a major step in implementation of reform in the health care system in Quebec. It sets out the fundamental objectives of health and social services and the rights of users. It also outlines the services to be performed by the various providers of health and social services and redefines certain procedures regarding health personnel, health facilities and other resources. The Bill also sets out new organizational structures for agency boards to facilitate mergers in order to streamline services.

ONTARIO

Ontario has conducted a series of studies looking into health care. Three committees were set up between 1985 and 1987:

1. to look into health promotion
2. to investigate goals
3. an overview committee to build on the other two and come out with recommendations.

The recommendations included more emphasis on health promotion and disease prevention, to be accomplished without too much remodelling of the system. A Premier's Council on Health Strategy (later changed to the Premier's Council on Health, Well-being and Social Justice when the New Democratic Party was elected to power) was established as a new mechanism for policy development — its task was to sift data from the studies mentioned above and prepare proposals. In response to these proposals, the Ministry of Health prepared a discussion paper called *Deciding the Future of our Health Care* (1989). The health goals sub-committee of the Premier's Council identified five goals:

1. shift emphasis to health promotion and disease prevention
2. foster strong and supportive families and communities
3. ensure a safe, high-quality physical environment
4. increase the number of years of good health by preventive measures
5. provide accessible, affordable and appropriate health services for all.

Other studies have been done on mental health, long-term care, hospital deficits and the use and provision of medical services and health promotion. The Premier's Council outlined the research done on the factors which determine our health in *Nurturing Health* and these have been summarized in a publication by the same title (1993). Ontario is currently embarking on reforming its system to implement these goals. A major study was undertaken to assess the health behaviours and health status of people in the province (1992).

Ontario has already moved to initiate decentralization of the system, with local boards functioning with regional funding envelopes so that they control the funds for health services in their local area. Rachlis and Kushner suggest that the delegation of financial responsibility, as well as decision-making authority, to the regional boards makes local communities more accountable for the funds spent on health care. The provincial ministries of health retain overall control through the establishment of minimum standards for personnel and facilities, such as the number of acute-care beds per population (Rachlis and Kushner, 1989).

A comprehensive regional planning demonstration in the London and South West Region is in progress and a restructuring of the delivery system is taking place. Examples of the restructuring include reorganizing mental health services, community clinic pilot projects, a reform of long-term care organization, controlling independent health facilities, restructuring of local government operations and conducting a corporate government review. The public is also being involved in discussions on the health care system.

MANITOBA

Manitoba set up a Health Advisory Steering Committee in 1988. Recommendations coming from the various Task Force groups of this committee were incorporated into a policy paper entitled *Quality Health for Manitobans: The Action Plan* (1992). The paper specified that the health services system must "be driven by [the] health status needs [of Manitobans] and [by] health outcomes . . . . [It must] consist of a full continuum of services to respond to individual and community needs." The province is embarking on a two-year plan to shift from institutional to community-based care. It is compressing acute care drastically by cutting beds and removing services from the hospital setting and transferring resources to more appropriate prevention and home care services in the community. Of particular interest to nurses is the store-front, nurse-operated Youville Clinic which has been highly successful in providing community health care services. A satellite Outreach program was established in 1986 at the Indian/Métis Friendship Centre in downtown Winnipeg (Crichton et al, 1994; Government of Canada, 1992; *CNA Today*, Nov/Dec 1992).

SASKATCHEWAN

Saskatchewan is busy restructuring its health services. The impetus for change came with the 1988 commission on health care which identified major problems in Saskatchewan. A policy paper soon followed issued by the prevailing government (Government of Saskatchewan,

1990). The government was not re-elected and *A Saskatchewan Vision of Health* (1992) was issued by the new government. This document stressed a wellness approach and suggested five strategies. The Ministry of Health has begun to implement these strategies. A shift in emphasis was initiated, moving away from institutional care and towards a more holistic approach with the provision of a wide range of services. The community is to be the base, but the emphasis on services will be on non-institutionalized care. Strategies to reach the wellness goal include:

1. public policies to promote good health with a provincial health council to advise on policies
2. emphasis on health promotion and disease prevention
3. the integration and coordination of services
4. the support of community-based services
5. better utilization of health services.

Already, a number of small hospitals (some with as few as nine beds) have been closed. The closures created a furore among people in the rural areas who had very strong feelings about what they saw as *"our* hospital" and a valuable asset to the community. Activities to provide more preventive care have resulted in a permanent breast cancer screening clinic, which opened in Regina in 1991, and two mobile units to service the southern and central parts of the province. Another permanent clinic was opened in Saskatoon with a satellite clinic in North Battleford. In addition, health boards were established in the cities of Regina and Saskatoon to operate health care services. The new boards replace those of hospitals, special care and home care. A pilot project with nurses playing a central role was recommended for Eastend, a rural community of 600 in rural southwest Saskatchewan (*CNA Today*, Nov/Dec 1992).

ALBERTA

A broad general study of the social needs of the province was followed by the establishment in 1988 of a Royal Commission on Future Care for Albertans. Its report, entitled *Rainbow Report: Our Vision for Health* (1990), made 22 recommendations. A policy paper entitled *Partners in Health* (November 1991) suggested five initiatives to be implemented immediately:

1. a health unit/health facility partnership initiative
2. establishment of a health services innovative fund to support research and evaluation for new ways of delivering services
3. establishment of the Alberta Family Life and Substance Abuse Foundation
4. development of a collaborative process to develop health goals for Alberta
5. commencement of a major initiative in coordination.

Another policy statement called *Future Directions for Mental Health Services in Alberta* (1992) emphasized the co-

ordination of services across a continuum of care. Emphasis is being placed on ensuring that people requiring mental health service will have access to the most appropriate services. A series of public forums in different areas of the province was held in 1992 for the purpose of discussing the reform process and health goals. For the time being, regional boards are not being established, although decentralization of services is in process (Crichton et al, 1994; Health and Welfare Canada, 1992).

BRITISH COLUMBIA

The Report of the Royal Commission on Health Services, *Closer to Home* (1991), was followed by a round of public consultations on its recommendations. In 1993, a policy document entitled *New Directions for a Healthy British Columbia* (1993) was published. The policy's outline was based on the principles of equity, partnership (with all participants in the health system), financial responsibility and sensitive implementation. The New Directions paper set out five goals for future health services in British Columbia:

1. Better health through fostering health promotion and disease prevention by such strategies as strengthening community action, creating supportive environments, developing personal health skills and targeting screening programs for high risk groups.
2. Greater public participation and responsibility at three levels: provincial, regional and community.
3. Bringing health closer to home through more local management of health services and the provision of more services in people's homes, local communities and regional areas.
4. Respecting the care provider with paid and volunteer care providers involved in planning health services.
5. Effective management of the new health system with clearly defined goals at all levels of service.

A Ministerial Advisory Committee and six working groups were established to advise on strategies for change: Better Management, Regionalization, Governance of Property and Financing, People with Special Needs, Services, and Care Delivery. Again, the "stakeholders" — professional organizations, administrators of service facilities and volunteer organizations — are being consulted.

At the time of writing, regionalization has been initiated with Regional Directors of Services (some of them nurses) appointed to facilitate the process. The number of acute care hospital beds is being decreased and community services, particularly home care, greatly expanded.

THE YUKON AND NORTHWEST TERRITORIES

Until fairly recently, health care services in the Yukon and the Northwest Territories have been handled primarily by the federal government, who provided direct care to First Nation people. We will discuss these services in Chapter 4. Meanwhile, the winds of change are also blowing in the North, as services are being taken over by territorial governments and by First Nation communities themselves.

KEY TERMS

welfare state p. 40

social safety net p. 40

welfare society p. 40

policy p. 40

public policy p. 40

healthy public
  policy p. 41

Family Allowance p. 44

Old Age Security
  (OAS) p. 45

Medicare p. 45

Canada Pension Plan
  (CPP) p. 45

quasi-governmental
  agency p. 47

national health services
  model p. 47

national insurance model
  p. 47

entrepreneurial
  model p. 47

Medicaid p. 47

comprehensiveness p. 48

IN REVIEW

In Canada, we believe that the government has a responsibility to provide adequate health services to all people and to provide assistance to those in need. In keeping with this philosophy, we have developed a "social safety net" that includes a national health insurance program covering both hospital and medical care, and social welfare programs such as unemployment insurance, universal old age pensions, contributory pensions for working people, a family allowance program and social assistance programs for those in need. Although Canadians today consider this social safety net a basic right, it came about as the result of a long and bitter struggle.

The British North America Act (BNA Act) of 1867, in setting out the terms of confederation, delegated responsibility for health and welfare matters to the provinces, but authority to collect revenues (including those to be used in the provision of health services) primarily to the federal government. During the early years of Confederation, public health laws were enacted in every province. These laws established provincial and local boards of health, but hospitals and care of the needy were mainly the responsibility of religious and charitable organizations. The work of the Roman Catholic nursing sisters, and that done by nurses of other denominations, was highly regarded, but conditions in secular hospitals were very poor, the premises dirty and the staff ill-trained. By the turn of the century, however, medical and nursing schools had been established and hospital conditions considerably improved. In addition, a number of voluntary organizations had emerged to provide services for the sick and the poor, for example, the Children's Aid Societies, the Red Cross Society and the Victorian Order of Nurses.

The first modern social security program in Canada was the Ontario Workmen's Compensation Act of 1914. The next major social legislation did not come about until passage of the federal Unemployment Insurance Act in 1941. This was followed by a Family Allowance Act of 1945 which is considered the first universal social program in Canada,

with every family, regardless of income, receiving an allowance for each child in the family.

Hospital insurance programs were established first in individual provinces, starting in Saskatchewan in 1948. Federal legislation for universal hospital insurance was enacted in 1957, with the federal and provincial governments sharing costs equally. Medicare came into being in the 1960s; and again Saskatchewan pioneered the way. The federal government enacted legislation for universal medical care insurance for all Canadians in 1966.

The 1950s and 1960s also saw the extension of social welfare programs including a universal Old Age Security (OAS) program (1951), a rehabilitation program for the disabled and a Canada Assistance Plan to provide a minimum income for those in financial need (1966). By the end of the 1960s, the social safety net was fairly comprehensive.

The 1970s and 1980s saw a restructuring of the safety net in response to concerns over the increasingly high cost of health care and, also, to accommodate changing views on health and its determinants. We have come to realize that health is determined as much by social, economic and environmental conditions as by biological, genetic and lifestyle factors. Further improvements in the health of people in Canada, it is felt, will only come about through measures to eliminate the root causes of illness which are often the social, economic and environmental problems in our society.

The Canadian national health insurance program was founded on five principles: public administration, comprehensiveness, universality, portability and accessibility. These principles were reconfirmed in the Canada Health Act of 1984. Within the guidelines of this Act, each province and territory has developed its own unique health care program. Currently, all provinces in Canada are engaged in restructuring their health services, both because of the need to curb costs and because of our changing perspectives on health and its determinants. The direction of change is towards home- and community-based care combined with a reduction in the number of hospital beds. Decentralization of policy-making and services is taking place, as is regionalization and increased public participation in policy-making, planning and management of key components in all provincial care plans. Other common trends are: increased intersectoral collaboration; efforts to ensure more equitable distribution of resources and services within provinces; more effective use of health personnel and attempts to curb hospital costs, the number of physicians and the costs of their services.

LEARNING ACTIVITIES

1. The interest of nurses in preserving the heritage of nursing has resulted in the development of both provincial history of nursing groups and a Canadian Association for the History of Nursing (CAHN). Explore what is happening in your province. Is there a provincial history of nursing group? If so, what is the group doing to preserve the history of nursing in your province? Who were some of the early nursing leaders in your province? When were the first hospitals established? Where? By whom? Who provided the nursing care? What were the conditions like in these early hospitals? Who carried out the first community health nursing in the province? When? Where?

2. What is the amount of the current budget for health services in your province? How much of the money for health services comes from the federal government? How much from the provincial treasury? How much has the budget increased in the past ten years? What portion of the provincial budget for health goes to hospitals? other institutions? physician services? the services of other health practitioners? drugs? community health? home care? other items?

3. What health care reforms are currently taking place in your province?

    a. To what extent has there been a movement to home- and community-based care in your province? What home and community services have been developed, extended or planned? Have additional funds been allocated for expansion of home and community services?

    b. Are hospital beds being closed? hospitals? If so, where in the province? What is the community reaction to these closures?

    c. Are regional health boards being established? If so, where? How will they be formed?

    d. What is your provincial government doing to foster public participation in policy-making, planning and management of health care? Are public meetings being held? Have community health planning groups been established?

    e. Are there examples in your province of intersectoral collaboration? For example, do you have mandatory seat belt legislation? If so, what departments of government were involved in passage of the legislation? Can you think of other examples of intersectoral collaboration?

    f. What efforts are being made in your province to reduce inequities between regions within the province and between specific groups within the population? For example, increasing services to northern regions, setting up community clinics or other services in low-income neighbourhoods?

    g. What attempts are being made to utilize health personnel more effectively? Are there pilot projects, such as primary health care projects, nurse-operated clinics or health centres, community health centres, extramural hospitals? If so, where are they? What stage are they at — planning, implementation, evaluation?

    h. What efforts are being made to control hospital costs?

    i. What is being done to decrease the rise in the number of physicians if this is a problem in your province? What is being done to cap expenditures on medical care?

REFERENCES AND READINGS

BOOTHE, P. and JOHNSTON, B. (1993, March). Stealing the emperor's clothes: Deficit offloading and national standards in health care. In C.D. Howe Institute *Commentary, 41.*

BOUDREAU, F. (1987). The making of mental health policy: The 1980s and the challenge of sanity in Quebec and Ontario. In *Canadian Journal of Mental Health, 6*(1), 24–47.

CANADIAN NURSES ASSOCIATION. (1968). *The leaf and the lamp.* Ottawa: Author.

CRICHTON, A., HSU, D., and TSANG, S. (1994). *Canada's health care system: Its funding and organization.* Ottawa: Canadian Health Association.

DU GAS, B. and BECKINGHAM, A. (1993). The emergence of gerontological nursing. In Beckingham, A. and Du Gas, B. *Promoting healthy aging.* St. Louis: Mosby, 70 – 79.

EPP, J. (1986). *Achieving health for all: A framework for health promotion.* Ottawa: Ministry of Supply and Services.

FRENCH, DORIS. (1988). *Ishbel and the Empire: A biography of Lady Aberdeen.* Toronto: Dundurn Press.

GIBBON, JOHN M. (1947). *The Victorian Order of Nurses for Canada: 50th anniversary 1897-1947.* Ottawa: Victorian Order of Nurses for Canada.

GOVERNMENT OF ALBERTA. (1988). *Caring and responsibility.* From the office of the Minister for Special Projects. Edmonton: Government Printer.

GOVERNMENT OF ALBERTA. (1990). *Rainbow report: Our vision for health.* Edmonton: Government Printer.

GOVERNMENT OF ALBERTA. (1991). *Partners in health.* Edmonton: Government Printer.

GOVERNMENT OF ALBERTA. (1992). *Future directions for mental health care in Alberta*. Edmonton: Government Printer.

GOVERNMENT OF BRITISH COLUMBIA. (1991a). *A guide for communities to enact health-promoting policies*. Victoria, BC: Queen's Printer. Prepared by the BC Ministry of Health Office of Health Promotion in collaboration with the Social Planning and Research Council of BC (SPARC).

GOVERNMENT OF BRITISH COLUMBIA. (1991b). *Closer to home: Summary of the Royal Commission on Health Care and Costs.* Victoria: Crown Publishing.

GOVERNMENT OF BRITISH COLUMBIA. (1993). *New directions for a healthy British Columbia*. Victoria: Ministry of Health and Ministry Responsible for Seniors.

GOVERNMENT OF CANADA. (1964). *Royal commission on health services.* (E. Hall, Chairman.) Ottawa: Queen's Printer.

GOVERNMENT OF CANADA. (1989). *Health and welfare in Canada.* Ottawa: Ministry of Supply and Services. (Catalogue No. H21–102/1989E)

GOVERNMENT OF CANADA. (1992). *Canada Health Act Annual Report 1991–1992*. Ottawa: Ministry of Supply and Services. (Catalogue No. H1–4/1992)

GOVERNMENT OF MANITOBA. (1992). *Quality health care for Manitobans: The action plan*. Winnipeg: Government Printer.

GOVERNMENT OF NEW BRUNSWICK. (1989). *Report of the Commission on Selected Health Care Programs.* Fredericton: Government Printer.

GOVERNMENT OF NOVA SCOTIA (Ministry of Health). (1990). *Health strategy for the nineties: Managing better care*. Halifax: Government Printer.

GOVERNMENT OF ONTARIO. (1987a). *Health promotion matters in Ontario*. A report of the Minister's Advisory Group on Health Promotion. Toronto: Government Printer.

GOVERNMENT OF ONTARIO. (1987). *A shared direction for health in Ontario*. Toronto: Government Printer.

GOVERNMENT OF ONTARIO. (1989). *Deciding on the future of our health care*. Toronto: Government Printer.

GOVERNMENT OF ONTARIO. (1992). *Ontario health survey 1990*. Toronto: Ontario Minister of Health.

GOVERNMENT OF ONTARIO. (1993). *Nurturing health*. Toronto: Government Publisher. Prepared by the Premier's Council on Health, Well-being and Social Justice. Other publications by the Premier's Council include: *A vision in health; From vision to action; Bringing health and social services together; Coordination and integration of health policies; Community services study; Funding and incentives study.*

GOVERNMENT OF QUEBEC. (1989). *Improving health and well-being in Quebec: Orientations*. Quebec City: Government of Quebec.

GOUVERNEMENT DU QUEBEC (Ministère de la santé et des services sociaux). (1990). *Une reforme axée sur le citoyen*. Québec: Gouvernement du Québec.

GOVERNMENT OF SASKATCHEWAN. (1990). *Directions in health care*. Regina: Saskatchewan Health.

GOVERNMENT OF SASKATCHEWAN. (1992). *A Saskatchewan vision of health*. Regina: Saskatchewan Health.

GUEST, D. (1985). Social security. In the *Canadian encyclopaedia*. Edmonton: Hurtig, 1723–1724.

HALL, D.C. (1989). *Primary health care — A nursing model*. A Danish–Newfoundland (Canada) project. St. John's, Newfoundland: Association of Registered Nurses of Newfoundland.

HALL, E.M. (1980). *Canada's national health program for the '80s*. Ottawa: Health and Welfare Canada.

LALONDE, M. (1974). *A new perspective on the health of Canadians*. Ottawa: Ministry of Supply and Services.

LARSEN, J. and BAUMGART, A. (1992). Overview: Shaping public policy. In *Canadian nursing faces the future: Development and change*. A. Baumgart and J. Larsen (Eds.). Toronto: Mosby, 469–494.

LEFORT, S.M. (1993). Shaping health care policy. *The Canadian Nurse, 89*(3), 23–30.

NAIR, C., KARIM, R. and NYERS, C. (1992). Health care and health status. A Canada–United States statistical comparison. *Health Reports 1992, 4*(2), 175–183. (Statistics Canada No. 82–003)

THE NOVA SCOTIA ROYAL COMMISSION ON HEALTH CARE. (1989). *Towards a new strategy*. Halifax: Government Printer.

NURSES AS A POINT OF ACCESS. (1993). In *CNA Today, 3*(2), 1.

NURSES PROVE THEMSELVES IN PRIMARY HEALTH CARE. (1994, April). *CNA Today, 4*(2), 1

PEDERSON, A.P., EDWARDS, R.K., MARSHALL, V.W., ALLISON, K.R. and KELNER, M. (1989). *Coordinating healthy public policy: An analytic literature review and bibliography*. Ottawa: Health and Welfare Canada. (Available from the Ministry of Supply and Services)

PRIMARY HEALTH CARE HAS ARRIVED. (1992). In *CNA Today, 2*(3), 4–5.

PRINGLE, DOROTHY M. and ROE, DONNA J. (1992). Voluntary community agencies: VON Canada as example. In A.J. Baumgart and J. Larsen (Eds.), *Canadian nursing faces the future*. Toronto: Mosby.

RACHLIS, M. and KUSHNER, C. (1989). *Second Opinion*. Toronto: Collins.

ROBICHAUD, J.B. and QUIVIGER, C. (1990). *Active Communities*. Ottawa: CSSD. (First published in French, 1990).

SINGH BOLARIA, B. and DICKINSON, H.D. (1988). *Sociology of health care in Canada*. Toronto: Harcourt Brace Jovanovich.

SOUTH FRASER VALLEY HEALTH COUNCIL. (1992). *Planning today for a healthy tomorrow*. (A statement of the philosophy, aims and organization of the Council). White Rock, BC: Author.

STEWART, J. (1993). Reform shaking up health care across the country. *Medical Post,* March 30, 1993.

SUTHERLAND, R. and FULTON, J. (1988). *Health care in Canada*. Ottawa: The Health Group.

TAYLOR, M.G. (1978). *Health insurance and Canadian public policy: The seven decisions that created the Canadian health insurance system*. Montreal: McGill-Queen's University Press.

TAYLOR, M.G. (1990). *Insuring national health care*. Chapel Hill: University of North Carolina Press.

VICTORIAN ORDER OF NURSES FOR CANADA (VON). (1983). *Missioners for Health*. Unpublished manuscript on the history of the VON.

Health Services:
The Continuum of Care

CENTRAL QUESTIONS

1. What is meant by the continuum of health care?

2. What is the philosophy underlying primary health care?

3. What strategies and mechanisms are outlined in the Epp Framework for Health Promotion?

4. What are the major responsibilities of federal, provincial and municipal governments and of the voluntary sector in health and welfare in Canada?

5. How do family and friends contribute to the health and welfare of people in our society?

6. What services are available for home care of people who are ill?

7. What is the role of voluntary and religious agencies in health and welfare?

8. What types of agencies provide health services in Canadian communities?

9. What are the differences among the following types of inpatient services:
   - acute care hospitals
   - rehabilitation agencies
   - long-term care facilities
   - personal care facilities
   - hospices/palliative care units

10. What roles do federal and provincial governments play in health and welfare?

11. Why do we need Workers' Compensation Boards when we have national health insurance?

12. Does the private sector play a role in health and welfare in Canada?

13. What are the functions of the principal members of the health team?

INTRODUCTION

We have the foundations upon which to build. Let us continue our efforts to achieve health and improve the quality of life of the people and communities of Canada.

Epp, 1986

At the present time, health care reform is sweeping the country. In every province and territory, the structure of health services is undergoing rapid change as our ponderous health care system — built up over the past 100 years — shifts from a disease-oriented, hospital-based system to one with a wellness orientation that is based in the community. The description of health services in this country used to be very straightforward — there were hospitals that cared for the sick and community health agencies that were concerned with health promotion and disease prevention. That dichotomy no longer holds true. Hospital walls are tumbling down as hospital nurses go out into the community to provide postpartum and postoperative care for early-discharge patients in their homes. The ambulatory services departments of hospitals (also called outpatient departments) provide health information and health counselling for people in the community, as well as screening clinics for those at risk for various diseases. Many hospitals have a palliative care team whose nurses provide support and comfort for terminally ill people in their homes so they can spend their last days with loved ones. Conversely, community health agencies are providing the whole spectrum of health services — from health promotion and protection (their traditional role) to acute and long-term care, rehabilitative and supportive care. Collaborative partnerships are being forged between community and inpatient health agencies to avoid duplication of services and to provide people with a continuum of care.

This continuum includes services to promote health, to protect the health of people through disease prevention and risk reduction, to restore the health of people who fall ill and to provide supportive services for people whose health is impaired and also for their families. The *continuum of care*, you will recall, was stressed in the health care reform packages put forward by all provincial and territorial governments. As the word *continuum* suggests, the range of health services can no longer be divided into neat compartments because each phase of care merges into the others. Let's look at the example of a person who is hospitalized briefly for a cholecystectomy (removal of the gall bladder). During the period when the individual's health is being restored post-surgery and through subsequent convalescence, the nurse, and probably the nutritionist and the physician, will help the patient to establish better dietary habits to promote his or her future health and to reduce the risk of further digestive — or possibly, circulatory—problems. No doubt, the patient's family will also be encouraged to adopt healthy nutrition habits, both to help the patient and to reduce the risks for themselves of developing similar problems.

In this chapter, we begin with a discussion of the philosophy of primary health care, which is providing the foundation on which health services are being restructured. Then we will discuss the mechanisms and strategies outlined in the Epp Framework for Health Promotion (1986) which give directions for implementing the philosophy. We will then look at the overall structure of health services in Canada — the foundation that is already in place — and go into more detail regarding the role of family and friends, the voluntary sector, the private sector and various community agencies in promoting and protecting our health. We will devote some time to a discussion of the role of hospitals and other inpatient facilities for care of the sick and conclude with a discussion of the people who provide the services.

THE PHILOSOPHY OF PRIMARY HEALTH CARE

In Canada, the term **Primary Health Care** was used in the *Report of the Committee on Nurse Practitioners* (The Boudreau Report, 1972) to refer to the first level of service in a comprehensive health care system. Subsequently, the meaning of the term has broadened to include an emphasis on a philosophy of care as well as on services. Primary health care was identified at an international conference sponsored by the World Health Organization in Alma Ata in the former U.S.S.R. in 1978 as an approach to ensure delivery of essential health care to the world's population (Shestowsky, 1992).

Primary Health Care

Primary Health Care is essential health care made universally accessible to individuals and families in the community by means acceptable to them, through their full participation and at a cost that the community and the country can afford.

SOURCE: World Health Organization, 1978, 34.

The Alma Ata Declaration states that "Primary health care is essential health care based on practical, scientifically sound and socially acceptable methods and technology made universally accessible to individuals and families in the community through their full participation and at a cost that the community and country can afford to maintain at every stage of their development" (WHO, 1978, 3). The Declaration goes on to say that primary health care is the initial point of contact for individuals and families with the health care system, and the first element of a continuing health process. It is seen as the central function and

COMPREHENSIVE HEALTH SERVICES
(Essential Health Services)

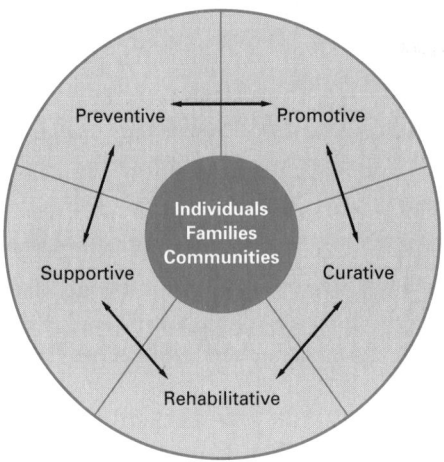

FIGURE 4.1 Primary Health Care. Comprehensive Health Services (Essential Health Services).

SOURCE: *Primary Health Care. A Nursing Model.* A Danish-Newfoundland (Canada) Project. (1990). St. John's Newfoundland: Association of Registered Nurses of Newfoundland.

main focus of the health system and an integral part of the overall social and economic development of a community (WHO, 1978). Figure 4.1 illustrates the comprehensive nature of primary health care as it is envisioned today.

Shestowsky explains the principles of Primary Health Care as follows:

The principles of primary health care mean that:
1. health services should be equally accessible to all
2. there should be maximum individual and community involvement in the planning and operation of health care services
3. the focus of care should be on prevention and promotion rather than on cure
4. appropriate technology should be used, i.e., methods, procedures, techniques and equipment should be scientifically valid, adapted to local needs and acceptable to users and to those for whom they are used
5. health care is regarded as only part of total health development; other sectors, such as education, housing and nutrition, are all essential for the achievement of well-being.*

If these principles sound familiar to you, they should. They are the same basic tenets enunciated in the Epp Report (1986), in *Nurturing Health* (Government of Ontario, 1993a) and in all of the health reform policy papers developed in various provinces. You will remember that WHO recommended the "healthy people" vision of the Alma

Ata Conference be implemented by all member nations and we noted (in Chapter 2) that the ways and means to do this in Canada became clear with the two reports on the health status of Canadians (1979 and 1985). The strategies and mechanisms to implement the approach were set out in the Epp Report, *Achieving Health for All — A Framework for Health Promotion* (1986), which we will discuss further in the chapter.

IMPLICATIONS OF PRIMARY HEALTH CARE FOR NURSING

Dr. Halfdan Mahler, the director-general of WHO at the time of the Alma Ata Declaration, foresaw an important role for nurses in the implementation of primary health care and he challenged them to "lead the way." Because they work so closely with people, nurses, according to Mahler, are the key to acceptance and expansion of primary health care. Mahler envisioned nurses becoming resources to people rather than assistants to physicians (Mahler, 1985).

In a good many countries of the world, nurses are, indeed, leading the way. They are the ones out in the villages working with the people, as, for example, in Fiji, a country that has won awards for its primary health care projects in various communities. It is nurses who staff the outpost nursing stations and health centres on the remote islands that make up the South Pacific country of Vanuatu (formerly the New Hebrides). Guyana had "sick nurse dispensers" (nurses with additional training in pharmacy) providing primary health care services for people living in the jungles of that South American country long before the term "primary health care" was used. In Suriname, outpost nursing stations dot the "hinterland." Nurses in these stations provide essential health care for the people of several villages — descendants of runaway slaves who re-established their African communities in the interior of the former Dutch colony. Case studies on the new and expanded

---

The Five Basic Principles of Primary Health Care

- accessibility
- public participation
- promotion of health and prevention of illness
- intersectoral cooperation
- appropriate technologies.

SOURCE: Making Primary Health Care Work for Canadians. A CNA Priority. In *CNA Today.* 2:3:1. Nov.–Dec., 1992.

---

* Shestowsky, B. (1992). Primary Health Care. Still relevant after 14 years. CNA *Today.* 2:3:3. Nov.—Dec., 1992.

role of nurses in the delivery of primary health care in Botswana, Colombia, Republic of Korea, Jamaica, Sudan and Thailand are documented in Health Manpower for Primary Health Care: The Experience of the Nurse Practitioner (Maglacas, Ulin and Sheps, 1987).

In our own country, Medical Services nurses in the Canadian North have been providing primary health care services for First Nations people since the 1950s. Now, these services are being transferred to the communities themselves, in keeping with the philosophy of primary health care as it is being extolled today and, also, with the movement to self-government by First Nations' populations. There are numerous examples of nursing projects in primary health care across Canada. We mentioned some of these in Chapter 3, in connection with innovative health care programs in the various provinces. The November/December 1992 and the April 1994 issues of CNA Today both describe a number of these projects.

IMPLEMENTING THE PHILOSOPHY: THE EPP FRAMEWORK FOR HEALTH PROMOTION

In Chapter 2, we talked about the Epp Framework for Health Promotion (1986) as a landmark document signalling a major shift in our thinking about health and health care. And we also said that this framework outlined the ways and means for implementing the new vision of health. We will examine the framework in a little more detail now because it is the

FIGURE 4.2 A Framework for Health Promotion

SOURCE: Epp, J. (1986). *Achieving Health for All: A Framework for Health Promotion.* Ottawa: Ministry of Supply and Services. Cat. No. H-39-102/1986 E.

Examples of Primary Health Care Nursing Projects in Canada

- **Newfoundland**. A total of six primary health care nurses meet the needs of 8800 people in 21 communities along the 150-mile south coast.

- **New Brunswick**. Nursing students from the University of New Brunswick have brought a wide variety of primary health care projects to communities across the province. The students assess community needs, then plan, implement and evaluate a primary health care (PHC) project such as a drop-in program at a shopping mall for fitness testing, blood pressure testing and health assessment.

  A clinic that opened in 1993 to serve the 2500 residents of McAdam, N.B., combines a 24-hour emergency facility with a community health clinic. Nurses are the entry point for both the emergency service and a health promotion and disease prevention public health program operated from the clinic, as well as one of five possible entry points for the shared care or community health clinic part.

- **Nova Scotia**. A primary health care project with a nurse coordinator is being operated out of the Sacred Heart Hospital in Cape Breton. Intended to meet the needs of residents of Cheticamp, a small Acadian community in an isolated area, it will be run by a community committee.

- **Prince Edward Island**. Two projects are mentioned: (1) a Farm Heart Health Project to meet the health needs of farming residents in the west central part of the island; (2) an Active Living Program being adapted to meet the stated needs of farming residents.

- **Quebec**. The Local Community Services Centres (CLSCs) were established in the early 1970s to provide primary health care for residents of communities in the Province of Quebec. They operate with a community board of directors and provide a wide range of health and social welfare services. Nurses in the CLSCs offer walk-in clinics that serve as a point of access to the health care system.

- **Ontario**. Street clinics operate in Toronto, catering to the needs of inner-city residents. One example is "Street Health" which we will describe later in the chapter. Another example of a primary health care project is the Centretown Community Health Centre in Ottawa.

- **Manitoba**. The store-front, nurse-operated Youville clinic, which is located in an urban shopping mall, has successfully offered primary health care services since 1984. A satellite Outreach Program was opened in 1986 at the Indian/Métis Friendship Centre to meet the specific needs of the aboriginal community where parenting classes, pre-and postnatal programs and individual counselling are among the services offered.

- **Saskatchewan**. An innovative pilot primary health care project was announced for the rural community of Eastend in response to an assessment of the health needs of its 600 residents. The project includes a Wellness Centre in which nurses are the key people in programs promoting healthy lifestyles and wellness.

- **Alberta**. The Boyle-McCauley Health Centre is an independently operated, inner-city street-front, walk-in clinic with a community board of directors. The total staff is 17, three of whom are nurses involved in a variety of programs, including maternal and child care, foot care, psychological assessment, alcohol recovery and nutrition.

- **British Columbia**. The nurse at a street clinic in Kamloops is involved in education, screening and some treatment for sexually transmitted diseases, HIV/AIDS, hepatitis B, tuberculosis and other health problems. She also does outreach work at the food bank and needle exchanges, first aid and referral to other services on the street.[*] Street clinics also operate in Vancouver, with nurses in blue jeans providing health care to hard-to-reach "streetpeople" much as the nurse in Kamloops does (Banks and Loftus, 1991).

- **Northwest Territories**. Aboriginal people serve as members of regional health boards and as community health representatives (front-line workers in First Nations communities) working with nurses in community health promotion, disease prevention, community development and related activities. The 43 outpost nursing stations operate on the PHC model.

- **Yukon**. Community health nurses provide primary health care to all residents outside Whitehorse. The Kwanlin Dun First Nation in Whitehorse opened its own health clinic in 1990 using a PHC model. It employs one nurse and two First Nations community health representatives and offers various programs geared to the needs of the local community.

[*] St. Michael, M. (1993). Letter to the Editor. *Nursing BC*. August/September 1993

SOURCES: Primary Health Care has Arrived! CNA *Today* 2:3:4,5. Nov/Dec, 1992; Nurses prove themselves in Primary Health Care. CNA *Today* 4:2:1, 2. April 1994 basis on which health care services in Canada are being re-structured. A diagrammatic representation of the Epp Framework for Health Promotion is shown in Figure 4.2.

Epp saw three major health challenges facing Canadians today:

- to reduce inequities between high- and low-income groups in our society
- to increase the prevention effort
- to enhance people's capacity to cope.

The Report suggests a way of addressing these challenges through an expansion of traditional "health promotion" strategies and mechanisms to complement and strengthen the existing system of care. **Health promotion**, used in this context, is defined by the World Health Organization as "the process of enabling people to increase control over, and to improve, their health" (WHO, 1984). In other words, it is helping people to help themselves to gain better health — helping a group of older adults to organize a Tai Chi program to improve their physical health,

Seniors' walking club having a picnic in the park

for example, or helping a community to mobilize its resources to build and staff a centre for teenagers (Government of British Columbia, 1992).

The focus in health promotion has shifted, then, from promoting the health of the individual to helping communities to create environments to promote health (RNABC, 1990).

The Epp Report suggests three mechanisms as intrinsic to health promotion:

1. Self-Care — The decisions and actions taken by individuals in the interest of their own health, for example, the decision you make to join a fitness class at the school or the choices you make in the foods you eat in the school cafeteria.

2. Mutual aid — The actions people take to help each other. For example, in Alberta, a group of older adults run a program called "Food for Life," designed to improve their nutritional status. The program includes "Smart Shoppers' Tours" to help people select the best nutritional food value for their dollar and a "Nutritious Meal Program" organized by volunteers but prepared, served and hosted by a group of older adults (Du Gas and Beckingham, 1993).

3. The creation of healthy environments — Communities and regions working together to create environments that are conducive to health. Activities may be as diverse as working with people in the community on a

---

Principles of Health Promotion

1. Health promotion involves the population as a whole in the context of everyday life rather than focussing on people at risk for specific diseases. This principle is the foundation of many public health programs, such as maternal and child health programs.

2. Health promotion is directed at the determinants of health, such as poverty and environment.

3. Health promotion combines diverse but complementary approaches including communication, education, legislation, fiscal measures, organizational change, community development and spontaneous local activities against health hazards.

4. Health promotion aims particularly at effective public participation with a view to having individuals take greater responsibility for their health and to empowering communities to take greater responsibility for and control over those things that affect health.

5. Health professionals have an important role in nurturing and enabling health promotion. This means that health professionals will work beyond the normal patient–provider relationship and participate in a more diverse range of activities.

SOURCE: World Health Organization. (1984). *A Discussion Document on the Concept and Principles of Health Promotion.* Cited in RNABC. (1990). Health Promotion: A Discussion Paper. Vancouver: Author. 3.

"cleanup campaign" to get rid of litter on the streets; ensuring that policies and practices are in place to encourage mothers of young children to participate in fitness programs, through the availability of child care for example; or lobbying for legislation to enforce stricter standards for food handlers (Government of British Columbia, 1992).

Three strategies to provide direction for promoting the health of Canadians are suggested in the Epp Report:

- fostering public participation
- strengthening community health services
- coordinating healthy public policy.

FOSTERING PUBLIC PARTICIPATION

Helping people to take control over the factors that influence their health is an essential component of all the provincial health care reform packages we talked about in Chapter 3. We mentioned there the regional and community health boards which are being established to decentralize and, hopefully, de-bureaucratize the system by putting the responsibility for and management of health services into the hands of people in the community.

The concept of empowering people to help themselves is illustrated in the description by Labonte of the experience of a group of young single mothers in a large Toronto housing project. The group decided to tackle the problem of healthful food and nutrition and determined that they had a problem getting nutritious food for their families because of a lack of control. Prices were too high in the local stores, there were no greengrocers in the neighbourhood, rents were excessive and welfare payments insufficient to cover rent and good, nutritious groceries. The group developed its own objectives which included: a community garden, community dinners, pick-your-own farm trips and a food co-op feasibility study. The project was so successful it was expanded to other housing projects. One goal of the expanded project is to increase the political strength of low-income groups so that they can lobby for policies to reduce hunger and end their dependence on foodbanks (Labonte, 1987, 1989).

In Chapter 11, we will look at the "Healthy Communities" concept and some of the projects that have been going on across the country the past few years. These projects provide excellent examples of public participation in health care. One example is the case of Granisle, British Columbia. The community was coping with the threat of closure of the mine which provided its economic base, and was concerned about the effect of these tensions on their young people. The community worked to establish the Granisle Youth Centre so they could have a place to call their own (Government of British Columbia, 1992). During the 1980s, the VON initiated a number of community development projects in Ontario to promote elders' participation in determining their own needs and developing programs to meet these needs. The project, given the acronym PEP (Promoting Elders' Participation), was targeted particularly at rural and underserviced areas. Programs developed included a Drop-in Centre for Seniors, Meals-on-Wheels, a Grief Reaction Support Group, Friendly Visitors, Handy Helpers, sitters for family relief, evening entertainment, volunteers for the rest home and a transportation network (VON, 1988).

STRENGTHENING COMMUNITY HEALTH SERVICES

The major shift in health care towards a health promotion and protection orientation requires that more resources — funds and people — are allocated to community health services. For example, a four million dollar initiative was launched in Victoria, British Columbia to improve the health of residents, particularly the elderly, living in the Capital Regional District. Programs that have ensued include: a series of seniors' wellness centres, an expanded Quick Response Team to prevent hospitalization of the elderly and programs to support family caregivers (RNABC, 1990).

The strengthening of community services also means providing more services for disadvantaged groups and taking more responsibility for planning and directing the community's own health care. It also implies greater intersectoral cooperation as communities work on fostering self-care, mutual aid and the creation of healthy environments. Such cooperation may include health and social services personnel working together with the business sector, the police, fire and other departments in community projects to promote health and protect people from illness. (Epp, 1986; Government of British Columbia, 1991; Government of Ontario, 1993a).

COORDINATING PUBLIC POLICY

As we discussed in Chapter 3, Canadians have become aware of the need for assessing the health impact of policy decisions made in all sectors of the economy. Epp suggests that "all policies — and hence all sectors — have a bearing on health" (1986, 10) and he states further that all policies that bear directly on health should be coordinated. This includes a long list of policies in different sectors of our society such as income security, employment, education, housing, business, agriculture, transportation, justice and technology. Policies in the agriculture sector, for example, on pesticides, have a direct bearing on the health not only of agriculture workers who apply the pesticides but also of people who eat the fruit and vegetables that have been sprayed with the pesticide.

THE OVERALL STRUCTURE OF HEALTH SERVICES

In Canada, as in all democratic societies, individuals are considered to be responsible for their own health and welfare. Primary support for both health and welfare comes from family and friends, who care for you when you are ill and support you when the going is rough. Backup is provided by religious and voluntary organizations and by local governments through their community services. Over and above these layers protecting our health and welfare, we have the provincial and federal governments. The provincial governments have primary responsibility for providing health and welfare services; the federal government, however, has considerable influence through legislation and through its sharing of the costs of services, as discussed in Chapter 3 (Health and Welfare Canada, 1989). Figure 4.3 outlines the major responsibilities of the federal, provincial and municipal layers of government and of the voluntary sector in health and welfare in Canada.

HEALTH AND WELFARE IN THE HOME

ROLE OF FAMILY AND FRIENDS

We cannot overemphasize the role of family and friends in helping each other to promote and maintain health and to care for those who are ill. *Nurturing Health*, the summary report of the Premier's Council on Health, Well-being and Social Justice in Ontario, suggests the following ways families and friends influence health:

- Provide the basic prerequisites of health (housing, food, etc.)
- Look after family members who are ill (90 percent of informal health care is provided in the home)
- Provide mental, physical and emotional support in times of distress
- Protect other family members (for example, buckle up a child's seat belt)
- Provide love and respect
- Support individual members in lifestyle changes.*

---

* Government of Ontario (1993a). *Nurturing Health*. Report of the Premier's Council on Health, Well-being and Social Justice (1987–1991). Toronto: Queen's Printer. Catalogue No. 01–93–20M.

HEALTH

FEDERAL
- contributions to provincial health programs
- native health services
- setting broad national standards
- funding research
- health promotion and protection

PROVINCIAL
- universal hospital and medical insurance
- dental and drug services

MUNICIPAL
- environmental and public health
- administration of hospitals

VOLUNTARY
- services related to specific diseases or conditions
- administration of hospitals
- fitness and recreational programs and activities

WELFARE

FEDERAL
- major income support programs
- cost-sharing provincial programs

PROVINCIAL
- social assistance programs and social services
- workers' compensation

MUNICIPAL
- some social assistance programs and social services

VOLUNTARY
- services such as family and child services, child care, homemakers, meals-on-wheels and food banks

FIGURE 4.3 Distribution of Major Responsibilities

SOURCE: Health and Welfare Canada (1989). *Health and Welfare in Canada*. Ottawa: Minister of Supply and Services. Catalogue No. 21–102/1989E, 11.

HOME CARE SERVICES

Anderson states that the current emphasis on home care and self-care is consistent with the ideology in Western culture that people should be self-reliant and productive members of society (Anderson, 1990). Indeed, the care of people at home when they were ill was the usual method of care and the principal area of practice for graduate nurses in Canada until the depression years of the 1930s when people could not afford the services of nurses at home and went to hospitals for care (Canadian Nurses Association, 1968).

During World War II, graduate nurses left the hospitals to join the armed services and hospitals were staffed mainly with student nurses. After the war, when the hospitals again had a full complement of graduate nurses and rapid advances were being made in medical and surgical treatment, the hospital was seen as the best place for care. The introduction of health insurance supported this view. Provincial insurance plans covered the costs of hospital care and care in physicians' offices but not home care.

The present return to home care is due to a number of factors. First, there is a trend towards making care less impersonal and more humanistic — patients have more control at home over the care they receive and they are able to enjoy a better quality of life with family and friends. Second, the cost of hospital care has escalated rapidly over the years and it is now considered cheaper to look after people at home. And finally, home care is becoming a part of essential health services covered by health insurance programs in most provinces and territories (Sutherland, and Fulton, 1988).

Home care services usually include: nursing, personal care and homemaker services, respite care and family relief.

1. **Nursing services.** Services may be provided by a Registered Nurse or a Licensed Practical Nurse depending on the level of service required. Virtually the whole range of nursing services can be provided in the home except those requiring equipment or services available only in a hospital. Thus, home nursing care may include health promotion as well as such diverse nursing interventions as intravenous therapy, dressings and other treatments including catheterization and enemas, the administration (and control) of medications and other therapeutic measures, nursing care for mothers and infants, postoperative care for early discharge patients or palliative care for the terminally ill.

2. **Personal care and homemaker services.** A wide range of care assistance is available, ranging from light housekeeping and meal preparation to personal care. Personal care includes assistance with bathing, grooming, dressing, walking, eating, oral medications, maintenance of dentures and glasses, and care of feet and nails. Depending on the level required, a Homemaker, Nurse's Aide or Health Care Aide may perform the service.

3. **Respite care and family relief.** Staff will come into the home to provide care for a patient to give the family caregiver relief. Some hospitals and other agencies provide adult day care and some have inpatient beds for people who are being looked after at home to give the family relief for a few days.

Home care services may also include one or more of the services listed below.

1. Household maintenance services, such as meal delivery, shopping, snow shovelling and heating (furnace) maintenance.

2. Health maintenance services such as nutrition counselling, physiotherapy, occupational therapy, podiatry (care of the feet), health teaching and speech therapy.

3. Health support services, including diagnostic services, transportation services, home equipment services, wheelchair and prosthetic appliance services.

4. Individual and family social services such as the provision of information about services and benefits available, counselling and referral as well as financial and employment and volunteer opportunity services.

5. Community liaison services such as educational services for school-age children, library services, visiting services, telephone assurance and telecheck services, child care, programs in seniors' centres and recreational activities.*

SOURCES OF CARE IN THE HOME

In Canada, home care programs are major providers of care. A number of agencies and services may provide these programs:

1. Provincial, metropolitan and regional community (public) health agencies. Manitoba, for example, has a province-wide home care program operated by the provincial government; so does British Columbia except for the metropolitan areas of Vancouver and Victoria where home care services are provided by municipal Departments of Health. In Ottawa, home care services are provided through the Ottawa–Carleton Regional Health Department.

2. Voluntary agencies such as the Victorian Order of Nurses, the Arthritis Society, the Canadian Red Cross Society, the Greater Vancouver Mental Health Service.

3. Private agencies such as ComCare, Paramed and others. Often, the services of private agencies like ComCare are contracted by government agencies to provide services.

4. Community Health Centres. In the Province of Quebec, home care is carried out by staff of the CLSCs. However, in some communities it has become a separate program.

5. Extramural hospitals. In New Brunswick, under the Extramural Hospital program, home care services are provided by hospital personnel.**

ISSUES IN HOME CARE

A wide range of services are available to assist with the care of people at home, yet there are differences in the utilization of these services by different groups in our society. Studies conducted in Great Britain showed that inequalities in health continued to exist, even after 15 years of the National Health Service. It was clear that people in higher-income groups knew how to access the system better and made better use of it than people in lower income groups (Grant, 1988). Both the Epp Report (1986) and the Ontario document, *Nurturing Health* (1993a), point out the need to redress similar health inequities that exist in our Canadian society.

Anderson (1990), reporting on research studies conducted to address policy issues in home care management and self-care, says that, despite the services available, the

---

* Adapted from a list of Types of Services provided at home or in support of care in the home. In R. Sutherland and J. Fulton, *Health Care in Canada*. Ottawa: The Health Group (1988) 229, 230.

** Sutherland and Fulton, 1988.

burden of care, that is, the ongoing monitoring and management of illness, still rests with families. She notes that new Canadians often find caring for ill family members particularly difficult for several reasons. There is a lack of services available to help families who do not speak English. Often, they are not aware of the services that are available. Then, too, many newcomers who are struggling to survive in their new environment require that both parents in a family work, leaving no one at home to care for a child or aged parent who is ill.

Roberts, in reviewing the literature on social support/network and help-seeking, suggests that the social network (of family, friends and trusted others) is an important influence on the process of seeking help for health-related problems. She further states that nurses in their day-to-day practice can and do provide the support needed to encourage people to utilize available services (Roberts, 1988).

ROLE OF VOLUNTARY AND RELIGIOUS AGENCIES

Voluntary agencies are established by the people in a community in response to a particular need. They are usually supported by donations, and the services they provide supplement or augment the functions performed by official agencies. In many instances, new services are pioneered by voluntary agencies and later taken over by government agencies. For example, the Victorian Order of Nurses, a voluntary agency established in 1898 to provide home nursing services in Canada, pioneered a number of home care programs which have subsequently been taken over by provincial and/or municipal government services (Du Gas and Beckingham, 1993).

Voluntary agencies usually provide services of a specific nature. They may be concerned with the preventive, curative and rehabilitative aspects of one disease, for example, provincial Heart and Stroke Foundations, the Canadian Liver Foundation and the Greater Vancouver Mental Health Service. Some voluntary agencies confine their attention to a particular segment of the population, such as the Volunteers for Seniors in Continuing Care, or the Shriners who operate hospitals for children. Dedicated volunteers have set up shelters for battered women in numerous communities. Volunteers also provide food, shelter and clothing in times of crisis for families in need — not only to battered women but, also, to the old and the young who are homeless, and to others who are in need of assistance.

Voluntary agencies also play a large role in the support of fitness and recreation programs. Many agencies today are concerned about environmental health hazards, spearheading movements to reduce pollution, to protect our waterways and preserve our wildlife habitats. Voluntary agencies may develop at the local, provincial or national

level. In Canada the major visiting nurse service has until recently been the Victorian Order of Nurses, a national voluntary agency. These services have been taken over in some provinces by government agencies and the VON has moved on to develop other innovative programs, such as foot care clinics and day care centres for the *frail elderly* (people who require nursing care or supervision). The role played by volunteers and by voluntary agencies in health and welfare in Canada is a very large one and we will be discussing it further in the section of this chapter on the people who provide health services.

Religious organizations have played a large role in the development of health and welfare services in Canada from the time of the early French settlers onward. They continue to play a very large role as, for example, in the Grace Hospitals run by the Salvation Army in most large cities in Canada and the hospitals run by orders of the Roman Catholic Church and other denominations. A large number of the hospitals formerly operated by religious groups are now under secular management. Most religious denominations, however, support, and many operate, a variety of services in their communities to help people in need. The basements of many churches are used for day-care centres for pre-schoolers and after-school care for older children. In inner-city neighbourhoods, religious organizations often provide shelter for the homeless at night. Religious groups work with alcoholics and provide meals for the hungry. In Vancouver, the Anglican Church helped to get a rehabilitation program started for "street kids," training and giving them practical experience in staffing and managing a restaurant that is open to the public five days a week.

COMMUNITY HEALTH SERVICES

Community health services are much more difficult to fit into neat categories than are hospital and other inpatient services. They are delivered in "homes, offices, clinics, the street, shopping centres, schools, workplaces, jails and recreation sites" (Sutherland and Fulton, 1988, 219). Community health services operate alongside, and, as recommended in the Health Promotion Framework, need to work closely with, other social networks in the community. These other social networks may include those involved with housing, urban planning, recreation, protective services and education.

OFFICIAL COMMUNITY HEALTH AGENCIES

The local government agency responsible for community health services is usually a municipal or regional health department, for example, the Vancouver Health Department, the Toronto Health Department or the Ottawa/Carleton (Regional)Health Department. Outside the large cities the

GEORGINA FANE POPE 1862–1938

Georgina Fane Pope, first matron of the Canadian Army Medical Corps, was also Canada's first recipient of the Royal Red Cross. The award, for conspicuous service in the field, was awarded in 1903 by the British Government for her outstanding work as a nursing sister in South Africa during the Boer War.

Cicely Jane Georgina Fane Pope was born in Charlottetown in 1862 to one of Prince Edward Island's most prominent families. Her father, W.H. Pope, was Colonial Secretary and became a Father of Confederation when Canada was formed in 1867. Georgina Pope trained as a nurse at Bellevue Hospital in New York, graduated in 1886, and worked in the United States for several years. During the Boer War, she was one of four nursing sisters who accompanied the first Canadian volunteer force to South Africa in 1899. The Canadian nurses served with great distinction in several locations at or near the front lines. In December 1900, after more than a year in South Africa, Sister Pope nursed the wounded on a troop ship returning to Canada. When fighting resumed in 1902, she returned once more with another band of nursing sisters and another contingent of troops.

Following the war, reorganization of the Canadian services was announced, first with a reserve unit of 25 nursing sisters, and then in 1906 with a permanent military nursing service. Nursing Sister Pope was selected from the reserves for this permanent group and in 1908 was named the first matron of the Canadian Army Medical Corps.

In World War I, Matron Pope (age 52) went overseas with the first group of nurses and served in Canadian army hospitals in the United Kingdom. In December 1917 she went with the No. 8 Canadian Hospital to France, where she fell ill and had to be invalided home. Despite a pensionable disability, Georgina Pope lived to age 76, died in her beloved PEI and was buried with full military honours.

Glennis Zilm

local government agency may be operated directly by a unit of the provincial health ministry. Other branches of a local government (for example, a school board) may also provide health services. Some municipalities and provincial governments also administer social assistance programs and provide social services. The health department of a municipality or a region usually develops its own health program, based on the needs of the people in the community and the resources available to meet those needs. The general community program usually includes the control of communicable diseases, a number of environmentally related health protection measures and a health promotion program. Many communities also provide other services.

Local government community health agencies also put a lot of emphasis on health promotion. Traditionally, this has involved health education and such services as prenatal, postnatal and well-baby clinics for mothers and infants, school health programs, wellness centres for older adults and similar activities. The health promotion role now encompasses community development and empowering people to assume more control over their own health services. We will discuss this concept in more detail in Chapter 11, Health and the Community.

Many official agencies at the local level also provide a number of specialized health services in addition to the general community programs. These services frequently include maternal and child care services, immunization clinics and,

Environmentally Related Health Protection Measures Carried Out by Local Official Community Health Agencies:

- examination of selected aspects of air and water quality
- testing of rural water and sewage systems
- food testing
- inspection of restaurants and other eating places and food premises
- control of insects and animals
- maintenance of cleanliness of public beaches and swimming pools
- inspection of public and residential buildings and spaces.

SOURCE: Sutherland, R. and Fulton, J. (1988). *Health Care in Canada*.

often, diagnostic, treatment and rehabilitative services for people on low incomes. Some municipalities also operate hospitals and other inpatient services for people who are ill or who need long-term care.

COMMUNITY HEALTH CENTRES

Community health centres provide primary health care services in an ambulatory setting. The common features of CHCs are shown in the box below.

Common Features of Community Health Centres

- emphasize health promotion
- are community-oriented
- offer a broad range of services
- are multidisciplinary
- do not rely on fee-for-service payments as primary source of income.

A number of different models have developed in Canada over the past 30 years. These include those designated as Community Health Centres (CHCs): Health Services Organizations (HSOs) and Comprehensive Health Organizations (CHOs), Health and Human Resources Centres (in British Columbia), Local Community Services Centres (CLSCs — in Quebec), multi-service centres, hospital-affiliated centres and physician-based centres. Most are funded by provincial governments and operate on a global budget — one which includes all services and salaries. Exceptions are the physician-based clinics you might find in local neighbourhoods (sometimes in shopping malls) that offer walk-in and after-hours services. Most HSOs are also controlled by physicians but they usually operate on a capitation basis (charging a fixed amount per person) rather than a fee-for-service basis.

Because most CHCs do not depend on fee-for-service as the major source of income, they can utilize the talents of nurses, social workers and whoever is best suited to do the work to achieve an integrated approach to assessment, care planning and service delivery. Most centres have a fairly extensive health team comprising Registered Nurses, community health nurses, nurse practitioners and social workers as well as physicians. The larger centres may have nutritionists, physiotherapists and occupational therapists, psychologists, mental health therapists and counsellors, pharmacists, health educators, optometrists, podiatrists or chiropodists, community developers, health records analysts and chiropractors (Sutherland and Fulton, 1988).

MULTI-SERVICE AGENCIES

As provincial governments begin restructuring their health services, Community Health Centres are being considered as a viable option for providing care that is convenient and comprehensive, and allows greater consumer participation and control of services. In Ontario, intersectoral cooperation between the Ministry of Health, the Ministry of Community and Social Services and the Ministry of Citizenship has resulted in the development of *multi-service agencies* (MSAs) to provide coordinated services for the following three groups:

1. Adults with physical disabilities
2. Elderly persons who need long-term care and support services
3. People of any age who require health services at home or at school, for example, people who need care at home after being hospitalized, those needing longer-term personal care at home and children who need professional health services to go to school.

The MSAs will serve as the single entry point (point at which an individual enters the health care system) for people needing long-term care services at home or in the community, and for those requiring care in a nursing home or a charitable or municipal residential facility for older people. The range of services to be delivered by MSAs includes visiting nurses, supportive housing, homemaking, friendly visiting, security programs, physiotherapy, nutrition counselling, meal programs and transportation as well as palliative care either at home or in the community. Care will be coordinated with other services such as hospitals (Government of Ontario, 1993b).

HEALTH MAINTENANCE ORGANIZATIONS (US)

The *health maintenance organizations* in the United States are essentially a form of prepaid group practice. They provide a comprehensive range of services on a fixed contract basis, which is paid for in advance by people enrolling in the organization. The emphasis in the HMOs, as in the Canadian CHCs, is on health promotion and protection. The range of services provided by HMOs covers both preventive and curative care and includes physician services, health counselling, inpatient and outpatient hospital services, and diagnostic and therapeutic services, including home care. Many nurses are employed in HMOs, including Nurse Practitioners in various fields, including midwifery.

STREET CLINICS

Street clinics, known also as "storefront" or "free" clinics, developed in the 1960s and 1970s in both Canada and the United States. Set up in poor or ghetto neighbourhoods, they provide services for the homeless, "street kids," alcoholics, prostitutes and drug addicts who are reluctant to use traditional agencies. The clinics offer readily accessible care, usually on a 24-hour free basis in a setting that is as devoid of "red tape" as possible. In the beginning, the clinics were staffed mainly by volunteers, but many of these clinics are now operated by official or other types of community health agencies. An example is Street Health, a community-based nursing organization in Toronto, currently operating four nursing stations in various drop-in centres and shelters for women and men who are homeless or underhoused. In order to document both the health problems and the barriers to services encountered by their patients in traditional health agencies, a comprehensive, rigorously executed research study was undertaken by Street Health. Findings of the study point to inadequacies in both the health and social services systems, providing the nurses with hard, reliable data that could be used to lobby for policy changes to improve the situation for the people they serve (Crowe and Hardill, 1993).

MENTAL HEALTH CENTRES AND OTHER COMMUNITY MENTAL HEALTH SERVICES

Mental health services have undergone tremendous change since the Second World War in Canada and elsewhere in the Western world. Most of the large asylums have been closed, the patients discharged and the care of people with mental illness transferred to the community. There has been a large and rapid increase in the number of psychiatric units within general hospitals and a network of community-based services, such as Mental Health Clinics, has developed. The hospital-based services provide treatment for the acutely ill under the care of psychiatrists. Community-based services are dominated by non-physician health professionals, such as psychologists, social workers and nurses (Dickinson and André, 1988). The types of services offered include the following treatment and support services:

- screening and referral
- assessment, diagnosis and treatment
- medication
- individual, couple, group and family therapy
- coordination of services
- rehabilitation services in self-care, leisure and work-related areas
- emergency services
- residential care.*

PHYSICIANS' OFFICES

A great deal of ambulatory care is provided in physicians' offices. The majority of physicians in Canada are in private

practice. They are reimbursed for their services on a fee-for-service basis by provincial or territorial government medical insurance programs. Physicians may work in either "solo" or group practice; the latter is becoming more common. In group practice, several physicians work together to provide more comprehensive care for individuals and families. For example, there may be one or two family practitioners in the group, an obstetrician, a pediatrician and a surgeon. Frequently, there is also a psychiatrist, and there may be other specialists as well. A large number of nurses are employed in physicians' offices; in a single large group practice, there may be several.

HOSPITAL AMBULATORY SERVICES/OUTPATIENT DEPARTMENTS

Five to ten percent of ambulatory health care is provided by hospitals (Sutherland and Fulton, 1988). The many services performed in emergency departments and outpatient departments have led to the latter being renamed "ambulatory care departments" in many institutions. These departments provide diagnostic, screening and treatment services, and often rehabilitative services. Many hospitals offer day programs for specific groups, such as those for seniors who are being cared for at home when caregivers need to work or have other commitments. They are also providing such services as one-day surgery and pre-admission clinics so that patients do not have to be admitted one or two days before surgery but can be admitted on the day of their surgery (LeNoble, 1993).

EMERGENCY SERVICES

We have become increasingly conscious in the past few years of the need for highly skilled personnel to deal with medical emergency situations in the community. Most large hospitals, and many small community ones, have well-staffed, well-equipped emergency rooms that are open 24 hours a day. A person does not usually wait to have a heart attack in the emergency unit — it may occur while the individual is shopping in a crowded mall, driving on a busy highway or even shovelling snow from the sidewalk in front of the house. Accidents and sudden attacks of illness may occur at any time and in any place. The first few minutes of care individuals receive are often crucial to their survival and subsequent recovery.

All provinces must provide ambulance services under their health insurance programs. In most provinces, the services are subsidized, so people pay only a small fee; in some, there is no charge. Ambulance drivers are being trained in emergency measures to provide initial treatment and in life support measures for people who have suffered an acute attack of illness until they can be treated in an acute

---

* As listed in a publication of the Greater Vancouver Mental Health Service.

care agency. Regrettably, not all ambulance drivers are fully trained as yet, particularly in rural parts of the country.

INPATIENT SERVICES

Hospitals, which began to flourish in the latter part of the last century, continue to dominate the health care scene. Despite the rapid de-institutionalization of services currently in progress, it is likely that there will always be people who are best cared for in a hospital or other inpatient facility. Those who require major surgery and those who need intensive care or recovery-room services, for example, need to be in a facility which has the high-technology equipment and teams of specialized personnel to provide skilled care. People whose aggressive behaviour threatens their own or others' safety also need the supervision available in an inpatient facility. The list of those who cannot be cared for in the community grows shorter, however, as alternative treatment delivery modes replace the dependence on hospital care for many people with health problems (Sutherland and Fulton, 1988).

Historically, older adults have utilized most hospital services and, as this segment of the population increases, it can be argued that the demand for hospital services will increase as well. In 1984, 51 percent of all hospital bed-days in this country were used by the elderly. Projections based on an extrapolation of current trends anticipate that it will be 74 percent by 2036, with a corresponding demand for more hospital beds (Hamilton and Trepanier, 1989). There are some indications, however, that the anticipated future demand for hospital beds may be offset by improvements in the health of people, particularly older adults, and by a reallocation of resources, including both money and people, to community-based services (Trepanna, 1990).

At the present time, in Canada, there are a number of different levels of inpatient services, including community, regional and teaching hospitals, rehabilitation centres, extended or long-term care facilities and supervised residences. Nurses are the largest component of professional staff in all inpatient services, with the exception of supervised residences, which may have predominantly lay staff with nursing services provided on a part-time basis. The need for skilled nursing care is often the major reason for admitting an individual to an inpatient facility.

HOSPITALS

The basic purpose of hospitals is the care of ill and injured people. They have traditionally performed curative, rehabilitative, preventive and rehabilitative functions, and are also involved in two additional areas of commitment: research and education. Hospitals provide a clinical laboratory for students of a good many health disciplines, including nurses, physicians, dietitians, laboratory workers and other skilled technicians and technologists. The hospital's role in research has expanded in recent years — from providing a field of study for health scientists to undertaking their own research on clinical practice, or collaborating with universities and government research teams on clinical studies. Most large hospitals now have a director of nursing research on their staff.

The functions of a hospital include

- care of ill and injured people
- education of health personnel
- research.

Hospitals vary considerably in size. In Canada we have had general hospitals of up to 1600 beds and psychiatric hospitals that housed 4000 or more people with mental illness, but today most hospitals are closing beds. Many small communities have had a hospital with between ten and 20 beds, but there is a trend towards making these small hospitals into multipurpose community health centres offering a wide range of services but retaining a few inpatient beds. Larger urban centres may have a medium-size hospital with up to 100 beds, while regional centres usually have a large hospital and offer such services as a high risk neonatal unit. When affiliated with a medical school, a hospital is designated as a "Teaching Hospital." Examples of teaching hospitals include the Ottawa General Hospital, the Ottawa Civic Hospital and the Children's Hospital of Eastern Ontario, all of which are part of the University of Ottawa Faculty of Health Sciences.

Control and Financing of Hospitals

Every province has a Public Hospitals Act and most have a Private Hospitals Act as well. In Canada, most hospitals are non-profit (public) general hospitals. The few private, for-profit, or *proprietary hospitals* are usually small and provide specialized mental health or addiction-related services. The *public general hospitals* vary in their ownership; they may be owned by religious groups, by municipalities, by a provincial government (for example, some hospitals in New Brunswick) or by the federal government (Sutherland and Fulton, 1988). The Canada Health Act specifies the services that hospitals must provide, although they may offer additional services over and above those deemed essential.

Provincial and territorial governments have both legal and financial control over public hospitals. The provincial statutes regulate the conduct of hospitals, and provincial hospital insurance provides the funding, usually through a global budget. The government also sets standards for all inpatient facilities, including those that are privately run. However, with the movement towards regionalization of health services, the control and operation of hospitals is being delegated in many instances to regional boards of health.

REHABILITATION CENTRES

Rehabilitation is the restoration of an individual who has been ill, from any cause, to the most complete level of social, physical and mental functioning that is possible for him or her. Rehabilitation should not begin when the patient has recovered from the acute phase of illness, nor should it be the responsibility of specialized agencies only. It should begin with the patient's admission to an agency for the care and treatment of an illness. The restoration of the individual to an active, functioning role in society, insofar as this is possible, should be the aim of all who care for that person.

Today, with the increasing prevalence of chronic and degenerative diseases and the vast numbers of people suffering injuries as a result of accidents, there is a growing need for long-term restorative services. For many people injured in accidents or crippled with degenerative disorders, restoration to their optimal level of functioning is a lengthy process that may take years of encouragement and require specialized care. Frequently these people need the help of members of a variety of health disciplines — physicians, nurses, occupational and physiotherapists, clergy, social workers and others — to assist in their rehabilitation. Often, they require facilities such as gymnasiums, swimming pools and outdoor recreation areas, as well as nursing units specially adapted to facilitate increasing independence in the activities of daily living.

In response to the growing need for these types of services, specialized agencies have developed whose primary purpose is rehabilitation, for example, the Rehabilitation Centre that forms part of the Health Sciences Complex in Ottawa and the G.F. Strong Rehabilitation Centre in Vancouver.

A rehabilitation centre coordinates the efforts of many disciplines in order to plan an approach designed to meet individual needs. The rehabilitation team meets regularly to discuss the patient's progress and revise the plan to the individual's changing needs.

Nurses play a key role in rehabilitation both while the patient is in the acute treatment agency and afterwards, in the specialized rehabilitation unit. When people are acutely ill, good nursing care supports their own resources in all areas of functioning and helps prevent the development of complications that can delay or prevent full recovery. For example, a person with a spinal injury who is paralyzed from the waist down can develop "foot drop," a condition which can hinder learning to walk again if adequate preventive measures, such as supporting the feet so they do not drop, are

not taken during the acute stage of illness by all who care for the individual. In both the acute care setting and in specialized rehabilitation units, nursing is the one constant in a variety of services needed to restore the individual to the optimal level of health. Nursing is there on a 24-hour-a-day basis, whereas other health workers come and go, spending varying amounts of time with the patient. It is frequently up to the nurse, then, to ensure that all aspects of the rehabilitation plan for the individual are carried through, and that there is continuity and consistency in the approaches used by all members of staff.

EXTENDED/LONG-TERM CARE FACILITIES

People with chronic or degenerative diseases and conditions need care over an extended period of time. As people get older, they tend to have more chronic and degenerative diseases and therefore more need of long-term services. However, we should point out that most older adults are functioning fully in the community — fewer than 10 percent are in residential facilities. The older generation are in good health mentally, physically and socially according to recent national and provincial health surveys and are taking better care of themselves than are younger Canadians. The findings of Canada's Health Promotion Study (1985) suggest that "to an even greater extent than among younger Canadians, positive preventive health measures are the norm among the older population" (Health and Welfare Canada, 1987, 4).

Most older people consider themselves well even if they have a chronic disease such as arthritis or hypertension — such individuals just need monitoring to make sure their arthritis is not interfering with the activities of daily living or that their blood pressure is not becoming too high. There are other groups in the population, however, who also need long-term care, such as children and adults with disabilities, people with long-term mental illness and those who are mentally handicapped. All need a continuum of care. The services available to help them live a normal lifestyle outside an institution are becoming more plentiful and, as outlined in the Ontario Government report, *Partnerships in Long-Term Care* (1993b), the services are becoming more coordinated and more sensitive to people's needs and wishes.

The philosophy of residential long-term care has changed also. The "warehousing" of older people in nursing homes and chronic hospitals, where physical needs were looked after but psychosocial ones neglected, is thankfully disappearing. Experts on aging contend, however, that we still have a long way to go to accommodate the needs of today's older population who are "healthier, better educated, more knowledgeable and therefore can be expected both to know their rights and to make them known to the service system" (Seymour, 1991, 27). The two Marys, Mary Buzzell and Mary Gibbon, who are well known across

A case manager assessing the long-term care needs of an older patient

term care. The range of facilities includes:

- communal residences, such as the Abbeyfield residences for small groups of nine to ten older people who can look after themselves, but who need the companionship and security of living in a residence
- group homes for the mentally handicapped, for people recovering from a mental illness and for disabled adults and children
- senior citizen apartment complexes designed to provide the safety and security measures needed by older people, such as "grab bars" in the bathroom and emergency call bells
- personal care homes for people who need help with dressing, grooming and other activities of daily living
- nursing homes and extended care units for people who need skilled nursing care
- multilevel facilities such as the Unitarian House (Centre) in Ottawa which combines single room and small apartment accommodation for people who are independent and a nursing unit for those needing skilled care, dining room service for those who want it, and kitchen facilities for people who wish to prepare meals or snacks for themselves.

HOSPICES/PALLIATIVE CARE

The purpose of both *hospices* and *palliative care units* (the terms are pretty well interchangeable) is to care for people who are dying, while enabling them to live as normally as possible with as much freedom from pain as possible. The terms *palliative care* and *hospice* are used to express both a philosophy of care and an agency for inpatient and home care services. Care is provided so that the dying person can be maintained at home as long as feasible, with nurses, physicians, clergymen and social workers on the palliative care team providing the assistance and support required by patients and their families. When it is no longer feasible to maintain dying patients at home, they are transferred to the inpatient facility, where they may move in and out as their condition warrants.

THE ROLE OF PROVINCIAL AND TERRITORIAL GOVERNMENTS

The primary responsibility for administering the national health insurance program in Canada is vested in the provinces. They are the insuring agencies and they are responsible for all aspects of the delivery of care. This includes setting standards for hospitals and long-term care agencies, negotiating fees and salaries for health care workers and determining the budgets for hospitals and all other

Canada for their outstanding work in the field of health care for older adults, point out the need to retain the "personhood" that makes each of us unique and to promote caring for the individual over caring for the illness in day-to-day practice (Buzzell and Gibbon, 1991).

A philosophy of restorative care for older people was pioneered by Vera McIver at four extended-care hospitals operating in Victoria in the mid-1970s. She introduced a method of care based on the belief that the older person is still a unique individual, working towards growth and self-fulfillment, and that a therapeutic and restorative environment can be achieved if this attitude is kept in mind (McIver, 1978). The **Priory Model**, as it has come to be called, has won international acclaim and has formed the philosophic background for gerontological nursing as it has developed in Canada (Mantle, 1992).

Implementation of the concept of restorative care is not equal across the country, by any means, but changes in our thinking about health and health care, as well as an increase in the number of nurses and other health workers with additional preparation in gerontological nursing, provide an optimistic scenario. The experience of the Queensway–Carleton Hospital in Nepean, Ontario, provides an example of how the concept of restorative care can be put into practice on an extended care unit in an acute care hospital. An interdisciplinary psychosocial approach was used to care for elderly on the unit, which made the resident "the centre of a caring community that fosters individual rights, respect and self-determination" (Carson and Ross, 1993).

A variety of new types of residential facilities are developing to meet the progressive needs of people for long-service agencies. Many provinces also have dental plans for children, and most have programs for senior citizens and other special groups to eliminate or defray the cost of prescription drugs.

Provincial governments assume a leadership and advisory role for local health agencies who, for the most part, operate the services. The provincial governments, however, also provide many direct services such as the operation of laboratories, the licensure of individuals and agencies, the dissemination of information and the provision of financial assistance to municipal and regional boards of health. Outside the large metropolitan areas, community health services have traditionally been organized and operated by provincial governments in Canada. As we noted in the previous chapter, however, many provinces are in the process of decentralizing and regional and community health boards are assuming increasing responsibility for the management and control of local health services. Provincial governments still operate some hospitals, such as psychiatric facilities and homes for people who are mentally handicapped (Health and Welfare Canada, 1989).

WORKERS' COMPENSATION BOARDS

Each province and territory has its own Workers' Compensation Act, but all are based on the same model. The Canadian model was derived from the German Accident Insurance Act, passed in 1884, which historians tell us was developed by Chancellor Bismarck as a political ploy to keep followers of Karl Marx from being elected to the German parliament. Be that as it may, the results have benefited workers in many countries of the world. Considered the first legislation in social welfare, Workers' Compensation laws are based on the principle that production costs should include the cost of any injuries sustained by workers in the making of a product. These costs should then be incorporated into the selling price — in this way, the consumer bears the cost burden (Eades, 1965).

Although earlier versions were passed in 1902 in British Columbia, and in the provinces of Alberta (1908) and Quebec (1909), it was the Workers' Compensation Act of 1914 in Ontario that provided the present basis for Canadian legislation (Eades, 1965). The legislation was, in effect, a compromise between labour and management, with labour giving up the right to sue an employer for negligence (the right of individuals under common law) in return for receiving benefits regardless of who was at fault. An exception is made where the injury was caused by serious and willful misconduct on the part of the worker, unless the individual is permanently or seriously disabled.

Workers' Compensation Boards in Canada operate under provincial statute, as quasi-governmental agencies (that is, created by government but autonomous in their operation). The Boards both collect and dispense funds. Money is collected from employers through an assessment designed to cover the costs involved in a particular industry. The rate of assessment for employers is determined by the Board. Under the scheme, industries are divided into rate groups reflecting industry and/or cost similarities. For example, logging has a higher cost history than does retail sales. Therefore, companies in the lumber industry would be assessed at a higher rate than department stores. The assessment levied on employers in each rate group is intended to cover the cost of health care, income replacement and survivor benefits for workers, including administrative costs and costs for accident prevention* and the rehabilitation of workers.

Most workers in Canada, except the self-employed, are covered by workers' compensation, although agricultural workers are not yet covered in all provinces. Workers' benefits include medical coverage, rehabilitation and income continuity for personal injury, disease or death arising out of and in the course of employment.

In the United States, as in Canada in the provinces, each state has its own Workers' Compensation legislation. The model that developed in the US, however, requires employers to be individually liable for providing coverage, as opposed to the Canadian "collective liability" system. In some states, this is done through private insuring agencies, in others the state is the insuring agency and still others have both private insurance carriers and a State Board (Workers' Compensation Board of British Columbia, 1993).

THE FEDERAL GOVERNMENT'S ROLE

The federal government exerts considerable influence over both health and welfare services in Canada through national legislation and through its financial contribution to the programs operated by the provinces. The federal government both funds and operates the national security program which includes Old Age Pensions, the Canada Pension Plan, Family Allowances and Unemployment Insurance. It also funds and operates health protection programs.

Through its numerous agencies, the federal government provides advisory and consultative services for municipal and provincial health agencies. Another federal responsibility is the maintenance of a national information service about health and social welfare matters. Statistics Canada is the agency with primary responsibility for collecting and disseminating information on a wide variety of topics. The individual ministries also collect and share information with their provincial counterparts across the country — through federal–provincial meetings of

---

* In some provinces, the Board funds accident prevention directly; in other provinces it provides the funds to another agency for this purpose.

Health Ministers and meetings of government nursing consultants, through the publication of papers on different topics and through news bulletins and journals such as *Canadian Social Trends*.

The federal government's role in research in all aspects of health and social welfare is also significant. The Extramural Research Programs Directorate is responsible for management of the National Health Research and Development Program (NHRDP). This program is the principal source of support for scientific research on national health issues. It also provides support for the development of research protocols and for the training and career development of health researchers. Some of your professors may be Career Scientists or Career Scholars whose positions are funded by the NHRDP program.

At the direct services level, the federal government is concerned with interprovincial hazards such as pollution, with the control of communicable diseases and with the setting of standards for drug control. The federal government is also directly responsible for the provision of health care services to certain segments of the population such as armed services personnel and their families, war veterans and the members of First Nations populations. Health Canada, through its Medical Services Branch, is currently in the process of transferring the provision of health care services to First Nations people (Health and Welfare Canada, 1989). We will be discussing this move in Chapter 12.

THE PRIVATE SECTOR'S ROLE

Although we tend to think of our health care system as being run by the government, the private sector is very much involved in the provision of health and welfare services in Canada. Many of these services, such as homemaker and home nursing services, as well as long-term care, are purchased by governments from private companies. Among the services provided by private companies are pharmaceuticals, home care, homes for the elderly, residential services for disabled persons and children and day care for children and disabled adults. The services of many health practitioners (such as physicians), also in private practice, are purchased by governments on a fee-for-service basis (Health and Welfare Canada, 1989).

THE PEOPLE WHO PROVIDE THE SERVICES

The provision of health care in Canada is estimated to employ between seven and eight percent of the labour force. In many communities, the health care sector is one of the largest employers (Trepanna, 1990). Thirty-one occupa-

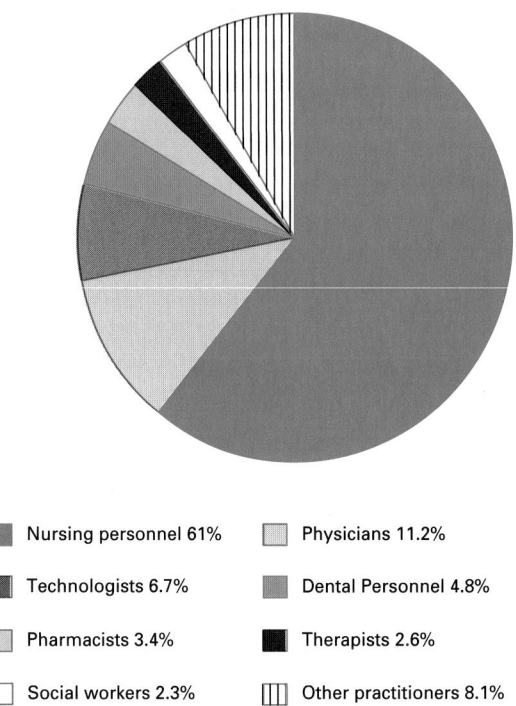

Nursing personnel 61% Physicians 11.2%

Technologists 6.7% Dental Personnel 4.8%

Pharmacists 3.4% Therapists 2.6%

Social workers 2.3% Other practitioners 8.1%

FIGURE 4.4 Health Care Practitioners in Canada, 1990

SOURCE: Health and Welfare Canada. (1992). *Health Personnel in Canada 1990*. Ottawa: Minister of Supply and Services. Cat. No. H1-9/1990. It should be noted that not all categories of health worker are listed in this publication.

tional groups of health care practitioners are listed by the publication, *Health Personnel in Canada 1990* (Health and Welfare Canada, 1992). Of the 531 664 practitioners enumerated in this document, more than one half are nurses (223 965 employed RNs, 82 281 LPNs/RNAs). If you add nursing orderlies (18 037) to this group, nursing personnel account for 61 percent of the total. The next largest group of health care practitioners are physicians, whose numbers total 59 409, followed by laboratory technologists (19 278) and then pharmacists (18 337). Approximately 25 000 people practise in the dental field, including 14 394 dentists, almost 8832 dental hygienists, 1772 dental assistants and 335 dental nurses/therapists. Figure 4.4 shows the relative numbers of Canadian health care practitioners in various categories in 1990.

COLLABORATION — AN ESSENTIAL COMPONENT OF NURSING PRACTICE

Regardless of where nurses practise, even if they are engaged in independent practice, they work in collaboration with other members of the health team. The health team of today is composed of a variety of personnel representing professional disciplines concerned with the health and welfare of people.

In addition to the traditional health professions of medicine, nursing, dentistry and pharmacy, a number of other, highly specialized positions in health care have developed. Many of the people in these specialties, such as physical therapists and occupational therapists, provide direct-care services to patients that are complementary to medical and nursing care. Some are technologists, such as respiratory technologists and renal dialysis (artificial kidney) technicians, whose occupations have evolved because of the need for people with specific skills in handling the complex machinery used in the care of patients. Several of the newer groups have emerged as a result of the delegation of certain functions by the major professionals. These include the licensed practical nurses/registered nursing assistants, dental hygienists, dental nurses, dental assistants and pharmacy assistants.

The provision of health care today requires a multidisciplinary team approach. In some instances, the team may consist of only three members — the physician, the nurse and the patient; in others, there may be a dozen or more health professionals involved in the care of one individual, a family or a community. All members of the team possess knowledge and skills unique to their discipline, and all contribute their special expertise to the care of the patient. There are also many areas of shared knowledge and skills. Students who have all or part of their educational program in the health sciences division of a community college, or in a university health sciences centre, may find themselves sharing common core courses with students in several other health disciplines. Most of the health professions require that their practitioners have a good foundation in the biophysical and social sciences and frequently students from several health sciences programs take classes together in such subjects as anatomy, physiology, microbiology, psychology and sociology.

Many skills are also shared among various members of the health team. Communications skills, for example, are needed by all health professionals, not only by those who work directly with patients. The nursing student and the medical student must both learn to give injections and to start intravenous infusions. The nurse must also learn to perform many of the common laboratory tests that are a part of the laboratory technologist's repertoire of skills.

The essence of the collaborative team concept is that all members work cooperatively with the patient — whether an individual, a family or a community. Together, they are able to make a concerted effort towards their common goal of attaining the highest level of health possible for that patient. The nursing team is an integral part of the overall health team; we will discuss the various members of the nursing team in Chapter 5, Nursing in Canada. In this section, we will look at other members of the health team with whom the nurse collaborates in community-based and in institution-based health services. We will also discuss the role of volunteers as part of a large and growing group of people working in the health field.

MEMBERS OF THE MEDICAL TEAM

Patients are admitted to a hospital in most instances under the care of their own private physician or a physician on the staff of the agency to which they have been assigned. The physician is usually responsible for directing the diagnostic and therapeutic plan of care for the patient. Most teaching hospitals and their related community agencies also have interns and resident physicians. Interns are recent graduates of medical school who have a planned program of clinical experience in the various services of these agencies in order to complete requirements for licensure as practising physicians. Residents are qualified medical practitioners who are preparing for practice in a medical specialty. If an agency is affiliated with a medical school, there will also be medical students receiving clinical instruction and experience in the various units of the agency. In Canada the numbers of specialist and family practice physicians are almost equal, with the balance slightly in favour of those in family practice.

In the United States (and in some other countries) a **physician's assistant** category of worker has developed. Designated by various titles, such as Medex, Primex or simply Physician's Assistant, he or she is usually employed by a physician and performs, under the supervision of the physician, many tasks traditionally considered a part of medical practice. These tasks may include taking the medical history and undertaking the initial physical examination of a patient, assisting in primary care and monitoring the progress of people under the care of the physician. Many physicians' assistants work in rural areas (where there is a scarcity of doctors) with physicians in solo practice, where they help to extend the range of medical coverage. Many are former military corpsmen, some are nurses and others enter the educational programs for preparation as physicians' assistants without previous experience in the health field. The course of studies, which is usually offered in a university setting in conjunction with a medical school, ranges from one to five years in length, depending on the individual's previous training and experience in the health field. The physician's assistant category did not develop in Canada.

MEMBERS OF THE HEALTH TEAM INVOLVED PRIMARILY WITH HEALTH PROMOTION

Health educators are responsible for the development of health education programs in the community. A large part of their work is in community development, working with people to identify community health needs and to take action to improve health conditions. The nurse and the health educator collaborate on many health promotion programs. The health educator usually has a baccalaureate or higher degree.

Recreation specialists are also members of the health team concerned with promoting health and physical fitness. Their responsibilities include the development of recreation, sports and physical fitness programs in the community. The recreation specialist is usually a graduate of a baccalaureate program in physical education (or recreation).

Nutritionists are on the staff of many community health agencies. They advise people about good dietary habits, counsel them about their nutrition problems and undertake nutrition education programs in the community. The nutritionist has usually had a four- to five-year program of studies at university, followed by a year of internship in various health agencies. The nutritionist who works in a hospital or other institutional setting is called a *dietitian*. The dietitian is usually responsible for planning meal service for patients and staff, supervising other workers in the preparation of food and counselling patients about their nutritional problems.

ENVIRONMENTAL HEALTH WORKERS

Environmental health workers have as their primary concern the improvement, control and management of our environment. *Public health inspectors* are the traditional workers in this field (called *sanitarians* in the United States). The responsibilities of these workers are principally the elimination or control of *nuisances* — factors in the environment that may endanger health, such as excessive noise, offensive odours; ensuring the safety of water, milk and food supplies; ensuring that garbage and sewage disposal is properly carried out; enforcing public health laws with regard to sanitation and assisting in the control of communicable diseases. In Canada, programs for public health inspectors are usually offered in institutes of technology or in community colleges. The sanitarian in the United States usually has a baccalaureate degree in the biological, physical or sanitary sciences.

A large number of new workers have emerged in the field of environmental health. There is, for example, the *industrial hygienist*, whose main concern is the detection and control of hazards in the work environment. There are also technologists specializing in water, in pollution and in other facets of environmental health.

OTHER HEALTH SERVICE PROVIDERS

Some of the other workers with whom the nurse will come in frequent contact are the social worker, the pharmacist, the physical therapist, the occupational therapist, the respiratory technologist, the medical laboratory technologist and the radiology technologist.

Social workers assist in evaluating the psychosocial situation of the patient and help people with their social problems. They usually have extensive knowledge of community agencies and frequently make arrangements for the patient to be cared for by the appropriate agency. The majority of social workers hold a bachelor's or master's degree in social work; many community colleges are now offering courses for assistant social workers.

The *pharmacist* is an individual whose primary area of responsibility is the preparation and dispensing of drugs and other chemical substances used in the detection, prevention and treatment of illness. Because drug therapy is an important part of the treatment of many illnesses, most hospitals and other health agencies in the community usually employ a staff of pharmacists. The pharmacist is an excellent source of information for nurses on the nature of medications — their composition, mode of action, method of administration, dosage and possible side-effects. Most pharmacists in North America complete a four-year course of studies at a university. A number of community colleges are developing courses for pharmacy assistants. In many countries of the world, new programs to prepare pharmacists (to replace the old apprentice type of training) are being located in community colleges and technological institutes as well as in universities.

Physiotherapists have specialized preparation in physical therapy in a three- to four-year program of studies, usually in a university. They assist in assessing the patient's functional ability, strength and mobility; carry out therapeutic treatments, particularly those dealing with the musculoskeletal system; and teach families and individuals exercises and other measures that can contribute to the patient's recovery and rehabilitation.

Closely allied to the physical therapist are two other occupational groups, the *remedial gymnast*, whose specialty is rehabilitation through exercise, and the *kinesiologist*, who is a specialist in human movement and human performance. Kinesiology is offered in baccalaureate programs, usually of four years' duration, in a university setting. Remedial gymnasts are often trained by kinesiologists in a certificate or diploma program at the community college or technological institute level.

Occupational therapists have a background similar to the physical therapist's. Many individuals, in fact, hold a combined degree (or certificate) in physical and occupa-

Physiotherapist teaching a patient how to transfer from bed to chair

tional therapy. The occupational therapist, however, is primarily concerned with the restoration of bodily functions through specific tasks or skills, rather than exercises and treatments. Occupational therapists frequently play a large role in rehabilitation by helping people to develop new skills or to relearn skills lessened or lost through illness.

Respiratory technologists (therapists) are experts in diagnostic procedures and therapeutic measures used in the care of patients with respiratory problems. They are skilled in handling oxygen therapy equipment, for example. Programs in respiratory technology are usually two to three years long and are offered in community colleges or other post-secondary educational institutions.

Many *clinical laboratory technologists* (also called *medical technologists*) assist in patient care in both the institutional and the ambulatory care setting. The medical technologist is responsible for collecting many of the specimens needed for laboratory tests; he or she treats and analyzes these specimens and advises physicians and nurses on the results of these tests. The technologist is also helpful in advising nurses on the nature of tests and the specific procedure for carrying these out if the nurse is to do this task. In Canada, courses in medical laboratory technology are offered in community colleges and technological institutes, and generally last two to three years. In the United States, clinical laboratory technologists are usually required

to have a baccalaureate degree in medical technology, chemistry or a biological science.

Radiology technologists carry out diagnostic and therapeutic measures involving the use of radiant energy. The radiology technologist's preparation is usually a two- to three-year program of combined academic work and clinical experience. The programs are usually conducted by post-secondary educational institutions, such as a community college or technological institute, with hospital affiliation.

MEMBERS OF THE HEALTH TEAM PRIMARILY CONCERNED WITH EMERGENCY SERVICES

Personnel in agencies providing emergency medical services require training that ranges from basic first aid to professional-level training in emergency care. In Canada, the St. John's Ambulance Society offers a 16-hour basic first aid course, which is often a pre-entrance requirement for nursing students. An advanced-level course is also offered in some provinces. Virtually all health professionals and others working in the clinical field today are required to become certified in cardiopulmonary resuscitation (CPR). As student nurses, you will probably take the six-hour CPR training as part of your introductory nursing course, unless this was a pre-entrance requirement. The CPR course is often taught by local branches of St. John's Ambulance or the Canadian Heart Association, and is also a regular offering of in-service educational programs in most health agencies today.

In Canada, people working as first aid personnel in industry (in industrial plants, canneries, logging operations, mining operations and the like) are usually required to have an Industrial First Aid Certificate. The program leading to this certificate consists of a 50-hour course which may be given in a concentrated two-week period, or extended over a period of several weeks. A "survival first aid" course of eight hours may be given to first aid attendants in work settings where the services of an industrial first aid attendant are not warranted (for example, when there are a small number of employees or when the probability of accidents requiring additional skills is minimal).

An advanced first aid course that includes CPR training is frequently incorporated into the basic training programs for police officers and fire fighters who, by the nature of their work, are often first on the scene in an emergency situation. This training is also often required for Civil Defence workers, who volunteer to assist in case of emergencies or civil disaster in their community.

Ambulance drivers and attendants in Canada are increasingly being trained as *Emergency Medical Technicians*. Programs leading to a certificate as an EMT are offered in many community colleges in Canada. They provide training in advanced life support skills so that the EMT can do basic and advanced first aid, CPR and can start intravenous infusions.

Nurses and physicians working in emergency services also need to have specialized training to be able to react quickly and without hesitation to carry out competently the care that is required. Emergency or trauma medicine has become a recognized specialty in the medical field. For nurses, a variety of continuing education courses are now being offered to assist those working in emergency units. The courses may be given on an inservice basis in a health agency, or offered as part of a continuing education program for nurses by an educational institution or other agency.

All emergency workers need to have their skills refreshed regularly. Most agencies granting certificates require that individuals be recertified annually.

PRACTITIONERS OF ALTERNATIVE MEDICINE

Today we are seeing a blending of Western and traditional medicine. A number of practitioners of alternative medicine are being recognized by the mainstream medical community as legitimate healers. For example, the services of **naturopaths** (practitioners of natural medicine) are covered under provincial health insurance in at least one province (British Columbia). We will discuss the topic of traditional — also called *alternative* or *complementary* — medicine more fully in Chapter 12, Health and Ethnicity.

VOLUNTEERS IN HEALTH CARE

Each year, volunteers contribute thousands of hours in unpaid services in the health field. According to a study undertaken by Statistics Canada, the factors motivating people to volunteer their services are: a desire to help others; working for a cause they believe in; doing something they like to do; and feeling that they have accomplished something (Duchesne, 1989).

Hospitals have traditionally looked to the Hospital's Auxiliary groups to furnish the funds for extra equipment. Volunteers provide enormous amounts of time and money to hospitals and, indeed, to all types of health agencies. The services they provide for patients are invaluable.

Services Provided by Volunteers in a Community Agency

- visit isolated seniors
- provide transportation and assistance to appointments
- assist at agency clinics
- provide labour support to pregnant teens
- organize shopping programs
- give public presentations
- participate in community organizations such as Stroke Clubs, Adult Day Cares, Neighbourhood Houses, Community Centres and Early Childhood Centres
- participate in planning new programs and facilitate community action and health promotion programs.

SOURCE: Vancouver Health Department, 1993

Services Provided by Volunteers in Acute Care Hospitals

- pre-admitting escort service
- admitting/discharge escort service
- flower delivery
- book/library service
- shopping carts
- craft carts
- activity assistants, especially with geriatric care, in occupational therapy
- one-to-one visiting
- emergency and outpatient departments—escort services and tea and coffee for patients and those waiting with them
- gift shops
- support aide services in surgical day care and cardiac units
- baby photos in maternity units
- recreational assistance in rehabilitation hospitals and children's hospitals, such as swim and exercise programs, arts and crafts, entertainment, meetings, etc.

SOURCE: Volunteer Vancouver, 1993

Services Provided by Volunteers in Palliative Care Units

- support to patients and families
- night sitters — sitting with patients during night so patient is not alone if there is no family or to provide respite to family
- marking of special events, such as birthdays, anniversaries
- outings, such as drives, visits to home or other special events.

SOURCE: Volunteer Vancouver, 1993

Services Provided by Volunteers in Long-Term Care Agencies

- program assistant — may help with crafts, general activities (e.g. bingo, checkers, bowling), outing, (group and one-to-one), gardening, special events like parties, lunches, teas, swim programs, exercise programs
- one-to-one visiting
- meal time helper
- hair care, manicure and pedicure
- entertainment — music, singalong programs

- music therapy
- pet therapy
- church services
- shopping service
- driving van or bus
- cooking programs with residents.

SOURCE: Volunteer Vancouver, 1993

KEY TERMS

IN REVIEW

As health care reform sweeps the country, health services are being restructured to provide a continuum of care that includes health promotion and health protection programs, health restoration services for the sick and supportive care for people with long-term or terminal illness. Primary health care, the foundation for this restructuring, encompasses both a philosophy of care and the services provided at the first level of the continuum. It includes preventive and health maintenance, diagnostic and therapeutic, as well as rehabilitative services, provided mainly on an ambulatory basis, for people in their homes or in the community. The basic principles of primary health care are accessibility, public participation, emphasis on health promotion and the prevention of illness rather than on cure, intersectoral cooperation and the use of appropriate technologies. The Epp Report outlined strategies and mechanisms for implementing the concept of primary health care. The three mechanisms identified were self-care, mutual aid and the creation of healthy environments. The strategies involved fostering public participation, strengthening community health services and coordinating healthy public policy.

In Canada, most health care and support for individuals is provided in the home by family and friends. Numerous services are available through government agencies and nongovernmental organizations to assist with care in the home. These services usually include nursing care, personal and homemaker services, respite care and family relief, and may also include various other health and support services. These services are provided by both governmental and nongovernmental agencies. Voluntary agencies, for example, provide services that are supplemental to those provided by government. These agencies are usually established in response to perceived needs in the community that are not being addressed by governmental services.

Health services in the community develop to meet the specific needs of people in a geographic area and, hence, vary greatly. They include services provided by official (government) agencies, by community health centres, street clinics, mental health centres, physicians' offices and clinics, hospital ambulatory services and emergency services.

Agencies providing inpatient services are regulated and funded, for the most part, by the government. They include hospitals that provide acute care services, rehabilitation centres, long-term care and personal care facilities and hospices/palliative care units. Rehabilitation and long-term care agencies are paying increasing attention to meeting the psychosocial as well as the physical needs of residents in these facilities. A variety of independent living residences have also developed to meet the individual needs of people who do not wish to, or are unable, to maintain their own homes.

The administration of health care programs is vested in provincial and territorial governments who provide a large portion of the funding for health services. They allocate funds, set standards of care, regulate facilities, determine budgets and negotiate salaries for health care workers. They also administer social assistance programs.

Workers' Compensation Boards operate under provincial or territorial statute as quasi-governmental agencies. They are financed through levies on employers and provide health care, rehabilitation services, income replacement and survivor benefits for personal injury, disease or death arising out of and in the course of employment. Workers' Compensation Boards also participate in accident prevention programs, either by funding these activities directly or by providing funds to another agency for this purpose. Under WCB legislation in Canada, most workers are covered except for the self-employed.

The Federal Government plays a major role in health and welfare in Canada, both through national legislation and through its financial contribution to programs. It also provides advisory and consultative services for provincial and municipal health agencies and maintains a national health information service through Statistics Canada which collects and disseminates information. The Extramural Research Programs Directorate of Health Canada administers research and educational funds for health scientists. The Federal Government also provides direct health services to certain segments of the population. It sets standards for drug control and for the control of communicable diseases and other hazards that cross provincial boundaries. The private sector provides many services in the health and welfare area. Some are purchased by government and others paid for on a fee-for-service basis.

Health care workers comprise approximately eight percent of the total Canadian labour force, totalling over half a million workers. Over one half of these are nurses, with physicians the next largest group. The remainder include pharmacists, dentists and other dental workers, physiotherapists and occupational therapists, laboratory and x-ray technologists, environmental health workers, emergency services personnel and many others. Volunteers also make a major contribution to health care in Canada. In health care today, a multidisciplinary team approach is needed, as each team member contributes his or her unique knowledge and skills, and all team members use shared skills, such as communication, to achieve the common goal of attaining the highest level of health possible for each person.

LEARNING ACTIVITIES

Nettie McLeod and her sister, Jean, live together in a small house in one of the suburbs of a large Canadian city. Nettie, who is 84, is a retired teacher. Jean (81 years old) was an accountant in a small business. Since her retirement, Nettie has devoted herself to looking after her sister who has had a series of health problems and has become a semi-invalid. Nettie herself had surgery for removal of a cancerous growth five years ago. She requires monitoring as well as occasional chemotherapy which necessitates an overnight stay at the cancer clinic in the city. Nettie does the shopping and manages most of the housework, including meal preparation for herself and her sister. She still drives the car, but only around the small community where they live. The two women do not have any family living in the province although they have a wide circle of friends, mostly older women like themselves, or older couples whom they have known for a long time.

From time to time, one or other of the sisters falls ill and, occasionally, Nettie has to go to the cancer clinic for an overnight stay for her chemotherapy. Jean was hospitalized recently for a removal of a kidney stone but has recovered quite well from that episode.

1. If Nettie and Jean lived in your community, what services would be available to help them to maintain their health and to stay in their own home as long as possible?

2. If Nettie or Jean developed a minor illness, sufficient to incapacitate but not to require hospitalization, how would they obtain care to help them in the home? What services might this include? Would they have to pay for these services? If so, what is the cost?

3. Once, Jean, who had a bout of diarrhea for several days and was not eating her meals, collapsed on her way to the bathroom in the middle of the night. What services could Nettie call on to get help? Where are the nearest emergency services in your area? How large is the nearest hospital? What services does the hospital provide?

4. Jean spent a week in hospital. What types of health workers would have been involved in her care? in the emergency department? when she was on the nursing unit? If she needed home care after her discharge, who would arrange for the services?

5. When Nettie feels she can no longer cope with the house and the meal preparation, the two sisters will have to consider alternative living arrangements. What is available in your community that might suit them? What would it cost these women per month? If the cost is more than they can afford, what other options are available for them?

REFERENCES AND READINGS

ANDERSON, J.M. (1990). Home care management in chronic illness and the self-care movement: An analysis of ideologies and economic processes influencing policy decisions. *Advances in Nursing Science, 12*(2), 71–83.

ASSOCIATION OF REGISTERED NURSES OF NEWFOUNDLAND. (1990). *Primary health care: A nursing model.* St. John's, Newfoundland: Author.

BANKS, J.W. and LOFTUS, P. (1991). Street smarts. *The Canadian Nurse, 87*(7), 25–27.

BOUDREAU, T. (1972). *Report of the committee on nurse practitioners.* Ottawa: Health and Welfare Canada.

BUZZELL, M. and GIBBON, M. (1991). Personhood. *The Canadian Nurse, 87*(6), 32–33.

CANADIAN NURSES ASSOCIATION. (1968). *The leaf and the lamp.* Ottawa: Author.

CARSON, M.M. and ROSS, M.M. (1993) Changing the model of practice: Geriatric extended care in an acute care hospital. *The Canadian Nurse 89(2),* 35–38.

CICELY JANE GEORGINA FANE POPE 1862–1938. (1986, July). *Gulf Wings, 30,* 4.

CROWE, C. and HARDILL, K. (1993). Nursing research and political change: The street health report. *The Canadian Nurse, 89*(1), 21–24.

DICKINSON, H.D. and ANDRE, G. (1988). Community psychiatry: The institutional transformation of psychiatric practice. In B.S. Bolaria and H.D. Dickinson (1988). *Sociology of health care in Canada.* Toronto: Harcourt Brace Jovanovich.

DUCHESNE, D. (1989). *Giving freely: Volunteers in Canada.* Labour Analytic Report No. 4. Ottawa: Minister of Supply and Services. (Catalogue No. 71–535)

DU GAS, B.W. and BECKINGHAM, A.C. (1993). The emergence of gerontological nursing. In A.C. Beckingham and B.W. Du Gas (1993). *Promoting healthy aging: A nursing and community perspective.* St. Louis: Mosby.

EADES, J.E. (1965). *Workmen's compensation in Canada and the United States.* Vancouver: Workers' Compensation Board of British Columbia.

EPP, J. (1986). *Achieving health for all: A framework for health promotion.* Ottawa: Minister of Supply and Services. (Catalogue No. 39–102/1986E)

GOVERNMENT OF BRITISH COLUMBIA. (1991). *Closer to home: Summary of the royal commission on health care and costs.* Victoria, BC: Crown Publishing.

GOVERNMENT OF BRITISH COLUMBIA. (1992). *Healthy communities 1991 yearbook.* Victoria, BC: Office of Health Promotion, British Columbia Ministry of Health and Ministry Responsible for Seniors. (Catalogue No. QP 92835 03/92)

GOVERNMENT OF ONTARIO. (1993a). *Nurturing health: Report of the Premier's council on health, well-being, and social justice (1987–1991).* Toronto: Queen's Printer. (Catalogue No. 01–93–20M)

GOVERNMENT OF ONTARIO. (1993b). *Highlights: Partnerships in long-term care.* Toronto: Ontario Ministries of Health, Community and Social Services and Citizenship.

GRANT, K.R. (1988). The inverse care law in Canada: Differential access under universal free health insurance. In B.S. Bolaria and H.D. Dickinson. *Sociology of health care in Canada.* Toronto: Harcourt Brace Jovanovich, 118–134.

HAMILTON, K. and TREPANIER, H. (1989, Winter). Hospital care in the 21st century. *Canadian Social Trends,* 31–34.

HEALTH AND WELFARE CANADA. (1987). *The active health report: Perspectives on Canada's health promotion survey.* Ottawa: Minister of Supply and Services. (Catalogue No. H39–106/1987E)

HEALTH AND WELFARE CANADA. (1989). *Health and welfare in Canada.* Ottawa: Minister of Supply and Services. (Catalogue No. H21–102/1989E)

HEALTH AND WELFARE CANADA. (1992). *Health Personnel in Canada 1990.* Ottawa: Minister of Supply and Services. (Catalogue No. H9–1/1990)

LABONTE, R. (1987, Summer). Community health promotion studies. *Health Promotion.* 5–10; 32.

LABONTE, R. (1989). Community and professional empowerment. *The Canadian Nurse, 85*(3), 23–26; 28.

LENOBLE, E. (1993). Preadmission clinics gaining ground. *Nursing BC, 25*(4), 20–24.

MAGLACAS, A.M., ULIN, P.R. and SHEPS, C.G. (1987). *Health manpower for primary health care: The experience of the nurse practitioner.* Chapel Hill, NC: World Health Organization / University of North Carolina.

MAHLER, H. (1985). Nurses lead the way. *WHO Features, 97* (June).

MAKING PRIMARY HEALTH CARE WORK FOR CANADIANS: A CNA PRIORITY. (1992). In *CNA Today, 2*(3), 1

MANTLE, J. (1992). Nursing practice in long-term care agencies. In A. Baumgart and J. Larsen. *Canadian nursing faces the future.* St. Louis: Mosby,135–151.

MCIVER, V. (1978). Freedom to be, part two: The priory method. *The Canadian Nurse, 74*(3), 23–26.

NICHOLSON, G.W.L. (1975). *Canada's nursing sisters.* Toronto: Samuel Stevens/Hakkert.

NURSES PROVE THEMSELVES IN PRIMARY HEALTH CARE. (1994). *CNA Today, 4*(2), 1–2.

PRIMARY HEALTH CARE HAS ARRIVED! (1992). *CNA Today, 2*(3), 4–5.

REGISTERED NURSES ASSOCIATION OF BRITISH COLUMBIA (RNABC). (1990). *Health promotion: A discussion paper.* Vancouver, BC: Author.

ROBERTS, S.J. (1988). Social support and help seeking: Review of the literature. *Advances in Nursing Science, 10*(2), 1–11.

SEYMOUR, M.D. (1991). Too old to care. *The Canadian Nurse, 87*(11), 26–27.

SHESTOWSKY, B. (1992). Primary health care: Still relevant after 14 years. *CNA Today, 2*(3), 3.

ST. MICHAEL, M. (1993, September). Letter to the editor. *Nursing BC.*

SUTHERLAND, R. and FULTON, J. (1988). *Health care in Canada.* Ottawa: The Health Group.

TREPANNA, K. (1990). *A view of the horizon: Regional trends.* Ottawa: Institute for Health Care Facilities of the Future.

VICTORIAN ORDER OF NURSES. (1988). *VON Health promotion project for seniors.* Final Report, March. Ottawa: Author.

WORKER'S COMPENSATION BOARD OF BRITISH COLUMBIA. (1993). Discussion with senior officials of WCB in Richmond, BC.

WORLD HEALTH ORGANIZATION. (1978). *Alma Ata 1978: Primary health care.* Geneva: Author.

WORLD HEALTH ORGANIZATION. (1984). A discussion document on the concept and principles of health promotion. Geneva: Author.

Nursing
in Canada

CENTRAL QUESTIONS

1. How has nursing education developed in Canada?
2. How are nurses currently prepared?
3. Why has the baccalaureate been recommended as entry level for professional nursing practice?
4. What continuing education opportunities are available for nurses in Canada?
5. What categories of nursing personnel are there in Canada?
6. Where are some of the various places nurses work?
7. What is meant by the caring paradigm of nursing?
8. How does Benner's "domains of practice" explain the nurse's role?
9. What is primary nursing?
10. What are some of the new models for practice and structures for care in inpatient facilities?
11. What are some of the career options nurses have?
12. How are nurses involved in the political process?

INTRODUCTION

Changes in all phases of life, including health care, are inevitable. Beneficent changes in the field of health care will be those reflecting the knowledge and experience injected through the political action of nurses.

Mussallem, 1977

Nursing is a dynamic profession and its practice is constantly changing. Throughout our relatively short history in this part of the world, nurses have played an important role in providing needed health services for people, a role that has been continuously reshaped by the changing needs of our society. In the preceding few chapters, we have discussed some of the changes that are affecting the current practice of nursing. Among these are:

1. population changes that include more older people as well as a more ethnically diverse society

2. a revision of our thinking about health and illness

3. recognition of the need to empower people so they can participate in planning, managing and evaluating their own health care

4. a change of focus that is shifting health care from an illness orientation to one stressing health promotion and the prevention of illness

5. a trend away from institutionalized and towards community-based services

6. the integration of services to provide a continuum of care.

These changes are having a profound effect on the practice of nursing. Nurses are being challenged to assume new roles, to work in new and different health care settings and to accept increasing responsibility in the provision of comprehensive health care.

In this chapter, we will discuss nursing resources in this country. We will start with a discussion of the development of nursing education in Canada from Confederation to the present. Next, we'll explain a little about the educational programs currently preparing nurses for practice. We will then look at the structure of the nursing workforce, the various categories of nursing personnel, their relative numbers and educational levels and also at the settings in which nurses practice. Then we will explore the domains of practice and the care paradigm that is becoming widely accepted as a basis for nursing practice. We will also look at modes of practice and at nursing's changing role in the current country-wide restructuring of care in hospitals and in the community. Finally, we will discuss the relationship between nursing and the political process.

NURSING EDUCATION IN CANADA

In Canada today, the education of the registered nurse takes place in three different types of educational program: in three-year diploma programs in a hospital school, in two- to three-year diploma programs in a community college or technological institute and in four-year baccalaureate programs in colleges and universities that grant a baccalaureate degree in nursing. In 1993 there were a total of 132 diploma programs: 16 in hospital schools of nursing, 116 in colleges or technological institutes and 21 generic baccalaureate programs in universities in Canada. There was also one generic master's program, at McGill University, for people holding a baccalaureate degree in another field (CNA, 1993).

Rapid change is occurring not only in health care in Canada today, but also in the education of nurses. Individuals familiar with the process of change maintain that it takes almost a full century to bring about a major revision in an educational system, and they cite as an example the incorporation of kindergarten into the public school system — which is still not an accomplished fact in all provinces (Du Gas, 1991). In nursing education, the change from hospital-based, service-oriented schools to programs integrated into the general educational system of the country has also taken 100 years — from the first insights into the need for change to the ultimate full-scale adoption of the change.

HISTORICAL PERSPECTIVE
THE HOSPITAL SCHOOLS

At the time of Confederation (1867) in Canada, care of the sick was mainly carried out in the home as the responsibility of the women in the family. Hospitals were basically charitable institutions operated by religious groups or other organizations for care of the poor, the homeless or those who, for one reason or another, could not be looked after at home. With the exception of the religious orders, nursing in Canada, as in other parts of the world at the time, did not attract a very high calibre of candidate. Most of the nurses in secular hospitals were poorly educated country girls who, in many instances, had never seen a hospital before. It was said of their situation that "the pay was a mere pittance, the work so repulsive and hopeless that there was little to attract a different class" (VON, 1983, 9).

The nursing sisterhoods of the Roman Catholic and other churches had an apprenticeship system for training new recruits but it is Florence Nightingale to whom we must give credit for ushering in a training system that permitted the eventual development of professional nursing education (Canadian Nurses Association, 1968). She raised the standards for women entering nursing and insisted on satisfactory evidence of good moral character. The elements of a basic educational program were prerequisites for admission to the Nightingale School of Nursing at St. Thomas' Hospital in London, England.

The first school of nursing in Canada based on the Nightingale model was the Mack Training School at the General and Marine Hospital in St. Catharines, Ontario in 1874. Schools of nursing followed in other cities across the country in rapid succession (Gibbon and Mathewson, 1947; CNA, 1968). There was no lack of candidates for the schools. Young women from good families considered it a privilege to be selected for the opportunity to enter their chosen vocation and cheerfully endured the rigorous, militaristic training imposed by their teachers. The students were well groomed, neatly uniformed, trained to be obedient and were well supervised. Nursing service was considerably improved by their presence. The graduates were proud of their "trained" status and, in the 1890s and early 1900s, the matter of "professionalism" was a serious issue concerning nurses. With the advent of the training schools, nursing entered a new phase as graduate nurses became part of the medical missionary movement taking their skills to the still sparsely populated settled areas of the country. In one highly publicized endeavour, four VON nurses travelled to the Klondike in 1898 to provide health services for the people flocking there for the Gold Rush (VON,

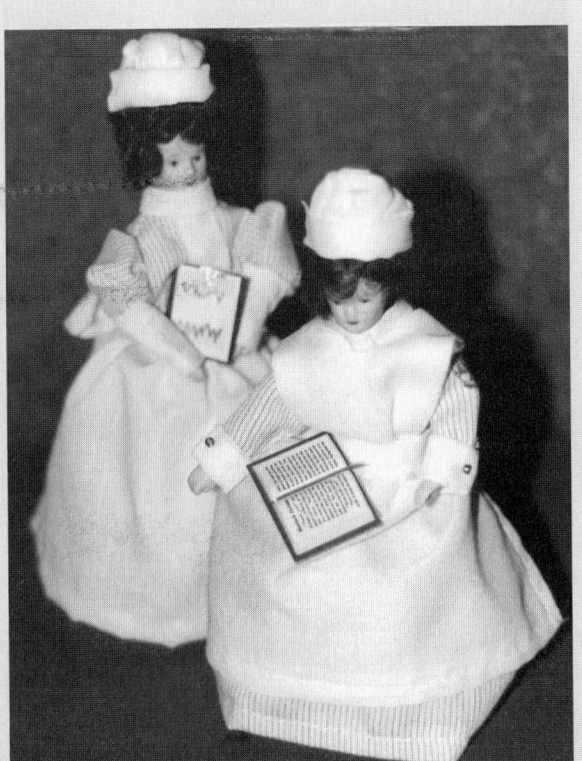

The student nurses' uniforms of the Winnipeg General Hospital, 1895 and 1897, as worn by Ethel Johns

1947). By the turn of the century, the nurse had an established role in Canadian society as an essential person in the care of the sick in hospitals and at home (VON, 1983).

DISSATISFACTION WITH THE SYSTEM

Regrettably, the Nightingale model for a school of nursing did not survive its cross-Atlantic voyage intact. Administrators of the rapidly proliferating hospitals in North America were quick to see the financial advantages of having a ready source of cheap labour in the nursing students. The schools, instead of being autonomous, as the Nightingale school had been, became an integral part of the hospital establishment (Mussallem, 1960). Dissatisfaction with the improperly imported system of nursing training started early. It was first vocalized in 1893 when nursing leaders in Canada and the United States came together in a historic meeting in Chicago to share their concerns. The result of this meeting was the formation of the American Society of Lady Superintendents of Training Schools. Its purpose was to promote the exchange of ideas and the establishment of high educational standards. Its main undertaking was to work for higher standards of nurse preparation. The Society later divided to become, in Canada, the Canadian Society of Superintendents of Training Schools for Nurses. In 1908, this became the Provisional Society of the Canadian Association of Trained Nurses — the forerunner of the Canadian Nurses Association. The first president of the Society, Miss Agnes Snively, took the Association into the International Council of Nurses in 1909 (CNA, 1968).

The desire to differentiate between trained and untrained nurses led to the development of provincial nursing acts regulating the preparation for and practice of nursing. Voluntary registration began in 1910 in Nova Scotia, followed by other provinces within the next few years (Gibbon and Mathewson, 1947). Detailed standard curricula for schools of nursing were established in different provinces and committees were set up by Graduate Nurses Associations (forerunners of present-day provincial Registered Nurses Associations) in attempts to improve training programs for nurses. Prominent nurses spoke out against the exploitation of nursing students. Ethel Johns, for example, when reporting on the findings of a Committee on Standardization of Training Schools at a national meeting in 1917 stated, "Anyone may start [a training school]. All that is necessary is to gather some sick people under a roof and call it a hospital. . . . There are no standards at all. . . . You just start a training school, and Providence and the patients do the rest" (Johns, 1917. Cited in Street, 1973, 90). Many of the small schools which had proliferated during and after the First World War were closed during the 1920s and 1930s in response to the lobbying efforts of the nurses.

MARY AGNES SNIVELY 1847–1933

Mary Agnes Snively was responsible for organizing nurses in Canada and making them a part of the international body of nurses. A teacher before she entered nursing, the Ontario-born woman graduated from New York's Bellevue Hospital School of Nursing in 1884 at age 37. She then accepted the position of Lady Superintendent of the Toronto General Hospital, where she remained until her retirement at age 63. One of her first priorities as superintendent was to improve the three-year-old nurses' training program; within 10 years the Toronto School's reputation was so high that there were 600 applicants for the 22 places in the program. To respond to the demand, the hospital became the largest in Canada and maintained a remarkable reputation for quality nursing care.

Through her friendships and professional networks with nurses in the United States, Mary Agnes Snively was a founding member of the American Society of Superintendents of Training Schools for Nurses (a joint Canadian–American group) and was a member of its first Board. She also was interested in a British proposal for an international organization. In 1899, she represented Canada as one of the leaders from countries still without national associations at the founding meeting of the International Council of Nurses (ICN) and was named its first honorary treasurer. After five years in that position, she became the Council's vice-president.

At home in Toronto, she had already formed an alumni association and worked to form a Graduate Nurses' Association of Ontario from the various alumni groups in the province. Through this organization, Mary Agnes Snively and others persuaded the provincial government to secure registration for nurses. She forged ahead with the idea of a national organization and, in 1908, was instrumental in bringing together representatives from 16 alumni associations from all parts of Canada to form the Canadian National Association of Trained Nurses (CNATN), which later changed its name to the Canadian Nurses Association (CNA). Mary Agnes Snively was elected its first president, from 1908–1912, shepherded it into full membership in ICN and established a sound professional infrastructure for Canadian nursing.

Glennis Zilm

THE WEIR REPORT

The problem of nursing education was of concern to nurses all across Canada. In 1927, the CNA struck a joint committee with the Canadian Medical Association to look into the problem of "the nurse in her relationship to the hospital, the medical profession and the public at large" (Cameron in Weir, 1932, 5). This committee appointed Dr. George Weir, head of the Department of Education at the University of British Columbia, to conduct a survey of nursing education in Canada. In his report, published in 1932, Dr. Weir recommended that nursing education be integrated into the general education system. Thus, some 40 years after the need for change in the education of nurses was voiced in Chicago, the direction of the needed change was determined (Weir, 1932). Sixteen years were to pass before an acceptable way was found to implement the recommendations of the Weir Report. Again, the Canadian Nurses Association took the lead and, with financing from the Red Cross, established a demonstration school of nursing in Windsor, Ontario. The Metropolitan School of Nursing (1948–1952), as it was

called, pioneered the independent school of nursing in Canada. The school was separated financially and physically from the hospital and the clinical practice of the students in hospitals and other institutions was under the direction of school authorities (CNA, 1968).

In the United States, a different solution was tried as Mildred Montag, in 1952, launched a two-year junior college program on an experimental basis (Donahue, 1985). This program set the pattern that came to be adopted throughout North America. Nursing education had finally found a niche in the educational system. The development of community colleges and the subsequent incorporation of nursing education into them took place a little later in Canada. Meanwhile, Dr. Helen Mussallem (1965) was asked to undertake a study of nursing education for the Royal Commission on Health Services. The Report of the Commission reinforced Weir's recommendation to transfer nursing education to post-secondary institutions (Hall, 1964). The first nursing education program in a post-secondary institution in Canada was established at the Ryerson Institute of Technology in 1963 but widespread acceptance of the idea had to wait for the development of the community college system in various provinces. Saskatchewan, in 1967, was the first province to transfer authority for schools of nursing from hospitals to the Department of Education (CNA, 1968). Quebec began the process in 1967 and by 1972 all hospital schools were closed and nursing education programs were offered in the community colleges (CEGEPS). Ontario transferred all diploma nursing education programs to the Colleges of Applied Arts and Technology in 1973. Community college programs developed rapidly in most other provinces during the 1970s and 1980s. In 1993 only four provinces still listed hospital diploma programs — Alberta had three; Manitoba, four; Nova Scotia, five; and Newfoundland, four (CNA, 1993).

DEVELOPMENT OF UNIVERSITY PROGRAMS FOR NURSES

Nursing education . . . cannot remain permanently apart from the stream of invigorating life and inspiration which the university can best supply. Sooner or later, the university, in affiliation with the well-equipped hospital, must face the problem of educating the nurse. Evolutionary trends all point in this direction.
Weir, 1932

When the Victorian Order of Nurses was founded in 1897, it was recognized that the nurses would need additional preparation to work effectively in the community. There were no programs providing this education in Canada at the time, so the VON set up their own programs in various cities across the country (VON, 1983).

Subsequently, the vision of a broader role for nurses, not only doing home nursing but also carrying out health promotion and disease prevention in the community, led to the establishment of a program for the preparation of public health nurses at the University of British Columbia. By 1919, the Department of Nursing and Public Health was established at UBC with Ethel Johns holding dual responsibilities as the head of the program and Lady Superintendent of the Vancouver General Hospital. The first class graduated from this program in 1920. The Bachelor of Applied Science in Nursing program was added as demand grew. The first three nurses graduated from this program in 1923 (Green, 1984). The program included two years on campus in university studies, followed by 24 (later 28, then 32) months at the Vancouver General Hospital. The final year of the six-year program was spent on campus where the students had the option of taking either public health nursing or teaching and supervision. Graduates of diploma schools of nursing could also enrol in the public health nursing or teaching and supervision courses, where they received a diploma in their respective field on successful completion of the one-year program. Similar "sand-

wich" type programs developed in other universities across the country (Gibbon and Mathewson, 1947).

Gradually, however, the university schools of nursing began to want more control over their students, instead of handing them over to the hospital for the entire clinical portion of the program. The Integrated Basic Degree Program was pioneered by E. Kathleen Russell in 1942 at the University of Toronto. This program gave students a broad foundation in the humanities and sciences as well as in nursing (Bajnok, 1992). During the 1950s and 1960s other universities began to follow suit. The Report of the Royal Commission on Health Services (1964), reflecting findings from the studies of nursing education by both Mussallem (1960; 1965) and Weir (1932), accelerated the movement by recommending expansion of university programs and criticized the "sandwich" program of studies. The integrated five-year (later reduced to four years) basic baccalaureate programs came to be the norm. In 1993, there were 21 basic degree and 28 post-basic baccalaureate degree programs in Canadian universities (CNA, 1993; Bajnok, 1992; Gibbon and Mathewson, 1947).

THE BACCALAUREATE AS ENTRY TO PRACTICE

Concerned about the increasing responsibilities that nurses were expected to assume in response to the changing demands of health care, the Canadian Nurses Association in 1982 recommended the baccalaureate as entry level for professional practice. Since then there has been a tremendous amount of activity in all provinces as nurses at all levels debated the issue and explored ways and means of accomplishing the target date of 2000 advocated by CNA.

The result has been a rapid increase in the number of baccalaureate programs in Canada. Some are new programs at universities but many are collaborative programs which combine diploma and baccalaureate programs. Some of the collaborative programs provide the option of diploma-level exit; some do not. Students exiting at the diploma level may write the examinations for registration as a nurse and enter the workforce at that point, with the option to complete their baccalaureate studies at a later date. At the time of publishing, the goal of the baccalaureate as entry level for professional nursing practice appears to be well underway in all parts of the country.*

Prince Edward Island has the distinction of having been the first province to move to baccalaureate preparation for all new graduates with the opening of a four-year baccalaureate program at the University of Prince Edward

---

* Information on the current situation with regard to the movement to baccalaureate education for nurses in this section is based on material from the CNA publication, *Entrance Requirements for Nursing Education Programs in Canada* (1993); from 1991, 1992 and 1993 issues of *Edufacts: The news in nursing education*, a CNA periodical reporting on news in nursing education; and from discussions with staff at CNA.

Island in 1992. The first collaborative program in Canada was established by the University of British Columbia and the Vancouver General Hospital Schools of Nursing in 1989. Now, all diploma nursing programs in British Columbia are involved in collaborative programs with a university. The majority of programs will offer both a diploma and a baccalaureate degree. The two exceptions in British Columbia are the VGH/UBC (Vancouver General Hospital/University of British Columbia) program and one at Trinity Western University in British Columbia which initiated a four-year baccalaureate program in nursing in September 1993. The RNABC has issued a policy statement to the effect that the diploma exit is to be phased out as soon as possible (RNABC, 1994).

In Alberta, the University of Alberta has collaborative programs with five diploma programs and the University of Calgary has collaborative programs with three. The collaborative programs in this province provide diploma level exit at the end of two years at the University of Alberta and at the end of three at the University of Calgary.

In Saskatchewan, a collaborative model has been developed for a four-year baccalaureate program that provides for a diploma exit after three years of study. It will be offered collaboratively by the University of Saskatchewan and the two nursing programs at the Saskatchewan Institute of Applied Sciences and Technology.

In Manitoba, the Health Sciences Centre and St. Boniface Hospital have entered into collaborative arrangements with the University of Manitoba School of Nursing so that all students will graduate with a baccalaureate in nursing from the university. The University of Manitoba also offers a Northern Bachelor of Nursing Program in le Pas at Keewatin College. Collaborative projects for the remainder of Manitoba's diploma nursing programs are being discussed with various universities.

In Ontario, a consortium has been formed to develop a province-wide approach to the restructuring of nursing education programs. Meanwhile, Laurentian University and the University of Western Ontario are collaborating with Cambrian and Fanshawe Colleges and Queen's University is collaborating with Saint Lawrence College, Loyalist College and Sir Sandford Fleming. The University of Ottawa, Algonquin College and La Cité Collegiale plan the implementation of a joint program in September 1995.

In Quebec, during the Quiet Revolution of the 1960s and 1970s, colleges and universities were restructured to form an educational continuum, with university programs building on those of the colleges. Students graduating from CEGEP diploma programs in nursing have access to degree programs at the Universities of McGill, Montreal, Sherbrooke, Laval and five campuses of the Université de Québec. The Order of Nurses of Quebec (a professional association of nurses) recognizes the need for baccalaureate preparation for all nurses in order to meet evolving health needs, and is supporting the development of basic nursing programs at universities which do not already have one.

The University of Quebec at Hull opened a basic program in 1994, one at the University of Quebec at Trois-Rivières admits its first class in the fall of 1995. Sherbrooke, Rimouski, Chicoutimi and Abiti-Temiscamingue are also potential sites for basic programs.

In New Brunswick, the Premier has given his support to baccalaureate education for nurses. Seven schools are working together to develop a curriculum. It is anticipated that there will be both an English multi-site program by the University of New Brunswick and a French multi-site program by L'Université de Moncton, possibly by September 1995.

In Nova Scotia, a new collaborative baccalaureate program will go into effect in September 1995 between Dalhousie University, the Victoria General Hospital and Camp Hill Medical Centre. The schools of nursing at St. Francis Xavier University and St. Martha's Regional Hospital are also planning a joint program.

In Newfoundland, with government support, a project is currently in progress to develop a single, province-wide nursing program that all schools would be able to deliver. Under this proposed program, students would be able to graduate with either a diploma or a baccalaureate degree in nursing.

NURSING PROGRAMS FOR PEOPLE OF THE FIRST NATIONS

"There are now more than 260 000 nurses in Canada, but only about 300 are of aboriginal ancestry" (Canada needs more. . .,1992). During the past decade, a number of programs have developed to help people of the First Nations to access nursing education. A new diploma program opened in September 1994 at Arctic College in the Northwest Territories to bring the programs closer to home for people of the Territories. Upgrading courses to prepare students for the first year of the course were started in September 1993. The program lasts two years, followed by a one-semester practicum. Students who wish to take further studies may do so at one of the southern universities. The University of Manitoba's Northern Bachelor of Nursing Program for Registered Nurses at Keewatin College was established in 1990. The program's goal is to provide aboriginal and northern nurses with the opportunity to gain advanced clinical and communication skills in order to meet the health care needs of isolated communities. In order to get more people of the First Nations involved in the health field, a National Nurses Access program was also developed. This program lasts nine weeks and is intended to orient First Nations students to nursing and to the intensity of a university progam. On successful completion of the program, access to a diploma or degree program of the student's choice is negotiated. Access programs are offered at the University of Saskatchewan, at Lakehead University in Northern Ontario, at both the le Pas and Thompson campuses of Keewatin College and at Red River Community College in Winnipeg. Other programs that provide special support for First Nations students include John Abbott College in St. Anne-de-Bellevue, Quebec, and the Indian Diploma Nursing Progam at the Saskatchewan Institute of Technology in North Battleford (CNA, 1993; Canada needs more. . ., 1992).

CONTINUING EDUCATION

"The Canadian Nurses Association considers continuing nursing education as vital to nurses in the maintenance of professional competence throughout their professional careers" (CNA, 1992). Continuing education includes self-study — the professional reading of journals, new texts and other literature and the gaining of new and varied clinical experiences — as well as the inservice educational programs run by agencies for their staff, short continuing education programs sponsored by various agencies, professional associations and educational institutions, and formal educational programs offered by educational institutions. These formal programs are often referred to as "post-basic education," particularly when they lead to a certificate, diploma or degree.

Early in the development of nursing education in this country, nurses recognized that *post-basic education* was necessary to practise in specialized fields. The earliest post-basic programs that developed were in community health nursing and in teaching and administration. But, hospitals also felt the need for nurses to have additional knowledge and skills in areas such as obstetric and neurosurgical nursing and the operating room. Most of the larger hospitals across the country developed post-basic courses in clinical nursing specialties. Graduates of the programs received a certificate attesting to their competence in a particular field. These *hospital postgraduate courses* unfortunately had the same flaw as the early hospital diploma programs and were accused of exploiting students. Although there were some very good programs, in many of them the postgraduate students were used simply as extra staff and given little in the way of education. When the diploma nursing programs moved into community colleges and other post-secondary educational institutions, the postgraduate programs were also transferred there, a move which has provided them with a more sound educational base.

A relatively recent movement has seen the predominantly college-based programs being accorded university transfer credit, and, in some instances, as at the University of Ottawa, incorporated into basic and post-basic baccalaureate programs (Du Gas and Casey, 1989). Another interesting program is a collaborative one between the B.C. Institute of Technology and the Open Learning Agency of British Columbia which permits nurses holding advanced diplomas in various clinical specialties to complete requirements for a baccalaureate degree in health sciences, with full transfer of credits (the equivalent of one year) for the post-basic program. A recent development has been the transfer of the Introduction to Nursing Management Distance Education Program, jointly operated by CNA and the Canadian Hospital Association, to McMaster University in the fall of 1993 (Collaborative project. . ., 1993).

An increased demand by nurses across the country for access to post-basic baccalaureate programs has led to the expansion of these programs by university nursing schools and to new and innovative ways of delivering courses. Currently, post-basic baccalaureate programs are offered at 28 universities, and many offer courses by distance education (CNA, 1993). The CNA regularly publishes a list of continuing education offerings for nurses at schools across the country (CNA, 1992). In addition, information is available from provincial nursing associations. Some, like the Registered Nurses Association of Ontario, produce an annual publication listing offerings by various schools, the association and/or other agencies in the province.

GRADUATE EDUCATION FOR NURSES IN CANADA

Master's Level Programs

In 1993, programs leading to a master's degree in nursing, or in nursing science, were offered at 13 universities in Canada. The programs are two years in length if taken on a full-time basis; provision is also made for those who wish to study on a part-time basis. Prior to 1965, the emphasis in master's level nursing programs in Canada was on teaching and administration — mainly in the hospital field. Since the early 1970s, the focus has changed to provide students with the opportunity to gain increased knowledge and skills in clinical specialties.

The number of applicants for master's level programs far exceeds the number of places available (see Figure 5.1), with the result that many nurses pursue graduate studies in other disciplines. As shown in Figure 5.2, approximately one half of the master's-prepared nurses in Canada hold master's degrees in disciplines other than nursing (Do we have enough. . ., 1993).

Doctoral Programs in Nursing

Doctoral programs in nursing were slow to develop in Canada. Nurses wishing to pursue studies at the doctoral level have until recently enrolled either in doctoral programs in the United States, which has more than 30 doctoral programs in nursing, or in doctoral programs in other disciplines, such as education, the social sciences and epidemiology or medical science. The first person to complete requirements for a PhD in Nursing at a Canadian university graduated from a conjoint program offered by McGill

Number of students

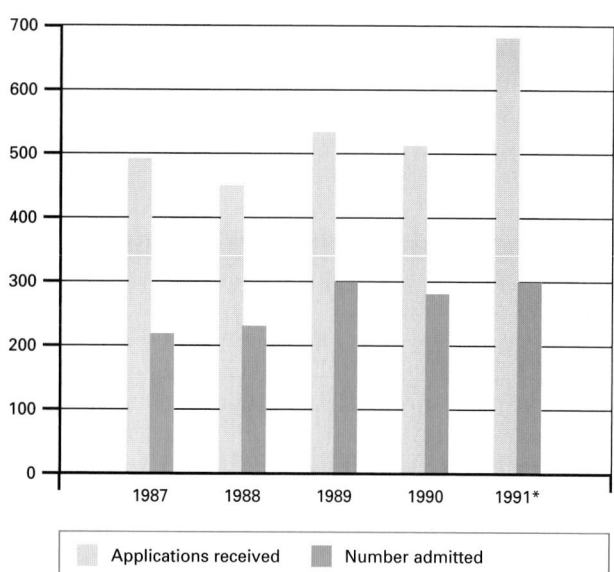

FIGURE 5.1 Applications received and number admitted into master of nursing programs from 1987–1991

* Quebec did not collect employment data in 1991; therefore Quebec is excluded from this total.

SOURCE: Research Department CNA. (1992, October). Cited in *Edufacts: The news in nursing education, 2*(4), 2.

Number of nurses

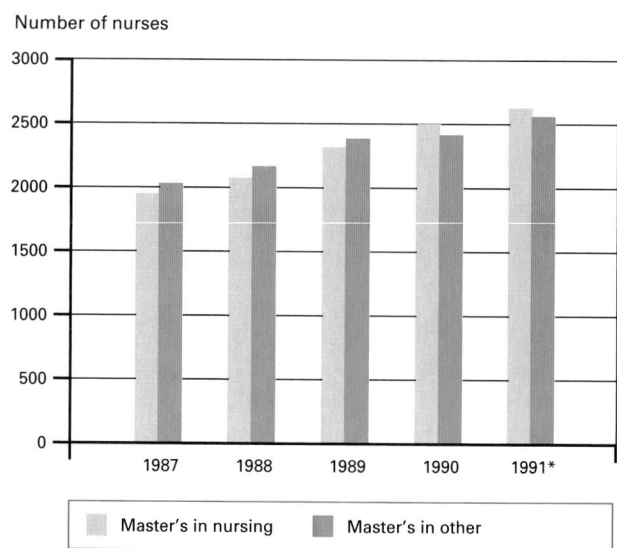

FIGURE 5.2 Registered Nurses employed in nursing holding a master's degree from 1987–1991

* Quebec did not collect employment data in 1991; therefore Quebec is excluded from this total.

SOURCE: Research Department, CNA. (1992, October). Cited in *Edufacts: The news in nursing education, 2* (4), 2.

University and the Université de Montréal in 1990 (Field, Stinson and Thibaudeau, 1992). In 1993, there were four programs offering a research degree with a focus on nursing at the doctoral level — Université de Montréal with McGill University, University of Alberta, University of British Columbia (approved in 1992) and University of Toronto (opened in 1993). The program of studies which includes formal course work and a major research study usually requires three to five years for completion (The PhD comes. . ., 1991; New PhD and master's. . ., 1993; Field, Stinson and Thibaudeau, 1988).

NURSING RESOURCES IN CANADA

Nurses constitute the largest single group of workers in the health field in Canada. Of the approximately three quarters of a million people employed in medicine and health occupations, over 60 percent are in nursing occupations (Statistics Canada, 1993). There were an estimated 263 683 nurses registered in Canada in 1992, of whom 234 128 were employed in nursing. These figures, representing professional nurses alone, constitute almost one third the total number of persons employed in health care. Registered Psychiatric Nurses, Licensed Practical Nurses/Registered Nursing Assistants, Certified Nursing Assistants and nursing aides, orderlies, and other attendants account for the

remaining numbers of nursing personnel. Nursing is still predominantly a women's profession in most countries of the world. And although the number of men in nursing has been increasing in Canada in recent years, men still account for less than four percent of the total number of registered nurses in the country, up from one percent in 1966 (Glasgow, 1992). Figure 5.3 illustrates the pyramid of persons employed in nursing occupations in Canada, arranged by level of preparatory educational program.

THE REGISTERED NURSING COMPONENT OF THE PYRAMID

The largest component of the nursing pyramid is made up of registered nurses. In 1964, the Royal Commission on Health Services reported that there was a severe shortage of skilled health personnel needed to implement the proposed national health care plan. Subsequently, educational programs for health professionals were expanded with the assistance of federal grants from the Health Resources Fund. Since then, the number of nurses in Canada has risen sharply, from 115 000 in 1966 to more than double that figure in 1992. The rate of growth of the nursing profession has been faster than the rate of growth of the population so that the proportion of nurses to population has increased. Indeed, Canada is in a very favourable position with regard to nursing resources vis-à-vis most other countries in the world. Our ratio of nursing personnel to population gives us one registered nurse for approximately 120 people (Statistics Canada, 1992 and 1993; Glasgow 1992).

The proportion of nurses holding baccalaureate or higher university degrees in nursing has also increased steadily, particularly in the past decade, from only five percent in 1966 to 10.1 percent in 1981 with a more rapid gain during the 1980s to 15.9 percent in 1992 (see Figure 5.4).

The number of nurses with master's level preparation is still relatively small, at a little over one percent of the total RN population. The numbers have, however, shown a steady increase in the past few years, growing from 1960 in 1987 to 2694 in 1991.

The first Canadian nurse to earn a doctoral degree was Sister Denise Lefebvre who received a Docteur de Pédagogie from the Université de Montréal in 1955. Since then, the number of nurses in Canada holding earned doctoral degrees has grown, albeit slowly. In 1989, according to the most recent survey (Stinson, MacPhail and Larsen, 1992) there were 257 nurses with doctoral degrees in Canada and 265 more nurses enrolled in doctoral programs (51 percent in Canadian universities).

FIGURE 5.4 Percentage of RNs with degrees in Canada, 1981-1991

* Quebec did not collect employment data in 1991; therefore Quebec is excluded from this total.

SOURCE: CNA Research Department as shown in *Edufacts: The news in nursing education*, 3(3), 2; Statistics Canada. (1993). *Registered Nurses 1992*. Ottawa: Author. (Catalogue No. 83–243)

REGISTERED PSYCHIATRIC NURSES

Registered Psychiatric Nurses are prepared in two-year community college programs in the four western provinces

FIGURE 5.3 Nursing resources in Canada, 1992

SOURCES: (1) Statistics Canada (1992). Nursing in Canada 1991 Registered Nurses. *Health Reports*. (Supplement No. 22). Ottawa: Canadian Centre for Health Information. (2) Statistics Canada (1993). Population 15 years and over by sex, work activity and detailed occupation. *The Nation*. Ottawa: Author. (Catalogue No. 93–332) (3) Health and Welfare Canada (1992). *Health personnel in Canada 1990*. Ottawa: Minister of Supply and Services Canada.

(British Columbia, Alberta, Saskatchewan and Manitoba). At Douglas College in British Columbia, graduates of the two-year RPN program also have the option of taking a third year of studies that leads to an Advanced Diploma in Psychiatric Nursing. They are then eligible to complete requirements for a Bachelor of Health Sciences degree (in Psychiatric Nursing) from the Open Learning Agency of British Columbia. A Bachelor of Science Mental Health Program is also available for graduates of RPN programs at Brandon University in Manitoba (Registered Psychiatric Nurses Association of British Columbia, 1993).

LICENSED PRACTICAL NURSES/REGISTERED NURSING ASSISTANTS/CERTIFIED NURSING ASSISTANTS

The total number of Licensed Practical Nurses/Registered Nursing Assistants/Certified Nursing Assistants employed in Canada in 1990 was 82 281 (Health and Welfare Canada, 1992). LPNs/RNAs/CNAs are prepared, for the most part, in one-year educational programs in a community college or in a vocational school. Many nursing schools provide access for graduates of these programs to enter registered nursing programs without loss of credit. LPN/RNAs/CNAs perform standardized nursing procedures and treatments, working under the direction of a registered nurse. The specific procedures which they may perform are detailed in provincial *Standards of Nursing Practice* established by provincial nursing associations.

ORDERLIES

According to Statistics Canada (1993) there were approximately 3500 *orderlies* employed in Canada in 1990, down from almost 5000 in 1985. Orderlies are nursing attendants who assist with the care of patients in hospitals, extended-care facilities, nursing homes and similar establishments. Although previously trained for the most part in on-the-job programs, an increasing number now graduate from formal training programs. In many health agencies, orderlies have been replaced by LPN/RNAs. The majority of orderlies listed in Statistics Canada census reports are employed in the Province of Quebec (Statistics Canada, 1993).

NURSE'S AIDES

The number of other nursing attendants has increased considerably in the past five years — from 77 000 in 1985 to more than 92 000 in 1990 (Statistics Canada, 1993). One reason for the rapid increase has been the expansion of home care as an insured service in various provinces (See Chapters 3 and 4). Designated by a variety of names, such as *nurse's aide*, *nursing attendant*, *personal care attendant* or *health care aide*, workers in this category are frequently trained on the job or in a formal course of a few weeks' duration. The nature of the tasks assigned to the nurse's aide varies considerably from one agency to another. In some agencies, nurse's aides perform tasks that are essentially

housekeeping in nature, while in others they assist with the care of patients.

SETTINGS FOR PRACTICE

At the present time, the overwhelming majority of professional nurses in Canada (64.2 percent) are employed in general and psychiatric hospitals. Another large number (10.8 percent) are employed in nursing homes and in rehabilitation centres that provide residential care for people. Relatively few (approximately 7.4 percent) work in nursing stations, in home care or in community health agencies. The expansion of community health services in every province has meant that more and more nurses are working outside of hospitals (see Figure 5.5) — in home care, in community health centres, clinics and other types of health services. Many nurses (approximately one percent of the total of employed nurses in the country) are employed in business and industry. Six thousand nurses (2.6 percent of employed RNs) are employed in educational institutions and an almost equal number in physicians' offices. A growing number of nurses are employed by private, for-profit and nonprofit entrepreneurial agencies that furnish home care and hospital replacement services, and still others are self-employed (Statistics Canada, 1993).

Most of the nurses with baccalaureate or higher degrees work in hospitals, but many are employed in community

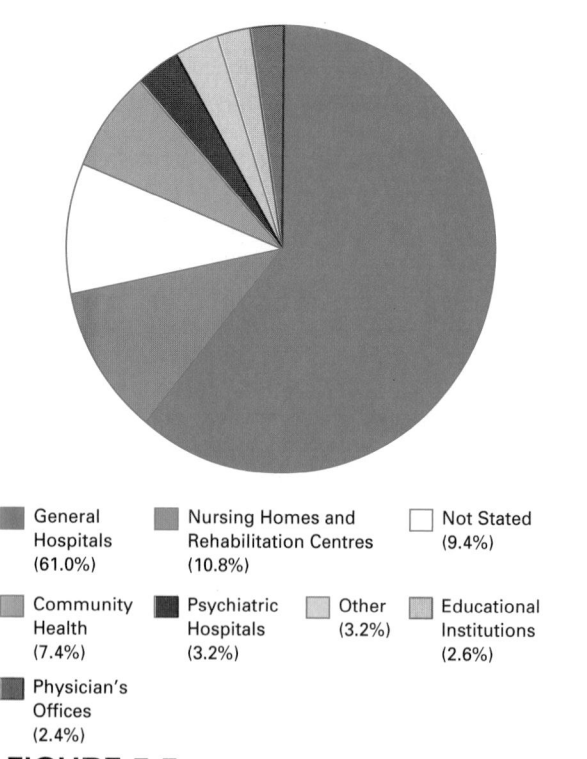

■ General Hospitals (61.0%) ■ Nursing Homes and Rehabilitation Centres (10.8%) ☐ Not Stated (9.4%)
■ Community Health (7.4%) ■ Psychiatric Hospitals (3.2%) ☐ Other (3.2%) ■ Educational Institutions (2.6%)
■ Physician's Offices (2.4%)

FIGURE 5.5 Settings for Practice: Registered Nurses in Canada, 1993

SOURCE: Statistics Canada. (1993, November). Health personnel in Canada. *Registered Nurses 1992*. Ottawa: Author. (Catalogue No. 83–243)

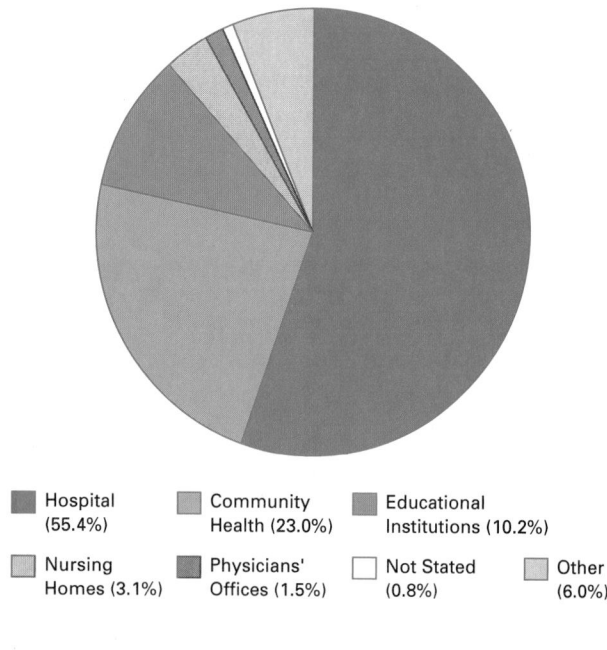

■ Hospital (55.4%) ■ Community Health (23.0%) ■ Educational Institutions (10.2%)
■ Nursing Homes (3.1%) ■ Physicians' Offices (1.5%) ☐ Not Stated (0.8%) ■ Other (6.0%)

FIGURE 5.6 Degree RNs (Bacc, Master's/higher by place of employment), 1991*

* Quebec did not collect employment data in 1991; therefore Quebec is excluded from this total.

SOURCE: Registered Nurses Management Data, Canadian Centre for Health Information, Statistics Canada. Cited in *Edufacts: The news in nursing education 3*(3), 2.

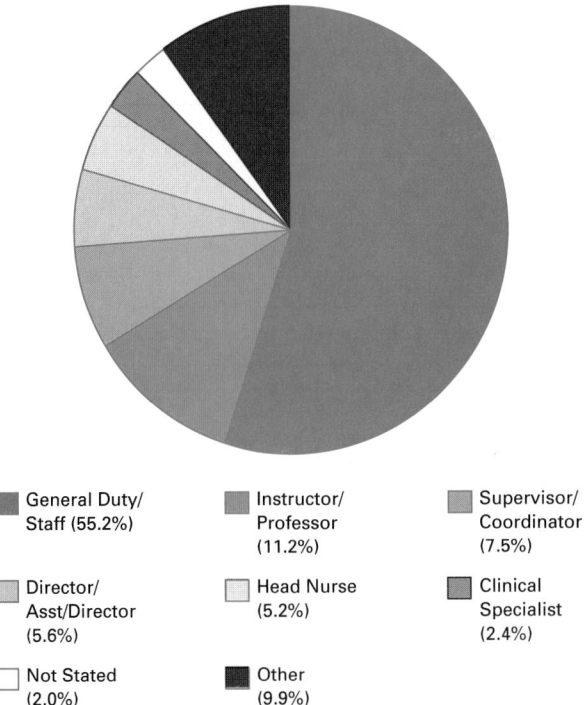

General Duty/ Staff (55.2%)

Instructor/ Professor (11.2%)

Supervisor/ Coordinator (7.5%)

Director/ Asst/Director (5.6%)

Head Nurse (5.2%)

Clinical Specialist (2.4%)

Not Stated (2.0%)

Other (9.9%)

FIGURE 5.7 Degree RNs (Bacc, Master's/higher) by position, 1991*

* Quebec did not collect employment data in 1991; therefore Quebec is excluded from this total.

SOURCE: Registered Nurses Management Data, Canadian Centre for Health Information, Statistics Canada. Cited in *Edufacts: The news in nursing education, 3*(3), 2.

health. The majority are involved in direct patient care as either general duty/staff nurses or as clinical specialists, although many are employed in administrative positions — as nurse managers, supervisors/coordinators or directors/assistants. See Figures 5.6 and 5.7.

NURSING'S ROLE IN HEALTH CARE

The International Council of Nurses has stated that "the fundamental responsibility of the nurse is fourfold: to promote health, to prevent illness, to restore health, and to alleviate suffering" (ICN, 1975).

In carrying out their responsibilities, nurses assist individuals, families and communities in the promotion of health and the prevention of illness; they minister to the needs of the sick, helping them to the fullest restoration of health compatible with their illness, or providing comfort and support in the event of incurable disease. In so doing, nurses work in close collaboration with patients and their families, with the members of other health disciplines and, increasingly, with people in sectors of the community other than health.

THE CARE PARADIGM

From its earliest beginnings, nursing has had a nurturing quality — the word *nurse* is in fact derived from the Greek word meaning *nurture* — and it is this quality that is dominating nursing literature at the present time. The caring, promoting growth and providing support implied by *nurturing* are referred to in the profession as the "care paradigm." This paradigm has been explored by numerous nurse theorists in the past decade. Theories that have emerged from these explorations include:

1. Dr. Madeline Leininger's Culture Care Theory of Nursing
2. Dr. Dorothea Orem's Self-Care Deficit Theory of Nursing
3. Dr. Jean Watson's Theory of Human Care
4. Sister (Dr.) M. Simone Roach's Theoretical Philosophy on the Nature of Human Caring.

Dr. Madeline Leininger was the first of the human care theorists in nursing. In studying different cultures, Dr. Leininger found that caring is a universal phenomenon, although the nurturant activities of people in different cultures vary considerably. Canadian mothers are noted for fostering independence in their children from infancy onwards, for example, by giving the child a spoon as soon as the hands can manipulate it and encouraging the child to feed himself or herself. In many other cultures, children are kept more dependent on their parents for a longer period of time. Dr. Leininger concluded from her studies that caring is a universal trait that is essential to human survival. In the mid-1950s, she identified caring as the "essence and central domain of nursing." The focus of her research was to discover the care phenomena (practices) of different cultures in order to provide people with culturally congruent care (Cohen, 1992; Leininger, 1977, 1978, 1991).

Dr. Dorothea Orem's Self-Care Deficit Theory of Nursing was based on the premise that individuals must continuously engage in activities for self maintenance and self regulation, such as feeding and dressing themselves, protecting themselves from illness and learning new and better ways of promoting their own health. She called these "self-care activities." Dr. Orem put forth the idea that the ability of people to meet their self-care needs varies both throughout the life cycle and with situational factors, such as illness or incapacity. The principal nursing interventions required to assist people with self-care deficits include such actions as teaching, guidance, physical or psychological support and providing an environment conducive to personal development (Orem, 1985; Morse, Solberg, Neander, Bottorff and Johnson, 1990).

Dr. Jean Watson calls her theory "Human Science and Human Care." She believes that the nurse's role is based on human caring for one who is ill and that nursing is "an art and a science directed toward the protection, enhancement and preservation of human dignity"(Watson, 1988, 35).

To Watson, the relationship between patient and nurse is the key to helping the individual to gain more self-knowledge, self-control and readiness for self-healing, regardless of the person's health condition. In her work, Watson emphasizes the psychological and emotional, as well as the spiritual, dimensions of nursing care. She states that "the interventions related to the human care process require an intention, a will, a relationship, and actions. The process entails a commitment to caring as a moral ideal directed toward the preservation of humanity" (Watson, 1988, 75).

Dr. Simone Roach, in her philosophical treatise entitled *The Human Act of Caring*, states that ". . . the desire to care is human, it manifests itself in the human mode of being" (48). Like Leininger, she sees caring as "an essential ingredient in human development and survival" (2) and, like Leininger and Watson, as the essence and core of nursing (11). She views nursing as the professionalization of human caring and states, as we did in Chapter 1, that most beginning students of nursing enter their professional schools with a sincere desire to help people. The knowledge, skills and attitudes they gain during their educational program enable them to provide the professional help people need to promote and protect their health, or to cope with health problems (Roach, 1992).

In answer to the question "What is a nurse doing when she or he is caring?" Dr. Roach suggests that in caring, nurses use the "Five Cs" of professional caring: compassion, competence, confidence, conscience and commitment.

Another "C"

Dr. Roach suggested that other "C"s might be added to this list. One of these is **comportment**, used here to mean bearing, demeanour, dress and language — all of which she feels are important in conveying an attitude of caring. A neat, well-groomed appearance conveys to the patient that you regard him or her as a person worthy of respect; it also means that you respect yourself. Although the starched white uniforms and crisp nurses' caps are no longer seen in most hospitals in Canada, studies have found that the traditional uniform conveyed an image of professional competence that is lacking in the informal dress code of today (Magnum, Garrison, Lind and Wyatt, 1991; Joseph, 1986). Campbell-Heider and Hart (1993) go so far as to say that the informality of dress and speech by nurses in today's health care agencies reinforces negative stereotypes of the nurse and diminishes the image of professional competence they wish to convey. In regard to language, the authors contend that social status is conveyed in the forms of address we use. Many people, particularly older people, do not like to be called by their first names — to them, it suggests a lack of respect and makes them feel robbed of their social status. Patients are also often confused by the implied social intimacy which they are not prepared for in a therapeutic re-

---

Attributes of Professional Caring — The Five Cs

- **Compassion** — a sensitivity to the pain and brokenness of the other, a quality of presence which allows one to share with and make room for the other
- **Competence** — having the knowledge, judgement, skills, energy, experience and motivation required to respond adequately to the demands of one's professional responsibilities
- **Confidence** — the quality which fosters trusting relationships
- **Conscience** — a state of moral awareness which grows with experience
- **Commitment** — a complex, affective response characterized by convergence between one's desires and one's obligations and by a deliberate choice to act in accordance with them

SOURCE: Roach, M.S. (1992). *The human act of caring: A blueprint for the health professions* (Revised ed.). Ottawa: Canadian Hospital Association Press.

---

lationship. If patients prefer to be called by "Mr.," "Mrs.," "Miss" or "Ms," nurses should respect their wishes. By encouraging patients and co-workers to call them by their first names, nurses may perpetuate a second-class role for themselves, in which they are seen as subservient to physicians who are, except in rare circumstances, always addressed by their professional title (see Figure 5.8).

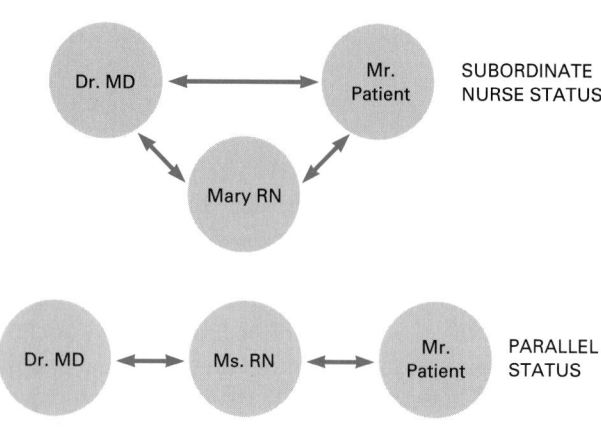

FIGURE 5.8 Communicating social status

SOURCE: Campbell-Heider, N. and Hart, C.A. (1993). Updating the nurse's bedside manner. *Image, 25*(2), 135. Reprinted with permission.

DOMAINS OF NURSING PRACTICE

Dr. Patricia Benner identifies seven aspects of the nurse's role, which she calls "domains of nursing practice":

- the helping role
- the teaching-coaching function
- the diagnostic and patient monitoring function
- effective management of rapidly changing situations
- the administering and monitoring of therapeutic interventions and regimes
- the monitoring and ensuring of the quality of health care practices
- organizational and work-role competencies*

To this list of nursing practice domains, we would add an eighth, relating to the nurse's role in primary health care: community development.

The Helping Role

From its inception, nursing's nurturing quality has been best evidenced in the helping aspects of the nurse's role. In the home and in the community, the nurse is a resource for patient and family, providing information about health matters and helping people to cope with developmental and emotional changes in their lives as well as the changes that illness brings. In caring for people who are ill, in the home or in an inpatient facility, the nurse assists the patient to carry out those activities that they would do for themselves if they were capable. Much of nursing action is thus concerned with the daily living of patients, helping them to meet their basic needs for water, food, rest and sleep and to maintain normal body functioning. A large part of the helping function is the provision of comfort and support for the patient and their family. Comfort and support may be offered through touch. Sometimes, it is just a matter of taking the other person's hand or helping him or her to walk down the hall. The gentle art of listening is also part of the provision of comfort and support, and sometimes, just being with the patient when, for example, they have to undergo a painful procedure, is enough to convey that you are there to help.

A large part of the nurse's helping role is concerned with assisting the person and the family to cope with illness and the stress and anxiety that accompany even the slightest deviations from health. In all of these activities the nurse works with the patients, helping them to regain their independence as rapidly as possible and to take control of their own health. Carrying out nursing activities with compassion, with empathetic understanding and with respect for the patient as an individual of worth and dignity is essential in the helping role of the nurse.

---
* Benner, 1984, 46.

The Teaching-Coaching Function

Teaching is a very important part of nursing care. It may involve such diverse activities as advising new mothers how to breast-feed their babies, teaching hygiene and nutrition to school children, helping people with diabetes to plan a diet compatible with their health problem, teaching deep-breathing exercises to a patient before surgery to prevent postoperative complications or helping a person to cope with the activities of daily living after he or she has been handicapped by illness. The nurse also teaches the patient and family members to carry out care at home.

The Diagnostic and Patient Monitoring Function

Many of the nurse's activities are concerned with the detection and treatment of illness. In the initial examination of an individual, the nurse assesses the patient's potential for wellness. Nurses carry out a good many diagnostic tests — many of them involving complex procedures. They must be able to explain the nature and purpose of the tests to the patient as well as being able to carry them out competently. Because nurses understand the particular demands and usual experiences of various illnesses, they are able to anticipate the patient's needs. They become very skilled at detecting significant changes in a patient's condition and taking appropriate action, either by intervening themselves or by alerting those who need to be made aware of the changes. The nurse's careful documentation of observations is invaluable for the continuity of care for the patient, as well as providing a legal record.

Effective Management of Rapidly Changing Situations

Because of the nature of their work, nurses often find themselves in life-threatening emergencies that require a rapid grasp of the situation and an ability to carry out emergency measures with skill and competence. Identifying and managing a patient crisis until physician assistance is available is something you will learn to do and will become comfortable in doing as you gain knowledge, skills and experience.

The Administering and Monitoring of Therapeutic Interventions and Regimens

Nurses carry out a good many of the therapeutic measures that are part of the plan of care for each patient. The administration of medications and the carrying out of treatments are illustrative of some of the therapeutic measures undertaken by nurses. Nurses also monitor the effects of therapeutic measures and must be alert to untoward reactions the patient may have to drugs or treatments that have been administered. Today, the nurse is responsible for carrying out and monitoring increasingly complex therapeutic regimens. Nurses are expected to start and maintain intravenous therapy with minimal risks to the patient, to administer total parenteral nutrition and to interpret the readings from cardiac monitors, among other tasks. They must also be skilled in the care of wounds and in combatting the hazards of immobility (all of these techniques are detailed in later chapters of this text).

The Monitoring and Ensuring of the Quality of Health Care Practices

In this domain of practice, the nurse acts as the patient's advocate. As the health care system has become more complex with a multitude of different agencies and an increasing variety of workers concerned with different aspects of health care, patients need someone who can speak for them and intercede on their behalf. This advocate role is an important aspect of nursing care.

In the community people often do not know about (or if they do know, they have difficulty accessing) the services that are available to help them with their problems. This is particularly true of people in low-income groups and new immigrants. The nurse, with knowledge of the services offered by government and various community agencies, and by virtue of professional contacts in these agencies, can facilitate the process of getting the patient to the appropriate people to provide help.

In an inpatient facility, the multitude of workers who do things for and to a patient seems never-ending. Some patients have reported as many as 50 employees who were in and out of their hospital room during one day. The patient needs one person to whom they can relate in a meaningful way and who can act as their spokesperson with other members of the health team.

Organizational and Work-Role Competencies

The coordinating aspects of the nurse's role have become increasingly important as health agencies have become decentralized, with more responsibility and authority vested in the individual nurse at the bedside, or in the staff nurse in the community. It is the nurse who establishes a plan of care for the patient and serves as coordinator for all activities concerned with it. In this, the nurse works in close collaboration with the patient, his or her family, the patient's physician and all other members of the health team. The nurse plans and supervises the care given by auxiliary nursing personnel, such as the LPN/RNA/CNA, the nurse's aide, and the various people who help with the provision of

Community health nurse discussing home care services with a patient who is about to be discharged.

home care services. In addition, the nurse consults with other professional workers regarding the care given to the patient. The nurse frequently needs to consult with the physician about the medical plan of care, and with the dietitian/nutritionist about the person's diet, with the physiotherapist about the patient's exercise program and with the community health nurse and the social worker about plans for home care, admission or transfer of the patient to another agency or facility.

The nurse sees that appointments are made for the patient's laboratory and other tests. If the patient is in hospital, the nurse makes sure that housekeeping staff have cleaned the room and that the dietary attendant has brought drinking water. In most health agencies that have inpatient services, nursing is the only service that is provided 24 hours a day, seven days a week. Other workers come and go, usually during the daytime and rarely on weekends.

Community Development

In the community, many nurses are now functioning in a community development role, helping people to identify their health concerns and to plan and organize actions relating to their concerns. In this role, the nurse works as a partner with community groups, rather than as a "doer-provider" of services, facilitating the process of identification of health needs and serving as a resource for information about programs and services to help communities to meet their health needs. In order to carry out this role, nurses identify and work with social networks in the community and with lay support groups such as the Enterostomy Association, the Multiple Sclerosis Society and other volunteer organizations and agencies in the community.*

MODES OF PRACTICE IN HOSPITALS

The vast majority of nurses in Canada still work in hospitals — and it is on the hospital wards that you will have much of your clinical practice as students. It is helpful, then, to understand how nurses function in hospitals. The most common mode of practice for nurses in hospitals today is "primary nursing," although other patterns are developing for the organization of nursing services.

Primary Nursing

Primary nursing is "a system of delivering nursing services where the nurse is responsible for planning complete 24-hour care for each patient" (What's the difference? CNA Today, 2(3), 2). It has become a fairly standard mode of practice in hospitals in this country in the last decade. In this type of nursing, each patient is assigned, on admission, to a specific (primary) nurse. Originally, this nurse was responsible for the patient's care throughout the hospital stay; in practical terms, however, the nurse cares for this patient throughout a tour of shifts, which may be four or five days depending on rotation patterns. The primary nurse plans for the patient's needs over the 24-hour period and gives direct care when on duty. Through the use of nursing care plans, conferences, referrals and collaboration with other nurses, the primary nurse guides and supervises the patient's care when not on duty. The primary nurse sees the patient with the physician when he or she is making rounds, confers with the physician about the patient's care and confers with other health team members, such as the physical therapist, who may be involved in the patient's care. The usual caseload for a nurse is three to four patients, although they may help with the care of patients assigned to other nurses.

Modular Nursing

In *modular nursing*, the nurse is assigned a group of patients, usually eight to twelve, whose beds or rooms are close together in the nursing unit. The nurse may have the same group of patients over a period of time. Often other personnel, such as a licensed practical nurse or registered/certified nursing assistant, are also assigned to the module so that it becomes, in essence, a small team. This method may be used in long-term care settings.

Shared Governance

Shared governance is a term used for the organization of hospital patient services in which staff nurses have more autonomy and decision-making authority than in the traditional structure. Sometimes called "participatory management," shared governance involves general staff nurses in making management decisions. The McKellar General Hospital in Thunder Bay provides one example of a hospital which has successfully implemented shared governance. Their process of change involved staff nurses from the outset, with staff and managers identifying together the changes they wanted made and then creating the desired structure. In the process, they learned to appreciate the special knowledge and skills each brings to patient care. The manager's role has shifted from one of controlling, planning and directing to one of coaching and facilitating. Staff nurses have gained skills in speaking up and expressing their opinions and have learned to take an active role in making management decisions (Changing structures: Sharing the power, raising the quality, 1992).

Alternative Modes

Another new mode is evolving at Sunnybrook Hospital in Toronto. The reorganization of patient services at this hospital is the first of its kind in Canada although similar changes are taking place in numerous hospitals in the United States. The reorganization at Sunnybrook involves three components: decentralization of authority, the establishment of patient service units and the development of multi-skilled employees. To reflect a patient-centred philosophy, decision-making is being decentralized and put into the hands of those closest to the patient. There are no middle management (supervisory) positions. The hospital is organized around the patient, rather than around departments, with a small number of clinical units, basically encompassing medicine, surgery, long-term care and psychiatry. Each clinical unit is composed of four or five patient service units. The patient service units are made up of like groups of patients, such as patients undergoing circulatory surgery. Each patient service unit becomes, in effect, a mini-hospital, with its own laboratory and basic x-ray equipment, where this is economically feasible, and its own budget. It is felt that nurses can coordinate their work better and get more satisfaction from their work in smaller care teams that focus on patients with similar health problems. The plan includes a system whereby a nurse and a multi-purpose worker are assigned to care for a group of

---

* The discussion of Domains 1–7 is adapted from Benner, P. (1984). *From Novice to Expert*. Menlo Park, CA: Addison-Wesley Publishing Company Inc. Domain 8. Community Development was developed from discussions with staff of the Vancouver Health Department, West Main Unit.

patients. The multi-purpose worker sees to all the non-nursing, non-professional activities that were carried out by a number of different workers, such as delivering meal trays to the patients, washing the floors and collecting the garbage. There would also be multi-skilled administrative personnel and clinical staff who can assist the nurse by doing tasks such as helping patients to ambulate (Hospitals in transition, 1993).

CAREER CHOICES FOR NURSES

Nurses graduating from educational programs in Canada today have a promising future. According to Employment and Immigration Canada projections, the demand for nurses, which has been growing steadily over the past 30 years, will continue to surpass employment opportunities for people in most other fields (see Figure 5.9).

The continually increasing demand for nurses is the result of a number of factors. There has been an increase in all-nurse staffing in hospitals. The role of nurses in health-care delivery is expanding and the increasing technical complexities of patient care require the services of a growing number of highly skilled nurses. Although the current downsizing of hospitals combined with the effects of a nation-wide recession has caused some concern over job opportunities for nurses, EIC projections anticipate a marked increase in the number of nursing positions becoming available over the next few years. Nurses holding university degrees and those with specialty training, such as intensive care, gerontological nursing and surgical nursing, will be in great demand (Job Prospects, 1992).

Nurses today have the opportunity to choose from a wide range of career options. We have selected a few to discuss here. These include hospital nursing (because the greatest number of nurses are currently working in this field), long-term care nursing, community health nursing, northern nursing, education, office nursing, occupational health nursing, independent practice, research, military nursing and midwifery.

HOSPITAL NURSING

Almost two thirds of all employed nurses in Canada work in general or psychiatric hospitals, most as general staff nurses (Statistics Canada, 1993). The duties and responsibilities of staff nurses vary, depending on the agency in which they are employed, although all are guided by the Standards of Practice established by provincial nursing associations and the College of Nurses of Ontario. In hospitals, they may work in any one of a number of areas, such as medical-surgical nursing, maternal-newborn, critical care or extended (long-term) care nursing, pediatric nursing, psychiatric nursing or in specialized units such as emergency, the operating room or critical care.

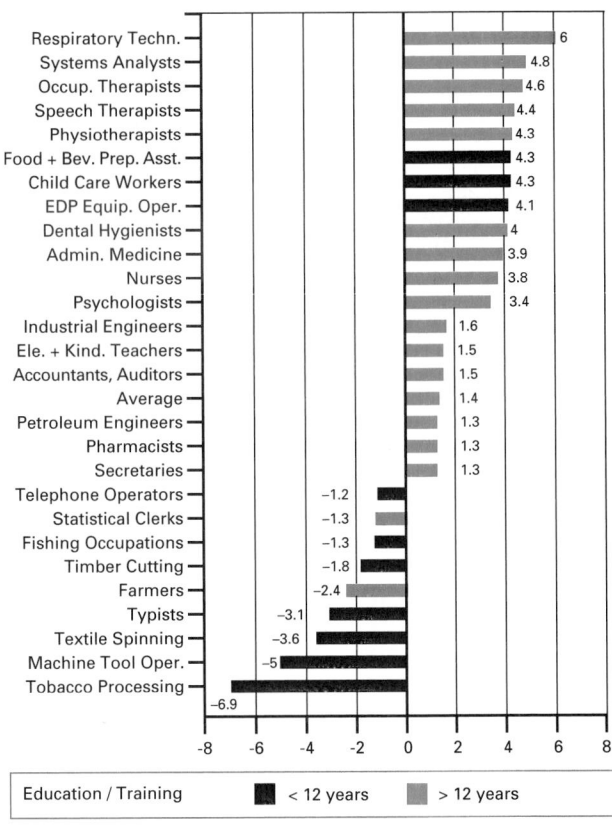

Occupations Contributing Most to Employment Growth, 1990-2000			
		1990-2000	
CODE Occupations	Employment	Average Annual Growth Rate	Share of total Employment Growth
3131 Nurses	250 743	3.8%	6.2%
2183 Systems Analysts	132 526	4.8%	4.3%
1137 Sales Management Occs.	264 162	2.6%	4.2%
1149 Office Managers	161 204	3.8%	4.0%
4133 Cashiers + Tellers	312 687	2.1%	3.9%
4143 EDP Equip Operators	135 841	4.1%	3.7%
4111 Secretaries + Stenographers	455 471	1.3%	3.5%
5135 Salespersons	667 140	0.9%	3.4%
6121 Chefs + Cooks	191 896	2.8%	3.3%
6147 Child Care Workers	107 184	4.3%	3.1%
1130 General Managers	189 916	2.3%	2.7%
4171 Receptionists	121 339	2.7%	2.0%
4131 Bookkeepers	403 913	0.9%	2.0%
1171 Accountants, Auditors	213 110	1.5%	1.9%
2731 Elementary + Kind Teachers	198 938	1.5%	1.8%
6125 Food + Bev Serving Occs.	247 154	1.2%	1.7%
6129 Food + Bev. Prep. Assistants	55 324	4.3%	1.6%
6143 Hairdressers	103 596	2.0%	1.2%
1142 Services Management Occs.	69 205	2.6%	1.1%
3135 Nursing Attendants	81 637	2.2%	1.1%
2333 Occs in Welf + Commun Serv.	68 769	2.4%	1.0%
2343 Lawyers + Notaries	54 004	2.7%	0.9%
3156 Medical Lab Technicians	41 340	3.4%	0.9%
1135 Managers-Financial	80 744	1.9%	0.9%
2331 Social Workers	53 902	2.5%	0.8%
All Occupations	12 571 791	1.4%	100%

FIGURE 5.9 Selected Detail Occupational Growth (Average Annual Percent Change) 1990–2000 and Occupations Contributing Most to Employment Growth, 1990–2000

SOURCE: Employment and Immigration Canada. COPS, 1991. Cited in Job Prospects. (1992). *Edufacts: The news in nursing education, 2*(2), 3.

THE CLINICAL CAREER

Many nurses who want to have a career in clinical nursing are choosing to increase their knowledge and skills in a particular field through further education. As we mentioned above, numerous courses are available in fields such as gerontology (care of the older adult), psychiatric/mental health nursing, critical care nursing, advanced obstetric nursing, nursing of the high-risk newborn and palliative care nursing (care of people with terminal illness). Increasingly, these courses are carrying university credits for transfer towards a degree in nursing. Nurses who wish to advance further in their chosen field through the clinical ladder may opt to become clinical specialists. The Canadian Nurses Association defines the clinical nurse specialist as "a registered nurse who holds a master's or doctoral degree in nursing with expertise in a clinical nursing specialty" (CNA, 1993). In 1992, there were a total of 310 clinical nurse specialists holding a master's or doctoral degree employed in Canadian health services (Statistics Canada, 1993).

"The clinical nurse specialist (CNS) is a registered nurse with expertise in a clinical nursing specialty; is an expert practitioner who provides direct care, education and consultation to patients, their families and other members of the health care team. The practice of the CNS is based on in-depth knowledge of nursing and other sciences gained through advanced education and practice with a clinical focus. The role of the CNS is to promote excellence in nursing practice and serve as a role model for nurses by acting in the interrelated roles of practitioner, leader, educator, researcher, consultant. The CNS bases nursing practice upon research and communicates and uses research findings. The CNS conducts research to improve the quality of patient care." (Approved by the Board of Directors of the Canadian Nurses Association, November, 1993.)

SOURCE: Canadian Nurses Association. Key policy concepts and supporting concepts.

In discussing clinical nurse specialists, we should say a word about Nurse Practitioners. The development of the position of Nurse Practitioner that took place in the United States in the 1970s was not paralleled in Canada. The Report of the Committee on Nurse Practitioners (1972) viewed the Nurse Practitioner's role as "an extension of the present nursing role with [the nurse's] unique skills in the care of the patient being developed and utilized more effectively" and as "complementary to that of the physician and other members of the health team" (5). Although a number of Nurse Practitioner programs were established in

Canada in the early 1970s, these programs were viewed as temporary measures until such time as preparation for an expanded role could be incorporated into basic educational programs.

There are, however, a number of graduates of nurse practitioner programs who have continued to practice and have formed an association. The Nurse Practitioner Association of Ontario defines the nurse practitioner as:

> . . . a nurse specializing in primary health care, with advanced knowledge and decision-making skills, built on basic nursing education preparation, and emphasizing health promotion and disease prevention.

In the same document, Primary Health Care was defined as:

> . . .[the] patients' first contact with the health care system and offers comprehensive and continuous care. Comprehensive primary health care may require collaboration with and referrals to other health professionals and health rsources. (Standards of Practice for Nurse Practitioners, March, 1993. Cited in Marchand and Goodine, 1993.)

There has recently been interest by provincial governments in the reestablishment of Nurse Practitioner programs. The Ontario Government has been working with nurses, colleges and universities and hopes to implement a program to prepare registered nurses for this role by 1995. It is expected that the Nurse Practitioners will usually be the first point of contact for people with the health care system and may work independently or as part of a health team (Haines, 1993; Ontario announces nurse practitioner plan, 1994, 14).

THE ADMINISTRATIVE CAREER

Some nurses opt to advance in nursing through the administrative ladder. More than 10 percent of employed nurses are in management or administrative positions as managers, supervisors or coordinators. They usually start as **nurse manager**, or charge nurse of a nursing unit. If they wish to advance further in administration, as a Director/Assistant Director of Nursing, a Vice-President, or Chief Executive Officer of Nursing, a baccalaureate or higher degree in nursing (or in administration of health services) is becoming the expected qualification, although at the present time less than one half of the nurses in CEO/Director positions hold an academic degree (Statistics Canada, 1993).

LONG-TERM CARE

The field of long-term care is an expanding one, first, because of the increased number of older persons in our society and second, because of the devastating number of people injured in motor vehicle and other accidents who require long-term care and rehabilitation. Long-term care includes both inpatient nursing services in nursing homes and rehabilitation centres and the provision of nursing services in the community to those who require direct care or monitoring over an extended period of time. The nurse's role in long-term care has many facets. In both community and inpatient facilities, it is usually registered nurses who undertake the initial assessment of the health care needs of individuals (and of family members) and it is the RNs who develop the plans of care, in conjunction with the members of other health disciplines, such as physicians, physiotherapists and social workers. Registered nurses provide high-level technical and complex care for those who need it, as well as palliative and bereavement care for individuals with terminal illnesses and their families. They also often have to sort out and manage the multiple medications taken by people in long-term care. They have a major teaching role with both the individual's family and with other care workers, teaching them to carry out a plan of care and to monitor procedures such as intravenous therapy. Another important function of nurses in long-term care is that of patient advocate (Blunt, 1992).

COMMUNITY HEALTH

The community health field is also one that is growing rapidly. At the present time, approximately 10 000 nurses are employed in community health agencies, and another 7000 in home care (Statistics Canada, 1993). These numbers are expected to increase considerably in the next few years. As hospitals are down-sized and community services expanded, provincial governments are encouraging nursing schools to offer courses in community health nursing to enable hospital nurses to make the transfer to community services. They are also encouraging nurses to enrol in post-basic courses. The role of the nurse in the community is discussed further in Chapter 11, Health and the Community. This is an exciting field in which nurses have an opportunity to be involved in a much broader role in the implementing of primary health care.

NORTHERN NURSING

Working in Canada's North has always had a special attraction for Canadian nurses — and for nurses from many other countries. In the North, community health nurses are employed in nursing stations and in health centres with and without treatment facilities. These nurses have a much broader scope of practice than in communities in southern Canada. In nursing stations and in health centres which provide treatment services, community health nurses are required to be knowledgeable and skillful in recognizing and managing common medical disorders and pediatric problems, as well as common obstetric conditions throughout the

maternity cycle for low-risk obstetric patients. They are also responsible for acute emergency care and initial management of problems requiring medical and surgical intervention, the temporary management of people with psychiatric problems and temporary management of patients with more serious medical, pediatric or obstetric problems. They also prepare patients for and manage them during emergency evacuations, when a medical or nursing escort is required.

All community health nurses in nursing stations, in health centres and in health centres with treatment facilities are expected to be able to provide the appropriate care, including referral, for an extensive list of community health program areas. Responsibilities include health education, promotion and prevention services in communicable disease control, maternal/child health, pre-school health, school health and adult health plus such areas as family violence, substance abuse, dental health and environmental health. The list of areas the nurse is expected to be able to be proficient in also includes nutrition, physical fitness, injury prevention, occupational health, disaster management and home nursing care.

Preparatory programs to enable nurses to practise in the extended role required by Northern health services is available through the National Clinical Training Program. The program is currently taught at McMaster University in a nine-month (one academic year) program of studies that combines theory with practical experience in a First Nations community and through the Dalhousie Outpost Nursing Program at Dalhousie University (Health and Welfare Canada, 1991, 1993).

EDUCATION

Almost 6000 nurses, roughly 2.6 percent of the number of employed nurses in Canada, are engaged in education (Statistics Canada, 1993). The field of education has three distinct sub-fields — all involve teaching, but to different groups of people:
1. patient education
2. inservice education for employees of health agencies
3. nursing education (that is, teaching students).

All three areas are growing. The emphasis on health promotion today, as well as on teaching people to protect their health and to cope with the complex therapies used in treatment when they are ill, has made patient education one of the most important aspects of care for people. Inservice education in a health agency involves a wide range of activities, including orientation programs for new employees, teaching new knowledge and skills to keep nurses and other health workers up-to-date with advances in their field, and holding conferences, teaching programs and other short, continuing education programs for people working in the agency and, often, in other agencies as well. For example, a regional hospital, such as the Prince George

Regional Hospital in central British Columbia, will often have inservice education programs for their nurses which they will share with nurses from smaller hospitals in the region. The majority of nurses engaged in teaching are, however, in schools of nursing. As the preparation of nurses moves into colleges and universities, the academic credentials of nursing teachers must meet the standards set for teaching faculty in other disciplines. This standard is usually a minimum of a baccalaureate degree, preferably a master's degree in colleges and, increasingly, doctoral preparation in university programs. As the current statistics show, the number of master's and doctorate-prepared nurses in Canada is woefully inadequate. Nursing education is a field that has been perennially short of qualified people.

OFFICE NURSING

Almost as many nurses (5600) work in physicians' offices as in teaching (Statistics Canada, 1993). The usual pattern is for the nurse to work in collaboration with one physician in solo practice or with two or more physicians in a group practice in the community. At the present time, most nurses are in a traditional "office nurse" role assisting the physician in his or her practice. We can anticipate, however, that an increasing number of nurses will become employed in collaborative practice (rather than purely as assistants) with physicians in the community, in doctors' offices, Community Health Centres and Health Service Organizations as these develop.

Two factors facilitate an expanded role for nurses in collaborative roles with physicians and in independent practice: first, the changes occurring in Health Practice Acts in various provinces that legitimize an expanded scope of practice for nurses and second, a clause in the Canada Health Act (1984) permitting "qualified health practitioners other than physicians and dentists" to be reimbursed for their services, providing this does not conflict with provincial legislation. This clause makes it possible for services provided by nurses to be insurable (Adaskin, 1988).

OCCUPATIONAL HEALTH

Approximately 2600 nurses are employed in business or industry in Canada. Traditionally, the *occupational health* nurse's role has included rendering emergency care to people who are injured or become ill at work, as well as providing health counselling, health promotion and health protection services for employees. An important aspect of their work has always been participating in safety programs to protect the health of people in their working environment. Although accident prevention, health protection and emergency care are still regarded as important, increasing attention is being paid to stress — both home- and work-related — as a major factor in employee productivity and absenteeism. This recognition of the role of stress, along with today's emphasis on health promotion, has shifted the emphasis in occupational health to wellness programs. Many corporations are hiring "wellness coordinators" whose role is to design and implement health promotion programs for employees. It should be noted that people from other disciplines, such as teachers, social workers and fitness experts, are vying for these positions too. Nurses, particularly community health and occupational health nurses, however, are in a good position vis-à-vis candidates from other disciplines, because of their preparation in health promotion and their broad background in health matters. Courses in occupational health nursing are offered at various schools across the country — at the University of Ottawa as a concentration in Community Health/ Occupational Health Nursing at the baccalaureate level and as a post-basic diploma or certificate program at some other schools. A 16-week post-diploma certificate program in Wellness and Lifestyle is offered at Centennial College in Toronto (Farr, 1990; Thomas, 1993).

INDEPENDENT PRACTICE

"A job is not only about money. A job is also about satisfaction and what you can do with your knowledge" (Mongeon-Meredith cited in Brown, 1993). The field of independent practice is attracting a growing number of nurses in Canada, although the ranks are still relatively small. There were an estimated 1080 self-employed nurses registered and employed in Canada in 1992. These nurses offer counselling, educational and administrative services on a consulting basis, as well as providing direct nursing care to the public on a fee-for-service basis. They offer a wide range of services, such as midwifery, mental health counselling, family counselling, sexual counselling, holistic nursing care and wellness education. They also offer consultant services in education (as curriculum development consultants, for example), in nursing administration and in research. Many Canadian nurses have served, and continue to serve, as consultants in various fields in international nursing with agencies such as the World Health Organization and the Canadian International Development Association.

RESEARCH

The number of nurses in research has grown steadily over the past decade. Although nurse researchers are still few in number in Canada, it is becoming evident that research is no longer the domain of academics only. Nurses in service agencies are questioning traditional nursing practices and are seeking to validate their actions through research (Brown, 1993). The benefits of research are also being recognized by hospitals and other health agencies. Administrators are encouraging nurses to use research as a method of developing more efficient and more effective nursing interventions. Of the 756 nurses who consider themselves researchers, more than one half were employed in general and psychiatric hospitals (Statistics Canada, 1993). These figures are slightly misleading, however, because research is also an essential component of the role of nurses on university faculty who consider themselves primarily to be teachers. At the present time, there are very few nurses qualified at the master's or doctoral level in Canada — the usual educational requirement considered necessary for research — but many hospitals and other agencies are making use of the few who have had preparation in research by having them act as research facilitators to enable staff nurses to conduct studies. The role of research in nursing practice is discussed further in Chapter 7.

MILITARY NURSING

A total of 364 nurses are currently serving with the Canadian armed services. They work in Department of National Defence hospitals and in field units in Canada and abroad. Canada has the distinction of being the first country to confer officer status on nurses serving with the armed forces. A Canadian nursing service became an integral part of the Army Medical Corps in 1901, and nursing sisters were accorded the rank, status and pay of lieutenant (Nicholson, 1975). The distinguished history of Canadian nurses in the Riel Rebellion, the Boer War, the First and the Second World Wars and in the Korean War makes for fascinating reading (Feasby, 1946; Gibbon and Mathewson, 1947; McPhail, 1925; Nicholson, 1975; Wilson-Simmie, 1981). Nurses also served with Canadian forces in the Gulf War, but their story is still to be written.

MIDWIFERY

Midwifery is the care of women and their families throughout the maternity cycle, which begins before pregnancy and ends approximately six weeks after birth. Its mandate is to provide care for normal, rather than high-risk pregnancies. Midwives refer high-risk women to family practice physicians or obstetricians for care. Until recently, Canada was one of the few countries in the world where midwifery was not a legal practice. Up to now, educational programs in midwifery have focussed mainly on preparing nurses to work in the missionary field abroad, in outpost nursing stations in the Canadian north or in other isolated parts of the country. At the present time, two university schools of nursing offer midwifery courses for nurses. At the University of Alberta, a Midwifery Certificate is offered in conjunction with the Master's in Nursing degree. At Dalhousie University in Halifax, a 15-month Outpost Nursing Program includes midwifery preparation with emphasis on comprehensive care throughout the maternity cycle.

The practice of midwifery has now been legalized as an autonomous discipline in the Provinces of Ontario, Alberta and British Columbia. There is no doubt that other provinces will follow suit. The Midwifery Act in Ontario permits the practice of midwifery by Direct-Entry practitioners as well as by nurse-midwives. The term "single-trained midwife" is also sometimes used instead of "direct-entry practitioner" to refer to an individual who has entered a midwifery program without having first qualified as a nurse. In some countries, midwives must be qualified nurses before they can enter a midwifery program; in other countries, there may be both direct-entry practitioners of midwifery and nurse-midwives. McMaster University's Faculty of Health Sciences, Laurentian University in Sudbury and Ryerson Polytechnic University in Toronto have collaborated on a program that will lead to a Bachelor of Health Sciences in midwifery. The first students were enrolled in the program in September, 1993. Nurses will be eligible for advanced credit in the program. The Government of Ontario has instituted a program for midwives who are in current practice to update their knowledge and skills in the field before applying for registration (Herbert, 1993).

NURSING AND THE POLITICAL PROCESS

Larsen and Baumgart liken the nursing profession to a sleeping giant in Canadian public life. The fact that nursing is "the largest nationally organized group in Canadian society made up predominantly of women" (469) provides it with the potential to wield a considerable amount of power (1992). Nurses have traditionally been uncomfortable with power; it is only recently that they have begun to appreciate the importance of taking an active part in the political process to influence public policy (Larsen and Baumgart, 1992).

Dr. Helen Glass (1985) suggested three approaches whereby nursing can influence public policy in the health field. The first is increased public representation by nurses, that is to say, getting nurses elected or appointed to positions on local, provincial and national committees and boards, and electing nurses to city councils, provincial legislatures and to parliament. The second is the integration of nurses into high-level government positions, for example, as Chief Nursing Officer in Ministries of Health. The present incumbent in that position at the federal level is Dr. Josephine Flaherty, a distinguished nursing author and ethicist. There are also Nursing Consultants in various branches of Health Canada (formerly Health and Welfare Canada) who wield considerable influence in their areas of expertise as, for example, in the development of national guidelines for infection control in hospitals. The third approach suggested by Glass was the use of professional power strategies to influence government decision-making. The Canadian Nurses Association and the various provincial associations are becoming much more skilled in using professional power strategies and in encouraging local groups and individual nurses to get involved in the political process.

Canadian nursing's political "coming of age" occurred in 1984 when the Canadian Nurses Association, in collaboration with the provincial nursing associations, succeeded in obtaining passage of a clause amending the Canada Health Act to permit nurses to have a broader role in primary health care (Adaskin, 1988). Since then, CNA has joined with six other national organizations to form a Health Action Lobby (HEAL) to preserve and protect the principles of the Canadian Health Care system. The other members of the alliance are the Canadian Hospital Association, the Canadian Medical Association, the Canadian Long-Term Care Association, the Canadian

Public Health Association, the Canadian Psychological Association and the Consumers Association. Members of the seven national HEAL organizations discuss issues that affect health care with consumers, politicians and government officials. They were involved, for example, during the 1993 election campaign when it appeared that some parties would institute user-fees for Medicare if elected. The Canadian Nurses Association also published an election handbook entitled *Nurses Know Nurses Can* which outlined why nurses should be involved in the political process and how they can get involved; gave some facts about nursing that could be helpful in presenting opinions to candidates; and suggested questions to ask of candidates (CNA, 1993). As nursing at the national level continues to press for health care reform, provincial nursing associations are making their voices heard and their influence felt in the restructuring of health services in their jurisdictions.

KEY TERMS

post-basic education p. 93	competence p. 98	modular nursing p. 101
hospital postgraduate courses p. 93	confidence p. 98	shared governance p. 101
orderlies p. 96	conscience p. 98	nurse manager p. 103
nurse's aides p. 96	commitment p. 98	occupational health p. 105
compassion p. 98	comportment p. 98	midwifery p. 106
	primary nursing p. 101	

IN REVIEW

Nursing is a dynamic profession whose practice is constantly evolving in response to societal needs. The rapid changes occurring in health care in Canada today are reflected both in changes to the nurse's role and in the preparation required for nursing practice. Over the past century, nursing has emerged from being subordinate to medicine to becoming an autonomous profession in its own right. Nursing education has evolved from apprenticeship-like training in hospitals to almost universal baccalaureate preparation in colleges and universities as the required entry level for practice. In 1993 only four provinces still listed hospital diploma programs; there were 21 basic and 28 post-basic baccalaureate degree programs, 13 masters' and four doctoral programs in Canada. Continuing education, which is vital for maintaining the professional competence of nurses, is available by numerous means, including self study, varied work experiences, inservice education and through formal programs at educational institutions.

Nurses are the largest group of health workers in Canada. In 1992, there were over 260 000 registered nurses and registered psychiatric nurses in Canada. Of these nurses, 15.9 percent hold baccalaureate or higher degrees. The number of nurses with master's and doctoral degrees is

still relatively small but is expected to increase over the next decade with the increase in the number of graduate education programs in nursing across the country. Other nursing personnel include Licensed Practical Nurses (or Registered or Certified Nursing Assistants as they are called in some provinces), orderlies and nurse's aides.

In Canada, almost two-thirds of all nurses are employed in acute or psychiatric hospitals; 10.8 percent in nursing homes and rehabilitation centers; 7.4 percent in nursing stations, home care and community health agencies; one percent in occupational health; 2.6 percent in education and the same percentage in physicians' offices.

The responsibility of nursing to health care is four-fold: to promote health, to prevent illness, to restore health and to alleviate suffering. The *care paradigm* of nursing has been explored by numerous nurse-theorists over the past decade. Sister Simone Roach, in her philosophical treatise on the subject, views nursing as the professionalization of caring. She includes as attributes of professional caring the qualities of compassion, competence, confidence, conscience and commitment. She also suggests the addition of comportment — the outward manifestations of bearing, demeanour, dress and language which help to convey an attitude of caring.

Benner identifies seven domains of nursing practice: the helping role, the teaching-coaching function, the diagnostic and patient monitoring function, the effective management of rapidly changing situations, the administering and monitoring of therapeutic interventions and regimes, the monitoring and ensuring of the quality of health care and practices and organizational and work-role competencies. To these, we added an eighth domain of community development to encompass aspects of the nurse's role in primary health care not covered in Benner's seven domains.

There appears to be a continually increasing demand for nursing services and today nurses have a multiplicity of career choices. Most nurses currently work in hospitals where both clinical and administrative career ladders are open to them. In hospitals, the most common mode of practice is primary nursing, although a number of alternative modes are developing for the organization of nursing services. Other possible career choices include long-term care, community nursing, northern nursing, education, office nursing, occupational health, independent practice, research, military nursing and midwifery.

Nurses have only in recent years become aware of their potential for influencing policy decisions about health care in Canada. Today, the Canadian Nurses Association and provincial nursing associations as well as nurses at the local level are becoming involved in the political process to press for health care reform and to make their voices heard in decisions regarding the restructuring of health services.

LEARNING ACTIVITIES

1. Explore the history of nursing education in your province:
   a. When were the first hospital schools of nursing started?
   b. Where were they located?
   c. What was the educational program like?
   d. Who were the most notable early nurse educators in the province?
   e. When did the educational preparation of nurses move from hospital schools and where did they move to?
   f. What changes are currently taking place in nursing education in your province?

2. You have been asked to talk at a career day for high school students in your community on basic education for nursing, specialty preparation and career options for nurses. You will be allowed 30 minutes. Outline your presentation.

3. Talk with two nurses — an older retired nurse and one who is in active practice in your community. Explore with each their education for practice and the nature of their practice in terms of the eight domains of practice discussed in the chapter.

4. Debate with your classmates the use of first names by and for patients and nurses.

5. What role is your provincial nursing association taking with regard to the restructuring of health care in the province? Are there particular issues affecting nursing?

REFERENCES AND READINGS

ADASKIN, E.J. (1988). Organized political action: Lobbying by nurses' actions. In A.J. Baumgart and J. Larsen. *Canadian nursing faces the future*. St. Louis: Mosby, 474–487.

BAJNOK, I. (1992). Entry-level educational preparation for nursing. In A.J. Baumgart and J. Larsen. (1992) *Canadian nursing faces the future*. (2nd ed.). St. Louis: Mosby, 383–420.

BELL, L. (1993). BC on target for BN. *Edufacts: The news in nursing education, 3*(2), 1.

BENNER, P. (1984). *From novice to expert*. Menlo Park, CA: Addison-Wesley.

BENNER, P. and WRUBEL, J. (1980). *The primacy of caring*. Menlo Park, CA: Addison-Wesley.

BLUNT, A. (1992). The registered nurse in long-term care. *Registered Nurse, 4*(3), 7.

BOUDREAU, T.J. (1972). *Report of the committee on nurse practitioners*. Ottawa: Health and Welfare Canada.

BROWN, L. (1993). Making it on her own. *Nursing BC, 25*(1), 15.

BUILDING A DEGREE PROGRAM IN PEI. (1992). *Edufacts: The news in nursing education, 2*(1), 4.

CAMPBELL-HEIDER, N. and HART, C.A. (1993, Summer). Updating the nurse's bedside manner. *Images, 25*(2), 133–139.

CANADA NEEDS MORE NATIVE NURSES. (1992). *Edufacts: The news in nursing education, 2*(3), 2–3.

CANADIAN NURSES ASSOCIATION. (1968). *The leaf and the lamp*. Ottawa: Author.

CANADIAN NURSES ASSOCIATION. (1992). *Continuing education in nursing: A directory*. Ottawa: Author.

CANADIAN NURSES ASSOCIATION. (1992). *Continuing nursing education position statement*. Ottawa: Author.

CANADIAN NURSES ASSOCIATION. (1993). *Entrance requirements for nursing education programs in Canada 1993*. Ottawa: Author.

CANADIAN NURSES ASSOCIATION. (1993). *Nurses know nurses can: An election handbook*. Ottawa: Author.

CANADIAN NURSES ASSOCIATION. (1994). *The clinical nurse specialist*. Ottawa: Author.

CANADIAN NURSES WITH PhDs. (1991). *Edufacts: The news in nursing education, 1*(1), 4.

CHANGING STRUCTURES: SHARING THE POWER, RAISING THE QUALITY. (1992). *Registered Nurse, 4*(3), 22–26.

COHEN, J.A. (1992). Janforum: Leininger's culture care theory of nursing. *Journal of Advanced Nursing, 17,* 1149.

COLLABORATION AMONG ALL SASKATCHEWAN NURSING SCHOOLS. (1992). *Edufacts: The news in nursing education, 2*(2), 4.

COLLABORATIVE PROJECT IN NOVA SCOTIA. (1993). *Edufacts: The news in nursing education, 3*(3), 3.

DALHOUSIE UNIVERSITY MASTER OF NURSING PROGRAM. (1992). *Edufacts: The news in nursing education, 2*(2), 1.

DONAHUE, M.P. (1985). *Nursing the finest art: An illustrated history.* St. Louis: Mosby.

DO WE HAVE ENOUGH MASTER OF NURSING PROGRAMS? (1993). *Edufacts: The news in nursing education, 2*(4), 2.

DU GAS, B.W. (1991). *The development of nursing education in BC.* Paper presented at the First Annual General Meeting of the History of Nursing Professional Practice Group of the RNABC.

DU GAS, B.W. and CASEY, A. (1989). Baccalaureates for RNs. *The Canadian Nurse, 85*(2), 31–33.

ETHICAL CONCEPTS APPLIED TO NURSING 1973. (1975, September). *ICN News Release. No. 6.*

FARR, M. (1990). Wellness at work. *The Registered Nurse, 2*(4), 13–17.

FEASBY, W.R. (1946). *Official history of the Canadian medical services 1939–1945. Volume 1: Organization and campaigns.* Ottawa: MDN.

FIELD, P.A., STINSON, S.M. and THIBAUDEAU, M.F. (1992). Graduate education in nursing in Canada. In A.J. Baumgart and J. Larsen. (1992). *Canadian nursing faces the future.* (2nd ed.).St. Louis: Mosby, 421–445.

GIBBON, J.M. and MATHEWSON, M.H. (1947). *Three centuries of Canadian nursing.* Toronto: Macmillan.

GLASGOW, M.S. (1992). Nursing in Canada. *Canadian Social Trends,* Spring, 27–29.

GLASS, H. (1985). *The future of health care in Canada and nursing's role within it.* Ottawa. (Available from the Canadian Nurses Association).

GREEN, M.M. (1983). *Through the years with public health nursing.* Ottawa: The Canadian Public Health Association.

HAINES, J. (1993). *The nurse practitioner: A discussion paper.* Ottawa: Canadian Nurses Association.

HALL, E.M. (1964). *Report of the Royal Commission on Health Services.* Ottawa: Queen's Printer.

HEALTH AND WELFARE CANADA. (1992). *Health Personnel in Canada 1990.* Ottawa: Minister of Supply and Services. (Catalogue No. H1–9/1–1990)

HEALTH AND WELFARE CANADA. (1991). *Scope of practice for community health nurses. (1) Nursing Station, (2) Health Centre, (3) Health Centre with Treatment.* Ottawa: Medical Services Branch Indian and Northern Health Services Nursing Division. (Currently under revision)

HEALTH AND WELFARE CANADA. (1993). Discussion with senior staff Health and Welfare Canada, Vancouver, BC.

HERBERT, P. (1993). Is midwifery education new to Canada? *Edufacts: The news in nursing education, 3*(2), 3–4.

HISTORY OF NURSING SOCIETY, SCHOOL FOR GRADUATE NURSES, MCGILL UNIVERSITY. (c1929). Pioneers of nursing in Canada. Montreal: Canadian Nurses Association.

HOSPITALS IN TRANSITION. *CNA Today, 3*(1), 1–2.

INTERNATIONAL COUNCIL OF NURSES. (1975). *Ethical concepts applied to nursing 1973.* ICN News Release No. 6.

IS MIDWIFERY EDUCATION NEW TO CANADA? (1993). *Edufacts: The news in nursing, 3*(2), 1, 4.

JENSEN, E. (1992, October/November). Founder of modern Canadian nursing. *Registered Nurse (RNAO Journal),* 16–18.

JOB PROSPECTS. (1992). *Edufacts: The news in nursing education, 2*(2), 3.

JOHNS, ETHEL M. (1917). Proceedings of the tenth annual convention of the Canadian society of superintendents of training schools, 12 and 13 June 1917. *The Canadian Nurse. XIII (September 1917),* 571–89. Cited in Street, M. (1973). *Watchfires on the mountains: the life and writings of Ethel Johns.* Toronto: University of Toronto Press.

JOSEPH, N. (1986). *Uniforms and non-uniforms: Communication through clothing.* New York: Greenwood Press.

LARSEN, J. and BAUMGART, A.J. (1992). Overview: Shaping public policy. In A.J. Baumgart and Larsen, J. (1992). *Canadian nursing faces the future.* (2nd ed.). Toronto: Mosby, 469–492.

LEININGER, M. (1977). *Caring: The essence and central focus of nursing.* New York: American Nurses Foundation.

LEININGER, M. (1978). *Transcultural nursing: Concepts, theories and practices.* New York: Wiley.

LEININGER, M. (1991). *Culture care diversity and universality.* New York: National League for Nursing.

MACPHAIL, SIR ANDREW. (1925). *History of the Canadian forces medical services 1914–1919.* Ottawa: MDN. Queen's Printer.

MAGNUM, S., GARRISON, C., LIND, C. THACKERAY, R. and WYATT, M. (1991). Perceptions of nurses' uniforms. *Image, 23,* 127–130.

MARCHAND, J. and GOODINE, W. (1993). Non-traditional roles for nurses. *Registered Nurse 5* (5), 10–12.

MORSE, J.M., SOLBERG, S.M., NEANDER, W.L., BOTTORFF, J.L. and JOHNSON, J.L. (1990). Concepts of caring and caring as a concept. *Advances in Nursing Science, 13*(1) 1–14.

MUSSALLEM, H.K. (1960). *Spotlight on nursing education: The report of the pilot project for the evaluation of schools of nursing in Canada.* Ottawa: Canadian Nurses Association.

MUSSALLEM, H.K. (1965). *Royal Commission on Health Services: Nursing education in Canada.* Ottawa: Queen's Printer.

MUSSALLEM, H.K. (1977). Nurses and Political Action. In B. Le Sor and M.R. Elliott. (1977). *Issues in Canadian nursing.* Scarborough: Prentice-Hall Canada, 154–181.

NEW BN EDUCATION — NOVA SCOTIA STYLE. (1992). *Edufacts: The news in nursing education, 2*(3), 1.

NEW BSCN PROGRAM FOR NURSES AT YORK UNIVERSITY. (1993). *Edufacts: The news in nursing education, 3*(1), 1.

NEW PHD AND MASTER'S PROGRAMS IN ONTARIO. (1993). *Edufacts: The news in nursing education2*(4), 1–3.

NICHOLSON, G.W.L. (1975). *Canada's nursing Sisters.* Toronto: Samuel Stevens Hakkert. Historical publication 13. Canadian War Museum, National Museum of Man, National Museums of Canada.

NURSING EDUCATION REACHES THE NORTH. (1993). *Edufacts: The news in nursing education, 3*(3), 1, 4.

NURSING MANAGEMENT PROGRAM MOVES INTO UNIVERSITY SYSTEM. (1993). *Edufacts: The news in nursing education, 3*(1), 4.

ONTARIO ANNOUNCES NURSE PRACTITIONER PLAN. (1994) News item. *The Canadian Nurse, 90*(3), 14.

ONTARIO EDGING CLOSER TO ENTRY TO PRACTICE. (1993). *Edufacts: The news in nursing education, 2*(4), 1, 3.

OREM, D.E. (1985). *Nursing: Concepts of practice.* (3rd ed.). New York: McGraw-Hill.

PERCENTAGE OF DEGREE NURSES RISES. (1993). *Edufacts: The news in nursing education, 3*(3), 2.

THE PHD COMES TO CANADA. (1991, June). *Edufacts: The news in nursing education, 1*(1), 1.

REGISTERED NURSES ASSOCIATION OF BRITISH COLUMBIA. (1944). *Position Statement: Education requirements for future nurses.* Vancouver, B.C.: Author.

REGISTERED NURSES ASSOCIATION OF ONTARIO (RNAO). (undated). *RNAO Responds.* Toronto: Author.

REGISTERED PSYCHIATRIC NURSES ASSOCIATION OF BRITISH COLUMBIA. (1993). Correspondence from the Coordinator of Membership Services.

REIGLER, N.N. (1992). *The work and networks of Jean I. Gunn, superintendent of nurses, Toronto General Hospital 1913–1941: A presentation of some issues during her lifetime 1882–1941.* PhD Thesis, University of Toronto.

ROACH, M.S. (1992). *The human act of caring: A blueprint for the health professions* (Revised ed.). Ottawa: Canadian Hospital Association Press.

SIMPSON, R.M. (1938). Mary Agnes Sniveley. *The Canadian Nurse, 34* (8), 401–403.

STATISTICS CANADA. (1980). Nursing occupations (selected tables). *Standard Occupational Classification.* Ottawa: Author.

STATISTICS CANADA. (1992). *Health Reports: Nursing in Canada 1992, registered nurses.* Ottawa: Author. (Statistics Canada Catalogue No. 83–243)

STATISTICS CANADA. (1993). Population 15 years and over with employment income by sex, work activity and detailed occupation (selected tables). *The Nation.* Ottawa: Author. (Statistics Canada Catalogue 93–332)

STEP BY STEP TO A BACCALAUREATE. (1993). *Edufacts: The news in nursing education, 3*(3), 1, 4.

STINSON, S.M., MACPHAIL, J. and LARSEN, J. (1992). *The Canadian nursing doctoral statistics: 1989 update.* Ottawa: Canadian Nurses Association.

STORCH, J.L. (1993, Summer). Calgary conjoint nursing programs. *Edufacts: The news in nursing education, 3*(2), 1.

STREET, M.M. (1973). *Watch-fires on the mountains: The life and writings of Ethel Johns.* Toronto: University of Toronto Press.

THOMAS, G. (1993, June). Working can be harmful to your health. *The Canadian Nurse, 89*(6), 33–38.

UNIVERSITY–COLLEGE COLLABORATION IN BC. (1992). *Edufacts: The news in nursing education, 2*(1), 3.

VANCOUVER HEALTH DEPARTMENT. (1993). Discussions with staff of the West Main Health Unit who are engaged in community development projects.

VICTORIAN ORDER OF NURSES FOR CANADA. (1947). *The Victorian Order of Nurses for Canada 50th anniversary 1897–1947.* Montreal: Southam Press.

VICTORIAN ORDER OF NURSES FOR CANADA. (1983). *Proud achievement: A history of the Victorian Order of Nurses.* (unpublished).

WATSON, J. (1988). *Nursing: Human science and human care.* Unknown: National League for Nursing.

WHAT'S THE DIFFERENCE? PRIMARY NURSING, PRIMARY HEALTH CARE, PRIMARY CARE. *CNA Today, 2*(3), 2.

WEIR, G.M. (1932). *Survey of nursing education in Canada.* Toronto: University of Toronto Press.

WILSON-SIMMIE, K.M. (1981). *Lights out! A Canadian nursing sister's tale.* Belleville: Mika.

The Ethical Basis of Nursing Practice

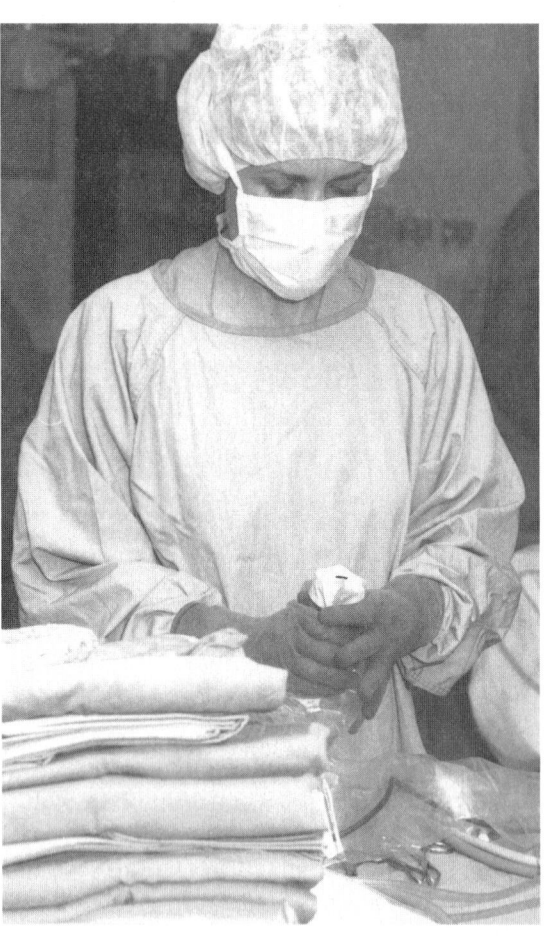

CENTRAL QUESTIONS

1. *What are the objectives of professional nursing associations at the national and international levels? Of nursing unions?*

2. *What ethical values does the Canadian Nurses Association hold?*

3. *What is the difference between licensure, registration and certification?*

4. *How are decisions made regarding the functions nurses are legally permitted to carry out?*

5. *What is the legal status of nurses?*

6. *What rights do Canadians have with regard to health care?*

7. *What mechanisms are in place to ensure that the quality of nursing care is maintained at a high standard?*

8. *What is an ethical dilemma?*

9. *What are the most common acts of negligence committed by nurses and how can they be prevented?*

10. *What is a Good Samaritan Law?*

11. *What is meant by informed consent?*

12. *What responsibilities do nurses have when dealing with confidential information? With wills?*

13. *What is the nurse's role regarding narcotic drugs and other controlled substances?*

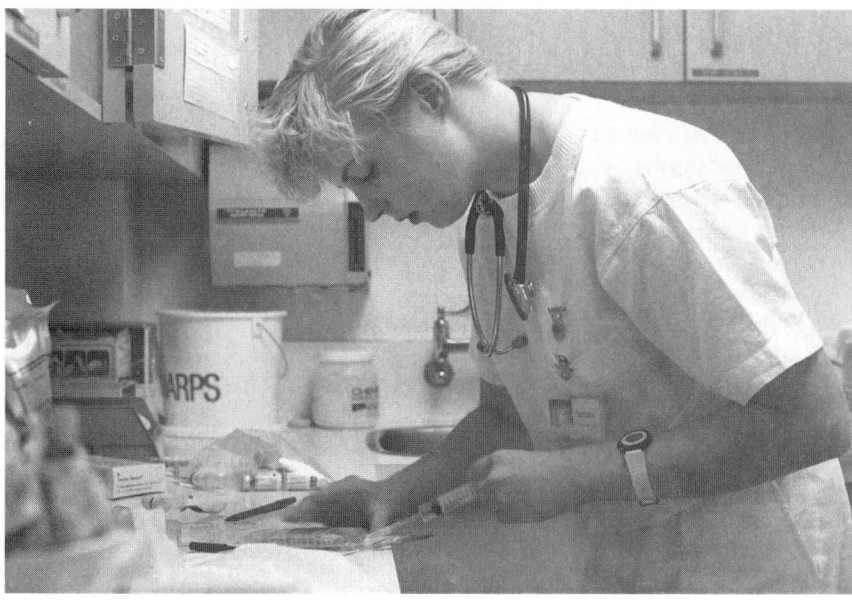

INTRODUCTION

The nurse, by entering the profession, is committed to moral norms of conduct and assumes a professional commitment to health and the well-being of patients. As citizens, nurses continue to be bound by the moral and legal norms shared by all other participants in society. As individuals, nurses have a right to choose to live by their own values (their personal ethics) as long as those values do not compromise care of their patients.

Canadian Nurses Association, 1991. Page one of the
Preamble to the Code of Nursing Ethics.

We all place a great deal of trust in health professionals. We expect them to be qualified to practise their profession, and to provide safe and competent care while respecting our basic rights as human beings. Although nurses are not responsible for all aspects of health care, they have a responsibility to ensure that, insofar as the nursing component is concerned, patients are assured of safe and competent care and that their fundamental rights, such as the right to courtesy, to privacy and to information, will be safeguarded during the process of care.

Most of the developed countries of the world have laws that regulate the practice of health professionals; these laws are intended to protect the public from unqualified practitioners. In some cases, the laws also define the scope of professional practice — that is, they specify the functions that the qualified practitioner may undertake. In many instances, however, the law has been vague in this respect, particularly in regard to the practice of nursing and medicine. Often it has been the professional associations that have undertaken to define the role and functions of the practitioner, based on currently accepted standards of practice.

In most democratic countries, an individual's basic human rights are protected, either in the constitution of the country or in its legally enacted laws. **Consumers' Bills of Rights** developed both in Canada and the United States have sought to further clarify an individual's basic rights as these are applicable to health care. Safeguarding the patient's rights is also an important aspect of the ethical codes adopted by each of the major health professions. These codes extend beyond the legal basis for practice and into the realm of social values to which members of the particular profession are committed. The professional associations have also become increasingly concerned with the need to develop standards to ensure that patients will receive safe and competent care. Both the Canadian Nurses Association and the provincial nursing associations, for example, have developed statements regarding standards that must be maintained in various fields of nursing practice in order to assure the consumer of quality nursing care.

Nurses should be familiar with the Canadian Nurses Association Code of Ethics for Nursing which describes values and obligations considered important in nursing

practice. They should also be familiar with the laws in their province concerning the provision of health care to the public, and particularly with the acts that control the practice of nursing. Nurses should be aware of their functions and responsibilities, both as defined by law and as delineated by their professional nursing associations. It is also important for nurses to be familiar with the various charters that outline consumers' rights in the health care system, and they should be aware of how the law protects the patient in this regard. Nurses should also be cognizant of their own legal status both as students and as graduate nurses.

PROFESSIONAL NURSING ASSOCIATIONS

Professional nursing associations in Canada and other countries, as well as the International Council of Nurses, have been instrumental in developing and promoting a sound legal and ethical basis for nursing practice. We will be referring throughout this chapter to statements made by the professional associations. It would seem important, then, for the beginning student of nursing to know a little about these organizations.

The International Council of Nurses is a non-political, self-governing organization, with headquarters in Geneva, Switzerland. It was founded in 1899 as a federation of national nurses' associations and has two primary objectives: 1) to develop and enhance the national nursing organizations, and 2) to promote favourable working and other conditions for nurses. The ICN holds an international congress once every four years which provides an opportunity for nurses from all member associations, now including over 80 countries, to meet to share common interests and discuss common problems. The 1993 Congress was held in Spain; the 1997 one will be held in Vancouver, British Columbia.

Each member association has one representative (usually its current president) on the Council of National Representatives, which is the policy-setting body of the ICN. The Council meets every two years. Its president, three vice-presidents and board of directors are elected at the previous ICN Congress (Splane and Splane, 1991).

The Canadian Nurses Association had its origins in a joint American–Canadian association called the American Society of Superintendents of Training Schools, which was concerned with the need to improve educational programs for student nurses. This group was established in 1894 and worked closely together for a number of years until 1908 when it divided to form the Provisional Society of the Canadian National Association of Trained Nurses (CNATN) — forerunner of the Canadian Nurses Association — and the National League for Nursing Education (in the United States).

The Canadian association was established at first to represent Canada at the International Congress of Nurses. It became a truly national organization only when the subsequently developed provincial associations joined. These provincial associations originally came into being in response to the need to differentiate between trained and untrained nurses. By 1922, all provinces had some form of Registration Act which set out educational requirements for admission to schools of nursing and delegated responsibility for maintaining the standards of practice in the province to the provincial nursing associations. By 1924, each province had a nurses organization with membership in the CNATN which in that year changed its name to the Canadian Nurses Association (CNA, 1968).

The CNA has retained its interest in the improvement of nursing education but has broadened its scope as befitted a national nursing association. Its objectives are stated as follows:

- To speak for Canadian nurses and represent Canadian nursing to other organizations on national and international levels
- To develop a national perspective on nursing and health-related issues
- To influence national health policy
- To promote high standards of nursing practice, education, research, and administration in order to achieve quality nursing care for the people of Canada
- To provide leadership in issues related to the working lives of nurses.*

The Canadian Nurses Association is a trilevel organization, that is, it is composed of national, provincial and district associations. All of the provincial and territorial associations (with the exception of the one in Quebec) belong to the CNA. The provincial associations are subdivided into district nursing associations, which provide all members with the opportunity to participate in the affairs of their professional association. An interesting trend is the increasing need for nurses in specialized areas of practice to keep up to date with the latest developments in their area by exchanging views with other nurses in the same field. This trend has resulted in the proliferation of Interest Groups within the provincial associations. These groups consist of nurses engaged in a specific area of practice, such as neurological nursing, home-care nursing and other specialized areas. In British Columbia, the interest groups have become Professional Practice Groups within the RNABC and, as of September 1994, had an elected representative on the board of directors of the association.

The Canadian Nurses Association represents nurses and serves as the official voice of nursing in relations with allied national and international organizations, governmental bodies and the public. The provincial associations function similarly within their jurisdictions. The Canadian Nurses Association publishes a monthly professional journal, *The Canadian*

Nurse/L'infirmière Canadienne. This journal serves as the principal resource for Canadian nurses in regard to national and international affairs affecting nursing. It also helps to keep nurses up to date with new developments in nursing through articles reporting on the latest in nursing research and clinical practice. The provincial nursing associations also publish monthly or bimonthly journals. Many of the provincial association journals started out as newsletters but they are rapidly becoming polished journals, along the line of *The Canadian Nurse*. Canada also has a student organization, the Canadian Student Nurses Association/L'Association des Étudiant(e)s Infirmiers et Infirmières du Canada (CSNA/AEIC). This association, to which students in all diploma and baccalaureate nursing programs may belong, is concerned with fostering high standards of nursing education to promote the highest quality nursing care.

CSNA/AEIC holds an annual national conference at which the association's business is accomplished and speakers on various topics are heard. Topics addressed have included women in health care, empowerment and assertiveness. At least one provincial nursing association, the Registered Nurses Association of British Columbia, permits undergraduates enrolled in RN programs to hold student membership in the Association for a nominal fee. Student members elect a student to sit on the Board of Directors, may participate in chapter and provincial activities, may serve on committees and may represent chapters as voting delegates to annual and special meetings.

The Canadian Registered Psychiatric Nurses Association (CRPNA) is composed of only four provincial associations, because there are preparatory programs for RPNs only in British Columbia, Alberta, Saskatchewan and Manitoba. These four provinces are also the only ones which recognize RPNs. The objects of the CRPNA, however, are similar to those of CNA and CAPNA — the promotion of high standards of psychiatric nursing care and the welfare of psychiatric nurses are its main purposes.

The Canadian Association of Practical Nurses and Nursing Assistants (CAPNA) is a national organization composed of provincial associations to promote practical nursing in Canada. As such, it is analogous to the CNA. Its purposes include promotion of the welfare of the Licensed Practical Nurse and the Nursing Assistant as well as promotion of the highest standards of health care. Membership is made up of all nurses who belong to their provincial association of practical nurses.

NURSING UNIONS

All professions must organize themselves to achieve three primary functions:

1. to protect the public
2. to advance the welfare of the professional
3. to promote the profession.

---

* Canadian Nurses Association, 1986.

Different professions and different provinces have organized themselves differently to accomplish these functions, establishing varying combinations of colleges, associations and unions. In 1973, however, the Supreme Court of Canada ruled that the professional association could not act as the bargaining agent for salaried nurses because the professional association was "management dominated." This meant that unions must become separate from associations. At present, there are provincial nursing unions and a union for nurses employed by the federal government, whose primary objective is to advance the social, academic and general welfare of the nurse (Jensen, 1992).

CODES OF NURSING ETHICS

Every profession is based on a code of ethics that commits its members to upholding certain social values. In 1985, the Canadian Nurses Association developed its Code of Ethics for Nursing. This was subsequently revised in 1991, and a commitment was made to review it again in five years. There are 13 values in the CNA Code of Ethics. They are as follows:

CODE OF ETHICS FOR NURSING

VALUE I. A nurse treats patients with respect for their individual needs and values.

VALUE II. Based upon respect for patients and regard for their right to control their own care, nursing care reflects respect for the right of choice held by patients.

VALUE III. The nurse holds confidential all information about a patient learned in the health care setting.

VALUE IV. The nurse is guided by consideration for the dignity of patients.

VALUE V. The nurse provides competent care to patients.

VALUE VI. The nurse maintains trust in nurses and nursing.

VALUE VII. The nurse recognizes the contribution and expertise of colleagues from nursing and other disciplines as essential to excellent health care.

VALUE VIII. The nurse takes steps to ensure that the patient receives competent and ethical care.

VALUE IX. Conditions of employment should contribute in a positive way to patient care and the professional satisfaction of nurses.

VALUE X. Job action by nurses is directed toward securing conditions of employment that enable safe and appropri-

ate care for patients and contribute to the professional satisfaction of nurses.

VALUE XI. The nurse advocates the interests of patients.

VALUE XII. The nurse represents the values and ethics of nursing before colleagues and others.

VALUE XIII. Professional nurses' organizations are responsible for clarifying, securing and sustaining ethical nursing conduct. The fulfilment of these tasks requires that professional nurses' organizations remain responsive to the rights, needs and legitimate interests of patients and nurses.*

Psychiatric and practical nursing associations in many provinces have also developed codes of ethics. The code of ethics developed by the B.C. Psychiatric Nurses Association and the one jointly developed by the B.C. Council of Licensed Practical Nurses and the Licensed Practical Nurses Association of British Columbia are shown below.

CODE OF ETHICS (FOR PSYCHIATRIC NURSES)

… The Code is divided into five sections representing areas of professional nursing obligation.…

THE REGISTERED PSYCHIATRIC NURSE AND THE INDIVIDUAL
• The Registered Psychiatric Nurse:
  • Respects and accepts an individual's uniqueness and integrity regardless of colour; race; national or ethnic origin; creed; sex; age; marital, family or legal status; lifestyle; or social status.
  • Is guided by consideration for the dignity, rights and independence of all patients.
  • Holds in confidence all information obtained in the nurse–patient relationship and uses professional judgement in sharing information when this is in the best interest of the patient and society.
  • Is obligated to inform patients about their care and to ensure informed consent prior to providing care.

THE REGISTERED PSYCHIATRIC NURSE AND PRACTICE
• The Registered Psychiatric Nurse:
  • Accepts responsibility for specific acts and functions based on the Standards of Practice prepared by the Registered Psychiatric Nurses Association ….
  • Provides competent care to patients based on the Standards of Practice and is accountable for outcomes of nursing actions.

* Canadian Nurses Association, 1991.

THE REGISTERED PSYCHIATRIC NURSE AND SOCIETY

- The Registered Psychiatric Nurse:

  - Shares with other citizens the responsibility for initiating and supporting action to meet the mental health needs of individuals and groups within our society.

THE REGISTERED PSYCHIATRIC NURSE AND COWORKERS

- The Registered Psychiatric Nurse:

  - Cooperates and collaborates with other health team members to meet patient needs for care.

  - Takes appropriate action when actions of any health team member are not in conformity with accepted standards of care.

THE REGISTERED PSYCHIATRIC NURSE AND THE PROFESSION

- The Registered Psychiatric Nurse:

  - Demonstrates knowledge of and practices within the boundaries defined by provincial legislation related to the practice of psychiatric nursing.

  - Takes responsibility for continuing individual growth and development.

  - Shares with the professional association, governments, educational facilities and employers the responsibility for ensuring that programs for professional development and continued quality of care are available.*

CODE OF ETHICS (FOR PRACTICAL NURSES)

The Licensed Practical Nurse is committed to conservation of life, prevention of illness, alleviation of suffering and promotion of health and wellness, and will:

a) function within the scope of practice for Licensed Practical Nurses as outlined in the Nurses (Licensed Practical) Act and Regulations and according to agency policy.

b) respect, promote and protect the physical, mental, emotional and spiritual health of the patient and their identified family.

c) be non-judgemental with regard to the patient's particular health care needs and values.

d) respect the patient's dignity and right to participate in decisions regarding their own health care.

e) respect the religious and cultural beliefs and practices of patients.

f) respect and protect the patient's right to confidentiality and disclosure of information.

g) adhere to high standards of personal and professional conduct and maintain optimum personal physical and mental health.

h) maintain and expand knowledge and skill to provide quality care.

i) accept responsibility and accountability for their own professional practice.

j) work collaboratively and cooperatively with all members of the health care team.

k) protect the integrity of the profession of practical nursing and the interests of the patient.**

ETHICS AND NURSING RESEARCH

One area of practice that has been of considerable concern to nurses from an ethical point of view is research that involves human beings as subjects. The Canadian Nurses Association (1994) has developed a position paper, *Ethical Guidelines for Nursing Research*, addressing this issue. The relationship of trust between patient and nurse has always been an essential element of the professional code of ethics. In research, the relationship of trust between subject and investigator requires that the investigator assume special obligations to safeguard the subject in several ways. Subjects in a research study must consent voluntarily to participate. Before obtaining this consent, the researcher must make sure that the subject understands the nature and purpose of the study and is fully aware of his or her role in it. The subject needs to know the risks involved and any potential physical or psychological discomfort that may ensue from participating. For example, in a study to examine the grieving process, asking the participant to discuss his or her reactions to the death of a loved one may bring back painful memories. Subjects also need to be made aware of the extent of any anticipated invasion of privacy. For example, when the study involves asking personal questions, the individual should know the areas to be covered by the questions and the amount of detail required in the answers. Additionally, the investigator must guarantee that no risk, discomfort, invasion of privacy or threat to personal dignity beyond that initially stated in describing subjects' roles in the study will be imposed without further permission being obtained. Finally, subjects must be assured that if they do not wish to participate in the study, neither will they be subjected to harassment nor will the quality of their care be influenced by this decision.

---

* Registered Psychiatric Nurses Association of British Columbia.

**B.C. Council of Practical Nurses and Licensed Practical Nurses Association of B.C., 1992.

NURSING PRACTICE ACTS

The laws in Canada derive from two main sources: the statutes passed by law-making bodies, such as Parliament, and the decisions of the courts. The latter are collectively known as common law. The law is a reflection of public opinion and of civic and social movements within a community. The law therefore is not static — it is constantly changing. Changes in the statutes and the decisions of the courts in cases involving nursing reflect changes in public thinking about nursing. In recent years, there has been an increasing awareness by nurses and by the public of the need to standardize the laws concerning the practice of both the professional and the practical nurse. The authority to control nursing, together with various other professions and occupations concerned with health and welfare, has been vested in the provinces. Thus, each province has enacted its own laws to control the practice of nursing. These laws are generally termed "nursing practice acts," although the exact title of the statute varies in the different jurisdictions. Because each province has set up its own law, it is understandable that the statutes vary somewhat. Nevertheless, the purpose of these laws is the same — that is, to protect the health of the public through the establishment of minimum standards that a qualified practitioner must meet in order to practise as a nurse.

LOOKING BACK

EUNICE HENRIETTA DYKE 1883–1969

Toronto's first "tuberculosis nurse" and first director of the Division of Public Health Nursing for the Toronto Department of Public Health was Eunice Henrietta Dyke. When she took on this challenge in May 1911 at age 28, she was committed to bringing under control the dreaded "white plague" — tuberculosis. Her first major duties were to "register" the cases of TB which, for the first time in Toronto, was made a "notifiable disease." Under her capable administration, she identified some 800 cases in the first year alone and soon had arranged for herself or another nurse to visit all positive and suspected cases.

Soon a small team of nurses was working under her direction, not only to carry out care in the home but also to educate the family and neighbours to prevent the spread of this highly contagious disease. Her public health nurses also visited schools and began to attack the serious problems of high infant mortality and morbidity. She introduced district offices both to cut down on transportation costs and to increase the presence of the health professionals in the neighbourhood. Under her capable and frequently outspoken direction, the city's public health service grew rapidly, soon becoming a model for other cities in North America.

Born in Toronto, Eunice Dyke graduated in 1909 from Baltimore's highly respected Johns Hopkins Hospital School of Nursing, which had an excellent reputation for preparing nurses to carry out public health nursing duties. Her nursing education was interrupted by a bout with tuberculosis and she spent a year as a patient in the Muskoka Sanatorium. Following graduation, she worked as a private nurse in Baltimore, then returned home to Toronto to care for an aunt who was dying of cancer.

Eunice Dyke's innovations as head of the nursing division led the League of Red Cross Societies in Geneva to second her for a four-month consultancy on public health nursing services in 1923. She then returned to Toronto's Department of Public Health until 1933 when she was forced to resign by the newly appointed medical director, with whom she had a serious dispute over the assignment of nurses. The local Council of Women appealed her dismissal to City Hall. Despite strong public support and a close vote in Council, she was not reinstated. However, the immediate offer of a Rockefeller Scholarship indicated the high regard in which she was held by the nursing and health communities nationally and internationally. Following her Rockefeller year and a cross-Canada tour to study public health nursing, she was appointed for a brief period to the Canadian Council of Child and Family Welfare in Ottawa as secretary of the maternal and child division.

After her retirement, she turned her attention to the needs for social and recreational services for the elderly. In 1946, she was instrumental in organizing the "Second Mile Club," where Toronto seniors were offered organized activities and a place to socialize and contribute to the community. Such a service marked her awareness of social needs and was considerably ahead of its time. In 1960, the Canadian Public Health Association made her an honorary life member. After several years of ill health and recurring episodes of cancer, Eunice Henrietta Dyke died in 1969.

Glennis Zilm

LICENSURE AND REGISTRATION

In Canada, with the exception of Ontario, provincial governments have delegated administration of the nursing acts to the provincial nursing associations. In Ontario the responsibility rests with a College of Nurses, which is separate from the nursing association. In Canada, nurses are not licensed; they are, rather, registered by their provincial nursing association and by the College of Nurses of Ontario. A *licence* is a permit granted by a government agency to an individual to engage in the practice of a profession and to use a particular title. The term "*registration*" means the listing of an individual's name on the official roster of a governmental or nongovernmental agency. Nurses who are registered are permitted to use the title "Registered Nurse"; nurses who have failed to register are not permitted to do so. In order to be registered, the nurse must have completed a basic course of nursing studies in a program approved by the registering body, and have passed the national qualifying examinations with an acceptable grade. Nurses from other provinces in Canada may be granted registration by endorsement, as may nurses from other countries, providing their qualifications meet the criteria established by the provincial registering body. Nurses wishing to return to practice after an absence from the professional work force may have their registration reinstated. Provincial agencies are beginning to demand that nurses take refresher courses to update their knowledge and skills if too many years have elapsed since they were last in active practice. Registration must be renewed on an annual basis in order to be valid. A nurse's registration may be revoked if, in the opinion of the disciplinary committee of the registering body, it is not safe to permit him or her to practise nursing. The three principal reasons for revoking a licence are professional misconduct, incompetence and negligence.

In the past few years, there have been a number of changes in registration regulations in Canada. Most of the provincial registered nursing acts now require that the nurse be registered with the provincial association in order to use the term "Registered Nurse" or the initials "R.N." There is a strong movement under way in Canada to make registration compulsory in all provinces. In addition to the laws controlling professional nurses, all provinces have practical nursing laws. Practical nurses, called Registered Nursing Assistants (RNAs) or Certified Nursing Assistants (CNAs)in some provinces, are granted licensure by provincial licensing bodies which administer the provisions of the act regulating practical nursing in that province. Psychiatric nursing is regulated under separate provincial legislation, and registration is mandatory for psychiatric nurses in the four provinces which recognize it as a separate branch of nursing. The regulatory body for psychiatric nursing is the provincial professional association. Graduates of RPN programs write the registration examinations for psychiatric nurses set by the provincial associations.

CONTINUING EDUCATION REQUIREMENTS

The speed with which new knowledge and technology are becoming available in nursing has created problems in keeping the practitioner up to date with the latest developments in the field. In Canada, although there has been considerable discussion about mandatory continuing education as a requirement for continued practice, no province to date has incorporated it into its registration renewal process. Instead, many associations now require nurses to have practised a minimum number of hours in the preceding year in order to renew their registration. Ultimately, it is up to the individual nurse to keep an up-to-date level of knowledge and skill.

CERTIFICATION

The many changes in nursing and in health care in Canada have made it very difficult for nurses to acquire all of the knowledge required to practise in all settings. Because of this, nursing practice is becoming increasingly specialized. There has been a lack of agreement and some confusion, however, over just what is a specialty, what the requirements to practise in the specialty should be and how continued competence in the specialty can be assessed and assured. In order to address some of these issues, the CNA developed a policy statement on specialization and certification (1982). In its statement, a *specialty* is defined as: "A specifically defined area of clinical and functional nursing with a narrowed, in-depth focus, necessary for the safe delivery of the full range of services required in that area of nursing" (CNA, 1982).

The CNA's *certification* process includes the designation of a specialty, the development of an examination by the Canadian Nurses Association Testing Services and the certification of individuals. Candidates must meet the eligibility requirements established for that specialty. On passing the examination in their selected specialty through the CNA certification program, an individual is certified for a period of five years. Recertification normally requires a specified minimum amount of time in practice, a certain number of continuing education hours and a satisfactory performance appraisal. The CNA distinguishes the nurse who acquires certification through this process from the *clinical nurse specialist*, who is a nurse with advanced preparation in a clinical area at the master's or doctoral level (CNA, 1993).

AREAS OF NURSING FUNCTION

Nursing practice, as we have already noted, is constantly changing in response to societal needs. Guidance on what constitutes nursing practice has come principally from two sources, the nursing practice acts and the statements of the professional nursing associations. Because of the interdependence of nursing and other health care professions, these professions frequently consult each other and often make joint statements on functions nurses may undertake. The opinions of provincial attorneys generally provide some additional assistance from the legal point of view, although these opinions usually pertain to specific situations (Philpott, 1985).

THE LAW AND NURSING FUNCTIONS

In the past few years, there have been an unprecedented number of changes in nurse practice acts in Canada, as nurses have felt the need to have imbedded in the law a more precise definition of nursing practice and a clearer description of their role and functions than previous statutes contained. Most nursing (and medical) practice acts in the past were written in broad, general terms. The general nature of the wording permitted both disciplines to enlarge the scope of their practice without the need for changes in the law each time and, also, made possible the orderly transfer of many procedural functions from medicine to nursing without recourse to the law. Not too many years ago, for example, only physicians were permitted to start intravenous infusions, yet today this is an accepted nursing procedure. One of the principal reasons for the need for a more precise definition of nursing practice has been the development and rapid proliferation of expanded roles for nurses. In some aspects of expanded role practice, as, for example, when a nurse practitioner initiates treatment on his or her own, the question of the legality of these actions has arisen. Another reason for precise definition has been the increasing concern by governments for legislation pertaining to all health personnel and government suggestions for changes in existing statutes. Examples of some definitions of nursing practice found in provincial nurse practice acts are as follows:

> Quebec: *"Every act the object of which is to identify the health needs of persons, contribute to methods of diagnosis, provide and control the nursing care required for the promotion of health, prevention of illness, treatment and rehabilitation, and to provide care according to a medical prescription constitutes the profession of nursing."*

(Nurses Act RSQ, Chapter 1, Quebec, 1989)

> British Columbia: *"The 'practice of nursing' means the performance for others of health care services that require the application of professional nursing knowledge and skills and includes (a) promoting, maintaining or restoring the health of the general public, (b) teaching nursing theory or practice,*

> *(c) counselling persons in respect of health care, (d) coordinating health care services, and (e) engaging in administration, supervision, education, consultation, teaching or research for any of the foregoing."*

(Nurses (Registered) Nurse Act Rules Part 1, British Columbia, 1988)

In addition to the definitions of nursing practice in provincial laws, the provincial nursing associations have issued guidelines from time to time regarding the additional functions that may be performed by nurses when these are delegated by a physician. Although statements made by professional associations lack the authority of legally enacted statutes, they are generally persuasive in that they reflect common practice (Philpott, 1985).

PROFESSIONAL VERSUS PRACTICAL NURSING FUNCTIONS

A **Licensed Practical Nurse (LPN)**, called a Registered Nursing Assistant (RNA) in Ontario and a Certified Nursing Assistant (CNA) in Alberta, is trained in basic nursing techniques and in direct patient care. The LPN/RNA/CNA practises under the supervision of a registered nurse or a physician in hospitals as well as other health care settings. They also provide nursing care in patients' homes with RNs giving direction and assuming responsibility for their care. Educational programs for this group are generally one year long. LPNs/RNAs/CNAs are licensed by their provincial licensing body after completing an approved educational program and passing a licensure examination.

THE LEGAL STATUS OF THE NURSE

The nurse in his or her practice can be classed as either an independent contractor or an employee. Private duty nurses, that is, nurses who are engaged by the patient to perform nursing service, come under the category of independent contractors. Nurses who are working in independent practice in the community (not in the employ of a community agency) would also be considered independent contractors. Nurses who work in hospitals or clinics, in public health agencies, in industry or for private physicians are considered employees. The distinction is a matter of authority. While all nurses are responsible to society, their professional association and their patients, independent contractors develop and are responsible for following their own policies and procedures. Employees, however, are also responsible to the employing institution and must follow the institution's policies. Nursing students, when assigned for clinical experience to a hospital or other health agency, are usually considered employees, since they are subject to the authority of nurse managers, clinical instructors and staff nurses and physicians (Philpott, 1985). In a hospital school of nursing, students are generally held to be employees of the hospital insofar as they perform services for the hospital and are supervised by its staff. Students in college or university schools of nursing may, however, be entirely under the supervision of the faculty of their school while in the practice area.

It is helpful for students to remember, however, that even though they may be responsible to others, they are still responsible for their own actions. Anyone who gives nursing care, whether student or graduate, assumes certain duties, and it is expected that these will be carried out with **reasonable prudence** under the circumstances. *Reasonable prudence* is taken to mean that the individual acts with the care that any reasonable person with his or her knowledge, education and experience would take. It is important to determine the status of the nurse because, under the law, not only are individuals liable for their own actions but their employers are also liable under the rule of *respondeat superior* (let the master answer). Thus, if a nurse is negligent and a patient is harmed, both the nurse and the employer can be sued. Nurses are not absolved of responsibility for their actions simply because they may be carrying out the orders of a physician. The law states that the nurse must understand the cause and effect of the treatment that is undertaken. If nurses carry out orders that they know are wrong, they are guilty of negligence. At all times the patient's safety must be paramount. If nurses undertake work that they know is beyond the scope of their education or experience — for example, performing an action or treatment that is defined as being within the province of medical practice — they may again be considered negligent or guilty of malpractice (Philpott, 1985).

CONSUMERS' RIGHTS IN THE HEALTH CARE SYSTEM

The art of healing has, from ancient times, been imbued with an aura of mystery, and magical powers have been attributed to those who practice the healing arts. Even modern practitioners of "scientific Western medicine" — nurses, physicians and other health professionals — have, until fairly recently, tended to perpetuate the belief that the average lay person could not possibly understand the complex workings of the human body or have the knowledge and experience to choose the best treatment. Through the use of technical jargon that is incomprehensible to anyone outside the health field, and in many other subtle (and some not-so-subtle) ways, health professionals usually managed

to convey to patients that they really should not question what was being done for them but simply trust in the experts to cure them of their ills. There is no doubt that trust

Consumer Rights in Health Care

1. Right to be informed
   - about preventive health care including education on nutrition, birth control, drug use, appropriate exercise
   - about the health care system, including the extent of government insurance coverage for services, supplementary insurance plans and the referral system to auxiliary health and social facilities and services in the community
   - about the individual's own diagnosis and specific treatment program, including prescribed surgery and medication, options, effects and side effects
   - about the specific costs of procedures, services and professional fees undertaken on behalf of the individual consumer

2. Right to be respected as the individual with the major responsibility for his own health care
   - right that confidentiality of his health records be maintained
   - right to refuse experimentation, undue painful prolongation of life or participation in teaching programs
   - right of adult to refuse treatment, right to die with dignity

3. Right to participate in decision making affecting own health
   - through consumer representation at each level of government in planning and evaluating the system of health services, the types and qualities of service and the conditions under which health services are delivered
   - with the health professionals and personnel involved in direct health care

4. Right to equal access to health care (health education, prevention, treatment and rehabilitation) regardless of the individual's economic status, sex, age, creed, ethnic origin and location
   - right to access to adequately qualified health personnel
   - right to a second medical opinion
   - right to prompt response in emergencies.

SOURCE: Consumers' Association of Canada, 1974.

is still a very important ingredient in the relationship between health professional and health consumer, but today's patient is viewed as an active member of the health team rather than a passive recipient of care. No longer is it felt that the physician or the nurse, or any other health professional, has a divine right to knowledge that is too far above the head of the average citizen. The average citizen of today is much more knowledgeable about the complicated mechanisms of the human body, and the things that can go wrong with it, than his or her parents or grandparents were. People learn from the popular media about the latest advances in medical treatment and surgical procedures. They also feel that they have a right to question the treatment they are being given, to have a say in the treatment and to be kept informed of their progress. There has been an active and growing consumer movement in the health field in recent years. Increasing public awareness of health issues, increased knowledge about health and illness, and the rising costs to the consumer of health services are three major factors that have contributed to this movement. Additionally, the fact that people have become more conscious of their rights generally — particularly women, people of the First Nations and members of minority ethnic groups — has had repercussions in the health field. Consumer bills of rights have been developed and widely publicized, in Canada by the Consumers' Association of Canada and, in the United States, by the American Hospital Association.

Charters on the rights of members of special groups have also been developed and made public. For example, declarations on the rights of the mentally retarded and those of disabled persons were adopted by the General Assembly of the United Nations in 1971 and 1975 respectively; the Dying Person's Bill of Rights was developed in 1975 at a workshop in Lansing, Michigan, on care of the terminally ill; and the Pregnant Patient's Bill of Rights was published by the International Childbirth Education Association in 1975. While these charters do not have the force of legally enacted statutes, they have been influential in raising the consciousness of consumers of health services so that they feel freer to express their dissatisfactions with the health care system and are less reluctant to demand their rights. The charters have also increased the awareness of health care workers of the fundamental rights of patients as human beings and as citizens.

ACCOUNTABILITY, SAFETY TO PRACTISE AND QUALITY ASSURANCE

One of the most pressing concerns of individual nurses and of professional nursing associations at present is to ensure that patients receive safe and competent nursing care re-

gardless of the setting or the circumstances under which that care is given. Health professionals have long been concerned about the need to maintain high standards of practice. However, the growing rise of consumerism in the health field and the generally increased sophistication of the public in relation to health care matters have put additional emphasis on the accountability of health professionals to the public they serve. Also, our elected representatives in government are becoming increasingly concerned about the quality of health care, since health care is taking more and more of provincial budgets. They too are demanding that the work of health professionals be monitored to ensure that high quality standards are maintained. We are hearing a lot these days about accountability, about safety to practise and about quality assurance. As beginning students, you are probably wondering what these terms mean, and how they affect you. **Accountability** means that a person is answerable (or accepts responsibility) for his or her own actions. Health professionals must be able to "account" for the care they give, to tell precisely what they did and why they did it. The term was initially used in the business world, but has now taken on a much broader meaning. Individual practitioners and health care institutions are being held accountable for both what they do and what they have said they will do, as well as for the process by which it is done (Quinn and Smith, 1987).

Safety to practise means simply what it says — the nursing profession, along with other health professions, makes sure that beginning practitioners have the knowledge and skills necessary to practise their profession competently and without harming the people to whom they render care. Ensuring that the practitioner remains "safe to practise" has become of increasing concern to the health professions. It used to be that once nurses, physicians or dentists had completed a basic educational program and passed qualifying examinations, their names would be inscribed on a permanent roster and they could practise throughout their lifetime — providing, of course, that they did not commit some flagrant offence that caused them to have their licence or registration revoked. The rapidity with which health care is changing, however, and the increasing emphasis on accountability have made it imperative that the professions develop mechanisms to ensure that practitioners remain competent and "safe to practise" throughout their professional careers.

Quality assurance, another term borrowed from the business world, refers to a program designed to ensure that health care provided to patients is consistently of good quality. In any situation in which health workers are providing services for the public, the quality of care the patient receives is dependent on at least the following four variables:

1. the providers of the care — the nurses, physicians and all others who contribute to patient care
2. the standards that are maintained in the agency providing care

3. the environment, or setting, in which the care is given
4. the recipient of care — the patients themselves.

In attempting to ensure that patients receive good nursing care at all times, the nursing profession has given a great deal of consideration to each of these four variables and has developed a number of mechanisms to try to ensure that the practice of nursing is consistently safe and of good quality.

THE PROVIDERS OF CARE

We have already mentioned several ways in which the nursing profession tries to ensure that its practitioners are competent and safe to practise. Perhaps it is time, however, to pull all of these together with others that we have not discussed so far. The quality of the providers of care (the nurses themselves) is assured by the following controls:

1. *Accreditation*/Approval of Basic Nursing Education Programs. Minimum standards for basic nursing education programs have been established in each province in Canada. All programs preparing candidates for registration are carefully monitored by the provincial nursing associations (or the College of Nurses in Ontario). Provincial approval is granted to schools of nursing meeting the minimum criteria. Another type of accreditation of schools of nursing is that done by the Canadian Association of University Schools of Nursing (CAUSN). This accreditation is concerned with optimum, rather than minimum, standards. In other words, accreditation by CAUSN certifies that an educational program has not only met minimum standards, but is considered "good" by national standards.

2. National Qualifying Examinations. The Canadian Nurses Association provides national testing services, which may be used by provincial registering bodies for the examination of candidates for the nursing profession. These examinations are available in both French and English. Appendix 3 contains further information on the CNA Nurse Registration/Licensure Examinations.

3. Licensing/Registration. The licensing/registration mechanism is the basic safeguard protecting the public from unsafe practitioners and assuring employers that the individual has met certain standards established by the licensing/registering body as minimum requirements for entry to practice.

4. *Disciplinary Bodies*. All professional nurse registering/licensing agencies in Canada have established disciplinary bodies that monitor the practice of nurses to whom they have granted registration/licensure. Depending on the severity of a nurse's infraction, the disciplinary body may reprimand the individual, suspend the individual's registration for a time or revoke the registration or licensure completely.

5. Continuing Education. The rapid expansion of knowledge in the health field means that all practitioners need to update their knowledge and skills on a continuing basis throughout their professional careers.

6. Certification. Certification provides yet another mechanism for ensuring the competence of practitioners — at a level higher than licensure. The Canadian Nurses Association has established a certification program for nurses who have achieved expertise in practice in specialized fields of nursing.

7. Assessment of Clinical Competence. A number of mechanisms have been developed that attempt to judge a nurse's competence in clinical practice:

   a) the traditional method has been the supervisor's rating of the nurse's performance in the work setting. Although numerous performance rating scales have been tried to make the ratings as objective as possible, it is difficult to eliminate the subjective bias from an assessment of one person's work by another.

   b) *peer review* is a method of assessing the quality of care provided by a practitioner through a review of his or her work by a group of peers. Methods used in this review may include looking at care plans or patient records written by the nurse, gathering evaluations from patients cared for by the nurse and from professional coworkers, and reviewing evidence of attendance at continuing education programs.

   c) a *nursing audit* is a method of evaluating nursing care through a review of patient records which document the care given. It may be used for evaluating a single nurse's clinical performance, or for assessing the quality of care on a given nursing unit or in an agency.

   d) the problem-oriented medical record (POMR) was hailed as an excellent means of evaluating the quality of care given by practitioners since it requires a detailed analysis of the individual patient's problems, a statement of the reasoning behind actions the practitioner takes, and precise documentation of those actions and their results. It did not, however, gain the wide acceptance in health care agencies that was anticipated.

STANDARDS OF CARE

In assessing the quality of care provided by individual health practitioners or by health agencies, it is essential to have objective criteria by which to judge whether the care given is good, adequate or unsafe. Such objective criteria both protect the public and regulate the practice of nurses. The national and provincial nursing associations have developed standards for nursing practice. An example of such standards are those from the Registered Nurses Association of British

Columbia which are classified according to the characteristics of a profession:

- STANDARD 1: The nurse bases practice on nursing science and on related content from other sciences and humanities.
- STANDARD 2: The nurse diagnoses actual or potential problems and strengths, plans interventions, performs planned interventions and evaluates outcomes.
- STANDARD 3: The nurse provides nursing services, coordinates activities and collaborates with others in providing health care services.
- STANDARD 4: The nurse adheres to the ethical standards of the nursing profession.
- STANDARD 5: The nurse assumes primary responsibility for maintaining competence and fitness to practise, and for acquiring new knowledge and skills.
- STANDARD 6: The nurse maintains standards of nursing practice and professional behaviour determined by the Nurses (Registered) Act, RNABC and the practice setting (RNABC, 1992).

In addition to the standards for practice developed by the professional nursing associations, individual health agencies have been attempting to determine standards that nurses in their agency consider important in the care of patients. This work has resulted in the development of standard nursing care plans for the care of patients with particular health problems, for example, patients who have had a cerebrovascular accident (stroke), who are unconscious, or who are undergoing different types of surgery. We will be discussing this topic at greater length in connection with the nursing process in Unit 2. The important point here is that these standard plans provide guidelines for nurses to assess, through reviewing documented records of patient care, whether everything that should have been done in the way of nursing care for a patient with a particular health problem was indeed done.

THE PRACTICE SETTING

In order for nurses to give good care to patients, the environment in which they work must permit and encourage good nursing care. In talking about the physical and social environments as determinants of health (in Chapter 3), we discussed some of their effects on individual and group health. Similarly, in considering the environment in which nursing is practised, one must take into account both the material things necessary to provide care and the social environment of the agency that encourages or discourages the maintenance of high standards of nursing care. Individual nurses and their professional nursing organizations have become increasingly concerned about such matters as ensuring that nurses have a safe environment in which to practise, that they have sufficient equipment in good working order to work with, that nursing units and community

health units are adequately staffed with competent personnel and that nurses are not required to work in areas for which they are not prepared, or in situations that conflict with their values.

THE PATIENT

The fourth variable in any health care situation is the patient. Because patients are human beings, in all their infinite variety, this is probably the least predictable element in the situation — and the most difficult to provide with adequate safeguards. The best prepared practitioner working in an agency with the highest standards and under the best possible conditions of work can still not guarantee the patient's response to care. The elderly woman whose mouth needs attention may spit the mouthwash the nurse has given her all over the bed. A "helpful" patient may lend his salt shaker to a neighbour who is on a salt-free diet. The emergency room patient "high" on drugs or alcohol may lash out at anyone who comes near, foiling the attempts of health personnel to provide the needed care.

ETHICAL CONCERNS OF NURSES

BASIC VALUES

Both ethical principles and laws are derived from the values to which people in a given society subscribe. Our National Health Insurance Plan legislation, as we mentioned in Chapter 3, has been based on the belief held by Canadians that everyone has the *right* to adequate health services, regardless of income, race, religion or geographic location. We mentioned earlier that the codes of ethics developed by different professional associations are based on the values to which members of that profession subscribe. Laws are concerned with setting minimum standards of behaviour; ethics provide us with ideal standards for right and wrong. Fowler, an ethicist, suggests that ethical standards may sometimes exceed or conflict with the law (1987 in Perry and Ericksen, 1993).

ETHICAL PRINCIPLES

If you have taken a course in philosophy or religion, you may have wrestled with such questions as "What is truth?" and "What is right?" Nurses, and other people who serve the public, are particularly concerned with one aspect of "What is right?" — namely, "What is right in terms of our responsibilities to others in society?" Four ethical principles that relate to this issue are autonomy, beneficence, nonmaleficence and justice.

Autonomy All people have the moral right to make decisions about themselves and their own behaviour in accordance with their values. **Autonomy** is the right to self-determination. This principle is incorporated in Value II in the CNA Code of Ethics.

Beneficence The principle of **beneficence** requires that the nurse do good and prevent harm. Promoting the highest level of independence for your patients exemplifies this principle. The nurse's actions should always be such that they promote the patient's well-being and prevent harm to the patient. It is important to keep in mind, however, that your perception of what is good for the patient may not necessarily be the same as the patient's perception. The good gained from wearing an incontinence pad, for example, may be offset by the blow to a patient's self-esteem in having to wear a "diaper" — "like a baby." (Perry and Ericksen, 1993).

Nonmaleficence **Nonmaleficence** means to do no harm. The nurse must carry out all interventions with meticulous care, bearing in mind that the patient's well-being is the most important priority. The principle of nonmaleficence is one of the issues in arguments for and against both abortion and euthanasia. The issues of abortion and euthanasia, and the termination of life support, are very controversial ethical issues (Simpson, 1992).

Justice The principle of justice is highly esteemed in Canadian society. Beauchamp and Childress (1989) suggest that there are essentially two principles of justice: minimal justice and material justice. In regard to health care, **minimal justice** would hold that the poor are as entitled to health care as the rich. **Material justice**, based on need, would see that scarce health resources, such as cardiac surgery, would be allocated according to the individual's need for service, rather than his or her ability to pay. The rising costs of health care in both Canada and the United States have provoked wide-scale debate on criteria for the allocation of our resources for health services (Perry and Ericksen, 1993).

ETHICAL REASONING

The 1991 revision of the CNA Code of Ethics for Nursing gave increased recognition to the nurse's role as patient advocate (Dunphy and Merger, 1993). In acting as patient advocate, nurses often find themselves in situations of conflicting values. Particularly problematic are situations where nurses must make decisions regarding care of the terminally ill. Regrettably, "the very technology that supports life has the capacity to prolong death" (Anderson, Gladue, Laurie, Skothiski and Tramer, 1991, 37).

If the patient has indicated to the nurse that he or she "just wants to be allowed to die with dignity" but aggressive treatment has been ordered, the nurse is faced with an *ethical dilemma* — a problem with two conflicting moral values (Yeo, 1991). On the one hand, the nurse has an obligation to support the treatment decisions made for the patient and to carry out the therapeutic measures ordered. On the other hand, the nurse also has an obligation to maintain the patient's right to make decisions regarding care, as well as an obligation to protect the patient from assaults on his or her dignity which may occur with aggressive treatment (Anderson et al., 1991).

Situations posing ethical dilemmas for nurses are very seldom clear choices between right and wrong — they are usually complicated by a number of intervening variables. The nurse's own cultural, religious and moral values may differ from those of the patient. Then too, nurses are both autonomous practitioners with obligations to uphold the ethical values of the nursing profession as well as employees who must adhere to policies laid down by the agency for whom they work. **Moral distress** is the term used to describe the situation of knowing the right thing to do, but being unable to pursue the right course of action because of agency constraints (Schattschneider, 1992).

In all situations where there are ethical dilemmas, the nurse has a responsibility to use sound reasoning based on the values set out in the CNA Code of Ethics. The nurse should also bring difficult ethical problems she or he

---

Knowledge Needed for Ethical Dilemmas

KNOWLEDGE OF THE SITUATION: A case history and knowledge of the roles and opinions of major participants helps to clarify the facts and the nature of the dilemma.

KNOWLEDGE OF ONESELF AND ONE'S VALUES: An understanding of one's own philosophy of nursing helps to clarify one's options and sometimes the nature of the dilemma.

KNOWLEDGE OF THE PROFESSION'S VALUES: In Canada, the CNA Code of Ethics defines the profession's expectations of the nurse.

KNOWLEDGE OF THE LAW: While ethical behaviour is not always consistent with legal behaviour, knowledge of the laws impinging on the dilemma aids in identifying consequences of alternative actions.

KNOWLEDGE OF PHILOSOPHY: Application of ethical principles as well as ethical theories provides a broader philosophical perspective to the problem at hand.

SOURCE: Perry, J. and Ericksen, J. (1993). Legal and ethical issues. In A. Beckingham and B. Du Gas. *Promoting healthy aging*. St. Louis: Mosby, 367. Reprinted with permission of the author.

encounters, where appropriate, for discussion with others whose opinions they trust. Many health agencies have an Ethics Committee whose responsibility it is to review the ethical implications of research projects and to give careful thought to ethical decisions that must be made by agency staff members.

A number of different frameworks exist for looking at ethical reasoning. However, regardless of the theoretical perspective, there are five components of knowledge considered essential to the resolution of ethical dilemmas (Perry and Ericksen, 1993). These are shown in the box on p. 125.

LEGAL ISSUES OF INTEREST TO THE NURSE

TORTS AND CRIMES

In addition to understanding their ethical responsibilities as professional nurses, nurses should be aware of their legal responsibilities as well. Nurses often become witnesses or defendants in various types of legal proceedings. Generally speaking, there are two types of court actions in which nurses may be involved. The first is called a *tort*. A **tort** is a legal wrong committed by one person against the person or property of another. The injured party may sue for damages and, if the suit is successful, is usually awarded money to be paid by the other party. Sometimes this is spoken of as a civil suit, as opposed to a criminal action.

A *crime* is also a legal wrong but, in general, it refers to a wrong committed against the public and is punishable by the crown. The punishment for a crime is either a fine or imprisonment. In a criminal action, the case is designated in the form Regina versus Mary Jones; in a tort, the form used is John Doe versus James Jones, or Mary Doe versus the Blank Hospital. Acts such as murder, manslaughter and robbery are considered crimes, whereas negligence and malpractice are usually torts. The case against Susan Nelles is an example of a criminal action. Ms Nelles was a nurse at the Hospital for Sick Children in Toronto and was wrongfully accused of a number of infant deaths on one of the wards at the hospital. After a lengthy investigation, she was cleared of all wrong-doing (Charbonneau, 1985; Grange, 1984; Dubin, Gilchrist, McDonald and Nadler, 1983; RNAO, undated; Hamilton, 1993).

NEGLIGENCE AND MALPRACTICE

It has already been noted that each individual is responsible for his or her own actions and that nurses can be held liable for their own negligent actions. **Negligence** is legally de-

fined as the omission to do something which a reasonable person, guided upon those considerations which ordinarily regulate the conduct of human affairs, would do, or doing something which a prudent and reasonable person would not do. The standards of care which a reasonable and prudent nurse would use in a particular situation are established by the courts through the review of nursing texts, nursing curricula, nursing standards and the testimony of expert witnesses.

The term *malpractice* is virtually synonymous with professional negligence. As a general rule, nursing negligence usually means failure by the nurse to take the appropriate action to protect the patient from harm. Negligence may involve either doing something that ought not to be done or failing to do something that ought to be done. Thus, if the nurse does not assess a patient's heart rate prior to giving digitalis, for example, and the patient dies, the nurse may be considered negligent. Similarly, failure to put up side rails on the bed of a confused patient could also be considered negligence on the nurse's part. Any individual, professional or nonprofessional may be sued for negligence; when the negligence is on the part of a professional person, it is deemed malpractice. It should be noted that, although the term is most frequently used in connection with cases involving negligence, malpractice may include other claims against a professional person (for example, breach of contract).

Because of the increase in the number of malpractice suits in general, and against nurses in particular, many authorities now recommend that each nurse carry malpractice insurance to cover the cost of lawyers' fees and possible damages. Several of the provincial nursing associations in Canada have made malpractice insurance available to their members at a reasonable cost or as one of the benefits of membership. Many nurses have the mistaken belief that, because they are employees, their employer will carry the burden of responsibility for their negligent actions. This is not so; the nurse can be sued as an individual as well.

COMMON ACTS OF NEGLIGENCE

Professional nurses may be called upon to testify in a legal proceeding in regard to some matter pertaining to their work. The most common incidents leading to legal proceedings involving a patient and a nurse are those in which negligence is a factor. The most common of such acts of negligence that have resulted in suits for damages involve burns, falls, medication, malfunctioning apparatus and abandonment. We shall look at each of these in turn.

Burns   Hot water bottles, heating pads, inhalators, steam radiators, enemas, douches and sitz baths can all cause a patient to be burned. Nurses may be held responsible if they have neglected to take the usual safety precautions, such as taking the temperature of the water used in a solution administered to a patient or keeping articles that might burn the patient out of reach.

Falls   Another common type of accident that may result in injury to the patient and subsequently a suit for damages is falling from bed. The usual safety precautions against falls include the use of side rails. Most health agencies have rules regarding the use of side rails for patients at risk of falling, for example, those who are recovering from anaesthesia and those under sedation. The nurse should remember, though, that the competent, alert patient has the right to refuse side rails as long as she or he has been informed about and understands the risks involved. The risk of falling must be balanced against the risk to the patient's dignity.

Wrong medicine, wrong dosage, wrong patient, wrong concentration   Another common area in which negligence occurs is in giving medications. Labels can be misread or may not be read at all. The nurse may fail to identify the patient correctly and consequently give a medication to the wrong person. Numerous errors are made in giving medicines. With the tremendous increase in the number of medications taken by patients and the numerous commercial names commonly used for the various drugs, safety precautions assume greater importance in ensuring that the right patient gets the right drug in the proper concentration at the right time and in the proper manner.

Defects in apparatus or supplies   Patients can be injured by the use of defective equipment. Nurses are not held responsible if patients are injured as a result of hidden defects, but if equipment or supplies are known to be faulty, nurses may be held liable. The use of unsterile gauze for a surgical dressing might be an example of negligence relating to defective supplies.

Abandonment   Instances in which patients have been left unattended and have injured themselves as a result have led to suits for negligence. If a nurse left a baby on a table and the baby fell in the nurse's absence, this might result in a negligence suit.

The above are by no means all the acts of negligence which have resulted in suits for damages. To guard against negligence, nurses should always use knowledge and judgement in providing care and follow established professional and agency guidelines and policies.

INCIDENT REPORTS

The nurse has an ethical and a legal responsibility to report to the health agency any accidents, losses or unusual occurrences. Most health agencies have special forms for this purpose. The primary purpose of reporting these incidents is to protect the patient and the nurse by ensuring that there is a record of the details of the incident and the subsequent action taken, in the event that legal proceedings are instituted. Incident reports are also useful as a source of information in research to improve the quality of care and the effectiveness of policies.

GOOD SAMARITAN LAWS

Some provinces have enacted legislation designed to protect the professional practitioner from all practice suits arising from care given to the injured at the scene of an accident or other emergency. Some of these statutes cover physicians only; others, all health care practitioners. In some instances, the law covers any individual who renders first aid at the scene of an accident, with the exception of persons who receive compensation for such acts, for example, ambulance workers or other emergency personnel. The laws are provincial rather than national; therefore, they tend to vary from one jurisdiction to another. These laws are usually referred to as **Good Samaritan laws** and are intended to encourage qualified people to give aid in an emergency. In general, these laws protect the individual who renders emergency care from civil liability for this care, unless he or she is guilty of gross negligence or extreme malpractice in giving the care.

In some provinces, there is specific legislation stipulating that no one may leave the scene of an automobile accident without first giving aid to those injured in the accident. The *Ontario Highway Traffic Act* also places an obligation on people directly or indirectly involved in an accident to render assistance to those who have been injured. In the absence of such a law, there is no legal compulsion for the nurse, or anyone else for that matter, to give assistance in an emergency. If aid is given voluntarily, the person giving the aid is under an obligation to give the best care possible under the circumstances, commensurate with his or her knowledge, training and experience. Thus if a nurse stops at the scene of an accident and gives emergency care as she or he has been taught (for example, applying pressure to stop bleeding), the nurse would be acting within accepted standards (Philpott, 1985).

ASSAULT AND BATTERY

In some instances, nurses have been involved in legal proceedings as a result of a charge of assault and battery by a patient. **Assault** refers to a threat to do physical harm to another, together with an apparent ability to carry out that threat. **Battery** is the actual touching of another person without consent. Assault and battery are considered criminal offences as well as torts. At all times, undue force is to be avoided in caring for patients. The law protects every individual against bodily harm by another person and also against any form of assault due to interference with his or her person. Therefore, a nurse cannot take a blood sample from a patient without consent. Nor may a person be operated on for any condition unless consent for the procedure has been obtained and the patient understands the significance of the procedure. Force-feeding a patient who refuses to eat may also be considered an assault.

The nurse may also be the victim of assault by a violent patient. If the assault results in injury, the nurse has a legal right, just as any other person, to sue the person who committed the assault. Although the problem of nurses (and other staff) being assaulted by patients is by no means new, it is receiving increased attention as health agencies become more concerned about safety in the workplace. Support services are being developed to assist staff who have been assaulted by patients. These services may include medical, psychological and legal services (Ryan and Poster, 1991).

INFORMED CONSENT

One of the most fundamental rights of patients is the right to consent to treatment. It is a well-established principle of law and ethics that competent individuals have the right to make their own decisions — including decisions about whether or not to have even life-saving treatment. Respect for this principle has led to the legal doctrine of informed consent. Informed consent is based on the ethical principle of autonomy.

Health professionals' belief that certain treatment is desirable for a person does not give them the right to go ahead with that treatment without the consent of the patient, except in an emergency. In an emergency, when treatment is a matter of life and death *and* the patient is unable to give permission, consent may be implied. In the past few years a number of lawsuits have centered on the issue of a patient's lack of consent to treatment. Although suits of this nature usually involve physicians or health agencies, the nurse may be called upon as a witness, for example, to attest to the patient's mental condition at the time consent was given to treatment. The nurse is also frequently asked to obtain the patient's signature on a consent form. She or he should be aware of the implications of these actions from a legal and ethical point of view.

Legally, *informed consent* means that the consent must be freely given, informed and specific to both the treatment and the caregiver (Philpott, 1985). In order for a consent to be valid, the patient must be of such mental capacity that he or she is capable of deciding whether or not to have the proposed treatment. In order to make that decision, the patient must be given sufficient information (in a language the patient understands) to give an informed consent. It is the physician's direct responsibility to inform patients about medical or surgical treatment — this is not a responsibility that can be delegated. The nurse may, however, present the form granting permission for medical or surgical treatment to the patient for a signature. In doing so, the nurse is simply verifying the identity of the patient — his or her signature does not require the nurse to determine whether the patient has had sufficient information to make a rational decision.

All health professionals should know, however, that the mere existence of a signed consent form does not by itself constitute a legal informed consent. Legally, there must be evidence that the patient is, indeed, informed. The ethical implications of witnessing a patient's signature on a consent form are, however, different from the legal implications. As a patient advocate, the nurse should ensure that the patient is informed about and understands what is being consented to. This does not mean that the nurse must supply the information — unless it is within the scope of nursing knowledge — but the nurse has an ethical obligation to make sure the patient gets the necessary information from the appropriate professional.

Professional nursing associations are concerned about the nurse's ethical responsibilities with respect to informed consent, and some have issued guidelines for nursing action in the form of policy statements. The Registered Nurses Association of British Columbia, for example, in their position statement on informed consent states that:

> *While registered nurses are responsible for explaining to the patient the care and treatment they give, physicians are legally responsible for informing patients of impending medical or surgical treatment. If a nurse should witness a consent form, this does not constitute obtaining the patient's consent. Nevertheless, nurses are ethically obliged to assess the patient's understanding of the proposed treatment and to inform the physician and/or the appropriate agency representative if there is reason to believe the patient has any misunderstanding regarding the nature, purpose, inherent risks or alternatives of his or her treatment.*

(RNABC, 1990)

In the case of children, either parent may give permission for treatments and operative procedures. The age when individuals are no longer considered minors and can give their own consent to medical treatment varies in different jurisdictions, from 14 years of age (in the province of Quebec) to 21 years in others. Canadian law is increasingly recognizing that age by itself does not signify competence; rather it is an individual's ability to understand the information and weigh the alternatives that matters. While it is unlikely that someone under the age of 13 would be able to demonstrate this, an older teenager may be able to do so. A teenager who no longer lives at home and is self-supporting may be legally deemed an *emancipated minor* and, as such, considered an adult for the purpose of giving consent for medical treatment. A *mature minor* is one who has demonstrated that he or she has the intelligence, understanding and independence to make decisions in regard to the acceptance or rejection of medical treatment. Many hospitals are in the process of revising both their procedures for obtaining consent from patients and the forms that are used. Nurses should familiarize themselves with those that are being used in the agencies they practice in. A general consent form and one used for specific operations or other special procedures are shown in Figures 6.1 and 6.2.

**LIONS GATE HOSPITAL
CONSENT
FOR EXAMINATION & TREATMENT**

I, the undersigned, do hereby certify that the purpose of this visit or admission to Lions Gate Hospital and the nature of the procedure(s) mentioned below have been explained to me by my physician.

I, hereby authorize Dr. _____ and/or such assistants as may be

selected by him/her to perform the following procedure (s) _____

_____

_____

_____

I recognize that, during the course of the operation, unforeseen conditions may necessitate additional or different procedure(s) than that/those set forth above. I, therefore, further authorize and direct the above named surgeon, his/her assistants or his/her designees, to perform such procedure(s) as are, in their professional judgement, necessary and desireable, including but not limited to, procedures involving pathology and radiology. The authority granted under this paragraph shall extend to remedying conditions that are not known at the time the operation is commenced.

I consent to the administration of any anaesthetics, blood transfusions or intravenous medications that the attending physician(s) consider necessary.

Dated this _____ day of _____, 199 _____

_____
Signature of Witness

(1) Signature of Patient: _____

(2) Signature of Guardian: _____
(or person authorized to consent for patient)

_____
(Reason patient unable to sign)

_____
(Relationship of above)

In situations where it is impossible to obtain a signature on line (1) or (2) above, two physicians shall certify by signing the following:

In the opinion of each of the undersigned physicians the treatment to be carried out is necessary and in the best interest of the continued health and well-being of the patient.

Dated this _____ day of _____, 199 _____

_____ M.D.

_____ M.D.

_____
Signature of Witness

_____
Signature of Witness

FIGURE 6.1   General Consent

SOURCE: Lions Gate Hospital, North Vancouver, B.C. Reproduced with permission.

AUTHORIZATION FOR SURGICAL OPERATION OR DESIGNATED SPECIAL PROCEDURE OR TREATMENT

RE: _____
(Name of Patient)

With regard to the above-named patient, I, the undersigned, do hereby consent to the following treatment or procedure

_____

_____

under the direction of _____, M.D./D.D.S.

The nature and anticipated effects of such treatment, surgical operation or special procedure as detailed above have been explained to me and I understand the explanation. I also consent to the administration of anaesthesia and to the use of such anaesthetics as may be deemed advisable.

I understand that for the purposes of medical education there may be students in attendance or observing.

Signed: _____ Signed: _____ _____
(by M.D. obtaining consent)   (Patient or person legally authorized to give consent)   (Relationship to patient)

Print name: _____ Print name: _____
(Physician obtaining consent)   (if not patient)

_____ / _____ hours
(Date and Time of Consent)

PATIENT UNDER 16 WHERE NO PARENT OR LEGAL GUARDIAN IS AVAILABLE:
We consider that the operation or special procedure described above is in the best interest of the continued health and well-being of the patient and that no legal guardian is available **OR** the patient has expressed the request that his/her legal guardian not be notified.

Signed: _____ M.D. Signed _____ M.D.
I st M.D.   2nd M.D.

Print name: _____ Print name: _____

TELEPHONE CONSENT:
I have discussed the above procedure and the nature of the anticipated effects of such treatment, surgical operation or special procedure outlined above

with _____ who is the patient's (state relationship) _____ and he/she has given verbal consent for the above named procedure.

Signature of M.D.: _____ Date: _____

Print name: _____

DECLARATION BY INTERPRETER:
This document was interpreted by me to the patient who acknowledged in my presence that he/she understood the explanation and consented to the procedure described above.

Signed: _____ Date: _____

Print name: _____

FIGURE 6.2 Consent to Operation or Special Procedures

SOURCE: Vancouver General Hospital

FALSE IMPRISONMENT

Individuals who are unjustifiably detained, or confined against their will and without a legal warrant for detention, may bring charges of **false imprisonment** against the individual or the agency that detained them. Most instances in which nurses have been involved in court proceedings on charges of false imprisonment have been in relation to patients with mental health problems. Canadian law provides for the detention without a warrant of persons who are mentally ill and who may hurt themselves or others, and also for the confinement of persons with selected communicable diseases that present a danger to society, for example, a person with tuberculosis in the highly contagious stage.

People cannot be prevented from leaving health agencies if they are of sound mind, even if health professionals feel that leaving would be inadvisable. If the patient insists on leaving, most agencies require that the patient sign a release stating that the agency will not be held responsible for any resulting harm. As with all patient decisions, the nurse and other health professionals should try to inform the patient in this situation of the risks and alternate courses of action. The use of force to hold someone against his or her will, or even the threat of forcible restraint made in order to detain a person, is considered assault. The nurse must therefore exercise caution in the use of restraints, as we have noted above.

INVASION OF PRIVACY

Under Canadian law, every individual has the right to withhold both self and property from public scrutiny. The right does not hold, however, if the individual has given consent for exposure; nor is there a tort when the person is a public figure or one who does acts of public interest (Philpott, 1985). A common instance in which the nurse must guard against invasion of a person's right to privacy is in the taking and use of photographs of patients. Consent must be obtained if these are to be used in any way not connected with the patient's treatment. Care must be taken by nurses also to avoid the exposure of a patient to roommates, visitors or others during the process of nursing care or when the patient is being transported from one area to another in the health agency.

Technology makes it more important than ever to take precautions to safeguard privacy. The use of tape recorders, videotapes and two-way mirrors without the patient's knowledge and consent could be taken as invasion of privacy.

DEFAMATION OF CHARACTER

Another area of the law the nurse should be aware of is that of suits arising from defamation of character.

Defamation of character occurs when a person's reputation is damaged by written or spoken words that tend to lower his or her esteem in the eyes of other people. If the defamation is in a published article or a letter to a third party, or is depicted in a cartoon that causes the person to be the subject of ridicule or contempt, the term **libel** is used (Picard, 1978). **Slander** refers to defamation of character through spoken words. The nurse should always be careful not to discuss patients except with others who are involved with their care. Not every negative mention of a patient is slander or libel, of course; these terms are used only when there is a threat to the individual's reputation. To state that a patient had a broken leg would not be defamatory. If, however, one added that the broken leg was the result of a fall down the stairs because the patient was intoxicated, this might be considered defamation of character.

THE NURSE AND CONFIDENTIAL INFORMATION

The right to privacy extends also to information about the patient. The patient's record contains confidential information; it should not be left where it might be read by unauthorized persons. In using information from patients' records (or any information obtained from the patient) for case studies or other types of classroom work, the student nurse should be careful not to reveal the patient's identity; nor should information about a patient be discussed carelessly with people who are not entitled to that information. The nurse should always be discreet in giving out information about patients. Care should also be taken to limit access to computerized information about patients.

The CNA Code of Ethics for Nursing (Value III) specifically states that the nurse has a responsibility to hold in confidence all information regarding a patient learned in the health care setting. Legally, the betrayal of a patient's confidence is covered under the area of professional misconduct and may result in discipline by the professional organization. Whether confidential information entrusted to the nurse by the patient is considered to be a privileged communication and therefore inadmissible as evidence in court proceedings has not been definitely settled. In Canada, the rule of privilege for confidential information is not absolute. Although the nurse and the physician should not disclose confidential information entrusted to them, they may be directed to do so if this is justified by public policy or if the law requires reporting of the matter or if the individual consents. The law requires that a witness in a court proceeding answer all questions that are relevant whether or not the answer is incriminating. The witness can, however, invoke the protection of the *Canada Evidence Act* in certain cases. Mark Siegler, an ethicist, reminds us, however, that it is the little indiscretions that the principle of confidentiality most probably arose to prevent (Siegler, 1982). Thus, the nurse should take care not to discuss patients in elevators, in the cafeteria, at home and so forth.

WILLS

Nurses are often asked to witness a will for a patient. A *will* is a declaration of an individual's wishes regarding what is to be done with his or her property after death. The individual making the will is called the **testator**. A will must ordinarily be in writing and must be signed by the testator. The law usually requires the signature of two or three competent witnesses in addition. Because an individual who may expect to benefit from a will should not act as a witness to its signing, the family and close friends of a patient are naturally reluctant to be witnesses. The nurse is therefore frequently called upon to act in this capacity, as the nurse is not an interested party. The nurse who is a minor should not agree to act as a witness, however. Minors — persons under the legal age as defined by the law of the particular province — are not usually acceptable as witnesses.

In most jurisdictions, all witnesses are required to be present at the same time and to sign the will in the presence of the person making it. Prior to signing the will, the witness should see the testator sign the will. If, however, the will has already been signed, the witness should either ask the testator to sign again or to declare that this is his or her will and signature and that the testator was competent to sign. It is not necessary for the witness to know the contents of the will, nor in most jurisdictions is it necessary for the witness to be told that the document is a will.

For a will to be valid, the person making it must be capable of understanding what he or she is doing. If the patient dies and the validity of the will is questioned, a nurse may be called upon to testify in court concerning the mental capacity of the individual at the time the will was made, even if the nurse was not a witness to the will. If the nurse is aware that a patient has made a will while in the hospital, it is a good practice to note on the patient's record the fact that a will was made, the date and time that it was signed, and the nurse's observations regarding the mental state of the patient at the time the will was made.

A *living will* is a form of what is called an advance directive in which an individual writes down preferences for treatment in the event that he or she cannot decide for him- or herself. Advance directives are increasingly common because people are afraid of what might happen if they become unable to make decisions for themselves. They often fear that they will be "hooked up to machines" when they would prefer to be allowed to die. At present, living wills have no legal authority in Canada, although there is considerable effort on the part of consumer groups to enact living will legislation. Nonetheless, a living will is often considered to be some evidence of a person's wishes. Patients should be counselled to discuss with their family members and physicians their preferences for treatment. Some agencies have policies about including a patient's living will in the patient's record.

CONTROLLED SUBSTANCES LEGISLATION

Another area of the law in which the nurse is involved is in the control and administration of narcotics and other potentially harmful drugs. In Canada, the control of narcotic drugs is under federal jurisdiction, the pertinent legislation being the Narcotic Control Act and Regulations. This legislation controls the use of a number of drugs classified as **narcotics** (substances which induce drowsiness, sleep, stupor or insensibility). Certain other drugs, for example, the barbiturates, have also been designated **controlled drugs** — those drugs which, under Canadian law, only certain persons are authorized to prescribe and dispense. Agencies develop policies based on these laws that nurses and other health professionals are responsible for upholding. These persons include physicians, dentists and veterinarians, but not nurses. Nurses are considered to be acting as agents of the physician when they administer controlled drugs. Nurses functioning as nurse practitioners in areas with few doctors usually prescribe and dispense medications (including controlled drugs) under *standing orders* from the physician, who is providing medical supervision, albeit on a remote basis. It is unlawful for nurses to have narcotic drugs in their possession. The attempt to obtain narcotic drugs by fraud or deceit is a violation of the law. Penalties for violation include fine or imprisonment or both. The nurse must be careful when handling narcotics to see that they have been ordered in writing by a duly licensed physician and that careful records are kept of their use.

KEY TERMS

consumers' bills of rights p.114

licence p. 119

registration p. 119

specialty p. 119

certification p. 119

clinical nurse specialist p. 119

licensed practical nurse
   (LPN) p. 120

reasonable prudence p. 121

accountability p. 122

safety to practise p. 122

quality assurance p. 122

accreditation p. 123

disciplinary bodies p. 123

peer review p. 123

nursing audit p. 123

autonomy p. 125

beneficence p. 125

nonmaleficence p. 125

minimal justice p. 125

material justice p. 125

ethical dilemma p. 125

moral distress p. 125

tort p. 126

crime p. 126

negligence p. 126

malpractice p. 126

good samaritan laws p. 127

assault p. 127

battery p. 127

informed consent p. 128

emancipated minor p. 128

mature minor p. 128

false imprisonment p. 131

defamation of character p. 131

libel p. 131

slander p. 131

will p. 132

testator p. 132

living will p. 132

narcotics p. 132

controlled drugs p. 132

IN REVIEW

Nurses have a responsibility to provide safe and competent care to their patients and to respect their patients' fundamental rights while doing so. Professional nurses associations have been instrumental in developing and promoting sound ethical and legal bases for nursing throughout the world. The International Council of Nurses (ICN) is a federation of national nursing associations. The Canadian Nurses Association (CNA) is a member of ICN. CNA is a tri-level organization composed of national, provincial (or territorial) and district nursing associations. In addition, there is a Canadian Student Nurses Association of Canada, a Canadian Association of Practical Nurses and Nursing Assistants, and a Psychiatric Nurses Association of Canada which has provincial associations in British Columbia, Alberta, Saskatchewan and Manitoba. Professional associations at all levels are concerned with both promoting the welfare of nurses and advocating high standards of nursing care. They also represent nursing and serve as the official voice for nursing in relations with other organizations, governmental bodies and the public.

In Canada, we also have nursing unions which serve as bargaining agents for salaried nurses. The unions are concerned with the social and financial welfare of their members.

In Canada, nursing is regulated by provincial/territorial *Nursing Practice Acts* with authority for administration delegated to the provincial/territorial nursing associations, except in Ontario where authority has been delegated to a separate College of Nurses. The *Nursing Acts* protect the health of the public by registering nurses to practice and by setting standards for practice. The functions nurses perform are outlined in provincial laws and are usually further delineated in professional nursing association guidelines.

Legally, all nurses are responsible to society, to their professional association and to their patients. *Reasonable prudence* is expected of all nurses and each nurse is accountable for his or her own actions. While student nurses are responsible to their supervisors, whether faculty or agency personnel, they are also responsible for their own actions. Nurses, graduate or student, are guilty of negligence if they carry out orders they consider wrong, or those which are beyond their level of competence.

Accountability, safety to practise and quality assurance are all matters of concern to nurses. Individual practitioners and health agencies are accountable both for what they do and for what they say they are going to do. The registration/licensure mechanism was designed to ensure that practitioners are competent. Quality assurance programs are established to ensure that patient care is consistently of good quality. Standards of nursing practice have been developed by national and provincial nursing associations and by many health agencies. In addition, a number of mechanisms have been developed to ensure that the quality of nursing care is maintained at a high standard.

The Canadian document on *Consumer Rights in Health Care* (1974) states that consumers have the right to be informed, to be respected as having the major responsibility for their own health care, to participate in decision making affecting their health and to have equal access to health care.

Professional Codes of Ethics are based on the values to which members subscribe or their standards of right and wrong. The CNA Code of Ethics commits its members to certain social values. Ethical principles of particular concern to nurses are those of autonomy, beneficence, non-maleficence and justice. When faced with ethical dilemmas, nurses have a responsibility to use sound reasoning based on the values set out in the CNA Code of Ethics.

Legal matters in which nurses could become involved include torts, crimes, negligence, malpractice, assault, battery, invasion of privacy, false imprisonment and defamation of character.

Informed consent is a fundamental right of the patient to consent to treatment (principle of autonomy). Legally this means informed, consensual, freely given and specific to both the treatment and the caregiver. The patient must be judged as being adequately informed and mentally competent. The nurse has the ethical responsibility to ensure that the patient is adequately informed before the consent form is signed.

A will is a declaration of an individual's wishes regarding the disposition of property after death. The person must be mentally competent for the will to be valid. Nurses may witness a will if they are of legal age in that jurisdiction. A living will is an advance directive regarding treatment preference in the case where a person is terminally ill and unable to make decisions. Although not a legal document in any jurisdiction in Canada, a living will indicates a person's preferences.

Narcotics and certain other substances are controlled under the Federal Government Narcotics Control Act and its regulations. Under this Act, nurses are not allowed to prescribe or dispense narcotics or controlled drugs and they must keep careful records on the administration of these substances.

LEARNING ACTIVITIES

1. What issues are currently of concern to CNA, your provincial association, your district association and the nursing union in your province?

2. Do you have a student association at your nursing school? Is it affiliated with the provincial/territorial nursing association? Does your class have a representative on it? What issues are of current concern to the student association?

3. What is the title of the provincial statute(s) regulating nurses in your province? When was it (were they) passed? How does it (they) define the functions of nurses? Does your professional association have guidelines delineating nurses' functions? Compare the functions of registered nurses, registered psychiatric nurses (if applicable in your province) and licensed practical nurses (registered or certified nursing assistants) as

these are specified in nursing acts and in professional association guidelines in your province/territory.

4. Discuss with your classmates the Susan Nelles case, using the following questions as a basis for your discussions:

   a) Why was Susan Nelles charged with the murder of infants at the Hospital for Sick Children in Toronto?

   b) What evidence led to her arrest?

   c) What were the findings of the Grange Inquiry?

   d) What were the recommendations of the Dubin Commission?

   e) How did the professional nursing association respond?

   f) What new evidence/theories have been put forth to explain the deaths of the infants?

REFERENCES AND READINGS

ANDERSON, M., GLADUE, S., LAURIE, M., SKOTNISKI, E. and TRAMER, D. (1991). Who has the right to choose? *The Canadian Nurse, 87*(10), 37–39.

B.C. COUNCIL OF LICENSED PRACTICAL NURSES and LICENSED PRACTICAL NURSES ASSOCIATION OF B.C. (1992). *Code of ethics.* Vancouver: Authors.

BEAUCHAMP, T.L. and CHILDRESS, J.F. (1989). *Principles of biomedical ethics.* New York: Oxford University Press.

CANADIAN NURSES ASSOCIATION. (1968). *The leaf and the lamp.* Ottawa: Author.

CANADIAN NURSES ASSOCIATION (1982). *Credentialling in nursing: Policy statement and background paper.* Ottawa: Author.

CANADIAN NURSES ASSOCIATION (1986). *Reports of biennial meetings 1981–1986.* Ottawa: Author.

CANADIAN NURSES ASSOCIATION (1991). *Code of ethics for nursing.* Ottawa: Author.

CANADIAN NURSES ASSOCIATION (1993). *Statement on the clinical nurse specialist.* Ottawa: Author.

CANADIAN NURSES ASSOCIATION.(1994). *Ethical guidelines for nurses in research involving human participants.* Ottawa: Author.

CHARBONNEAU, L. (1985). The Grange Report: Nurses criticize commission's report for lack of answers. *Canadian Nurse, 81*(3), 14–18.

CONSUMERS ASSOCIATION OF CANADA. (1974). *Consumer rights in health care.* Toronto: Author.

DUBIN, C.L., GILCHRIST, J.M., MCDONALD, H.D. and NADLER, H.L. (1983). *Report of the Hospital for Sick Children Review Committee.* Toronto: Alan Gordon, Queen's Printer of Ontario.

DUNPHY, E. and MERGER, M. (1992). The revised code of ethics: an overview. The *Canadian Nurse, 88*(10),19–21.

EUNICE HENRIETTA DYKE (1960). *Canadian Journal of Public Health, 51*, 287.

EUNICE HENRIETTA DYKE. (1990). In *Herstory* [Annual Calendar]. Toronto: Women's Press, 6; 112.

GRANGE, S.G.M. (1984). *Report of the Royal Commission of Inquiry into certain deaths at the Hospital for Sick Children and related matters.* Toronto: Ontario Ministry of the Attorney General. (Available by mail through Publications Services, 5th Floor, 880 Bay Street, Toronto, Ontario)

HAMILTON, G. (1993). The nurses are innocent. *The Canadian Nurse, 89*(11), 27–32.

JENSEN, P.M. (1992). The changing role of nurses' unions. In A.J. Baumgart and J. Larsen (1992). *Canadian nursing faces the future.* St. Louis: Mosby, 557–573.

NURSES (REGISTERED) ACT RULES, Part 1. (British Columbia,1988).

NURSES ACT RSQ Chapter 1. (Quebec, 1989).

PERRY, J. and ERICKSEN, J. (1993). Legal and ethical issues. In A. Beckingham and B.W. Du Gas. *Promoting healthy aging.* St. Louis: Mosby, 353–369.

PHILPOTT, M. (1985). *Legal liability and the nursing process.* Toronto: W.B. Saunders.

PICARD, E. (1978). *Legal liability of doctors and hospitals in Canada.* Toronto: Carswell.

QUINN, C.A. and SMITH, M.D. (1987). *The professional commitment: Issues and ethics in nursing.* Toronto: W.B. Saunders.

REGISTERED NURSES ASSOCIATION OF BRITISH COLUMBIA (1990). *Position statement: Informed consent.* Vancouver: Author.

REGISTERED NURSES ASSOCIATION OF BRITISH COLUMBIA (RNABC). (1992). *Standards for nursing practice in British Columbia.* Vancouver: Author.

REGISTERED NURSES ASSOCIATION OF ONTARIO (RNAO). (undated). *RNAO responds. A nursing perspective on events at the Hospital for Sick Children and the Grange Inquiry.* Toronto: Author.

ROYCE, MARION. (1983). *Eunice Dyke: Health care pioneer: From pioneer public health nurse to advocate for the aged.* Toronto: Dundurn Press.

RYAN, J. and POSTER, E.C. (1991). When a patient hits you. *The Canadian Nurse, 87*(8), 23–25.

SCHATTSCHNEIDER, H. (1992). Ethics for the nineties. *The Canadian Nurse, 88*(10), 16–18.

SIEGLER, M. (1982). Confidentiality in medicine: A decrepit concept? *New England Journal of Medicine, 301,* 1518–1521.

SIMPSON, R. (1992). Nursing ethics and euthanasia. *The Canadian Nurse, 88*(11), 36–38.

SPLANE, R. and SPLANE, V.H. (1991). International nursing: Looking beyond our borders. In *Canadian nursing: Issues and perspectives* (2nd ed.). J. Kerr and J. MacPhail (Eds). Toronto: Mosby, 353–365.

YEO, M. (1991). *Concepts and cases in nursing ethics.* Peterborough: Broadview Press.

Research and Nursing Practice

CENTRAL QUESTIONS

1. *What is meant by research-based practice?*

2. *What is my role as a student in research-based practice?*

3. *How do we know things?*

4. *Why do nurses do research?*

5. *What kinds of research are Canadian nurses doing?*

6. *What is involved in critiquing a research report?*

7. *How can I understand research reports?*

8. *What is the purpose of the abstract?*

9. *What is a problem statement? Hypothesis? Assumption?*

10. *What kinds of research design are there?*

11. *What do the terms "sample," "population," "independent variable" and "dependent variable" mean?*

12. *How do I interpret the results of research findings?*

13. *What is the purpose of a statistical analysis of data?*

14. *How can I tell from the analysis whether the findings of the study are valid?*

15. *What can I learn from the discussion section of a report?*

16. *What does "clinical significance" mean?*

17. *What does the term "scientific merit" mean?*

INTRODUCTION

Research is central to the development of theories for nursing practice. It stimulates growth of the body of knowledge upon which the practice of nursing is built.

Canadian Nurses Association, 1990

We said at the beginning of this text that research-based practice is an imperative for all who practise nursing in Canada today. You will, no doubt, have one or more courses on research methodology and on statistics at a more senior level in your program. In this chapter, we are concerned with helping you to gain an appreciation of the role of research in nursing practice, so that you can base practice on a solid research foundation from the first clinical assignment. In order to do this, it is essential to have some understanding of the research process and of the kinds of research that nurses in Canada and in other parts of the world are doing. You must also develop beginning skills in reading research reports, interpreting the findings and assessing the usefulness of these for your practice.

In this chapter, then, we will talk first about the meaning of the term, *research-based practice*, and your role as students in regard to its various components. We will then discuss some basic concepts, such as ways of knowing, the goals of research and the kinds of research nurses are doing in Canada. The major portion of this chapter will be devoted to learning to read and understand research reports. As you gain skill in reading reports, you will also gain some understanding of the process a researcher follows in conducting a study.

RESEARCH-BASED PRACTICE

HISTORICAL PERSPECTIVE

The idea of basing one's clinical practice on nursing research is a radical change from even 10 years ago. Although nurses have in the past made extensive use of research done in other fields, particularly in the social and the biomedical sciences, there has until recently been a dearth of nursing studies. Nursing research was slow to develop in Canada for several reasons. First, there has been a scarcity of nurses qualified to undertake research. Courses in research and statistics are recent additions to nursing undergraduate programs. Research courses were generally reserved for graduate programs, and graduate programs in nursing in research methodology and the statistical treatment of data were few in Canadian universities. The first master's level program in nursing at a Canadian university was established at the University of Western Ontario in 1959. Nurses wishing to

undertake graduate studies prior to that time entered programs in other disciplines such as education or public health, or they went to American schools of nursing (Field, Stinson and Thibeaudeau, 1992). Although there are now 13 master's level programs in nursing in Canada, the number of places in these programs is still inadequate to meet the demand by nurses for graduate study. And we still have only four doctoral programs in nursing at Canadian university schools.

Then, too, research takes time and nurses in clinical practice have always been too busy to undertake studies. It was not considered part of the practising nurse's role; research was done by scientists in universities. Nowadays, however, most large hospitals and community health agencies have nurse researchers on staff to carry out studies and to help other nursing staff formulate research questions and undertake studies relevant to their practice area.

Nurses have also had to overcome a lack of self-confidence in their ability to undertake research. Research has traditionally been associated with the academic world; it was considered by many to be beyond the realm of ordinary nurses educated for the most part in hospital schools of nursing. And most highly qualified nurses, those with master's or doctoral degrees, were teaching in university or collegiate schools of nursing; they were not practising on the nursing units of hospitals. That picture has changed dramatically in the past decade, as we noted in Chapter 5. There are many nurses in both hospital and community agencies with baccalaureate, master's and doctoral degrees. The number of clinical nurse specialists is increasing and agencies are employing people with doctoral degrees in senior positions. In many agencies, nurse researchers hold workshops and conferences for nurses at all levels. These workshops help them not only to use the research that is being done but also to formulate questions worthy of research from situations they encounter in practice and to carry out studies to resolve problems they have identified (Brown, 1993; RNABC, 1990).

Components of research-based practice

"Research-based practice" includes three components:

1. the conduct of studies
2. the dissemination of research findings
3. the utilization of research in practice.

CONDUCTING NURSING RESEARCH

One of the questions frequently asked by students is, "Are all nurses expected to do research these days?" The answer is that not all nurses design and conduct research studies

EVALINE MARY PEMBERTON CIRCA 1875–1949

Canada's first "Registered Nurse" was Evaline Mary Pemberton of Halifax; hers was the initial signature on the official Register when Nova Scotia enacted the first nursing legislation in Canada in April 1910. As president of the Graduate Nurses Association of Nova Scotia, she had been one of the growing number of nurses in Canada who, in the early 1900s, lobbied their provincial governments for protection of the public through registration. Before that time, no legislation in Canada had recognized the need for standards for nursing practice.

Although nursing education had shown great strides in the preceding 35 years, legislation to register nurses and have nurses set standards for practice was something entirely new in Canada. The Graduate Nurses Association of Nova Scotia was not the first provincial organization of nurses; the Graduate Nurses Association of Ontario had been formed from hospital nurses' alumnae groups in 1904 and by 1910 several provinces had associations. However, the small group of Nova Scotia nurses organized in 1909 under president Evaline Pemberton was determined to achieve official status for properly educated "graduate" nurses who would be certified as safe practitioners. They were the first to get a provincial body to act.

Little is documented about Evaline (also spelled Eveline) Pemberton's personal life. She graduated in 1894 in the sixth class of the School of Nursing of Western Hospital of Montreal (later part of Montreal General) and was immediately placed in charge of the Women's Hospital in Montreal. Her records show that she also at some time received a certificate in Home Economics from Battle Creek (Michigan) Sanatorium and took a course at New York's Bellevue Hospital. She then moved to England, where she attended Queen Victoria's Jubilee Institute for Nurses and was appointed a Queen's Nurse in 1897. She stayed at least eight years in England, finally working as nurse-in-charge of the Victoria Nursing Station in Grantham, Lincolnshire. When she returned to Canada, she became matron of the Edgehill Church School for Girls in Windsor, Nova Scotia, at which time she became active in forming the Graduate Nurses Association of Nova Scotia. She remained active in the Association for many years. In 1922, when the Act of 1910 was amended, the Association issued official Certificates of Registration and awarded Certificate Number One to Evaline Pemberton as first president and charter member, thus making her "Canada's first Registered Nurse."

Glennis Zilm

but all nurses are expected to be aware of research being done in their area, to be able to read and interpret research findings and to use relevant findings in their practice. Because one of the basic societal functions of a university is to push back the boundaries of knowledge, it is understandable that a considerable amount of research in nursing is being conducted by people in university schools of nursing — master's and doctoral level students and faculty. Completion of an "original" research project (either as a thesis or as a smaller study) is one of the requisites for a master's degree in nursing as it is in most other disciplines. The doctorate (in any field) is considered a research degree; completion of a dissertation (the report of a major research study) is always a requirement and the major focus of doctoral studies. Except in a few instances, all university faculty members are required to undertake research in their field as an ongoing part of their workload. In addition, there are the research "scholars" and "fellows" who have received funding to enable them to devote themselves full-time or part-time to conducting studies.

As we mentioned in our discussions on the role of government in Chapter 4, a major source of funding for nurses is Health Canada's National Health Research and Development Program. Other major sources include The Canadian Nurses Foundation, provincial governments and provincial nursing association foundations as well as private organizations. The Medical Research Council and the Social Sciences and Humanities Research Council of Canada (SSHRC) are also potential sources of funds for nursing research. There is considerable competition, however, and nurses must compete with scientists from other fields. The increasing number of nursing research fellows and scholars attests to the quality of studies being undertaken by nurses.

In addition to nursing studies conducted in universities, a considerable amount of research is taking place in clinical agencies and by staff nurses with the help of agency staff who are skilled in research methodology or with the help of faculty members from a university school of nursing.

SOLO AND COLLABORATIVE RESEARCH

Master's and doctoral candidates are required to undertake *solo research* — research that is done independently by one person. Other nurses may conduct their own studies as independent researchers or they may do **collaborative research** — research done in teams with colleagues, people in other agencies, people in other provinces or countries or with members of other disciplines. Research teams are becoming common in nursing, as in many other disciplines, with the faculty and associated clinical staff of one agency collaborating on one particular area of enquiry and several people undertaking studies on various aspects of it. For example, at the University of Ottawa School of Nursing several colleagues have been involved in research in patient decision-making, exploring beliefs, values and social influences on decisions to quit smoking or decisions concerning suicide, toxic cancer treatments, immunization for Hepatitis B and influenza and the duration of breast feeding (CNA, 1991).

A large amount of inter-agency research is also being done; collaboration between university faculty and staff of an affiliated hospital is very common, as are university and community agency research teams. Collaboration between hospitals is also occurring more and more, as in the case of the Calgary District Hospital Group who have completed several studies on different aspects of caring for the elderly. We are also seeing interprovincial collaboration on research projects, as for example, the Western Consortium of Cancer Nurses who have carried out a project on the prevention and treatment of chemotherapy-induced mouth sores with researchers from all four western provinces examining various aspects of the problem (CNA, 1991,1992; Church, Thurston, Tenove and Weisgerber, 1991; RNABC, 1991).

INTERNATIONAL COLLABORATION

Many Canadian University and Collegiate Schools of Nursing are engaged in international projects to help with the development of nursing education in third world countries. For example, the University of Ottawa School of Nursing has had a project with the Tienjin Medical College School of Nursing in China for several years to help faculty with their baccalaureate program. The School of Nursing at Dalhousie University has had a project with a school in Tanzania and the University of Manitoba School of Nursing one in Chengdu, China — and there are many more. Many faculty from Canadian universities are collaborating on research with their colleagues in these countries.

Some collaborative international research is done by students meeting requirements for a master's or doctoral degree. A student from China studying at the University of Manitoba may wish to do research for a master's degree on a nursing problem in China or, as travelling fellowships for nurses become more common, Canadian nursing students may undertake to collect data for their study in another country. There may also be collaboration between experienced researchers in different countries as in, for ex-

ample, the Denmark–Newfoundland project on primary health care (Hall, 1989). Participating in this project are the Nurses Association of Denmark and the Association of Registered Nurses of Newfoundland (Canadian Nurses Association, 1991, 1992; Church et al., 1991).

Many Canadian nurses are also seconded by international agencies to undertake studies in other countries, in collaboration with nurses in that country. To cite one example, Dr. Linda Ogilvie of the University of Calgary undertook a study for the World Health Organization to examine forces shaping nursing contributions to primary health care in Nepal (1993).

MULTIDISCIPLINARY COLLABORATION

Also becoming more common is multidisciplinary research. The investigation of falls and the trial of intervention to prevent them carried out by staff of the University of Victoria School of Nursing and the Capital Regional District is an example of multidisciplinary collaboration (RNABC, 1991). Another example of a multidisciplinary research project is a study directed towards the prevention of preterm births which looked at the health promotion practices of health professionals in eastern Ontario. This study involved nurse researchers, a public health physician and a statistician (Davies, Niday, Nimrod, Stewart, Sprague and Dulberg, 1993).

THE STUDENT'S ROLE IN CONDUCTING RESEARCH

As beginning students, you are able to examine the practice of nursing uninfluenced by the dogmas and rituals of the past. From your first clinical experience, you should begin to think of ways of improving nursing practice and articulate your ideas. The ideas may seem unconventional at first but often can be developed into original ideas for research.

In some senior courses, you may be expected to undertake a small study; probably it will be a small group project. As beginning students, you are not likely to be asked to do research. You should, however, be aware of and begin to develop an appreciation for the research that has been done in the area of practice in which you are having clinical experience. You should also be aware of completed research that has contributed to the knowledge you are gaining from other courses you are taking. In this, you will be guided by reading lists for each course, but you will also want to explore other avenues. You will find research articles in all refereed and many other professional journals. **Refereed journals** contain articles that have been reviewed, assessed for accuracy, scholarliness and scientific merit and accepted for publication by an editorial board of nursing experts (RNABC, 1990). The two major Canadian refereed journals that publish nursing research reports are *Canadian Journal of Nursing Research (Nursing Papers)* and *Canadian Journal of Public Health*. You will also find articles reporting on nursing research in *The Canadian Nurse* and in many of the provincial nursing journals and the journals of interest groups, such as the *Canadian Journal of Nursing Administration*. You may also look at the American, British and Australian journals you will find on your reading lists.

Some of you may have the opportunity to work as research assistants for your instructors during the summer vacation period or as part-time assistants during the term. This type of work experience is not only interesting, it also gives you valuable insight into the actual process of research.

As students at any level, you may be asked to participate in research being conducted by others. Your participation may take the form of being a *subject*, that is, a member of a given population under study, or you may be asked to assist in collecting data. Most of you will have considerable clinical practice in teaching hospitals and community agencies affiliated with a university Health Sciences Centre. There may, therefore, be numerous research projects involving your patients. You can use this situation as an additional learning experience by finding out the nature of the research being undertaken and the methodology being used. Researchers and their assistants are usually very willing to share what they are doing with an interested student.

The ethical guidelines developed by the Canadian Nurses Association (1994) stress that the relationship between subject and researcher is the most important component in the ethical dimension of the study. The relationship must be one of mutual trust in which the subject is aware of and satisfied with his or her involvement and protection during the course of the study.

The guidelines point out that, although researchers have the primary responsibility to build a trusting relationship with subjects in their study, it is every nurse's responsibility to collaborate in fostering relationships that will facilitate the ethical conduct of research.

If you are involved in a particular study, as a data collector or as a subject's caregiver, you should be aware that the investigator is obligated to provide you with information that clarifies the roles of everyone involved, that is, the researcher, the research subject, the data gatherer and the care giver. You will also want information about the purpose of the study.

It is the responsibility of all nurses to ensure that the health and the rights of the patient who is a subject in a research study are safeguarded. All universities and most hospitals and other health agencies now have an Ethics Committee which reviews all research proposals to ensure that patient rights are not jeopardized by the conduct of a study.

THE DISSEMINATION AND USE OF RESEARCH FINDINGS

The process of disseminating, and subsequently using, research findings in practice has been studied in many fields including education, anthropology and rural sociology. Two of the most eminent researchers in the diffusion and adoption of innovations, as this branch of research has been called, are E.M. Rogers and R.G. Havelock. Rogers maintains that people in any social system go through a similar process from first awareness of a new idea or practice, through seeking information about it, to making a decision to adopt it in practice. Both Havelock and Rogers have used the concept of **change agents** in their theories. These are outside consultants who are called in to assist with the dissemination of information about new ideas and/or practices in an organization (or in a social system) and with their adoption in practice (Burns and Grove, 1993). A classic Canadian nursing study showed that nurses in a given community did, indeed, follow a definable pattern similar to that found in other groups as they sought information about new ideas and practices and made decisions to adopt or not adopt the innovation. The channels of communication used by nurses to find out about new ideas and practices may be expected to vary somewhat from one jurisdiction to another. In this study, the channels used included the nursing journals, continuing education courses (conferences, seminars or formal courses), nursing consultants from government and from the professional nursing association, as well as nursing faculty from schools of nursing and other colleagues. One of the most important findings in this study, and in diffusion and adoption studies in all disciplines, is the importance of personal communication — nurses talking to other nurses about their work (Du Gas, 1969).

The RNABC has developed a *Workbook on Nursing Research* which lists various ways to interest nurses in research. These ways include a good sampling of "channels of communication" that may be used by nurses to disseminate information about nursing research activity, as well as ways to encourage the conduct of research in agencies and the utilization of research findings.

THE STUDENT'S ROLE IN THE DISSEMINATION OF RESEARCH FINDINGS

As students, you have a wonderful opportunity to learn about the latest findings of nursing research. You can attend the research seminars, "brown bag" lunch discussions of research and many other continuing education programs that are held regularly by different departments in health sciences centres and teaching hospitals. You can also attend

---

Examples of Ways to Motivate Nursing Research Activity

- Nursing Research Committees in Health Care Agencies
- Research Interest Groups
  - agency-based, inter-agency–based
  - nursing and interdisciplinary
  - brown bag discussions on research topics
- Journal Clubs
- Research Awareness Days in Agencies
  - nursing units can submit problems and questions that might be studied
  - competitions between nursing units for examples of how research was used to solve a problem
- Professional Association Annual Research Days
  - paper and poster presentations
  - colloquiums or workshops on research and practice
- Professional Practice Group Activities
  - newsletters
  - meetings
  - networking

SOURCE: Registered Nurses Association of British Columbia. (1990). *Nursing research: From question to funding. A workbook.* Vancouver: Author, 2. Reproduced with permission.

---

nursing conferences where research reports are given — registration for students is usually at a much reduced rate from that charged other registrants. The annual meetings of provincial nursing associations and the Canadian Nurses Association are also good places to find out about new ideas and practices, to exchange information with students from other schools and to talk with experienced nurses about their views on some of the new ideas.

The most reliable way of disseminating new knowledge and practices in nursing, as in any other field, is through the education process. Many heads of nursing departments in clinical agencies will tell you that they always question new graduates, particularly those coming from other parts of the province and other provinces or countries, on new practices they have been taught in their basic nursing programs. As students you and your faculty guides are sources of new knowledge for staff of the agency in which you are gaining experience.

USING RESEARCH FINDINGS

Much of nursing research focusses on resolving problems nurses have encountered in practice or on ways to improve practice. For example, a major concern of nurses caring for people in an inpatient facility is the problem of patients falling out of bed, or falling while walking on legs made unsteady by age, illness or infirmity. A study at St. Joseph's Hospital in London, Ontario, set out to identify the risk factors associated with patients' falls in acute and long-term care. A study with a similar focus on preventing falls was conducted by the University of Victoria School of Nursing and the Greater Victoria Capital Region. Another study at the Calgary Children's Hospital was designed to help nurses to facilitate the transition for parents coping with their child's admission to the Intensive Care Unit.

The findings of all of these studies can be used by nurses in numerous health agencies. If nurses can identify the risk factors associated with patients' falls, for example, they can take preventive measures to eliminate (or minimize) the factors wherever possible. Similarly, the findings of the study on parents' coping behaviours could be useful to nurses in pediatric units and in emergency departments in general hospitals as well as to nurses in children's hospitals all across the country (CNA, 1991; Church et al., 1991; RNABC, 1991).

Unfortunately, the adoption of new ideas and practices is a lengthy process which usually takes a number of years. In seeking to help nurses to use research findings in their practice, Grinspun and others at Mount Sinai Hospital in Toronto found that several barriers to the use of research in clinical practice have been identified. These include: "(1) limited access to research findings, (2) difficulty interpreting published research reports, and (3) attitudes" (46). Believing that organizational support and a knowledgeable staff are necessary to promote the utilization of nursing research, the nursing research committee at Mount Sinai made the use of research their priority, rather than the conduct of research itself (Grinspun, MacMillan, Nichol and Shields, 1993).

THE STUDENT'S ROLE IN THE UTILIZATION OF RESEARCH FINDINGS

As students, you may be involved in identifying problems that can be researched, gathering data for studies, evaluating research reports, utilizing findings from credible studies in the practice field and sharing research findings with colleagues.

In an educational program, you reap the benefits of others' research in learning up-to-date nursing interventions which, increasingly, are being based on research findings. It is important to know which of the nursing interventions you are learning are based on sound research, which are *empirically* based (rooted in experience) and which are unsubstantiated.

You can also offer a fresh outlook on the way things are done and can question your professors on the rationale behind various nursing interventions and routines. Don't hesitate to ask your professors, "Why do they do it this way?" Usually, there is a valid reason. If not, you may have a potential researchable question. During your clinical experience in various agencies, you will want to look for possible researchable questions that you may be able to develop into a study later in your program.

BASIC CONCEPTS

WAYS OF KNOWING

Nursing research is the scientific investigation of nursing practice problems to generate new knowledge that is essential to the quality of nursing care (CNA, undated). The knowledge generated by research is important but Benner points out that "mere techniques and scientific knowledge are not enough" in nursing (Benner, 1984, 4). She suggests that *caring* is what makes the nurse take note of those interventions that help the patients and guide their future actions. Nor has all of the body of knowledge that nursing encompasses been derived from research. Henderson suggests that clinical nurses develop knowledge through the practice of nursing (Henderson in Benner and Wrubel, 1980).

Much of our knowledge has come from the experience of nurses who have gone before us, some of it from common sense, some learned by trial and error in the process of giving care, some passed on by tradition and some from scientific enquiry. As the number of clinical nursing studies has expanded, many traditional nursing techniques have been questioned — often resulting in the discovery that there is, indeed, a scientific basis for traditional nursing interventions. For example, the evening back rub has been used in hospitals by many generations of nurses who found that it helped patients to relax in preparation for sleep. Nowadays, we are aware that there is a scientific reason for the back rub; the slow, gentle massage has the effect of stimulating the thick nerve fibers in the spinal cord that help to mitigate pain. In other cases, research has led to new knowledge and to new nursing interventions. Dr. Dolores Krieger's research on faith healing, for example, led to the development of therapeutic touch techniques which are being used by many nurses today.

LoBiondo-Wood and Haber (1990) suggest that the numerous ways of gaining knowledge can be classified into two broad categories: structured and unstructured. Unstructured ways of gaining knowledge include empathy, intuition, trial-and-error experience, tradition and authority and meditation. Structured ways include scientific enquiry, critical thinking and logical reasoning.

The nursing process follows the logical sequence of a scientific enquiry/research process:

1. statement of the problem (hypothesis, assumptions)
2. the gathering of facts already known about the problem
3. development of a theoretical framework on which to base the study
4. selection of methodology to gather more facts (research design)
5. analysis of data collected

TABLE 7.1 Comparison of the scientific enquiry/research process and the nursing process

THE SCIENTIFIC ENQUIRY/RESEARCH PROCESS	THE NURSING PROCESS
1. statement of the problem	assumption that patient needs nursing assistance
2. the gathering of facts already known about the problem	data collection about individual, the family or other group or community
3. development of a theoretical framework on which to base the study	identification of specific problems (stated as nursing diagnosis)
4. selection of methodology to gather more facts (research design)	development of a plan of care
5. analysis of the data collected	implementation of the plan
6. interpretation of the results of the data analysis	evaluation of the results
7. the communication of findings	communication to other members of health team

SOURCE: Adapted from LoBiondo-Wood, G. and Haber, J. (1990). *Nursing research: Methods, critical appraisal and utilization.* (2nd ed.). St. Louis: The C.V. Mosby Company, 29. Adapted with permission.

6.   interpretation of the results of the data analysis
7.   the communication of findings.

In the nursing process, you start with the assumption that the patient needs nursing assistance. Specific problems are identified following the gathering of data about the individual (or it may be a family or other group, or a community). Inferences are made about these problems (a nursing diagnosis is made); a plan of care is developed and carried out and the results of the intervention are evaluated and communicated to other members of the health team.

GOALS OF GENERATING RESEARCH-BASED KNOWLEDGE

In conducting research, nurses use their curiosity, imagination and reasoning to adapt the methodology of scientific enquiry to gain fresh knowledge and to find solutions to practical problems.

Some authors make a distinction between *nursing research* and *research in nursing*. Nursing research, these authors feel, is a systematic, logical enquiry into the processes of health care, and the clinical problems and issues encountered in the practice of nursing. It is a process by which the knowledge base for nursing practice grows. Research in nursing, on the other hand, they feel, is the broader study of people and the nursing profession, including historical, policy and ethical studies. Others feel that dividing the research that is being done in the nursing field into two categories is an arbitrary distinction; in the final analysis, research into all

aspects of nursing will strengthen nursing practice.

The position of the Canadian Nurses Association (CNA, 1985) is that the results of research provide guidance to nurses in all practice areas and indicate what nurses should do, what they could try and what they should question and research.

The four principal goals of nursing research, as set forth by the Canadian Nurses Association, are:

1.   building the knowledge base of nursing
2.   describing and explaining phenomena, predicting the results of interventions and controlling undesirable outcomes
3.   strengthening accountability in patient care
4.   ultimately improving the quality of human life.

RESEARCH BEING DONE BY CANADIAN NURSES

Nursing is a dynamic profession and its knowledge base is constantly changing as new information is discovered. The motivation for this search for new information comes from recognition of the gaps that exist in current knowledge. Research plays a critical role in enlarging the scientific foundations of nursing knowledge. Much of the early research in nursing in Canada was on nursing education. As graduate programs began to develop in nursing administration, nursing education and community health in Canadian universities, these areas became the main foci for research by nurses. From the early 1970s, however, the

---

The Goals of Nursing Research

BUILDING THE KNOWLEDGE BASE
Nursing must build its own knowledge base, rather than falling back on tried and true practices. The search for new knowledge is part of nursing's commitment to high quality care. What is learned through nursing research can be used to:

• help people and their families develop constructive lifestyles

• promote the maintenance and restoration of health

• care for individuals and families through periods of health crisis

• improve the quality of community health care delivery.

PREDICTION AND CONTROL Along with other scientific disciplines, nursing research aims to *describe* and *explain* phenomena, *predict* the results of interventions and *control* undesirable outcomes.

ACCOUNTABILITY Nurses who base their clinical decisions on scientifically documented evidence are nurses who are being accountable to the patients they serve.

QUALITY OF LIFE The ultimate goal of nursing research is to improve the quality of human life by helping people to learn healthier lifestyles, restore their health or deal positively with a terminal illness.

SOURCE: Canadian Nurses Association. (undated). *Nursing research: A solid foundation for nursing practice.* Ottawa: Author.

principal focus has been on issues related to nursing practice (Ritchie, 1992). In looking at current trends in Canadian nursing research, the CNA (1991) identified that a considerable amount of research is currently being carried out in the following areas:

1. women's health
2. HIV infections
3. nurses' roles in the health of Canadians
4. care of families with chronically ill children
5. promoting and maintaining health in the elderly
6. systems to deliver health care
7. the development of nursing.

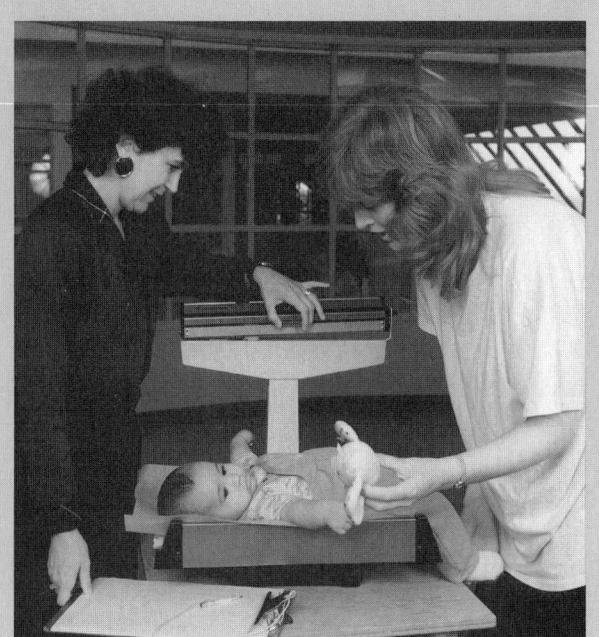

A considerable amount of research is being done in maternal and child health.

LEARNING TO READ AND INTERPRET RESEARCH REPORTS

As beginning students, the primary role in nursing research is that of research consumer. In order to become an intelligent consumer of research literature and, ultimately, to be able to use research findings in your clinical practice, you need to develop skills in reading research reports and in assessing research for scientific merit and clinical applicability. These skills require learning to critique research reports — an activity you will be given plenty of practice in during your nursing courses. The following section is an introduction to critiquing research reports.

WHAT IS A CRITIQUE?

A *critique* is a critical assessment of a piece of research involving a systematic appraisal according to specified criteria (Woods and Catanzaro, 1988). Conducting a good critique of a research study, proposal or report of findings requires not just a list of pertinent questions to ask, but criteria or standards against which to evaluate answers to the questions and comprehension of the rationale for asking them in the first place (Ryan-Wegner, 1992; Downs, 1984; Burns and Grove, 1993). In order to critique a research study, you will need to engage in three activities:

1. Analysis of the study to identify the component parts and the procedures used by the researcher, as well as to understand the reasons given for their use.
2. Evaluation of the study by appraising the strengths and weaknesses of those areas identified in the analysis.
3. Expression of your judgement about the merit or worth of the study. This assessment should be based on the analysis and evaluation. Remember, a critique identifies both strengths and weaknesses.

As you can see, a critique is not a summary of the study, although the opening sentence or paragraph of a critique should briefly summarize the whole article and emphasize a major strength. Nor is a critique a checklist identifying whether an element of a study is present or absent. While these two aspects are part of a critique, the main focus should be on providing evidence to support your evaluation and on suggesting improvements that could be made to the research study.

> A critique is an objective evaluation of the quality of the written report or article, the strength of the research design and the adequacy of the author's interpretation of the findings.

GUIDELINES FOR WRITING A CRITIQUE

Although the terms *critique* and *evaluation* are frequently perceived as having negative connotations, when used to describe research procedures, they imply only an objective assessment. The tone of a critique can convey either a negative or positive view. The term *evaluation* implies a comparison against accepted standards which apply to all types of research. Objectivity is important in a critique. Always keep in mind that you are making evaluative comments about the study and not about the researchers.

In a critique you should strive to be readable, concise, rational, accurate, sensitive and impartial; explanations for the judgements that you make must always be given. You should convey respect for the investigator's activities; it is often easier to critique than to create. To soften the tone of your delivery, use conditionals such as *could, would, should, might.*

To start the process of critiquing a research report or research article, it is helpful to read the entire report through once, quickly and objectively, to gain a perspective of what was done, why and how it was done, and the results of the study. Following this first assessment, a more in-depth evaluation of each section of the research report can then be accomplished.

THE ELEMENTS OF A RESEARCH REPORT

The headings commonly used to divide a research report can be useful in organizing a critique of a research study or report of findings. These usually follow the steps the researcher followed in conducting the study. Understanding the logic behind the organization of the report whether you are merely critiquing the research or contemplating its use in practice, is important. As a reader, you must raise critical questions and find satisfactory answers from the information communicated in the report.

At the end of each section below describing the content of elements in a research report, we have suggested some basic questions that should be asked about each particular element and could be used as a guide for critiquing that section of the report. A summary of these questions is included at the end of the chapter. In addition to the questions, we suggest looking at the excellent worksheet prepared by Davies and Logan to assist nurses (and others) in clinical practice to read research articles. You can find this worksheet in the CNA publication by Davies and Logan (1993) entitled *Reading research: A user-friendly guide for nurses and other health professionals*.

Like the nursing process, the format for research report writing and communicating is a problem-solving one, with subdivisions using research process labels which relate to each step of the research process.

TYPICALLY, A RESEARCH REPORT WILL HAVE THE FOLLOWING HEADINGS:
- Title
- Abstract
- Introduction
- Review of the literature and theoretical framework
- Hypothesis, assumptions and objectives
- Research methods, design and procedures
  - population
  - data collection
- Data analysis and results
- Discussion.

Let us examine each of the components of a research report more closely.

TITLE AND ABSTRACT

Typically, a research article begins with a title to introduce the major topic or area of study. Following the title is an *abstract* which is intended to give the reader a brief summary of the entire study. An abstract usually provides the following information about the study: its purpose, objectives or hypotheses; a description of the subjects or sample members; a brief explanation of the data collection methods and analysis procedures; and a summary of important findings.

QUESTIONS TO ASK ABOUT THE TITLE AND ABSTRACT
1. Does the title of the research accurately reflect the problem under study?
2. Does the abstract present a succinct overview of the study?

INTRODUCTION

The introduction provides a brief overview of the research topic. It is a summary statement of what the research is about, why it was done and how it is important to nursing. The introduction describes the nature of the research and should briefly explain why the study was undertaken. It also usually includes a short rationale for addressing the topic which should let the reader know whether the research is relevant to his or her practice arena.

In the introductory section, the investigator also describes the preliminary research steps which specify the general focus of the study, presents background information and the need for the study, and then states the purpose of this particular investigation. Consider, as an example, a large hospital that is planning to introduce primary nursing which it is hoped will help nurses in their clinical practice. Some nurses like the idea; others have expressed doubts it. In order to develop a relevant teaching program for the nurses, the nursing education unit of the hospital would like to investigate why some nurses like and some do not like the idea of primary nursing. They hope to use their findings to plan a program to overcome negative attitudes and foster interest and enthusiasm among all the nurses for primary nursing. The purpose of the research would be to examine (investigate) the reasons for nurses' anxiety towards primary nursing in order to design a program to help them to feel comfortable in learning how to implement it. From the stated purpose (also called sometimes a *problem statement* and, sometimes, the *research question*) the reader should be able to clearly identify the general problem under study.

QUESTIONS TO ASK ABOUT THE INTRODUCTION
1. Do you have a clear idea of what the research is all about?
2. Do you understand why the research is being done?

3. Is the significance of the problem discussed and the research justified?
4. Is the problem substantiated with adequate background information?
5. Is the problem statement clear? Concise?

REVIEW OF THE LITERATURE AND THEORETICAL FRAMEWORK

A literature review is the next section of a research report (and next step in the research process). It is a discussion of previous relevant studies that the investigator or others have conducted, as well as a review of the current knowledge about the concepts under study. The literature review serves multiple purposes and provides essential information for many of the other components of the research process. In general, there are three purposes of the literature review:

1. to validate knowledge
2. to avoid unintended duplication
3. to review methods used in previous research.

The first purpose of a literature review is to allow the researcher to **validate the knowledge base** (assess the extent of current knowledge about the subject). The literature forms the background and framework for the study. This background information helps the reader to understand how the study relates to and builds on previous research and theory in the field. Gaps in existing knowledge should become apparent as you read the literature review.

The second purpose of a literature review is to determine if the proposed study has already been done. Prior to conducting the study, the researcher needs to identify how different or similar other studies are to the proposed study, and determine whether replication with a different sample and in a different setting is needed. Replication is the repetition of a study in different settings with different samples taken from the same or different populations (LoBiondo-Wood and Haber, 1990, 371). If the researcher finds that the proposed study differs significantly enough from previous studies to warrant pursuing the project, the researcher may use the previous studies to build the framework for the proposed study. If, to return to our example, it had been established in a previous study that a large number of nurses employed in the hospital were worried about the introduction of primary nursing, the proposed study to identify reasons for anxieties could build on the framework of the previous study.

Finally, the third purpose for performing a literature review is to identify methods other researchers have used in their investigations on the topic of interest. The researcher may uncover new research tools or measures that can be used for data gathering in the proposed study, variables he or she had not considered or unanticipated problems in

data collection or analysis. A careful look at these aspects of previous work can help the researcher to avoid problems others have had, thus strengthening his or her own research.

The literature review also helps the reader to determine how the study being reported relates to current theoretical knowledge on the topic. Knowledge of the literature available on a subject allows subsequent placement of the problem in a theoretical context — an important step in the eventual integration of findings.

QUESTIONS TO ASK ABOUT THE LITERATURE REVIEW

1. Does the literature review support the significance of the selected problem?
2. Is the relationship of the problem to previous research clear?
3. What is the theoretical base for this study? What are the major concepts used? For example, change theory, diffusion/adoption theory and theories on attitudinal change are all possibilities to use as a foundation for the study on nurses' anxieties and attitudes about the introduction of primary nursing.
4. Does the researcher indicate how they have used previous knowledge in developing this study?
5. Is the literature review well organized? What topics are addressed?
6. Is there a sufficient review of the literature so that the reader can be assured that the investigator has considered a broad spectrum of possibilities for investigating the problem?
7. Are the references up to date, that is, most of them less than 10 years old?
8. Has reference also been made to classic studies (early studies in an area of research), to original and up-to-date work by experts in the field, as, for example, Leininger's work over the years in studies involving cross-cultural nursing.

HYPOTHESES, ASSUMPTIONS AND OBJECTIVES

From the review of the literature, the researcher narrows down the field of enquiry and refines the problem statement into a more specific research question. You will very often find a section entitled Operational Definitions in a report. An **operational definition** specifies all the relevant aspects of the concept to be measured. It defines a concept so that later researchers will be able to measure the same thing in the same way. Thus, the concept of "close friend" might be operationally defined in a particular study as a person you can talk to if you need help or have a problem (Health and Welfare Canada, 1987). When concepts have been operationalized, they are called *variables*.

As the word suggests, a **variable** is something that changes. In research the term is used to designate a quality, characteristic or property of an object, a person or a situation that can and does change in different circumstances (Burns and Grove, 1993). The fact that it changes implies that it can be measured. A variable may be concrete and directly measurable, for example, height, weight or pulse rate, or it may be abstract and only indirectly observable, for example, anxiety, pain or grief. In the latter case, the elements may be called **research concepts** rather than variables.

Research often attempts to determine the relationship between variables, that is, whether differences in one variable are related to differences in another (for instance, whether a person's age is related to the number of close friends he or she has). Relationships between variables do not necessarily imply **causality**, that is, that one variable is the cause of the other. However, if there is no relationship between the variables (if a study showed that there was no difference in the number of close friends older and younger people had), the researcher can rule out the possibility of a causal relationship. Conversely, the possibility of a causal relationship increases as the relationship strengthens, although it should be noted that two variables can be closely related without one being the cause of another (Burns and Grove, 1993).

Variables are categorized as *dependent*, *independent* or *intervening*. The **dependent variable** is also sometimes called the *outcome* variable. It is the characteristic that the study or experiment intended to measure. In the case of the nurses' anxiety about the introduction of primary nursing, the dependent variable is their level of anxiety. The dependent variable is related to (depends on) the independent variable.

The **independent variables** are also sometimes called *experimental* variables or *intervention* variables. These are the characteristics that may be changed (manipulated) by the investigator. Many drug experiments involve giving different groups of subjects varying amounts of a medication. In this case the amount of medication would be the independent variable. Independent variables can also refer to things which the experimenter cannot change, but which nonetheless differ — the subjects may themselves vary in certain characteristics. Age and sex are two important (demographic) independent variables that play a role in many studies. The values of independent variables are established by the researcher ahead of time. They constitute the input of an experiment and precede the measurement of the dependent variable. It is possible to have both more than one dependent variable and more than one independent variable, but all must be operationally defined. The variables (including the population under study) to be examined, and others that may affect the study, should be introduced in the hypothesis section of the report.

Intervening variables are sometimes called *confounding* variables or *extraneous* variables. These are characteristics that are not under study but might influence the results

of the study. The researcher tries to think of all the variables that might possibly have an influence and tries to negate their effect through the design of the research or through statistical techniques (Davies and Logan, 1993).

In the case of the nurses' anxieties about the introduction of primary nursing, a nurse's employment status (permanent or casual) and/or personal problems that are causing anxiety might be intervening variables that could affect the results of the study. The former could be controlled by having only permanent staff members participate in the study, but it would be difficult to control for personal circumstances that could be influencing a nurse's attitude to something new in the work situation.

Once the variables have been identified, the researcher normally formulates a hypothesis (or hypotheses), develops objectives, or assumptions or states the research questions in more precise detail than the general statement made in the introductory section of the report. The **hypothesis** suggests solutions or answers by translating the problem into a precise prediction of expected outcomes.

While we usually think of research as aiming to give evidence that a particular relationship exists, frequently, it has the opposite aim. Researchers sometimes expect their studies to show that a particular relationship doesn't exist. In these cases, it is the negative or **null hypothesis** that is tested (RNABC, 1990). For example, if the *hypothesis* has been defined as: Nurses' anxiety about the introduction of primary nursing decreases with the amount of inservice training they receive, the *null hypothesis* might be: There is no significant difference in anxiety between those groups who received extra instruction and those who did not.

Assumptions, objectives and research questions are used in more descriptive studies where precise prediction of results is not the ultimate goal. **Assumptions** are provisional suppositions; the researcher might assume, for example, that there is a relationship between age and response to medication.

When the primary purpose of the research is to gather new knowledge about a phenomenon, objectives may be developed to provide guidance for the study, or the original research question (problem statement) may be refined into more precise questions. For example, is age related to response to medication? Is gender related to it? Is expectations about results a factor? By developing hypotheses, assumptions, objectives or specific questions prior to the conduct of a study, the researcher provides specific direction for subsequent aspects of design, as well as data collection and analysis.

QUESTIONS TO ASK ABOUT HYPOTHESES, ASSUMPTIONS, OBJECTIVES AND RESEARCH QUESTIONS

1. Has the initial problem statement been refined? Is the research question now more precisely stated?

2. What dependent and independent variables has the researcher identified?

LOOKING BACK

1600 1650 1700 1750 1800 1850 1900 1950

ETHEL JOHNS 1879–1968

Ethel Johns was the first director of the first baccalaureate degree program in nursing in Canada. One of Canada's foremost nursing leaders, she was appointed in 1919 to be both Superintendent of Nurses at Vancouver General Hospital and head of the newly approved Department of Nursing at the University of British Columbia (UBC). A dynamic leader, she had already helped shape the forces that led to the introduction of nursing education at the university level. She believed strongly that nurses needed a strong, science-based, liberal education in the university system, paid for from educational rather than hospital budgets, and she accepted the challenge of trying to bring such a program into being.

Ethel Mary Johns was born in England on May 13, 1879, and moved with her family to Canada at age 13. She graduated from the Winnipeg General Hospital nursing program in 1902. During the early part of her career, she was involved with the launching of the Manitoba Association of Graduate Nurses and championed the movement underway in Eastern Canada for nurse registration; Manitoba was, in 1913, the second province to achieve a Nurse Registration Act. In addition, she spoke and wrote prolifically on the need for standardization of nursing educational programs and for standardized provincial nursing examinations. She spent one year at Teachers College, Columbia University, where she studied under Mary Adelaide Nutting, Annie Goodrich and Lavinia Dock. Unfortunately, finances did not allow her to complete her degree, but through her efforts she initiated a new pathway for nursing education.

She headed UBC's baccalaureate program for only six years, during which she established the program securely. She then became Field Director of Nursing in Europe for the Rockefeller Foundation and filled other influential positions in the United States before returning to Canada in 1933 to become editor of *The Canadian Nurse*. A life-long writer and influential speaker, she wrote three books, a series of 16 pamphlets, and hundreds of memorable reports, articles, editorials, speeches and presentations. Among her many awards were an honorary doctorate from Mount Allison University and the Mary Agnes Snively Memorial Medal from the Canadian Nurses Association. She died in Vancouver in 1968.

Glennis Zilm

---

3. Are the variables specified in the refined research question? What is the dependent variable? independent variable(s)?

4. What possible intervening variables has the researcher considered? Can you think of others?

5. Will the hypotheses or data collected to prove assumptions, attain objectives or answer specific research questions solve the research problem?

6. If a hypothesis is stated, is it specific to one relationship between the variables? If more than one hypothesis is stated, is each specific to one relationship?

METHODOLOGY (DESIGN OR PROCEDURES)

In the section of a research article entitled *Methodology* (or *Design* or *Procedures*), the investigator explains, in detail, exactly how the study was conducted. The investigator should provide an explanation of the type of research design used in conducting the study, who participated in the study, what tools or instruments were used to collect data, what data were collected, what procedures the participants were required to do, and the methods used for data analysis.

THE RESEARCH DESIGN

The *research design* refers to the structure of an investigation, and explains *how* the answers to research questions are sought. The design section of the report gives the reader a description of the investigator's overall plan for organizing the study and some predictions about how data might be treated.

There are numerous designs for conducting research, and, according to Davies and Logan, none is perfect (1993). In general, research designs can be divided into two major groups: *quantitative* and *qualitative*.

In **quantitative** studies (which involve the analysis of numbers to answer research questions) the criteria are derived from the tenets of the scientific method, measurement theory, statistical principles and ethical standards. In **qualitative** studies, which analyze words instead of numbers for their meanings to answer the research questions, the ethical standards still apply, but in this case there is no statistical analysis of data. In both types of study, researchers want to ensure *reliability* (that the instruments used give consistent results) and *validity* (that they measure what they are supposed to measure), but in qualitative studies, the terms used for these principles may be *confirmability, dependability* or *trustworthiness* (Davies and Logan, 1993).

Field and Morse (1985) state that although the purpose of both quantitative and qualitative research is to generate nursing knowledge, there is a basic difference in the approach of the two methodologies. In quantitative research, knowledge is derived **deductively**, that is to say, the investigator works from existing theory and hypothesizes relationships that are then tested by experimental or non-experimental means. An example of an experimental study is one that was done by a multidisciplinary team at the University of Ottawa. The research team evaluated the effectiveness of a diabetic education program for nurses to assist patient self-care in the community. Two randomly selected teams of nurses were used with one group receiving a one-hour briefing, the other a two-day workshop with additional case management assignments. Both groups had access to the same resources in the agency (Davies, Leiterman, Dulberg, Closs and McDonald, 1993). The numerous health surveys undertaken by Statistics Canada are examples of quantitative studies done on a non-experimental basis. We have referred to a number of these in earlier chapters. Another example, on a smaller scale, was a study by nurses in Fort McMurray and district in northern Alberta who used a survey to collect data on the health behaviours of pregnant women (Ali, Dow-Clarke and MacCalder, 1993).

In qualitative research, on the other hand, knowledge is developed **inductively** from the data. The studies are usually descriptive and are used when not much is known about a topic. In the course of the study, phenomena and concepts are identified and possible relationships are suggested. In other words, qualitative research identifies variables in order to generate a theory, which may subsequently be tested in further quantitative studies.

There are three major types of qualitative studies: *grounded theory* (used to develop theories), *phenomenology* (used to describe experience) and *ethnomethodology* (used to examine cultures).

Grounded theory studies
The term **grounded theory** refers to theory that has been grounded in reality. The theory is derived from data systematically obtained from social research and must provide an explanation of events as they occur (Field and Morse, 1985).

An example of a study using grounded theory methods is one undertaken on the health-seeking behaviour patterns among older women with ovarian cancer in northern Alberta in which transcribed interviews with a sample of older women was a major source of data.

The findings gave some insight into the care-seeking activities of the groups under study. The authors were able to suggest (theorize) that all women went through a similar process. The authors identified three stages in the process, which they described as: (1) developing awareness, (2) monitoring and (3) "getting the run-around." At each stage of the process, the women sought confirmation of their diagnosis (Olson, Honore, Van der Klauw, Berkel and Goedke, 1993).

Phenomenological studies
The purpose of **phenomenological** studies is "to describe experience as it is lived" (Munhall and Oiler, 1986, 70). They are not done for the purpose of generating theory or developing general observations. The researcher, rather, is concerned with how people perceive experiences such as being in pain, recovering from an illness or giving birth (Field and Morse, 1985).

The phenomenological investigator starts with no preconceived notions, attempting only to describe accurately the phenomenon being studied. It has been suggested that empathy could be studied by phenomenological methods because it is so little understood and yet is considered a very important trait for nurses to have (Field and Morse, 1985). One area in which phenomenological study methods have been used is examining the meaning of health to homeless persons, as this is a subject on which very little empirical data exists (McCormack and Gooding, 1993).

Ethnomethodological studies
Ethnography is the scientific description of human races. The research methodology developed by anthropologists to generate cultural theory through the examining of different cultures has begun to be used in nursing as transcultural nursing has come into prominence. The purpose of **ethnomethodological** (ethnographic) studies is to undertake a descriptive analysis of a culture or sub-culture which can be used as a basis to develop theories about that culture. For example, Dr. Madeleine Leininger, who is recognized as the founder of transcultural nursing, has studied human care phenomena in 54 cultures (Cohen, 1992). From these studies she developed her theories of the diversity and universality of cultural care which we will discuss further in Chapter 13.

In nursing, the ethnomethodological approach is also used to look at questions such as "What does it mean to be a member of a mixed-ethnic family," "What are the rules for appropriate behaviour among teenage girls in Sikh–Canadian society?" and other questions that are relevant to holistic nursing. In ethnomethodological studies, the researcher has to become to a certain extent a part of the community under study for a while in order to gather the data and gain insight into the behaviours of people in the group. Methods used to gather data include interviewing people in the community who are knowledgeable about the culture and willing to talk with the researcher and **participant observation** in which the researcher takes part in the activities of the group. The participation may range from full involvement to pure observation (LoBiondo-Wood and Haber, 1990; Field and Morse, 1985; Munhall and Oiler, 1986).

Quantitative Design

Experimental and Non-Experimental

Experimental designs have three essential characteristics:

- Randomization of subjects when choosing the sample to be studied
- A control group for comparison with the experimental group
- Manipulation of a special treatment (e.g. early discharge, teaching program, etc.)

Non-experimental designs lack one or more of the above three characteristics.

Common Quantitative Designs

Experimental

- Pre-Test/Post-Test
- Clinical Trial

Non-Experimental

- Survey
- Correlation

Qualitative Design

There are some important differences to note when reading about a qualitative study. The standards for choosing a sample, sample size and data analysis methods are not the same.

The sample is selected by different means, for example, purposive (not random) or nominated (named by knowledgeable others).

The number of participants (usually not called subjects) in a qualitative study will be much smaller (8-20 subjects). Since there is no statistical analysis of numbers to be done, large samples are not required.

The procedures to ensure reliability and validity should be described but the terms used may be different (e.g. confirmability, dependability, trustworthiness).

Analysis of qualitative data involves coding and categorizing to form themes and generate theoretical concepts. The categories must be defined. Quotes or examples from the data should be provided.

Common Qualitative Designs

- Grounded Theory—To develop theory
- Phenomenology—To describe experience
- Ethnomethodology—To examine cultures

SOURCE: Davies, B. and Logan J. (1993). *Reading research. A user-friendly guide for nurses and other health professionals.* Ottawa: Canadian Nurses Association, 7. Reprinted with permission.

QUESTIONS TO ASK ABOUT THE STUDY DESIGN

1. What research design was used in this study? Quantitative: experimental? or non-experimental? Or qualitative: grounded theory? phenomenological? or ethnomethodological?
2. Is the method appropriate for studying the problem? Does it follow clearly from the problem statement and research questions?

THE POPULATION UNDER STUDY

The term **population** refers to the participants in a study. This is a well-defined group of people who have certain characteristics in common; they may be nurses who work in the Intensive Care Unit of a hospital, for example, or people with a specific disease. The reader needs a full description of the subjects who participated in the study and the process by which they were selected, because the conclusions of most studies are valid only for people who are similar to the subjects in the study (Brink and Wood, 1989).

In some studies, a *total population* may be used, for example, all the senior nurse administrators in public general hospitals in a province. Most times, however, it is not feasible to survey a total population and it is necessary to use a **sample** of the total. The way the sample is selected is a critical aspect in determining the extent to which the findings from a study sample may be generalized to the larger population. The procedures for selecting the sample of study subjects should be carefully described by the investigator, as should the size and the characteristics of the sample. Failure to report sampling procedures greatly weakens any research report.

There are several appropriate and legitimate ways in which samples can be selected from a population. The population that is a feasible source of sample members is termed the **accessible population**. In most types of quantitative studies, the investigator wants to ensure that each element in the accessible population has an equal and independent chance of being selected. In order to ensure this, **probability sampling**, in which participants are selected randomly from within the accessible sample, is used. Probability sampling is also called **random sampling**. **Simple random sampling** using a table of random numbers is the most widely used and acceptable method of obtaining a random sample for quantitative studies. However, there are many variations that may be used.

Stratified sampling involves making a random selection from each of different sub-groups within the population (for example, diploma RNs, baccalaureate graduates and nurses with master's and higher degrees among a population of nurses). **Cluster sampling** involves taking progressively larger random samples from different units within a population. **Systematic sampling** is done by taking every nth member of the population, for example, every tenth name on the list of RNs in the various counties of eastern Ontario. In experimental research, the investigator selects a *control* group that can be compared with the experimental group; the characteristics of the control group should be similar to those of the experimental group. The control group is not part of the experimental *manipulation*; they are used only as a basis for comparison, to ensure that the effects of the research variables are genuine. For example, if recovery rates for a control group were just as high as for a group who received increased medication, it would be clear that it wasn't the medication that was improving recovery, but some other factor altogether.

In qualitative research, it is important to ensure that participants are knowledgeable about the information the investigator wants to collect, so non-probability (non-random) methods of sampling the population are used. Convenience, quota and purposive sampling are three types of non-probability sampling.

Convenience sampling (or **accidental sampling**) allows the entry of any available (convenient) subjects into the study until the desired sample size is reached. The study of health perceptions of homeless people, McCormack and Gooding (1993), used a convenience sample of 29 individuals from among the homeless who made use of shelters and hostels.

Quota sampling is done by selecting participants by proportional representation of different groups or strata within the total population. For example, in a hypothetical study of the adjustment to school of New Canadian children in Toronto, one might want to use quota sampling to be sure to include in the sample children of different ethnic groups, with the sample size for each group proportionate to their numbers in the total population of newcomers to the school system. That is to say, if 100 children from different ethnic groups entered the Toronto public school system in a given year and 30 came from China, 25 from Korea, 20 from the Philippines, 15 from Peru and 10 from Scotland, the quota sample of the population would be proportionate with 30 percent Chinese children, etc.

In **purposive sampling** the investigator uses his or her knowledge of the population under study and the elements of the study to select subjects. For example, a researcher collecting data about health-seeking behaviours in a particular ethnic group of older adults might establish the following criteria for the sample to be chosen: (1) speaks English fairly fluently (so that the participant is able to understand and answer a questionnaire, or participate in an interview), (2) is over the age of 50 years, (3) lives in neighbourhood. These participants have been selected by purposive methods (LoBiondo-Wood and Haber, 1990; Field and Morse, 1985; Davies and Logan, 1993).

QUESTIONS TO ASK ABOUT THE POPULATION UNDER STUDY

1. What are the common characteristics of the population under study?
2. How was the study population selected — were sampling techniques employed?

3. If sampling was used, what method was used for obtaining the sample? Is it appropriate for the type of study that was done?
4. Is the number in the sample sufficient? How does the researcher justify the sample size? Selection process?
5. In your opinion, is the sample representative of the defined population?
6. How did the researcher control for bias in selecting the sample?

Safeguarding the Rights of the Population Under Study

Ethical issues require careful attention when research of any type is conducted. These issues relate to the rights of research subjects, the recruiting of subjects, the confidentiality of responses and the disclosing of the actual purpose of the research to the respondents. Today, research proposals are under close scrutiny by human-subject review committees in most universities, hospitals and other health agencies. Such committees are made up of groups of representatives of various departments or disciplines with the purpose of reviewing ethical concerns about research proposals. The major concern is the protection of the rights of the participants in the research study. The role of the researcher is to communicate clearly in writing to the review committee how subjects will be used in the research and whether or not subjects are at any risk as a result of participating in the research. The researcher is responsible for carrying out these plans as directed or approved by the committee. The Research Committee of the Canadian Nurses Association has developed *Ethical Guidelines for Nursing Research Involving Human Subjects* (1994) which all introductory nursing students would do well to read.

QUESTIONS TO ASK ABOUT MEASURES TO SAFEGUARD THE RIGHTS OF SUBJECTS IN THE STUDY

1. What measures were taken to ensure that the rights of subjects were protected?
2. Does the researcher make available to the reader the information given to subjects about the research?
3. Does the researcher discuss possible benefits of the research for the subjects in the study?

DATA COLLECTION

The term **data** is used to describe the information the researcher (also called the *investigator*) collects from subjects or participants in the research study, or about objects in a non-human study (note that *data* is a plural noun). To collect data, for quantitative studies where one wants to obtain numerical values, the investigator will use some sort of **instrument**. This might be a questionnaire, a structured interview (in which all participants are asked the same questions) or an instrument such as a sphygmomanometer (to measure blood pressure). Whatever the instrument used to collect the data, the researcher should describe exactly how the measurements were done and report on the instrument's validity and reliability. If modifications to the instrument are made for the purpose of the study being reported, the researcher should also explain how the original instrument was modified.

In qualitative research, both interview and observation methods are used. In an interview, the researcher gathers information from the research subject by means of verbal communication. The interview may be unstructured, or "open-ended," or it may be guided by the interviewer. The interview may or may not be recorded on audio- or video-tape. Short-answer questionnaires are used in some studies. A variety of observational strategies may also be used.

Measurement by observation tends to be more subjective than measurement by other means (using a sphygmomanometer, for example). Hence, the researcher needs to include safeguards to ensure consistency. As with interviews, observations may range from totally unstructured, with the researcher simply observing the subjects' behaviour in their natural setting, to structured. Structured observation techniques include the use of tools such as categories, checklists and rating scales. In using categories, observed behaviours are recorded in previously defined categories of activity. With checklists, the observer indicates simply whether listed behaviours occurred or did not occur. With rating scales, the observer judges the behaviour observed on a predetermined scale (Burns and Grove, 1993). In studying other cultures, participant observation is commonly used.

Videotapes may also be reviewed to study different behaviours. Other methods of gathering data for qualitative studies include studying life histories. In historical research on nursing, there is usually considerable perusal of old records, as well as interviews with people who were practising in the early years of the century and/or with their daughters, sons or grandchildren. Letters are also a rich source in historical research. For example, in one aspect of an International Council of Nurses Centennial Project (the ICN will be 100 years old in 1999), Barbara L. Brush of the University of Pennsylvania and Dr. Meryn Stuart of the University of Ottawa School of Nursing examined international women's history theory and the concepts of "difference" and "unity." Focussing on the ICN's longevity and power and reviewing its purpose, the study used ICN Board minutes, financial records, Congress notes and personal correspondence, as well as numerous secondary source materials (Brush and Stuart, 1992).

QUESTIONS TO ASK ABOUT DATA COLLECTION METHODS USED IN THE STUDY

1. What data were collected?
2. Were the data collected the right data to answer the research question?
3. How were the data collected?
4. Were the measures used to collect data appropriate for the study?
5. Did the researcher use a standard protocol for gathering data during the research?
6. If others besides the principal investigator collected data (e.g. interviewed subjects or informants, administered questionnaires or other instrument) how were they trained?
7. Does the researcher show evidence of having established the reliability and validity of the procedures used for data gathering?

DATA ANALYSIS AND RESULTS

The data analysis section of a research report explains how the data that were collected were processed and interpreted. In qualitative studies, the process of data analysis occurs as data are collected. There are few or no numbers to be analyzed or reported. Instead, analysis is focussed on categories or themes and may suggest possible causal relationships which can be tested in further studies. A number of computer programs have been developed to assist people with qualitative analysis. These programs help the investigator to process, store, retrieve, catalogue and sort data that have been collected. The researcher does the actual analysis. You may note in the Data Analysis section of a qualitative study, for example, that the investigator has used the CATS (Computer Assisted Topical Sorting) or another program to assist with one of the tasks mentioned above (Davie and Logan, 1993; Burns and Grove, 1993).

In quantitative studies, data are collected and then subjected to analysis. The data collected are numerical and, therefore, lend themselves to statistical analysis. The term *statistics* refers to the "systematic collection, organization, analysis and interpretation of numerical data" (*Taber's Cyclopedic Medical Dictionary* (16th ed.), 1989, 1744). Most basic nursing education programs today include a course in statistics as well as courses in research methodology. We will not, therefore, go into a detailed description of statistical techniques in this chapter. Instead, we will talk about the purpose and methods of using statistics to assist in data analysis. We have also provided at the end of the chapter an explanation of some of the more common statistical terms you may find in reports. A knowledge of these terms is basic to understanding how data were handled in many research studies and in other professional reports.

In quantitative research studies, statistics are used to find those numbers that most accurately communicate the nature of attitudes, processes, events and achievements that need to be described; using statistics makes numbers more manageable and casts light on data. Statistical methods assist researchers in describing data, in drawing inferences to larger bodies of data and in studying causal relationships.

There are two types of statistical analysis that are done on numerical data. The first type is **exploratory** or **descriptive data analysis**. This type of analysis is usually performed first, to get an overall impression of the data. The second type is called **confirmatory data analysis.** At this stage, inferential statistics are used. Researchers make an *inference* (generalization) about a population or a process based on data collected during the study.

Exploratory or **descriptive statistics** represent the end result of the tabulating, depicting and describing of collections of data. The data might include measures of blood pressure, anxiety, weight, medical diagnosis, gender or nationality or any other type of data that have been systematically collected and can be represented numerically. Generally speaking, large masses of data must undergo a process of summarization or reduction in order to make them more comprehensible. For example, the large masses of data collected by Statistics Canada about university students in the country are much easier to understand when they are put into tables, graphs or histograms as exemplified in Figure 7.1 than in the original *raw data* form, which is also available from Statistics Canada. Descriptive techniques serve as tools to describe, summarize or reduce to a manageable form the properties of an otherwise unwieldy accumulation of data. In some studies, descriptive analysis is all that is done.

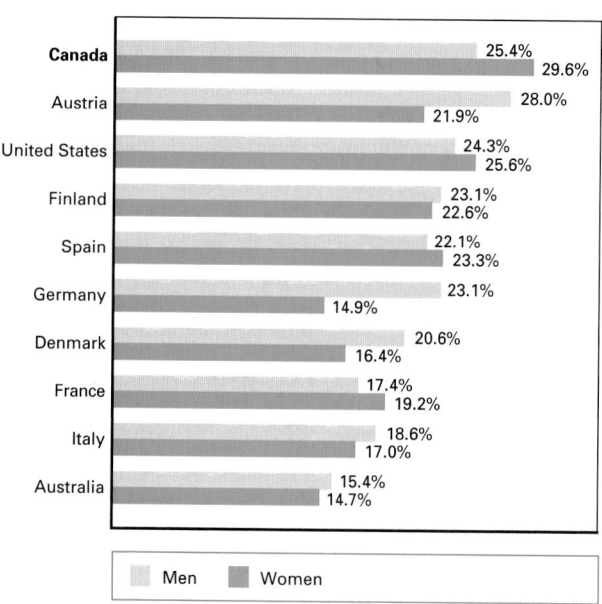

FIGURE 7.1 Ten OECD (Organization for Economic Cooperation and Development) countries with the highest percentage of young adults enrolled* in university, 1988

---

* Full-time and part-time enrolment converted to full-time equivalents. Population is those of theoretical university enrolment age (18–25 in Canada).

SOURCE: OECD, 1992. In *Canadian Social Trends, 30*(3), 9. (Statistics Canada Catalogue Number 11-008E) Reprinted with permission.

Confirmatory statistical treatment of data (using inferential statistics) involves the use of various techniques in order to:

- test proposed relationships between variables
- ascertain (infer) that the findings from a sample are representative of the total population
- examine causality (that a specific change in *a* caused reaction *b*)
- predict (that under similar circumstances, *a* will probably cause *b* again)
- infer from the sample to a theoretical model.*

The results of a study are translated and interpreted, a process that yields the study *findings* — in statistical form (Burns and Grove, 1993). These may be reported in the text, summarized in tables or presented visually in figures or graphs.

In qualitative research, after the initial process of data analysis (sorting, categorizing and ordering the data), the investigator develops concepts and hypotheses that are supported by the data they have observed. The concepts and hypotheses put forth by the researcher provide a basis for further studies by indicating possible directions for subsequent data collection (Field and Morse, 1985). These will be postulated by the investigator in a *results* or *findings* section of the report.

In quantitative studies of a non-experimental nature, the findings of the study are often shown in tables, graphs or histograms. Because it is difficult to interpret the findings from inferential statistical techniques without a course on statistics, we will not go into great detail here. However, at the very least, you will need to be able to understand from reading research reports whether the findings show that there is a significant relationship between the variables. Davies and Logan suggest that, for consumers of research, the key point to look for in the report is the p (for probability) value of statistical significance of the results. These are stated in terms of p which indicates the probability of the results being *not true*. If p is less than 0.05 (or less than 0.01), it means that the probability of the results being *not true* is less than five percent (or one percent). To put that statement in the positive, a low p value indicates more likelihood that the findings from the study were due to the experimental manipulation of the variable by the researcher — that is, that the experimental manipulation did have an effect (Davies and Logan, 1993).

In experimental studies, the investigator should report on whether or not the hypothesis was supported. When support for the hypothesis is obtained, the researcher must be cautious in generalizing the results. Factors related to validity, methodological problems and limitations of the research design must be taken into account when generalizing study results. Often, however, hypotheses are not

---

* Burns and Grove, 1993.

supported or findings are contradictory to those of similar studies. In such cases, the researcher should attempt to identify probable reasons for the findings.

Contradictory findings may be the result of lack of precision or methodological problems. A common problem is the imprecise definition of variables. If this is the case, it may well be that the method of measuring variables has affected the results. Finally, there may be nothing wrong with the study, but contradictory findings may have identified an intriguing aspect of ambiguity which opens a whole new field of investigation. The important point to remember is that while it may be difficult to identify the actual basis for the unusual findings because of lack of information, the investigator should always discuss them.

QUESTIONS TO BE ASKED ABOUT DATA ANALYSIS AND RESULTS

1. Does the researcher inform you of the steps taken to process and interpret the data?
2. Do the methods selected to analyze the data seem appropriate?
3. Are reasons given for decisions to analyze the data in the manner that they were?
4. Are the primary findings of the study clearly presented?
5. Are the results clear?
6. Are conclusions logical?
7. Is there a statement on whether the data support the hypothesis(es) or assumptions?
8. Did the researcher identify methodological problems?

DISCUSSION

Whereas the section on results presents a report of how the statistical analysis turned out, the discussion section explains what the results mean with regard to the purposes of the study and relates them to a theoretical context. Sometimes the discussion section is called *Conclusions*.

In reading a research report, you must decide whether the discussion and conclusions articulated represent a logical outcome of the procedures, methods, design and analysis of data; they should also be consistent with the focus of the problem and variables under study. In the Discussion section, the researcher points out what the results mean in terms of the problem being studied and identifies the extent to which additional knowledge about the purpose of the study has been gained. Thus, the investigator relates the findings to the theoretical position in the study. At this time, findings should be discussed in light of results from related research. One must keep the research problem in mind when writing the discussion section in order to ensure that no subtle re-interpretation of the problem has taken place. As readers of research reports, you should be aware of these considerations as well.

In addition to the statistical significance of the findings of a study, you will want to consider their **clinical significance** — whether the study is going to be useful in clinical practice. Looking at a specific example, Rosenbaum's 1991 study on *Widowhood Grief* among older Greek–Canadian women should enable community health nurses to provide more culturally sensitive care to older women members of the Greek–Canadian community in Canada.

Sometimes, the clinical significance is reported in a separate section entitled Implications, in which the investigator explains in more specific terms how the findings can be implemented. Clinicians would want to know the area of practice where the findings could be used, for instance, in the assessment of patients, in the improvement of nursing interventions or interpersonal relationships or in the modification of factors in the environment or in the work life of nurses. For example, the research may have involved the trial of a new procedure for skin care. The researcher would indicate the specific situations in which this procedure might be used, such as the protection of skin around a wound, the prevention of decubitus ulcers (bedsores) and other situations where there is a risk of skin breakdown.

In the section discussing clinical significance, the researcher should also indicate the ease with which the findings can be implemented. Does the implementation involve changes in routines or in record forms, for example, or will it involve an extensive educational program, for example, teaching all staff a new procedure. The clinician will be concerned also with whether the findings are compatible with the agency's present policies, procedures and standards — or do they require major changes in these areas. Above all, clinicians will want to know about safety. Can the findings be implemented without jeopardizing the safety of patients, staff or visitors? Do they it provide more safeguards than present procedures?

The resources required to implement the change(s) suggested in the findings of the study are also of concern. Would the implementation require the purchase of new equipment, more staff or a major investment of time or money (Davies and Logan, 1993)?

It is also important to consider whether or not the study contributes to the general body of nursing knowledge. Some studies in nursing — historical studies, for example — may not be directly applicable in clinical practice but they contribute to our base of nursing knowledge. In the Discussion section of the report, the investigator should show how the findings of the study contribute to the field (Burns and Grove, 1993).

Most investigators identify areas where knowledge is inadequate and further research is required. These recommendations for further research should arise directly from the problem and findings. Such recommendations are either included in the Discussion section of the article, or these may appear in a separate section.

It is a convention in research to present a general summary of the study at the end of the article or report. It may be labelled Summary, or it may be included in a section titled Conclusions. This section is very similar to the abstract found at the beginning of the study, although the summary frequently emphasizes the findings more than the methodology. It is important to ensure that the summary is consistent with the focus of the study and that no deviations from the original purpose have taken place.

QUESTIONS TO ASK ABOUT THE DISCUSSION

1. Is the discussion clearly presented?
2. Is it reported logically? Is it well organized?
3. Are conclusions drawn from the data rather than the speculation of the researcher?
4. Are omissions and limitations of the study noted by the researcher?
5. Are the implications of the study clearly stated?
6. Do they seem plausible to you?
7. Is it clear how the study will extend previous findings?
8. Does the author give a concise, inclusive summary?

The Scientific Merit of a Study

Funding agencies who allocate monies for proposed research projects use *scientific merit* as one criterion in their evaluation of the worth of a project. Experts at the RNABC have identified the following as the basic elements for judging the scientific merit of a research project.

SCIENTIFIC MERIT — THE BASICS

* The proposal must be grounded in previous knowledge and relevant literature.
* The hypothesis and/or research question must be relevant, clear and crisp.
* The research design must be elegant — complete yet direct and simple.
* The methods proposed to test the hypothesis or answer the questions must be clearly described and appropriate.
* The study must be scientifically valid.
* The study must generate knowledge not yet articulated; or corroborate previous findings which need further study.

SOURCE: RNABC. (1990). *Nursing research: From question to funding — A workbook.* Vancouver, B.C.: Author. Reprinted with permission.

Selected Research Terminology

HYPOTHESIS A hypothesis is the statement of relationships the researcher expects to find between independent and dependent variables in a study. The hypothesis is usually a declarative statement and may be designated by the symbol H. If the researcher is going to test the reverse of his or her hypotheses, H_o represents the null hypothesis which is a statement that no relationship other than chance exists between or among a study's concepts or variables.

INSTRUMENTS Instruments are the devices used to record the data obtained from subjects. Two important qualities of research instruments used to measure variables in a research study are their reliability and validity. Reliability means that the instrument will produce consistent results, or data, on repeated use. For instance, if temperature is measured several times under unchanged conditions and the same readings are obtained, the measure is said to be reliable. Validity refers to the property or characteristic of a psychosocial instrument that means the instrument measures what it purports to measure.

FREQUENCY DISTRIBUTIONS A *frequency distribution* is an analysis method that involves determining how often scores or values appear in a data set. This procedure produces a **graph** showing how many times each score has occurred, that is, displaying the frequency of each score.

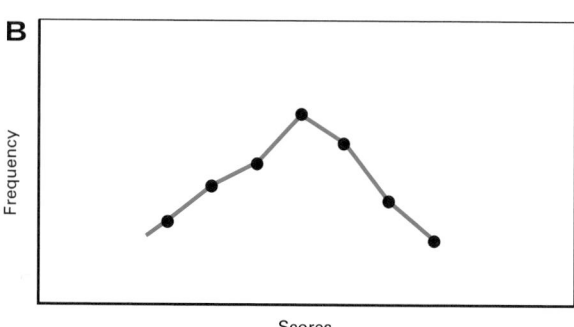

FIGURE 7.2 A. Histogram and B. Frequency polygon

The graph illustrates what is called the distribution of scores. An example of a frequency distribution is a **histogram**, which is a graphic display of a frequency table using rectangular bars with heights equal to the frequency in a particular class. Figure 7.2 shows a histogram and a polygon. The range is the simplest measure of dispersion. It represents the difference between the smallest and largest numbers in a distribution.

Measures of Central Tendency A measure of central tendency is a statistic that summarizes the data into one representative value. There are three measures of central tendency: the mean, median and mode.

- *Mean* (also called the average) is the measure of central tendency derived by dividing the sum of the values in a data set by the total number of values, scores or subjects in it. It is represented by the symbol x, read as *x bar*. The mean score is a balance point. If the scores were weights on a scale, the mean would be the spot at which the scale would balance.

- *Median* is the measure of central tendency that corresponds to the middle score. The median is obtained by rank ordering the scores. If there exists an uneven number of scores, exactly 50 percent of the scores are above the median, and 50 percent are below the median. If there are an even number of scores, the median is the average of the two middle scores. Thus, the median may not be an actual score in the data set.

- *Mode* is the category or class that has the highest frequency. It is the simplest measure of central tendency. The mode is the score or numerical value that occurs with the greatest frequency. A data set can have more than one mode. If two modes exist, the data set is referred to as bimodal. Thus, the mode does not necessarily indicate the centre of data set. Figure 7.3 shows the mean, median and mode all having the same value in a normal distribution. Figure 7.4 shows a bimodal frequency distribution where there are two large clusters of scores, one at the upper end of the of the curve, the other at the lower end. Figure 7.5 shows a skewed curve where a few high scores distort the value of the mean.

Standard Deviation The standard deviation is the most widely used measure of variability when a frequency distribution approximates a normal curve. It is the average of the deviations from the mean. The standard deviation of a group of scores is a number indicating whether most of those scores cluster closely around their mean or are spread out along the scale.

Correlation The Pearson Moment Correlation (r) is a statistic that shows the extent to which values of one variable are related to values of another variable. A correlation can be described in terms of the direction of the relationship. For example, a direct relationship is a pos-

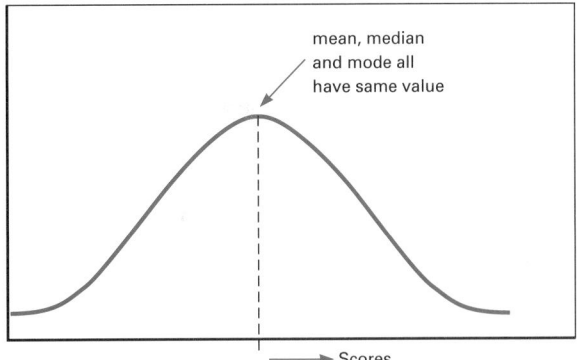

FIGURE 7.3   Measures of central tendency in a normal distribution

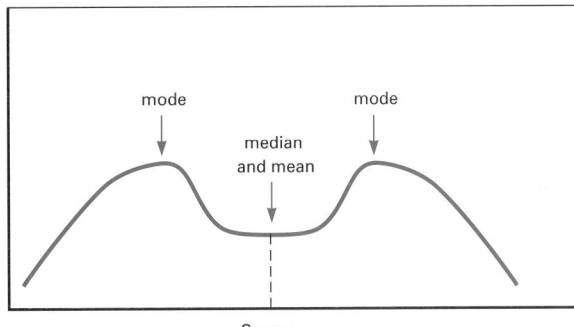

FIGURE 7.4   Bimodal frequency distribution

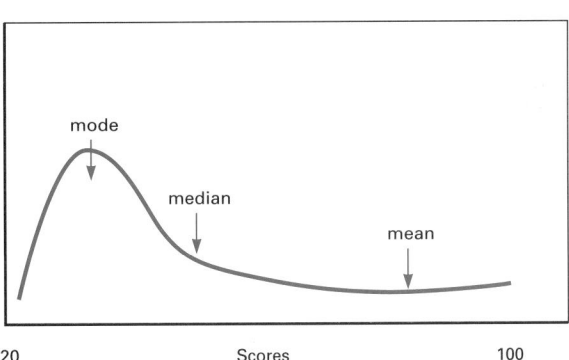

FIGURE 7.5   Skewed frequency distribution*

* In this situation, a very few students received extremely high scores, whereas the majority received very low scores. This means that the mean tends to give too high a picture of the typical score, and the mode gives a marked underestimate of the typical score. The median is the best indication of the typical score.

itive correlation between two variables. On the other hand, an indirect relationship (inverse relationship) is a negative correlation between two variables.

Guidelines for A Research Critique

TITLE AND ABSTRACT

1. Does the title of the research accurately reflect the problem under study?

2. Does the abstract provide a succinct overview of the study?

INTRODUCTION

1. Do you have a clear idea of what the research is all about?

2. Do you understand why the research is being done?

3. Is the significance of the problem discussed and the research justified?

4. Is the problem substantiated with adequate background information?

5. Is the problem statement clear? Concise?

REVIEW OF THE LITERATURE AND THEORETICAL FRAMEWORK

1. Does the literature review support the significance of the problem?

2. Is the relationship of the problem to previous research clear?

3. What is the theoretical base for this study? What are the major concepts used?

4. Does the researcher indicate how he or she has used previous knowledge in developing this study?

5. Is the literature review well organized? What topics are addressed?

6. Is there a sufficient review of the literature to assure the reader that the researcher has considered a broad spectrum of possibilities for investigating the problem?

7. Are the references up to date that is, are most of them less than 10 years old?

8. Has reference been made to classic studies in the area being investigated?

HYPOTHESES, ASSUMPTIONS AND OBJECTIVES

1. Has the initial problem statement been refined? Is the question now more precisely stated?

2. What variables has the researcher identified?

3. Are the variables specified in the refined research question? What is the dependent variable? Independent variables(s)?

4. What possible intervening variables has the researcher considered? Can you think of others?

5. Will the hypothesis(es) or data collected to prove

assumptions, attain objectives or answer research questions solve the basic research problem?

6. If a hypothesis is stated, is it specific to one relationship between variables? If more than one hypothesis is stated, is each one specific to one relationship?

THE RESEARCH DESIGN

1. What research design was used in this study? Quantitative: experimental? or non-experimental? Or Qualitative: grounded theory? phenomenological? or ethnomethodological?

2. Is the method appropriate for studying the problem? Does it follow clearly from the problem statement and research questions?

THE POPULATION UNDER STUDY

1. What are the common characteristics of the population under study?

2. How was the study population selected — were sampling techniques employed?

3. If sampling was used, what method was used for obtaining the sample? Is it appropriate for the type of study that was done?

4. Is the number in the sample sufficient? How does the researcher justify the sample size? Selection process?

5. In your opinion, is the sample representative of the defined population?

6. How did the researcher control for bias in selecting the sample?

SAFEGUARDING THE RIGHTS OF SUBJECTS IN THE STUDY

1. What measures were taken to ensure that the rights of subjects were protected in this study?

2. Does the researcher make available to the reader the information given to subjects about the research?

3. Does the researcher discuss possible benefits of the research for the subjects in the study?

DATA COLLECTION

1. What data were collected?

2. Were the data collected the right data to answer the research question?

3. How were the data collected?

4. Were the measures used to collect data appropriate for the study?

5. Did the researcher use a standard protocol for gathering data during the research?

6. If others besides the principal investigator collected data, how were they trained?

7. Does the researcher show evidence of having established the reliability and validity of the procedures used for data gathering?

DATA ANALYSIS AND RESULTS

1. Does the researcher inform you of the steps taken to process and interpret the data?

2. Do the methods selected to analyze the data seem appropriate?

3. Are reasons given for the methods used to analyze the data?

4. Are the primary findings of the study clearly presented?

5. Are the results clear?

6. Are conclusions logical?

7. Is there a statement on whether the data support the hypothesis(es) or assumptions?

8. Did the investigator identify methodological problems?

DISCUSSION

1. Is the discussion clearly presented?

2. Is it reported logically? Is it well organized?

3. Are conclusions drawn from the data rather than the speculation of the researcher?

4. Are omissions and limitations of the study noted by the researcher?

5. Are the implications of the study clearly stated?

6. Do they seem plausible to you?

7. Is it clear how the study will extend previous findings?

8. Does the researcher give a concise, inclusive summary?

9. What recommendations would you make to the author to improve this research? Note: These recommendations should follow logically and clearly from your assessment of the study.

10. How can you utilize this research in your studies or in your clinical practice?

KEY TERMS

research-based practice p. 138
solo research p. 139
collaborative research p. 140
refereed journal p. 140
subject p. 141
change agent p. 141
empirical p. 142
critique p. 145
evaluation p. 145
abstract p. 146
problem statement p. 146
research question p. 146
validate the knowledge base p. 147
operational definition p. 147
variable p. 148
research concepts p. 148
causality p. 148

dependent variable p. 148
independent variable p. 148
intervening variable p. 148
hypothesis p. 148
null hypothesis p. 148
assumptions p. 148
research design p. 149
quantitative p. 149
qualitative p. 149
reliability p. 150
validity p. 150
deductive p. 150
inductive p. 150
grounded theory p. 150
phenomenological p. 150
ethnography p. 150
ethnomethodological p. 150

participant observation p. 150
population p. 151
sample p. 151
accessible population p. 151
probability sampling p. 151
random sampling p. 151
simple random sampling p. 151
stratified sampling p. 151
cluster sampling p. 151
systematic sampling p. 151
control p. 152
convenience sampling
 (or accidental sampling) p. 152
quota sampling p. 152
purposive sampling p. 152
data p. 152
instrument p. 152

IN REVIEW

Nursing research was slow to develop in Canada for a number of reasons: a scarcity of qualified nurse researchers, a paucity of graduate programs offering courses in research methodology and a lack of incentive for practising nurses to do research. Until recently, most research in nursing has been undertaken in university schools of nursing by graduate students, faculty, research scholars and fellows. Today almost every large health agency, both hospital and community, has nurse researchers on staff who undertake studies and who help other staff to carry out research relevant to their practice areas.

Over the past decade, research-based practice has become an imperative for nurses. The components of this practice include the conduct of studies, the dissemination of findings and the utilization of research in practice. As students you can begin to identify researchable nursing practice problems. You may also be involved in gathering data for studies, evaluating research reports, using the findings of credible studies in your practice and sharing the findings of research with colleagues. You also have a responsibility to safeguard the health and the rights of clients who are subjects in a research study.

Nursing knowledge is gained both through unstructured means such as empathy, trial and error, intuition and tradition and through more structured research using scientific enquiry, critical thinking and logical reasoning. The scientific enquiry/research process involves the sequential steps of: (1) stating the problem, (2) gathering facts already known about the problem, (3) forming a theoretical framework for the study, (4) designing the research, (5) collecting data, (6) analyzing the data, (7) interpreting the results and (8) communicating the findings.

The goals of nursing research are to increase the knowledge base of nursing, to describe and explain phenomena, to strengthen accountability in client care and to improve the quality of human life. As beginning students your primary role is that of research consumer. This role includes learning to read and interpret research reports. These reports usually follow a format that includes: title, abstract, introduction, literature review, hypothesis/assumptions/ objectives, methodology, research design, population, data collection, data analysis and results and discussion. A critique involves a critical assessment of a study for its scientific merit and contribution to the nursing field. All elements of a research report should be assessed, using pre-determined criteria.

LEARNING ACTIVITIES

1. Explore the research being done in your school and in the clinical agencies affiliated with your school of nursing.

   a) What research projects are currently being carried out by school faculty? By graduate students? By nursing staff in the clinical agency (agencies)?

   b) Do the projects involve solo, collaborative or multidisciplinary research? International collaboration?

2. Compare the ethical guidelines suggested by the Canadian Nurses Association with those established by the research committee of your school/university or of a clinical agency with which the school is affiliated.

3. What sources are available to you for information on recent nursing research findings? What research journals are available in the library? Are there research seminars or conferences to which you can go? Is there a research interest group in the school or health agency? What other sources are available?

4. Select a research article on a topic of interest to you from one of the nursing research journals in the library. Do a critique of the article, using the guidelines at the end of the chapter.

REFERENCES AND READINGS

ALI, D., DOW-CLARKE, A. and MACCALDER, L. (1993). Health behaviours of pregnant women. In M. King, S.M. Stinson and K. Mills (Eds). (1993). *Proceedings of the First International Conference on Community Health Nursing Research. Edmonton, Alberta, Canada. September 26–29, 1993.* Edmonton: Edmonton Board of Health.

BENNER, P. (1984). *From novice to expert.* Menlo Park, CA: Addison-Wesley.

BENNER, P. and WRUBEL, J. (1980). *The primacy of caring.* Menlo Park, CA: Addison-Wesley.

BRINK, P.J. and WOOD, M.J. (1989). *Advance design in nursing research*. Newbury Park, CA: Sage.

BROWN, G. (1993). The sacred cow contest. *The Canadian Nurse, 89*(1), 31–35.

BRUSH, B.L. and STUART, M. (1992). Unity amidst difference? The I.C.N. project and writing international women's history. In *Visionaries: Proceedings of the First International Nursing History Conference, June 17–20, 1992, Saint John, New Brunswick, Canada*. The Canadian Association for the History of Nursing and the American Association for the History of Nursing.

BURNS, N. and GROVE, S.K. (1993).*The practice of nursing research. Conduct, critique and utilization*. (2nd ed.). Philadelphia: Saunders.

CANADIAN NURSES ASSOCIATION. (undated). *Nursing research: A solid foundation for nursing practice*. Ottawa: Author.

CANADIAN NURSES ASSOCIATION. (1985). *Statement on research in nursing*. Ottawa: Author.

CANADIAN NURSES ASSOCIATION. (1990). *Submission to the Royal Society of Canada University Research Committee*. Ottawa: Author.

CANADIAN NURSES ASSOCIATION. (1991). *Current trends in Canadian nursing research*. Ottawa: Author.

CANADIAN NURSES ASSOCIATION. (1992) *Index of Canadian nursing research. Including 1992 supplemental data*. Ottawa: Author.

CANADIAN NURSES ASSOCIATION. (1994). *Ethical guidelines for nursing research involving human subjects*. Ottawa: Author.

CHURCH, J., THURSTON, N., TENOVE, S. and WEISGERBER, R. (1991). *Nursing research in Canadian teaching hospitals*. Calgary: Foothills General Hospital Department of Nursing and Faculty of Nursing, University of Calgary.

COCHRAN, W.G. (1977). *Sampling techniques*. New York: Wiley.

COHEN, J.A. (1992). Janforum: Leininger's culture care theory of nursing. *Journal of Advanced Nursing, 17*. 1149.

DAVIES, B. and LOGAN, J. (1993). *Reading research. A user-friendly guide for nurses and other health professionals*. Ottawa: Canadian Nurses Association.

DAVIES, B., LEITERMAN, J., DULBERG, C., DONBROOK, C., CLOSS, C. and MCDONALD, B. (1993). In M. King, S.M. Stinson and K. Mills (Eds). (1993). *Proceedings of the First International Conference on Community Health Nursing Research. Edmonton, Alberta, Canada. September 26–29, 1993*. Edmonton: Edmonton Board of Health.

DAVIES, B., NIDAY, P., NIMROD, D., STEWART, P., SPRAGUE, A. and DULBERG, C. (1993). Prevention of preterm birth: A population survey of health professionals. In M. King, S.M. Stinson and K. Mills (Eds). (1993). *Proceedings of the First International Conference on Community Health Nursing Research. Edmonton, Alberta, Canada. September 26–29, 1993*. Edmonton: Edmonton Board of Health.

DOWNS, F.S., (1984) *A source book of nursing research*. (3rd ed.). Philadelphia: F.A. Davis.

DU GAS, B.W. (1969). *An analysis of certain factors in the diffusion of innovations in nursing practice in the public general hospitals of the province of British Columbia*. Unpublished doctoral dissertation, the University of British Columbia, Vancouver.

ETHEL JOHNS PAPERS. (undated). University of British Columbia Main Library Special Collections.

EVALINE MARY PEMBERTON: REGISTRATION INFORMATION. Various unpublished documents. Registered Nurses Association of Nova Scotia.

FIELD, P.A. and MORSE, J.M. (1985). *Nursing research. The application of qualitative approaches*. Rockville, Maryland: Aspen Publishers, Inc.

FIELD, P.A., STINSON, S.M. and THIBEAUDEAU, J. (1992). Graduate education in nursing in Canada. In A.J. Baumgart and J. Larsen. *Canadian nursing faces the future*. Toronto: Mosby, 421–445.

GRINSPUN, D., MAC MILLAN, K., NICHOL, H. and SHIELDS, D.(1993). Using research findings in the hospital. *The Canadian Nurse, 89*(1), 46–48.

HALL, D.C. (1989). *Primary health care–A nursing model*. A Denmark–Newfoundland (Canada) project. Report available farom Registered Nurses Association of Newfoundland.

LOBIONDO-WOOD, G. and HABER, J. (1990). *Nursing research. Methods, critical appraisal and utilization*. (2nd ed.). St. Louis: Mosby.

MCCORMACK, D. and GOODING, B.A. (1993). Homeless persons communicate their meaning of health. *Canadian Journal of Nursing Research, 25*(1), 33–50.

MOSES, F.M. (1979). *RNANS 1909–1979: A brief history of the years from the beginning of the Association in 1901 through 1934*. Halifax: Registered Nurses Association of Nova Scotia.

MUNHALL, P.L. and OILER, C.J. (1986). Nursing research. A qualitative perspective. Norwalk, CT: Appleton–Century–Crofts.

OGILVIE, L. D. (1993). Nurses and primary health care in Nepal. In M. King, S.M. Stinson and K. Mills (Eds). (1993). *Proceedings of the First International Conference on Community Health Nursing Research. Edmonton, Alberta, Canada. September 26–29, 1993*. Edmonton: Edmonton Board of Health.

OLSON, K., HONORE, I., VANDER KLAAUW, A., BERKEL, J. and GOEDKE, H. (1993). Ovarian cancer among older women in Northern Alberta. In M. King, S.M. Stinson and K. Mills (Eds). (1993). *Proceedings of the First International Conference on Community Health Nursing Research. Edmonton, Alberta, Canada. September 26–29, 1993*. Edmonton: Edmonton Board of Health.

REGISTERED NURSES ASSOCIATION OF BRITISH COLUMBIA (RNABC). (1990). *Nursing research: from question to funding. A workbook*. Vancouver, B.C.: Author.

REGISTERED NURSES ASSOCIATION OF BRITISH COLUMBIA (RNABC). (1991). *Current nursing research projects in BC (1991). A compendium*. Vancouver: Author.

RITCHIE, J.A. (1992). Research issues. In A.J. Baumgart and J. Larsen. *Canadian nursing faces the future*. Toronto: Mosby, 307–324.

ROSENBAUM, J.N. (1991). Widowhood grief: A cultural perspective. *Canadian Journal of Nursing Research, 23*(2), 61–76.

RYAN-WENGER, N.M. (1992).Guidelines for critique of a research report. *Heart and Lung, 21*(4), 394–401.

STREET, M.M. (1973). *Watch-fires on the mountains: The life and writings of Ethel Johns*. Toronto: University of Toronto Press.

TABER'S CYCLOPEDIC MEDICAL DICTIONARY. (16th ed.). (1989). Philadelphia: F. A. Davis.

THE WESTERN HOSPITAL OF MONTREAL, 1974–1924: A HALF CENTURY OF SERVICE. (1929). Montreal: Nurses' Alumnae Association of the Western Hospital of Montreal.

WOODS N.F. and CATANZARO, M. (1988). *Nursing research*. St. Louis: Mosby.

Dimensions of Health

Health and Basic Needs

CENTRAL QUESTIONS

1. What is the nature of Maslow's hierarchy of needs?

2. What five basic needs did Maslow postulate?

3. How did Kalish adapt Maslow's hierarchy of needs?

4. Describe briefly Freud's Theory of Psychosexual Development.

5. What are the four stages of Piaget's Theory of Cognitive Development?

6. Describe briefly Kohlberg's Theory of Moral Development.

7. What are the stages and conflicts in each stage of Erikson's Theory of Psychosocial Development?

8. What are the different Passages of Adulthood described by Sheehy?

9. What are Peck's developmental tasks of middle-aged and older adults?

10. How do cultural values and beliefs influence social and psychological growth and development?

11. What are the stages of fetal growth and development?

12. What needs require special attention during pregnancy and what factors affect these needs?

13. Outline the development of an individual through the various stages of the life cycle from birth to old age.

14. What factors affect basic needs during each stage of the life cycle?

INTRODUCTION

In Unit 1, we discussed some of the basic concepts that underlie our current beliefs about health and illness. If we accept the premise that optimal health, or wellness, is the ability to function at one's highest level physically, mentally, spiritually and socially, it seems appropriate to look at the conditions that foster optimum functioning. What is needed for individuals to attain their optimal level of well-being? This leads us to a consideration of basic human needs.

There are certain basic needs common to all human beings which must be fulfilled if individuals are to attain their optimal level of well-being. The subject of basic needs has been studied in depth by social scientists looking for the motivating forces underlying human behaviour, and by people in the health field seeking to identify factors causing health problems. Early theorists felt that all human needs could be categorized under two headings: physiological and psychological. Another group of theorists classified needs on the basis of whether their origin was internal or external. Still others felt that basic human needs couldn't be categorized, and simply identified long lists of them.

Abraham Maslow's theory of a hierarchy of needs is used in many nursing schools as a conceptual framework for the consideration of human needs. Not everyone agrees with all aspects of his theory, and some have suggested modifications to his hierarchy, but the basic principles outlined in the theory are fairly well accepted.

Maslow suggested that there are five basic categories of human needs and that these may be arranged in order of priority for satisfaction. According to Maslow's theory, lower level needs must be satisfied (or, at least, mostly so) before the individual can attempt to satisfy needs of a higher order. The types of needs identified by Maslow, in order of priority, are:

1. Physiological needs
2. Safety and security needs
3. Needs for love and belonging
4. Esteem needs
5. Needs for self-actualization (Maslow, 1970).

Much of nursing is concerned with helping people to meet their basic needs and to achieve optimal health or wellness. This part of nursing is embodied in the caring aspects of the nursing role and includes basic nursing measures that are applicable in the care of individuals of all ages.

It is generally agreed that people have the same basic needs throughout the life span. However, the expression of these needs and their relative importance to an individual's well-being vary with a person's age and his or her stage of physical and psychosocial development A growing child's nutritional needs are different from those of a middle-aged adult; the child needs more protein, for instance, to build bones and muscle tissue.

Both the very young and the very old have increased safety needs. The very young have not yet learned to be aware of danger, and so need the help of others to protect them from harm. The elderly have bones that are more fragile and break more easily than those of younger people. Their sensory faculties are also usually not as efficient in alerting them to danger in the environment. Therefore, they are more likely to trip over something in their path and suffer a broken wrist or ankle as a result.

In this chapter, we will explore the nature of basic human needs. We will also look at some of the theories of growth and development that contribute to our understanding of differences in basic needs at various stages in the life cycle. Finally we will try to put it all together in a discussion of changes that occur as individuals grow and develop throughout life, and look at the needs requiring particular attention at each stage.

THE NATURE OF BASIC NEEDS

MASLOW'S HIERARCHY OF NEEDS

The basic needs identified by Maslow were listed at the beginning of this chapter. Maslow believed that there is a prioritization to these needs, hence his concept of a hierarchy. According to Maslow, the more fundamental needs must be satisfied before a person can proceed to seek satisfaction for needs of a higher order.

Physiological needs, of course, take precedence over all others because they are essential for survival. These include the need for water, for food, for air, for elimination, for rest and sleep, for temperature maintenance and for the avoidance of pain. When a person is starving, life revolves around the need to obtain food. Similarly, a person deprived of water for a long period of time is concerned above all else with relieving his or her thirst. The fulfillment of certain physiological needs is so essential that if there is interference with the attainment of them, life itself is threatened. If there is interference with breathing, for example, and a person's air supply is cut off, prompt measures must be initiated to restore adequate respiration or the person will die within a matter of minutes. The relief of pain is also a primary physiological need. If pain is severe, the sufferer cannot rest, sleep or think of anything else until the pain is relieved.

Next in order of priority, according to Maslow, are the *safety and security* needs. These include adequate shelter from the elements and protection from harmful factors in the environment. But people must also *feel* that they are secure and protected from both real and imagined dangers. People usually feel more secure when they are in familiar surroundings, with accustomed routines and with those they can trust. Conversely, they feel threatened when they are in strange places, when their usual pattern of living is disturbed or when they are among strangers or have no familiar objects around them. Often, inanimate objects assume a symbolism that represents safety and security for an individual. Linus's blanket (in Charles Schulz's cartoon "Peanuts"), which he carries everywhere with him, has become a symbol of security that is recognized by most North Americans. Almost all children have a toy or other object that gives them a sense of security; they often like to take their favourite teddy bear or pillow with them wherever they go. The familiar object helps to give them a feeling of security when they are in strange surroundings or unfamiliar situations. Many adults, too, have lucky charms, talismans or other objects that they feel give them special protection against harm. Maslow has suggested that many of our religious rituals, our superstitions and our traditions have their origins in this basic need for safety and security.

Maslow placed the needs for **love and belonging** as next most fundamental. There is little question that these are very basic needs indeed. Infants deprived of love and affection do not thrive, even if all of their physiological and safety needs are met. Adults also need love and affection. They need to have people who are close to them to share their joys and sorrows, their anxieties and their doubts. People who do not have close ties with others often have pets on whom they lavish all the love and affection they do not have the opportunity to share with other people.

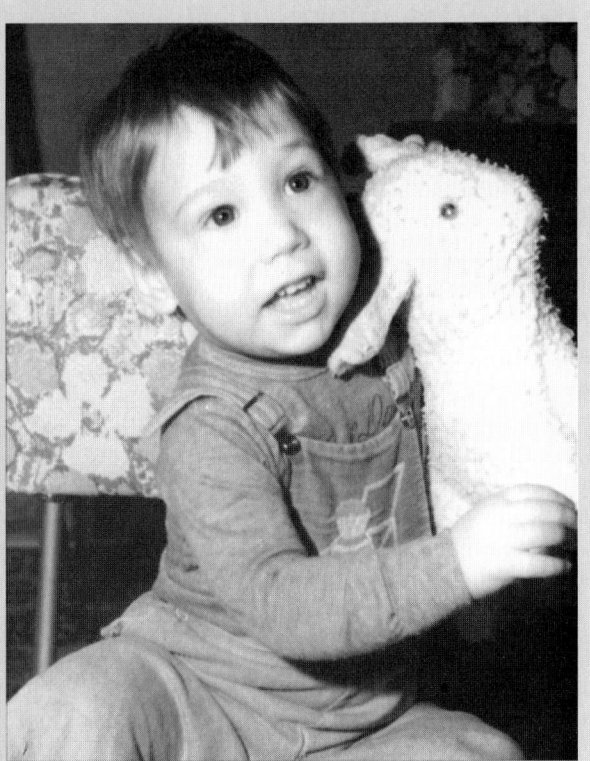

Most children have a favourite toy that gives them a sense of security. This little boy takes "Buppy," his favourite lamb, wherever he goes.

Next in the hierarchy Maslow put the **esteem** needs. People have to feel that they are worthwhile human beings — that is, they must have self-esteem — and they must also feel that they are considered persons of worth and dignity. Maslow has suggested that many of the problems in our depersonalized society, particularly in big cities, are due to failure to satisfy the two basic needs of love and belonging and of esteem. If these needs are not satisfied, people have a low regard for themselves, and feelings of inadequacy, frustration, alienation and hopelessness result (Bourne and Ekstrand, 1979).

Finally, in Maslow's hierarchy, are the needs for **self-actualization**. These include the need to attain one's highest potential and achieve one's ambitions in life. Maslow also included here the need for knowledge and aesthetic needs.

KALISH'S ADAPTATION OF MASLOW'S HIERARCHY

Subsequent theorists have suggested modifications to Maslow's hierarchy. Richard Kalish (1966), for example, believed that the need for knowledge, as exemplified by human curiosity, is a more fundamental need than Maslow depicted in his hierarchy. He placed it second, after physiological needs, and included in this category sex, activity, exploration and novelty. Again, to use an example drawn from childhood, infants who do not have sufficient opportunity to explore their surroundings and to manipulate objects, or who are kept in a monotonous environment, do not attain their optimal development physiologically, emotionally or socially. Older children and adults will often forgo safety and security in a desire to obtain stimulation or, sometimes, just to satisfy their curiosity.

The sex drive is also, of course, very fundamental, since it is essential for the survival of the species. However, it is a drive that can be sublimated; that is, it can be channelled into other forms of activity, such as a career. Or, its gratification can be delayed. It may sometimes be delayed indefinitely, as in the case of people in some religious orders who take vows of chastity.

GROWTH AND DEVELOPMENT

THEORIES ABOUT GROWTH AND DEVELOPMENT

In Maslow's hierarchy (and in others subsequently developed) individuals are seen as constantly striving to fulfill their basic needs. As one set of needs is gratified, others of a higher order emerge and become more powerful. People who have fulfilled the first four levels of needs may spend

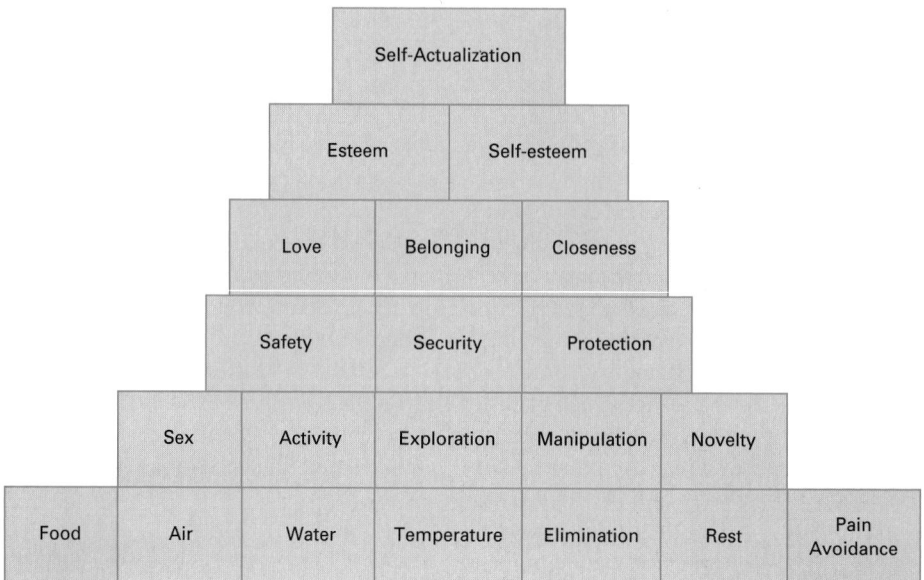

FIGURE 8.1   Maslow's hierarchy of needs adapted by Kalish

SOURCE: Kalish, R.A. (1966). *The Psychology of Human Behavior.* Belmont, California: Wadsworth.

their lives developing their self-actualizing needs by hunting for rare art objects (aesthetic needs) or by becoming scholarly authorities on particular subjects (knowledge needs).

The concept that is presented in Maslow's theory, then, is not of human beings as static entities, trying simply to maintain their equilibrium in a changing world, but of individuals as developing beings, constantly reaching for things beyond their immediate grasp. This concept embodies the idea of continuous growth and development of the human organism, which begins at the moment of birth and continues until death.

The study of human development has received a great deal of attention in recent years from educators and social scientists, as well as from people in the health field. Our knowledge of physical growth and development has increased tremendously with advances in scientific technology that permit us to measure, with a great deal of accuracy, the changes occurring in most body tissues and processes throughout the life span. Our understanding of social and psychological development, however, has to be derived from studies of observable behaviour. A wide variety of theories exist to account for our social and psychological development, each one stressing one or more aspects of it.

FREUD AND PSYCHOSOCIAL DEVELOPMENT

One of the pioneers in the field of personality development was Sigmund Freud. His theory of psychosexual development shocked the scientific and lay community of the early 1900s and still evokes controversy today. According to Freud, individuals progress through five stages of development from infancy through puberty, and it is the quality of their experiences in each stage that determines their adult personality. Deprivation, or overindulgence, of the individual's needs in any one of the stages may cause him or her to become "fixated" at that stage. The five stages identified by Freud were:

- **Oral Stage** (birth to 18 months) Freud believed that during this stage infants derive their greatest sensual satisfaction through their mouths. Behavioural traits that may develop as a result of too little or too much oral satisfaction in infancy, he felt, included aggression, a preoccupation with food or drink, cigarette smoking and nail biting.

- **Anal Stage** (18 months to 3 years) Freud felt that toddlers' greatest pleasures come from moving their bowels. The management of toilet training during this stage is therefore crucial to one's development. If this training is not handled correctly, the individual may show behavioural characteristics as an adult that include hoarding, an obsession with cleanliness, or conversely, a tendency towards slothfulness. If training is too rigid, Freud felt, the parent might stifle the child's creativity.

- **Oedipal Stage** (3 to 6 years) During this stage, according to Freud, the child identifies with and derives sensual satisfaction from the parent of the opposite sex, and views the parent of the same sex as a rival. Behavioural traits that Freud felt may develop from overindulgence or deprivation at this stage include competitiveness, seductiveness and a preoccupation with older partners.

- **Latent Stage** (6 to 11 years) The child at this stage identifies with the parent of the same sex, and learns to assume his or her appropriate social role. Behavioural characteristics that Freud believed were formed at this stage include the development of a conscience as well as the seeds for later rebellion if this stage is not handled properly by parents.

- **Genital Stage** (11 to 14 years) Freud believed that adolescents derive their most pleasurable experiences through their genital organs. Personality traits felt to result from mishandling of this stage include a tendency to rationalization and a preoccupation with sex.

The terms coined by Freud are still widely used, although most people feel that his theory of psychosexual development is too restrictive, focussing as it does on only one aspect (sexual) of growth and development (Freud, 1972).

PIAGET AND INTELLECTUAL DEVELOPMENT

Looking at growth and development from a different perspective, Jean Piaget formulated a theory of cognitive, or intellectual, development based on four sequential stages. Subsequent studies have confirmed that although the rate of development may vary, children do indeed seem to progress through the stages of intellectual development in a sequence similar to the one Piaget outlined. These stages are briefly described as follows:

- **Sensorimotor Stage** (birth to 2 years). During this stage children are concerned mainly with actions and sensations that affect them directly. They begin to relate to outside events, at first tentatively, then actively experimenting with their environment. They develop *object permanence* (knowledge that an object exists even when it is not visible to them). At birth, the infant's response range is basically limited to reflex actions. By the age of two he or she is capable of thinking through a problem before taking action.

- **Preoperational Stage** (2 to 7 years). At this stage a child's thinking is still *egocentric*. That is, children are concerned mainly with themselves. They believe that everyone sees the world as they do. Language becomes an important vehicle of communication. Piaget has divided this stage into two distinct periods:

  - **Preconceptual Period** (2 to 4 years). Children at this point are not yet capable of reason, although they are able to form general concepts. They may call all soft, stuffed toys "bear," for example, or they may use a face cloth (with which they have just wiped their face) to polish the furniture.

  - **Perceptual (Intuitive) Period** (4 to 7 years). Children at this stage are capable of reason, yet it is not a logical, adult form of thinking. They can only concentrate on one aspect of an object or idea at a time. For example, if a child at this stage put an equal number of candies in two jars, one tall and narrow, the other short and stout, he or she would think there were more candies in the tall narrow jar because the level of candies would be higher.

- **Concrete Operational Stage** (7 to 11 years). During this stage, children's reasoning becomes logical but is limited to their own experiences. They are now able to understand concepts and to concentrate on more than one aspect of an object or idea. For example, if you asked a seven-year-old boy to describe a coin, he could probably tell you that it is round, that it is shiny and that it is a form of money. At this point the children acquire the ability to reverse their thinking, learning the relationship of cause and effect.

- **Formal Operational Stage** (11 to 16 years). During this stage individuals acquire the ability to develop abstract concepts for themselves. Their thinking is oriented towards problem-solving and transcends concrete experience. They no longer have to experience things before they can understand them. Science fiction has a great appeal for people at this stage.

Piaget's Theory of Cognitive Development is currently well accepted, although some feel that it is incomplete because Piaget believed that the highest level of cognitive development is reached by the end of adolescence. Subsequent studies indicate that individuals do not reach their full mental capacity until about age 25, and that they continue to learn throughout their life span. Another criticism of Piaget's theory is that he does not give enough consideration to the effects of environmental factors on intellectual development (Piaget, 1963, 1969).

KOHLBERG AND MORAL DEVELOPMENT

Looking at a different aspect of psychological development, Lawrence Kohlberg presented a theory of *moral* development, defining three levels that, like Piaget's, are inflexibly sequential, but are attained at varying rates. According to Kohlberg, the individual's progression through these levels occurs as conflict is encountered, often through interaction with a person at a higher level. Progression through these levels of moral development is not necessarily age-related; in fact, it may be more dependent on socioeconomic status. According to one study, more middle-class adolescent boys reached levels two and three than did their lower-class peers (Munsinger, 1975). Kohlberg's levels are as follows:

- **Preconventional** At this level, individuals are primarily concerned with themselves. They are occupied only with satisfying their own needs, without regard to others. An individual at this level will obey an authority figure, although only to avoid punishment.

- **Conventional** At this level, individuals are concerned mainly with pleasing others and maintaining order. They show great respect for rules and socially accepted authority figures, such as policemen.

- **Postconventional** At this level, an individual's morality is based on personal conscience, dictated by the desire to avoid self-condemnation. The individual shows a profound respect for human dignity and life. He or she is able to think abstractly and to take another's point of view (Kohlberg, 1984).

ERIKSON AND PSYCHOSOCIAL DEVELOPMENT

Erik Erikson formulated a theory of psychosocial development that, like Kohlberg's theory of moral development, is based on conflicts. According to Erikson's theory, however, people encounter the conflicts within themselves. Although, ideally, individuals resolve each conflict as it is encountered, failure to do so does not mean that they will forever be burdened with it. It is possible to resolve the conflict at a later stage. According to Erikson, there are a number of developmental tasks related to the principal conflicts that an individual must complete at each stage.

Resolution of the conflicts during the stages of infancy through the preschool years is largely dependent on one's parents. During middle childhood and the adolescent years this responsibility is shared with the child's teachers. Beginning in adolescence and continuing through the adult years, individuals assume responsibility for their own development. A brief outline of Erikson's stages of development, including the principal conflict and some related developmental tasks, is given below.

- **Infancy** (birth to 18 months)
Principal Conflict: Trust vs. Mistrust. During this stage infants develop either a basic trust or mistrust of others, depending on the relationship they develop with their mothers (or other principal caregivers) and the quality of care they receive.
Tasks: Mother and infant adjust to each other. Infant learns to take solid foods, to walk and to talk.

- **Early Childhood** (18 months to 3 years)
Principal Conflict: Autonomy vs. Shame. During this stage children either develop a sense of pride in their independence and new accomplishments or they develop feelings of shame and doubt concerning their abilities to deal with other people and the world.
Tasks: The child seeks independence in his or her actions, learns to control elimination, learns to communicate through language and learns to differentiate between right and wrong.

- **The Preschool Years** (3 to 6 years)
Principal Conflict: Initiative vs. Guilt. In this stage children learn to initiate activities, and it is the response

they receive to these activities that determines whether their sense of initiative will remain intact or whether they will feel a sense of guilt for their actions.
Tasks: The child establishes relations with his or her peers, begins to form concepts based on reality, refines his or her motor control and learns a social role based on gender identification.

- **Middle Childhood** (6 to 11 years)
Principal Conflict: Industry vs. Inferiority. During this stage children divide their time between home and school. A negative response received at home to their new sense of industry can be neutralized by a positive response at school, or vice versa. If children encounter consistent failure or discouragement, however, they will experience feelings of inferiority.
Tasks: The child learns autonomy, refines his or her coordination, learns cooperation and self-control, develops social skills, learns to view the world objectively and forms values.

- **Adolescence** (11 to 18 years)
Principal Conflict: Identity vs. Role Confusion. During this stage adolescents ideally develop a positive and stable sense of identity, or self-image, in relation to their past and future. Lacking this, they will experience a sense of confusion with regard to their social role.
Tasks: The adolescent accepts his or her changed physique, seeks and achieves independence from adults, forms close peer relations, defines his or her social role and reasons logically.

- **Early Adulthood** (18 to 35 years)
Principal Conflict: Intimacy vs. Isolation. During this stage individuals establish close relationships with others of the same and opposite sex. If individuals develop no close emotional ties they will experience feelings of isolation.
Tasks: The individual decides on a career path, chooses a marriage partner, raises children and assumes social responsibilities.

- **The Middle Years** (35 to 65 years)
Principal Conflict: Generativity vs. Self-absorption. Generativity means being concerned with the future of society and the world in general. Persons lacking in this quality are overly concerned with themselves.
Tasks: Individuals adjust to physical and physiological changes, accept the needs of their children and of their aging parents and attain their career and social goals.

- **The Later Years** (65 plus)
Principal Conflict: Integrity vs. Despair. During this stage most adults take stock of their lives and their accomplishments. If they are content with what they have done, they experience what is called "integrity," or a sense of "wholeness." People who are dissatisfied with life, who wish they could do it over again, yet know that it is impossible, succumb to despair.

Tasks: The individual accepts the aging process, adjusts to retirement and adjusts to the death of his or her spouse and friends (Erikson, 1963).

SHEEHY AND THE PASSAGES OF ADULTHOOD

Erikson was one of the earliest of the developmentalists to go beyond the realms of childhood to incorporate changes occurring during adulthood into his life cycles theory of growth and development. His work has subsequently been extended by others in the field. Notable among those who followed Erikson is Gail Sheehy (1976), who has contributed much to our understanding of the nature of the inner changes taking place as a person passes through the various turning points of adulthood. Sheehy preferred to call these turning points "passages," rather than crises, because *crisis* has negative connotations. The passages, Sheehy felt, are very normal and highly predictable. Although individuals experience a period of instability as they pass each turning point, it is not necessarily a "bad" experience. Rather, each passage represents an essential factor in their growth and development.

Early Adulthood   In her research, Sheehy found that, although men and women both reported going through the same passages in adult life, they did not necessarily do so at the same ages or in the same sequences. A woman who has spent her young adult years at home raising a family, for example, may be just entering the labour force at the age of 40. On the other hand, a man who has been the bread-winner of the family since his early 20s may feel that he has reached just about the peak of his career at age 40 and will be looking for something else to round out and enrich his life. Sheehy divides the early adult period (from 18 to 35 years) into four stages or passages:

1. **Pulling up Roots** (after age 18) — Moving away from the family and family home for higher education or career and beginning independence.
2. **The Trying Twenties** — A time of goal achieving, career, relationships, child bearing and rearing.
3. **Catch 30** (approaching age 30) — The need to reassess and change the direction of one's life — a marriage or divorce, a child where there was a decision to be childless, a promotion or a new career.
4. **Rooting and Extending** (to age 35) — Stabilizing and putting out roots. Community involvement and family promotion, plus all-out career efforts.

Later Adulthood   Erikson grouped together the years from age 35 to 65, calling them the "middle years." Sheehy, however, divides these years into two distinct "passages." The period from age 35 to 45 she calls the "Deadline Decade." It is a crossroads, a time when individuals must come to terms with themselves and set a life course before time runs out. Levinson (1978) has coined the term "BOOM" (becoming one's own man) to describe this maturational crisis stage. According to Sheehy, women often feel this push around age 35, and men feel it around age 40.

"Renewal or Resignation" is the term Sheehy uses to describe life after age 45. If individuals have felt and responded to the urge to reorganize life during the preceding decade, they will experience a feeling of happiness or renewal during the remainder of adult life. If they have simply continued on in an unsatisfactory course set earlier, they may experience a feeling of stagnation, becoming resigned to the idea that now it is too late to change.

PECK'S DEVELOPMENTAL TASKS OF MIDDLE AGE AND OLDER

Robert Peck's (1960) research shows that the middle aged are more concerned with a reassessment of self than with Erikson's concepts of intimacy and generativity. To Peck, the middle-aged and older individuals are faced with four additional developmental tasks:

1. Valuing wisdom versus valuing physical power: Finding identity from values and judgements based on wisdom from life experiences as one's physical strength declines.
2. Socializing versus sexualizing: Redefining the male–female relationship away from sexual objectives.
3. Cathectic or emotional flexibility versus cathectic impoverishment: Adjusting to the losses of middle and older age and investing in new interpersonal adventures.
4. Mental flexibility versus mental rigidity: Problem-solving and finding new solutions to old problems, option-hunting versus doing things from habit.

OTHER THEORISTS

Neugarten (1968), Gould (1975), Berger (1993) and Schuster (1992) all offer other theories about the developmental stages of the middle-aged and older person. Healthy development through involvement in continuing education, extending family pursuits, second careers and changing life style patterns are discussed. Retirement planning in early adulthood is proving to be another key to healthy, happy and active aging.

CULTURAL INFLUENCES ON GROWTH AND DEVELOPMENT

Cultural groups in any one society offer a wealth of diverse beliefs and practices. It is essential to consider these differences as they relate to health behaviours and thus to the

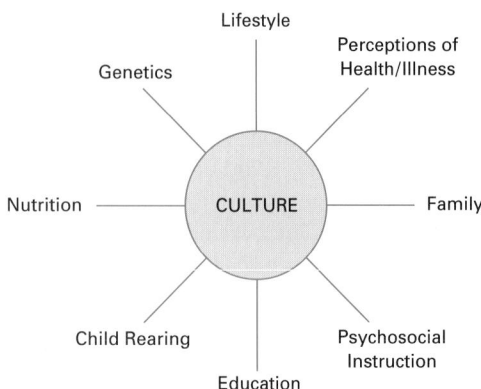

FIGURE 8.2 Cultural influences on growth and development

SOURCE: Developed by Vukic, A. and adapted by Fraser-Davey, H. (1993). *Culture/Health*. Halifax, Nova Scotia: Dalhousie University, School of Nursing. Reproduced with permission.

growth and developmental patterns of individuals. Each culture has different emphases on family, on child-rearing practices, on nutrition, on health care and on education. The culture will influence the lifestyle and the socialization of its members.

Even genetically, there are health-related differences among people. Different races may have a greater tendency to some diseases and disorders than others in the same country of residence. Asians have a predisposition to adult lactose intolerance and African Americans a higher incidence of anemia.

It is a part of the nurse's task to understand and adapt to the cultural status of an individual. In the young, growth and development tests commonly used must only be applied when culturally specific. Although some would dispute the possibility of developing tests that are entirely "culture-free," it is possible to use tests that are not culturally biased. In a verbal test, for example, a picture-matching technique may be used when the child's first language is not English. At the other end of the age spectrum, the elderly tend to depend on and get comfort from their traditions and practices. No matter what the age, in times of stress, illness, loss and separation, it is not unusual for people to call on all their cultural values and beliefs to sustain them.

PRENATAL GROWTH AND DEVELOPMENT

There is a great deal of controversy, particularly in regard to the debate over abortion, as to whether the fetus is a human being. Regardless of one's views on this matter, **gestation** — the term used to describe the development of new life that takes place in the womb between conception and birth — begins at conception when the male sperm unites with the

female ovum (or ova) during its journey down the fallopian tube. This development normally takes nine months and is divided into three stages.

Zygote Stage (Fertilization to 2 Weeks)

During this stage, the cells of the fertilized ovum, now called a **zygote**, multiply rapidly and the new cell mass moves down the fallopian tube and into the uterus. Approximately two weeks after fertilization the zygote attaches itself to the uterine wall.

Embryonic Stage (2 to 8 Weeks)

After the zygote has attached itself to the uterine wall, the cells continue to multiply, forming three distinct layers. The **ectoderm**, or outer layer, will later form the nervous system and sense organs; the **mesoderm**, or middle layer, becomes the skeletal, muscular and circulatory systems; the **endoderm**, or inner layer, becomes the digestive system.

It is during the embryonic stage that the amniotic sac and the placenta are formed. The **amniotic sac** is a protective membrane filled with fluid that surrounds the developing embryo, providing warmth, moisture and relative freedom of movement. The **placenta** is an organ that attaches to the uterine wall and to the fetus by means of the **umbilical cord**. Through the umbilical cord, the unborn child receives nourishment and oxygenated blood, and disposes of wastes. The placenta serves as a barrier protecting the developing child from potentially harmful agents.

By eight weeks, the embryo is recognizably human, with distinct arms, legs, fingers and toes, although the head comprises about half its length. It is only about two and a half centimetres long, but already its systems are beginning to function.

Fetal Stage (8 Weeks to Birth)

The most striking change that occurs during the fetal stage is the dramatic increase in size from approximately two and a half centimetres to an average length of 45 to 50 centimetres at birth. The systems that began to form in the embryonic stage increase in complexity and maturity. The fetus begins to move by the third month, although this is not usually felt by the mother until the fourth or fifth month when its actions become more vigorous. By the sixth month, the eyelids open and the fetus begins to take amniotic fluid into its lungs as a rudimentary form of breathing.

The greatest brain development occurs during the last few months of the fetal stage. Until the seventh month, the fetus is virtually incapable of living outside the womb owing to the immaturity of its nervous system.

The seven-month fetus is neurologically mature enough to survive in the extrauterine world in a controlled environment. It can breathe, although the lungs are not fully developed until approximately 36 weeks, or just before birth in a full-term infant. Also, the fetus at seven months has not accumulated the layers of fat so noticeable in a full-term baby, which protect the fetus from temperature changes and enable him or her to go without nourishment for the first day or two after birth.

The eighth and ninth months of fetal development are devoted primarily to maturation of the lungs and nervous system and to the accumulation of fat. Towards the end of the ninth month, activity often diminishes as the fetus becomes cramped for space. Shortly before the onset of labour the fetus becomes "engaged" in the pelvic cavity, normally with its head down, in preparation for birth.

During its period of development inside the womb the fetus is totally dependent on the mother to satisfy its basic needs. She provides nutrients, oxygen, warmth and protection and disposes of fetal wastes. Although the placenta provides some protection from harmful agents, many others pass through the placental barrier to the fetus. As the fetus is very vulnerable to infection and the effects of noxious stimuli, particularly in its early developmental stages, the mother must take care to protect her unborn child from such dangers. Studies have suggested that maternal emotions might affect the developing fetus, too, and can have long-range effects on personality. To date, the results of such studies have been inconclusive, largely owing to the difficulty of collecting data over a period of several years, and of separating out other influences that may affect a person's psychological make-up.

PREGNANCY

Pregnancy occurs traditionally during the stage of early adulthood. Just as there are three stages of growth and development of the fetus, there are three stages of pregnancy for the mother-to-be. While the unborn child grows and develops inside the womb of the mother, many other changes are occurring that affect the pregnant woman herself. The duration of an average pregnancy is 38 weeks from conception (or 40 weeks from the last menstrual period), divided into trimesters of three months each.

Pregnancy

NEEDS REQUIRING PARTICULAR ATTENTION	FACTORS RELATED TO THESE NEEDS
Nutrition	Growth of new tissue, requiring additional nourishment Fetal nutritional needs are met through proper maternal intake
Elimination	Hormonal changes affecting kidney and bowel function and digestion Expansion of uterus in pelvis and into abdominal cavity
Circulation	Increase in total fluid volume Increased body mass
Comfort, rest and sleep	Weight gain, increasing body bulk Altered body proportions, making some resting positions difficult
Pain management	Medications may cross placenta and have harmful effects on the fetus
Movement and exercise	Awkwardness due to weight gain; increase in fluid volume; shift in centre of gravity, affecting balance; and relaxing of ligaments Slowing down of body processes
Safety	Fetal well-being dependent on mother Shift in centre of gravity, affecting balance
Hygiene	Hormonal changes affecting skin texture and secretions
Infection control	Placenta only a partial barrier to harmful agents
Love, security and self-esteem	Possibility that strong emotions may affect the fetus
Sexuality	Hormonal and psychological changes as well as altered body proportions, affecting sexual expression New motherhood role requires psychosocial adaptation

FIRST TRIMESTER

A woman's first indication that she is pregnant may be the cessation of menses, or swollen and tender breasts. Or, she may just feel generally "out of sorts." During the first trimester of pregnancy there is a marked increase in the production of hormones, particularly estrogen and progesterone. These hormonal changes account for many of the early signs of pregnancy. The newly pregnant woman usually (but not always) misses a menstrual period. She may feel tired and her breasts may swell, tingle and feel tender as the milk glands prepare to produce milk. She may experience nausea and vomiting, especially upon arising in the morning (usually called *morning sickness*).

At this stage, the pelvic structure begins to widen to accommodate the growing uterus. During pregnancy, the uterus will increase in weight from approximately 60 grams (pre-pregnant weight) to approximately 1100 grams at full term. Many women feel the need to urinate more frequently owing to pressure of the uterus on the bladder as well as to hormonal changes. The increase in progesterone has a relaxing effect on smooth muscle, which causes bowel irregularity and, in many cases, constipation.

The degree to which these changes are felt depends on the individual — on her physiological make-up and on her emotional response to her pregnancy. While one woman may experience nausea every day for the first trimester, another may simply feel tired, while yet another may feel no change at all. No two pregnancies are exactly alike, as any woman with more than one child will tell you.

SECOND TRIMESTER

During the fourth to the sixth month of pregnancy, the future mother usually experiences a feeling of overall well-being. Her body has adjusted to the hormonal changes and she has more energy. And she can now feel the baby move, which usually has a positive effect. Many women take on a "radiant glow" at this time.

By the fourth month, weight gain is usually evident. There is a thickening of the waist as the uterus expands and rises out of the pelvis. The amount of body fluid increases by approximately seven litres, about three litres of which is increased blood volume. The cervix softens and is closed by a mucous plug. The breasts, including the nipples, enlarge and may begin to produce *colostrum* (a thin, yellowish substance rich in maternal antibodies). The nipples may become darker, and a vertical line of dark pigment, called the *linea nigra,* appears between the pubic area and the navel. Some women develop *stretch marks* (reddish streaks) on their breasts and abdomen.

THIRD TRIMESTER

During the third trimester, the future mother again often experiences fatigue and a new feeling of heaviness. A general

The expectant couple share the joy of pregnancy as they anticipate the birth of their baby.

relaxation of all body ligaments occurs in late pregnancy, and the continually enlarging uterus pushes her centre of gravity backward. The enlarged uterus is responsible for much of the discomfort the woman feels at this time. It may press on the lungs or the diaphragm or both, causing shortness of breath; on the bladder, causing urinary frequency; or on the stomach, causing indigestion.

Approximately two weeks before birth the baby "drops" as its head settles into the pelvic cavity. This makes the mother generally more comfortable, although the uterus may now be pressing on the bowel, causing constipation. During this stage *Braxton-Hicks contractions*, that is, tightening of the uterine muscles in preparation for labour, often occur.

The loss of the mucous plug (often called a "show") and the appearance of amniotic fluid are generally good indications that labour is imminent. **Labour** is the process by which the baby is expelled from the uterus. It consists of a series of strong contractions, and can be divided into four stages.

During *first stage labour* the cervix shortens and becomes thinner (*effacement*) and opens (*dilation*) to allow the baby to pass through. *Second stage labour* begins as the baby's head "crowns" or becomes visible, and ends with the birth of the infant. During *third stage labour* the placenta is expelled. The *fourth stage of labour* is a time of critical adaptation and bonding of the mother (and father) and newborn.

During pregnancy and labour many women sense a diminution of their self-image, a loss of respect from others for their needs and wishes. All too often, especially during labour, the pregnant woman's wishes have been overruled or ignored in favour of the convenience of hospital personnel. It should be remembered that while the health and safe delivery of the infant are important, so are the needs and wishes of the parents. For these reasons, many couples are seeking alternative birthing arrangements either in the hospital setting or at home.

INFANCY (BIRTH TO 18 MONTHS)

The first sight of a newborn baby comes as a shock to most of us. Expecting to see a plump, rosy-cheeked, bright-eyed infant (as often depicted on television), we are instead presented with a squalling bundle with reddish or blue-tinged wrinkled skin, a puffy face, a flat nose and, often, a misshapen head. Newly born infants are covered with a creamy white substance called *vernix*, which protected their skin in the womb and eased their passage through the birth canal. They may also be covered with *lanugo*, a thick downy hair, and they may be splattered with blood. Upon closer inspection you may notice that their skin is peeling in some places or they may be bruised from a forceps delivery. In addition, their legs may be bowed and their toes bent in odd ways from their cramped position in the womb.

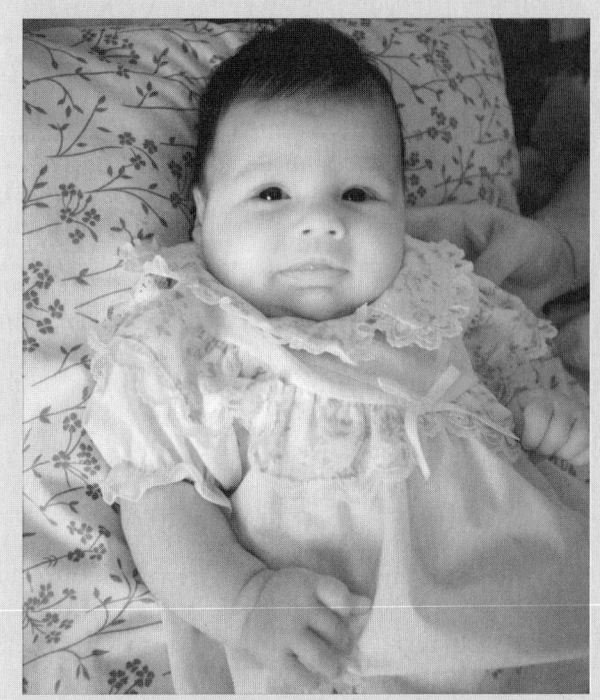

Emily relates to the world primarily through the use of her senses.

Infancy

NEEDS REQUIRING PARTICULAR ATTENTION	FACTORS RELATED TO THESE NEEDS
Nutrition	Immaturity of gastrointestinal system Rapid growth of all body tissues, requiring increased nutrition Appearance of teeth
Elimination	Immaturity of gastrointestinal system Immaturity of neuromuscular structures necessary for control
Temperature regulation	Immaturity of temperature regulation system
Comfort, rest and sleep	Rapid growth, requiring increased rest and sleep
Sensory stimulation	Quality of environment Mobility status
Movement and exercise	Neuromuscular development Opportunity for exploration of environment
Protection and Safety	Lack of experience to perceive danger Inability to protect self
Hygiene	Vulnerability to infection Sensitivity of skin
Infection control	Maternal antibodies in young infants — prolonged by breast-feeding Immunization schedule
Security and self-esteem	Mother-infant adjustment of primary importance
Love and belonging	Mother-infant "bonding" important Quality of care, extent of cuddling, affection important

At birth, newborns must make immediate adjustments in order to survive. Accustomed to having their needs met automatically in the womb, they are now forced to rely on their own systems to satisfy many of their basic needs, such as nutrition, elimination, oxygen and circulation. Newborns typically fall into a deep sleep shortly after birth, and this sleep can last up to 12 hours. During the first few months of life in this world, many babies spend most of their time sleeping.

The first 18 months of life are a period of rapid growth. By the end of their first year, most infants have tripled their birth weight and increased their length again by half. Normally born without teeth, they begin teething at around five or six months. Most infants have six to eight teeth by one year and four to six more by 18 months. Babies have a relatively immature gastrointestinal system at birth. For the first few months they can handle only breast milk or formula; anything else passes through them without being absorbed. By 18 months, however, the gastrointestinal system has matured to the point at which toddlers can handle most adult foods.

Newborns and young infants generally have very sensitive skin. It breaks down easily, providing an ideal site for bacteria and other organisms to grow. Skin rashes on the face and especially in the diaper area are common. Young babies are also very sensitive to even mild fluctuations in temperature, as their temperature regulating system is immature and does not adapt quickly. They do not shiver; instead they produce heat when they are cold by increasing their metabolic rate and burning calories.

Infants receive some protection from disease during their first two to three months through the mother's antibodies that remain in their system. It is also possible to confer some passive immunity through breastfeeding, as some maternal antibodies are present in breast milk. In Canada, the recommended immunizations are usually begun when infants are two or three months old, and are continued throughout their childhood years.

Newborn babies have very little motor control; most of their movements are **reflexes**, that is, automatic responses to stimuli. They will withdraw from a pinprick, turn towards a sound, grasp your fingers or startle at a loud noise. When their cheeks are stroked babies will turn their heads in the direction the stroking is coming from and begin sucking movements. This reflex is called *rooting*, and allows babies to begin sucking when they come in contact with the breast. Many of the reflexes present at birth disappear as the infants achieve control over their actions. They progress from simple movements, such as watching their mother move around a room, to complex skills within a relatively short time. By 18 months, infants are capable of negotiating stairs, for example, or turning the pages in a favourite book. Development of motor skills appears to progress in a head-to-foot, central to peripheral direction (see Figure 8–3). By 12 months most infants have learned to walk, and by 18 months they are running and climbing.

In the area of communication, infants progress from crying to smiling in a few short weeks. Soon they begin to vocalize. By one year, most infants have two or three words with many meanings; at 18 months they may have an "understandable" vocabulary of about a dozen words. Infants can understand their own name by about eight months, and by one year they know and can say the names of those close to them. They are capable of understanding more than they can say and enjoy being read to, although their attention span is very short.

Erikson identified the principal conflict of this stage as *Trust vs Mistrust*. Perhaps the most important task during infancy is the adjustment that mother (and father) and child must make to each other. The **bonding**, or attachment, that occurs between parent and newborn is important in creating a sense of security in the infant. When the parents care for their infant in a loving and consistent manner, meeting his or her needs as they arise, the infant develops a sense of trust in others. This sense of trust also appears to be a motivational force. Studies have shown that in

ANATOMIC PROGRESSION	AGE AND MOTOR SKILL
	Birth (full term) Suck, breathe, and swallow in a coordinated fashion
	3 Months Direct vision — reaching for objects with eyes
	6 Months Sit with head erect when hips, are supported; reach for objects, though grasp of them is immature **9 Months** Sit unaided indefinitely; grasp, using opposition of thumb and fingers (pincer grasp) **12 Months** Walk unaided

FIGURE 8.3 Mnemonic for motor development

SOURCE: Sells, C.J.(1978). Infancy — The First Two Years. In D.W. Smith, E.L. Bierman and N.M. Robinson (Eds). *The Biologic Ages of Man*. 2nd ed. Philadelphia: Saunders, 113.

institutions such as orphanages, where there is not always sufficient staff to deal with each infant's needs on an individual basis, the infants are generally anxious and display little curiosity about their environment. This passivity can have the effect of slowing their rate of development.

EARLY CHILDHOOD (18 MONTHS TO 3 YEARS)

During the early childhood stage, children continue to grow, although not quite so rapidly as during infancy. The proportions of their body begin to change — the head does not appear quite so large, and the limbs begin to lengthen in relation to the trunk. The body systems continue to mature, and mental functions increase in complexity. For example, between 18 and 24 months, most children have the neuromuscular capacity for sphincter control; that is, they are capable of controlling elimination. This is the time when most parents initiate toilet training.

Language plays an important role for children at this stage. They are learning to make their wants and needs understood by others. By two years of age, children have a vocabulary averaging 50 to 100 words; by the age of three they are capable of forming complex sentences to express their ideas.

Motor coordination improves greatly during this stage. Children can hold a crayon to draw, and they can manipulate buttons to put on and take off their clothes. There is a new sense of mobility as they learn to ride a tricycle or push themselves on the swings.

Small wonder, then, with all their new abilities, that children seek to employ them. This stage is often referred to as the "Terrible Twos" as the charming and compliant one-year-old child is transformed into a veritable monster. At this stage they seem to have limitless energy. Their new abilities, combined with an insatiable curiosity about their world, turn them into little dynamos, busily exploring everything within their reach. They want to do things themselves, without another's help, and they can be very

Early Childhood

NEEDS REQUIRING PARTICULAR ATTENTION	FACTORS RELATED TO THESE NEEDS
Nutrition	Continued growth and maturation of systems
Elimination	Proportional fluid constituency of body is great compared with that in adults Achievement of control of elimination
Sensory stimulation	Increased mobility and improved motor control, making exploration further afield possible Developing sense of autonomy Independence of movement
Movement and exercise	Increasing neuromuscular maturation Improved motor control Development of motor skills
Protection and safety	Developing independence Insatiable curiosity Improved motor control Inability to understand danger
Hygiene	Parental teaching Toilet training
Infection control	Increased contact with other children Immunization schedules
Security and self-esteem	Developing sense of autonomy Home atmosphere
Love and belonging	Quality of parent-child interactions Stability of relationships with parents and siblings Development of trust
Sexuality	Gender identification

Toddlers enjoy toys that are active and that they can play with independently.

vocal when expressing their disapproval of interference. Unfortunately, children of this age have little concept of danger, and even less understanding of cause and effect. It is often necessary to curtail their activities for their own protection.

Erikson identified the principal conflict of this stage as *Autonomy vs. Shame*. Children are actively seeking independence, yet they also need approval for their actions. It is important, then, in setting limits, to help the child to understand the distinction between right and wrong, without discouraging them in their activities.

Before age three, children take little notice of one another. They will play side by side (*parallel play*), but there is little interaction. Around age three, however, children begin to have more contact with others their age, and they learn to play together as a sense of cooperation emerges. The primary influence on children of this stage, however, is still the immediate family. They learn mainly through observation and imitation of their parents and siblings. The home atmosphere has a profound effect on a child's image of him- or herself.

THE PRESCHOOL YEARS (3 TO 6 YEARS)

During the preschool years, the rate of growth begins to slow down, although children will continue to gain two to three inches a year until they reach puberty. In appearance, their proportions resemble more closely those of an adult. Their bones become harder and their muscle control and co-

ordination improve noticeably. In general, boys of this age have better large muscle control and may enjoy such sports as soccer or baseball. Girls usually have better fine motor coordination and may be more interested in crafts such as painting or doing jigsaw puzzles.

By the age of three, most children have all their primary teeth. Their body systems have reached functional maturity. For example, they can handle adult foods, and they are capable of controlling their elimination and taking care of their various toilet needs. Although infants are capable of seeing at birth, full visual maturity does not occur until about age five.

At this stage, children begin to develop active immunity through exposure to disease. From the time they start playing with other children on a regular basis, at preschool or kindergarten, for example, they seem to catch whatever is going around, be it a cold, the flu or a disease such as measles, mumps or chicken pox. Immunization programs, usually begun in infancy, continue throughout the childhood years. Although inoculations do not guarantee that a child will not succumb to a particular disease, they usually mean a less severe attack and a quicker recovery.

The preschool stage is a time when children begin to socialize actively with each other. Many children attend preschool or nursery school at age three or four, and almost all school systems now incorporate a kindergarten class for five-year-olds. The child's world expands beyond the home and family, although the family is still a major influence on his or her development. During this stage, children begin to identify with the parent of the same sex, learning a social role based largely on imitation of this parent. They prac-

Preschoolers enjoy experiences in which they can use their active imaginations.

The Preschool Years

NEEDS REQUIRING PARTICULAR ATTENTION	FACTORS RELATED TO THESE NEEDS
Nutrition	Continued growth and maturation of systems
Elimination	Functional maturity of systems
Sensory stimulation	Maturation of vision Improved muscle control making exploration easier
Movement and exercise	Improved neuromuscular control Developing motor skills
Protection and safety	Lack of awareness of danger Expanding horizons
Infection control	Increasing contact with others Development of active immunity to infection Immunization schedule for communicable diseases Nutritional status affects vulnerability to infection
Sexuality	Gender identity with parent of same sex
Love and belonging	Home environment Development of initiative Parents' and siblings' attitudes towards child
Security	Development of initiative Support and guidance from parents Stability of home Accustomed routines
Self-esteem	Interaction with peers Family atmosphere Relationships with parents and siblings important

tise these new-found social skills during play with their peers; the physical differences between the sexes become apparent.

Language development continues to play a major role throughout this stage. It is a means by which children can capture the attention of others and assert themselves. As their horizons broaden and they are capable of doing more and more for themselves every day, children want to tell people about it. Sometimes children of three and four can't seem to stop talking. They have fertile imaginations and often get reality and fantasy mixed up. Children at this stage are highly impressionable; that is, they will take to heart what others, particularly adults, tell them. It is important to recognize, in talking with young children, that they are not always capable of detecting sarcasm.

According to Erikson, the principal conflict of this stage is *Initiative vs. Guilt*. The delight of children as they explore the world and discover their own emerging capabilities is truly wonderful to see. They are so proud of their accomplishments. However, not all their endeavours may fall into the category of "acceptable behaviour," and often it may be necessary to redirect their energies. Children of this age are mainly motivated by a sense of discovery, and it is important to discourage unacceptable behaviour without discouraging initiative or making the child feel guilty.

MIDDLE CHILDHOOD (6 TO 11 YEARS)

During middle childhood, the child's growth continues at a slow and steady rate. Boys are generally heavier and taller than girls of the same age. The child's body is now in proportion to that of an adult. There is further maturation of the body's systems and brain development is virtually complete by puberty. Neuromuscular coordination is further refined, and team sports become a major activity for children of this age. As they continue to develop their active immunity, school-age children are prone to various "childhood diseases." Immunization schedules generally continue throughout this stage.

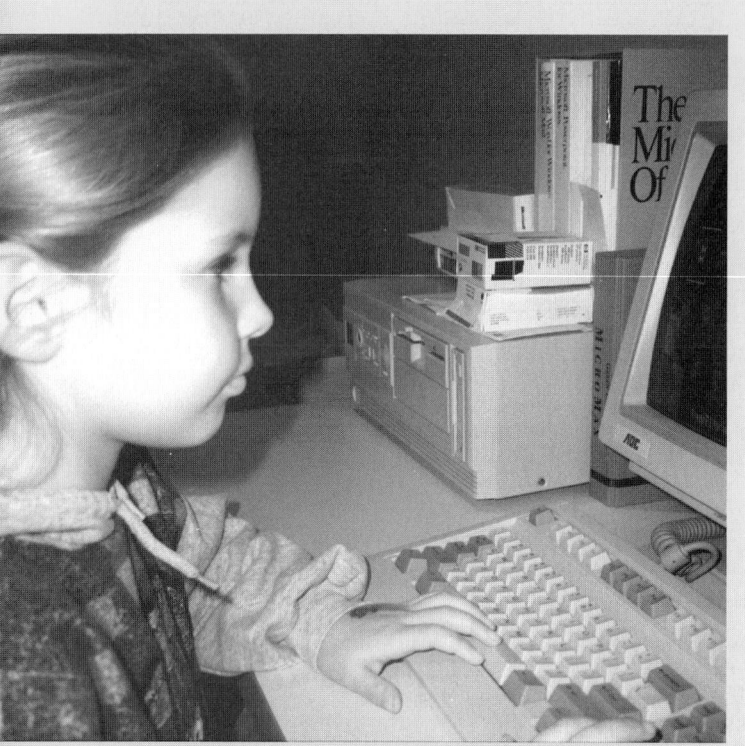

Today's school-age children enjoy high-tech games.

In the schoolroom and through participation in team activities, children develop an attitude of cooperation and self-control. Their thinking and actions are no longer so completely self-centred as they learn that not everyone shares their viewpoint. They begin to think about things that do not necessarily affect them directly and to express their thoughts and feelings about themselves and others. They learn that there is a relationship between cause and effect.

The period of middle childhood is a critical one in terms of psychosocial development. During this time children firmly establish their sense of independence and define their social role. According to Erikson, the principal conflict of middle childhood is *Industry vs. Inferiority*. Children are on a quest of discovery throughout both their inner and outer selves. They ask many questions, seeking to understand every aspect of the world. They may want to know where they came from, for example, or who made the world. They might enjoy taking things apart to see what makes them work. (They may not be so successful in putting things back together again, though.)

If children are encouraged to try new things and taught to learn from their mistakes, they will develop a positive image of themselves and their capabilities. If, on the other hand, they are continually discouraged in their endeavours through failure or negative comments from others, they

Middle Childhood

NEEDS REQUIRING PARTICULAR ATTENTION	FACTORS RELATED TO THESE NEEDS
Nutrition	Continued growth and maturation of systems
Movement and exercise	Further refinement of neuromuscular control
Protection and safety	Understanding of relationship of cause and effect
Infection control	Increased contact with others (school and extracurricular) Development of active immunity Immunization schedule Nutritional status
Sexuality	Adoption of social role based on sex
Self-esteem	Establishment of independence Home atmosphere and school atmosphere Relations with peers, adults outside home Success in endeavours
Security	Parental support Teachers' support
Love and belonging	Stability of home environment Continuity of school environment Routines and schedules
Sexuality	Development of social role based on gender Role model (parent or parent-substitute of same sex)

will soon feel incapable of anything worthwhile, assuming what is commonly called an "inferiority complex." Success in any endeavour, no matter how small, is necessary for individuals to feel good about themselves.

As mentioned above, children during this stage establish their independence from their family. They spend a large part of their day now away from home. As well as attending school, they may also participate in community activities or team sports. Although the home and family remain a primary factor in their development, other adults and their peers are beginning to play an important role in their life, too.

These students appear to be enjoying their visit to the school health room.

ADOLESCENCE (11 TO 18 YEARS)

Much has been written about the turbulent adolescent years. The notion that adolescence is an unsettling (or unsettled) period in one's life, however, seems to be peculiar to the modern Western world. In many other parts of the world, for example, Samoa, where adult roles are clearly defined, the transition from childhood to adulthood is gradual and serene (Papalia and Olds, 1986). Even in our own Western society less than a century ago, children gradually assumed adult responsibilities at home and then apprenticed at an early age in a vocation that, as often as not, was chosen for them. Perhaps the number of options available to adolescents today can be unsettling.

Adolescence has been defined as "the period of psychobiologic maturation during which the secondary physical growth spurt is completed and sexual maturity and the ability to reproduce are achieved" (Smith, Bierman and Robinson, 1978). It is a stage involving many changes for the individual. There is a growth spurt during adolescence, including an increase in both height and weight. Girls usually attain their maximum height earlier, but boys are generally taller. There is also a rapid increase in the vital capacity of the lungs during adolescence, greater in boys than in girls.

Adolescence

NEEDS REQUIRING PARTICULAR ATTENTION	FACTORS RELATED TO THESE NEEDS
Nutrition	Growth spurt Maturation of systems
Oxygen	Rapid increase in vital capacity of lungs
Movement and exercise	Change in body proportions
Safety	Risk-taking behaviour
Hygiene	Excessive sebum production Attainment of puberty
Infection control	Sexual experimentation
Sexuality	Maturation of reproductive system Establishment of social role
Self-esteem	Physical appearance Peer relations Attainment of independence Establishment of identity

During adolescence, body proportions change — girls develop breasts and hips, and boys' shoulders become broader. Other physical changes are apparent as the reproductive system matures. There is an increased production of the hormones *testosterone* in males and *estrogen* in females, which are primarily responsible for the appearance of the secondary sex characteristics. **Puberty** is marked by *menarche* (the onset of the menstrual cycle) in girls, and by the production of sperm in boys. The increased production of hormones also results in the secretion of excess amounts of *sebum*, a thick, oily substance that can plug the hair follicles, often resulting in skin eruptions called *acne*.

Most adolescents enjoy general good health, having already established immunity to most contagious diseases. The principal infections suffered by adolescents these days are sex-related. For instance, in 1991, 33.7 percent of reported cases of chlamydia, 24.4 percent of gonorrhea and 9.6 percent of early symptomatic syphilis involved people between the ages of 15 and 19 (Health and Welfare Canada, 1991).

As adolescents take on the appearance of adults they want to be treated as adults. They can be very critical of their parents, partly because they are frustrated at still being dependent on them, partly because they feel parents do not understand them. This is a common complaint of adolescents. And yet, as they seek independence, they also desire parental guidance and approval.

Communication with parents is often difficult at this stage, and adolescents tend to turn to their peers. The importance of peer relations during adolescence cannot be overemphasized. The peer group provides the individual with a sense of belonging. Conformity is the order of the day, as no one wants to be "different." Peer pressure is an important influence on an adolescent, affecting many aspects of his or her life. For example, the attitude of the group usually decides the degree to which individuals will engage in sexual experimentation, the leisure activities in which they will participate, how long, or short, they will wear their hair and what style of clothes they will buy. Adolescents are particularly concerned with their physical appearance, often spending hours in front of a mirror.

Adolescence is characterized by experimentation as individuals seek to gain knowledge about themselves and about the world around them. During this stage, many adolescents engage in risk-taking behaviour, often pushing themselves and each other to test their limits. For example, they may drive at high speeds, experiment with drugs or alcohol or engage in sex without taking precautions against pregnancy or disease. Experimentation with their new-found sexuality is a major concern of most adolescents, both boys and girls, although boys have the stronger sex drive at this stage of development.

Adolescents also experiment with their own self-image, trying on various roles in an effort to establish a true sense of self. For example, parents may watch their teen-age son drive off with his friends in a great roar on his motorcycle one moment, and find this same son strumming his guitar

Teenagers' appearance and the clothes they wear are important in establishing their sense of identity.

and singing quiet folk songs the next. Erikson has defined the principal conflict of this stage as *Identity vs. Role Confusion*. The individual who does not have the opportunity to try on different roles may ultimately be unable to settle on one identity. This leads to role confusion and can disrupt one's relationships with others.

In the area of intellectual development, adolescents differ from younger children in their ability to think and reason in a logical manner. Also, they are capable of understanding and forming abstract thoughts. Values acquired in childhood are questioned and new ones formed. Adolescents are often critical of the state of the world in general, and actively seek to change it.

EARLY ADULTHOOD (18 TO 35 YEARS)

As they enter adulthood, most people have reached their physical maturity and their body systems are functioning at their optimum level. Sensory and intellectual perception and muscular strength are at their peak.

Young adults comprise the healthiest segment of our population. They rarely succumb to contagious diseases, and when they do, their illness is generally brief and without complications. As with adolescents, however, the major causes of infection are sexually transmitted diseases. According to Health and Welfare Canada (1991) in the report *Notifiable Diseases Annual Summary*, over 60 percent of chlamydia, gonorrhea and early symptomatic syphilis oc-

Early Adulthood

NEEDS REQUIRING PARTICULAR ATTENTION	FACTORS RELATED TO THESE NEEDS
Nutrition	Continued growth and development in early adult years
	Establishment of own dietary habits (early training and habits formed in childhood important here)
	Time and work pressures
Movement and exercise	More sedentary lifestyle
	Development of own lifestyle
	Gradual decline in physical performance from peak fitness
Safety	Feelings of indestructibility
	Risk-taking behaviour common
Infection control	Strength of sexual drive
	Choice of sexual partners
Sexuality	Self-image
	Ability to establish close relationships
	Choosing a marriage partner
Security and self-esteem	Decline in physical performance
	Relationships with others
	Ability to make major decisions
Love and belonging	Ability to form close ties with others

curred in the young adult age group. A major concern in young adults is AIDS. In 1990, 937 men died from AIDS compared to 45 reported deaths of women. The majority of men who succumbed to this disease were over 30 years of age (Duman and Lavoie, 1992).

Young adults have a tendency to view themselves as indestructible and as having limitless physical capabilities. The feeling that "It won't happen to me" is very prevalent among this age group. Consequently, as with adolescents, there is much risk-taking. High-risk activities may also provide a release for individuals from the many stresses they encounter at this stage of their life.

Initiation to adulthood involves many major decisions. Young adults, often for the first time, set goals for the future. Whether to continue one's education, whether to find a job immediately after high school, whether to remain at home or move out are but a few of the decisions facing a young adult. They are also faced with the questions of whether to settle down, choose a marriage partner and have children.

The numerous major decisions young adults must face can make this stage of life an extremely stressful one. Often young people have to leave their home, family and friends as they move to a different city to pursue their education or a career goal. Or, they may be unable to make a definitive career choice. They may want to travel, yet feel pressured by their family and friends to settle down and get married. A major factor contributing to the stress individuals experience at this stage in their life is their own conviction that

the decisions they make at this time, once made, are irrevocable. They want to be sure to make the right decision now.

Another cause of stress for individuals in the later years of this stage may be the realization that their physical

Young adult poised to begin his career

performance is diminishing. They can no longer match the strength and endurance of which they were capable just a year or two ago. If they are unwilling to accept these new physical limitations in their activities, they may push themselves too far, causing more harm than good in many cases. Acceptance of such limitations may make people feel that they have compromised their self-image.

According to Erikson, the principal conflict of this stage is *Intimacy vs. Isolation*. Individuals need to establish a close relationship with one or more persons with whom they can share their innermost thoughts and feelings, and who will accept them as they are. Many individuals achieve such closeness only with their marriage partner. Others may have several good friends on whom they can rely for emotional support. A person who has no one to share his or her intimate thoughts may experience a feeling of profound loneliness or isolation. He or she may feel worthless and lacking in positive qualities. Individuals' relationships with others, that is, family and especially friends, during this stage are important in the development of their self-esteem. They look to others for advice and support as they seek to establish their own personal lifestyle.

THE MIDDLE YEARS (35 TO 65 YEARS)

During the first decade of this period (Sheehy's "Deadline Decade"), the physical changes accompanying the aging process may be almost imperceptible. Individuals who have participated in a regular exercise program, maintained good nutritional habits and had a generally healthy lifestyle throughout their young adult years often look, feel and are remarkably fit in their late 30s and early 40s. Many young adults, however, are too busy — climbing the corporate ladder, raising children or just earning a living — to look after their health. They are often suddenly brought up short by the realization that the waistline has thickened or wrinkles have suddenly appeared around the eyes or mouth. People may also notice a decrease in the perception of taste and smell, or find that they need to wear glasses for the first time in their life. Sometimes, the change in health status is more serious. For example, there has been an alarming incidence of heart attacks among men around the age of 40. As part of the general reassessment of one's lifestyle that is often done some time between the ages of 35 and 45 years, health is usually an important consideration. An increasing number of people in this age group are joining fitness programs as they begin to realize that their health is not indestructible and that it is time to take action to safeguard it.

The physical changes of the aging process inevitably catch up with people in the late middle years. The "change of life" may occur as early as the mid-40s in some women and as late as the mid-50s in others. Generally, this means the *menopause* or end of the childbearing years for women. The onset and duration of menopause varies with each individual. It may start and end abruptly, or it may be a gradual process. There is a decrease in the production of estrogen, causing

The Middle Years

NEEDS REQUIRING PARTICULAR ATTENTION	FACTORS RELATED TO THESE NEEDS
Nutrition	More sedentary lifestyle
Sensory	Greater intensity of stimulation required
Movement and exercise	Decline in physical performance Awareness of preventive value of regular exercise program Availability of programs
Hygiene	Decrease in skin integrity
Sexuality	Elimination of fear of pregnancy for women Decrease in fertility Self-image
Self-esteem	Attainment of career and social goals Decline in fertility and sexual function
Security	Visual signs of aging process Mid-life crisis
Love and belonging	Decline in sexual function Teen-aged children Aging parents

the ovaries to cease releasing ova. Other changes directly related to decreased estrogen production are "hot flashes," a thinning of the vaginal linings and urinary dysfunction.

Some women experience other symptoms such as fatigue, dizziness or nervousness, for example, which, although not directly attributable to estrogen reduction, may result from a combination of factors at this stage in a woman's life. We do not seem to be hearing so much about the dreaded female menopause these days, however. Many women, indeed, look forward to the cessation of menstruation as a blessed end to an inconvenience, and view the last child's leaving home as an opportunity to assert their individuality and seek their own fulfillment. Perhaps the new lease on life being experienced by so many women as they go back to school or work in their late 30s (and on through the 40s and 50s) has taken the sting out of nature's withdrawal of the ability to reproduce.

Although the phenomenon of "male menopause" does not exist, men do experience a decrease in the production of testosterone, which reduces fertility and the ability to achieve orgasm. Impotence can also be a problem. In our youth-oriented North American society, many men seem to have difficulty accepting the "change of life" process. They may feel the need to compensate by wearing loud clothes, driving flashy sports cars and seeking involvement with younger people — particularly of the opposite sex. It is not unheard of for a man in this age group to abandon his wife of many years and all he has worked hard to achieve for a new life with a younger woman.

The middle years may offer leisure rewards

There are other adjustments associated with the middle years. Often, individuals at this stage are caught in the middle of three generations. While coping with the problems of teen-aged children and adjusting to their eventual independence, the middle-aged individual is often faced with the realization that his or her own parents are getting old. They may now need help and support with their physical, emotional or financial problems.

In spite of the many changes and adjustments one experiences, the late middle years are often referred to as the "prime of life." It can be a time of general good health and relative stability, when individuals attain the goals they have set for themselves. This is often the most productive period in a person's life. Through their various life experiences, individuals have achieved a measure of self-assurance and will feel satisfied as they reach the peak of their career and earning power and attain their most influential role in society. As the children grow up and leave home, many married couples find that they have more time to devote to leisure activities and more time for each other. Many women report having a renewed interest in and considerably more enjoyment from sex at this time of their lives than at any other.

THE LATER YEARS (AGE 65 PLUS)

The final stage in an individual's development has been called the "golden age." It is a time when individuals no longer have to strive to achieve, when they can relax and enjoy the fruits of their labour. In Canada, we believe that the state has a responsibility to care for its older people, who have already made their contribution to society. Through our social security program, older people are assured of an income sufficient to meet their basic needs, at least minimally.

Senior citizens in Canada are also provided with health care, largely at government expense. This is particularly important because our health typically diminishes as we get older. This is characterized by a general decline in the functioning of all body systems. The body, in this respect, is rather like a motor that begins to show the effects of long usage. Body parts start to wear out (luckily, an increasing number of them can be replaced these days) and our internal systems become unable to tolerate the wear and tear they once did. Individuals may have to be more selective in the foods they eat, for example, or pay the penalty of indigestion. Like a vintage model car, the older person's body needs gentle handling and preventive maintenance to ensure that all systems are kept functioning as well as possible, for as long as possible. Physiological needs, then, assume a great deal of importance for people in their later years.

Mrs. Julia Hemphill being "piped in" to her ninetieth birthday party

prepared for their withdrawal from the work force can find it a very rewarding period. In an article on Pre-Retirement Counselling, Diekelmann (1978) has suggested that there are six areas individuals should consider as they plan for their later years:

- income
- activities
- living arrangements
- role change
- health
- legal matters

Income affects many aspects of a person's life — the food one eats, the activities in which one participates and one's self-esteem, to name a few. Most people contribute to pension or retirement plans during their working years in order to supplement the state-provided pension. In most communities in Canada, senior citizens also benefit from a number of financial concessions such as reduced fares for transportation; special rates for admission to movies, concerts, sports events and other entertainment; and reduced (or waived) tuition fees at colleges and universities. Financial considerations such as these help people to stretch a fixed income and also enable them to participate in a great many activities they would otherwise not be able to afford. The secret of a happy old age, according to many in that age bracket, is to keep active, and certainly there is no shortage of activities for people over 65 these days.

Living arrangements are also an important consideration for older people. It is important for them to retain their independence as long as they are physically capable

Protection and safety needs are also increased during the later years. There is a diminishing of sensory perception with aging, and people become less alert to danger. There is also a lessened physical ability to cope with it. The reflexes are not as fast as they were, for example, and coordination is not as good. Thus, reactions to dangerous situations are slower and less effective. Combined with these changes is an increased fragility of the bones. This is due to a loss of cartilage (which in many parts of the body provides a cushion to protect bony structures) and a loss of calcareous material from the bones. The elderly are more likely to suffer fractures when they fall than younger people are. Healing is also slower, largely because circulation is less efficient, and the elderly do not bounce back from illness as rapidly as younger adults do.

In the psychosocial realm, the later years are marked by many lifestyle changes. Retirement involves a major adjustment. Most companies in Canada require that their employees retire by age 65 (some now 70). Even though it is expected, many people find retirement a traumatic experience. Often, it means a reduced income, a loss of self-esteem (as one no longer feels useful) and diminished social status — ours is, unfortunately, not a culture in which old people are revered for their wisdom. It may also mean dependence on one's family or on the state for financial, physical or emotional assistance.

Increasingly, however, companies are helping their employees to prepare for retirement. Those who have

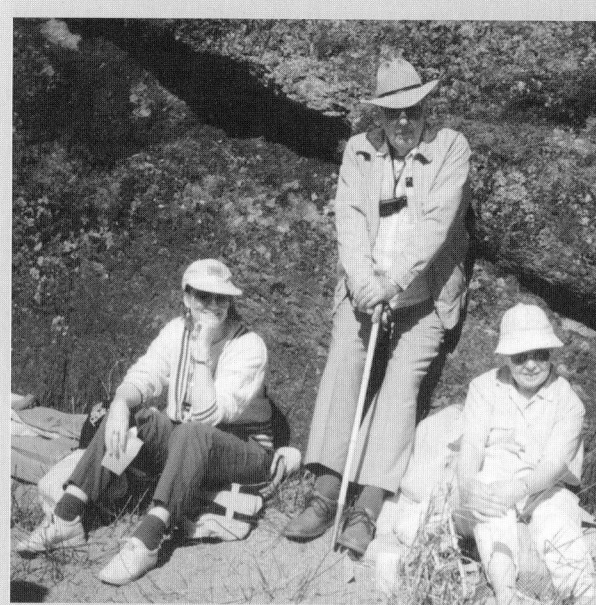

Older adults enjoying a river rafting expedition with their coordinator

The Later Years

NEEDS REQUIRING PARTICULAR ATTENTION	FACTORS RELATED TO THESE NEEDS
Nutrition	Fixed or diminished income Reduced caloric intake Oral problems Loneliness, depression
Elimination	More sedentary lifestyle Loss of muscle tone Poor eating habits
Circulation	Slowed heart rate Fatty deposits around heart Chronic conditions
Oxygen	Decrease in vital capacity of lungs Chronic conditions
Temperature regulation	Diminished adaptation to extremes of heat and cold
Comfort, rest and sleep	Alteration of sleep patterns
Pain management	Reduced sensitivity to pain
Sensory	Diminished perception in all areas
Movement and exercise	Loss of muscle tone, mass Loss of cartilage Limited range of motion Slower coordination
Safety	Loss of cartilage Bones more fragile Presence of osteoporosis Slower reflexes Diminished sensory perception
Hygiene	Loss of skin integrity Loss of teeth Dentures, gum disease
Infection control	Loss of skin integrity Decreased isoimmunity Immunosuppressive drugs Chronic conditions
Sexuality	Privacy Past sexual patterns
Self-esteem	Financial status Leisure, social activities Dependency status Attitudes of family, others
Security	Financial, social status Dependency status Death of spouse, friends Attitudes of family, others
Death, loss and grieving	Death of spouse, friends Inevitability of own death

of doing so. An increasing number of services are helping people to remain in their own homes, such as "meals on wheels," homemaker services, "good neighbour" programs and the like. Inevitably, however, the stairs become too much to climb, the house becomes too much to keep up or illness strikes, and the older person is no longer able to manage alone. Many people, at this stage, decide to go into a smaller house or an apartment, or they may move in with relatives. A wide variety of alternative housing arrangements for senior citizens have developed in recent years, including the very expensive, privately developed "retirement communities" complete with golf course, swimming pool and other amenities; the publicly financed low-

rent apartment complexes; the housing projects sponsored by church groups and service clubs; and boarding and personal care homes both private and state-run. Regardless of the type of accommodation, however, the move is always a difficult one for the older individual. It is less painful if the individual can retain an essence of privacy and if steps are taken to ensure that he or she is always treated with dignity and respect.

One of the major adjustments for the older person is the reversal of roles that takes place with one's children, as the older individual becomes more dependent on them. Another role change that many elderly people must face is that of being widowed. The sense of loss experienced by

LOOKING BACK

DOROTHY PERCY 1901–1992

Dorothy Percy was the first nurse to be hired in Canada's fledgling Department of National Health and Welfare when it was set up in 1947, and the first to become Canada's "chief nursing consultant" in 1954. This chief nursing officer (CNO) position represented the increasing importance of nursing in the government bureaucracy. The position was created partly as a response to lobbying efforts by the Canadian Nurses Association and partly in response to the increasing importance of the nursing role in provincial health care systems. Until Dorothy Percy's appointment, advisory roles to government on health care had been filled mainly by physicians. Her sound knowledge, frankness, clarity of thought and diplomacy made her a key contributor in the development of Canada's social service programs, including the implementation of nation-wide hospital insurance and later, medical care insurance. Her role went largely unrecognized because she believed wholeheartedly in public service employees remaining in the background.

After undergraduate study at Queen's and Carleton universities, she graduated in nursing from Toronto General Hospital in 1924 and obtained a diploma in public health nursing from the University of Toronto. She then returned to her home town of Ottawa to be a nurse at the Ottawa Civic Hospital and with the Victorian Order of Nurses, moving quietly up the administrative ladders. In 1934, she was appointed lecturer at the University of Toronto School of Nursing.

She volunteered for duty as a nursing sister during World War II, serving overseas in Britain, and was discharged in 1945 with the rank of Captain. Among her awards for duty overseas are the Red Cross Medal of Honor, the Defence of Britain Medal, and the Jubilee and Coronation medals. Following the war, she took the position of executive secretary for the Welfare Council of Toronto before joining government service.

In 1953, she received a one-year fellowship from the World Health Organization and took a leave of absence to observe and study nursing throughout the world. During her years as chief nursing consultant, she acted as a liaison between the national and provincial nursing organizations in Canada. She also established strong international ties with her counterparts in other nations as well as with the World Health Organization and the International Council of Nurses. Upon her retirement, the position of chief nursing consultant was discontinued, but reinstated as a Principal Nursing Officer position under the Deputy Minister of Health. This PNO position has since been filled by Verna Huffman Splane, Rose Imai, Hugette Labelle and Josephine Flaherty.

Dorothy Percy's 43 years of service to nursing were acknowledged in 1967 when she was the first recipient of an honorary Doctorate of Nursing awarded by the University of Ottawa. That same year, the University of Toronto established a scholarship in her name. In 1977, Governor General Jules Léger presented her with the Florence Nightingale Medal, given by the International Committee of the Red Cross — one of the highest international awards in nursing. She was the thirteenth Canadian to be so honored. She died peacefully in Ottawa in 1992.

— Glennis Zilm

an elderly person at the death of a spouse is often over-whelming. Although the support of family and friends can be a great comfort, the surviving spouse may never recover from his or her despair. Many who have become widowed do, however, recover and remarry, and indeed weddings in senior citizen communities are becoming quite common.

As people age, they must accept not only the death of those close to them, but the inevitability of their own death as well. In preparation for this eventuality, many individuals make out a will. Often, older people are able to discuss the disposal of their worldly assets with relative equanimity, but their family may become upset at the thought of the parent's death. Many older individuals like to have a "squaring up" of their accounts, to get all their affairs in order.

Often, too, there is a renewed interest in religion as one gets older and faces the prospect of death. The individual's spiritual counsellor can usually provide much solace and support. Counselling in matters related to death and dying has been developed in recent years largely as a result of work done by Elisabeth Kübler-Ross. This matter will be further discussed in Chapter 36. As science continues to extend the time we mortals spend on this earth, we are becoming wiser about how to enrich the later years.

In your clinical experiences on the medical-surgical wards of acute-care hospitals, in nursing homes and extended care units and in your work in community agencies, you will undoubtedly meet many 90-year-olds and even 100-year-olds. If you take the time to talk with some of your older patients, you will find that a rapidly growing number of people continue to lead full, active and interesting lives long after the traditional retirement age of 65 years.

KEY TERMS

physiological p. 166	esteem p. 167	mesoderm p. 172	labour p. 174
safety and security p. 166	self-actualization p. 167	endoderm p. 172	reflexes p. 176
love and belonging p. 167	gestation p. 172	amniotic sac p. 172	bonding p. 176
	zygote p. 172	placenta p. 172	puberty p. 182
	ectoderm p. 172	umbilical cord p. 172	

IN REVIEW

There are certain basic needs common to all human beings which must be fulfilled if individuals are to attain optimal health or wellness. Much of nursing is concerned with helping people to meet basic needs and to achieve their optimal level of functioning. Needs vary as individuals grow and develop throughout their lifetime. Cultural influences result in diverse beliefs and values which affect health behaviours and needs such as nutrition, health care and child-raising, lifestyles and the socialization of family members.

Maslow's theory of a hierarchy or priority of needs states that fundamental needs must be met before a person can proceed to higher needs. Physiological needs take precedence over others as they are basic necessities of life. Safety and security needs include shelter and protection from harm. The need for love and belonging includes the need for a significant other with whom to share one's feelings. Esteem needs involve a person's feelings of worthiness both in his or her own regard and that of significant others. Self-actualization needs are those a person fulfils by attaining a feeling of success in his or her endeavours.

Kalish adapted Maslow's model to place the need for knowledge as the second most important need. He included sex, activity, exploration, manipulation and novelty in his definition of this need.

Growth and development in the physiological sphere are well understood. However, various theories have been put forth to explain the spheres of personality, psychosocial, cognitive and moral development. Early theorists include Freud, who identified stages of childhood psychosocial development; Piaget, who formulated a theory on cognitive development; and Kohlberg, who developed a theory of moral development. Erikson formulated a psychosocial developmental theory that embodies a person's whole life. Gestation, infancy, early childhood, preschool, middle childhood, adolescence, early adulthood, middle years and the later years are the stages outlined by Erikson, who gave each stage a developmental task which must be completed for satisfactory progress. Sheehy described "passages" through which each adult passes during the early and middle adult years and Peck refined the theory for the middle and later years by adding more developmental tasks.

LEARNING ACTIVITIES

1. Reflect on the basic needs of a patient you recently cared for in clinical practice. How did the person's illness alter his or her basic needs? How did these compare with Maslow's priority of needs? How did the patient's illness and/or the constraints of the hospital environment affect the patient's fulfilment of their psychosocial needs?

2. Think about your own growth and development through the years. What were some of the major influences on your social, psychological, moral and spiritual development? In what ways did your family's cultural values and beliefs influence your growth and development?

3. From your own family or the family of friends or neighbours, select an individual from each of the different age groups and observe his or her physical, psychosocial, psychosexual, cognitive, moral and spiritual development. Compare your observations with the theories discussed in this book.

4. Visit a preschool or playground in your neighbourhood. Observe the social interactions of the children. Describe behaviours that characterize the emotional and social development of preschool children. What is the importance of social interactions in the preschool child's psychosocial development?

5. Talk to a school nurse about working with school-age and adolescent children. What are the common health problems of school-age children and adolescents? Ask the nurse to share strategies he or she finds effective in working with children in these age groups.

6. Talk with young or middle-aged adults and ask them to share some of their current problems and concerns. As a young or middle-aged adult, what are your concerns? How would illness or injury disrupt the psychosocial development of young and middle-aged adults?

7. Visit a community centre in your neighbourhood. What programs and activities are offered to promote healthy living for older adults?

REFERENCES

AVARD, D. and HANVEY, L. (1989). *The health of Canada's children: A CICH profile*. Ottawa: Canadian Institute of Child Health.

BARROW, G.M. (1989). *Aging, the individual and society* (4th ed.). New York: West Publishing.

BERGER, K.S. (1991). *The developing person through childhood and adolescence* (3rd ed.). New York: Worth Publishers.

BERGER, K.S. (1993). *The developing person through the life-span* (3rd ed.). New York: Worth Publishers.

BOMAR, P. (Ed) (1989). *Nurses and family health promotion*. Baltimore: Williams and Wilkins.

BOURNE L.E. Jr. and EKSTRAND, B.R. (1979). *Psychology: Its principles and meanings* (3rd ed.). New York: Holt, Rinehart and Winston.

DIEKELMANN, N. (1978) Staying well while getting old: Pre-retirement counselling, part 2. *American Journal of Nursing, 78,* 1337–1338.

DROEGEMULLER, H.A., MISHELL, D. and STENCHEVER, M. (1987). *Comprehensive gynecology*. St. Louis: Mosby.

DUMAN, J. and LAVOIE, Y. (1992). *Statistics Canada 1992 report on the demographic situation in Canada*. Ottawa: Minister of Supply and Services.

DWORETZKY, J.P., and DAVIS, N.J. (1989). *Human development — A lifespan approach*. New York: West Publishing.

EDELMAN, C.L. and Mandle, C.L. (1990). *Health promotion throughout the life-span* (2nd ed.). St. Louis: Mosby.

EBERSOLE, P. and HESS, P. (1985). *Toward healthy aging: Human needs and nursing response* (2nd ed.). St. Louis: Mosby.

ERIKSON, E.H. (1963). *Childhood and society* (2nd ed.). New York: Norton.

FREUD. S. (1972). *A general introduction to psychoanalysis*. New York: Pocket Books.

GEE, E.M. and KIMBALL, M.M. (1987). *Women and aging*. Toronto: Butterworths.

GOULD, R. (1975). Adult life stages: Growth towards self tolerance. *Psychology Today, 8*(9), 74–78.

GRESS, L.D. and BAHR, R.T. (1984). *The aging person: A holistic perspective*. St. Louis: Mosby.

HEALTH AND WELFARE CANADA. (1991). *Notifiable diseases annual summary*. Ottawa: Minister of National Health and Welfare.

HEGNER, B.R. and CALDWALL, E. (1991). *Geriatrics: A study of maturity* (5th ed.). Delmar Publishers Inc.

HOW KIDS GROW: HEALTH PSYCHOLOGY AND VALUES. (1991, Summer). *Newsweek Special Edition*.

KALISH, R.A. (1966). *The psychology of human behavior*. Belmont, CA: Wadsworth.

KAPLAN, P.S. (1993). *A child's odyssey, child and adolescent development* (3rd ed.). New York: West.

KOHLBERG, L. (1984). *The psychology of moral development*. New York: Harper and Row.

LEVINSON, D.J. (1978). *Seasons of a man's life*. New York: Ballantine Books.

MARSHALL, V. (1987). *Aging in Canada* (2nd ed.). Markham: Fitzhenry and Whiteside.

MASLOW A.H. (1970). *Motivation and personality* (2nd ed.). New York: Harper and Row.

MCPHERSON, B.D. (1990). *Aging as a social process* (2nd ed.). Toronto: Butterworths.

MUNSINGER, H. (1975). *Fundamentals of child development* (2nd ed.). New York: Holt, Rinehart and Winston.

NEUGARTEN, B.L. (1968). *Middle age and aging*. Chicago: University of Chicago Press.

NOVAK, M. (1988). *Aging and society: A Canadian perspective*. Scarborough: Nelson Canada.

PAPALIA, D.E. and OLDS, S.W. (1986). *Human development* (3rd ed.). New York: McGraw-Hill.

PECK, P.F. (1960). *The psychology of character development.* New York: Wiley.

PERCY, D.M. (1967). Historical aspects of the role and function of nursing services in the Department of National Health and Welfare. *Medical Services Journal Canada, 23*(11), 1461–1486.

PESMAN, C. (1984). *How a man ages.* New York: Ballantine, Esquire Press.

PIAGET. J. (1963). *The origin of intelligence in children.* New York: Norton.

PIAGET, J. (1969). *The theory of stages in cognitive development.* New York: McGraw-Hill.

RICE, P.F. (1992). *Human development: A life-span approach.* Toronto: Maxwell-MacMillan.

SCHROEDER, B.A. (1992). *Human growth and development.* New York: West Publishing.

SCHUSTER, C.S. and ASHBURN, S.S. (1992). *The process of human development: A holistic life-span approach* (3rd ed.). Philadelphia: Lippincott.

SHEEHY, G. (1976). *Passages: Predictable crises of adult life.* New York: Bantam Books.

SHERIDAN, M.D. (1988). *From birth to five years: Children's developmental progress.* Oxford, UK: NFER—Nelson.

SPLANE, R.B. and SPLANE, V.H. (1994). *Chief nursing officer positions in national ministries of health: Focal points for nursing leadership.* San Francisco: University of California San Francisco School of Nursing.

STENGER, L.A. and SMITH, C.M. (1985). *Healthy moves for older adults.* Washington DC: Eric Clearinghouse of Teacher Education.

STEVENS-LONG, J. (1984). *Adult life* (2nd ed.). Los Angeles: Mayfield.

SCHWARTZ, A.N., SNYDER, G.L. and PETERSON, J.A. (1984). *Aging and life: An introduction to gerontology* (2nd ed.). Toronto: Holt, Rinehart and Winston.

SMITH, D.W., BIERMAN, E.L. and ROBINSON, N.M. (Eds.). (1978). *The biologic ages of man* (2nd ed.). Philadelphia: Saunders.

THURBER, F. and BERRY, B. (1990). Children with AIDS—Issues and future directions. *Journal of Pediatric Nursing, 116*, 168–178.

TURNER, J.S., and HELLMS, D.B. (1984). *Contemporary adulthood.* Philadelphia: Saunders.

VARIOUS NEWSPAPER CLIPPINGS. Ottawa: Canadian Nurses Association Archives, Vertical files.

Health and
the Individual

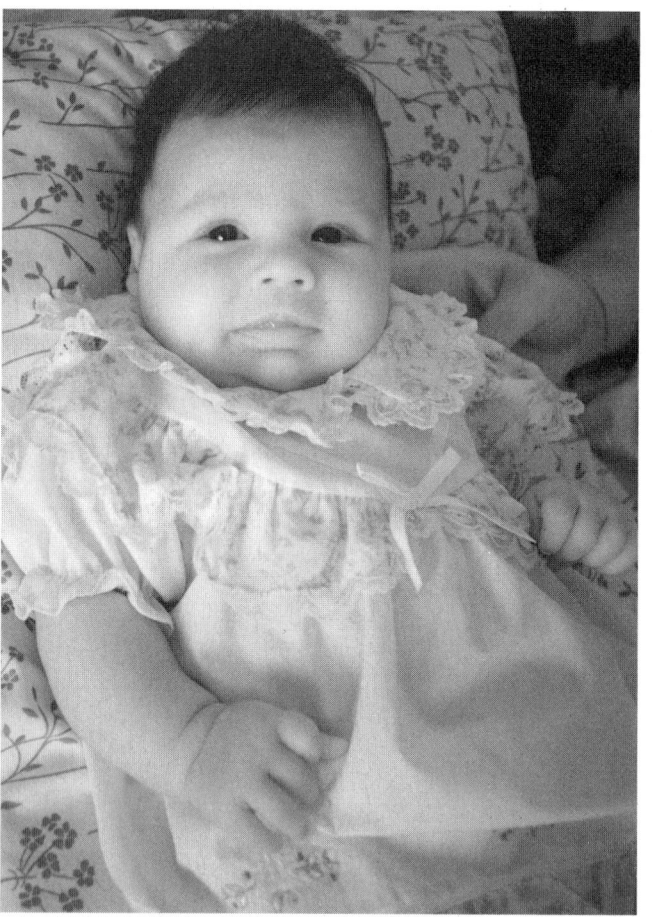

CENTRAL QUESTIONS

1. *Why is a person's health viewed as a spiral?*

2. *How is systems theory used to explain the structure and functioning of the human body?*

3. *What do the terms "equilibrium" and "homeostasis" mean?*

4. *What is involved in physiological homeostasis? Psychosocial equilibrium? Ecological equilibrium? How do they interact on an individual's health?*

5. *What is stress? Is all stress harmful?*

6. *What are the common stressors affecting an individual's health?*

7. *How do people react to stress?*

8. *How can a person minimize the emotional and physiological effects of stress?*

9. *What is "learned resourcefulness"?*

10. *What personality characteristics differentiate stress-resistant people from others?*

11. *How do people determine their health status?*

12. *What is the nurse's role in the admission of an individual to a health agency? In the discharge of an individual?*

13. *What is the nurse's role in the care of the individual in health promotion? In health protection? In health restoration and supportive care?*

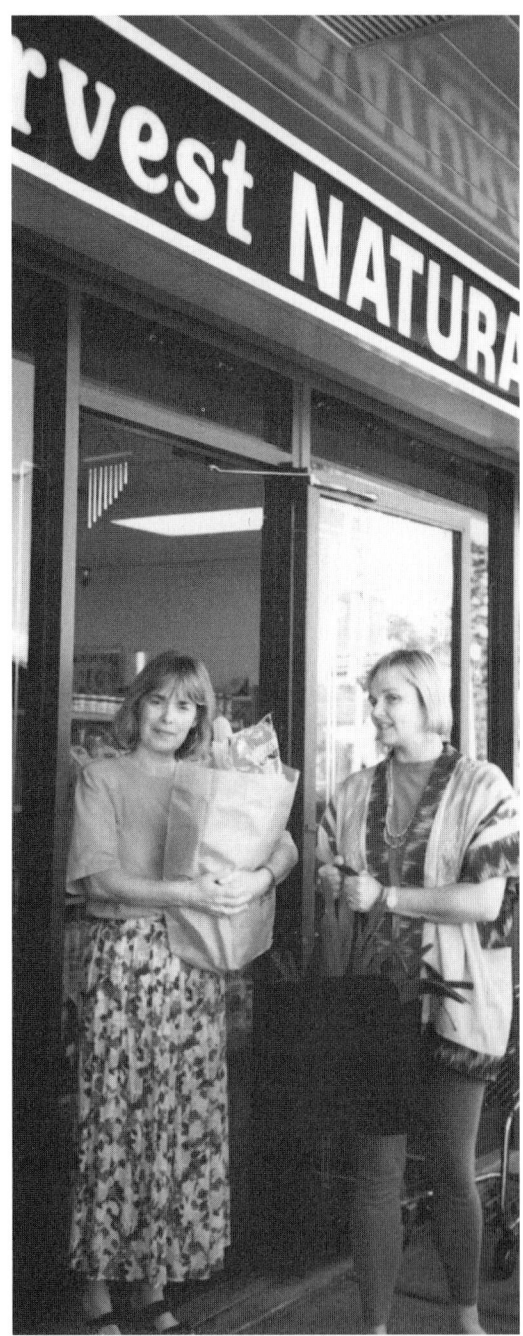

INTRODUCTION

An individual's health is more than a personal phenomenon. As we discussed in Chapter 2, health is affected by myriad inter-related aspects of our lives, including living and working conditions and social support networks, as well as genetic endowment and individual behaviours.

Health can be depicted in terms of a spiral. In this analogy, human beings are seen as a system composed of numerous subsystems which interact internally. The system is also constantly interacting with external forces in the surrounding environment, in a series of ever-widening circles that include an individual's family, school or workplace, community and country.

In order to understand the health of the individual, then, it is essential to have some knowledge of systems theory. We will, therefore, deal with this concept at the beginning of the chapter. Then we will look at some of the other basic concepts that are important to an understanding of health. These include the concepts of equilibrium and homeostasis, stress and stressors and an individual's coping capabilities. In connection with coping we will explore hardiness which is considered an important factor in rendering some people more resistant to stress than others.

The next section of the chapter deals with the personal experience of health as it affects the individual and the personal experience of illness. In connection with the experience of illness, we will also discuss admission to an inpatient health care facility and discharge from the facility. In the last section of this chapter we will discuss the role of the nurse in health care for the individual.

GENERAL SYSTEMS THEORY

In recent years there has been a renewed interest (in both nursing research and nursing practice) in systems theory as a theoretical basis for examining the phenomenon of the individual as a human system interacting with other systems in the surrounding environment. Systems theory has been particularly useful in understanding the individual as a member of a family and of the community.

General systems theory provides a way of examining knowledge pertaining to the world or to certain phenomena of interest. A *system* consists of two or more connected elements or parts which mutually interact to form an organized whole. Each part has a function and the system as a whole has a function. The focus in systems theory is on the interaction among the various parts rather than on describing the functions of the parts themselves (Auger, 1976; von Bertalanffy, 1968). The human individual can be viewed as a system whose parts interact as a unified whole, which in turn interacts with the environment. A change in one part of the individual will create a change in the whole individual. For example, if a person undertakes a weight reduction program, the resulting loss of weight will affect physical appearance. This, in turn, may enhance the individual's self-esteem which will spill over into increased confidence in social interactions with others. This view of the whole person interacting with their environment forms the basis of holistic health care.

General systems theory was introduced by Ludwig von Bertalanffy in the 1960s as a universal theory that could be used in many fields of study. Indeed, general systems theory provides the framework for understanding a large number of physical as well as social and psychological phenomena. Principles of systems analysis are being used in the behavioural, social and physical sciences, and have been applied to educational systems, cybernetics (the science of systems of control), information theory and computer sciences, to name a few.

In nursing, systems theory provides an approach to understanding the multitude of elements that make up the individual human system — the biological and physiological functions, as well as the interaction of the psychological, cognitive, social and spiritual dimensions that constitute a unified whole. It also allows an examination of the individual interacting as part of a larger system, namely the family, the community and society as a whole. This aspect will be dealt with further in Chapter 10, Health and the Family.

In systems theory, the human system is seen as comprising parts with specific structure and function. *Structure* refers to the arrangement of the specific parts of the system (what it is). For example, the body is made up of cells, organs and organ systems. *Function* is the dynamic interaction among these component parts (what it does). In a smoothly functioning system, all of the body systems (for example, the respiratory, cardiovascular and nervous systems) interrelate and affect one another, such that we are not consciously able to distinguish the function of one part from that of another (Auger, 1976).

The parts of living systems exist in a hierarchy of order. At each level, a part may be examined as a separate system having specific function to the whole or as a component of another system at the same level of functioning, called a *subsystem*. In human beings, for example, the respiratory system may be examined as a separate system made up of cells, tissues and organ structures all interrelating for the effective exchange of oxygen and carbon dioxide. The respiratory system, in turn, may be examined along with the circulatory system, endocrine system, nervous system and others as subsystems of the larger physiological system. Each of these subsystems, then, may be scrutinized as whole entities with interrelated parts that have functions specific to the subsystem, functions specific to the other subsystems and functions that relate to the physiological system as a whole (Auger, 1976). At a higher level, the whole individual is viewed as a part of larger systems, such as the family or the community. These are called *macrosystems*. Figure 9.1 depicts the hierarchical nature of living systems.

ALICE GIRARD (b. 1907)

The first Canadian to become president of the International Council of Nurses (ICN) was Alice M. Girard, taking office at the meeting in Frankfurt, Germany, in 1965 and serving until 1969. As Canada's representative to this prestigious post, she was a dynamic leader. But this was just one of a number of "firsts" for this diplomatic, yet outspoken nursing leader. She was the first woman to be appointed a dean at the University of Montreal, when she became "doyenne fondatrice" (founding dean) of the Faculty of Nursing Education (1963–1972). She was also the first bilingual president of the Canadian Nurses Association (1958–1960). And she was the only woman named to the seven-member 1961 Royal Commission on Health Services.

Born in Waterbury, Connecticut, she received most of her education in Canada and graduated in nursing from the St. Vincent de Paul Hospital in Sherbrooke, Quebec. After several years as a staff nurse with the Metropolitan Life Insurance Company and then as a nurse assistant to a physician, she took a public health nursing certificate at the University of Toronto in 1939, a baccalaureate in nursing science from the Catholic University of America in Washington, D.C., and a master's degree in nursing education from Columbia University in New York. She returned to Metropolitan Life as the national director of nursing service. During her travels across Canada, she encouraged the development of municipal and provincial public health services, effectively putting herself out of a job as the company gradually decreased the nursing services it had offered for more than 40 years.

Alice Girard was then approached to help set up a university hospital at the French-language Université de Montréal. When political pressures delayed this project, she took further courses in hospital administration at the Johns Hopkins University in Baltimore, then became Director of Nursing and later, Assistant Administrator at St. Luke's Hospital in Montreal. In 1962, the Université de Montréal once again called upon her to establish the nursing program. She proceeded to establish not only a basic program, but in 1965, the world's first master's level nursing program in the French language. She retired in 1973.

Always active in provincial and national nursing organizations, Alice Girard was named an honorary member of both the Ontario and Saskatchewan registered nurses associations and in 1974, was honoured by the Canadian Nurses Association for her long and outstanding career in nursing. She received the Florence Nightingale Medal from the International Red Cross and is a Commander of the Order of St. John and Dame Commander of the Order of St. Lazarus. She has received two honorary doctorates, from the Universities of Toronto and Montreal. She is an honorary citizen of the City of Montreal and has been a member of the Order of Canada since 1968.

— Glennis Zilm and Kirstine Griffith

The parts of a system are surrounded by imaginary or actual lines, called **boundaries,** that separate the system from its environment. A boundary may be a cell membrane that separates structures within the body, the skin that physically separates the body from the external environment or abstractions like attitudes, values and beliefs that regulate human interaction with other systems in the environment. Boundaries regulate the exchange of information, energy and matter between the individual and the environment. A boundary might be envisioned as a filter which permits varying degrees of exchange between the system and the environment (Auger, 1976). Systems that freely exchange energy, matter and information are termed **open systems**. All living systems are open systems because their survival depends on a continuous exchange of energy, matter and information with the environment. The more porous the boundary, the greater the degree of interaction between the system and its environment. Conversely, systems that limit interaction with their environment are **closed systems**. A family that isolates itself from the community in which it lives by building a fence around its property and by avoiding social contacts is an example of a closed system.

In order to function effectively, open systems receive energy, matter and information from the environment, known as **input**. The system must then transform the input into meaningful forms that it can use for its survival. This process is termed *transformation*. For instance, food taken into the body must first be transformed, through the process of digestion, into carbohydrates, proteins and fats that the body can use. The system not only takes input from the

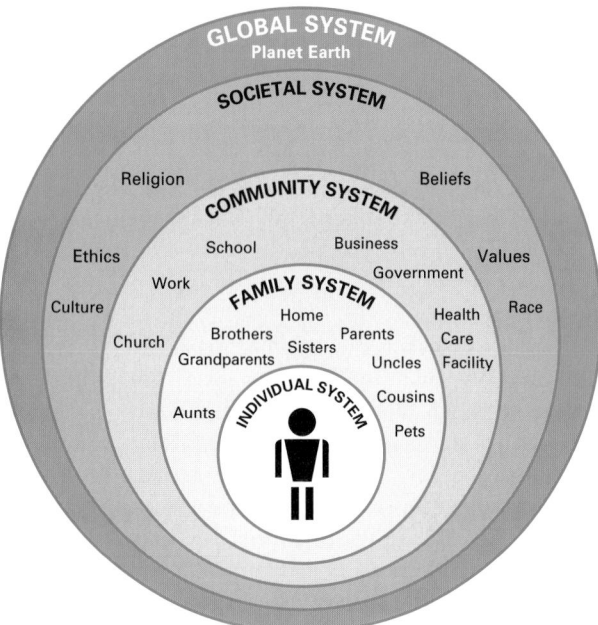

FIGURE 9.1   The hierarchy of living systems

SOURCE: Berger and Williams.(1992). *Fundamentals of nursing: Collaborating for optimal health.* Norwalk, CT: Appleton-Lange, 144. Reprinted with permission.

environment, it gives similar forms of energy, matter and information back to the environment. This is called **output**. For example, energy and intestinal wastes are the output from the intake and digestion of food. The output of a system creates a process of **feedback** which permits the system to maintain stability of its internal function (shown in Figure 9.2). In the body, the constant interplay between the sympathetic and parasympathetic nervous systems in regulating heart rate is but one example of the use of feedback.

Open systems function to maintain a constant state of equilibrium or balance between the system and its surroundings. Disruption in the stability of the system results in tension or stress, which triggers an adjustment in function and energy distribution. For example, when body temperature rises above normal for any reason, the thermoregulatory mechanisms are mobilized to bring the temperature back to its normal limits.

EQUILIBRIUM AND HOMEOSTASIS

Throughout life, individuals must continuously adjust to changes both within themselves and in their relationships with the world around them. Their basic needs must be met, and at the same time they must maintain equilibrium in a constantly changing world.

As these children compete in a relay race, changes occur constantly as their bodies adjust to the demands of running interspersed with waiting.

PHYSIOLOGICAL HOMEOSTASIS

The nineteenth century French biologist Claude Bernard is credited with being the first to understand the body's need to maintain a certain consistency in its internal environment. He described the process of physiological homeostasis, although he himself did not use the term. It was Walter Cannon, an American physiologist of the twentieth century, who coined the word *homeostasis*. Cannon wrote of the "wisdom of the body" in bringing into play certain mechanisms if changes in its internal environment threaten to go beyond safe limits (1932). These are frequently referred to as "adaptation mechanisms"; they are the body's counterbalances.

As people carry out the functions of daily living, changes are constantly occurring within the body as it adjusts to demands made upon it. One's temperature, for example, rises during waking hours and falls again during sleep. The heart beats faster when a person exercises and returns to a lower rate when at rest. Muscles alternately tense

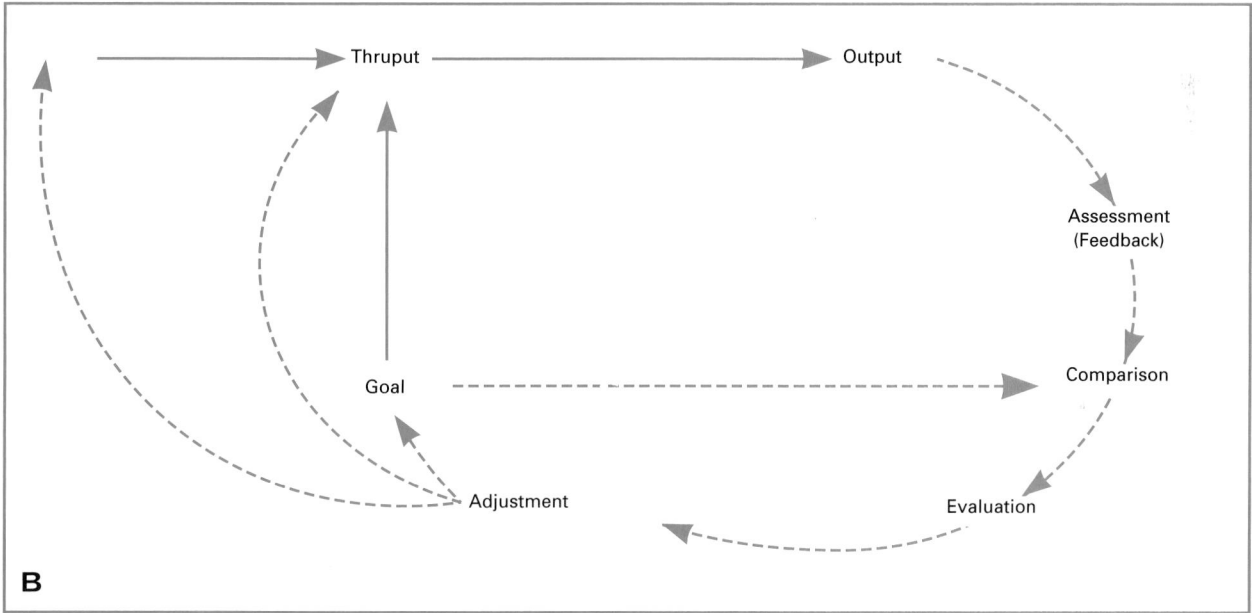

FIGURE 9.2   A. Basic systems model B. Systems model with a cybernetic loop

SOURCE: Stevens, B.J. (1985). *The nurse as executive.* (3rd ed.). Rockville, MD, 328; 329. Reprinted with permission.

and relax as individuals engage in various activities. In fact, an infinite number of minor adjustments are continuously being made in the body during the normal process of living. However, these adjustments must be kept within certain limits if the individual is to survive. The process whereby the body maintains a state of relative balance of the internal environment is called **homeostasis.** Homeostasis is an automatic, self-regulating process that occurs within the cells, organs and organ systems of the body. Its purpose is to maintain the internal environment (see Figure 9.3).

If body temperature threatens to go too high, the individual usually becomes very flushed and breaks out into a profuse sweat. Both of these reactions are attempts on the body's part to lower its internal temperature. Increased circulation to the tissues underlying the skin (which causes the appearance of flushing) helps to expose more blood to the cooling effects of the surrounding atmosphere. The perspiration from the profuse sweating evaporates on the surface of the skin and, in the process, also helps to carry heat away from the body. The body has a number of adaptation mechanisms, and we will be discussing many of these in later chapters of this text in conjunction with specific body processes.

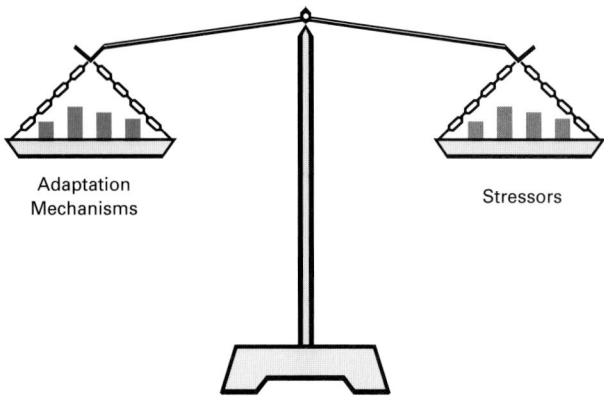

FIGURE 9.3 Homeostasis

SOURCE: Du Gas, B.W. (1983). *Introduction to patient care.*
Philadelphia: Saunders, 14.

PSYCHOSOCIAL EQUILIBRIUM

Contact with other human beings is essential to our well-being. We are constantly interacting with family, friends and neighbours — all of the people who inhabit our social world. Most of us have learned to achieve a balance in our relationships with other people, so that our *psychosocial equilibrium* remains intact. We have learned to use emotional outlets when stress becomes too great. We may use physical exercise, yoga or meditation, for example, to get rid of tensions caused by an unpleasant day with people at work or at school. Or, we may go to a movie to forget temporarily our troubles with the family.

ECOLOGICAL EQUILIBRIUM

Just as the body must maintain a relatively constant internal environment and the individual must maintain equilibrium in the psychosocial sphere, the human organism must also achieve a balance in its interactions with the physical environment. The physical environment consists of the natural elements such as the land we inhabit, the forests, the oceans, mountains, lakes, rivers and streams and the wildlife therein, as well as the structures that we have built upon the earth.

We have learned both to adapt to the physical environment and to change the environment to suit human needs. In a cold climate, for example, the human basal metabolic rate increases in order to maintain the body temperature at a constant level. People living in such climates must eat more energy-giving foods and wear warm clothing to protect themselves from the cold. But we have also modified the environment to meet our needs by building well insulated and heated houses in cold climates and well ventilated houses in hot climates.

There are many aspects of our interaction with the physical environment that are currently giving cause for concern. *Ecology*, the study of organisms and how they relate to their environment, is a major area of study in universities across the country. Many people fear that the delicate balance between human beings and nature is being disturbed. Assessing the ecological implications of large projects such as the building of hydroelectric dams is now a mandatory requirement prior to approval of these projects. We will discuss *ecological equilibrium* (environmental equilibrium) in more detail in Chapter 11, Health and the Community.

THE INTERPLAY OF FACTORS

In discussing health and the individual, it is impossible categorically to separate physiological homeostasis from psychosocial equilibrium and from ecological equilibrium. Each affects the others. A computer programmer, for example, may be under considerable pressure at work. His or her psychosocial equilibrium may be disturbed by constant pressure at the office — but the hypertension the programmer develops indicates a resultant disturbance in physiological equilibrium. On the other hand, when a person is physically ill, relationships with other people undergo a change. A sick person is less inclined to interact socially with others. The physical environment also affects physiological and psychosocial equilibrium. A lack of adequate housing, for example, can be a major contributing factor in both physical and mental illness (Ambrosio, 1991).

STRESS AND STRESSORS

The late Hans Selye, a professor of endocrinology at the University of Montreal, is internationally renowned for his work on stress. He used the term *stress* to refer to the response to any demand, physical or mental, made upon the body (Selye, 1980. Cited in Martin, 1993, 305). Demands of any kind upset the delicate balance of the human organism, which reacts by altering certain structures, processes or behaviours to restore equilibrium. A person may restore physical equilibrium, for example, by increasing fluid intake after perspiring profusely on a very warm day.

The term *stressor* is used to designate any factor that disturbs equilibrium. There are a number of ways of categorizing stressors. We have opted to classify them as physiological, psychosocial and ecological. Common stressors in each category are shown in the box.

Potential Physiological, Psychosocial and Ecological Stressors

PHYSIOLOGICAL STRESSORS
- Chemical agents such as drugs, poisons, alcohol
- Physical agents like heat, cold, radiation, electric shock, trauma
- Infectious agents such as bacteria, viruses, fungi
- Faulty immune mechanisms
- Genetic disorders
- Nutritional imbalance

PSYCHOSOCIAL STRESSORS
- Commonly occurring frustrations or day-to-day stressors like the traffic jam that makes you late for class
- Major occurrences that may involve large groups such as war, terrorism
- Stressors that fall in between — occur less frequently and involve fewer people — such as death of a spouse, loss of a job or other life event

ECOLOGICAL STRESSORS
- Pollution
- Noise
- Earthquakes, floods and other natural disasters
- Inadequate housing
- Lack of recreational facilities

SOURCES: (1) Brunner, L.S. and Suddarth, D.S. (1988). *Textbook of medical-surgical nursing.* (6th ed.). Philadelphia: Lippincott, 88;89. (2) Government of British Columbia. (1992). *Health indicator workbook.* (1st ed.). Victoria: Office of Health Promotion, B.C. Ministry of Health and Ministry Responsible for Seniors. (Catalogue No. QP 92835–03/92)

Ten Most Frequent Hassles and Uplifts[*]

HASSLES
1. Concerns about weight
2. Health of a family member
3. Rising prices of common goods
4. Home maintenance
5. Too many things to do
6. Misplacing or losing things
7. Yard work or outside home maintenance
8. Property investment or taxes
9. Crime
10. Physical appearance

UPLIFTS
1. Relating well with your spouse or lover
2. Relating well with friends
3. Completing a task
4. Feeling healthy
5. Getting enough sleep
6. Eating out
7. Meeting your responsibilities
8. Visiting, phoning or writing someone
9. Spending time with family
10. Home (inside) pleasing you

[*] (N=100; items listed by frequency)

SOURCE: Black, J.M. and Matassarin-Jacobs, E. (1993). *Luckmann and Sorensen's medical-surgical nursing. A psychophysiologic approach.* Philadelphia: Saunders, 48. Reproduced with permission.

MAJOR LIFE EVENTS AND LIFE'S DAILY HASSLES

The various types of stressors and the physiological and psychosocial responses to them have been investigated by many medical scientists and social psychologists over the years. A number of lists on the stresses of major life changes and on the irritating, distressing and frustrating demands of everyday life (daily hassles) have been developed, along with rating scales to assess stress-load.

The popular Social Readjustment Rating Scale developed by Holmes and Rahe ranks major life events on a scale from 0 to 100. The death of a spouse is considered to be the change causing the greatest disturbance in a person's life. Other stressful events include losing one's job, changing jobs, moving from one part of the country to another, or

even from one neighbourhood to another, and changes in lifestyle. Happy events, such as marriages, getting a promotion, taking a vacation and even Christmas, also bring their stresses. If people have too many changes in their lives in too short a period of time, they may become candidates for major illness (Holmes and Rahe, 1967). Although the scale has been found not to correlate as significantly as originally thought to illness (Kobasa, 1979), it can be used to get an indication of the amount of stress a person has experienced.

Lazarus, a social psychologist, was particularly interested in the effects of **daily hassles** on a person's health. He postulated that these daily stressors are more likely to cause illness than are major life events, possibly because the minor frustrations and irritations tend to accumulate to create a chronic state of stress. Lazarus felt that there are things in a person's daily life that help to balance these stressors, circumstances such as relating well to one's spouse or lover, relating well to friends, completing a task or feeling healthy. He called these buffers **daily uplifts** (Lazarus, 1981).

STRESS, DISTRESS AND EUSTRESS

Not all stress is unhealthy. Selye coined the term **eustress** to refer to "good" stress and used **distress** to refer to harmful stress. Other writers differentiate between necessary or appropriate stress (for example, the kind that makes one study for an exam) and unwanted, undesirable or excess stress. Existential philosophy suggests that, because life is constantly changing, stress is an integral part of life and, further, that "persons can rise to the challenges of their environment and turn stressful life events into opportunities for growth and benefit" (Kobasa, 1982. Cited in Martin, 1993, 6).

Life would indeed be very dull if we did not have some challenges. Boredom has, in fact, been called the worst enemy of wellness (Martin, 1993). Most of us like some excitement in our lives. Some people seem to enjoy a high level of stress and deliberately seek it out. Often they have high achievement needs and set themselves increasingly difficult goals. Sometimes referred to as "**Type A Personalities**" or "workaholics," these people often drive themselves to the brink of exhaustion by ignoring the need for rest and relaxation.

THE INDIVIDUAL'S RESPONSE TO STRESSORS

Each individual responds differently to stressors. Physiological responses to stress are modulated by the emotions attached to the stressor. This individual reaction is called the **stress response**. The physiological aspects of the stress response were first studied by Hans Selye who, in his early work, was looking only at the body's reaction to physiological stressors. He postulated first the General Adaptation Syndrome to account for the generalized reaction of the body, then the Local Adaptation Syndrome to explain the localized reaction when a specific area of the body is affected. Although Selye's early work focussed only on the body's general response to physiological stressors, subsequent studies have indicated that the stress response is evoked by psychological or social factors as well as physical ones. More recent research has explored the specific physiological changes that occur in the body and the mind–body interaction that modulates the individual's responses to stress.

THE GENERAL ADAPTATION SYNDROME

In his research on stress, Selye found that there is a general response that occurs when the body's equilibrium is disturbed. He described this originally as the phenomenon of "just being sick" and later elaborated on it in his theory of the **general adaptation syndrome** (GAS). This syndrome, he believed, is the response of the body to any agent that causes physiological stress. The response may be divided into three stages: the alarm reaction, in which the body's defence mechanisms are mobilized; the stage of resistance, when the battle for equilibrium is most active; and the stage of exhaustion, which occurs if the stressor is severe enough, or is present over a period of time long enough to deplete the body's resources for adaptation (Selye, 1972).

The early signs and symptoms of disease are remarkably similar for many illnesses; this fact may account for Selye's original "just being sick" phenomenon. These symptoms usually include a slight rise in temperature, a loss of energy, a lack of interest in food and a general feeling of malaise. It is in the second stage of this syndrome, the "stage of resistance," that the signs and symptoms of the body's reaction to specific disorders are seen: a rash may erupt on the skin of the child with measles, or localized pain in the chest and difficulty in breathing may occur in pneumonia. If the stress is not relieved, or if it is of sufficient intensity to cause extensive damage to tissues, the body's adaptive mechanisms may not be able to restore equilibrium and exhaustion will set in.

THE LOCAL ADAPTATION SYNDROME

In addition to the generalized reaction that occurs in the body as a result of stress, localized reactions occur when a specific part or organ is affected. Probably the most common example of a localized reaction is inflammation, which represents an attempt on the part of the body to barricade or "wall off" the area that has been damaged to prevent the spread of the harm-producing agent to other healthy sections of the body. Thus, if you prick your finger with a contaminated needle, you will probably soon have a swollen, painful finger. The finger may be very uncomfortable, but the localization of the inflammation will help to prevent the infection from entering the blood stream and travelling to other parts of the body (Selye, 1972).

Selye called this local reaction the **local adaptation syndrome** (LAS). It follows the same three-stage pattern as the GAS. First, there is a generalized reaction — in the case of a swollen finger, the whole hand becomes slightly reddened and a little swollen. This is followed by a more localized reaction in the specific finger, which becomes very painful, reddened and swollen. The inflammation will gradually subside unless the infection is sufficiently potent to overcome the defences marshalled to stop it. In the latter case, it will overcome the "barricade" and travel up the arm, spreading to other parts of the body.

COGNITIVE APPRAISAL

Evidence suggests that we become ill not so much from the presence of the stressor itself but, rather, from the way we react to it. As Selye himself put it, "it is not so much what happens to you but the way you take it" that is important in producing stress (1977, 35). Lazarus and Folkmann, who coined the term **cognitive appraisal** to describe this phenomenon, suggest that the individual's perception of a situation as harmful or potentially harmful is the stimulus that triggers the chemical changes that occur in the brain and the body (1984). "The brain appears to be the mediating physical structure between the body and the mind" (Black and Matassarin-Jacobs, 1993, 47). The cognitive appraisal of a situation involves both an interpretation of a situation as threatening or non-threatening and the assessment of an individual's capacity to deal with it. Lazarus and Folkmann (1984) see this process essentially as a transaction between the person and the environment. The process is as follows:

- Let us suppose that you are hiking up Mount Seymour and you see a brown bear on the trail further up the mountain.
- The stimulus (visual image of a brown bear) is received in the cortex, the centre of logical thinking in the brain which interprets it as a potentially harmful stimulus.
- A message is sent to the limbic system which adds an emotional tone, (fear). The limbic system is a series of brain structures that influence both the endocrine system and the autonomic nervous system.
- A message is sent by the limbic system to the hypothalamus which regulates the autonomic nervous system and sets into motion a chain of reactions to prepare the body to respond to the threat. Messages are sent:
  - to the pituitary gland that regulates hormones
  - to the medulla of the adrenal glands to release adrenaline and noradrenaline which contribute to increased heart rate, elevated blood pressure, dilated pupils, palpitations and pain and tightness in the chest
  - to the pons in the lower brain which regulates heart beat, respiration and other basic body functions.
- The hypothalamus also stores neuropeptides, the special proteins in the brain that turn physiological responses on or off in response to a stimulus and the emotion it provokes.
- The anterior lobe of the pituitary gland secretes ACTH which travels to the outer cortex of the adrenal glands.
- The posterior lobe of the pituitary gland releases ADH, the antidiuretic hormone which causes the retention of water in the kidneys, thereby raising blood volume and blood pressure.
- The adrenal cortex releases corticosteroids into the circulation, including the mineralcorticosteroids of which Aldosterone is the principal one and the glucocorticosteroids, mainly cortisol, which together have the effect

of decreasing urinary output, increasing blood pressure and increasing the amount of sucrose in blood serum. In addition to raising blood sugar levels, the glucocorticosteroids increase fat in the blood, increase protein metabolism, reduce inflammation and reduce the responsivity of the immune system.*

This is a rather simplified version of the stress response, dealing with the short-term effects of stress, which are instantaneous and extensive. There is a mobilization of the body's physiological defence mechanisms as the body prepares for instant action, either flight or fight. The heart beats more forcefully and faster, breathing is increased in rate and depth, blood is withdrawn from surface vessels and the viscera and is shunted into the muscles, the unneeded gastrointestinal tract goes into a temporary slow-down, blood pressure increases and the muscles become tense in preparation for action. This is the body's emergency mechanism, designed to protect the individual from real or imagined danger.

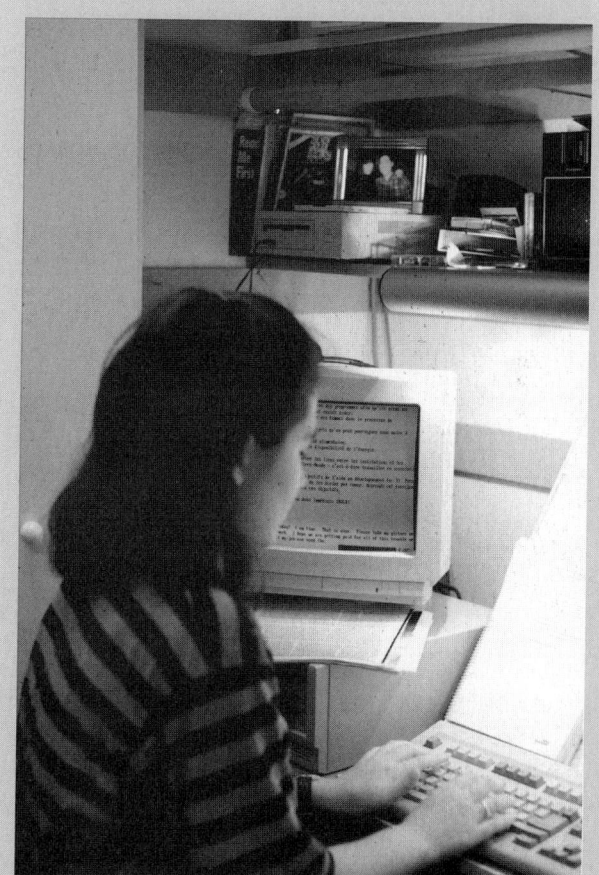

The pressure of writing term papers is a major source of stress for many students.

---

* (Green and Shellenberger, 1991).

MANIFESTATIONS OF STRESS

People react to stress in different ways. If you are having lunch in the cafeteria, for example, and one of your classmates comes along and says, "The mid-term exam results are posted," you may suddenly find that your appetite is gone. You leave your lunch until after you have seen the grade you received — and, if the grade is not up to your expectations, you may find that you still have no interest in eating. On the other hand, most of us know of people who eat to relieve tension. We also know people who chatter incessantly when they are tense. They feel they just have to talk to someone immediately about the grade they received. Other people just want to withdraw and be alone.

Reactions to stress are highly individualized. They include physical, emotional, spiritual, mental and interpersonal relationship symptoms. Everyone, of course, does not exhibit all of these symptoms. A person's reaction depends on his or her cognitive appraisal of the situation, on basic personality characteristics and on past experience in coping with stressful situations.

The physical manifestations may be readily apparent as, for example, drumming the fingers on the table or foot-tapping, or they may be internal responses such as digestive upsets, headaches and fatigue. Emotional reactions to stress may vary from mild anxiety and irritability to profound depression. In the spiritual realm, people under stress often say they are discouraged or they have a lack of direction and express self-doubt.

Although mild stress may increase alertness, prolonged stress may dull the mental processes and the sufferer may complain of lethargy, of boredom or of feeling "spaced out." Some patients say their mind is "going in a dozen different directions" and they have trouble concentrating. Often people who are under a great deal of stress want to isolate themselves to work out their problems and they may be intolerant of others (Martin, 1993).

COPING CAPACITIES

Lazarus and Folkmann (1984) have defined coping as the individual's attempts to manage situations that are perceived as harmful or potentially harmful. The stress management process is two-pronged: first, to minimize, avoid, tolerate or accept the situation and second, to achieve control over the situation. The first approach suggests an emotion-focussed mode of attacking the problem, by relieving it of its harmful meaning and minimizing its impact on the body. The second is a problem-oriented approach to resolve the situation by doing something about it. For example, if you are worried about a mid-term examination coming up, you want to modify your anxiety (the emotional reaction) so

that it does not overwhelm you. And, you will want to take some action to resolve the problem by taking control of the situation, for example, by setting up a study schedule for yourself.

THE EMOTIONAL BUFFERS

All people develop individual coping strategies that work for them. Some of the strategies that people commonly use in their day-to-day lives to buffer the emotional impact of a stressful situation are well known to psychologists as *defence mechanisms*. These are often referred to as "mental mechanisms" because they represent intellectual processes, or changes in thought behaviour; we use them to protect ourselves from stressors that threaten our self-esteem. If people are frustrated in attempts to fulfill their basic needs, they usually become angry and may retaliate with aggression towards the person or object that is thwarting their goal-attainment. Open aggression is not generally acceptable in our society, and by the time we have reached adulthood, we have usually learned to control hostility. Adults seldom attack people in a physical sense, as children often do, but they resort to more subtle forms of aggression, such as verbal attacks, against the person or group of persons blocking them from attaining their goals.

If a person fails to gain an objective on the first attempt, he or she may try again, fighting a little harder this time or seeking alternative means to achieve the same goal. A person who wants to be promoted, for example, may not get the coveted position on first application. This person may then decide to upgrade his or her qualifications and enrol in an evening course to improve chances for the next opening. Or, such a person may decide to use every means available, fair or unfair, to get the next promotion. Alternatively, of course, he or she may decide to stop trying and move to a different company, or to settle for a less prestigious position in the same company.

If people have used socially unacceptable means to achieve their goals — for example, the executive who has ridden roughshod over others to reach the top — or if they have failed to achieve their goals either by withdrawing from the field completely or by accepting a lesser, more achievable goal, they must somehow find a way to protect their self-esteem. In order to make their behaviour acceptable to themselves and to others, they frequently make use of defence mechanisms.

Rationalization   One of the most commonly used defence mechanisms is *rationalization*, in which a person gives socially acceptable reasons for a particular behaviour. A student who goes to a movie, for example, instead of staying in to study for exams, may rationalize the behaviour by saying that, after all, everyone needs a little relaxation.

Displacement of affect   If the individual later gets angry at the teacher for not assigning a high enough grade, the student may not be able to express hostility directly at the teacher. Instead, he or she may become annoyed with a best friend, or go home and take the anger out on parents or siblings. This is a form of ***displacement of affect***, in which emotional reactions associated with experiences (affect) are not directed at the offending person (or object), but are shifted to a substitute. If the hostility is frequently directed at one particular person or group of people, it is called ***scapegoating***. In a family situation, there is often one member, child or adult, who seems to bear the brunt of the other members' anger. He or she is the family scapegoat.

Projection   Oftentimes, we ascribe our own unacceptable feelings or attitudes to other people. We may say, for example, that somebody else doesn't want a group home for people with mental health problems in the neighbourhood when, in actual fact, these are our own feelings that we dare not admit to ourselves. This is called ***projection*** and is another form of defence mechanism by which we protect our feelings of self-worth.

Identification   When people have not achieved their own goals, they may tend to identify themselves with someone who has. They may adopt this person's form of dress or mannerisms and suffer acute distress when their idol is attacked. Children, of course, identify with parents of the same sex as themselves, and this is a necessary part of their development. Students, too, will frequently select one particular teacher as an example of the person they want to become when they graduate, and then try to model themselves upon the image they have of this person. ***Identification***, like the other defence mechanisms we use, is often very helpful in goal achievement.

Compensation   ***Compensation*** can also be a constructive defence mechanism. With compensation we attempt to make up for real or imagined inferiorities by becoming highly competent in a sphere of endeavour different from the one in which we feel we are not competent. The child who has poor motor coordination and does badly at sports in the early school years, perhaps because of growth patterns, may compensate by achieving success in the academic field.

Sometimes, compensation takes place in the same sphere as the inferiority. This same child may feel that he or she has to make good at sports whatever the cost in time and energy, and will practise night and day to overcome physical problems and become skilled at some form of sports. Such a child may choose a highly individualized sport where skills can be developed at his or her own rate, and become an expert tennis player, a ping-pong champion or long-distance runner. Or, this person may become a physical education teacher

with an unconscious (or expressed) desire to help children with problems similar to the ones he or she had.

Denial   When we have feelings or desires that we cannot accept consciously, or when we encounter problems that we do not feel capable of resolving, there are a number of defence mechanisms we use to deal with the situation. We may deny that we have the forbidden motive or problem and unconsciously refuse to acknowledge that it is there, in which case we are using ***denial***. We may state, for example, "I would never do that sort of thing," when we may subconsciously be tempted to do just that. A person's first reaction on learning of a serious health problem may be to deny that the words they are hearing are true. Sometimes the denial persists for a long time, and the person has to work through the acceptance of the diagnosis before undergoing treatment.

Reaction formation   At times, a person may attempt to remove a subconscious, and forbidden, motive or desire by vigorously attacking it. Witness the ex-smoker who denounces the evils of smoking to those who are still smoking. Or the person who jokes about unacceptable feelings, for example, fear, thereby giving the impression that only the weak are afraid, and that he or she certainly is not. Such behaviours as proclaiming too loudly against other people's sins and temptations and joking about unacceptable feelings or actions are termed ***reaction formation.***

Sublimation   Socially unacceptable motives are, however, often channelled into acceptable forms of behaviour. This is called ***sublimation***. A person may sublimate strong aggressive feelings by participating in sports where these feelings are acceptable, for example, football, where kicking the ball and attacking opponents physically are within the rules of the game.

Repression   When we have problems that we cannot resolve or experiences we would prefer to forget, we may unconsciously put them out of our minds; this is called ***repression***. Without knowing we are doing so, we forget all about the appointment we do not want to keep, or completely eliminate from our minds all memory of unpleasant events. This has sometimes been called the "old oaken bucket" phenomenon, from the song in which fond memories of the songwriter's childhood are recalled. Unpleasant memories, for most of us, are often removed from memory by the subconscious mechanism of repression.

Suppression   If, however, we consciously decide to forget about something, the behaviour is called ***suppression***. An example of suppression is Scarlett O'Hara in *Gone With the Wind*, saying "Tomorrow is another day," clearly putting off focussing on her present problems.

Fantasy   Most of us use *fantasy* in the form of daydreaming to escape temporarily from the realities of our everyday problems. In fantasy we can indulge our secret desires, achieve our goals and forget our troubles. Daydreaming can, of course, be very productive. When lost in reverie, we may work out the solution to an impossible problem or develop long-range plans to achieve our goals; sometimes it is very difficult to separate thoughtful reverie from unproductive daydreaming.

Regression   On occasion, in attempting to reach our goals, we may revert to a form of behaviour that was acceptable at one stage of our development but is no longer considered appropriate. The expression "you are acting like a child" succinctly describes this type of mental mechanism, which is called *regression* in technical terminology. People, when they are ill, are often forced to sacrifice their independence in regard to caring for themselves. Having someone else do for them the things they are accustomed to doing, such as feeding or bathing, is often seen as a form of regression to an earlier dependent stage of development.

Somatization   Emotional discomfort or psychosocial stress, rather than being expressed openly, is often channelled into bodily symptoms or physical language. This behaviour is called *somatization.* The child who does not want to go to school because some bigger children are bullying him or her on the schoolground may develop a stomachache, which offers a legitimate excuse for not going to school. The stomachache is real; the child may vomit and have diarrhea, but its cause is emotional. Sometimes, somatization involves both vocal expression of emotion and body language, as when you hold your nose and turn away from a disgusting sight (Burgess, 1990).

THE USEFULNESS OF DEFENCE MECHANISMS

Psychological defence mechanisms serve a useful purpose. They help to reduce the anxieties caused by conflicts or frustration in our attempts to fulfill basic needs; they help us to maintain our equilibrium. If, however, defence mechanisms are overused, or used inappropriately, illness may ensue. As with disturbances of physiological functioning, abnormalities in the use of defence mechanisms may be viewed as quantitative changes that blend imperceptibly into one another and into the normal.

MEASURES TO MINIMIZE THE STRESS RESPONSE

As we noted in talking about the cognitive appraisal of stress, a number of physiological reactions are triggered in the stress response, including elevated blood pressure, increased heart rate and other manifestations to prepare the

Emotional Buffers — Psychological Defence Mechanisms

- Rationalization: giving socially acceptable reasons to defend one's actions
- Displacement: the type of behaviour in which one transfers anger at one person to another person or object
- Projection: ascribing one's own unacceptable feelings to others
- Identification: modelling oneself on a successful person
- Compensation: over-achieving in the same sphere or one different from that in which we feel inferior
- Denial: refusal to acknowledge a threat
- Reaction formation: protesting too much against something for which one secretly yearns
- Sublimation: channelling socially unacceptable motives into acceptable forms of behaviour
- Repression: unconsciously forgetting that which we do not want to remember
- Suppression: deliberately putting something unpleasant out of one's mind
- Fantasy: day-dreaming
- Somatization: expression of emotional discomfort and psychosocial through physical symptoms or body language

body for emergency action. If the stress is prolonged, these manifestations become destructive and render the person vulnerable to serious illness, such as a stroke (cerebrovascular accident) or a heart attack, to name just two of the many stress-related illnesses. Activities that are particularly useful in helping to minimize the harmful effects of stress are physical activities and exercise. Exercise can release much of the muscle tension and generalized physical readiness to "fight or flight" that accumulates when the stress response is prolonged (Charlesworth and Nathan, 1984). Often a brisk walk is enough to lower stress level after a difficult day. Many people find physical fitness activities helpful, for example, a good work-out of aerobic exercise at the gym. Other activities many people enjoy are swimming, cycling, dancing, gardening and games such as tennis, volleyball, basketball and the like, all of which are good tension-reducers. As students, you will want to ensure that you take time to engage in a regular program of physical activity to relieve the stresses of studying.

There are also specific *relaxation techniques*, such as meditation, deep breathing, progressive relaxation, massage and biofeedback training which are all being widely

LOOKING BACK

1600 1700 1800 1900
1650 1750 1850 1950

LYLE MORRISON CREELMAN (b. 1908)

Canada's first nurse to serve with the World Health Organization (WHO) was Lyle Morrison Creelman, whose dedication to health for all at the international level remains an inspiration to Canadian nurses two generations later. In 1950, she was invited to become a nursing consultant in maternal and child health in WHO's newly formed Nursing Unit and, in 1954, she became WHO's second Chief Nursing Officer, a position she held until her retirement in 1968.

Her international role began at the end of World War II, when she was invited by the United Nations Relief and Rehabilitation Administration (UNRRA) to be chief nurse in the British Zone of occupied Germany. Her job was to organize nursing services to help care for millions of people of many nationalities who had been displaced during the war. After an intense two-year period in this work, she returned to working with public health services in British Columbia.

Born in Nova Scotia, she moved with her family to British Columbia as a child. Her first brief career was as a teacher, but when she graduated from the nursing program at the University of British Columbia in 1936, she immediately entered the pubic health sector. A Rockefeller scholarship in 1938 took her to Teachers College at Columbia University in New York for a master's degree. During the early 1940s, she worked with Metropolitan Health in Vancouver, first as a supervisor then as director,

and served on the board of directors and as President of the Registered Nurses Association of British Columbia. Following her work with UNRRA, she was the field director for an extensive study of public health services in Canada conducted by the Canadian Public Health Association and was co-author, with Dr. J.H. Baillie, of a highly acclaimed report used for many years as a reference for public health professionals in Canada.

During her work with WHO, she visited many countries and collaborated with nurses from many nations. She also recruited many well-prepared nurses to initiate international projects that could later be carried on independently by the host country. She recognized the importance of national self-sufficiency in health care and used her superb administrative abilities to put this philosophy into practice. She was a frequent advisor to the International Council of Nurses and on her retirement from WHO, an editorial in *ICN Calling* recognized her many contributions, stating: "In these fourteen years, she has probably achieved more for nursing throughout the world than any other nurse of her time."

Following her retirement, she was commissioned by WHO to help study maternal and child health services in South-East Asia. Although she now lives quietly, she continues to be consulted by visitors from other countries. She has received many tributes, including recognition from nurses associations at provincial, national and international levels and honorary doctorates from the Universities of British Columbia and New Brunswick. The Government of Canada awarded her the Canada Centennial Medal and the Medal of Service — Canada, and she is a member of the Order of Canada.

— Glennis Zilm

---

used to combat stress today. Many relaxation techniques such as deep breathing and progressive relaxation are incorporated into physical fitness programs for people of all ages. Stress has been called the disease of the 90s and we are all beginning to appreciate the importance of learning to relax to preserve well-being (Martin, 1993; Green and Shellenberger, 1991).

NEGATIVE COPERS

Some people choose ineffective coping strategies, which have been called **negative copers**. Some of these are listed here:

NEGATIVE COPERS

- Physical: smoking tobacco, using drugs (caffeine, alcohol, tranquilizers, sedatives, etc.), overeating (fats, sugars, etc.), overspending, becoming ill.
- Mental: blaming, criticizing (self or others), punishing.
- Emotional: throwing a tantrum, taking revenge, worrying, becoming stubborn, sulking, pouting, becoming depressed.
- Social: fighting, abusing, withdrawing, being passive.
- Spiritual: blaming God, withdrawing.*

---

* Tubesing, D. Stress talk worksheet. In A.C. Beckingham and B.W. Du Gas. (1993). *Promoting healthy aging.* St. Louis: Mosby. Reprinted with permission.

HEALTHY COPING STRATEGIES

Rosenbaum (1983) has suggested that there is a learned repertoire of skills that people use to regulate their lives and overcome the stresses of life. He coined the term *learned resourcefulness* to cover this repertoire of skills, which he felt was a major factor in health and wellness. They include (1) cognitive coping skills, (2) problem-solving skills, (3) delayed gratification and (4) self-efficacy (cited in Green and Shellenberger, 1991, 190).

Cognitive coping skills   These skills are the mental processes used to regulate the emotional and physiological responses to stress by attempting to see at least some part of a stressful situation in a positive way (Martin, 1993). They include using positive imagery and positive thoughts, setting positive expectations for oneself and engaging in positive self-talk. For example, regarding the mid-term exam you are worried about, you might say to yourself "I am going to get an "A" or "I can do it if I try" — expressions which include both a positive expectation and some positive thinking. Your chances of being successful in achieving the grade you desire will be much better than if you had started with the negative "That teacher never gives me better than a 'C+' anyway, so why should I bother trying?" Indeed, negative thinking hinders achievement (Green and Shellenberger, 1991; Martin, 1993).

Problem-solving skills   Problem-solving skills include being able to

1. acknowledge that a problem exists and assess its dimensions
2. plan a course of action
   a) identify possible alternative courses to resolve the problem;
   b) anticipate the possible consequences of carrying out each of these alternative courses of action;
   c) select one course of action that would best resolve the problem with the most beneficial and least harmful consequences
3. implement the plan
4. evaluate the results of your action
5. if necessary, revise the plan and try again.*

Delayed gratification   *Delayed gratification* is the ability to put off immediate rewards in order to achieve long-term goals. You have probably all learned to do this in order to enter the school of nursing. For example, you probably denied yourself the pleasures of spending all the money you made in your part-time job in order to save enough for your expenses at college or university. And, you probably stayed in many nights to study in order to get good grades to meet the school's admission criteria when your friends were out partying. The ability to delay gratification is essential if you

---

* (Green and Shellenberger, 1991; Martin, 1993).

are to achieve long-term goals; it is also important in health and wellness. For example, if you want to achieve physical fitness, you usually have to suffer a few minor muscular aches and pains when you start an exercise program.

Self-efficacy   "*Self-efficacy* is a belief in personal responsibility for one's own behaviour and in one's ability to influence events" (Martin, 1993, 324). One of the leading researchers in the field of self-efficacy is Albert Bandura, a psychologist at Stanford University in California (1977; 1986). He maintains that when people feel that they have some control over a situation, their efforts are much more likely to be successful. They will work longer and harder to get something done and they can successfully overcome their fears. The feeling of self-efficacy enables us to have confidence that we can accomplish what we set out to do (Green and Shellenberger, 1991; Martin, 1993).

Healthy Coping Skills

Healthy people use a repertoire of skills to regulate their lives successfully and to cope with the stresses of everyday life. Termed *learned resourcefulness*, these skills include:

- cognitive skills — using positive thinking
- problem-solving
- delayed gratification
- self-efficacy.

Physical Health and Stress Resistance

People who are physically healthy are better able to resist stress than those who are not. In our discussions of stress and ways of coping with stress, then, we should not overlook the importance of physical fitness. To maintain good physical fitness requires good nutrition, a regular program of exercise, adequate amounts of rest and relaxation and the avoidance of known health risks. In this connection, our own personal behaviours and health practices are important. These behaviours include the choices we make in the food we eat, the amount of exercise we do, the amount of rest we get and the health risks we take or avoid such as smoking, the excessive use of drugs or alcohol, driving recklessly or taking unnecessary risks in sports.

Social Support and Coping

The Premier's Council on Health, Well-being and Social Justice in Ontario has said, "The support we get from family and friends from birth throughout life is an important determinant of a healthy long life" (1993, 18). Many studies in recent years have demonstrated the positive relationship between social support and good health. Social support has many dimensions, as we noted in Chapter 2. It includes our social networks — our family and friends, the people we work with and go to school with and a supportive community. Social support can also buffer some of the economic stresses and strains of everyday life, through such systems as national health insurance, unemployment insurance, Workers' Compensation and the Canada and Quebec Pension Plans.

Of all the components of social support, the one that has been found to have the highest correlation with health and longevity, however, is the number of social ties that a person has (Green and Shellenberger, 1991). In Chapter 4, Health Services, we talked about the role of families and friends in exerting a positive influence on health. Of particular importance in our discussion of stress and coping strategies is the role of family and friends in providing mental, physical and emotional support in times of distress. When something doesn't go well, it is to family and friends that we look for support. They can often help to relieve the stressor of its emotional force so that you are able to look at it from a different perspective. Frequently, it helps just to talk things through with a family member or a close friend. As you talk about the stressful situation, you very often work through the problem-solving process to find your own solution to a dilemma, or to allay your fears (see Chapter 16 on Communication Skills).

Much of the research on social support has focussed on the role of social support in directly protecting a person, and in serving as a buffer from the effects of life's stressors. For example, a study cited in *Nurturing Health* found that older women with few social contacts are three times more likely to die than are older women with many contacts. With men, the risk is doubled if they have few friends and acquaintances (Government of Ontario, 1993, 18).

The Concept of Hardiness

Some people seem to be able to resist stress much better than others. They never become ill or collapse when faced with life's challenges; instead, they seem to grow stronger. The question of why some people are more stress-resistant than others has intrigued social psychologists and people involved in stress research in the health field for many years. Much of the work on stress has shown that there is a definite link between stress and illness. Some people, however, seem better able to cope with stress than others. Studies by psychologist Suzanne Kobasa (in 1979, 1982, 1983 and 1985), and by others, found low correlations between scores on one of the popular social readjustment rating scales and illness. Indeed, some people had high scores and yet few illnesses (Kobasa, 1979; Neugebauer, 1984 in Green and Shellenberger, 1991).

In the course of subsequent studies, Kobasa identified a particular constellation of personality characteristics that helps people to stay healthy despite facing stressful life events (Tartasky, 1993). She coined the term **hardiness** to describe these characteristics. Hardiness includes:

1. **Commitment.** This is a belief in the rightness and importance of what one is doing that gives a person a sense of purpose in life. People who feel they have a purpose in life are better able to make decisions than those who do not. The commitment may be to work, family, friends, religion, a political party, an altruistic endeavour or other major interest.

2. **The ability to view change as a challenge.** People who are hardy can turn change into a challenge. They feel confident that they can handle situations rather than helpless when faced with stressful life changes.

3. **A sense of personal control over their lives.** This is essentially the same as Bandura's concept of *self-efficacy*. People who have a sense of having some control over events feel they can make their own decisions; they are not passive recipients of whatever life deals out. These people can incorporate stressful life events into their ongoing life plans. For example, a pregnant student in a master's program in nursing decided in consultation with her faculty advisor that, rather than drop out of the program completely, she would forego summer school and also stay at home with her new baby (expected in September) during the fall term. She would then return to school in the winter term to complete her course work and master's thesis. She graduated that summer — a little later than originally planned but with all course work and thesis completed.

Promoting Stress-Resistance

- Eat a well-balanced diet
- Engage in a regular exercise program
- Develop a regular pattern of daily activities for
  - eating
  - sleeping
  - activity and rest
  - recreation
- Avoid known health risks, such as smoking, excess consumption of caffeine or alcohol or the use of drugs
- Develop a positive outlook on life
- Practise stress management skills
- Maintain your social contacts with friends and family.

Personality Characteristics Associated with Hardiness

- Commitment: a belief in the rightness and importance of one's actions
- The ability to view change as a challenge
- A sense of personal control over one's life.

THE PERSONAL EXPERIENCE OF HEALTH

We all interpret our own health status according to a particular perspective. The way we view our health status tends to vary with a number of factors. These include cultural background, religion, socioeconomic status, educational level, experience, gender, role and situational factors.

Cultural background   Personal perspectives on health are considerably influenced by social and cultural factors. In assessing a person's health, it is important to understand the social context in which he or she lives. All societies, as well as sub-groups within these societies, have certain norms, or standards, with regard to health and illness. In some cultures, for example, obesity is considered a healthy and desirable state, whereas in others it is regarded as an affliction.

The customs, traditions and mores of a society also dictate acceptable behaviours in regard to health. Individuals are expected to take all measures necessary, as approved by that society, to promote and protect their health. The beliefs about health and about ways of preventing and treating illness in other cultures do not always coincide with those of Western medicine. In the culture of First Nations people, for example, a healthy individual is seen as one who is in harmony, or balance, with the universe. The traditional Oriental medicine belief in the principles of Yin and Yang is also based on a balance theory. Differing health beliefs and practices are discussed in Chapter 12, Health and Ethnicity.

Religion   In many cultures, health behaviours are closely intertwined with religious beliefs and practices. Many religious groups hold strong beliefs about a number of things that affect a person's health. Some have strict dietary rules, for example, that forbid the use of tea, coffee or other beverages containing caffeine. Many prohibit the eating of pork. In some religions, the giving or receiving of organ transplants is not permitted. Some religions, for example, the Roman Catholic Church, prohibit abortion and permit only natural contraceptive methods. A belief about the cause of illness common to many religions is that the afflicted individual is being punished for his or her sins. This

belief will, of course, affect a person's reaction to illness. Such people may feel guilty about being sick, or feel that they have to atone for their sins through suffering, and sometimes may feel that they do not deserve to get better. Some religious sects believe in the total efficacy of prayer to help the individual either overcome or accept his illness, and do not believe in intervention by physicians or other health practitioners. We will discuss the intertwining of religious and health beliefs in more detail in Chapter 12.

Socioeconomic status and level of education
Socioeconomic status influences the way people perceive their health, as does their level of educational attainment. People in higher socioeconomic brackets are usually much more knowledgeable about the signs and symptoms of illness than are people in lower socioeconomic brackets. They are also much more inclined to seek the help of a health professional on the basis of symptoms. People in lower socioeconomic groups are just as concerned about health as those in higher socioeconomic groups, but often they lack knowledge about health and about the services available. Often, too, they do not trust the prevailing health care system. Sociologists point out that there is a wide social gap between physicians who are at the top of the socioeconomic scale and most of their patients. This social disparity makes it difficult to achieve the "partner" relationship which is being advocated today (Grant, 1988; Epp, 1986).

Age   Age has a great deal to do with how we view our health. Healthy young people tend to take good health for granted and often take more risks than older people do. Older people usually value health as one of the most important assets in life, but they do not expect to enjoy the same level of health as they did when they were younger. The findings of Canada's Health Promotion survey indicated that older people are much more likely to engage in positive health promotion practices than are younger people. Older people are more likely to eat breakfast regularly, less likely to smoke or drink excessively, less likely to drink and drive and more likely to use seat belts (Government of Canada, 1989).

Gender   In most cultures, men are not encouraged to express pain as much as women are permitted to; hence, they may tend to ignore the early signs and symptoms of illness. Also, women may have more access to health-related information as they are often the ones who attend well-baby clinics and the like. It is usually the mother in the family who sets the tone for health care, and her attitudes and practices greatly influence those of her children.

Situational factors   Situational factors also play a role in the perception of health. The mother in a family, for example, frequently does not become ill, even when one after another of the children, and the father, take to their beds with a cold or the flu; she is literally too busy looking after everyone else to become ill. Often, it is after a crisis is past that a person succumbs to illness, when the stresses and strains that have forced the body to maintain its healthy status have subsided and the individual has time to rest.

CRITERIA FOR JUDGING HEALTH

We all have our own standards for assessing the state of our health. The World Health Organization defines health as a dimension of our "quality of life" — a resource for every-day living that enables people to satisfy their needs, achieve their aspirations and cope with the environment (1984). And, indeed, people tend to view their health mainly in terms of the way they feel and their ability to carry out their daily activities. In Canada's Health Promotion Survey of non-institutionalized adults over the age of 15 years (1985), respondents were asked to rate their health on four measures: (1) their perceptions of their health status vis-à-vis that of others of their age, (2) their health-related activity limitations, (3) their assessment of the level of stress in their lives and (4) their assessment of their happiness. The survey indicated that most Canadians, including most older adults, perceived themselves as healthy, despite reported problems that limited their activity. Adults over the age of 55 tended to report lower stress levels than did younger adults. They were also less likely to say they were very happy and a little more likely to say they were not happy than younger adults (Government of Canada, 1989).

THE PERSONAL EXPERIENCE OF ILLNESS

THE SICK ROLE

Numerous studies have been undertaken by sociologists and social psychologists about the health and illness behaviours of people. There appears to be general agreement that heath and illness behaviours are socially learned responses. Society has established acceptable and unacceptable behaviours for sick people. In most societies, the sick person is not expected to carry out usual responsibilities; he or she can be excused from work or school, for example. Usually, sick people are not considered responsible for their illnesses, although we are learning more and more about the role we can play in protecting our health. People who are ill are expected to take "appropriate" action to restore themselves to a healthy state; they are expected to want to get well. If they solicit help from a health professional, they are also expected to cooperate with the treatment suggested (Parsons, 1972; Bolaria, 1988).

> ## *Characteristics of the Sick Role*
> * Exempted from usual responsibilities
> * Not considered responsible for the illness
> * Expected to want to get better
> * Expected to take appropriate action to get better
> * Expected to cooperate with treatment.

Many of the studies on health and illness behaviours have focussed on the stages of illness. Some researchers divide illness into three stages, some into five. For ease of discussion, we have opted to use a three-stage approach which includes: (1) the experience of symptoms, (2) the dependent role and (3) recovery and rehabilitation.

STAGE 1. THE EXPERIENCE OF SYMPTOMS

During the initial stages of an illness, sufferers may experience many of the discomforts that Selye described as "just being sick." They usually do not feel well, they may have distressing symptoms and they often find that they cannot keep up with their normal workload without tiring or, perhaps, cannot enjoy their usual leisure-time activities. People are usually irritable when they do not feel well. This irritability may show itself in tears that come at the slightest provocation or in anger.

People react to the early signs of illness in a variety of ways. Some attempt to deny that they are ill and "keep going" despite their fatigue, or may even try to do more than usual to prove to themselves that they are not really sick. Some people respond to the threat of illness with anger; others become very quiet and withdrawn. A few seem to enjoy their symptoms and the attention they receive from other people. The individual's reaction depends to a large extent on the way the person perceives the situation and the social ramifications that go with it (King, 1962, cited in Bolaria, 1988, 7).

STAGE 2. THE ACUTE PHASE OF ILLNESS

The acutely ill have disturbances in all areas of functioning. If the problem is a physical one, not only are they physiologically in a state of disequilibrium, their emotional balance is also threatened, and their relationships with other people are upset. Physically, they are often weakened by the illness and simply do not have the strength to cope with the daily activities of living, let alone withstand additional stress.

The nurse cares for an acutely ill patient

They are particularly vulnerable, then, to assault by such stressors as shock, fluid and electrolyte imbalance, or infection. Particular care must be taken to protect the patient from further harm. Extra precautions must be taken against infection, for example, and the patient's physiological responses carefully monitored to assess progress of the disease and the effects of therapy.

Mentally, the patient's energies are focussed on the illness. He or she will likely be much more concerned with bodily processes and will want to know what his or her temperature and blood pressure are, and will anxiously await the outcome of tests and examinations. The interests of the acutely ill are narrowed; the patient is much more concerned with the immediate environment than with anything that goes on outside the sickroom. Frequently, defence mechanisms the individual has found useful in coping with the initial stages of illness, such as denial, rationalization and repression, continue to be used. It is important that the nurse respect these behaviours and not challenge them. It is essential that the patient maintain integrity and a feeling of having some control over the situation. The nurse and the patient work together as partners to enable the patient to get better.

In the social realm, there are certain expectations that go along with being ill. People are expected to stay at home, for example, and not engage is social activities while ill. They are also supposed to want to get well since illness is not a desirable state of being. They are expected to cooperate with those who are helping them in the process of getting better, and to assume increasing responsibility for their own care.

Acutely ill patients often find themselves highly dependent on others for things they used to do on their own. They may need help to bathe, for example, to change po-

sition in bed, or to have a dressing reinforced. They may even need help in maintaining such a vital body function as breathing. People who have been independent all their lives may find it difficult to accept this help, and the nurse will need to be very careful to ensure that the person is able to maintain self-respect and dignity. It is very important, too, that the individual be allowed to retain a sense of control over the situation. Often, the patient's family can be very helpful during the acute stage in helping the sick person, and the nurse should support them in their efforts.

STAGE 3. RECOVERY AND REHABILITATION

The Convalescent Stage

During the convalescent stage of an acute illness, the patient is recovering physical and psychosocial balance. Soon, he or she will leave the sickroom and move back into the everyday world. This is a transition period and, for many patients, a difficult time. Most people recovering from an acute illness are irritable. Their strength has not fully returned, yet often new demands are being put upon them. Patients recovering from hospitalizations for such conditions as diabetes will probably have to adjust to many lifestyle changes. They may have to learn to give themselves insulin injections, to do various tests to estimate their insulin needs and to modify their eating habits to keep the diabetes under control. Often, people worry about their ability to learn everything they need to know to look after themselves. They may be fearful, too, about resuming normal activities.

A convalescent patient learns to use a walker

The primary focus of nursing during the convalescent stage is to enhance the patients' ability to care for themselves. The nurse's teaching role is important at this stage. Not only must the nurse help the patient to gain new knowledge and skills, he or she must also provide the support and encouragement needed to foster a good learning environment. The patient's family or significant others are resources that should be tapped for assistance during the convalescent stage. This effort involves the nurse in working with the family, as well as the patient, and supporting them in their efforts to help. Many people require a lengthy rehabilitation program to restore their health to an optimal level. As we mentioned in Chapter 4, much rehabilitation takes place in the community with the patient at home, but there are also specialized rehabilitation units — sometimes a unit within a general hospital and sometimes a separate facility — where programs are tailored to each individual's needs for physical and social rehabilitation.

The Stage of Restored Health

After the convalescent stage is over and the recovered patient returns to normal activities, he or she enters a stage of restored health. For people who have had a self-limiting illness, such as a bout of pneumonia or surgery to remove a diseased gallbladder, restoration to health ideally means a return to a state of balance in all areas of functioning. For those who have a chronic health problem, such as newly diagnosed diabetes, and those with a terminal illness such as leukemia (often called cancer of the blood), it means restoration to a state of optimal functioning for that individual.

All will, however, require continued supervision by health personnel to make sure that health, once restored, is maintained. The person who has had an episode of acute illness, with no residual problems, will probably need a checkup in a few weeks and, then, perhaps, another in a few months to make sure that all is going well with the healing process. After that, he or she can usually return to a regular health maintenance program. A person with a long-term health problem will require supportive health care throughout the remainder of his or her lifetime — to assess responses to therapeutic regimens, to help institute changes as needed and to detect the early signs of any developing imbalance before it reaches critical proportions. The person with a terminal illness requires supportive care to help maintain an optimal level of functioning for as long as possible and to provide comfort and support for the individual (and family) as health deteriorates.

In the stage of restored health, the nurse's focus is again primarily on enhancing the patient's self-care abilities. Once the patient is discharged from a health agency and begins to resume normal daily activities, doubts and fears may arise. The person with diabetes, who was doing well with injections under the nurse's supervision, may lose self-confidence when he or she is at home, and require reinforcement of those skills learned while the patient was an inpatient. Convalescing patients may also need help in fitting an exercise schedule into their daily routine, or assistance in utilizing health information services in the community. For example, many communities have "Dial-a-Dietitian" services available to help with any uncertainties about diet. The nurse should alert patients to the services available.

Today, there are many services available in the community to help people with long-term health problems and those who have been discharged from the hospital — some still in the acute stage. We discussed a number of these when we were talking about the structure of health services in Chapter 4.

SECTORS OF HEALTH CARE

Helman (1990) describes three sectors of health care that are used by people in any society when they feel ill: (1) the popular sector, (2) the folk sector and (3) the professional sector.

The Popular Sector

The majority of minor illnesses are diagnosed and treated in the home, which Helman states is the "real site of primary heath care in any society" (1990, 56). Most people who think they are coming down with an illness follow similar patterns. They first try to treat themselves. They may take extra Vitamin C and drink more fluids, for example. The treatments people use vary considerably, depending on their beliefs about the structure and functioning of the body and the causes of health and ill-health. People can buy a wide variety of medicines in the drugstores to treat themselves. There are numerous folk remedies that are tried before further help is sought, for example, eating a clove of garlic to cure a cold, wearing a copper bracelet to ward off arthritis or eating chicken soup to cure a multitude of ailments.

If the self-treatment is not effective, certain family members or friends may be consulted who, primarily because of their experience, are considered good resources. Among them are nurses and pharmacists who are family members or friends, as well as people with relevant experience, such as a mother who has had several children. If the ill person has a long-term condition, such as diabetes or arthritis, he or she may consult with someone else who has the same health problem. Self-help groups such as the diabetes and arthritis societies are good resources . The leaders of such groups are usually very knowledgeable and a good source of information. In some religious cults and churches, people share experiences about their illnesses, as in some Pentecostal religions and spiritualist churches where there is a belief in "occult" or "divine" healing (Helman, 1990).

If self-treatment and remedies suggested by friends fail to cure, an ill person will usually seek the advice of healers from the folk or professional sector. Some of the specific situations that encourage a person to seek a higher level of health advice include:

1. other people calling attention to symptoms (remarking about a rash, for example, a raspy cough or a limp in the walk)
2. the symptoms interfering with social activity
3. other people sanctioning the person's need to see someone
4. the person perceiving the symptoms as threatening
5. comparing the nature and quality of present symptoms with those experienced previously or with those of other people indicating the need for further advice.*

The Folk Sector

After the popular sector, the next level of care people turn to is the folk sector. This sector includes practitioners who deal with the spiritual world and those who heal by secular means. The first group includes the shaman (medicine man/woman or "witch doctor") and the "divine healers" of some religious groups, such as the healers of the Christian Science Church. The secular practitioners include herbalists; people who practise acupuncture, acupressure and other forms of Eastern medicine; lay midwives and others whom we will talk about in Chapter 12, Health and Ethnicity. Practitioners in the folk sector have had special training in their fields or are believed to have been appointed by divine authority.

Although practitioners in the folk sector have been widely consulted in many countries for thousands of years, Western medicine has until recently been highly skeptical of these healers. For many people growing up in rural parts of developing countries, however, where Western medicine is not widely available, "folk medicine" is often the only type of medical care they have known. Many recent immigrants to Canada from developing countries in Asia, Africa and Central America have brought with them traditional health practices and practitioners to whom they turn when they are ill. An increasing number of non-immigrant Canadians are also turning to practitioners such as herbalists, naturopaths and others who use diet, herbs and natural substances, massage and other non-invasive techniques to treat illness.

In addition to treating people with non-invasive techniques, practitioners in the folk sector provide other advantages. They usually use a more holistic approach than many traditional physicians do. That is to say, they tend to look at the whole person, rather than only at the problem. They look at social environment, interpersonal relationships, and involve the whole family in diagnosis and treatment. Usually, the practitioner in the folk sector is from the same culture as the patient and has the same sort of social background which can make patient–practitioner relationships more satisfactory (Heiman, 1990).

* (Zola, 1964, cited in Bolaria, 1988, 7.)

The Professional Sector

The professional sector is made up of the organized health care system. It includes physicians, dentists, nurses, physiotherapists and other legally sanctioned health professionals.

Although some people use the folk sector to meet most of their health needs, not everyone does. The majority of people in Canada still turn to the professional sector when self-treatment and home remedies fail to effect a cure. Often, both the folk and the professional sectors are used; a person may take vitamins recommended by a naturopath and go to a physician for major health problems.

ADMISSION OF AN INDIVIDUAL TO A HEALTH AGENCY

The rapid changes taking place in the health care system across the country are having an impact on all aspects of care. The admission of patients to a health agency and their discharge from an agency is no exception.

ADMISSION TO A COMMUNITY AGENCY

In the community, people may take advantage of health promotion services that are available or they may not. Expectant parents may register for prenatal classes being given by the community health nurse but they do not have to do so; the choice is theirs. Similarly, with health restoration and supportive services, the individual has the right to decide whether or not to take advantage of them. Referrals for home care of an individual may come from any one of a number of sources: the physician, the community liaison nurse in a hospital or the patient's family, friends or concerned neighbours. Patients may also make the initial contacts themselves (Government of Ontario, 1993). Whatever the source of the original contact, it is important to remember that the patient has the right to self-determination. Unless the patient has been declared incompetent, he or she must make the decision to receive care.

Once this decision has been made, a Case Manager usually goes into the home to undertake an initial assessment. The Case Manager is most often a nurse but, in some cases, may be someone from another discipline such as a social worker. The Case Manager assesses the patient and the home situation, decides on the type and amount of care needed and makes arrangements for the various services. These include nursing, physiotherapy, homemaker services and other types of services, as described in Chapter 4. In the case of nursing services, the Case Manager specifies the level of care required. For example, the situation may require a Registered Nurse to do dressings, injections or other intervention or, on the other hand, may only involve bathing and other activities of daily living, which could be

NURSES AT WORK

Our aging population and philosophy of deinstitutionalization is changing the face of our communities and, as a result, the roles of community nurses. As a Case Manager (Community Nurse Assessor) in the Continuing Care Division of the Ministry of Health, I help patients with chronic health problems to remain independent as long as it is possible for them to do so. Working with patients, I assess needs and plan how and what resources families and communities can provide. I use the services of health care providers such as home nursing care, rehabilitation services, home support, adult day care, respite or mental health services. I use these services in conjunction with community organizations such as meals on wheels, handidart, community volunteer organizations and seniors centres. I frequently link patients to the services of specific groups such as the Multiple Sclerosis Society and social, recreational and cultural resources. I also help patients access information about other provincial and federal government services which are available to help with their financial, housing or legal needs.

When patients and their families feel they can no longer cope, or when available home resources cannot meet their needs, I help them work through the difficult process of having to place a family member in a care facility. I provide information and counsel them about what care facilities might best meet the patient's needs. After the patient and family have viewed and selected a future home, I place the patient's name on the waiting list of the chosen care facility.

My patients range from 19 to 96 years of age. The greatest percentage of them are elderly women over the age of 80, who have minimal resources and supports. I help them learn to cope with physical disabilities, memory loss and social isolation. I have developed expertise in helping patients cope with chronic illness or disabilities such as strokes, Parkinson's disease, Alzheimer's and osteoporosis. I help patients to realize their strengths and personal coping styles or strategies. I also help them to use these skills to meet the challenges they face as they try to remain independent and live with dignity.

My role involves educating patients about their disease process, counselling them about lifestyle changes they might need to make. I help them access the services that can best assist them to cope and be independent. I am ever mindful of the potential for patient abuse and neglect. My practice is greatly influenced by family dynamics and societal expectations about women's roles as caregivers. I find that wives and daughters carry the largest burden for providing support and need be proactive about their right to receive help to prevent burnout.

I frequently have to educate family members and other health professionals about the patients' rights to self-determination and the right to choose how and where they want to live. I strive to always respect the reality of what the patient is experiencing and to see the person rather than the disease or the disability. I respect and support the choices that patients make. I have patients who have experienced ageist, sexist and racist barriers in their efforts to access services and health care. I am an adamant advocate of my patients' rights to receive appropriate assessment, treatment and services.

— Cherry Nettleton, RN, BScN.

---

done by someone with less training. Waring (1994) points out in an article in the *Canadian Nurse Journal*, "The responsibility for admission, discharge and the amount and kind of care [an individual receives] is held by the primary Home Care nursing and rehabilitation staff" (24).

ADMISSION TO AN ACUTE CARE HOSPITAL

Patients are usually admitted to acute care hospitals through either the Admitting or Emergency Department. In the case of elective surgery, however, an increasing number of hospitals have preadmission clinics for people who are slated for day-care, short-stay or inpatient services. The clinics serve as surgical outpatient units. People report to the clinic seven to fourteen days before surgery for various administrative procedures, laboratory tests and preadmission assessment and counselling. Some of the services that may be included are shown in the box below.

Services Commonly Provided in Preadmission Clinics

- clerk interviews for patient demographics
- nursing interviews/preoperative assessments
- diagnostic preoperative testing — blood tests, electrocardiograms, X-rays, respiratory tests, etc.
- screening of test results for early detection and treatment of abnormalities
- discharge planning
- patient teaching and support
- anesthetic consultations and medical examinations.

Some preadmission clinics also admit patients on the day of surgery and prepare them for the operating room. They are transferred postoperatively to another surgical unit. The preadmission clinics have many advantages. Family members are welcomed. Patients and families become familiar with the hospital surroundings, routines and procedures, which helps to reduce stress and anxiety. Teaching sessions are a major focus in most preadmission clinics and these also help to relieve a considerable amount of anxiety. Patients are taught postoperative exercises and have a chance to practise them. Some units have generalized teaching sessions for all patients, followed by specialized sessions for specific types of surgery (LeNoble, 1993).

For people entering hospital through the usual routes, that is, through the admitting or emergency department, there are also certain admitting formalities. Although each agency has its own admission procedure, there are some commonalities that the nurse will find in all agencies. The patient's first impression of a hospital is often formed in the admitting department. It is essential that nurses and other admitting staff treat patients as people of worth and dignity and do what they can to make them feel welcome. Hospitals are busy places and personnel are often rushed, but it does not take extra time to be kind or to convey welcome.

Staff in the admitting department usually explain hospital policy to the patient and/or family regarding personal effects and advise that clothing and valuables be sent home whenever possible. Specific information is gathered from the patient (or from the person accompanying, if the patient is unable to communicate). The information usually requested includes: medical insurance number and additional coverage; demographic data, such as full name and address, date of birth, next of kin, religion and usual employment; as well as physician's name and the reason for admission. Most hospitals have an admission form which becomes part of the patient's record. Most require patients to sign a consent form during the admitting procedure. This form usually gives the hospital staff permission to perform any diagnostic and treatment procedures considered necessary during the patient's stay.

After the admission formalities are completed, the patient is taken to a nursing unit. The reception provided by the staff here is again of the utmost importance. A sincere welcome helps to ease adjustment to the new environment. The new patient should be greeted by name and asked how he or she would like to be addressed. Nurses should also introduce themselves. Any family or friends who have accompanied the patient to the hospital should also be made welcome.

The patient's room or bed unit should be ready, so that he or she feels expected. The nurse admitting the patient to the unit should explain the use of equipment such as the call system, the bed controls and over-bed table, and, if the patient is to be up and walking around, show them the location of bathrooms and showers, as well as other facilities, such as telephones and the patients' lounge. It is also helpful to give directions to the cafeteria or coffee shop, and to describe other services for patients and visitors. The nurse should also explain hospital routines such as meal-times, visiting hours and restrictions on smoking. Many hospitals have patient information pamphlets.

Introductions to staff are important. All nurses who enter the patient's room should introduce themselves, and it is also helpful if the admitting nurse tells the patient who will be looking after him or her. If the patient is in a room with other people, introductions are in order.

The nurse should also find out if the patient has any particular needs or wishes that would make the stay in hospital more comfortable. A detailed nursing history will be taken later but it is useful to know right away whether the patient has any specific dietary requests so that the dietitian can be alerted. If applicable, an "allergy alert" should be posted on the patient's record and entered into the computer file (if the agency has a computer-based information management system).

Once the initial orientation to the hospital has been completed, the patient is usually examined by the hospital physician. This examination includes a medical history, a physical examination and routine screening tests. In many hospitals, these tests include a urinalysis and routine blood work. The nurse should explain to the patient what to expect and who will be coming in to do the various tests.

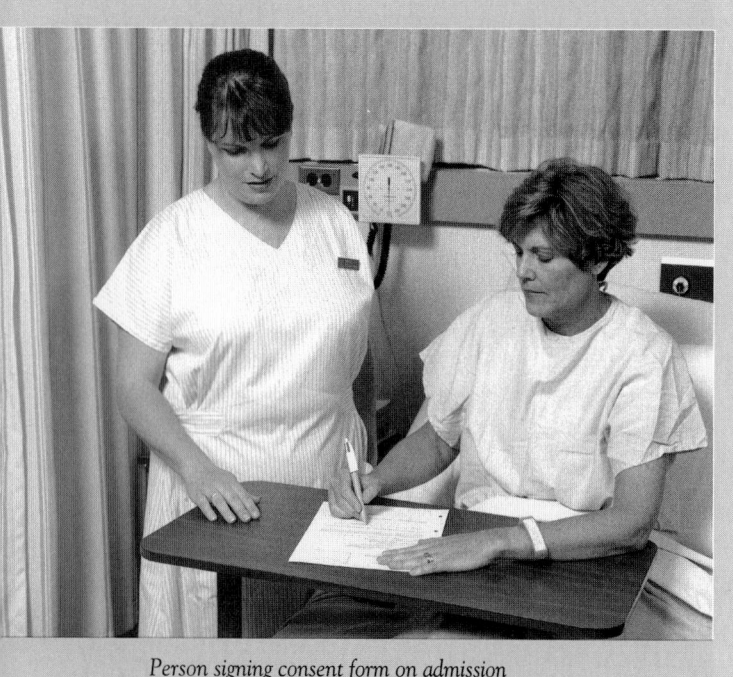

Person signing consent form on admission

DISCHARGE FROM A HEALTH AGENCY

Preparation for discharge begins with the patient's admission to an agency. Whether the individual is being cared for in a home situation or an inpatient facility, the goal of care is to enable the patient to take control of his or her own health. This does not negate the provision of supportive care as required; it does, however, mean helping patients to gain the knowledge and skills needed to provide this self-care insofar as this is possible to develop confidence in their ability to do so.

Hospitals provide a protective environment for patients and many are genuinely concerned about their discharge. They wonder how they will manage at home. They worry about being a burden to their families and about their ability to contribute as a functioning member of the family and the community. Patients are usually discharged from the hospital when they no longer need the services it offers. If they need the services of another agency, such as a rehabilitation unit, a long-term care agency or home care, arrangements are made prior to discharge. Most hospitals have a nurse or other staff member who is responsible for making arrangements and coordinating the services needed by patients on discharge. The social worker may also see the individual if there is a need for financial assistance or for homemaker service.

THE NURSE'S ROLE IN THE CARE OF INDIVIDUALS

The nurse works in all phases of the health care continuum — helping people to promote health, to protect themselves from illness and disease and, if need be, to restore health in the case of an acute episode of illness or to provide supportive care in the case of long-term or terminal illness.

NURSING AND HEALTH PROMOTION

In keeping with the World Health Organization definition of health promotion as "the process of enabling people to increase control over, and to improve their health" (WHO, 1984), the nurse's role in health promotion for the individual is one of helping people to help themselves to attain their optimal state of health and wellness. In health promotion, the nurse and the individual work as partners, with the process based on the specific needs of the individual as they are perceived. Health promotion, then, is patient-driven, rather than being controlled by the nurse. In health promotion, the nurse is a resource for the patient. In this capacity, the nurse may:

1. assist in procuring information. For example, in one hospital, computer programs are available for patient (and family) use in the hospital library so patients can learn about their condition. This may include learning about the disease process, its possible causes, recommended treatment and home care. Nurses direct patients and/or families to the library to study these.

2. encourage patients to explore health habits and practices and to look at possible alternatives to maximize patients' potential for wellness.

3. assist in making healthy choices from the alternatives available.

4. assist in planning a course of action to implement patients' choices if requested to do so by the patient.

NURSING AND HEALTH PROTECTION

Health protection has always been a core component of the work of community health nurses but it is an equally important part of the nurse's role in caring for people in inpatient facilities. The traditional role of the nurse in health protection in the community is to help healthy people to prevent illness through such measures as:

- the control of communicable diseases, for example, immunization programs for protection against those diseases for which there are known vaccines or other immunity-producing agents
- screening programs to detect illness in its early stage
- environmental safety programs.

The nurse is responsible for helping patients (both at home and in inpatient facilities) to protect their health by:

- maintaining their regular patterns of functioning. This includes a nutritious diet, good hygiene practices, normal patterns of elimination and sufficient rest and sleep to increase stress resistance. In so doing, the nurse helps patients to maintain normal activities of daily living insofar as this is possible within the limitations of their illness.
- implementing measures to prevent complications such as infection, constipation and the loss of muscle tone due to bed rest.

Many nursing interventions for people who are ill are basically health protection measures — to ensure that general health does not deteriorate during the course of treatment for an illness. For example, someone who has had a fall that necessitates hospitalization with surgery to correct a fracture in one wrist may have difficulty using the other hand as well because of painful bruises and swelling. This patient will need help with meals to prevent development of a nutrition deficit. The hazards of bed rest are discussed in Chapter 28, Movement and Exercise Needs, as are measures the nurse can take to prevent these. Interventions to protect the health of the individual are included in the chapters dealing with basic needs, that is, Chapters 19 to 36.

NURSING AND HEALTH RESTORATION

The nurse's role in health restoration includes not only helping a patient to recover from episodic illness but, also, providing supportive care for those with long-term or terminal illnesses. As we discussed in Chapter 4, in talking about the continuum of care, health restoration services in the community blend imperceptibly with those for health support. To try to separate them would seem to be an exercise in semantics, rather than being helpful in the provision of nursing care. We have therefore not attempted in this text to separate nursing measures for health restoration from those for supportive health care.

What is more important is the reorientation of nursing care to a health promotion model that permeates all aspects of nursing care from health promotion and health protection through health restoration and supportive care. This implies that the nurse and the individual work together in a collaborative (rather than provider/recipient) relationship.

HOME CARE

The focus in home care is on helping patients and their families to learn to manage the acute, chronic, rehabilitative and palliative care needs of the individual. The Case Manager in the initial home visit and, subsequently, the nurses and other health personnel involved in care of an individual assess the capacity of the patient (or the family) to manage his or her own care or to learn to manage it. The nurses and other clinicians in home care work in a collaborative role with patients and their families, serving as consultants on health matters, rather than as "doer–providers" of care. They share their knowledge with patients and explain their professional perspective, encouraging patients to share with them their own view of their health and their health goals (Waring, 1994; Government of Ontario, 1993).

Waring (1994), in a recent article in *The Canadian Nurse*, described the changing role of the nurse in home care with the Vancouver Health Department. In this home care program nurses act as Case Managers and are the "gatekeepers" to services. They are responsible for admission and decisions as well as the amount and kind of care the patient receives. The care focusses on health and health promotion. It is provided within a family-community context in which the nurse is "ally and consultant" to the patient and the patient's family who provide much of the "hands-on" care. The nurses foster a climate in which the patient's ability to take control of health-related decisions is nurtured. To undertake their role as independent practitioners, Waring feels that the nurses need a strong generalist clinical background and that they must be sensitive to cultural issues.

ACUTE CARE

In Chapter 5, we discussed the various aspects of the nurse's role, using Benner's "domains of nursing practice" as a framework (1984). These domains can be used to explain the nurse's role in health restoration and supportive care for people in an acute care facility.

The helping role   The helping role involves helping people who are ill to carry out those activities that they would do for themselves if they were capable, such as feeding themselves, bathing and the like. It also means letting people make as many decisions and retain as much independence as possible. It involves helping patient and family to come to terms with illness and helping the patient to regain as much independence as possible and take control of his or her own health.

The teaching-coaching function   People who are ill have many learning needs and patient teaching is one of the nurse's major functions in acute care. We mentioned earlier the teaching sessions that are part of the preadmission clinics for surgical patients. Nurses on the nursing unit follow up on these, and incorporate other teaching as needed, as does the nurse who goes into the home on followup visits. People with medical conditions, such as a weak heart, must learn to cope with their illness which, in many cases, means restructuring their lives. Far too often in the past, patient teaching was based on the nurse's perceptions of what the patient needed to know. The emphasis has changed to focus on the patient's perceptions which are often quite different from those of the nurse and other health professionals. We discuss this aspect of the nurse's role further in Chapter 17, Teaching and Learning Skills.

The diagnostic and monitoring function Nurses today are responsible for carrying out many complex diagnostic procedures. They also monitor the condition of patients in situations where highly technical equipment is being used, for example, in the intensive care unit. In order to carry out these tasks, the nurse needs considerable skill in manipulating equipment and in interpreting the readings on various machines (such as cardiac monitors), as well as the knowledge base required to take appropriate action when necessary. It is important to note, however, that, in the midst of all the machines and highly specialized equipment, it is the nurse who provides the human link for patients and their families, always remembering that the patient is a person, not an inanimate object in a bed. The nurse is alert to the feelings of the patient and family and sensitive to their reactions to all that is going on.

Effective management of rapidly changing situations   People are unpredictable and, as you go about your daily work on clinical assignments, you will find you have to adjust your plans innumerable times in many situations. As you become more experienced you learn to handle the unexpected with calm assurance and to take charge in emergency situations with skill and competence.

Administering and monitoring therapeutic interventions and regimens People tend to think of the nurse as the person who gives medications and injections and, indeed, this is an important aspect of nursing care. Equally important, however, is monitoring the reactions of people to medications and treatments. Another aspect of this part of the nurse's role — which is receiving increasing attention — is teaching people (patients and families) to administer their own medications and treatments in the home situation.

Monitoring and ensuring the quality of health care practices In home care, the Case Manager coordinates all aspects of the individual's care. This concept is also being tried in the acute care hospital. The Case Manager is in an ideal position to monitor the care the patient receives from all practitioners. Every nurse, however, has a responsibility to the patient to see that they receive the best care possible. In doing so, the nurse frequently acts as the patient's advocate, speaking for the patient or interceding with others on his or her behalf.

Organizational and work-role competencies In the busy work situation of the acute care hospital, the nurse needs good organizational skills. Often responsible for the care of several patients, the nurse must juggle seeing to the patients' personal care needs with administering medications and treatments, supervising auxiliary staff, monitoring the work of other staff and responding to unexpected interruptions and special requests from patients or families.

LONG-TERM CARE

Many people do not need the services of an acute care hospital but, because of physical or mental frailty or disability, are unable to function in the community. These are the ones who require long-term care. The majority of these people are older adults, most of whom require care for months, years and often until they die (Mantle, 1988).

Nursing in long-term care agencies has changed dramatically in recent years. Formerly patterned on the acute care hospital model, the focus was on physical care of the patients. Nursing homes and other long-term care agencies were essentially custodial institutions. Today, these agencies are considered communal residences for people which take the place of the individual's own home when he or she can no longer maintain independent living. A major player in bringing about change in the long-term institutional care field was Vera McIvor who introduced the Priory Method in four extended care hospitals operated by the Juan de Fuca Hospital Society in Victoria (Du Gas and Beckingham, 1993). The Priory Method is based on the belief that the older person is still a unique individual, working towards growth and self-fulfillment, and that a therapeutic and restorative environment can be achieved if this attitude is kept in mind (McIvor, 1978). The Priory Method has become a model for care of the elderly across the country.

In long-term care agencies today, people are called *residents*, rather than *patients*. As Mantle so aptly describes it, "A primary goal of long-term caregivers is to create environments that facilitate healthy living and dying even though the residents are experiencing varying degrees of illness" (1992, 142).

PALLIATIVE CARE

Another term for **palliative care** is *hospice care*, a term derived from the original model at St. Christopher's Hospice in London, England. Both terms refer to the provision of humane, compassionate care of the dying. "It is the link between the needs of the terminally ill and their families and a staff that employs the medieval concept of hospitality in which a community assists the traveller at dangerous points along his journey" (Death education, 1978, cited in Ebersole and Hess, 1990, 740). In this analogy, the dying are the travellers at a point in their journey along the continuum of life when they need the comfort and support of their community of family and friends, and the specially trained palliative care team. These teams may be community or institution- based, with the individual often moving from one to the other as needed. The role of nurses in palliative care is discussed in Chapter 36 (Death, Loss and Grief).

KEY TERMS

system p. 194
structure p. 194
function p. 194
subsystem p. 194

macrosystems p. 194
boundaries p. 195
open systems p.1 95
closed systems p.195

input p. 195
output p. 196
feedback p. 196
homeostasis p. 197

IN REVIEW

Systems theory provides a theoretical basis for examining the phenomenon of the individual as a human system interacting with other systems in the surrounding environment. The focus in systems theory is on the interactions among the various components of the system and between the system and its environment. Physiological homeostasis, psychosocial equilibrium and environmental equilibrium all play a role in maintenance of an individual's equilibrium. Alterations in any one of these areas affects the person's interaction with the others — a basic concept in holistic nursing.

Physiological, psychosocial and environmental stressors all upset the delicate balance that is maintained in the human system. Stressors can be positive or negative and can vary from minor to major in their effect on the human system. A person who experiences many life changes in a short period of time may become a candidate for major illness. This may also be true for the person with constant "daily hassles." These may become chronic stressors unless balanced by interspersed uplifts.

Stressors in themselves do not cause illness but our reaction to them can. Cognitive appraisal is our perception of a situation as harmful and the assessment of our ability to cope with it. When danger threatens, a number of physiological changes occur as the body prepares for fight or flight. Stress reactions are very individualized, being dependent on a person's cognitive appraisal of a situation, basic personality characteristics, past experiences and previous coping strategies.

The response of the body to physiological stress was described by Hans Selye who referred to it as the general adaptation syndrome (GAS). It consists of the alarm reaction, the stage of resistance and finally exhaustion when the body has depleted its ability to adapt and can no longer restore its equilibrium. There may also be local reaction to stress which Selye called the "local adaptation syndrome" (LAS).

People use various coping strategies or buffers to protect themselves from the emotional impact of stress. Defence mechanisms are used constantly in daily living to protect an individual's self-esteem. They help to reduce anxiety and therefore help to maintain equilibrium. Overuse of defence mechanisms may lead to illness. Physical activity, exercise and relaxation techniques are often effective in minimizing the stress response. Ineffective coping strategies, or negative copers, include the use of tobacco and alcohol, withdrawal behaviour and worrying.

Healthy coping strategies, or "learned resourcefulness," include a repertoire of skills such as the cognitive coping skills, the ability to problem-solve, delayed gratification and self-efficacy. Physical fitness and social support from family and friends bolster a person's ability to cope. Some individuals are better able to cope with stress than others. Characteristics associated with the "hardy" personality include: a sense of commitment, the ability to view change as a challenge and a sense of personal control over one's life.

Perceptions of health are influenced by cultural background, religion, socioeconomic status, education, age, gender and situational factors. Illness behaviour is socially based — learned behaviours guide us through the stages of symptom awareness, acute illness, recovery and rehabilitation. People usually engage in self-treatment first when they feel ill and if this is not effective, they then seek various sources for assistance. These sources may include the popular sector of friends, family and neighbours, the folk sector of spiritual and traditional healers, and the professional sector of physicians and other professionally trained practitioners.

People may admit themselves to a community health agency or they may be referred by any one of a number of different sources, such as a physician, a nurse or their family or friends. People are usually admitted to an acute-care facility though the Admitting or Emergency Department although many hospitals have established Preadmission Clinics, particularly for those undergoing surgery. Preliminary paperwork, laboratory work, preoperative examinations and teaching are some of the services offered in these clinics. Discharge teaching and planning begins in the admitting units and continues through the stay in an inpatient facility with follow-up in the community.

The nurse's role in the health of the individual includes health promotion, health protection, and restorative and supportive care. In health promotion, nurses work in partnership, helping people to help themselves attain optimal health. In health protection nurses are involved in the control of communicable diseases, in screening programs and in environmental safety. Their role in health protection also includes helping people to maintain normal body functioning and to prevent complications when they are ill. The nurse also carries out interventions to help patients recover from episodic illness and to provide support when they are chronically or terminally ill.

LEARNING ACTIVITIES

1. Think of one of the most stressful events in your life.
   a) What physical signs and symptoms do you remember having?
   b) What emotional response did you have?
   c) What action did you take?
   d) Do you think you coped well?

2. What defence mechanisms are you aware of having used? What ones have you seen friends, family members or other people using?

3. Think of two people among your friends or acquaintances who have undergone a considerable amount of stress in the past few years, one who has coped well and one who has coped not so well. Compare the characteristics of the two individuals, using as a basis for comparison Kobasa's characteristics of a "hardy" personality.

4. Talk with someone who has had an illness requiring medical care in the past few weeks or has recently undergone surgery. Ask about their experience of illness.

   a) What made them think that they were ill?
   b) What self-treatment did they try?
   c) Whom did they consult in the early stages of their illness?
   d) What made them seek further consultation?
   e) Did they consult anyone in the folk sector? If so, whom did they consult? Did they try herbs or other remedies or treatments?
   f) What made them seek professional help?
   g) What professional help did they choose?

5. Discuss with a patient in hospital his or her thoughts and feelings about the admission procedure in the admitting or emergency department or in the preadmission clinic and about his or her preparation for discharge.

6. Talk with a community health nurse and with a hospital nurse. What do these nurses see as their roles in health promotion? Health protection? Health restoration and/or health support?

REFERENCES AND READINGS

AMBROSIO, E. (1991). Poor housing, poor health. *The Canadian Nurse, 87*(5), 22–24.

AUGER, J.R. (1976). *Behavioural systems and nursing.* Englewood Cliffs, NJ: Prentice-Hall.

BANDURA, A. (1977). Self-efficacy: Towards a unifying theory of behavioral change. *Psychological Review, 84,* 191–215.

BANDURA, A. (1986). *The social foundations of thought and action.* Englewood Cliffs, NJ: Prentice-Hall.

BENNER, P. (1984). *From novice to expert.* Menlo Park, CA: Addison-Wesley.

BLACK, J.M. and MATASSARIN-JACOBS, E. (1993). *Luckmann and Sorenson's medical–surgical nursing: A psychophysiological approach.* Philadelphia: Saunders.

BOLARIA, B.S. (1988). Sociology, medicine, health and illness. In B.S. Bolaria and H.D. Dickinson. (1988). *Sociology of health care in Canada.* Toronto: Harcourt Brace Jovanovich, 1–14.

BRUNNER, L.S., and SUDDARTH, D.S. (1988). *Textbook of medical–surgical nursing* (6th ed.). Philadelphia: Lippincott.

BURGESS, A.W. (1990). *Psychiatric nursing in the hospital and the community* (5th ed.). Norwalk, CT: Appleton & Lange.

CANADIAN NURSES ASSOCIATION. *Vertical files, 1991.*

CANNON, W.B. (1939). *The wisdom of the body.* New York: Norton.

CHARLESWORTH, E.A. and NATHAN, R.G. (1984). *Stress management: A comprehensive guide to wellness.* New York: Atheneum.

DIER, K. (1992). Nursing practice in international areas. In A.J. Baumgart and J. Larsen (Eds). *Canadian nursing faces the future.* Toronto: Mosby, 200–217.

DU GAS, B.W. and BECKINGHAM, A. (1993). The emergence of gerontological nursing. In A. Beckingham and B. Du Gas. *Promoting healthy aging.* St. Louis: Mosby.

EBERSOLE, P. and HESS, P. (1990). *Toward healthy aging: Human needs and nursing response* (2nd ed.). St. Louis: Mosby.

EPP, J. (1986). *Achieving health for all: A framework for health promotion.* Ottawa: Health and Welfare Canada.

FELICITAS, M. (1967). Meet the president. *International Nursing Review, 14*(1), (reprint, not paginated).

GIRARD, A.M. [biographical file]. (1991). *Who's who in Canada.* Toronto: Global Press.

GOVERNMENT OF BRITISH COLUMBIA. (1992). *Health indicator workbook* (1st ed.). Victoria: Office of Health Promotion. B.C. Ministry of Health and Ministry Responsible for Seniors. (Catalogue No. QP 91029).

GOVERNMENT OF CANADA. (1989). *The active health report on seniors.* Ottawa: Health and Welfare Canada.

GOVERNMENT OF ONTARIO. (1993). *Highlights. Partnerships in long-term care: A new way to plan, manage and deliver services and community support.* Toronto: Ontario Ministries of Health, Community and Social Services and Citizenship.

GOVERNMENT OF ONTARIO. (1993). *Nurturing health.* Premier's Council on Health, Well-being and Social Justice 1987–1991. Toronto: Queen's Printer. (Catalogue No. 01.93.20M).

GRANT, K.R. (1988). The inverse care law in Canada: Differential access under universal free health insurance. In B.S. Bolaria and H.D. Dickinson. *Sociology of health care in Canada.* Toronto: Harcourt Brace Jovanovich, 118–134.

GREEN, J. and SHELLENGBERGER, R. (1991). *The dynamics of health and wellness: A biopsychosocial approach.* Philadelphia: Harcourt Brace College.

HELMAN, C.G. (1990). *Culture, health and illness* (2nd ed.). London: Butterworths.

HISTORY OF NURSING GROUP, REGISTERED NURSING ASSOCIATION OF BRITISH COLUMBIA. *Biographical files.*

HOLMES, T.H. and RAHE, R.H. (1967). The social readjustment rating scale. *Journal of Psychosomatic Research, 11,* 213–218.

KOBASA, S. (1979). Stressful life events, personality and health: An enquiry into hardiness. *Journal of Personality and Social Psychology, 37,* 1–11.

KOBASA, S.C. (1982). The hardy personality: Toward a social psychology of stress and health. In G.S. Sanders and J. Suls (Eds). *Social psychology of health and illness.* Hillsdale, NJ: Erlbaum, 3–32.

KOBASA, S.C. (1985). Stressful life events, personality and health: An inquiry into hardiness. In Monat and Lazarus (Eds). *Stress and coping: An anthology* (2nd ed.). New York: Columbia University Press.

KOBASA, S.C. and PUCETTI, M.C. (1983). Personality and social resources in stress resistance. *Journal of Personality and Social Psychology, 45,* 839–850.

LAZARUS, R.S. (1981, July). Little hassles can be hazardous to health. *Psychology Today,* 58–62.

LAZARUS, R.S. and FOLKMANN, S. (1984). *Stress, appraisal and coping.* New York: Springer.

LENOBLE, E. (1993). Preadmission clinics gaining ground. *Nursing B.C., 25*(4), 20–24.

MANTLE, J. (1992). Nursing practice in long-term care agencies. In A.J. Baumgart and J. Larsen. *Canadian nursing faces the future* (2nd ed.). Toronto: Mosby, 134–151.

MARTIN, L. (1993). Stress, distress and eustress. In A.C. Beckingham and B.W. Du Gas. *Promoting healthy aging.* St.Louis: Mosby, 303–331.

McIVER, V. (1978). Freedom to be (Part two): The priory method. *The Canadian Nurse, 74*(3), 23–26.

PARSONS, T. (1972). Definitions of health and illness in the light of the American values and social structure. In E.G. Jaco. *Patients, physicians and illness* (2nd ed.). New York: Free Press, 107–127.

ROSENBAUM, M. (1983). Learned resourcefulness as a behavioral repertoire for the self-regulation of internal events: Issues and speculations. In M. Rosenbaum, C.M. Franks and Y. Jaffe (Eds.) *Perspectives on behavior therapy in the eighties.* New York: Springer.

SCHWARTZ, R. (1986), The internal dialogue. On the asymmetry between positive and negative coping thoughts. *Cognitive Therapy and Research, 10,* 591–605.

SELYE, H. (1972). Stress and the nation's health. In *Proceedings of the National Conference on Fitness and Health. Ottawa, December 4, 5 and 6, 1972.* Ottawa: Health and Welfare Canada.

SELYE, H. (1977). A code for coping with stress. *AORN Journal, 25* (1), 35–42.

SPLANE, R.B. and SPLANE, V.H. (1994). *Chief nursing officer positions in national ministries of health: Focal points for nursing leadership.* San Francisco: University of California School of Nursing.

TARTASKY, D.S. (1993, Fall). Hardiness: Conceptual and methodological issues. *Image, 23*(3), 225–229.

VON BERTALANFFY, L. (1968). *General systems theory: Foundations, development, applications.* New York: Braziller.

WARING, J. (1994). The new emphasis of home care. *The Canadian Nurse, 90*(2), 22–26.

WORLD HEALTH ORGANIZATION (WHO). (1984). *Health promotion glossary.* Copenhagen: WHO Regional Office for Europe.

Health and the Family

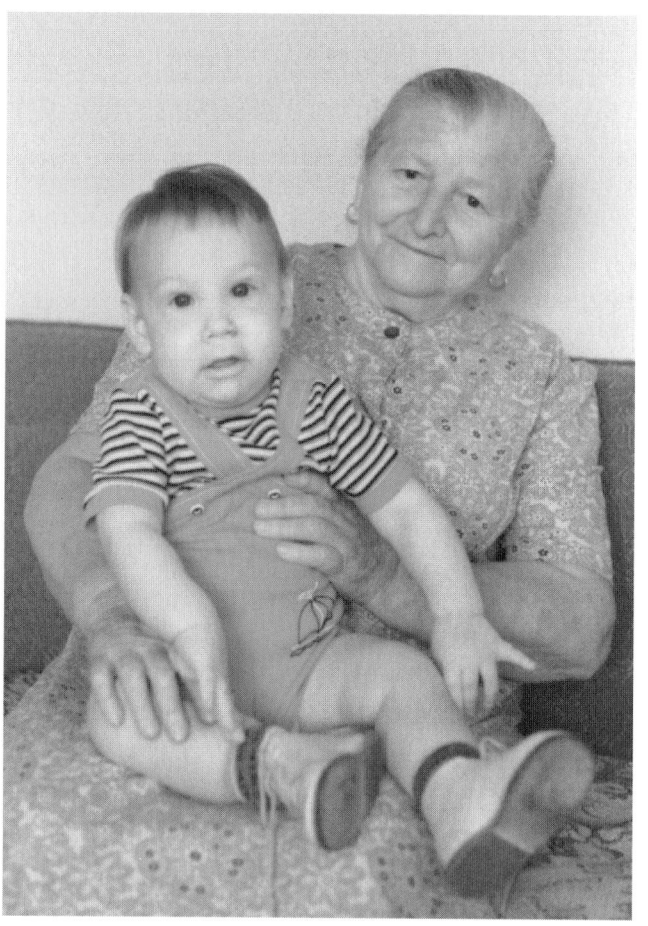

CENTRAL QUESTIONS

1. *What is the meaning of family?*

2. *What is the relationship between health of the individual and health of the family?*

3. *What are the different types of family forms in Canada?*

4. *What are the theoretical perspectives of the family systems framework, the structural-functional framework and the family developmental framework?*

5. *How can nurses use concepts from the selected frameworks when working with families?*

6. *How does the meaning of family health differ from the meaning of health?*

7. *What are the main determinants of family health?*

8. *What are the criteria for judging family health?*

9. *What is family stress and crisis?*

10. *How does illness in a family member impact on family functioning?*

11. *How is the family conceptualized in the three types of nursing practice with families?*

12. *What are the categories of the Calgary Family Assessment Model and how is it used in family assessment?*

13. *What intervention strategies can nurses use in assisting families to promote and protect family health?*

14. *What intervention strategies can nurses use in helping families to cope with family stress and crisis?*

INTRODUCTION

Behavioural scientists tell us that few people can live in isolation. By interacting and associating with other human beings, we develop our personality and our humanness. Our initial interactions with others most often occur within the family. How we lead our lives and give meaning to all that happens to us is usually rooted in experiences we have had with our families. And when we are in need of human support and affection, it is often our families that we turn to because we know that they will provide us with unconditional love and accept us for who we are.

In many parts of the world, the family is recognized as society's most basic institution. Consisting of individuals bound together by emotional ties and a sense of belonging, the family persists as the major unit for reproduction, socialization and the perpetuation of sociocultural traditions. As a social unit, the family is believed to exert the greatest influence on the growth and development of its members, namely its children. It is through the family that children first learn about the social world into which they are born and it is with the family's ongoing nurturing and support that they grow up to be productive and self-sustaining members of society. Children develop their sense of identity and self-worth, and learn rules of conduct, values and adult social roles largely through the family. How we behave socially, our sense of self and our career choices are the result of influences from our families. For example, children who grow up with family expectations that they will excel in whatever they do and become strong, competitive individuals soon develop a sense of the kind of person they must endeavour to be.

The family is viewed by some as a mediating agent or a "buffer" between society and the individual. As such, it transmits and modifies social values, goals and expectations while at the same time fostering the growth of individuals so that they will become capable members of society. Other groups, such as the school, the church or youth clubs, may have a mediating function as well. However, these groups do not consider the total needs of the individual. For example, the school focusses on the child's scholastic achievement and cooperative spirit in work and play, while other facets of the child's life, such as health and safety, remain the concern of the family. The family must provide transportation, lunches and snacks, and proper clothing and footwear, for instance, to ensure the child's physical well-being at school in addition to fostering attitudes and values that ensure positive, productive learning behaviours (Friedman, 1992).

The family plays a vital role in the health of its members. Some health professionals believe that the family is "probably the most significant factor in the state of health and well-being of individuals" (Ramshorn, 1978, 248) and "constitutes perhaps the most important social context

within which illness occurs and is resolved" (Litman, 1974, 495). The family is a significant factor in the health of individuals because it provides the physical and social environment, or the living conditions, in which health and illness occur.

A family's health beliefs, practices and socioeconomic capabilities influence the lifestyle and living conditions for individual members. It is difficult to maintain a healthy lifestyle if one does not have enough money to afford good housing and nutritious food. Individuals whose families live in poverty, for example, often lead unhealthy lifestyles, lack adequate social support and generally experience more illness than do those individuals who come from more privileged families. Poverty is a significant threat to health because it limits options available to the family for creating living conditions that promote health and prevent illness.

The family is also a primary resource for its members in its ability to provide support and care in health and in illness. Families care for one another. Parents care for their children, spouses care for each other, and adult children become caregivers for their aging parents. The support and care a family gives to an ill member can be a powerful ally in that person's ability to cope with his or her illness and to recover. For example, educating a diabetic patient about diet would not achieve a successful outcome unless his or her spouse was committed to purchasing and cooking foods that are low in sugar content. Individuals have shown that they respond to treatment and heal more effectively when they have the support of a caring family.

There is a reciprocal relationship between the health and well-being of the family and its members. The health or illness status of one family member affects all other family members, which in turn affects the health and well-being of the family as a whole. When two-year-old Angie goes into hospital for open heart surgery, the whole family worries about the outcome. In addition, her older sibling feels neglected because the mother spends all of her time in hospital with Angie.

Sometimes the family itself is at the root of problems for the individual. For instance, poor family communication and interaction may lead an adolescent to use drugs and alcohol. In this case, care for the individual would involve an assessment of family dynamics and intervention for the whole family. Because of this interrelationship between family health and the health of family members, nurses often care for families as well as individuals. In this chapter we will outline the nature of Canadian families and discuss concepts of family life as a foundation for nursing care of families. Family health will be defined and described along with family stress and the impact of illness on the family. We will present a model for family assessment as well as nursing interventions for helping families promote family health and cope with family stress and illness.

LOOKING BACK

1600 1700 1800 1900
1650 1750 1850 1950

SISTER DENISE LEFEBVRE 1907–1993

The first Canadian nurse to obtain a doctoral degree was Sister Denise Lefèbvre, who received a Docteur de Pédagogie from the Université de Montréal in 1955. Although nursing education had moved into universities in Canada in 1919, a lack of advanced academic qualifications for nurses had plagued the profession. Without doctorally prepared academics, nursing could not achieve status within universities; and without status in the campus communities, the discipline could not introduce programs to enable nurses to achieve academic qualifications. Sister Lefèbvre was the first to break this cycle and pioneer the movement to doctoral preparation for Canadian nurses.

The first doctoral nursing program (PhD Nursing) did not open in Canada until the University of Alberta began enrolling students in January 1991. At that time, three "special case" students (Joan Bottorff, Joy Johnson and Paulette Paul) and one direct admission student (Ginette Rodger) were admitted to the Alberta program. The "special case" programs — with three students at McGill University and three at the University of Alberta — started in 1988. These programs were a direct result of strong lobbying by the nursing profession to ensure that doctoral education in nursing was finally available in Canada.

Marie-Denise Lefèbvre was born in Saint-Benoît, Québec, into a staunch Christian family that already had several members in the Grey Nuns Community. She was admitted to the novitiate at the Mother House of the Grey Nuns of Montreal in 1926. During the latter part of her career, from 1973 to 1981, she was Superior General of the Order. Beginning in 1981, she was assigned to preparing the case of Marguerite d'Youville, the founder of the Order, for canonization, which was realized in 1991. Sister Lefèbvre graduated as a nurse from St. Boniface (Manitoba) Hospital School, then attended the University of Saint Louis, Missouri, for a bachelor of science in nursing. She also held a baccalaureate degree in nursing education from St. Louis University in Missouri and a master of science in nursing education from the Catholic University of America in Washington, D.C.

For 20 years, she was director of the Institut Marguerite d'Youville, a French-language nursing school, which soon developed a baccalaureate program in conjunction with the Université de Montréal. In 1967, this program was integrated with the newly created Faculty of Nursing Science at the University of Montreal. After this integration, the Institut Marguerite d'Youville closed after 33 years, although Sister Lefèbvre remained on faculty at the university. Sister Lefèbvre also worked with the World Health Organization as a member of several of its committees, including one on nursing specialists. She wrote numerous articles, especially in the areas of advancement of nursing science and improvement of teaching methods in nursing.

Among the many awards for her contributions to the education of nurses and to the improvement of care for the ill was a Centennial Medal of Confederation in 1967 from the Government of Canada. In 1984 the government also awarded Sister Lefèbvre the Thérèse Casgrain prize and appointed her to the Order of Canada. Also in 1984, the Canadian Nurses Association presented her with the Jeanne Mance Award, its highest honour. She also holds an honorary doctorate from the University of Moncton and has been recognized by the Nursing departments at Université de Montréal and McGill University for her services to nursing.

— Glennis Zilm

THE CANADIAN FAMILY

There was a time in Canada when an immediate household comprising a married man and woman living with their children or an entire group of kinfolk related by blood, marriage or adoption was synonymous with *family*. This no longer is the case. Even though the family is the fundamental social unit of society, its form and character varies greatly throughout the world. Because Canadian families are made up of Canadian-born descendants of immigrants from many different countries, of recent migrants and of Aboriginal people, family structure is diverse. In addition, a number of changes have taken place — and are still taking place — in Canadian society that are influencing family form. For instance, the women's movement, high cost of living, rising divorce rates, increased personal freedom, growing acceptance of out-of-wedlock births, and increased disclosure of sexual preference are contributing to the evolution of family structure and the resulting diversity in form.

Because of this diversity in family form, a definition of *family* must encompass a broad meaning. Therefore, **family** is defined as two or more people, who may or may not be related by blood, marriage or adoption, bound by strong emotional ties, a sense of belonging and a commitment to live with and care for one another over time. This broad definition covers the wide range of forms the family can take. It includes, for example, a family comprising an unmarried mother and her offspring, a married but childless couple or two gay males and their adopted child. Each of the family forms has its own set of distinctive characteristics which may help or hinder family life. As nurses, we must have an awareness and an understanding of the characteristics of the various family forms so that we can assess, plan and implement care to meet the unique needs of families. The types of family forms that are common in Canada today are outlined in the following pages and summarized in Table 10.1.

The nuclear family remains the predominant family form in Canada.

TYPES OF FAMILY FORMS

NUCLEAR FAMILY

The **nuclear family** consists of a husband and wife with their own or adopted children, who share a residence, divide their labour and cooperate economically (Baker, 1990). This form had traditionally been accepted as the "ideal" family in which the father was the sole provider and the mother was the full-time homemaker. The mother was primarily devoted to supporting her husband in his career and bringing up the children. However, due to increased costs of food, shelter, education and living in general, and to women's desire to pursue their own careers, many married women have made the transition to working outside of the home.

In 1991, 63 percent of women with children under the age of 16 combined a job or a career with raising a family (Ghalam, 1993). This movement created a new family structure called the *dual-career* family. Rapaport and Rapaport define the **dual-career family** as "the type of family in which both heads of the household pursue careers and at the same time maintain a family life together" (1971, 18). In this new family structure the traditional husband–wife roles of provider and homemaker give way to a contemporary relationship of equal power and decision-making along with shared economic and domestic responsibility. The careers of husband and wife are viewed as equally important. Similarly, housekeeping duties and child-rearing are equally divided. While dual-career families enjoy the economic advantages of two incomes, they also face a number of difficulties. For example, there might be competition in relation to career importance as well as conflict and strain in assuming family versus career roles. Women, in particular, sometimes find that it is not easy trying to be a wife, a mother and a career woman, along with maintaining a household. When a child is ill, for example, it is often the mother who must take time off work to provide necessary care. While she fulfills her role as mother, she feels guilty because her work-related tasks are put on hold. Dual-career couples may need support and assistance in establishing a balance in their pursuit of a satisfying family life and fulfilling careers.

Not all nuclear couples have children. Known as the **nuclear-dyad**, this type of family comprises a couple without children. Some married couples choose not to have children; others are childless because of infertility or because their children have grown up and left home. While the nuclear-dyad does not completely fit the definition of nuclear family because of the absence of children, these couples are recognized as families, nonetheless.

The nuclear family still predominates as the most common family form in Canada. However, fewer Canadians are living in nuclear families today than were 20 years ago. At the same time, those living in single-parent families, blended families and cohabiting (common-law) families are gradually becoming more numerous.

EXTENDED FAMILY

The **extended family** is a wider network of two or more related nuclear families, known in everyday language as *relatives* or *kinfolk*. This family unit consists of grandparents, aunts, uncles and cousins, who may live near by or far away from one another. Regardless of proximity, it is a network of relatives who visit or correspond regularly, and who, in good times or bad, give social, emotional, physical and economic support to each other. In some cultures extended families still live together in a single household. In South

Relatives get together for special occasions such as this fiftieth wedding anniversary party.

Asia, for example, often brothers and their nuclear families live with their parents, sharing economic resources and living a collective lifestyle (Assanand, Dias, Richardson and Waxler-Morrison, 1990). Extended family units, with three or more generations living together, also predominate in certain Canadian communities such as the Inuit, Cree, Hutterites and Amish (Ramu, 1989).

SINGLE-PARENT FAMILY

A *single-parent family* refers to a mother or a father living with one or more dependent children. The majority of single-parent families are headed by women. According to Statistics Canada, in 1991, 12.9 percent of all families were single-parent families. Of these, 82 percent were headed by women, a high proportion of whom were divorced or separated. Widowed and never-married mothers made up the balance of female-headed, single-parent families (La Novara, 1993).

Having to assume responsibility as both provider and homemaker, single mothers, in particular, often encounter financial burdens and experience difficulty providing adequate food, housing and child care. Because of their dual role, single parents spend less time with their children than do married parents. They may also feel stress, loneliness in a couples-oriented society and weakened self-esteem. All of these conditions can combine to create a negative influence on the health and well-being of the family as a whole. Single parents often need help and support from their extended families (particularly their parents) and from the communities in which they live in order to succeed as parents and achieve satisfaction in other facets of their lives.

BLENDED FAMILY

The **blended** or **reconstituted family**, also known as the *step-family*, consists of a husband and wife, at least one of whom has been married before. The blended family can include one or more children from a former marriage as well as offspring from the new union, creating a constellation of step-children, step-parents and step-siblings. Also associated with the blended unit is the **binuclear family**, in which children are members of two family households as a result of joint-custody arrangements by their parents following divorce (Bohannan, 1985). Blended families may experience the same kinds of problems faced by nuclear families, particularly if both adults work. In addition, blended families encounter the challenges of integrating family members and establishing satisfying relationships. For example, children do not always accept their step-parents right away. They need time to adjust to new patterns of interaction and authority, which can create stress and disharmony in the family unit.

COHABITING FAMILY

The **cohabiting family** consists of a man and a woman living together without being legally married. Also known as *common-law* relationships, these unions are common among young adults as a prelude or "trial run" to marriage. Cohabiting unions can provide the social, emotional and economic support provided by legal marriages but without the binding commitment of marriage. There is also testimony suggesting that common-law unions are a growing alternative to marriage and remarriage following divorce or death of a spouse. For some Canadians, particularly those who have gone through the emotional trauma and financial burden of divorce, a common-law union may be more desirable than another legal marriage. In 1990, 21 percent of Canadians whose first marriage ended in divorce were living in common-law relationships. Overall, cohabitation doubled in Canada during the 1980s. By 1990, 12 percent of all couples were in common-law relationships, up from six percent in 1981 (Stout, 1991).

GAY OR LESBIAN FAMILY

The **gay** or **lesbian family** is a form of cohabitation in which individuals of the same sex live together, with or without children, and share a sexual relationship (Caudle and Grover, 1992). Even though the nature of homosexuality is becoming more clearly understood and social acceptance of homosexual coupling is increasing, gay and lesbian families still encounter a number of problems. The first is stigmatization. Because of continued homophobia (the strong, irrational fear of homosexuals), lesbian women and gay men may be the subjects of jokes, disparaging remarks and verbal and even physical abuse. Gay men and lesbians may face isolation and lack of support from their families of origin (their parents and siblings) who, for personal, cultural or religious reasons, do not regard homosexuality as an acceptable lifestyle.

A second problem gay and lesbian couples may experience relates to the law. These couples may have difficulty obtaining benefits for one another because the Canadian legal system does not recognize gay and lesbian unions. For example, in Vancouver in 1993, a Supreme Court of Canada decision ruled against a gay man's allegation of discrimination because he was denied paid leave to attend the funeral of his partner's father. The court judgment was based on the legal ground that gay and lesbian couples do not constitute a family under the Canadian Human Rights Act (Vancouver Sun, 1993). However, there is growing acknowledgment of the gay couples' right to receive the same marital benefits as heterosexual couples. Many employers throughout Canada now grant health benefits to same-sex partners if the couple have been living together for two years. In addition, at the time of writing, legislative proposals had been put forth at both the provincial and federal levels to change laws regarding same-sex families.

The law also discriminates against sexual orientation in cases of child custody and adoption, especially for gay men. According to Harry, "in contested custody cases where parents' sexual orientation is an issue, lesbian mothers win in about 15 percent of the cases, with gay fathers winning less frequently" (1983, 225).

Concerns about custody often revolve around unfounded fears that children of gay or lesbian parents will become homosexuals and around the worry that the children will be harassed by their peers (Baker, 1990). Evidence reveals, however, that this is not the case. Parental homosexuality has been shown to have no effect on the sexual identity of children. Children of homosexual parents develop their sexual identities and orientations in the same manner that all children do (Williamson, 1986). Furthermore, Harry found that, while the lives of gay and lesbian parents and their children are not without problems, harassment is uncommon, and manageable when it does occur (1983). It is important for nurses working with gay and lesbian families to realize that homosexuality is a sexual orientation or a lifestyle preference. Sexual orientation is only one aspect of these individuals' lives, and they have the same physical and emotional needs as do all human beings.

COMMUNAL FAMILY

The *communal family* is an intimate network of unrelated adults and their children who make a commitment to live together as one large family unit. Communal families are like extended family systems in that they fulfill similar functions of affection, interdependence, and social, physical

TABLE 10.1 Types of families and their defining features

FAMILY TYPE	DEFINING FEATURES
Nuclear	Husband and wife who are married with biological or adopted children
Dual-career	Nuclear family in which husband and wife pursue active careers, in a relationship of equal power and decision-making, and shared economic and domestic responsibility
Nuclear-dyad	A married couple who are childless because of choice or infertility, or because their children have left home
Extended	Network of relatives of the nuclear family such as grandparents, aunts, uncles, cousins
Single-parent	A mother or father living alone with biological or adopted children
Blended	Husband and wife, one or both of whom were previously married, living with children from previous marriages and/or children from the new union
Cohabiting	Unmarried heterosexual couple living together, with or without children
Gay or Lesbian	A cohabiting couple of the same sex living together, with or without children
Communal	An intimate network of unrelated adults and their children who make a commitment to live together as one large family

and economic support (Scanzoni, 1976). "People choose to belong to communes because of some common attraction, which may vary from a desired geographic location to a strong commitment to a particular ideology of religious doctrine" (Logan and Dawkins, 1986, 421). Control over communal members can be so strong that friendships and relationships outside the group may be difficult or even impossible. Communal families can vary in structure and function. For example, in some communes married couples may retain their nuclear structure, sharing separate dwellings and economic independence, whereas in others, all adults are considered to be married to each other. The children belong to the whole group. Personal possessions are relinquished and economic resources are pooled for use by all.

Although communal living may be seen as a reasonable alternative to the traditional nuclear family, such forms may have negative consequences for their members. For example, decision-making can be very complicated leading to resistance, rivalries and conflicts of interest. Multiple caretaking and sharing of tasks may need ongoing negotiation and clarification of roles. Children, although they may benefit from having various teachers and socializing agents, may suffer from the lack of someone special to care for them, to stand up for them or simply to be there when they are in need. Communal family members may also experience lack of privacy and feel they are constantly under scrutiny, making it hard to resolve problems and difficult relationships (Logan and Dawkins, 1986).

CULTURE AND THE FAMILY

The family has been called society's transmitter of cultural practices and traditions. Traditions, attitudes, values and beliefs are passed down from one generation to the next. Family structure, communication patterns, coping strategies, lifestyles, dietary habits and eating patterns, health practices and behaviours, and religious beliefs are reflected in one's cultural and ethnic background. Nurses must be sensitive to the influence of cultural values and beliefs on the family's personal views of health and family functioning. A nurse's culturally-based health beliefs and values can help or hinder his or her work with families. Nurses must be culturally aware of their own health beliefs and values and avoid imposing these on the patient and family. The influence of culture and ethnicity on health and the implications for nursing care are examined in Chapter 12, Health and Ethnicity.

CONCEPTUAL FRAMEWORKS OF THE FAMILY

Conceptual frameworks are used to guide nursing practice. In family nursing, conceptual frameworks give us a perspective on family life. They also provide a basis for assessing families, interpreting their needs and planning their care. The conceptual frameworks of family that we use in nursing practice come from a variety of disciplines, such as sociology, anthropology, public health and family therapy. Each framework provides a distinct perspective on family life. For instance, the structural-functional framework looks at how family members are arranged and at the relationships between them, whereas the developmental framework looks at the life cycle of the family and the changes that occur as members grow and mature. As much as the frameworks focus on different aspects of family, they also overlap in some of their concepts. For example, concepts such as communication patterns and interaction among members run through all of the frameworks.

Nurses working with families may select a single framework or they may use a combination of concepts from several frameworks to guide their care, depending on their focus of practice. Some nurses prefer a pluralistic approach, in which they use selected concepts from a number of frameworks. This is because they often find that not all aspects of a particular framework explain the relevant phenomena of the families they work with. Three frameworks that are commonly used in family nursing will be described here. These are the *systems*, *structural-functional* and *developmental* frameworks.

FAMILY SYSTEMS FRAMEWORK

The family systems framework was derived from the general systems theory introduced by von Bertalanffy (1968). He defined a system as "a complex of elements in interaction" (1968, 83). While various authors have altered this definition somewhat, "it is generally agreed that a system consists of two or more connected elements which form an organized whole and which interact with each other" (Clemen-Stone, Eigsti and McGuire, 1991, 191). Further, the actions of a system are goal-directed. In order to achieve its goals, the system functions in a dynamic state of adaptive interaction with its environment. In Chapter 13 we note that a number of general conceptual models of nursing are based on systems theory, for example, the Roy and Neuman models. In this section we will discuss the basic concepts of general systems theory as they apply to family.

The family systems framework characterizes the family unit as it relates and interacts with itself and with other units in a larger society. In the systems framework, the family is viewed as a social system comprising a small group of people who share common goals and functions, and who interact and interrelate with each other and their environments as a whole.

The interrelationships among family members are characterized by mutual dependence. Children are dependent on their parents for food, shelter, affection and an education. At the same time, parents may be dependent on their children for personal gratification or the satisfaction gained from watching their sons' and daughters' achievements as they grow and develop. Elderly parents may rely on their adult children for physical and emotional support. The relationships among family members are intertwined in such a way that whatever happens to one member will invariably affect the entire family. For example, when a mother is hospitalized, her husband may have to take time off work to care for their preschool son, placing the family under financial stress. Further, the child will be upset by his mother's absence and may react by wetting his bed and refusing to eat, adding to the new demands on the father's time.

According to family systems theory, a family is made up of members who interrelate as subsystems or hierarchies. Two or more interrelating family members can form *subsystems*, such as the spousal subsystem, the parent-child subsystem or the sibling subsystem. "Any one family member is a part of several subsystems in which the members have different functions and levels of power and influence" (Janosik and Miller, 1979, 7). For example, parents usually hold the power in the family and have substantial influence over their children. The subsystems keep the family organized and provide the capacity to carry out its functions. The family system, in turn, is part of a wider social system which includes, for example, the school, church, community or the country, all of which make up the suprasystem. The *suprasystem* comprises the physical, social and cultural environment with which the family interacts in order to sustain its life, continuity and growth (Friedman, 1992).

Boundaries encompass the family and individual family members, and also the subsystems within it. *Boundaries* are physical demarcations such as the family's property line or a member's bedroom, or abstract entities like rules, norms, attitudes and values which separate families and subsystems from their environments, and which regulate human interaction inside and outside the family. Boundaries filter the flow of inputs from the environment and outputs to it. *Input* refers to the energy, information and resources that the system receives and then processes in order to achieve its goals or outputs. *Output* refers to the energy, information and resources that are released back to the environment. For example, Mary Martin is a community health nurse in Halifax who wants to return to work but who is having difficulty finding child care after school. She brings her concern to the school's Parents' Association, where it is discovered that there are a number of families who would support an after-school care program. For Mary, the *input* was the knowledge of inadequate child care facilities in her community. Her decision to approach the Parents' Association in support of her family's need constituted the *process*. The *output* was the establishment of an after-school care program which met not only the Martins' needs but also the needs of other families in the community. This exchange of energy is crucial to the survival of the system. Boundaries promote equilibrium in the system and allow the exchange of energy with the environment.

Systems are typified by the degree of interaction with their surrounding environment. The family is viewed as an *open system*, because it exchanges energy, resources and information with its environment. As an open system, the family takes in what is needed from the environment for its own survival and growth, and, in turn, gives back energy, information and materials to support the environment's more global needs.

An important element in the functioning of family systems is *feedback*. Janosik and Green describe feedback

Grandparents look forward to visits with their grandchildren.

as "a continuous process of input and output exchanges between families and the community that surrounds them" (1992, 14). An example of feedback might be neighbours reacting negatively to heavy metal band practices next door. Feedback fosters family functioning and stability by alerting the family to behaviours that comply with or deviate from community norms. It is an important process that helps a family identify its strengths and evaluate how well it is achieving its goals. Feedback may be informal, such as a neighbour's reaction to loud music, or it may be formal, such as a phone call to parents from the school, for example, reporting that their son's excessive talking disrupts class activities. Both of these are examples of negative feedback, but feedback can be positive as well. Positive feedback tells the family to carry on with its existing standards and patterns of behaviour. Negative feedback indicates to the family that it needs to modify its current behaviours. The family can adapt by accepting or rejecting the incoming feedback, or by modifying it to suit its particular needs.

While the family is an open system, the degree of openness varies according to the nature of its boundaries. Open families, for example, invite people into their home, encourage their children to bring friends in and interact freely with neighbours. These families welcome change as a normal process in life, and reach out to the larger community for support in solving their problems and maintaining their well-being. Closed families, on the other hand, resist change. They believe that people are not trustworthy and that interactions and relationships must be kept under strict control. Closed families might keep fences around their property and lock their gate. They avoid discussing matters with people outside their immediate family. Families who keep highly rigid boundaries are often isolated and deprived of necessary information and resources required for optimal growth and well-being (Friedman, 1992).

Nurses can use concepts from the family systems framework to assess family functioning and determine family needs. Because the systems framework considers the family as a whole, it provides the basis for a holistic approach to nursing practice. Functional and dysfunctional patterns of behaviour are regarded as the result of systems functioning as opposed to individual member functioning. Family structure, functions and processes are examined for adaptive or maladaptive behaviours within families. Blame is shifted away from individual members, while attention is centred on the family system and how it must change in order to function successfully.

STRUCTURAL-FUNCTIONAL FRAMEWORK

The structural-functional framework was developed by anthropologists and sociologists, who viewed the family as a social system interacting with other social systems such as the school or the health care system (Duvall, 1977). The essence of this framework is family structure and function. *Family structure* refers to the way a family is organized. It identifies how family members are arranged and how they relate to each other as a unit.

Friedman (1992) identifies four basic components of family structure:

1. role structure
2. value systems
3. communication patterns
4. power hierarchy.

The first component, family *role structure*, defines the behaviours expected of members in designated positions. For example, the oldest child in the family has expectations placed upon him or her, by virtue of being the first born. The oldest child might be the one who carries the money, buys the tickets and treats, and looks out for the younger siblings when they all go to a Sunday afternoon movie. Roles are important in family functioning because it is through the execution of family roles that family functions are fulfilled.

The second component of family structure is the value system. Every family creates its own system of values primarily from its culture and secondarily from the society in which it lives. *Values* are the ideas, attitudes and beliefs about the worth of an entity that bind together the members of a family in a common culture (Parad and Caplan, 1965. Cited in Friedman, 1992, 240). Family values serve as guides to judge behaviour and develop norms and rules for conduct. For example, families who believe in self-responsibility for problem solving actively seek out information and necessary resources to deal with their problems. On the other hand, families who believe in fate might accept and cope with problems as "God's will." Family values are affected by such variables as religion, spiritual beliefs, social class, age and developmental stages of family members. A family's value system is not static. Rather, it is a dynamic system that evolves over time as the family and its members interact with different subcultures, adjust to changes in society or respond to particular needs in their lives. For example, a family belonging to the Jehovah's Witnesses faith, which prohibits blood transfusions, might grant permission for a life-saving blood transfusion if their child sustained a near-fatal injury in an accident.

Values are important in the context of family structure because a family's attitudes and beliefs affect the behaviour of family members. Thus, it is important for nurses to identify a family's value system in order to understand the behaviours of family members. As nurses, we must also be aware of our own value system. Differences in values between the nurse and the family can interfere with the nurse–family relationship which ultimately will affect the care a family receives (Friedman, 1992; Ross and Cobb, 1990).

Communication patterns and processes are key components in family structure. **Communication** is the process by which individuals transmit information to one another through verbal and nonverbal messages or cues. The meaning of these messages is influenced by the roles and value systems of the members. Communication patterns directly influence family interactions and family functioning. When messages among members are clearly conveyed and understood, the family communication patterns are considered to be functional. Alternately, communication patterns are dysfunctional when messages are ambiguous or blocked, or when there is no communication among family members at all.

Power hierarchy, the fourth component of family structure, is defined as the actual or potential ability of individual members to control, influence or change the behaviour of other family members (Friedman, 1992). The power structure of a family determines who makes the decisions and who has the most influence in the family. In other words, it defines the authority figure and the "pecking order" of family members. **Authority** is the status attributed to individuals or groups giving them the power and right to command and be obeyed. In the family, authority is often vested in a particular member on the basis of family and cultural values and social factors. For example, in traditional mid-European families, the father is usually the authority figure who makes decisions unilaterally and holds firm control on family behaviour. This highly patriarchal family structure is becoming less common in Canada, but in many nuclear families it is still the husband or male partner, who, as head of the family, holds the major decision-making power.

However, with changing social influences, we are also finding a more egalitarian distribution of power in Canadian families. Power and decision making are often shared jointly by parents, with the participation of family members. The power structure is important for family functioning because it affects communication patterns and interactions inside as well as outside of the family unit. That is to say, families who interact openly and freely among themselves are more apt to interact in the same manner with other social institutions or groups, for instance, other families, the church or the neighbourhood.

Family functions are those activities a family performs in order to meet the needs of both individual family members and society as a whole. Friedman (1992) has identified five basic family functions:

1. Affective function: for meeting the psychological needs of family members for affection and understanding.
2. Socializing and social placement function: primarily for teaching children how to function, making them productive members of society; and conferring status on family members, that is, passing on values, traditions and social class privileges.
3. Reproduction function: for insuring family continuity over the generations and producing new members for society.
4. Economic function: for providing sufficient economic resources and allocating them effectively.
5. Health care function: for providing physical necessities, such as food, clothing, shelter, health care.

The structural-functional framework provides a valuable guide for assessing families because it analyzes the internal and external forces which influence individual members as well as the family as a whole. The nurse in a medical setting, for instance, can use the structural-functional approach to assess the impact of illness on family functioning. She or he could evaluate how illness of the husband/father, which required a lengthy hospital stay, would affect the family's economic resources and the role of the wife/mother. Would she have to obtain employment outside the home to maintain the family financially and, if so, what assistance would she need for child care? How is the family adjusting to the father's illness? Does it continue to function effectively, or is it experiencing stress? Answers to questions such as these would determine the nursing interventions, for example, support and mobilization of resources, that this family may require to meet its needs.

FAMILY DEVELOPMENTAL FRAMEWORK

The developmental framework examines the family as it continues over time, following the chronological and sequential changes in growth, development and dissolution or decline throughout the entire life cycle of the family (Duvall, 1977). This framework describes the changes that occur in family roles and relationships as individual members grow

and mature, moving from one life stage to the next. Duvall developed an eight-stage model of the family life cycle, each stage of which has a set of distinctive developmental tasks.

The family developmental tasks refer to the growth responsibilities that must be accomplished by a family during each stage of its development in order to fulfill its biologic function, its cultural obligations and its own aspirations and values (Duvall, 1977). Family developmental tasks parallel individual developmental tasks, such as Erikson's stages of emotional development (Erikson, 1963). Like individual developmental tasks, family developmental tasks must be successfully achieved in each stage before proceeding to the next. Further, family members must achieve both individual and family developmental tasks in order to function effectively as a family unit. Failure to achieve a developmental task leads to unhappiness in the family, social disapproval and difficulty accomplishing later developmental tasks (Duvall, 1977). Duvall's family life cycle and developmental tasks are outlined in Table 10.2. In this model, Duvall uses the age and school placement of the oldest child to define life-cycle stages.

The developmental framework is a very useful guide for assessing families and determining their health needs. The common, general features of family life for the different stages of the life cycle provide a basis for knowing what to expect. These common features, however, are based on the premise of the normal nuclear childbearing family. As we discussed earlier, not all families fit into these typical family life-cycle stages (Friedman, 1992). For example, the never-married single-parent family begins with Stage 2, the early childbearing stage. Parental adaptation includes the performance of both maternal and paternal roles, while providing a healthy environment for family growth and development. Family life-cycle patterns are altered for childless couples, single-parent families and reconstituted families. Nurses working with these families need to be aware of the modifications in the respective family life cycles in order to make accurate assessments of their health needs.

FAMILY HEALTH

WHAT IS FAMILY HEALTH?

Family health can be defined from the perspective of a number of theories and frameworks dealing with the family. For example, if we were to use the developmental framework as a perspective, which identifies family developmental tasks that must be accomplished according to the family life-cycle, family health would be defined as the ability of family members and the family as a whole to achieve stage-specific developmental tasks. Or, if we subscribed to Roy's (1984) nursing model, family health would be viewed as a state and a process of being or becoming an integrated and whole family system (Loveland-Cherry, 1989).

TABLE 10.2 Family life cycle and developmental tasks

FAMILY STAGE	TIME PERIOD	DEVELOPMENTAL TASKS
1. Married couple	Marriage to birth of first child	Establishing a mutually satisfying marriage Adjusting to the kin network Family planning
2. Childbearing	Birth of oldest child to 30 months of age	Adjusting to parenthood Maintaining a satisfying home Facilitating infant's developmental tasks
3. Preschool-age	Oldest child is 2 to 5 years of age	Promoting growth and nurturing children Integrating new children Learning to separate from children Coping with energy depletion and lack of privacy as parents
4. School-age	Oldest child is 6 to 13 years of age	Socializing children and promoting educational achievement Fitting into the community of school-age families Maintaining a satisfying marriage
5. Teenage	Oldest child is 13 to 20 years of age	Balancing teenage freedom with responsibility Establishing postparental interests
6. Launching	From time first child leaves home to time last child leaves home	Releasing children as young adults Extending the family upon marriage of children Developing postparental interests Assisting aging and ill parents
7. Middle-age	From time last child leaves home to retirement	Rebuilding marital relationship Enhancing leisure activities Maintaining a healthy environment Maintaining family ties with older and younger generations
8. Aging	Retirement to death	Maintaining satisfying housing Adjusting to retirement, reduced income, aging, loneliness, death

SOURCES: Duvall, 1977; Friedman, 1986; Janosik and Green, 1992.

In this book, our perspective on family health is reflected in the World Health Organization's (1984a) definition of health. You will recall from Chapter 2 that health is defined as the extent to which an individual or group is able to realize aspirations, to satisfy needs and to change or cope with the environment (WHO, 1984a). The family, as society's most basic unit, provides the physical, cultural, spiritual, psychological and social foundation for the health and well-being of individual members. Since health and illness behaviours are primarily learned and, for the most part, performed within the family, the family is both a resource and an environment for the health and well-being of individual members. Therefore, family health is:

> . . . a resource for everyday life, not an object of living. It is a positive concept, emphasizing social and personal resources, as well as physical capabilities. Family health is the extent to which a family and its members are able to realize aspirations, to satisfy needs and to change or cope with the environment (adapted from WHO, 1984a).

Family health, like health in general, is not static in nature. It is a dynamic process in which families create adaptive patterns of interaction with each other and with an ever-changing physical and social environment. This is done in order to manage stress, survive crisis, handle conflict and organize themselves so as to satisfy their needs and achieve their goals. Family health is an enabling process with a focus on the quality of life as opposed to correcting disease or infirmity. For example, a family who has effectively adapted its lifestyle around nurturing a child with diabetes may not see itself as having a health problem — even though others might view it that way because of the child's disease. Family health and wellness is gauged not by the presence or absence of illness in members; rather, it is measured by the amount of love and joy members share, and on collective feelings of purpose, growth, unity and control over lifestyle and living conditions.

DETERMINANTS OF FAMILY HEALTH

Wellness and illness do not happen on their own. An individual's health is influenced by sociological and environmental factors, as well as health-promoting and health-protecting beliefs and practices of his or her family. Social and environmental factors are instrumental in family health because they impact on the family's economic resources and housing and on family dynamics. **Family dynamics** are the interrelationships among members, namely their roles, relationships and communication patterns.

Social factors play a large role in family health. Families in which parents are well educated and have ample financial resources to afford adequate housing, transportation and good nutrition tend to practise healthier lifestyles. These families are often located towards the wellness end of the wellness-illness continuum. On the other hand, families who live in poverty place lower priority on healthy lifestyles. Because of unemployment or low-paying jobs, parents often lack the resources for adequate housing, nutrition and family care. They are therefore at risk for location at the illness end of the continuum (RNABC, 1992).

The family environment influences the health of family members. Danielson, Hamel-Bissell and Winstead-Fry (1993) reviewed a number of studies dealing with family influences on individual health and illness behaviours. They found that a family's ethnic background, social class and satisfaction with life influenced nutritional status and health-promoting practices. For example, obesity in children was attributed to family nutrition and eating patterns. Another study showed that children as young as four years of age understood health behaviours and practised them in their lives. Furthermore, parents who, as children, were taught and encouraged to engage in self-care practices were especially effective in bringing up children who actively

promoted their own health. Whether or not adolescents engaged in negative behaviours such as smoking cigarettes or marijuana and drinking alcohol was related to the family's ability to solve problems. Research indicated that "excessive demands within the family may have caused stress for the adolescent and could be ameliorated if the adolescent and family could communicate and resolve conflicts and differences" (1993, 12). It is interesting to note that adolescent peer support did not prevent these negative behaviours nor did complaining about family members to friends or other adults. The important factor was the ability of the adolescent and his or her family to communicate and resolve differences in a satisfying manner (Danielson, Hamel-Bissell and Winstead-Fry, 1993).

Family values also influence health protecting practices and use of health care services. For example, whether an infant is immunized or taken to the community health clinic for health assessments depends on the parent's beliefs and attitudes regarding use of health care services.

The health status of family members and the family mutually influence one another. Illness of one member affects the whole family and its interactions, while the family in turn affects the health status and course of illness of its members (Friedman, 1992). The following case depicts this relationship.

Irfan Virani is a 28-year-old self-employed truck driver who sustains traumatic injury including loss of a leg in an accident. Irfan's family will play a large part in his healing and return to health, and in turn, his recovery will influence the health of the whole family. The family can help Irfan directly by giving care and providing support, or indirectly by participating with health care professionals in decisions regarding treatment and care. For example, Irfan's healing process requires prolonged convalescence. In collaboration with the health care team, Irfan and his wife, Mina, decide that he will convalesce at home. Mina will be taught necessary physical care and, in addition, will drive Irfan for daily physiotherapy. Clearly, this father's injury has affected the whole family. In order to care for Irfan, Mina has to make adjustments in family schedules and routines. The children's swimming lessons are put on hold and alternative transportation is arranged to get the children to and from their weekly religion classes. The family is now without a regular income because Irfan was the sole wage earner. Mina finds little time to spend with her children and even less time for herself, which, when combined with the financial burden of lost income, leaves her feeling tired and depressed.

How well this family can support Irfan's recovery and at the same time facilitate the growth and well-being of its members will depend on its coping strategies and its strengths and capabilities as a unit. We will follow Irfan and Mina in the next section to see how they mobilize their strengths to cope with this health challenge.

CRITERIA FOR JUDGING FAMILY HEALTH

Research on families and family behaviour points to a number of similarities in how healthy families maintain their health and cope with life's problems. Spradley (1990) outlines six important characteristics exhibited by healthy families:

1. There is a facilitative process of interaction among family members.
2. They enhance individual member development.
3. Their role relationships are structured effectively.
4. They actively attempt to cope with problems.
5. They have a healthy home environment and lifestyle.
6. They establish regular links with the broader community.

These characteristics of healthy families will be described more fully.

Facilitative process of interaction In healthy families, communication is open and supportive. Ideas, feelings and concerns are shared with one another on a regular basis, through a variety of forms. Verbal communication is often used — healthy families telephone or write to one another when they are separated. These families also use nonverbal techniques in an effective manner to transmit feelings, thoughts, love and affection or show consideration for each other. For example, a mother smiles warmly and gives her son a hug when he achieves an A in mathematics. On the other hand, she frowns in disapproval when he asks to play out on the street with friends. Spradley maintains that in healthy families, members are sensitive to each other. They watch for cues and confirm messages so as to ensure understanding. These families also recognize and resolve conflicts and problems as they arise. Members learn to share and to work cooperatively with each other in meeting individual and family needs.

Open and facilitative patterns of interaction enable families to meet their needs and achieve their goals. Families must communicate in order to show affection and acceptance, to promote identity and affiliation and to guide behaviour through socialization and social controls. Families who communicate openly and effectively with each other will also be better prepared to communicate outside themselves. That is, they will be better able to interact with other families and groups, or with society as a whole (Spradley, 1990).

Enhancement of individual development Healthy families are responsive to the needs of individual members and provide the freedom and support that is necessary to foster the growth of each member. In the case of Irfan Virani, the truck driver who lost his leg in an accident, family responsiveness and support would be shown through efforts to aid his emotional and physical adjustments and by encouraging him to move forward with a new career opportunity.

The healthy family understands and promotes the growth and development needs of children. This kind of family provides opportunities for increasing freedom and autonomy and permits developing differences in opinions and lifestyles. It shows unconditional love, affection and approval, as well as respect for the unique rights of each member. Families vary in how they promote the development of individual members, depending on their cultural orientation. For example, the Virani family, being Indo-Canadian, may express autonomy differently than an Italian-Canadian family would. Nonetheless, each family facilitates freedom and autonomy of its members in some way (Spradley, 1990).

Effective structuring of role relationships Healthy families are adaptive and flexible. That is, they can alter their roles and tasks to meet changing needs over time. The needs of families change according to their life-cycle stages or because of forces such as loss of a job, illness or sudden death of a member. Healthy families are able to adapt their roles and tasks in response to forces beyond their control. The Virani family, for example, are adjusting to the effects of Irfan's accident by changing their roles and tasks. Mina obtained a job outside the home, while Irfan took on more of the household and child-care duties. This family shows flexibility and the ability to restructure its roles and relationships in order to meet the demands of their situation.

In healthy families, roles and tasks are also altered to fit the developmental needs of members. For example, children are given increasing responsibility and assigned more complex household tasks as they become more mature. Parents may adapt the rules of conduct, giving the children more freedom as they learn to manage their own behaviour in a positive, constructive manner.

Effective coping with problems Families who try to solve their problems in an effective, creative manner are considered to be healthy. Not only do these families take responsibility for problem solving, but also they ensure mutual involvement of family members in identifying problems and making decisions (deChesnay, 1986). Healthy families try to find solutions and overcome their problems by themselves; however, they may seek outside help if necessary. Using the Virani family as an example once again, Irfan and Mina dealt with their financial difficulty by deciding that Mina would get a job until Irfan was established in a new occupation. Irfan enrolled in evening courses at the community college so that he was free to care for the children after school. Because money was still a problem, they decided to move into a suite in Irfan's parent's home, while renting out their own house in order to keep up mortgage payments.

Healthy home environment and lifestyle

Healthy families maintain a safe, healthy home environment and lifestyle. For example, a young childbearing family removes potential hazards such as sharp objects or toxic solutions from the reach of infants and toddlers. These families also ensure good hygiene and cleanliness in order to reduce infection and the spread of disease. Healthy families foster a healthy family lifestyle. They advocate a nutritious diet along with adequate rest, exercise and relaxation. The emotional environment of a healthy family is positive and supportive, and one in which members feel welcome and accepted. Members share a strong sense of values, which may or may not be coupled with a religious orientation (Spradley 1990). The home environment provides a strong influence on health practices and lifestyles of individuals. It is not unusual for young adults to continue eating nutritiously and living healthy lifestyles after they leave home.

Maintain links with the broader community

Families do not live in isolation but are members of a suprasystem — the neighbourhood in which they live, the school their children attend, the church they choose for religious affiliation and the larger community from which they derive services. Healthy families maintain regular, open ties with the broader community. They are active participants in community groups, such as the school's parents' association, the church choir or the local Boy Scouts group. They select external resources most suited to the family's needs. For example, a family who recognizes their daughter's talent in playing the saxophone might join the local Youth Band, in which one of the parents might serve as secretary-treasurer.

It is not unusual for healthy families to assume leadership positions in the community groups they join. Healthy families keep themselves informed of events in the world around them. They attempt to know and understand current social, economic and political issues that impact on their lives. As a result, healthy families possess a wide range of options and a variety of resources that are available to them for meeting their needs (Spradley, 1990).

FAMILY STRESS AND ILLNESS

All families face a certain degree of stress as they strive to meet their needs for every-day living and cope with changes in their physical and social environments. Some stress-producing events, such as loud music or traffic noise, may be mild and even go unnoticed, whereas others, for example, illness in the family, divorce or death of a family member, may be devastating. The family's perception of the stressful event, the availability of resources and its coping abilities determine the degree of stress a family actually experiences. When families cannot resolve stressful events because of inadequate coping abilities or lack of appropriate resources they experience crisis.

FAMILY STRESS AND CRISIS

Family stress is defined as a state of imbalance in the family, or as Boss puts it, "an upset in the steady state of the family. . . anything that . . . causes uneasiness or pressure on the family system" (1987, 695). Life events or demands that impact on the family and disturb the family's equilibrium are called *family stressors*. Family stressors may emerge from within the family system itself or from external sources.

Internal family stressors originate from individual members or from relationships between and among family members. The developmental transition of children from school-age to adolescence is an example of an internal stressor. This transition imposes a change on all other family members, particularly the parents who must now adjust their control over the adolescent as they allow increasing freedom and responsibility so as to foster individual growth and development. Other examples of internal stressors include financial pressures when a parent becomes unemployed, birth of a baby with a congenital defect, children leaving home, family adjustments in newly blended families, arguments between family members or illness of a family member.

External family stressors originate outside of the family. They involve situations such as conflicts at work, disagreements with neighbours or friends and social stressors such as racism or prejudice.

A stressor produces tension — a response in the family which signals the need for change. "Stress emerges when this tension is not reduced or brought within manageable limits" (Danielson, Hamel-Bissell and Winstead-Fry, 1993, 30). The amount of stress varies, depending on the family's perception of the stressor, the resources and capabilities of the family to handle stress, and the physical and psychological well-being of individual members at the onset of the stress-producing event. Families respond to stress in the same way that individuals do. That is, when the stressor is perceived as an unpleasant or hazardous event that creates hardships, the family experiences *distress*. An example of distress might be the changes required in family functioning when the mother is absent from the home for a few days because of travel responsibilities associated with her work. Events that are perceived as pleasant bring *eustress*, or good stress, to the family. For example, even though the birth of a baby is a joyous occasion for most families, there is a certain amount of stress brought about by the challenges of integrating this new person into the family unit.

The family's ability to resolve stress depends on its strengths, or resources for managing a stressor. Crucial resources include economic stability, family cohesiveness, flexibility, hardiness, shared spiritual beliefs, open communication, traditions, family routines, patterns of problem solving and coping strategies. Family problem solving refers to the process of organizing a stressor into manageable parts, identifying alternative courses of action and initiating steps to resolve the issues. Family coping refers to the strategies and behaviours designed to maintain or strengthen the family as a whole, to maintain emotional stability and well-being of members, to use family and community resources and to resolve the hardships created by the stressor. The goal of family adaptation to stress is to manage the stressor without creating major or lasting changes in the family's established patterns of functioning (Danielson, Hamel-Bissell and Winstead-Fry, 1993).

Effective family adaptation to a stressor is exemplified by the case of Sara, a single parent who has lost her evening babysitter. This is particularly problematic because Sara, who is a waitress, works morning and evening shifts. She deals with this situation by inviting a cousin, who is a college student, to live with her in exchange for evening babysitting. This arrangement proves effective because it causes minimal disruption to the family's usual routines.

In many situations, families are able to respond to stressors with minimal adjustments in the family unit. Some stressors, however, such as loss of family home and belongings by fire, create numerous problems that demand significant change. Families in these situations often face difficulty resolving the stressor. Stress that is unresolved progresses to crisis. *Family crisis* is defined as a state of disorganization in the family unit (Danielson, Hamel-Bissell and Winstead-Fry, 1993).

Stressors such as loss of a family home or sudden death of a family member move quickly into crisis because families do not have enough time to mobilize their adaptive resources. Emotional turmoil and disorganization quickly follow and, as a result, the family's usual approaches to problem solving and decision making may not be effective. Boss (1987) states that when families can no longer cope, they exhibit the following characteristics:

1. they cannot perform their customary roles
2. they are unable to maintain their structural boundaries
3. they become immobilized as a system.

Danielson, Hamel-Bissell and Winstead-Fry state that crisis signals family disorganization and a demand for changes in patterns of family functioning in order to restore stability, order and a sense of coherence and well-being. The family's move to begin changes in its patterns of functioning indicates the start of family adaptation to the crisis (1993). When the crisis is resolved, families may not necessarily return to their pre-crisis level of functioning. Some, having been weakened from the experience, will function below their pre-crisis state, whereas others, having developed strengths because of it, will function at a higher level (Boss, 1987).

IMPACT OF ILLNESS ON THE FAMILY

Illness in the family is a stressful event, which may lead to a crisis if the family is not able to adjust its coping strategies with ease. When a family member is ill the total family unit is affected.

If the ill person is the breadwinner, there is a natural concern about the loss of ability to maintain financial responsibility for the family. Both patient and family may worry about how long the patient will be unable to work and the using up of sick leave from the place of employment. There may be additional concern over the costs of illness, such as medications, equipment, medical supplies and surcharges for diagnostic and medical services. The head of the household may not be in a position to make decisions about family matters while ill. Someone else may have to take over the responsibility for this.

When the single mother is sick, not only does the family encounter financial worry but household routines and child care are also disrupted. Other family members must take over the shopping, the planning and cooking of meals, the washing and the ironing in addition to looking after the children. Relatives are often thousands of miles away, and the family may have to rely on friends or homemaker services to provide help.

There is also much concern when an older member of the family is ill. It may be the first member of the household to be seriously ill and the family is reminded of the fragility of human life. There may be additional worries over who will care for the patient, and again the costs, particularly of prolonged illness, may be a matter of considerable concern.

When one of the children is sick, parents are usually very anxious. They may feel guilty of being in some way responsible for the child's illness. Often they feel helpless, and their anxiety and feelings of helplessness may be expressed in hostility and criticism directed towards those who are caring for the child. Hospitals today permit open visiting on children's wards and encourage parents to share in the care of their children. If nurses understand some of the reasons behind the parents' behaviour and that of family members, and also realize that their own feelings about this behaviour are normal, they are better able to accept hostility and criticism without showing anger and hostility in return.

Admission to hospital has many implications for the patient and for their families. While at home, responsibility for their care probably fell to other family members. After entering a hospital, the responsibility for care is transferred from the family to hospital personnel. This transfer of responsibility often produces emotions of mixed relief and guilt on the part of the family. They feel relief because trained people will now provide professional care, and perhaps guilt because they think the patient would be happier at home or that they have passed on responsibilities that they should be accepting as a family. These feelings are sometimes expressed verbally to hospital personnel or they may be expressed in activities such as bringing food to the patient or by criticizing the personnel and the institution. If the nurse recognizes the needs of family members and solicits their help in appropriate areas of patient care, such as assisting the patient to eat, the family will feel more comfortable and will be better able to assist in the patient's healing.

NURSING CARE OF THE FAMILY

Nurses care for families in almost every area of nursing practice. This may be in hospitals, extended care agencies, old age homes, hospices, clinics and doctor's offices; and in the workplace, the home and the community. Regardless of where it is practised, nursing of families focusses on involving families in health care and on helping families to promote, protect or restore their family health. Various terms are used to describe nursing care of the family. Some of these are *family-centred nursing* (Wright and Leahey, 1984), *family-focussed nursing* (Janosik and Miller, 1980), *family interviewing* (Wright and Leahey, 1984), *family nursing* (Wright and Leahey, 1990; Gilliss, 1991; Friedman, 1992), *family systems nursing* (Wright and Leahey, 1990) and *nursing of families* (Feetham, Meister, Bell and Gilliss, 1993; Wright and Leahey, 1994).

TYPES OF NURSING PRACTICE WITH FAMILIES

According to Friedman (1992), there are three types of family nursing practice. These are conceptualized as *family as context, family as sum of its parts* and *family as patient* (see Figure 10.1).

Family as Context

In the first type of nursing practice with families, the family is conceptualized as the social environment or context for the individual. The nurse is concerned primarily with the needs of the individual family member. The family, as the patient's primary social group, can act as either a stressor or a resource to the patient. For example, in one family, parents taught their adolescent son the dangers of using drugs and alcohol and discouraged him from using these substances. Yet, they openly related stories of their own social use of marijuana. When the son was discovered to be using marijuana, he argued that it was O.K. because his parents used the substance, too. In this case, the family, specifically the behaviour of the parents, is initially the stressor. But, the family can then become a resource, a source of support, if the parents participate in a drug rehabilitation program with their son. Many nursing theories and most of the nursing specialties view the family as a crucial social environment and a primary resource for the patient (Friedman, 1992). Pediatric nursing is one specialty that ". . . considers and treats the child in the context of the family and recognizes the family as the primary and continuing provider of care for the child" (Friedman, 1992, 22).

Family as Sum of its Members

In the second type of nursing practice with families, the family is viewed as the sum of the individual family members. As such, "care is made available to or provided for all of the family members" (Friedman, 1992, 22). This type of nursing might be carried out in an intensive care unit where the nurse is concerned about the response of family members to their father's heart attack. The family's coping strategies and care-giving abilities in addition to the father's needs become the focus of assessment and planning for optimal care of the father once he goes home.

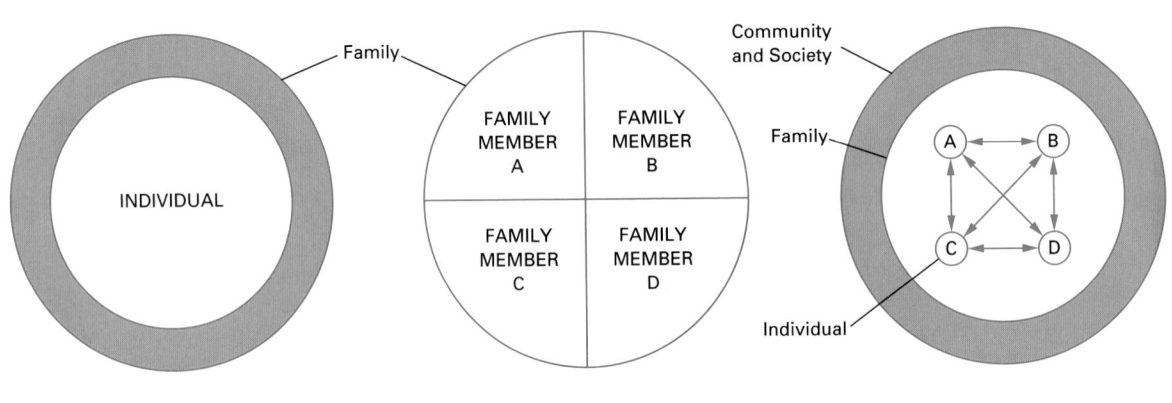

FIGURE 10.1 Types of nursing practice with families

SOURCES: Adapted from Friedman, 1992; Wright and Leahey, 1990.

I'm a staff nurse at the British Columbia Children's Hospital. During the course of a day at my job, I interact with many different people, employ a wide range of nursing skills and enjoy the rewards of "hands-on" care. In this tertiary care hospital, children come to our neurosurgical unit from all over the province, with a wide variety of diagnoses such as head injury, seizure disorders, non-accidental trauma, spina bifida (a tumour caused by a defect in the walls of the spinal canal resulting in a protrusion of the membranes of the spinal cord) and brain tumours. Frequently, they have already been seen or treated in a community hospital and come to Children's Hospital for more specialized care.

A typical shift on our unit begins at 0700 or 1900 hours and lasts 12 hours. Each nurse is assigned three to five clients, depending on the complexity of each child's care. After studying my assignment for the shift and participating in a detailed nursing report, I spend about 15 minutes assessing each client's condition briefly while taking vital signs. Pouring and administering medications is followed by breakfast and morning care. Our clients range in age from birth to 17 years and within this span, development varies from severely delayed to normal. The task of feeding four infants at once can be overwhelming! On the other hand, it is much easier to bathe an infant than to convince a toddler that she needs a bath, or to manoeuvre a comatose teenager into a Century tub.

It is a particular challenge to meet children's nutritional needs. Hospital food may be unfamiliar or unap-pealing to them. We keep a large stock of popsicles, ice cream, yogurt, pudding and juice and we also encourage parents to bring favourite treats from home. During the day, I do ongoing assessment of nutritional and fluid intake, seizure activity, intravenous sites and rates, dressings, level of consciousness, as well as arranging school and playtimes. Probably the hospitalized child's greatest need is for love and security. To this end, the hospital actively promotes family-centred care. Parents and siblings are a constant presence on the ward. Because of this, I do a lot of teaching and a lot of listening.

This large teaching hospital attracts specialists and students from around the world. As a staff nurse, it is my job to facilitate their work while acting as an advocate for the client and family. I make decisions about when to contact the physician about the client's condition and which physician to contact. I ensure that orders are carried out safely and on time. I intervene when the family is overstressed from too many visitors or is attempting to cope with a catastrophic diagnosis. As the family nurse, I also coordinate the activities of physiotherapists, the Child Life Department, social services and pastoral care.

I see many sick children during a day. The rewarding part of my job is watching so many of them heal so quickly. Most children don't lie in bed for long. They are in a hurry to get out of bed and get on with the business of growing.

— Anne Gasson, BA, RN,
Staff Nurse, B.C. Children's Hospital

Community health nurses also practice this second type of family nursing but a distinction has to be made in their target of practice. In community health nursing, the target of practice is health of a community. Community health nurses attempt to enhance and maintain the health of the community by providing care to families. In the community health setting, the nurse would still be attentive to the health needs of the family but the focus would be on common community problems that are relevant to the particular family. For example, in caring for a young childbearing family, the community health nurse would be concerned with such aspects as immunizations and family planning along with the unique health needs of the family (Friedman, 1992).

Family as Patient

The third type of nursing care with families is called *family systems nursing*. Family systems nursing views the whole family as a unit of care, such that the family *is* the patient.

"Family systems nursing is the integration of nursing, systems, cybernetic and family therapy theories" (Wright and Leahey, 1990, 149). The focus of assessment and care is on family interactions and relationships, and on the reciprocity between family functioning and health and illness. The impact of illness on the family and the influence of family interaction on health, illness and healing are primary factors considered in plans for care. In family systems nursing, the nurse concentrates on the family system and individual systems simultaneously, and may also include the interaction of the community and society. Wright and Leahey offer a clear example of the nurse's involvement at all systems levels. They state:

> … if the presenting problem is electrolyte imbalance, then the primary unit of treatment would be the individual patient with attention to the cellular level. If the presenting concern is a husband's understanding of the diabetic regimen, then the primary unit of treatment would be the family for health teaching about diet, exercise and insulin. If the patient is a

school-age child, then the primary unit of treatment might also include, in addition to the family, the community (i.e., school) because this is where the child spends a large majority of time (1990, 150).

The type of family care the nurse chooses to practise depends largely on the clinical setting, the context of the health challenge and on his or her expertise as a practitioner. For instance, when the primary focus of care is the illness or health challenge of a family member as may occur in emergency rooms, intensive care units or medical-surgical areas, the conceptualization of family as context would be the appropriate choice for practice. This type of nursing with families is typically used by nurse generalists at the baccalaureate level. Wright and Leahey prefer the term *nursing of families* to describe this level of practice (1994). On the other hand, when the focus of care is the interaction and reciprocity of family members, family systems nursing would be more suitable. For example, family systems nursing might be used in helping a family resolve problems created by the pregnancy of an unwed adolescent daughter. According to Wright and Leahey (1994), family systems nursing requires specialization at the graduate (master's or doctoral) level.

As a beginning graduate you will need interviewing theory and skills in order to work with families. The communication skills and interviewing techniques that you will need for family interviewing are outlined in Chapter 16. Here, we will outline a family assessment model and discuss nursing interventions for enabling families to promote their health and cope with stress and crisis in their lives.

FAMILY ASSESSMENT

There are several assessment frameworks that can be used for assessing family health and well-being. Many combine family theory and nursing conceptual frameworks in order to identify the unique focus of family health in relation to nursing practice. Here we will present one such framework — The Calgary Family Assessment Model (CFAM).

THE CALGARY FAMILY ASSESSMENT MODEL

The Calgary Family Assessment Model, developed by Lorraine Wright and Maureen Leahey, is an integrated conceptual framework which combines concepts from nursing and family therapy to provide a clear, systematic model for assessment. The model, which was originally adapted from the assessment model produced at the Family Therapy Program, University of Calgary, places emphasis on a method of continuous family assessment rather than on family diagnosis. As such, it focusses on the use of an open-ended and changing problem list rather than a finite schema of family classification (Tomm and Sanders, 1983).

The CFAM is a multidimensional model which incorporates structural, functional and developmental theory and is based on a systems–cybernetics–communication–change theory foundation. Individuals are viewed as bio–psycho–social–spiritual beings where the person as a whole is seen to be greater than and different from the sum of its parts.

Five predominant systems concepts are used in the CFAM. These are:

- A family system is part of a larger subsystem and is also composed of many subsystems.
- The family as a whole is greater than the sum of its parts.
- A change in one family member affects all family members.
- The family is able to create a balance between change and stability.
- Family members' behaviours are best understood from a view of circular rather than linear causality.

There are two primary cybernetics concepts in the CFAM:

- Families possess self-regulating ability through the process of feedback.
- In families, feedback processes can occur simultaneously at several different systems levels.

At this point, it is necessary to differentiate cybernetics from systems theory. Conceived by mathematician Norbert Weiner, the term **cybernetics** refers to the science of communication and control theory. In cybernetics, both parts and wholes are looked at in terms of their patterns of organization (Keeney, 1982). **Systems theory**, you will recall, is a science of wholeness. As such, it examines the interconnections of two or more parts which form an organized whole and which interact with each other. The whole is greater than the sum of its parts.

Even though systems theory speaks of feedback from a similar perspective, cybernetics distinguishes feedback as positive or negative. Positive or negative feedback occurs in a family system as information about the output. With positive feedback, information serves to increase the output, whereas, with negative feedback, the same information serves to decrease the output. For example, if nagging a withdrawing husband increases his withdrawal behaviour, then positive feedback has occurred. On the other hand, if nagging causes the husband to withdraw less, then negative feedback has occurred (Wright and Leahey, 1984). With cybernetics, feedback may occur at several levels simultaneously. Therefore, the communication pattern between a nagging wife and withdrawing husband, for example, would be examined in greater scope and involve the couple's relationship to their families of origin.

The four communication concepts used in the CFAM are:

- All verbal communication is meaningful.
- All communication has two major channels for transmission: digital and analogic. **Digital** refers to verbal communication and **analogic** refers to usual nonverbal

communication such as body posture, facial expression and tone, as well as creative expression such as music, poetry and painting. If there are discrepancies between the digital and analogic channels, then the analogic is seen as more valid and reliable.

- A dyadic relationship has varying degrees of symmetry and complementarity. A relationship is symmetrical when the two people behave as if they have equal status, for instance, a pre-adolescent peer relationship. In a complementary relationship, the two people are of unequal status, where one appears to initiate action and the other follows. A basic example of a complementary relationship is a mother and an infant.

- All communication consists of two levels: content and relationships. Content refers to what is being said. Relationship defines the nature of the relationship between those interacting, for example, is it loving or conflictual.

The CFAM uses seven change concepts. These are:

- Change is dependent on the perception of the problem.
- Change is dependent on context.
- Change is dependent on coevolving goals for treatment. Goals are set collaboratively between the nurse and the family once the family has gained a different view of its problem and the changes it desires.
- Understanding alone does not lead to change.
- Change does not necessarily occur equally in all family members.
- Facilitating change is the nurse's responsibility.
- Change can be due to a myriad causes.

In the CFAM, families are seen to be a group of individuals who are bound by attributes of affection, strong emotional ties and a sense of belonging. A family evolves an ecology of beliefs which helps each individual to define thoughts (cognitions), behaviours and emotions. Individuals and families are seen to be unique and autonomous, possessing the strengths and abilities necessary to solve their own problems. The focus is on "family" even when only one person is involved in treatment because individuals are best understood within the context of their families.

Health is viewed through relationships and communication with other human beings. Distinctions such as "health" and "illness" are believed to be subjective judgements made by observers about adaptation. When individuals or families are seen with problems that have been identified, this model seeks to invite new ways to view the situation (in order to broaden the range of solution options) without making judgements about the problem or solution.

We mentioned earlier in this section that CFAM incorporates structural, functional and developmental theory. CFAM considers each of these approaches separately,

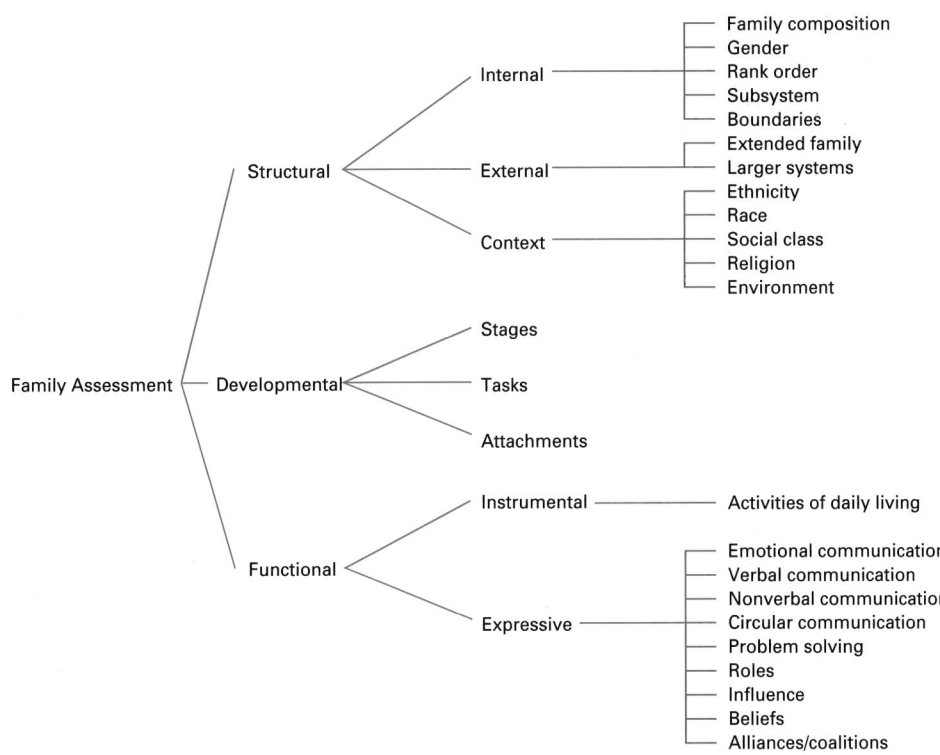

FIGURE 10.2 Branching diagram of CFAM

SOURCE: Wright, L.M. and Leahey, M. (1994). *Nurses and families: A guide to family assessment and intervention.* (2nd ed.). Philadelphia: F.A. Davis Company, 38. Reproduced with permission.

The Calgary Family Assessment Model

STRUCTURAL ASSESSMENT

INTERNAL STRUCTURE

Internal structure includes the notions of family composition, rank order, subsystem and boundary.

FAMILY COMPOSITION   *Family composition* refers to all members living in the home. This definition includes nuclear families, single-parent families, homosexual couples, boarders, grandparents, step-parents and children. A family is a small social system made up of individuals related to each other by reason of strong reciprocal affections and loyalties and comprising a permanent household that persists over years.

GENDER   *Gender* refers to the set of beliefs about or expectations of male and female behaviour and experiences that have developed by cultural, religious and family influences. Gender is an important consideration because differences in how males and females experience the world is at the heart of therapeutic conversation.

RANK ORDER   *Rank order* refers to the position of the children in the family with respect to age and gender. It is believed that sibling position influences personality and levels of motivation and achievement as well as vocational choices.

SUBSYSTEMS   *Subsystems* in a family are delineated by generation, sex, interests and function, according to Minuchin (1974). Each family member belongs to several subsystems that differentiate the level of power and skills. Examples of non-typical subsystems include a step-parent who lacks power over the children, or a child who has power over the parent.

BOUNDARIES   *Boundaries* refer to the rule defining which family members participate in functions and how. Boundaries protect the family members by obtaining, containing, retaining and disposing of information, products or people. For example, a family may prevent members from bringing in drugs or using vulgar language, or it may prevent members from divulging the family information to outsiders. Boundaries can be diffuse or rigid and the degree of permeability may change over time.

EXTERNAL STRUCTURE

This includes two subcategories: extended family and larger systems.

EXTENDED FAMILY   The *extended family* includes grandparents, aunts, uncles and cousins who may live near or far away.

LARGER SYSTEMS   The subcategory of *larger systems* refers to social agencies and personnel with whom the family has meaningful contact. Such systems generally include work systems. For some families they may include welfare, child care, foster care, courts and ambulatory clinics. They may also include services for special populations such as people with mental or physical disabilities or frail older adults.

CONTEXT

Context means the whole situation or background relevant to the family. Each family system is part of broader systems such as neighbourhood, social class, religion, community and country.

ETHNICITY   *Ethnicity* refers to the concept of a family's "peoplehood" which is derived from a blend of cultural heritage, race and religion. It pertains to the ancestral roots or origins of a population and depicts a commonality of conscious and unconscious processes that are transmitted by the family over generations. Ethnicity is an important factor influencing family life as well as family health beliefs and practices.

RACE   *Race* refers to a distinct group of people who share certain physical characteristics such as skin colour or body frame that are transmitted genetically. Its influence on family life is mediated by variables such as social class, religion and ethnicity. Racial attitudes, stereotyping and discrimination are powerful influences on family interaction, and if they are not addressed, they can have negative effects on nurse–family relationships.

SOCIAL CLASS   *Social class* status and mobility strongly influence the family value system. The adults' educational attainment, income and occupation usually determine values that influence the family's lifestyle and behaviour patterns.

RELIGION   *Religion* refers to the family values, size, health care practices and socialization practices. It includes level of community involvement and maintaining of certain traditions, both religious and hygienic.

ENVIRONMENT   *Environment* refers to both the general neighbourhood and the home. The type of neighbourhood, proximity of stores, transportation, recreation and health facilities are considered. In the home, the amount of space and privacy along with access, safety and security are important.

DEVELOPMENTAL ASSESSMENT

The family development level is based on the family developmental framework outlined earlier in this chapter and on Falicov's definition of family development. According to Falicov, "... family development is an overarching concept, referring to *all* transactional evolutionary processes connected with the growth of the family ..." (1988. Cited in Wright and Leahey, 1994, 57). In addition, she states:

> Although there is a regularity and internal logic to many of the processes subsumed under family development ... each family is different precisely because each can be said to have its own developmental path, which evolves from all the different settings in which development takes place, including each family's construction of its past and present (1988. Cited in Wright and Leahey, 1994, 58).

STAGES

There are eight stages to the family development assessment. *Stages* refer to the identifiable periods which occur during the length of marriage and are noted by the age of the eldest child. The cycles are repeated as later children reach the identified stages. Family theorists stress that families do not move smoothly or automatically through one stage to another and that there are stressful transition points along the way.

TASKS

The *tasks* are considered general maintenance responsibilities such as employment, spending, education and socialization which are necessary to achieve a satisfactory resolution of the stages. The tasks are outlined for each of the stages.

ATTACHMENTS

Attachments are the unique and relatively enduring emotional ties between two family members. They are looked at from an adaptive and maladaptive perspective at each of the eight stages.

FUNCTIONAL ASSESSMENT

Family functions include the actual behaviours of family members in relation to daily activities and their emotional interactions. There is an instrumental function and an expressive function.

INSTRUMENTAL FUNCTIONING

Instrumental functioning includes activities of daily living in a family.

ACTIVITIES OF DAILY LIVING *Activities of daily living* are the patterns of functioning such as working, eating, sleeping and cooking meals. These are what the family members do together and what they do alone and they constitute the more frequent everyday activities. The instrumental function may include the tasks involved in caring for an ill or elderly family member.

EXPRESSIVE FUNCTIONING

Expressive functioning involves emotional communication, verbal communication, nonverbal communication, circular communication, problem solving, roles, influence, beliefs and alliances/coalitions.

COMMUNICATION *Communication* between family members includes verbal and nonverbal as well as the range and types of emotions and feelings expressed in interaction. Circular communication refers to the reciprocal communication between members or the patterns they establish in the relationship which are adaptive or problematic.

PROBLEM SOLVING *Problem solving* refers to the family's method of identifying and solving problems. That is, how are decisions made and who is called upon to make them.

ROLES *Roles* of family members are their established patterns of behaviour as they interact with one another. Each member can have overlapping roles. These roles may be assumed or assigned, formal or informal. What function have these roles in family interaction?

INFLUENCE *Influence* refers to the methods that family members use to affect each other's behaviour. Instrumental influence refers to the use of objects or privileges (for example, the use of money, watching television or going to a movie) as reinforcers. Psychological influence refers to communication and feelings (for instance, words, affection or the withholding of these) to control members.

BELIEFS *Beliefs* refer to the expectations, attitudes, values and priorities that the family holds. Are different views tolerated by other family members? What are the family myths?

ALLIANCES/COALITIONS *Alliances/coalitions* refers to the direction, balance and intensity of relationships among family members.

SOURCES: Wright, L.M. and Leahey, M. (1984, 1994).

and consists of the following three major categories:

1. structural
2. development
3. functional.

Each assessment category contains several subcategories. It is important for the nurse to decide which subcategories are relevant and appropriate for families at particular points in time. That is, not all subcategories need to be assessed at the first meeting and some may never have to be used. Wright and Leahey conceptualize the three assessment categories and the many subcategories as a branching diagram adapted from Tomm and Sanders (1983). This diagram is depicted in Figure 10.2 (on page 241). Although the family may be examined by looking at specific parts, each part interacts with others and changes the whole family configuration.

The CFAM is very useful during assessment because it can be applied to various types of families such as single-parent, blended and communal families. It also includes extended family members. Another advantage of this model is that it integrates sociocultural, ethnic and community data. The nurse poses questions to the family to assess each of the categories.

THE GENOGRAM AND THE ECOMAP

The genogram and the ecomap are two tools commonly used in working with families. They are particularly helpful to the nurse in outlining the family's internal and external structures.

The *genogram* is a diagram of the family constellation. It shows the structure of the intergenerational relationships of a family. The *ecomap*, on the other hand, is a diagram of the family's contact with others outside the immediate family. It pictures the important connections between the family and the world. Both the genogram and the ecomap are simple to use and require only a piece of paper and a pencil.

GENOGRAM

The skeleton of the genogram tends to follow conventional genealogical charts. It is useful to include at least three generations. Family members are placed on horizontal rows that signify generational lines. For example, a marriage or common-law relationship is denoted by a horizontal line. Children are denoted by vertical lines that are rank-ordered from left to right beginning with the eldest child. Each individual is represented. Ages are noted as are illnesses and deaths. A blank genogram is shown in Figure 10.3.

Authors differ slightly in the symbols that they use for details of the genogram. The symbols depicted in Figure 10.4 are generally agreed upon by the majority of family therapists (Wright and Leahey, 1984). The person's name and age

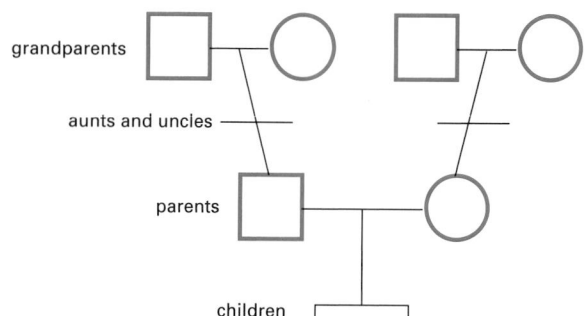

FIGURE 10.3 Sample of a blank genogram

SOURCE: Wright, L.M. and Leahey, M. (1984). *Nurses and families: A guide to family assessment and intervention*. Philadelphia: F.A. Davis Company, 31. Reproduced with permission.

should be noted *inside* the square or circle. Significant data, such as "depressed" or "overinvolved at work," should be noted *outside* the symbol.

The genogram is an important tool that can be used when conducting a family interview. At the beginning of the interview, the nurse can tell the family that they will be asked a few background questions that will help to gain an overview of their situation. The nurse uses the structure of the genogram to spell out the family's composition and boundaries. Initially, the interviewer starts out with a blank sheet of paper and draws a square or circle for the first person with whom he or she is talking. After inquiring about the immediate family, the nurse continues to inquire about

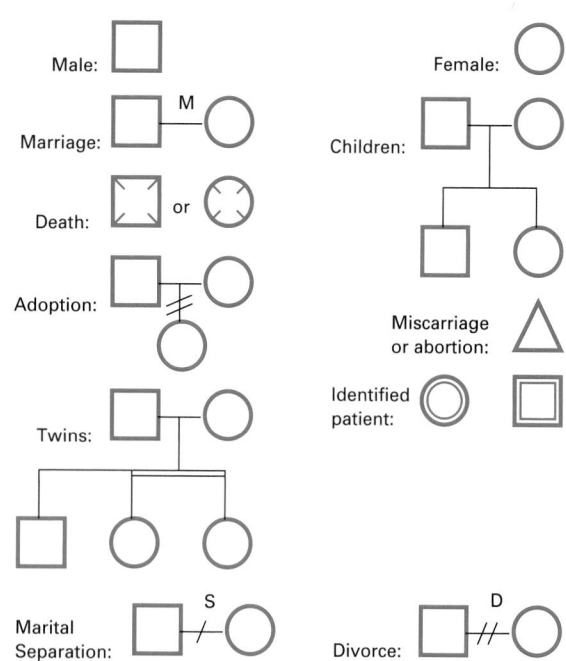

FIGURE 10.4 Symbols used in genograms

SOURCE: Wright, L.M. and Leahey, M. (1984). *Nurses and families: A guide to family assessment and intervention*. Philadelphia: F.A. Davis Company, 31. Reproduced with permission.

the extended family. It is important to gain an overview of the family structure without getting sidetracked and inundated by a volume of information. Most families are extremely cooperative and interested in completing the genogram.

ECOMAP

As with the genogram, the primary value of the ecomap is in its visual impact. The purpose of the ecomap is to depict the family members' contact with their outside world. It demonstrates the flow of resources or the lacks and deprivations thereof. The mapping procedure highlights the points of conflict to be mediated, bridges to be built and resources to be sought and mobilized. As with the genogram, family members can actively participate in working on the ecomap during the assessment process. An ecomap is depicted in Figure 10.5.

The family genogram is placed in the centre of the ecomap (see the circle in the centre Figure 10.5). The outer circles represent significant people, agencies or institutions within this family's context. Lines are drawn between the family members and outer circles to show the nature of the connections that exist. Straight lines depict strong connections, dotted lines depict tenuous connections and slashed lines depict stressful relationships. Arrows can be drawn beside the lines to indicate the flow of energy and resources.

FAMILY INTERVENTION

FAMILY HEALTH PROMOTION AND PROTECTION

In keeping with the *Ottawa Charter for Health Promotion* (WHO, 1986), family health promotion is the process of enabling families to increase control over and improve the quality of life and well-being. Families promote health by creating living conditions in which family members' experiences of health and well-being are increased. They do this

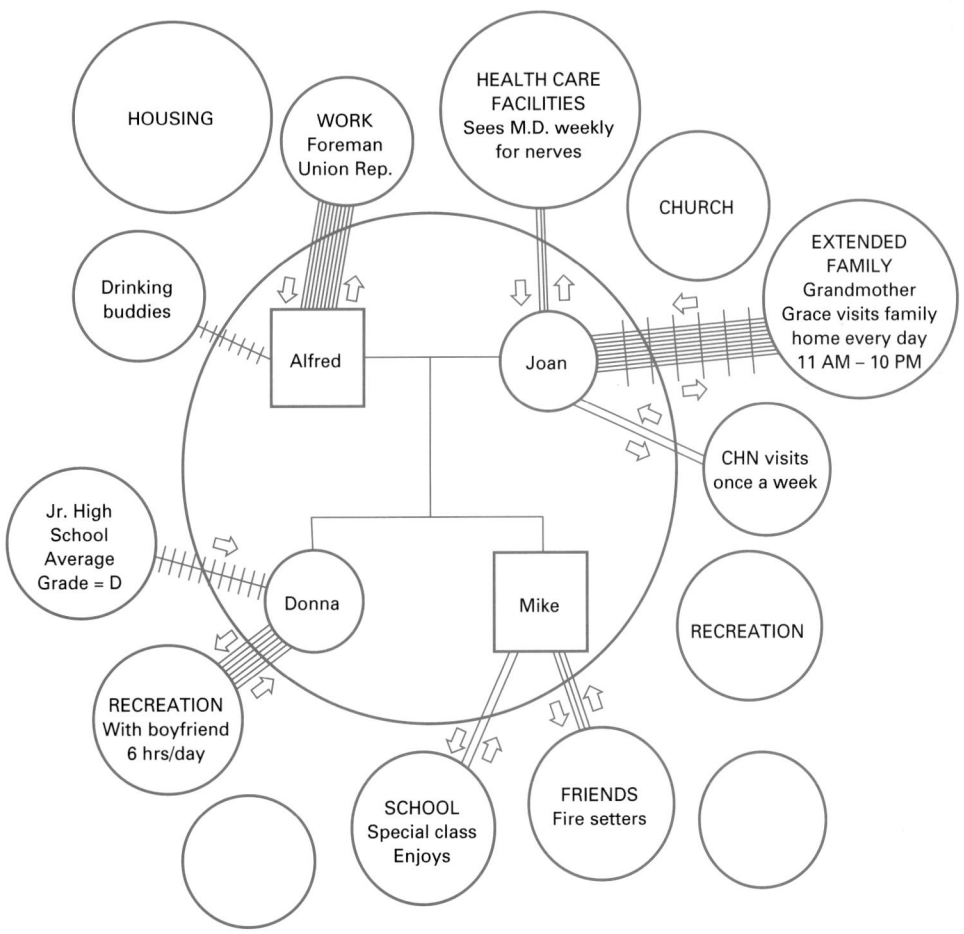

FIGURE 10.5 Ecomap

by teaching and fostering health practices, such as washing hands before handling food or eating, and by managing health resources, such as providing a safe, clean dwelling. Families also protect their health by promoting activities that prevent or decrease the risk of disease, as, for example, avoidance of smoking, alcohol or drugs. Nursing interventions for family health promotion and health protection are based on the assumptions that families are the best judges of their health needs and that they are capable of assuming responsibility for health and those things that affect their health. As such, families are seen as collaborative partners with health professionals in promoting health and wellness of members. Collaboration implies the sharing of information and equal participation in decision making and assumption of responsibilities (Lancaster, McCance and Vanderschmidt, 1986). Families are asked what their health care needs are as opposed to being told. In addition, their opinions regarding health care are considered along with those of the health care professional.

The nurse's role in family health promotion is to help in enhancing family resources (that is, their strengths and capabilities) so that they can increase control over and improve their health. Nurses do this by appraising families' personal meanings of health, determining their strengths and capabilities and educating them about health and healthy living. Nurses also promote family health by facilitating use of health resources and fostering active family involvement in health-promoting programs and policies in the community.

Appraising Family Meanings of Health

In order for nurses to effectively intervene in family health promotion they must have an understanding of a family's personal definition of *health*. Health means different things to different families. For a retired couple, health might mean having the finances and the physical capabilities to live in their own home, drive their automobile, get out and visit with friends and relatives and continue with leisure activities such as walking, swimming or golfing. A young childbearing family, on the other hand, might define its health as the ability of all members to eat nutritiously, to express themselves freely, to be actively involved in school activities and sports and to participate together in leisure activities. These examples point to the fact that a family's view of health changes as it progresses through the family life cycle. A family's personal meaning of health is also influenced by its health beliefs, its past experiences with health and its cultural and ethnic background.

Some families have a clear idea of what health means to them, others do not. It is not unusual to find people who say that they do not really think about their health beliefs or practices. They simply behave according to past traditions and norms without too much thought about the effect these might have on their overall health. It is not until they have reflected upon and considered their personal beliefs and practices that they might see a need for improvement or change. Therefore, an appraisal of the family's personal definition of health assists both nurse and family. This appraisal helps the family become aware of its own health beliefs and practices, and at the same time helps the nurse gain knowledge of the family's views and perceptions. The nurse can view the family through the "eyes of the family," so to speak.

Communication and interviewing techniques such as discussion, exploration, values clarification and critical reflection are tools the nurse uses in helping families define health. These are discussed in Chapter 16.

Determining Family Strengths and Capabilities

Family strengths and capabilities are central to interventions which enable families to take responsibility for and control over the health of their members. Duffy states that "health promotion in the family is the result of an interaction between the internal environment of the family and the external environment which impinges upon it" (1988, 112). The internal environment mainly refers to structure and function. Family structure includes composition, subsystems, boundaries, social class, roles and power, and occupation and income of adult members. Family function refers to things like activities of daily living, allocation of tasks, communication, problem solving and decision making.

The external environment involves a wide range of influences outside of the family, for example, the kinship network, religious affiliations, type of neighbourhood and community resources including health promotion facilities. A study done by Blaxter and Patterson (1983) found that an environment of poverty, rather than the health attitudes and behaviours of mothers, contributed to accidents in families. Poverty is said to be "the greatest threat to health promotion since it decreases the family's options, thus contributing to many of the health problems faced by the poor" (Duffy, 1988, 112).

An analysis of family structure and function will determine a family's strengths and capabilities for healthy living as well as its weaknesses. Once these are established, the nurse and the family can work together to plan activities that support existing strengths. In addition, resources can be appropriated to fulfill health needs within the economic constraints of the family.

Educating Families about Health and Healthy Living

In order for people to analyze their health behaviours and determine their health needs, they must have knowledge about health and healthy living conditions. For instance, many of us considered eggs to be an excellent dietary source of protein until we learned of their high fat and cholesterol content. Similarly, a pregnant woman may think an occasional social drink is acceptable until she discovers the potential harmful effects of alcohol on her growing fetus.

Dunn identified education of individuals and families about health and healthy living as an important approach for promoting high-level wellness (Dunn, 1980). Through education, families are provided with information which assists them to cope more effectively with life, life changes and stresses of daily living. Having useful information helps families feel a sense of control and enables them to explore options and solve their own problems (Watson, 1985). Because nurses interact directly with families in hospitals, in community clinics and at home, they play a large role in educating families about health and health self-care. Using principles of teaching and learning as outlined in Chapter 17, nurses educate families in a number of ways. They can give information through verbal interaction, handouts or pamphlets. They may suggest books or videos the family could obtain from the library. Nurses also teach care-giving skills through role-modelling or demonstration, as, for example, instructing a new childbearing family in bathing techniques and infant care.

Facilitating Family Use of Health Resources

"Many families are in need of supportive services at various points of their lives; at other times a supportive environment is all that is necessary to enable a family to function effectively" (Lundy, 1992, 4). Many healthy families actively seek out health resources in their community, with little need for assistance from health care professionals. There are others, however, who are not able to do this for themselves. These people either lack knowledge of available resources or perceive themselves as being unable to pursue assistance. They also may not know how to go about obtaining needed resources. People of low socioeconomic status and people with low self-esteem or self-confidence often fall into this category.

Nurses provide support to these families by helping them find and then access the resources they require to meet their needs. Because these people often feel helpless, it is important for the nurse to bolster their sense of self-esteem and self-confidence so that they feel empowered to take action for themselves. To illustrate, one nurse helped an elderly family find respite care to ease the burden of the spouse in caring for his wife.

Cora, who has been living with diabetes and Parkinson's disease for the past 20 years, is no longer able to look after herself. Her spouse, Elmer, takes care of her and maintains the household. He doesn't go out very often because he can't leave Cora alone. When Cora is in hospital, Elmer confides to the nurse that he is finding it more and

more difficult to care for Cora. In further discussion with Elmer, the nurse finds out that Elmer is not aware of services in the community that may be able to provide assistance to him, such as adult day care or respite programs. When the nurse suggests some options to Elmer, he is reluctant to pursue them because he doesn't know how to go about doing such things. With Elmer's consent, the nurse places a phone call which starts the process of arranging respite care. In this case, all that was needed was a community health care aide who would come into the home and spend time with Cora so that Elmer could get out for some exercise, do the shopping or spend time with friends at the recreation centre.

There is a wide range of resources in the community offering education and support to families in meeting their health needs. Local, regional or provincial social services and human resources agencies provide financial assistance, housing and child care, in addition to health services, such as adult day care for seniors or homemaker services for families in need.

Community organizations offer educational programs dealing with family life such as marriage counselling and positive parenting. There are supportive networks for new parents, teen parents and gays and lesbians. Community health departments also provide well-baby clinics which offer programs for screening infant growth and development, immunization and teaching of infant needs and care. There are also a host of educational programs such as "quit smoking" or "eating for healthy heart" directed towards health protection.

Many communities provide drop-in centres for all age groups, seniors' centres, women's resource centres, teen centres and family centres. Transition houses for battered and abused women and children are available in urban centres in Canada. In large cities where language and cultural beliefs of different ethnic groups may pose problems to families, interpreters and other resource persons for the new immigrants are available through neighbourhood and community centres, local drop-in centres or churches. Communities often modify programs and facilities to meet the ever-changing health needs of individuals and families. Therefore, it is important for nurses to keep up to date with the various health resources in their communities.

Fostering Active Involvement of Families in Healthy Communities

Canadian families have the opportunity to participate in decision making and public policy regarding health promotion issues in their communities. Through what is known as the *Healthy Communities* initiative, municipal governments and residents can work together to resolve their health issues and create supportive environments for health (Office of Health Promotion, 1992). Providing safe streets and roads, adequate and affordable housing, recreational activities for teens, clean environments and smoke-free flying are but a few examples of health issues for which communities created solutions and set policies that would promote healthy living for their residents.

The healthy communities concept arose from the World Health Organization's emerging definition of health and health promotion (Ottawa Charter, 1986), which recognized the importance of public policy, particularly at the municipal levels, in creating a physical and social environment that promotes health for the community as a whole (Office of Health Promotion, 1990). Families may become directly involved in the health of their communities by identifying issues and by participating in the development of programs and public policies. Nursing's participation in health promotion at the community level will be discussed in Chapter 11.

In family nursing, the nurse's role is to give information, nurture and empower families to take action on health issues in their communities. Information and guidelines on the process of establishing health-promoting policies in communities may be obtained from the Office of Health Promotion, Ministry of Health, in each province.

CRISIS INTERVENTION WITH FAMILIES

The family bears a very distinct position in our society. It is the most common source of support and understanding which many of us turn to when we are in trouble, yet it can also be the domain in which we encounter our most intense distress. All families have problems at one time or another and all families deal with problems in their own ways. Some are more successful than others in solving their problems. Much of their success depends on the resources available to them and their usual strategies for coping (Hoff, 1989). Nursing intervention for families experiencing stress and crisis in their lives focusses on helping them to identify their strengths and resources and mobilize their coping strategies. This involves establishing communication and rapport, determining the family's meaning of the stressor event, facilitating use of social supports and resources and supporting family coping strategies. **Empowerment**, that is enabling families to assume control over their stressor events, meet their needs and re-establish their health and harmony, is central to crisis intervention with families.

Establishing Communication and Rapport

Interventions for family stress and crisis are dependent upon the establishment of rapport and effective communication. Hoff argues that crisis interventions are not likely to work unless we can establish rapport and communicate effec-

tively with families. She maintains that communication is the medium through which:

- we struggle to survive (for example, giving away prized possessions or stating "I don't care anymore" conveys a "cry for help" following serious loss)
- meaningful human interaction is developed and maintained (such as giving and receiving support during stress and crisis)
- we bring stability and organization into our lives (such as sorting out the chaotic elements of a traumatic event with a caring person)
- social and political struggles at the national and international level are negotiated.*

Hoff also maintains that when communication fails, people may feel alone, abandoned, worthless and unloved, or conflict and tension may be created in interpersonal relationships. "The most tragic result of failed communication is violence toward self and others; at the societal level it translates into war. Such destructive outcomes of failed communication are more probable in acute crisis situations" (Hoff, 1989, 113). Nurses need skills in communication in order to work with families in stress and crisis.

Inasmuch as nurses need communication skills in crisis intervention, they must also establish a relationship in which the family will accept their help. The quality of the relationship, in particular the empathy, caring and sincerity displayed by the nurse, has been shown to affect the outcome of work with people in crisis (Hoff, 1989). Hoff says that in trying to establish rapport and use our relationship with people in crisis we should strive for two objectives:

1. We should make the distressed person feel understood. We can convey understanding through our response by using reflective statements such as "You seem to be very hurt and upset by what has happened" and "Sounds like you're very angry." If our perception of what the person is feeling is incorrect, the words "seem to be" and "sounds like" provide an opening for the person to explain his or her perception of the traumatic event. The expression "I understand" should generally be avoided as it may be perceived as presumptuous; there is always the possibility that we do not truly understand. Parents who suffer the loss of a child say that *no* one but a similarly grieving parent can truly understand.

2. If we are unclear about the nature or extent of what the person feels or is troubled by, we need to ask questions or make a comment that will convey our desire and *attempt* to understand, for example, "Could you tell me more about that?" "How do you feel about what has happened?" "I'm not sure I understand — could you tell me what you mean by that?"**

---

* Hoff, 1989, 113.

** Ibid

Determining Family Meaning of the Stressor Event

A family's ability to cope with a stressful event is influenced by its perception of the problem. Even though family responses to stressful events vary, there is evidence to support the theory that distress increases when people encounter a number of stressors at once, when they experience the stressor for a prolonged period of time and when they are exposed to a stressor with little time to anticipate problem solving. Distress also increases when people encounter events that are highly ambiguous, or when they present hardships or serious consequences, such as death. As stress increases, people develop a distorted view of the stressor. They often experience such feelings as helplessness, hopelessness, anxiety, fatigue and depression (Clemen-Stone, Eigsti and McGuire, 1991).

In order for a stressor to become problematic, "it must be perceived as a threat or loss to needs satisfaction or as a challenge" (Caplan, 1964. Cited in Clemen-Stone, Eigsti and McGuire, 1991, 235). Caplan believes that there are two major variables that affect how people perceive life events. These are personality and sociocultural factors. "These variables determine the type of life experiences one has, prescribe the limits of acceptable behaviour when dealing with stress, and influence how one feels about one's abilities to handle changes in life" (Clemen-Stone, Eigsti and McGuire, 1991, 235). By way of example, let's consider two childrearing families, both of whom lost the father, about six months ago. Both fathers were the families' sole providers.

In the first family, the Whites, the mother is distraught. She can barely look after her two school-aged children. Her home is untidy, she cries all the time and cannot see how she will cope with the future. Her husband made all of the decisions for the family. Mrs. White is concerned because her husband's insurance is not quite adequate for the family needs. She married at a young age and has never worked because it was the family belief that women should stay at home and care for the family. She is afraid to consider work outside the home because she thinks she is not good enough to do anything besides clean the house, cook meals and raise a family.

In the second family, we see a different picture. Five months after her husband's death, Mrs. Storly perceives that while she is still grieving, she is managing well. She arranged day care for her preschool daughter and obtained a job at a local A & W restaurant, where she had worked as a teenager. She is planning to enrol in nursing at a community college. Money will be a problem; however, she will seek financial assistance from the Welfare Department. In addition, Mrs. Storly's parents have offered to help pay for her education.

Both of these families have experienced similar stressor events in that both lost a significant other who was the sole family provider. In the White family, the mother was immobilized by sociocultural beliefs regarding her role and a lack of confidence in her abilities to work outside the home and provide for the family. Mrs. Storly, on the other hand, took control of her situation and became actively involved in assuming her provider role. Having worked as a teenager, she was more confident in her abilities to succeed. The life experiences of both women provided them with differing perceptions of their roles, which influenced their sense of control over the stressor events.

Facilitating Use of Family Social Support and Resources

"Whether or not stressful events lead to crisis depends on a family's resources for handling such events" (Hoff, 1989, 147). In times of difficulty, many people turn to someone with whom they have a meaningful relationship for strength and support. The network of social relationships through which resources may be derived is known as social support (Kane, 1988). A family's social support network may include relatives, friends, neighbours, colleagues, health care professionals, social workers, employers, teachers, school counsellors, clergy and lawyers.

Kane maintains that "family social support is a pattern of social interaction characterized by interdependence in social relationships" (1988, 20). For example, when Janice's husband suffered a near fatal heart attack at the age of 44, she sought help from her younger sister, Julie, someone with whom she shares a special relationship. Both sisters have always "been there" for one another in times of need. For families, social support comes from long-term relationships and the things they have in common (Kane, 1988). Social supports provide a *buffer* against stressor events and have a *mediating effect* which fosters effective coping strategies (Clemen-Stone, Eigsti and McGuire, 1991).

Nurses can assist families by helping them to identify and obtain social supports. When first confronted with a situational crisis, as, for example, when a family member is admitted to the emergency or critical care unit, families often experience a period of distress and disorganization. During this time, a calm sensitive manner, reassurance and an atmosphere that enables expression of feelings will help reduce tension and foster a sense of control. The nurse might also help the family contact their support people by providing access to a telephone or making the call for them.

Supporting Family Coping Strategies

During times of disequilibrium, people need supportive relationships that enable then to verbalize feelings, sort out the realities of their situation and begin to solve their problems (Clemen-Stone, Eigsti and McGuire, 1991). When first confronted with a crisis, people often have a distorted view of the situation and want to place blame on someone else for their problem. Furthermore, initial shock and anxiety can cause difficulty in understanding and storing information accurately. Clear, simple explanations, focussing only on aspects that will relieve immediate concerns, are necessary at this point. The nurse should give the family members time to ventilate feelings and help them place existing circumstances into perspective. Reassure families that their reactions are common and predictable. Figley maintains that "normalizing" a family's situation is an effective supportive technique (1989). Avoid and discourage blaming behaviours as these only inhibit family growth and successful problem-solving.

Effective support for family coping strategies is based on the assumption that families possess a "natural resourcefulness" for solving their own problems. All families have strengths and resources to help them deal with stressful events. As nurses, we can support families in crisis by empowering them to identify their strengths and coping strategies. We can explore coping mechanisms the family has found effective in the past. If these are not adequate for the current situation, then we can assist further by exploring new coping mechanisms. Help might also be needed in mobilizing community resources such as financial assistance or home care services. Figley explains the benefit of empowerment in crisis intervention. He states:

> I try to empower the family by creating the kind of intervention context that results in the resolution of the traumatizing experience but, just as importantly, that results in the family's giving themselves most of the credit for the accomplishment. Moreover, this approach makes the family feel more confident to face any future traumatic experience equipped with the necessary information, skills, and problem-solving methods (1989, 42).

KEY TERMS

family p. 226
nuclear family p. 226
dual-career family p. 226
nuclear-dyad p. 226
extended family p. 226
single-parent family p. 227
blended or reconstituted family p. 227
binuclear family p. 227
cohabiting family p. 227
gay or lesbian family p. 227
communal family p. 228
subsystems p. 230

suprasystem p. 230
boundaries p. 230
input p. 230
output p. 230
open system p. 230
feedback p. 230
family structure p. 231
role structure p. 231
values p. 231
communication p. 231
power hierarchy p. 231
authority p. 231
family functions p. 232

family dynamics p. 234
family stress p. 236
family stressors p. 236
distress p. 236
eustress p. 236
family crisis p. 237
cybernetics p. 240
systems theory p. 240
digital p. 240
analogic p. 240
genogram p. 244
ecomap p. 244
empowerment p. 248

IN REVIEW

In most societies the family is the basic institution for reproduction, socialization and perpetuation of sociocultural traditions. The family plays a vital role in the health of its members. A family's health beliefs and practices and its socioeconomic conditions influence the lifestyle and living conditions of family members which in turn contribute to health or illness. The family is a primary resource for its members in its ability to provide support and care in health and illness. Some authors believe that the family is the most significant factor in the health and well-being of individuals. Family support and involvement in an individual's care has been shown to be a powerful ally in healing.

There are many types of families in Canada — nuclear, extended, single-parent, blended, cohabiting, gay or lesbian and communal. Nurses must be aware of the characteristics of the various family forms so that they can implement care to meet the unique needs of families. In addition, nurses must be sensitive to the ethnic and cultural differences in families and avoid imposing their personal health beliefs and values on patients and families.

Conceptual frameworks of the family give a perspective on family life and provide a basis for assessing families, interpreting their needs and planning interventions. Three frameworks commonly used in nursing with families include the family systems framework, the structural-functional framework and the family developmental framework.

Family health is determined by the family's beliefs and practices, the impact of internal and external social and environmental factors, their economic resources and their coping strategies. Healthy families enhance individual development. They have open supportive communication, an effective structure of role relationships, effective coping methods, a healthy home environment and lifestyle and regular links with the broader community.

A state of imbalance in the family, or family stress, signals a need for change. Continuing unresolved stress can lead to a crisis or a disorganization in the family unit and a state of immobilization. The illness of a family member may cause such a crisis.

Nursing care of a family varies with the situation and depends on whether the family is the stressor or a resource. Nurses promote family health by educating families about health and healthy living, empowering families to create living conditions conducive to a good quality of life and well-being and facilitating family support and use of community resources. Nursing interventions with families experiencing stress and crisis in their lives focus on helping them to identify their strengths and resources and to mobilize their coping strategies and to facilitate an effective level of functioning.

LEARNING ACTIVITIES

1. When working with families, the nurse brings along a unique set of beliefs about family based on personal life experiences. It is important for the nurse to be aware of his or her values and attitudes about family and effective family functioning and to ensure that these are not unconsciously imposed on the patient. Clarify your beliefs and values of family through reflection, talking with classmates and reading professional literature on the subject. Find a values clarification tool in the literature (Pender, 1987, 162–181 gives one) and, by yourself or in a group, complete a values clarification exercise.

2. Explore the concept of family health. How does the meaning of family health differ from the meaning of health? In what ways do families promote and protect the health of family members? What health practices did you learn from your family? What programs are available in your community aimed at family health promotion (for instance, positive parenting classes at the neighbourhood community centre)?

3. Complete an assessment of a family using CFAM. You might consider doing this over three visits and explore one major category per visit. Then draw the information together into an integrated database of the family. What family strengths and problems are evident in the data?

4. Using sources in the reference list (Wright and Leahey, (1994); Danielson, Hamel-Bissell and Winstead-Fry, (1993); Friedman, (1992)), explain and illustrate with examples the difference between nursing intervention with families and family therapy.

REFERENCES AND READINGS

ASSANAND, S., DIAS, M., RICHARDSON, E. and WAXLER-MORRISON, N. (1990). The South Asians. In N. Waxler-Morrison, J. Anderson and E. Richardson. *Cross-cultural caring*. Vancouver: University of British Columbia Press, 150–152.

BAKER, M. (1990). *Families: Changing trends in Canada* (2nd ed.). Toronto: McGraw-Hill Ryerson.

B.C. MINISTRY OF HEALTH (Office of Health Promotion). British Columbia supports healthy communities. *Health Promotion in Action, 1*(3), 1–4.

B.C. MINISTRY OF HEALTH (Office of Health Promotion). (1992). *Healthy Communities 1991 Yearbook*. Victoria, BC: British Columbia of Ministry of Health and Ministry Responsible for Seniors. (Catalogue No. Q 92835)

BLAXTER, M. and PATTERSON, E. (1983). The health behaviours of mothers and daughters. In N. Madge (Ed). *Families at risk*. London: Heinemann, 174–196.

BOHANNAN, P. (1985). *All the happy families: Exploring the variety of family life*. New York: McGraw-Hill.

BOMAR, P.J. (1989). Family stress. In P.J. Bomar (Ed). *Nurses and family health promotion*. Baltimore: Williams and Wilkins, 103–114.

BOSS, P.G. (1987). Family stress. In M. Sussman and S. Steinmetz (Eds). *Handbook on marriage and the family*. New York: Plenum, 695–723.

CAUDLE, P. and GROVER, S. (1992). Care of the family patient. In Clark, M.J. *Nursing in the community*. Norwalk, CT: Appleton & Lange, 396–417.

CHRISTIE-SEELEY, I. (1984). *Working with the family in primary care: A systems approach to health and illness*. New York: Praeger.

CLEMEN-STONE, S., EIGSTI, D.G. and MCGUIRE, S.L. (1991). *Comprehensive family and community health nursing* (3rd ed.). St. Louis: Mosby.

DANIELSON, C.B., HAMEL-BISSELL, B. and WINSTEAD-FRY, P. (1993). *Families, health and illness*. St. Louis: Mosby.

DeCHESNAY, M. (1986). Promoting healthy family functioning in acute care units. *Journal of Pediatric Nursing, 1*(2), 96–101.

DUFFY, M.E. (1988). Health promotion in the family: Current findings and directives for nursing research. *Journal of Advanced Nursing, 13*, 109–117.

DUNN, H.L. (1980). *High level wellness*. Thorofare, NJ: Charles B. Slack.

DUVALL, E.M. (1977). *Marriage and family development* (5th ed.). Philadelphia: Lippincott.

ERIKSON, E.H. (1963). *Childhood and society*. New York: Norton.

FEETHAM, S.L., MEISTER, S.B., BELL, J.M., and GILLISS, C.L. (1993). *The nursing of families: Theory, research, education and practice.* Newbury Park, CA: Sage.

FIGLEY, C.R. (1989). *Helping traumatized families.* San Francisco, CA: Jossey-Bass.

FRIEDEMANN, M. (1989). The concept of family nursing. *Journal of Advanced Nursing, 14,* 211–216.

FRIEDMAN, M.M. (1986). *Family nursing: Theory and assessment* (2nd ed.). Norwalk, CT: Appleton-Century-Crofts.

FRIEDMAN, M.M. (1992). *Family nursing: Theory and practice* (3rd ed.). Norwalk, CT: Appleton & Lange.

GHALAM, N.Z. (1993, Spring). Women in the workplace. *Canadian Social Trends.* Ottawa: Minister of Supply and Services, 2–6. (Statistics Canada Catalogue 11–008E)

GILLISS, C.L. (1991). Family nursing research, theory and practice. *Image: Journal of Nursing Scholarship, 23*(1), 19–22.

HARRY, J. (1983). Gay male and lesbian relationships. In E. Macklin and R. Rubin (Eds). *Contemporary families and alternative lifestyles.* Beverly Hills, CA: Sage

HILL, R. and MATTESSICH, P. (1979). Family development theory and life-span development. In P. Baltes and R. Brown (Eds). *Life-span development and behaviour.* New York: Academic Press, 161–204.

HOFF, L.A. (1989). *People in crisis.* Redwood City, CA: Addison Wesley.

JANOSIK, E.H. and GREEN, E. (1992). *Family life: Process and practice.* Boston: Jones and Bartlet.

JANOSIK, E.H and MILLER, J.R. (1979). Theories of family development. In D.P. Hymovich and M.U. Barnard (Eds). *Family health care: Volume one* (2nd ed.). New York: McGraw-Hill, 3–15.

JANOSIK, E.H and MILLER, J.R. (1980). *Family-focused care.* New York: McGraw-Hill.

KALBACH, W.E. (1983). The Canadian family: A profile. In Ishwaran, K. (Ed). *The Canadian family.* Toronto: Gage.

KANE, C.F. (1988). Family social support: Toward a conceptual model. *Advances in Nursing Science, 10*(2), 18–25.

KEENEY, B. (1982). What is an epistemology of family therapy. *Family Process, 21,* 153–168.

LANCASTER, J., MCCANCE, K. and VANDERSCHMIDT, H. (1986). A curriculum project for clinical prevention: The role of the nurse. *Family, Community and Health, 8*(4), 48–53.

LANOVARA, P. (1993, Summer). Changes in family living. *Canadian Social Trends.* Ottawa: Minister of Supply and Services, 12–14. (Statistics Canada Catalogue 11–008E)

LANSBERRY, C.R. and RICHARDS, E. (1992). Family nursing practice paradigm perspectives and diagnostic approaches. *Advances in Nursing Science, 15*(2), 66–75.

LASKY and EICHELBERGER. (1985). Cited in C.B. Danielson, B. Hamel-Bissell and P. Winstead-Fry. (1993). *Families, health and illness.* St. Louis: Mosby.

LITMAN, T.J. (1974). The family as a basic unit in health and medical care: A social-behavioral overview. *Soc Sci Med, 8,* 495. In S. Clemen-Stone, D.G. Eigsti and S.L. McGuire. (Eds). *Comprehensive family and community health nursing* (3rd ed.). St. Louis: Mosby, 188.

LOGAN, B.B. and DAWKINS, C.E. (1986). *Family-centered nursing in the community.* Menlo Park, CA: Addison-Wesley.

LOVELAND-CHERRY, C.J. Family system patterns of autonomy and cohesiveness: Relationship to family members' health behaviour. *Nursing Research, 33*(1), 51–52.

LOVELAND-CHERRY, C.J. (1989). Family health promotion and protection. In P.J. Bomar. *Nurses and family health promotion.* Baltimore: Williams and Wilkins, 13–25.

LUNDY, T. (1992). *Healthy families in healthy communities: Tools for action.* British Columbia: British Columbia Council for the Family.

MERCER, R.T. (1989). Theoretical perspectives on family. In C.L. Gliss, B.L. Highley, B.M. Roberts and I.M. Martinson (Eds). *Toward a science of family nursing* Menlo Park, CA: Addison Wesley, 9–36.

MINUCHIN, S. (1974). *Families and family therapy.* Cambridge: Harvard University Press.

MOORE, M. (1987, Winter). Women parenting alone. *Canadian Social Trends.* Ottawa: Minister of Supply and Services, 31–35. (Statistics Canada Catalogue 11–008E)

NETT, E.M. (1988). *Canadian families: Past and present.* Toronto: Butterworths, 17–28.

RAMSHORN, M.T. (1978). The individual in the family system. In L.A. Hall and D. Collins (Eds). *Psychiatric nursing: Theory and application.* New York: McGraw-Hill, 248.

RAMU, G.N. (1989). *Marriage and the family in Canada today.* Scarborough: Prentice-Hall Canada Inc.

RAPAPORT, R. and RAPAPORT, R.N. (1971). *Dual-career families.* Harmondsworth: Penguin Books.

REGISTERED NURSES ASSOCIATION OF BRITISH COLUMBIA (RNABC). (1990). *Health promotion: A discussion paper.* Vancouver: Author.

REGISTERED NURSES ASSOCIATION OF BRITISH COLUMBIA (RNABC). (1992). *Determinants of health: Empowering strategies for nursing practice.* (RNABC Publication No. 24). Vancouver: Author.

RICE, H.R. and ZINK, M.R. (1991). Theories as a framework for practice. In M.H. Oermann. *Professional nursing practice.* Philadelphia: Lippincott.

ROSS, B. and COBB, K.L. (1990). *Family nursing.* Redwood City, CA: Addison Wesley.

SCANZONI, L. (1976). *Men, women and change: A sociology of marriage and family.* New York: McGraw-Hill.

SMITH, J.A. (1983). *The idea of health: Implications for the nursing professional.* New York: Teachers College Press, Columbia University.

SPENCER, M. (1985). *Foundations of modern sociology* (4th ed.). Englewood Cliffs, NJ: Prentice-Hall Inc.

SPRADLEY, B.W. (1990). *Community health nursing: Concepts and practice* (3rd ed.). Glenview, IL: Scott, Foresman.

SPRADLEY, B.W. (1991). *Readings in community health nursing* (4th ed.). Philadelphia: Lippincott.

STATISTICS CANADA. (1988, March). Census of population: Mobility, labour force, education. *The Daily.* Ottawa: Minister of Supply and Services, 7–9. (Statistics Canada Catalogue 11–001)

STATISTICS CANADA. (1992). Families: Number, type and structure. *The Nation.* Ottawa: Minister of Industry Science and Technology. (Statistics Canada Catalogue 93–312)

STOUT, C. (1991, Winter). Common-law: A growing alternative. *Canadian Social Trends*. Ottawa: Minister of Supply and Services, 18–20.

STUART, M.E. (1991). An analysis of the concept of family. In A.L. Whall and J. Fawcet (Eds). *Family theory development in nursing: State of the science and art*. Philadelphia: F.A. Davis.

TOMM, K. and SANDERS, G. (1983). Family assessment in a problem oriented record. In J.C. Hansen and Keeney (Eds). *Diagnosis and assessment in family therapy*. London: Aspen Systems Corporation, 101–122.

VANCOUVER SUN, February 26, 1993.

VON BERTALANFFY, L. (1968). *General system theory: Foundations, development, applications*. New York: Brazillicer.

WATSON, J. (1985). *Nursing: The philosophy and science of caring*. Denver, CO: Colorado Associated University Press.

WHALL, A.L. (1991). Family systems theory: Relationship to nursing conceptual models. In A.L. Whall and J. Fawcett (Eds). *Family theory development: State of the science and art*. Philadelphia: F.A. Davis, 317–341.

WHITE, P.M. (Summer 1989). Ethnic origins of the Canadian population. *Canadian Social Trends*. Ottawa: Minister of Supply and Services. 13–16. (Statistics Canada Catalogue 11–008E)

WILLIAMSON, M. (1986). Lesbianism. In J. Griffith-Kenney *Contemporary women's health*. Menlo Park, CA: Addison Wesley.

WORLD HEALTH ORGANIZATION. (1986). *Ottawa Charter for Health Promotion*. Geneva: Author.

WORLD HEALTH ORGANIZATION. (1984a). *Health Promotion Glossary*. Copenhagen: WHO Regional Office for Europe.

WRIGHT, L.M. and LEAHEY, M. (1984). *Nurses and families*. Philadelphia: F.A. Davis.

WRIGHT, L.M. and LEAHEY, M. (1990). Trends in nursing of families. *Journal of Advanced Nursing, 15*, 148–154.

WRIGHT, L.M. and LEAHEY, M. (1994). *Nurses and families: A guide to family assessment and intervention*. Philadelphia: F. A. Davis.

Health and
the Community

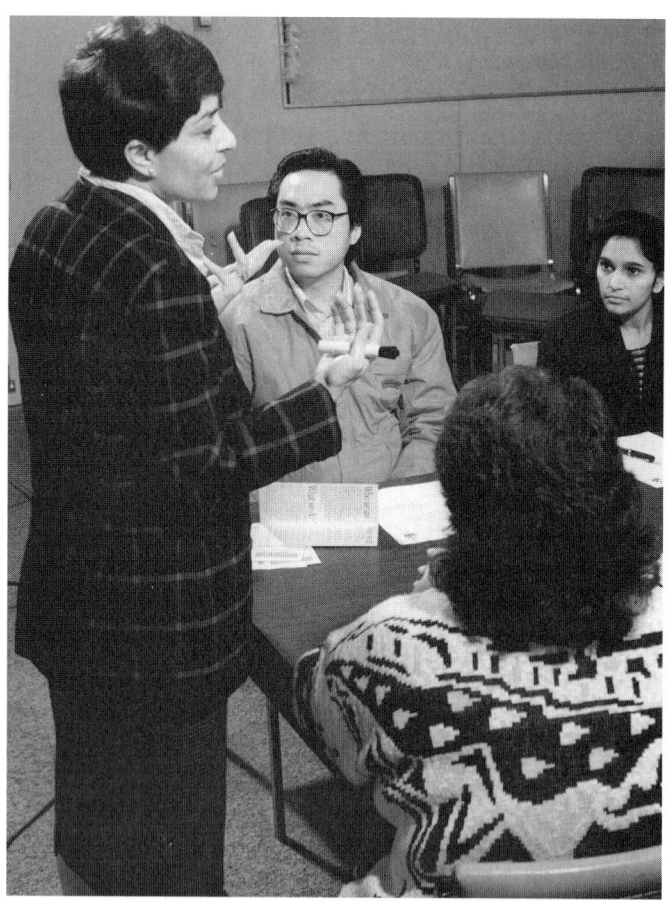

CENTRAL QUESTIONS

1. *How has the concept of community developed in Canadian society?*

2. *How is the science of epidemiology used to assess the health of a community?*

3. *What is the Healthy Communities concept and how does it differ from the epidemiological approach in looking at the health of a community?*

4. *Why do people live in communities?*

5. *What factors affect the healthy functioning of a community?*

6. *What are the major stressors affecting the health of communities?*

7. *What community ills can result from these stressors?*

8. *What is the nurse's role in community health?*

INTRODUCTION

One of the major factors in the improvement of health in Canada and, indeed, in all of the developed world in the past century and a half has been the reduction of environmental hazards brought about by the application of known public health measures. These measures have traditionally been instituted at the local level in organized communities by municipal or city councils. They include provisions to ensure safe water, food and milk supplies, sewage treatment, standards for housing and the control of communicable diseases. All too often, a lack of safe drinking water, inadequate sewage disposal and improper handling of food and milk supplies are major contributors to high infant and early childhood mortality rates as well as the spread of communicable diseases — problems that still plague many developing countries.

In Canada today, the emphasis in health care is once again on the community. As our health-care system shifts from a disease orientation to focus on health and its socioeconomic determinants, the base for services is shifting from hospitals to the community. Nurses at all levels are expected to be able to function in community settings as well as in hospitals. It is important for you as beginning students to develop an understanding of how communities function and the factors affecting the health of the people in communities, as well as the various facets of the nurse's role in community health.

In this chapter, we are going to examine the concept of community and the reasons for its prominence in the restructuring of health services underway in all provinces and territories. We will look at methods for assessing the health of communities, at the various functions of a community and at the factors affecting these functions. We will also discuss the stressors that can disrupt the healthy functioning of a community and the ills that can result. We will then look at the nurse's role in community health as it is being practised in Canada today.

HISTORICAL PERSPECTIVE

Human beings are social creatures. As far back as we have historical records, we know that families have tended to live together in organized groups for mutual protection and social support as well as for the sharing of skills needed for survival. In Canada, we developed a strong sense of community as an integral part of our social structure. Ours is a vast country with wide expanses of land and a relatively small number of inhabitants. Until well into the middle of this century, most Canadians lived in small, rural communities in which they were often cut off from their neighbours during the severe Canadian winters. People in these small communities were dependent on their own resources for food, protection from the elements, social interaction and health care. Neighbour had to help neighbour in order to survive. A strong sense of community developed and, along with it, an assumption of collective responsibility for matters of common concern, such as health and social welfare (Du Gas and Beckingham, 1993).

This assumption of collective responsibility for the common good is evident in many aspects of Canadian life, for example, in the cooperatives that developed in fishing communities in the Maritime Provinces, in the farming cooperatives of the prairies — and, today, in credit unions that provide an alternative to the chartered banks for financial services. In the health field, the principle of collective action for the common good is illustrated in the passage in Saskatchewan of a Rural Municipality Act in 1916 which enabled communities to raise funds by local levy to pay for the services of a physician for people of the community. This legislation was a forerunner of our national health insurance program pioneered by the same province that has initiated so many of our health care reforms.

In Canada, the community is now being viewed as the basic unit for health care. *Closer to Home* is the title of a Royal Commission report on health services in the Province of British Columbia (1991) which strongly recommended shifting health care from an institutional to a community base. In Ontario, the report of the Premier's Council on Health, Well-being and Social Justice, entitled *Nurturing health: A framework of the determinants of health,* states that "Health is created in our homes, schools, workplaces and communities" (1993, 20).

The potential of communities for dealing with health matters in a democratic way is being explored in all provinces. Communities are participating in the planning and management of their health care, rather than merely accepting the provision of community health services guided and directed exclusively by bureaucratic departments of health. We will explore the concept of participation in more detail when we discuss the healthy communities approach to community health. First, however, we will talk about types of communities and then discuss two conceptual frameworks for looking at health in the community — the epidemiological model and the healthy communities model. We will also look at the stressors and subsequent illnesses that afflict communities, the role of the nurse in community health care and measures to promote, protect or restore the community to a healthy state.

TYPES OF COMMUNITIES

We usually think of community as a group of people living in one locality. There are other types of communities, however. The term *community* is broadly used in the English language to refer to any group of people with a common bond, who interact with one another and share collective responsibility for common concerns. The communities most familiar to us are those with defined geographical and jurisdictional boundaries, that is, villages, towns and cities. The term *community* can, however, also be used to refer to smaller, local areas such as neighbourhoods which may or may not be defined in municipal by-laws. Community Centres provide social, recreational and educational services for people within a specific local area. If you live in a large city or town, your community may be a specific neighbourhood. If you practise in a rural area, you may have many miles to cover to service your community in your daily rounds.

A *community* can also be made up of people who may not necessarily live in the same area but who share a common interest. A university is often referred to as a "community of scholars," for example. Or, you might use the term "nursing community" to refer to all the nurses who practise in Canada. A large hospital often is like a community, almost like a small town, with a wide diversity of workers and patients sharing common goals, as well as all the services and amenities needed to meet their needs.

In our discussions of health and the community we will be using *community* in its most familiar sense as a group of people living in a given geographical area (which may not necessarily be defined by legislation) who interact with one another and work collectively on matters of common concern.

CONCEPTUAL FRAMEWORKS FOR LOOKING AT COMMUNITY HEALTH

The two conceptual frameworks we will discuss for looking at community health are the *epidemiological model* and the *healthy communities model*. The healthy communities model is being widely used across the country as nursing moves beyond the Lalonde "health fields concept" (introduced in Chapter 2) to a broader approach to community health.

THE EPIDEMIOLOGY APPROACH

The traditional way of looking at health in the community has been through an epidemiological approach. *Epidemiology* is "the study of the distribution and determinants of various health-related states or events in specified populations and the application of this study in the control of health problems" (Last, 1988, 42). Historically, epidemiology has been concerned primarily with the study of disease. Until this century, it was the communicable diseases such as cholera, typhoid, plague, smallpox, and yellow and typhus fever which posed the most serious

threats to human life. As these communicable diseases were brought under control through widespread immunization programs and effective control measures, attention turned to the frequency and determinants of the non-infectious and the chronic diseases such as heart conditions, hypertension, arthritis and cancer, which are major problems in our present-day societies.

Now, the field of epidemiology has been expanded to include the study of the health status of people and the factors that determine health. The federal government's *Active Health Report* (1987) presented the results of the first national survey on how Canadians felt about their own health. Whereas previous surveys had studied the nature and causes of health problems, this report provided a comprehensive picture of the health knowledge, attitudes, behaviour and intentions of Canadians (Health and Welfare Canada, 1987).

The *epidemiological model* of community health has served us well in the past and continues to do so. The basic components of this model are the systematic collection of health data through epidemiological surveys and the search for causes of various states of health. The methodology used includes both observational and experimental studies.

Observational studies measure the amount and distribution of disease (or other states of health) within a given population by looking at the number of persons affected, where the cases are located and when they occur (that is, they look at person, place and time). For example, a study may find that 40 percent of the elementary school children were absent with the flu during the week of January 18–25 in Weyburn, Saskatchewan whereas there were no cases reported during the week of May 3–7. One would gather from this data that there was a flu epidemic in January.

Surveys in which people gather data about various characteristics of the population are the most common type of observational study done in epidemiology. Health departments routinely gather information on illnesses occurring among the school population, for example, and the incidence of communicable diseases in the community. Statistics Canada regularly collects a large amount of information about the health of Canadians, such as births, deaths and the occurrence of illness in the population, as we discussed in Chapter 2. It also undertakes special surveys at the request of Health and Welfare Canada on particular aspects of health such as, for example, the data reported in the *Active Health Report*.

In *experimental studies*, the researcher intervenes and changes one variable, then observes what happens. For example, in order to find out if "flu shots" are effective, a possible study might involve giving one group of older people in a community flu shots at the beginning of winter. The question under study would be, "Do people who had the flu shots report fewer cases of flu than a comparable group of older people who did not have the preventive inoculations?" The investigators would, of course, have to take into consideration the ethical dimension of giving some people and not others the opportunity to protect themselves from the flu.

This type of experimental study would probably not be done; instead, the research team would probably collect observational data on the number of cases of flu among those who voluntarily chose to have or not to have the flu shots.

A more common type of experimental study in epidemiology is a **demonstration project** that involves studying a new method of delivering health care in the community. For example, the Ministry of Health in British Columbia funded a two-year demonstration project of a nursing centre to serve as a point of entry for the public into the health care system (*RNABC Newsline*, April, 1993). The centre, located in the Comox Valley on Vancouver Island, opened in 1994. Using a primary health care approach, the centre will provide an alternative method for delivering health care in line with the New Directions for Health Care program in the province. Other examples of demonstration projects involving nurses in key roles in the delivery of health services include the McGill Workshops, which were based on the Allen family-oriented nursing model, and the Denmark–Newfoundland project, "Primary Health Care — A Nursing Model" (Hall, 1989).

At some point in your career you are likely to participate in epidemiological studies, either as part of a population under study and/or as a member of an investigative team. You will also want to be able to interpret data stemming from these studies. Therefore, you need to understand the meaning of the key terms used. We discussed some of the common terms, such as mortality and morbidity rates, causes of death and number of potential years of life lost, in Chapter 2. A few more are listed in the box on p. 259.

EPIDEMIOLOGY AND ITS USES

The systematic collection of health data and the search for causation of health and illness have been of inestimable value in helping us to tackle health issues for a number of reasons.

Development of a health profile   The systematic collection of health data enables us to develop profiles of the health status of people living in different geographical areas or of people in different socioeconomic groups. We can then compare the profile of one group with that of another. In Chapter 2 we discussed some comparisons between countries on a few of the common health status indicators such as life span, causes of death, and infant and maternal mortality rates. We also looked at trends over time, such as, for example, the lengthening of the life span in Canada. Canada's 1985 Health Promotion Survey provided data for comparisons between different socioeconomic groups in the country. The *Active Health Report* on the findings of this survey showed clearly that "not all Canadians have equal likelihood of being healthy or have equivalent access to the resources required for health. In particular, the socially disadvantaged are much more likely to be living in poor health than are others" (Health and Welfare Canada, 1987, 7).

Identification of health problems   Epidemiology also enables us to identify health problems. This knowledge helps in the determination of priorities for the allocation of resources, including the need for continuous monitoring as well as the need for specific programs. For example, data collected on the incidence of communicable diseases have alerted health authorities to the alarming increase in the number of cases of Hepatitis B in Canada over the past 10 years. This has led to widespread immunization programs for people who are most at risk, namely, children and health workers. Most nursing schools now require students to be immunized against Hepatitis B before beginning clinical practice.

Control of epidemics   The continuous monitoring of communicable diseases enables health authorities to take quick action to avoid epidemics. The report of measles in one child in a daycare centre, for example, alerts the community health nurse to watch for symptoms in other children at the centre as well as in the child's siblings and playmates. If several cases develop, health authorities would have to consider whether or not a major immunization program should be mounted for children in the area. The systematic collection of data about health-related problems in a population also provides scientists with a more complete picture of the manifestations of disease. It also enables them to differentiate between variations of a disease, for example, the identification of the different types of Hepatitis — A, B, C, D and E (Tyler and Last, 1992).

Identification of risk factors   Epidemiology enables us to identify the risk factors associated with specific health problems and to take appropriate action. For example, the high incidence of low birth weight among the infants of women who smoke and the incidence of fetal alcohol syndrome in infants of mothers who consume excessive alcohol have stimulated the development of programs advocating the avoidance of smoking and drinking alcohol during pregnancy.

Evaluation of health services   Direct cause and effect relationships (causalities) are difficult, some say impossible, to establish when dealing with the multiplicity of variables involved in a person's health. Still, it is possible, by means of epidemiological surveys, to assess the impact of health programs on overall health, some more definitively than others. For example, widespread immunization programs for children have dramatically reduced the incidence and number of deaths from communicable diseases in most countries. Although heart disease is still the leading cause of death in Canada, mortality from both heart disease and stroke has been reduced by half over the past 20 years (1971–1991), as found by Statistics Canada (see Chapter 2). The reduction is felt to be due in large part to people changing their lifestyles in response to health promotion programs.

Research Terminology

CAUSALITY — the "relating of causes to the effects they produce" (Last, 1988, 21). The establishment of a link between specific factors (such as smoking or eating a high-fat diet) and the development of health problems might be an example of *causality*.

Down through the ages, disease has been attributed to many causes including divine intervention, malevolent mists or other harmful substances in the environment and, more recently, to single, specific agents such as bacteria or foods (Clark, 1992). We now believe that disease is *caused* by a multiplicity of factors. Many people in a room may be exposed to tuberculosis germs, for example, but only one, or perhaps none at all, will develop the disease, depending on a number of factors including each individual's resistance and state of health at the time of exposure. The recent resurfacing of TB as a major health problem is felt to be due to many factors, including poverty, overcrowding and poor nutrition as well as inadequate immunization and control measures (Friedman, 1987). Causality is therefore often hard to determine, and is rarely, in the case of disease, attributable to a single source.

RISK — "the probability that an event will occur, for example, that an individual will become ill or die within a stated period of time, or [at a specific] age" (Last, 1988, 115).

Although a variety of factors are involved, as we noted above, if there is diabetes in your family, you are more *at risk* of developing the disease than others without a family history of the disease. Fatigue and stress render you more vulnerable to, or *at risk* of, developing a cold or the flu than when you are in good physical and emotional condition.

POPULATIONS AT RISK — groups of people who, because of certain risk factors, are more likely to develop a disease or condition.

Nurses and other health workers are more at risk of developing tuberculosis than people in the general population because of their close contact with patients and the potential exposure to the disease from undiagnosed cases. They are also at risk for diseases like Hepatitis B and AIDS (Acquired Immunodeficiency Syndrome) that can be transmitted through body fluids and may enter the bloodstream through a puncture of the skin with an infected needle.

INCIDENCE — "the number of instances of illness commencing, or of people falling ill, during a given period in a specific population" (Last, 1988, 63). For example, the first case of AIDS was diagnosed in Canada in 1979. Since then, the *annual incidence*, or number of new cases, has risen rapidly.

PREVALENCE — "the number of instances of a given disease or other condition in a given population at a designated time" (Last, 1988, 103). In other words, *prevalence* tells us the total number of people in a specific group who are affected at any given time. Malaria, for example, is still *prevalent* in many provinces in China (and in many other parts of the world) and travellers are advised to take precautionary measures when going into these areas.

Although a number of factors must be taken into consideration in the reduction of infant mortality rates in any country, including improvements in the overall socioeconomic well-being of people, there is no doubt that community health nursing services play a large role. Primary health care provided by nurses in the rural villages and on the outer islands of Fiji, for example, includes prenatal monitoring, midwifery services and well-baby clinics and these services have been a significant factor in cutting the infant mortality rate in half in less than 20 years (Government of Fiji, 1986).

In the Canadian North, infant mortality rates have also shown a dramatic decline — from 79.0 to 17.2 per 1000 live births between 1960 and 1986 (Bobet, 1989). The expansion of the Northern nursing program that was started in the 1950s and continued during the 1960s and 1970s by the Medical Services Branch of Health and Welfare Canada is credited with being a significant factor in lowering the infant mortality rates in the North. As recommended by the Royal Commission on Health Services (*Hall Report*) of 1964, each community of 150 persons or more was allocated a nursing station, with at least one Registered Nurse assigned to carry out primary health care (Health Canada, 1993).

Public policy development   "Epidemiology is essential to the development of scientifically responsible public health policy" (Tyler and Last, 1992, 37). Surveillance of the health status of a community and investigation into specific problems provide the baseline data needed for decisions by policy makers. For example, differences in health indicators such as higher-than-average infant mortality rates and a shorter life span in rural and remote areas of British Columbia have led to policies designed to provide better health service to these parts of the province (Government of British Columbia, 1993).

The search for the causes of disease and other health states has enabled us to take action to eliminate many causes of poor health and to reinforce those factors that contribute to good health. For many years, the search for causality focussed on disease entities and the research done in this connection has been of inestimable value in helping to reduce many health problems. The majority of communicable diseases have been brought under control in large part because epidemiologists have traced the *etiology* (science of the causes of disease) of the different diseases. For example, knowledge of the etiology of malaria helped to bring about changes in environmental policy to assist in curbing the disease, by doing such things as draining swampy areas where mosquitoes breed.

The *New Perspective on the Health of Canadians* (Lalonde, 1974) was based on findings from epidemiological studies. Now, studies such as those discussed in the *Active Health Report* are showing that "... health is affected by social and environmental concerns as well as lifestyle and medical factors. Health is inextricably linked to the living and working conditions Canadians enjoy" (Government of Canada, 1987, 3). And, our attention is turning to ways and means of improving the living and working conditions of the socially disadvantaged as a health priority.

THE HEALTHY COMMUNITIES CONCEPT

The *Active Health Report* emphasized that health is affected by social and environmental concerns as well as lifestyle and medical factors. As we discussed in Chapter 2, we tend today to look at health as a much broader concept than we did 20 years ago. Health is seen as a social issue as much as a biological phenomenon. An individual's health is determined not only by biological inheritance and health services but also by the circumstances of our daily lives, our culture and beliefs and by social, economic and physical aspects of our environment. The WHO definition states that health is "the extent to which an individual or group is able, on one hand, to realize aspirations and satisfy needs; and, on the other hand, to change or cope with the environment. Health is, therefore, seen as a resource for everyday life, a dimension of our "quality of life," and not the object of living; it is a positive concept emphasizing social and personal resources as well as physical capabilities" (WHO, 1984).

Recognizing the importance of public policy, particularly at the municipal level, in creating a physical and social environment that promotes health for the community as a whole, the World Health Organization in 1985 launched a five-year Healthy Cities project in Europe as a vehicle for achieving its health promotion goal of "Health for all by the Year 2000" (Boothroyd and Eberle, 1990). In 1988, a similar project was initiated in Canada entitled the Canadian Healthy Communities Project. The project was funded for a three-year period by Health and Welfare Canada. Some Canadian cities, such as Toronto, have kept the WHO ter-

minology of Healthy Cities for their project. However, the Healthy Communities framework is common to all.

The philosophy behind the healthy communities concept is that communities have the ability to identify their own health needs and to plan and manage their own health care — and to do so in a democratic way that involves the whole community. In British Columbia, for example, it is envisioned that management of health services will be delegated to "Community Health Councils" and "Regional Health Boards." Each community will have a "Community Health Council," with members elected by the public and by individuals appointed by the Ministry of Health.

The Community Council will be responsible for planning and coordinating health services in the local area and identifying local health priorities. Regional Health Boards will be composed of representatives from community councils and individuals appointed by the Minister of Health. Initially, these Boards will be responsible for regional health planning and service coordination. In the future, it is anticipated that the Regional Boards will also be responsible for allocation of a regional global budget for health services (Government of British Columbia, 1993). The province of Saskatchewan is also planning to delegate financial responsibility for health services to the local level. Although not all provinces are moving in this direction at the present time, all are involved in major reforms to shift health care to the community.

THE HEALTHY COMMUNITIES PROCESS

In many neighbourhoods, towns and cities across the country, people are using the "healthy communities" process to identify and resolve local health issues. In this context, the community is seen not as the focus of action for health providers but as the *agent* of action. The emphasis is on the democratic process of people, health care providers and community organizations working together to bring about change. Collaboration between different departments of government, voluntary and official health agencies, professional associations and citizen groups is the key to the successful implementation of change. The "healthy communities" process includes conducting surveys, neighbourhood discussions, public forums and holding interviews with key leaders to gather information on health needs and to monitor progress towards the goal of a healthier community (Government of British Columbia, 1992a, b).

Between June 1989 and June 1990, the Town of Princeton experienced an unusual increase in suicide. In response, the town mounted a crisis line staffed by volunteers. The committed response from volunteers is what has made the crisis line work. Unemployment rates in Princeton are high. Making the crisis line work is one way that the residents of the town have banded together to support one another. The challenge now is to build partnerships with other sectors in the community to develop a comprehensive approach to suicide prevention. This has started with discussions between crisis line workers and the hospital health committee.*

DETERMINANTS OF COMMUNITY HEALTH

A healthy community is "one in which all organizations — from informal groups to governments — are working effectively together to improve the quality of all people's lives" (Boothroyd and Eberle, 1990, 7). This definition of the healthy community was formulated in line with the WHO definition of health as "the ability to realize aspirations and satisfy needs and, on the other hand, to change or cope with the environment."

In order to look at the determinants of health in a community we need to examine first the functions of a community. We need to ask ourselves such questions as Why is it that most people prefer to live in communities rather than in isolation? What is the purpose of a community? Why does it exist? When we understand the functions, then we can look at the factors that affect the health of a community by supporting or hindering its ability to perform its various functions. The following sections of this chapter — on functions of a community (and factors affecting these functions) and on community stressors — were developed from material contained in the *Health Indicator Workbook; A tool for healthy communities* (First edition) published by the Office of Health Promotion of the B.C. Ministry of Health and Ministry Responsible for Seniors (1992b).

FUNCTIONS OF A COMMUNITY AND THE FACTORS AFFECTING THESE FUNCTIONS

The "Healthy Communities" projects in British Columbia have identified the following six functions of a community: (1) production, (2) consumption, (3) maintenance of the physical environment, (4) management, (5) growth and development and (6) social support. (Government of British Columbia, 1992b).

Production

Communities produce the goods and services needed to promote good health. A healthy community supports people in their ability to obtain the necessities of life and provides opportunity for them to gain the knowledge and skills needed to cope with and/or change the environment. A thriving business sector and the ready availability of goods and services contribute to the health of a community by providing employment opportunities and a sound economic base for community development.

A community's production capacity is enhanced by the presence of schools, colleges, universities and libraries and by the availability of other educational programs. As we move into the era of the knowledge-based society, it is increasingly apparent that education is one of the most powerful tools at our disposal in developing and maintaining a healthy economy in our communities. A well-educated work force is essential in the new competitive environment of the global economy. And, it is education that provides us with the skills to manage our environment, for example, to develop better ways of controlling — and, ideally, reusing — our human and industrial waste to enhance rather than pollute our environment.

> ### Factors Affecting the Production Function of Communities
> - the soundness and extent of a community's economic base
> - the availability of a wide range of education services

Consumption

A community not only produces goods and services, it also uses them. Our physical and social abilities are strongly influenced by the availability and affordability of goods and services. Food, housing and energy to heat our homes in winter, for example, are essential for good health. But there are also items people purchase that are detrimental to health, such as cigarettes, alcohol, foods with a high fat content and illegal drugs. In looking at the factors affecting health in a community, then, one must consider both aspects of consumption, that is to say, both those things we consume that are good for us and those that are detrimental to our health.

> ### Factors Affecting Consumption in a Community
> - the availability and affordability of goods and services that contribute to good health, for example, nutritious food and adequate housing
> - the ready availability of goods and services detrimental to health, for example, alcohol, drugs and high-fat foods

* Princeton (B.C.) *Healthy Communities 1991 Yearbook.* Victoria, B.C: Office of Health Promotion, British Columbia Ministry of Health and Ministry Responsible for Seniors, 26. Reprinted with permission.

Maintenance of the Physical Environment

As we mentioned in Chapter 2, our physical environment affects our health in many ways, both directly and indirectly. The quality of the air we breathe and the water we drink, the safe handling of our food supplies and of our garbage and sewage all affect us directly. Less direct, but also important, is the quality of the soil on which our fruit and vegetable supplies are grown, the noise level in a community, the availability of recreational sites and the diversity of wildlife.

Factors Affecting Maintenance of the Physical Environment

- the quality of the air we breathe
- the safety of food and water supplies
- the safe disposal of waste
- the availability of recreational sites
- wildlife preservation

Management

Good management is essential for the smooth, efficient functioning of all aspects of community health. A well-managed community identifies its priorities, adapts services to the needs of changing situations and makes the most of resources. In a democratic society, it is essential that people take an active part in local government to ensure that wise and effective decisions are made to meet their needs and to promote a healthy community in which to live and bring up their children. We cannot all be city councillors or other elected office-holders, but we can all vote in elections and on referendums. We can express our opinions at town meetings and through participation in local action groups, on local planning committees and community boards.

It is easy to express our views on what is wrong, but much more difficult to put things right. In order to tackle health problems in the community, priorities must be established and a plan of action developed if things are to be accomplished. Long-range planning in a community is important in order to protect green space, for example, or to ensure the maintenance of water and sewage systems. A community also has to make plans to cope if disaster strikes. Planning is also needed to ensure safe, affordable housing for people, and to see that health and education services are maintained at a high level. The list of planning needs is long and communities usually have to set priorities for action based on what is possible within a given time-frame, and with the resources of the community.

Factors Affecting the Management Function of Communities

- citizen participation in governance
- short- and long-range planning

Growth and Development

A very important function of any community is the promotion of human growth and development of the people who live there. Most communities include a diversity of age groups. Healthy, well-nourished children who are growing and developing normally are essential for the continued renewal of a community.

Also important is a healthy economy that attracts new business into the community. Nor should we forget the importance of the cultural sector in contributing to the intellectual and spiritual growth and development of a community. Early immigrants to Canada knew the importance of cultural stimulation when they established the Chatauqua program that took eminent speakers, well-known musicians and theatrical offerings to rural communities and frontier towns in the late 1890s and early 1900s as part of a continuing education program for people living in rural areas.

Factors Affecting the Promotion of Growth and Development Function of Communities

- the availability and accessibility of health promotion and health protection services for people of all ages
- a business climate conducive to attracting new businesses
- an active cultural sector

Social Support

As pointed out in the Epp Report (1986) and in the Nurturing Health document (1993), health is considerably affected by social relationships. After family and friends, it is the community in which we live that provides us with the most important source of social contacts. A supportive nurturing community also provides people with opportunities for social interaction through recreation programs, clubs, churches, libraries and schools. In supportive communities, you will find that there is no problem recruiting volunteers for community projects. You will probably also

Communities need adequate recreation facilities.

find numerous community associations and projects such as Neighbourhood Watch and Block Parents advertised in the windows of various houses in residential areas.

Community support is also evident in the accessibility of adequate health services — emergency, restorative and palliative — and in the range of social services that are available and accessible to all citizens. A supportive community protects its citizens from violence and other criminal activities.

Factors Affecting the Support Function of Communities

- the availability of affordable and accessible recreation facilities
- opportunities for social interaction (clubs, churches and adult education programs)
- adequate and accessible emergency, restorative, rehabilitative and palliative health services
- an effective social services network
- effective law enforcement

COMMUNITY STRESSORS

We all know communities that are healthy, thriving places where people like to live and bring up their children and others from which people are anxious to move away as soon

as they can. What makes the difference? Why do some communities seem to grow and develop at a rapid rate while the streets of others are lined with empty houses, closed stores and playgrounds where there are no children playing?

There are many stressors that can affect communities negatively and many ways to categorize these stressors. We have opted to discuss the following stressors that can have a negative impact on communities and their ability to carry out their normal functions: (1) economic stressors, (2) population pressures, (3) excessive consumption of harmful substances, (4) physical and chemical stressors and (5) biological stressors. Let us take a look at some of the stressors and the effect they have on the community's ability to perform its major functions.

ECONOMIC STRESSORS

Tough economic times can have a devastating effect on every one of the six major functions of a community. The "Great Depression" of the 1930s that crippled North America, or a business recession such as the one much of Canada experienced in the early 1990s, have a tremendous impact on individual communities throughout the country. When markets slump, the production of goods and services declines. Factories and stores close and people lose employment. They cannot afford to buy the things they need to maintain their health — let alone luxuries — and the consumption of goods and services is decreased. This causes more stores and manufacturing plants to close, creating a further downward spiral of the economy.

When the economy is poor and people are out of work, a strain is put on the support services in a community. Governments have to make more funds available for unemployment insurance and for social assistance. Money left over for environmental services is decreased and the renewal of highways, the development and maintenance of the water supply system, and even the building of needed sewage disposal plants may be postponed. When budgets are tight, all departments, including the health department of a community, must share in cost-cutting. The growth and development function of a community may be jeopardized by the cutting of health promotion and protection services. The cultural sector is always the first place governments look when they are trimming the budget but schools usually suffer too as programs are cut and "non-essential" staff are laid off.

Unemployment is bad for a person's health (Government of Ontario, 1993). Health suffers, not only because of the lessened income but, also, because of the loss of self-esteem. Unemployment affects not only the worker but also the family. Children are likely to worry about who will pay the bills, and whether they will lose their home. Even the insecurity caused by the threat of unemployment can be enough to cause ill health (Government of Ontario, 1993). As we noted in Chapter 2, poor people have more health problems than people with an adequate income. There are also more mental health problems among the children of the poor (Sutherland and Fulton, 1988). Some people turn to alcohol or drugs to provide temporary solace from their problems. And crime often increases as people become desperate for money.

**Potential Community Problems
Resulting from Economic Stressors**

- poverty
- crime and violence
- mental and physical illness
- decaying community infrastructure (highways, water supply systems, etc.)

POPULATION PRESSURES
POPULATION INCREASES

In Canada we have seen rapid increases in population in many of our cities and towns in the past few years. Two factors have contributed to this growth. One is the trend towards urbanization which we mentioned in Chapter 1. The other is immigration. Both factors have put tremendous pressure on all community services from the sheer increase in number of people to be served. We should point out, however, that the growth of a community has both positive and negative effects. Population growth benefits the economy in contributing to the number of new housing starts and to the establishment of more shops and factories to cater to the needs of the increased population. Thus, there is a positive effect on both the production and consumption capacities of communities. Also, many newcomers bring with them specialized skills and knowledge that contribute to the economy. Canadian culture has been considerably enriched by the talents of artists, musicians and writers from many other lands.

Both urbanization and the wave of new immigrants into many of the cities have, however, put tremendous pressures on all community services — health, education, social services and protection services, to name a few. There is a great need for more inpatient and community health services, as well as a need to offer these services in different languages, keeping in mind the cultural differences in health beliefs and customs of people from different countries (see Chapter 12, Health and Ethnicity). There is considerable pressure on the schools as they try to keep up with the demand for classroom places and for qualified teachers. One of the greatest needs is for courses in English as an additional language. There is currently also a great need in most parts of the country to expand post-secondary educational

facilities to prepare the skilled work force needed for today's economy. Immigrants often need help to adjust to their new environment, thus the demand for social services grows. There is also a need for long-time residents of the community to accept the newcomers and to develop tolerance for other people's customs and beliefs. Racial prejudice is unfortunately a problem that many communities must confront and take steps to overcome.

**Potential Community Problems
Resulting from Population Increases**

- lack of affordable housing
- crowded schools
- insufficient post-secondary educational facilities
- racial tensions and conflicting values
- mental health problems
- insufficient services, for example, water and sewage lines, telephone and hydroelectric services, transportation services

---

POPULATION DECREASES

As some communities grow, others get smaller. One of the major reasons for the exodus of people from a community is loss of its economic base. In many parts of Canada, the economy is still largely resource-based and when the mines run out, when crops are poor several years in a row, or there are no more fish on the cod banks, people must leave their home community to seek work elsewhere. You have probably all visited a "ghost town" that was once a thriving community. When the economic base of a community is lost and people have to move elsewhere, it is the younger people who go first, the older ones being more reluctant to give up their homes and cherished possessions. The result is a smaller community with an older population. This puts tremendous pressures on those who stay to maintain all community functions. The tax base created by businesses and working people for the funding of services is decreased, and the human resources to staff services are no longer there.

**Potential Community Problems
Resulting from Population Decreases**

- decreased production capacity
- decreased consumption of goods and services
- decaying infrastructure due to loss of tax base

EXCESSIVE CONSUMPTION OF HARMFUL SUBSTANCES

Cigarettes, alcohol, drugs and greasy, high-fat foods are all detrimental to our health. The dangers of smoking have been well documented in numerous studies and reports. And, there has been a tremendous reduction in the number of smokers in Canada. Still, many continue to smoke, and our health care system is burdened with people whose health has been damaged by smoking.

Damage resulting from the excessive consumption of alcohol affects not only the individual but also the family and the wider community in which they live. We have already talked about the devastating effects of alcohol-related accidents on mortality rates and hospital and rehabilitation needs. Excessive drinking also contributes to family violence and other community problems. The abuse of illegal drugs not only undermines the individual user's health, but is also devastating to families and a major factor in promoting crime in communities.

With regard to the overconsumption of harmful foods, a good many people have changed their eating habits in recent years and are consciously purchasing foods that are lower in fat and cholesterol content and higher in fibre (Government of Canada, 1987; Government of Ontario, 1993). Still, French fries and gravy are a common lunch, as you can observe in many hospital and school cafeterias. As we have pointed out in earlier chapters, poor dietary habits are an important factor in a number of health problems, such as diabetes, heart disease and other circulatory problems that put a strain on our health services.

When we talk about the problems resulting from the excessive consumption of harmful substances, however, we must be careful not to fall into the trap of "blaming the victim." The underlying causes are complex. People who drink too much alcohol, continue to smoke in spite of all the dire warnings, those who are dependent on drugs and people who overeat all need help and *support* from the community — not condemnation. We need to ask why people are making these choices and what can we do to help them to make healthier choices. As pointed out in the Epp Report, lifestyles cannot be changed in isolation without considering the social, economic and environmental context in which people live.

PHYSICAL AND CHEMICAL STRESSORS

Among the physical stressors affecting communities are factors such as pollution, radiation, noise, workplace hazards, severe weather conditions and the forces of nature.

Most of us are aware of the dangers of environmental degradation these days. It is frequently a leading topic in our newspapers, on television and radio. Both indoor and outdoor atmospheric pollution are problems in many communities. Heavy traffic on the highways, and smoke from mills, manufacturing plants and incinerators combine to create the "smog" that hangs over many large cities. This smog can become so bad that people with asthma and other respiratory problems may experience difficulties in breathing. Our water, food and milk supplies can also become polluted. On the West Coast, it is not unusual for a warning to be issued, advising people not to eat the shellfish coming from specific areas because of the contamination. The emptying of waste products from lumber mills into the ocean near the fishing grounds has been blamed in some instances for contamination of the fish. All levels of government have a responsibility to control pollution in areas under their jurisdiction. The Federal Government, for example, sets standards in regard to matters such as the content of water supplies, foods and drugs. Provincial governments are taking steps to restrict the amount of chlorine and other noxious substances in the effluent of mills and manufacturing plants. There is a need for the establishment of regulations regarding the safe disposal of noxious products and, also, a need for constant monitoring to ensure that manufacturing plants, mills and other industries are adhering to the regulations. Many municipalities have established safety levels for air pollution in their community and building standards for allowable smokestacks and other possible sources of air pollutants.

People are concerned about the depletion of the ozone layer, a phenomenon which results in increased levels of harmful ultraviolet (UV) rays. Overexposure to UV rays is linked to skin cancer; many weather-monitoring stations now report the UV index (a measure of the strength of UV rays) on a daily basis during the summer season and advise people on the length of time they can stay in the sun before skin starts to burn.

Radiation is an increasing problem in our technological age. The use of atomic fuel as a source of energy is a controversial issue. It is a clean and efficient fuel source but there are worries about its manufacture and use.

Potential Community Problems Resulting from Excessive Consumption of Harmful Substances

- crime and violence
- excessive mortality and hospitalization rates
- family disintegration
- excessive number of health problems, such as heart conditions, stroke, lung cancer and chronic lung disorders, obesity, diabetes, etc.

Although we have been assured that the production process in atomic energy plants in Canada is safe, people worry that a disaster like the one at Chernobyl in Ukraine or at Three Mile Island in the United States, due to leakage or an explosion at a nuclear plant, may occur here as well. There is also much concern about the health risks involved in the disposal of nuclear wastes.

Also unknown are the effects of computers, microwaves, cellular telephones and other common factors in our daily lives. Too much radiation can cause genetic defects. People who work with radioactive materials must constantly be monitored to ensure that they do not receive too much radiation. Nurses and other health workers also need to take special precautions when caring for patients who are receiving treatments involving radiation, or the use of radioactive substances. The hydroelectric lines running over residential communities are also a concern to many because of the unknown long-term effects of electromagnetic fields. In newer communities, these are now being placed underground.

Noise, which is a common characteristic of many workplaces and city streets, is another pollutant that must be kept under control. The hustle and bustle of city streets and the noise of traffic on the highways is something we have learned to live with, but excessive noise can be harmful in that it actually destroys some of the 15 000–20 000 sensitive hair cells lining the cochlea. Repeated noise will destroy the nerve fibers leading to these cells, causing deafness. One should beware, then, of the dangers of turning the volume too high on radio and stereo sets.

There are also hazardous chemical products that we encounter in our everyday living — in the home and in the workplace. There are numerous other workplace hazards besides noise, radiation and air pollution that are of concern to workers, unions, employers and health authorities. The Workers' Compensation Boards, or in some provinces, the Department of Labour, have developed safety standards for most industries and these are enforceable by law.

Nor should we forget the effects of severe weather conditions and natural phenomena such as earthquakes, hurricanes (typhoons), floods and the like which put such tremendous stress on communities. In Canada we have learned to dress appropriately to withstand the bitter cold of our northern winters and to build houses that will keep us warm in the winter and cool in the summer. Still, a prolonged "cold snap," a heavy snowfall, torrential rains or a prolonged hot spell can cause havoc in a community. Excessively severe weather can cause floods, violent windstorms and the like.

There is much concern currently about the effects of the weather on people's health. Infants, older people, people with cardiovascular disease and the chronically ill are particularly at risk when environmental temperatures are extremely high or low. The problem is more acute when there is a prolonged period of heat combined with high humidity. Many people find that moods are affected by the weather; most of us feel more cheerful on a sunny day than on one that is dull and grey. *Seasonal affective disorder (SAD)* is the term given to a depression induced by insufficient exposure to sunlight.

A *Public Health Inspector monitoring the noise levels at a construction site*

Potential Community Problems Resulting from Physical and Chemical Stressors

- atmospheric pollution
- pollution of water, food and/or milk supplies
- health problems — respiratory, gastrointestinal, genetic and other problems
- civic disaster

BIOLOGICAL STRESSORS

Biological stressors are those caused by living organisms. Included in this category are plants, insects and animals, and the infectious agents that cause disease.

Plants are an essential element in renewal of oxygen in the atmosphere and, thus, the promotion of a healthy environment. Many plants are used in the preparation of medicines, prescription and over-the-counter drugs as well as herbal remedies. However, some plants are poisonous.

Poison ivy and poison oak, for example, can cause severe skin conditions. Other plants are poisonous when eaten, such as, some varieties of mushrooms, holly, honeysuckle and the spider plant (Clark, 1992).

Insects and animals frequently serve as both reservoirs and carriers of disease-causing agents. Flies, fleas, cockroaches, mosquitoes and animals such as rats, cats and dogs often bring disease into a community. The malaria that caused so many deaths among soldiers building the Rideau Canal from Ottawa to Kingston in the early 1800s was carried by the swarms of malaria-carrying mosquitoes that infested the marshy lands through which the canal was built. Rats are thought to have been the principal carriers of the Plague that devastated Europe in the Middle Ages.

The draining of swampy marshes and other measures used to eradicate mosquitoes have rid us of the malaria problem in this country but it is still a problem in many parts of the world. Rats and other rodents still infest some communities in Canada, particularly the sea ports. We should not forget that dogs, cats and other household pets can also be vectors (carriers) of disease. Not only are there insects that can bring disease, but some, such as grasshoppers and locusts, can destroy crops, which can destroy the economic base of a farming community. Destruction of crops can devastate both the production and consumption functions of a community as well as the physical environment.

Other biological factors are the infectious agents that cause disease. They may be transmitted by air currents, by person-to-person contact, by animals and insects (as we have noted above) or by other vectors. It is estimated that, worldwide, 80 percent of all communicable diseases are transmitted by infectious agents in water (Page, 1987, 105–138).

Potential Community Problems Resulting from Biological Stressors

* pestilence
* disease
* epidemics
* economic distress

HEALTH CARE IN THE COMMUNITY

The following was written by a nurse currently practising in the field of community health in Vancouver, British Columbia:

The role of the nurse in community settings requires continual consideration of the overall health of the community, and the strengths and capabilities of those within it.

Health is now understood to be a resource for everyday living, and health promotion as "a process which enables people to increase control over, and improve their health" (Ottawa Charter, 1986). Community health nurses who understand their primary role to be one of promoting health have good success when they build on the capacity of the local community to support an acceptable quality of life for individuals, families and neighbourhoods. The nurse must consider the ability of the community to support healthful living. The most effective strategies for health promotion in the community focus on forming partnerships. Collaboration with citizens, professionals, associations, agencies, and other individuals and groups help to identify and resolve health issues. The process increases opportunities for people to have control over their health.

Nurses work in a variety of community settings such as homes, workplaces, community health centres, public health units, clinics and schools. Nursing interaction in each of these settings includes working with individuals, families, groups and the community as a whole. A nurse's role in promoting health varies with the setting, the health issues identified, the level of interaction (individual or group) and the strengths and abilities of those involved. Despite these variables, however, the common role is that of the skilled facilitator who may, for example, be working in partnership with a person who is managing a chronic disease, or a group of citizens who are concerned about the safety of the streets in a neighbourhood. Utilizing additional health promotion strategies in community settings further builds on the strengths of those involved, and in turn, increases resources for everyday living.

P. Lynn Buhler, RN, BSN, MSc
Manager
Health Promotion and Prevention Programs
Vancouver Health Department
West Main Health Unit
October 1993

ASSESSMENT OF THE HEALTH OF A COMMUNITY

In your nursing program you will have courses on community health nursing. This chapter is intended as merely an introduction to the field of community health nursing. We will not, therefore, describe a detailed assessment tool but will, instead, suggest ways in which you, as a beginning student, can look at the health of a community. The basic methods you can use include gathering information by (1) reviewing statistical data and literature related to the community, (2) direct observation and (3) talking with people who live and/or work in that community. Other methods that are used in the "Healthy Communities" process to gather information on a community's health needs and to monitor its progress towards a healthier state include surveys, neighbourhood discussions, public forums ("town hall" type meetings) and interviews with community leaders.

When gathering information about a community, it can be useful to focus on how well it is carrying out its major functions of production, consumption, maintenance of the physical environment, management, growth and development and social support.

GATHERING BASELINE DATA ABOUT A COMMUNITY

The data collected, compiled and analyzed by Statistics Canada and by the Vital Statistics Departments of provincial Ministries of Health can provide a lot of valuable information about a community. Census data, for example, gives basic information about a given population, such as total number of people, age and sex distribution, ethnic origin of inhabitants, population density (number of people per square kilometre) and birth rates. Government health departments — federal, provincial and municipal — usually collect and publish basic health statistics, such as life expectancy rates; maternal, infant and child mortality rates; leading causes of death and major illnesses. These statistics are often broken down to the county or municipal level. A good source of information on specific topics such as the health of people who live in the North or trends in child mortality is the Statistics Canada Quarterly entitled *Canadian Social Trends*.

COLLECTING INFORMATION BY DIRECT OBSERVATION

You can learn a lot about a community by walking about the streets. If you keep in mind the community functions we talked about and look for evidence of the factors affecting these functions which we discussed above, you will be able to develop a focus for your observations.

The factors affecting the *production function* of a community are the soundness and extent of the community's economic base and the availability of a wide range of educational services. The businesses, manufacturing plants, shops and offices, banks and other places where people are employed are all relevant. Important, too, are the number and types of schools and colleges in the area. Regarding the *consumption function*, the price of groceries, for example, and whether there is a good supply of fresh foods and vegetables can be very revealing. The type of housing in the area — single-family homes, apartments, high rises etc. — their state of repair and the number of "For rent" and "For sale" signs can be important indicators of the consumption function within a community. The state of the physical environment of the community can also be assessed on a preliminary basis by wandering around it. How clean are the streets? Are there trees in residential areas, parks and other recreational sites? Are these clean or littered with empty bottles, beverage cans, paper and the like? A Public Health Inspector might be able to provide specific information about the safety of food and

water supplies. You can assess, on your own, however, the cleanliness or lack of it, in stores, in restaurants and fast-food outlets in the neighbourhood — and you can note garbage on the streets or in the alleyways. People from countries where waste disposal is more of a problem than it is here are often both amused and impressed by the neatly tied green garbage bags sitting at the curb on garbage pickup days in Canadian cities. Indications of a healthy physical environment can also be observed from the parks and other recreation sites in the community, as well as the wildlife living in them.

How well the *management function* of a community is operating can be difficult to assess just by walking around a community. However, attending, as an observer, a meeting of the community/town council or other elected body can provide some information.

Although more precise data from other sources should be gathered, one can also observe in "walkabouts" the *growth and development function* of the community. Are there many mothers with small children in the grocery stores, strolling the streets or playing in the parks? Are there a lot of older people in the neighbourhood? Do you see notices regarding health promotional activities such as the services of a health unit, well-baby clinics or "wellness centres" for older people? Many large grocery stores now have "smart shopper" or similar programs with a nutritionist helping people select the most nutritious foods of the choices available. In the context of cultural growth and development, is there evidence of cultural activities in the community — art galleries, theatres, playhouses? Is there advertising for concerts, plays by a local theatrical group in neighbourhood stores or on bulletin boards in the grocery store? Does the community look prosperous enough to support cultural activities?

With regard to the *support function*, is there a community centre? If so, what sorts of programs do they have for different age groups in the community? Is the community centre busy with groups of people doing different things, such as a group of older adults playing cards, a pre-school group colouring, older children playing basketball in the gym or swimming in the pool? Are there many churches in the neighbourhood? Do you see "Neighbourhood Watch" or "Block Parent" signs in the windows of many houses?

The location of health services in the community is also an important indicator of a community's overall functioning. Are there other health agencies in the community — physicians' offices and those of other health practitioners such as physiotherapists, massage therapists, naturopaths? Do you see any local social service agencies? Are there many police officers on the streets and/or patrolling the neighbourhood in cars? In Canada, there are three levels of police: municipal, provincial (in some provinces) and the Royal Canadian Mounted Police (RCMP) who provide police services in communities and rural areas without a provincial or municipal service. At all levels, police officers work in partnership with community groups, in talking in the schools about street safety or running programs to teach children the rules of the road by driving miniature cars.

DR. SHIRLEY M. STINSON (b. 1929)

Shirley Stinson, one of Canada's most distinguished nurses, has a number of "firsts" among her many contributions to health care generally and to nursing and nursing research in particular. In 1972, she was the first nurse (and the first woman) to receive a Senior National Health Scientist Award (National Health Research and Development Program (NHRDP)). She completed only one year of the term of the award as she took a position as Acting Director of the University of Alberta's Nursing program. However, she was then selected to serve on several NHRDP Review Committees that helped select those to receive the Senior National Health Scientist Award.

Dr. Stinson also was the founding chair of the first nursing research foundation in Canada to be funded by provincial or federal monies, the Alberta Foundation for Nursing Research, which was established in 1982. This foundation was the culmination of her efforts between 1972 and 1982 to achieve such status for nursing.

Born in Arlee, Saskatchewan, Shirley Stinson was raised in Alberta and received a bachelor of science in nursing from the University of Alberta in 1953. She took a master's degree in nursing service administration from the University of Minnesota in 1958 and a doctorate in higher education in nursing from Columbia University, New York, in 1969. Except for a four-year stint as Associate Director of Nursing Services with the Hospital for Sick Children in Toronto, she was associated for most of her career with the University of Alberta. In 1969, she was the first nurse in Canada to be given a joint appointment to teach in both the Nursing and the Health Sciences Administration departments. During her appointment with the Faculty of Nursing at the University of Alberta, she served for various terms as Acting Director and Associate Dean for Graduate Education. She was the principal developer of Canada's first doctoral nursing (PhD Nursing) program in 1991 and in 1988, she started working with three "special case" nursing students who were working towards this doctoral degree.

While teaching at the University of Alberta, she also held several other joint teaching appointments, with the Faculty of Medicine at the University of Alberta and with the Faculty of Nursing at the University of Calgary. She also carried out a large amount of nursing research of her own, including major studies on nursing education needs in Canada and investigations into doctoral preparation for nursing, including several national studies on doctoral preparation for nurses. During this time, she also served as an officer with nursing associations provincially, nationally and internationally, including a term as president of the Canadian Nurses Association from 1980 to 1982.

Upon her retirement from the University of Alberta at the end of 1993, she was described as "Alberta's most distinguished nurse." Her honours and awards are many, including the Jeanne Mance Award from the Canadian Nurses Association, the Ross Award for Leadership from the Canadian Nurses Foundation, and the Alberta Achievement Award for Excellence from the Government of Alberta. She holds honorary doctorates from the University of Calgary and Memorial University. Following her retirement, she had plans to serve as visiting professor at various universities, including at least one appointment in Australia.

— Glennis Zilm

GATHERING INFORMATION BY TALKING WITH PEOPLE

A good way to learn how people perceive the community's ability to carry out its major functions is to meet and talk with them informally — in the community centre, in the grocery store, in the coffee shop. As you gain skills in interpersonal relationships and in communication, you will find it much easier to elicit information from people about business and educational facilities in the community. You will want to find out about the availability of affordable housing, for example, and the cost of living in that community. You will want to find out where people go when they are sick. How do they feel about the health services that are available? Once you have gained their trust, people will usually talk about their concerns.

Many of these concerns will probably not be "traditional" health concerns. One community health council's survey of health needs in four communities in the Fraser Valley (outside Vancouver) found that the issues varied in the different communities. The major concerns were similar, the issue of affordable and accessible health care the

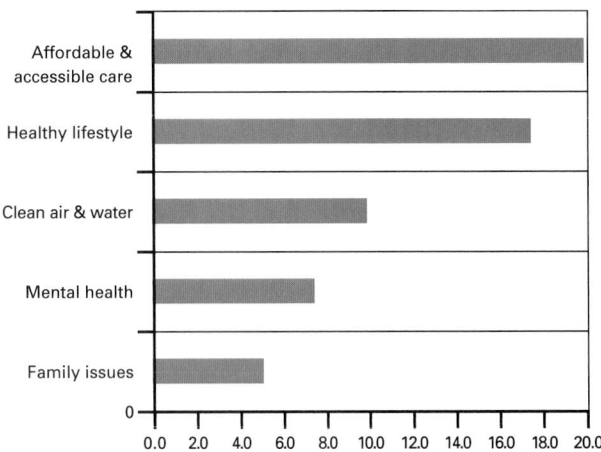

FIGURE 11.1   Most important health issue

SOURCE: South Fraser Valley Health Council. *Regional and Community Health Profile: An Initial Perspective July 1993*. White Rock. Author, 12. Reproduced with permission of the Council.

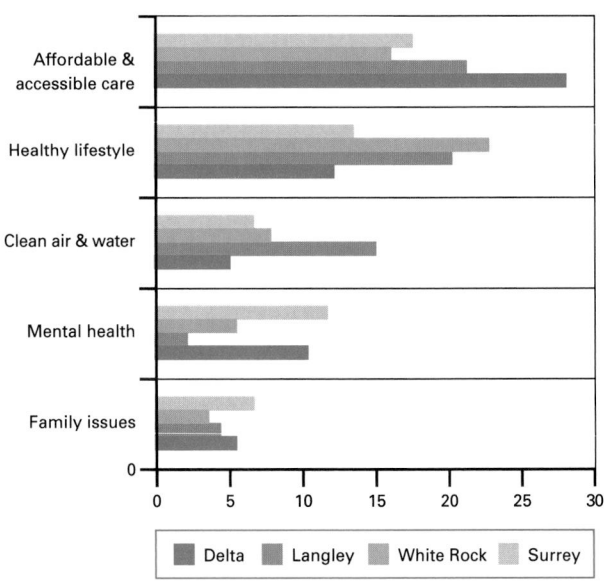

FIGURE 11.2   Most important health issue, by community

SOURCE: South Fraser Valley Health Council. *Regional and Community Health Profile: An Initial Perspective July 1993*. White Rock. Author, 12. Reproduced with permission of the Council.

most important concern (see Figure 11.1). You will note, however, in Figure 11. 2, that some issues were of more concern than others in each of the four communities (South Fraser Valley Health Council, 1993). It should be noted that this survey was not an official research project, but provides an example of what a community group can do to get the "feel" of their community regarding health issues.

INTERPRETING THE RESULTS

Once you have collected the data, you will want to try to identify problems in the community. If you are acting as a resource person for people in a community in a Healthy Communities or similar project, analysis of the data might be accomplished by the group. Statistical data for individual communities can be compared with national and provincial data and with that of other communities in the province. For example, you will probably find a difference in infant mortality rates in regions across a province and different rates of crime and violence in specific communities. Average income of families in the community will certainly vary, as will the number of people with high school completion or post-secondary education. You can compare your community with that of other communities in the city, if you live in a major urban centre, in the province and also with the national average.

You can also collate the impressions you have gained by walking around the neighbourhood or community and the data you have picked up from talking with people. These can be grouped under the six major functions of the community to create a community profile.

For those working in Healthy Communities projects wishing to do a more specific analysis, the Office of Health Promotion of the B.C. Ministry of Health and Ministry Responsible for Seniors has developed a *Health Indicator Workbook* (First edition, 1992) as a tool to assist commu-

nities to gather information about their health needs and to monitor the community's progress towards a healthier community. They point out that there are numerous criteria that could be developed. The ones shown in the workbook are examples of criteria that have been found useful in Healthy Communities projects.

NURSING INTERVENTIONS IN THE COMMUNITY

The distinction is rapidly blurring between institutional and community health care. Many hospitals are becoming "hospitals without walls," as nurses and other health professionals take services out to people in the homes. For example, an enterostomy service that has been strictly hospital-based may be extended to have the nurses doing preoperative counselling and follow-up visits to teach people to care for their "ostomies" at home. Another example is the Early Postpartum Discharge program of the Lions Gate Hospital in North Vancouver, British Columbia. Patients who meet specific criteria are discharged home within 24 hours of giving birth. Nurses employed at Lions Gate Hospital make home visits on Days 2, 3, 5 and 10 postpartum. During their visits, they assess the health status of both mother and baby, provide education on aspects of self and infant care, and provide emotional support and counselling to the new parents as they cope with integrating the new baby into the family. This usually involves a reintegration of the family, a redefinition of the roles of members and changes in their relationships as they return to family lifestyles and the activities of daily living.

Community agencies and hospitals are also getting together in partnerships to offer people more continuity of care. We have come a long way since the VON assigned the first "Liaison Nurse" to the Montreal General Hospital in 1955 to discuss discharge plans with patients and coordinate the services needed (VON, 1983).

In the community, nurses are at work in all phases of the health care continuum — in health promotion and health protection activities, in providing restorative and rehabilitative services involving direct care in the home and in providing comfort and support to people with chronic and terminal illness.

HEALTH PROMOTION ACTIVITIES

A major portion of the community health nurse's work has always been in health promotion activities — helping people learn how to live a healthier life. Traditionally, this has involved activities such as prenatal classes for pregnant women (fathers are now included), visits to new mothers, well-baby clinics, and school and employee health programs. Since the Lalonde Report in 1974 pointed out the link between lifestyle and the major causes of death (heart disease, strokes and accidents), health promotion has become a large part of the work of national, provincial and municipal health agencies. A Health Promotion Directorate at Health and Welfare Canada and similar units in Provincial Ministries of Health and Municipal Departments have been established.

As we mentioned in Chapter 3, Health Care in Canada, our ideas about health promotion have broadened considerably over the years since the Lalonde Report (1974). By the mid-1970s, health promotional activities had expanded from teaching people to adopt a healthy lifestyle to include education, training and research, legislation, policy coordination and community development. The Ottawa Charter defined health promotion as "the process of enabling people to increase control over, and to improve, their health" (1986). A key word here is *empowerment* — the health professional's task is to help people to take control of their own health. It is essential that people take an active role in developing programs to suit individual and community needs.

NURSES AT WORK

I am a Community Health Nurse with the City of Vancouver Health Department. Three years ago, the West Main Health Unit in Vancouver made a decision to assign a Community Health Nurse to work with residents in the Little Mountain neighbourhood. This is a middle class neighbourhood in which many recent immigrants have settled over the past few years. The role of this Community Health Nurse (CHN) was to work with local residents to address issues affecting the livability of Little Mountain. I volunteered to undertake the project.

In the first few months, I identified key informants who could provide me with some background information about the area and activities that were taking place. The steering committee for a Community Awareness Survey invited me to be a member. This survey was a tool to collect demographic data and to identify interested residents who would like to participate in organized actions aimed at strengthening community networks.

After completion of the survey, I helped to establish the Little Mountain Healthy Communities Initiative and secure funding from the Ministry of Health. Residents decided to use the funds to hire a community development worker. I then worked closely with the residents and the community development worker to set up community meetings. At these meetings, the residents debated issues that were important and formulated action plans to address some of these concerns. Examples of these included:

1. traffic

2. the need to increase community cohesiveness

3. a business sector that was not reflecting the needs of the residents

4. petty crime.

The residents set up small committees to examine some of these issues more closely. Many of these neighbourhood concerns have been solved through the cooperation between residents, social agencies and civic government.

In this project, I maintained the role of a facilitator at community meetings and a resource person to liaise with the different levels of government. The community identified the issues and decided on the approach to address them. This approach differs from the traditional medical model that employs a top-down approach to problem-solving. In the Healthy Communities framework, the role of health professionals changes depending on the needs of the community in question. This bottom-up approach allows residents to become experts in their particular communities and me to maintain a supportive role.

— Vanessa Lam, BScN, RN

It is also important for people to be able to make choices regarding the programs they want to participate in to improve their health (Epp, 1986, 3). The Epp Report suggests three mechanisms for promoting health:

1. self-care, the decisions and actions individuals take in the interest of their own health
2. mutual aid, the actions people take to help each other
3. healthy environments, the creation of conditions and surroundings conducive to health.

The implementation of these three mechanisms involves nurses in many non-traditional activities to promote the health of people in the community. The Victorian Order of Nurses has been instrumental in pioneering many programs for various groups in the community. One example is the Foot Care Clinics which have enabled many older adults with painful feet to participate in walking and other exercise programs. Another program initiated by the VON, but taken over in many communities now by official or other voluntary agencies, is Meals-on-Wheels which ensures the recipient of at least one good hot meal a day. In line with the newer definition of health promotion to enable people to take control of their own health, the VON initiated community development programs to encourage older adults to participate in developing their own programs. This program was titled PEP, an acronym for Promoting Elders' Participation, and was targeted primarily for rural and underserviced areas. The VON provided a Coordinator to establish the group. The PEP undertakes needs assessments and explores ways and means of supplying the needed services (Du Gas and Beckingham, 1993; VON, 1988, 1991).

HEALTH PROTECTION ACTIVITIES

Among the activities of nurses in the health protection segment of the health care spectrum are those involving the control of communicable disease, screening programs to detect the early development of health problems in people at risk for specific disorders and environmental safety programs.

The Control of Communicable Diseases

Nurses are very involved both in preventing the spread of infection of communicable disease and in carrying out immunization programs to increase the resistance of people to these diseases. The nurse is very often the person who identifies the disease, for example, when examining school children. The nurse is often responsible for identifying people who have been exposed to a disease, informing them that they have been exposed and referring them to the appropriate agency for testing and treatment (Clark, 1992). Nursing interventions in the prevention of communicable disease include teaching people precautions that should be taken to prevent other members of a family and other people from developing the disease. As we mentioned in Chapter 2, most of the infectious diseases that were the leading causes of death at the beginning of this century have been virtually eliminated. One of the main reasons has been the development and widespread use of vaccines and other immune-producing agents. Today, immunization is available for many communicable diseases including the childhood diseases of measles, mumps, rubella, diphtheria, pertussis and polio. Immunization is also available for hepatitis B, diseases caused by the *Hemophilus influenzae* Type B bacteria (Clark, 1992). Nurses often carry out immunization programs in a community.

Screening Programs

Screening is done to detect disease in its early stages. It is "a preliminary examination or testing of a person to determine whether or not he or she might have a particular condition and whether further diagnostic testing is indicated" (Clark, 1992, 435). A woman with a family history of cancer of the breast may be advised to have a mammogram (an X-ray of the breast) on a yearly basis as a screening procedure whereas other women without family histories of the disease would not have this diagnostic procedure done as often. The screening, which includes a thorough physical examination of the breast, is often carried out by nurses. For many years, a routine chest X-ray was included in the admission procedure to hospitals to screen for tuberculosis (the procedure is no longer part of the admissions routine). Screening may also be carried out for sexually transmitted diseases, for example, in people who have been exposed to chlamydia, gonorrhea or HIV, the human immunodeficiency virus that causes AIDS (Clark, 1992).

The eye examinations and hearing tests carried out on children starting school in the public school system are other examples of screening programs.

Environmental Safety Activities

The nurse collaborates with a number of other health workers and with workers from other sectors in carrying out environmental safety activities in the community. Among the others concerned with environmental safety are Public Health Inspectors, whose main focus is environmental safety, the Medical Officers of Health, whose mandate concerns all possible sources of ill-health in the community, social workers concerned with the living conditions of people (among other things) and the Fire Department who carry out fire prevention programs in the community. In the workplace, the nurse and the Occupational Safety Officer work in collaboration. During home visits, nurses have a good opportunity to observe conditions in the household and to advise on measures to make the house a safer place. In families with young children, for example, parents may want some help in "child-proofing" the house. A great many devices are available to make home environments safer for older people and those with disabilities. These include "grab-bars" for bathtubs, handrails for walls and numerous other adaptations to normal household equipment.

NURSING INTERVENTIONS IN RESTORATIVE AND SUPPORTIVE CARE

The interventions nurses carry out in the community to help people to restore their health or to cope with long-term or terminal illness include direct "hands-on" nursing care, monitoring the health of people with various illnesses, counselling and providing emotional support for patients with long-term and terminal illness and their families, coordinating care given by others and teaching and supervising other caregivers (Bullough and Bullough, 1990).

Direct Care

Home nursing has been part and parcel of community nursing in Canada from the early 1700s when the Grey Nuns began visiting the sick in their homes in Montreal. However, it did not become an integral part of secular nursing until the establishment of the VON in the latter part of the 19th century. Today, with early hospital discharge, the tremendous increase in "day surgery," and the increased provision of services in the home, there has been considerable expansion of the need for highly skilled nurses in the community (Bullough and Bullough, 1990).

Direct nursing care is also needed by many people with long-term illnesses and by people who are terminally ill. In providing direct care in the home, nurses may assist patients with hygiene measures, they may carry out treatments, such as dressings, or injections and they may administer medications. Many patients have intravenous and other types of therapy which the nurse administers, or teaches patients or family members to administer (Bullough and Bullough, 1990).

Monitoring Health Status

Many people with acute or long-term illness need a nurse to check on their progress at regular and frequent intervals. The postoperative patient's incision needs to be looked at to make sure the wound is healing, for example, and the new mother and infant need to be monitored to see that both are doing well. The nurse can use the visit to answer questions, perhaps incorporate some new health teaching as well as follow up on the teaching carried out in the hos-

pital. People with illnesses that are of long duration, such as hypertension, diabetes and arthritis, need regular visits. In the case of the hypertensive patient, the nurse would visit to check the blood pressure; with the diabetic patient, to make sure the disease is not getting out of control; and with the arthritic patient, to see that he or she is coping adequately with the activities of daily living and is not troubled with too much pain. If things are not proceeding normally, the nurse can then take appropriate action to have the problem taken care of before expensive hospitalization is needed.

Coordinating Home Care Services

Many nurses serve as coordinators, or "Case Managers," for people needing care in the home. In this capacity, they undertake the initial assessment of the patient's needs and develop a plan of care. They also make arrangements for the services of nursing, physiotherapy or occupational therapy, for "homemaker" services or whatever is needed. They monitor the care given and intervene if problems occur. Here, it is the nurse, rather than the physician, who acts as a "gatekeeper" for health care services (Bullough and Bullough, 1990; Clark, 1992).

Teaching and Supervising Other Caregivers

Paid caregivers in the home include a variety of workers: Registered Nurses, Licensed Practical Nurses (Registered/Certified Nursing Assistants), Long-term Care Aides, Attendants and Sitters/Companions. In addition, a family member or a friend may be the principal caregiver for a person needing nursing care, personal care or supervision in the home. The Registered Nurse is often responsible for teaching basic nursing techniques to paid caregivers who have not had formal preparation, such as Attendants and Sitters/Companions before they are assigned to cases. The nurse is also available to teach the family member or friend who is a principal caregiver. Family members providing care in the home are not infrequently on 24-hour duty, seven days a week, as in the case of someone caring for a spouse who has Alzheimer's Disease (a chronic organic mental disorder). It is important to remember that volunteer caregivers need relief or they too will become ill. A variety of caregiver relief services are available, including daycare centres and day programs for the elderly and the handicapped. We discussed a number of these programs in Chapters 3 and 4. The nurse who is going into the home is well suited to assess the caregiver's needs, suggest ways and means for respite and, if needed, make the necessary referrals.

Providing Counselling for People with Long-term Illness

People with long-term or terminal illness and their families need help in coping with the illness. In addition to the physical problems associated with both long-term and terminal illness, the mental anguish that accompanies them needs to be addressed. There is a need for people to come to terms with illness — to adjust to decreasing physical, and sometimes mental, ability. If patients have to depend on others to do things for them, they feel keenly the loss of the independence they have cherished. People need to be able to talk through their feelings. Often, they do not want to distress family members by discussing these feelings with them and feel more comfortable talking with a nurse. We will be returning to this topic in Chapter 16, Communication Skills, and also in Chapter 36, Death, Loss and Grief. Many nurses work on palliative care teams, providing comfort and support to people who are terminally ill and to their families.

KEY TERMS

community p. 256

epidemiology p. 257

epidemiological model p. 257

experimental studies p. 257

demonstration project p. 258

causality p. 259

risk p. 259

populations at risk p. 259

incidence p. 259

prevalence p.2 59

etiology p. 260

seasonal affective disorder (SAD) p. 266

screening p. 272

IN REVIEW

A major factor in the improvement of health in the Western world over the past 150 years has been the reduction of environmental hazards through the institution of public health measures by local governments. Today, the community is viewed as the basic unit in health care and so it is important for nurses to understand how a community functions as well as the factors that affect the health of the people in communities and the nurse's role in community health.

The science of epidemiology has been used extensively to assess the health of communities. The methodology of epidemiology includes the systematic collection of health data and the search for causes of various states of health. Until fairly recently, epidemiological studies were concerned primarily with the causes of disease, but the focus has now expanded to include the health status of people and the factors determining health. Epidemiological studies have been very useful in adding to our knowledge of the manifestations of specific diseases and in the identification of risk factors. They have also been used to develop health profiles of communities, to identify health problems, to control epidemics, to determine the impact of health programs and to assist in the formulation of public health policy.

The "healthy communities" approach looks at the health of a community by assessing its ability to carry out its various functions. These functions include production, consumption, maintenance of the physical environment, management, growth and development and social support. Healthy communities are those in which all functions are carried out well. Through assessing the functioning of their community, people can identify their community's health needs and then plan, prioritize and manage their own health care.

The nurse's role in community health is primarily that of promoting health, through enabling people to assume control of and improve their own health. Nurses are therefore concerned with the community's ability to support healthy living as well as with the health of individuals, families and other groups. They work in collaboration with citizens, professional agencies and other individuals and groups to identify and resolve health issues.

Community health nurses work in all phases of the health care continuum. Health promotion activities include helping people to live healthier lives (self-care), to help each other (mutual aid) and to create an environment that is conducive to healthy living (community development). The nurse's health protection activities include the control of communicable diseases, screening programs and environmental safety programs. In restorative and supportive care, nurses provide direct care, they monitor the health of the acutely ill and those with long-term illness and they assist people and their families to cope with acute, long-term and terminal illnesses. In addition, they coordinate home-care services and they teach and supervise other caregivers in the home.

LEARNING ACTIVITIES

Select a city neighbourhood or a small rural community to which you have access and see what you can find out about the health of that community from a literature search, from direct observation and from talking with people in the community. Some questions are suggested to help you to organize your plan for gathering information (you may want to add more).

1. Review statistical data and literature in the area.
   a) How many people live in the community?
   b) What is the approximate age distribution of the population?
   c) What is the population density?
   d) What are the predominant ethnic groups?
   e) What statistical data have been collected on the health status of people in this community?
   f) Are there brochures or pamphlets about the community in the library or a community centre?

2. Walk around the streets and look around. Look for evidence of community functioning in regard to:

   a) *Production*
   - What businesses, manufacturing plants, shops and offices do you see?
   - Do these look prosperous or shabby?
   - What types of schools and colleges are there? What other educational programs exist there?
   - Is there a public library? If so, is it busy?

   b) *Consumption*
   - Is there a good supply of fresh fruits and vegetables in the local shops?
   - Is the price of groceries high, average or low in the shops?
   - What type of housing is there in the area: single family dwellings, apartment blocks, townhouse complexes?
   - What is the state of repair of the residences?
   - How many "For rent" and "For sale" signs do you see?

   c) *Maintenance of the Physical Environment*
   - How clean are the streets?
   - Are there trees in the residential areas? Are there parks or green spaces or other recreational sites?
   - How clean are the shops, restaurants and fast food outlets? The parks and recreational areas?

   d) *Management*
   If possible, attend a meeting of the community council.
   - Is there a good representation of both men and women, people of different age groups, various ethnic groups and people representing different interests?
   - What issues are of concern?

   e) *Growth and Development*
   - Are there many mothers with small children in the grocery stores, in the parks or strolling on the streets?
   - Are there notices regarding health promotional activities?
   - Does the community have an art gallery, a theatre or any other evidence of cultural activity?

   f) *Social Support*
   - Is there a community centre? If so, what types of programs does it offer?
   - Is there a "Senior Citizen" centre?
   - Are there many places of worship in the area?
   - Do you see many "Neighbourhood Watch" or "Block Parent" signs in the windows of residences?
   - Are there police officers on the streets?
   - What health services are available in the community?

3. Talk with some residents of the community informally to supplement the information you have obtained from your literature search and your observations. Some of the questions you might ask are:
   - Do you think this is a good neighbourhood to live in?
   - What are your reasons for saying yes (or no)?
   - What are business opportunities like here?
   - Are there good educational facilities?
   - What are real estate prices like?
   - Where do you go when you are ill?
   - How do you feel about the health services and the recreational facilities in the community?
   - Is there much crime in the community?
   - Do you think this is a healthy community? Why or why not?
   - Do you think the community is well run?
   - What are your major concerns about this community?

4. Summarize your impressions of the health of the community. Compare your findings with those on other communities done by your classmates.

REFERENCES AND READINGS

BOBET, E. (1989, Winter). Indian mortality. *Canadian Social Trends, 15.* 11–14.

BOOTHROYD, P. and EBERLE, M. (1990, August). Healthy communities: What they are, how they're made. *CHS Research Bulletin.* British Columbia: UBC Centre for Human Settlements.

BRITISH COLUMBIA ROYAL COMMISSION ON HEALTH CARE AND COSTS. (1991). *Closer to home.* (Vols. 1 – 3). Victoria, B.C.: Crown Publications.

BULLOUGH, B. and BULLOUGH, V. (1990). *Nursing in the community.* St. Louis: Mosby.

CANADIAN PUBLIC HEALTH ASSOCIATION. (1986). *International Conference on Health Promotion.* Ottawa. Author.

CLARK, M.J. (1992). *Nursing in the community*. Norwalk, CT: Appleton & Lange.

DU GAS, B.W. and BECKINGHAM, A. (1993). The emergence of gerontological nursing. In Beckingham, A. and Du Gas, B. (1993). *Promoting healthy aging*. St. Louis: Mosby.

EPP, J. (1986). *Achieving health for all: A framework for health promotion*. Ottawa: Minister of Supply and Services.

FRIEDMAN, G.D. (1987). *Primer of epidemiology* (3rd ed.). New York: McGraw-Hill.

GOVERNMENT OF BRITISH COLUMBIA. (1992a). *Healthy Communities Yearbook 1991*. Victoria: Office of Health Promotion, B.C. Ministry of Health and Ministry Responsible for Seniors. (Catalogue No. QP 92835 03/92)

GOVERNMENT OF BRITISH COLUMBIA. (1992b). *Health indicator workbook* (1st ed.). Victoria: Office of Health Promotion, B.C. Ministry of Health and Ministry Responsible for Seniors. (Catalogue No. QP 91029 01/92)

GOVERNMENT OF BRITISH COLUMBIA. (1993). *New Directions for a Healthy British Columbia*. Victoria: B.C. Ministry of Health and Ministry Responsible for Seniors.

GOVERNMENT OF FIJI. (1986). *Ministry of Health Annual Report for the years 1985–86*. Suva: Ministry of Health.

GOVERNMENT OF ONTARIO. (1993). *Nurturing health. Report of the Premier's Council on Health, Well-being and Social Justice*. Toronto: Queen's Printer. (Catalogue No. 01–93–20M)

HALL, D. (1989). *Primary health care — a nursing model: A Denmark–Newfoundland (Canada) Project*. (Report available from the Registered Nurses Association of Newfoundland.)

HALME, S. (1993). Major force behind Nursing PhD set to retire. *Folio, 31*(7), 4.

HEALTH AND WELFARE CANADA. (1964). *Report of the Royal Commission on Health Services. (Hall Report)*. Ottawa: Author.

HEALTH AND WELFARE CANADA. (1987). *Active health report — Perspectives on Canada's health promotion survey 1985*. Ottawa: Minister of Supply and Services. (Catalogue No. H39–106/1987E)

HEALTH CANADA. (1993). Telephone conversation with Ann Wiehler, Acting Regional Nursing Advisor, October 3, 1993.

LABONTE, R. (1987, Summer). Community health promotion strategies. *Health Promotion, 26*(1), 5–10.

LALONDE, M. (1974). *A new perspective on the health of Canadians*. Ottawa: Information Canada.

LAST, J.M. (1988). *A dictionary of epidemiology* (2nd ed.). Toronto: Oxford University Press.

LETTER [to Glennis Zilm] and Curriculum Vitae files supplied by Shirley Stinson and the University of Alberta Faculty of Nursing, April, 1994.

PAGE, G.W. III. (1987). Water and health. In M.R. Greenberg (Ed). *Public health and the environment*. New York: Guilford Press. As cited in Clark, M.J. (1992). *Nursing in the community*. Norwalk, CT: Appleton & Lange, 348.

REGISTERED NURSES ASSOCIATION OF BRITISH COLUMBIA (RNABC). (1993, April). Government backs plan for new nursing centre. *RNABC Newsline*.

SOUTH FRASER VALLEY HEALTH COUNCIL. (1993). *Regional and community health profile: An initial perspective July 1993*. White Rock, B.C.: The Council.

SUTHERLAND, R. and FULTON, J. (1988). *Health care in Canada*. Ottawa: M.O.M. Printing. (Distributed by the Canadian Public Health Association, Ottawa.)

TYLER, C.W. and LAST, J.M. (1992). Epidemiology. In Maxcy, Rosenau and Last. *Public health and preventive medicine* (13th ed.). Norwalk, CT: Appleton & Lange.

VICTORIAN ORDER OF NURSES FOR CANADA. (1983). *Missioners for health*. Unpublished manuscript.

VICTORIAN ORDER OF NURSES FOR CANADA. (1988, March). *VON Health promotion project for seniors: Final report*. Ottawa: Author.

VICTORIAN ORDER OF NURSES FOR CANADA. (1991, May). The VON Footcare Project: Keeping Canadians on their feet: Final report. Ottawa: Author.

WORLD HEALTH ORGANIZATION (1984). *Health promotion glossary*. Copenhagen: WHO Regional Office for Europe.

CHAPTER 12

Health
and Ethnicity

CENTRAL QUESTIONS

1. How is the ethnic composition of the Canadian population relevant to health care?

2. What do the terms culture, ethnicity, socialization and acculturation mean?

3. What is the difference between the integration of immigrants in the United States and those in Canada?

4. What are some of the beliefs about health, illness and death held by major religious groups?

5. What are the basic tenets of the following types of alternative medicine: shamanism, naturopathy, Ayurvedic medicine, Chinese/Oriental medicine, faith healing, therapeutic touch, chiropractic medicine, aromatherapy, reflexology?

6. What are some of the barriers to health care for non-immigrant and new Canadians?

7. How can these barriers be crossed?

8. What are some of the health care concerns for the people of the First Nations?

9. What is the role of nurses in health services in Canada's North?

INTRODUCTION

Canada is often called a nation of immigrants (Royal Bank Letter, 1992). People have come in successive waves from all over the world to settle here. The people of the First Nations, the North American Indians and the Inuit are believed to have come from Asia. The earliest settlers to join them were the French. Then came the British, followed for the most part by Europeans until the latter part of this century when people from Asia began to dominate the immigration ranks. Over the years, Canada has also been the destination of a large share of the world's refugees from numerous war-torn countries, so that there are now over 100 distinct ethnic groups listed by Statistics Canada.

As people have come, they have brought customs and traditions from their native lands and often-times, healers or traditional practitioners of the healing arts have come as well. It has been the policy of the Canadian government to help people retain and take pride in their heritage and Canadian culture has been enriched by the contributions of people from many different lands.

The latest wave of immigration poses many challenges for nurses as they try to practise culturally sensitive care and adapt interventions to meet the needs of people of various ethnic backgrounds. Particularly important is a knowledge of clients' religious customs and of the types of medical treatment in which they have faith. Many religious customs have a direct bearing on health care, as for example, the dietary restrictions followed by Muslims and many other religious groups. It is also helpful to know if the clients come from communities where non-Western medicine is the common mode of practice and to know about treatments they have received.

Of particular interest to Canadian nurses is health care for people of the First Nations. This field of practice has

Learning to practise culturally sensitive care can be very rewarding.

always attracted Canadian nurses and the adventure of "nursing in the North" has lured nurses from around the globe. In line with the movement towards self-government for people of the First Nations, the federal government is rapidly transferring the control of health care to the people — a process that will permit the incorporation of traditional customs and healing practice into the care.

In this chapter, we will first define the basic concepts of culture and ethnicity. Then we will look at the ethnic composition of the Canadian population. Next, we will review some of the differing beliefs about health and illness held by various religious groups and look at some alternative health care practices. Then, we will discuss some of the barriers to health care both for segments of the general population and for new Canadians and we will look at ways to overcome these barriers. Finally, we will talk about health care for people of the First Nations and the transfer of health services from government to the people that is currently in progress to provide First Nations people with more integrated, culturally relevant health programs.

BASIC CONCEPTS

Ethnicity

Statistics Canada defines **ethnicity** as "the ethnic or cultural group(s) to which an individual's ancestors belonged; it pertains to the ancestral roots or origins of the population and not to place of birth, citizenship, nationality or language" (Renaud and Badets, 1993, 280).

Culture

The word *culture* has many different meanings in the English language. We are using **culture** in our discussions as it is used in sociology and anthropology to refer to the basic beliefs, values and lifeways of groups of people. These are the characteristics that differentiate one group from another (Leininger, 1978). We have mentioned in earlier chapters some of the beliefs and values shared by people in our country that distinguish us as Canadians. We believe, for example, that everyone has the right to adequate health services regardless of race, colour, creed or ability to pay and we value the health care system that provides us with universal access to health services. As Canadians, we also believe in free speech and the democratic process, and value the political system that enables everyone to voice opinions. And, in great numbers, we exercise our right to vote in municipal, provincial and federal elections.

The examples mentioned above are just a few of many characteristics Canadians have in common. Within the overall common culture that identifies us as Canadians, however, there are numerous sub-cultures in which people have differing ideas on nutrition, hygiene, child-rearing, and other health-related issues. As people have come from other lands, it has been the policy of the Canadian government to help them to retain their cultural identity within the overall Canadian whole.

Socialization

The process by which people learn the beliefs, values and lifeways of a culture is called *socialization*. The process starts in the home as children are socialized into behaviour patterns that are acceptable in the family. It continues through school and through work and social settings as people move into different environments and learn the customs and conventions (the social mores) characteristic of the new community. In this chapter, we will be concerned with the socialization of newcomers into Canadian society and the difficulties encountered when the traditions, practices and values learned in other cultures differ from those of the dominant group in our society.

Acculturation

Acculturation refers to the process whereby individuals learn the beliefs, values and lifeways of a culture other than the one into which they were born, and accept these as their own. As newcomers settle into Canada, they learn one or both of the two official languages, and they gradually adopt behaviour patterns similar to those of other people in the community. Children adapt very quickly but older people sometimes find it more difficult to become accustomed to Canadian ways. Particularly troublesome are situations where there is a conflict of cultural values. In families coming from a culture where young women are not allowed to mix with members of the opposite sex except in closely chaperoned situations, for example, the free and easy comradeship of teenage boys and girls in this country is often a cause of dissension in the family.

Assimilation and Integration

The United States has been called a *melting pot*, and Canada a *cultural mosaic,* or an *ethnically plural* society, because of the different ways the two countries have absorbed immigrants. The United States has encouraged the blending of the various nationalities into a homogeneous American identity. Canada, on the other hand, has opted to assist people to retain a more distinct sense of their own cultural identity. This policy was formalized and incorporated into legislation in the Canadian Multiculturalism Act (1988) which states:

> The Government of Canada recognizes the diversity of Canadians . . . as a fundamental characteristic of Canadian society and is committed to a policy of multiculturalism de-

signed to preserve and enhance the multicultural heritage of Canadians while working to achieve the equality of all Canadians in the economic, cultural and political life of Canada.

(Multiculturalism and Citizenship Canada, 1990)

Porter (1979) suggests that neither *melting pot* nor *cultural mosaic* is entirely appropriate for these two countries. In the United States, many immigrant groups are beginning to assert their cultural heritage. And in Canada intermarriage between racial groups is becoming more common, so that a blending of cultures would appear to be inevitable (Porter, 1979).

THE COMPOSITION OF THE CANADIAN POPULATION

The composition of the Canadian population can be looked at from a number of different perspectives. In discussing the multicultural nature of our society, we are concerned particularly with the following aspects: (1) the immigration patterns that have shaped the present composition of our population, (2) the ethnic origins of people in our society, (3) their language(s) and (4) their religions.

IMMIGRATION PATTERNS

The first immigrants to this country are said to have been the ancestors of the people of the First Nations who, it is believed, migrated to North America from Asia many hundreds of years ago. Anthropologists believe that various waves of migration occurred over the centuries. In a well-researched and carefully documented text on the Dene and the Na-Dene, Ethel G. Stewart (1991) presents an interpretation of the history of the Athapaskan or Dene people whom early European explorers found living from Alaska to New Mexico, and the Na-Dene people living on the coastal islands of British Columbia. The ancestors of these linguistically related people originated from a region in northwest China, near the border of present day Kazakhstan. They reportedly followed early routes of the fur hunters from northeast Asia along the Aleutian Island chain as they fled from the Mongol armies of Genghis Khan in the thirteenth century. Many were from royal descent, the ruling classes, military leaders or caravan traders. These disparate groups joined together for the expedition to the Great Land. Coming from multi-ethnic groups and from a highly developed region, they had to learn to become hunters and gatherers in the new undeveloped area where they settled. As their numbers grew, they dispersed southward and eastward in search of grazing lands (Stewart, 1991).

The next group of settlers to come to Canada were the French, some hundreds of years later. Although they settled mainly in Quebec, New Brunswick and Nova Scotia, they also moved westward, establishing settlements in various parts of Ontario, the Prairie provinces and British Columbia. The defeat of Montcalm on the Plains of Abraham above Quebec City in 1769 put Canada under British rule and stimulated a wave of settlement by people from England, Ireland, Scotland and Wales. During the nineteenth century, immigrants came mainly from Britain and other parts of Western and Eastern Europe to help open up the land.

During the twentieth century, there have been three major waves of immigration which have helped to shape the present composition of the population. The first occurred in the early years of the century, between 1901 and 1912, when almost three million people arrived, mainly from the British Isles, and other countries in Europe. The second wave came after the Second World War when hundreds of thousands of people were displaced from their homeland or were refugees. Canada accepted a total of 1 222 000 immigrants between 1946 and 1955, with most of them again coming from the British Isles and other European countries.

The third wave started in 1977 and continues at the present time. Between 1977 and 1990 more than two million immigrants were accepted into Canada. The largest group have come from Asia, Eastern European and other countries, with the British Isles contributing less than 10 percent and France only two percent. This latest wave of immigration is rapidly changing the demographics of Canada, as you can see from Figures 12.1 and 12.2 (Renaud and Badets, 1993; Badets, 1993).

REFUGEES

Since the end of World War II, a considerable proportion of immigrants — more than half a million in total — have been refugees from various troubled countries. They came from Hungary in 1956, Czechoslovakia in 1968, and, more recently, from Southeast Asia, the Middle East, South and Central America and from Africa; from countries such as Vietnam, Lebanon, Poland, Iran, Chile, El Salvador, Sri Lanka, Guatemala, and more recently from Bosnia and Somalia. Table 12.1 shows the 10 leading countries of birth for recent immigrants and for all immigrants.

PROVINCIAL DISTRIBUTION OF IMMIGRANTS

In 1991, the immigrant population of Canada, that is, those who were not born here, accounted for 16 percent of the population, approximately the same proportion as in 1971 and less than the 22 percent in 1911. The provinces of Ontario, British Columbia, Quebec and Alberta continue to attract the largest number of immigrants. More than 90 percent of all immigrants, according to 1991 census figures, live in these four provinces. With regard to the ethnic composition of the population of specific provinces, the Atlantic provinces are the only ones where people of British origin are now the majority ethnic group, while Quebec retains French as the dominant ethnic origin of the majority of its population. Table 12.2 shows the provincial distribution of people of various ethnic origins in 1991.

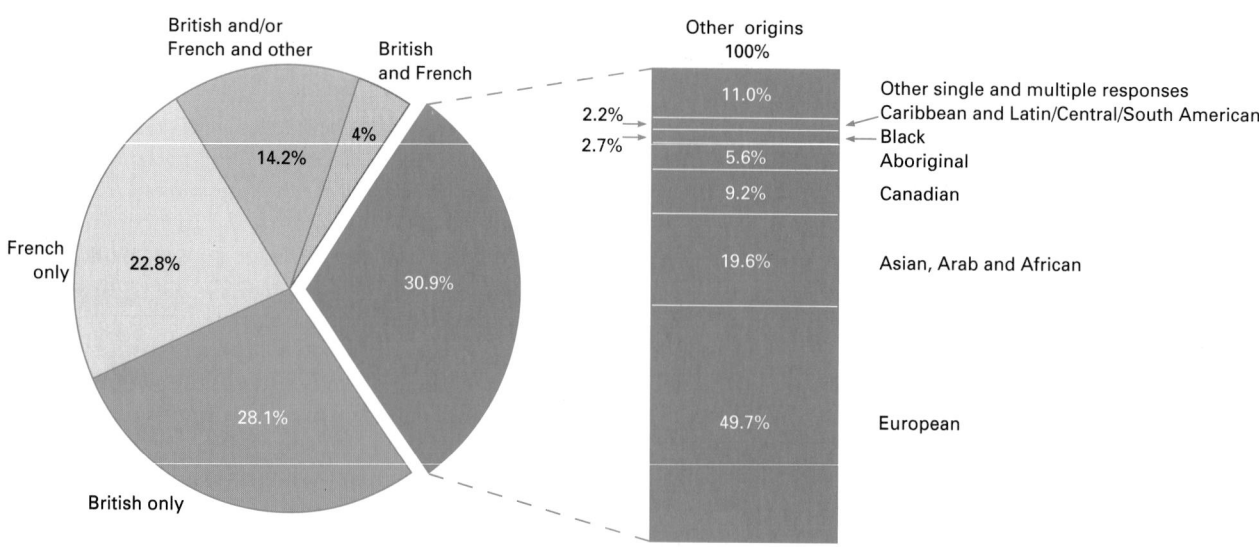

FIGURE 12.1   Ethnic composition of Canada's population, 1991

SOURCE: Renaud, V. and Badets, J. (1993, Autumn). Ethnic Diversity in the 1990s. *Canadian Social Trends, 30,* 20.

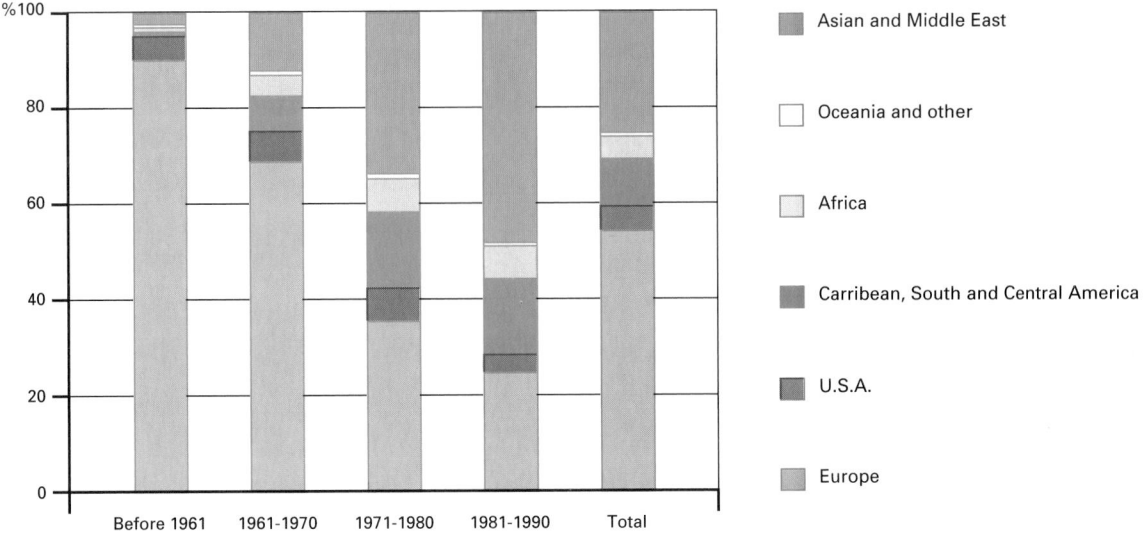

Definitions *Immigrant population* refers to people who are not Canadian citizens by birth, but who have been granted the right to live in Canada permanently by Canadian immigration authorities. Most have taken out Canadian citizenship, but some have not. Some have resided in Canada for a number of years, while others are recent arrivals.

Canadian-born population refers to people who are Canadian citizens by birth. Most are born inside Canada, but there are some who were born outside Canada to Canadian parents.

FIGURE 12.2   Immigrant population by place of birth and period of immigration, 1991

SOURCE: Badets, J. (1993, Summer). Canada's immigrants. Recent trends. *Canadian Social Trends, 29*, 11.

TABLE 12.1   Top 10 countries of birth for recent immigrants and all immigrants, 1991

RECENT IMMIGRANTS*	NUMBER	%		ALL IMMIGRANTS	NUMBER	%
1. Hong Kong	96,540	7.8	1.	United Kingdom	717,745	16.5
2. Poland	77,455	6.3	2.	Italy	351,620	8.1
3. P.R. of China	75,840	6.1	3.	United States	249,080	5.7
4. India	73,105	5.9	4.	Poland	184,695	4.3
5. United Kingdom	71,365	5.8	5.	Germany	180,525	4.2
6. Viet Nam	69,520	5.6	6.	India	173,670	4.0
7. Philippines	64,290	5.2	7.	Portugal	161,180	3.7
8. United States	55,415	4.5	8.	P.R. of China	157,405	3.6
9. Portugal	35,440	2.9	9.	Hong Kong	152,455	3.5
10. Lebanon	34,065	2.8	10.	Netherlands	129,615	3.0

* Immigrants who came to Canada between 1981 and 1991.

SOURCE: Statistics Canada (1991, Summer). Census of Canada. Cited in J. Badets. Canada's immigrants. Recent trends. *Canadian Social Trends, 29*, 11.

TABLE 12.2 Ethnic origins, 1991

TOTAL	BRITISH ONLY	FRENCH ONLY	BRITISH AND FRENCH	BRITISH AND/OR FRENCH AND OTHER	OTHER	OTHER MAIN GROUPS (% OF TOTAL POPULATION)	
Newfoundland							%
%　　100.0	88.3	1.7	3.9	3.6	2.5	Aboriginal	0.9
Number　563 940						German	0.2
						Canadian	0.2
Prince Edward Island							
%　　100.0	65.6	9.4	12.3	8.7	4.0	Dutch	1.0
Number　128 100						Canadian	0.6
						German	0.5
Nova Scotia							
%　　100.0	58.2	6.3	9.0	15.5	10.9	German	2.8
Number　890 950						Black	1.2
						Canadian	1.1
New Brunswick							
%　　100.0	44.0	33.5	9.2	8.3	4.9	Canadian	1.3
Number　716 495						German	0.6
						Aboriginal	0.6
Quebec							
%　　100.0	5.1	74.6	2.7	3.7	13.9	Italian	2.6
Number　6 810 300						Jewish	1.1
						Aboriginal	1.0
						Greek	0.7
Ontario							
%　　100.0	34.9	5.3	4.6	15.5	39.7	Canadian	5.3
Number　9 977 055						Italian	4.9
						German	2.9
						Chinese	2.7
Manitoba							
%　　100.0	24.8	5.0	2.9	19.8	47.4	German	8.7
Number　1 079 390						Aboriginal	6.9
						Ukrainian	6.9
Saskatchewan							
%　　100.0	23.4	3.1	2.5	25.2	45.8	German	12.4
Number　976 040						Aboriginal	6.8
						Ukrainian	5.7
Alberta							
%　　100.0	27.7	3.0	3.3	24.6	41.5	German	7.4
Number　2 519 185						Ukrainian	4.1
						Canadian	3.7
British Columbia							
%　　100.0	35.2	2.1	3.3	21.7	37.7	Chinese	5.6
Number　3 247 505						German	4.8
						East Indian	2.7
						Aboriginal	2.3
Yukon							
%　　100.0	29.6	3.2	4.2	28.6	34.4	Aboriginal	13.7
Number　27 655						German	3.8
Northwest Territories							
%　　100.0	14.7	2.4	2.5	16.1	64.3	Aboriginal	51.2
Number　57 430						Canadian	1.8
Canada							
%　　100.0	28.1	22.8	4.0	14.2	30.9	German	3.4
Number　26 994 040						Canadian	2.8
						Italian	2.8
						Chinese	2.2

SOURCE: Statistics Canada. (1991). Census of Canada. In V. Renaud and J. Badets (1993, Autumn).
Ethnic diversity in the 1990s. *Canadian Social Trends. 19.*

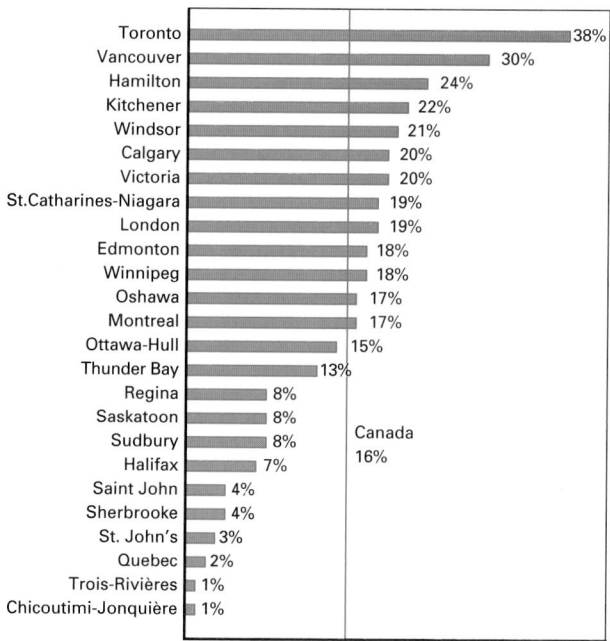

FIGURE 12.3 Immigrants as a percentage of census metropolitan areas, 1991

SOURCE: Statistics Canada. (1991). Census of Canada. In J. Badets (1993, Summer) Canada's immigrants. Recent trends. *Canadian Social Trends, 30,* 10.

Most immigrants live in urban, rather than rural parts of Canada, with more than one half (57 percent) in the three largest metropolitan areas of Canada — Montreal, Toronto and Vancouver. Toronto is the most multicultural, with 38 percent of its population (1.5 million) composed of immigrants, although Vancouver runs a close second (Statistics Canada, 1993b). Figure 12.3 shows the percentage of immigrants in the census population of metropolitan areas

ETHNIC ORIGINS

PEOPLE OF THE FIRST NATIONS

The small bands who originally found their way across the Bering Sea flourished in the new land, growing to an estimated 200 000 in Canada by the time the first French settlers arrived. Although Canada did not have the Indian wars that decimated the aboriginal people in the United States, the numbers of First Nations people dwindled considerably during the eighteenth and nineteenth centuries due, it is felt in large part, to the new diseases the Europeans brought with them. During the past half century, the aboriginal population has begun to grow again as infant and child mortality rates have declined. At present, the growth rate of First Nations people is greater than the overall Canadian rate (Bobet, 1989).

In the 1991 census, approximately one million people reported either single Aboriginal origin or Aboriginal origin in combination with other ethnic origins. The aboriginal population, however, cannot be looked upon as a single, homogeneous group. According to a 1991 Aboriginal Peoples Survey, there are over 15 languages spoken among people of the First Nations. The **First Nations** population includes approximately 40 000 Inuit, who live mainly in the Arctic, almost half a million Native North American Indians (status or single origin) and more than 135 000 Métis (of mixed ethnic origin). There are also those who name another ethnic group as their primary origin but claim some First Nations people among their ancestors (Statistics Canada, 1993a). The North American Indian group includes some 600 tribes. The **Inuit** occupy small communities north of the treeline in Canada's Far North stretching from the Mackenzie River Delta, through the Arctic Islands and Baffin Island, along the coast of Hudson Bay and Ungava Bay in Quebec, to the east coast of Labrador (Siggner, 1989).

THE FRENCH

The first French colonists arrived on Canadian shores in the early 1600s and established settlements in the areas we know as Quebec, Nova Scotia and New Brunswick. The large families that were common in Quebec up until the Quiet Revolution of the 1960s helped to ensure perpetuation of the French language and culture in Canada. The current low birth rate in Quebec is, however, causing concern as it is now below replacement level. In 1991, the population reporting ethnic origin as French only was an estimated 23 percent of the total population, down slightly from 24 percent in 1986. Another four percent of the population reported mixed French and British origins — again down slightly from 4.6 percent in 1986. The greatest number of people claiming French as their ethnic origin or as one of their ethnic origins are concentrated in Quebec and the next largest group is in New Brunswick, although communities of ethnic French people are found in almost all provinces (Statistics Canada, 1993b).

THE BRITISH

The British conquest of Canada in 1769 marked the beginning of wide-scale settlement by people from England, Ireland, Scotland and Wales. A century later, at the time of Confederation, 61.5 percent of the estimated 5.7 million people in Canada were of British origin. Today, the percentage of people of British origin, including both single and multiple origin, has dwindled to 28 percent.

FIGURE 12.4 Proportion of population reporting origins other than British or French, 1991

SOURCE: Statistics Canada. (1991). Census of Canada. In V. Renaud and J. Badets. (1993, Autumn). Ethnic diversity in the 1990s. *Canadian Social Trends, 30,* 21.

OTHER GROUPS

A larger proportion of people (31 percent) reported on the 1991 census that their ethnic origin was other than British or French than those of either of the two founding nationalities. This figure represents an increase of six percent from 1986. This number includes people of the First Nations, as well as a fairly large number (almost one million people) who gave Canadian as their only ethnic origin and another one percent who gave Canadian in combination with other origins. Figure 12.4 shows the proportion of the Canadian population reporting origins other than British or French.

LANGUAGE

During the 1991 census, all Canadians were asked for their mother tongue, defined as "the first language that a person learned at home in childhood and still understands" (Statistics Canada, 1993d). A total of 126 languages were reported, including 23 aboriginal languages. English was the most common language, with almost two thirds of the population reporting it as either their first language (mother tongue) or one of their mother tongues. Second most common was French which 25 percent of the population reported. A single mother tongue other than English or French was reported by 15 percent of the population. The most common languages listed as mother tongue (other than one of the two official languages) were, in order, Italian (1.8%), German (1.7%), Chinese (1.0%), Native Indian (0.3%) and Arabic (0.2%) (Statistics Canada, 1993). Approximately 10 percent of couples in Canada are mixed-language couples. Most commonly, these are English and

French, English and **Allophone** (other than English or French) or French and Allophone (Turcotte, 1993). Table 12.3 shows the most common primary languages in Canada and the approximate number of people in the country speaking them.

In 1991, according to the latest census, 308 500 people (a little more than one percent of the total population) over the age of five were unable to speak either one of the two official languages. This is a larger number than at any other time in the century, a situation that puts a strain on services, such as English/French language training and translation services and can cause problems in the delivery of

TABLE 12.3 Most common primary languages of Canadians

CANADA		POPULATION 27 296 560
Single language	**Total:**	**26 571 050**
	English	16 516 180
	French	6 505 565
	Non-official	3 549 305
Multiple language	**Total**	**725 810**
	French and English	216 585
	English and other	405 085
	French and other	47 270
	English, French and other	29 155
	Other	27 715

SOURCE: Statistics Canada (1993). *The Nation: Mother Tongue.* Ottawa: Statistics Canada, 8. (Catalogue No. 93–313)

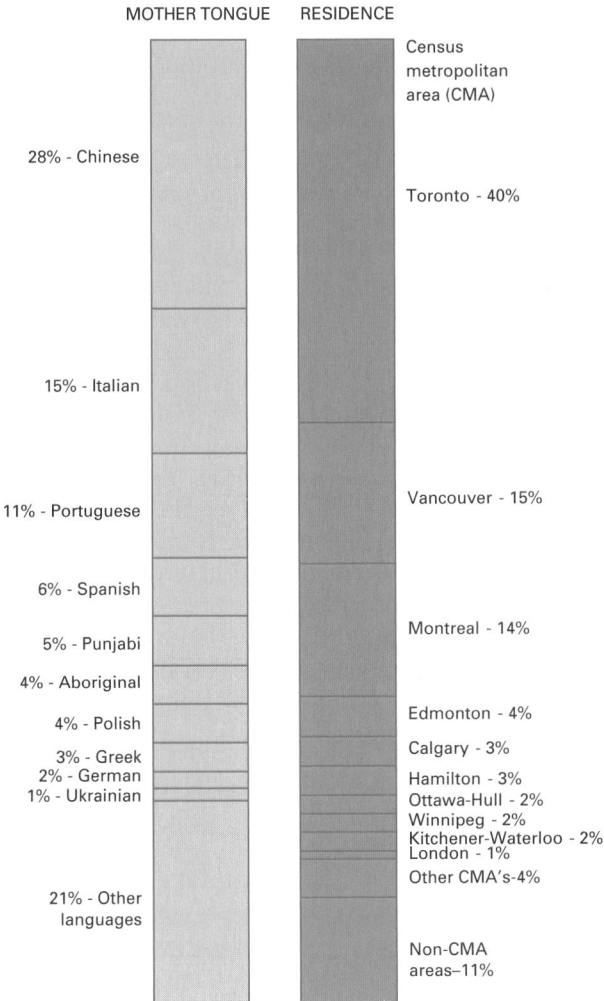

FIGURE 12.5   Distribution of people* unable to speak English or French, 1991

---

* Age 5 and over

SOURCE: Statistics Canada (1991, Winter). Census of Canada. In *Non parlo ne' inglese ne' francese. Canadian Social Trends*, 3, 27.

health care. Most people who cannot speak either one of the two official languages live in large households in urban areas where there is a sizable ethnic community. Many have been in the country for over 10 years. They are mainly women who because of domestic responsibilities and limited labour force participation have not had many opportunities to meet with other people outside their own ethnic community or to have access to language training programs. Chinese has been the fastest growing language group in Canada and was the mother tongue of the largest number of people not speaking English or French. Figure 12.5 shows the distribution of people unable to speak English or French in 1991 in major urban centres in Canada (Turcotte, 1993; Statistics Canada, 1993a, 1993d, 1993e).

RELIGION

More than 100 denominations were named by Canadians as religious affiliation on the 1991 census. Historically, the major religions in this country have been Christian, either Catholic or Protestant. A 1990 General Survey undertaken by Statistics Canada indicated that a larger proportion of Canadians (46.5 percent of the population) were Roman Catholic than Protestant (30 percent). The most common other religions reported were: Judaism (one percent), Islam, Hinduism, Sikhism and Buddhism. The last four named constitute the majority of the three percent reporting other than Christianity or Judaism. Approximately 12 percent of the people in Canada reported that they had no religious affiliation (Colombo, 1992; Royal Bank Newsletter, 1992).

DIFFERING BELIEFS AND HEALTH CARE PRACTICES OF MAJOR RELIGIONS

People acquire beliefs about health and health practices for the most part in the home as part of the cultural heritage that is passed on from generation to generation. Although these beliefs and practices may be modified by education and by exposure to other beliefs and practices in later life, there is a tendency when one is ill to revert to the beliefs and practices that were learned first. As the influence of thoughts and beliefs on healing is increasingly being recognized, it is essential that nurses and other health workers are aware of the health beliefs and practices of people coming to them for care.

Health beliefs and practices are more closely tied to religion and to medical philosophy than to country of origin or ethnicity. But, in caring for people of different cultures, it is important to remember that no matter the country of origin or the religious beliefs, the patient must be assessed and treated as an individual as the diversity between people of similar backgrounds is likely to be greater than the similarities (Wexler-Morrison, Anderson and Richardson, 1990).

Religious beliefs tend to reflect the different wants and needs of different people. Based on faith and extended study, these beliefs are not always well understood by non-believers. Among the major world religions, there are many minor divisions with great differences in belief and practice. Many of these beliefs and practices have implications for health care. As a nurse, for example, you will want to know if the religion your patient subscribes to has any particular beliefs or practices regarding such matters as cleanliness, modesty, diet, burial and faith healing, as well as any taboos that might interfere with the acceptance of treatment.

The religions of the world can be divided basically into two major groups — Western and Eastern. The birthplace of the Western group of religions was the Near East; in Palestine, the Arabian Peninsula and Iran. The Western religions include Christianity, Judaism, Islam, Baha'i and Zoroastrianism. People adhering to these religions believe that each person has an individual relationship with God and they believe in a life after death. The major Eastern religions in Canada are Hinduism, Sikhism and Buddhism. Common beliefs of people adhering to these religions include a belief in reincarnation and in non-violence (Bentley, 1986).

WESTERN RELIGIONS

Although different in many respects, the Western religions all share some common themes or beliefs, such as the following:

- God is the creator of the world
- He is the final judge of the people he created
- He forbids the worship of false gods
- human beings were created by God and have a duty to obey God
- humans have only one life to live in this world
- prophets reveal God's will
- the Holy books or Scriptures contain revealed truth
- a moral code, or code of conduct (for example, the Ten Commandments), must be adhered to.*

We will look at the Western religions in the order in which they developed historically.

ZOROASTRIANISM

This religion is not among those with a large number of members in Canada. It is, however, the oldest monotheistic religion practised today. It originated in Persia (now Iran), predating both Christianity and Islam, and has many followers in India and Iran. *Zoroastrianism* provides an interesting bridge between the religions of the West and the East. It has a highly moral belief system where salvation is the reward for those who follow "good thoughts, good words and good deeds." There is one god, Ahura Mazda. Immortality in heaven is believed to be attained by striving for spiritual and physical perfection through expanding one's knowledge and understanding. The spiritual leaders are priests whose titles are inherited. Their Scriptures are the Gathas and Avesta. There are no particular beliefs or practices that relate specifically to health care (Bentley, 1986).

JUDAISM

Judaism is the mother religion of both Christianity and Islam. It began before written history in the Eastern Mediterranean. There are over 15 million Jews in the world. There are three main branches of Judaism: Orthodox, whose adherents maintain traditional ways of worship and rituals, including dietary laws; Reform whose members are not as strict and may not adhere to dietary rules; and Conservative which falls between the traditional and the reform.

The Jewish place of worship is the **synagogue**; the spiritual leader (a teacher, not a priest) is called a **rabbi**. Jewish people set aside Saturday as their holy day (from sunset Friday to sunset Saturday). Festivals include: Rosh Hashanah (New Year's Day), Yom Kippur (Day of Atonement — considered the most holy day), Hanukkah (festival of lights) and Passover (festival of freedom). Their Holy Scriptures are: the Tanach (the Old Testament of the Bible), the Torah (teachings of Moses), and the Talmud (oral law).

Sacraments include: (1) Grace (meal-time prayers) is given after meals; (2) a glass of wine is taken with the main meal on holy days (a religious act); (3) Bar Mitzvah (for boys at age 13) and Bat Mitzvah (for girls at age 13).

Beliefs and practices affecting healt hcare include:

1. **Clothing**: Men wear the Yarmulke (traditional head covering) as a sign of respect.

2. **Food**: For Orthodox and others who maintain dietary laws, food must be specially prepared in a Kosher kitchen, according to ritual:
   a. Meat must come only from animals with a split hoof who chew the cud (no pork); only fish with fins are eaten (no shell fish); no predatory birds are eaten
   b. Animals must be killed in a Kosher manner by a specially trained person and prepared by ritual
   c. Milk and meat cannot be served at the same meal
   d. Two sets of dishes are used for preparing and serving food — one for meat, one for milk dishes.

3. **Contraception** is limited to females and only allowed for medical reasons.

4. **Circumcision**: All male infants are circumcised on the eighth day of life.

5. **Burial**: The right to die is not recognized. The body is buried intact within 24 hours of death; neither autopsy nor cremation is permitted. Transplants and the donation of body organs or parts are also prohibited.**

CHRISTIANITY

Christianity has more followers than any other religion of the world, with an estimated one billion adherents.

---

* (Bentley, S., 1986).

** Ibid

Christians believe that Jesus is the Messiah and the son of God. He is called the prophet of the Christian religion, who proclaimed a New Covenant between God and all humankind. There are over a thousand different denominations within the Christian Church, with Roman Catholic the largest, claiming over 600 million members.

Christians share many beliefs including the belief in Jesus as the son of God. Their Holy Scriptures are the Bible, both Old and New Testament. God is perceived to be a God of mercy and grace which are mediated through the church. The sacraments are signs and seals of God's expressions to His people, and through them a believer attains a state of grace, which is necessary for salvation. A Christian attains forgiveness of sins or salvation through God's grace. In response to God's forgiveness, Christians are meant to forgive those who sin against them.

All Christians celebrate Christmas as the birthday of Christ and Easter as the day of His resurrection. There are many variations in the sacraments performed in the different denominations of the Christian church. The two principal sacraments, shared by Roman Catholics and by most Protestants, are baptism and communion. *Baptism* is considered by most to be essential for salvation although the age at which baptism is performed varies. In this ritual, the individual is immersed in or sprinkled with water as a sign of purification and of admission to the Church; it is usually accompanied by the giving of a name. *Communion*, or Eucharist, is a ritual in which believers partake of bread and wine. The bread represents the body of Christ; the wine His blood. Some consider this rite to be a cleansing of sin from the soul. The sacraments vary in the different denominations, as do many of the beliefs and practices pertaining to health (Bentley, 1986).

The Roman Catholic Faith

Roman Catholics celebrate Sunday as the holy day of the week. A number of other days are celebrated as well. Fasting and penitence are practised during Lent in commemoration of Christ's fasting in the wilderness. Lent lasts for 40 days, from Ash Wednesday until Easter Eve. The rosary is an important religious symbol to all Catholics and is used for saying prayers. Some Roman Catholics wear a religious medal, which may be a cross or a medal of one of the saints.

There are seven sacraments in the Roman Catholic Church: baptism, communion, confession, confirmation, anointing (or unction) of the sick, holy matrimony and holy orders. Those of most concern to nurses are baptism, communion and the anointing of the sick.

Baptism is the first of the sacraments to be administered; it is usually performed when an infant is one to several months of age. Because Catholics believe that it is necessary for an infant to be baptized in order to receive salvation, it is very important to see that an infant in danger of death is baptized. According to Roman Catholic doctrine, an infant has a soul from the minute of conception; therefore a fetus at any stage of development must be baptized if it is born.

A nurse can perform a baptism by pouring water on the head of the child and saying, "I baptize thee in the name of the Father, and of the Son and of the Holy Spirit." Most hospitals have forms to record baptism of an infant.

Holy communion is often requested by people who are seriously ill or dying. When it is requested, a priest from the church the patient attends should be notified or, if the patient is in an inpatient facility, the sacrament can be performed by the Roman Catholic chaplain of the agency. A clean white cloth, such as a towel, is used as a cover for the bedside table on which the nurse places a glass of water and a spoon. Because people may wish to confess their sins at this time, it is important to ensure that the patient and the priest have privacy for the sacrament. Dietary rules regarding fasting before communion are not as strict as they once were; it is sufficient for the patient to abstain from food and alcohol for 15 minutes prior to receiving communion.

The *Anointing of the Sick* is a sacrament many people request when they are ill. Formerly known as Extreme Unction, or last rites, it used to be given only to the person who was dying. Now, however, it is interpreted as an aid to healing and a source of strength. It may therefore be received by a patient one or more times during an illness. Prayers, the anointing with oil and faith are believed by Catholics to restore health but these do not rule out medical treatment. It is felt that the sacrament of anointing the body should be administered when the patient is conscious, although it can be administered to an unconscious person as well. It can be performed any time of the day or night. In this sacrament, the priest anoints the eyes, ears, nostrils, lips, hands and feet with oil, for which cotton balls have been provided. Even if a patient of the Roman Catholic faith dies without receiving the Anointing of the Sick, a priest should be called. He can administer the sacrament immediately following death. Nothing should be done to the body until all sacraments have been completed. The body is treated with respect and honour. All body parts must be left intact for burial or cremation.

The Roman Catholic Church does not permit abortion nor does it allow artificial contraception.

The Protestant Denominations

The sacrament of baptism is practised in most Protestant denominations. In some, baptism is performed in infancy; others baptize at the age of understanding, often when a child is 12 years old. For a few Protestant denominations, baptism is a necessity before death. Some Protestant denominations hold Holy Communion. Some consider this rite to be a cleansing of the soul from sin. A few Protestant churches also practise the ritual of anointing. Some Protestant religions have dietary customs. Some forbid the eating of certain meats or espouse vegetarianism and some prohibit the drinking of tea and coffee. Others prohibit smoking or the consumption of alcoholic beverages because of religious doctrine. During Lent, some Protestants practise a variety of dietary restrictions. Generally, however, most Protestants' eating habits are not restricted by religious doctrine. Particular denominations whose beliefs and practices affect health care are noted below:

Church of Christ the Scientist   Christian Science was founded in 1879 by Mary Baker Eddy because of a personal healing experience. A fundamental belief of this religion is that healing occurs through divine power. There is no need, therefore, for medical intervention except in the case of births or fractures for which conventional medical care is sought. The church has its own health practitioners who devote themselves full-time to healing. Members do not believe in physical examination or immunization, although they will comply with the law in this regard (Bentley, 1986).

The Baptist Church   The Baptist Church was one of the earliest Protestant denominations. It was founded in 1525, shortly after the beginning of Protestantism. It is the largest Protestant group in the United States where many Baptists fled in the early 1600s to avoid religious persecution in Europe. Although the beliefs and practices of most Baptists do not affect health care, it is helpful to know that many Baptists like some quiet time to read the Bible. Many Baptists believe in healing by the laying on of hands. The artificial prolongation of life is discouraged (Zumbro Valley Medical Society, 1975).

Jehovah's Witnesses   This religion was founded in 1884 by Charles Taze Russell and has over two million followers throughout the world. Jehovah's Witnesses withdraw from society to a certain extent, refusing to salute the flag or participate in worldly politics. There are no holy days, no sacraments and Jehovah's Witnesses do not believe in faith healing. Drug therapy is considered acceptable, if necessary. They refuse blood transfusions because the Bible says that people should not "eat" blood. Abortion and artificial insemination are both prohibited. Autopsy is permitted only if legally necessary. Euthanasia and the receiving or giving of organ transplants are not permitted (Bentley, 1986).

Mormon Church (Church of the Latter Day Saints)   The Mormon Church was founded in the United States by Brigham Young in 1830. It is estimated that there are over five million followers. Laws in this religion are very strictly adhered to. The use of alcohol, tobacco and other addictive substances is prohibited. Mormons do not drink tea, coffee or cola drinks because caffeine is addictive. Mormons believe in baptism by immersion and the laying on of hands to heal the sick by those who have the authority to act in Jesus Christ's name. They also believe that spiritual growth continues after death. They do not permit euthanasia or birth control (Bentley, 1986; Zumbro Valley Medical Society, 1975).

ISLAM

Islam means "peaceful submission to the will of Allah" (Bentley, 1986). A **Muslim** is one who practises Islam. Muslims believe that life is but a stay on earth during which people are tested, purified and developed. This religion began in Arabia over 1400 years ago and it has spread throughout the world. It teaches the equality of all humans in the eyes of God. The Islamic God is Allah and Mohammed was his prophet.

The Holy Scriptures of the Islamic religion are the **Koran**, containing the revelations of Allah, and the Hadith which is an interpretation of the Koran by the Prophet Mohammed containing his wisdom and explorations. There are two major sects in the Islamic religion — the Sunni and the Shiites. There are no priests and no baptism in this religion. The mosque is the house of worship; when **Muezzins** call the faithful to prayer five times a day, they must kneel, if possible, facing Mecca. The sabbath day is Friday. Muslims celebrate Eid El Fita which is the first day of Ramadan (the ninth month of the Islamic year) and Eid El Adha, the Feast of Sacrifice, for the pilgrimage to Mecca which all Muslims are required to make once in a lifetime.

Islamic dietary laws prohibit the eating of pork and shellfish and the use of alcohol. During the month of Ramadan, Muslims fast from dawn until sunset.

Modesty is very important to Muslims. If at all possible, their health care should be given by people of the same sex. Orthodox Muslim women must always be covered from neck to ankles and men from waist to knees. The typical hospital gown is therefore considered indecent. Many Muslim women still wear a veil and in some countries women do not go outside the home. They need the consent of the family leader (a man) for treatment, medications and the like.

Muslims always wash, preferably with running water, in preparation for prayers and after going to the bathroom. The importance of cleanliness requires that Muslims have a full shower after seminal discharge or menstruation.

Muslims are fatalistic, accepting what happens (for example, the birth of a crippled child) as the will of Allah. They believe in life after death and in burial, rather than cremation. After death, the body should only be handled by Muslims; it is usually looked after by family members. Burial should take place within 24 hours after death. Faith healing may be used to supplement a physician's efforts. The "right to die" is not accepted (Bentley, 1986; Zumbro Valley Medical Society, 1975).

BAHA'I

Baha'i is a fairly new religion, founded in 1844 in Persia (Iran) by Baha'u'llah whom Baha'is believe is the latest of God's prophets. The fundamental belief of the Baha'i is that everyone is a part of one human race; they teach the unity of all religions and the unity of all human beings. The world centre for this religion is Mount Carmel in Haifa, Israel. The sacred Baha'i literature was written by the

NURSES AT WORK

It's a crispy cool Saturday afternoon in Arctic Red, one of the satellite towns our nursing station is responsible for. It's October, and I've been here now for almost two weeks. Arctic Red will be completely cut off from civilization for the seven or eight weeks when the road is closed. The road depends on ferry crossings in the summer and ice roads in the winter. During the between-times, there is no way into Arctic Red except by skidoo or helicopter.

It finally happened yesterday. I went to work as usual and watched the first ferry crossing while I ate my breakfast at the health centre. It seemed to be having a bit of trouble dodging the big pieces of ice that floated down the river. Some of these "floaters" are about a quarter-mile long with jammed-together pieces of ice. Anyway, the ferry got hit broadside by a "floater," which apparently did some damage, and for about an hour, I watched a most interesting drama of "rescue the ferry." By afternoon, it was running normally again. According to the ferry patrol, today is the last day it is in the water. Tonight they will be down there winching the ferry up onto the shore. I guess that should be worthy of a few pictures. Right now, I can see the ferry has a "cat-digger" on board and he's hanging over the edge, breaking up the ice for the ferry as it goes along.

My nursing duties are mainly preventive in nature — that is, until a medical emergency occurs that I must deal with. This week, I was invited to the "school feeding" program. They actually had a Thanksgiving dinner

with all the trimmings for the kids and all the town. There must have been 100 people there.

The next day I was invited to the adult education pot-luck lunch that they do every Wednesday. I had no warning, so I had no one to take but my dog, Misha. The kids had a splendid time with her.

I also went to the school this week to do the physicals and the eye and hearing checks. My problem is that the kids all seem to have several names. At the school, they are registered under one name, and in the health care system, they are under their birth registered name, so it gets pretty confusing sometimes.

The coldest we have had here in Arctic Red so far is –28° C. People here don't seem very conscious of the temperatures, but one old-timer told me you can tell how cold it is by watching the birds. He went into an amazing spiel about how they fly differently in different temperatures, how they huddle, how they eat. I found it amazing when all we do is look at a thermometer. He did say that beyond –45°C it was hard to know 'cause the birds don't move at all.

—Caroline Wiebe*

---

* This excerpt was taken from a letter contributed to an on-going research project into Northern nursing experiences. Research and analysis of descriptions of experiences in the many letters collected by this project will be used to document and validate the role of nurses in Canada's North.

---

founder in the mid 1800s. There are no clergy or other spiritual leaders. Rather, there is a spiritual assembly, democratically elected by the congregation. They read the scriptures of all religions. Baha'is pray daily and fast from sunrise to sunset for 19 days of the year.

The use of alcohol and narcotics is prohibited. Canadian Baha'is have been active in international affairs to promote world unity. At the local level, they are active in community development projects (Bentley, 1986; Martin, 1985).

EASTERN RELIGIONS

The three most common Eastern religions in Canada are Hinduism, Sikhism and Buddhism.

HINDUISM

Hinduism is more than a religion to 80 percent of India's population; it is a social system and a way of life. There are many Hindu gods and goddesses; the main ones are Vishnu, Shiva and Brahma. A number of holy days are observed.

The most important festival is Dewali (festival of the lights). There are holy writings — the four oldest being the Vedas, which were written in Sanskrit and are believed to be more than 4000 years old. There are no major prophets and many ways to follow one's religion. However, the following beliefs are common to all Hindus:

- there is one supreme spirit
- there is an immortal soul in all living beings
- people are reincarnated after death
- Karma (fate) is the reward or punishment for one's acts and thoughts
- there is a clear code of dutiful and right behaviour
- violence is unacceptable
- the supreme duty is to seek truth.

The Hindu family is often an extended one with several generations living together. The obligation for all family members to care for those who are ill or elderly is very strong. It is usually the eldest granddaughter who looks after grandmother when she is ill or incapacitated. The father is traditionally the breadwinner and the mother custodian of family beliefs, values and religious teaching.

Many of the Hindu practices and beliefs are relevant for health care. Hindus are modest about their bodies. Women keep their upper arms, legs and breasts covered in the traditional *sari* and blouse or long tunic and loose trouser (*salwar kameze*). A long scarf is usually worn as well which can be used as a head covering. Hospital gowns are embarrassing for devout Hindus who should be provided with a long gown, or gown and pyjama bottoms. A man's body must be covered from waist to knees. For examinations, only one part of the body should be exposed at a time. It is considered improper to touch the body of a member of the opposite sex, except one's spouse.

Washing is done before prayers and after using the toilet. Food is eaten with the fingers and Hindus wash their hands both before and after meals. Running water is necessary to purify the body; still water is believed to be unclean.

Many Hindus are vegetarian. The cow is considered sacred; therefore, beef is not usually eaten; milk and milk products are also not consumed. A devout Hindu may refuse food if he or she does not know what the ingredients are. Fasting is common, and may be done several times a week.

Death at home is preferred, if at all possible. After death, relatives wash and prepare the body. Non-Hindus should not touch the dead body of a Hindu person. The dead are cremated, rather than buried. Cremation occurs as soon after death as possible in a special ceremony. In India, the ashes of the dead are often scattered on the holy Ganges River (Henley, 1983a).

SIKHISM

Sikhism is an offshoot of Hinduism which originated in the 16th century. There are now ten to twelve million Sikhs in the world, most of whom are from Punjab State in northern India. Sikhs believe in one God and in reincarnation. Their New Year is April 13 (Baisakh), celebrated with special sweets prepared in the temple. The Holy Scriptures are the Guru Granth Sahib, named after the founder of Sikhism. There are no ordained priests; any initiated Sikh can lead prayers and readings, as all Sikhs are equal. Family ties are strong — extended families often live together and duty to all family members is emphasized. Sikh men wear a turban to cover their long hair, which the faith requires not be cut.

In addition to the turban worn by men, there are five signs of Sikhism worn by all Sikhs, both men and women:

- *Kosh* — uncut hair. Hair must be kept clean and neat. If shaving is necessary, the patient should be consulted; a depilatory cream may be preferred
- *Kanga* — a comb worn in the hair
- *Kara* — a steel bangle, worn on the right wrist, that should never be removed (it should be taped if possible)
- *Kirpan* — a symbolic dagger, worn under the clothes, as a symbol of readiness to fight

- *Kaccha* — special undershorts. These are worn 24 hours a day by members of both sexes. They are a reminder of modesty and sexual morality for women. During childbirth and surgery, women often prefer to keep Kaccha on one leg or one ankle.

Modesty is very important to Sikhs. Upper arms, legs and breasts are covered by a sari and blouse or salwar kameze. A long scarf is usually worn by Sikh women. Washing is done before prayers, after lavatory and before and after eating.

The Sikh diet is often vegetarian. Pork is not eaten as the pig is considered a scavenger, and beef is seldom eaten. Fasting is not usual.

Death is considered a part of life. Hymns and prayers are said for the dying person. After death, family members wash and prepare the body. Cremation is done as soon as possible (Henley, 1983b).

BUDDHISM

Buddhism is a world-wide religion which was founded in the fifth century BC in the area now known as Nepal. It has spread throughout Asia to the rest of the world. There are no gods in this religion, no priests and no sacraments. In Canada, Sunday is usually observed as the sabbath. There are several special holy days but no specific rituals. This religion encompasses various philosophical beliefs and ethical systems.

A central belief common to all branches is that the ultimate state is one of self-enlightenment. Buddhists are agreeable to all pursuits that enhance one's ability to attain enlightenment. They believe in faith healing, and feel that the spiritual peace and liberation from anxiety that comes from awakening to Buddha's wisdom will hasten healing and recovery, but most will take medications and treatment as needed. Buddhists are fatalistic, accepting life's events with imperturbable calm. Death is likewise accepted. Since the body is considered only a shell after death, there are no restrictions on handling the body. Burial may be by cremation or interment (Zumbro Valley Medical Society, 1975).

ALTERNATIVE MEDICINE

Throughout the world, millions of people rely on traditional healers when they are ill or injured. Although many people who immigrate to this country are city-dwellers who have been exposed to Western medicine, many others have never known anything but the folk medicine used in their villages. Many of these folk medicines, remedies and traditions have their roots in antiquity and have survived because they work.

In this section we will briefly discuss shamanism, herbalism, Ayurvedic medicine, natural medicine, Chinese/Oriental medicine, faith healing and therapeutic touch, chiropractic medicine and two other health systems that are currently receiving attention: aromatherapy and reflexology. All of these forms of medicine and many more are practised in Canada today. Most of these health care practices and their modifications work together in a complementary way with "Western" medicine (Grossman, 1985).

SHAMANISM

When spirits are considered to be the cause of a health problem, traditional rituals are used to exorcise the spirit. This is accomplished by the **shaman** who occupies an important position in the group because he or she deals with the spirit world. Since a person will heal more quickly when he or she believes in the effectiveness of the remedy, regardless of what that remedy is, rituals play a large part in the psychological aspect of the cure (Frideres, 1988).

Practitioners of alternative medicine have long been aware of the importance in health of the connections between body and mind. Western scientific medicine, however, has traditionally emphasized the physical aspects of disease. The importance of the body–mind connection has only recently been explored. Through the work of Selye and others, we have learned much about the phenomenon of stress and its effects on the body. And we have learned to control the stress response through the use of various relaxation techniques, as we discussed in Chapter 9. At the present time, considerable research is being undertaken by scientists exploring connections between the mind, the endocrine system and the immune systems to see if we can use the mind to control other bodily processes to prevent disease (Guiness and Rutherford, 1993).

The traditional health practices of people of the First Nations are rooted in shamanism. We will explore their health beliefs and practices a little more in a separate section on health care for the people of the First Nations.

HERBALISM

In a shamanistic society, there is usually another health worker, the **herbalist**, who deals with the physical aspects of disease, treating the afflicted with potions, salves and brews made from various plants. In prescientific times, herbalists were usually women who, because of limited mobility due to childbearing, became the harvesters and prepared the concoctions. It usually became a specialized function of one member of the group, with mothers passing down knowledge to their daughters. Plant medicine, as it is sometimes called, has been used through the ages by almost all societies throughout the world. The first known record of using herbs was made approximately 3000 years ago in China in a "Canon of Herbs" which deals with 252 herbs. Although the synthetic preparation of drugs during the present century caused herbal remedies to be dismissed as folk

Natural food stores specialize in organically grown fruits and vegetables and stock a wide variety of herbal remedies.

remedies for a while, there has been a reawakened interest in their use in recent years. Much of the renewed interest is due to increasing concern over the side effects of synthetic drugs, a renewed awareness of ecology and the fact that people are taking more responsibility for their own health. Health food stores which specialize in organic fruits and vegetables (those grown without the use of pesticides and other chemicals) and stock a wide variety of herbal medicines have been highly successful in most communities. Plant substances also form the basis of many conventional prescription drugs such as those used to treat asthma, depression, heart disease, pain and many other disorders. In fact, 37 percent of all prescription drugs are derived from plants (Bremness, 1989).

AYURVEDIC MEDICINE

Ayurvedic medicine is the oldest form of health care that considers natural phenomena, rather than spirits, to be the cause of illness. Records of the use of Ayurvedic medicine go back 2500 years in India where it is believed to have originated. Treatment is based on a belief in the body's innate ability to heal itself. Illness is felt to be a result of internal disharmony resulting from improper diet, activities that are out of place for the season (such as swimming in the river in the midst of winter) or other lifestyle indiscretions.

Central to Ayurvedic medicine is the concept of the Triumvirate of health which holds that each person has three life forces or *doshas* which must be kept in balance. The doshas are (1) Vata, symbolized by air, which produces movement, (2) Kaffa, allied with the earth, which is the stabilizing force and responsible for body structure and (3) Pitta, the fire dosha, which is responsible for regulatory functions, such as heat maintenance, digestion and hydration and also serves as the interface between the two other Doshas. People are born with varying proportions of the three elements and these proportions must be determined for each person and treatment adjusted to restore individual balance.

There is a dual emphasis in Ayurvedic medicine on treatment and prevention. Treatment is carried out by physicians, trained in a five-and-a-half-year program in India or in a short, postbasic course for physicians wishing to specialize in this field in North America. Prevention is initiated on noting a disturbance in functioning, and can involve altering diet or exercise routines or initiating changes in thought and emotional patterns to restore balance between the three doshas.

This type of medical practice is highly complex; one must learn to assess the proportions each person has of the three doshas and to diagnose imbalances. A wide range of treatments are used, including many herbal remedies and "panchakarma," to cleanse the body of its accumulated wastes. Cleansing methods include herbalized steam treatments, oil massage, nasal purging, laxatives and medicated enemas. Many people in India, and people of East Indian descent in Canada, make use of both Ayurvedic medicine and Western medicine (Guiness and Rutherford, 1993).

NATUROPATHY

At the time of writing, British Columbia is the only province in Canada to license naturopaths. Practitioners of **naturopathy** use a combination of natural therapeutic and healing techniques that are a mixture of traditional folk wisdom and modern science.

Through drugless therapy, the naturopath attempts to address the underlying causes of a person's health problems, focussing particularly on unhealthy lifestyles. Treatment relies heavily on diet management and herbal remedies, the cleansing of the gastrointestinal tract through enemas and on exercise (Olson, 1990).

CHINESE/ORIENTAL MEDICINE

Traditional **Chinese** and other **Oriental medicine** is preventive rather than curative. It revolves around theories of energy and elements. Important concepts to understand are the basic principles of Yin and Yang, Chi and the five elements of the universe.

The principle of **Yin Yang flow** affects all of Chinese thought and action. These are two opposing but complementary forces which Chinese philosophers believe balance everything in the universe. **Chi** is the finite amount of energy we are endowed with at birth. It flows from one *meridian* or channel to another in the body. It is our dynamic force and is determined by heredity and lifestyle. It can be enhanced by the right foods, proper exercise and clean air. The five elements of the universe are fire, wood, earth, water and metal/air. These elements interact with body energy and all must be balanced. Balance results in health and imbalance is a sign of illness (Olson, 1990; Grossman, 1985).

Chinese medicine encompasses the following three basic types of intervention:

1. **Herbal medicine.** The herbal remedies are similar to those used in shamanism. They are derived from plants native to China; Ginseng root is one of the most commonly known.

2. **Acupuncture.** Originating in China, Acupuncture is now practised extensively in Canada. It is based on the principle that, as Chi flows through the body, many factors can block or slow its flow, thus creating an energy imbalance. To correct the imbalance, needles are inserted on **meridians** (energy channels) and the needles are rotated. In China this is done by hand; Western medical practitioners attach electrical charges which rotate the needles.

   a. **Acupressure** is a massage technique which uses manual pressure to stimulate energy points on the body. Light to moderate pressure is used on the same points that are used in acupuncture.

   b. **Shiatzu** is a Japanese form of acupressure in which pressure is applied to the body along the meridians. It combines the use of touch with a traditional form of Oriental massage.

   c. **Qui Gong** is the healing art of building up energy. Based on the same principles of energy flow as acupuncture and acupressure, it uses visualization and breathing exercises to unblock the channels of energy flow.

3. **Exercise.** Probably the most common form of exercise practised by the Chinese (and many other Asians) is Tai Chi. One of the gentlest of the martial arts, it is a form of meditation in motion, used as both part of a spiritual quest and a lifestyle health practice. **Tai Chi** consists of a series of dancelike, gentle turning movements that loosen the joints and the spine and relax tension points. Because it does not involve jarring movements that might tear muscles, it can be practised by people of any age and with varying degrees of disability.*

---

* (Olson, 1990; Shaw, 1986)

FAITH HEALING/THERAPEUTIC TOUCH

There is an increasing amount of interest (in medical and lay circles) in the power of the mind to heal the body, in the healing relationship, and in the use of touch in healing. Let us then examine these three concepts and the relationship of one to another.

Faith healing has existed from time immemorial. It is based on a belief in the healing power of an object or place or the healing ability of an individual. An example of belief in healing places is the annual pilgrimage that thousands of people have made to the Roman Catholic shrine in Lourdes (France) and the many who have experienced miraculous cures there. According to Frank (1974) who studied the phenomenon of faith healing, the patient's state of mind is the key factor in the healing process (Frank cited in Kennison, 1987).

In the case of the healing power of an individual, the healing relationship is the crucial factor. This relationship is based on trust in the "healer" and the belief that this person can help you. The spiritual element of the faith healing process is more important than the physical — the person has to have faith that the cure will work. There is also a strong emotional commitment involved.

Many religious faiths have practised faith healing through the centuries. It is the essence of the shaman's healing power. There are many stories in the Christian Bible of Jesus healing the sick. The anointing of the sick in the Roman Catholic theology is a present day example of the use of faith healing. Members of the Christian Science Church believe that illness is caused by wrongful thoughts and that a person can be cured by faith healing alone. They have their own practitioners and reject conventional treatment.

Touch is very often used in conjunction with faith healing and is generally referred to as the "*laying on of hands*." Touch, in itself, can convey a sense of comfort and support. Touch has been used to relieve pain, to reassure the anxious and to comfort the dying.

Therapeutic touch was developed as a nursing tool by Dolores Krieger (1975). She was sent as a young graduate student to observe a faith healer who was holding a session in town. Her professor told her to observe the performance and see if anything appeared to be happening as a result of the laying on of hands. Krieger came to the conclusion that, indeed, believers were being healed, and she set out to study the phenomenon.

In experimental studies on patients who had been treated with therapeutic touch, Krieger found that in addition to increased relaxation and reduced anxiety, there was a significant rise in hemoglobin levels. Krieger believes that the energy fields surrounding the body play a part in the healing process and that through the laying on of hands the practitioner supplies the energy to boost hemoglobin levels. Therapeutic touch is practised by many nurses in Canada. A non-invasive technique, it is often used in conjunction with other therapies (Krieger, 1975, 1979; Guiness and Rutherford, 1993).

CHIROPRACTIC MEDICINE

Chiropractic medicine is the third largest primary health care specialization after medicine and dentistry in the Western world. It is primarily concerned with the examination and treatment of the spine. Used mainly for mechanical dysfunctions, "its central modality is adjustment of the spinal column to rehabilitate normal nervous system functioning" (Olson, 1990, 119).

Some practitioners confine their practice to manual manipulation of the spine; others make use of a wide range of therapies to treat their patients. Chiropractic medicine does not use drugs or surgery. Once frowned upon by orthodox medicine, chiropractic medicine is now accepted as a legitimate treatment mode by most Western physicians. Chiropractors are not to be confused with osteopaths, who are medical doctors with additional preparation in disorders of the musculoskeletal system. Osteopathic physicians are concerned with the structural elements of the body.

OTHER THERAPIES

A number of other therapies are used by practitioners of alternate medicine. Two that are receiving attention currently are aromatherapy and reflexology.

Aromatherapy makes use of aromatic essences extracted from wild or cultivated plants for therapies similar to those used in herbal medicine. The oils are administered by massage, through baths or through inhalation and produce a wide range of therapeutic responses (Olson, 1990).

Reflexology, also known as "zone therapy," is the study of the reflexes of the foot, which are believed to correspond to specific parts of the body. Massaging the reflexes of the feet reduces tension and helps the body to seek its own equilibrium (Shaw, 1986; Eastman, 1985).

BARRIERS TO ACCESSING CARE

The Epp Report (1986) documented the poor health status of certain segments of the Canadian population. Particularly at risk are people in low socioeconomic groups, new immigrants and other minority groups including the people of the First Nations. One major cause is poverty and the inability to purchase the things needed for good health, such as nutritious food, good housing and the like. We have discussed this aspect in previous chapters. Other factors contributing to the poor health of various groups are the barriers they meet when they seek health care. In Canada, although we have universal health care, for various reasons, many people find it difficult to access this care.

ATTITUDES OF HEALTH CARE WORKERS

A major barrier to accessing health care for some people is the attitude of health care workers. Even though an increasing number of health workers in this country are second, third and fourth generation Canadians of both European and non-European descent, their backgrounds are considerably different from those of new immigrants. Most health workers have gone through the Canadian educational system and are well socialized into Canadian ways. Many have lost their native language; it may not have even been spoken in the home in which they were raised.

Although many physicians came from other countries to Canada in the middle years of the century, when we were short of Canadian trained physicians, few are admitted now that we have a more than adequate supply. Those who are admitted have difficulty obtaining licensure to practise in Canada; the process is a lengthy one. Credentials must be examined for equivalency to those of educational programs here. The individual is usually required to write Canadian qualifying examinations. Often the person has to learn English or French first. There is also a shortage of places, over and above those allocated for graduates of Canadian medical schools, for the internship that is required of out-of-country physicians. Nurses coming from other countries are often required to take additional clinical courses. Another problem in nursing is the difficulty in recruiting students into nursing schools whose families have come from countries where nursing has a low status. Brisson and Deslauriers (1992) in a study on the proportion of immigrants in nursing in Canada found that the proportion had dropped from 7.7 percent to 0.4 percent between 1967 and 1977.

Physicians, nurses and other professionally trained health workers in this country have all been educated in the Western medical model with its emphasis on the biophysical causes of disease and the scientific treatment of it. It is only in very recent years that alternative forms of medicine have been accepted in Canada as having some validity — and even so, are greeted with much skepticism by many. The biomedical model assumes certain attitudes towards health care and those who come for care. These attitudes are deep-rooted; their foundations are in cultural values and beliefs that have been acquired in the home and molded by education, religion and personal experience. We are often not aware of our own values and beliefs because they are obtained subconsciously. They determine, however, the way in which we view the world and the way we relate to other people (Grypma, 1993).

SPECIAL PROBLEMS FOR THE GENERAL POPULATION

Unequal distribution of resources   Some problems people have in accessing health care are due to disparities in the health care system itself. Tertiary care hospitals and most of the highly qualified health professionals, such as specialist physicians and nurses with advanced preparation, are located in major urban centres in the southern parts of Canada. People living in northern and rural areas have long been underserved. Provincial governments, in planning health care reforms, are aware of the problem and in several provinces, steps are already underway to address the disparities.

Other reasons   The poor, the homeless, people with mental health problems and those who are mentally handicapped, alcoholics and drug addicts frequently experience difficulties accessing care regardless of whether they live in urban Toronto or in Inuvik. The barriers to care for these groups come in part from the attitude of health workers towards them and the low self-esteem they often have. These factors are often compounded by a lack of information about the health care system and how to access services.

SPECIAL PROBLEMS FOR IMMIGRANTS AND REFUGEES

Health insurance regulations   People coming into the country in most provinces are not eligible for health insurance until they have completed three months' residency. Meanwhile, their immigration sponsors are responsible for their welfare, so they need to take out private insurance. In the case of refugees, financial help is available from Employment and Immigration Canada in the event of a critical situation.

Language   In many cases, there is a language barrier to overcome when immigrants seek the help of health professionals. As we noted above, a large number of immigrants can speak neither English nor French, which are often the only languages the health care workers do speak (*Non parlo ne inglese ne francese*, 1993).

Low self-esteem   Many immigrants, even people who have been professionals in their home country, often have to take low-paying, low-status jobs. Many of the people who have come from Central or South America, Somalia or Bosnia, for example, are refugees who were victims of torture for their political or religious beliefs, or for their ethnic identity. Both of these situations can contribute to feelings of low self-esteem. Any lack of sensitivity on the part of health workers can cause further insecurity in people whose self-esteem is already low.

Lack of culturally relevant treatment   In our Western medicine oriented health agencies, people from different cultures may experience conflict with their religious beliefs or cultural values. One example is a Chinese man who was admitted to the emergency department of a large hospital. The patient did not speak English and became very agitated when the nurse tried to take a sample of blood that had been ordered. The patient eventually had to be restrained and was put in isolation. When an interpreter arrived on the scene, it was learned that the patient was objecting to the invasion of his body and he was not going to submit to it. When the procedure and the reasons for it were explained, he relaxed and allowed the nurse to take the blood sample.

Culturally sensitive care is particularly important for people with mental health problems. Often hidden because of the stigma attached to them, mental health problems are common among immigrants — for many reasons. One is the instability caused by moving to another part of the world and getting settled in a new community. Another is the stress of the immigration process itself. The problems are more pronounced in refugees who often suffer from depression and anxiety, constantly wondering if they are ever going to be safe.

Cultural differences in attitude towards treatment   In some cases, services such as social assistance are considered unacceptable because any form of charity is a disgrace. Community health services may also be looked upon as charity because in the person's home country, one has to pay for health care. Wife-beating is considered a family matter in some cultures and not a matter for health authorities. In most Eastern cultures, it is the duty of the family to care for aging parents, aunts and uncles. Having to put them in an extended care facility — because there is no one at home to care for them or for any other reason — causes the family a tremendous burden of guilt.

Inconvenient hours for services   The nine-to-five office hours of physicians and clinics are often a deterrent for people who work long hours and are unable to take time off because they are paid on an hourly basis. Immigrants usually start in the lowest paying jobs and work long hours. Not infrequently, both husband and wife work to make enough money for the family to survive. In these situations, it is difficult for parents to take a child to the clinic for immunization or to make time to go to the physician themselves.

Racial tensions   Sometimes, racial conflict can create a barrier to health care. A patient may not want to be cared for by a physician or nurse of a certain race, or colour.

Or, a visiting health worker may be reluctant to go to the home of a person of a different race (Hong Fook Mental Health Association, 1984).

CROSSING THE BARRIERS

Dr. Madeline Leininger, the acknowledged founder of transcultural nursing, believes that nursing is basically a transcultural care profession. Its primary focus is the provision of "human care to people in a way that is meaningful, congruent and respectful of cultural values and lifestyles" (Luna and Cameron, 1989, 228). The transcultural nursing concepts and cultural care theory developed by Leininger over the past three decades have given nurses a new insight into better ways to understand individuals, families and cultures (Leininger, 1978).

Numerous researchers have subsequently extended Leininger's work through comparative studies of cultural care patterns, values and practices of people of different cultures to add to our nursing knowledge and thereby improve nursing practice. The terms, **cultural sensitivity**, *cross-cultural competence*, *intercultural effectiveness* and *ethnic competence* have all been used to describe the ability to work effectively with people of different cultures in a way that people of these cultures find acceptable.

Lynch and Hanson, in their book entitled *Developing cross-cultural competence*, have suggested that this competence includes five elements: an awareness of one's own cultural limitations; openness, appreciation and respect for cultural differences; a view of intercultural interactions as learning experiences; the ability to use cultural resources as interventions; and an acknowledgement of the integrity and value of all cultures. We will look at each of these in turn (Lynch and Hanson, 1992).

An awareness of one's own cultural limitations   The first step in overcoming the barriers in caring for people of other cultures is to become aware of our own beliefs and values. Most of these we have acquired subconsciously and they may therefore be difficult to identify. What, for example, are your beliefs about abortion? Breastfeeding? The right to die? How do these influence your reaction to a patient who has just had an abortion, refuses to breastfeed her infant or has requested "do not resuscitate" orders?

Openness, appreciation and respect for cultural differences   Cultural values, customs and beliefs are an integral part of an individual. If each patient is to receive "humane, personalized culturally sensitive care with due regard for spiritual, physical and emotional needs in addition to the full spectrum of patients' rights" as suggested by Berube (1990), we must first establish the role of

---

Cultural Sensitivity

"Cultural sensitivity, cultural competence, intercultural effectiveness and ethnic competence . . . all refer to ways of thinking and behaving that enable the members of one cultural, ethnic or linguistic group to work effectively with members of another. . . . it does not mean knowing everything there is to know about another culture. It is, instead, respect for the difference, eagerness to learn and a willingness to accept that there are many ways of viewing the world."

SOURCE: Lynch, E.W. and Hanson, M.J. (1992). *Developing cross-cultural competence*. Baltimore: Paul H. Brooks, 357. Reprinted with permission.

---

the patient's ethnicity in their beliefs about health and illness. Do they belong to a group that follows strict rules in regard to their diet, bathing, clothing, prayers, and the like?

There is a tremendous diversity of beliefs and practices within each major religious/cultural group. It is necessary, then, to ask the patient about individual preferences in order to determine whether there are any differences in viewpoint about health and illness and, if so, what these are. Some religions have strong views on medical-surgical procedures such as blood transfusions, abortion, transplants and the prolongation of life; some have none. Holy days have varying meanings for each individual and their significance should be ascertained. Respect for the patient's beliefs is essential and, insofar as possible, the patient should be assisted to maintain traditional rituals of prayer, washing, and diet. Religious objects, such as holy scriptures and prayer beads, should be handled with respect.

A view of intercultural interactions as learning opportunities There is a wealth of knowledge about different cultures among patients in all health care agencies in Canada today. In the process of care for your patients, you have a wonderful opportunity to expand your knowledge about the world.

The ability to use cultural resources in interventions Both in Vancouver and in Toronto, the Health Departments have established a separate division to assist in providing culturally sensitive health care to people of different ethnic groups. A number of cultural resources have been developed in different centres across the country. These include health promotion material, such as pamphlets and videotape, in a number of languages and the use of cultural media for health education programs. Additionally, there is the important task of training interpreters for hospitals and other health care needs.

Continuing education sessions are being held to sensitize health care workers to the needs of people of different cultures. Health education can be incorporated into English as a second language classes (ESL) with the cooperation of the teacher. Ethnic community organizations can be approached for people to help, for example, with interpretation. Volunteers can also be useful in helping with the organization of clinics for pregnant women and new mothers or for seniors and the establishing of health education programs. With some ethnic groups there are now third and fourth generations in Canada who are also usually willing to assist newcomers, although many may have lost their mother tongue and cannot be called upon as interpreters.

An acknowledgment of the integrity and value of all cultures As you learn more about the beliefs, the values and the customs of other people, you will gain a greater appreciation of the heritage of people coming from different lands. Koreans will proudly tell you that their ancestry goes back four thousand years as a race separate from the Chinese and the Japanese. Our Canadian heritage is a brash newcomer, compared to the cultures of people from the Middle East, Asia and Europe (Lynch and Hanson, 1992; Berube, 1992; Wexler-Morrison, Anderson and Richardson, 1990; Vancouver Health Department, 1993).

HEALTH CARE FOR PEOPLE OF THE FIRST NATIONS

HISTORICAL PERSPECTIVE

The traditional health care system of people of the First Nations was rooted in their religious beliefs. It was felt that people brought illness upon themselves by actions such as breaking a taboo, thus allowing an evil spirit to enter the body. There were basically three types of illness:

1. those that were visible, such as a fracture or a bleeding leg resulting from physical injuries

2. those caused by an invisible external agent such as infectious agents including smallpox, pneumonia and measles

3. a group of residual diseases that did not fit into either of the other two categories, for example, mental illness.*

The people of the First Nations had a wide variety of medicines, including many herbal remedies, that were developed to treat different diseases. Acting on the belief that most illnesses had a biological basis, the medicines were administered at the onset of an illness. If the ill person did not respond to the medications, it was assumed that the

---

* (Frideres, 1988).

disorder in question was rooted in spiritual, rather than biological causes. Shamanistic methods might then be tried. The task of the shaman or medicine man (or woman) was to drive out the foreign object or evil spirit that had invaded the ill person's body. These methods might involve such practices as incantations and/or prayers to the spirits (Frideres, 1988; Jilek, 1982; Tucker, 1965).

Regrettably, the traditional health care system of the people of the First Nations disintegrated as colonization by the Europeans proceeded. The new settlers brought not only Western style medicine but also a new way of life and new diseases. The people of the First Nations were decimated by epidemics of smallpox, diphtheria, measles and influenza, along with the ever-present tuberculosis. In addition, high rates of mental illness and alcoholism resulted from attempts to cope with the rapid changes that were taking place in their society (Frideres, 1988).

In 1945, the Department of Health and Welfare assumed responsibility for the provision of direct health care services to all people of the First Nations. At first, this was in a separate unit called "Indian Health." In 1962, this unit was merged with other federal health programs, to form the Medical Services Branch of the Department. During the 1960s and 1970s, a network of hospitals, nursing stations and community health centres was developed by Medical Services to provide health care to people of the First Nations, including those living on reserves within provincial boundaries and those living in the northern territories. The structure is still in place, with services provided by physicians, nurses, health educators, dental therapists and community health representatives.

THE CURRENT SITUATION

Nurses have played the greatest role in the delivery of these health services — first with the missionary services provided by church groups and later by the federal government (Keith, 1971). The network of services consists of base hospitals from which satellite nursing stations and community health centres (also staffed by nurses) fan out, supported by community health workers at the local level.

LOOKING BACK

ALICE KATHERINE SMITH (b. 1910)

Alice Katherine Smith, the first Chief Nursing Consultant with Indian Health Services (later renamed Indian and Northern Affairs and still later the Medical Services Branch of Health and Welfare Canada), was a major contributor to the development and success of the health care programs for Canada's remote areas from 1950 to 1975 and a major force behind the development of Canada's northern health services.

Alice Katherine Smith was born in Cartwright, Manitoba, in 1910, the eldest daughter in a family that lost the father during World War I. She received her nursing diploma from the Winnipeg General Hospital in 1933 and took a certificate in public health nursing at the University of Toronto in 1938. She then joined the Manitoba Department of Health as a staff nurse in rural areas, eventually becoming the nursing consultant responsible for rural cancer education programs from 1942 to 1948. As a young public health nurse in rural and northern areas, she recognized the importance of primary nursing services in the many areas of Canada where doctors are not available.

In 1948, she was asked by the Canadian Nurses Association to go to Great Britain to study the effects on nursing of the new national health insurance plan that had been launched in that country. She received her baccalaureate degree in nursing education from Teachers College, Columbia University, in 1950. She then joined the newly reorganized Indian Health Services, part of the Department of National Health and Welfare in Winnipeg. She took her master's of public health degree at Yale University in 1957.

In her 25 years with the federal government, during which she achieved increasing influence as a Chief Nursing Consultant, she initiated continuous refinements in the medical services under her supervision. She saw drastic improvements in health care for the Inuit and the North American Indian peoples, especially the dramatic decreases in maternal and infant mortality rates and the reductions in incidence of tuberculosis. She found many practical ways for northern nurses to upgrade their credentials and improve practice in their remote health facilities. As well, she provided opportunities for universities to work with remote nursing stations to increase their field experience and understanding of primary nursing needs. Her efforts helped establish ever-better guidelines for health care delivery in Canada's remote areas.

— Glennis Zilm

The standard nursing station has two or more nurses, and may have a few inpatient beds, cribs and bassinets.

The nurses are responsible for providing primary health care for a community of 200 to 800 people and possibly the people in one or two surrounding smaller communities. The nurses provide treatment services for those who are ill and promotive and preventive services for people in the community, including school health services, pre- and post-natal clinics and home visits. The nurses diagnose and treat common illnesses and follow certain standard drug protocols. They also have access to medical support at the base hospital through radio-telephone and can evacuate patients if necessary to the base hospital or to other centres for treatment. Physicians make regular visits to all the nursing stations to see people who require additional care.

By 1988, Medical Services Branch staff consisted of more than two hundred doctors (eleven of them First Nations people), over a thousand nurses (150 of whom were First Nations) and over five hundred Community Health workers (Frideres, 1988). In addition to the nursing and medical services described above, the Indian and Northern Health Services provide non-insured health benefits to Inuit and Registered Indians. These services include drugs, medical supplies, medical equipment, vision care, dental care, medical transportation, health insurance premiums and co-insurance fees.

The governments of the Northwest Territories (and the Yukon) have taken over administration and delivery of non-insured health benefits for Inuit and registered Indians in the territories under agreements with the Federal Government. Other programs include a National Native Alcohol and Drug Abuse Program which was established to provide culturally relevant, community-based preventive and treatment services, as well as a program directed at minimizing family violence. Medical Services also has a Native Career Development Program to prepare First Nations people for careers in the health field.

There is no doubt that the health care provided by Medical Services did a great deal to improve the health status of First Nations people — one has only to look at the considerable decline in infant and child mortality from the 1950s to the 1980s to appreciate this fact. However, the rate is still more than double that of the rest of Canada and other health statistics strikingly attest to the need for improved health conditions.

Keeping in mind the *Active Health Report* (1987) which documented the poor state of health of people in low income brackets, it is important to note that First Nations people as a group occupy the lower status positions in Canadian society. Nearly half of the adults have less than a Grade 9 education, and more than half do in the North (see Figure 12.6).

The unemployment rate among people of the First Nations has been excessively high (around 60 percent ranging to 90 percent in some parts of the country). Income is correspondingly low, with most of those who work occupying low status jobs (see Figure 12.7). Much of the income comes from government transfer payments although it should be noted that the income figures do not include income-in-kind from hunting, fishing and similar activities. Housing, which is looked upon as one of the main determinants of the level of welfare of a population, is well below that of the average non-First Nations Canadian (Maslove and Hawkes, 1989; Frideres, 1988).

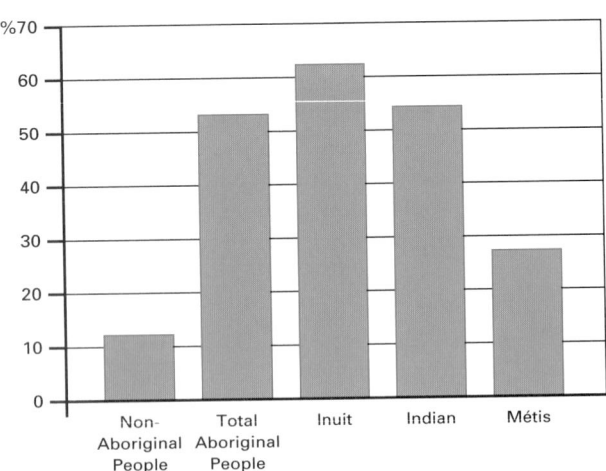

FIGURE 12.6 Proportion of Northern Aboriginal and non-Aboriginal people aged 15 and over with less than Grade 9, 1986

SOURCE: Maslove, A. and Hawkes, D. (1989, Winter). The northern population. In *Canadian Social Trends, 15,* 5.

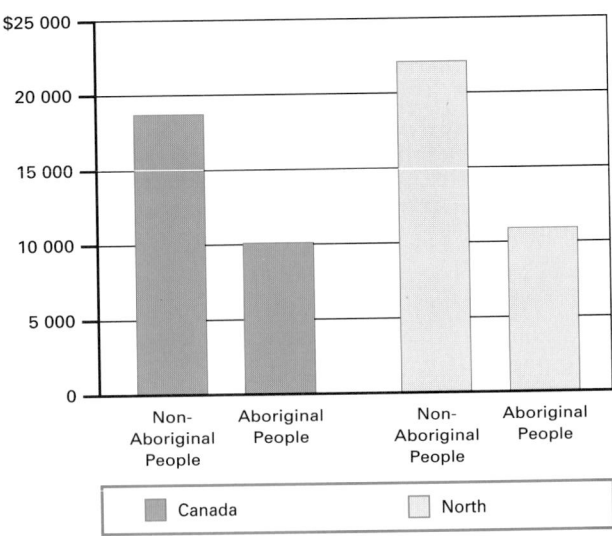

FIGURE 12.7 Average income of Canadian and Northern Aboriginal and non-Aboriginal people, 1985

SOURCE: Maslove, A. and Hawkes, D. (1989, Winter). The northern population. In *Canadian Social Trends, 15,* 6.

THE TRANSFER OF SERVICES

The transfer of health services to First Nations people can be viewed as part of a devolutionary process that has been going on for the past 20 years. This process started in the 1970s when the Federal Government turned educational control over to local First Nations authorities. It continued through the 1980s and into the 1990s with the transfer of child and family services and with the development of economic institutions for people of the First Nations that have continued to progress (Gibbons and Associates, 1992).

The push for a transfer of health services was accelerated by passage of the Constitution Act of 1982 and the subsequent movement towards self-government. Between 1983 and 1986, Medical Services funded community health demonstration projects in 31 communities as an experiment with the administrative transfer of health services. The Health Transfer Initiative was announced by Health Minister Jake Epp in 1986. Following a period of consultation with all North American Indian bands in the country, the Treasury Board of Canada in June, 1989, approved authorities and resources for the transfer of Indian health services from the Federal Government to First Nations wishing to assume responsibility. The long-term goal of the transfer, as stated in a discussion paper that was sent to all Indian Chiefs in Canada, is "a more integrated, culturally relevant community health program and improved health conditions for Indian people" (Health and Welfare Canada, 1986; Gibbons and Associates, 1992).

The transfer process was designed to have three phases:

1. research into the health needs of the community and the resources available to meet these needs with subsequent development of a community health plan

2. negotiation between the First Nations community and government. During this phase, any outstanding issues are resolved and a Transfer Agreement is signed

3. the actual transfer implementation. As part of the agreement, the community must prepare an annual report for community members and an evaluation of the program to be used for future planning.*

The whole process takes approximately one to two years, or more, in some cases. The Health Transfer process is going on at the same time as many Indian bands are becoming self-governing. The Health Transfers appear to be most successful in communities where the two processes are taking place together or where self-government is already in effect.

Early reports indicate that most communities feel they have benefited from the transfer process. At the local level, there has been a development of new skills in planning and management and few negative consequences. People of the First Nations are involved in the health care of their own communities as members of community and regional health councils and they are involved as front line workers, as community health representatives and increasingly as professional health workers in these communities.

Health Care Transfer

Health transfer enables First Nations to

- design and manage health programs according to specific community priorities;

- mobilize community participation leading to improved health status

- become recognized as equal participating health care providers within the Canadian Health Care System

- be autonomous and accountable to their memberships

- enhance self-government.

SOURCE: Health and Welfare Canada. (1992). *Health Transfer. Year End Report 1991–1992*. Ottawa: Medical Services Branch.

---

* (Health and Welfare Canada, 1992).

KEY TERMS

IN REVIEW

Canada is a multicultural society whose people have come from many different countries. Starting with the people of the First Nations who are believed to have migrated from Asia, future Canadians came from France, then from Britain in successive waves of immigration predominantly from European countries until the latter part of this century. From the 1970s onward, people from Asian countries have dominated the immigration ranks. Ontario, British Columbia, Quebec and Alberta attract the largest number of immigrants, most of whom settle in urban areas: Toronto, Montreal and Vancouver have the most new Canadians.

Although two-thirds of the population named English as their first or second mother tongue and one-quarter listed French, a total of 126 mother tongues were named by Canadians in the last census. Twenty-three of these were aboriginal languages. Just over one percent of the population, mainly new immigrants and the elderly, speak neither English nor French, a fact which can sometimes put stress on health care and other services.

National policy encourages immigrants to retain their own culture within the overall framework of Canadian society. The multicultural nature of this society makes it imperative that nurses become skilled in the practice of culturally sensitive care. People bring their beliefs about health and their health practices with them when they immigrate. These beliefs and practices are more closely related to religious beliefs and to the family's traditional health doctrine than to ethnic origin. They may be modified by the dominant culture over time, but when people are ill they often fall back on the time-honoured ways of home.

The religions of the world can be divided into two groups, Western and Eastern. The majority of Canadians subscribe to one of the three major Western religions: Catholic (46.5%), Protestant (30%) and Judaism (one percent). These religions share the belief that each individual has a personal relationship with God and that there is a life after death. The most common Eastern religions in Canada, subscribed to by three percent of the population, are Hinduism, Sikhism and Buddhism which share a belief in reincarnation and advocate non-violence.

The religious groups differ on their Holy Days, their Holy Scriptures, their religious holidays, food taboos and rules regarding addictive substances, clothing, cleanliness, baptism, transplantation of body parts, abortions, autopsy and care of the dead. The nurse should always check with the patient and/or family about any religious preferences.

All cultures have developed their own healing practices. Those that were effective have been handed down from generation to generation and are still being used in many parts of the world. Among the most common of the traditional practices are: shamanism, herbalism, Ayurvedic medicine, naturopathy, Chinese/Oriental medicine, faith healing and therapeutic touch, chiropractic medicine and others like reflexology and aromatherapy. Many of these are being used in conjunction with Western medicine as practitioners acknowledge that there is a role for traditional medicine in modern health care.

Although we have universal health care in this country, many people have difficulty accessing this care. Among the general population, the factors that limit access include the unequal distribution of health resources as well as the negative attitude of some health care workers towards people who are not of the dominant culture, who hold views other than their own or who belong to certain segments of society such as the poor, the homeless, alcoholics or drug abusers. In addition to these barriers, immigrants and refugees often have further problems such as health insurance regulations, lack of a common language, low self-esteem, conflict with traditional beliefs and practices, insecurity, cultural attitudes holding that treatment should be free, inconvenient hours for health services and racial tensions.

Crossing the barriers to effective health care for all people involves an awareness of one's own cultural limitations; openness, appreciation and respect for other viewpoints; viewing intercultural interactions as learning experiences; using cultural resources as interventions; and acknowledging the integrity and value of all cultures.

The traditional health care of people of Canada's First Nations made use of both herbalism and shamanism.

Colonization by Europeans brought new diseases which decimated the aboriginal population. At the same time, their traditional health care practices were discontinued with gradual assumption of health care for them by the federal government. There has been considerable improvement in the health of the people of the First Nations since the government set up its network of hospitals, nursing stations and community health centres across northern Canada with nurses playing the major role in delivery of services. Still, much remains to be done to improve the social conditions which contribute to poor health. The current transfer of health services to people of the First Nations is intended to provide them with more culturally relevant health programs that will better meet community needs.

LEARNING ACTIVITIES

1. Who were the first members of your family to settle in Canada? What country did they come from? When did they arrive in Canada and where did they settle first?

2. Examine your own health beliefs and practices.
   a. What do you think causes illness?
   b. What health practices (preventive and curative) are traditionally used in your family?
   c. Are there religious traditions or taboos that might influence a hospital stay by someone in your family?
   d. What influence has your background (ethnicity, religion and education) had on your health beliefs and practices?
   e. Do your beliefs and practices concur or conflict with concepts being taught in your nursing program?

3. In discussion with classmates, compare backgrounds of ethnic origin, religion, health beliefs and practices and modifications to these that have occurred or are occurring.

4. If possible, talk with someone among your friends or acquaintances who comes from a different ethnic background than your own. Explore with this individual:
   a. what it was like growing up, either in his or her homeland or in Canada, as a member of an ethnic group different from your own.
   b. what experiences have family members had with the Canadian health care system:
      - How did the individual enter the health care system? Through a family physician? The Emergency Department? A clinic or hospital visit? A Community Health Nurse?
      - How did the person and the family feel about the experience?
      - What comparisons did they make to the care they were used to receiving in their country of origin?
      - Did they encounter any difficulty getting care? If so, what were the problems? How were these problems resolved?

5. Talk with a nurse who has worked or is working in the North about his or her experiences there. If this is not possible, read the articles in the March 1994 issue of The Canadian Nurse on nursing in the North (Bates; Brumwell and Janes; Edgecombe; Graham; and Morewood). Write a short report outlining the benefits and drawbacks of working in a nursing station, community health centre or hospital in the North.

REFERENCES AND READINGS

BADETS, J. (1993, Summer). Canada's immigrants: Recent trends. *Canadian Social Trends, 29*, 8–11.

BATES, V. (1994). What is a northern nurse? *The Canadian Nurse, 90*(3), 26–31.

BENTLEY, S. (1986). *Religions of our neighbours.* (Vols. 1–8). Coquitlam, B.C.: Bentley West Publishing Co.

BERUBE, J. (1990). *Delivering culturally sensitive care.* Vancouver: B.C. Health Association.

BOBET, E. (1989, Winter). Indian Mortality. *Canadian Social Trends, 15*, 11–14.

BREMNESS, L. (1989). *The complete book of herbs.* Montreal: The Readers Digest Association (Canada).

BRISSON, D.P. and DESLAURIERS, C.L. (1992). Les groupes minoritaires visibles. *The Canadian Nurse, 88*(3), 33–35.

BRUMWELL, A. and JANES, C. (1994). Primary health care in Rae-Edzo. *The Canadian Nurse, 90*(3), 37; 38.

CANADA'S FAMILY TREE: CELEBRATING OUR DIVERSITY. (1992, Spring). *Royal Bank Reporter.*

COLOMBO, J.R. (Ed.) (1992). *1993 Canadian Global Almanac.* Toronto: Macmillan.

EASTMAN, Y. (1985). *Reflexology.* Campbell River, B.C.: Ptarmigan Press.

EDGECOMBE, N. (1994). Northern nurses' petition. *The Canadian Nurse, 90*(3), 39.

EPP, J. (1986). *Achieving health for all: A framework for health promotion.* Ottawa: Minister of Supply and Services.

FRIDERES, J.S. (1988). Racism and health: The case of the native people. In B.S. Bolaria and H.D.Dickinson *Sociology of health care in Canada.* Toronto: Harcourt Brace Jovanovich, 135–147.

GIBBONS, A. and ASSOCIATES. (1992). *Short-term evaluation of Indian Health Transfer.* Victoria, B.C.: Author.

GRAHAM, K. (1994). Inservice education for northern nurses. *The Canadian Nurse, 90*(3), 33–36.

GROSSMAN, R. (1985). *The other medicines.* Garden City, NY: Doubleday.

GRYPMA, S. (1993). Culture Shock. *The Canadian Nurse, 89*(8), 33–36.

GUINESS, A.E. and RUTHERFORD, A.P. (1993). *Family guide to natural medicine.* Montreal: The Reader's Digest Association (Canada).

HEALTH AND WELFARE CANADA. (1986). *A discussion paper on the transfer of Indian health programs for consultation with the Indian people.* Ottawa: Author.

HEALTH AND WELFARE CANADA. (1992). *Health transfer. Year end report 1991–1992.* Ottawa: Medical Services Branch, Health and Welfare Canada.

HENLEY, A. (1983a). *Asians in Britain: Caring for Hindus and their families — religious aspects of care.* Cambridge, England: National Extension College.

HENLEY, A. (1983b). *Caring for Sikhs and their families: Religious aspects of care.* Cambridge: National Extension College.

HONG FOOK MENTAL HEALTH ASSOCIATION. (1986). *Assessment and treatment of Chinese patients: A holistic model.* Toronto: Author.

JILEK, W.G. (1982). *Indian healing.* Surrey, B.C.: Hancock House.

KEITH, C.W. (1971). Leadership in nursing north of sixty. *Nursing clinics of North America, 6*(3), 479–488.

KENNISON, M.M. (1987). Faith: An untapped health resource. *Journal of Psychosocial Nursing, 25*(10), 28–30.

KRIEGER, D. (1975). Therapeutic touch: The imprimateur of nursing. *American Journal of Nursing,* 784–787.

KRIEGER, D. (1979). *Therapeutic touch: How to use your hands to heal.* Englewood Cliffs, NJ: Prentice-Hall.

LEININGER, M. (1978). *Transcultural nursing: Concepts, theories and practices.* New York: Wiley.

LOYER, M. (1975). Remarks on presentation of Honorary Doctorate to Alice Katherine Smith, University of Ottawa. Unpublished paper. Available University of Ottawa, Ottawa.

LUNA, L. and CAMERON, C. (1988) Leininger's transcultural nursing. In J.J. Fitzpatrick and A.L. Whall. *Conceptual models of nursing.* Norwalk, CT: Appleton & Lange, 227–240.

LYNCH, E.W. and HANSON, M.J. (1992). *Developing crosscultural competence.* Baltimore: Paul H. Brooks.

MARTIN, J.D. (1985). Baha'i Faith. *The Canadian Encyclopaedia.* Edmonton: Hurtig.

MASLOVE, A. and HAWKES, D. (1989, Winter). The northern population. *Canadian Social Trends, 15,* 2–7. (Statistics Canada Catalogue No. 11–008E)

MOREWOOD, N. (1994). Nursing in the Northwest Territories. *The Canadian Nurse, 90*(3), 26–31.

MULTICULTURALISM AND CITIZENSHIP CANADA. (1990). *The Canadian Multiculturalism Act — A Guide for Canadians.* Ottawa: Author.

NON PARLO NE' INGLESE NE' FRANCESE. (1993, Winter) *Canadian Social Trends, 31,* 26–28.

OLSON, K.G. (1990). *The encyclopedia of alternative health care.* New York: Simon and Shuster.

PORTER, J. (1979). *The Measure of Canadian Society: Education, equality and opportunity.* Toronto: Gage.

RENAUD, V. and BADETS, J. (1993, Fall). Ethnic diversity in the 1990s. *Canadian Social Trends, 30,* 17–22.

SHAW, E. (1986). *60 second Shiatzu.* New York: Mills and Sanderson.

SIGGNER, A.J. (1989, Winter). The Inuit. *Canadian Social Trends, 15,* 8–10.

SMITH, A.K. (1992). *Biographical information profile.* Unpublished paper. Available from the History of Nursing Professional Practice Group, Registered Nurses Association of B.C., Vancouver.

STATISTICS CANADA. (1993a). *1991 Aboriginal peoples survey: Language, tradition, health, lifestyle and social issues.* Ottawa: Author. (Catalogue No. 89–533)

STATISTICS CANADA. (1993b). Ethnic Origin. *The Nation.* Ottawa: Author. (Catalogue No. 93–315)

STATISTICS CANADA. (1993c). Immigration and Citizenship. *The Nation.* Ottawa: Author. (Catalogue No. 93–316)

STATISTICS CANADA. (1993d). Knowledge of Languages. *The Nation.* Ottawa: Author. (Catalogue No. 93–318)

STATISTICS CANADA. (1993e). Mother Tongue. *The Nation.* Ottawa: Author. (Catalogue No. 93–317)

STEWART, E. (1991). *The Dene and Na-dene Indian migration 1233 AD: Escape from Ghenghis Khan to America.* Columbus, GA: Institute for the Study of American Cultures Inc.

TUCKER, P. (1965). *Cultures of the North Pacific Coast.* San Francisco: Chandler Publishing.

TURCOTTE, P. (1993, Summer). Mixed-language couples and their children. *Canadian Social Trends, 29,* 15–17. (Statistics Canada Catalogue No. 11–008E)

VANCOUVER HEALTH DEPARTMENT. (1993). Discussions with G.C. Mumick, Multicultural Health Education Consultant, Vancouver, B.C.

WEXLER-MORRISON, N., ANDERSON, J. and RICHARDSON, E. (1990). *Cross Cultural Caring.* Vancouver, B.C.: University of British Columbia Press.

ZERR, S.R. (1993). *Interview with Alice Smith and Kay Keith* [Oral History tape]. Available Library, Registered Nurses Association of B.C., Vancouver.

ZUMBRO VALLEY MEDICAL SOCIETY. (1975). *Religious aspects of medical care.* Rochester, MN: The Catholic Hospital Association.

UNIT 3

Skills Basic to Nursing Practice

CHAPTER 13

Theories and Conceptual Frameworks for Nursing Practice

OUTLINE

Introduction

The Nature of Nursing Knowledge

The Evolution of Nursing Theories

Theoretical Pluralism

The Value of Theories and Conceptual Models For Nursing Education,
  Research and Practice

CENTRAL QUESTIONS

1. What do the terms theory, model, conceptual model, conceptual framework, grand theory, mega theory and metaparadigm mean?

2. What is the difference between a concrete and an abstract concept?

3. What concepts are considered central to nursing?

4. What are the three levels of nursing theory?

5. How have developments in the humanities and in the biological and physical sciences influenced the development of nursing theory?

6. What differentiates one conceptual model of nursing from another?

7. What is the value of nursing theories for nursing practice, education and research?

8. How do you use a nursing model in clinical practice?

INTRODUCTION

Theory is the process by which nursing becomes a science and a special way of human caring.

Roach, 1992.

The caring professions are as old as humankind. There have always been healers and wise men and wise women who have assisted in the birth of infants, have cared for the sick and gathered medicinal herbs from which they concocted medicines to heal ailments. In some societies, the healer and the care-giver were one and the same. In others, the healers became a specialized group known variously as *wizards*, *witches*, *shamans*, and later, *doctors* or *physicians*. And those who nurtured the sick — the "care-givers" — became another specialized group: the *nurses*, from the Greek word for *nurture*.

Behavioural psychologists tell us that the knowledge and skills of both groups were probably learned initially through a process of trial and error, with medicines and techniques found to be effective passed down from one generation to the next. There are others who believe that there is a collective consciousness, or "collective knowing," that is imprinted in the subconscious memory of the human race which provides us with an intuitive understanding of what needs to be done for the survival of the species. Those who subscribe to the latter theory believe that we can tap into this archetypal knowledge if we open ourselves up to it (Agan, 1987).

Whichever theory you subscribe to, there is evidence to support the view that, as the knowledge and skills of healing and of caring for the sick became more clearly defined, an apprenticeship form of training evolved. Self-selected, chosen by the master or, sometimes, by the community, apprentices learned by observing and by listening, and then, by carrying out procedures and preparing medications themselves under the watchful eye of their role model. Both nursing and medicine went through the same process.

In nursing, the apprenticeship type of preparation for practice lasted well into the second half of the nineteenth century when Florence Nightingale opened the first truly educational program for nurses at St. Thomas' Hospital in London, England, in 1860. For the better part of a century, most nurses were prepared in hospital schools modelled on the Nightingale school. There are many who say that nursing really did not progress from the apprenticeship method of training until the middle of the twentieth century, however, because the hospital schools that followed in the wake of the Nightingale school gave higher priority to service by students than to the educational component of the programs.

Be that as it may, nursing managed finally to emerge from the apprenticeship mode and into the realm of professional education based on an emerging nursing science.

As with the evolution of knowledge in other fields, the development of nursing science is a history of shifting ideas. Many traditional nursing procedures have been discarded, others have been modified and the value of some reaffirmed in studies undertaken by nurse researchers.

An example of a modified traditional procedure is the back rub — a nursing intervention used over the years by thousands of students and practitioners. Nurses used to rub the patient's back with alcohol after a bed bath and also as part of the "evening care" routine in most hospitals. There was probably good reason to use rubbing alcohol in the days when infections were rampant and there was a need to cool the skin of feverish patients. The practice has long since been replaced by back rubs for bedridden patients using emollient creams or lotions that do not have such a drying effect on the skin. Practitioners no longer do things simply because it is the traditional way of doing them but, rather, with an understanding of the rationale behind their actions. Students learn not only to carry out nursing interventions with skill and dexterity, they also learn why these interventions are implemented, through a process of logical reasoning.

The importance of certain aspects of traditional practice has been reaffirmed in the current emphasis on the caring aspect of the nurse's role in numerous texts and treatises. We now seem to realize that the human aspect of caring for patients is just as important in developing nursing expertise as are the knowledge and skill components. This caring aspect was historically passed along from expert to novice in good apprenticeship programs but was almost lost sight of when we became enamoured with science.

Leininger says that human caring is a universal phenomenon and she feels that it is the "central, dominant and unifying feature" for the body of nursing knowledge (1988, 152). The focus of nursing is on people and on how people cope with their state of health, while the focus of medicine has historically been on people's illnesses. Nursing theory is what differentiates the focus of nursing from that of medicine and other disciplines. It also facilitates the identification of nursing problems and provides nurses with a rational basis for their actions. It guides the nurse in making decisions during the process of giving care. Increasingly, nurses in clinical practice are using theoretical models not only to provide direction for their practice but also to develop standards for evaluating the quality of care (Campbell, 1987; Casey, 1989).

Credit for the tremendous advances in nursing that have come about in the past few decades belongs to the nurse researchers who have pushed back the boundaries of knowledge in the field, to the nurse clinicians whose expertise provides us with clues about the nature of nursing practice and to the nurse theorists who have contributed the framework on which to base further nursing knowledge. In this chapter, we are going to talk about the nature of nursing knowledge, the evolution of nursing theories and the value of theories for education, research and practice.

In your readings, you will come across a number of different terms used in talking about nursing theories. *Theory, model, conceptual model, conceptual framework, grand theory, mega theory, metaparadigm* are all terms that are used to describe theoretical frameworks. Different theorists ascribe different meanings to some of the terms. We will try to sort out the terms and provide you with workable definitions as the words are used in this text.

THEORIES AND CONCEPTUAL MODELS

The terms *theory* and *conceptual model* are used interchangeably in much of the nursing literature and we will use them interchangeably in this text. Strictly speaking, however, they are not the same. According to Watson, "A theory is an imaginative grouping of knowledge, ideas and experience that are represented symbolically and seek to illuminate a given phenomenon" (Watson, 1988, 1). In other words, a **theory** is a supposition, or system of ideas that has been proposed to explain a given happening in the world. For example, Newton proposed the theory of gravity concerning the gravitational pull of the earth's centre to account for the apple always falling from tree to ground rather than the other way round.

A **conceptual model** is the diagrammatic representation of a theory. You have probably seen a number of conceptual models, particularly in courses such as chemistry and physics where models have been used for many years to describe various theories. Most nurse theorists develop diagrammatic representations of their theories, and the term *conceptual model*, or simply, *model*, has, by common usage in nursing, come to refer to both the diagram and the theory. The models are also often spoken of as **conceptual frameworks**.

Sometimes you will see conceptual models in nursing referred to as *grand* or *mega theories*. Some theorists, for example, Fawcett, use the term *metaparadigm* to refer to the grand theories (conceptual models), reserving the term *theory* for smaller, testable suppositions (Fawcett, 1989, 21). We prefer to use the generic term *theory* as defined above. The term *metaparadigm* comes from two Greek words, *meta* meaning *with* and *paradigm* meaning *pattern*. Thus, **metaparadigm**, **grand theory** and **mega theory** are terms used to describe the essential pattern of a discipline. Basically, they imply a global statement that identifies phenomena (concepts or ideas) that are of interest to the discipline.

Theories and conceptual models are found in all disciplines. They can be classified into three levels:

1. *Descriptive* — These theories classify or describe phenomena of concern to a discipline, for example, the descriptions of person, health, environment and nurs-ing stated explicitly or implicitly inferred in all conceptual nursing models. They are needed when there is nothing or not much known about the phenomenon.

2. *Explanatory* — These specify relationships among phenomena. Orem, for example, identifies linkages between person, environment and nursing when she talks about the role of the nurse in helping the person to cope with developmental changes.

3. *Predictive* — These move beyond explaining relationships to predicting precise relationships among certain characteristics of a phenomenon or specific differences among groups. Predictive theories deal with the principle of cause and effect. This type of theory may be used to suggest interventions. Nursing does not as yet have very many prescriptive theories that tell us what interventions are best in which situation because there is still much basic descriptive research on phenomena and their relationships that needs to be done.*

The concepts considered to be central to nursing — the ones discussed in all nursing theories (although not always explicitly defined) — are four in number:

1. *person* — the individual, family, group or community that is the recipient of nursing care

2. *environment* — including both the social environment (the patient's family, friends and significant others) and the physical environment, that is, the surroundings

3. *health* — the patient's state of wellness/illness

4. *nursing* — the actions taken by the nurse on behalf of, or in conjunction with, the patient.**

CONCEPTS

In discussing theories and conceptual models, it is important to have a clear understanding of the term *concept*. A **concept** is a complex mental formulation of an object, a property (characteristic) or an event that is derived from an individual's perceptual experience. Some concepts, such as *chair, apple* and *book*, are concrete, or **empirical**. They can be observed, touched or seen and there is a high level of agreement on their meaning. An apple, for example, is an apple to most people (unless it is a computer), whether it is a red Macintosh, a Granny Smith, or any one of a number of other varieties.

Other concepts are **abstract**, however; their meaning is inferred from direct or indirect evidence in the real world. Abstract concepts are more general in nature and are related to an event or to a property of something. Examples of abstract concepts include the emotions — *love, hatred,*

---

* (Fawcett, 1989; Fawcett and Downs, 1986)
** (Fawcett, 1989, 21)

prejudice or *anxiety*, for example, and events, such as *Christmas*, *Passover* or *Ramadan*, as well as properties, or characteristics, such as *normalcy* and *abnormality*. Some abstract concepts can be observed indirectly and some are more intangible. *Pain* is an example of an abstract concept that is indirectly observable — from the patient's facial expression, for example, or attempts to protect an injured part of the body. As we discussed in Chapter 2, health is an intangible concept that each individual views according to his or her own perspective.

There is usually less agreement about the meaning of abstract concepts than there is about concrete ones. There is a need to confirm, or validate, with people exactly what they mean when they use an abstract term. The four concepts of major concern to nurses — person, environment, health and nursing — are abstract concepts. Like other abstract concepts, the terms have different meanings for different people. Later in the chapter, we will take a look at the different meanings ascribed to the basic concepts of person, environment, health and nursing by some of the theorists. Other concepts within the domain of nursing have been identified in diagnostic systems and categories which have evolved as part of the nursing process. We will be discussing diagnostic systems and categories in Chapter 14.

THE EVOLUTION OF NURSING THEORIES

Numerous authors have traced the development of nursing theory and it is not the purpose of this text to duplicate their work. Nor do we believe that, as beginning students, you need exposure to all the nursing theories that have been articulated over the past few decades. We will, therefore, limit our discussion to major trends in the development of nursing theory, illustrating these with conceptual frameworks that have been adopted in Canadian nursing schools and health agencies.

THE BEGINNING — A PHILOSOPHY FOR NURSING

Florence Nightingale is often spoken of as the first modern nurse theorist. Long before the nurses of this century began questioning what nursing is and is not, Nightingale had articulated her views on the subject. These views are recorded in her well known *Notes on Nursing*, first published in 1859 following her experience in the Crimean War. In these *Notes*, Nightingale proposed a philosophy for nursing that outlined the basic premises on which nursing should be practised and the functions nurses should undertake (Chinn and Kramer, 1991, 34). Nightingale felt that nursing was quite distinct from medicine, the focus of nursing being to put "the patient in the best condition for

nature to act upon him" (Nightingale, 1859. Cited in J. George, 1990, 36).

The nurse's responsibility was to provide a clean, safe, quiet, pleasant environment and to provide an adequate diet to promote the patient's recuperative powers. Nightingale's emphasis on a clean, sweet-smelling environment is understandable when one considers that sanitary conditions in most towns and cities of the late nineteenth century were deplorable. Secular hospitals were with few exceptions dirty, foul-smelling places, staffed by slovenly workers who no doubt lived in deplorable conditions themselves. The first Public Health Law in England was enacted in 1875. This law established standards for sanitation, quarantine regulations for communicable diseases, and measures to ensure safe water and food supplies. Most Canadian provinces subsequently passed laws modelled after the English one during the latter years of the nineteenth century.

Using today's terminology, we might say that Nightingale focussed on the interaction between the recipient of nursing care (the patient) and the environment, with nursing interventions directed at manipulating the environment in order to promote the person's return to health.

EARLY 20TH CENTURY NURSING THEORY

The period following Florence Nightingale's era — the first half of the twentieth century — was not a positive one for nursing. It saw the hospitals become the primary focus for health care and physicians the dominant force in the provision of health services. Nursing schools, which Nightingale had envisioned as separate educational institutions, became instead part of the nursing service of hospitals. Students were looked upon as a source of cheap labour in most hospital "training schools." Most courses were taught by physicians, and most hospitals were administered by physicians — nursing was viewed simply as an extension of (and subordinate to) medicine. Nursing was considered a vocation for women, whereas the medical profession was for men, with very few exceptions. Indeed, nurses were considered to be "handmaidens to the physician."

It was not until the 1950s and early 1960s that nurses began to assert their independence. A number of factors were involved in this movement, including feminism, the increasing number of nurses prepared in university schools and the emergence of graduate programs in nursing to prepare nursing leaders. Struggling to find their own identity separate from medicine, nurses kept asking, "What is nursing?" Eventually, some nurses began to articulate their views on just what nursing was all about. Gradually, the four basic concepts emerged as common themes in the descriptions of nursing by the early theorists. In developing their views on nursing, these theorists also began to explore the relationships between the four concepts, for example, how the environment affected the person and his or her health and what actions nurses could take to help bring about changes in the health status of the person they were caring for (Chinn and Kramer, 1991; Whall, 1989).

THE INFLUENCE OF THE HUMANISTS

Many of the early nurse theorists were influenced by developments taking place in the behavioural sciences of psychology, sociology and education (often referred to as the human sciences). These humanist disciplines provided a perspective from which to explore ideas central to nursing. Three of the humanists whose work was particularly influential in the development of nursing theory were Carl Rogers, Edward Thorndike and Abraham Maslow.

During the 1940s and 1950s, Rogers' non-directive approach to counselling had revolutionized the field of psychology. This approach was based on the premise that all people have the capacity to solve their own problems, given the opportunity to work them through with an empathetic counsellor who permits the patient to direct the therapeutic process (Rogers, 1961).

Thorndike was the author of *Human nature and the social order* (1940) and is well known for his work in the field of education. He postulated a set of "laws of learning" which has been widely used in courses on the nature of learning.

Abraham Maslow's primary contribution to nursing theory is found in his hierarchy of human needs, which we discussed in Chapter 8. His prioritization of needs is of direct relevance to nurses, who are responsible for attending to a patient's many, and often conflicting, needs (Maslow, 1970).

Two of the most influential of the early nursing theorists of the twentieth century were Hildegarde Peplau and Virginia Henderson. Hildegarde Peplau's work shows the influence of the humanists, in particular, that of Rogers. Her work embraces his emphasis on patient-directed therapy. Peplau saw nursing as a "significant, therapeutic, interpersonal process" and coined the term "therapeutic use of self" which has subsequently been incorporated into our nursing language. She viewed the nurse's role in the therapeutic process as assisting the individual to solve problems through increasing interpersonal and problem-solving competencies (Peplau, 1952; Forchuk, 1990).

Virginia Henderson has had considerable influence on nursing in North America and around the world. She is well known for her *Textbook on the Principles and Practice of Nursing* (co-authored with Canadian Bertha Harmer), subsequent texts on the nature of nursing (1966) and numerous scholarly papers. She defined nursing as assisting "...the individual, sick or well, in performance of those activities ... that he or she would perform unaided if he or she had the strength, will or knowledge, ... to gain independence as rapidly as possible" (Henderson, 1966. Cited in Fitzpatrick and Whall, 1989, 110).

Henderson's work reflects the influence of Thorndike and Maslow, both of whom saw the person as an integrated whole. Henderson believed in the uniqueness of the individual and in the inseparability of mind and body. Henderson's well-known definition of nursing and list of fundamental needs extended Thorndike's research in the field of psychology to apply to the person in hospital (Fitzpatrick and Whall, 1989).

Henderson identified 14 fundamental needs. These are the need to:

1. Breathe normally
2. Eat or drink adequately
3. Eliminate body wastes
4. Move and maintain desirable postures
5. Sleep and rest
6. Select suitable clothes — dress and undress
7. Maintain body temperature within normal range by adjusting clothing and modifying the environment
8. Keep the body clean and well-groomed and protect the integument
9. Avoid dangers in the environment and avoid injuring others
10. Communicate with others in expressing emotions, needs, fears or opinions
11. Worship according to one's faith
12. Work in such a way that there is a sense of accomplishment
13. Play or participate in various forms of recreation
14. Learn, discover or satisfy the curiosity that leads to normal development and health and use the available health facilities.*

The nurse's actions should be directed to promoting the patient's optimum independence in meeting these needs (Henderson, 1966). We are indebted to Evelyn Adam, a Canadian nurse theorist, for presenting Henderson's philosophy of nursing in the structure of a conceptual model (Chong Choi 1989; Adam 1991).

One can see in Henderson's work the foundational ideas that Orem used in her self-care conceptual framework which is also based on a needs approach. Dorothea E. Orem is another early American nurse theorist whose work has continued to evolve over the past two decades. The major theme of Orem's conceptual theory is that human beings have self-care needs. These needs may be universal; they may be developmental, changing as the individual passes from one stage of life to the next; or they may be related to the individual's health status.

Orem saw nursing as a helping service and the nurse's role as helping individuals to achieve the maximum independence of which they are capable. She identified the

---

* (Adam, E., 1991, 14–15)

following five methods nurses use for helping people:

- acting for or doing for another
- guiding another
- supporting another (physically or psychologically)
- providing an environment that promotes personal development in relation to becoming able to meet present or future demands for action
- teaching another.*

THE SCIENTIFIC ERA

In Chapter 1, we talked about the explosion of knowledge that has characterized the biomedical sciences in the latter half of this century. We are living in a technological age and nurses have to become skilled in many highly technical diagnostic and therapeutic procedures in the course of their work. Nursing theory has not been immune to the prevailing emphasis on science. A number of nursing theories put forth in the 1960s and 1970s were based on advances in the biomedical sciences. Nursing theories that developed in this era were also influenced by Selye's work on stress (discussed in Chapter 2) and by Dunn's ideas of "optimal wellness."

Faye Abdellah is credited with ushering in the "scientific" era in nursing theory. We are indebted to her for changing our way of thinking about nursing. She has moved us from the medical model's focus on the signs and symptoms of disease to a separate nursing model with a singular focus — the pa-

---

* (Orem, 1985, 138)

tient — and a unique body of knowledge generated from nursing phenomena. Abdellah's approach to nursing, as outlined in the text *Patient-Centred Approaches to Nursing* (1960), revolutionized nursing curricula, changing the emphasis of nursing courses from a disease and body systems orientation to one focussed on patient needs. This was the beginning of patient-centred nursing practice as we know it (Fitzpatrick and Whall, 1989).

Like Henderson and Orem, Abdellah used a needs approach as her conceptual framework. She classified the problems that could be helped by nursing action into 21 categories which she called **nursing problems**. Abdellah felt that it was the nurse's responsibility to help patients (individuals and/or families) to meet their needs using a problem-solving approach. This approach included an assessment of individual patients receiving nursing care, a determination of the nature and extent of their problems (this step is now referred to as **diagnostic reasoning**) and actions taken within the province of nursing to help to resolve these problems. The problem-solving approach is now called the **nursing process** and the steps are labelled slightly differently but, basically, it is the same process that Abdellah introduced to our thinking more than 30 years ago (Abdellah and Levine, 1986).

Although in this book we have divided the evolution of nursing theory into separate periods to illustrate changes in ideas about nursing over the years, the divisions are not clear cut. Nurse theorists have continued to develop their original ideas over the years, incorporating newer ways of thinking as they went along. Orem, for example, has used the more recent concept of the nursing process in elaborating on her conceptual model.

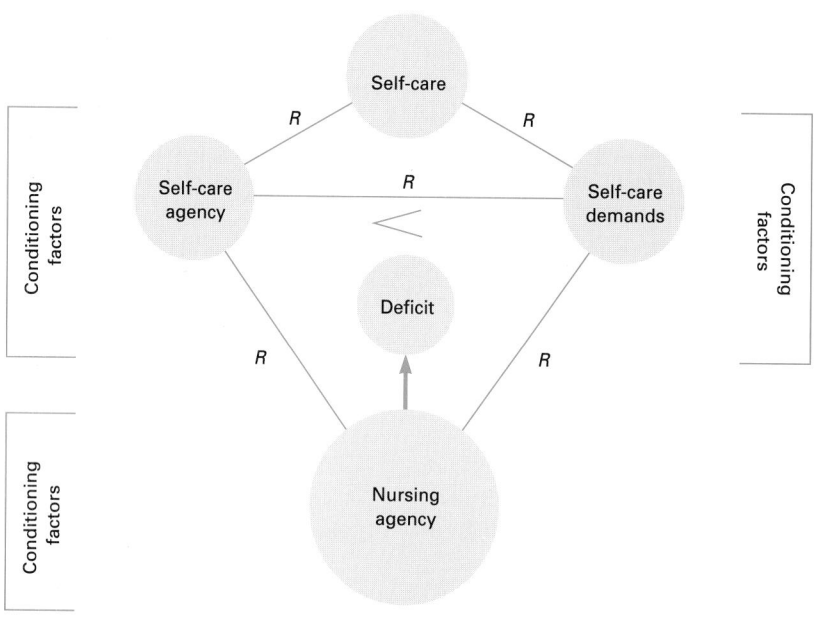

FIGURE 13.1 Orem's conceptual framework for nursing

SOURCE: Orem, D.E. (1991). *Nursing: Concepts of practice* (4th ed.). St. Louis: Mosby Yearbook, 64. Reprinted with permission.

SYSTEMS THEORY

Among the many theorists who were influenced by the biomedical and psychosocial sciences were those who based their conceptual frameworks on general systems theory.

The University of British Columbia (U.B.C.) Model for Nursing, developed in the 1970s by Dr. Margaret Campbell for the U.B.C. School of Nursing, reflects both the humanist approach of earlier theorists and the scientific approach ushered in by Abdellah. According to this model, the patient is an individual who has the following nine basic needs:

1. mastery
2. love, belongingness and dependence
3. respect of self by self and others
4. collection and removal of accumulated wastes
5. intake of food and fluid, nourishment
6. safety and security
7. balance between production and utilization of energy
8. intake of oxygen
9. stimulation of the senses.*

The individual can be looked at as a behavioural system with nine subsystems, each consisting of one of the basic needs and the ability to meet that need (inner personal region) and the psychological environment (need-related goals and the forces influencing their attainment).

In this model, the nurse's role is seen as nurturing "individuals experiencing critical periods so that they may develop and use a range of coping behaviours that will permit them to satisfy their basic human needs, to achieve stability, and to reach optimal health" (Campbell, 1987, 10). The critical period may be either maturational events, such as puberty, or unpredictable events, such as the death of a loved one. Optimal health is the highest level of behavioural system stability achieved by the individual at any given time. Figure 13.2a illustrates the interrelatedness of the

---

* (Campbell, 1987, 7)

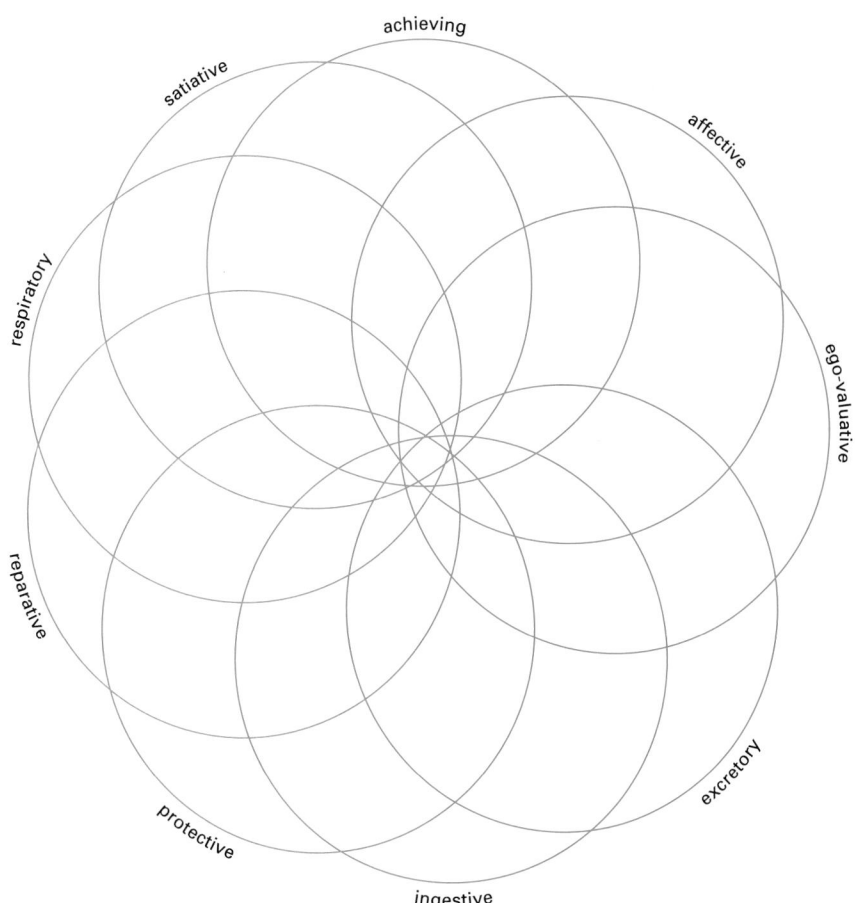

FIGURE 13.2A The individual as a behavioural system

SOURCE: Campbell, M.A. (1987). *The U.B.C. model for nursing: Directions for practice.* Vancouver: University of British Columbia School of Nursing, 32. Reprinted with permission.

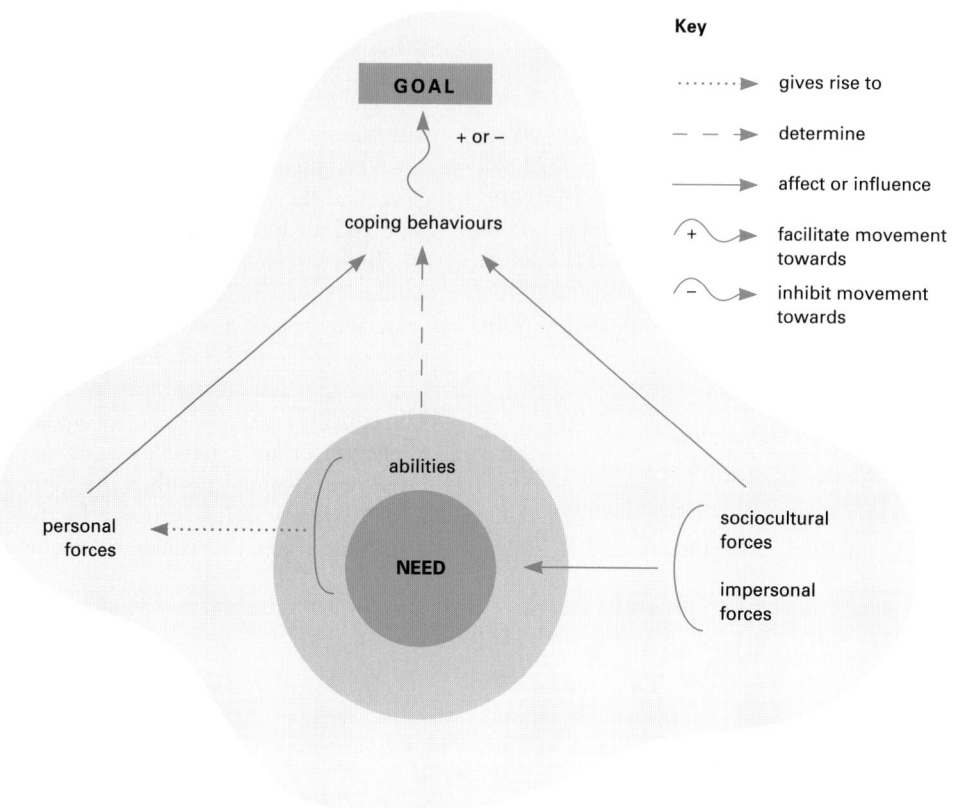

FIGURE 13.2B Structure of a subsystem: Interrelationship of the parts

SOURCE: Campbell, M.A. (1987). *The U.B.C. model for nursing: Directions for practice.* Vancouver: University of British Columbia School of Nursing, 32. Reprinted with permission.

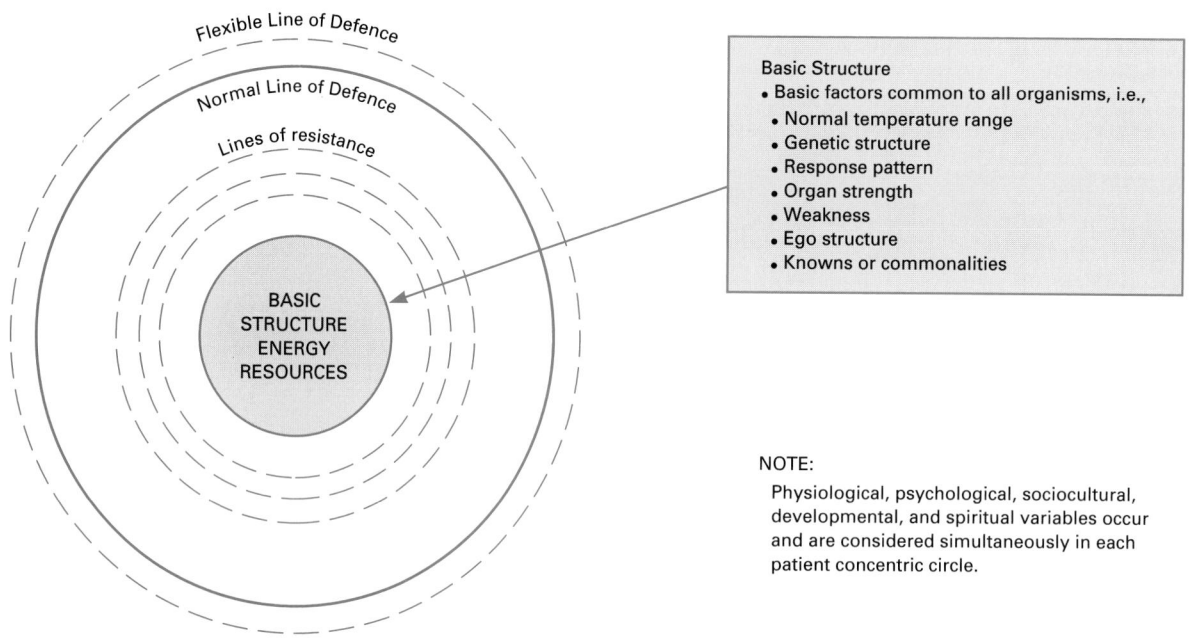

FIGURE 13.3 Neuman's systems model

SOURCE: Neuman, B. (1989). *The Neuman systems model* (2nd ed.). Norwalk, CT: Appleton & Lange, 34. Reprinted with permission.

various subsystems that make up the behavioural system of the individual. Figure 13.2b shows the structure of a subsystem and the interrelationship of its parts.

Betty Neuman and Sister Calista Roy are two other nurse theorists who based their models on systems theory, viewing the human being and the environment as interacting systems.

Neuman's conceptual model is often referred to as a *holistic* model, focussing as it does on the total person, the person's reaction to stress and on factors influencing the person's ability to cope with stress and restore equilibrium. Neuman uses the term **patient system** to refer to either an individual or a group. Neuman sees her model as "a comprehensive, systems-based conceptual framework for nursing … (which) illustrates the composite of five interacting variables — physiological, psychological, sociocultural, developmental and spiritual — ideally functioning harmoniously or stable in relation to internal and external environmental stressor influences upon the patient, as a system, at a given point in time" (Neuman, 1989, 25). Neuman considers nursing to be primarily concerned with appropriate nursing action to facilitate optimal wellness in patients by assisting them to achieve system stability (Neuman, 1989, 25). Neuman's model is shown in Figure 13.3.

In her conceptual model, Roy makes use of general systems theory and of Selye's work on stress. The major theme of Roy's theory is adaptation with a holistic focus on the person in an adaptive system. According to Roy, *person* may refer to either an individual, family or group, a community or a society. The person is also viewed as an adaptive system interacting with the external system of the environment. The adaptive system that is the person is further divided into two major internal processor systems, one

working mainly through the central nervous system, the other through the autonomic nervous system. Roy saw nursing's role as promoting adaptation in the patient (individual or group) to promote wellness. Roy's model is illustrated in the description at the end of this chapter of how the nursing staff at one hospital used a conceptual model to move into theory-based practice in their agency (Roy, 1984; Roy and Andrews, 1991). Figure 13.4 is a diagrammatic representation of Roy's Adaptation Model.

ENERGY FIELDS

Martha Rogers and, more recently, Rosemary Parse, used developments in modern physics to take nursing theory beyond the concepts of equilibrium used in earlier systems models (Chinn and Kramer, 1991). Rogers, in her "Science of Unitary Human Beings," portrays humankind as a unified whole whose fundamental unit is the human energy field. The human energy field is an open system constantly exchanging energy with the environment (Rogers, 1970, 1980; Quillin and Runk, 1989). Rogers says that nursing is unique among the sciences because it is the only one that deals with the person as a whole. She sees the goal of nursing as promoting harmonious interaction between the person and the environment (Rogers, 1980, 1986; Barrett, 1990).

Parse, in explaining her Man-Living-Health model (1981, 1987), expresses the view that nursing is both an art and a science. She sees the individual as a unitary, indivisible human being existing together with the universe and free to make independent decisions. The role of nursing she sees as assisting the patient to participate in making decisions in situations involving the person's health.

FIGURE 13.4 The person as an adaptive system

SOURCE: Roy, C. (1984). *Introduction to nursing: An adaptation model* (2nd ed.). Englewood Cliffs, NJ: Prentice Hall, 30. Reprinted with permission.

RETURN OF THE HUMANIST INFLUENCE

By the late 1970s, nurses, and many people in other fields, were beginning to question the widespread reliance on empirical science as the sole basis for knowledge. The 1980s saw a shift towards a broader view that encompassed personal knowledge, as well as ethics and esthetics as a basis for nursing knowledge. There has been a reawakened interest in the writings of humanists. We see this return to humanism in the later writings of some of the nurse theorists we mentioned earlier, but it is in the work of Madeleine Leininger and of Jean Watson that this trend is probably best exemplified.

Leininger (1978, 1991), working with people of different cultures in the mid 1970s, came to the conclusion that human care is universal — it is seen in all cultures. She feels that caring is the essence of nursing and defines *care* as "action towards assisting, supporting or enabling another individual (or group) with evident or anticipated needs to ameliorate or improve a human condition or lifeway" (Leininger, 1988, 156). Leininger sees the person as a cultural being. She feels that human beings have survived because of their ability to care for infants, younger and older adults and their ability to adapt to different environments and different ways. She sees the environment as a broad concept encompassing the total context in which a person lives, including the physical, social, ecological and global setting.

A diagrammatic representation of Leininger's Sunrise Model is shown in Figure 13.5.

Watson's work shows the influence of Carl Rogers, both in her definition of the self and in the inclusion of the soul in her description of the recipient of nursing care. She feels that nursing is a human science and that caring is the moral ideal of nursing (Watson, 1988, 6). She defines nursing as "an art and a science directed toward the protection, enhancement and preservation of human dignity" (Watson, 1988, 35) and sees the nurse's role as helping the person gain more self-knowledge, self-control and readiness for self-healing regardless of the external health condition.

TOWARDS A HEALTH ORIENTATION

Many of the nurse theorists whom we have discussed have continued to develop their conceptual models over time. Many of the earlier models viewed patients as being somewhat incapacitated and needing the nurse's help to regain health and independence. Now, as our health care system shifts towards a health- rather than an illness-oriented model, we see in the work of nurse theorists increasing emphasis on health promotion and health protection (rather than illness prevention — a subtle distinction but one that underscores the changes taking place) and on the concepts of self-knowledge and self-healing. Watson's and Leininger's work both show evidence of this trend.

One Canadian theorist whose work reflects this reorientation to health is Moyra Allen. Her nursing model serves as the curriculum model of the McGill School of Nursing and is sometimes referred to as the McGill Model. The model, which has been evolving over a period of some 20 years, was designed to serve as a means for generating a knowledge base about nursing through accumulating basic knowledge about the nature of healthy living. Much of the data was gathered through a series of health workshops funded by Health and Welfare Canada.

Allen suggests that the search for healthy living is a natural quest of human beings and she sees nursing as a professional response to this search. Health is viewed as a way of living, rather than as a state of being. It is something that is learned over time. The basic unit in Allen's model is the family or other social group in which learning about health and healthy behaviours take place. The nurse and the patient (patient–family) are viewed as equal partners in the search for healthy living. The nurse's role is to assist families to enhance their problem-solving skills and to use their own (individual, family and community) potential to make the best decisions possible about the various options open to them. The process involves learning how to select from among available resources, when to ask for help and where and how to get it (Allen, 1974, 1982, 1986; Kravitz and Frey, 1989).

Nursing theory continues to evolve. The questioning and testing of existing knowledge by clinicians, researchers and theorists stimulates the development of new ideas. As new ideas emerge, they are used to build on previous thinking. Thus, there is a synthesis of knowledge that adds to, refines and changes the existing body of knowledge (Casey, 1989).

As we look at the evolution of nursing theory, it is easy to see the emergence of different schools of thought. The differences in conceptual frameworks that have emerged reflect the theorists' interpretations of the major concepts considered central to nursing and the linkages between them. Table 13.1 provides a comparison of how some of the different theorists view *person, environment, health* and *nursing*.

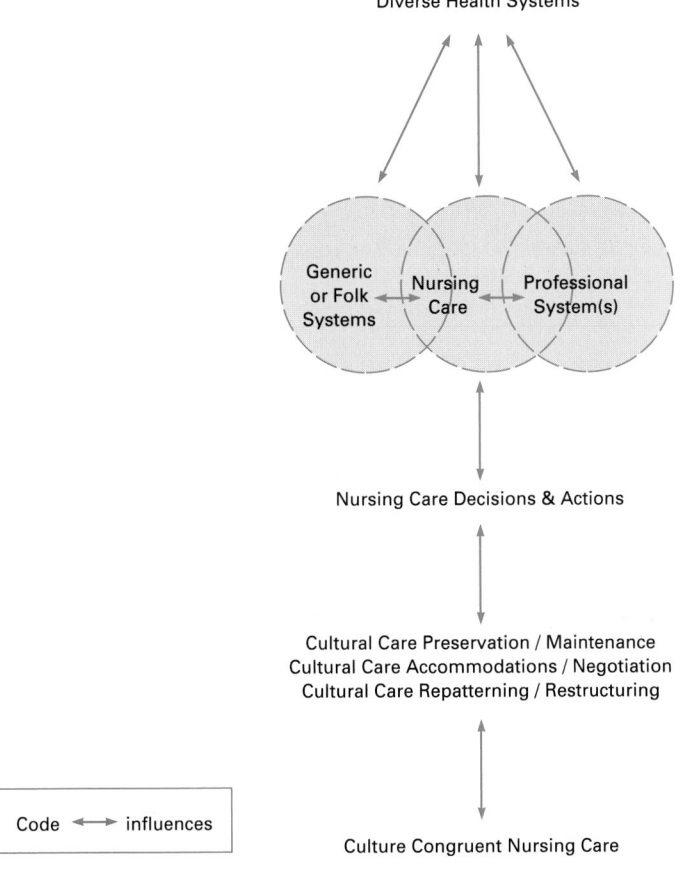

FIGURE 13.5 Leininger's Sunrise Model

SOURCE: Leininger, M.M. (Ed.). (1991). *Culture care diversity and universality: A theory of nursing.* New York: N.L.N.E. Press, 43. (Publication No. 15–2402) Reprinted with permission.

TABLE 13.1 The Basic Elements of Selected Conceptual Models

	FLORENCE NIGHTINGALE	HILDEGARDE PEPLAU	VIRGINIA HENDERSON	DOROTHY OREM	FAYE ABDELLAH	SISTER CALISTA R
Major Theme	Unique Role of the Nurse	Interpersonal Process within the Nurse-Patient Relationship	Basic Needs	Self-care Needs	Patient's/Nursing Problems	Adaptation
Person	An individual who has the recuperative powers within self to restore own health	An individual with the capacity for growth through increasing interpersonal and problem-solving competencies	A unique individual in whom mind and body are inseparable who has 14 fundamental needs	A unity functioning biologically, symbolically and socially, who has three categories of self-care needs: 1. universal 2. developmental 3. caused by health deviations	Patient or the patient's family with an overt or covert problem which the nurse can assist in solving through the performance of professional functions	A biopsychosocial being in constant interaction wit the environme who has four modes of adaptation: 1. physiologica needs 2. self concept 3. role function 4. interdepend
Environment	Involves those external conditions that affect life and the development of the individual, with a focus on ventilation, warmth, odours and light, and diet	Significant others with whom the person interacts	Not defined specifically	Environmental elements are seen as external to the person and composed of both physical and psychosocial components	Societal and environmental needs are contributing factors to actual and/or anticipated problems. These include not only need-satisfaction problems the patient has in hospital but also at home in the community	All conditions, circumstances and influences surrounding ar affecting the development and behaviour of persons or groups, having both internal and external components ar constantly changing

...TY ...JMAN	MARTHA ROGERS	ROSEMARY PARSE	MADELEINE LEININGER	JEAN WATSON	MOYRA ALLEN	MARGARET CAMPBELL (U.B.C. MODEL OF NURSING)
...ms	Interaction Between Person and Environment	Man-Living-Health	Transcultural Care Diversity and Universality	The Human to Human Process of Caring	The Nature of Healthy Living	The person as a behavioural system with interacting and interdependent subsystems, each representing a basic human need
...teracting ... system that ...namic and ...osed of five ...acting ...bles — ...iological, ...hological, ...cultural, ...lopmental ...spiritual	A four-dimensional energy field characterized by organization and pattern that functions as a unified whole within an open system, exchanging energy with the environment	May be an individual or family. The person as a unitary indivisible human being in constant interchange with the environment, who is free to make decisions and choices about health behaviours based on past or present experience	Human beings (individuals, families and cultural groups) who have survived because of their ability to care for infants, young and older adults in a variety of ways and places	A living, constantly growing totality comprising mind, body, emotion and soul	The family or other social group in which learning is initiated, nurtured and directed	An individual with nine basic human needs, constantly striving to satisfy these needs by using a range of coping behaviours, both innate and acquired
...both external ...internal ...ponents; the ...rnal includes ...ndividual's ...nal lines of ...nce, his or her ...ng patterns, ...yle, family ...economic ...s and ...ational level; ...nternal includes ...ines of resistance ...nding basic ...tures	Also a four-dimensional energy field, with organization and pattern, that is specific for each individual and includes all that is outside the person's own energy field	A constantly changing energy field that surrounds the person and is an integral part of the state of being	The total context within which the individual, family or cultural group live including the physical, ecological, social and world-view aspects	The external reality of the person	The social context in which learning takes place. This may be at home, the workplace, community group, a hospital or a clinic	That which lies outside the boundary of the system

**TABLE 13.1   The Basic Elements of Selected Conceptual Models   *(continued*

	FLORENCE NIGHTINGALE	HILDEGARDE PEPLAU	VIRGINIA HENDERSON	DOROTHY OREM	FAYE ABDELLAH	SISTER CALISTA R
Health	Absence of disease and the ability to use one's own abilities to the highest potential, with emphasis on the reparative process of getting well	Health is represented by forward growth of personality	Optimum health is achievement of the desired measure of independence in carrying out activities of daily living	A state of integrity of human beings. Wellness is equated with the ability to maintain self-care	An optimum state of need satisfaction including the ability to satisfy one's own needs	Health is a function of the degree of change and th state of the pe experiencing change
Definition of Nursing	A profession for women, separate and distinct from medicine, using nature's laws of health in the service of humanity	An interpersonal process between nurse and patient that is goal-oriented	An independent, unique health profession carrying out activities with or on behalf of the patient that contribute to health or recovery (or to a peaceful death) that the patient would perform unaided given the necessary strength, will or knowledge	A human service helping people to overcome self-care deficits related to health	An art and a science that focusses on helping people to solve their health problems	The science and practice of promoting adaptation in individuals, or groups in order to help them achieve health
Goal of Nursing	To place the patient in the best condition for nature to act by providing an environment conducive to healthy living and a nourishing diet	To assist the patient to solve problems through new learning and positive change	To assist humankind to regain optimal health or, in the event of incurable illness, to achieve peaceful death	To assist the individual to achieve the maximum independence of which he or she is capable, in caring for own health and that of dependent others	Satisfaction of patient health needs is the objective of nursing function and nursing activity	To assist the patient to achieve a higher level of wellness

TTY EUMAN	MARTHA ROGERS	ROSEMARY PARSE	MADELEINE LEININGER	JEAN WATSON	MOYRA ALLEN	MARGARET CAMPBELL (U.B.C. MODEL OF NURSING)
alth or wellness quated with tem stability	Health and illness are seen as cultural values denoting behaviours of high and low value as defined by individuals and cultures	A continuously changing state of being, or "becoming," as experienced by the person	Culturally determined beliefs, values and patterns of action used to preserve and maintain the well-being of persons	Unity and harmony within mind, body and soul of the person	A social process, a way of living rather than a state of being. Similar in meaning to health behaviour, it is something that can be measured and can be modified	Optimal health is the highest level of behavioural system stability perceived by an individual as achievable at any given time
nique profession ussing on the al person tient system) and or her, or group, ctions to stress d on factors uencing constitution	A profession with a focus on compassionate concern for the maintenance, promotion, protection and restoration of health in people	An art and a science focussing on the living unity that characterizes all people	A learned humanistic art and science concerned with personalized care behaviours, functions and processes	A human art and science directed towards the protection, enhancement and preservation of human dignity	A professional response to the person's natural search for healthy living	The nurturing of individuals experiencing critical periods in the life cycle, so that they may develop and use a range of coping behaviours that permit them to satisfy their basic human needs, to achieve stability and to reach optimal health
promote system bility	To promote harmonious interaction between the patient and the environment	To facilitate optimal wellness in the patient by assisting him or her to achieve system stability	To assist, support or enable another person (individual or group) with existing or potential needs to ameliorate their health through preservation, accommodation or repatterning of culturally determined beliefs, values and patterns	To help people gain more self-knowledge, self-control and readiness for self-healing regardless of the external health condition	To assist people to enhance their problem-solving skills in dealing with health matters	To nurture the behavioural system that is the person

THEORETICAL PLURALISM

Many schools and health agencies have adopted one or another of the conceptual models that have been developed as their particular framework for nursing practice. Watson's science of human caring is being used in many schools and health agencies. Henderson's model, as outlined by Archer, has also been widely used in many educational programs and clinical agencies. Still other schools and agencies are committed to Roy's model, to Neuman's model or to one of the others. Still others subscribe to **theoretical pluralism** — the belief that there is value in several different models.

Those who espouse theoretical pluralism might include a variety of models in their educational programs. For example, Watson's model of human caring might be taught in introductory and medical-surgical nursing courses, Roy's adaptation model in psychiatric nursing, and Orem's self-care model or Neuman's systems model in courses on community health nursing.

Similarly, nurses in some health agencies feel that there is no one model that suits all fields of nursing practice and, in one agency, several different conceptual frameworks may be used. On one nursing unit, such as a rehabilitation unit, for example, the nurses might prefer to use Orem's model of self-care while in the outpatient clinic the nurses might prefer Neuman's systems model. In this text, we are not going to select any one model for students to use, but will instead take the generic approach of theoretical pluralism in subsequent units of the text.

THE VALUE OF THEORIES AND CONCEPTUAL MODELS FOR NURSING EDUCATION, RESEARCH AND PRACTICE

In any given discipline you will usually find more than one conceptual framework on which people may base their practice. The theories underlying an individual's pattern of practice depend on the theories espoused by teachers in their professional training programs or theories which practitioners have subsequently decided best suit their beliefs and values and the situations encountered in their practice.

Psychiatry is one field in which you are likely to encounter practitioners who hold widely divergent views on both diagnostic measures and treatment regimens, depending on the theory they espouse. Some psychiatrists, psychologists and mental health counsellors believe in the *fundamental objective* school of thought, based on stimulus-response theory, and in behaviour modification by conditioning. Others espouse psychoanalytic theory and believe that the subconscious has to be probed to find the root of a problem before it can be treated. And you will no doubt encounter many practitioners whose beliefs lie somewhere between these extremes.

The Canadian Nurses Association Standards for Nursing Practice (1987) states that "...nursing practice requires that a conceptual model(s) for nursing be the basis for that practice" (Canadian Nurses Association, 1987, 3). Most Canadian schools of nursing and many health agencies have now adopted specific nursing models or have developed their own. The acceptance of theory-based practice by both academics and clinicians has been slow and fraught with resistance. The early theories provided rather general descriptions of nursing and were criticized for presenting an overly idealistic view that did not reflect real life. They were also often couched in esoteric language which the average nurse found difficult to understand. Nurse educators were the first to make use of the conceptual models as a framework for curriculum, but they were considered of little value for the nurse in day-to-day practice. As the theories have been expanded and explained by the original author or by others, they have become more widely accepted. Today, the health agency that does not base practice on a conceptual framework is the exception, rather than the rule.

The value of the models commonly used in schools and agencies across the country is first and foremost in providing us with a nursing perspective. All members of the health team are concerned with the patient but all view the patient from a different perspective. The physician, for example, sees the patient as someone with a health problem, which it is their responsibility to diagnose and treat. The nutritionist is concerned with the patient's diet and nutritional status; the physiotherapist focusses on the patient's musculoskeletal system and mobility.

The conceptual frameworks in nursing help practitioners to look at the patient as a whole person, not just as a health problem, a nutritional problem or a mobility problem. Indeed, Rogers call her theory "The Science of Unitary Human Beings." Orem defines the person as a unity functioning biologically, symbolically and socially while Neuman talks of five interacting variables (physiological, psychological, sociocultural, developmental and spiritual) impinging on a person's health. These are just three examples but you will find that all of the nursing models treat the person as a multifaceted being and acknowledge that all of these facets must be taken into account in caring for that person.

In addition to providing us with a distinctive nursing perspective and helping us to look at the whole person, the assessment tools that have developed from the models provide a framework for the organization of nursing care. They offer guidance for the collection of data and the identification of nursing problems. The models also give us a common language which can be used to describe the patient's health status and to communicate nursing's concerns. For example, if an agency has adopted Orem's conceptual model as the basis for practice, the nurses will talk in terms of the patient's "self-care deficits." These will be identified and described in the nurse's assessment of the patient and nursing interventions planned to overcome the deficits. To illustrate, a nurse may have noted in assessing Mrs. Singh that she had had a mild stroke which resulted in a weakness of the left arm. As a result, she has difficulty dressing and feeding herself. The nurse would note that Mrs. Singh has a self-care deficit in regard to certain activities of daily living. All nurses would be alerted through nursing orders that Mrs. Singh needs help, for example, with dressing and undressing and also needs help at meal-time.

USING THEORIES AND CONCEPTUAL MODELS IN EDUCATION

As we mentioned earlier, it was the nurse educators who adopted the theories (conceptual models) first, using them originally as a framework for curriculum, and later to provide the structure for individual nursing courses. The use of nursing models provided a distinctive approach that served to differentiate nursing education programs from medical ones.

Nursing education programs up to, and including, the early 1950s tended to look very much like mini-medical schools, with heavy emphasis on the basic sciences and little on the social sciences. Clinical courses were taught predominantly by physicians, with follow-up lectures on nursing care of patients with various diseases given by the nurse educator responsible for the course. The use of specific nursing models as the structure for clinical nursing courses has enabled nurse educators to change the focus of their teaching to matters that

are important to nursing. The medical school course pattern of etiology, epidemiology, diagnosis and treatment of diseases has been replaced by a focus on the process of nursing care with structure provided by a specific nursing theory. For example, a new caring curriculum, based on the principles of health promotion, has been developed at the University of Victoria in collaboration with eight community colleges.

USING NURSING THEORIES (CONCEPTUAL MODELS) IN RESEARCH

The nursing theories that have evolved in the past few decades have provided a fertile field for nursing scholars, as they expand on the original concepts in two important ways. First, they describe other phenomena that are part of nursing (in addition to the four basic concepts of person, health nursing and environment). For example, Benner has explored the nature of caring in studies focussing on the daily practice of expert nurses (Benner, 1984).

Second, they have led to the development of midrange theories that can be used more directly to guide nursing care than can the "grand theories" (conceptual models). Orem's model, for example, has given rise to a "theory of self-care" which states that the care of oneself and the care of dependent family members (or significant others) are behaviours which human beings learn in order to regulate their structural identity, functioning and development (Orem, 1985). New mothers, for example, need to learn how best to care for their babies and a teaching program, based on this midrange theory, can be developed to help them. One might then study the effectiveness of various teaching strategies on the mothers' subsequent behaviour with their offspring.

There is a definite reciprocal relationship between theory and research. The theories must be tested (validated) in research. Other researchable questions on the self-care theory cited above, for instance, might be: How do people learn to care for themselves? For dependent others? Who are the care-givers? What teaching strategies are best to help new mothers learn to care for their babies?

Research of nurses' practice has also generated new theories as noted in the example cited above of Benner's work. Many other concepts with which nursing is concerned are also being explored as focusses for theory development, for example, the nature of social support, prenatal maternal attachment, pain control and coping mechanisms for stress (Chinn and Kramer, 1991).

Nursing Theories in Practice at Mount Sinai Hospital

Nursing care based on knowledge drawn from a nursing perspective is an essential contribution of our discipline to the health care system and to those in need of nursing services. Provision of quality care, based on a sound body of nursing knowledge, enables us to meet our social mandate and empowers us to influence health care policy. It is in this context that theory-based practice has become a popular theme in nursing practice settings throughout North America (Mayberry, 1991; Sorrentino, 1991) and elsewhere (Perry, 1985).

The use of nursing theories in the practice setting was encouraged in Ontario by the College of Nurses who, in 1984, stated that nursing practice should be guided by a conceptual framework. Several hospitals have since adopted nursing theories as guiding frameworks for their practice. In Toronto alone, the models of King, Orem, Watson, Peplau, Parse and Roy have been incorporated into different practice settings.

Nursing is a discipline that provides holistic care. Theory-based practice supports and fosters holistic care. Theory-based practice encourages nurses to a higher level of conceptual thinking, assisting us in broadening and deepening the mental image that we have of "what nursing is" and providing some specific characteristics and direction to our nursing practice. Theories also assist us in articulating the meaning of nursing for ourselves and for others.

The process of implementing a conceptual framework at Mount Sinai Hospital began in the Fall of 1984. A nursing theories committee explored 20 conceptual frameworks during a period of 10 months. Following this extensive review, four conceptual frameworks were chosen as possible options. These were again reviewed in five half-day workshops with participation of outside speakers who had worked with these models. The decision to choose the Roy Adaptation Model was based on the belief that this conceptual framework offered the best fit with the values held by the department of nursing. In the Winter of 1987, we began piloting the model in four units. It was only in 1994 that hospital-wide implementation was completed.

The Roy Adaptation Model is a highly developed and widely used conceptual description of nursing. As in all other models, the major concepts of the Roy Adaptation Model are *person, environment, nursing* and *health* (Roy, 1984). According to Roy, the recipient of nursing care can be an individual person, a family, a group, a community or society as a whole. Roy considers nursing first in terms of its goal to promote adaptation. Adaptation, a key concept in the model, is "a process involving holistic functioning to affect health positively" (Roy, 1984, 36). Adaptation is the process of promoting health. Roy defines health as a state and a process of being and becoming an integrated and whole person. Thus, Roy believes that health is a dynamic process of evolution and growth.

The following is a description of how the Roy Adaptation Model could contribute to the plan of care of a person who has suffered a cerebro-vascular accident (CVA):

Focal stimuli for the patient who has suffered a CVA will be the impact and implications of the CVA physiologically (physiological mode), in the way this patient feels about him- or herself (self-concept mode), the patient's relationships with others (interdependence mode) and his or her ability to effectively function as a parent or in other important roles (role function mode). As the nurse, during the initial assessment phase, identifies areas of ineffective responses (for example, a poor relationship between the patient and spouse), the nurse will conduct a more in-depth, second-level assessment.

During the second-level assessment, the nurse will explore with the patient the impact of the focal stimuli (what is immediately confronting the patient), the contextual stimuli (what else is occurring in the patient's life that affects the way he or she responds) and the residual stimuli. Residual stimuli include general stimuli that have a life-long and permeating effect on behaviours. These include culture, socio-economic status, religion, ethnic group, education level, family structure and stage of growth and development of the patient. Some of these stimuli may contribute to promote adaptation while others may hinder adaptation. For example, a well-constituted family structure might contribute to the patient's adaptation process. A history of addiction to drugs may hinder adaptive responses. One of the purposes of nursing assessment will be to determine which stimuli are predominant in each case. Effective adaptation will contribute to the patient's long-term quality of life, which should be the goal of nursing intervention. In order to tailor nursing intervention to promote adaptation, one must identify factors that assist in or detract from promoting adaptation in all four modes.

As we can learn from this example, nurses practising from a Roy perspective aim at assisting people to respond in a positive way to stimuli and to move to a state of health (being and becoming an integrated and whole human being). These can be done by changing the stimuli and/or by enhancing the coping mechanisms.

Our experience of practising nursing based on a conceptual framework at Mount Sinai Hospital has been a positive one. Its impact has been significant for patients and their loved ones, as well as for nurses. Formal and informal evaluations attest to a genuine change towards holistic nursing care. We have integrated theoretical thinking and the Roy Adaptation Model in all aspects of our practice — the nursing process documentation, unit-based primary nursing rounds (held every two weeks) and hospital-wide primary nursing rounds (held every two months). It is important to note that our focus at Mount Sinai Hospital has been on "thinking nursing," "practising nursing" and "documenting nursing." We very strongly believe that the model has contributed positively to our nursing practice and to the quality patient care we so proudly provide.

— Doris Grinspun, RN, MSN, CRRN,
Program Director, Nursing

KEY TERMS

theory p. 311

conceptual model p. 311

conceptual framework p. 311

metaparadigm p. 311

grand theory p. 311

mega theory p. 311

descriptive theory p. 311

explanatory theory p. 311

predictive theory p. 311

person p. 311

environment p. 311

health p. 311

nursing p. 311

concept p. 311

empirical p. 311

abstract p. 311

nursing problems p. 314

diagnostic reasoning p. 314

nursing process p. 314

holistic p. 317

patient system p. 317

care p. 318

theoretical pluralism p. 324

IN REVIEW

Until the middle of the nineteenth century, nursing knowledge was traditionally passed down from one generation to the next through a process of apprenticeship training. Articulation of this knowledge into a formal structure of nursing science developed from the need to differentiate nursing's role and functions from those of other health caregivers. Florence Nightingale recorded her views on this subject in 1860 but it was not until the early 1950s that nurses in North America began to express their ideas on what nursing was all about. In developing their conceptual frameworks, nurse theorists were influenced by events occurring in other fields, using their nursing perspective to develop theories pertinent to their field of practice.

The four major concepts considered central to nursing and included, explicitly or by implication, in all nursing models, are *person, environment, health* and *nursing*. As the original theories have been expanded and explained, by the original author or by others, the models have been used first by nurse educators as a framework for curriculum and course construction and, increasingly, as a basis for nursing practice in health agencies. The existing theories are being tested by nurse researchers and new theories are emerging from studies of nursing practice. The Canadian Nurses Association Standards for Nursing Practice require that a conceptual model(s) for nursing be the basis of nursing practice. All Canadian schools of nursing and most health agencies have either adopted specific nursing models or they have developed their own.

The value of the models for nursing education, practice and research is multifaceted. They provide us with a distinctive nursing perspective for looking at the patient and a common language and specific tools for identifying nursing concerns in care of the patient and for selecting measures to alleviate these concerns. They also help us to look at the patient as a whole person, not just as someone with a health problem, and to consider all the factors, both internal and external, that are affecting the patient's health.

In education, the models are now used as frameworks for curricula and also for clinical courses. They provide the students with a nursing perspective which the medical model previously used in most nursing schools did not. Research studies are needed to validate the theories proposed in conceptual models, to explore related phenomena that are part of nursing, to develop theories that can be used to guide nursing care more definitively and to study the effectiveness of various nursing interventions.

LEARNING ACTIVITIES

1. What conceptual models are used in your school of nursing as a framework for the curriculum and/or nursing courses?

2. What conceptual models are used in the clinical agencies that are affiliated with your school?

   a. in community agencies

   b. in inpatient facilities (hospitals, rehabilitation centres or other specialized units, or long-term care facilities)?

3. Explain how the uses of conceptual models in practice discussed on p. 324 are illustrated in Grinspun's description of the use of the Roy Adaptation Model at Mount Sinai Hospital in Toronto.

REFERENCES AND READINGS

ABDELLAH, F.G., BELAND, I.L., MARTIN, A. et al. (1960). *Patient-centered approaches to nursing.* New York: Macmillan.

ABDELLAH, F.G. and LEVINE, E. (1986). *Better nursing care through nursing research* (3rd ed.). New York: Macmillan.

ADAM, E. (1991). *To be a nurse* (2nd ed.). Toronto: Saunders.

AGAN, R.D. (1987). Intuitive knowing as a dimension of nursing. *Advances in Nursing Science, 10*(1), 63–70.

ALLEN, M. (1974). Query and theory. *Nursing Papers, 6*(1), 43–44.

ALLEN, M. (1982). A model of nursing: A plan for research and development. In *Research: A base for the future proceedings of the international conference on nursing research.* Edinburgh: University of Edinburgh.

ALLEN, M. (1986). A developmental health model: Nursing as continuous inquiry (audio cassette). In series *Theory congress — Theoretical pluralism: Directions for a practice discipline.* Markham, ON: Audio Archives of Canada.

BARRETT, E.A.M. (Ed.). (1990). *Visions of Rogers science-based nursing.* New York: National League for Nursing.

BENNER, P. (1984). *From novice to expert.* Menlo Park, CA: Addison-Wesley.

CAMPBELL, M.A. (1987) *The U.B.C. Model for Nursing: Directions for practice.* Vancouver: The University of British Columbia School of Nursing.

CANADIAN NURSES ASSOCIATION. (1987). *A definition of nursing practice: Standards for nursing practice.* Ottawa: Author.

CASEY, A. (1989). *An introduction to conceptual frameworks: Unit objectives and course notes.* Ottawa: University of Ottawa School of Nursing.

CHINN, P. and KRAMER, M.K. (1991). *Theory and nursing (a systematic approach)* (3rd ed.). St. Louis: Mosby.

CHONG CHOI, E. (1989). Evolution of nursing theory development. In Marriner-Tomey. *Nursing theorists and their work.* St. Louis: Mosby.

FAWCETT, J. (1984). *Analysis and evaluation of conceptual models for nursing.* Philadelphia: F.A. Davis.

FAWCETT, J. and DOWNS, F.S. (1986). *The relationship of theory and research.* Norwalk, CT: Appleton-Century-Crofts.

FAWCETT, J. (1989). Nursing knowledge and nursing practice: Essential tension. *Proceedings of the National Conference on Putting it All Together: Nursing theory, nursing diagnosis and nursing interventions.* Ottawa: University of Ottawa Service for Continuing Education, 20–29.

FITZPATRICK, J.J. and WHALL, A.L. (1989). *Conceptual models for nursing: Analysis and application.* Norwalk, CT: Appleton & Lange.

FORCHUK, C. (1990). Peplau's interpersonal theory. In A. Bauman, A.N. Johnston and D. Antai-Otong. *Decision-making in psychiatric and psychosocial nursing.* Toronto: B.C. Decker.

GEORGE, J.B.(Ed.). (1990). *Nursing theories: The base for professional nursing practice* (3rd ed.). Norwalk, CT: Appleton & Lange.

HARMER, B. and HENDERSON, V.(1955). *Textbook of the principles and practice of nursing* (5th ed.). New York: Macmillan.

HENDERSON, V. (1966). *The nature of nursing: A definition and its implications for practice.* New York: Macmillan.

KRAVITZ, M. and FREY, M.A. (1989). The Allen nursing model. In J.J. Fitzpatrick and A.L. Whall. *Conceptual models of nursing.* Norwalk, CT: Appleton & Lange, 313–330.

LEININGER, M.M. (Ed.). (1991). *Culture care diversity and universality: A theory of nursing.* New York: N.L.N.E. Press. (Publication No. 15–2402)

LEININGER, M.M. (1978). *Transcultural nursing: Concepts, theories and practices.* New York: Wiley.

LEININGER, M.M. (1988) Leininger's theory of nursing: Cultural care diversity and universality. *Nursing Science Quarterly, 1,* 152–160.

MASLOW, A.H. (1970). *Motivation and personality* (2nd ed.). New York: Harper and Row.

MAYBERRY, A. (1991). Merging nursing theories, models, and nursing practice: More than an administrative challenge. *Nursing Administration Quarterly, 15*(3), 44–53.

NEUMAN, B. (1989). *The Neuman systems model* (2nd ed.). Norwalk, CT: Appleton & Lange.

NIGHTINGALE, F. (1859). *Notes on nursing: What it is and what it is not.* (Commemorative edition, 1992). D.P. Carroll (Ed). Philadelphia: Lippincott.

OREM, D.E. (1985). *Nursing: Concepts of practice* (3rd ed.). New York: McGraw-Hill.

OREM, D.E. (1991). *Nursing: Concepts of practice* (4th ed.). St. Louis: Mosby.

PARSE, R.R. (1981). *Man-living-health: A theory of nursing.* New York: Wiley.

PARSE, R.R. (1987). Parse's man-living-health theory of nursing. In R.R. Parse (Ed). *Nursing science: Major paradigms, theories and critiques.* Philadelphia: Saunders, 181–204.

PEPLAU, H.E. (1952). *Interpersonal relations in nursing.* New York: Putnam.

PERRY, J. (1985). Has the discipline of nursing developed to the stage where nurses do "think nursing"? *Journal of Advanced Nursing, 10,* 31–37.

QUILLIN, S.I.M. and RUNK, J.A. (1989). Martha Rogers' unitary person model. In J.J. Fitzpatrick and A.L. Whall. *Conceptual models of nursing* (2nd ed.). Norwalk, CT: Appleton & Lange.

ROACH, M.S. (1992). *The human act of caring: A blueprint for the health professions* (Revised ed.). Ottawa: Canadian Hospital Association Press.

ROGERS, C.R. (1961). *On becoming a person.* Boston: Houghton Mifflin.

ROGERS, M.E. (1970). *An introduction to the theoretical basis of nursing.* Philadelphia: F.A. Davis.

ROGERS, M.E. (1980). *A science of unitary man.* In J.P. Riehl and C. Roy (Eds). *Conceptual models for nursing practice* (2nd ed.). New York: Appleton-Century-Crofts.

ROGERS, M.E. (1986). Science of unitary human beings. In V.M. Kalinski (Ed). *Explorations on Martha Rogers' science of unitary beings.* Norwalk, CT: Appleton-Century-Crofts.

ROY, S.C. (1984). *Introduction to nursing: An adaptation model* (2nd ed.). Englewood Cliffs, NJ: Prentice-Hall.

ROY, S.C. and ANDREWS, H.A. (1991). *The Roy Adaptation Model: The definitive statement.* Norwalk, CT: Appleton & Lange.

SORRENTINO, E. (1991). Making theories work for you. *Nursing Administration Quarterly, 15*(3), 54–59.

THORNDIKE, EDWARD. (1940). *Human nature and the social order.* New York: Macmillan.

WATSON, JEAN. (1988). *Nursing: Human science and human care.* New York: National League for Nursing.

WHALL, A.L. (1989). Nursing science: The process and the products. In A.L. Whall and J.J. Fitzpatrick. *Conceptual models of nursing: Analysis and application* (2nd ed.). Norwalk, CT: Appleton & Lange, 1–14.

Nursing Process

CENTRAL QUESTIONS

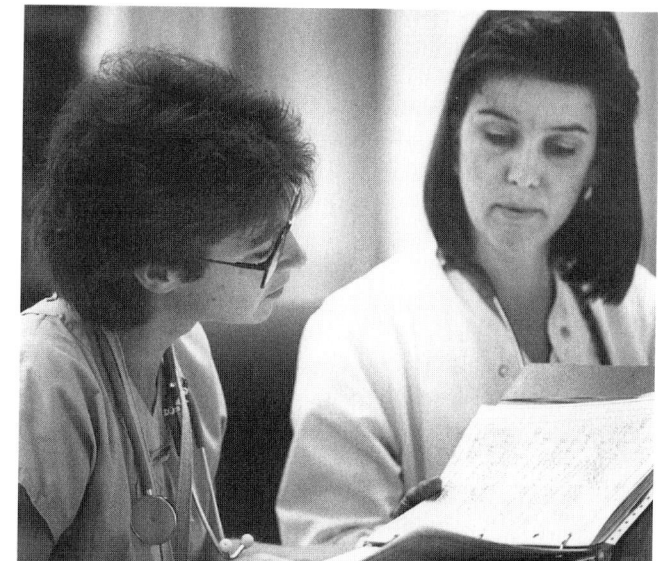

1. What is the nursing process and why is it used?

2. What are the steps in the nursing process and how do they relate to one another?

3. What are the purposes of data collection and what information does the nurse collect during assessment?

4. What sources are used for data collection?

5. What is diagnostic reasoning and how is it used in the assessment phase of the nursing process?

6. What is the difference between subjective and objective data?

7. What are some frameworks the nurse can use for organizing assessment data?

8. How does the nurse document and communicate the information collected?

9. How does the nurse use the diagnostic process to identify client problems and strengths?

10. How do nursing diagnoses differ from collaborative problems?

11. What are the parts of the diagnostic statement and how would the nurse write diagnostic statements for actual, potential and possible nursing diagnoses and for collaborative problems?

12. How does the nurse determine priorities among the identified problems?

13. How are goals and expected outcomes developed?

14. What types of interventions does the nurse carry out in giving care?

15. How does the nurse determine nursing interventions?

16. What is a nursing care plan and how does the nurse develop one?

17. What knowledge and skills does the nurse need to implement a plan of care?

18. What methods does the nurse use in evaluating the effectiveness of care?

INTRODUCTION

Nursing care may range from the simple act of cleansing and bandaging a child's cut finger to the highly complex measures involved in caring for a patient in the intensive care unit of a hospital, or in helping a family with multiple problems to meet their health needs in a community setting. The process of nursing is the same, however, whether the nursing care given is a basic first aid measure or a sequence of complicated nursing activities.

The term *nursing process* designates a systematic and organized approach to practice which embodies a series of interrelated steps the nurse takes in identifying and making decisions about nursing care. Based on the problem-solving, or scientific, method, the process provides a consistent framework which all nurses can use in planning and giving care. Moreover, the terminology that has evolved can be readily understood by all nurses as well as by other members of the health care team.

The essential elements of the nursing process are that it is planned, it is patient-centred, it is problem-oriented and it is goal-directed. The term *patient* is used here to denote the recipient of care and can mean an individual, a family or a community. Five basic steps are involved in the process:

1. Assessment — gathering and organizing information.
2. Diagnosis — analyzing and synthesizing the information to identify strengths and actual or potential problems.
3. Planning — establishing goals and developing a plan of action.
4. Implementation — carrying out the plan of action.
5. Evaluation — determining if the goals have been achieved.

The steps in the process follow logically one after the other. As a basis for making decisions about nursing actions, the nurse must first assess the need for action. During assessment the nurse gathers all pertinent information (commonly referred to as data) about the patient and then groups the information into meaningful categories or clusters. This prepares the information for the next step, diagnosis.

In diagnosis, the data is analyzed and a judgement is made about the patient's health status. This may include a patient's strengths, level of wellness and actual or potential health problems that are amenable to independent nursing intervention or those that require referral to other health care professionals. In order to diagnose accurately, the nurse must have a thorough understanding of the nature of health and illness; of the physiology, pathophysiology and signs and symptoms of illness; and of human behaviour. Nursing diagnoses provide a focus and give direction in planning goal-directed care.

In planning, the nurse and the patient together set patient-centred goals (also referred to as *expected outcomes*) and develop a plan of action (called the *nursing care plan*) to help patients promote and protect their health or re-solve problems. The next step is implementation in which the specified measures (nursing interventions) outlined in the plan of action are carried out.

The final step is evaluation. In evaluation, the results of the action taken are reviewed to determine if the expected outcomes have been attained. The last step may result in new information that leads to modification in the nursing diagnoses, changes in the plan of action, or a restatement of patient goals. Thus, the process is a sequential, yet circular, one that involves a continuing dynamic set of activities on the nurse's part. Figure 14.1 depicts the nursing process.

Although the nursing process is viewed as a series of deliberate steps that are separated and studied individually, it must be pointed out that in practice the steps are continuously interacting and overlapping with one another in such a way that one step may contain elements of the next. Or, in some situations, especially emergencies (as when a patient stops breathing), all of the steps may occur simultaneously.

Assessment and diagnosis overlap significantly, as illustrated by the following example: During a physical examination, the nurse finds that the patient feels warm, looks flushed and has a rapid pulse. The patient also reports anorexia and nausea. From his or her knowledge of pathophysiology, the nurse assumes that the patient has a fever and focusses the data-gathering activity on validating this assumption. In this example we see that as the data were being collected, the nurse grouped the information and began to make an assumption about the meaning of this information. In other words, a nursing diagnosis was being made even before data gathering was complete. This overlap in the thinking process between assessment and diagnosis describes what a number of authors refer to as "diagnostic reasoning" (Carnevali, Mitchell, Woods and Tanner, 1984; Kelly, 1985; Gordon, 1987; Carnevali and Thomas, 1993).

Diagnostic reasoning is the process of critical thinking in which the nurse uses his or her clinical knowledge and experience to collect information, interpret the information collected and make a judgement about the patient's health status. This judgement is the nursing diagnosis. The reasoning process will be discussed in more detail later on in the chapter.

Some authors, Yura and Walsh, for example, do not see assessment and diagnosis as two distinct steps of the nursing process. Rather, they view diagnosis as an integral part of assessment and advocate a four-step model in which diagnosis is seen as the conclusion of the assessment phase (Yura and Walsh, 1988). Furthermore, particularly as nurses become more advanced in their abilities, diagnostic reasoning is carried out with little conscious awareness of the mental activities involved. Students, however, with beginning levels of the knowledge and skills needed for data collection and limited experience in diagnostic reasoning, may find it easier to learn the processes involved by carrying out these steps as separate operations (Carnevali and Thomas, 1993).

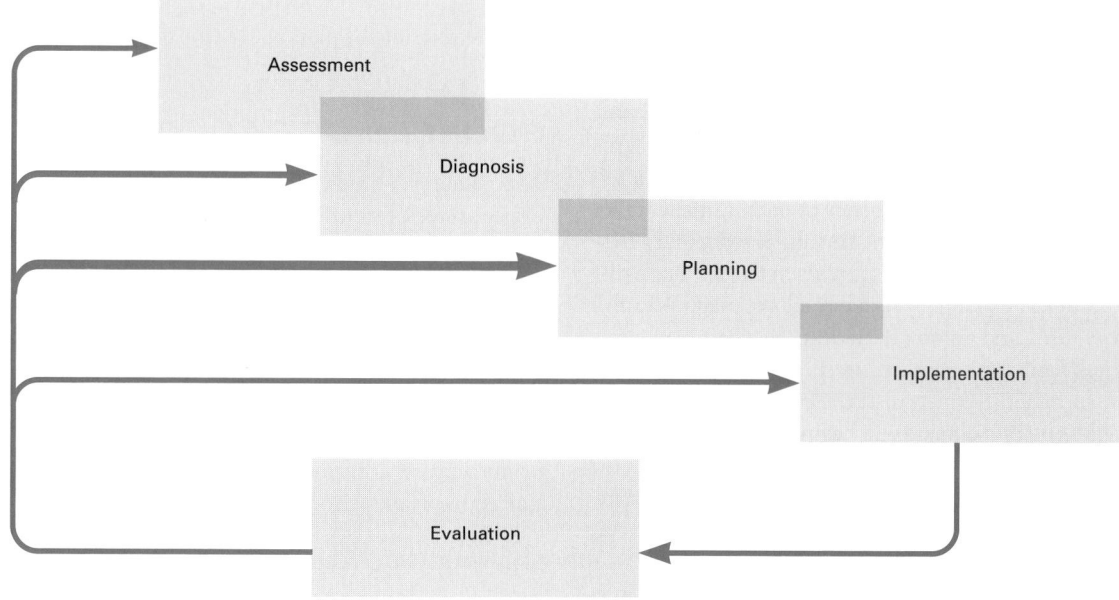

FIGURE 14.1   Relationships among the steps of the nursing process*

* Each step of the nursing process is dependent on the accuracy of the preceding step. The steps are also overlapping because the nurse may have to move more quickly for some problems than for others. Evaluation involves examining all previous steps of the nursing process, but focusses especially upon goal achievement (given that the diagnoses were accurate and the goals were appropriate).

SOURCE: Alfaro, R. (1990). *Applying nursing diagnosis and nursing process* (2nd ed.). Philadelphia: Lippincott, 9. Reproduced with permission.

Diagnosis and planning may also overlap. In the situation described above, for example, if the patient's temperature were found to be 40°C and the patient expressed severe headache, the nurse would first take action to deal with the fever and pain, and then continue with analysis and synthesis of all of the assessment data. Similarly, planning and implementation overlap because there are times when actions have to be implemented before the entire plan for care is developed. Thus, the nursing process is a dynamic series of steps that provides a framework for giving quality care, yet is open and adaptable to the unique and changing needs of the patient.

ASSESSMENT

As the first step in the nursing process, *assessment* refers to the collection and interpretation of clinical information (Gordon, 1987). The systematic collection of information for a specific purpose is called "data gathering." The information collected is used to develop a *data base*, which can be analyzed in a number of different ways depending on the purpose for which the information was collected in the first place.

As a nursing function, assessment focusses on the patient's health status and responses to illness as opposed to medical assessment which focusses on the pathology underlying illness and is the responsibility of a doctor. The information collected during assessment forms the basis on which nursing diagnoses and treatment decisions are made. Therefore, it is essential that the information is complete and relevant to the patient's situation and that it is sorted and organized into a format that can be analyzed. In addition, the information has to be recorded and communicated to other appropriate health team members. Assessment involves three components:

1. collecting information — gathering data about the patient's health status and responses to illness
2. organizing the information — grouping or clustering the data into meaningful patterns
3. documenting the information — recording of relevant data.

COLLECTING INFORMATION

In order to develop a solid base for identifying health problems and planning nursing care, the nurse needs to know 1) the purpose for which the information is being collected, 2) what information is needed, 3) what sources can be used to obtain data, 4) how these sources can be tapped, and 5) how to interpret and use the information collected.

PURPOSE OF DATA COLLECTION

The nurse's objective in collecting information about a patient is to identify areas in which nursing intervention is required. There are two types of data collection for this purpose: data base assessment and focus assessment (Alfaro-LeFevre, 1994). The **data base assessment** is conducted on admission to a health care agency or upon initial contact with the patient. It includes the nursing history and physical assessment, the physician's report on the patient's history and physical examination, the results of diagnostic and laboratory tests, and reports from other health team members. The information gathered in the baseline assessment gives a comprehensive picture of the patient's health status and enables the nurse to make a beginning plan of care for the patient. Information collected by the nurse may also identify problems that require intervention by other members of the health team, such as the physician, the social worker or the physical therapist.

In addition to the baseline assessment, information is collected on an ongoing basis to determine changes in the patient's health status and the need for change in the nursing plan for care. This is called a **focus assessment**. As the name suggests, data collection is directed to specific problems or needs. For example, the nurse who periodically examines the colour and respiratory pattern of a newborn baby or observes the wound drainage of a postoperative patient is conducting a focus assessment.

INFORMATION NEEDED BY THE NURSE

Virginia Henderson, in the well-known and often-quoted definition of nursing, has stated, "The unique function of the nurse is to assist the individual, sick or well, in the performance of those activities contributing to health or its recovery (or to peaceful death) that he [she] would perform unaided if he [she] had the necessary strength, will or knowledge" (Henderson, 1966).

We might rephrase this to say that nursing care of individuals, families and groups is primarily concerned with assisting them to cope with the activities of daily living in such a way as to promote their optimal functioning or, in the case of incurable disease, to cope with terminal illness. In order to identify areas in which individuals (or families or groups) require such nursing assistance, the nurse needs to know:

1. basic data about the individual as a person.
2. his or her usual abilities (or lack of abilities) in coping with activities of daily living (health patterns).
3. the nature of any health problems that are interfering with the ability to cope (illness patterns).
4. current status in regard to these abilities.
5. health-promoting and health-protecting practices.
6. any potential risk factors.
7. the physician's plan of care for the individual.

SOURCES OF DATA COLLECTION

The primary source of information is always the patient. Other sources, termed secondary sources, include other people such as family members or "significant others" with whom the individual has had a close relationship. In the case of a child or an unconscious or irrational patient, much of the information the nurse needs must be obtained from someone other than the patient.

The patient's health record is also a valuable source of data for the nurse, and today an increasing number of health team members contribute to it. If a record has already been started, or if old records are on file, the nurse should review these, if possible, before the first encounter with the patient. This review helps to avoid duplication in information gathering and gives the nurse the benefit of data gathered by others. The physician, for example, is usually responsible for taking the patient's medical history, for identifying medical problems and for developing diagnostic and therapeutic plans for the individual, if such are warranted. The results of the physician's findings and the medical plan of care are incorporated into the patient's record. In addition, the nurse will find other sources, such as reports on radiography and ultrasonography, as well as laboratory and other diagnostic tests on the patient's record. This information is necessary for developing a nursing plan of care.

Other members of the health team also contribute to the nurse's understanding of the patient's health status. Observations and interpretations may be communicated by the social worker, the nutritionist (dietitian) or the physical

The primary source of information is always the patient.

therapist, to name only a few, through written notes on the patient's record, in consultations with the nurse or in conferences and other meetings of various members of the health care team.

If the individual has a known medical problem the nurse may want to increase his or her knowledge of it by reading available literature in the library. Students might review notes they have taken in class or through independent study that will contribute to their understanding of the particular problem.

HOW TO COLLECT INFORMATION

Whether conducting a data base assessment or a focus assessment, the nurse uses the same methods of gathering data about a patient. These are the interview (talking to the patient, family or significant other), the physical assessment (observation and examination), consultation (with other members of the health care team) and records (and other written material).

Interview

The nurse conducts an interview to obtain information from patients or from their family or significant other. Interviewing goes on during every phase of the nursing process and is a component of both data base and focus assessments. An interview must be conducted in a deliberate, systematic manner to ensure that all necessary information is obtained. In order to carry out an effective interview, nurses need to have knowledge and skill in communication, such as listening, questioning and observing, and in basic interviewing techniques. These skills are discussed in Chapter 16.

The Nursing Health History

A primary tool for collecting baseline data which relies on skillful interviewing techniques is the health history. The **health history** provides a guide for systematically obtaining information which can help the nurse to plan and modify care to suit the individual patient's preferences and usual living patterns, as well as to establish a baseline from which to evaluate the results of nursing action.

The history is taken as soon after the patient's admission to the agency as is feasible, preferably by the nurse who has primary responsibility for planning the patient's care. The technique for obtaining the history is a **structured interview**, that is, one in which the nurse controls and directs the interview for the purpose of gathering specific information. Information commonly gathered in a nursing history includes:

1) Events leading up to admission to the agency — the reasons for admission, basic social data about the patient.

2) Usual patterns of daily living — habits in regard to eating, eliminating, rest and sleep and hygiene practices.

3) Health and illness patterns — perception of usual patterns of physiologic, psychosocial and spiritual functioning and an exploration of changes in these patterns.

4) Health promotion and protection patterns — what he or she does or does not do to remain healthy.

5) Environmental factors that may affect health — the patient's family, where the patient lives and works.

6) Concerns and expectations of care — things the patient is worried about, what he or she expects to happen and the care anticipated from health care personnel.

Many agencies use a specific form commonly called a *health history*, a *nursing history* or a *patient profile* to assist nurses in gathering data and to provide a written record of the information obtained. Today, most agencies have patterned their health history form on a nursing model (see Chapter 13) to ensure that the central concepts of nursing are integrated into the data collection. The views of the nurse and the agency about the patient, the patient's environment, health and the purpose of nursing govern how the nurse will carry out the nursing process. Establishing a data base on those views sets the foundation for optimal care. Figure 14.2 gives an example of a nursing history form based on Roy's adaptation model.

Physical Assessment

The physical assessment is conducted by using observation and examination techniques. **Observation** refers to the collection of information through the use of the physical senses (sight, sound, touch, smell and taste). For instance, upon approaching the bedside of a postoperative patient, the nurse will look at the patient's posture and facial expression and listen to the sound of the patient's voice in order to detect signs of emotional distress or physical discomfort. Or, the nurse might touch the patient's skin to feel moisture and temperature. Then, the nurse will inspect the equipment (such as an intravenous line or drainage tubing) for proper functioning and visually scan the surrounding area for potential hazards to patient safety. Skillful observation is vital in data collection. Observation provides information about patients' physical, emotional, developmental and social behaviour, as well as their physical and social environment. It is a process that occurs in every nurse–patient encounter, be it during an interview or physical examination, or when giving and evaluating care. These basic skills are discussed further in Chapter 15.

Examination is an objective, systematic assessment of the patient's physical status, performed in conjunction with, or after, the nursing interview. It involves the use of four

NURSING/PATIENT/FAMILY PROFILE
Nursing Department
MOUNT SINAI HOSPITAL
600 University Avenue, Toronto, Ontario M5G 1X5
MS 589 (11/93) Page 1 of 6

| Obtained from: | | | Reviewed by: | Unit: | Date: |
| Conducted by: | Unit: | Date: | Reviewed by: | | |

Age:	Sex:	ADMISSION VITAL SIGNS					
		Temperature	Pulse	Respirations	Blood Pressure	Height	Weight

Allergies:

| Admitting Medical Diagnosis: | | Admission Date: | Related Diagnosis: |

Surgical Procedure: | Date: | Admitting Physician:

"Why are you here?" | Previous hospitalization? When? Where? Why?

Current Prescription and Non-prescription medications (type, dose, frequency and time taken at home, reason)

Language spoken: | Translator:

Significant other: | Phone # (Home): (Work): | Do they know you are here? ☐ Yes ☐ No ☐ Notified

Where do you anticipate going after discharge?

SELF-CONCEPT MODE

1. How would you like to be addressed? ___
2. How do you feel about being in the hospital? ___ Why? ___

No Yes
3. Has there been a marked change in your mood in the previous 3 - 4 months? ☐ ☐
4. Are you depressed? ☐ ☐
5. Are you having problems with anxiety? ☐ ☐
6. What, if any, cultural or spiritual/religious practices are important to you or your family while you are here? ___

PHYSIOLOGICAL MODE

Oxygenation No Yes | If yes, describe: | Update*
1. Any problems with your breathing? ☐ ☐
2. Do you smoke? ☐ ☐
3. Do you use alcohol/drugs? ☐ ☐

*See progress notes
Developed by Documentation Committee of Conceptualization Nursing Program 1993, Kathleen Tong R.N. BScN./Chairperson

FIGURE 14.2 Nursing health history form patterned on Roy's adaptation model

SOURCE: Nursing Department, Mount Sinai Hospital, Toronto. Reproduced with permission.

NURSING/PATIENT/FAMILY PROFILE
MS 589 (11/93) Page 2 of 6

PHYSIOLOGICAL MODE continued

Oxygenation continued   No Yes If yes, describe: |Update*
4. Any problems with: ☐   ☐

   – your blood pressure?   ☐   ☐

   – your circulation?   ☐   ☐

5. Any bleeding problems?   ☐   ☐

Nutrition/fluids and electrolytes
1. Any recent weight loss or gain? ☐ ☐

2. How has your appetite been?   ☐   ☐

3. When did you last eat or drink? ☐   ☐

4. Special diet/intolerances?   ☐   ☐
5. Dental appliances or problems? ☐   ☐

Elimination
1. Any problems with urinating?   ☐   ☐
2. Any problems with your bowels? ☐   ☐

3. What is your normal bowel pattern? ☐ ☐

4. Date of last bowel movement?   ☐   ☐
5. Any ostomy appliances?   ☐   ☐

Activities of Daily Living (ADL) and Rest
1. Are you able to manage ADL independently? ☐ ☐
2. Assistive devices for above?   ☐   ☐

3. ** *Risk for falls assessed?*   ☐   ☐
   If yes, followup with Standards for
   Fall Prevention
4. Any problems sleeping lately?   ☐   ☐
5. Do you take/do anything to help you sleep? ☐ ☐
Protection
1. Any problems with your skin?   ☐   ☐

2. ** *High risk for skin breakdown?*
3. If yes, inspect: (check if intact)
   ☐ Heels ☐ Head ☐ Hips ☐ Coccyx ☐ Elbows ☐ Nails ☐ Back ☐ Ears ☐ Other
   Describe affected areas: _____
   If yes to 2 or 3, utilize Standards for Potential or Actual Impaired Skin Integrity
1. Senses and Neurologic function
   Any changes or difficulties with the following:
   ☐ Vision ☐ Hearing ☐ Memory ☐ Smell ☐ Taste ☐ Sensation ☐ Speech
   Describe:_____
Assistive devices:
2. ** *Mental Status:* ☐ Alert ☐ Oriented ☐ Disoriented ☐ Confused ☐ Semi Conscious ☐ Comatose
   Describe:_____

*** Must be assessed by Nurse; do not ask patient   *See progress notes*

FIGURE 14.2 Continued

NURSING/PATIENT/FAMILY PROFILE
MS 589 (11/93) Page 3 of 6

	No	Yes	If yes, describe:	Update*

3. Do you have pain? ☐ ☐
   Where?_____ Describe: _____ When did it start?_____ _____
   Rating (0-10)_____ What helps it?_____ How long does it last? _____ _____
   What makes it worse? _____

4. Have you noticed any changes from the
   way you usually think, feel, behave? ☐ ☐ _____ _____

Endocrine function
1. Do you have: If yes, describe:
   Diabetes? ☐ ☐ _____ _____
   Thyroid problems? ☐ ☐ _____ _____
   Other hormonal problems? ☐ ☐ _____ _____
   Sexual functioning problems? ☐ ☐ _____ _____

Other
2. Communicable diseases? ☐ ☐ _____ _____

ROLE FUNCTION

1. Secondary role (occupation, marital status, etc.): _____
   Significant relationships: (list) _____ _____

2. Tertiary role (hobbies, interests, life style): _____
   _____ _____

3. Do you foresee any financial concerns ☐ No ☐ Yes
   in relation to your illness? _____ _____

INTERDEPENDENCE MODE

1. What are your living arrangements?

   ☐ Alone   ☐ Shared   If shared, with whom:_____

   ☐ House   ☐ Apartment   ☐ Other (describe):_____

2. Of your significant others, who would you like to be included in decisions about your care and/or teaching?
   _____

3. Do you anticipate any difficulty caring for yourself after leaving the hospital? ☐ No ☐ Yes   If yes, how?
   _____

4. Are there any nurses or agencies visiting you in the home? ☐ No ☐ Yes _____
   _____

5. Are you currently involved with other health care related services? ☐ No ☐ Yes _____
   (eg., clinics, chiropractor) _____

   Are there any other issues related to your health or hospital stay that you ☐ No ☐ Yes
   would like to discuss? _____

General Impressions/Second Level Assessment

_____
_____
_____
_____

   What are your main goals while here? (See Care Plan) _____

*See progress notes

FIGURE 14.2   Continued

sensory techniques: inspection through critical visual observation; palpation by touching and feeling with the fingers; percussion by tapping with the fingers and listening for sounds; and auscultation by listening for sounds directly or with a stethoscope. These techniques are outlined in Chapter 15.

The physical examination is carried out in a systematic manner. There are a number of ways of conducting a physical examination. The nurse can use a head-to-toe format, a systems approach or a needs approach. In the head-to-toe method, the nurse begins by assessing the head and neck, and then continues down the body to the chest and thorax, the abdomen, the perineum and then the arms, legs and feet. In the systems approach, each of the body systems is examined separately. The nurse first assesses the respiratory system (nose, mouth, throat and lungs), and then continues methodically with the cardiac and circulatory system, neurological system, gastrointestinal system, genitourinary system, musculosketetal system, integumentary system, and so on.

The patient needs approach uses a biopsychosocial format that includes an analysis of biological, psychological, developmental, social, cultural, religious and spiritual factors, organized around needs such as oxygen, nutrition, self-esteem or safety. A physical examination can also be organized around a nursing model. For example, when using Orem's model the patient would be examined for self-care capabilities and deficits. Use of a nursing model is beneficial because it directs the examination towards a particular nursing perspective and clearly points out the nurse's role in patient care. The approach that a nurse uses in conducting a physical examination depends on personal preference and agency requirements.

Review of Resources

Resources are reviewed to ensure that information about a particular patient is complete. The nurse should check the patient's chart, scan the baseline or focus data, review laboratory and diagnostic test results, talk to family members or significant others if appropriate or consult with other health team members for any additional information that may be required for making nursing diagnoses and planning care.

HOW TO INTERPRET AND USE INFORMATION COLLECTED (DIAGNOSTIC REASONING)

The information collected during assessment is of no value unless it means something within the context of the patient's situation. During and after data collection, the nurse assigns meaning to data and makes judgements about the patient's health status and abilities to function in daily living. This critical thinking process, or diagnostic reasoning, is the basis for establishing nursing diagnoses and making decisions for care.

Diagnostic reasoning is a complex mental process which combines data-collecting activities with the deliberate use of knowledge, experience and logic to identify and classify the findings in a patient situation and then form a conclusion about the patient's state of health. In many cases, this process goes on without the nurse's conscious awareness of the mental operations involved. An experienced nurse, for example, can make an observation, form a conclusion and take immediate action for the problem without thinking about the underlying reasoning process.

Diagnostic reasoning, however, is a learned skill. As in learning all skills, the beginning practitioner has to learn the elements of diagnostic reasoning and carry out the mental operations in their logical order. To understand diagnostic reasoning one should know something about the nature of information and how meaning is derived from this information. We will begin by looking at the types of information collected, and then move on to an examination of specific pieces of information (cues) and how to derive meaning from these cues (inferences).

Subjective and Objective Data

There are two types of information that the nurse gathers through assessment. **Subjective data** refers to information reported primarily by the patient, but it can also come from the patient's family or significant other. It includes feelings and perceptions about one's state of health and abilities to cope with activities of daily life. "I feel short of breath," "I feel hopeless," "I have a stomachache" are examples of subjective information expressed by the patient. Subjective data obtained from a family member, for example, may include a mother's perception of her child's stomachache and how she herself is feeling about her child being sick. Subjective data, also called *symptoms* or *covert* data, cannot be observed directly but are obtained by asking questions.

Objective data refers to information about a person that can be observed, perceived or measured by another through the use of sense organs or instruments. The colour of skin, vital signs, changes in behaviour and laboratory tests are examples of objective data — also called *signs* or *overt* data.

Recognizing Cues and Making Inferences

Interpreting information is knowing the meaning of what is being perceived from the environment. In order to do this, one has to notice a piece of information, put a name to it and attach meaning to it. The pieces of information that one perceives from the environment are called **cues**.

Subjective and objective data are cues. The nurse's interpretation of these cues is called an *inference*. For instance, the nurse notices a grimacing look on a patient's face (a cue) and infers that the patient is anxious or in pain (the inference). Or, a patient who looks flushed and reports feeling chilled (cues) leads the nurse to infer that the patient has a fever. Inferences are subjective interpretations of cues and, therefore, are influenced by the nurse's level of knowledge and experience as well as by personal attitudes and values. It is important to validate cues and inferences with the patient to avoid making the wrong interpretation.

Interpreting data involves two cognitive skills: recognizing the cue or inference as significant and assigning meaning to the significance (Carpenito, 1993). The nurse recognizes the significance of cues or groups of cues on the basis of knowledge of patterns or features of phenomena. Meaning is assigned to cues by comparing them to patterns or features of normal, healthy or abnormal, unhealthy states retrieved from memory or obtained from reference materials. The inference mentioned above about a patient's rising temperature was made by associating the cues (flushed skin and feeling chilled) to knowledge of the signs and symptoms and pathophysiology of infection.

Knowledge and experience enhance the nurse's ability to make accurate inferences about patient states. Inferences that nurses make are aided by their:

• knowledge of normal functioning, derived from courses in basic biophysical and social sciences
• understanding of normal and abnormal factors that may affect functioning in a particular area
• awareness of common problems, signs and symptoms that accompany various health problems.

As a beginning student in nursing, you will not have an extensive knowledge base from which to draw. You will, however, be able to identify many deviations from normal and relate these to the knowledge you do have. As your knowledge increases and your clinical experience grows you will be able to determine the significance of your findings more readily and with greater depth of understanding. At all times, however, it is important that you communicate your findings and interpret them honestly at your level of understanding.

An important feature about information cues is that they are variable and uncertain. That is to say, cues can mean different things in different situations. A single cue can have different meanings whether by itself or in combination with other cues. For example, a young woman who gave birth to a baby two days ago is found crying. This cue, that she is crying, could mean a number of things. Perhaps she is crying because she is overjoyed with the birth. On the other hand she may be feeling disappointment over the sex of the baby. She may be experiencing baby blues, a common response caused by hormonal readjustment after childbirth. Or she may be crying because she is in pain or because she just received some sad news from home. Obviously,

more information is needed to make an inference about the cause of this woman's crying.

Cues can also mean different things when combined with other cues. Take, for example, the cue of hot and flushed skin. When combined with signs of infection, this cue is a fairly strong indicator of fever; whereas in a diabetic person, hot and flushed skin combined with signs of high blood sugar indicates an altered nutritional state. Thus, cues vary in their relation to the patient's circumstances.

Some cues give irrefutable grounds for making inferences; for example, if a patient's temperature is 39°C, one can infer absolutely that the patient has a fever. Gordon calls this type of cue a *diagnostic cue* (Gordon, 1987, 191). When a diagnostic cue is present in the assessment findings, the nurse can be quite sure of the condition it represents. Other cues are not so clear. The hot and flushed skin, in the example above, may not stand alone as a diagnostic cue, but is valuable in assuring certainty of the patient's state when combined with other cues. These variable indicators are called *supporting cues* (Gordon, 1987, 191).

Validating Inferences

Because inferences are often based on cues that are variable and uncertain, there is a risk of error in the conclusions reached. Nurses can decrease the chance of error by validating the inferences and the information they collect. One way of doing this is by comparing objective and subjective data. For example, if a patient states, "I feel very warm" and the nurse observes a temperature of 39°C, the nurse's observation validates the inference of fever made on the basis of what the patient is experiencing. If there is a discrepancy between the nurse's observations (objective data) and what the patient states (subjective data), however, data collection must continue until a valid inference is established. Inferences may also be validated by reexamining data or reassessing the patient, by consulting sources, such as a nurse teacher, a clinical nurse specialist or an experienced nurse, or by referring to a textbook.

ORGANIZING THE INFORMATION

In order to critically examine data in the diagnosis step of the nursing process, the nurse will find it helpful to group the information by categories, commonly referred to as *clusters*. Putting information into a logical and systematic order makes the mass of data more meaningful and manageable. It brings together related information which helps the nurse see patterns and identify problems and strengths.

There are a variety of frameworks the nurse can use for clustering the assessment data. A nursing model provides designated categories for data that give meaning to the information from a nursing perspective. Frequently the

TABLE 14.1   Frameworks for Organizing (Clustering) Data

ROY (1984)*	BODY SYSTEMS	HUMAN NEEDS
Adaptive modes	Integument	Physiological needs
Physiologic mode	Head and neck	Oxygen
Exercise and rest	Special senses	Nutrition
Nutrition	Thorax and lungs	Urinary elimination
Elimination	Heart and blood vessels	Bowel elimination
Fluid and electrolytes	Breast	Fluid, electrolyte,
Oxygen and circulation	Abdomen	and acid-base balance
Regulation:	Extremities	Temperature regulation
temperature	(Musculoskeletal)	Comfort, rest, and sleep
Regulation: the senses	Extremities	Pain management
Regulation: endocrine	(Neurological)	Activity needs
system	Genitourinary	Sensory
Self-concept		Movement and exercise
Physical self		Protection and Safety needs
Moral-ethical self		Safety
Self-consistency		Hygiene
Self-ideal and		Control of infection
expectancy		Psychosocial needs
Role function		Sexuality
Interdependence		Security and self-esteem
		Death, loss and grieving

*SOURCE: Roy, C. (1984). *Introduction to nursing: An adaptation model* (2nd ed.). Englewood Cliffs, NJ: Prentice-Hall.

model used for the nursing history of a data base assessment can also serve as an organizing framework for data clustering. Frameworks based on human needs also help keep a nursing focus and, in addition, lead logically to nursing diagnoses. A body systems approach is useful because it helps the nurse identify problems that should be referred to the physician (Alfaro, 1990). Table 14.1 illustrates three frameworks for organizing assessment data: Roy's model, human needs, and body systems. The needs framework is reflective of the needs approach we have taken in this book. These needs follow the 13 functional areas described by McCain (1965) and are organized according to Maslow's (1970) hierarchy of needs.

COMMUNICATING THE INFORMATION

The last phase of assessment is communicating and documenting the data that have been collected. Any findings that point to problems requiring immediate attention (for example, abnormal vital signs, breathing problems, severe pain) that the nurse is not qualified to deal with independently must be reported to an appropriate health team member (head nurse, physician or supervisor) before documentation occurs. As a nursing student you will want to report to your primary nurse or supervisor, or your teacher. In this way significant

problems can be examined by appropriately qualified health team members and treatment measures can be instituted without delay.

Documentation procedure for the patient's baseline data varies. Many agencies now use admission forms or patient profiles for recording the nursing history as well as pertinent observations and examinations. Focussed assessments are entered onto the patient's record according to charting procedure. General guidelines for charting are presented in Chapter 18, Information Management.

DIAGNOSIS

As the second step in the nursing process, *diagnosis* is defined as a deliberate, systematic process of data analysis and synthesis that ends with a clinical judgement. During assessment, the nurse gathers and organizes data into clusters depicting patterns of health and illness. In diagnosis, these patterns are examined (analyzed) and pulled together (synthesized) to identify patient problems and strengths. The problems form the basis of the nursing care plan and the strengths are used in developing the most effective plan for the patient. There are three components involved in diagnosis: 1) Identifying patient problems and strengths, 2) Formulating the diagnosis, and 3) Writing the diagnostic statement.

IDENTIFYING PATIENT PROBLEMS AND STRENGTHS

In diagnosis, the nurse examines the data clusters identified during assessment to determine what they mean in the context of the information available. In identifying problems and strengths the nurse goes "beyond the information contained in the inferences, cues or cue clusters to generate a set of possible diagnostic meanings" (Gordon, 1987, 220). The nurse formulates hypotheses of probable diagnoses by comparing observed patterns of functioning in the data clusters to knowledge of significant deviations from normal. What is unusual in the findings about this patient? In what way does the status of the patient's functional abilities compare with known health problems? How important are the deviations from normal?

Problems are identified by comparing the clusters of data to knowledge of lists or categories of signs and symptoms (objective and subjective data) or risk factors that depict the hypothesized problems. These lists or categories are called *defining characteristics* (Carpenito, 1993). If, for example, a nurse hypothesizes that a patient's problem is dehydration, he or she will look for defining characteristics of dehydration. If the data in the cluster are similar to the defining characteristics for dehydration, the nurse will conclude that the patient has an *actual problem* of dehydration or fluid volume deficit. If the data in the cluster are not similar to the defining characteristics the problem is rejected and alternative explanations are considered.

The presence of risk factors in a data base without the accompanying defining characteristics of a hypothesized problem indicate a *potential problem*. For instance, the patient who experiences fever, vomiting and diarrhea faces the potential problem of developing fluid volume deficit because fluid loss would likely be greater than intake. Problems may also be defined in the absence of adequate defining characteristics. In this case, there are some data to support a diagnosis but they are insufficient to say the patient has an actual problem. For example, a nurse might consider the possibility that ineffective breastfeeding in a young mother might occur because she has not taken prenatal classes. This problem is called a *possible problem*. It indicates that more information is needed to validate that a problem actually exists.

Once a problem has been identified, the nurse's next task is to determine the causative etiology or the contributing factors of the problem (Carpenito, 1993). For example, in an identified problem of patient anxiety, the contributing factor might be "insufficient knowledge of diagnostic test procedure." It is important to determine the cause of the problem because knowing the cause helps to select appropriate nursing interventions. For example, the problem statement "anxiety" gives no indication of actions needed. But, "anxiety related to insufficient knowledge of diagnostic test procedure," on the other hand, tells the nurse what actions will be necessary to treat the problem.

Alfaro LeFevre offers the following questions the nurse can ask to help identify the factors causing or contributing to a problem:

- What factors does the patient (or significant others) identify as causing or contributing to a problem?
- Are there factors related to developmental age, disease or changes in lifestyle that could be contributing to the problem?
- Do other resources for data collection (medical records, other health care professionals, literature review) identify factors that might be causing or contributing to the problem?*

In addition to identifying health problems, the nurse also has to determine patient strengths. *Strengths* refer to the physical and psychosocial capabilities, the cultural and religious values and beliefs and the spiritual dimensions of persons or families which enable them to cope with the challenges of daily living. Strengths can help patients and families adjust to their health problems and assume responsibility for their own care. Knowledge of patients' strengths helps the nurse determine the amount of assistance they will require in meeting their needs.

Physical strengths include good physical health, regular exercise, a nutritionally well balanced diet, appropriate weight for body size, and strong muscles and endurance. Psychosocial strengths include effective coping abilities, strong motivation to live optimally with a chronic condition, relatives who are available to help with home care, ability to use resources in the community, or a positive

---

Example of Problem Identification

DATA CLUSTER	DEFINING CHARACTERISTICS
Temperature 38.4°C	Insufficient fluid intake
Nausea and vomiting	Less intake than output
Not drinking or eating	Dry skin, mucous
Diarrhea	membranes
Dry skin, decreased	Decreased, concentrated
turgor	urine
Concentrated urine	

Interpretation: Data cluster similar to defining characteristics

Actual problem: Fluid volume deficit

---

* (Alfaro-LeFevre, 1994, 103.)

health attitude (belief in eating well, balancing rest and exercise, avoiding alcohol or nicotine). Together with the patient and/or family, the nurse makes a list of strengths that will help in planning care for the identified problems. A benefit of this process is that it may also indicate opportunities in which the nurse can assist patients and families in achieving higher levels of wellness.

FORMULATING THE DIAGNOSIS

Nursing Diagnosis and Collaborative Problems

A *nursing diagnosis* is a clinical judgement about individual, family or community responses to actual or potential health problems or life processes which provides the basis for selecting interventions to achieve outcomes for which the nurse is accountable (NANDA. Cited in Carpenito, 1993). The nursing diagnosis describes a health problem which nurses are responsible for identifying and treating by nurse-prescribed interventions. However, nurses are also responsible for identifying complications that occur or may occur in association with specific pathology and treatment which they must monitor or refer to the physician for treatment (Carpenito, 1987; 1993). These are called *collaborative problems*. As an example, if a patient were at risk for fluid volume deficit following surgery because of the possibility of bleeding, the collaborative problem would be described as

Potential Complication: Bleeding. Table 14.2 provides a comparison of nursing diagnoses with collaborative problems.

Alfaro (1990) outlines a number of guidelines the student may use in identifying collaborative problems. These are:

1. Consider your patient's medical diagnosis and determine the signs and symptoms of the most frequent and most dangerous complications.
2. Be aware of recent diagnostic or treatment modalities, and determine whether there are associated potential complications.
3. If the situation is complex, check with a reference or a more qualified professional (for example, ask the attending physician or a clinical nurse specialist).
4. Consult policy, procedures, protocols and standards that address your patient's diagnostic or treatment situations (for example, management of chest tubes), because they will often list associated potential complications.*

NANDA Diagnoses

The North American Nursing Diagnosis Association (NANDA) is composed of nurses from the United States and Canada who represent all constituents of the profession: practice, education and research. Its first meeting was held in 1973 to identify nursing knowledge and develop a classification system that could be computerized. Since its inception the group has developed a classification of diagnostic categories to describe health problems that are identified and treated

---

* (Alfaro, 1990, 83.)

TABLE 14.2   Comparison of Nursing Diagnoses with Collaborative Problems

	NURSING DIAGNOSES	COLLABORATIVE PROBLEMS
Assessment	Focus is on human responses to actual and potential health problems or life changes	Focus is on pathophysiologic response of body organs and systems
Problem Identification	Nurse identifies and validates existence of problem independently	Nurse may identify problem but refers to the physician for validation
Treatment	Nurse initiates interventions independently	Nurses are responsible for detecting and reporting signs and symptoms that may indicate a need for medical intervention. Nurse collaborates with physician to initiate treatment measures. Nurse may have standing orders from physician or through agency policy to initiate diagnostic studies or treatment measures for the problem without physician's order.

SOURCE: Alfaro, 1990, 67; Alfaro-LeFevre, 1994, 89.

through independent nursing function. The latest list approved by NANDA at its tenth conference in 1992 is presented in Table 14.3. The diagnoses provide a common language which facilitates communication among nurses and a knowledge base which nurses can use in diagnosing existing and potential problems. A solid, consistent base of knowledge also helps students in learning the complex nursing diagnostic process.

There are three components to NANDA diagnoses: 1) the label, which describes the actual or potential health

---

TABLE 14.3   North American Nursing Diagnosis Association (NANDA) Accepted Nursing Diagnoses

Activity Intolerance
Activity Intolerance, Risk for*
Adaptive Capacity: Intracranial, Decreased#
Adjustment, Impaired
Airway Clearance, Ineffective
Anxiety
Aspiration, Risk for*
Body Image Disturbance
Body Temperature, Risk for Altered
Bowel Incontinence
Breastfeeding, Effective
Breastfeeding, Ineffective
Breastfeeding, Interrupted
Breathing Pattern, Ineffective
Cardiac Output, Decreased
Caregiver Role Strain
Caregiver Roe Strain, Risk for*
Communication, Impaired Verbal
Community Coping, Ineffective#
Community Coping, Potential for Enhanced#
Confusion, Acute#
Confusion, Chronic#
Constipation
Constipation, Colonic
Constipation, Perceived
Coping, Defensive
Coping, Ineffective Individual
Decisional Conflict (Specify)
Denial, Ineffective
Diarrhea
Disorganized Infant Behaviour#
Disorganized Infant Behaviour, Risk for#
Disuse Syndrome, Risk for*
Diversional Activity Deficit
Dysreflexia
Energy Field Disturbance#
Environmental Interpretation Syndrome, Impaired#
Family Coping: Compromised, Ineffective
Family Coping: Disabling, Ineffective
Family Coping: Potential for Growth
Family Process: Alcoholism, Altered
Family Processes, Altered
Fatigue
Fear
Fluid Volume Deficit

Fluid Volume Deficit, Risk for*
Fluid Volume Excess
Gas Exchange, Impaired
Grieving, Anticipatory
Grieving, Dysfunctional
Growth and Development, Altered
Health Maintenance, Altered
Health Seeking Behaviours (Specify)
Home Maintenance Management, Impaired
Hopelessness
Hyperthermia
Hypothermia
Infant Feeding Pattern, Ineffective
Infection, Risk for*
Injury, Risk for#
Knowledge Deficit (Specify)
Loneliness, Risk for#
Management of Therapeutic Regimen: Community, Ineffective#
Management of Therapeutic Regimen: Families, Ineffective#
Management of Therapeutic Regimen: Individual, Ineffective#
Memory, Impaired#
Mobility, Impaired Physical
Noncompliance (Specify)
Nutrition: Less than Body Requirements, Altered
Nutrition: More than Body Requirements, Altered
Nutrition: Potential for More than Body Requirements, Altered
Oral Mucous Membrane, Altered
Organized Infant Behaviour, Potential for Enhanced#
Pain
Pain, Chronic
Parent/Infant/Child Attachment, Risk for#
Parental Role Conflict
Parenting, Altered
Parenting, Risk for Altered*
Peripheral Neurovascular Dysfunction, Risk for*
Personal Identity Disturbance
Poisoning, Risk for*
Post-Trauma Response
Powerlessness
Protection, Altered

Rape-Trauma Syndrome
Rape-Trauma Syndrome: Compound Reaction
Rape-Trauma Syndrome: Silent Reaction
Relocation Stress Syndrome
Role Performance, Altered
Self-Care Deficit, Bathing/Hygiene
Self-Care Deficit, Dressing/Grooming
Self-Care Deficit, Feeding
Self-Care Deficit, Toileting
Self-Esteem, Chronic Low
Self-Esteem, Situational Low
Self-Esteem Disturbance
Self-Mutilation, Risk for*
Sensory/Perceptual Alterations (Specify: visual, auditory, kinesthetic, gustatory, tactile, olfactory)
Sexual Dysfunction
Sexuality Patterns, Altered
Skin Integrity, Impaired
Skin Integrity, Risk for*
Sleep Pattern Disturbance
Social Interaction, Impaired
Social Isolation
Spiritual Distress
Spiritual Well-being, Potential for Enhanced#
Suffocation, Risk for*
Swallowing Impaired
Thermoregulation, Ineffective
Thought Processes, Altered
Tissue Integrity, Impaired
Tissue Perfusion, Altered (Specify: renal, cerebral, cardiopulmonary, gastrointestinal, peripheral)
Trauma, Risk for*
Unilateral Neglect
Urinary Elimination, Altered
Urinary Incontinence, Functional
Urinary Incontinence, Reflex
Urinary Incontinence, Stress
Urinary Incontinence, Total
Urinary Incontinence, Urge
Urinary Retention
Ventilation, Inability to Sustain Spontaneous
Ventilatory Weaning Response, Dysfunctional (DVWR)
Violence, Risk for: Self-directed or directed at others

New diagnoses added in 1994
* Diagnoses with modified label terminology in 1994
SOURCE: North American Nursing Diagnosis Association. (1994). *NANDA nursing diagnoses: Definitions and Classification 1995-1996.* Philadelphia: Author.

problem; 2) related factors, the pathophysiological, treatment-related, situational, and maturational factors that cause or contribute to the problem; and 3) defining characteristics, the cluster of signs and symptoms that point to the diagnosis. The related factors for potential problems are the risk factors themselves.

In terms of NANDA, there are four types of nursing diagnosis: *actual*, *high-risk*, *wellness* or *syndrome*. An **actual diagnosis** represents a problem that has been validated by the presence of major defining characteristics. NANDA specifies major and minor defining characteristics for the diagnoses. A **high-risk diagnosis** describes a potential problem. Prior to 1992, these diagnoses were labelled

"potential for." A **wellness diagnosis** is "a clinical judgement about an individual, family or community in transition from a specific level of wellness to a higher level of wellness" (Carpenito 1993, 17). Two cues must be present for a wellness diagnosis. First, the patient must express a desire for a higher level of wellness; and second, present status or function must be effective (Carpenito, 1993). A **syndrome diagnosis** consists of a "cluster of actual or high-risk nursing diagnoses that are predicted to be present because of a certain event or situation" (Carpenito, 1993, 20). Two currently approved NANDA syndrome diagnoses are *Rape Trauma Syndrome* and *High Risk for Disuse Syndrome*. Figure 14.3 shows a decision schematic for differentiating among the types of diagnoses.

FIGURE 14.3 Decision tree differentiating among actual, high-risk and possible nursing diagnoses (© Lynda Juall Carpenito)

SOURCE: Carpenito, L. J. (1993). *Nursing diagnosis: Application to clinical practice* (5th ed.). Philadelphia: Lippincott. Reproduced with permission.

WRITING THE DIAGNOSTIC STATEMENT

Nursing diagnoses provide a focus and give direction in planning goal-directed care. Therefore, to be useful, diagnostic statements must describe the problem in a manner that will help the nurse make intervention decisions. Review the diagnoses below:

- Fluid volume deficit related to decreased oral intake manifested by dry skin and mucous membranes.
- Fluid volume deficit related to decreased oral intake secondary to difficulty in swallowing manifested by dry skin and mucous membranes, takes only sips of juice, states it hurts to swallow.

The first statement describes the problem but tells nothing about why the nurse chose that particular diagnosis, nor does it give any direction to intervention choices. The second statement, on the other hand, describes why the patient has the particular problem and indicates what the nurse should do to treat the problem.

Stating an Actual Nursing Diagnosis

An actual nursing diagnostic statement consists of three parts: the *problem*, the cause or *etiology*, and the *manifesting signs and symptoms* (defining characteristics). These three parts are linked in the written statement as:

> Problem RELATED TO etiology MANIFESTED BY *defining characteristics.*

> Example: *Impaired physical mobility* RELATED TO *pain from surgical incision* MANIFESTED BY *reluctance to move in bed, moaning and stating "it hurts."*

The *problem* should describe the state that exists as specifically as possible. For example, the diagnosis *Knowledge deficit* does not specify in what area the patient has a learning need. However, *Knowledge deficit in diet for diabetes* indicates exactly what it is the patient has to learn.

The **etiology** should specify one or more causes of (or contributors to) the health problem. To be useful it should not only tell why the problem is occurring but give direction in determining nursing interventions. For instance, the problem *Ineffective family coping* may be related to conflict between husband and wife, to lack of mutual decision making or to economic difficulties. Nursing interventions would vary considerably for these etiologies. Etiologies may include physiological, psychological, sociological, environmental and spiritual factors believed to cause or contribute to the problem.

Sometimes the cause of a problem may occur at two levels. For example, *Fluid volume deficit* related to decreased oral intake may be due to two (or more) factors. In this case, the etiology is stated in two parts, such that the second part explains the first. Notice how the diagnosis *Fluid vol-ume deficit related to decreased oral intake* SECONDARY TO *difficulty swallowing* clearly indicates the nature of the patient's decreased intake.

The defining characteristics are the signs and symptoms of the problem which, in the diagnostic statement, serve to validate the nursing diagnosis. They should include the clinical cues, that is, the subjective and objective data that confirm the health problem exists. NANDA's defining characteristics are separated into major and minor categories. "Major defining characteristics are defined as critical indicators present 80% – 100% of the time; minor defining characteristics, or supporting indicators, occur 50% – 79% of the time" (Carpenito, 1993, 13).

Stating a Potential or Possible Diagnosis

Potential and possible diagnoses may often have no defining characteristics. Potential diagnoses are made because of factors in patient situations that may leave them vulnerable to specific problems. For example, a newborn baby is always at risk for ineffective thermoregulation or infection. Possible diagnoses may be made to identify suspected problems that require more investigation. Potential and possible diagnoses direct the nurse to continue assessing and monitoring the patient. These diagnoses are written in two-part statements which outline the problem and possible etiology.

> Example: *Potential for or high risk for infection related to laceration and blood loss; Possible altered parenting related to lack of support from partner.*

Stating the Collaborative Problem

The nurse uses the collaborative problem statement to describe a potential complication that may result because of the disease process, trauma or diagnostic tests and treatment. This type of problem identification helps the nurse focus on nursing assessments and the need for referral to the physician. A collaborative problem is written as a potential complication, abbreviated as "PC," linked to its cause.

> Example: *PC: pulmonary edema secondary to congestive heart failure.*

PLANNING

In the planning step of the nursing process, the nurse prepares for intervention. Goals are set and strategies are selected to achieve the goals. A care plan is written to outline the individualized care needed to promote, protect or restore the patient's health. It is based on the nursing diagnoses and collaborative problems identified in assessment and diagnosis. During planning, the nurse sets priorities, develops goals, selects strategies, collaborates with the patient and family or other health team members and writes the nursing care plan. Because patients and families are now assuming greater responsibility for decisions regarding their care, their active involvement in every phase of planning for their care is essential.

SETTING PRIORITIES

Once nursing diagnoses and collaborative problems are identified, they are placed in order of importance. It is not possible to attend to all of the patient's problems at the same time. Therefore, it is necessary to determine those problems which require treatment now and those which can be attended to later.

A helpful guide in priority-setting is Maslow's hierarchy of needs which we introduced in Chapter 8. Basic physiological needs are given the highest priority, followed by safety, and then love, esteem, and self-actualization needs. When physiological and safety needs are not threatening a patient's well-being, priority is given to psychosocial, cultural, developmental and spiritual needs.

However, physiological and safety needs are often the most urgent. Patients may have multiple physiological and safety needs that must be prioritized. In this case, "priorities for treatment depend on 1) the urgency of the problem, 2) the nature of the treatment indicated, and 3) the interactions among diagnoses" (Gordon, 1987, 315). Actual or potential problems that are life-threatening are given highest priority. Examples are ineffective breathing patterns or violence directed at self or others. Similarly, when patients are physiologically unstable, intervention for physiological needs may take precedence over attending to knowledge or emotional needs. For example, the nursing diagnosis of *Knowledge deficit of diet and drug therapy for hypertension* would not be given priority until the patient's physiological state (in this case, high blood pressure) had been stabilized.

And finally, the interaction of diagnoses also influences priority setting. For a woman who had just given birth and was diagnosed with situational low self-esteem and knowledge deficit of infant care, teaching her about infant care would be the priority because improved knowledge and skill in caring for the baby would help the woman reestablish her self-esteem.

Priorities should also be set according to the patient's or family's perception of what is important. When physiological or safety problems take precedence, however, the nurse should clearly explain the rationale for these priorities.

DEVELOPING GOALS AND EXPECTED OUTCOMES

Goals are the statements of expected outcomes of nursing intervention. Intervention is planned to assist or enable the patient to achieve these outcomes. The ***expected outcomes***

describe the behaviour the patient is expected to achieve. For example, "Mr. M. will dress himself without help every morning" might be one goal for a partially paralyzed patient. Expected outcomes provide the criteria for evaluating the effectiveness of care. Therefore, they must be observable and measurable.

Goals for Nursing Diagnoses

A goal statement usually includes:

1. the healthy response, or desired patient behaviour (for example, "dresses himself")
2. the conditions, if any, under which it is to occur (for example, "without help")
3. a criterion of performance, or standard for judging the performance (for example, each morning).

Some agencies ask that a target date be included (for example, "by April 10, the patient will dress himself without help every morning"). By following a number of guidelines, the nurse can correctly develop a goal and its outcome criteria. These are outlined in Table 14.4 along with examples of correct and incorrect goal statements.

Goals originate from the nursing diagnoses and should reflect improvement in the identified problems. The easiest way to derive a goal is to convert the problem component of the nursing diagnosis into a description of the state of health that would exist if the problem were absent. For example, if the nursing diagnosis is *Activity intolerance related to congestive heart failure*, then the goal should be stated as: "The patient will demonstrate progressive activity tolerance." The outcome criteria are then listed in the goal statement using the phrase "as evidenced by." Thus, a goal statement for the nursing diagnosis above might be, "The patient will demonstrate progressive activity tolerance as evidenced by sitting in the chair for 15 minutes t.i.d. without chest pain by Monday."

Outcome criteria can also be derived from the etiology component of the diagnosis, because the best way to treat the problem is to reduce or eliminate the etiology or contributing factors. For example, if the patient's problem is stated as "altered nutrition: more than body requirements related to poor eating habits and lack of physical activity," the outcome criteria would focus on the patient's learning proper nutrition and exercising.

Goals should be realistic and attainable both in terms of the patient's potential and of the ability of nurses to help. For example, to set as a goal that Mr. T. will regain complete motor functioning may not be realistic for a patient partially paralyzed by a stroke. But Mr. T. may be able to achieve independence in feeding and dressing himself, and these are goals the nurse can help him achieve. Whenever possible, goals should be set mutually with the patient and family and other members of the health care team. This will ensure that the goals are compatible not only with the

TABLE 14.4   Guidelines For Writing Goals and Outcome Criteria

GUIDELINE	EXAMPLE
1. Focus the goal statement on expected patient behaviours and responses.	**Correct:** The patient will walk... **Incorrect:** The nurse will help the patient walk...
2. Base the goal statement on the nursing diagnosis.	Nursing diagnosis: Ineffective airway clearance related to incisional pain. **Correct:** The patient will keep his or her airway clear... **Incorrect:** The patient will support his or her incision when coughing...
3. Use observable verbs to state the outcome criteria. These must describe an expected action or response that can be seen or heard by the nurse.	Goal: The patient will keep his or her airway clear as evidenced by: **Correct:** 1. deep breathing and coughing ... 2. changing positions... **Incorrect:** 1. knowing how to cough and turn... 2. relief of incisional pain...
4. State outcome criteria in measurable terms, such that they give a standard against which the patient's activity or response can be compared. Use modifiers to describe what, when, where, and how the activity or response will take place.	Goal: The patient will keep his or her airway clear as evidenced by: **Correct:** 1. deep breathing and coughing 5 times q.h. without incisional pain... **Incorrect:** 1. deep breathing and coughing frequently...
5. Specify a time frame for goal achievement. This helps to keep patient priorities in perspective. Terms like "by discharge" or "continued" are acceptable.	**Correct:** 1. The patient will walk down the hall t.i.d. with the aid of a walker by Friday. 2. The patient will show continued intact skin.

patient's (and family's) expectations for care but also with other treatment measures, such as physiotherapy, occupational therapy or diagnostic testing.

There are short-term and long-term goals. When expected outcomes can be met in a relatively short period of time — a week or less — they are called *short-term goals* (STG). Those that will be achieved over a long period of time, sometimes weeks or months, are called *long-term goals* (LTG). Long-term goals are used in discharge planning from an acute care agency (see Chapter 9) and are very useful in ensuring the continuity of care when patients are discharged to home care or to community settings such as long-term care and ambulatory services. They are also used for patients receiving mental health services both in institutions and in community settings.

Because long-term goals may span weeks or months and patient progress may be slow, short-term goals are often used as stepping stones to reaching long-term goals. By breaking down the long-term goals, the nurse is better able

to assess the patient's progress in achieving the final desired outcomes. Both short- and long-term goals are written in the same format as described in Table 14.4.

Goals for Collaborative Problems

Goals for collaborative problems are different from goals for nursing diagnoses. Because the nurse is not responsible for diagnosing and prescribing interventions for collaborative problems, setting patient goals for collaborative problems is not appropriate. Rather, collaborative problems involve nursing goals, which reflect nursing accountability in situations requiring physician-prescribed and nurse-prescribed interventions. This accountability includes:

- Monitoring for physiologic instability
- Consulting standing orders and protocols or a physician to obtain orders for appropriate interventions

- Performing specific actions to manage and reduce the severity of an event or situation
- Evaluating patient responses.*

Nursing goals for collaborative problems can be written to indicate that the nurse will minimize or manage the problem (Carpenito, 1993). For example, if the patient's collaborative problem is *PC: Postoperative hemorrhage*, the nursing goal would be, "The nurse will manage and minimize postoperative bleeding."

SELECTING NURSING STRATEGIES

Nursing strategies are the specific actions or interventions the nurse performs to achieve the patient outcomes. These include activities to assist and enable individuals to promote, protect and restore their health or to experience a peaceful death. Nursing interventions are based on the nursing diagnosis and take into account the patient's strengths, preferences and level of ability as well as the physician's orders for care.

Types of Intervention[s]

Nursing interventions are any direct care measures that nurses perform on behalf of patients. These interventions include nurse-initiated measures that result from nursing diagnoses, physician-initiated treatments that result from the medical diagnosis and performance of essential daily functions for patients who are unable to do these (Bulechek and McCloskey, 1989). Bulechek and McCloskey identified six types of nursing activities the nurse carries out in the course of giving care. These are:

1. Assessment activities to make a nursing diagnosis.
2. Assessment activities to gather information for a physician to make a medical diagnosis.
3. Nurse-initiated treatments in response to nursing diagnoses.
4. Physician-initiated treatments in response to medical diagnoses.
5. Daily essential function activities (for example, bed-making, help with meal trays) that may not relate to either medical or nursing diagnoses but are done by the nurse for the patient who cannot do these things for himself/herself. These do not include deficits in performing the activities of daily living (ADL) such as bathing or combing the hair. When patients cannot perform these activities by themselves they would be diagnosed as having a self-care deficit and care would be done as nursing treatments in 3. above.
6. Assessment activities to evaluate the effects of nursing and medical treatments.**

Determining Nursing Interventions

In determining interventions for nursing diagnoses, the nurse selects activities to reduce or eliminate the cause or contributing factors; for collaborative problems the activities focus on managing or minimizing the problem. Alfaro (1990) maintains that to determine nursing interventions for actual and potential nursing diagnoses, the nurse has to identify the etiology and decide what needs to be done to eliminate or reduce it. Thus, for a diagnosis of *Fluid volume deficit related to decreased oral intake secondary to difficulty swallowing*, the nurse would select activities to reduce or eliminate the problem with swallowing.

There are three basic methods of selecting interventions. These include thinking, using standardized care plans and collaborating with the patient and members of the health care team (Hickey, 1990). "*Thinking* should be the nurse's first action when planning care" (Hickey, 1990, 111). Using reflection and remembering, devising and brainstorming, the nurse generates possible ways to achieve the expected outcome. *Standardized care plans* and professional reference books and journals can be consulted for general solutions to the problem. The nurse must examine the general solutions in light of the patient's needs, level of ability, strengths and preferences to determine the interventions most suited to the patient. After formulating a list of possible interventions, the nurse *collaborates with the patient and other health team members*. Knowledgeable members of the health care team — those who have cared for the patient or who have expertise in the problem area — will provide valuable information and advice on the planned interventions. The final information on the interventions most suitable for them based on their values, beliefs and preferences comes from patients and families. Involving patients and families in selecting interventions for their care will promote patient and family well-being and make implementation easier for the nurse.

Writing the Nursing Care Plan

To facilitate the implementation of nursing action, many agencies have developed a system of nursing care plans. The nursing care plan is a written guideline for nursing care. It includes the nursing diagnoses, the goals and outcome criteria, and the specific strategies for care. The care plan is formulated as soon after the patient's admission as sufficient data are available on which to base a plan. It is developed by the nurse who has the primary responsibility for the patient's care; or, in some agencies, it is developed jointly by the nursing team responsible for caring for the patient.

---

* (Carpenito, 1993, 66–67)
** (Bulechek and McCloskey, 1989, 24)

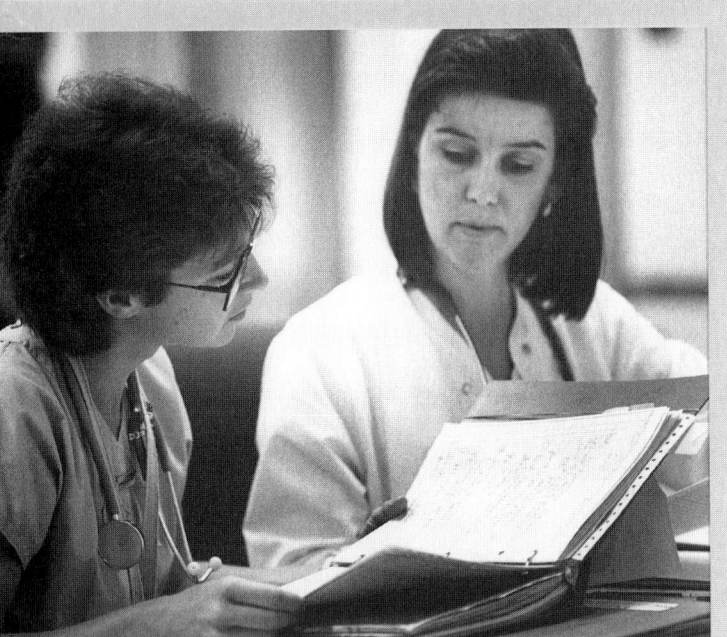

Nurses developing a plan of care for their patients

Because patients' problems may change from day to day when they are acutely ill, the nursing care plans for sick people are constantly subject to revision. Care plans for patients in ambulatory settings and for those in long-term facilities also need frequent revision but usually not as often as for patients in acute-care settings.

In some agencies, the nursing strategies are written in terms of nursing orders, which are prescribed and followed through in the same way as doctor's orders. In other agencies, the terms "nursing approach," "nursing actions" or "nursing directions" may be used to identify the specific strategies prescribed for care of the patient. Nursing orders must be sufficiently detailed and sufficiently specific to enable all personnel to carry them out in the same manner at the designated times.

The nursing care plan is a means of communicating in writing, to other nursing personnel and to other members of the health team, the nursing diagnoses, the expected outcomes of care, and the specific actions to be taken in the care of the patient. In many agencies, the care plans are incorporated into the patient's record; in some, they form part of the Kardex report. Sometimes, a separate notebook is kept for nursing care plans. An example of a nursing care plan used in an acute care agency is presented in Figure 14.4.

Standard Care Plans

Because nurses have found that patients with similar conditions have many problems in common, a number of agencies have developed standard care plans for use with patients who have a particular type of condition. There might be a standard care plan for all medical patients, for example, supplemented by a plan for all patients who have suffered a stroke. There might be another standard care plan for all surgical patients, supplemented by one for patients who are having one particular type of surgical intervention. Space is usually left on these standard plans for unusual problems — problems that are not anticipated and are unique to the patient.

IMPLEMENTING

Once nursing care plans have been developed, the next step is to put them into action. Implementing is the step of the nursing process in which nurses use their knowledge and skills to carry out the planned interventions. The nurse may give direct care to patients or engage in indirect activities that contribute to their care. This may include giving patients a bath, administering their medications or supervising others in these activities. Nursing care encompasses a variety of interventions. As students progress through their educational program, they will learn many types of interventions; and they will continue to do so throughout their career.

The knowledge and skills needed for implementing a plan of care focus on:

- Performing ongoing assessments to determine the status of existing nursing diagnoses and identify new ones
- Setting daily priorities to facilitate optimum treatment of a number of different problems during the course of the day
- Directly performing activities for patients
- Assisting patients or families in performing activities for themselves
- Teaching patients and families about their health care and management of a disorder
- Counselling patients and families in making decision about their own health care and using health care resources
- Monitoring patients for potential complications or problems
- Charting or documenting according to the legal specifications of the agency.*

Documenting Care

Agencies vary in their requirements for documentation. In some, the nursing care plan is supplemented by a record that lists the nursing orders (taken from the care plan) and provides space for the nurse to tick off as each intervention is carried out. This type of record acts as a checklist that the nurse responsible for the patient's care on each shift can review to see what was done and what was omitted.

---

* (Alfaro, 1990)

NURSING/PATIENT/FAMILY PROFILE
NURSING/PATIENT CARE PLAN

MS (12/93) Pg 1 of 2

PRIMARY/ASSOCIATE NURSE SIGNATURE AND INITIALS			Discharge Plans:
Jaqueline Maley, R.N.			

Teaching Focus:

INITIATION DATE	NURSING DIAGNOSIS and/or CLINICAL FOCUS	PATIENT OUTCOME	NURSING INTERVENTIONS/STRATEGIES	PATIENT OUTCOME REVIEW	RESOLUTION DATE	INITIAL
	Actual altered skin integrity (buttock sinus): (F)* Immobility Inability to communicate when wet or uncomfortable (C) Incontinent Nutritional status (R) Age History of skin breakdown	Buttock sinus will heal within one month. Patient pressure areas and perineum will remain intact.	1. Dressing change of Hygeol 1:20 packing TID 10 - 16 - 22. 2. Inspect pt's skin for potential pressure areas and document q shift. 3. Pressure reducing strategies: a) foam mattress x 2 b) change pt q 3 h for incontinence. Provide skin care using sween and peri creams to coccyx, buttocks, groin, and heels at this time. c) increase protein intake in diet by using protein supplements. d) reposition pt q 3 h while in bed. e) when up in chair, return pt to bed q 3 h for skin care. 4. Consultation with Duoderm company re alternative dressings sinus evaluated with rep re depth, any tracking of sinus, and potential for healing. Rep recommended Duoderm dressing with Duoderm paste q 3 h days. 5. Duoderm dressing q 3 h days. Please cleanse sinus, with N/S to remove old paste. Check sinus with Q-tip for any deep tracking of sinus over 1/4" then fill sinus with paste evenly and cover with large triangular Duoderm. 6. Duoderm dressing q 5 days with continued monitoring.	evaluated original dressing regime, sinus clean but slow to granulate After 1 month decrease duoderm to q 5 days. Sinus granulating well.		
	Risk for sleep pattern disturbance r/t altered hs routine (previous hospitalization)	Patient will show decrease agitation and settle hs with consistent hs routine	1. Provide hs care between 2030-2100 2. If time allows spend 15-20 min with patient. Give her milk and cookie. N.B. Please give kiss. Leave at least one light on in patient's room all night (consistent with home routine). 3. Document consistently the effectiveness of care plan and R/A patient's potential need for sedation (Haldol).			

FIGURE 14.4   Nursing Care Plan   *(continued on the next page)*

SOURCE: Nursing Department, Mount Sinai Hospital, Toronto, Ontario. Reproduced with permission.

NURSING/PATIENT CARE PLAN

MS (12/93) Pg 2 of 2

INITIATION DATE	NURSING DIAGNOSIS and/or CLINICAL FOCUS	PATIENT OUTCOME	NURSING INTERVENTIONS/STRATEGIES	PATIENT OUTCOME REVIEW	RESOLUTION DATE	INITIAL
	Risk for failure to thrive:	Patient will interact with staff and family	1. In am - 0800 - up to bathroom using high walker. Needs assistance of two. Not requiring help to actually walk ++ encouragement needed will say no all the time.			
	(F)* Loss of independence Change in environment	Patient will increase independence in ADL. To include:	2. Allow her to sit on toilet for *5-10 mins* it takes her a few tries to empty her bladder.			
	(C) Inability to communicate Fluctuating dementia	a) ambulation b) toileting	3. Sit her in wheelchair and allow patient to wash as much of herself as possible. Dress patient in her own clothes.			
	(R) No previous hospitalizations	c) AM care	4. Ambulate patient to nursing station. She will sit here all day. She needs to use bathroom @ A-1000, B-1300, C-1730.			
			5. Encourage interaction with patient during the day by periodically spending 5-10 mins with patient. Communicate by writing on board, looking at magazines with patient, or just sitting quietly with patient.			
			6. Balance patient's reorientation to environment with patient's need to believe she is at home. Patient will become agitated and upset with persistent reorientation.	Family verbalizes patient "is		
			7. Encourage Kelly to visit regularly to spend time with patient.	herself".		
			8. Patient can go to bed at 1900 if tired. Try to avoid putting her to bed before this time.	Decrease agitation noted		
			9. At night toilet her at 2200, 0200 (if awake) and 0500.	during day as documented		
			10. No fluids after 2100.	on chart.		
			11. If routine not followed patient will become agitated.			

FIGURE 14.4   Continued

*The Roy Framework encourages the breakdown of causative or contributing factors to Focal, Contextual and Residual stimuli.

Another type of form, similar in purpose to the checklist described above, is the flowsheet. When a specific intervention or a group of related interventions are to be done on a regular basis, it is helpful to have a special form that details the intervention specifically and documents the results of that intervention. See Chapter 18 for more details about documentation.

EVALUATING

Evaluation is a continuous process in which nurses assess and reassess the progress patients have made towards reaching the pre-established goals. Implicit in this reassessment is the need for constant revision of nursing care plans as new problems emerge, some are resolved, and some change. Priorities may need to be reordered, goals modified and new goals established. In addition, new decisions may have to be made in light of new information, changes that have occurred in the patient's condition, and success or failure of the interventions that have been tried.

Evaluating Patient Goal Achievement

Evaluation is the process of determining the extent to which the expected outcomes have been attained. It implies measurement against predetermined standards. If the outcome criteria have been carefully thought out and stated as observable and measurable standards, the nurse has a standard for comparing the patient's achievements. For example, in the case of an outcome criterion for a problem of impaired physical mobility stated as *Will maintain prescribed position at all times, except when necessary to turn on side for care*, the physician prescribed the position explicitly. In evaluating the patient's achievement of the outcome criterion, the nurse checks through the points enumerated regarding the position. Is the patient (Ms. J) flat in bed? Is she on her back? Does she have two pillows under her head? Is one supporting her shoulders? Does she have a pillow under her knees? Is she maintaining this position at all times, except when it is necessary to turn on her side for a back wash or rub or a linen change?

In evaluating the patient's goal achievement, the nurse compares the patient's activities and responses to the standards set out in the outcome criteria of the goal statement.

Progress can be noted and, if a particular nursing strategy does not appear to be effective, an alternative course of action can be recommended. The attainment of certain short-term goals may mean that the patient is ready for more far-reaching ones. The patient who has learned to dress without assistance, for example, may be ready to learn another activity of daily living.

Stating outcome criteria in question form helps the nurse to be objective and look for specific indications that expected outcomes have been met. Questions are not always written down, but beginning nurses may find it easier to develop the habit of asking themselves the questions implicit in the outcome criteria for the patient if they do put them onto paper.

Nurses evaluate the effectiveness of care through observations of the patient. Is the paralyzed arm in good anatomical position, or is the hand in a dependent position? It is also necessary to ask patients if nursing actions have been effective. Is the patient more comfortable or free from pain?

Revising the Plan of Care

In addition to evaluating the effectiveness of nursing strategies in relation to the patient's achievement of expected outcomes, the nurse critically examines the nursing care plan. Does it contain enough information for effective nursing diagnosis and care planning? Were all relevant factors taken into consideration in making the nursing diagnoses? Were diagnoses omitted for which care would have helped the patient? Were the established priorities, indeed, correct? Was the nursing care plan a logical outgrowth of the nursing diagnoses? Were unique factors in regard to the patient taken into consideration? Was the plan consistent with the physician's plan of therapy? Were expected outcomes logical, realistic and attainable? Were the nursing orders clearly stated? Was the plan successful? Were there factors that interfered with its success? What factors contributed to its success? Is the plan current and up to date? Have some of the problems resolved? Have new ones emerged?

As we stated in the beginning of the chapter, the nursing process is a circular one. Evaluation means reassessment and a gathering of additional new information. On the basis of reassessment, the nurse may identify new problems, modify the care plan or decide to try alternative interventions for the goals that were unsuccessful.

KEY TERMS

IN REVIEW

The nursing process is a problem-solving approach to practice which embodies a series of interrelated steps the nurse takes in planning and giving care. The steps in the process (assessment, diagnosis, planning, implementation and evaluation) follow one another in a logical, sequential order.

Assessment is the collection and interpretation of clinical information. It includes collecting, organizing and documenting the information on a nursing history or patient profile. Data are gathered through interviews with patients and/or families, observation and physical examination, consultations with other health team members and reviews of records. A data base assessment is performed on admission to a health care agency. It provides a comprehensive picture of the patient's health status and enables the nurse to make a beginning plan of care. Focus assessments are conducted on an ongoing basis and are directed to specific problems or patient needs.

The nurse uses diagnostic reasoning to interpret the data collected and make judgements about patients. There are two types of data collected by assessment. *Subjective data* are any information reported by the patient; *objective data* are observed, measured or perceived by another person through the use of sense organs or instruments. Subjective and objective data are cues the nurse uses to make inferences or judgements about the patient's health status. Nurses can decrease the chance of error in their inferences by validating the data collected. Organizing the data into clusters of related material helps to reveal patterns and identify problems and strengths. Frameworks for organizing data can be based on nursing models (such as Roy's model) or on human needs or body systems approaches.

Diagnosis is a deliberative process that involves the analysis and synthesis of data to identify patient problems and strengths. The nursing diagnosis describes a health problem which nurses are responsible for identifying and treating by nurse-prescribed interventions. It includes the diagnostic label which describes the actual or potential health problem, the etiology and the defining characteristics. The nursing diagnosis must describe the problem in a way that directs intervention decisions. Nurses also diagnose collaborative problems or potential complications which they must monitor or refer to the physician for treatment.

The planning step of the nursing process involves setting priorities, establishing goals, selecting strategies or interventions to achieve the goals, and writing the nursing care plan. Problems are prioritized so that the most pressing ones are dealt with first. Maslow's hierarchy of needs offers a helpful guide to priority setting. Goals are statements of expected outcomes derived from the nursing diagnoses. They outline behaviours the patient is expected to achieve as a result of intervention. Goals should be attainable, measurable and agreed upon by the patient and family. They may be short-term or long-term. Collaborative problems require other health professionals' orders. The nursing goals in these cases can be written to indicate that the nurse will minimize or manage the problem.

Nursing interventions are any direct care measures the nurse performs to achieve expected outcomes. These include assessment activities, nurse-initiated and physician-initiated interventions, essential daily functions for patients who are unable to do these, and evaluation activities of all interventions. Interventions are chosen by thinking, using standardized care plans or collaborating with the patient and other health care team members.

Nursing care plans are developed as soon as sufficient data are available and are updated in accordance with changes in the patient's health status. These plans include the nursing diagnoses, the goals and outcome criteria and the specific strategies for care. Care plans function as a means of communication among members of the health care team.

Implementing is the step of the nursing process in which the planned interventions are carried out. Implementation includes direct care, ongoing assessment and monitoring of problems, supervision of care given by other staff, the patient or the family, as well as teaching, counselling and documentation of care.

Evaluation is a continuous process of assessment and reassessment to determine the patient's progress towards reaching the goals. Revisions are made in the nursing care plan as some problems are resolved, some change and new ones emerge. Priorities may need to be reordered, goals reestablished and new strategies selected.

LEARNING ACTIVITIES

In consultation with your teacher, select a patient who has recently been admitted to the agency in which you are doing your clinical practice.

1. Review the patient's record to identify how and where the steps of the nursing process are documented.

2. Examine the patient's baseline data. Identify the information that would be helpful in planning nursing care.

3. Determine how focus assessment data are recorded. How does information gathered by focus assessment differ from baseline data? What factors might determine what information is gathered in the focus assessment?

4. State the nursing diagnoses you can identify from the data in the patient's record.

5. Arrange these problems in a list according to priorities as you see them.

6. Develop expected outcomes for each of the diagnoses.

7. Compare your diagnoses and expected outcomes with those on the nursing care plan prepared by experienced nurses. Did you identify the same problems? Did you miss any? Did you identify ones not listed? Did you use similar wording in the diagnostic statements? Did you rank priorities in the same order? If not, why do you think it was different? Were your goal statements similar?

8. Review the nursing interventions prescribed in the nursing care plan and flowsheets or other forms used to facilitate care. Relate these interventions to the nursing diagnoses and to principles underlying care.

9. Describe how you would evaluate the effectiveness of the nursing care plan.

REFERENCES AND READINGS

ALFARO, R. (1990). *Applying nursing diagnosis and nursing process.* (2nd ed.). Philadelphia: Lippincott.

ALFARO-LEFEVRE, R. (1994). *Applying nursing process: A step-by-step guide* (3rd ed.). Philadelphia: Lippincott.

BULECHEK, G. and McCLOSKEY, J. (1985). *Nursing interventions: Treatments for potential nursing diagnoses.* Philadelphia: Saunders.

BULECHEK, G. and McCLOSKEY, J. (1989). Nursing interventions: Treatments for potential nursing diagnoses. In M. Carroll-Johnson (Ed). *Classification of nursing diagnosis: Proceedings of the eighth national conference.* Philadelphia: Lippincott.

CARNEVALI, D., MITCHELL, P.H., WOODS, N.F. and TANNER, C.A. (1984). *Diagnostic reasoning in nursing.* Philadelphia: Lippincott.

CARNEVALI, D.L. and THOMAS, M.D. (1993). *Diagnostic reasoning and treatment decision making in nursing.* Philadelphia: Lippincott.

CARPENITO, L.J. (1987). *Nursing diagnosis: Application to clinical practice* (2nd ed.). Philadelphia: Lippincott.

CARPENITO, L.J. (1993). *Handbook of nursing diagnosis* (5th ed.). Philadelphia: Lippincott.

GORDON, M. (1976). Nursing diagnosis and the diagnostic process. *AJN, 76,* 1298.

GORDON, M. (1987). *Nursing diagnosis: Process and application* (2nd ed.). New York: McGraw-Hill.

HENDERSON, V. (1966). *The nature of nursing: A definition and its implications for practice, research and education.* New York: Macmillan.

HICKEY, P.W. (1990). *Nursing process handbook.* St Louis: Mosby.

IYER, P.W., TAPTICH B.J. and BERNOCCHI-LOSEY, B. (1986). *Nursing process and nursing diagnosis.* Philadelphia: Saunders.

KELLY, M.A. (1985). *Nursing diagnosis source book: Guidelines for clinical application.* Norwalk, CT: Appleton-Century-Crofts.

LA MONICA, E.L. (1985). *The humanistic nursing process.* Monterey, CA: Wadsworth.

LEDDY, S. and PEPPER, J.M. (1993). *Conceptual bases of professional nursing.* Philadelphia: Lippincott.

MASLOW, A.H. (1970). *Motivation and personality* (2nd ed.). New York: Harper and Row.

McCAIN, R.F. (1965, April). Nursing by assessment — Not intuition. *AJN.* 82–84.

MILLER, E. (1989). *How to make a nursing diagnosis work.* Norwalk, CT: Appleton & Lange.

MORITZ, D.A. (1982). Nursing diagnosis in relation to the nursing process. In M.J. Kim and D.A. Moritz (Eds). *Classification of nursing diagnoses: Proceedings of the third and fourth national conferences.* New York: McGraw-Hill, 53–57.

NORTH AMERICAN NURSING DIAGNOSIS ASSOCIATION. (1994). *NANDA nursing diagnoses: Definitions and Classification 1995-1996.* Philadelphia: Author.

ROY, C. (1984). *Introduction to nursing: An adaptation model* (2nd ed.). Englewood Cliffs, NJ: Prentice-Hall.

SHOEMAKER, J. (1984). Essential features of a nursing diagnosis. In M.J. Kim, G.K. McFarland and A.M. McLane (Eds). *Classification of nursing diagnoses: Proceedings of the fifth national conference.* St. Louis: Mosby, 109.

YURA, H. and WALSH M. B. (1988). *The nursing process.* Norwalk, CT: Appleton & Lange.

Clinical Assessment Skills

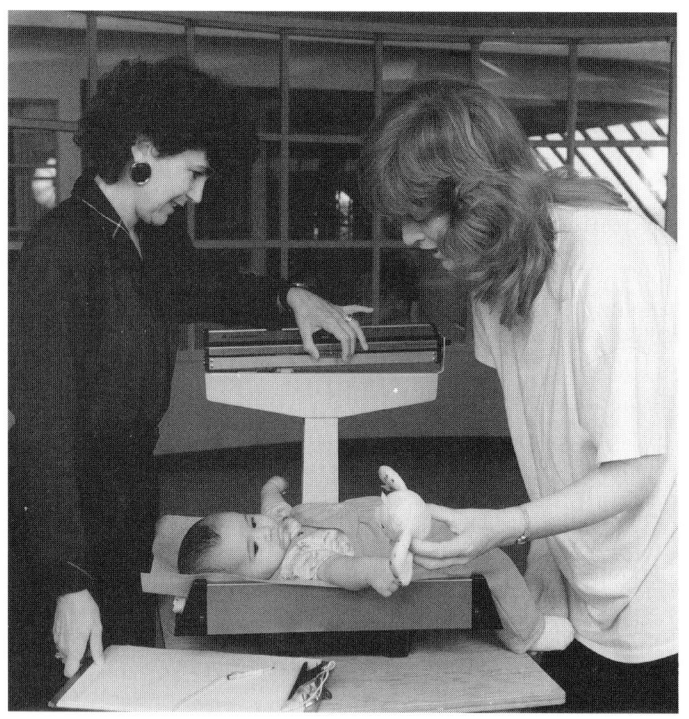

CENTRAL QUESTIONS

1. What are the components of a health history?

2. What are the four basic techniques used during physical examination and how does the nurse perform these techniques?

3. What sequence might a nurse use for a head-to-toe examination?

4. What is included in a beginning assessment of basic needs or functional abilities?

5. How does the nurse measure temperature, pulse, respirations and blood pressure?

6. What are the nurse's responsibilities when assisting with a physical examination?

7. What are some common positions patients are asked to assume for examination or treatment?

8. What are the responsibilities of the nurse when assisting with diagnostic tests and examinations?

INTRODUCTION

In the assessment phase of the nursing process, the nurse gathers subjective and objective data to develop an informed base on which to make judgements or diagnoses about a person's health status and to plan, implement, and evaluate care. Subjective data are collected through the use of interviewing techniques and by taking a health history. Objective data are gathered through observation and examination techniques and by conducting a physical examination. Data from the history and physical examination are combined with laboratory and diagnostic studies to form the patient's data base.

Nurses need skills in interviewing to collect a health history; and in observation, examination, and measurement techniques to perform a physical examination. The development of assessment skills begins early in a nurse's education program and continues to expand during his or her course of studies and throughout his or her professional career. The key to these skills is the ability to make intelligent observations. Intelligent observations are based on the nurse's knowledge of the biomedical, physical, and social sciences. As knowledge increases through education and experience, the nurse develops increasing skill in observing significant factors in the patient's appearance and behaviour, as well as his or her physical, occupational, and social environment. The nurse learns what to inspect for and how to differentiate the normal from the abnormal. Skill in assessing requires a knowledge of what is normal, the ability to identify and describe deviations from normal, and the expertise to determine the significance of these deviations.

Basic interviewing skills are outlined in Chapter 16, Communication Skills. The health history, the use of the four classical examination techniques (inspection, palpation, percussion and auscultation) and the measurement of vital signs (temperature, pulse, respirations and blood pressure) are the focus of this chapter. The assessment of specific basic needs and functional abilities are introduced here and enlarged upon in each of the basic needs chapters. For example, assessing an individual's nutritional status will be described in the chapter on nutritional needs, and similarly, assessing respiratory status in the chapter on oxygen needs.

It must be noted at this point that the assessments described in this book are at an introductory level of skills development. These assessments include basic skills such as taking vital signs, observing colour or listening to bowel sounds and depend on the student's knowledge of the structure and functioning of the body and the ability to detect readily observable deviations. More advanced skills, such as listening to heart sounds or conducting a neurological assessment, are not addressed in this text. Some schools offer a separate course on physical assessment. We recommend that students purchase a book specifically on physi-

cal examination and health assessment which they can use as a reference throughout their program.

Besides taking health histories and conducting physical examinations, the nurse often assists other health care team members in carrying out diagnostic procedures that are part of the medical assessment of a patient's health status. It is the nurse's responsibility to prepare patients physically and mentally for the various diagnostic tests and procedures. Collection of specimens for laboratory tests may be necessary. Nurses perform many of the tests and procedures as collaborative functions on orders from the physician or, more and more often today, as independent functions based on their own judgements. Information of a general nature about the more common measures used in the detection of illness has been included in this chapter. More detailed information about diagnostic tests and examinations used in assessing various body systems is included in the chapters on specific needs.

THE NURSING HEALTH HISTORY

INTERVIEWING

The primary purpose of interviewing is to obtain a health history and to explore the patient's symptoms and perceptions of health problems. During a successful interview, the nurse gathers a complete and accurate data base about a person's health status. The interview is the first and most important part of data collection because it allows patients to express what they are feeling, what their symptoms are, and what they perceive their health status to be (Jarvis, 1992). The interview is an important step before physical assessment. Information elicited about symptoms determines the focus of examination and the use of assessment techniques.

In order to conduct a successful interview, the nurse must first establish rapport and a climate of trust with the patient. People are not apt to share relevant information or ask questions about their health unless they trust the examiner. Through the interview (by asking questions and receiving explanations), patients develop a better understanding of their health status, which enables them to participate more fully in identifying strengths and weaknesses. Furthermore, the rapport that is established in the initial interview will form the basis of a continuing working relationship and "set the tone for future interactions" (Gehring, 1991).

There are a number of things the nurse can do to foster good communication during the interview. These include introductions; an explanation of the purpose and process of health assessment; and the provision of a quiet uninterrupted, private environment. In addition, the nurse should make sure the patient is comfortable before beginning the interview.

COMPONENTS OF THE HEALTH HISTORY

The health history is the first element of the patient's data base. It is considered to be the single most important element in determining a patient's problems and needs. A comprehensive health history describes people's past and present health and illness patterns and records their responses to health problems. It provides a complete picture of the person as a whole and how that individual interacts with the environment. It identifies usual patterns of daily living, strengths and coping capabilities, and what the patient does or does not do to stay healthy (health promotion and health protection patterns). "Thus it records not only weaknesses and abnormalities but also the strengths that will support therapy and care" (Malasanos, Barkauskas, and Stoltenberg-Allen, 1990, 109).

The health history yields information which the nurse uses to plan and modify care that conforms with the patient's individual preferences and usual patterns of living. The nurse also uses this information to identify opportunities for teaching and for enabling individuals and families to satisfy their needs and to achieve optimum health and wellness.

A health history consists of several components or parts, each of which has a specific goal or set of goals that must be clear to the examiner. The parts of a history follow a standardized sequence which may be grouped or labelled differently depending on the system or nursing model used in an agency. An example of a health history form may be found in Chapter 14. A standardized sequence or plan of history-taking is followed to ensure that no omissions occur. The parts of a health history are as follows:

1. Demographic data
2. Chief concern
3. History of present problem
4. Past medical history
5. Family history
6. Social and experiential history or patient profile
   a. personal status
   b. social data including habits
   c. home and work environment
   d. travel
   e. religious preferences
7. Review of systems or functional abilities.

The purpose of each component of the health history is presented in Table 15.1. In the review of systems or functional abilities, symptoms relating to the various systems

TABLE 15.1　Purposes of Health History Components

COMPONENT	PURPOSE
Demographic data	Provides biographical facts about the patient, such as age, sex, address, language spoken, employment status, type of health care coverage.
Chief concern	Identifies, in the patient's own words, the reason for seeking health care.
History of present health problem	Aids in differential diagnosis through a narrative account of the problem. Includes events leading up to the patient's admission to the agency.
Past medical history	Determines other illnesses experienced in the past, relapses, and recurrences.
Family history	Used to rule out hereditary and genetic influences. Identifies health status of relatives, as well as home environment, roles and relationships, and family support. Can use genograms.
Social and experiential history	Determines daily lifestyle and usual patterns of living. Includes education, financial circumstances, work habits, relationships, coping strategies.
Review of systems	Provides subjective data pertaining to health and illness patterns and the present health problem. Questions pertaining to health promotion and protection patterns reveal what a person does or does not do to stay healthy. Provides opportunity for health teaching.

and regions of the body are explored. Such a review often reveals related or new information the patient may have forgotten when giving the history of the present illness. It takes the form of direct questions asked by the nurse that the patient answers usually with a yes or no. The systems review can be done separately or as the patient is examined. For example, while examining the head, the nurse might ask about headaches, dizziness, convulsions. The data collected are recorded on the respective health history and physical examination forms according to agency protocol. The review of systems or functional abilities includes a long and difficult-to-remember list of symptoms. The student nurse may find a pocket reference card to be most useful.

SYMPTOM ANALYSIS

When the history of present problems and the review of systems are discussed with the patient, it is important to get a full description of symptoms. The four *Ws* — *what*, *when*, *where*, and *why* — will remind the nurse of the types of questions to be asked.

Questions the Nurse May Ask to Analyze Symptoms

What   What caused it? What makes it worse? What makes it better? What does it feel like, sound like, look like? What has it done to your lifestyle, daily activities?

When   When did you last feel well? When did it begin, end?

Where   Where is it? Does it spread? Point to it.

Why   Why do you have it? Why are you seeking medical attention now?

THE PHYSICAL EXAMINATION

The physical examination is a systematic, objective assessment of a patient which makes use of four basic techniques: inspection, palpation, percussion, and auscultation. The nurse is equipped with all the tools necessary for a fairly comprehensive and detailed examination. Use of the senses is necessary for inspection. Specific instruments such as the **ophthalmoscope** (for examining the eyes) and **otoscope** (for examining the ears) enhance the inspection process. The hands and fingers are the main tools for palpation and percussion. Although several specific instruments, such as the

stethoscope and tuning fork, refine the examination, it is important to remember that few of them can replace the human tools of skill, knowledge and interpretation. An organized approach to physical examination is presented here.

PREPARATION FOR PHYSICAL EXAMINATION

The nurse will use the techniques of physical examination in a variety of settings and situations. For example, preplacement screening by occupational health nurses assists employers in determining suitability of an applicant for a job. It is usually the nurse who is responsible for the initial intervention with ill or injured patients. By carrying out physical examination techniques appropriately, the nurse collects information which is necessary for making decisions regarding further care. The nurse should always be aware of normal findings and report deviations from normal.

The physical assessment should be carried out in an organized fashion to avoid omission of necessary components. The beginning student is advised to develop a sequence for the complete basic physical examination and stay with this sequence until it becomes a habit. This will give the student a systematic way of approaching assessments and avoid possibly missing portions of the examination. Here is a suggested sequence for conducting a basic physical examination.

1. *Observe body movement*, gait and general status of patient on entry.
2. Take *history* (seven components). *Observe* for state of health, alertness, mood, intelligence.
3. Record *vital signs*
4. *Body as a whole*: Have patient undress. *Inspect* gait, balance, spine, body build, height, weight.
5. Throughout the examination, note skin colour, condition, pigmentation.
6. Now Proceed from Head to Toe.
   HEAD:

Face	• inspect eyebrows, mouth, sensation, hair.
Skull	• shape, masses, tenderness.
Eyes	• bulging, lids, conjunctiva, sclera, cornea, equality of pupils and their reaction to light.
Ears	• pinna, canal, mastoids, hearing.
Nose	• shape, septum, mucosa.
Mouth	• colour, breath, teeth, gums, tongue, symmetry, palate, tonsils, gag reflex.
Neck	• Range of motion (R.O.M.), trachea, lymph glands, thyroid, jugular distention.

UPPER EXTREMITIES
- for each joint: inspect, palpate, R.O.M., tone, strength and resistance, coordination, sensation, reflexes, pulses.

CHEST
- contour and shape of thorax, chest deformities, accessory muscles, visible pulsations, respirations, breathing pattern, audible breath sounds, tactile fremitus (palpable vibration), percussion, adventitious breath sounds.

HEART
- apical impulse (thrust noted over the apex), heart sound.

BREAST
- nipples, masses, axillary nodes.

ABDOMEN
- respirations, contour, umbilicus, scars, auscultate per quadrant, percussion, light, deep palpation, fluid, hernia.

LOWER EXTREMITIES
- for each joint, inspect, palpate, R.O.M., tone, strength and resistance, coordination, sensation, pulses, reflexes.

GENITALIA
- inspect and palpate.

ANAL AREA
- inspect.

Equipment Used in a Physical Examination

- Tongue blades
- Two rulers
- Measuring tape
- Percussion hammer (reflex hammer)
- Tuning fork (either 128, 512 or 1024 cycles/second)
- Wristwatch with a second hand
- Penlight
- Thermometer
- Safety pins
- Cotton swabs
- Stethoscope with bell and diaphragm
- Nasal speculum
- Alcohol swabs
- Sphygmomanometer
- Ophthalmoscope
- Otoscope

INSPECTION

Inspection is the most valuable, least mechanical, and most difficult technique to learn. It involves the use of the senses — primarily vision — to assist in making judgements, comparisons, and decisions. Because inspection is a highly subjective process, it requires skill, repetition and practice to establish reliable findings for distinguishing among ranges of normal, borderline and abnormal.

One of the criteria of thorough inspection is the conscious systematic use of one's senses. Adequate lighting and adequate exposure of the area to be inspected are also essential criteria. A diagnostic set which includes an ophthalmoscope, an otoscope and a nasal speculum is necessary to examine the internal eye structures, the inner ear, and the internal nose, respectively. An ophthalmoscope and an otoscope are depicted in Figure 15.1. It is important to care for the battery housing of both instruments to ensure complete, dependable service.

A   **B**

FIGURE 15.1   A. The ophthalmoscope illuminates and magnifies the interior of the eyes, permitting examination of the internal structures. B. The otoscope illuminates the external ear canal, permitting examination of the canal and the tympanic membrane.

SOURCE: Block, G.J. and Nolan, J.W. (1986). *Health assessment for professional nursing* (2nd ed.). Norwalk, CT: Appleton-Century-Crofts, 138; 155. Reproduced with permission.

Care and Maintenance of Equipment with Rechargeable Batteries

1. New rechargeable batteries should be charged overnight before use.

2. A regular recharging schedule should be established. Leaving handle in uncharged condition is harmful to batteries. The method to follow is to recharge once a week whether or not instrument is used regularly. Completely discharge a battery before recharging to lengthen the life of the battery.

3. If a battery fails during an examination, a few minutes of charging will restore sufficient current to complete the exam.

4. When rechargeable battery no longer accepts a charge (approximately two years) it may be replaced by unscrewing the bottom cap, shaking out the old and replacing with a new one.

5. Lamp replacement is done from the base of the head by pulling the old one out, and pushing the new one into place.

6. All the equipment should be kept in its case, charged and cleaned regularly. Speculum tips should be cleaned at the end of each examination or discarded if the disposable type is used.

PALPATION

Palpation is the use of touch to detect both superficial and deeper characteristics of the body. It is combined with inspection because in many instances it validates visual impressions. It is used to examine all accessible parts of the body. A thorough knowledge of anatomy is essential in differentiating palpation of normal body structure from abnormal. Light pressure and firm pressure yield different types of data.

Light Palpation is especially helpful in determining temperature, muscular resistance, superficial organs, masses and abdominal tenderness. It should be done in a gentle manner to help reassure and relax the patient. Complete relaxation of the patient is essential to good palpation. *Deep Palpation* is used to locate organs, determine their size, feel masses, check for tenderness and rigidity.

PALPATION TECHNIQUE

To relax your patient's muscles
• warm your hands
• instruct the patient to breathe through the mouth
• place a pillow under the head and shoulders.

A

B

FIGURE 15.2   A. A percussion hammer is used to test deep tendon reflexes. B. A tuning fork is used to determine a gross conductive or a perceptive hearing loss.

SOURCES: A. Block, G. J. and Nolan, J. W. (1986). *Health assessment for professional nursing* (2nd ed.). Norwalk, CT: Appleton-Century-Crofts, 138; 155. Reproduced with permission. B. Burns, K. R. and Johnson, P. J. (1980). *Health assessment in clinical practice.* Englewood Cliffs, NJ: Prentice-Hall, 89. Reproduced with permission.

FIGURE 15.3   Correct placement of the hands for percussion

SOURCE: Norton, B. A. and Miller, A. M. *Skills for professional nursing practice.* Norwalk, CT: Appleton-Century-Crofts, 1986.

TABLE 15.2   Five Percussion Sounds

SOUND	INTENSITY	PITCH	DURATION	EXAMPLE
Resonance	Loud	Low	Long	Normal lung
Dullness	Medium	Medium	Medium	Liver, cardiac area
Tympani musical	Loud	High	Medium	Gastric air bubble – Puffed-out cheek Abdomen
Flatness	Soft	High	Short	Thigh
Hyper-resonance	Very loud	Lower	Longer	Emphysematous lung

Light palpation   Using the pads of your fingertips of one hand in a gentle, dipping motion, indent the skin 1.25 cm (1/2 in). Avoid sudden short jabs. Palpate all body surfaces. Identify any organs, masses, tenderness or increased resistance. If resistance is present, try to determine whether it is a voluntary or an involuntary spasm.

Deep palpation   Increase fingertip pressure by placing one hand on top of the other to indent the patient's skin more than 1.25 cm (1/2 in). Be sure to press with your top hand and feel with your lower hand.

PERCUSSION

Percussion involves striking or tapping the body surface to produce sounds that correlate with the type of underlying tissue density. The skin's surface is struck, setting the organs below into motion. The result of this action causes a vibration known as a percussion note. The notes vary in quality according to the density of the underlying structures. Percussion is used to differentiate the density and size of underlying structures. It is also used to stretch certain tendons of the body with a percussion hammer and obtain a deep tendon reflex such as the knee jerk (Patellar reflex).

PERCUSSION TECHNIQUE

Place the nondominant hand, as illustrated in Figure 15.3, over the area to be percussed, making sure that only the middle finger (pleximeter) is in contact with the skin surface. Use a quick, sharp but relaxed wrist motion to strike the middle finger of the nondominant hand, at the distal in-

terphalangeal joint with the middle finger (plexor) of the dominant hand. Use the tip of this finger rather than the pad. This necessitates short fingernails on the examiner. The two fingers should almost be at right angles. The movement is at the wrist, not in the finger.

Five percussion notes   The percussion technique can invoke five percussion notes or sounds. Each sound has its own intensity, pitch and duration. Table 15.2 differentiates the five percussion sounds. The principle of percussion can be understood by remembering that the more solid a structure, the lesser the vibrations produced. For example, the solid thigh vibrates very little, hence you hear a flat sound. The liver vibrates slightly more, thus a dull sound is heard. The air-filled lung vibrates even more, creating a resonant sound. The stomach filled with an air bubble vibrates considerably, hence the tympanic or musical sound heard. Normal percussion notes over the thorax and abdomen are resonance, dullness and tympany. Abnormal percussion notes are flatness and hyper-resonance. Percussion will not produce vibrations in structures more than 4–5 cm deep or less than 4–5 cm in size.

AUSCULTATION

Auscultation is similar to percussion in that it involves the evaluation of body sounds. It differs, however, in that the examiner listens for sounds produced by the body arising from the heart, lungs and abdomen, and not for those that are produced exogenously. The main instrument used for auscultation is the stethoscope (see Figure 15.4).

Diaphragm   Bell

FIGURE 15.4   Stethoscope

The *stethoscope* can yield valuable information only if it meets certain criteria and is utilized properly. The following points should be followed to promote optimum sound transmission.

1. The *eartips* must fit the external auditory meatus snugly yet comfortably while occluding it. Clean these often as they become occluded with wax.

2. The *binaural curvature* is directed anteriorly towards the nose when the eartips are in the ears.

3. The *tubing* should be 30 to 38 cm long and 3 mm in diameter to decrease sound distortion.

4. The correct chest piece must be used. The chest piece has two components. The *diaphragm*, which is flat and broad, transmits high pitched sounds. It should be held firmly against the skin. The *bell*, which is dome-shaped, transmits low pitched sounds. It should be held very lightly against the skin.

AUSCULTATION TECHNIQUE

Be sure the tubing at the junction of the diaphragm or bell is turned in the correct direction to allow sound to be transmitted to your ears. It is a good idea to insert the ear tips and tap the side you want to use to check for patency. It is not uncommon to hear accidental sounds while auscultating. Three causes of accidental sounds while auscultating are: movement of the tubing against the skin; breathing heavily on tubing, which produces a roaring sound; and friction of the stethoscope on hairs. Practice, knowledge, and concentration are required to develop skill in using the stethoscope.

ASSESSING FUNCTIONAL ABILITIES

NUTRITIONAL STATUS

In assessing an individual's nutritional status, the nurse may have information about *height, usual weight,* and *present weight* from the nursing health history. It is customary practice in most health agencies to take height and weight measurements for all newly admitted patients, and this is usually a nursing responsibility. Many agencies use a combination height and weight measuring scale. Patients are asked to remove their shoes and to stand on the scales. It is a good hygienic measure to use a fresh paper towel on the scales for each patient. The nurse usually measures the height first (with the patient's back to the measuring scale), and then weight. If the patient is too ill, the height and weight measurements might not be taken on admission. A portable scale that can be wheeled to the bedside is used if it is important to monitor the weight of a patient confined to bed. Height and weight may be compared with the average for the patient's age, sex, and type of body frame to aid in assessment of his or her nutritional status. Tables showing desirable weights for individuals of different ages are included in Chapter 19.

In addition to noting patients' height and weight, the nurse also observes their general appearance — do they look *obese, plump, average* in build, *thin,* or *emaciated?* What are their usual eating habits? Do they usually have a small, average or big appetite? The nurse should also know about special diets patients have been following as well as any dietary restrictions they observe for cultural or religious reasons or because of allergies. Observations can be made regarding the individual's *present response to food* and eating. Normally people enjoy food, although they do not always eat enough of the proper nutrients.

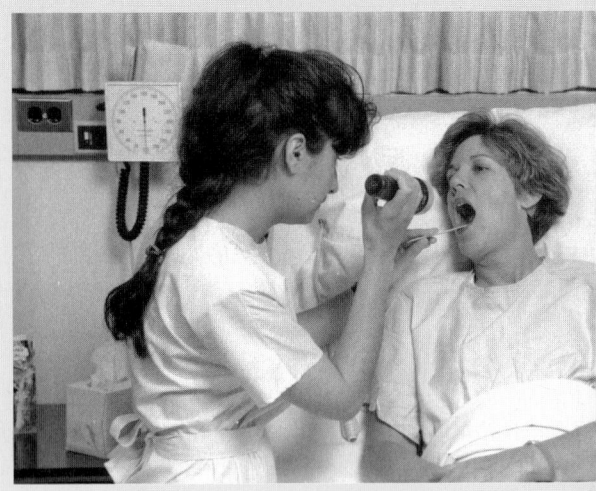

The nurse examines the condition of the patient's mouth and throat

Abnormalities that should be noted in the person's ability to eat or in response to food include: *nausea* (a queasy feeling in the stomach); *anorexia* (loss of appetite); refusal to eat; difficulty in swallowing; *distention* (enlargement of the abdomen due to internal pressure of gas or liquid); or *distorted tastes*. The nurse should also note if the patient has any difficulty in swallowing (dysphagia). The nurse notes the amount of food or fluids that the individual takes. If the patient takes only small amounts of food or fluids, this too should be noted.

ELIMINATION STATUS

Data about an individual's elimination patterns are usually included in the health history. In assessing the individual's current elimination status, the nurse makes observations about the following:

Emesis   Emesis is the vomiting of contents of the gastrointestinal tract through the mouth. Vomiting is always an abnormal condition. The nurse should make observations about the *amount* (it should be measured or approximated) and the *contents* of the emesis. Common terms used to describe the latter include: *bloody* (containing red blood); *liquid* (primarily liquid in consistency); *undigested food* (recognizable particles of food); and *bile* (a thick, viscid fluid varying in colour from yellow to brown or green, and having a bitter taste).

Bowel status   Significant observations about current bowel status include the date and time of the individual's last bowel movement, the colour of the stools, and the frequency of bowel movements. Normal stool is brown, soft, and formed. Abnormal findings should be noted, such as *clay-coloured* stools; *tarry* stools (black or blackish-brown viscous semi-liquid or liquid stools).

Common problems with bowel functioning that the individual may report are *diarrhea* (frequent bowel movements; stools of more or less fluid consistency); *constipation* (infrequent passage of feces or difficult defecation; stools are unduly hard and dry); and *flatulence* (gas in the digestive tract). When individuals are unable to control the movement of their bowels, they are said to have *involuntary* bowel movements (incontinence). The term *impacted* bowel refers to a condition in which there is an accumulation of feces in the rectum pressed firmly together so as to be immovable.

Urinary status   Normal urine is clear and straw coloured. Assessments should include colour, clarity and amount. Common terms used to describe abnormalities are: *cloudy, dark orange, pink, red, frothy* or *containing sediment*. Common problems in urinary functioning that the individual may report include: *frequency* (urinating at short intervals); *urgency* (the need to void suddenly, with an inability to retain urine without acute distress); *burning* (a

scalding sensation on voiding); and *dribbling* (an intermittent flow of urine). A person is said to be *incontinent* of urine when he or she is unable to control urination.

SENSORY PERCEPTION

The abilities to see, to hear, to feel, to taste and to smell are vitally important in coping with the daily activities of living. In making observations relating to an individual's sensory perception, the nurse is concerned with the integrity of the anatomical structures needed for functioning in these areas: the eyes, the ears, the nose, the mouth and throat, and the skin, as well as any disturbances in the functioning of these structures. Deviations from the individual's normal abilities, as indicated in the baseline data collected about that person, should be noted for all sensory areas.

Vision

In assessing current visual status, the nurse makes observations about the condition of the eyes, the eyelids, and the pupils, as well as asking about any visual disturbances the patient may be experiencing. When observing the individual's eyes, the nurse should look first at the condition of the eyelids. They may be *reddened* and look irritated, or they may appear *swollen* (puffy enlargement). The individual may experience *itching* or *burning* of the eyes or lids; frequent rubbing of the eyes is often indicative of this feeling. The nurse should also look for *tearing* or *exudate* from the eyes. In addition, he or she should ask the individual about having any visual disturbances such as *blurring* (seeing objects as vague or lacking in outline), or *diplopia* (double vision, seeing two objects when there is only one). In noting comments about the eyes the nurse should record which eye is affected — right, left or both.

The nurse also observes the pupils of the eyes. The average normal pupil is four to five millimetres in diameter. If the pupils are excessively large, they are said to be *dilated*; very small pupils are termed *pinpoint*. It is often important also to observe the reaction of the pupils to light. Normally an individual's pupils contract when exposed to a strong light. A flashing light directed at the eyes is used to observe this reaction. The nurse should note if both pupils react at the same time (consensually), as well as watch the separate reactions.

Hearing

The average individual can hear a normal conversation from a distance of approximately five metres. Hearing is one of the senses that becomes less acute as one grows older. Men lose the ability to hear high sounds first (women's voices, for example), whereas women find the low tones more difficult to hear as they grow older. Long-standing deficits in hearing are included in the data collected about an individual.

The nurse observes the condition of the ears. Normally, these are clean and free from discharge. Abnormalities that should be noted include the presence of *cerumen* (earwax), a sticky substance, usually brownish in colour, and any discharge coming from the ear. These may be described as *watery* secretions, *purulent* (yellowish), or *bloody* (usually red in colour). The amount of discharge should be noted as scant, moderate, or copious. The nurse always records which ear is affected (right, left or both).

The nurse also asks if the individual has noticed any disturbances in hearing, such as a buzzing or ringing in the ears *(tinnitus)*, or any *dizziness* or *loss of balance*.

Smell

The nose is not only instrumental in the ability to smell, but it is also an important part of a person's respiratory apparatus. Common abnormalities include *nasal discharge* (secretions from the nose), or bleeding *(nosebleed)*. Disturbances in the sense of smell, such as an *absence of this sense*, or *distorted odours* (odours usually considered agreeable are unpleasant, and vice versa), should also be noted.

Taste

The condition of a person's mouth and throat is important not only to the sense of taste but also to the ability to take food and fluids, thereby affecting nutritional status. Pertinent observations include noting if the mouth looks dry. A *dry mouth* is evidenced by a lack of saliva, and often one can see fine cracks in the surface of the lips or mucous membrane lining of the oral cavity. A mouth that is *not clean* has a collection of mucus and food particles around the teeth and gums or adhering to the mucous membranes. Sometimes the oral cavity appears *red* and inflamed. Any *bleeding* in the mouth should be noted; it usually occurs in the gums around the teeth.

The nurse also observes the condition of the tongue. The term *coated tongue* is used to describe the presence of a thick, furry covering, which may be variously coloured. The mouth may also have a *foul odour*. Another abnormality to look for is *lesions* in the mouth, such as sores or fever blisters. The nurse notes whether the individual's teeth are in good condition. *Dental caries* (decayed teeth) may be observed. If the individual wears dentures, the nurse should note this fact and also their condition. A person without teeth is said to be *edentulous*.

Disturbances in taste that the individual may describe include a *bad taste* in the mouth, an *absence of taste* or *distorted taste* (misinterpretation of tastes). Or the patient may report an *increased acuteness* of this sense or, conversely, *decreased ability* to distinguish tastes. When looking at the mouth, the nurse should observe the throat; it may appear *reddened* or *swollen*, and the person may report having a *sore throat*.

Touch and Feeling

Touch and feeling are subjective experiences, and the nurse must rely on the individual's observations regarding deviations from the normal in this sensory area. Disturbances in feeling, such as *numbness*, *prickling* or *tingling*, are most commonly noted in the extremities or in the facial area. Sometimes there is a *heightened sensitivity* to touch (pressure), heat or cold, or, conversely, a *decreased sensitivity*.

THE SKIN AND ITS APPENDAGES

The intact skin provides a protective covering for the body. Normal, healthy skin is clear (free from blemishes), intact (unbroken), warm to the touch and has a characteristic colour, depending on the person's ethnic background and inherited complexion tones. Although each individual's skin colouring varies to a certain extent, the nurse may observe common abnormalities such as *flushing* (redness of the skin, particularly noticeable in the face and neck), *pallor* (lack of colour), *cyanosis* (bluish or greyish cast to the skin, particularly noticeable in the lips, earlobes, and nailbeds), and *jaundice* (yellow colour of the skin or whites of the eyes).

The nurse should also look for blemishes and breaks in the skin. Common blemishes include *rashes* (eruption of the skin, usually reddish in colour); *bruises* (superficial discolourations due to hemorrhage into the tissues from ruptured vessels); *reddened areas* (diffuse red discolouration); *weeping areas* (oozing a watery secretion); *dry, itching areas* (rough and scaly skin which the individual has a desire to scratch); and *mottled areas* (marked with blotches of different shades of colour). *Scabs* (crust of a sore, wound, ulcer, or pustule) and *lesions* (open areas or breaks in the skin surface) should be noted, as well as scars on the body or incisions from surgical operations. The presence of *lumps* under the skin (abnormal masses that perform no physiological function) should also be observed. Both the location (specific area of the body on which the blemish or lesion appears) and its size should be recorded.

Other observations that the nurse may make about the skin are the presence of excessive perspiration, which may be seen on the forehead, upper lip, palms of the hands and/or soles of the feet, in the axillary area, or covering the entire body. If the entire body is bathed with perspiration, the term *diaphoresis* is used. The nurse may also notice abnormalities in the temperature of the skin. For example, it may feel *hot* (abnormally warm) or *cold* (abnormally cool) to the touch.

MOTOR STATUS

A normal individual can sit, stand, walk and perform a great number of movements, provided that the bones and muscles, circulation and nerve supply are intact. Limitations in mobility due to chronic health problems, such as paralysis, weakness or difficulty in movement of one or more limbs (or parts of limbs), should be included in the data collected about the individual. Nursing observations pertaining to present motor status focus on the integrity and functioning ability of the extremities. Abnormalities to which the nurse should be alert in the extremities include disturbances in circulation or sensory perception, limitation of movement and abnormal muscular movements.

An important observation the nurse should make relative to circulation is the *presence or absence of distal* (peripheral) *pulses* — that is, whether a pulse can or cannot be obtained by compressing the arteries at the points farthest from the heart in any of the extremities. Other pertinent observations include the presence of *swelling* (abnormal localized enlargement) or edema (an excessive amount of tissue fluid) in any part or all of an extremity. Sensory disturbances that the individual may tell the nurse about include paresthesia, that is, an abnormal sensation without objective cause, such as *numbness, prickling* or *tingling,* or a *heightened sensitivity* (to pressure, heat or cold) in any part, or all of one or more limbs.

The nurse should also observe the limbs for deficiencies in range of motion of a part or of the whole extremity. *Weakness* (that is, a lack of strength in any area) should be noted, especially a marked decrease in the ability to grasp an object *(weak hand grip).*

Abnormal muscular movements include: contractures, a permanent fixation contracture of a muscle in a fixed position due to spasm or paralysis; tremors, a quivering or involuntary convulsive muscular contraction; and *muscle spasms,* involuntary convulsive muscular contractions. *Missing limbs,* or parts of a limb, absent as a result of a birth defect, trauma or surgery, should be noted if not already reported.

The nurse includes observations relating to the individual's response to activity. Some common terms that people use to describe abnormal responses to activity are feelings of: *dizziness,* a whirling sensation in the head that gives the affected person a tendency to fall; *faintness,* a feeling of weakness; *fatigue,* a feeling of tiredness or weariness; and *shortness of breath,* slow, rapid respirations on exertion. It should be noted that these observations are predominantly subjective. The nurse must ask the individual if he or she has noticed any of these symptoms in response to normal activities, such as walking, climbing stairs and the like.

The individual's mobility should also be determined. Aids to mobility required at the present time, such as crutches, a cane, a walker, a wheelchair or persons to assist the individual, are noted. If restrictions have been placed on activities because of a current illness (such as bed rest or bathroom privileges only), these are included also.

STATE OF REST AND COMFORT

The individual's usual patterns of rest and sleep are noted in the nursing health history. Problems that the person is currently experiencing should also be noted, for example, insomnia or excessive drowsiness. The nurse notes the presence of any pain, since it is one of the most common causes of disturbances in rest and sleep. Pain is, of course, a subjective experience, and the nurse must rely on the patient's observations of pain. The exact location of the pain and its nature are recorded, if the patient is able to describe these. People use a variety of expressions to describe pain that they are experiencing. Common terms which the individual may use include: *sharp,* (acute or cutting); *aching* (dull, generalized, persistent); *cramp-like* (severe paroxysmal type); *throbbing* (pulsating); *constant* (continuous, unchanging); and *intermittent* (coming and going at intervals). The nurse also notes whether the pain reacts to therapy — whether the severity or intensity of the pain is, or is not, appreciably alleviated by the ministrations of the nurse or by the medication or treatment specified.

REPRODUCTIVE STATUS

Age, sex, and marital status are vital statistics about the individual that are noted in the patient's record. Other information about reproductive status that is collected in the nursing or medical history of a female patient includes data about usual menstrual pattern, and, if applicable, the age of menopause and of menarche, the number of pregnancies and of live births, the number and ages of children, and information about contraceptive methods used.

Assessment data about an individual's reproductive status also include the date of last menstrual period (if female) and the presence of any discharge from the genitals (both sexes). If the patient reports, or the nurse observes, discharges from the vagina or penis, it is important to note the colour and amount of the discharge. Common types of discharge include *bloody, white,* or *yellow* discharges. An intermittent bloody discharge is termed "*spotting.*" If a discharge has a *foul odour,* this also should be noted.

MENTAL STATUS

Normally, during the waking hours, a person is alert and responsive. In appraising the mental status of patients, the nurse should observe their movements. If they are slow or sluggish in moving, or appear to suffer from abnormal drowsiness, they are said to be *lethargic.* If they appear bewildered and perplexed, and/or give inappropriate answers to questions, the term *confused* is commonly used to describe their mental state. *Disoriented* individuals perceive themselves and/or their environment incorrectly in relation to time, place or person. They may not know who they are (or recognize familiar people), where they are or what day it is.

People are said to be *inattentive* when they are unable to focus their minds on an idea or on some aspect of their surroundings or on reality. The term *forgetful* is used when a person has a temporary loss of memory, for example, they cannot remember what you asked them a few minutes ago, or whether they have eaten lunch. When individuals make no response to sensory stimulation, for example, they do not answer or obey simple commands such as, "Please raise your hand," or they do not turn their head away from a bright light or react to touch, they are said to be *unresponsive*.

EMOTIONAL STATUS

People are not happy all the time. Most people experience a range of emotions in their day-to-day lives. These emotions are communicated to other people both by what the individual says and by his or her actions. In assessing an individual's emotional status, the nurse needs to identify both the individual's feelings as he or she expresses them in words and his or her observable behaviour. These feelings include: *depression* (a feeling of sadness or melancholy); *nervousness* (easily excited, irritated, jumpy, uneasy or disturbed); *anger* (strong feelings of displeasure or antagonism); and *fear* (unpleasant emotion caused by anticipation or awareness). The patient may claim to *want to die* or may have feelings of *anxiety* concerning possible ill effects from his or her present state of health, or from surgery.

Some common types of observable *behaviour* include: *restless* (continually moving the body or parts of the body); *crying* (weeping or lamenting); *withdrawn* (socially detached and unresponsive); *underactive* (not moving about as much as is desirable); *combative* (physically striking or attempting to strike others); *abusive* (harshly attacking others verbally); and *noisy* (talking loudly, shouting or banging objects).

SOCIAL STATUS

People normally are gregarious; they enjoy the company of other people. The ability to make contact and to exchange communication with other members of the human race not only makes life more interesting and enjoyable, but is essential to daily living. People convey messages to others by speaking, by writing, and through their behaviour. Deviations from the normal in regard to an individual's social status may be observed through their speech, writing and behaviour.

Verbal communication Normally a person has the ability to carry on a conversation with another person and to respond to questions in such a way that the meaning is clear. This, of course, assumes that there are no language

problems. Two common abnormalities of speech that the nurse can identify by listening to a person talking are *stuttering* (stumbling and spasmodic repetition of the same syllable), and *slurring* (sliding or slipping over word sounds that would normally be heard). A person who is unable to make meaning clear (provided everyone is speaking the same language) is said to be *incoherent*. When an individual who previously was able to speak normally is unable to speak at all, the term *aphasia* (or aphasic) is used. *Dysphasia* is a general term used to refer to difficulties in speaking.

In observing an individual's speech, the nurse should note willingness to communicate. He or she may, for example, be *reticent* (inclined to be silent and uncommunicative); *evasive* (avoids answering people directly); or *verbose* (extremely talkative). If the individual is unable to write, this fact should be noted.

Social response People respond to other people in an infinite variety of ways. Behaviour that is normal for one individual may be abnormal for another. If the individual is ill, however, the nurse should note his or her response to the presence of others.

It is important to note, for example, whether the individual wants to be alone (to have minimal or no contact with *anyone*) or does not want to be left alone, but desires or needs constant companionship. The nurse should also record his or her observations if the patient becomes *upset by contact* with family, friends, staff, visitors or roommates.

THE VITAL SIGNS

Temperature, pulse and respirations have traditionally been referred to as the ***vital signs,*** or *cardinal signs*, of life. Together with blood pressure and heart rate, they indicate basic physiological functioning, specifically in the functional areas of temperature status, circulatory status and respiratory status. In making observations about an individual's current functional abilities, the nurse frequently starts with the vital signs.

DETERMINANTS OF VITAL SIGNS

Age, exercise, hormones levels, circadian rhythms, stress and the environment have an impact on vital signs. In assessing vital signs, it is important to remember that individuals each have their own ***circadian (diurnal) rhythm,*** or a 24-hour biological time clock, that regulates the daily events in their life. The rhythm is evident in biological functioning such as body temperature, sleep and blood pressure, and the nurse will note differences in the vital signs of patients at different times of the day. Normally, a person's temperature, for example, is lowest in the early morning hours and highest in the late afternoon or early evening. Blood pressure, in most individuals, is also highest after the individual has been active for a good part of the day.

Although temperature, pulse, respirations and blood pressure readings vary between and within individuals, there is a range that is generally considered to be normal for each of these signs. Normal ranges for individuals in different age groups are included in each of the following sections on temperature, pulse, respirations and blood pressure.

Because of the variable nature of vital sign measurements — from one individual to another, and within the same individual at different times of the day and in various states of health and illness — it is important to establish baseline data for each patient. The patient should be made aware of these signs and work towards a lifestyle that promotes normal findings. A series of readings, undertaken systematically and in a consistent manner, helps to determine what is normal for a particular individual, to identify deviations from the normal and to pick up trends in the early stages of illness. For example, if a patient's temperature is usually around 36.1° C before breakfast but, one morning, you find it to be 37.5° C and, by noon, it is 37.8° C, you would suspect that the patient is developing a fever, even though all temperature readings fall within the "normal" range.

It is important, too, for the nurse to interpret vital sign readings in relation to other information about a patient. A sudden drop in blood pressure, an increase in pulse rate (or irregularity of rhythm or weakness of the pulse), or a lowered body temperature, with or without rapid and deep respirations, would alert the nurse to a change in status and should be reported promptly to the physician.

TEMPERATURE

PHYSIOLOGY

The surface temperature of the body fluctuates with the temperature of the surroundings. In a cool room, for example, exposed skin surfaces soon feel cold and are cold to the touch. The deep body, or core, temperature, on the other hand, is precisely regulated and maintained within a very narrow range. Body temperature measurements taken to determine a person's temperature status reflect core temperature. Under normal conditions it does not vary more than a degree or so from the mean, or average, for that person. Variances greater than that are usually indicative of disturbed functioning of the body's heat regulating system.

The temperature regulating system is one of the principal homeostatic mechanisms, whereby the internal climate of the body is maintained at an optimal level for functioning. The centre for controlling the internal temperature of the body is located in the hypothalamus, in the lower portion of the brain. In health, this centre maintains a fairly precise balance between heat production and heat

loss. Heat is continually being produced in the body as a byproduct of metabolism. It is also constantly being lost through *evaporation* (perspiration from the skin); *radiation* (the transfer of heat in the form of electromagnetic waves), for example, from the body to cooler objects in the environment; *conduction* (the transfer of heat from a warmer to a cooler substance by direct contact), for example, from the body to the surrounding air; and *convection* (movement of air), as currents around the body carry away heat that has been conducted to the air from the body surface. The factors affecting heat production and the processes by which heat is lost from the body are described in more detail in Chapter 24.

DETERMINANTS OF BODY TEMPERATURE

The **body temperature**, as measured by a clinical thermometer, reflects the balance between heat production and heat loss. It usually varies slightly during the course of a 24-hour period in any one individual, being lowest during the early morning hours before a person wakens and highest in the evening. The cycle may be reversed in persons who work at night and sleep during the day. Many people who are ill have an elevated temperature; it is often one of the first observable indications of disturbed body function. In addition, a temperature below normal may be indicative of ill health. **Pyrexia** and **fever** are two terms used to refer to an elevated temperature. The term **hypothermia** refers to a temperature that is below normal.

Factors other than disease processes, however, can affect body temperature. The activity of the individual can make some difference — the active person usually has a higher temperature than the sedentary person. Exercise can cause a marked, but temporary, elevation in body temperature. Age also affects temperature; for example, infants and older adults often have a body temperature lower than the young adult, as discussed in Chapter 24. Emotions and stress can increase the basal metabolic rate of an individual and thereby elevate temperature.

ASSESSING BODY TEMPERATURE

Sites

An estimate of the body's core temperature can be obtained from the mouth, the rectum, the axilla or the ear. The site that is used most commonly in everyday clinical practice is the mouth (*per os*). The small blood vessels on the underside of the tongue are supplied with blood by branches of the external carotid artery, that are close to the bifurcation with the internal carotid artery (Clemente, 1985). When a thermometer is placed in the posterior pocket under the tongue, and the mouth is closed, it is possible to obtain a reasonably accurate estimate of the body's internal temperature. The normal body temperature when taken orally ranges from 35.8° C to 37.3° C (Bates, 1991). The oral method of temperature assessment is the most convenient for patients who are awake, alert and can follow directions. It is unsafe for young children and for adults who are disoriented, confused, unconscious or experiencing seizures. Accurate readings require that hot or cold foods or fluids have not been taken 15 minutes prior to measurement.

An axillary temperature, taken by placing a thermometer in the axilla (under the arm), is a very safe method of temperature-taking because it is noninvasive. Major arteries situated near the area provide accurate readings, providing the thermometer is kept in place long enough. The axilla is the site of choice for taking temperatures in newborns and preschoolers but it can be used for people of all ages and conditions. It is an appropriate alternative for patients with conditions of the mouth which contraindicate use of an oral thermometer, such as infections or oral surgery. Axillary temperatures measure approximately 0.5° C lower than oral temperatures; however, readings may vary considerably. A drawback of this site is that it takes longer to register a temperature and therefore its use requires valuable nursing time in order to obtain an accurate reading.

The rectal site is used for adults when it is considered either unsafe or inaccurate to take the temperature by mouth, as when a patient is unconscious, disoriented or irrational. Rectal temperatures should not be taken as standard practice in newborns and infants because of the danger of damage to the rectal mucosa with a thermometer and, in preschoolers because of the fear of intrusive procedures. When a rectal temperature is necessary, care must be taken to prevent rectal trauma and fear in the child (Pillitteri, 1995). On the average, rectal temperatures are approximately 0.5° C higher than core body temperatures. The rectal method should not be used for people with diseases of the rectum, those with diarrhea or those who have had rectal surgery.

The ear, particularly the tympanic membrane, is an excellent site for taking core temperature. True core temperature exists within and near the hypothalamus, which holds the central thermoregulators. The ear is an ideal site for temperature assessment because it lies close to the hypothalamus and receives its blood supply from branches of the external carotid artery. The tympanic membrane is even more desirable because it shares its blood supply with the hypothalamus, from the anterior cerebral artery, a branch of the internal carotid (Tourangeau, MacLeod, and Breakwell, 1993).

Temperature measurements are made from either the ear canal or the tympanic membrane. These sites may be used for all patients, regardless of age or condition. Ear thermometry is noninvasive and causes little discomfort. Temperature assessment is quick, taking up to 15 seconds or less. Its major disadvantage is that improper technique can give inconsistent and inaccurate readings. For instance, nurses may think that they are taking a tympanic membrane temperature but, because of improper placement of the probe, they may in fact be reading the temperature of the ear canal.

The ear canal, like the oral cavity, is subject to variant effects. For instance, a higher reading would be obtained if the temperature were taken in the ear the patient has just slept on, or lower if taken in the outside ear and a fan were blowing overhead. The presence of an ear infection or excess ear wax may also affect the reading. Nurses must be cautious when using ear thermometry. First, they should know how the thermometer works. That is, does the device use a scanning or shutter method to sense the infrared heat rays? Is the thermometer designed to read tympanic membrane or ear canal temperature? Second, they must use a consistent technique, which ensures that the ear canal is straightened and the probe sensor is placed far enough in the ear canal to exclude the outer ear. In a tympanic temperature, this would mean making sure that the probe sensor is pointing at the tympanic membrane. The techniques for taking temperatures from the various sites are outlined in Procedure 15.1.

Preparing the Patient

Inform the patient that his or her temperature will be taken and explain the method that will be used. The patient needs to know what is expected in order to be able to participate in the procedure. If an oral temperature is to be taken, find out if the patient has been smoking, or has just had a hot or a cold drink. If so, wait about 15 minutes before measuring the temperature.

Assembling Equipment

Several types of thermometers are available for measuring body temperature. These are the glass mercury thermometer, the electronic predictive thermometer, and the infrared ear thermometer. Disposable thermometers and commercially marketed temperature-sensitive tapes are also available. These are particularly useful in the home (and in some health agencies) for infants and small children. The tape is usually applied to the child's abdomen and will change colour if the temperature is above or below normal. If deviations are noted, the temperature should be taken with a standard thermometer to obtain a more accurate measurement.

The glass mercury thermometer
The mercury thermometer is an elongated glass tube (called the *stem*) calibrated in degrees Celsius (centigrade) or degrees Fahrenheit. Within the tube is a column of mercury, which expands or contracts in response to the heat of the body. The scale on the Celsius thermometer generally starts at

A

B

FIGURE 15.5   Glass mercury thermometers. A. Oral thermometer B. Rectal thermometer

about 34° C and terminates at 42.4° C. As depicted in Figure 15.5, each long line represents 0.5 degrees; each short line represents 0.1 degrees. The Celsius scale is the only one used in health care agencies; however, the Fahrenheit scale may still be found in some Canadian homes. The formulas for converting centigrade and Fahrenheit scales are given in the box below.

Centigrade and Fahrenheit Conversion formulas

To convert Fahrenheit to centigrade:
$$C = (F - 32) \times 5/9$$
To convert centigrade to Fahrenheit:
$$F = (C \times 9/5) + 32$$

The contact surface of a thermometer, called the bulb, differs depending on whether it is for oral (and axillary) or rectal use (see Figure 15.5). The oral mercury thermometer has a long thin bulb that provides a substantial surface for contact with blood vessels under the tongue or in the axilla. The bulb of a rectal thermometer is short and blunt (pear-shaped); its purpose being to prevent injury to rectal tissue on insertion. Rectal and oral thermometers are sometimes differentiated by the colour of the bulb. Oral bulbs are often silver in colour and rectal bulbs are blue.

The glass mercury thermometer is usually kept in a small vial containing a disinfectant. Various kinds of disinfectants are used to soak the thermometers, for example, synthetic phenols or isopropyl alcohol (70 percent). Because thermometers are soaked in a disinfectant when not in use,

they need to be rinsed with cool water and wiped with a tissue before use. Clean thermometers are wiped from the bulb towards the fingers. This prevents the spread of microorganisms from dirtier to cleaner areas.

Electronic thermometer   Electronic thermometers are widely used today. With these, it is possible to get an accurate temperature reading in a few seconds and to monitor temperature over a period of time. An electronic thermometer consists of a heat-sensitive probe that is inserted into the body site, a digital display unit, and a connecting cord (see Figure 15.6). It can be set to work in two modes: predictive and monitor mode. In the predictive mode, a heat sensor (thermistor) in the probe detects heat from the site through a change in its characteristics with regard to temperature. This change is transmitted to a computer chip in the unit, where a temperature reading is computed and displayed. Using a mathematical formula, the unit electronically calculates an equilibrium temperature. For example, from the initial rate of change in probe characteristics, it predicts what an oral temperature would be if the probe were kept in the sublingual pocket for an optimal period of time. Oral and rectal temperatures are obtained with the thermometer in the predictive mode. The circuitry of electronic thermometers in predictive mode temperature calculations is designed to account for the characteristics of the oral and rectal mucosa. Axillary temperatures, on the other hand, should be taken in monitor mode. The axilla does not have the same characteristics as the mouth and rectum. Therefore, the use of the predictive mode for axillary temperature will not yield accurate readings.

The thermometer is set in *monitor* mode for axillary temperatures or when a continuous reading is needed. This might happen in an emergency unit, for instance, when a

FIGURE 15.6 Electronic thermometer, and probe covers

Source: Courtesy of the IVAC Corporation, San Diego, CA.

person is admitted in a state of hypothermia and the physician orders a continuous rectal temperature. In monitor mode, the thermometer provides a display of the temperature it is actually sensing; there is no predictive computation in between. Simply stated, the predictive mode computes the temperature based on a sampling and the monitor mode provides a direct temperature readout. There is a switch on the back of the unit for selecting the mode.

Most electronic thermometers have a different probe for the oral/axillary sites and for the rectal site. Oral/axillary probes are blue in colour, while rectal probes are red. The probe is capped with a disposable plastic cover every time a temperature is taken and, therefore, does not require cleaning. However, because the unit is battery-powered, it should be promptly put back on its charging unit after use.

Infrared ear thermometer The infrared (IR) ear thermometer is the latest development in temperature assessment instruments. It consists of a hand-held device with a sensor probe, similar to an otoscope, which is placed in the external opening of the ear canal (see Figure 15.7). The sensor measures the invisible heat rays emitted by the tympanic membrane and surrounding ear canal tissue. These infrared heat rays travel in a straight line from the source and are absorbed into the thermopile sensor in the thermometer.

Most IR thermometers have a thermistor which measures the temperature of the probe itself. These readings are converted into an electrical impulse and are sent to a computer which interprets the information and displays a reading on a screen. Some of the IR thermometers may be programmed to make a second conversion and display the readings in equivalent oral, rectal or core readings. This practice is less common now as practitioners become more familiar with the technology. As well, there is some indication that this second conversion results in reduced accuracy of the reading (Terndrup, 1992).

Most of the IR thermometers on the market use a shutter design, much like a camera, that opens when the examiner presses a button. The infrared heat sensed by the unit in that split second is used by a computer in the thermometer to predict the temperature. It is essential that the tympanic membrane is in the "picture"; otherwise the reading may be falsely low.

In another design, a series of measurements are taken while the probe is gently moved from side to side in the ear. This is called scanning. The maximum temperature observed in the scan is interpreted by the unit to be the tympanic membrane temperature. There are no computer conversions in this design. The highest temperature sensed is displayed, so, again, the tympanic membrane must be scanned to ensure tympanic membrane assessment. Although this design tends to result in more accurate readings, the scanning process is less comfortable for the patient than the simple shutter process.

The effectiveness of IR tympanic thermometry is based on the premise that the probe sensor is aimed at the tympanic membrane. If the tympanic membrane is not included in the "picture" or scan, the reading obtained will reflect the ear canal rather than the tympanic membrane temperature. The design of the probe in shutter models has a wide field of view and will "see" the tympanic membrane and

FIGURE 15.7 Infrared tympanic thermometer

Source: Courtesy of the IVAC Corporation, San Diego, CA.

Robichaud-Ekstrand, S, and Davies, B. Comparison of electronic glass thermometers: Length of time of insertion and type of breathing. *The Canadian Journal of Nursing Research*, 21(1), 61–73.

Robichaud-Ekstrand and Davies (1989) conducted a study in which they compared electronic and glass mercury thermometers in assessing oral temperatures. The purpose was to determine differences in temperature readings between electronic and glass thermometers with respect to length of time of insertion in the mouth and type of breathing (mouth or nose). In addition, it sought to establish the optimal placement time for glass thermometers. Forty-eight university nursing students participated in the study. The sample was divided into two groups — mouth and nose breathing. There were no significant differences between groups in terms of the extraneous variables affecting oral temperature readings, such as age, stress level or food consumption or exercise before the experiment.

The participants were assigned to groups of two: a subject and a partner. The role of the partner was to ensure proper placement and insertion technique of the thermometers, proper mouth or nose breathing, and to double-check and record the readings. In a timed sequence, temperatures were first taken with an electronic thermometer probe inserted into the right sublingual pocket of the participant. At the audible sound (beep) of the thermometer, the reading was recorded. A glass thermometer was shaken to 35° C and inserted into the same right sublingual pocket. The temperatures were read and recorded at 3, 5, 8, 10 and 12 minutes from starting time. Five seconds were allotted for participant and partner to read and double-check the reading and re-insert the thermometer. Another electronic temperature reading was taken at the completion of the glass thermometer readings. The experiment was then repeated with the participants reversing roles.

The results showed that the average electronic thermometer readings were 0.12° C higher than the average glass thermometer readings. The difference between the two types of thermometer readings was 0.09° C for mouth breathing and 0.14° C for nose breathing. The optimum placement times for glass thermometers were found to be five minutes for mouth-breathing subjects and five to eight minutes for nose-breathing subjects. In examining the effect of type of breathing, mouth-breathing subjects recorded temperatures 0.19° C and 0.14° C lower than nose-breathing subjects for electronic and glass thermometers respectively. For the glass thermometer, significant differences were found between mouth and nose breathing at 8 and 12 minutes but not at 3 and 5 minutes.

According to the researchers, "...in this study, conservative statistical tests indicating statistical significance did not imply clinical significance because of the existence of small variances among and within subjects..." (69). Given the results of this study the researchers recommendations were:

1. Health professionals can rely on the accuracy of oral temperature readings obtained from either glass or electronic thermometers to guide their interventions.

2. For afebrile patients, glass thermometers should be left in the sublingual site for three minutes.

3. When a patient's temperature is elevated or at borderline levels, a glass thermometer should be left in place for at least *five minutes* or an electronic thermometer should be used.

4. Electronic thermometers give more precise readings than glass thermometers for mouth-breathing patients when the glass thermometer is left in the oral cavity for only three or five minutes.

surrounding ear canal. Even when properly positioned, the resulting reading is an average of what is in its field of view. For that reason, these thermometers are called "infrared (IR) ear thermometers" rather than tympanic thermometers.

The scanning thermometers tend to have a smaller field of view and are more likely to capture the true tympanic membrane temperature. The probe tips are currently designed for the adult ear canal. This fact should be kept in mind when using IR thermometry with neonates, infants

and children. At this point, there is only one scanning type IR thermometer on the market with a probe suitable for neonates and infants (Ototemo™ Pedi-Q). Ear thermometry is a new and complex technology. As with any new technology, we can expect more growth and change before an efficient and effective thermometer is developed. Like electronic thermometers, the ear probe is capped with a disposable cover for each use and is stored in a charging unit when not in use.

Measuring Body Temperature

ACTION	RATIONALE
1. Wash hands.	Prevents the spread of microorganisms.
2. Gather appropriate thermometer:	Facilitates efficiency and economy of time.
• Glass thermometer, tissue, lubricant for rectal thermometer	
• Electronic thermometer, blue probe for oral/axillary method, red for rectal method, probe cover	
• Ear thermometer, probe cover	
• Clean gloves as necessary	When using glass thermometers, gloves should be used if there is visible blood in the patient's oral secretions or in the feces. The risk of transmission of non-blood borne pathogens, such as pulmonary tuberculosis, infectious diarrhea and Hepatitis A, can be reduced by wearing gloves (Timby and Lewis, 1992).
3. Prepare the patient.	Promotes well-being and facilitates patient participation in care.
4. Ready the thermometer:	
Glass: Hold the stem horizontally at eye level and rotate it until the scale becomes visible.	Brings the temperature scale into view.
Read the mercury level. If it is above the 34° mark, grasp the stem between the thumb and forefinger and, with a snapping wrist motion, shake down the mercury.	Ensures the thermometer reading is below body temperature. Brisk shaking downward lowers the mercury level.
Electronic: Slide a probe cover on the probe until it locks in place.	Prevents the transmission of microorganisms from patient to patient.
Infrared ear: Apply a probe cover on the probe as directed by the manufacturer.	
5. Take the patient's temperature.	
Oral Method: Glass Thermometer	Heat from the superficial blood vessels in the sublingual pocket warms the thermometer which registers a temperature reading.
• Place the bulb of the thermometer in the right or left posterior sublingual pocket under the base of the tongue.	

Posterior
sublingual pocket   Tip of thermometer

PROCEDURE 15.1
continued

ACTION	RATIONALE

• Instruct the patient to hold the thermometer between closed lips and avoid biting it.

Maintains proper position and ensures accurate measurement. Prevents trauma and mercury poisoning should the thermometer break.

• Leave the thermometer in place for 3 minutes. If the temperature is borderline or elevated above normal, leave it in place for 5 minutes.

Optimum placement times ensures accuracy. Optimum placement times are recommendations from the research by Robichaud-Ekstrand and Davies, (1989).

• Remove the thermometer and wipe it from the fingers towards the bulb, using a twisting motion.

Prevents the spread of microorganisms from dirtier to cleaner area. A twisting motion facilitates mechanical removal of mucus and secretions.

• Read the temperature.

Oral Method: Electronic Thermometer

• Place the probe in the right or left posterior sublingual pocket under the base of the tongue.

As for oral glass thermometer.

• Instruct the person to keep the the mouth closed.

• Hold the probe in place until an audible signal occurs and a temperature reading appears on the digital display. Note the temperature.

Ensures accurate reading.

• Remove the probe from the patient's mouth. Eject the cover into a waste paper basket.

Rectal Method: Glass Thermometer

• Draw curtains and help the patient assume a side-lying position with the upper leg flexed. Drape with bed linens.

Makes the rectal area accessible for the procedure. Provides privacy and reduces embarrassment.

• Apply clean gloves as necessary.

Protects the nurse from contamination with patient's body substances.

• Lubricate the bulb end of the thermometer.

Facilitates insertion and reduces irritation or injury to the rectal mucosa.

• Ask the patient to take a deep breath and then breathe out slowly.

Helps to relax the patient.

• Using the nondominant hand, lift the upper buttocks, and with the dominant hand, insert the thermometer about 7.5 cm for adults and not more than 1.25 cm for infants and 2.5 cm for young children.

Exposes the anal opening.
Ensures sufficient contact with blood vessels in the rectal wall.
Ensures adequate contact time to register an accurate temperature.

• Hold the thermometer in place for 2 to 3 minutes.

Facilitates reading the thermometer.

• Remove the thermometer and wipe off lubricant and fecal material.

• Read the temperature.

Continued on the next page

ACTION	RATIONALE
Rectal Method: Electronic Thermometer	
• Prepare and position the patient as when using the glass thermometer.	
• Ask the patient to take a deep breath and then breathe out slowly.	Helps to relax the patient.
• Using the nondominant hand, lift the upper buttocks, and with the dominant hand, insert the probe as for a glass thermometer.	Exposes the anal opening. Ensures sufficient contact with blood vessels in the rectal wall.
• Hold the probe in place until an audible signal occurs and a temperature reading appears on the digital display. Note the temperature.	Ensures accurate reading.
• Remove the probe and eject the cover into a waste paper basket.	
Axillary Method: Glass Thermometer	
• Pull curtains and remove the gown from the arm and dry the axilla, if moist.	Provides privacy and exposes the axilla. Moisture conducts heat.
• Place the bulb of the thermometer in the centre of the axilla, lower the arm over the thermometer, and position the arm across the patient's chest.	Maintains proper contact of the thermometer against blood vessels in the axilla.

ACTION	RATIONALE
• Keep the thermometer in place for 5 to 10 minutes. If the patient is alert, ask him or her to hold the thermometer in place. If the patient is not alert or is confused, hold the thermometer in position.	Ensures sufficient time to register an accurate temperature reading.
• Remove the thermometer, wipe it with tissue. Read the temperature.	
Axillary Method: Electronic Thermometer	
• Pull curtains and remove the gown from the arm and shoulder. Dry the axilla, if moist.	Provides privacy and exposes the axilla. Moisture conducts heat.
• Put the thermometer in monitor mode according to the manufacturer's instructions.	

ACTION	RATIONALE
• Place the probe in the centre of the axilla, lower the arm over the thermometer, and position the arm across the patient's chest.	Maintains proper contact of thermometer against blood vessels in the axilla.
• Hold the probe in place for 5 to 10 minutes. Note the temperature reading appearing on the digital display.	Ensures accurate reading.
• Remove the probe from the patient's axilla. Eject the cover into a waste paper basket.	

Ear thermometry:

ACTION	RATIONALE
• Hold the thermometer in the right hand to take the temperature in the right ear and in the left hand to take the temperature in the left ear.	Avoids crossing over of the hands which promotes dexterity and accuracy in positioning the probe.
• Grasp the pinna firmly at the midpoint, then pull up and back.	Straightens the ear canal.
• Insert the probe completely into the ear canal, pointing the tip midway between the eyebrow and the sideburn on the opposite side of the face. Make sure the probe seals the ear canal from ambient air.	Ensures the beam of infrared light points on the tympanic membrane. Prevents inaccurate readings due to environmental conditions.

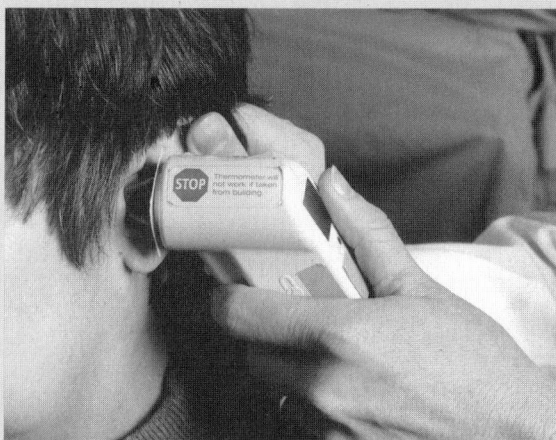

ACTION	RATIONALE
• **Shutter design**: Hold the thermometer in place until a reading is displayed.	
• **Scanning design**: Gently wiggle the probe in the ear until a reading is displayed.	Scans the tympanic membrane using a gentle side-to-side motion.
• Note the temperature and discard the probe cover.	
6. Leave the patient comfortable.	Promotes patient well-being.

Continued on the next page

ACTION	RATIONALE
7. Return **electronic** and **infrared ear thermometers** to their charging units.	Maintains battery charge.
Wash **glass thermometers** in cold soapy water. Rinse in cold water, dry, and return them to their storage container.	Maintains cleanliness and prevents the transmission of microorganisms. Any protein left on the thermometer will interfere with disinfection.
8. Document the temperature and the site on the patient's graphic flowsheet (Figure 15.8) according to agency guidelines.	Provides a data base for ongoing evaluation of patient status.
9. Report temperature elevations immediately to the charge nurse and physician. Document the patient's temperature in the nurses' notes and that the patient's physician was notified.	Temperature elevation may require immediate treatment. Fulfills requirements for nurse accountability and facilitates continuity of care.

PULSE

PHYSIOLOGY

When the left ventricle of the heart contracts, a wave of blood surges through the systemic arteries. This wave of blood, called a *pulse*, can be palpated at various sites on the body where an artery crosses over a bony prominence.

At rest the heart is required to pump only four to six litres of blood per minute. This volume is increased as much as five times during exercise. Normally each ventricle pumps 70 ml of blood with each contraction, although wide variations in the amount are compatible with life. This volume of output is reflected in the rate, rhythm, size (volume) and tension (elasticity) of the pulsations that can be felt. The *rate* of the pulse is the number of ventricular contractions or heartbeats per minute.

DETERMINANTS OF PULSE RATE

Deviations from the normal *pulse rate* are frequently seen in illness. Many medications affect the pulse rate. A number of factors other than disease processes and medications may also affect the pulse rate. Pulse rate varies according to age, sex, size and physical and emotional activity, for example. The pulse rate decreases as a child grows and continues to decrease until extreme old age. Men generally have a slower pulse rate than women. Exercise increases the rate of cardiac contractions, and when a person is experiencing strong emotions, such as anxiety, fear or anger, the heart usually beats faster also. The normal range and average of pulse rates for human beings at various ages are shown in the Table 15.3.

TABLE 15.3 Normal Pulse Rates for Specific Ages*

AGE	NORMAL RANGE	AVERAGE
Newborn	70–170	120
1–11 months	80–160	120
2 years	80–130	110
4 years	80–120	100
6 years	75–115	100
8 years	70–110	90
10 years	70–110	90
12 years	70–110	85
14 years	65–105	85
16 years	60–100	85
18 years	50–90	80
Adult	50–90	80
Elderly	60–90	70

*These averages vary with the sex of the individual.

Sources: Pillitteri, 1995; Berger and Williams, 1992; Tackett and Hunsberger, 1981.

ASSESSING PULSE RATES

Pulse rates are assessed by palpation of selected sites located in the periphery of the body (for example, the wrist, neck or foot) and by auscultation of the central pulse located at the apex of the heart. These are called the peripheral pulse and the apical pulse respectively.

FIGURE 15.8   Example of a graphic flowsheet for temperature, pulse, respiration, and blood pressure. Note the symbols used to identify the methods of assessing temperature and pulse rates. Other agencies may use different symbols.

SOURCE: Courtesy of Lions Gate Hospital, North Vancouver, BC.

Assessing a Peripheral Pulse

When taking a peripheral pulse, the rate, rhythm, size (volume) and tension (elasticity) of the pulse are noted. The normal pulse rates are given in Table 15.3. If the pulse rate is greatly accelerated (for example, over 100 beats per minute in adults), the condition is referred to as **tachycardia**. A very slow pulse rate (under 60 beats per minute in adults) is called **bradycardia**.

Pulse rhythm refers to the pattern of the beats. In health the rhythm is *regular;* that is, the time between beats is essentially the same. The pulse is *irregular* when the beats follow each other at irregular intervals.

The *size*, or amplitude, of a pulse wave (the **pulse volume**)reflects the *volume* of blood pushed against the wall of the artery in the ventricular contraction. A *weak* pulse lacks a feeling of fullness and a definite beat; it may feel thready. When a pulse cannot be felt or heard, it is said to be *imperceptible*. A bounding pulse is one in which the volume reaches a higher level than normal, then disappears quickly. A scale for describing pulse volume is given in the box below.

Scale for Describing Pulse Volume

SCALE	DESCRIPTION
0	Absent, not palpable
+1	Threadly, weak, difficult to palpate, easily obliterated with pressure
+2	Normal, easily palpated, may be obliterated by strong pressure
+3	Strong, forceful, not easily obliterated by pressure
+4	Bounding, difficult to obliterate.

SOURCES: Alder, 1979; Berger and Williams, 1992.

Pulse tension (elasticity) refers to the compressibility of the arterial wall. If the pulse is obliterated by slight pressure, it is a pulse of low tension. A pulse that is obliterated only by relatively great pressure is a pulse of high pressure. The words *soft* and *hard* are used to describe pulse tension.

To assess a person's pulse, the examiner places the second, third and fourth fingers lightly on the skin at a location where an artery passes over underlying bone. The thumb is not used because the examiner might feel the pulsations of the radial artery of his or her own thumb. Usually, counting the rate for 30 seconds and then multiplying by two gives an accurate record of beats per minute. Some people prefer to count the rate for 15 seconds and multiply by four. If the pulse is irregular in any way it is counted apically for a full minute.

Locating peripheral pulse sites There are numerous sites on the body from which a pulse may be obtained (see Figure 15.9). When a person is lying on the back, one can normally observe pulsations from the carotid artery and, also, from the jugular vein. The carotid pulse shows as a brisk, localized throbbing; the jugular pulse is slow and undulating. In emergency situations, the **carotid pulse** is convenient for assessing cardiac functioning. Care must be taken, though, to make sure that one does not inadvertently cut off, or seriously slow down, carotid circulation. Palpation should be done high in the neck, to avoid undue pressure on the carotid sinus, which is located just above the bifurcation of the artery into its external and internal branches. Excessive pressure on the artery is to be avoided and only one carotid artery should be palpated at a time.

In non-emergency situations, the peripheral pulses located in the head and the extremities are commonly used for assessment of a person's circulatory status. Of these, the radial and the brachial pulses are the ones most frequently used by nurses. The radial site is used to assess the pulse, and the brachial site is used in taking the blood pressure. Other peripheral sites may be used for pulse assessment if the radial pulse is obscured, or if there is a need to test the circulation of blood to a specific area. The temporal, femoral and dorsalis pedis pulses are three that are used most often.

The **radial pulse** is located on the inner aspect of the wrist on the thumb side where the radial artery passes over the radius. With slight pressure, the artery may be held against the radius so that the pulsations of blood may be felt. The **brachial pulse** is located on the anterior surface of the arm, just below the elbow, where the brachial artery passes over the ulna. The **temporal pulse** is felt anterior to the ear at the mandibular joint, where the temporal artery passes over the temporal bone. It can also be felt at the temple, that is, to the side of the eyebrow just in front of the hairline. The **femoral pulse** may be taken at the point in the middle of the groin where the femoral artery passes over the pelvic bone. The **dorsalis pedis pulse** (usually taken to assess circulation in the foot) can be felt on the dorsum of the foot in a line between the first and second toes, just above the longitudinal arch.

Other peripheral pulses that are sometimes used include the **ulnar**, which is on the opposite side of the wrist to the radial, the **posterior tibialis**, on the inner aspect of the ankle, and the **popliteal pulse**, which can be felt on the *apical pulse* is the beat of the heart auscultated at its apex. The apex is considered to be the *point of maximal impulse* **(PMI),** also called the apical impulse. The apical site is located in the fifth intercostal space, 7 cm to 9 cm to the left of the midsternal line, just below the left nipple. By listening with a stethoscope in this area, the apical pulse can usually be heard.

To determine the apical pulse, the bell or diaphragm of the stethoscope is placed over the apex of the heart and the beats are counted for a full minute. A heartbeat is heard as "lub-dup." The "lub" represents the closure of the atrioventricular or tricuspid and mitral valves (S_1 sound); it occurs at the onset of systole (the contraction of the heart). The "dup" represents the closure of the semilunar (aortic and pulmonic) valves (S_2 sound) at the end of systole. The rhythm of the heart beat can also be assessed by noting the interval between beats. Procedure 15.2 outlines how to take an apical pulse.

Assessing an Apical-Radial Pulse

In health, the apical and radial pulse rates are the same, but in illness they sometimes differ, as when some apical beats are not transmitted to the radial artery. An *apical-radial* pulse is taken when it is necessary to determine whether such a difference exists. Two nurses are needed for this technique. One nurse counts the patient's radial pulse at the same time that the second nurse counts the apical beats of the heart. Both nurses must use the same watch. Each pulse is counted for a full minute. The difference between the apical rate and the radial rate is termed the *pulse deficit*.

Preparing the Patient

Inform the patient of the procedure and tell him or her what to do to facilitate accurate assessment of the pulse. Generally, the patient should lie or sit quietly for a few minutes before the pulse is counted. Exercise, a change in activity or posture, or anxiety can accelerate the pulse rate to the extent that it does not reflect the normal rate at rest.

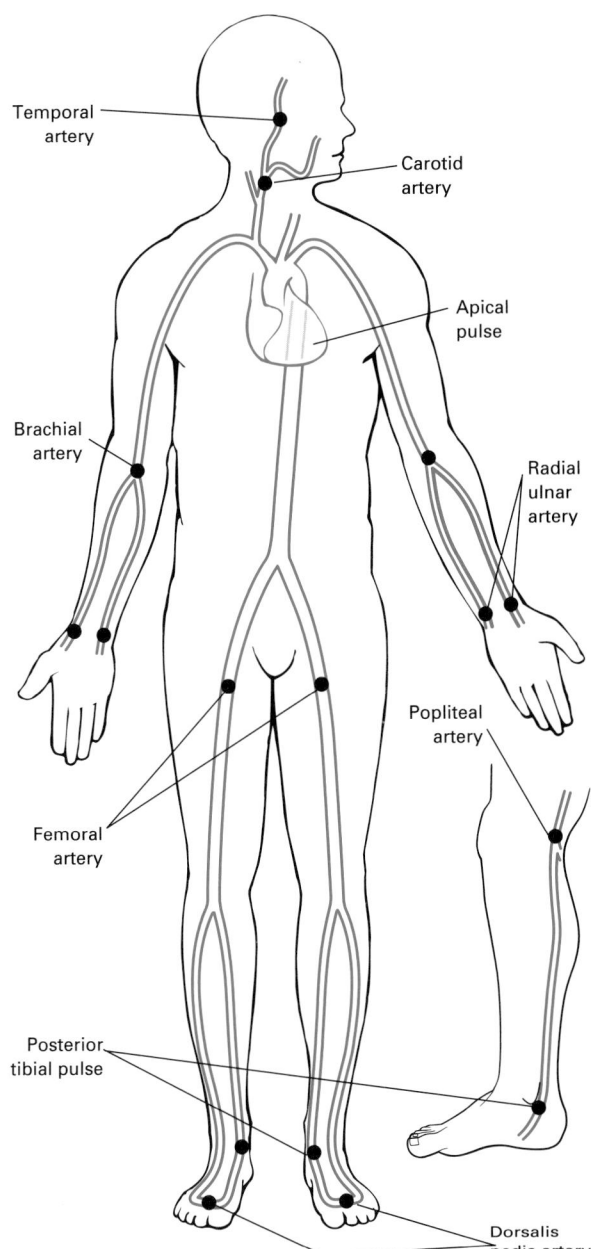

FIGURE 15.9 Peripheral pulse sites

inner aspect of the back of the knee. The technique for assessing a peripheral pulse is detailed in Procedure 15.2.

Assessing an Apical Pulse

It is often necessary to assess the heartbeat by listening to the heart sounds rather than palpating a peripheral pulse. The

Assembling Equipment

The nurse will need a watch with a second hand to count the pulse rate. A stethoscope is needed if an apical pulse is being taken.

Assessing Peripheral and Apical Pulses

ACTION	RATIONALE
1. Wash hands.	Prevents the spread of microorganisms.
2. Gather equipment • Watch with a second hand • Stethoscope if needed	Facilitates efficiency and economy of time.
3. Prepare the patient.	Promotes well-being and facilitates patient participation in care.
4. Take the patient's pulse.	

Peripheral sites:

• If taking a **radial pulse**, have the patient in a sitting or lying position with the arm resting at his or her side or across the abdomen or chest. The wrist should be slightly extended with the palm facing downward.	Promotes comfort for the patient and convenience for the nurse. Exposes the artery for palpation.
• Place the first, second, and third fingertips lightly on the skin along the artery at the selected site.	Sensitivity of fingertips to touch permits palpation of pulsations.
• Feel the sensations, assess the rhythm and the volume by noting the pattern and strength of the beats.	
• If the pulse is regular, count the beats for 15 or 30 seconds and multiply by 4 or 2 respectively.	Determine the rate of beats per minute.
• If the pulse is irregular, count the beats for one full minute. Note if the irregularity occurs randomly or in a pattern. If there is any doubt about the pulse assessment take an apical pulse.	Provides more accurate assessment of rate, rhythm, and volume.

Apical Pulse:

• Pull curtains and assist the patient into a supine position with head elevated or a sitting position. Expose the left side of the chest.	Provides privacy and facilitates access to the point of maximal impulse (PMI).
• Warm the bell or diaphragm of the stethoscope by holding it in the palm of the hand.	Prevents variations in the pulse from the patient being startled by a cold stethoscope.
• Place the diaphragm or bell of the stethoscope over the fifth intercostal space, about 7 to 9 cm to the left of the midsternum, just below the left nipple.	Positions the instrument over apex and the PMI.

ACTION	RATIONALE
• Listen for normal S$_1$ and S$_2$ sounds and note their strength and regularity.	Determines length of time needed to accurately assess rate.
• If the rhythm is regular, count the heartbeats for 30 seconds and multiply by two. If it is irregular, count the beats for one full minute.	Ensures accurate measurement of rate.
5. Leave the patient comfortable.	Promotes patient well-being.
6. Document the pulse rate on the patient's graphic flowsheet (see Figure 15.8) according to agency guidelines. Record changes in rhythm, volume, and tension of peripheral pulses and changes in rhythm and strength of apical pulses in the nurses' notes.	Provides a data base for ongoing evaluation of patient status.

RESPIRATIONS

PHYSIOLOGY

Respiration is a term used to cover both the exchange of oxygen and carbon dioxide that takes place in the lungs, and the exchange of these gases that takes place in the tissues (between the blood and body cells). The former is technically called *external* respiration, the latter *internal* (or *tissue*) respiration. When we are assessing respiration as one of the vital signs of body functioning, it is the external process we are measuring.

External respiration, or breathing, involves two principal movements: **inspiration** *(inhalation)*, the act of breathing in, and **expiration** *(exhalation)*, the act of breathing out. Breathing is carried out by the diaphragm and the chest muscles. The process is controlled primarily by the respiratory centre in the medulla oblongata. This centre is influenced by several factors, including chemical changes in the body (for example, a high carbon dioxide level, which stimulates respiration), alterations in blood pressure (for example, increased blood pressure, which inhibits respirations), and stimuli arising from the muscles (for example, exercise, which increases respiration). A more detailed discussion of the factors affecting respiration will be found in Chapter 23.

Respirations controlled in this manner are automatic. Their rate and depth are regulated within a range that meets the metabolic needs of the body for oxygen. Any activity that necessitates increased oxygen supply will result in more rapid and usually deeper respirations. It should be noted, however, that the rate and depth of respirations are to a certain extent under voluntary control. A person can take deep breaths or shallow breaths, or breathe more quickly or slowly, within the limitations imposed by the body's needs for oxygen.

ASSESSING RESPIRATIONS

Respirations are assessed for rate, depth, rhythm and character, or sounds of breathing. The accessory muscles involved in breathing are also examined.

The **respiratory rate** is the number of breathing cycles per minute. An inhalation and an exhalation comprise one cycle. Normal respiratory rates vary with age. The average rate for adults is 12 to 20 per minute (Malasanos, Barkauskas, and Stoltenberg-Allen, 1990). For newborns at rest it is 30 to 50 per minute, slowing to 20 to 40 at one year. The average respiratory rate for children is 20 to 30 per minute at two years, slowing down gradually to 17 to 22 at 10 years. By 20 years of age, the average respiratory rate declines to 15 to 20 per minute (Pillitteri, 1992). An abnormal increase in the respiratory rate is called **tachypnea** *(polypnea)*, and an abnormal decrease is technically referred to as **bradypnea.** Normal breathing, which is effortless, regular, and noiseless (quiet), is called **eupnea**. An absence of breathing is termed **apnea**.

The **respiratory depth** refers to the amount of air inhaled and exhaled with each breath movement. It is observed by watching the chest movements. Normal respirations result in deep and even movements of the chest. In *shallow* respirations, the rise and fall of the chest and abdomen are minimal. If the respirations are shallow and rapid, the person is said to be *short of breath*. The term *air hunger* is frequently used to describe respirations that are abnormally deep and accompanied by an increased respiratory rate.

The **respiratory rhythm** refers to the regularity of inhalation and exhalation cycles. Normal respirations follow one another evenly, with little variation in the length of the pauses between inspiration and expiration. *Symmetry* refers to the synchronous movements of each side of the chest. *Asymmetrical* breathing may be observed in some individuals.

The *respiratory character* refers to digressions from normal, effortless breathing. **Dyspnea**, which refers to difficult or laboured breathing, for example, involves active participation of accessory inspiratory and expiratory muscles. In normal breathing the principal muscles concerned are the diaphragm and, to a lesser extent, the external and internal intercostal muscles. If, for any reason, respiration becomes difficult, all the muscles attached to the thoracic cage are brought into play. These include the major and minor pectoral muscles, the sternomastoid, the scalene, and the subclavius. Difficulty in breathing accompanied by whistling sounds is called *wheezing*. On auscultation with a stethescope, fine sounds that resemble hair being rubbed between fingers are called *crackles*; bubbling sounds in air cells (alveoli) or bronchial tubes, are termed *gurgles*. Another descriptive term that is commonly used for noisy breathing due to secretions in the trachea or large bronchi is *stertorous* respirations.

When assessing respirations, the nurse counts the rate, watches the chest movements, and listens for the character of breath sounds. Respirations must be assessed unobtrusively because people usually find it difficult to maintain their normal breathing pattern when they are aware their respirations are being observed. Thus, respirations are often assessed after taking the pulse, while the nurse has his or her fingers on the wrist. Procedure 15.3 outlines how to assess respirations.

Preparing the Patient

For the reason described above, the patient is not informed that his or her respirations will be assessed. However, if the nurse observes factors in the patient that have altered their normal pattern, for instance, signs of anxiety, distress, pain, exercise, crying or coughing, assessment should be deferred until the patient is in a resting state.

PROCEDURE 15.3

Assessing Respirations

ACTION	RATIONALE
1. Wash hands.	Prevents the spread of microorganisms.
2. Gather equipment: • Watch with a second hand	Facilitates efficiency and economy of time.
3. Take the patient's respirations: • Observe the rise and fall of the chest, noting the rhythm.	Determines length of time needed to accurately assess rate.
• If regular, count the respiratory cycles for 15 seconds and multiply by 4 or for 30 seconds and multiply by 2.	
• If irregular, count the cycles for 1 full minute.	Accounts for variations in respiratory rate and pattern.
• While counting, watch the chest movement to note the depth of respirations and listen for breath sounds.	
• Sometimes it is impossible to see a person's chest movements or hear the breathing. When this happens, place a hand on the patient's chest and count the cycles by feeling the rise and fall of the chest.	
4. Document the respiratory rate on the graphic flowsheet (see Figure 15.8) according to agency guidelines. Record changes in rhythm, depth, and character in the nurses' notes.	Provides a data base for ongoing evaluation of patient status.

BLOOD PRESSURE

PHYSIOLOGY

Blood pressure refers to the pressure of the blood within the arteries of the body. When the left ventricle of the heart contracts, blood is forced out into the aorta and travels through the large arteries to the smaller arteries, arterioles and capillaries. The pulsations extend from the heart through the arteries and disappear in the arterioles. The *systolic pressure* reflects the force exerted against the arterial wall as the left ventricle contracts and pumps blood into the aorta. It is the maximum pressure that is exerted on the vessel wall. The **diastolic pressure** reflects the arterial pressure during ventricular relaxation, when the heart is filling. It is the minimum pressure in the arteries. Blood pressure is measured in millimetres of mercury (mm Hg) and the values are separated by a slash mark. For example, the blood pressure in a young adult might be 120/80, signifying a systolic pressure of 120 and a diastolic pressure of 80. The difference between the systolic and diastolic pressure is the *pulse pressure.*

The blood pressure is determined by cardiac output and peripheral vascular resistance. The **cardiac output** is the amount of blood ejected from the heart with the force of each ventricular contraction. The force of the contractions depends on the pumping action of the heart. The greater the strength of the pumping action, the more blood is ejected with each contraction. The amount of cardiac output is also affected by the total *volume of blood* circulating in the body. A decrease in blood volume, such as occurs in hemorrhaging, will result in less cardiac output, hence a lowered blood pressure.

Peripheral vascular resistance is "the resistance to blood flow primarily caused by friction with the vascular walls" (Martini, 1989, 913). Normally, the pressure in the large blood vessels is high, and the pressure in the smaller vessels (the arterioles and capillaries) is low. Blood, as any other liquid, tends to flow from areas of high pressure to areas of low pressure. Peripheral resistance is created by the size of the lumen (the inner channel) of arterioles and capillaries and by the elasticity of vessel walls. Peripheral resistance increases as the size of the lumen decreases, assuming the blood volume remains constant. Thus, the smaller the lumen, the higher the blood pressure. Factors that decrease the lumen of the blood vessels affect the smaller vessels proportionately more than the larger ones, and increase the amount of pressure required to pump the blood through them. Any constriction of the vessels, as when deposits occur on the lining of the vessels, increases the peripheral resistance and, therefore, the blood pressure.

The *elasticity* of the muscular walls of the blood vessels contributes to vascular resistance and the maintenance of blood pressure. Elasticity refers to compliance, or the ability of the vessel wall to expand or contract in response to the pressure of blood exerted upon it. For instance, arteries normally expand during systole and contract somewhat during diastole to maintain a relatively constant blood pressure. When blood vessels lose their elasticity, as happens with aging, for example, blood pressure goes up.

Blood pressure is also affected by the *viscosity* (thickness) of the blood, which is dependent on the number of red blood cells and on the amount of plasma protein it contains. Blood pressure increases as the blood flowing through the vessels becomes thicker. Viscosity may be altered by disturbances of fluid balance.

DETERMINANTS OF BLOOD PRESSURE

A number of variables affect the arterial blood pressure. At the outset, the normal blood pressure increases with age. At birth, the blood pressure averages 80/46 and gradually rises to 130/85 by young adulthood. As a person grows older, blood vessels become less compliant and blood pressure continues to rise. The normal blood pressure ranges (over the brachial artery) for individuals of different ages are listed in the box below.

An individual's blood pressure varies from hour to hour and from day to day. It falls during sleep and is highest late in the day or early in the evening. Stress, activity and exercise cause the blood pressure to rise. It may be strikingly elevated by strong emotions, such as fear and anger. Position also affects the blood pressure. When a person is lying down, blood pressure is lower than when sitting or standing. Also, the pressure may differ in the two arms of the same patient. Therefore, before taking the blood pressure, the nurse should check (a) the patient's baseline value, (b) the time of day, (c) the arm used and (d) the position the patient was in for the previous reading.

Normal Blood Pressure For Age

Age	Systolic (mm Hg)	Diastolic (mm Hg)
Newborn	80±16	46±16
1 year	96±30	66±25
3 years	100±25	67±23
6 years	100±15	56±8
10 years	111±17	58±10
13 years	118±19	60±10
16 years	118±20	60±10
Adult	100–140	60–90
Older Adult	Maximum 160	60–90

SOURCE: Pillitteri, 1995, 1861; Fuller & Schaller-Ayers, 1994, 67.

MEASURING BLOOD PRESSURE

Blood pressure is measured indirectly by auscultation. The technique requires a sphygmomanometer and a stethoscope. A *sphygmomanometer* consists of an inflatable cuff, an inflation bulb with a release valve, and a mercury manometer or an aneroid pressure gauge. The most common site used is the upper arm, although it is sometimes necessary to take a blood pressure reading on the thigh.

In the auscultatory method, the examiner listens, with a stethoscope, for a series of sounds created as blood flows through an artery after it has been occluded with a cuff and then the cuff pressure gradually released. At the same time, the blood pressure registers on the manometer or gauge of the sphygmomanometer. The pattern of sounds the examiner hears are called Korotkoff sounds; they are depicted in Figure 15.10.

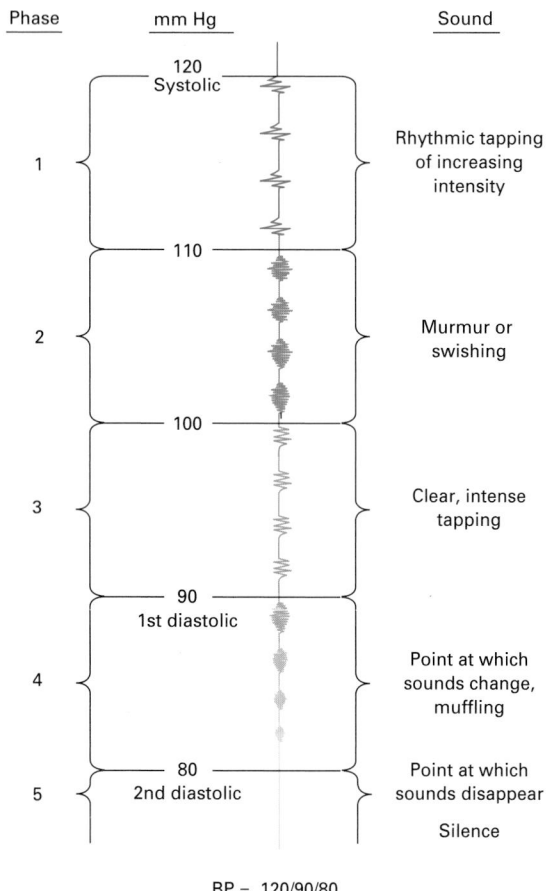

BP = 120/90/80

FIGURE 15.10 Phases of the Korotkoff sounds

To take the blood pressure, a deflated cuff is wrapped smoothly and firmly around the patient's upper arm so that the lower border of the cuff is 2.5 cm above the antecubital space. The bell or diaphragm of the stethoscope is placed over the site of the brachial pulse and the cuff is pumped to 30 mm of Hg above the pressure at which the pulsation in the brachial artery disappears. At this stage, the artery is occluded by the pressure of the cuff and no blood is flowing through it. Then, as the pressure is gradually released, the examiner watches the manometer or gauge for the level at which the Korotkoff sound changes are heard.

The *systolic pressure* is the reading at which Korotkoff sounds are first heard. This is Phase 1, which is characterized by an initially faint, clear, rhythmic tapping or beat that increases in intensity. With the continual lowering of the pressure in the cuff, the sounds continue to be heard as the artery alternately collapses and fills. Phase 2 sounds like a murmur or swish; and Phase 3 a crisp, more intense tapping. Eventually the sounds diminish in intensity as the artery no longer collapses; weakened beats are usually heard for a few seconds and then disappear altogether.

The onset of muffling (point at which the sounds change) is the beginning of Phase 4. It is used by many clinicians as the index of *diastolic pressure* and is frequently called the first diastolic pressure. Phase 5, or the point at which the Korotkoff sounds disappear entirely, is the second diastolic pressure. Some authorities prefer to record Phase 5 as the diastolic pressure for adults. The problem with this is that, in some individuals the fifth sound does not subside until well below their true diastolic pressure. Thus, in many agencies, three values are recorded: the systolic pressure, the point of muffling of Korotkoff sounds (first diastolic pressure) and point of silence (second diastolic pressure). For instance, a blood pressure reading might be recorded as 130/86/60 (Malasanos, Barkauskas, and Stoltenberg-Allen, 1990; Hill and Grim, 1991).

It usually takes practice to learn to distinguish the systolic and diastolic points of pressure with ease and accuracy, and in some patients they are very difficult to discern. Care should be taken, however, to avoid repumping the sphygmomanometer repeatedly within a short space of time. Procedure 15.4 outlines the technique for measuring blood pressure by auscultation.

Preparing the Patient

The nurse informs the patient that blood pressure will be taken. The size of the patient's upper arm should be looked at to determine the size of blood pressure cuff that will be necessary.

FIGURE 15.11 A. Mercury sphygmomanometer B. Aneroid sphygmomanometer mounted on a wall

Assembling Equipment

There are three basic types of sphygmomanometers for measuring the blood pressure: mercury, aneroid, and electronic (see Figure 15.11). The electronic unit is discussed later. The mercury manometer uses liquid mercury within a glass tube calibrated in millimetres. The blood pressure is indicated by the level of the meniscus, or the concave surface of mercury as it descends in the tube. The mercury must be read at eye level, otherwise the value may be distorted. The aneroid gauge is a circular dial calibrated in millimetres and a needle that registers blood pressure as it descends the calibrations on the dial.

The blood pressure cuff consists of an inflatable rubber bladder that is covered with self-securing fabric. A tube connects the cuff to the manometer; another connects it to the inflation bulb. The cuffs come in various sizes to fit infants, children and adults; sizes for the thigh as well as the arm are available. For best accuracy, the cuff should be approximately 20 percent wider than the diameter of the extremity on which it is being used. Using a cuff that is too small will yield a false high reading because it is not big enough to adequately compress the artery. A cuff that is too big, on the other hand, will give a false low reading. Thus, for a very obese patient, it may be necessary to use a thigh cuff rather than an adult arm size one.

The equipment should be checked before use to ensure proper functioning. The release valve on the inflation bulb should open and close freely. The cuff must be free of residual air and the manometer or gauge must register zero.

Measuring Blood Pressure

ACTION	RATIONALE
1. Wash hands.	Prevents the spread of microorganisms.
2. Prepare the patient.	Promotes well-being and facilitates patient participation in care.

3. Gather equipment:
  • Sphygmomanometer
  • Stethoscope
	Facilitates efficiency and economy of time.

4. Help the patient assume a lying or sitting position, with the arm supported at heart level, and the palm turned up.	If the arm is above heart level, readings can be falsely low; if it is below heart level, readings can be falsely high.
5. Position the sphygmomanometer so that it is at eye level and in direct view; check that the mercury manometer or aneroid gauge is at zero.	Readies the equipment for accurate reading.
6. Expose the upper arm and palpate brachial pulse.	Locates the artery for the placement of the cuff.
7. Fold the cuff's bladder in half. Position the cuff so that the centre of the bladder lies directly over the brachial artery and the lower boarder about 2.5 cm above the antecubital space. Then wrap the cuff snugly and evenly around the upper arm.	Finds the cuff's true centre. Promotes the most accurate blood pressure reading. A loose and unevenly placed cuff may cause a false reading.
8. Palpate the brachial artery with fingertips, close the valve of the inflation bulb, and inflate the cuff until the pulse disappears. Note the point on the manometer or gauge where the pulse disappears. Deflate the cuff and wait 15 seconds.	Avoids misinterpreting an auscultatory gap and recording a falsely low systolic or a falsely high diastolic pressure (Hill and Grim, 1991). Allows the blood to circulate through the arm before continuing.
9. Place the stethoscope ear pieces in the ears and the bell or diaphragm over the brachial artery.	

ACTION	RATIONALE
Inflate the cuff until the mercury manometer or aneroid gauge registers 30 mm Hg above the point at which the pulse disappeared.	Ensures ample time to accurately hear the systolic pressure.
10. Carefully open the valve and slowly release the air at a rate of 2 to 3 mm Hg per second. While releasing the air, watch the mercury manometer or aneroid gauge and listen for the Korotkoff sounds.	
Note the point at which the first clear sound is heard.	Indicates the systolic pressure.
Continue to deflate the cuff, noting the point at which the first muffled sound appears, and finally, the point at which the last sound is heard.	Indicates the first diastolic pressure. Indicates the second diastolic pressure.
11. Rapidly deflate the cuff. If the reading must be repeated, wait at least 30 seconds.	Reestablishes blood circulation through the veins.
12. Remove the cuff and return it to storage. Assist the patient to a comfortable position.	Promotes well-being.
13. Document the blood pressure on the graphic flowsheet (Figure 15.8) according to agency guidelines. Record variations in technique, position, or extremity used in the nurses' notes.	Provides a data base for ongoing evaluation of patient status and promotes continuity of care.

MEASURING BLOOD PRESSURE WITH AN ELECTRONIC SPHYGMOMANOMETER

Electronic sphygmomanometers are available which give a digital readout of the blood pressure (see Figure 15.12). A cuff with a built-in pressure transducer is placed on the upper arm as is done with the ordinary sphygmomanometer. The machine is then turned on. A flashing light or a beeping sound indicates that systolic and diastolic pressures have registered. These machines may also be set to take blood pressure measurements at precise intervals. Some instruments are designed to provide a print-out of the blood pressures so that they can be examined and recorded appropriately. The electronic instruments help to give a more accurate reading, since they eliminate the human error possible when one has to interpret sounds and coordinate hand and eye movements at the same time.

FIGURE 15.12 Electronic unit for measuring vital signs. It includes a sphygmomanometer, thermometer and pulse meter.

Source: Courtesy of the IVAC Corporation, San Diego, CA.

EXAMINATIONS AND DIAGNOSTIC TESTS

A comprehensive health assessment often includes a large number of tests and examinations that may be performed by many other health care workers. The first step in the assessment is usually a complete physical examination, performed by a physician or by a nurse practitioner. In conjunction with the examination, laboratory tests are usually ordered, and x-rays and other special examinations may be scheduled. The gamut of specialized tests and procedures used in the detection of illness today includes not only the standard x-ray with which most of us are familiar but also its sophisticated offspring, the CAT scan, as well as the ultrasonic scan, nuclear medicine studies, electrodiagnostic studies, magnetic resonance imagery, thermography, cardiopulmonary laboratory examinations and tissue biopsies. The neuropsychiatric field also has a number of specialized tests to help in assessing an individual's mental status.

Examinations and diagnostic tests create a good deal of anxiety in many people. Of primary importance to anyone undergoing them is what the results will mean in terms of prognosis (medical opinion of the final outcome of a health problem) and treatment. Some of the questions that run through a person's mind are: Will the results indicate that I have an incurable disease? Will I be crippled? Do I have to have surgery? These questions often preoccupy even the person who is just going to have a routine chest x-ray or blood test. Patients also want to know the reasons for the tests, and when they will be able to have the results.

Diagnostic testing is part of a comprehensive health assessment.

Under present rules of ethical practice, the nurse does not give the patient the results of examinations or tests. This is the responsibility of the attending physician. However, the nurse can provide the patient with information about the tests and with emotional support before, during and after many procedures. This is done by confirming and explaining what the physician has said about the "whys" of the test or examination and by giving the patient pertinent information. Nurses explain how the procedure is to be carried out, in terms the patient can understand, and answers questions to the best of their ability.

The patient often feels a need to help in the procedure, and the nurse can assist by explaining what he or she can do before, during and after the test to facilitate the examination. The nurse can also communicate to the patient an understanding of his or her anxiety and need to have confidence in the measures that are being taken for the patient's care. If the nurse feels that the patient does not understand what is being done, he or she has an important responsibility as a patient advocate to communicate this to the physician. The nurse also has an important coordinating function in regard to diagnostic tests and examinations. This may include assisting in the scheduling of many of these, carrying out some of the tests and assisting other members of the health team in carrying out many others.

ASSISTING WITH A PHYSICAL EXAMINATION

The responsibilities of the assisting nurse usually involve gathering the necessary equipment and supplies, preparing the examining room or patient's unit and helping both the examiner and the patient with the physical examination. Most patients want some explanation about the examination — what is to be done and why. The patient will need to fully or partially undress and may need help in putting on the gown provided; the gown may be removed during parts of the examination. It is important to ensure the patient's privacy and also to make sure that he or she is not cold. If the patient lies on a bed for the examination, a light blanket may be used. During the examination the nurse is usually responsible for draping the patient as appropriate for comfort and modesty, and helping the patient, as needed, to assume the best position to facilitate the examination.

The nurse does not always stay throughout the entire physical examination, although many agencies today, and also many physicians, request that a female nurse be present during the examination if the patient is female and the examiner male. The reason for this is twofold: it contributes to the psychological comfort of the patient and also provides legal protection for the examiner. The nurse should also consider the patient's age, mental alertness, balance and cooperativeness in judging whether to stay with the patient throughout the examination.

If the patient is ambulatory, a general inspection is often done with the patient standing; that is, one assesses posture and general appearance and notices abnormalities. Alternatively, it is done with the patient lying in a **supine position** (on the back). Most examiners prefer to have the patient sitting up for examination of the head and neck and the chest and lungs (back and front). The supine position is the usual choice for examination of the breasts, heart and abdomen. The examiner may also look at the extremities when the patient is lying down but will often want to do a further examination with the patient sitting and, also, standing. For examination of the rectum, a male patient may be asked to bend over the examining table. For a bed patient, or a female patient, Sims' position or a knee-chest position may be used (see Figure 15.13). **Sims' position** is also known as the semi-prone or three-quarter prone position. It is a position that is frequently used for people who are unconscious and is described in detail in Chapter 25.

In the *knee-chest position*, the patient kneels with the buttocks upward. It is important that the patient who assumes this position be adequately draped. Many health agencies have special rectal drapes that completely cover the buttocks of a patient except for a circular cutout over the anus. The patient will generally need additional covering for the shoulders and a pillow for the head.

If the health agency does not have special drapes, the nurse can improvise with a cotton drawsheet. The drawsheet is placed across the patient so that the lower edge just covers the buttocks. The corners are tucked around the medial aspect of the patient's thighs. By raising the fold of the sheet, the anal area is exposed.

During this procedure, the examiner needs a rectal glove, lubricant and kidney basin. The examiner inserts a lubricated gloved finger into the patient's rectum, palpating for abnormalities such as hemorrhoids and fissures.

The **lithotomy position** (see Figure 15.13) is used chiefly for examinations and operations involving the reproductive and urinary tracts for both sexes. In this position patients lie on their backs with a small pillow for their heads. The patient's hips are flexed and slightly abducted and the knees are also flexed. The patient needs support for the feet to maintain this position for more than a few minutes. The stirrups provide a means for supporting the feet.

A

B   **C**

FIGURE 15.13   Positions used in examinations and treatments: A. Sims' position B. Knee-chest position C. Lithotomy position

Because this position is embarrassing for most people, it is important that adequate drapes be provided. One way of draping the patient is to place a drawsheet across the patient so that the lower border is 10 cm below the symphysis pubis. Then each of the lower corners of the drawsheet is brought to the medial aspect of the patient's thighs and tucked around the patient's legs. When the upper fold of the drawsheet is lifted the patient's perineum is exposed. The nurse should also provide the patient with a covering for the upper part of the body. Another method is to place a bath blanket diagonally over the patient. The opposite corners (at each side of the patient) are wrapped around the legs and anchored at the feet. The lower corner can be drawn back and tucked under the top layer of the bath blanket to expose the perineum.

For a vaginal examination the examiner requires gloves, lubricant, a vaginal speculum, a kidney basin and a good light. This equipment is sterilized after use in order to prevent the transmission of infection. The physician may also want a tongue blade and a microscopic slide in order to take a sample of the cervical secretions, which are then sent to the laboratory for examination for abnormal cells. This is called a Papanicolaou smear.

LABORATORY TESTS

In conjunction with a physical examination, various laboratory tests are usually ordered. These generally include blood tests and a urinalysis in the initial assessment of an individual's health status, or a periodic health checkup. In the blood work, the tests commonly ordered include white blood cell count (WBC) and differential, hematocrit (Hct), a red blood cell morphology (RBC) and platelet examination and a hemoglobin (Hgb) estimate. In many places where laboratory data systems are computerized, it is now common practice to order a battery of tests, instead of ordering them singly. Analyses on one sample of blood can provide an assessment of nutritional status, liver and kidney function, tissue injury and parathyroid function. In a routine urinalysis, the urine is tested for pH, specific gravity, albumin and sugar, and a microscopic examination is done. If abnormalities are found in the blood tests or urinalysis, further laboratory investigation or other special tests are undertaken.

Frequently, the nurse is responsible for collecting specimens from patients. These may include specimens of blood, urine, sputum and drainage from wounds. For these tests, patients usually need explanations as to what they can do to help. Most patients like to be able to assist, and often the success of a test is dependent upon the patient's willingness to provide a specimen or perform some activity at a particular time.

Various specimens are sent for microbiological examination in the laboratory. Specimens of a patient's secretions, excretions and any exudates are frequently examined in order to isolate and identify an infecting organism. A

secretion is a product produced by a gland (for example, bile); an *excretion* is a substance excreted or discharged by the body (for example, urine). An *exudate* is an inflammatory fluid, such as pus, that is discharged from an infected area of the body.

For most specimens, a sterile container is required, and precautions must be taken to avoid contaminating the specimen with organisms in the environment. A smear or culture may be needed. If a specimen is required for a smear, clean (preferably new) slides and a sterile, cotton-tipped applicator are needed. The specimen is gathered with the applicator, which is rolled over the centre of the slide. The smear is covered with another glass slide. The slides are appropriately labelled and sent to the laboratory.

For cultures, the specimen is placed in a sterile container. Urine, blood, ascitic fluid, and the like are usually put in sterile test tubes. For cultures of specimens of wound discharge, many agencies furnish sterile test tubes that are equipped with sterile applicators suspended from the cork that seals the tube. When the cork is removed the applicator is removed with it. The applicator tip is touched to the area of discharge and then returned carefully to the sterile container. Sputum specimens are collected in wide-necked sterile containers or on Petri dishes. Sputum is collected early in the morning, when the patient is most able to cough up sputum from the lungs.

When stools are sent for culture, it is seldom necessary to send the entire specimen. Normally a sterile applicator dipped in the feces is sufficient. If the feces are to be examined for amebae, the specimen is sent to the laboratory while it is warm and it is examined within 30 minutes after it is obtained. Only a small quantity (approximately 3 ml) of feces is needed for this examination.

Nursing Functions for Specimen Collection

1. Explain the procedure to the patient and gain their participation
2. Collect the right amount of specimen at the correct time
3. Place the specimen in the correct container
4. Label the container accurately (this usually includes the patient's full name and identification number, the date, the physician's name, and, if in a hospital, the number of the nursing unit) and place it in a plastic bag.
5. Complete the laboratory requisition (this specifies what tests are to be carried out and gives pertinent data about the patient)
6. Record anything unusual about the appearance of the specimen

It may be necessary to test a culture for differentiation and sensitivity. *Differentiation* is accomplished by means of Gram's stain, which divides bacteria into two classes: gram-negative organisms stain red; gram-positive organisms stain purple. *Sensitivity* refers to the effect of specific antibiotics upon bacteria. The organisms are streaked on nutrient plates, various antibiotics are then added to the plates, and the plates are placed in an incubator. The areas where the growth of the bacteria is inhibited indicate the particular antibiotics to which the bacteria are sensitive.

X-RAYS

Radiation is a highly publicized and emotionally charged word these days, and many people are afraid that having any kind of an x-ray will harm them. Excessive radiation is most certainly dangerous, and special precautions are taken to ensure that people who work in x-ray departments or in places where radiation therapy is used (such as in a cancer clinic) are not exposed to excessive amounts. You may have noticed the monitors that workers in the x-ray department wear on their uniforms. These monitors, which look something like metal pencils, are carefully checked on a regular basis to make sure that the worker has not had a dangerous level of radiation exposure. The amount a person receives during diagnostic tests, however, is minimal. A person does not receive enough radiation to destroy tissue unless this is being done therapeutically, as for treatment of a tumour.

X-rays today are used in diagnosis and therapy on virtually every system of the body. In diagnosis, their purpose is to assist in the visualization of internal structures of the body, so that pictures of these structures can be put on film. X-rays, which are also called *roentgen rays*, are electromagnetic radiations, or energy waves, of short wave length.

When x-rays are passed through the body, denser structures, such as bone tissue, absorb more of the rays and, hence, register heavier shadows on the photographic film. Less dense structures, such as soft organs (like the stomach), permit the rays to pass through them more easily. These structures register lighter shadows on the film. It is the contrast between light and dark shadows (because of the differing density of tissues and, hence, the differing amount of rays they absorb) that enables the person reading the x-ray to find abnormalities.

In order to visualize softer structures within the body, such as the gastrointestinal tract, a substance (called a contrast medium) is often used to make the structures radiopaque so that they will show on photographic film. The contrast media usually used are either metallic salts or gases. Barium sulfate, for example, is the contrast medium used for the gastrointestinal tract. If the upper part of the tract (the esophagus, stomach and duodenum) is to be visualized, the patient drinks the barium solution; to allow visualization of the lower part (colon and rectum), the barium is given as an enema. For x-rays of the ventricles of the brain, oxygen is injected into the spinal canal. Organic soluble iodides are used to visualize the gallbladder, urinary tract and blood vessels.

The ordinary diagnostic x-ray is like a still photograph and provides a permanent record. Sometimes, however, it is desirable to observe body organs or systems in motion, as, for example, the filling and emptying of the stomach. Then, *fluoroscopy* is used. In this procedure, x-rays are passed through the body and images of the moving internal structures are projected onto a fluorescent screen. Again, a contrast medium may be used to aid in the assessment.

The CAT scan (also known as CT and CAT) is another form of x-ray. The initials stand for *computerized axial tomography*. In this procedure, x-rays are passed through the body in the region of the structure to be "scanned." A 180° sweep of the structure, at three or four different planes, is used. The x-rays are fed into a computer, which records the *absorption potential* of different tissues at varying planes within the structure. The computer prints out a visual representation of these. Photographs are also taken of the image on the screen. Usually these are in black and white, although colour photography is also possible.

NUCLEAR MEDICINE STUDIES

Radioactive isotopes, which are also known as *radionuclides* or *radiopharmaceuticals*, are another form of radiation that is used in both diagnosis and treatment. These substances give off radioactivity in known, predictable quantities as they decay, and they can thus be traced in the body by a monitor that picks up radioactivity. Certain radioactive substances have a particular affinity for specific parts of the body; for example, radioactive iodine taken orally (it is usually given in a drink) will find its way to the thyroid gland, where it tends to accumulate. Given in large doses, it will destroy tissue in much the same way as radiation therapy using x-rays does. In smaller doses (called tracer doses) it can be used to identify abnormalities in the thyroid gland. The radioactivity given off by the iodine as it decays can be picked up by a scanner (much like a form of Geiger counter) and the emissions transformed into electrical impulses, which can then be counted. Or, a camera, called a gamma camera, may be used to take photographs of the accumulation and distribution of the radioactive iodine in the body. It is possible, using radioactive substances, to detect abnormalities or malignant tumours in such tissues as the brain, bone, lungs, liver, kidneys, spleen, pericardium and thyroid.

ELECTRODIAGNOSIS

Various organs of the body, including the heart, the brain, the stomach, the muscles and the skin, constantly emit electrical impulses as they function. These impulses can be picked up on a machine and transformed (transduced) into a set of tracings that provides a graphic representation of the impulses. The tracings are then "read," or interpreted, by an expert to assess the functioning of the particular organ. In this way, graphic representations can be made of the electrical impulses emitted by the heart (*electrocardiogram*, also called an ECG or EKG), brain (*electroencephalogram*, or EEG) and muscles (*electromyogram*, or EMG).

ULTRASONIC SCAN

Auscultation, the listening for sounds within the body, is one of the basic methods of observation we discussed at the beginning of this chapter. The *ultrasonic scan* is a diagnostic tool that utilizes this basic methodology. Sound waves of too high a frequency to be heard by the human ear are directed at the organ or structure of the body that is to be assessed. The vibrations that come back are transformed (transduced) into tracings, called *oscilloscope tracings*, which can be read to detect pathological changes in tissues of the muscles and joints, the brain, or the heart. Ultrasonic scans are commonly used to assess fetal development.

THERMOGRAPHY

Thermography is the assessment of the temperature of various body areas for the purpose of detecting underlying pathological processes. It is basically a technique using self-emanating infrared radiation to portray surface temperatures of the body photographically. It is frequently used in the detection of tumours of the breast, for example, and may also be used in assessment of blood vessels and inflammatory processes.

MAGNETIC RESONANCE IMAGING

Magnetic resonance imaging (MRI) identifies abnormalities by creating sectional images of the body. MRI provides clear images of internal structures in response to the magnetic field created by harmless, low-energy radio waves. MRI is used to detect and localize malignancies of the central nervous system, spine, head and musculoskeletal system.

TISSUE BIOPSIES

It is sometimes important to examine a sample of living tissue from a particular structure of the body. Usually this is done to look for either abnormal cells that may indicate the presence of a tumour or structural changes indicative of an infectious process. The procedure for obtaining a specimen of tissue from the body is called a **biopsy**. The specimen is sent to a pathology laboratory for microscopic examination. There are basically three ways that a tissue biopsy may be obtained: (1) by use of a needle for punc-

ture or aspiration; (2) by endoscopy; and (3) by surgical excision.

A sample of bone marrow may be obtained by inserting a hollow needle through the surface tissue of the body and into the marrow cavity of a bone. A small amount of the marrow is aspirated to obtain the specimen. The sternum is the most common site for this procedure, although the iliac crest, the posterior superior ilium, and the spine are also used.

Endoscopy is the examination of body cavities and openings through the use of specially designed instruments that enable the examiner to observe tissues more clearly. The instruments are called scopes and usually come equipped with a small light at the inserting end and, often, a small mirror to make visualization easier. If a tissue sample is wanted, a narrow instrument is inserted through the scope to pick up cells for the biopsy.

For obtaining a sample of tissues that are imbedded in a body structure, for example, from a lump in the breast, it may be necessary to use surgical excision to get specimen cells for laboratory examination.

CARDIOPULMONARY LABORATORY TESTS

Many tests and examinations have been developed to aid in the assessment of functioning of the heart and lungs — so many that there are now specialized laboratories devoted to this diagnostic area. The electrocardiogram mentioned above is a procedure commonly ordered as part of a complete physical examination for all patients over the age of 40 years. In addition, various x-ray techniques may be used to visualize the size, positioning and functioning of the heart, lungs and blood vessels. A number of specialized tests may also be done, such as the stress tolerance test and treadmill test that assess cardiac functioning, and the pulmonary function tests that measure lung volumes, capacities and flow rates. We will be discussing the more commonly used diagnostic tests for cardiopulmonary functioning in Chapter 23.

TESTS OF MENTAL STATUS

In some cases, particularly when it is considered important to establish a psychiatric diagnosis, specialized psychological tests may be used. These include the objective tests, such as the intelligence tests with which most of us are familiar, the vocational interest and aptitude tests and the personality tests (for example, the Minnesota Multiphasic Personality Inventory). These may be supplemented by projective tests, such as Draw-a-Person, the Rorschach ink blot test or the thematic apperception test. The latter two call for the individual to interpret different shapes of ink blots and pictures of people in different situations, respectively. The projective tests are said to reflect a person's fantasies and modes of adaptation. They are always administered and evaluated by a skilled psychologist.

Guidelines for Assisting with Tests and Examinations

Before the procedure:

1. Prepare the patient
   - Explain the procedure, what exactly is to be done and why it is being done, in terms the patient can understand
   - Explain how the patient can help with the examination
   - Provide the patient with a gown and assist him or her in getting into it, if necessary
   - Provide privacy for the patient to dress and undress and to wait for the examination
   - Help the patient to assume the position required for the examination
   - Drape the patient for comfort and to facilitate the examination

2. Practise body substance precautions

3. Prepare the equipment
   - Obtain all the equipment needed for the examination
   - Maintain the sterility of the equipment before and during the examination, as necessary
   - Obtain the containers needed for specimens and label these with the patient's name, the examiner's name and the date

4. Prepare the examining room
   - Close the windows and eliminate drafts
   - Ensure privacy
   - Place equipment so that it is convenient for the examiner
   - Provide a chair for the examiner when this is indicated

During the procedure:

1. Provide emotional support for the patient
2. Provide physical support for the patient as needed, for example, when they must keep very still in one position
3. Assist the examiner with equipment as necessary
4. Observe the patient for reactions to the examination

After the procedure:

1. Carry out measures for the patient's comfort, for example, cleaning lubricant off the skin or drying areas that may have been dampened
2. Observe the patient closely for any untoward reactions
3. Send labelled specimens to the laboratory
4. Clean and dispose of equipment as necessary
5. Enter details of the examination on the patient's record, such as date, time, exactly what was done, and whether and for what purpose specimens were sent to the laboratory

KEY TERMS

ophthalmoscope p. 360
otoscope p. 360
inspection p. 361
palpation p. 362
percussion p. 363
auscultation p. 363
stethoscope p. 364
vital signs p. 368
circadian (diurnal) rhythm p. 368
body temperature p. 369
pyrexia p. 369
fever p. 369

hypothermia p. 369
pulse p. 378
pulse rate p. 378
tachycardia p. 380
bradycardia p. 380
pulse rhythm p. 380
pulse volume p. 380
pulse tension p. 380
carotid pulse p. 380
radial pulse p. 380
brachial pulse p. 380
temporal pulse p. 380

femoral pulse p. 380
dorsalis pedis pulse p. 380
ulnar pulse p. 380
posterior tibialis pulse p. 380
popliteal pulse p. 380
apical pulse p. 381
point of maximal impulse (PMI) p. 381
external respiration p. 383
inspiration p. 383
expiration p. 383
respiratory rate p. 383

IN REVIEW

Clinical assessment involves the collection of data to develop a comprehensive base on which to make informed judgements and decisions about patient care. Data are collected through the use of interviewing techniques and by taking health histories and performing physical examinations. Tests and examinations performed by other health care professionals also make up the patient data base.

Interviewing is done to obtain a health history and to explore patients' symptoms and perceptions of their health problems. The health history is the first element of patients' data bases and an important factor in determining problems and needs. It provides a complete picture of the person as a whole and how he or she interacts with the environment, including patterns of daily living, strengths and coping capabilities, as well as health promotion and health protection patterns. The nurse uses this information to plan or modify care to conform to patients' preferences and usual patterns of living. The health history usually follows a sequential list of questions and then a review of body systems to avoid omissions. A symptom analysis, following the pattern of what, when, where and why, will remind the nurse of the types of questions to ask.

The physical examination is a systematic assessment of a patient using inspection, palpation, percussion and auscultation techniques. It should be carried out in an organized manner to avoid omission of necessary components. Inspection involves the conscious systematic use of one's senses to distinguish normal versus borderline and abnormal findings. Palpation is the use of touch to detect superficial and deeper characteristics of the body. It may be light or deep depending on the part of body being examined. Percussion involves striking or tapping the body surface to differentiate the density and size of underlying structures. It produces five tonal notes depending on the density (solidness) of the structure. Auscultation is the listening for body sounds with a stethoscope. Knowledge, practice and experience are necessary to develop skill in using these examination techniques.

Functional abilities — the status of nutrition, elimination, sensory perception, skin and tissue integrity and motor ability — are also assessed in a sequential fashion. Also noted are the state of rest and comfort and the reproductive, mental, emotional and social status of the patient. Verbal communication and social responses are observed.

The vital signs are temperature, pulse and respirations. Together with blood pressure and heart rate, they provide an indication of basic physiological functioning. Vital signs vary in any individual over a 24-hour period and in different states of health and illness. A consistent systematic series of readings establishes a normal baseline for each patient. Sudden changes in temperature, pulse, respirations or blood pressure should be reported immediately.

The temperature-regulating system is the principal homeostatic mechanism for maintaining the body at an optimal level for functioning. The balance is maintained between heat gain through metabolism and heat loss through evaporation, radiation, conduction and convection. Body temperature measurements can be obtained from the mouth, rectum, axilla or ear.

The pulses of the body are the result of the surge of blood sent through the systemic arteries when the left ventricle contracts. Peripheral pulses can be felt wherever an artery crosses a bony prominence; the apical pulse is the beat of the heart auscultated at its apex. The pulse rate is the number of ventricular contractions per minute. This rate varies with age, sex, size, physical and emotional activity, medication and illness. A peripheral pulse is assessed for rate, rhythm, size and elasticity. The apical and radial pulses are the same in health but may differ in illness. Both are taken when a difference is suspected and the difference is referred to as the pulse deficit.

Respiration covers both the external respirations (the exchange of oxygen and carbon dioxide in the lungs), and internal respiration (the exchange of these gases between the blood and the body cells). In taking vital signs the external respirations are measured. External respiration involves inspiration and expiration and is controlled by the respiratory centre in the medulla oblongata. The respiratory centre is influenced by chemical changes in the blood stream, increased blood pressure and exercise. Changes in respiration are automatic but can also be voluntary. Respirations are assessed for depth, rhythm and character.

Blood pressure is the pressure of the blood within the arteries. The systolic pressure is the pressure exerted when the left ventricle contracts and the diastolic pressure is the pressure exerted when the left ventricle rests. The difference between these pressures is the pulse pressure. Blood pressure is determined by cardiac output and peripheral vascular resistance. Cardiac output is affected by the strength of the pumping action of the heart and by the amount of circulating blood. Peripheral vascular resistance is caused by the size of the lumen and elasticity of the vessels. Blood pressure is affected by age, sex, stress, activity and position.

A comprehensive health assessment often includes a number of tests and examinations performed by other health care professionals. Although the results of the tests are disclosed to the patient by the physician, the nurse can help immeasurably to alleviate anxiety by providing information and support before, during and after many procedures. The nurse also acts as an advocate in communicating the patients' concerns to the physician. In assisting examinations, the nurse ensures patients' privacy and preserves their modesty. Blood work, urinalysis, x-rays and sometimes specimens may ordered. In all cases explanations and the patient's understanding and cooperation are to be encouraged.

LEARNING ACTIVITIES

In consultation with your teacher, select a patient who has recently been admitted to the agency in which you are having clinical practice.

1. Review the patient's data base, paying particular attention to the nursing health history and the physician's medical history and progress notes.

2. Undertake a clinical assessment of the patient's functional abilities, including:
    • temperature, pulse, and respirations
    • blood pressure
    • nutritional status
    • elimination status (bowel status, urinary status)
    • sensory perception (vision, hearing, smell, taste and touch)
    • motor status
    • state of rest and comfort
    • reproductive status
    • mental status
    • emotional status
    • social status (verbal communication and social response).

3. Identify deviations from the normal that you observed in the patient's functional abilities.

4. How important are these deviations in terms of planning nursing care for this patient?

5. What diagnostic tests and examinations have been ordered for this patient? Was a complete physical examination done? What laboratory tests were ordered? Roentgenography? Other? Why were they ordered? Are the results back on any of these yet? Do they show deviations from normal? What are the implications in terms of nursing care?

REFERENCES AND READINGS

ALDER, J. (1979). Patient assessment: Pulses. *American Journal of Nursing, 79*(1), 115–132.

ASSESSING VITAL FUNCTIONS ACCURATELY. (1977). (Nursing Skillbooks Series). Horsham, PA: Intermed Communications.

ASSESSING YOUR PATIENTS. (1980). (Nursing Photobook Series). Horsham, PA: Intermed Communications.

BAIRD, S.C., WHITE, N.E. and BASINGER, M. (1992, August). Can you rely on tympanic thermometers? *RN. 55* (8), 48–51.

BATES, B. (1991). *A guide to physical examination and history taking* (5th ed.). Philadelphia: Lippincott.

BERGER, K.J. and WILLIAMS, M.B. (1992). *Fundamentals of nursing: Collaborating for optimal health.* Norwalk, CT: Appleton & Lange.

BLACK, J.M. and MATASSARIN-JACOBS, E. (1993). *Luckmann and Sorensen's medical-surgical nursing* (4th ed.). Philadelphia: Saunders.

BLOCK, G.J. and NOLAN, J.W. (1986). *Health assessment for professional nursing* (2nd ed.). Norwalk, CT: Appleton-Century-Crofts, 138; 155.

BRAVERMAN, B.G. (1990). Eliciting assessment data from the patient who is difficult to interview. *The Nursing Clinics of North America, 25*, 743–750.

BROWN, M. (1991). How do you spell assessment? *American Journal of Nursing, 91*(9), 55–56.

BURNS, K.R. and JOHNSON, P.J. (1980). *Health assessment in clinical practice.* Englewood Cliffs, NJ: Prentice-Hall.

CLEMENTE, C.D. (1985), *Gray's anatomy of the human body* (30th ed.). Philadelphia: Lea and Febiger.

EARNEST, V.V. (1993). *Clinical skills in nursing practice* (2nd ed.). Philadelphia: Lippincott.

ERICKSON, R.S., and YOUNT, S.T. (1991). Comparison of tympanic and oral temperatures in surgical patients. *Nurs Res, 40*(2), 90–93.

FALLIS, W.M. (1993). Determination of oral temperature accuracy in orally intubated critical care patients utilizing oral, rectal and pulmonary artery temperatures. Unpublished master's thesis. Faculty of Nursing, University of Manitoba, Winnipeg, Manitoba.

FITZGERALD, M. (1991, November). The physical exam. *RN, 54*(11), 34–39.

FULLER, J. and SCHALLER-AYERS, J. (1994). Health assessment: A nursing approach (2nd ed.). Philadelphia: Lippincott.

GEHRING, P.E. (1991). Physical assessment begins with a history. *RN, 54*(11), 26–38.

HEIDENREICH, T. and GIUFFRE, M. (1990). Postoperative temperature measurement. *Nurs Res, 39*(3), 153–155.

HILL, M.N. and GRIM, C.M. (1991). How to take a precise blood pressure. *AJN, 91*(2), 38–42.

INFRARED EAR THERMOMETRY: GUIDANCE ARTICLE. (1991). *Health Devices, 20,* 431–441.

JARVIS, C. (1992). *Physical examination and health assessment.* Philadelphia: Saunders.

MALASANOS, L., BARKAUSKAS, V. and STOLTENBERG-ALLEN, K. (1990). *Health assessment* (4th ed.). St. Louis: Mosby.

McCONNELL, E. (1988). Seeing your patient as a mosaic. *Nursing '88, 18*(12), 50–51.

MENGEL, A. (1982). Getting the most from patient interviews. *Nursing '82, 12*(11), 46–49.

PILLITTERI, A. (1995). *Maternal and child health nursing: Care of the childbearing and childrearing family* (2nd ed.). Philadelphia: Lippincott.

ROBICHAUD-EKSTRAND, S. and DAVIES, B. (1989). Comparison of electronic glass thermometers: Length of time of insertion and type of breathing. *The Canadian Journal of Nursing Research, 21*(1), 61–73.

ROGERS, J., CURLEY, M., DRISCOLL, J., LEBLANC, G., LIBMAN, M., McCARTY K. and KERRIGAN, T. (1991). Evaluation of tympanic membrane thermometer for use with pediatric patients. *Pediatric Nursing, 17,* 376–378.

SACKSTEDER, M., WILLIAMS, B. S. and SHULKO, P. (1992). History and physical examination in assessment. In L.O. Burrell (Ed). *Adult nursing.* Norwalk, CT: Appleton & Lange, 31–41.

SANTO-NOVAK, D. (1988). Seven keys to assessing the elderly. *Nursing '88, 18*(8), 60–63.

TACKETT, J.J.M., and HYNSBERGER, M. (1981). *Family-centered care of children and adolescents.* Philadelphia: Saunders.

TERNDRUP, T. An appraisal of temperature assessment by infrared emission detection thermometry. *Annals of American Medicine, 21,* 1483–1492.

TIMBY, B.K. and LEWIS, L.W. (1992). *Fundamental skills and concepts in patient care* (5th ed.). Philadelphia: Lippincott.

TOURANGEAU, A., MACLEOD, F. and BREAKWELL, M. (1993). Tap in on ear thermometry. *Canadian Nurse 89*(9), 24–27.

C H A P T E R 16

Communication Skills

OUTLINE

CENTRAL QUESTIONS

1. *What are the five basic characteristics of a helping relationship?*

2. *What are the three major phases of the nurse–patient relationship?*

3. *What are the main aspects of the process of contracting with a patient?*

4. *What is the SMCR model of the communication process?*

5. *Which factors can interfere with elements of the communication process? Give examples.*

6. *What factors should the nurse consider when conveying a message?*

7. *How must characteristics of language be considered by the nurse in communications with patients?*

8. *How do people communicate nonverbally? Give examples.*

9. *What are some of the ways of fostering an open climate for nurse–patient communications?*

10. *What role does the interview play in nurse–patient communications?*

11. *How are various media used for information exchange between members of the health team?*

INTRODUCTION

The fundamental core of nursing is the relationship that is established between the nurse and the patient. This is a professional relationship, based on trust and mutual respect. Individuals who comes to a health agency are there because they need help with some aspect of their health; nurses and other health professionals are there to provide that help. The relationship that develops between the nurse and the patient is collaborative — nurse and patient work together to promote the patient's optimal level of health. In order to develop relationships whereby nurses can help patients, nurses must develop skills in communicating, since, without communication, relationships are not possible.

Communication is the process by which people convey thoughts, feelings and ideas to each other. It is a tool that provides a means for one person to understand another, to accept and be accepted, to convey and receive information, to give and accept directions and to teach and learn. The nurse communicates with the patient and the patient with the nurse. Communication is always a two-way process. The nurse also communicates with patients' families and friends, with visitors to the agency, with other members of the health team and other personnel and with a host of other people during the course of a day. Nurses should, therefore, know something about the process of communication.

THE NURSE–PATIENT RELATIONSHIP

Nursing is one of the helping professions. Nurses help people to promote and maintain optimal health, to protect them from disease, to restore health following an episode of illness, and to cope with the exigencies of chronic or terminal illness. The relationship that is established between nurse and patient is a *helping relationship*. This relationship is the basis of nursing practice, and it is woven into the fabric of every interaction that occurs between nurse and patient. In the health field, the helping relationship is often referred to as a **therapeutic relationship**, because it is a key element enabling the health professional to administer care to the patient.

Several characteristics of the helping relationship have been identified by different authors. One essential element is **empathy**: the ability to recognize and understand another person's feelings. Empathy requires imagining yourself in another person's place and looking at things from that point of view. For example, the removal of a mole from the face may seem like a minor surgical procedure compared to open heart surgery, but, to the person who is having it done, there are all sorts of frightening possibilities. In order to have empathy, the nurse should consider the patient's thoughts and feelings. If the doctor had said the mole was probably just a harmless little growth, but was going to send

it to the laboratory just to make sure, the individual might well wonder: What if it turns out to be cancer? Will it grow back? Do moles spread? It is important to try to think of the implications of any procedure from the point of view of the person who is having it done. Questions to ask yourself include: How would I feel if I were facing this situation? How would I wish the information to be given to me? What questions would I want to ask? What words and actions on the part of others would I find helpful, reassuring and comforting?

Another commonly cited characteristic of the helping relationship is mutual *respect*. Demonstrating **respect** means treating the patient as a person of worth and dignity, and observing the social courtesies that indicate respect. Patients should be called by the name and title they prefer. Some older people may not like to be addressed by their first name. It is always a good idea to ask people how they like to be addressed. In Oriental cultures, age is highly respected and deference is shown in many ways. A younger person asks permission of an older person to sit down, or to speak. In some cultures, a young girl is expected to keep her eyes cast down and not look directly into the face of an elder when speaking. Nurses are not expected to observe the traditions of other cultures, but an awareness and understanding of these traditions is an important part of the nurse–patient relationship.

Western societies also have courteous ways of addressing people and of asking them to do something — ways that show respect for the other person. Respect can be demonstrated by asking permission to use a patient's time for an interview, for example, and by introducing yourself by name and explaining what you are doing. Autonomy and independence is respected by inquiring about the patient's concerns and preferences. Bearing in mind that not only are people's bodies being treated, but that their thoughts and feelings are also affected, compassionate involvement should always be offered to the patient. Patients have the right to participate in decisions regarding what shall be done with their bodies.

Nurses need to have the respect of patients if the relationships are to be effective — that is, if nursing interventions are to be related to positive patient outcomes. Your nursing education qualifies you to help others with regard to health problems; these qualifications in themselves engender respect from others who have not had this professional training. Competence in carrying out the nursing interventions, whether teaching preoperative exercises, putting on a dressing or taking a blood pressure, reinforces the inherent respect for the professional felt by the lay person. The confidence of the patient in the nurse is promoted by the demonstration of self-respect by the nurse. Self-respect is evidenced by such things as personal grooming, good posture, confident tone of voice and deliberative, well-planned actions.

Both empathy and mutual respect contribute to fostering a **climate of trust**, which is a very basic element in the helping relationship. Patients must be able to trust nurses as people who are concerned first and foremost with patient welfare. Patients must be confident that the nurse will not betray their confidence before they will feel free to discuss personal matters or express their feelings. Once sure of the nurse's competence, patients are able to trust that complex, invasive measures can be carried out safely. As the patient develops trust in the nurse, the nurse is able to assess the patient's readiness to accept responsibility in regard to personal health care. Trust usually develops slowly as rapport is built. Rapport can be facilitated by attention to small things such as remembering to make the phone call the patient asked you to make, and reporting back to the patient, by being honest and giving only reliable information, and, again, by demonstrating competent nursing care.

Genuineness, or **authenticity**, is another characteristic of the helping relationship that creates a climate of trust. Spontaneity of response, self-disclosure, and a lack of defensiveness on the nurse's part all contribute to authenticity. The nurse's willingness to disclose opinions and feelings, will model, for the patient, the ability to express private concerns and anxieties. The nurse may disclose similar feelings, such as grief that he or she may have experienced in the past because of the death of a family member, but care must be taken not to burden the patient with the nurse's personal problems. It should be remembered that the purpose of self-disclosure is limited to promoting the development of a therapeutic relationship whereby the patient feels that the nurse is a real human being who has a sincere interest in the patient's welfare. Remember that the patient's concerns are the focus of the relationship.

Once the patient's concerns have been established, the nurse uses **specificity** to clarify the exact nature of the patient's problem; ambiguity and vagueness are replaced by clarity as the nurse constantly communicates an understanding of the patient's concerns and seeks to validate that this understanding is accurate. As problems are accurately identified, appropriate interventions can be initiated.

Studies of the nurse–patient relationship have identified three major phases in the relationship. There is first of all an introductory, or *orientation*, phase, when nurse and patient get to know and trust each other, then a *working phase*, and, finally, a *termination phase*. Some authors subdivide these phases, and some identify more than three, but since the components coincide, we will discuss them under the three major headings (Peplau, 1991, 1992; Forchuk and Brown, 1989; Forchuk, 1992).

ORIENTATION

The time it takes for nurse and patient to get to know and begin to trust each other is referred to as the **orientation phase**. Under normal circumstances, they start off as strangers. The nurse, however, usually has the advantage of having some information about the patient before the initial meeting. If a nurse is assigned a patient in the clinical area, for example, relevant information can be obtained from the patient's record. The nurse will also be able to obtain a verbal report from the charge nurse (or the primary nurse) before meeting the patient.

The nurse takes the initiative in the relationship that is being established. It is up to the nurse to set the tone for the encounter (or series of encounters). Both nurse and patient are identified by name, and roles are clarified during this introductory, or orientation, phase. Both parties come with preconceived ideas about the nature of the relationship. The patient may have been conditioned by the media to have certain beliefs about hospitals and nurses, and comments about the agency or hospital may have been offered by friends or relatives. Experiences with the health care system will influence expectations of the care to be received.

The nurse comes to the encounter with expectations formed by previous clinical experiences and by the knowledge attained during education. Nurses should be sensitive to the possibility that expectations may not coincide. It is imperative that during this orientation phase, expectations about the nature of the working relationship be clarified between the two parties. The patient, for example, may expect the nurse to do everything while he or she simply lies in bed getting better. The nurse, on the other hand, may believe in promoting as much self-care as the patient is capable of. The importance of exploring the patient's expectations and resolving differences between the nurse and the patient was discussed in Chapter 14.

An orientation to the nursing unit or health agency is usually part of the introductory phase. It is important that the patient be introduced to people who will be participating in his or her care and that the nurse's roles be explained. Taking the nursing history is often a part of this phase and is sometimes the first opportunity the nurse has to get to know the patient. During this phase of the relationship there may be some testing, as both parties attempt to develop trust while exploring the possibilities and limitations of the relationship.

WORKING PHASE

The **working phase** of the nurse–patient relationship begins when the nurse has gathered data and is beginning to draw up a tentative plan of care in collaboration with the patient. Increased emphasis on accountability and responsibility for both providers and consumers of health services has led to the premise that both are equal partners in the process of health care. It is this premise that guides the nurse in the working phase of the relationship with the patient. The nurse and the patient share in developing mutually agreeable goals, and both have a definite role to play in achieving these. There is a division of responsibility, and it is important to clarify at the beginning of the working phase who will be responsible for which aspects of care.

Patient Contracting

One structured type of communication between the nurse and patient is the patient contract. Steckel and Swain (1977) defined a ***patient contract*** as a systematic agreement between the patient and nurse that grants reinforcement to the patient for performing a specific, desirable behaviour.

The contract may simply be a verbal agreement, for example, "I will teach you how to do the deep-breathing exercises before surgery, but I would like you to consider doing them four times a day on your own." Or, the contract may be a written statement that is signed by all parties concerned (a family member or significant other may also be involved, and there may be more than one nurse or other health care provider in the development of the contract).

Herje (1980) specified several characteristics central to an effective patient contract — the contract must be:

1. realistic (are the goals specified attainable for the patient?)

2. measurable/capable of being evaluated (are the goals concrete? can progress be evaluated?)

3. positive (what goals would the patient like to attain? what existing patient strengths can be built on?)

4. time-dated (when can the contract be started? how much progress is expected in a given time frame?)

5. written (have the patient and nurse both signed and retained a copy of the written contract?)

6. rewardable (is the desired patient behaviour rewardable? is the reinforcement desirable to the patient?)

Hayes and Davis (1980) have identified five steps in the process of contracting, and these provide good guidelines for nurses wishing to initiate the process:

1. Identification of the problem/priority ranking

   (Patient and nurse discuss the patient's perception of his or her health and create a problem list that is prioritized)

2. Contract development

   (Includes the behaviour that is expected from the patient and what reinforcement the patient will receive in return for this behaviour)

3. Contract implementation

   (Patient and nurse attempt to perform the goals/behaviours that were specified in the contract)

4. Contract evaluation

   (Together the patient and nurse periodically evaluate the contract's success to assess whether the stipulated goals are being attained. It is important to note that the contract may have to be periodically re-evaluated depending on patient progress)

5. Contract termination

   (It is useful to include a pre-determined termination date in the contract).

Hayes and Davis stress the importance of making the contract very specific to ensure that the terms of the agreement are clearly understood by all concerned. It should contain not only specific daily activities but also the variables of the activity. For instance, in the verbal contract described above, the nurse would specify the number of times the patient would be helped with deep-breathing exercises and the times of the day the patient should practise alone before surgery. More than one nurse is often involved in the patient's care; they would all need to be agreeable to the arrangements if the contract is to be fulfilled. The patient's primary physician should also be involved in the contract design. Depending on the nature of the activity, the physician's orders may need to be included, and the contract must be consistent with the overall plan of care for the patient.

Nurses have an important motivating role during the working phase of the nurse–patient relationship, in addition to their responsibilities in carrying out specific nursing care measures. Nurses encourage patients to take increasing responsibility for their own care (to the extent that they are able), and help the patient work towards the goals that they have established together. A review of the progress made each day and honest praise for accomplishment of the various tasks help to keep the patient motivated. Family and friends, who often are very concerned, can also provide support in motivating the patient to work towards the established goals.

TERMINATION PHASE

The nurse–patient relationship terminates when the patient is discharged from the agency or the nurse leaves for another assignment, or for any other reason ceases to provide care for the patient. Sometimes the relationship is of short duration, as when the nurse has had the responsibility of caring for the patient for one shift only. For the nurse working in an acute-care setting, the relationships are usually short, extending over a few days or a few weeks. In long-term care facilities, in which the patients are often residents, the nurse may work with one group of residents for several months. The community health nurse may have people he or she works with over a period of years. Whatever the length of the relationship, there is an inevitable sense of loss when the relationship is terminated. This feeling is more acute, of course, the longer the relationship has been.

It is helpful during this ***termination phase*** to review with the patient the progress that has been made in achieving previously established goals. When the relationship has been of longer duration, feelings of loss can be mediated by drawing the patient's attention to the goals that have been met. In this way the patient is able to accept more readily that the nurse's care is no longer needed. When patients have been adequately prepared for the termination of the relationship, a sense of mutual satisfaction may exist between the patient and the nurse. Sometimes, it is necessary to hand over the care of a patient to another person. In these situations it is always helpful to introduce the patient to the new care-giver. If the patient is to be transferred to another agency he or she needs to be prepared for the transfer. Reviewing progress to date and giving the patient information about the new agency will help to make the transfer easier. If the patient is being moved from an acute care hospital to an extended care unit, for example, fears and concerns should be fully explored. Knowing where the agency is located, the type of accommodation and the care provided will be greatly appreciated by the patient. If a member of the family can visit the facility and describe in detail to the patient what can be expected, the transfer will be facilitated.

THE PROCESS OF COMMUNICATION

Communication involves both the sending and the receiving of a message. If the message is not received, no communication has taken place.

Because communication is such an essential component of most work, as well as a basic social process, it has received a great deal of study. Numerous models have been developed to illustrate the process. The Source, Message, Channel, Receiver (SMCR) model of the communication process (Rogers and Rogers, 1976) is one that illustrates the process simply, contains all the basic elements, and is easily understood (see Figure 16.1). The essential elements in the communication process are:

1. a *source* (sender) — someone who sends a message to another person
2. a *message* — the thought, feeling or idea that the sender wishes to convey
3. a *channel* — the means by which the message is conveyed
4. a *receiver* — the person for whom the message is intended.

Let us consider an example. The nurse in a doctor's office wishes Ms. Lim to go into the examining room and tells her so. The *source* is the nurse. The *message* is "Please go to the examining room." The *channel* is the spoken word. The intended *receiver* of the message is Ms. Lim. The desired effect on the receiver is that she gets up from the chair and

FIGURE 16.1 The SMCR model of communication

SOURCE: Rogers, E.M. and Rogers, A. (1976). *Communication in organizations.* New York: The Free Press.

proceeds to the examining room. If she does, the nurse will know that she received the message. If she does not, the nurse will assume that the message was not received. The *effects* on the receiver provide the sender with **feedback**, since they enable the person who has sent the message to know if it was received or not. If it was not, communication has not taken place and the sender should try again.

FACTORS AFFECTING COMMUNICATION

Effective communication means that the message the sender intended to convey reached the intended receiver, was received and was interpreted correctly, and that the receiver was able to respond in some meaningful way to indicate that the message was received. Difficulties can occur anywhere along the way in the communication process.

THE SOURCE (SENDER)

The sender may have trouble putting the message into a form that can be communicated. This is called coding the message. Some people are very skilled at translating their messages into drawing, painting or music. Most of us, however, communicate with words, both spoken and written, and with nonverbal behaviour, such as facial expression, gestures, body postures and touch. We can communicate some ideas quite eloquently using nonverbal means, but, in order to convey most messages, we need to be able to attach symbolic meanings — in the form of words — to those messages. People must also be able to arrange these symbols (words or signs) to form messages that can be understood by others, and they must be able to send these messages clearly.

Consider the person who is in a foreign country, for example, and is unable to speak the language. Getting along is possible to a certain extent by pointing and using gestures, but, when it comes to asking directions or ordering a meal, it may be difficult to get the meaning across accurately without the use of words. It is at this stage that difficulties will be encountered. Likewise, a person who has suffered brain damage and is unable to speak, or cannot convert thoughts into verbal expression that can be understood by others, will also have trouble coding messages intelligibly. A person having difficulty making vocal sounds will experience problems communicating and must depend on written forms of communication, gestures or other nonverbal expressions to get messages across.

An individual's physical well-being and emotional state also affect the ability to communicate. A person who is ill may find trying to communicate too much of an effort, or thought processes may not function well enough to enable a coherent message to be put together. A person's emotional state can make communication easier, may hinder self-expression or may prevent communication completely. When a person is at ease emotionally and feels comfortable with another person, it is usually much easier to communicate. Nervousness and anxiety often interfere with the ability to put together a clear message and send it. The nervous applicant at a job interview, for example, frequently finds it difficult to say the right thing in the way it should be said.

Many different emotions can affect the sender's ability to communicate. A person can be so overwhelmed with happiness that the appropriate words cannot be found for self-expression. Extreme anger and fear can similarly impair communication. But, on the other hand, the clenched fist, the pounding on the table, or the slamming of a door can convey anger as eloquently as words can. All of these emotions can affect the communication, by impacting (positively or negatively) on the effectiveness of the source.

THE MESSAGE

The message itself may not be clear. Sometimes two conflicting messages are being sent simultaneously. For example, a nurse may say to a patient, "I am glad that you came, even if it is late," but the impatient tapping of a foot, or the surreptitious glances at a watch, may convey an entirely different meaning to the patient. Noise or other distractions can also interfere with message exchange.

In order to convey the meaning intended by the sender, the message must be sent in a form the receiver can understand. If Ms. Lim does not speak English, the communication process breaks down, unless the nurse is able to put the message into a language the individual does understand, or can convey the intent of the message by nonverbal means. Even with someone who speaks the same language as the nurse, the terminology must be at a level that the person can understand, or again the message will be unclear. If the intent of the message is not completely and explicitly stated, for example, if directions on how to get to the examining room are not included with the request to go there, the message is not complete.

THE CHANNEL

The channel chosen for sending a message must be appropriate. There are three main channels by which we communicate with other people: oral (speech), written, and nonverbal communication.

For oral communication, we have a number of tools at our disposal: talking directly with a person in a face-to-face meeting, recording messages on tape (audio or video), telephoning, or communicating by radio or television. All are media for the spoken word. There are also many forms of written communication: notes, letters, interoffice memos, records and forms, newspapers, books and magazines all convey messages in written form.

Messages are also conveyed nonverbally. It has often been said that a person communicates true feelings more in actions and mannerisms than in words. A whole area of study in recent years has been on "body language" — that is, the interpretation of messages people send through facial expressions, gestures, postures, ways of walking and so forth.

Other nonverbal forms of communication include the various sign languages (the most common being American Sign Language, or ASL) used by the deaf community. Sign languages can range from simple gestures to forms similar to ASL. These more complex forms are highly developed languages in which body language combines with a complex system of gestures to communicate messages.

Pictures and diagrams are often useful as an adjunct to, or in place of, words. Consider the use of diagrams, slides, videos and films in educational programs, for example. It is possible to learn to make a bed by listening to a description and reading the directions, but it is much easier to learn by watching your instructor make a bed, by watching a video or filmstrip or by following an illustrated manual.

The medium chosen must be appropriate for the message and must make the intent of the message clear to the intended receiver. Touch can sometimes convey more empathic understanding than words to someone who has suffered a loss. Direct face-to-face talking is often a more effective means of communication than telephoning, or writing a message. On the other hand, some people have difficulty expressing themselves orally and can put their thoughts and feelings down on paper more easily. When there is a long list of instructions for someone to follow, the written channel (supplemented with oral clarification as needed) is more appropriate.

THE RECEIVER

Problems in communication can also occur at the *receiving* end of the process. The message may reach someone other than the intended receiver. If Ms. Lim is the intended receiver but Mrs. Armani gets up and moves in the direction of the examining room while Ms. Lim continues to sit in her chair, the nurse knows that the wrong person received the message. An individual who is hard of hearing may have difficulty receiving spoken messages. A person who cannot read or write is unable to receive communications sent in written form. The intended receiver must not only receive the message but also be able to interpret it.

Many physical and psychosocial factors can affect a person's ability to understand communications. Age, for example, must be taken into consideration. Children often will not understand messages that are directed to them by an adult, either because their language skills have not developed sufficiently for them to be able to symbolize in the same terms as the adult, or because their intellectual development has not reached a level where they can comprehend the idea the adult is trying to convey. The integrity of the anatomical structures and physiological processes involved in interpreting messages must also be intact. When mental faculties have been impaired by brain damage, or are affected temporarily by drowsiness, by alterations in the level of consciousness, or by alcohol or drugs, for example, the ability to receive and interpret messages is decreased.

Emotional state may also interfere with both the ability to receive messages and the ability to interpret them. The frightened individual attends only to those messages that concern the object causing fear. Other messages may not be received or may be misinterpreted. The patient who is afraid that an injection will be painful may perceive the nurse's smile as threatening rather than reassuring.

It has often been said that people hear only what they want to hear. Receiving and interpreting messages is an active process. A woman who is told that she has inoperable cancer may not hear the message because she has "turned off." Nurses and other health professionals may have difficulties processing the significance of messages being given by their patients for a number of reasons: environmental distractions, multiple demands, personal presumptions, cultural differences, personality issues and lack of skill or attentiveness in decoding messages.

THE NURSE AS SENDER IN THE COMMUNICATION PROCESS

There is an old rhyme that says, "I have six honest serving people who taught me all I know. Their names are *Who* and *What* and *When*, and *Where* and *Why* and *How*." In thinking about communication and how to get a message conveyed to an intended receiver so that the message is correctly interpreted, the nurse may find it helpful to ask the six questions contained in the rhyme. We will start with the *what*, since the first thing the nurse must do is to get the message clear in his or her own mind before deciding how to send it.

- What is to be communicated?

  Is it directions, such as how to get somewhere or how to do something?

  Is it information, such as what is going to happen in the x-ray department or for a series of tests?

  Is it an attitude, such as a feeling of warmth and acceptance?

- Who is the intended receiver?

  Do I know much about the patient as an individual?

  Do I know anything about the patient's background?

What is likely to be the patient's point of view?

- Why is this message to be communicated?

  Does the patient need to know something in order to become oriented to the agency?

  Does the patient need help to overcome the fear of surgery?

  Does the patient need this message for safety? To increase independence?

- How should it be communicated?

  Should I speak with the patient, should I give information (or directions) in writing, or would nonverbal communication be best for this particular message?

- Where should the communication take place?

  In the patient's room, in the nursing station, in a classroom outside the nursing unit, in the patient's home?

- When should it be communicated?

  Is the person receptive to the message?

  Does he or she need the message now?

  Should it be delayed?

  Should others such as family members be present?

The nurse will probably think of many more questions that could be asked, but, if the six basic ones are remembered, it will help to keep in mind some of the fundamental elements of the communication process when the nurse is the sender in the process.

THE SPOKEN WORD AS A MEDIUM OF COMMUNICATION

In sending messages, either in speech or in writing, the language level chosen for the message should be simple and clear. Some people have a tendency to over-communicate. The message gets lost somewhere among the explanations, embellishments, or general extra verbiage that the sender feels should be included. Some people under-communicate, so that the message is incomplete, and the receiver has to ask for further clarification. If a person has something important to communicate, the message should be sent in the simplest language and with as few words as possible (but as many as necessary to get the meaning across), if the individual wants to be certain the message will be interpreted correctly.

The choice of words is another important consideration. Although many people in our health-oriented society are quite knowledgeable about health matters, such as the causes and treatment of illness, they often do not understand the technical terms that health workers use. Each line of work has its own *jargon* — that is, technical terms that are used in that particular field but are not in common use outside the field.

The terminology that nurses learn in order to be able to communicate effectively with other health professionals is often not understood by patients. Effective communication with others depends on the use of common terminology. It is important that nurses talk to patients in terms that they can understand. The nurse must assess the patient's language level and use appropriate words to express meaning clearly. For example, a nurse might ask a public health inspector or a medical officer of health "what measures are taken for vector control?" and expect a satisfactory answer. If an average homeowner were asked the same question, he or she probably would not know what the nurse was talking about. On the other hand, if the nurse were to say "do you have screens on the doors and windows to keep out insects?" the person would be able to understand the question more clearly.

Health workers commonly use technical terms to refer to vital bodily functions. The words *void* and *defecate*, for example, are used for urination and bowel elimination, but terms such as *pass water*, *pee* and *bowel movement* are probably more readily understood by most people. In working with children it is important to find out the particular terms for bodily functions that they have been taught.

NONVERBAL COMMUNICATION

Feelings and attitudes are conveyed not only in the words a person says, but also in nonverbal behaviour. Nurses should be aware that their facial expression, tone of voice, gestures and posture all convey in subtle ways their regard and feeling for another person. At the same time, the nurse should be aware that clues about the patient's feelings, attitudes and physical condition can be picked up through observations of nonverbal behaviour.

Facial expression   Facial expression is perhaps the most common way in which feelings are expressed by people nonverbally. One conveys feelings of happiness, fear, surprise, anger, disgust (contempt) and sadness by using facial muscles. Facial expressions speak a universal language. In cross-cultural experiments, psychologists have found remarkable agreement in people from different countries in interpreting emotions expressed in photographs (see Figure 16.2). Both literate and illiterate cultures have been tested, with remarkably similar results (Ekman, Friesen, O'Sullivan and Chan, 1987; Matsumoto, 1992).

Human beings, as opposed to the lower animals, can use the muscles around their eyes and mouths to express their feelings. Actors on the stage are aware of the impact of facial expression and learn to control their muscles to such an extent that the audience is able to tell, merely by looking at their faces, the emotions they wish to convey. Perhaps the nurse does not need as much skill in facial expression manipulation as the actor, but the nurse does need to be able to control nonverbal expressions of dislike, hostility and disgust. The nurse can begin to accomplish this by examining personal motivations and feelings.

Posture   Body posture is also a means of communicating. An erect, upright posture usually indicates a feeling

	Happiness	Fear	Surprise	Anger	Disgust Contempt	Sadness
Japan	87	71	87	63	82	74
Brazil	97	77	82	82	86	82
Chile	90	78	88	76	85	90
Argentina	94	68	93	72	79	85
United States	97	88	91	69	82	73

FIGURE 16.2   Judgements of emotion in five literate cultures

SOURCE: Ekman, P. (1975, September). Facial muscles talk every language. *Psychology Today, 9,* 36.

FIGURE 16.3   The dejected walker

SOURCE: Calero, H.H. *How to Read a Person Like a Book*. New York: Hawthorn Books, 1971.

FIGURE 16.4   Tension indicated by folded arms and clenched fists.

SOURCE: Calero, H.H. *How to Read a Person Like a Book*. New York: Hawthorn Books, 1971.

of self-esteem and a considerable degree of inner poise. Sadness, depression or a low regard for oneself usually makes a person stoop or slouch (see Figure 16.3). It is not uncommon, for example, to see a severely depressed person sitting slumped over in a chair or shuffling along with head down and shoulders rounded.

Grooming   Grooming also conveys meaning. A neat, well-groomed look indicates pride in appearance. The attitude of the patient towards grooming is often indicative of his or her state of well-being. Very ill people often do not have the strength or the desire to keep up their grooming. The request of a patient for a mirror has often been noted as an indication that the patient is feeling better.

Gestures   People are often unaware of the gestures they use, but gestures play an important role in conveying thoughts and feelings. The welcoming gesture as you ask a person to sit down helps to put the patient at ease. A hurried manner with quick gestures on the part of the nurse evokes a feeling that the nurse does not have much time and, as a result, the patient becomes reluctant to ask questions or to confide fears and worries. The patient's gestures are equally important. Lowered eyes or an averted glance usually indicate a wish to avoid communication on a topic. A person who sits with folded arms, occupying as little space as possible, is often tense (see Figure 16.4).

Intonation   A wide variety of subtle meanings are conveyed by the tone of one's voice. There is an adage that it is not so much what you say as how you say it. Small children in particular respond much more to the tone of a person's voice than to the actual words. Adult patients, however, are also sensitive to coldness or warmth as conveyed in the tone of the nurse's voice.

Tone of voice is often indicative of an individual's feelings of well-being. A person who is ill usually speaks more slowly and in a lower tone than usual. With excitement, the voice often rises and is more highly pitched. Myriad feelings may be expressed simply by changing the intonation of one's voice as, for example, in saying "Good morning." People are seldom aware of how their voice sounds to others. Listening to a tape recording of one's voice is often useful in helping to hear oneself as others do.

Touch   Touch can also convey the nurse's thoughts and feelings to patients. Past research has revealed that when one individual touches another in a non-obtrusive manner, positive reactions generally occur, even between strangers (Crusco and Wetzel, 1984).

CREATING A CLIMATE FOR OPEN COMMUNICATION

In order to foster an atmosphere of openness in which the patient feels free to communicate, the nurse must convey a feeling of warmth and acceptance.

Warmth implies a genuine liking for people. Acceptance involves the ability to understand another person's point of view and to respect the right of each individual to be different. Acceptance means being nonjudgemental. This is not an easy task. We all have conscious and unconscious attitudes, biases and prejudices that reflect our social background and our learning and life experiences. We all tend to evaluate other people and events from our own personal perspective.

A member of one of the helping professions, however, must learn to understand patients in the light of their backgrounds and experiences. Learning to be nonjudgemental is a conscious undertaking for most people. It is helpful for the nurse to first become aware of personal attitudes and to understand how they were acquired. Attitudes, biases and prejudices are all learned. They can all, therefore, be unlearned or at least modified by additional learning and life experiences. Taking courses in psychology can help a nurse to gain an increased understanding of self and also greater insight into individual differences and the factors motivating behaviour. Courses in sociology and anthropology help in developing an appreciation of cultural and social influences on behaviour. Working with people from other cultures and from different social backgrounds, and getting to know them as individuals, also helps to change attitudes previously held, consciously or unconsciously.

GIVING INFORMATION

Communication is always a two-way process and, in order to keep the communication channels open, both the nurse and the patient must contribute. The nurse is an important source of information for the patient, as we have noted before. The nurse should always answer the patient's questions, both those that have been verbalized and also, where possible, the unspoken ones. Answers should be specific, with as much information as can be provided and in terms that the patient can readily understand. The patient, for example, may say to the nurse, "Dr. Leroux said he was sending in a referral for a neurologist to investigate this ringing in the ears I've been having. What, exactly, did he mean?" The nurse might answer, "He has asked Dr. Mei to come in and check you over. He thinks the problem may be related to the nerves that are involved in hearing. Dr. Mei is one of our top-flight specialists in this field. She will probably be in to see you later this morning." Or, the patient may say, "I hear they are going to operate on me tomorrow. I wish I knew what time." The nurse might say, "I have just seen the schedule for tomorrow's surgery. Your operation is down for eight o'clock in the morning" or, "I don't know just yet. They make up the schedule in the afternoon and we usually have it by three o'clock. As soon as it comes, I will let you know."

LEARNING TO LISTEN

In any nurse–patient communication, the patient's problems, interests, feelings and activities are the primary focus. In order to help the patient, the nurse must learn to listen. Most people will communicate quite readily if they have an attentive listener who is not going to impose personal values on them, nor proffer unwanted advice. The techniques of being a good listener can be learned. Although most beginners tend to feel a little self-conscious using the techniques described below, they soon become a habitual way of responding.

One of the first things to learn is to listen attentively. To patients this conveys that someone is interested and is willing to devote time and energy to hearing what they have to say.

Posture   The nurse's posture is important in conveying to the patient that he or she is listening attentively. Much nurse–patient communication occurs during the process of giving care, and the nurse, particularly in a hospital setting, is usually standing at work. For an interview (such as taking the nursing history), a discussion of problems the patient has, negotiating a contract, or the like, it is always better if the nurse can sit and talk with the patient. Sitting down to talk implies a more relaxed and less hurried manner than standing. Getting out from behind a desk and sitting in a comfortable chair (with the patient also in a comfortable chair) helps to create a more relaxed atmosphere for both the nurse and the patient in a community health setting. Sitting at the same level also helps to convey that you and the patient are equal partners in this relationship. When nurse and patient are on the same level, good eye contact can be maintained. It should be remembered, however, that in some cultures, it is considered disrespectful to look another person directly in the eyes.

The nurse should sit facing the patient directly — this helps to indicate a willingness to listen. Neither arms nor legs should be crossed, as these actions tend to portray a defensive posture. Openness is fostered by a non-defensive posture. It helps for the nurse to lean slightly forward, towards the patient, when talking. Most people do this automatically in conversational situations.

Personal space   The distance between the nurse and patient is also important. Each of us likes to have a certain amount of space around us. It is a natural protective instinct, and we feel threatened when other people intrude upon it. If you are in a crowded elevator, for example, and a number of people get off at one floor, you will almost automatically move to put more space between you and the next person. The amount of room a person likes as **personal space** varies, depending on personal idiosyncrasies, on cultural mores, on how a person feels at the time and on the intimacy of the situation. Some people prefer not to be touched (except in intimate family situations) because they feel that their personal space is being violated. Other people use demonstrative affectionate gestures, like hugging, even among people they do not know very well. Some people when they are ill do not want anyone near them while others are comforted by the presence of others close by.

Studies have been done on the distances most commonly maintained in various types of social interaction. A knowledge of these ranges is useful for nurses to use in judging the space to keep between themselves and patients in different situations, so that both parties feel comfortable.

For *intimate interaction* 7.5 to 45 cm is the average range. This distance is used for confidential information — a whisper can be heard at this distance by most people. It is also used in nonverbal communication, such as putting an arm around the shoulder to comfort someone or cuddling an infant. For *personal interaction*, when you are discussing personal matters, the range is from approximately 0.4 to 1.2 metres. At this distance, a soft voice can be heard by the person with normal hearing but people at a farther distance cannot overhear the conversation. This is the distance to maintain when you are discussing personal matters with the patient. You should be near enough to shake hands or touch the patient's shoulder.

Distances from 1.2 to 3.7 metres are used for most *social interactions* (as in small group discussions). The normal speaking voice is used, but it is important to remember that it can be heard by others within the range. This distance is suited to discussions on non-personal matters. In *public interactions*, such as teaching in a classroom or giving a talk to a fairly large group of people (more than 10 to 12), the distance may be beyond four metres. One has to be careful in these situations to speak in a loud, clear voice and enunciate words clearly. Six to seven and a half metres is usually as far as the average person can project the voice indoors without the use of a microphone, although they may be able to do so up to 30 metres outdoors (Smith and Cantrell, 1988).

Many of the measures nurses use in caring for patients necessitate being in the intimate range of interaction. People often feel uncomfortable at this distance with someone they do not know well, and they may react with a reflex withdrawal. The nurse should, whenever possible, alert the patient beforehand as to what he or she is going to do, so that the patient isn't alarmed by sudden actions at close range.

Listening attentively is an active process. The patient must have the nurse's undivided attention. Some people feel that the nurse should not take notes when talking to a patient to obtain information; others, however, feel that taking notes does not hinder the communication process. Certainly, if a lot of information is needed from the patient, it is difficult to remember everything that has been said without the benefit of notes. It may be reassuring too for the patient to know that details about likes and dislikes, and particular concerns, have been noted and will not be forgotten. Attentive listening is also indicated by the responses the nurse makes.

RESPONSES THAT HELP

Minimal responders   Sometimes just a word or a nod of the head is sufficient to give the patient the feeling that the nurse is interested in what is being said and that the nurse would like the patient to continue. Words or utterances such as "Mmm," "Yes," "I understand," and so forth, have been termed **minimal responders** and are frequently used to reassure the patient of attentiveness.

Silence   Sometimes it is best not to say anything, particularly if the nurse feels that the patient has something to add to an earlier statement. Most of us feel uncomfortable when conversation lapses and, if a pause lasts too long, we want to rush in to fill the space. Often, however, people need to think about what they are going to say and, given a little time, will continue with their train of thought. On the other hand, the person may decide that he or she does not want to pursue the matter any further and will introduce a new topic. The nurse should not press, nor give the appearance of prying into the patient's private affairs. Some people just do not like to talk about personal matters, and the nurse should respect their wishes in this regard. Sometimes, just sitting quietly with the patient or walking together down the corridor is enough to convey that the nurse understands the patient's feelings.

Touch   Touch is a very important form of nonverbal communication for nurses. We use our hands in so many of our nursing measures. Touching the patient's hand or shoulder or holding the sobbing child can convey empathy and attentiveness. There is often no need for words. Touch is something that has to be used with discretion, however, because, as we have already mentioned, some people find touch distressing.

Reflecting feelings   Another way of indicating interest and attention is through the reflection of feelings the patient has expressed. People sometimes express their feelings directly in words, for example, "I was so angry that I…." Sometimes a description of actions allows the nurse to identify the feelings behind the actions. For instance, if a patient says, "I banged on the door," he or she is obviously expressing feelings of frustration and probably hostility towards whoever was on the other side of the door.

The nurse may also pick up clues about the patient's feelings from nonverbal behaviour, as discussed earlier in this chapter. The nurse might respond in words that acknowledge the feelings as, for example, by saying, "I understand that you were angry [or annoyed, or hurt]" or "I can see that this bothers you." Although it can be useful to use the patient's own words in response, it is more important to reflect his or her feelings. Repeating the individual's words can sometimes make the nurse's response sound mechanical, as if parroting a learned response.

Repeating key words or phrases   At times, though, it is helpful to repeat key words or phrases that the patient has used, particularly if a number of thoughts have been expressed at one time. To use an example, a person might say, "Nothing seems to have gone right since I had that operation a year ago. I can't seem to work the way I used to. I haven't been able to go to the club either and I miss that. The club members are a very nice group of people." Here it might be useful for the nurse to pick up the key phrase "since I had that operation a year ago," rather than responding to the specific mention of the club. The nurse could then explore how things have changed for the patient rather than becoming side-tracked on a discussion of the various club members. Repeating a key word or phrase helps to keep the conversation focussed on important issues rather than irrelevant items.

Using open-ended questions or statements

If the nurse wishes to obtain more information about a specific point, it is often helpful to repeat a part of a question or statement that gives the patient an opportunity to say more. The nurse might say, "You said that you had an operation a year ago, perhaps you could tell me more about it." Or, the nurse might simply ask, "You had an operation a year ago?" Sometimes the nurse can use an open-ended statement or question, such as "You were going to say…" or "Would you like to tell me more about it?" to elicit more information from the patient.

Asking for clarification

Sometimes it is difficult to identify feelings or to understand the meaning of a person's words. The nurse might sometimes need to ask for clarification. Phrases such as "you mean that you were angry?" or "am I right in thinking that you felt guilty [or depressed, or sad]?" are examples of responses the nurse could make to verify impressions. Asking for clarification also helps to indicate to the patient that the nurse is trying to understand his or her point of view.

Exploring alternatives

Sometimes the nurse can help patients explore possibilities for resolving problems that they have identified. An awareness of factors in the situation that the patient may not be aware of can be useful when selecting strategies to enable the patient to work through problems to create solutions. The nurse should be careful, however, not to give personal opinions on what the patient should do, but rather to enable consideration of all factors and possible alternatives in the situation.

RESPONSES THAT HINDER

Dismissive reassurance

Responses that hinder the flow of conversation can be made if the nurse does not think about the impact of his or her words. One of the most common ways of cutting off communication is the use of dismissive reassurance. Nurses want to make the patient feel better and, therefore, often say things such as "don't worry, everything is going to be all right," "everybody feels like that," or "we haven't lost a patient yet" (from a simple or routine procedure). Comments such as these may be said with the intention of reassurance, but they may convey to the patient that the nurse is minimizing their problem.

Social clichés

Closely allied to dismissive reassurance as hindering responses are the social clichés that seem to come almost automatically to our lips when we are not thinking about what we are saying. Expressions such as "you'll feel better after a good night's sleep," "your doctor knows what is best for you," and "everything will work out in time" are examples of common clichés, that is, pat answers that are trite and have lost their meaningfulness through overuse. They tend to convey to the patient that the nurse isn't really listening.

Hostility

People who are anxious frequently react with anger and hostility to those around them. Nurses and other health workers often bear the brunt of this anger from patients and their families, and it can be difficult not to be hostile in return. A hostile response made by a nurse, such as "you shouldn't say things like that," can humiliate the patient and, most certainly, will hinder the progress of the nurse–patient relationship. A statement along the lines of "this experience must be terribly difficult for you" can enable the patient to express anxiety directly. In turn the nurse will be able to offer support in an effective manner.

Imposing values

The nurse should be careful not to impose personal values on the patient. "It was wrong of you to do that," or "if I were you, I would have done this or that," are examples of evaluative responses that are best avoided, since they neither support the self-esteem of the patient nor do they facilitate effective problem-solving by the patient.

Giving advice

Giving advice implies to patients that the nurse knows better than they do what they should do. If your advice is being requested on matters pertaining to the patient's health, this is an area in which you are expected to have more knowledge, and advice may be appropriate. Advising people on the conduct of personal matters other than health is generally not acceptable. For example, statements such as "I would tell your sister to stop bothering you," or "If I were you, I'd sell the house and move to a condominium" are likely to cut off communication. Most people don't want advice, unless they specifically ask for it. Even if a patient asks for your opinion, it is wise to refrain from giving advice in areas in which you are not an acknowledged expert. Even when it is a matter of health, it is preferable to help patients to explore alternatives, so they can make their own decisions, rather than giving cut and dried answers.

Probing

We have already mentioned that the nurse should avoid probing into a patient's private life. Exceptions to this rule exist in the area of psychiatric and mental health nursing. In this area the patient will often expect and accept that feelings about personal matters will be explored. Questions such as "why do you feel this way?" or statements such as "tell me more about your relationship with your sister" tend to be probing unless the patient's specific problem necessitates exploration of this nature. Often, the patient may not know the answer, or may resent the intrusion. Patients can be placed in uncomfortable positions when they are asked to explain their actions. Silence can often be used with an attentive manner to enable patients to explore their feelings, without causing them to feel as if their privacy has been invaded.

Belittling Belittling the feelings or actions of another person engenders resentment and diminishes self-esteem. Saying things such as "other people don't seem to feel this way" conveys to patients that there must be something wrong with them to be reacting in this fashion. Telling patients about other people's accomplishments (or problems that are greater than theirs) makes them feel small and insignificant. If a postpartum patient says, "My stitches hurt" and the nurse answers, "You have to expect a little pain. My sister told me she couldn't sit down for a week after she had her baby," the patient is not likely to confide further in the nurse.

Rejection The nurse can cut off communication, consciously or unconsciously, by rejecting the patient's feelings, thoughts or actions. Statements such as "you shouldn't feel like that," "I don't want to hear about it" or "how could anyone do that?" give the impression that the patient's thoughts, feelings or actions are unworthy. The patient is likely, then, to avoid talking further about that subject, and may be hesitant to bring up other matters. Rejection can also be communicated by nonverbal means. Turning away from a person, averting the eyes and subconsciously backing away can all indicate rejection.

A CASE IN POINT

The following example shows how the nurse can affect the patient's well-being through communication.

Mr. Antonio Niccolini is a 64-year-old widower who was admitted to the hospital suffering from difficulty in breathing and pain in his chest, left arm and back. Mr. Niccolini emigrated from Italy 50 years ago and, although he is fluent in English, he can still communicate in Italian. He lives with his daughter and son-in-law and their four teenage children in a predominantly Italian neighbourhood. He is a baker, head of the family business, which he runs with his three sons, who live in the same neighbourhood. Mr. Niccolini's working day is usually from 0400 to 1800 hours, six days a week. He smokes about a pack of cigarettes a day. He enjoys food and is consequently overweight. He drinks what he considers a moderate amount of wine every day. He has never been hospitalized before and appears very anxious about being separated from his family.

Mr. Niccolini is sitting up in bed playing solitaire and muttering to himself when the nurse walks in.

N.: Good morning, Mr. Niccolini. How are you feeling this morning?

Mr. N.: What's good about it? I feel fine. Why can't I go home? I just sit here all day. Why can't I have a cigarette and some decent food? How can you expect me to eat these meals? Now, what I would like is a good steak, some decent bread, and a little wine. I can't even taste the food you give me here.

N.: You seem to be upset this morning, Mr. Niccolini.

(reflecting feeling)

You say you want to go home?

(picking up key words)

Mr. N.: Yes, I want to go home. Nobody's doing anything for me here. They just take my temperature and my blood pressure now and then, and expect me to lie around like this. I have better things to do with my time.

N.: You feel you have a lot to do.

(reflecting feeling and asking for clarification)

Mr. N.: Yes, like who's looking after the bakery, for example? They need me there.

N.: Do your sons work in the bakery with you?

(asking for clarification)

Mr. N.: Yes, yes, my sons. But they all have their own jobs to do — who's going to make the bread? I always make it myself every morning. They need me.

N.: I'm sure they do need you. Mr. Niccolini. Is someone making the bread now while you are in the hospital?

(accepting the patient's feelings and helping him to explore the situation)

Mr. N.: Yes, my oldest boy. But he has his jobs to do too. And who will mind the counter when everyone is busy?

N.: You mind the counter as well as make the bread?

(picking up key phrase)

Mr. N.: My daughter does most of the time, but I help out when things get busy. Luigi comes in and helps on the weekends.

N.: Luigi?

(asking for clarification)

Mr. N.: He's my oldest grandson. He seems to like the bakery or maybe he just likes the money he earns.

N.: Could Luigi come in and help after school?

(helping the patient to explore solutions)

Mr. N.: That might be an idea. Luigi is 17 now and should be taking more responsibility. I'll call my daughter and see about it.

When the nurse comes back a little later, Mr. Niccolini seems a little more cheerful.

N.: Well, Mr. Niccolini, you look as if you are feeling a little bit better now. Did that conversation with your daughter help?

(showing interest in the patient)

Mr. N.: Yes, it did, but I just remembered something.

N.: What's that, Mr. Niccolini?

(encouraging the patient to elaborate)

Mr. N.: I'm supposed to give a speech at the baker's association meeting next week. I've never missed a meeting. I guess that's how I became president. Now I won't be able to go on the day I'm supposed to give my speech.

N.: Do the members of the association know you are in the hospital?

(picking up key words and helping patient to explore the situation)

Mr. N.: No. But my sons will tell them at the meeting tonight. Two meetings in a row I'm going to miss.

N.: Would you like to talk with one of the other members? The vice president perhaps?

(helping patient to explore the possibilities to resolve problem)

Mr. N.: Yes, I would, but not until tomorrow. Otherwise, they might decide to let someone else give my speech, and I want to give it myself later on, when I'm out of hospital.

INTERVIEWING

The interview has been called a "talk with a purpose." It is a basic tool of communication that is used a great deal by health workers, although its use is not, of course, limited to the health field. Most nursing students will have had experience with interviews. If you have applied for a summer or full-time job, for example, you have probably had an interview with your prospective employer.

In the health field, the interview is used for a number of different purposes, by most health professionals. Nurses, in their practice, may use interviewing for gathering information or for verifying it, for assessing the results of nursing care, in counselling people about health matters, in planning with individuals their care and as a therapeutic tool.

When planning an interview, the nurse should take into account not only its purpose, but also the time and the setting for the interview. The nurse should be familiar with some of the basic techniques of interviewing, such as those used in beginning and ending an interview, and in eliciting specific information. As with other skills, interviewing requires practice. Many textbooks and articles have been written on interviewing, and the nurse will probably want to supplement the introductory material presented here with additional readings from the list of references suggested at the end of the section.

SETTING THE TIME AND PLACE FOR THE INTERVIEW

An adequate amount of time should be set aside for the interview; how long is considered adequate will depend on the purpose and nature of the interview. Judgement must be exercised about both the length of time allotted for the interview and the time at which it takes place. If a patient is seriously ill and many new and frightening things are happening, or if the patient has just been admitted to the hospital and is having numerous tests and examinations, it may be best to delay an interview until the immediate crisis is over. Also, if the patient appears to be fatigued, it is wise to terminate an interview and complete the session at another time. Interviews should be scheduled for a time when both the patient and the nurse are free from other commitments. They should not conflict with appointments the patient has for x-rays, laboratory tests, treatments or visiting hours. Nor should the nurse feel hurried or rushed because of other commitments. In short, the nurse should strive to create a relaxed, unhurried atmosphere.

It is always best to have a quiet and private room in which to conduct an interview. This is, however, not always possible in our busy and often crowded health agencies. It is important, though, that the person being interviewed has the undivided attention of the nurse and that confidentiality is being respected. A corner of a lounge or office can be used, or the curtains can be pulled around the bed if the patient is in the hospital and not in a private room.

BEGINNING AN INTERVIEW

An interview is essentially a conversation between two people. Often, as when the patient has just been admitted to the agency, it is a conversation between two strangers. The nurse, as the interviewer, has a responsibility to put the other person at ease. For the beginning student, who may be a bit apprehensive about interviewing someone, it is helpful to remember that the patient, too, is probably anxious. Most people who seek the help of health professionals are either ill or in some way concerned about their health. Even those who are well and attending a health maintenance clinic usually have some minor worries. They are all, therefore, at least a little anxious. It helps if the nurse observes the common courtesies of greeting people — by name, with a smile or a hand shake, by offering a seat (in an ambulatory setting) or asking permission to sit down and talk (if the patient is in an inpatient facility). The nurse should also introduce him- or herself by name. These ate concerns, that is, the patient's feelings and perceptions about the subject of the interview, without interjecting too many questions in the beginning. If the nurse does not allow the patient to speak freely, there is a possibility that important factors may be missed.

It is usually considered most useful, in asking questions, to start with the general and then proceed to specific details. People usually respond much better to impersonal questions at first. The nurse should leave the more personal ones until the patient has had a chance to get to know the nurse a little during the course of the interview. In this age of information, most people are used to filling in forms and answering questions about their name, age, education and place of employment. These are considered relatively impersonal items. An individual's likes, dislikes and feelings are more personal. If the specific information to be elicited requires asking such questions, these should be left until after the general questions have been answered.

ENDING AN INTERVIEW

When the purpose of the interview has been accomplished, the nurse should take some time to ask if the patient has any questions, or if there are other things that he or she is concerned about that were not discussed. Patients often feel that the nurse is too busy and are sometimes reluctant to take up the nurse's time. Taking a few minutes to listen to patient concerns often saves the nurse time in the long run, since patients are less apt to make frequent requests later if they have been reassured that the nurse is concerned about them.

In terminating an interview, it is again important to observe social courtesies. Thanking patients for their time, saying that you will see them again, and assuring them that they can call on you if they are concerned about anything, are all ways of conveying that they are worthy of respect (Braverman, 1990; Justice, 1986; Cameron, 1982; Haselfeld, 1990).

Nurses may use interviews for a number of different purposes in a variety of situations.

courtesies convey a feeling of respect for the person who is being interviewed and help to put him or her at ease.

The nurse should also state the purpose of the interview and the approximate amount of time it will take. This information helps to set the climate for the interview. A patient will feel more comfortable knowing what to expect and what the purpose of the interview is. The nurse might say, in an initial assessment interview, for example, that the purpose is to learn something about the patient so that care can be planned to suit individual needs and preferences.

ELICITING SPECIFIC INFORMATION

Although the nurse often has specific information to obtain from the patient during the interview, it should not be conducted as a strict, one-way question and answer session. It may be a structured interview in the sense that the nurse controls and directs the conversation, as when gathering information in the assessment interview, but the patient should feel free to discuss feelings and concerns. Most people will give all the information needed, and more, if an open climate is created.

When there is specific information that the nurse wants to obtain, some direct questions will have to be asked. In such cases it is probably a good idea to start with immedi-

COMMUNICATING WITH OTHER MEMBERS OF THE HEALTH TEAM

Nurses very seldom work in complete isolation. Even in a remote nursing station where the nurse may be the sole provider of health care for a community, there is almost always telephone, or, at least, radio contact with a base hospital where communication with other members of the health team is possible. More usually, the nurse is employed in a busy, urban health agency with many nurses and a variety of other health personnel. Irrespective of the setting, nurses, by virtue of their roles, must be excellent communicators.

Communication with other members of the health team is an important part of the nurse's work. It is essential for facilitating the process of patient care. Information gathered by all team members provides the basis for planning comprehensive care for the patient. Sharing information helps to avoid duplication of effort in gathering data and also enables each team member to benefit from the information others have collected. Communication is also essential in the planning of patient care; it ensures that everyone shares the same goals for the patient and that care is coordinated and people are not working at cross-purposes.

The actual implementation of health care today is also very much a team effort. The provision of comprehensive care requires the skills and talents of many different disciplines. The physician and the nurse have always worked closely together in many aspects of patient care and continue to do so. With the number of specialized workers in the health field today, however, it is more than ever essential that all coordinate their efforts in caring for patients. There must be adequate, effective communication channels for the achievement of this coordination.

Communication between members of the health team takes place in many ways. A great deal of information is exchanged informally, through face-to-face meetings and telephone conversations. But there are also more formal channels, both oral and written, that help to facilitate the exchange of information.

The patient's record is one very important tool that helps to keep all team members up-to-date on the latest information about a patient and the most recent developments regarding the patient's progress. Patient records will be discussed in detail in Chapter 18, so we will not say more about them at this point. Other common communication media that the nurse will use frequently are reports, both oral and written, consultations, conferences, referrals and patient rounds.

REPORTS

Reporting information to other members of the health team is essential if they are to be briefed on events that have taken place (or are likely to take place), be told of developments that have occurred in regard to patients' progress and be alerted to things to watch for in the care of specific patients. Reports may be given either orally or in writing. At the end of each shift, members of the nursing team usually report orally to the team leader on the progress of each patient. The team leader (or primary nurse, if this system is used) reports to the nurse manager, who uses this information to prepare a change-of-shift report for the nurses who are coming on duty.

The change-of-shift report is usually a fairly formal report, in which the nurse on completing a tour of duty "hands over" the care of patients on the unit to those who will be responsible for their care on the next shift. At this time, the progress of each patient on the unit is reviewed, and the nurse who is leaving briefs the newly arrived staff on treatments or other activities that are still in progress, and on events that are likely to occur on the next shift. The nurse may, for example, say that Dr. X will be phoning Mr. Smith's medication orders this evening, or that the Admitting Department has called to say that the unit will be receiving a new patient.

As part of the change-of-shift report, the Nurse Manager or Charge Nurse often makes rounds with the nurses coming on duty, thus exchanging information about each patient in the process. Many agencies are now using tape recorders to make the change-of-shift report less cumbersome. Each nurse who has been responsible for the care of a group of patients can dictate the report about those patients. Nurses coming on duty then need to receive only a brief report from the Nurse Manager or Charge Nurse going off duty and can obtain direct information about each patient from the tape-recorded report. The Charge Nurse reports to the Nurse Manager about the patients on the unit. The Nurse Manager in turn conveys important information to Nursing Administration and to the chief medical officer responsible for the unit. This is often a written report, supplemented by an oral report as needed.

In addition to patient care reports, most health agencies have a large number of other reports and forms that nurses use. These vary from agency to agency and nurses must familiarize themselves with those used in the agency in which they are working. There are usually forms for requesting laboratory, x-ray and other types of diagnostic tests, forms for recording the administration of narcotics and other controlled drugs (a count has to be kept of these), forms for ordering drugs and other supplies and a good many others. We have already mentioned (in Chapter 6) the accident (incident) report, which is completed whenever an unusual occurrence takes place.

CONSULTATIONS

Often nurses feel the need to consult with other health practitioners about the care of patients. Nurses usually consult informally with peers, or with the Charge Nurse, or with the Nurse Manager, or with both. Nurses also consult with physicians about the patient's plan of care and progress. If there is a Clinical Nurse Specialist available, the nurse may want to consult with him or her about the patient's plan of care, or about unusual problems the patient has. Nurses consult with the physical therapist frequently and with the nutritionist and the social worker — in fact, with all who are involved with the patient's care.

Physicians consult with other physicians; they frequently call in specialists to see patients and give opinions regarding diagnostic or therapeutic measures. The nurse will note the requests for specialist consultations and the specialist's report on the patient's record.

CONFERENCES

Members of the nursing team usually meet daily in a team conference to exchange information about their patients and to review and revise their care plans. Common too are team conferences, at which various members of the health team meet to review their findings about a physician, to develop a combined plan of care or to review the patient progress. Until very recently team conferences have been used most frequently in rehabilitation settings, in community health agencies, in psychiatric settings and in agencies providing long-term care for people who are ill. However, they are common in all types of health care settings.

REFERRALS

Referrals are basically of two types: those requesting the services of another department within an agency in the care of a patient, and those referring a patient to another agency for care. In a multiservice ambulatory health care agency, such as a Community Health Organization (CHO), a Community Health Centre (CHC) or the Outpatient Department of a hospital, patients are frequently referred from one service to another for specialized care. A patient might be referred to the dental or eye clinic, for example, or to the nutritionist or social worker from a generalized service. In a hospital setting, a referral might be made to such departments as social service, physiotherapy or inhalation therapy (respiratory technology) for specialized services for the patient.

Patients may also be referred from one agency to another. A Community Health Organization or Community Health Centre might refer an individual to a hospital for inpatient care (the patient would be admitted under the care of their attending physician) or a hospital might refer a patient to a CHO or CHC. If a patient is being discharged from hospital and requires home care services, a referral would be made to the appropriate agency. Referrals may be made by a community health nurse (or a school nurse) for individuals to receive care from any number of agencies in the community.

A referral system is important to assure continuity of care. It is essential that the agency to which the patient is being referred have sufficient information to assure that continuity. Most agencies have referral forms on which summary information about a patient is written; it is often the nurse who is responsible for completing these forms, although policies vary. In a hospital, the patient's record would be available to the member of the department being called in to see a patient; therefore, the referral is usually simply a request for services.

PATIENT ROUNDS

Another means of communicating information about patients is through patient rounds. We have already mentioned one type, where nurses make the rounds on a nursing unit during the change of shift report. The nurse usually makes rounds with the physician when visiting patients on a hospital nursing unit. A considerable amount of information is exchanged at this time, as opinions are shared regarding the patient's progress and plans are discussed for care. Often, nursing rounds are made by the Nurse Manager on a unit with a supervisor, with the Clinical Nurse Specialist, or with staff nurses on the unit. Teaching rounds are also made for the benefit of students; both medical and nursing schools use patient rounds as learning experiences for students.

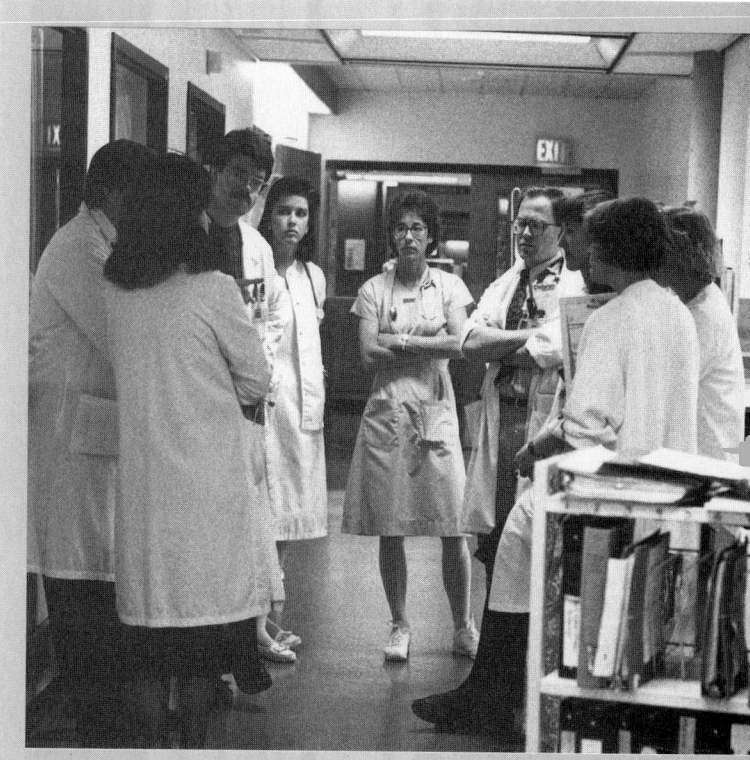

An interdisciplinary team preparing to make rounds on a nursing unit.

KEY TERMS

therapeutic relationship p. 402

empathy p. 402

respect p. 402

climate of trust p. 402

authenticity p. 403

specificity p. 403

orientation phase p. 403

working phase p. 403

patient contract p. 404

termination phase p. 404

source p. 405

message p. 405

channel p. 405

receiver p. 405

feedback p. 405

jargon p. 407

personal space p. 410

minimal responders p. 411

IN REVIEW

The nurse–patient relationship is the core of nursing. It is a professional helping relationship, based on trust and mutual respect, in which nurse and patient work collaboratively to achieve the patient's optimal level of health. Often referred to as a therapeutic relationship, it includes the elements of empathy, respect and authenticity. The nurse uses *specificity* to clarify and validate patient concerns.

The nurse–patient relationship has three phases: the orientation phase, the working phase and the termination phase. During the working phase, a verbal or written contract may be negotiated that provides the patient with reinforcement for the performance of a specific behaviour.

Fundamental to the nurse–patient relationship is the process of communication. The process involves four basic elements: a source, a message, a sender and a receiver, each of which may be influenced by a number of factors that may adversely affect the process. In their communications with patients, colleagues and others, nurses should keep in mind the questions, *who, what, when, where, why,* and *how.* Most messages are sent and received verbally by oral or written means. However, feelings and attitudes are often conveyed by non-verbal means, such as facial expression, posture and grooming, by gestures, by touch and by the tone of one's voice.

To create a climate for open communication, the nurse must convey a feeling of warmth and acceptance. A genuine liking for people and a nonjudgemental attitude towards them is important. Nurses are sources of information for the patient but they must also learn to listen to the patient's problems, interests, feelings and activities with interest and without imposing personal values or offering advice.

To foster open communication, the nurse's posture should be such that good eye contact can be maintained with the patient without infringing on personal space. Some responses that have been found helpful in nurse–patient communication are the minimal responders such as "Mmm," silence, the use of touch instead of words, reflecting the patient's feelings, repeating key words or phrases, using open-ended questions or statements, asking for clarification and helping the patient to explore alternatives. Responses that hinder communication include dismissive reassurance, using social clichés, expressing hostility, imposing one's own values, giving advice, probing, belittling what the patient says or rejecting the patient's feelings, thoughts or actions.

The interview is a basic tool of communication which nurses use to gather information or to verify it, to assess the results of nursing care, to counsel people about health matters, to plan care with individuals and as a therapeutic tool. The nurse communicates with other members of the health team both informally in conversation and through more formal means such as the patient's record, written and oral reports, through consultations, conferences and referrals and through patient rounds.

LEARNING ACTIVITIES

1. With the help of your instructor, select a patient from the clinical area in which you are working. Arrange a time to visit the patient, and, using the agency's form, take a nursing health history. Use the techniques outlined in the "Learning to Listen" section of this chapter to find out about the patient as a person.

   a. Write a short narrative report describing the patient as a person.

   b. List the techniques you found helpful in establishing a climate that encouraged the patient to communicate freely.

   c. Did the patient request information from you? If so, what information? How did you handle the request? What information did you volunteer?

   d. What listening techniques did you use to facilitate conversation between you and the patient?

   e. How did you terminate the interview?

REFERENCES AND READINGS

BRAVERMAN, B.G. (1990). Eliciting assessment data from the patient who is difficult to interview. *Nursing Clinics of North America, 25,* 743–750.

CAMERON, J.E. (1982). "Giant leap forward" begins with the nurse interview. *Australian Nurses Journal, 12,* 47–48.

CRUSCO, A.H. and WETZEL, C.G. (1984). The Midas touch: the effects of interpersonal touch on restaurant tipping. *Personality and Social Psychology Bulletin, 10,* 512–517.

EKMAN, P. (1975, September). Face muscles talk every language. *Psychology Today, 9,* 35.

EKMAN, P., FRIESEN, W., O'SULLIVAN, M. and CHAN, A. (1987). Universal and cultural differences in the judgments of facial expressions. *Journal of Personality and Social Psychology, 53,* 712–717.

FORCHUK, C. and BROWN, B. (1989). Establishing a nurse–patient relationship. *Journal of Psychosocial Nursing and Mental Health Services, 27,* 30–34.

FORCHUK, C. (1992). The orientation phase of the nurse–patient relationship: How long does it take? *Perspectives in Psychiatric Care, 28,* 7–10.

HASELFELD, D. (1990). Patient assessment: Conducting an effective interview. *AORN Journal, 52,* 555–557.

HAYES, W.S. and DAVIS, L. (1980). What is a health care contract? *Health Values, 4*(2), 82–89.

HERJE, P.A. (1980, February). Hows and whys of patient contracting. *Nursing Educator.* 30–34.

JUSTICE, L.A. (1986). Skill sharpening methods in conducting patient interviews. *Today's OR-Nurse, 8,* 32–35.

MATSUMOTO, D. (1992). American–Japanese cultural differences in the recognition of universal facial expressions. *Journal of Cross-Cultural Psychology, 23,* 72–84.

PEPLAU, H.E. (1991) *Interpersonal relations in nursing: A conceptual frame of reference for psychodynamic nursing.* New York: Springer.

PEPLAU, H.E. (1992). Interpersonal relations: A theoretical framework for application in nursing practice. *Nursing Science Quarterly, 5,* 13–18.

ROGERS, E.M. and ROGERS, A. (1976). *Communication in organizations.* New York: The Free Press.

SMITH, B.J. and CANTRELL, P.J. (1988). Distance in nurse–patient encounters. *Journal of Psychosocial Nursing, 26,* 22–26.

STECKEL, S.B. and SWAIN, M.A. (1977). *Hospitals, 51.* 81–84.

CHAPTER 17

Teaching and Learning Skills

CENTRAL QUESTIONS

1. Why is teaching such an important part of the nursing role?
2. How do we learn?
3. Why are teaching and learning considered reciprocal processes?
4. What factors need to be taken into consideration in helping people to learn?
5. What are the three main domains of learning?
6. What teaching strategies are most suitable for learning tasks in each domain?
7. How do you assess a person's learning needs?
8. Are there specific nursing diagnoses related to learning needs?
9. How do you plan, organize and implement a teaching and learning program?
10. How would you assess the success of the program?
11. How can you evaluate your teaching skills?
12. How can you get maximum benefit from your clinical learning experiences?

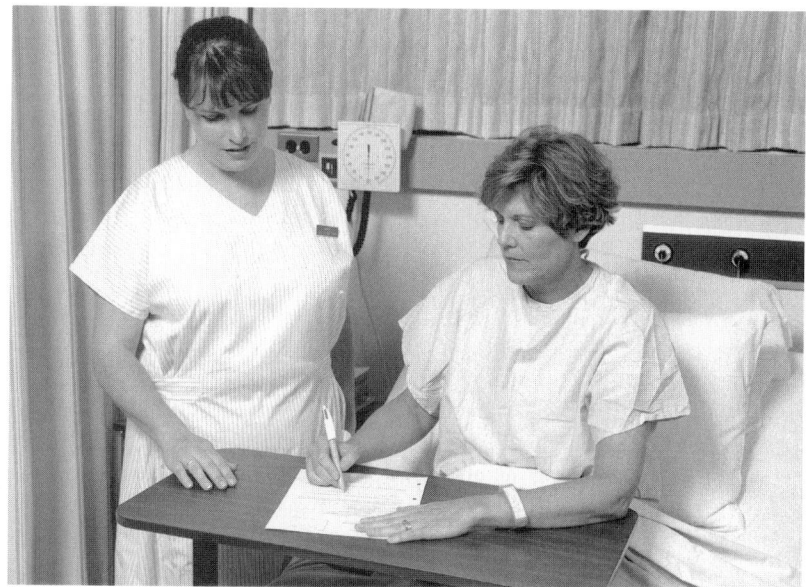

INTRODUCTION

The central goal of nursing is to maintain, strengthen, and develop the patient's health by actively engaging him or her in a learning process.

The McGill Model of Nursing, described in Gottlieb and Rowat, 1987.

An integral component of nursing care is helping individuals and families learn what they need to know to promote, protect and restore their health, or to maintain their comfort and independence in the case of chronic or terminal illness insofar as this is possible. Teaching is a part of the nurse's role through all stages of the life span and in all phases of the health continuum. In Chapter 5, Nursing in Canada, teaching/coaching was identified as one of the major domains of nursing practice. As people assume increasing responsibility for the promotion and protection of their own health, and as more and more restorative and supportive care is transferred from hospital to home, they need to gain the knowledge and skills that will enable them to meet their health needs competently and with confidence. One of the major complaints people have had about professional health care is that they were never given enough information. Today, however, more than ever before, health professionals are sharing their knowledge and skills so individuals and their families can make informed decisions about their health and can take control of their own health care.

Nurses play a key role in teaching about health matters. Nurses are regarded by the public as being knowledgeable about health; their opinion is respected and their advice sought on matters that concern health. As we mentioned in Chapter 9, Health and the Individual, family members or friends who are nurses are among the first people sought for advice when a person becomes ill. By now, you have probably found that your friends and family — and other people too — ask you questions about health matters, even though you are just at the beginning of your nursing program. You cannot possibly expect to be able to teach everybody all they want or need to know about health at this stage of your career, or even after you have completed your nursing course. But you can help them learn how to access the information they seek.

Teaching should be incorporated into the nursing care of every patient. The teaching aspects of care, then, need to be incorporated into the steps of the nursing process as you work through these in providing care. In order to be able to incorporate teaching in your nursing care, you need to understand both the learning and the teaching processes, as well as the factors that influence an individual's ability to learn. These topics are covered in the first section of this chapter. The next section discusses the assessment of learning needs, nursing diagnoses involving learning needs, the planning of teaching and learning sessions, interventions to implement these plans and evaluation of the effectiveness of teaching and learning programs. The third and final section of the chapter discusses ways you as a learner can get maximum benefit from your clinical practicums.

THE LEARNING PROCESS

Learning is an active process that continues from birth to death. Throughout our lifetime, we are constantly learning as we gain information, develop skills, acquire attitudes and apply these in adjusting to new life situations. Learning takes place either informally, through the ordinary activities of living, or formally, through a series of selected learning experiences designed to achieve specific goals.

We learn a great deal about health and illness through informal means. In the home, for example, parents usually teach children basic hygiene measures, such as washing hands before meals and using tissues. Children also learn measures to protect their health: "Don't go outside without your coat on — you'll catch cold" or "Wear your rubber boots — you don't want to get your feet wet and take a chill."

Care during illness is also a part of childhood learning experiences. The child is put to bed when a fever strikes. The parent has certain remedies for a cold, and these are passed on to the child through informal teaching methods. Dietary habits too are learned in the home. The learning that occurs in the family is supplemented by informal talks with people in the popular health sector, such as a neighbour who is a nurse, the person who works in the local health food store and others considered knowledgeable about health.

Other sources, such as books, newspaper and magazine articles or radio and television shows about health matters, contribute to informal learning. Additionally, people who are ill and need the help of health professionals for restorative and supportive care usually learn much about their health problems and how to care for themselves informally through the actual experience of being ill.

There are, however, situations in all phases of the health care continuum where more structured teaching is needed. In today's world, we place a high social value on health and our thirst for knowledge about health matters appears unquenchable. *Wellness centres* are popular, particularly among members of the rapidly growing older segment of the population. *Wellness programs* are also developing in corporations, industrial plants and other places of business as the cornerstone of occupational health programs. In wellness centres and wellness programs, the promotion and protection of health are the primary focus. In restorative and supportive care of people who are ill, patient education is a recognized part of total care.

Many hospitals and long-term care agencies, as well as community agencies, have separate patient education departments. The fact that an agency has a separate department, however, does not eliminate or negate in any way the individual nurse's role in teaching. The departments gather and prepare resources that can be used by nurses and by patients and their families, such as pamphlets, copies of articles by experts about specific conditions, and other reference materials including textbooks, video- and audiotapes and interactive computer programs. Staff of a patient education department may engage in direct patient teaching, for example, by running a series of classes for newly diagnosed diabetic patients and/or by providing guidance, teaching aids and other resources for staff on the nursing units. In home care, a great part of the nurse's role is helping people to take as much responsibility for their own (or a family member's) health as they possibly can.

THE PHENOMENON OF LEARNING

Theories have been postulated by numerous educators over the past century to explain the phenomenon of learning. Most theories have been based on studies that have measured the ease with which learning takes place (how much was learned? how long did it take?), the extent of learning retention (how much was retained? for how long?) and observations of changes in the thinking patterns of children as they develop. You are probably familiar with many of these learning theories from your introductory courses in psychology. Among the schools of thought which have influenced North American education are:

1. **The Behaviourist School**. Proponents of this school believe that all learning is manifested in observable changes in behaviour and that learning can be controlled by manipulating factors in the environment. Also known as operant conditioning, this stimulus–response–reinforcement model has been used in numerous behaviour modification programs to help people substitute desirable behaviours for undesirable ones.

2. **The Cognitive School**. Believers in the cognitive model think that learning is not necessarily always observable; it is an intellectual process using cognitive skills. Learning, according to the cognitive theorists, can be thought of as information processing. Programmed learning texts and computer learning packages are based on this model of learning.

3. **The Humanist School**. Humanists believe that learning is more than a mechanistic exercise; meaningful learning must involve the whole person including both the intellect and the emotions.*

As we noted in Chapter 1, there has been a growing disenchantment with science and a return to humanism in many fields of endeavour. In education, the scientific, tech-

nological view of learning as operant conditioning or as information processing is giving way to the humanistic approach. One of the main proponents of this approach is Carl Rogers, a humanist whose work has influenced many nurse theorists. Rogers believed that it is impossible to teach another person directly: one can only facilitate the learning (Rogers, 1969. Cited in Knowles, 1990, 79).

The trend to humanism in education is in line with the broadened definition of health we discussed in Chapter 2, as a "resource for everyday living, encompassing social and personal resources, as well as physical capabilities." The humanist school of thought in education views the learner as a whole person and is concerned more with the overall growth of the individual in both cognitive and affective areas than with the content of what is taught per se. The role of the teacher has shifted, too, from one of "instructor" to one of "facilitator" (Yelon and Weinstein, 1977), in much the same way that the role of the nurse has shifted from care-provider to collaborator with the individual in health care.

The fact that humanism has become the dominant philosophy in education does not negate the work by people of other schools of thought who have contributed greatly to our knowledge of the process of learning. In the process of teaching, most of us use concepts derived from behavioural theory, from cognitive theory and from humanist theory. Everyone does better when efforts are rewarded — when there is reinforcement of learning. This would happen, for example, when content and presentation are structured (as the cognitive theorists recommend) and we apply the humanist principles of respect for the total person (Yelon and Weinstein, 1977). Goodwin Watson developed a list of "what we know about learning" which incorporates findings from the research of educators from different schools of thought. Malcolm Knowles (1990), one of the leading figures in adult education, suggests that Watson's list could serve as "guidelines for the facilitation of learning."

THE TEACHING PROCESS

Teaching and learning are collaborative processes. The teacher's role is to assist learners to acquire the knowledge, skills and attitudes they need to learn. Teaching facilitates the learning process. It is not just a matter of imparting information, of giving someone the ability to do something or of changing opinions or feelings. The behavioural changes all have to take place in the learner, and the teacher can only guide and direct the learning process, so that it takes place more easily and more effectively (Benoliel and Soule, 1988). There is an adage in the education field that says if the student hasn't learned, the teacher hasn't taught. This saying sums up the reciprocal nature of teaching and learning.

* Yelon and Weinstein, 1977.

Guidelines for the Facilitation of Learning

1. Behaviour which is rewarded — from the learner's point of view — is more likely to recur.

2. Sheer repetition without reward is a poor way to learn.

3. Threat and punishment have variable effects upon learning, but they can and do produce avoidance behaviour — in which reward is the diminution of punishment possibilities.

4. How "ready" we are to learn something new is contingent upon the confluence of diverse — and changing — factors, some of which include:

   a. adequacy of previous experience on which to build (we can learn only in relation to what we already know)

   b. significance and relevance of the material to be learned to the learner's own purposes (we learn only what is appropriate to our purposes)

   c. freedom from discouragement, the expectation of failure, or threats to physical, emotional or intellectual well-being.

5. Whatever is to be learned will remain unlearnable if we believe that we cannot learn it, or if we perceive it as irrelevant, or if the learning situation is perceived as threatening.

6. Novelty (per 4 and 5 above) is generally rewarding.

7. We learn best that which we participate in selecting and planning ourselves.

8. Genuine participation (as compared with feigned participation to avoid punishment) intensifies motivation, flexibility and rate of learning.

9. An autocratic atmosphere (produced by a dominating teacher who controls direction via intricate punishments) produces in learners apathetic conformity, various — and frequently devious — kinds of defiance, "scapegoating" (venting hostility on a colleague), or escape. . . . An autocratic atmosphere also produces increasing dependence upon the authority, with consequent obsequiousness, anxiety, shyness and acquiescence.

10. "Closed," authoritarian environments (such as are characteristic of many conventional schools and classrooms) condemn most learners to continuing criticism, sarcasm, discouragement and failure so that self-confidence, aspiration (for anything but escape) and a healthy self-concept are destroyed.

11. The best time to learn anything is when whatever is to be learned is immediately useful to us.

12. An "open," non-authoritarian atmosphere can be seen as conducive to learner initiative and creativity, encouraging the learning of attitudes of self-confidence, originality, self-reliance, enterprise and independence; all of which is equivalent to learning how to learn.

SOURCE: Adapted from Watson, 1960–61. In M. Knowles (1990). *The adult learner: A neglected species.* Houston: Gulf, 81–82. Reprinted with permission.

TEACHING STYLES

The style a teacher uses — the way of conducting classes and guiding other learning experiences — reflects the teacher's leadership role with the students. At one end of the continuum is the *autocratic* style, in which all decisions are made by the teacher, and there is little or no opportunity for the student to have a voice in the goals to be achieved or in the nature of the learning experience, or to take any responsibility for its direction. An extreme example of the autocratic style of teaching is the nurse who tells the patient, "these are the things you need to know," and proceeds to give a nonstop talk about the patient's medical condition, or whatever else it was the nurse set out to teach. This type of teaching gives the impression that nurses feel they know better than the patients what the patients need to know, a perception that can engender resentment.

At the other end of the continuum is the *laissez-faire* style of teaching, in which decisions about what is to be learned and how it is to be learned are left entirely up to the students. While this style may be effective with a group of well-motivated and well-educated adults, it is all too easy for a group to be sidetracked and to deviate from its original goals.

The middle style on the continuum is the *democratic* style, in which the learner participates in establishing goals, assumes some responsibility for the conduct of the learning session, and feels free to participate in decisions regarding the direction of the experience. The humanists believe that this style is most effective in facilitating learning (Yelon and Weinstein, 1977).

However, it is important to remember that the styles represent a continuum; teachers may display varying degrees of these styles, and students will respond better to some styles than to others according to their own background and preferences (some feel more comfortable in a more structured learning situation, others react against it). And while it can be difficult to develop a style that pleases all students, it is usually wise to strive for a middle-of-the-road, democratic approach in teaching patients.

Recent research on the specialization of different areas of the brain and on the concept of dominance — that is, the tendency to favour the use of one hemisphere of the brain over the other — has had considerable implications for the use of different teaching styles. Brain dominance and specialization affect our general behaviour, as well as our learning styles.

On the whole, people whose thinking is dominated by the left hemisphere of the brain are more verbal, logical and analytical, and tend to use sequential thinking. They usually prefer a structured learning environment, with lectures and textbooks, and they take to programmed learning easily. People with right-sided dominance are more intuitive and creative, preferring pictures to words. They use simultaneous and holistic thinking, rather than sequential thinking. These people prefer a more experiential approach, with case studies and group interaction rather than more traditionally structured learning (Covey, 1990).

Knowledge of the specialization of the brain combined with the concept of dominance has introduced researchers to a multiplicity of possibilities regarding the different ways people learn. This knowledge means that each individual must be considered "as a unique learner with learning preferences and avoidances different from other learners" (Knowles, 1990, 241). It means too that people respond differently to different methods of teaching. It is important to find out how a patient learns best and to adjust your teaching strategies accordingly (for more on the concept of brain dominance and its implications for structuring teaching and learning, refer to Hermann, 1987, as cited in Knowles, 1990, 241–249).

DETERMINANTS OF TEACHING AND LEARNING

A number of factors affect the reciprocal processes of teaching and learning. The most important variables in these processes are the characteristics of the learner, the characteristics of the teacher, the nature of the material to be learned and the social climate of the situation in which teaching and learning take place.

CHARACTERISTICS OF THE LEARNER

"The chief factor that influences the nurse's teaching is the nature of the learner, the physical and emotional state, the age, social and cultural background, education and experience, the voluntary nature of the patient's relationship to the nurse as teacher" (Pohl, 1981, 53). In developing an educational program it is important to know something about the learner or learners.

> ### *Foundation Stones of Modern Adult Learning Theory*
>
> - Adults are motivated to learn as they experience needs and interests that learning will satisfy; therefore, these are the appropriate starting points for organizing adult learning activities.
> - Adults' orientation to learning is life-centred; therefore, the appropriate units for organizing adult learning are life situations not subjects.
> - Experience is the richest resource for adults' learning; therefore, the core methodology of adult education is the analysis of experience.
> - Adults have a deep need to be self-directed; therefore, the role of the teacher is to engage in a process of mutual enquiry with them rather than to transmit his or her knowledge to them and then evaluate their conformity to it.
>
> SOURCE: Knowles, M. (1978). *The adult learner: A neglected species* (2nd ed.). Houston: Gulf, 31.

Age   Age is a factor that affects both learning and the teaching done to facilitate learning. Young children do not think in abstract terms. They need the concrete — something they can see, do, feel, touch, taste or smell or something they have experienced. They usually have fertile imaginations, but their imagery is based on past experience. If imaginary situations are used in teaching, then, they need to be based on experiences familiar to the child, such as going to the store, playing with friends, helping Mummy or Daddy, or, for teaching about health, blasting germs with ray guns (Rankin and Stallings, 1990; Redman, 1993).

Adults are usually more goal-oriented in their learning than children are and more selective in what they learn (Cantor, 1992). With adult learners, it is well to remember Malcolm Knowles' "foundation stones of modern adult learning theory" shown in the box above.

Communication skills   Teaching patients is essentially a communication process, with the interaction between nurse and patient at its core (Rorden, 1987). The individual's ability to communicate needs to be taken into account when planning patient teaching. For example, both hearing and vision become less acute with advancing age. If you are teaching a group of older adults, you will probably find that you have to talk a little louder than you normally would, enunciate your words more clearly, and perhaps provide written material in larger print.

Lack of a common language can be a considerable barrier to teaching and learning. If the patient speaks only a language that is foreign to you, you can use nonverbal

The library is a learning resource for patients and their families as well as for health agency staff.

communication to a certain extent — gestures, pantomiming, diagrams or printed material in the patient's language. When there are complicated instructions, or complex material to be learned, an interpreter is needed. Often, a family member or friend accompanying the patient can help. Many agencies whose clientele includes people of different ethnic origins have staff members who speak one or more of the languages commonly used by patients and are often called upon to assist in interpreting. Many agencies also have phrase books in different languages for use in departments such as Emergency and a wide range of teaching materials which have been translated into the languages used by different ethnic groups in the community. The Canadian Translators and Interpreters Council is also a good resource for interpreters or people to help with translating learning materials. (Translators work in written material, interpreters with oral speech.) The provincial branches each maintain a directory of qualified translators and interpreters for their jurisdiction.

Even when you share a common language it is important to ensure that the words you use are understandable to the patient. You would use different terms in teaching adults and children, for example. You would probably expect a college graduate to understand terms that a person with less education would not. However, many people without a college degree have extended their formal education through reading, attendance at continuing education classes, or life experience and have gained an extensive vocabulary. One should never make the mistake of "talking down" to people just because they have not had much formal education. Conversely, education does not guarantee familiarity with

medical terminology, and dealing with those in stress may require stating things simply and repeating important points.

Cultural background   As we discussed in Chapter 12, Health and Ethnicity, the cultural background of the patient is another factor to be considered. It is important to assess the individual's subjective beliefs and perceptions as well as looking at more objective characteristics of the learner (Rorden, 1987). Customs and mores vary from one ethnic group to another, from one part of the country to another, and from one socioeconomic group to another.

In one particular instance, new mothers in a hospital in northern India scoffed at a nurse's demonstration of bathing a baby. When asked why they laughed, they said they could bathe six babies in the time it took the nurse to bathe one. On further questioning, they said they would not use a basin, soap and a washcloth as the nurse did. They would sit on the mud floor of their one-room home in the village and, holding the baby between their ankles with one hand, pour water from a jug over him or her with the other, letting the water flow off the baby into an open drain in the floor. The nurse did a little research with a community health nurse and, in the next round of classes, demonstrated a "safer" method for the procedure the mothers had described. The nurse also showed them the basin method while sitting on a mat on the floor. This time the teaching was accepted with no scoffing. It should be pointed out that the nurse was from the same geographic region as the mothers, but from a different socioeconomic group.

State of health   In health teaching, the state of the patient's health must be considered. When we are ill we usually have a shorter attention span than when we are well. Teaching sessions for ill patients need to be short and gauged to the patient's ability to participate. One should not attempt to teach any more than patients need to know for their own safety when they are seriously ill. Hence, deep-breathing exercises should be taught preoperatively, when patients are feeling relatively well, rather than postoperatively, when they may be in considerable pain, not as alert as they normally would be owing to effects of the anesthetic or medication and generally not feeling well.

It is important, too, to find out what patients already know about their health status to determine the base of experience on which new learning can be built. People today are much more knowledgeable about health matters in general and their own health problems in particular than they were 20 years ago. Health information is much more readily available today. A patient may, in fact, sometimes know much more than the nurse about a particular health problem, and the nurse will have to do some extra studying in order to help the individual extend his or her knowledge and skills. However, the nurse should never assume that patients know everything they want or need to know about tests and procedures, or want to know about their health and health problems. It is always wise to ask patients both what they know and what they want to know.

Motivation The individual's **motivation** for learning is also vitally important. As we discussed earlier, in the guidelines for the facilitation of learning, to be most effective, learning must be in response to what the learners perceive as *their* needs; the learners must feel that what is being taught is relevant to *their* purposes. Someone who has participated in a hypertension screening clinic and been told that his or her blood pressure is a little elevated is much more motivated to learn about hypertension and what can be done to bring blood pressure down than would be the person whose readings are normal. Confirmed smokers may not be motivated to learn techniques for breaking the nicotine habit until they have a sore throat that will not go away or they find they are having trouble breathing. For some people, it is only when they see noticeable changes in their health that they really feel the need to stop.

CHARACTERISTICS OF THE TEACHER

The teacher is, of course, a key figure in the process of teaching and learning. We can all think of memorable teachers who influenced us, from whom we feel we learned the most and, with their guidance, most easily.

Knowledge of subject matter A good knowledge of the subject matter is basic (Cantor, 1992). If you are going to help a group of overweight individuals — or even one individual — to learn how to control their diet to lose weight, you will need to have a good knowledge of foods and the nutrients they contain, as well as their caloric content. You should be familiar with the Canada Food Guide put out by the federal government in Canada. It is also helpful to have guides for estimating the number of calories expended during various types of activity, such as swimming, jogging, bicycling, resting and various types of housework.

You, as a knowledgeable health professional, are a resource for the group you are teaching and you will want to be prepared to answer their questions and have materials available for them. It is a good idea, when you are planning a teaching session, to think of questions people might ask. If, during the actual teaching session, you find you do not have the answer to someone's question, don't be afraid to say, "I don't know, but I will see what I can do to find the answer to your question next session." Or, you might give patients references so they can research a particular issue further on their own. If you feel confident in your mastery of the subject matter on other points, you will feel more comfortable in saying this. Even the best of teachers are not expected to have all the answers.

When you are teaching skills, you must be sure of your mastery of these before you attempt to teach someone else. It is always helpful to practise the skill beforehand, even if you think you know it well, just to refresh your memory. You might enlist the help of one of your classmates to observe, so you can have the point of view of someone watching you perform the procedure.

Using strategies and assessing needs Knowledge of the subject matter is, however, not enough to guarantee effective teaching. The teacher also has to have skill in using teaching strategies to communicate the material effectively. We will discuss strategies commonly used in teaching patients in the next section of the chapter. A knowledge of the various methods that can be used will help you to select the one best suited to meet a particular patient's needs. Skill in using the different strategies will come with practice, as is true of any other skill. A wide range of teaching aids, including models, charts, diagrams, audio- and videotapes on a wide variety of health topics, is available to help you in your teaching. You will need to become skilled in handling the various types of audiovisual equipment to use them successfully.

The teacher must also have skill in assessing the learner's needs and in planning and organizing the material to be taught. In thinking about teaching, the fundamental questions are: What is the patient going to have to do? What does the patient therefore need to learn? We will discuss these questions in detail later in this chapter.

Planning and organizing skills When the material to be learned has been identified, the teacher needs planning and organizing skills. How much material should be included? Can it all be taught in one session, or are several sessions needed? What should be presented first? Are there things that need to be taught before something else can be learned? Where should the teaching be done? Do I need to prepare the place beforehand? What materials do I need? Are there teaching aids I can use? These are some of the questions to ask yourself when you are planning and organizing a teaching program.

THE SOCIAL CLIMATE

Another important factor that affects teaching and learning is the **social climate**. Teachers need good interpersonal skills to be able to foster a climate that is conducive to learning. People cannot learn easily if they feel threatened (Watson, 1969 in Knowles, 1990; Waines, 1993). Many patients view the nurse as an authority figure and it is important to dispel any threats the patient may feel. In this regard, the material in Chapter 16, Communication Skills, on creating an open climate for communication is relevant in the process of teaching and learning.

In teaching, both on a one-to-one basis and in groups, it is important to have an atmosphere in which each person feels free to participate and the communication channels remain open. When you are teaching a group of patients, you will find that there is interaction not only between you as teacher and the learners but also among the learners. People feel more comfortable in a group when they know who the other members are and why they are there. It is helpful at the beginning of a teaching session to have everyone introduce themselves and, perhaps, tell a little about their background and why they are there attending the program.

The authority inherent in the nurse's role is made less threatening if the nurse sits as a member of the group, rather than standing at the front of the room behind a lectern. A more relaxed, informal atmosphere is promoted if everyone can sit around a table. In many situations, however, this is not feasible. If the group is large or if you need to use aids such as flip-charts or a blackboard, you should stand where everyone can see you and you can see everyone in the class. It is important that both you and the learners feel comfortable and at ease, and that everyone is within sight and hearing range.

NATURE OF THE MATERIAL

Basically, there are three basic domains of learning tasks: one involves the acquisition of knowledge (the **cognitive domain**), one, the development of skills (the **psychomotor domain**) and one the development, or changing, of attitudes (the **affective domain**).

During your educational program, you will acquire a considerable amount of *knowledge* through the classes you attend, the reading you do, the projects you undertake, and the assignments you are asked to do, as well as from your experience in the clinical area. You will also develop a repertoire of nursing *skills*. In the course of your program, you will probably change your *attitude* about a good many things. For example, you may overcome a fear of the operating room once you have had experience there. You may even begin to enjoy getting up in the early morning hours to be on duty by seven o'clock in the morning. It is during your clinical experiences that you learn to apply your knowledge and skills, and put the attitudes you have acquired into practice in the real-life situations that constitute nursing.

Additionally, in teaching patients, the nurse's primary concern is that the patients use their knowledge and skills in day-to-day living. This application involves the integration and application of knowledge, skills and attitudes. A person may learn all about nutrients and calories, for example, and may develop skill in planning meals that contain nutritious, low-calorie foods, but is not likely to lose weight — the purpose of the learning — unless he or she actually carries through with the planned menu at home and does not deviate by adding additional snacks or increasing quantities.

Many patient learning needs can be categorized as "knowledge to be gained." As we have stated before, this is a need that is frequently expressed by patients. People want to know what is happening to them, what the test or examination is all about (and what the results are as quickly as possible), and what they can do to become more physically fit, to hasten their recovery or to meet whatever goal led them to seek help from the health agency.

Patients also often need to learn new skills. A patient with a spinal cord injury who is not in traction may need to learn the skill of log-rolling for turning in bed, for example. The diabetic must learn to test urine or blood samples for sugar and acetone and the new parent needs to learn the skill of bathing a small infant.

Often, before other learning can occur, attitudinal changes need to take place. Patients have to recognize the need to take their medications on time and appreciate the significance of skipping a dose. If people feel that the material to be learned is not important or relevant to them, they are likely to adopt an attitude of "why bother?" Attitudes are very important in the application of learning.

TEACHING AND LEARNING STRATEGIES FOR DIFFERENT LEARNING TASKS

Various teaching and learning strategies are particularly suitable for each type of learning task.

STRATEGIES FOR ACQUIRING KNOWLEDGE

A newcomer in the field of patient education that is proving to be very useful in helping people to acquire knowledge is the interactive computer program, which may well revolutionize patient teaching. It is used extensively, for example, in patient teaching at the British Columbia Children's Hospital. Families can gain confidence in decision-making, through having the opportunity to consider various alternative courses of action.

In keeping with the philosophy of the learner as an active participant in identifying learning needs and seeking the information needed to meet these needs, the hospital has established a Family Resource library. Learning resources have been developed by staff and materials collected from other sources for use by patients and their families.

The library holdings include reference books, articles and other written materials on various health problems and other relevant subjects, as well as videotapes that can be borrowed for in-agency or home use. A major part of the holdings is a collection of interactive computer programs. Discharge planning is facilitated because families can go to the library and use the computer programs to learn about the care the child requires at home, the danger signals they need to be alert to and other matters about which they would like more information. Printouts can be made from the computer for people to peruse at their leisure and to keep as reference material. Other pamphlets and written material are also available for patients and their families in a number of different languages (British Columbia Children's Hospital, 1994).

Written materials are available from your local health department and from numerous other agencies concerned with specific health problems, such as the Arthritis Society and the Lung Association. There are pamphlets on smoking, nutrition, exercise, hypertension, heart disease and a great many other topics that will be useful in teaching patients. The health agency in which you are gaining clinical experience may have developed patient teaching handouts for patients with problems that are common in the area. Handouts are very useful to supplement teaching by other means. They can be taken home and kept at the bedside, to be read and reviewed at leisure, or referred to at a later date. Some samples are shown in Figure 17.1.

Interactive computer programs and written materials may be used separately or in conjunction with other forms of teaching. Information, for example, may be presented in the form of a lecture, or short talk, or during the course of a conversation. Conversation is suitable when you are dealing with one patient, or a very small group (two to four patients). For most groups, the *lecture* or *talk* is usually more appropriate. A straight **lecture**, or uninterrupted talk, however, does not involve much activity on the part of the learner, except through the sense of hearing, and it depends on the ability to listen attentively. If you are giving a talk, it is wise to remember that the attention span of the average adult is only about 20 minutes. It is less for children and for old people, and usually less for those who are ill. In order to ensure that this span will not be exceeded, one should vary the techniques used in teaching, and intersperse lecturing with other techniques such as discussion and looking at diagrams or other visual aids.

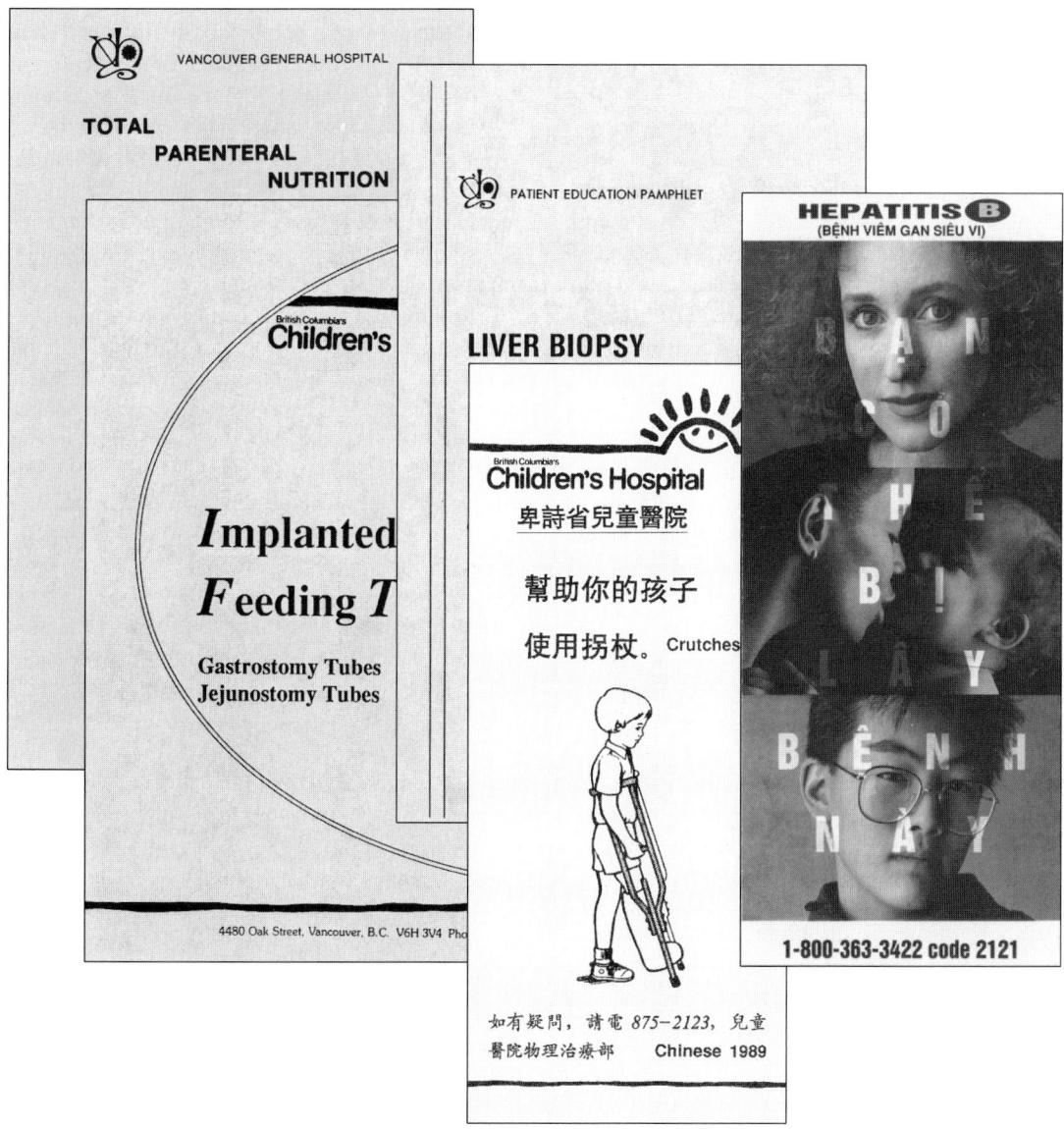

FIGURE 17.1   Sample patient teaching materials

SOURCE: The Vancouver Hospital and Health Sciences Centre, the British Columbia Children's Hospital and the Canadian Liver Foundation. Reprinted with permission.

Discussion, which involves participation on the part of the patient, facilitates the retention of learning. In conversation and in group discussions, the participants have to have some knowledge of the subject at hand in order to discuss it intelligently. There also needs to be some structure to the session, that is, someone guiding and directing it, for it to be effective. The combination of a short talk followed by discussion is often a good way of structuring a teaching session.

Audiovisual materials are also useful adjuncts to teaching. Illustrating a talk with diagrams or pictures on a blackboard, flip-chart or piece of paper, will often help you to get points across that are difficult to grasp through words alone. Models are also useful supplements for teaching. Models of various portions of food, for example, are often used in teaching people to estimate the size of a portion that weighs a certain number of grams. There are also various anatomical models available, of the eye, for example, the uterus and other anatomical structures.

Many slides, audio- and videotapes about common health problems have been developed to help in teaching patients. When using audiovisual aids in teaching, it is a good idea to review these ahead of time, in order to assess their suitability and relevance to the class and to become familiar with the content. The actual presentation should be introduced with an explanation of the purpose of viewing the slide or video and the points to watch for during the presentation. Opportunity should be provided for discussion during or after the presentation to clarify a point or to emphasize basic concepts or key points that are illustrated.

Storytelling is a useful technique for presenting information to children. Given the nature of children's imaginations, situations used in the story should be based on things familiar to the child. A number of illustrated children's books are available on the market to help children prepare for a hospital experience, and cartoons and comic strips have been developed to help children learn about health topics such as nutrition, brushing their teeth and other hygiene measures.

STRATEGIES FOR DEVELOPING MOTOR SKILLS

Complex movements, such as those involved in skill development, involve the establishment of a series of connections in the neural pathways between the brain and the muscles. In order to develop skill in carrying out a procedure, it is necessary to go through the movements of doing it and to practise these movements until proficiency is achieved.

Patients learning to give themselves an injection of insulin, for example, have to go through the motions of sterilizing the syringe and needle (or unwrapping the package), assembling the equipment, disinfecting the top of the insulin container, drawing up the correct amount, selecting an injection site, cleansing it and giving themselves the injection. A complicated series of sequenced movements is involved in the skill.

Appropriate methods for learning various skills are used extensively in nursing education programs, and you are probably already familiar with the demonstration (or lecture-demonstration), the return demonstration, and skill practice.

In demonstrating a specific skill, the nurse should wherever possible use the type of equipment the patient will be using at home. Is the individual or caregiver going to use disposable syringes, for example, or glass ones that will need to be sterilized? (The disposable ones are expensive if you are on a minimal income.) Many health agencies have standard trays of home care equipment consisting of common household items. Nurses can use these to advantage in demonstrating many nursing measures to patients.

In giving a *demonstration*, the nurse should first explain what is going to be done and why it is to be done in this way (referring to basic principles or concepts is helpful). The nurse should always be sure that the learner can see exactly what he or she is doing. For example, the learner should be able to see the numbers on the syringe when learning to draw up a liquid. An overview of the procedure is given first; then the procedure is broken down into steps. Key points are stressed while the nurse is demonstrating. The material that is being taught can often be related to something that is familiar to the patient, so that the learning can be transferred from the familiar to a new area. A person who is familiar with canning procedures will find it easier to learn to sterilize equipment when similarities in the procedures are pointed out.

Audiovisual materials can be used advantageously in teaching many skills. A short videotape can help the learner to visualize the procedure and can often be used as a substitute for an actual demonstration by the teacher. A written outline of the procedure, with diagrams illustrating key points, is also helpful, particularly if there are several steps involved in the procedure. These provide a set of directions

A community health nurse and new mothers at a breastfeeding clinic.

to which learners can refer when they are returning the demonstration or practising on their own.

The patient should have an opportunity to perform the procedure in a **return demonstration** soon after the nurse has demonstrated it — preferably immediately afterward. It is helpful to guide and direct patients through the various steps when they are returning your demonstration, so that they perform them correctly and in the right sequence. In learning a skill, accuracy is more important than speed in the beginning. Efficiency and speed will come with practice. Sufficient practice sessions should be arranged so that the patient feels confident before having to perform the skill alone.

STRATEGIES FOR ATTITUDINAL CHANGES

Learning experiences to help people change their attitude about something are, perhaps, the most difficult to structure. Attitudes often develop over a long period of time; many we acquire almost subconsciously. A person's attitude towards the importance of having regular meals, for example, is usually acquired in the home through early childhood experience.

Attitudes can be changed, however, through a variety of teaching strategies. To use a familiar example, through an intensive educational program over the past few years on the part of the Canadian government and private health associations, we are changing from a nation of armchair athletes to one where millions of people consider a regular exercise program an essential part of their lives. We have changed our attitude about exercise. We have also changed our attitude towards smoking. A generation ago, learning to smoke was almost a rite of passage in nursing schools. Today, very few nursing students smoke. The proportion of smokers in the general population has declined substantially. The strategies used to bring about these changes have included a massive campaign that has used every available form of mass communication, including radio and television programs, newspaper articles, and the wide distribution of pamphlets and other written materials, the development of physical fitness testing centres, and the holding of clinics and workshops on common health problems across the country.

Attitudes towards the material to be learned will affect whether or not patients actually put their learning into practice. Patients have to recognize the need to take their medications on time, and appreciate the effect of skipping a dose, if they are to maintain a regular schedule. If the material learned does not seem important or relevant, they are not likely to apply it.

Often, attitudinal changes come about with increased knowledge. A hypertensive person who understands the effects of obesity on blood pressure, for example, will be more likely to recognize the importance of losing weight and more likely to participate in a weight-reduction pro-

gram. An awareness of the potential problems of high blood pressure, such as heart disease, a stroke or kidney failure, will help them to realize the importance of keeping to their treatment regimen.

In helping people to change their attitude and apply their knowledge and skills, it is important to remember two of the basic guidelines for the facilitation of learning:

- To be meaningful, learning must be in response to what the learner perceives as needed.
- Learning is made easier when learners achieve a reward as a result of their behaviour.

In changing attitudes, as well as in helping people to acquire knowledge and develop motor skills, it is important to know something about the patients' needs and priorities. What things are important to them? What are the things that give them satisfaction? What do they find rewarding? (Cantor, 1992).

THE APPLICATION OF LEARNING

The nurse's primary concern is that patients apply the knowledge and use the skills they have learned. Having the information, and being able to perform the skills, is not enough; they must apply these. To learn to apply their knowledge and skills, the learners must be actively involved. Some teaching strategies are particularly useful in helping people to apply their learning.

Problem-solving   The *problem-solving* method has been suggested by educators as very appropriate for learning to apply knowledge. This method is useful in teaching patients. The steps in problem-solving include:

1.   perceiving a learning need
2.   exploring possible solutions
3.   selecting one solution to be tried
4.   putting the solution into action
5.   evaluating the results of this action, reconsidering, and possibly trying other solutions.

The nurse's role in problem-solving is one of supportive assistant. The nurse helps the patient to identify the learning need, gather information, and assess the relative merits of various alternative courses of action. The nurse may help the individual (or family) to select and try one course of action, and assist in evaluating this action.

For example, an older man who has been hospitalized for a kidney condition has been told by his physician that he should stay on a salt-free diet. The nutritionist, or dietitian, has given this patient information regarding foods that are low in salt, and he appears to accept the idea of salt substitutes to flavour his food. He seems worried about being able to stay on the diet at home. The nurse may help him to identify the problem. The individual and his wife are older and they live alone. His wife does the cooking. He is afraid that it is going to give her extra work to cook his meals without salt.

The nurse helps him to work through possible solutions. Has he talked to his wife about his concerns? It would seem that the wife, who does the cooking, should be consulted in solving the problem. Together the patient and his wife might examine possible solutions. The patient's food could be cooked separately, in which case there would be two meals to prepare and two sets of pots and pans to wash. Or, food for both could be cooked together without salt, and the patient's wife could add salt to hers later. Many people find food tasteless when salt is not added during the cooking, and the wife may not like her food cooked this way. Both alternatives should be explored and a decision reached. The couple may decide to try cooking meals for both together without salt. If this solution does not work, then they can try the alternative.

There are many examples that could be cited of situations in which problem-solving seems the logical method for helping patients to understand their disease processes and make realistic plans to care for themselves. The patient's family needs to be included, since many problems related to health and illness involve adjustments in family living. Family members, particularly wives, mothers and daughters, are very frequently the caregivers in a family.

Case study The **case study** is another method that is often used in helping people to apply knowledge. The case study includes a description of a person with the same problem the patient has, and a series of questions or points to consider in a discussion. Potential real-life situations may be described and the patients asked to tell what they would do. The use of an imaginary person is helpful because it is less threatening to the individual concerned. It is a strategy that is often useful in helping to bring about attitudinal changes. People often feel freer to express their feelings and opinions about an imaginary person than about themselves.

Role-play **Role-play** is another useful strategy in helping people to apply knowledge and skills. Again, an imaginary situation is used. People in a weight-reduction program, for example, might be asked to think of going to the market and selecting foods to feed themselves and their families. The situation might then be acted out by participants — or they might actually go to the market. This strategy is helpful in encouraging people to express feelings and attitudes or to work through difficult situations. It is most effective when it is relatively unstructured, and the participants are permitted to develop the situation as they go along. Not everyone feels comfortable with role-play, however, and it is time-consuming.

Children usually love role-playing, and this is a strategy that can be used very effectively with them. It is a good way to help them acquire new information, with the nurse in the role of teacher, storekeeper, TV character or other

suitable figure. And role-playing can also be used for demonstrations, return demonstrations and practice sessions in learning new skills. It can also be very effective in helping children put into practice material they have learned in a simulated situation that is close to real-life situations they may encounter (Redman, 1993).

Behaviour modification **Behaviour modification** is a strategy that is frequently used in helping people to replace behaviours that are undesirable with new ones that are desirable. Originally used in mental institutions to bring about changes in the behaviour of mentally retarded individuals, it is now being used in many situations where lifestyle patterns need to be changed. The process involves the substitution of healthy habits (or behaviours) for unhealthy ones. In order to do this effectively, the desirable behaviour has to be learned first. The behaviour modification technique is used in many programs designed to help people to stop smoking, for example, or to stop overeating. It is also used in helping children to "unlearn" behaviour that is undesirable, such as bullying or fighting with other children, and to substitute desirable behaviour, such as playing cooperatively, helping smaller children, and the like.

Behaviour modification is based on rewarding the desirable behaviour and extinguishing the undesirable through a lack of reinforcement. The child is rewarded for good behaviour with praise, stars on a chart or other suitable tangible rewards. The undesirable behaviour is ignored and is extinguished because it is not reinforced (Redman, 1993). Sometimes an aversive response to the undesirable behaviour, such as separating the child from a group of children temporarily when the child is disrupting it, may be used in combination with rewards for good behaviour.

Methods used for helping people to stop smoking often use behaviour modification, such as substituting a new habit, like walking around the block, instead of the usual coffee and cigarette after dinner. In one "last resort" method, smokers are encouraged to smoke continuously for a period of time until they get to the point where they cannot stand the sight or smell of cigarettes. Pleasure in smoking is replaced by distaste. Behaviour modification has also been used in some instances in treating alcoholics. A substance to induce vomiting is put into alcoholic drinks, so that every time the alcoholic takes a drink, he or she vomits. The technique involves substituting an unpleasant response to alcohol consumption for the pleasurable effect it had for the individual.

INCORPORATING TEACHING IN NURSING CARE

People who seek the help of professional health care providers all have learning needs. Teaching and learning interventions should therefore be incorporated into all nursing-care plans.

I am an Enterostomal Therapist in a regional hospital in northern British Columbia. I have had formal post-basic education in the management of "ostomies," wounds (including pressure sores and leg ulcers) and incontinence.

This morning I visited patients on the surgical ward who have undergone ostomy surgery. One of the patients, Mrs. Gopal, is recovering from colostomy surgery for a ruptured bowel, caused by an acute inflammatory condition of the colon. She had never heard of a colostomy before her surgery and feels overwhelmed by the thought of wearing a pouch. Her ostomy is temporary but she is concerned about how she will manage pouch care because she has limited hand dexterity due to arthritis. I discussed the nature of the surgery and the results with Mrs. Gopal, and I think she has a better understanding of her condition and the reasons for the surgery. I also left some of our Patient Teaching pamphlets with her and arranged to have a member of the United Ostomy Association visit to give her some moral support and help her with the day-to-day concerns of living with a colostomy.

This afternoon, I will see patients in the Ostomy Outpatient Clinic. Mr. Kucera, I know, is slated for surgery and is coming in for his preoperative assessment. He has had Crohn's disease (a chronic inflammatory condition of the small intestine) for 10 years and has had two bowel resections. He still has extensive Crohn's disease in the anal canal. He is exhausted with pain and has elected to have a permanent ileostomy. During the preoperative session I have with him, I will:

- assess the level of his understanding about the surgery, based on what his physician has told him

- use some simple diagrams to show him the structure of the gastrointestinal tract, the section that will be involved in the surgery and the alteration that will be done
- describe in simple terms the stoma, the output and appliance management
- reassure Mr. Kucera that he can resume his activities of daily living after surgery; he does not have to give up his favourite sports of fishing, hunting and curling. Mr. Kucera has discussed with his surgeon possible sexual implications of the surgery
- discuss dietary implications with him and give him a patient teaching handout on this topic
- give Mr. Kucera a list of local ostomy supply retailers and discuss with him the procedure for obtaining financial assistance for these supplies if he should need it
- provide him with a contact number for the United Ostomy Association.

It is also my responsibility to mark the stoma site with indelible pen in the right lower quadrant of the abdomen, below the belt line and within the patient's range of vision. After I have done this, I will tell Mr. Kucera that I will see him in the hospital after his surgery. There, my role will be to promote Mr. Kucera's independence in ostomy self-care so that he can successfully return to the community.

Another part of my role as an enterostomal therapy nurse is to act as a resource consultant to the United Ostomy Association and to other hospitals and agencies in northern British Columbia.

—Lenore Du Gas, R.N., E.T
Prince George Regional Hospital

In this section of the chapter, we review the steps of the nursing process the nurse would carry out in meeting teaching and learning needs in a specific situation: that of surgical patients with a colostomy or ileostomy (the opening of some portion of the colon or ileum to the outer surface of the abdominal wall; the opening is called the stoma).

ASSESSMENT OF LEARNING NEEDS

In assessing learning needs, the basic question is what does the patient need (or want) to be able to know or do? It is important to clarify your perception of needs in relation to the perception of the individual who is to do the learning,

to be sure that you, as teacher, and the patient, as learner, are both headed in the same direction. The two patients described by the Enterostomal Therapist in the box entitled Nurses at Work would appear to have similar needs. Both need to learn more about their condition, the type of surgery they have had, or are going to have, and how to care for themselves at home. The nurse would verify with the patients that these are indeed the things they want to learn and they might add other points. Some health agencies have developed a questionnaire that is given to patients to identify their particular learning needs. A sample questionnaire is shown in Figure 17.2.

In addition to knowing exactly what the patients' learning needs are, it is important to assess the factors that may affect their learning. You will want to assess the level of

Please check off as many of the items as you like. Thank you for helping us to help you.

I would like to know more about:

_____ the nature of my medical condition and its causes

_____ the reasons for the surgery

_____ what was done during the surgery

_____ what will my abdomen look like after it has healed

_____ pouch care

_____ care of the skin around the opening

_____ diet considerations

_____ daily living with an ostomy

_____ what to do if something unusual happens

Other things I would like to know:

_____

_____

_____

_____

_____

FIGURE 17.2 Questionnaire on learning needs for a patient with a colostomy or ileostomy

SOURCE: Adapted from a questionnaire on learning needs for a diabetic patient in Haggard, A. (1989). *Handbook of patient education.* Rockville, MD: Aspen, 33. Adapted with permission.

Guidelines for assessing a patient's learning needs

- What does the patient perceive as their learning need(s)?
- What is the patient's motivation for learning? (Why does he or she want to learn?)
- How old is the patient?
- What is the patient's state of health?
- What is the patient's level of education?
- What is the patient's cultural background: ethnic origin, language(s) spoken, religion practised?
- What is the patient's lifestyle like?
- What are the patient's coping capacities?
- How does the patient think that he or she learns best? Group discussion? Individual instruction? Programmed instruction? Written materials?

their knowledge about and past experience in promoting and protecting their health or about the disease or condition that they have. It is helpful to know how strong their motivation is to learn (Why do they want to learn this?). Also helpful is information about age, educational level and ethnic and/or religious background. Ability to communicate is also important; you will want to know if patients speak English (or French) fluently enough to participate in discussions and, if not, what their mother tongue is, so that an interpreter can be available to assist with the teaching process. It is helpful to know something about lifestyle, particular strengths and likes and dislikes in regard to learning methods.

NURSING DIAGNOSES AND LEARNING NEEDS

According to Jenny, **knowledge deficit** is not a nursing diagnosis since it "does not represent a human response, alteration, or pattern of dysfunction but rather a related factor" (Jenny, 1987, cited in Carpenito, 1993, 474). Individual (or family) teaching, then, is a part of nursing interventions for all nursing diagnoses. For example, if the nursing diagnosis for an individual is *sleep pattern disturbance*, teaching interventions would be indicated to help the person to reestablish a normal sleep pattern. If a lack of knowledge is the principal cause of a diagnosis, the diagnosis might be stated as *anxiety related to insufficient knowledge of preoperative routines*. Other examples might be *high risk for infection related to lack of knowledge of safety precautions in handling contaminated equipment* or *ineffective management of therapeutic regime due to lack of knowledge regarding medications ordered by physician*. With Mrs. Gopal (from the Nurses at Work box) possible diagnoses might be:

> *High risk of ineffective management of therapeutic regimen, related to insufficient knowledge of ostomy care*
>
> *Anxiety related to concern over managing ostomy care at home*
>
> *Self-concept disturbance related to sudden change in body structure following surgery* (Carpenito, 1993, 482, 483).

With Mr. Kucera, we might add:

> *Anxiety related to possible lifestyle disturbance as a result of surgery.*

Once the diagnoses have been established, they need to be placed in order of priority. What is most important to be achieved first — because of its critical nature (for the learner's or other people's safety)? In this case, the diagnoses are probably in the correct order unless Mrs. Gopal's anxiety was too overwhelming and needed to be dealt with first.

PLANNING TEACHING AND LEARNING INTERVENTIONS

Once the nurse has identified the nature of the learning needs, verified these with the individual, and developed diagnostic statements, the next step is to develop outcome criteria (goals or objectives). For example:

> *Mrs. Gopal will demonstrate skill in changing the pouch/stoma dressing before she is discharged from the hospital*

> *Mr. Kucera will relate less anxiety related to managing ostomy care at home before he leaves the hospital.*

When you have identified the outcome criteria, you will want to analyze the learning tasks involved in achieving them. These include the knowledge, skills and attitudes the learner needs to gain. The questions in this case are: What does the person need to know in order to manage ostomy care effectively at home? To reduce anxiety? To restore a healthy self-concept? What does the patient need to be able to do? What skills need to be learned? Are there attitudinal components that need to be considered? In your written plan, it is helpful to list the learning needs under the headings of knowledge, skills, and attitudes, so that you do not overlook any in planning your teaching.

DEVELOPING A TEACHING PLAN

Once the learning tasks have been identified, the next step is developing a teaching plan. First of all, the learning tasks should be organized into logical groups and arranged in sequential order. For example, all content dealing with the patient's condition could be taught as one group of knowledge components and information about equipment and supplies in conjunction with a demonstration of the skills of dressing change and/or pouch care could be taught as a separate grouping. Skin care would logically follow the dressing or pouch change. It is helpful to ask: What must be learned before other behaviours can be learned? Do any of the tasks (or outcomes) involve something the patient may find frightening? (It is usually wise not to try to tackle these first.) What are the key, or most important, behaviours the person must learn?

The next step is to identify suitable learning experiences so that the learners can achieve the desired outcomes. The appropriate strategies, such as a lecture or short talk, discussion, demonstration, return demonstration or others we have discussed will need to be selected. It is also a good idea at this stage to identify teaching aids that could be helpful, such as videotapes, diagrams, handouts and the like.

The teaching plan may be brief, including simply the expected outcomes and the method to be used in teaching. Or, it may also include the content in brief or key points.

Many agencies have developed teaching plans for patients with specific problems. Figure 17.3 is a copy of a patient teaching flowsheet for patients with a colostomy or ileostomy used in one hospital. Flowsheets help to ensure that all material that people need to learn is covered. On the flowsheet various health professionals may be indicated as responsible for teaching, with the physician and the enterostomal therapist, or RN, explaining the nature of the medical condition, its causes and the aims of treatment. The enterostomal therapist or registered nurse is responsible for the remainder of the teaching. Note also the stated objectives (which have been abbreviated for the written teaching plan), the grouping of learning tasks and the sequence of content indicated. Teaching aids are listed at the beginning of the plan and referred to by number in the plan.

All teachers develop their own style of lesson plan. The important thing to remember is that the plan is to help the teacher to keep in mind the expected outcomes (reasons for teaching) and to serve as a reminder of what needs to be covered (Carpenito, 1993; Redman, 1993; Rankin and Stallings, 1990; Rorden, 1987).

IMPLEMENTING THE PLAN

Selecting the time and place for teaching

Much teaching in the community is done in the patient's home, usually in the living room or the kitchen, wherever the individual feels most comfortable. Some may take place in a classroom in the local community centre, or in the health room at a school. With patients coming into a hospital and those who are already inpatients, some of the teaching will be in a class or conference room, some in an office in the ambulatory services or outpatient department and some at the patient's bedside. It is important, when discussing personal matters, to ensure privacy for the individual; if the patient is not in a private room, it might be a good idea to take him or her to a conference room or lounge on the unit, or draw the curtains around the bed.

All teaching, if it is to be worthwhile, takes time. Some of the nurse's teaching may be done informally, during the process of talking with the patient, but when specific material is to be taught, a definite plan should be developed and sufficient time should be allocated for carrying it out. A time that is suitable for both the learner and the nurse — when neither feels rushed and the learner is not overly tired — should be selected. The choice of time varies, depending upon the learner's activities and the nurse's schedule. In an ambulatory care setting, there may be definite times allocated when classes are scheduled for people with common concerns, for example, the prospective parenthood classes run

B.C. CHILDREN'S HOSPITAL

PATIENT TEACHING FLOWSHEET—COLOSTOMY/ILEOSTOMY	Addressograph

Teaching Aids / Key

Key	Title
1	Children with an Ostomy
2	Teaching Doll
3	These Special Children
4	Nutritional Care
5	Convatec Booklet - Parents Guide
6	Convatec Booklet - Teenage Guide
7	Hirschprung's Pamphlet
8	ET Business Card
9	UOA Pamphlet

Req'd Yes/NO	Objective Knowledge/Skills	Key	Date & sign when teaching done.	Comments & concerns (indicate further teaching required, referrals, notes on chart)
	Anatomy & Physiology Is familiar with: - normal anatomy and physiology - nature of medical condition - causes of medical condition - aims of treatment	1, 7		
	Physical Management Stoma Care - able to describe what a stoma is, its purpose, appearance, location and type of construction - is familiar with types of ostomy pouches and products, such as: - paste - barrier - pouch - powder - observes pouch/stoma dressing change - demonstrates pouch/stoma dressing change - empties pouch and suggests alternate methods	1, 2, 5, 6		
	Skin Care - prepares skin for changing pouch - reviews signs of skin problems requiring attention, such as: - yeast/fungal infection - severe excoriation - ulceration			

FIGURE 17.3   Patient teaching flowsheet

(continued on the next page)

B.C. CHILDREN'S HOSPITAL

PATIENT TEACHING FLOWSHEET—COLOSTOMY/ILEOSTOMY		Addressograph

Teaching Aids / Key

Key	Title
1	Children with an Ostomy
2	Teaching Doll
3	These Special Children
4	Nutritional Care
5	Convatec Booklet - Parents Guide
6	Convatec Booklet - Teenage Guide
7	Hirschprung's Pamphlet
8	ET Business Card
9	UOA Pamphlet

Req'd Yes/No	Objective Knowledge/Skills	Key	Date & sign when teaching done.	Comments & concerns (indicate further teaching required, referrals, notes on charts)

	Nutrition
	
	- reviews general information concerning:
	  - food blockage
	    gas
	    odour
		4		

	Potential Problems Outlines signs and actions to take re: - obstruction, dehydration, constipation, diarrhea, prolapse, parastomal hernai, stomal bleeding, and stomal swelling	1		
	Daily Activities Review general points concerning: - hygiene/bathing - play/sports - school/work - travel	1, 5, 6		
	Psychosocial Has had opportunity to discuss: - body image/loss - telling others - sex, pregnancy, birth control	5,6		
	Discharge Planning Reviews procedures for ordering supplies - has list of equipment/supplies - states follow-up clinic appointment - is familiar to UOA - aware of how to contact ET	8		

FIGURE 17.3

Continued

SOURCE: The British Columbia Children's Hospital.

by some agencies, or classes for people with diabetes or other specific health problems. There may also be regularly scheduled classes in an inpatient facility to accommodate people with similar problems, for example, in a preadmission clinic for those slated for the same type of surgery.

Often, however, the teaching needs to be done on an individual basis. In inpatient facilities, the period in the morning after treatment and care have been completed, or the early afternoon, are often good times for teaching. For the sick, teaching periods are kept relatively short because most people, during illness, have a decreased attention span, and the nurse must be careful not to try to cover too much in any one session.

Whenever possible, one nurse should initiate and carry through the teaching plan. Patients usually prefer to have the same person teaching them, and the nurse can develop a more effective relationship with the patient and provide continuity by carrying through the complete teaching plan. If this is not feasible, however, a team approach in which each nurse is responsible for one aspect of teaching can be used quite effectively.

Preparing for the teaching session   The nurse will need to prepare the material to be taught and to decide how much material to include; it should all be appropriate to the goals of the learners and relevant to their needs. Far less theoretical content would be needed for teaching people enrolled in a home nursing course to take temperatures, for example, than is included in university or college nursing classes. The best criterion for selecting content is what is important to the learner and what can be covered in the time allotted. Research or extra studying is always a good idea to ensure thorough knowledge of the subject matter and mastery of skills.

The place where the teaching is to be done may need to be prepared ahead of time. It is always a good idea to check that everything that will be needed (blackboard, flip-chart or audiovisual aids) is there in the room ahead of time. It is important to check that there are enough chairs, and a place to put notes, materials and equipment. Equipment, such as a slide projector or VCR, should be checked to make sure it is in working order. Whenever possible, it is helpful to go through the entire session in a "dry run," either alone or with another person. A classmate or family member can be helpful in this regard.

Conducting the teaching session   In conducting a teaching session, whether for one person or a group of people, it is important that the learners are clear on the expected outcomes. These should be reviewed at the beginning of the session. The session should then proceed logically from one point to the next. The learners should understand one step, or point, before the teacher moves on to the next. Feedback techniques, such as asking the patient (or group) if everything is clear or if there are any questions, are useful in making the decision whether to go on with the next point.

Asking learners to restate in their own words what they have just heard is another useful technique. It is always a good idea, too, to watch for signs of a lack of interest or irritability that may indicate that learners are not ready to go on to new material. At the end of the session, the learners should be left with a clear idea of the main points of the teaching session.

EVALUATING THE LEARNING THAT HAS TAKEN PLACE

Evaluation is the assessment of how far the learner has come along the road towards attainment of the pre-established goals. If the expected outcomes (objectives) have been stated specifically in terms of what the learner is expected to be able to do at the end of the teaching program, the task of evaluating the effectiveness of the learning is relatively simple. For example, one objective mentioned in the Nurses at Work box for both Mrs. Gopal and Mr. Kucera is that they demonstrate skill in changing the pouch/stoma dressing. The extent of Mrs. Gopal's and Mr. Kucera's learning would be evaluated through the nurse's observations of their actually changing their pouch or stoma dressing.

Methods of evaluating learning will vary with each of the four types of learning task. If the task has been one of acquiring information — for example, learning more about action to take if there are untoward complications when the patient is back at home — questioning the patient is a good method of finding out the extent of knowledge. Can the patient list the complications? Does he or she understand the significance of them? Does the patient know what to do about them?

The acquisition of skills can be assessed by observing the ability to carry out the specific procedures, as we noted above. Some other questions might be: Do Mrs. Gopal and Mr. Kucera use good skin care techniques around the stoma of their ostomy? Do they know how to prepare the equipment for pouch/stoma dressing change, handle it and maintain good technique while doing it? Questioning the patient while he or she is performing the procedure helps to ascertain whether the patient understands the principles involved. In assessing attitudes, it is important to look at not only whether a person applies knowledge and skills but also the way they apply them. For example, is the patient careful to maintain good technique in handling the pouch or dressing? Attitudes can also be assessed through talking with the patient. For example, if Mrs. Gopal tells the nurse that she is less anxious about how she is going to manage on her own, then the teaching can be considered successful.

In assessing the application of knowledge and skills, observing what the patient does in a given situation is the best way of measuring this type of learning. In assessing how well Mrs. Gopal and Mr. Kucera manage their ostomy care at home, the nurse must either pay a follow-up visit to the patients at home or rely on the patients' reporting of how they are managing when they come in for post-surgery appointments at the Outpatient Department. If the hospital Enterostomal Therapist does not make home visits, the liaison between hospital and community agency is vitally important to ensure the needed follow-up in the home. Indeed, one of the most important responsibilities of the community health nurse is helping people to apply their knowledge in day-to-day living.

EVALUATING TEACHING

The questions shown in the box below can be used to help evaluate how well a teaching session with one patient or a group of patients was conducted. As a nursing student, you can apply these questions to your own teaching sessions. The questions are organized under headings that correspond to the skills of the teacher which affect teaching and learning (these were discussed earlier, although not in this order).

DOCUMENTING PATIENT TEACHING

In patient teaching, it is essential that all members of the health care team are familiar with the plan for teaching and all know their responsibilities in carrying it out. The communication tools used by nurses for patient teaching include the patient's record, nursing care plans and forms that have been designed specifically for patient teaching, such as the patient teaching flowsheet shown in Figure 17.3. It can be a

---

Guide for evaluation of your teaching

Planning Skills

1. Did you have a written plan?
2. Did you state the objectives for the session clearly and specifically, in behavioural terms?
3. Were the objectives attainable in the time available for the session?
4. Was the content relevant to the patients' needs?
5. Was the content appropriate considering what the patients already knew or were able to do?
6. Did you include appropriate material and strategies?

Organizing Skills

1. Were the time and place for the teaching adequate? Appropriate?
2. Did you make sure the place for teaching was ready?
3. Did you have all your equipment and supplies ready before the session?
4. Did you make sure that all participants had a clear, unobstructed view of equipment and materials used?
5. Did you make the objectives clear to participants at the beginning of the session?
6. Did you develop the lesson logically and sequentially?
7. Did you stop to see if the participants understood and were clear on one point before you proceeded to the next?
8. Did you emphasize key points in your conclusion?
9. At the end of the session, did the participants have a clear understanding of what it was all about?

Skill in Using Teaching Strategies

1. Do you feel the strategies you used were effective in gaining and holding the attention of participants?
2. Do you feel the strategies were appropriate for the content of the session?
3. Did you use teaching aids effectively (blackboard, diagrams, audiovisuals)?
4. Was the language you used clear and precise? Was it appropriate for the participants?
5. Did you explain technical terms?
6. Did you project your voice clearly so that everyone could hear you?
7. Do you think the participants found the session interesting?
8. Were the patients attentive?
9. Did the patients participate in the session?
10. Did you use appropriate techniques to evaluate the extent of the patients' learning?

Mastery of Subject Matter

1. Was subject matter correct in terms of current theory and practice?
2. Did you explain basic concepts clearly and simply?
3. Did you explain to the patients how this session related to the total program? How it was related to their needs?
4. Did you use approved technique in demonstrating a skill?
5. Do you feel you answered the patients' questions appropriately?

good idea to have a copy of the teaching plan in the patient's room and one in the nursing station to ensure that everyone is aware of the plan and their specific responsibilities in carrying it out (Haggard, 1989; Rankin and Stallings, 1990).

The teaching that is done needs to be recorded on the patient's chart just like any other intervention in nursing care. In some agencies, the patient teaching flowsheet becomes a part of the permanent record. In others, both the teaching plan and the individual's response to it are included on the patient's record.

APPLYING YOUR OWN LEARNING IN THE CLINICAL SETTING

The goal of your educational program is to use the knowledge, skills and attitudes you acquire during the various courses in the nursing program in your subsequent practice as a nurse. Your learning experiences in the clinical area are designed to help you to apply what you have learned in the classroom and the laboratory. To this end, you will probably have clinical experience in a variety of patient care settings — in an acute care agency, probably in an extended care facility or nursing home, and in various community health agencies. In these experiences, you will be assisted and guided by your clinical instructors and also by staff of the agency. The following section of the chapter is intended to offer some practical suggestions for getting the most out of your clinical experiences. These are particularly relevant to experience in inpatient facilities — where a large portion of your clinical time will be spent, and where the majority of graduate nurses work — but it will also be applicable in community agencies.

1. *Always be punctual for clinical assignments.* Few things feel worse (or are more annoying to people who are waiting for you) than being late before you get started. The day starts early in most inpatient health agencies, and it is up to you to arrange your personal life so that you arrive at the right place, dressed in the approved attire and looking neat and professionally well groomed, ready to start work at the appointed hour.

2. *Become familiar with the physical layout of the unit.* You will probably have an orientation tour, but it is hard to remember where everything is — particularly if you have clinical experience in a number of different agencies. Do not hesitate to ask if you are not sure where the linen cupboard is or where supplies are kept. It will save you considerable time if you don't have to search on your own.

3. *Make sure you know the names of key personnel on the unit,* such as the nurse manager or nurse responsible for patients

you will be caring for, and other staff with whom you will be working. It is always helpful to write the names down.

4. *Find out all you can about the patient,* or patients, to whom you will be giving care, before you start your care. Your instructor will probably give you a brief review, and you may have been present at the change of shift report, but you will want to supplement this information with looking at the patient's record and the Kardex (if it is used on the unit), or at the computer file on the patient. In some programs, students are expected to go to the nursing unit the evening before clinical practice to prepare for the next day's assignment. If this is the case in your program, it is wise to go when the unit is not too busy. The early evening hours are a good time in many units. Don't forget to introduce yourself to the nurse in charge of the unit, explain why you are there, and ask permission to look at charts and other records. You will need identification if the charge nurse does not know you; you should carry your student identification card with you. In many situations, however, it is not practical or feasible for students to go to the unit in advance of clinical practice. Your instructor may give you time at the beginning of the clinical practice period to review patient records and plan your activities, or you may have to incorporate these activities into your own plan.

5. *Make sure you know exactly what you are supposed to do in your assignment.* Uncertainties frequently arise. Are you supposed to help with serving meals and gathering up meal trays, for example, or is this done by staff from the food service department? Are you expected to take your patient's temperature, pulse and respirations as part of morning care, or is this task assigned to one staff member? Are you supposed to fill the humidifier at the patient's bedside, or is this done by a respiratory technologist? Should you empty a drainage bag, or, if it is full, alert the team leader to this fact? Do you throw the contents away? Most of these things will probably have been explained to you by your instructor (or primary nurse whose patients you are caring for), but routines vary from one agency to another. Or, you may not remember exactly what was said. Don't hesitate to ask!

6. *Take the initiative in getting as much experience as you can.* If there are procedures you have not been supervised in doing, and they are available on the unit, ask if you can do them. Instructors cannot remember everything that everyone has done, particularly if they have several students to supervise. They will check with their group, to make sure all procedures included in the objectives for the assignment have been done, but there may have been something that has been left over from an earlier assignment. There may not have been opportunity for you to have had the experience. Some procedures that you will be expected to do as a graduate are not done very frequently any more — catheterization is one example. You have to take a certain amount

of responsibility for your own learning. If a treatment you would like to see is being performed on the unit, ask your instructor if it can be arranged for you to watch it.

7. *Always be courteous in asking questions.* You will get a better response if you are polite and respectful when you are asking questions, asking for assistance or requesting the opportunity to do something. Address the person by name, phrase your request in proper language, and do not forget to thank the person for his or her assistance. Try not to interrupt when people are busy unless the matter is urgent, if you need help with a patient right away. The patient's safety is paramount in any situation.

8. *Learn to organize your activities so that you complete your assignments on time.* In nursing, there are always unexpected things happening — the patient's physician may come in when you are in the midst of giving the patient a bed (blanket) bath, the operating room schedule may have been rearranged and you find that the time your patient is scheduled to go to surgery has been advanced. It is not always possible to adhere to the plan you have made, but you should have a plan. It is a good idea to list all the things you are going to have to do during the clinical practice period, and arrange them in the order in which you will be doing them. If you have just one patient to care for, things are less complicated and reasonably straightforward. You will need to put into your plan the times when you must do certain activities, such as giving a medication or helping a patient to ambulate.

If you have two or more patients to care for, you will need a little more organizing skill. At this point, we will introduce you to a technique that is borrowed from ad-

ministration courses. It is called the *critical path* technique. You will find that you can use the basic methodology of this technique in coordinating all your morning activities. The idea of the *critical path* is that you have a given starting time, a given finishing time, and a certain number of things to accomplish between these times.

For example, if you need to be in class by 0800 hours, you have to set your alarm clock for 0600 hours to allow time to get up, have a shower, get dressed, listen to the early morning news, eat breakfast, organize your books and other things to take with you, start your car (or get out the exact change for the bus) and allow sufficient time to get wherever you are going. You have probably found that you can do some things at the same time as others. You can listen to the news while getting dressed, for example. Or you may have the coffee perking or breakfast cooking while you take a shower. Some things need to be done before others. You have to get washed before getting dressed. Most people have their morning activities down to a science — some to the split second. Others just never seem able to get themselves organized. Figure 17.4 illustrates a critical path for organizing your morning routine.

The critical path can, of course, be applied to your care routine as well. In applying the same methodology to organizing care for two or more patients, as with one patient, it is helpful to list all the activities you need to do for each patient. Note the time when specific tasks need to be done, such as giving medications, taking vital signs and carrying out treatments. These are the critical points in your overall plan. Estimate the amount of time needed to do the various activities. It is always wise to allow a little extra time, so that you do not feel rushed, and to allow for the unexpected. Identify priorities for the activities you have to do.

FIGURE 17.4   Critical path for organizing morning routine

SOURCE: Du Gas, B.W. (1983). *Introduction to patient care: A comprehensive approach to nursing.* Philadelphia: Saunders, 211.

A good general rule is to look after the sickest patient first, but other considerations may also determine your priorities. For example, if you know that Mr. S goes down for occupational therapy every morning at 0930 hours, he needs to be given morning care, be dressed and be up in his wheelchair ready to go by that time. Some activities may need to be done before others, such as taking a patient's temperature, pulse and respiration before starting your care, or helping patients with a bath before they get up for the first of their scheduled walks down the corridor.

Whatever the case, you should make up a tentative time schedule for getting everything done. You may be able to do some things simultaneously, such as getting Ms. J started with her bed bath while Mr. Y is sitting up in a chair. It is a good idea, especially when you are starting out, to write out your time schedule and keep it handy in your pocket while you are working. When you are busy, you may forget things, and it is wise to check your schedule when you have finished one activity, to remind yourself of what you should be doing next. In the days when student nurses wore aprons, the inside hem of the apron often served as a memo pad (with the writing in pencil). Today, most agencies provide a form for nurses to use in planning and organizing their activities. Figure 17.5 illustrates a critical path for planning the care of two patients.

You may find that you have to rearrange your time schedule if an activity takes longer than you anticipated, or if priorities change, as when one of your patients vomits and you need to change the bed right away.

9. *Get help when you need it.* Many times, nurses will try to do things themselves when they really should have help, such as lifting a heavy person up in bed. Remember that your own health is at stake, as well as the patient's, because you may injure yourself performing these tasks alone. You will learn techniques for lifting and moving patients. Use them. Some of them, such as placing a semi-helpless patient in a wheelchair, require two or more people to be done properly. Be sure to wait until you have assistance before undertaking these tasks.

If you are not sure how Mr. J's sling is supposed to go on — you may have never seen that particular kind before — be sure to get someone who knows the proper method to help you with it.

Whom do you ask for assistance? Your instructor is a good person to ask when you are doing procedures you are not sure of. Even if you have been supervised in a procedure once, you may have not developed sufficient skill to feel comfortable doing it yourself. Or, an agency may have equipment that is different from the equipment with which you

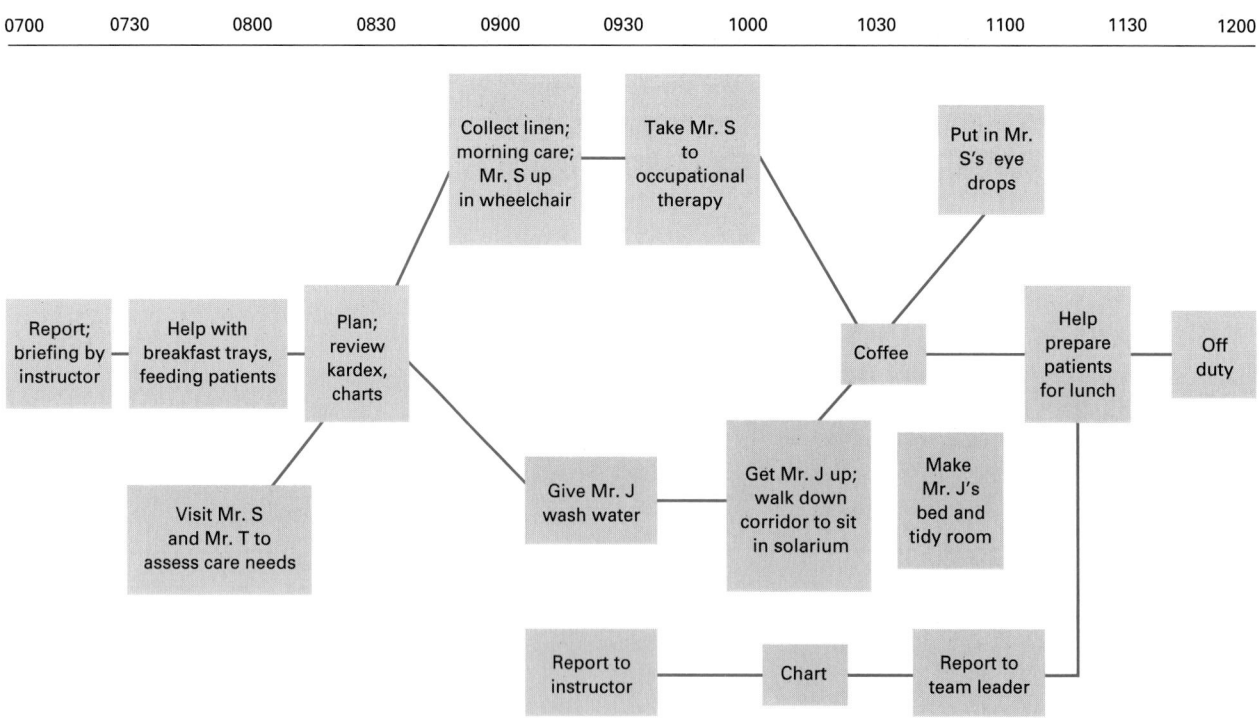

FIGURE 17.5   Critical path for planning care for patients

SOURCE: Du Gas, B.W. (1983). *Introduction to patient care: A comprehensive approach to nursing.* Philadelphia: Saunders, 211.

have had previous experience. The primary nurse responsible for your patients is another good source of assistance, as are other nurses working in the same area.

10. *If you are concerned about a patient who seems to be having difficulty, get help at once.* Reasons for summoning help may include that the patient is bleeding, having difficulty breathing, in severe pain, displaying sudden erratic behaviour, having an ashen colour, falling out of bed or failing to respond to sound, light or touch. A stopped intravenous or an equipment failure may also indicate a need to summon help. Pressing the call bell in the patient's room is the best way to get help. Only if this fails to bring help, and if you think the patient can be left safely, should you leave the room to get help. Remember that the patient's safety is the most important consideration.

11. *If you make an error, such as giving the wrong medication or putting drops in the wrong eye, tell someone at once.* Again, it is the patient's safety that is most important. Fill in an incident report with exact details of what happened.

12. *Be sure to follow basic health rules yourself.* Eat a good breakfast. Nursing involves hard physical work. If you don't eat breakfast, waiting for coffee break may become the most important part of the morning. Make sure you engage in a regular schedule of exercise. You really need to be in top physical condition to accomplish all the activities involved in the hard physical work of lifting and moving patients, making beds and being on your feet for several hours at a time. (You will be glad to be able to sit down and do your recording at the end of the morning.) Be sure to maintain a balance of work and recreation.

13. *Enjoy the rewards of helping people.* That is why you came into nursing, after all. Even if your contribution is small, you will enjoy the feeling of at least doing something to make a patient feel more comfortable. The rewards in nursing come from helping people. You will find your life enriched by the infinite variety of people you will meet in the course of your work.

14. *Avoid coffee room chatter about patients and don't discuss your patient's personal affairs with your classmates, family or friends.* You may be excited about something you have done on the nursing unit or in a home visit and want to tell everybody about it at coffee break or lunch in the agency cafeteria. Remember, however, that most agency cafeterias are open to patients and to visitors as well as to staff. The unthinking remark that Mrs. X has inoperable cancer, or that Mr. B is a very difficult patient, may be overheard by Mrs. X's daughter or Mr. B's wife. Snatches of coffee-time conversations among nurses (or other health professionals) can be very disturbing to patients, relatives and other visitors.

KEY TERMS

behaviourist school p. 423

cognitive school p. 423

humanist school p. 423

autocratic p. 424

laissez-faire p. 424

democratic p. 424

motivation p. 427

social climate p. 427

cognitive domain p. 428

psychomotor domain p. 428

affective domain p. 428

lecture p. 429

storytelling p. 430

demonstration p. 430

return demonstration p. 431

problem-solving p. 431

case study p. 432

role-play p. 432

behaviour modification p. 432

knowledge deficit p. 434

IN REVIEW

Helping the patient to meet learning needs is a primary responsibility of nurses. In order to accomplish this, nurses need an understanding of the teaching and learning process. Three major schools of thought have influenced our thinking about teaching and learning over the past century: the behaviourist school (operant conditioning); the cognitive school which focussed on information processing; and the humanist school which stressed involvement of the whole person in learning. Although all of these schools of thought have contributed to our knowledge of the teaching and learning process, the dominant philosophy in education currently is the humanist school.

The teacher today is viewed as a facilitator, rather than an instructor. Teaching styles vary on a continuum that ranges from laissez-faire to autocratic. Although individual learners vary in their response to different styles of teaching, a democratic, "middle of the road" approach is recommended for patient teaching. It is important to find out how patients feel they learn best and adjust teaching strategies accordingly.

The most important variables in the learning process are the characteristics of the learner, the characteristics of the teacher, the educational setting and the nature of material to be learned. In planning patient teaching, nurses need to consider the patient's age, ability to communicate, cultural background, state of health and motivation for learning. Nurses also need a good knowledge of the subject matter as well as skill in assessing the patient's learning needs, in using appropriate teaching strategies and in planning and organizing teaching and learning activities. Additionally, good interpersonal skills help to promote a relaxed, informal atmosphere which is conducive to learning.

There are three domains of learning: the cognitive, the psychomotor and the affective, each with different teaching and learning strategies. To help patients gain knowledge (the cognitive domain), information may be provided in books, pamphlets, journals and other written materials; through audiovisual aids, such as slides, transparencies, audio- and videotapes, television programs and computer programs; or orally in lectures, informal talks or conversation, storytelling and role-playing.

To develop psychomotor skills needed, for example, when giving an injection, patients need to observe a demonstration of the correct technique by someone skilled in using it. Patients need to demonstrate the ability to carry out the correct movements involved in the skill in the proper sequence. Once they have mastered the correct movements, they need to practise to develop competence in performing the skill efficiently and without error.

Changing attitudes is a slower process than gaining new knowledge or skills and it is more difficult to structure learning experiences to help people with this domain. Increased knowledge about a subject often helps people to change attitudes; for example, knowing more about the causes of illness can act as an incentive in helping people to change unhealthy lifestyles.

Most important in patient teaching, however, is the application by patients of the knowledge, skills and attitudes they have learned. Useful strategies to promote the application of learning are problem-solving, case study and role-play. Behaviour modification may also be used to help people replace undesirable behaviours with desirable ones.

Teaching and learning interventions should be incorporated into all nursing care plans. The initial assessment of patients should include an assessment of learning needs and factors that may affect learning. Teaching should be a part of the interventions planned for all nursing diagnoses. Outcome criteria should be specified for identified learning needs, a teaching plan should be developed and implemented, and the patient's learning should be evaluated. It is important to evaluate how well the teaching has been carried out. As with all nursing interventions, patient teaching should be documented in the patient's record.

LEARNING ACTIVITIES

1. Lee, who is eight years old, has an infected cut on his thigh. He is at home where he is being looked after by his grandmother, since both his mother and his father work outside the home. As the community health nurse in the area, you have been asked to visit the home and teach Lee's grandmother how to apply hot compresses to the cut. Lee's grandmother is Chinese and speaks only a few words of English.

    a. What factors would you consider before initiating any teaching?

    b. What strategies would be best to use for teaching Lee's grandmother?

    c. What factors might inhibit learning?

    d. What aids could you use to facilitate learning?

    e. In developing a teaching plan, what specific outcomes would you anticipate?

    f. How would you evaluate what Lee and his grandmother have learned?

REFERENCES AND READINGS

BENOLIEL, J.Q. and SOULE, E.S. (1988). Some reflections on learning and teaching. *Journal of Nursing Education, 27*(8), 340–341.

BRITISH COLUMBIA CHILDREN'S HOSPITAL. (1994). Discussions with Director of Patient Education.

CANTOR, J.A. (1992). *Delivering instruction to adult learners.* Toronto: Wall and Emerson.

CARPENITO, L.J. (1993). *Nursing diagnosis: Application to clinical practice* (5th ed.). Philadelphia: Lippincott.

COVEY, S.R. (1990). *The seven habits of highly effective people.* New York: Simon and Schuster.

DU GAS, B.W. (1983). *Introduction to patient care: A comprehensive approach to nursing.* Philadelphia: Saunders.

GOTTLIEB, L. and ROWAT, K. (1987). The McGill model of nursing: A practice-derived model. *Advances in nursing science, 9*(4), 51–61.

HAGGARD, A. (1989). *Handbook of patient education.* Rockville, MD: Aspen Publishers, 33.

KNOWLES, M. (1978). *The adult learner: A neglected species* (2nd ed.). Houston: Gulf.

KNOWLES, M. (1990). *The adult learner: A neglected species* (4th ed.). Houston: Gulf.

POHL, M.L. (1981). *The teaching function of the nursing practitioner* (4th ed.). Dubuque, IA: Wm. C. Brown.

RANKIN, S.H. and STALLINGS. (1990). *Patient education: Issues, principles, practices* (2nd ed.). Philadelphia: Lippincott.

REDMAN, B.K. (1993). *The process of patient education* (7th ed.). St. Louis: Mosby.

RORDEN, J.W. (1987). *Nurses as health teachers: A practical guide*. Philadelphia: Saunders.

WAINES, R. (1993, February). AIDS education from a front line worker's perspective. *Canadian Journal of Public Health*, 31–33.

YELON, S.L. and WEINSTEIN, G.W. (1977). *The teacher's world: Psychology in the classroom*. New York: McGraw-Hill.

CHAPTER 18

Information Management

CENTRAL QUESTIONS

1. *Why is documentation of nursing care important?*

2. *What information is kept on the patient's record?*

3. *What is a nursing audit?*

4. *What are the advantages and disadvantages of:*
   - *narrative charting?*
   - *the Problem-Oriented Medical Record?*
   - *PIE charting?*
   - *focus charting?*
   - *charting by exception?*
   - *electronic documentation?*

5. *How are flowsheets used?*

6. *What standards have been established regarding the documentation of nursing care?*

7. *What information is considered essential for nurses to document on patient records?*

8. *What basic guidelines should be kept in mind when documenting nursing care?*

INTRODUCTION

Precision of communication is important, more important than ever in our era of hair-trigger balances, when a false or misunderstood word may create as much disaster as a sudden thoughtless act.

James Thurber (1961)

Documentation is the communication in writing of essential facts in order to maintain a continuous history of events over a period of time. **Reporting** is the communication of information to another individual (or group of individuals) and may be either written or oral. A number of different records and report forms are kept by various health agencies, and the nurse will find that these vary from one agency to another. All types of health agencies maintain patient records or charts. The form of the record usually depends on the type of agency. Hospitals use one type of record, community health agencies another and extended care institutions yet another.

No matter what form of charting is used in the agency in which you work, a knowledge of basic standards in nursing documentation is imperative. In this chapter, we present the basic elements of nursing documentation of patient care. Professional nurses should be able to adapt these elements to fulfill their responsibilities in whatever agency they may be employed.

PURPOSE OF DOCUMENTATION OR CHARTING

Documentation, or charting, in the patient record serves a number of functions. It provides a means of communication among health care workers and a legal record of patient care. In addition, the record is used for education and research, and for the **nursing audit** — the evaluation of the quality of nursing care.

Communication   The documentation on the **patient record** serves as a means of communication among health care providers. It is an account of the patient's history, present health status, treatment and response to treatment. "Since the provider of care has a duty to the [patient] to provide the care in a reasonable and prudent manner and to take reasonable steps to minimize reasonably foreseeable risks, communication of information becomes an integral part of that duty" (Rozovsky and Rozovsky, 1984, 6).

The nursing care provided should be reflected by documentation of the nursing process, including assessment, nursing diagnosis, plan, implementation and evaluation. Through documentation of the care plan and the patient's response to care, continuity of care is established and maintained.

Legal record   Because the patient's record is recognized as a legal document, accurate record keeping becomes a professional responsibility. In a majority of malpractice suits involving patient care, the patient record serves as an invaluable account of actions concerning the issue in question (Iyer and Camp, 1991).

In 1970 the Supreme Court of Canada ruled that:

Hospital records, including nurses' notes made contemporaneously, by someone having the personal knowledge of the matters being recorded and under a duty of care to make the entry or record should be received as prima facie proof of the facts stated therein.

(Ares vs. Venner, 1970; RNABC, 1992, 1)

As a legal record, the chart is the property of the agency or the medical professional responsible for the patient's care. However, the patient has a right to access the information on the chart (RNABC, 1992, 6).

Education and research   The patient record is used by all disciplines in teaching rounds, for conferences and for study purposes. Trends in specific disease entities identified from chart reviews provide information for the treatment of the individual patient.

When patient records are used for education or research purposes, it is essential to ensure the confidentiality of these records. The third value in the CNA Code of Ethics for Nursing states:

An affirmative duty exists to institute and maintain practices that protect patient confidentiality — for example, by limiting access to records or by choosing the most secure method of communicating patient information.

(Canadian Nurses Association, 1991, 6)

Audit   An audit is a methodical review of the medical record for the purposes of collecting data. The nursing audit consists of a review of patient records to evaluate the quality of nursing care as documented in the record. The nurse must remember that if the care has not been documented, it is assumed that the care has not been given. The audit may be retrospective, that is, looking back at the care received by patients who have been discharged, or concurrent, looking at care that is currently being given.

The process of care, as documented in the record, is compared with standards for nursing care as determined by members of the nursing profession. Criteria for evaluation are established through such aspects of care as the data base, the identification of problems, the expected outcomes of care, the selection of nursing interventions and the degree to which the plan of care was carried out as evidenced by the nurses' notations on the patient's record.

A nursing audit may be undertaken to evaluate either the quality of care given by individual nurses or the quality of care provided by an entire agency. In either case, it is the individual patient records that are reviewed. A nursing

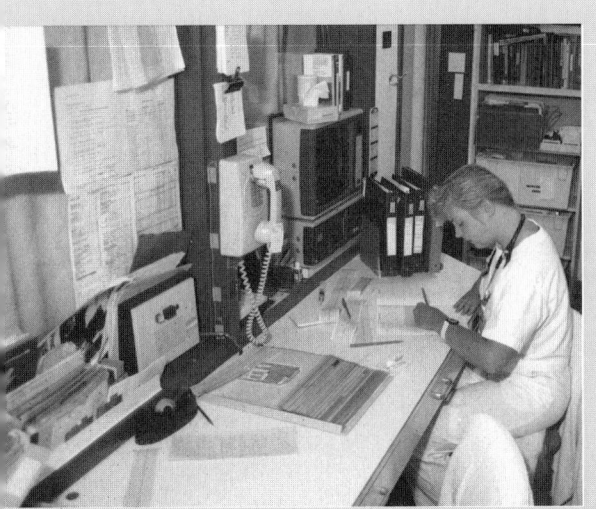

The documentation of patient care is an important nursing responsibility.

audit committee within the agency is responsible for determining the standards of care to be met. If the agency's quality of nursing care is being evaluated, an outside committee is established. Representatives on this committee might include members of the provincial nurses association, nurses from an accrediting agency and possibly nurses employed by a government agency. Because an audit is done by members of the same professional group, it is often referred to as "peer review."

FORMS OF CHARTING

Many forms of charting are currently in use in Canadian health agencies. Following is a brief overview of six charting systems.

NARRATIVE

Narrative charting (also known as *source-oriented medical recording*, is the most traditional approach to documentation. The progress notes are written in simple paragraph form and in chronological order as patient issues are presented. There is little structure to these notes unless documentation guidelines and standards have been established by the health care agency. In some agencies, all disciplines document in the same progress note. This allows for concentration of patient information in one area. However, in agencies where each discipline has its own progress note, information about the same patient problem could be scattered throughout the record. Narrative notes tend to be lengthy and cluttered with accounts of routine care and assessment (RNABC, 1992; Iyer and Camp, 1991).

With the use of flowsheets, the documentation of routine care and treatments is removed from the narrative note.

The purpose of the **flowsheet** is to show in graphic form interventions or observations in respect to one particular problem. Flowsheets are usually developed for use for a designated period of time. They may cover a week or a 24-hour period. The Vital Signs Record used in most hospitals is an example of a flowsheet that is used to record temperature, pulse, respiration and other vital signs for a week at a time. When it is necessary to monitor vital signs more frequently than every four hours, as allowed for on the usual Vital Signs Record, a seperate flowsheet may be used. The minute-to-minute monitoring of vital signs of patients in the intensive care unit of a hospital would be charted in this way.

This leaves a more pure narrative that refers to significant findings and specific patient problems. Flowsheets were developed originally by nurses in intensive care units but are also used in other units for the following reasons:

- to save time
- to document routine care
- to prevent duplication in charting
- to ensure a systematic assessment and
- to provide the greatest amount of patient information in one area of the record.

Flowsheets can be used with other forms of charting as well as with narrative charting.

Figure 18.1 is an example of a flowsheet used at the Vancouver Hospital and Health Sciences Centre.

A narrative note, combined with flowsheet documentation, should provide the information needed for all disciplines to make informed patient care or patient treatment decisions (Iyer and Camp, 1991). An example of a narrative note follows:

Feb. 6, '94, 1930 hours: Pt. complaining of lower abdominal pain in area of abdominal incision; also has sense of "fullness" and need to void. Scant, old, dried, dark brown drainage noted on abdominal dressing. Wound is clean, no fresh drainage noted. Fresh dressing applied. Urinary catheter tubing repositioned; clear yellow drainage in tubing and bag. Pt. instructed re. urinary catheter and its purpose; reassured that voiding on her own not necessary. Medicated for pain with morphine per MD's order. Repositioned to R side.
— Jane Doe, RN

Feb. 6, '94, 2000 hours: Pt. indicates she is more comfortable; able to do coughing and deep breathing exercises with nurse's encouragement; cough is nonproductive. Turned to L side. No further comments re. urge to void. Catheter continues to drain well.
— Jane Doe, RN

PROBLEM-ORIENTED MEDICAL RECORD (POMR)

In the **Problem-Oriented Medical Record (POMR)** all patient data are organized according to patient problems. A problem list is established and members of all disciplines

VANCOUVER GENERAL HOSPITAL
BRITISH COLUMBIA'S HEALTH CENTRE

ACTIVITIES OF DAILY LIVING FLOWSHEET

B = Breakfast	2P = 2 person assist	SM = Small
L = Lunch	1P = 1 person assist	M = Moderate
D = Dinner		L = Large
T = Total	W = Well	NN = See Nurses's Notes
P = Partial	I = Intermittent	Blank space = not applicable
S = Self	Pr = Poor	

DATE   NURSING UNIT

MR., MISS, MRS.   UNIT NUMBER

SURNAME   GIVEN NAME

DOCTOR   (PLEASE BLOCK CAPITALS)
          SEX   AGE

Month _____ Year _____

Day

Time

	No nursing observation/intervention required ✓		
D I E T	Diet Change	Time	
	Tolerated ✓	Amount Taken %	B
			L
			D
		Snack	
	Assistance	T, P, S,	
H Y G I E N E	No nursing observation/intervention required ✓		
	Tub/Shower	T, P, S,	
	Sink/Basin	T, P, S,	
	Bedbath	T, P, S,	
	Mouthcare	T, P, S,	
	Pericare	T, P, S,	
A C T I V I T Y	No nursing observation/intervention required ✓		
	Assistance & # (T, 2P, 1P, S)	Last Time Walking	
		BRP	
		Chair	
		Dangle	
	Bedrest	✓	
	Sleep	W, I, Pr,	
E L I M I N A T I O N	No nursing observation/intervention required ✓		
	Bowel Movements		
	Loose	SM, M, L	
	Soft	SM, M, L	
	Hard	SM, M, L	
	Absent	✓	

INITIAL

FIGURE 18.1 Activities of Daily Living flowsheet

are involved in documenting issues concerning problems relevant to their disciplines. The POMR has five components: data base, problem list, initial plan/orders, progress notes and discharge summary.

The **data base** includes the physician history and physical exam and the nursing history and functional health pattern assessment. The *problem list* is generated from the data base. Updates occur as problems are solved and/or new problems develop. A **plan of care** is developed from the problem list. The medical plan of care is documented in the **progress notes**; the nursing care plan is usually in a separate format that includes the nursing diagnoses, expected outcomes and interventions. Progress notes are recorded by all disciplines on the same sheet and are numbered to correspond with the problem from the problem list. Information is organized in the **SOAPIE format**, an acronym for:

S = Subjective data (what the patient tells you)
O = Objective data (what the clinician observes)
A = Assessment (nursing, medical diagnoses)
P = Plan (plan of action based on above information)
I = Interventions (actual interventions implemented)
E = Evaluation (patient's response to plan and changes needed).

The Problem-Oriented Medical Record (POMR) system was seen as a tremendous improvement over traditional patient records when it was introduced two decades ago. It focussed on patient problems with a format that could be used by all disciplines and in all types of agencies. It was felt that the use of POMR would foster collaboration among all members of the health team since all plans would be recorded on the same form. It was felt that it would also help to bring about greater uniformity in recording in different agencies.

However, the SOAPIE format can be redundant with plan and interventions noted both on the care plan and in the progress notes. If flowsheets are included, charting duplication occurs. Because each problem requires an entry, problems tend to overlap, causing repetition. A final potential drawback is that integration with other disciplines may cause resistance from individual clinicians (Iyer and Camp, 1991). The SOAPIE format is illustrated in Figure 18.2.

PIE CHARTING

PIE charting (problems, interventions and evaluation of nursing care) was developed to simplify documentation by eliminating the traditional care plan and incorporating it into the daily documentation. It is a problem-oriented approach similar to SOAPIE charting. However, PIE charting was developed from the nursing process whereas SOAPIE charting originated from the medical model. The system consists of a 24-hour, daily assessment flowsheet. The nurse initials the portions specific to the patient. Deviations from

the normal are flagged with an asterisk; the deviation is then described in the progress notes. Each problem, using the NANDA (North American Nursing Diagnosis Association) list, is labelled with a P and numbered (P#__). The intervention is labelled IP#__, (the number corresponds to the previously identified problem number). The problem is then evaluated each shift and labelled EP#___ (Iyer and Camp, 1991). An example of PIE charting is given in Figure 18.3.

The overall planning component of the nursing process may not be addressed in PIE charting. The nurse will need to assure that patient outcomes are considered, probably through the addition of standardized or individualized care plans.

FOCUS CHARTING

Focus charting is a type of charting that can be used as an alternative to the more traditional narrative nurses notes. It provides more specificity than the narrative notes and records nursing concerns rather than the medically oriented problems listed on the POMR.

In **Focus charting**, the nurse identifies a patient *concern* rather than a problem. The nurse focusses on a behaviour, a change, an event or a nursing diagnosis. The progress notes are organized into three columns; the date and time in one, the focus in another, and the patient care note in the last. The patient care note is further organized into three sections: data (subjective or objective), action (nursing interventions) and response (patient's response to interventions). Assessment forms and flowsheets, developed by the individual agency, support and are necessary to Focus charting (Iyer and Camp, 1991; RNABC, 1992). Figure 18.4 shows a focus progress note. Chart audits of focus charting have revealed that nurses tend to revert to narrative charting, because they have some difficulty documenting the correct information under the appropriate focus charting sections (Kozier, Erb and Olovieri, 1993).

CHARTING BY EXCEPTION (CBE)

The **Charting by Exception (CBE)** system documents only significant findings or exceptions to the norm. There are several components to this system:

- Flowsheets — Nursing/physician order flowsheet, graphic record, teaching record and discharge note.
- Standards of practice — A checkmark indicates that previously developed standards of care have been met.
- Nursing data base
- Nursing diagnosis-based care plans
- SOAPIE progress notes
- Accessibility of forms — All flowsheets are kept at the patient's bedside, negating the need for transcription of data (Burke and Murphy, 1988).

PROBLEM LIST:

1. Post operative pain
2. Bladder discomfort

DATE/TIME	PROBLEM	PROGRESS NOTES
Feb. 6, '94	Abd. pain	S: "I'm having pain in my stomach."
1900 hours	postop	O: Pt. is 4 hours postop abd hysterectomy. Last med for pain 3 hours ago in the RR. Pt. lying on her back, tense posture, guarding abd. On scale of 1-10, rates pain at 6. Scant old, dried, dk. brown drainage on abdominal dressing. Wound is clean, no fresh drainage noted. Fresh dressing applied.
		A: Alteration in comfort: acute pain secondary to surgical trauma today.
		P: Medicate pt. according to MD's orders. Instruct pt. to request pain med before pain is severe. Check pt. in 1/2 hour to 45 min to assess for relief. ——— Jane Doe, RN
	Bladder discomfort	S: "Please bring me a bedpan. My bladder feels full and I want to use the bedpan."
		O: Pt. has indwelling foley cath; cath draining freely of clear, yellow drainage.
		A: Knowledge deficit: unaware of cath placement. Urinary Elimination, Alteration in patterns related to foley cath placement.
		P: Reposition foley cath. Assess for relief of discomfort in 45 minutes. Instruct pt. re foley cath placement.
		I: Foley cath repositioned to promote optimum drainage. Pt. instructed that foley cath placed during surgery, would remain in place through the night, and that cath is positioned in bladder allowing continuous drainage and negating need for pt. to void on her own. Pt. remembers now preop instruction re. cath insertion. ——— Jane Doe, RN
Feb. 6, '94	Abd. pain	I: Pt. medicated with morphine re MD order. Pt. positioned in R side. Pt. instructed to put on call light if pain continues or when relief begins to wear off. ——— Jane Doe, RN
1915 hours	postop	
Feb. 6, '94		E: Pt. indicates she is more comfortable; rates pain at 2. Pt. able to do coughing and deep breathing exercises with nurse's encouragement. Repositioned on L side.
1945 hours		
	Bladder discomfort	E. Cath continues to drain well. Pt. has no further complaints of discomfort. ——— Jane Doe, RN

FIGURE 18.2   SOAPIE format for documentation

DATE	TIME	PROGRESS NOTES	
Feb. 6, '94	1900	P#1	Alteration in comfort: acute pain secondary to surgical trauma today.
		P#2	Knowledge deficit: unaware of urinary cath placement during surgery. Wants to void.
			—— Jane Doe, RN
Feb. 6, '94	1915	IP#1	Pt. medicated for pain. Instructed to call RN if pain persists or as relief wears off. Call light within reach. Abd. wound assessed. Scant dk. red, dry drainage on dressing. DSD applied. Pt. positioned on R side.
		IP#2	Pt. instructed re foley cath placement during surgery. Pt. also instructed re purpose of cath and position in bladder. Cath tubing repositioned to encourage optimum drainage.
			—— Jane Doe, RN
Feb. 6, '94	1945	EP#1	Pt. indicates she is more comfortable. Able to do coughing & deep breathing exercises with Nurse's encouragement. Pt. repositioned on L side.
		EP#2	No further comments re need to void. Cath draining appropriately.
			—— Jane Doe, RN

FIGURE 18.3   PIE charting

DATE	TIME	FOCUS	PROGRESS NOTES
Feb. 6, '94	1900	Alteration in comfort: acute pain secondary to surg. trauma today.	D: Complaining of pain in abd. Lying on back. A: Abd. incision site assessed: site clean; scant dk. red, dry drainage on dressing. DSD applied.
		Knowledge deficit: Unaware of urinary cath. placement.	D: Wants to void. A: Pt. instructed re urinary cath placement during surgery., that cath will remain in place thru the night, that cath is positioned in bladder allowing cont. drainage and negating need to void. Cath. repositioned to promote optimum drainage. —— Jane Doe, RN
Feb. 6, '94	1915		A: Pt. medicated with morphine per MD orders. instructed to call RN if pain persists or as relief wears off. Call light placed within reach. —— Jane Doe, RN
Feb. 6, '94	1945		R: Pt. indicates she is more comfortable. Able to do coughing and deep breathing exercises. Cath. draining appropriately. No further comments re need to void. States she now remembers pre-op instruction re cath placement. —— Jane Doe, RN

FIGURE 18.4   Focus progress note

Educating staff to document only the abnormal findings has proven difficult. Charting by Exception was pilot-tested at St. Luke's Hospital in Milwaukee, Wisconsin, under a grant from the Aurora Health Centre. The purpose of the project was to teach nurses to document selectively in order to reduce the amount of time spent on charting. The project was successful in reducing charting time. However, educating staff to document only the abnormal findings proved difficult because nurses have traditionally been taught to record all pertinent observations (both normal and abnormal) about a patient. Some nurses were concerned about checking standard care boxes on a flowsheet instead of writing a narrative note because they were unsure of their accountability when they made such an entry. For these reasons, orientation to CBE involves a major educational effort (Iyer and Camp, 1991).

For more in-depth information about CBE refer to *Charting by Exception* by L. Burke and J. Murphy (1988).

ELECTRONIC DOCUMENTATION

Increasingly, health care facilities are using computerized systems to document patient care. These systems are commonly referred to as "*Patient Care Information Systems*" *(PCIS)* and are an integral component of the health care

organization's information system. In hospitals this is called the HIS (Hospital Information System). The PCIS can be accessed by care providers in multiple locations, including the bedside and the physician's office. Previous visit information about the patient, as well as intra-agency information, may be retrieved, thus creating a continuous health record "from crib to grave." There are many other features of a PCIS that contribute to more timely, reliable and complete patient documentation. Figure 18.5 illustrates a computer screen in a PCIS.

PCIS Process

Patient data are collected and retrieved using a variety of different methods in a PCIS. These include keyboards, light pens, touch screens, bar code readers, a point-and-click mouse and hand writing or voice recognition. Data are entered and retrieved on a terminal, a workstation and by hand-held or palm-top devices. Patient information is stored in the computer (on line) and can be printed and placed on the patient chart (hard copy). The approach varies between agencies depending on the type of PCIS they are using and the extent of the health record that is stored electronically.

The components of most PCISs include: order entry and results reporting, medication administration record-

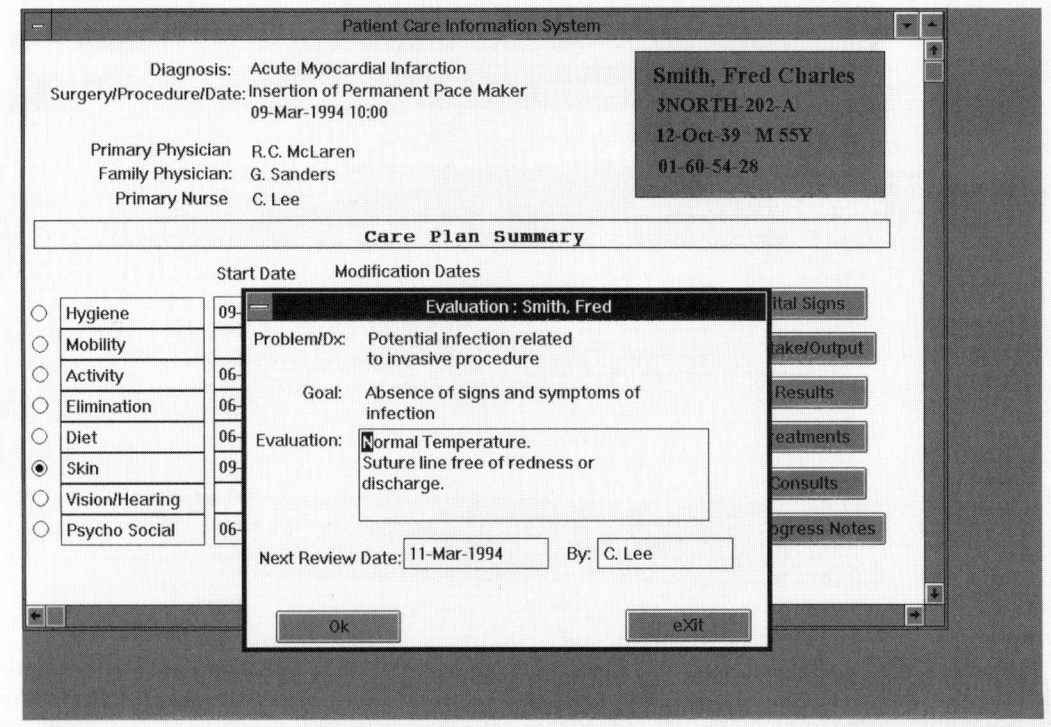

FIGURE 18.5   Patient (Client) Care Information System. This is a simulation of a computer screen in a patient (client) care information system. In this screen, the nurse is able to view a current summary of the patient's care plan and chart the patient's response to a specific intervention. The nurse could also "click" the buttons on the right or left sides of the screen to access other sections of the care plan or the chart.

SOURCE: Diagram developed by Susan Ball, Christina Beckett and Pat Jesselon.

ing, care planning and charting. Ideally, these components are designed for multi-disciplinary use and integrated across the functions. For example, order entry is used by physicians to enter diagnostic and treatment orders and by nurses to enter nursing orders. When the charting function is used, information that was entered into the Orders and Care Planning functions prompts the nurse on required charting. The patient information stored in the data base is then available for patient acuity and workload requirements. All PCISs have the ability to produce many different types of reports that can be used by nurse care providers, nurse educators, nurse administrators and nurse researchers.

Information can be sent and received between the PCIS and other systems in the Health Information System (HIS) via electronic interfaces. For example, orders for lab tests are communicated immediately and directly to the lab system and when the test results are obtained, the data are sent immediately from the lab system to the PCIS. In addition, the PCIS can automatically capture data recorded by other equipment, such as intravenous infusion pumps, analgesia pumps, heart monitoring devices, thermometers and urometers.

The PCIS supports the immediate capture of data, thus eliminating the need for paper notes, duplicate recording and transcription of information. Once data are entered into the system they can be displayed wherever appropriate. For instance, allergy information may be displayed on different screens and/or reports as well as communicated to other systems that require it, such as the one used by the pharmacy.

Uses of PCIS

The PCIS provides a variety of options to review patient information for care providers. Some screens show summary information with the ability to "drill down" to details as required. Data such as results and vital sign can be viewed in columnar or graphical formats. Care providers can also control the information display in terms of picking exactly what they want to see at any given time. For example, the nurse may want to view certain lab results and medication records simultaneously, and in another case the nurse may wish to see care plan interventions that have an impending review date. Access to information may be from points where patient care is provided such as the bedside, in clinics and in diagnostic or treatment areas, as well as locations remote from the point of care, such as the physician's office.

The PCIS supports the nursing process by storing large amounts of data for a variety of purposes and linking up related information. Standards of care and individualized care plans are retained in the system. As orders are entered, results reported and care documented, the care plan is automatically updated to reflect the "new" information. Interventions are automatically added or suggested as the care plan is created and the patient assessment is charted.

Quality Assurance programs are supported by the PCIS through the use of "rules" which can be incorporated into the program to prompt the nurse to provide additional information in specific situations. For example, if a patient's vital signs exceed the normal ranges, the system prompts the nurse to increase the frequency of vital signs monitoring. Teaching materials can be printed for patients from the PCIS. As well, diagnostic procedure preparation information for nurses can also be made available on-line. Many PCIS include access to databases, such as CINAHL (on-line journal search) and MICROMEDEX (pharmaceutical and trauma database). Some health care agencies have all their manuals on-line, as part of their PCIS.

In response to tightened health care funding and increased public accountability, a shift is occurring which combines clinical guidelines and standards of care into Critical Paths. Critical Paths are built around "**CMGs**" (*Case Mix Groups*) — called "DRGs" (Diagnosis Related Groups) in the United States. The **Critical Path** outlines the care to be provided the patient for each day (or at more frequent intervals) of their stay in hospital by all physicians, nurses and other allied health professionals. Care is recorded against this Critical Path in much the same way as was indicated in the section on Charting by Exception. Administrators can review the care delivered and determine when and where there were deviations from the Critical Path. This allows them to better monitor budgets and care delivery, physician practices, resource utilization (patient costing) and outcome of care delivered.

Discharge planning is facilitated by the PCIS, by automatically or with little additional effort including information already in the system in a patient's discharge plan. Some hospitals have links with the community, allowing the discharge plan to be sent electronically to the community agency.

Concerns About PCIS

The issues of privacy, confidentiality and security of electronically stored patient information are paramount. Nurses must continue to be patient advocates in this area. They must ensure the integrity and security of patient information held in computer information systems to the same degree they do paper charting. To this end, passwords should never be shared under any circumstance and terminals and workstations should never be left unattended while logged-on. All agencies with computerized systems have policies and procedures to ensure the security of patient records. Most PCISs have elaborate and sophisticated security systems within the software, which can restrict access to patient information on a "need to know" basis.

In summary, the PCIS is a valuable information tool to support the process of providing patient care. Many of the features of computerized documentation can significantly enhance the quality and timeliness of patient information, thus allowing the care providers to enhance the quality of care delivered. PCIS features provide advantages such as:

- reducing the number of phone calls to various hospital departments and physicians

- eliminating duplicate recording of information in multiple locations
- assuring that patient documentation is more thorough, relevant and complete
- facilitating the development and updating of patient care and discharge plans
- significantly reducing medication errors, order entry errors and charting omissions
- eliminating errors resulting from misinterpretation of illegible writing
- providing accurate and current patient acuity and workload information
- giving immediate access to pertinent patient information by multiple care providers at multiple locations.
- creating faster turnaround time between information collection and retrieval
- developing a data base to support nursing administration, research and education

There are also disadvantages to computer documentation. These are:
- The initial investment is costly.
- If terminals are not at the bedside, there are not enough terminals or space in the nursing stations.
- Downtime due to routine service or failure is disruptive and frustrating.
- Some nurses have difficulty giving up the old system.
- The legal issue of confidentiality is yet to be clarified.*

STANDARDS FOR DOCUMENTATION

Standards for charting have been developed to ensure that essential information is consistently documented. All health care agencies have their own standards regarding the content to be included in documenting patient care. The health care professional must be oriented to the standards of charting in the agency and must chart according to the system that is in place. However, professional nurses can develop their own standards and adjust these to correspond to whatever area they work in.

General charting standards have been established by professional nursing organizations. It is important for the practitioner to become familiar with the general standards of the nursing profession. Nurses will also find it helpful to have access to specific standards of the area or specialty in which they work. From standards that have been formally developed, one usually finds specific references to documentation expectations. Following are some examples of charting standards:

CANADIAN NURSES ASSOCIATION:

Standards II.1: Nurses are required to collect data in accordance with their conception of the patient (CNA, 1987).

ONTARIO COMMUNITY HEALTH NURSES:

Standard 2 Planning: The nurse develops a written care plan which assigns priorities and prescribes nursing strategies or measures to achieve the short and long term goals for each nursing diagnosis (Registered Nurses Association of Ontario, 1985, 9).

QUEBEC COMMUNITY HEALTH NURSES:

Standard 2: The community health nurse knows and uses a scientific process in her work with her patientele and when preparing health programs.

2.6: The community health nurse puts in writing:
- the information collected
- the priorities established
- the objectives defined
- the planned interventions
- the results of the evaluation of the interventions.

2.7: The community health nurse keeps her charts up to date (Ordre des infirmières et infirmiers du Quebec, 1986, 17; 21).

BRITISH COLUMBIA RESIDENTIAL CARE SERVICES/FACILITIES (CONTINUING CARE DIVISION):

Standard 4.1, Resident Care Services: Individualized Care Planning: There shall be a current, individualized, written plan of care developed and implemented for each resident (Government of British Columbia, 1992, xviii).

ESSENTIAL DOCUMENTATION

Following is a description of essential documentation that should be carried out in accordance with charting standards.

1. An admission note will be written at the time of admission on the approved form by the nurse admitting the patient. The admission note will include date and time of admission, mode of transportation and person accompanying the patient. The note will also include

---

* Brunner et al., 1986; Iyer and Camp, 1991; Meyer, 1992.

the reason for admission as stated by the patient, if appropriate, and a brief description of the patient's presenting signs and symptoms. Allergies, medications the patient is currently taking and assistive devices (such as dentures and eyeglasses) will be noted. The nurse will document the patient's perception of reason for admission, past health problems and problems or concerns in need of immediate attention.

2. An assessment by functional health patterns and an initial care plan will be written for each patient by a registered nurse within 24 hours of admission. Each agency usually has developed its own nursing assessment form. In some agencies, a discharge planning form is often part of the patient record and is initiated on admission.

3. A progress note will be written at least once a shift and as often as the patient's condition warrants, by the nurse caring for the patient. Progress notes will reflect continued assessment of patient condition, planning, mutual goal setting, interventions and patient outcome evaluation. Patient response to nursing interventions for resolution of nursing diagnoses or collaborative problems will be the focus. Patient teaching and patient response to that teaching are also written in the progress notes.

4. Nursing activities generated by the medical plan of care and patient response to those interventions (for example, medications, treatments, etc.) will be recorded on the approved forms.

5. A transfer note will be written when a patient is transferred from one unit to another by the nurse transferring the patient. The note will include date and time of transfer, unit of acceptance and mode of transport and status of current patient problems. The nurse accepting the patient will write a note to include date and time patient is received and a statement of the patient's condition. A notation is made when a patient leaves and returns from a procedure that necessitates a consent and/or premedication (for example, the operating room). Date, time of transfer and mode of transport, scheduling procedure, and patient's condition including response to medications are all included.

6. A discharge note is written upon discharge by the nurse discharging the patient. It includes patient condition, person accompanying the patient, mode of transportation, prescriptions and follow-up appointments.

A notation of resolution of nursing diagnoses should be added.

CHARTING GUIDELINES

Entries are written in black or blue ink and signed with full name and registration status. In some agencies, student nurse notes are countersigned by a registered nurse. Each note must be dated with the exact (24-hour clock) time. If initials are used on a flowsheet, the nurse's full signature with initials should appear somewhere on the flowsheet.

Errors in documentation are corrected by putting a single line through the incorrect information, writing "charting error" above it, and initialling it. No whiting out or erasures are permitted.

Chart entries must be made in chronological order. Nothing should be written between the lines. Out of order notes (recorded in the progress notes by another person before the nurse has had a chance to write) should be written after the last charted note. The words "out of order entry" should precede the note. The time the entry is made and the time the care was given must be recorded. There should be no attempt to insert a note between other notes. Late entry notes (notes made after the fact) are written after the last charted note and are preceded by "late entry note." Lines should not be left blank. If a blank line is present, a line should be drawn through it to prevent someone from inserting a note (RNABC, 1992). Only the abbreviations used by the agency in which you are working should be used. Commonly used medical abbreviations are listed in all medical dictionaries. Most agencies have selected one set of abbreviations for use in all departments.

The nurse must check the agency's policy for verbal orders. Usually registered nurses can take verbal orders, signing their name and indicating the physician responsible for giving the order. The physician then signs the verbal order within a specified time.

Notes and entries must be made promptly. If the nurse must document the care given by someone else (for example, a nurse's aide or family member), the name and status of the individual involved must be recorded (RNABC, 1992). Notes should be concise, without repetition and free of jargon; writing must be legible and words spelled correctly. Generalizations should be avoided.

KEY TERMS

documentation p. 448

reporting p. 448

nursing audit p. 448

patient record p. 448

narrative charting p. 449

flowsheet p. 449

Problem-Oriented
Medical Record (POMR) p. 449

data base p. 451

plan of care p. 451

progress notes p. 451

SOAPIE format p. 451

PIE charting p. 451

Focus charting p. 451

Charting by
Exception (CBE) p. 451

PCIS (Patient Care
Information System) p. 454

Case Mix Groups (CMGs) p. 455

Critical Path p. 455

IN REVIEW

The basic purpose of the chart is to maintain a legal record of treatment received by a patient and of the patient's response to that treatment while under the care of a health agency or private health practitioner. It also serves as a channel of communication among health professionals, as a tool for education and research and as a means for assessing the quality of care through the nursing audit. Documentation of patient care is a professional responsibility. By documenting the care given to patients and the patient's response to that care, the nurse supports the goal of continuity of care. Nurses have an ethical responsibility to maintain the confidentiality of patient records. As a legal record, the chart is the property of the health agency or medical professional responsible for the patient's care. However, the patient has a legal right to access the information on the record.

Forms of charting used in Canadian health agencies include the traditional narrative charting (also known as source-oriented medical recording), the Problem-Oriented Medical Record (POMR), PIE charting (problems, intervention and evaluation of nursing care), focus charting, charting by exception (CBE) and electronic documentation. There are advantages and disadvantages to each system. Nurses must become familiar with the system used in their agency. With the increasing number of agencies installing computer networks, it is important for nurses to become computer literate and to learn how to use electronic documentation to the best advantage in nursing care.

All health care agencies have their own standards regarding content to be included in patient records. In addition, the Canadian Nurses Association, other professional nursing associations and some government agencies have developed general standards regarding nursing content in patient records. Essential documentation by nurses includes an admission note; an initial assessment and care plan; progress notes once a shift and as often as necessary to record nursing interventions and patient response to these interventions; continuing assessment and reevaluation of the plan of care; nursing activities generated by the medical plan of care (and the patient's response to these); and transfer and discharge notes.

Certain basic guidelines must be followed regardless of the agency or form of charting used. The full signature and registration status of the person making an entry on the chart is mandatory. Notations must be made promptly in blue or black ink and with a record of date and time (using the 24-hour clock). Entries must be in chronological order with no lines left blank on the record. Care given by the patient's family or other person must be recorded with the name and status of care-giver. Entries on the record should be concise, and repetition, jargon and generalizations should be avoided.

LEARNING ACTIVITIES

1. Mrs. Rose Wong is a patient who has undergone abdominal surgery. She has been on the nursing unit three days postoperatively. Her orders from the physician include dressing changes once a day as necessary and Demerol, 50–100 milligrams (mg.) intramuscularly (IM) or Tylenol #3, every four hours (q4h), as needed (p.r.n.) for pain.

    Her dressing is soaked through with reddish brown fluid and she complains of pain. As her nurse you give her 50 mg. of demerol and change her dressing. The following questions should be answered for recording on each of the different charting methods (narrative nurses' notes, a problem-oriented medical record, PIE documentation, focus charting, charting by exception and electronic documentation).

    a. Where should you check for Mrs. Wong's orders?

    b. Give a sample of the charting for Demerol, including what should be recorded about the patient.

    c. What should be included in recording the dressing change? Give an example.

    d. Where are these data recorded?

    e. How would a change in the physician's orders be indicated to nursing personnel? A change in nursing orders?

REFERENCES AND READINGS

BRUNNER, ET AL. (1986). *The Lippincott manual of nursing practice* (4th ed.). Philadelphia: Lippincott.

BURKE, L. and MURPHY, J. (1988). *Charting by exception*. New York: Wiley.

CANADIAN NURSES ASSOCIATION (CNA). (1987). *A definition of nursing practice standards for nursing practice*. Ottawa: Author.

CANADIAN NURSES ASSOCIATION (CNA). (1991). *Code of ethics for nursing*. Ottawa: Author.

GOVERNMENT OF BC. (1992). *Standards for residential care services (facilities)*. BC: BC Ministry of Health and Ministry Responsible for Seniors, Continuing Care Division.

IYER, P.W. and CAMP, N.H. (1991). *Nursing documentation: A nursing process approach*. St. Louis: Mosby.

KOZIER, B., ERB, G. and OLIVIERI, R. (1993). *Techniques in clinical nursing* (4th ed.). Redwood City, CA: Addison-Wesley.

MEYER, C. (1992). Bedside computer charting: Inching toward tomorrow. *American Journal of Nursing, 92*(4), 38–44.

ORDRE DES INFIRMIERES ET INFIRMIER DU QUEBEC. (1986). *Standards and criteria of competence for community health nurses in Quebec*. Quebec: Author.

REGISTERED NURSES' ASSOCIATION OF BRITISH COLUMBIA (RNABC). (1992). *Nurse to nurse information for nurses. Charting: A review of nursing documentation*. BC: Author.

REGISTERED NURSES ASSOCIATION OF ONTARIO (RNAO). (1985). *Standards of nursing practice for community health nurses in Ontario*. Ontario: Author.

ROZOVSKY, L. and ROZOVSKY, F. (1984). *The Canadian law of patient records*. Toronto: Butterworths.

THURBER, J. (1961). Friends, Romans, countrymen, lend me your earmuffs. *Lanterns and lances,* 38. Quoted in *International Thesaurus of Quotations*. (1970). New York: Thomas Crowell Co., 93.

Physiological Needs

Nutritional
Needs

CENTRAL QUESTIONS

1. What is the role of food in meeting basic human needs?

2. What are the processes involved in the digestion, absorption and metabolism of carbohydrates, proteins and fats?

3. What are the functions of vitamins and minerals in the body?

4. What are the nutrient and energy requirements of healthy people?

5. How do nutritional needs vary throughout the life cycle?

6. What are the main determinants of nutritional status?

7. How do nutritional needs change in illness?

8. What are some common nutritional problems?

9. What basic principles would the nurse apply in assisting individuals to meet nutritional needs?

10. How does the nurse assess an individual's nutritional status?

11. What are the common nursing diagnostic statements for individuals with nutritional problems?

12. How would the nurse develop a plan of care for individuals with nutritional problems?

13. What strategies might the nurse implement in helping individuals, families or groups to promote optimum nutritional status and protect nutritional functioning?

14. What health restoring and supportive strategies might the nurse implement in the care of individuals with nutritional problems?

15. How would the nurse evaluate the individual's response to nursing interventions?

INTRODUCTION

The term *nutrition* is derived from the Latin root *nutr-*, which means to *nurture* or *nourish* (Williams, 1989). Nutrition is concerned with the foods people eat and how the body uses these foods to sustain life. Food and the partaking of meals also have a significance in human society that goes beyond the provision of nourishment for the body. In addition to fulfilling a basic physiological need, food may also help to satisfy one or more of an individual's many other needs. It has long been recognized, for example, that food is closely related to feelings of security. This security comes not merely from the presence or absence of food in sufficient quantity to satisfy hunger, but from the availability of specific foods. For many people, milk is a basic security food; for others, it may be meat, potatoes, rice, or some other familiar food that helps most to foster feelings of security. When people are ill, it is sometimes necessary to deprive them of certain foods. Individuals may feel threatened if foods which hold strong security meanings for them are absent from their diet. By the same token, a person's emotional health, especially in the stress of illness, may be "enhanced by significant 'comfort foods' that hold special meaning for the person and help to heal both the body and the spirit" (Williams, 1989, 12).

Food is often used to promote a feeling of social acceptance. Sitting down to eat with another person conveys to the person that he or she is considered an equal. Offering someone a cup of tea or coffee — the "ritual of hospitality" — can do much to foster an atmosphere of warmth and friendliness that is often difficult to attain in other ways.

Some people use foods for their prestige value, to enhance feelings of self-esteem. In many cultures, bread is a prestige food. For many years, steak and roast beef were considered prestige foods in North America. Now that the world has become a "global village," however, people have been introduced to the delights of cooking from other countries, and more exotic fare has become prestige food. Food may also be used to express creativity. Many women and men enjoy using their creative talents to prepare gourmet meals to please their families and friends.

The sharing of food in one form or another plays an important role in many religious ceremonies. In the Christian ceremony of Communion, for example, food has great significance. At Communion, one partakes of bread, which symbolizes the flesh of Christ, and of wine, which symbolizes His blood. In some religions, as for example in Judaism and in Islam, the preparation of food is in itself a ritual. There are also many food taboos associated with specific doctrines of other religions. The devout Muslim will not eat pork, for example, nor the Hindu, beef.

Food is, in fact, intertwined with the traditions, superstitions, and prejudices of virtually every culture. The

Being together for meals can help strengthen family ties.

Easter ham in our country and the Devali[*] gift of sweets in India are but two examples of the incorporation of food into traditional customs. To spill salt is considered by many people to be bad luck — a common example of a superstition involving food. Most of us have prejudices against certain foods; yet these foods may be eaten with great enjoyment by others. Few North Americans would have eaten snails 25 years ago; today they are selected by many as an appetizer in expensive restaurants. The fruit bat is considered a delicacy in Guam, but few "state-side" Americans relish it.

Mealtime, in many parts of the world, is a significant aspect of family life. In many cultures, eating is considered a private affair, to be shared and enjoyed only with one's family or intimate friends. Meals often play an important role in reaffirming solidarity within the family group. The traditional gathering of a family for Thanksgiving or Christmas dinner serves to strengthen ties within the extended family unit. Meals, too, may provide a time when family roles are defined and clarified, as when father (or mother, in many single-parent families) sits at the head of the table, a tangible symbol of the role as head of the family.

In addition, mealtime is often considered a pleasant time — a period of relaxation, when one can enjoy the company of others and engage in social conversation. Health agencies today are doing much to make mealtimes more pleasant for patients. Food is arranged attractively on trays; there is usually a menu from which patients may select the foods that they like; and many hospitals now have small dining areas next to the nursing units, where patients who are able may gather to eat their meals.

Thus, nutrition is vital to all aspects of health. As well as having psychological, social, cultural, and spiritual sig-

---

[*]   Devali, the "Festival of Lights," is a major religious festival in India.

nificance in a person's daily life, food is essential for physical health and well-being. Because all cells in the body require adequate nourishment for optimal functioning, all systems of the body may be affected by nutritional problems. When a person is ill, nutrition and diet therapy are primary factors in restoring health. A person's state of health may be restored without medicine, but the body cannot heal without proper nutrition (Poleman and Peckenpaugh, 1991). Whether well or ill, people may need assistance to maintain an adequate nutritional state, to achieve an even better state, or to correct a poor one. The responsibility for assisting individuals meet their nutritional needs rests with the physician, the dietitian, and the nurse. This chapter is intended to provide the nurse with basic knowledge of nutrition and diet therapy which will enable him or her to do the following:

1. assess the nutritional needs of individuals in health and illness
2. assist individuals in maintaining adequate nutrition and hydration during illness
3. provide restorative care to individuals experiencing nutritional problems
4. assist individuals in promoting optimal nutritional health for themselves and their families.

NUTRITIONAL NEEDS IN HEALTH

A person cannot exist for long without taking some form of nourishment. Food is the fuel which provides the energy for human metabolism. In order for people to function at their optimal level, they must consume adequate amounts of foods containing the essential nutrients for human life. A **nutrient** is defined as any chemical substance found in foods that functions in the growth, maintenance and repair of muscles, bones and other tissues, in the synthesis of enzymes and hormones, and in the regulation of body processes. The amount of nutrients required varies from one individual to another, depending on age, sex, current physical status, lifestyle, physical environment and many other factors. The essential nutrients are carbohydrates, proteins, fats, vitamins, minerals and water. Before discussing these important nutrients, we will review the physiological and biochemical processes involved in nutrition — digestion, absorption and metabolism.

DIGESTION, ABSORPTION AND METABOLISM

The food we eat is of no benefit to us unless it is in a form the cells of our bodies can use. To be usable, the nutrients that are taken into the body, normally via the gastrointestinal tract, must be digested and then absorbed into the blood stream for delivery to the cells. Metabolism, which refers to the chemical processes that sustain life and health, takes place in the cells. Figure 19.1 depicts the organs of the digestive system and summarizes their functions in digestion and absorption.

Digestion

Digestion is the process by which complex food forms are changed into simpler, soluble chemical parts so that they can be absorbed into the circulation for use by the body. Two simultaneous activities are involved in digestion — one is mechanical, the other chemical.

Mechanical or physical digestion pertains to the neuromuscular activities that break down food into smaller particles, mix them with digestive juices and propel the contents through the digestive tract so that digestion and absorption can take place. The rhythmic wave-like muscular contractions that move food down the gastrointestinal tract are called **peristalsis**.

Chemical digestion is carried out by the actions of several gastrointestinal secretions. Specific *enzymes* in digestive juices change food nutrients, namely carbohydrates, fats and proteins, into simple, soluble forms that can be absorbed. The chemical breakdown of nutrients occurs through the process of **hydrolysis**. Under the actions of digestive enzymes, nutrients are split into simpler elements by the addition of water to molecules. Carbohydrates are converted to simple sugars (glucose, fructose and galactose), fats to fatty acids and glycerol, and proteins to amino acids.

Enzymes have specific actions which occur under relatively specific conditions. For example, *pepsin*, which begins the breakdown of complex proteins in the stomach, is activated by hydrochloric acid. *Trypsin*, on the other hand, which acts on proteins in the small intestine, functions best in an alkaline medium. Thus, *hydrochloric acid* is secreted in the stomach and *buffer ions* (bicarbonate) are secreted in the pancreatic and intestinal juices to maintain the proper pH environment for the specific enzymes. Large amounts of *mucus* are secreted by the mouth, stomach and small intestine to lubricate and protect the lining of the entire gastrointestinal tract during its digestive activities. Other substances, such as bile from the liver and certain hormones, also aid in digestion. The secretions of the gastrointestinal tract are influenced and controlled by a number of factors, which include hormones, nerves, food passage, sensory stimuli and emotions (Williams, 1989). These factors are summarized in Figure 19.2.

Absorption

Absorption is the process whereby soluble nutrients pass through the intestinal wall into the blood or lymphatic circulation. Nutrients are mostly absorbed in the small intestine. The extremely large surface area of the small

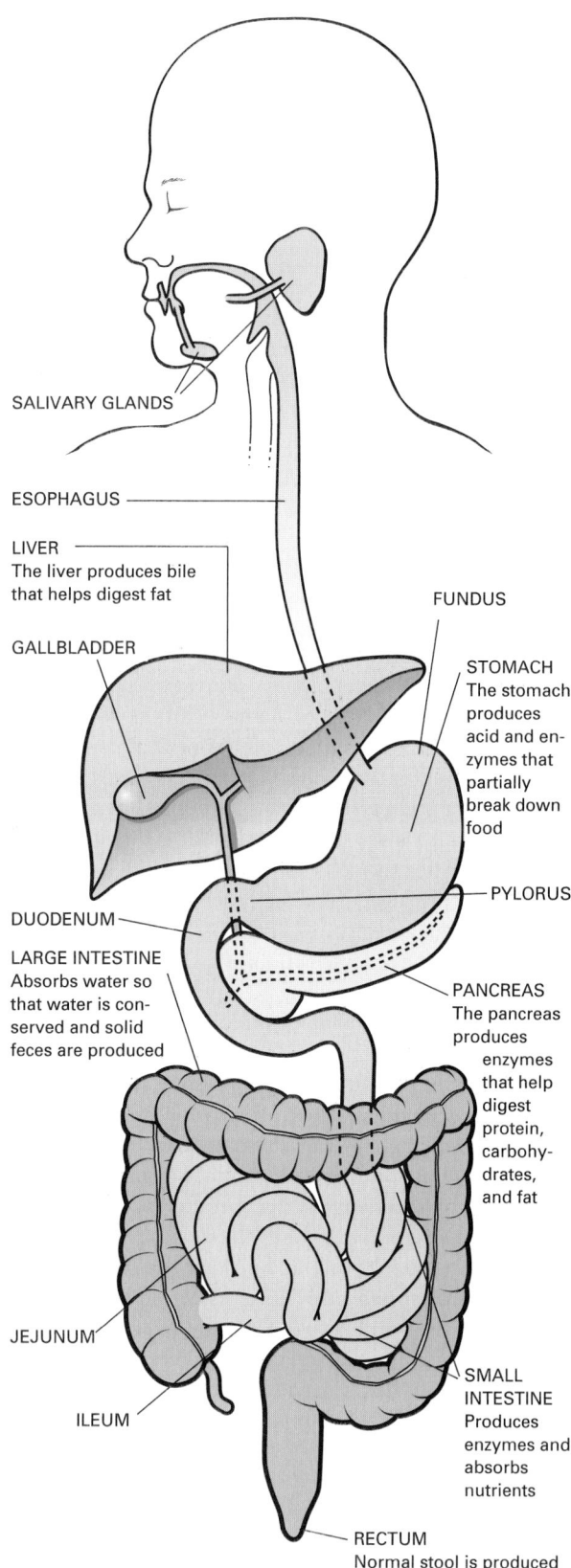

SALIVARY GLANDS

ESOPHAGUS

LIVER
The liver produces bile
that helps digest fat

GALLBLADDER

FUNDUS

STOMACH
The stomach
produces
acid and en-
zymes that
partially
break down
food

PYLORUS

DUODENUM

LARGE INTESTINE
Absorbs water so
that water is con-
served and solid
feces are produced

PANCREAS
The pancreas
produces
enzymes
that help
digest
protein,
carbohy-
drates,
and fat

JEJUNUM

ILEUM

SMALL
INTESTINE
Produces
enzymes and
absorbs
nutrients

RECTUM
Normal stool is produced

FIGURE 19.1 The digestive system

SOURCE: Poleman, C.M. and Peckenpaugh, N.J. (1991). *Nutrition: Essentials and diet therapy* (6th ed.). Philadelphia: Saunders, 61. Redrawn with permission.

intestine and its unique absorptive inner lining facilitate the process. The mucosal surface of the small intestine has a multitude of folds, called **mucosal folds**. Within these folds there are tiny finger-like projections called **villi**. Each villus contains vascular capillaries and a lacteal (a lymphatic vessel) to receive the absorbed nutrients. The surface of a villus consists of numerous absorptive cells which are capped by smaller projections referred to as *microvilli*. The villi trap the nutrient particles, which are then taken in by the absorptive cells. The mucosal folds, villi, and microvilli together increase the inner surface area of the small intestine about 600 times beyond that of the outer serosa (Williams, 1989).

Nutrients in the form of simple sugars, some fatty acids, amino acids, minerals and water soluble vitamins enter the blood stream through capillary beds that lead to the portal vein. The absorbed nutrients pass through the portal vein and into the liver where they are processed before reaching the general circulation. Other fatty acids, certain fat molecules and fat-soluble vitamins enter the lymphatic circulation via the lacteals. Also, water is absorbed from the large intestine.

Metabolism

"**Metabolism** is a general term covering all physical and chemical changes that food nutrients undergo after their absorption from the gastrointestinal tract, as well as the use of simple sugars, amino acids and glycerol by the body cells" (Poleman and Peckenpaugh, 1991, 64). There are two basic metabolic activities: catabolism and anabolism. In **catabolism**, compounds are broken down or oxidized for energy. In **anabolism**, this energy is used in the synthesis of enzymes and proteins needed by the body cells. The restructuring of amino acids to form protein elements of the body is a particularly important part of anabolism.

ESSENTIAL NUTRIENTS

Carbohydrates

As the name implies, **carbohydrates** are organic compounds that contain the elements carbon, hydrogen (and oxygen) in varying combinations. For the most part, they are starches and sugars produced in green plants through the process of photosynthesis. Some carbohydrates, such as lactose, come from milk produced in animals. The primary function of carbohydrates is to supply a source of energy for the body. Because of their availability and ease of production, carbohydrates are the most common nutrients in the diets of a vast majority of people throughout the world.

There are many forms of carbohydrates with varying degrees of complexity. The simple forms are called simple sugars and the more complex forms are called com-

Sucrose, or common table sugar, is the most common dietary disaccharide. Lactose is the sugar found in milk products. Maltose, like galactose, does not exist free in nature. It is found in malt and malt products, and, as such, is not a significant source of dietary carbohydrate. Maltose plays an important role in nutrition as an intermediate product formed when starch is changed to sugar during digestion.

Complex carbohydrates, or *polysaccharides*, are composed of many monosaccharide units, mainly glucose. They include starch, glycogen, dextrin and dietary fibre. Dietary sources of complex carbohydrates are commonly known as *starches*. The major foods containing starch are grain products such as wheat and rice, legumes such as beans and peas, potatoes and other vegetables. *Glycogen* is a form of animal starch which is stored in liver and muscle tissues. It is extremely important in energy metabolism as a source of glucose needed to maintain normal blood sugar levels during periods of fasting, such as when a person sleeps, and during high-intensity and high-endurance exercise. *Dextrin* is an intermediate polysaccharide formed from the breakdown of starch in the body.

Dietary fibre refers to the nondigestible residues of plant foods such as cellulose and pectin. Some fibres, such as cellulose, are water-insoluble. Their presence in the bowel adds bulk which stimulates peristalsis. Water-soluble fibres, such as pectins and gums, absorb and hold water in the intestine which further increases bulk and softens the stool, easing elimination. Dietary fibre has been receiving a lot of attention lately, as scientists have discovered that "there is considerable epidemiological evidence and some experimental evidence that increased fibre intake may help reduce the incidence rates of colon cancer and other intestinal disorders. In addition, some studies have also reported reduced cholesterol levels in the blood following a diet high in soluble fibres" (Williams, 1993, 100).

Dietary carbohydrates, with the exception of fibre, are easily digested and eventually converted to glucose which is easily absorbed into the bloodstream. The digestion and metabolism of carbohydrates are illustrated in Figure 19.3. Several things can happen to blood glucose. It may be metabolized directly by tissues, for instance, the brain and nervous system, for energy or it may be stored in the liver or muscles as glycogen. Some excess glucose is excreted in the urine, but the bulk of it is converted to fat and stored in adipose tissue.

Fats

Fats, or *lipids*, are compounds that are insoluble in water. They too are composed of carbon, hydrogen and oxygen, but in different ratios than in carbohydrates. They function primarily as a source of heat and energy to the body, and because they contain less oxygen, they release their energy more quickly and in greater quantity than do carbohydrates.

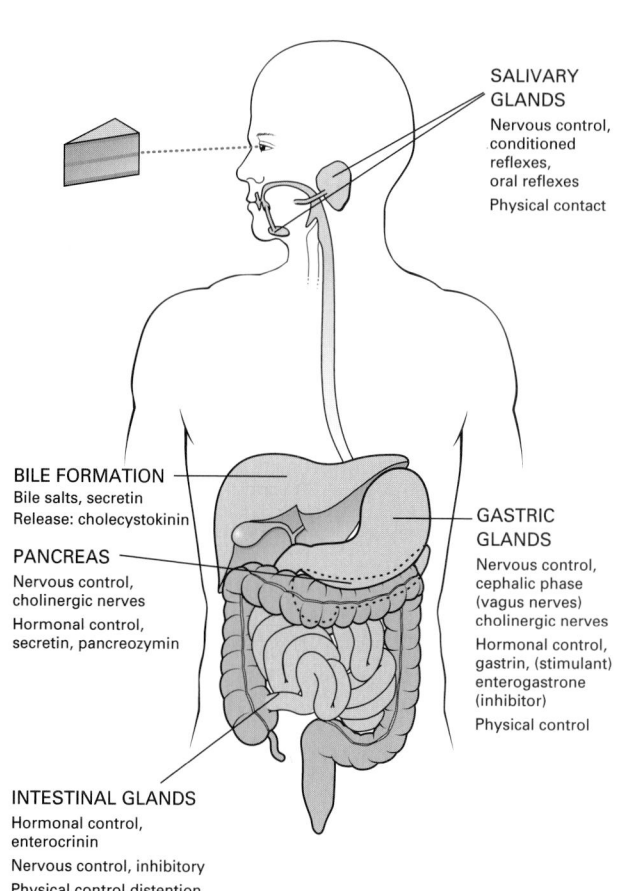

SALIVARY GLANDS
Nervous control, conditioned reflexes, oral reflexes
Physical contact

BILE FORMATION
Bile salts, secretin
Release: cholecystokinin

PANCREAS
Nervous control, cholinergic nerves
Hormonal control, secretin, pancreozymin

GASTRIC GLANDS
Nervous control, cephalic phase (vagus nerves) cholinergic nerves
Hormonal control, gastrin, (stimulant) enterogastrone (inhibitor)
Physical control

INTESTINAL GLANDS
Hormonal control, enterocrinin
Nervous control, inhibitory
Physical control distention

FIGURE 19.2 Factors influencing secretions of the gastrointestinal tract

SOURCE: Williams, S.R. (1989). *Nutrition and diet therapy* (6th ed.). St. Louis: Mosby. Redrawn with permission.

plex carbohydrates and dietary fibre. *Simple sugars* include monosaccharides (meaning one molecule or unit) and disaccharides (meaning two monosaccharides combined). The most common monosaccharides are glucose, fructose and galactose. Glucose and fructose occur naturally in fruits, honey and some vegetables. Galactose does not exist free in nature; it is found only in mammary glands. It occurs in the body as a by-product of lactose metabolism since it is attached to glucose in sugars that are found in milk.

Glucose is the major monosaccharide in the body. It is the end-product of all carbohydrate digestion and the form that is absorbed into the blood. Because it is the major sugar found in the bloodstream, glucose is also referred to as *blood sugar* or *dextrose*. In intravenous fluid therapy, dextrose is used as the carbohydrate fuel source. Sucrose, maltose and lactose are the most common disaccharides found in foods.

FIGURE 19.3 Digestion and metabolism of carbohydrates

SOURCE: Poleman, C.M. and Peckenpaugh, N.J. (1991). *Nutrition: Essentials and diet therapy* (6th ed.). Philadelphia: Saunders, 70. Reproduced with permission.

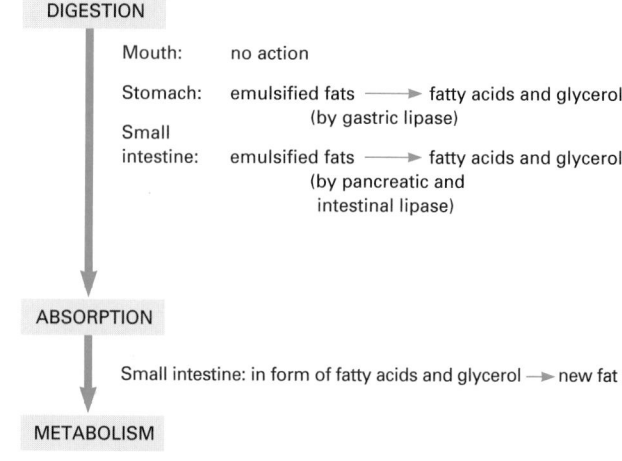

FIGURE 19.5 Digestion, absorption and metabolism of fats

SOURCE: Poleman, C.M. and Peckenpaugh, N.J. (1991). *Nutrition: Essentials and diet therapy* (6th ed.). Philadelphia: Saunders, 91. Reproduced with permission.

Moreover, they furnish essential fatty acids for the body, spare the burning of protein for energy, promote absorption of fat-soluble vitamins and insulate vital organs. Fats add flavour to foods and enhance satiety (the satisfied feeling of fullness) after eating by slowing the digestive process, thereby retarding the development of hunger (Poleman and Peckenpaugh, 1991). Fats are found naturally in animals and in plant seeds. The most common sources of fats in our diets are butter, margarine, nuts, eggs and oils used for cooking and in salad dressings.

There are two important lipids in human nutrition: triglycerides and cholesterol. **Triglycerides** are compounds made up of three fatty acids to one glycerol base. Glycerol is a sugar alcohol that is similar to carbohydrate. Fatty acids are chains of carbon atoms linked to hydrogen atoms. When all of the carbon atoms are linked to hydrogen atoms, the fatty acid is said to be **saturated**. In other words, it cannot

take up any more hydrogen atoms. Saturated fatty acids come primarily from animal food sources. They usually remain solid at room temperature, as, for example, butter or the fat that often surrounds a pork roast.

Fatty acids that come from plant sources are called **unsaturated** because not all of their carbon atoms are attached to hydrogen atoms, but are linked to each other by double bonds. This makes them capable of absorbing more hydrogen. Unsaturated fatty acids are classified as monounsaturated or polyunsaturated fatty acids, depending on the number of carbon-carbon double bonds they contain (see Figure 19.4). *Monounsaturated fatty acids* contain one carbon-carbon double bond which makes them capable of absorbing two or more hydrogen atoms. Olive and canola oil are sources of monounsaturated fatty acids. Fatty acids that contain two or more carbon-carbon double bonds are called *polyunsaturated fatty acids*. They can absorb four or more hydrogen atoms. Soybean, corn and most vegetable oils contain a good percentage of polyunsaturated fatty acids. Unsaturated fats are usually liquid at room temperature. They can be converted from liquid to solid states by the addition of hydrogen to some of the unfilled bonds (hydrogenation). The conversion of canola and corn oils into margarine is but one example.

There are three fatty acids essential to human health that are not synthesized by the body and must be obtained from food. These essential fatty acids, found in vegetable oils, are linoleic acid, linolenic acid, and arachidonic acid (LaQuatra and Gerlach, 1990). Essential fatty acids help to maintain skin and cell membrane integrity, lower serum

FIGURE 19.4 (A) Saturated fatty acid (B) Unsaturated fatty acid cholesterol levels and prolong blood clotting (Williams, 1989). They are also "precursors of prostaglandins, compounds that are important in the regulation of blood pressure and blood aggregation and that are intermediates in pain sensation" (LaQuatra and Gerlach, 1990, 32).

Cholesterol is a fat-like substance (sterol) that is necessary for the production of hormones such as estrogen and testosterone and the formation of bile (a principal emulsifier in fat digestion). It is also an essential component in the formation of cell membranes. Some cholesterol may be obtained from animal foods (for example, egg yolk); however, most of it is manufactured in the liver from fatty acids and products derived from carbohydrates and protein. Epidemiological studies have associated an excessive intake of saturated fats and cholesterol to heart disease and certain types of cancer. However, valid cause and effect relationships have not been established through experimental research (Health and Welfare Canada, 1990; Williams, 1993).

Figure 19.5 illustrates the digestive breakdown, absorption, and metabolism of dietary fats. Fats are mostly digested in the small intestine by pancreatic and intestinal juices after emulsion by bile and bile salts. They are changed to fatty acids and glycerol and absorbed from the small intestine. They may then be oxidized for energy, stored as fatty tissue, or combined with phosphorous to form phospholipids (essential cell elements).

Proteins

Like carbohydrates and fats, **proteins** are composed of carbon, hydrogen, and oxygen, but with the added element of nitrogen. These four elements are combined to form **amino acids**, the specific compounds (or building blocks) that are then linked together to make protein. The nitrogen component of an amino acid is responsible for protein's unique function in the human body — the building and repair of tissues. It is also essential for the production of body compounds such as digestive enzymes, hormones and glandular secretions; the formation of hemoglobin, antibodies and other blood proteins; and the regulation of water balance, nitrogen balance and nutrient transport. It can also be used as a source of energy. Protein is found in nature in animals and plants. The most common dietary sources are dairy products, meat, fish, eggs, legumes (such as peas and beans), nuts and seeds.

There are 22 amino acids that are known to be necessary for the building and repair of body tissues and for life-sustaining physiological processes. Most amino acids can be synthesized within the body or found in food. There are nine amino acids that cannot be manufactured in the body and must be acquired from dietary sources. These are called essential amino acids. They are isoleucine, leucine, lysine, methionine, phenylalanine, threonine, tryptophan, valine and histidine (for children). The amino acids formed in the body are termed nonessential amino acids. It must be stressed, however, that all 22 amino acids are necessary and

FIGURE 19.6   Digestion, absorption and metabolism of proteins

SOURCE: Poleman, C.M. and Peckenpaugh, N.J. (1991). *Nutrition: Essentials and diet therapy* (6th ed.). Philadelphia: Saunders, 81. Reproduced with permission.

must be present concurrently for the optimal maintenance of body growth, repair and function. Additionally, amino acids are not stored by the body as are carbohydrates. Thus, the body requires a constant supply of protein foodstuffs to meet ongoing needs.

Foods that contain all of the essential amino acids in amounts and proportions for proper use in the body are termed **complete proteins**. In order to ensure a balanced supply of amino acids, a diet should include proper amounts of complete proteins. As a general rule, animal sources of protein are complete proteins. Most vegetable and plant sources are not complete proteins and, therefore, do not meet the total protein needs of the body unless they are combined to form a complete protein. This poses a challenge to people who choose to avoid animal sources of protein in their diets. They must plan their diets to ensure the proper combinations of vegetable and plant sources of protein needed to supply an adequate balance of all the essential amino acids. For instance, legumes (kidney beans, soybeans, garden peas, black-eyed peas, lentils and lima beans), when combined with grains (wheat, barley) in a meal, provide a complete protein. This balance of intake is of extreme importance in strict vegetarian or vegan diets in which all foods of animal origin are avoided.

The digestion, absorption and metabolism of proteins are depicted in Figure 19.6. After digestion, amino acids are absorbed and used for synthesis of body tissues and protein substances. Excess protein may be stripped of nitrogen and converted to glucose. Waste products are excreted in the urine.

Vitamins

Vitamins are a natural component of most foods. They are necessary for promoting and regulating chemical processes that convert food into energy, build and repair tissues and protect cells. Vitamins are designated as A, B, C, D, E and K, and are classified into two main groups — the fat-soluble and the water-soluble vitamins. The *fat-soluble vitamins* (A, D, E and K) are transported throughout the body in fats. The *water-soluble vitamins* (the B complex and C) use water as their vehicle. For this reason, foods containing these vitamins are most effective when eaten raw, since cooking tends to remove the vitamins. Some vitamins may be synthesized in the body, such as vitamin A from beta-carotene, vitamin D from the action of sunlight on the skin, and vitamin K from the action of bacteria in the bowel (Williams, 1993). However, most vitamins must be supplied from food.

A summary of the major vitamins, their functions, some food sources and primary symptoms of deficiency or excess is outlined in Table 19.1. Some vitamins, such as the B vitamins, serve as coenzymes in chemical reactions. *Coenzymes* are essential elements needed for the activation or control of enzyme activity which regulates physiological processes in the body such as digestion, energy production, and carbohydrate, fat and protein metabolism (Williams, 1993). Other vitamins, such as C, E, and beta-carotene (a precursor to vitamin A), function as antioxidants. Antioxidants are agents that help to prevent DNA alteration caused by electron-seeking (oxidizing) substances. The antioxidants interfere with this oxidative process by donating electrons. Vitamin E also delays or prevents the destruction of cell membranes by protecting polyunsaturated fatty acids from oxidizing compounds (Wardlaw, Insel, Seyler, 1992; Williams, 1989). Vitamin D has been found to act as a hormone (Williams, 1989).

Minerals

Minerals are necessary to the body in the building and maintenance of bones, teeth and the various body systems. The main essential minerals are considered to be calcium, iron, phosphorus and magnesium. Other minerals, called trace minerals, are equally essential, but are needed in much smaller amounts. Some of these other minerals required by the body are copper, iodine, manganese, zinc and fluorine.

Calcium is important for the proper formation of teeth and bones, for muscle tone and nerve transmissions and for the coagulation of blood. The main sources of calcium in most diets are milk and other dairy products, but calcium is also found in dark green leafy vegetables, fish with edible bones, eggs, meat and cereals.

Phosphorus aids in the formation and strengthening of bones. It can be obtained from dairy products, meat, fish, poultry, nuts, whole grains and legumes.

Magnesium is an important factor in the regulation of the body's temperature, nerve conduction, and muscle contractions. Common dietary sources of magnesium are green leafy vegetables, nuts, whole grains and beans.

Iron is important for building hemoglobin in red blood cells and for preventing nutritional anemia. The best sources are liver, red meats and egg yolk, but it is also found in lentils, green leafy vegetables, whole grain and enriched cereals, flours, bread and pastas.

Water

Water is the single most important nutrient in the human body. It is a component of most foods, both liquid and solid. Water is a vehicle of absorption for most nutrients in the body and is present in all body excretions and secretions. Approximately 60 to 70 percent of the adult body is composed of water. Because of its importance in the regulation and maintenance of all body tissues and processes, water is discussed in more detail in Chapter 22.

ENERGY REQUIREMENTS

Dietary requirements are generally considered in terms of both specific nutrients and energy requirements. The body's needs for energy and the energy value of foods are usually expressed in calories (a term taken from the physical sciences), which measure heat units. A *calorie* is the amount of heat required to raise the temperature of one gram of water by one degree Celsius. The large calorie, or kilocalorie (kcal), is used in nutrition to indicate that it represents 1000 of the calories used in the physical sciences. As such, a *kilocalorie* is the amount of heat needed to raise the temperature of one kilogram of water by one degree Celsius. The energy value of food is also expressed in kilojoules (kJ) such that 1 kilocalorie is equal to 4.184 kilojoules. The energy values of the principal foods are 4 kcal per gram (17 kJ) of carbohydrates, 9 kcal/gm (38 kJ) of fat and 4 kcal/gm (17 kJ) of protein.

ENERGY USE BY THE BODY

The body uses energy for three basic purposes. These are
• basal metabolism
• physical activity
• the thermic effect of food.

In addition, there may be a small energy expenditure when a person is cold and the body produces heat through shivering (Wardlaw, Insel and Seyler, 1992). Growing individuals and pregnant women also require extra energy for the synthesis of new tissue.

Basal Metabolism

The **basal metabolic rate** (BMR) represents the minimum energy requirements of the body when the individual is awake and at digestive, physical and emotional rest (Williams, 1989). It is the amount needed for the internal work of the body, which includes maintaining a heartbeat, circulation, respiration, temperature and muscle tone. In adults living in Western countries, basal metabolism accounts for approximately 60 to 70 percent of a person's total caloric expenditure (Katch and McArdle, 1988). A BMR test, conducted in a laboratory or hospital setting, is required to get an accurate BMR value for an individual. However, a less accurate estimate can be obtained by multiplying one's weight in kilograms by 0.9 (calories) for a woman and 1.0 (calories) for a man and then by 24 (number of hours in a day).

A person's basal metabolic rate is influenced primarily by body composition and lean body mass. Lean body mass consists of muscles, bones and body organs such as the heart, liver and kidneys; it represents the body weight minus fat. The influence of lean body mass on metabolism is the result of higher metabolic activity in tissues such as muscles and the liver. Other factors such as surface area, sex and age only determine basal metabolism as they relate to the lean body mass (Williams, 1989). These are outlined in the box in the next column.

Physical Activity Needs

To the basal metabolic requirements are added the energy needs for work, movement and exercise. It is primarily the work of body muscles that demands the energy. Mental activity consumes very little extra energy, because the brain is always active and is therefore accounted for in the basal metabolic rate. However, emotional states may increase energy needs as a result of restlessness, agitated activity or muscle tension. Physical activity is estimated to account for 20 to 30 percent of an adult person's total energy use by the body (Katch and McArdle, 1988).

Energy expenditure for physical activity varies widely among individuals. The amount of energy used depends upon the vigor with which a person works and the amount of time per day he or she spends at the activities. A person would not expend as much energy in dancing a slow waltz, for example, as in a fast square dance. People who play a leisurely game of tennis for an hour two or three times a week would not have energy expenditures per hour as great as the professional who puts full effort into every point. There is also a wide variety of energy expenditure involved in the specific jobs that might be found in any given line of

work. A person living alone in a small apartment usually would not use as much energy in housework as one who has to clean an eight-room house and cook for a large family. A cabinet maker whose work involves small detail would not expend as much energy as a carpenter building houses. Table 19.2 presents the expenditures in various types of work and recreation.

Thermic Effect of Food

When food is taken into the body, the body uses energy to digest, absorb, transport and further process the nutrients. This overall stimulating effect of food is called **dietary thermogenesis** (Williams, 1989) and accounts for about

---

Factors That Determine Basal Metabolic Rate

FACTOR	INFLUENCE ON BMR
Lean body mass	The greater the body mass, the higher the BMR.
Body surface	The greater the area, the greater the heat loss.
Gender	Males average higher energy rates because of greater lean body mass.
Age	BMR rises during the first five years of life, levels off, rises again just before and during puberty, and then declines with advancing age in adults.
Body temperature	Fever increases BMR about 7 percent for each .83° C rise.
Thyroid hormone activity	Higher levels increase metabolic rate.
Nutritional state	Eating less slows metabolic rate.
Pregnancy and lactation	Metabolic rate increases.
Caffeine and tobacco use	Metabolic rate increases.

SOURCES: Wardlaw, Insel and Seyler (1992), 343; Williams (1989), 201.

TABLE 19.1 Essential Vitamins

VITAMIN NAME (OTHER TERMS)	MAJOR SOURCES	MAJOR FUNCTIONS IN THE BODY
Fat-Soluble Vitamins		
Vitamin A (retinol; provitamin carotenoids)	Retinol in animal foods: liver, whole milk, fortified milk, cheese. Carotenoids in plant foods: carrots, green leafy vegetables, sweet potatoes, fortified margarine from vegetable oils.	Maintenance of epithelial tissue in skin and mucous membranes; formation of visual purple for night vision; bone development.
Vitamin D (calciferol)	Vitamin D fortified foods like dairy products, margarine, and fish oils. Action of sunlight on the skin.	Acts as a hormone to increase intestinal absorption of calcium and promote bone and tooth formation.
Vitamin E (tocopherol)	Vegetable oils, margarine, green leafy vegetables, wheat germ, whole grain products, egg yolks.	Functions as an antioxidant to protect cell membranes from destruction by oxidation.
Vitamin K (antihemorrhagic vitamin)	Pork and beef liver, eggs, spinach, cauliflower. Formation in the human intestines by bacteria.	Essential for blood coagulation processes.
Water-Soluble Vitamins		
Thiamin (vitamin B_1)	Ham, pork, lean meat, liver, whole grain products, fortified breads and cereals, legumes.	Serves as a coenzyme for energy production from carbohydrate; essential for normal functioning of the central nervous system.
Riboflavin (vitamin B_2)	Milk and diary products, meat, fortified grain products, green leafy vegetables, beans.	Functions as a coenzyme involved in energy production from carbohydrates and fats; maintains healthy skin.
Niacin (nicotinamide, nicotinic acid)	Lean meats, fish, poultry, whole grain products, beans. May be forced in the body from tryptophan, an essential amino acid.	Functions as a coenzyme for the aerobic and anaerobic production of energy from carbohydrate; helps synthesize fat and blocks release of FFA; needed for healthy skin.
Vitamin B_6 (pyridoxal, pyridoxine, pyridoxamine)	Protein foods, liver, lean meats, fish, poultry, legumes, green leafy vegetables.	Functions as a coenzyme in protein metabolism; necessary for formation of hemoglobin and red blood cells; needed for glycogenolysis and gluconeogenesis.
Vitamin B_{12} (cobalamin; cyanocobalamin)	Animal foods only, meat, fish, poultry, milk, eggs.	Functions as coenzyme for formation of DNA, development of RBC, and maintenance of nerve tissue.
Folic acid (folacin)	Liver, green leafy vegetables, legumes, nuts.	Functions as coenzyme for DNA formation and RBC development.
Biotin	Meats, legumes, milk, egg yolk, whole grain products, most vegetables.	Functions as a coenzyme in the metabolism of carbohydrates, fats, and protein.
Pantothenic acid	Beef and pork liver, lean meats, milk, eggs, legumes, whole grain products, most vegetables.	Functions as part of coenzyme A in energy metabolism.
Vitamin C (ascorbic acid)	Citrus fruits, green leafy vegetables, broccoli, peppers, strawberries, potatoes.	Forms collagen essential for connective tissue development; aids in absorption of iron; helps form epinephrine; serves as antioxidant.

DEFICIENCY SYMPTOMS	SYMPTOMS OF EXCESS CONSUMPTION
Night blindness, intestinal infections, impaired growth, xerophthalmia.	Nausea, headache, fatigue, liver and spleen damage, skin peeling, pain in the joints.
Rare. Rickets in children and osteomalacia in adults.	Loss of appetite, nausea, irritability, joint pains, calcium deposits in soft tissues such as the kidney.
Extremely rare. Disruption of red blood cell membranes, anemia.	General lack of toxicity with doses up to 600 IU.
Increased bleeding and hemorrhaging.	Possible clot formation (thrombus), vomiting.
Poor appetite, apathy, mental depression, pain in calf muscles, beriberi.	General lack of toxicity.
Dermatitis, cracks at the corners of the mouth, sores on the tongue, damage to the cornea.	General lack of toxicity.
Loss of appetite, weakness, skin lesions, gastrointestinal problems, pellagra.	Nicotinic acid causes headache, nausea, burning and itching skin, flushing of face.
Nervous irritability, convulsions, dermatitis, sores on tongue, anemia.	Loss of nerve sensation, impaired gait.
Pernicious anemia, nerve damage resulting in paralysis.	General lack of toxicity.
Fatigue, gastrointestinal disorders, diarrhea, anemia.	May prevent detection of pernicious anemia caused by B_{12} deficiency.
Rare. May be caused by excessive intake of raw egg whites. Fatigue, nausea, skin rashes.	General lack of toxicity.
Rare. Only produced clinically. Fatigue, nausea, loss of appetite, mental depression.	General lack of toxicity.
Weakness, rough skin, slow wound healing, bleeding gums, scurvy.	Diarrhea, possible kidney stones, rebound scurvy.

TABLE 19.2   Energy Expenditure Per Hour During Various Activities*

LIGHT ACTIVITIES (120-150 KCAL/HR)	LIGHT TO MODERATE ACTIVITIES (150-300 KCAL/HR)	MODERATE ACTIVITIES (300-420 KCAL/HR)	HEAVY ACTIVITIES (420-600 KCAL/HR)
Personal care Dressing Washing Shaving **Sitting** Rocking Typing Writing Playing cards Peeling potatoes Sewing Playing piano **Standing or slowly moving around** **Billiards**	**Domestic work** Making beds Sweeping floors Ironing Washing clothes **Yard Work** Light gardening Mowing lawn (power mower) **Light Work** Auto repair Painting Shoe repair Store clerk Washing car **Walking** 2 to 3 mph on level surface or down stairs **Recreation** Archery Bicycling 5 1/2 mph on level surface Bowling Canoeing 2 1/2 to 3 mph	**Yard work** Digging Mowing lawn (not motorized) Pulling weeds **Walking** 3 1/2 to 4 mph on level surface Up and down small hills **Recreation** Badminton Calisthenics Ballet exercises Canoeing 4 mph Dancing (waltz, square) Golf (no cart) Ping-Pong Tennis (doubles) Volleyball	**Yard work** Chopping wood Digging holes Shovelling snow **Walking** 5 mph Up stairs Up hills Climbing **Recreation** Bicycling 11 to 12 mph or up and down hills Cross-country skiing Jogging 5 mph Swimming Tennis (singles) Water-skiing

* Energy expenditure will depend on the physical fitness (that is, amount of lean body mass) of the individual and on the continuity of exercise.

SOURCE: Williams, S.R. (1989). *Nutrition and diet therapy* (6th ed.). St. Louis: Mosby, 203. Reproduced with permission.

10 percent of the body's total energy needs in adults (Katch and McArdle, 1988). For example, in a person whose daily caloric requirement is 2400 kilocalories, about 240 kilocalories would be needed for the thermogenic effect of food.

DAILY ENERGY REQUIREMENTS

The body's energy requirements vary considerably from one individual to another, depending principally on body composition (lean body mass and body fat), age, sex and the kind and amount of daily activity. Thus, there is no fixed level of energy intake that is required by all individuals of the same age, sex, and size. Rather, there is a wide range of energy intakes that can be considered adequate, depending on the level of activity performed, on what is considered desirable in the society in which they live, and on

their degree of adaptation to environmental stresses, such as changes in temperature or food intake, and emotional tension (Health and Welfare Canada, 1990). Table 19.3 outlines estimates of average energy requirements according to age, sex, and physical activity. These estimates are based on average desirable weights for each age and sex category.

RECOMMENDED NUTRIENT REQUIREMENTS

Recommended daily requirements of specific nutrients have been established in Canada, as in many other countries. International standards have been issued by the United Nations Food and Agriculture Organization and the World

TABLE 19.3 Daily Energy Requirements According to Age, Sex, and Activity (kcal/day)[a]

	19-24 YEARS		25-49 YEARS		50-74 YEARS		75 YEARS+	
	M	**F**	**M**	**F**	**M**	**F**	**M**	**F**
Weight	69	58	67	58	65	56	64	54
BMR	1735	1349	1654	1337	1472	1237	1351	1163
Light activity[b]	2700	2100	2600	2100	2300	1900	2100	1800
	(39/kg)	(36/kg)	(38/kg)	(36/kg)	(35/kg)	(34/kg)	(33/kg)	(34/kg)
Moderate activity[c]	3100	2200	2900	2200	2600	2000	2400	1900
	(45/kg)	(38/kg)	(44/kg)	(38/kg)	(40/kg)	(36/kg)	(37.5/kg)	(35/kg)
Heavy activity[d]	3600	2500	3500	2400	3100	2300	2800	2100
	(53/kg)	(42/kg)	(52/kg)	(42/kg)	(48/kg)	(40/kg)	(44/kg)	(39/kg)

a. 1 kcal is equivalent to 4.184 kJ.
b. Calculated on the basis of average expenditure = 1.55 BMR for men and 1.56 BMR for women.
c. Calculated on the basis of average expenditure = 1.78 BMR for men and 1.64 BMR for women.
d. Calculated on the basis of average expenditure = 2.10 BMR for men and 1.82 BMR for women.

SOURCE: Health and Welfare Canada. (1990). *Nutrition recommendations: The report of the Scientific Review Committee.* Ottawa: Minister of Supply and Services, 24. (Catalogue No. H49–41/1990E). Reproduced with the permission of the Minister of Supply and Services Canada, 1994.

Health Organization (FAO/WHO). Food guides have also been developed to help people select foods that will ensure an adequate supply of essential nutrients in their daily diets. These are discussed later on in the chapter.

The latest edition of national nutrition guidelines for Canadians was completed in 1990 by the Scientific Review Committee in a Report entitled *Nutrition Recommendations*, made to the Minister of National Health and Welfare. Their purpose is to provide guidance in the selection of a dietary pattern that will supply adequate amounts of essential nutrients to promote and maintain health and reduce the risk of nutrition-related diseases (Health and Welfare Canada, 1989). *Nutrition Recommendations for Canadians* is summarized in the box. A summary of recommended daily intakes of nutrients is presented in Tables 19.4 and 19.5.

NUTRITIONAL NEEDS THROUGHOUT THE LIFE CYCLE

Major factors affecting nutritional needs throughout the life cycle were included in the discussion of needs requiring particular attention at each stage of the life cycle in Chapter 8. In this section, we will discuss how changes in growth and development affect specific nutrient requirements in each age group.

Nutrition Recommendations for Canadians

- The Canadian diet should provide energy consistent with the maintenance of body weight within the recommended range.
- The Canadian diet should include essential nutrients in amounts recommended.
- The Canadian diet should include no more than 30% of energy as fat (33 g/1000 kcal) and no more than 10% as saturated fat (11 g/1000 kcal).
- The Canadian diet should provide 55% of energy as carbohydrate (138 g/1000 kcal) from a variety of sources.
- The sodium content of the Canadian diet should be reduced.
- The Canadian diet should include no more than 5% of total energy as alcohol, or two drinks daily, whichever is less.
- The Canadian diet should contain no more caffeine than the equivalent of four regular cups of coffee per day.
- Community water supplies containing less than 1 mg/litre should be fluoridated to that level.

SOURCE: Health and Welfare Canada (1990).

TABLE 19.4 Summary of Recommended Nutrient Intakes Based on Energy Expressed as Daily Rates

AGE	SEX	ENERGY KCAL	THIAMIN MG	RIBOFLAVIN MG	NIACIN NE[b]	N-3 PUFA[a] G	N-6 PUFA G
Months							
0-4	Both	600	0.3	0.3	4	0.5	3
5-12	Both	900	0.4	0.5	7	0.5	3
Years							
1	Both	1100	0.5	0.6	8	0.6	4
2-3	Both	1300	0.6	0.7	9	0.7	4
4-6	Both	1800	0.7	0.9	13	1.0	6
7-9	M	2200	0.9	1.1	16	1.2	7
	F	1900	0.8	1.0	14	1.0	6
10-12	M	2500	1.0	1.3	18	1.4	8
	F	2200	0.9	1.1	16	1.2	7
13-15	M	2800	1.1	1.4	20	1.5	9
	F	2200	0.9	1.1	16	1.2	7
16-18	M	3200	1.3	1.6	23	1.8	11
	F	2100	0.8	1.1	15	1.2	7
19-24	M	3000	1.2	1.5	22	1.6	10
	F	2100	0.8	1.1	15	1.2	7
25-49	M	2700	1.1	1.4	19	1.5	9
	F	1900	0.8[c]	1.0[c]	14[c]	1.1[c]	7[c]
50-74	M	2300	0.9	1.2	16	1.3	8
	F	1800	0.8[c]	1.0[c]	14[c]	1.1[c]	7[c]
75 +	M	2000	0.8	1.0	14	1.1	7
	F[d]	1700	0.8[c]	1.0[c]	14[c]	1.1[c]	7[c]
Pregnancy (additional)							
1st Trimester		100	0.1	0.1	1	0.05	0.3
2nd Trimester		300	0.1	0.3	2	0.16	0.9
3rd Trimester		300	0.1	0.3	2	0.16	0.9
Lactation (additional)		450	0.2	0.4	3	0.25	1.5

a. PUFA, polyunsaturated fatty acids
b. Niacin equivalents
c. Level below which intake should not fall
d. Assumes moderate physical activity

SOURCE: Health and Welfare Canada. (1990). *Nutrition recommendation: The report of the Scientific Review Committee*. Ottawa: Minister of Supply and Services, 203. (Catalogue No. H49–41/1990E). Reproduced with the permission of the Minister of Supply and Services Canada, 1994.

A community health nurse provides counselling for a pregnant woman.

THE PREGNANT WOMAN AND THE FETUS

Although a good pregnancy outcome cannot be guaranteed by diet alone, proper nutrition does significantly influence the health of the mother and her fetus (Chez, 1991). The developing fetus is totally dependent on his or her mother for nourishment. Inadequate nutrition can seriously impair fetal growth and can result in low birth weight, growth retardation, congenital defects and neonatal mortality. Malnutrition in the first few weeks of pregnancy (two to eight weeks), when organs and structures are developing, may cause irreversible abnormalities. Growth retardation is the effect of nutritional deprivation later in pregnancy, once organ formation is complete.

In order to ensure that the nutritional needs of the fetus are met, the mother must maintain a well-balanced diet with the addition of extra nutrients. In particular, more carbohydrates are needed for maternal and fetal energy, protein for fetal tissue development and growth, and calcium for mineralization of the fetal skeleton. As well, increased amounts of folic acid (folacin) and iron are essential for red cell formation required to ensure adequate hemoglobin levels in both mother and fetus. Maternal demands rise in response to the need for greater red cell production owing to the increased blood volume during pregnancy. In addition to needing iron for building red blood cells and hemoglobin, the fetus also stores iron in the liver to sustain him or her through the first three months of life when intake from milk is low. The recommended nutrient intakes for pregnant women are included at the end of Tables 19.4 and 19.5.

THE BREASTFEEDING MOTHER AND THE INFANT

The woman who is breastfeeding her infant has higher requirements for most nutrients, including energy, proteins, minerals and vitamins, than the expectant mother. These nutrients are needed to cover the demands made on the mother's body for the production of the milk as well as the nutrients secreted in the milk that provides nourishment to the infant.

The diet recommended for lactating mothers is essentially the same as for pregnant women and should include plentiful supplies of milk and alternate calcium and protein sources. The nursing mother needs a lot of fluids to provide for the water content of breast milk; two to three litres are suggested.

The normal newborn generally loses five percent of his or her birth weight during the first two to three days of life, owing to adjustments in total body water. With adequate nutrition (120 kcal per kg per day), the normal healthy infant should gain one kg per month from one to three months of age, 500 g per month from three to six months of age, and 250 g per month from six to twelve months of age (Health Promotion Directorate, Health and Welfare Canada and Canadian Pediatric Society, 1988). Adequate nutrition during infancy is important for optimal growth and development of body tissues. Fatty acids are necessary for neurological growth and development.

The gastrointestinal tract of infants is relatively immature. Breast milk, which is the baby's natural food, provides the most easily digested source of nourishment. Breast milk is also the most complete food, needing only to be supplemented by vitamin D for the first few months. However, many babies have been raised to healthy adulthood on goat's milk and formulas made from other substances (soybeans, for example). The formula used must be tailored to the needs of each individual infant.

It is now generally recommended that solid foods not be introduced until six months of age. More rapidly growing infants may, however, need solids after four months (Hewat, 1987). Until that time the tongue extrudes, which makes swallowing food difficult. It is also believed that exposure to certain foods (especially those high in protein) in early infancy may lead to food allergies later in life. Solids should be introduced gradually, with one new food at a time, in soft, or pureed, form.

During the first year of life, the infant's rate of growth and development is quite remarkable. It slows down during the second year, however, and the mother may notice that the one-year-old's appetite is not as great as it was. She should be reassured that the loss of appetite of the typical one-year-old is normal. It is during the second year of life, too, that the child moves from breast or bottle feeding and soft food supplements, to drinking from a cup and eating table foods.

THE CHILD

In the toddler and preschool years the child's physical and social skills related to eating develop rapidly. A summary of their skills from approximately three months to six years is

TABLE 19.5 Summary of Recommended Nutrient Intakes Based on Age and Body Weight Expressed as Daily Rates

AGE	SEX	WEIGHT KG	PROTEIN G	VIT. A RE[a]	VIT. D µG	VIT. E MG	VIT. C MG
Months							
0-4	Both	6.0	12[b]	400	10	3	20
5-12	Both	9.0	12	400	10	3	20
Years							
1	Both	11	13	400	10	3	20
2-3	Both	14	16	400	5	4	20
4-6	Both	18	19	500	5	5	25
7-9	M	25	26	700	2.5	7	25
	F	25	26	700	2.5	6	25
10-12	M	34	34	800	2.5	8	25
	F	36	36	800	2.5	7	25
13-15	M	50	49	900	2.5	9	30[e]
	F	48	46	800	2.5	7	30[e]
16-18	M	62	58	1000	2.5	10	40[e]
	F	53	47	800	2.5	7	30[e]
19-24	M	71	61	1000	2.5	10	40[e]
	F	58	50	800	2.5	7	30[e]
25-49	M	74	64	1000	2.5	9	40[e]
	F	59	51	800	2.5	6	30[e]
50-74	M	73	63	1000	5	7	40[e]
	F	63	54	800	5	6	30[e]
75 +	M	69	59	1000	5	6	40[e]
	F	64	55	800	5	5	30[e]
Pregnancy (additional)							
1st Trimester			5	0	2.5	2	0
2nd Trimester			15	0	2.5	2	10
3rd Trimester			24	0	2.5	2	10
Lactation (additional)			20	400	2.5	3	25

a. Retinol Equivalents
b. Protein is assumed to be from breast milk and must be adjusted for infant formula.
c. Infant formula with high phosphorus should contain 375 mg calcium.
d. Breast milk is assumed to be the source of the mineral.
e. Smokers should increase vitamin C by 50%.

SOURCE: Health and Welfare Canada. (1990). *Nutrition recommendation: The report of the Scientific Review Committee.* Ottawa: Minister of Supply and Services, 204. (Catalogue No. H49–41/1990E). Reproduced with the permission of the Minister of Supply and Services Canada, 1994.

TABLE 19.5 continued

FOLATE µG	VIT. B$_{12}$ µG	CALCIUM MG	PHOS-PHORUS MG	MAG-NESIUM MG	IRON MG	IODINE µG	ZINC MG
25	0.3	250[c]	150	20	0.3[d]	30	2[d]
40	0.4	400	200	32	7	40	3
40	0.5	500	300	40	6	55	4
50	0.6	550	350	50	6	65	4
70	0.8	600	400	65	8	85	5
90	1.0	700	500	100	8	110	7
90	1.0	700	500	100	8	95	7
120	1.0	900	700	130	8	125	9
130	1.0	1100	800	135	8	110	9
175	1.0	1100	900	185	10	160	12
170	1.0	1000	850	180	13	160	9
220	1.0	900	1000	230	10	160	12
190	1.0	700	850	200	12	160	9
220	1.0	800	1000	240	9	160	12
180	1.0	700	850	200	13	160	9
230	1.0	800	1000	250	9	160	12
185	1.0	700	850	200	13	160	9
230	1.0	800	1000	250	9	160	12
195	1.0	800	850	210	8	160	9
215	1.0	800	1000	230	9	160	12
200	1.0	800	850	210	8	160	9
200	0.2	500	200	15	0	25	6
200	0.2	500	200	45	5	25	6
200	0.2	500	200	45	10	25	6
100	0.2	500	200	65	0	50	6

TABLE 19.6   Development of a Child's Physical and Social Skills

AGE	PHYSICAL SKILLS	SOCIAL SKILLS
3-6 months	Tongue projects so swallowing food is difficult. Fingers foods.	
6-12 months	Uses hands. Uses tongue and lips when eating. Chewing movements start. Takes juice and water from cup but spills when cup is removed.	Perceives size, shape, weight, and texture. Reads facial expressions and gestures. Very demanding of person who feeds him or her.
12-18 months	Grasps and releases finger foods. Grasps spoon, inserts in dish but filling poor. Spoon often upside down when reaches mouth. Release of cup and spoon poor and drops frequently.	Demands everything in sight at table. Refuses milk from bottle. Loves an audience.
18 months-2 years	Drop in appetite. Uses both hands when feeding. Drinks well from cup but release still poor. Tongue can lick off chin. Turns spoon in mouth.	Ritualistic. Refusals and preferences. Easily distracted.
2-3 years	Drinks with small glass held with one hand. Spoon is grasped between thumb and index finger and goes into mouth without turning. Considerable spilling.	Finicky and fussy eaters. Spotless eaters may demand to be fed. Messy eaters won't accept help. Food jags. Ritualistic. Dawdles. Demanding: • of whole foods; • of between-meal-snacks; • of candy if in home. Dislikes: • food mixtures; • vegetables. Food is the most important part of second birthday.
3-4 years	Holds cup by handle. Tilts head back to empty cup. Pours from pitchers. Uses fork. Little spilling. Little assistance needed. Chews more foods.	Conforming and assenting. Fair appetite: • milk intake increase; • vegetables are slowly accepted. Asks for favourite foods. Able to choose between two alternatives. Birthday cake is important part of third birthday party.
4-5 years	Use knife and fork. Tilts cup to empty it.	Assertive. Lively mind. Very social. Fair to very good appetite. Food jags or strikes. Reacts to incentives, e.g., "eating to be big." Sets table and cooks.
5-6 years	Able to feed self.	Influenced by group and social pressures outside home. Still prefers plain foods.

SOURCE: *Selected nutrition teaching aids.* (1976). Ottawa: Department of National Health and Welfare.

outlined in Table 19.6. Children need the same types of foods as adults, with quantities adjusted to meet their smaller size (these were shown in Tables 19.4 and 19.5). Because their independence is also rapidly developing, small children much prefer foods that they can manage themselves, usually foods that can be eaten with the fingers. Good eating habits can be established at this time, with a pattern of regular meals and a sufficient but not excessive intake of nutritious food.

Malnutrition in childhood results in growth failures and renders the child more susceptible to infections. In addition, iron-deficiency anemia can occur.

Excess intake of vitamins, particularly vitamins A and D, has become a common problem, presumably because many mothers mistakenly believe that their children can only benefit from consuming large amounts of vitamins. A good diet can provide the minerals and vitamins children require, although physicians and baby clinics may recommend supplements in special situations. This may be, for instance, when children are going through a growth spurt, when their appetite is poor during illness, or if certain foodstuffs are not eaten because the child does not like them (or cannot tolerate them) or because some foods are not available or too expensive, as, for example, fresh fruits and vegetables at certain times of the year.

School-age children's rates of growth are slower than they were in infancy or will be again in adolescence. However, it is critically important that their nutritional needs be met to promote optimal growth and development. A nutritious breakfast that includes a good source of protein is particularly important for the school-age child to ensure good work performance and good concentration in the late morning hours. Teachers of special education classes for children with emotional problems have found that the most troublesome youngsters were those who had come to school without eating breakfast.

School-age children are also developing their social skills and enjoy inviting another child home to share meals with them. At this age children also begin to enjoy experimenting with different food tastes and add to the variety of foods they will eat, although they still prefer plain foods and those they can eat with their fingers.

Among the common problems of childhood, iron deficiency is the most prevalent deficiency, and deficiencies in calcium and vitamins C and D are also problems in many children's diets. Socioeconomic factors play a large part in the dietary sufficiency of children, with those from higher income families generally having a more adequate intake of essential nutrients, and those with the least income and education having the most problems. Obesity is fairly common in all racial groups, and among rich and poor, during the pre-adolescent stage. It is often caused by poor eating habits such as eating too many non-nutritious snacks and overeating, particularly rich, high-fat foods. There is, however, some feeling now that one cannot rule out heredity as a factor in obesity.

THE ADOLESCENT

During adolescence, both boys and girls undergo growth spurts, and their nutritional needs are greatly increased. They still require the same essential nutrients as adults, with increased quantities of those particularly required for growth. They especially need larger quantities of food items from the milk food group. Parents may be amazed at the amount of food teen-agers, especially boys, can consume and, if they are active, remain slim. Adolescents, as they begin to assert their independence from parental control, often begin to make decisions about the foods they will eat. Peer pressure is a very strong influence, and diet fads may be taken up by a group (or sometimes just by one adolescent) who may become vegetarian, or adopt a diet that contains only organically grown foodstuffs.

Obesity is a major health problem in this age group. Obese adolescents, as a general rule, tend to be less active physically than those of normal weight, and this seems to be especially true of girls. Some adolescents, particularly girls, develop an obsession with being thin, and a condition known as *anorexia nervosa* (a psychological loss of appetite and self-starvation due to an emotional disturbance in body image and a fear of becoming fat) has become a serious problem in this age group. It may be caused by other problems, such as anxiety or depression (which may, or may not, be related to obesity). If unchecked, anorexia nervosa can lead to abnormal water and temperature regulation and deranged hormonal changes. If severe, the anorexia can lead to death, as the teen-ager literally starves herself to death.

Teen-age girls are particularly vulnerable to *iron-deficiency anemia,* as the monthly loss of blood begins to occur with puberty. Adolescents, both boys and girls, experience a rise in gastric acidity, which is felt to be caused by hormonal changes. They are also prone to abdominal pains of vague origin. It is not wise, however, to ascribe them always to "growing pains." Persistent or severe abdominal pain should always be investigated.

THE ADULT

Growth continues into the early years of young adulthood, although not at such a rapid rate as during adolescence. The young adult needs a good supply of proteins, minerals and vitamins, although not in such large quantities as teenagers. This is the age when good eating habits need to be strengthened to maintain health and to prevent illness in the future. Young adulthood is often a turning point, when individuals are setting up housekeeping away from parental influences. They are on their own, then, to make decisions regarding the foods they will eat or not eat, and to establish their own eating habits. Many young adults, because of pressures of work or other commitments, slip into poor dietary habits that will affect their future health. Good nutritional counselling is an important measure in helping young adults protect themselves against problems such as obesity, heart attacks, and hypertension in their middle and later years.

Caloric needs usually decline, as does the need for extra supplies of protein when people reach full adulthood, but their vitamin and mineral requirements do not. A large number of Canadians are overweight, presumably not because they eat too much, but because they are too sedentary (Health and Welfare Canada, 1990). Anemia, due to inadequate intake of iron, is a common problem in women.

During the middle years there is usually a gradual slowing down of activity, and individuals require fewer calories than they did in their young adult days. Often, people tend to eat the same amounts, however, with the result that they put on weight, and obesity is a major problem. As a person gets older, there is a decrease in digestive enzymes, and heartburn (dyspepsia) is a common problem among middle-aged and older adults. If good oral hygiene has not been practised, problems with teeth and gums may develop and lead to poor nutrition. With the aging process, there is a loss of skeletal calcium (a condition known as *osteoporosis*), and a good intake of calcium and vitamins is required. Women are particularly prone to this problem after the menopause because of changes in hormonal secretions.

OLDER ADULTS

The nutritional needs of older adults are the same as those of other adults, although they do require fewer calories, again, because of lessened activity. Their nutritional problems usually stem from a lack of adequate intake. Older adults often have deficiencies of proteins, vitamins and minerals in their diet. Calcium (for the reason noted above) is particularly important. A lack of Vitamin D leads to a condition called *osteomalacia* (softening of the bones). Vitamin D-fortified milk and margarines help to combat this problem.

The failure of many older adults to eat an adequate diet may be due to a number of factors including a lack of money for food; out-of-date nutrition information; physical handicaps that make shopping or cooking difficult; feelings of loneliness, rejection or apathy; and physical changes such as a loss of appetite, poorly fitting dentures and troubles with constipation. Good nutrition counselling is very important. Older adults can be helped to get the most out of their dwindling food dollar and to prepare nutritious meals simply. They should be encouraged to share meals with friends and to engage in activities that will stimulate the appetite, such as walking in the fresh air or mild exercise. The development of *Meals on Wheels* programs has been a boon for the housebound elderly and those who find preparing a substantial meal difficult. Volunteers who have participated in these programs often remark that the friendly visit of the person delivering the meal seems to mean as much to the individual as the food. It is sometimes difficult for the volunteer to get away and deliver the rest of the meals on time.

DETERMINANTS OF NUTRITIONAL STATUS

A person's nutritional status reflects the balance that is maintained between the body's requirements for nutrients and energy and the actual intake of food. It depends on three major factors:

1. the requirements of the individual for nutrients and energy
2. the intake of food
3. the efficiency of bodily processes for absorbing, storing, utilizing and excreting nutrients.

Nutrient and energy requirements in health throughout the life cycle have been discussed in the previous section. Here, we will focus on food intake and health status factors.

INTAKE

If people eat more food than the body requires, or, conversely, they do not eat enough to meet their energy and nutritional requirements, problems develop. A number of factors — socioeconomic, physical, psychological, cultural and religious — affect food intake.

Socioeconomic

An analysis of apparent nutrient intake patterns of Canadians by Campbell and Horton (1991), using Statistics Canada's Family Food Expenditure Survey of 1984, revealed the influence of income, family composition, and education on nutrient intake. Although the majority of apparent intake patterns were found to be adequate, there were differences in apparent intake of calories, proteins, fats, carbohydrates and a number of vitamins and minerals between households with differing sociodemographic characteristics. The apparent intake for all nutrients increased with income. Households in the lowest economic decile consumed fewer calories than did those in the highest decile. Interestingly, however, the proportion of calories from carbohydrates and fats did not change with income. Canadians consume an average of 40 percent of their calories from fat and 47 percent from carbohydrates. The difference in calories did, however, mean that people in the lowest income decile had apparent protein intakes below the "Recommended Nutrient Intakes for Canadians" (RNI). With respect to essential vitamins and minerals, diets were found to be most inadequate in folate, thiamin, iron, calcium and riboflavin for all income groups. However, the proportions of diets with inadequate amounts of these nutrients decreased with increasing income.

Family composition, the presence of a spouse and work status of the wife were found to make a difference in the adequacy of nutrient intake. Dietary patterns in senior households were higher for all nutrients and significantly so for all but folate. "Single-parent households with children had markedly greater proportions of diets apparently inadequate than those with two parents" (376). As well, "households where the wife worked outside the home had lower apparent intakes (especially when the wife worked full time outside the home), and had a greater likelihood of dietary inadequacy" (377). The limited amount of time these individuals have for shopping and food preparation may be the critical limiting factor.

Levels of education of the head of the household beyond high school were found to be important over and above income-related effects. "Higher levels of education were associated with lower intakes of fats and higher levels of Vitamin C, folate and calcium" (379). This finding supports the importance of knowledge in promoting proper nutrition and suggests that educational programs must reach those with less education (Campbell and Horton, 1991).

Physical

Among the physical factors affecting food intake, the condition of a person's teeth, gums, and the mucous membranes of the oral cavity may affect a person's nutritional status. A person with no teeth or with poorly fitting dentures, or one whose mouth is in poor condition, will have difficulty in biting or chewing food effectively. Other physical factors to be considered are the person's general state of health and specific health problems they may have (these are discussed in more detail in subsequent sections). There are also biological variations in the ability to tolerate certain foods. Many people have allergies to specific foods. Milk, chocolate, shellfish and berries are some of the foods to which many people are allergic.

The need for milk and milk products to provide sources of protein and calcium is not the same for people in all racial groups. Adults in many racial and ethnic groups suffer from lactose intolerance — the inability to tolerate milk. The problem is caused by the absence of lactase, the enzyme which digests the milk sugar, lactose. Without this enzyme, lactose in milk ferments in the gastrointestinal tract, and the individual may complain of diarrhea, a bloated feeling, and discomfort due to the formation of gas. It is felt that one reason for the deficiency may be the dropping of milk from the diet after childhood in many cultures. It has been estimated that between 50 and 75 percent of African Americans, Asians, Inuit and American Indians show lactose intolerance, as do approximately 10 to 25 percent of adults of European descent (Overfield, 1977). However, even though some groups experience more lactose intolerance than others, almost anyone is prone to it. "Probably 70 percent of adults worldwide experience a large decrease in their abilities to synthesize lactase as they age. This loss of lactase activity is not due to disease; it happens naturally" (Wardlaw, Insel and Seyler, 1992, 141). To improve nutrition for these people, sharp cheese (aged over 60 days), yogurt, and tofu (soy bean curd) may be used, since the lactose in these foods has been converted to lactic acid, which can be digested.

Psychological

A person's emotional status will also affect his or her intake of food. We have already mentioned this point in connection with anxiety, such as the "knots" and "butterflies" in the stomach and the pre-examination nausea or vomiting. In one psychiatric hospital setting, the dietetic staff observed interesting correlations between food intake and the general anxiety level of both patients and staff. When they were upset by changes in their environment, such as staff changes, hospital policy changes and holidays, the consumption of such "security foods" as bread and milk went up, as did the amount of food left on plates. When things settled down, eating patterns returned to normal (Chappelle, 1972).

Some people use food as a source of comfort and security; they may eat excessively because of their anxieties or because of a lack of fulfillment of the basic needs of love and belonging. Other emotions besides anxiety will also affect a person's appetite and, hence, their intake of food. The depressed patient does not want to eat; the happy individual usually does, unless he or she is too excited by happiness to eat. The attractiveness of a meal and the environment in which it is served also contribute to a person's enjoyment of food and encourage people to eat, as all restaurant managers realize.

Culture and Religion

As we noted at the beginning of this chapter, cultural, moral and religious values play a considerable role in the food people eat. Food habits are learned, and eating habits vary considerably in different cultures and among different religious groups. They also vary from one family to the next, and from individual to individual.

Among cultural groups, food habits usually have their origins in the types of food available in the part of the world in which the group lived. Potatoes are plentiful in many parts of North America; hence, they form a staple of the diet in many homes. In many countries, rice is the staple food and forms a part of the culture. When people from one culture move to another part of the world, they usually carry their food habits with them. In Canada, where people from all over the world have settled, it is important for the nurse to be aware of the cultural food heritage of patients and of their religious backgrounds as well, since many religions have specific food-related rules.

Vegetarianism   Many people are vegetarian because of religious beliefs or personal preference (it is not unusual in an East Indian household, for example, to find both vegetarian and non-vegetarian family members). Orthodox Hindus subscribe to the doctrine of *ahimsa*, which means "not killing." Many other religious groups also espouse vegetarianism. The largest group in North America are members of the Seventh Day Adventist Church. Other people are also becoming vegetarians for moral reasons (not wanting to kill animals for food), for health reasons (to reduce saturated fat and cholesterol or because of a declining tolerance of meat with advancing age), for environmental reasons (deforestation to create cattle grazing lands) or simply for personal preference. It is possible to have a vegetarian diet that fulfills, or even exceeds, recommended nutrient requirements providing foods are selected very carefully.

There are different forms of vegetarianism. Some people do not eat red meat, but will eat poultry and fish. Some will not eat any animal products, including poultry, fish, milk and eggs. Because the cow is sacred in India to both Hindus and Sikhs, cow's milk and products made from it are not consumed by these people (milk from the water buffalo is used instead in India). It is important in caring for people to find out the particular foods they do eat, as well as those they do not. The most common nutritional problems among vegetarians include deficiencies of iron and vitamin D.

Acceptable sources of protein include milk and dairy products (if eaten) and meat alternatives. Soybeans and peanuts (and foods made from these) are a very important source of dietary protein in many parts of the world. To ensure an adequate intake of iron, the use of eggs (if permitted), fruits and vegetables containing iron and whole grain and enriched cereals should be encouraged. To increase the Vitamin D content of vegetarian diets, eggs and vitamin D-fortified milk and margarine, or a regular intake of vitamin tablets, may be suggested. Children and expectant and lactating mothers are particularly vulnerable to nutritional disorders because of their additional nutrient needs. In addition to the problems mentioned above, they may have a deficiency of calcium if milk and milk products are not included in their diet. It is often necessary to use calcium tablets as a supplement.

Other dietary restrictions Various cultural groups have other dietary restrictions as well. Many religious groups — for example, people of the Islamic, Jewish, Seventh Day Adventist religions — do not eat pork. Non-vegetarian Hindus and Sikhs will usually not eat beef or veal because of the sacredness of the animal from which these meats come.

Food preparation is also a concern for some groups. For people of some religious faiths, the preparation of food is a ritual. Orthodox members of the Jewish religion will only eat foods that are *kosher*, that is, prepared according to prescribed ritual. Many Islamic people will eat meat only if the animal has been ritually slaughtered. Kosher meat may, however, be acceptable.

Besides following formal restrictions, many people limit their diets to food prepared in styles customary to their own culture. In most Asian countries, meat, poultry and fish are usually cut up into small pieces and cooked with vegeta-

bles. A large steak, or piece of chicken or fish, may not be acceptable to the Oriental patient. Many people from other cultures are used to foods that have been highly spiced, such as the Indian curries, the hot Mexican chilies, and the kimchee* of Korea. People from these cultures often find the typical North American diet very bland and unappetizing. They usually like to add a very hot sauce to most foods to improve the flavour.

Food habits vary from one family to another, even if all other factors are constant. In some households, breakfast is a sketchy or non-existent affair, whereas in others it is considered one of the main meals of the day. The patterns of eating that children learn in the home have a considerable influence on the food habits they maintain later in life, and are handed down from one generation to the next.

There is, however, also the matter of individual differences in taste and preference for food, as anyone from a large family knows. From the moment of birth, various factors, such as good or poor digestion, allergies, and differences in taste, imagination, education and the food habits in the home, will influence the individual's set of eating habits.

Health Problems

Health problems also affect a person's intake of adequate nourishment. In addition to allergies and poor digestion, most physical and emotional problems affect food intake in some way, often by bringing on anorexia or nausea and vomiting. These will be discussed later in this chapter. Three common health problems that can interfere with a person's intake of sufficient nourishment will be outlined here. These are *alcoholism, drug addiction,* and *smoking.*

Alcoholics often drink instead of eating, and their nutritional status suffers as a result. Serious nutritional problems are found in many alcoholics, and these require prompt intervention. Drug addicts too can have serious nutritional problems. Addicts may opt to buy drugs instead of food with their limited funds, or they may not feel the need for food when they are "high" on drugs. Smokers often substitute coffee and a cigarette for food at mealtime. Smoking diminishes the sense of taste and leaves a person with a bad taste in the mouth. People who have stopped smoking often remark on how good food tastes again.

EFFICIENCY OF THE BODY IN PROCESSING FOOD

Any factor that interferes with the body's ability to retain, absorb, store, utilize or excrete nutrients will adversely affect a person's nutritional status. Disease processes, congenital problems or injury to any part of the gastrointestinal system may therefore result in nutritional problems. Probably

---

* Kimchee is known as the Korean salad and contains a mixture of vegetables and large amounts of garlic and spices.

the most common type of illness affecting the gastro-intestinal tract is infection, especially gastroenteritis, which is a major cause of death in many underdeveloped countries, and a very common cause of illness in Canada. A number of other disorders, which the student will learn about in more advanced courses, are also specific to the gastrointestinal system. Congenital problems are usually discussed thoroughly in pediatric nursing courses, so we will not discuss these at this point, except to note that they include both congenital malformations, that is, defects or abnormalities in the anatomical structures of the system, and congenital disorders affecting the physiological processes involved in the digestion and absorption of food.

Illnesses involving parts of the body other than the gastrointestinal tract may also cause disturbances in the processing of food, as well as altering the body's needs for energy and for specific nutrients. This aspect of nutrition will be discussed in the next few paragraphs.

NUTRITIONAL NEEDS IN ILLNESS

Food as a source of nourishment is particularly important for those who are ill. Nearly all sick persons have some disturbances in gastrointestinal functioning. They may lose their appetites or be unable to tolerate food and fluids, or there may be a problem in the digestion of food or in the absorption of nutrients from the gastrointestinal tract. Whatever the problem, the sick person's nutritional needs are usually different from those of the healthy individual. Lack of exercise because of illness may decrease the body's need for energy-giving foods but, at the same time, there is a greater need for tissue-building nutrients.

In the well person, the processes of anabolism and catabolism are normally equal. In the sick, particularly those who are incapacitated, the catabolic activities are increased, which leads to a breakdown of cellular materials and a subsequent deficiency of protein. Additional protein foods are important for almost all sick people. There are, of course, some conditions in which a high-protein diet is contraindicated, but the foregoing statement is a good general rule.

There are certain conditions, too, in which metabolic activity, both anabolic and catabolic, is increased, as in patients with fever or certain cancers, and in these cases there is a need for additional energy-giving foods as well as proteins.

In many disease conditions, the patient may be unable to tolerate food or fluids, or may lose these through vomiting, diarrhea or other means. When food is not available as a source of energy, the body can draw on stored resources to sustain its needs for life. Liver and muscle glycogen, the stored form of carbohydrates, is the most readily available source of stored energy. Through the process of **glycogenolysis**, glycogen is converted to glucose and made available to the body. These sources, however, are only able to satisfy basal kilocalorie demands for a few hours and are readily used up if not replenished by the intake of food. If starvation continues for more than 24 hours and glycogen stores are depleted, the body begins to convert protein into glucose through the process of **gluconeogenesis**. The amino acids which make up protein break down and release nitrogen into the urine in the form of urea and ammonia. As well, in an effort to conserve protein, fatty acids are mobilized from the body's *adipose* (fatty) tissue and used as fuel to meet energy requirements. Fatty acids break down to ketone bodies which leads to **ketosis** — an abnormal accumulation of ketones in the body resulting from a deficiency or inadequate utilization of carbohydrates. Without an adequate supply of calories from food, the body's nutrient stores are used up quickly and a state of protein-calorie malnutrition results. In these cases, the replacement of lost fluids and nutrients is an important part of the patient's therapeutic care. In some disease conditions, there is interference with the absorption of food. These cases require special adaptation of the diet.

TYPES OF DIET FOR THE ILL

As a part of the patient's therapeutic regimen, food is usually prescribed in the form of a diet. There are many kinds of diet. For example, the average patient is on a *regular* (also called *house, full,* or *general) diet.* This diet includes practically all foods people normally eat that are easy to digest and simply prepared. Generally, fried and highly seasoned foods are not served to patients because of the difficulty many people normally have in digesting them. A modification of the regular diet is the *light diet.* The foods on this diet are cooked simply, with an avoidance of fried foods, rich desserts and other fat-laden foods. Coarse gas-forming foods, such as corn, turnips, radishes, onions, cabbage, cauliflower and cucumbers, are also usually avoided.

A third type of diet is the *soft diet.* This diet consist of food that requires little chewing and contains no harsh fibre or highly seasoned foods. Because soft-diet foods are easily digested, they are often indicated for people who have gastrointestinal disorders or difficulty in masticating food. A fourth kind of diet is the liquid diet of which there are two types. A *clear liquid diet* permits water, tea with lemon, coffee, juices, clear bouillon, carbonated beverages and clear gelatin desserts. A *full liquid diet* is free of irritating condiments and cellulose. Often included in a full liquid diet are all the foods on a clear liquid diet plus such others as strained soups, simple puddings or custards, refined cooked cereals and milk.

Therapeutic diets are special diets designed for the needs of the individual patient and vary greatly in their composition and purpose. Many special diets are planned to eliminate substances that are irritating to the gastrointestinal tract. The amount and kind of nutrients may be varied or certain non-nutritive compounds eliminated. For example, restrictions may be placed on the flavouring or seasoning used or on the amount of cellulose to be consumed. There are also diets that restrict the amount of sodium, sugar or protein. There are high-calorie diets and low-calorie diets, high-protein diets and low-protein diets. There are also diets which control the quantity and type of fats. Each therapeutic diet is ordered by the physician to meet the patient's specific needs. The quantity of each kind of food is calculated by the dietitian or nutritionist, and each meal contains the prescribed amounts of specific foods.

Regardless of the kind of diet, it is important that patients understand why they are served certain foods. A patient's acceptance of the specified food as part of the prescribed therapy and of his or her commitment to following the diet will be enhanced if the benefits or reasons for it have been fully explained.

COMMON PROBLEMS

MALNUTRITION, STARVATION AND OBESITY

On a global basis, the most common problems associated with nutrition throughout the world are malnutrition, starvation and obesity. Although malnutrition is often regarded as an affliction of only underdeveloped and poor countries, it is also of great concern to health workers in North America.

Malnutrition is a state of "failing health that results from a long-standing dietary intake that either fails to meet or greatly exceeds nutritional needs" (Wardlaw, Insel and Seyler, 1992, 568). Malnutrition can manifest itself as anemia or obesity, or in close association with diseases related to poor nutrition, such as heart disease, hypertension, stroke, diabetes, severe dental and periodontal disease and digestive diseases. Especially vulnerable to malnutrition are young children, adolescents, young pregnant women, families of the poor, handicapped persons and people over 65 years of age.

There are many causes of malnutrition. In poor and underdeveloped nations, the climate and terrain may be such that those crops that do grow well are neither sufficient in quantity nor nutritionally adequate for the resident population. Overpopulation is often a concomitant factor in such cases. If little land is available for agriculture, many foods will have to be imported and will, therefore, be costly, so that only the very rich can afford to eat well. Indeed, the situation in some countries is so extreme that many people starve to death. The United States and Canada, with other countries and international organizations (such as UNESCO, UNICEF and WHO, for example), are participating in food distribution programs to countries in need and providing agricultural specialists to advise on food cultivation and processing.

Nutritional problems are a major concern in industrialized nations as well. In countries where food is abundant, many people suffer from inadequate nutrition, often in the form of obesity. *Obesity* may be caused by simple overeating, but more often than not it is a symptom of malnutrition. Contrary to popular belief, people do not necessarily choose naturally the foods their bodies need. In fact, most people choose their foods according to cost and preparation time. The convenience foods, which are relatively expensive, are highly processed and take little or no preparation. They are also usually high in carbohydrates and low in protein. Foods rich in carbohydrates occur abundantly in nature and therefore are usually inexpensive in comparison with protein-rich foods, such as meat and dairy products. With the escalating cost of living, therefore, the average person is likely to eat more rice and potatoes and less meat, and more canned and fewer fresh fruits and vegetables.

People who are ill face an increased risk of starvation and malnutrition. Many common diagnostic tests and treatments for the ill interrupt normal dietary patterns, and as a result ill people may not have a sufficient intake of essential nutrients and energy-giving foods. Meals may be withheld for tests that are ordered, the patient may be allowed nothing by mouth for long periods of time and maintained on low-calorie infusions or a nutritionally inadequate diet may be required as part of the treatment. The term *hospital malnutrition* has been applied to this increasingly prevalent nutritional problem. The nurse working in an acute care facility needs to be aware of the need for a careful assessment of his or her patients so that remedial measures can be instituted promptly.

INDIGESTION, ANOREXIA, NAUSEA AND VOMITING

Among the most common eating-related problems nurses will encounter in patients in their day-to-day practice are indigestion, anorexia, nausea and vomiting. Indigestion is often the first indication that something is wrong with gastrointestinal functioning. A loss of appetite or desire for food often leads to nausea and vomiting, unless the source of stress is removed and the body's normal equilibrium is restored. The inability to take in food and fluids, or the body's rejection of them, poses a serious threat to homeostasis and involves all areas of functioning of the human body. Indigestion is common among people of all ages, but most prevalent in older adults. It is one of the annoying and, often, distressing accompaniments of the aging process.

Gastroenteritis, which is a common cause of anorexia, nausea and vomiting, still remains one of the most common types of short-term illness in North America. It is a very common problem in infants and small children. It is also a distressing problem for many international travellers, whose gastrointestinal tracts are exposed to foods and fluids that are not a part of their normal diet. In addition, anorexia, nausea and vomiting frequently accompany so many health problems that the nurse should be acquainted with the physiological mechanisms involved in these disturbances, and be able to take appropriate action to assist patients with these problems.

Physiological Considerations

Indigestion is characterized by pain and distress in the epigastric region. It may be accompanied by other symptoms, such as eructation (burping) or flatulence (the excessive formation of gases in the stomach or intestine; *flatus* is the term used for gas expelled through the anus). Many pregnant women and older adults complain of heartburn, which is characterized by a burning pain located behind the sternum. It is caused by a regurgitation of acid contents of the stomach into the esophagus, the burning sensation being due to irritation of the mucous membrane lining the esophagus.

Anorexia, nausea and vomiting are varying degrees of distress of the upper gastrointestinal tract. **Anorexia** means loss of appetite, or lack of desire for food, and it involves the subjective perception of a distaste for food. The individual often expresses this by saying, "I don't feel like eating." Anorexia may precede nausea. In **nausea**, not only is there a distaste for food but the mere thought of food becomes repelling. In addition, the individual usually complains of an uncomfortable sensation in the region of the stomach. **Vomiting**, the forceful ejection of the stomach's contents, is usually preceded by nausea. Although anorexia, nausea and vomiting are considered by many to be sequential stages of the same physical phenomenon, any one of the three may occur by itself in the absence of the other two.

Anorexia has been defined as a loss of appetite. **Appetite** is the pleasant sensation of a desire for food. Although appetite and hunger frequently occur together, they are not the same. **Hunger** is an uncomfortable sensation that indicates a physiological need for nourishment, whereas appetite is a learned response. As such, appetite is closely related to cultural and social values. To a large extent, one's appetite is conditioned by previous pleasant experiences with food. A number of different stimuli will arouse the appetite. These include olfactory stimuli, such as the pleasant odour of something cooking; visual stimuli, such as an attractively served meal; auditory stimuli, including the clatter of pots and pans in the kitchen as dinner is being prepared; or gustatory stimuli, as when one tastes a sample of food and finds it agreeable, and the appetite is whetted for more.

When people lose their appetite, specific visceral changes occur. There is usually a hypofunctioning of the stomach; gastric tone is lessened and the secretion of hydrochloric acid is decreased. These same physiological findings have been observed in individuals suffering from nausea, except that in the case of the nauseated person, they are more pronounced. In nausea, there is a relaxation of the walls of the stomach, and gastric secretions and muscular

contractions cease. Because of this relaxation, the stomach is usually situated lower in the abdominal cavity than it normally is. At the same time as the muscles of the stomach are in a relaxed state, the muscular wall of the intestine shows increased contractility, and contents from the duodenum may be regurgitated back into the stomach. *Retching* — an unproductive attempt at vomiting — may occur several times before vomiting actually takes place.

The act of vomiting involves a sequence of events that culminates in the forceful ejection of the stomach's contents. Initially there is a relaxation of the upper portion of the stomach, including the cardiac sphincter. This is followed by strong contractile waves in the lower portion of the stomach, which effectively close off the pyloric sphincter and prevent the stomach contents from passing into the duodenum. Subsequently, the diaphragm and the abdominal muscles contract. The strong contractions of these muscles during the act of vomiting account for the feeling of "soreness" that many people experience as an aftereffect of vomiting. With the simultaneous contraction of the diaphragm and the abdominal muscles, intra-abdominal pressure is greatly increased and the stomach is literally squeezed between the two sets of muscles. The contents in the relaxed upper portion of the stomach are then forced upward through the esophagus and out through the mouth. Normally, the glottis is closed and respirations cease during the act of vomiting in order to prevent the vomitus from being aspirated (entering the lungs).

Common Causes of Indigestion, Anorexia, Nausea and Vomiting.

Indigestion is caused by the body's inability to process the foods that are taken into it. It may result from diminishing ability to chew food properly. Or, it may result from putting too much of a load on the system by overeating, by eating too quickly or by eating highly spiced foods or foods that are foreign to the gastrointestinal tract. It is often associated with eating certain foods. Foods that contain a lot of fat or are cooked in fats or oils are particularly troublesome to many people, as are gas-forming foods (lettuce, cabbage, and beans, for example) and milk for those unable to tolerate it. Smoking may also be a factor because it stimulates the secretion of acid gastric juices in the stomach.

The primary centre controlling vomiting is located in the medulla oblongata. It is thought that stimulation of this centre may give rise to anorexia, nausea or vomiting, depending on the degree or intensity of the stimulus. Thus, a person who does not feel like eating may become nauseated at the sight of food and may vomit if he or she tries to eat it. However, vomiting is not always preceded by nausea, and it is believed, therefore, that only certain areas in the vomiting centre are directly involved with nausea. The vomiting centre may be stimulated by a number of factors. These include chemical stimuli (drugs and other toxic substances), impulses from the cerebral cortex (strong emotions) and impulses arising from receptors in the viscera (internal factors).

Drugs and other toxic substances   Two of the most common causes of nausea and vomiting the nurse may see in community practice and in the emergency unit of acute-care facilities are food and drug poisonings. Toddlers and small children are particularly vulnerable to both because they will often eat or drink food that is left on a counter or table, or ingest household products (such as bleach or insecticides) or their parents' pills, if these are within reach.

A number of different chemical agents may give rise to anorexia, nausea and vomiting. Many common drugs also cause anorexia, nausea and vomiting, including digitalis (frequently used in the treatment of people with heart conditions); a number of the narcotics, such as morphine; and many drugs used as anesthetics. When giving a patient any medication, in fact, it is important to note whether nausea and vomiting are listed as possible side effects of the drug, and, if so, to watch for these symptoms in the patient. Other toxic substances that are circulating in the blood stream, such as bacterial toxins in infections or in food poisoning, may also stimulate the vomiting centre.

Food poisoning   Every year, a number of deaths from food poisoning receive a great deal of publicity, but countless more cases occur, many of them unreported. Food poisoning is always a potential problem in large gatherings, such as picnics, where food may be held for long periods of time at temperatures conducive to the growth of bacteria.

If food poisoning is suspected, it is important to find out what the person has eaten and also whether any other person who ate the same food is affected as well. The symptoms of food poisoning usually occur within one to five hours after the contaminated food is eaten. They usually develop abruptly and may include nausea, vomiting, abdominal cramps and diarrhea. Most cases of food poisoning last no more than five to six hours, or 24 hours at the most. They will usually subside on their own as the body rids itself of the offending substance. The individual should be watched for signs of shock and for the development of neurological symptoms, which occur with certain types of food poisoning, including botulism, shellfish poisoning, and mushroom poisoning. Shock may be caused by excessive fluid loss (from vomiting and diarrhea), by bacterial toxins or by an allergic reaction to the food ingested.

Botulism (caused by the *Clostridium botulinum* organism) is the most serious food poisoning because it can be fatal. Although cases receive a great deal of publicity, its occurrence is relatively rare. The most frequent cause is improperly home-preserved vegetables, although preserved fruits, fish and meat products may also be sources of botulism.

The botulism organism releases gas as it grows and is sometimes evidenced by a bulging can or lid of a jar. The symptoms of botulism usually develop 4 to 36 hours after the food has been eaten, but may be delayed up to four days. The early symptoms are similar to those of other food poisonings, with the addition of weakness, dizziness, visual disturbances and dryness of the mouth and throat. Often the person will complain of headache. Other neurological symptoms, such as paralysis, limitation of eye movements, dilated pupils, decreased tendon reflexes and impaired speech, often follow. When botulism is fatal, the cause of death is usually respiratory paralysis. If botulism is suspected, the person should be referred for emergency medical treatment immediately.

Shellfish poisoning can also cause neurological symptoms, through the transmission of toxins from the plankton on which they feed. Particularly dangerous are shellfish harvested during the so-called "red tide." Fortunately, the mortality rate is not as high as with botulism, although rates ranging from 5 to 18 percent have been reported in some outbreaks. The symptoms may develop as soon as 20 minutes after eating, with *paresthesia* (abnormal sensations such as prickling or tingling) of the hands and mouth, weakness of the arms and legs, and a feeling of floating. The person may also notice *ataxia* (a failure of muscle coordination), headache and vomiting. Respiratory or *bulbar paralysis* (due to effects of the toxin on motor centres in the medulla oblongata) may ensue. Prompt medical attention is important. No specific treatment is known as yet; the measures used are those for respiratory paralysis. If the person survives the first 12 hours, he or she is likely to recover.

Another common type of food poisoning, particularly in the spring, late summer and early fall, is that caused by certain "wild" varieties of mushrooms. In mushroom poisoning, the individual usually has an acute attack of nausea, vomiting and diarrhea starting about two to three hours after eating. Hallucinations and intoxication reactions may follow. Some varieties of mushrooms are more poisonous than others and may lead to kidney and renal failure. It is important, therefore, to find out what kind of mushrooms were eaten, how many and where. If possible, the nurse should get a sample of the mushrooms or save any *emesis* (vomited contents) for analysis. The individual should be hospitalized so that he or she can be watched for delayed reactions. Often, the stomach is washed out, and a strong laxative is given to speed the mushrooms through the gastrointestinal tract.

Psychosocial stressors   Indigestion may be caused, or aggravated, by psychosocial factors. A meal that is taken when a person is under stress, for example, is not easily digested. When people are angry, or worried about something, they may feel that their stomachs are "tied up in knots," excessive acid secretion may ensue, and they may also suffer from excessive gas formation and resultant distention in the stomach and intestines.

Stressful situations may give rise to anorexia, nausea or vomiting. The event or situation need not necessarily be unpleasant. An individual may be "too excited to eat." Infants and toddlers will often vomit if overstimulated, particularly after a meal. Older children, too, may become nauseated or vomit if excited or fearful. However, it is in connection with unpleasantly stressful situations that the symptoms of anorexia, nausea, and vomiting are most often noted. Worry over a pending examination, pain, anxiety and fear may all give rise to these symptoms. Similarly, other psychic factors such as the sight of something particularly abhorrent, unpleasant odors or even extremely loud noise can also take away one's appetite, make one feel nauseated or cause vomiting.

Internal factors   The parts of the body containing receptors that initiate vomiting are the stomach, duodenum, uterus, kidneys, heart, pharynx and semicircular canals of the ear. The stimuli that give rise to anorexia, nausea and vomiting include irritation of the receptors, such as, for example, the tickling of the back of the throat to induce vomiting; the eating of irritating foods; stretching of the organ, as occurs when a child stretches his stomach by overeating and promptly vomits; or pressure on the receptors. Irritation of the gastrointestinal tract by infectious, chemical or mechanical agents, and distention of, or trauma to, other viscera also affect the vomiting centre.

A disturbance in motion, as one experiences with the rolling motion of a ship at sea or with any rapid change in direction of the body, stimulates receptors in the labyrinth of the ear. These receptors send out impulses that are carried by the vestibular nerve to the cerebellum, and thence to the vomiting centre in the medulla.

Indigestion is often caused by problems in the gastrointestinal tract, where a disturbance in structure or functioning, inflammations, or new growths (such as tumours), either in the tract itself or in its accessory organs, may interfere with the body's ability to process and utilize foodstuffs. In older persons particularly, chewing may be difficult if the person gradually loses teeth or if ill-fitting dentures prevent proper mastication. The motility of the gastrointestinal tract also lessens with age — food is not processed as quickly.

ASSESSING NUTRITIONAL STATUS

In order to assess the nutritional status of an individual, the nurse needs information about all of the factors that affect an individual's state of nutrition. The parameters of data collection include a nutritional history and physical examination, as well as anthropometric measurements (size, weight and body proportions) and laboratory tests. Information about the patient's disease process is furnished by the medical history. Medical management and special diet orders will be found in the patient's record.

NURSING HEALTH HISTORY

A nutritional history is taken as part of the health history. The nurse obtains data such as age and stage of development, sex, height, usual weight and present weight. Usual habits with regard to daily activities and current activity level, usual dietary pattern and any recent deviations from it, and present status with regard to food and fluid intake are explored. Information is gathered about the patient's (and/or family's) socioeconomic status and lifestyle. The person's general physical condition, emotional status, and any health problems he or she may have that could cause alterations in nutritional needs or interfere with digestive processes are determined. The person's religious affiliation, ethnic origin, any special beliefs about food, and his or her attitudes towards food are also investigated. If the patient is female, the nurse should obtain information about her menstrual history and determine if she is pregnant or a nursing mother.

Indigestion, anorexia and nausea are subjective feelings; hence, their identification is highly dependent on the individual's ability to express discomfort. The person who has indigestion may report pain in the epigastric region. The nurse should identify the location of the pain, its nature, its intensity, when it occurs and its frequency. Is it related to eating certain foods? Is it relieved by any particular measures? Often the patient claims to have "a little indigestion" or "heartburn." The patient may report a "burning" feeling or a bloated feeling in the abdomen, "gas in the stomach," or flatulence.

Patients with anorexia may say that they are not hungry or that they "just don't feel like eating." The nauseous person may complain simply of "feeling sick" or may specifically locate the sensation of nausea as being in the epigastric region. An uncomfortable feeling in this area is usually accompanied by other symptoms of a distressing nature. Frequently there is increased perspiration and greatly increased salivation. Patients may state that their mouths are full of saliva. Some people feel faint, and some report vertigo (dizziness) or tingling sensations in the fingers or toes. After vomiting, a person often complains of a soreness in the stomach area.

The nursing history provides an essential base for identifying nutritional problems and planning individualized care. An evaluation of the patient's (and family's) health promoting and protecting patterns aids in identifying potential problems and opportunities for health teaching. A guide for obtaining a nutritional health history follows.

MEASUREMENTS

An important parameter of a person's nutritional status is weight. Being underweight or overweight are considered risk factors in many diseases, such as hypertension,

Nutrition

Health and Illness Patterns

USUAL DIETARY PATTERN AND EATING HABITS

- Are you on a special diet? If so, what kind? Do you understand the purpose for it? Do you adhere to it? If not, why?
- What is your basic eating pattern?* Number of meals per day? Snacks? Typical times?
- Do you eat regularly? Do you skip meals? If so, how often?
- Do you often eat when you are not hungry? If so, for what reason? Stress? Anger? Nervousness? Boredom? Habit?
- What foods do you usually eat?* Milk and milk products? Meats and alternatives? Grains? Fruits and vegetables? How much of each in a typical day?
- Do you drink fluids with meals? Between meals? If, so what type? How much?
- Do you have any cultural, religious, or moral beliefs and values that influence your eating pattern and food preferences? If, so what are they?
- What foods do you especially like? Dislike?
- Are there certain foods you avoid because they cause unpleasant reactions such as headache, gas, indigestion, diarrhea or constipation?
- Do you have any food allergies? If so, what are they?
- Do you use vitamin and mineral supplements? If so, what kinds? How often?
- What is your usual weight?
- Do you need help with your meals? If so, what kind of help?
- In your opinion, are you eating a well-balanced diet? An unbalanced diet? Would you like help to plan a well-balanced diet?

RECENT CHANGES IN DIETARY PATTERN AND EATING HABITS

- Have there been any recent changes in your usual food intake and eating habits? Have you noticed that you are eating and drinking more or less than usual? Do you know the cause of these changes? If so, what are they?
- Have you noticed a change in your weight? Loss or gain? How much over the past week? Past month?

- Have you had a recent illness that affected your food intake and eating habits?
- Have you experienced loss of appetite, nausea, vomiting or abdominal pain?
- Has there been a change in your activity patterns? Why?
- Have you noticed unusual fatigue, tiredness, muscle weakness or recurrent fever lately?

PRESENTING HEALTH PROBLEM

- Describe the symptoms you are experiencing now. (Use questioning techniques as necessary to explore symptoms.)
- When did the symptoms begin?
- Are the symptoms related to a specific cause, such as eating habits, particular foods, medications, personal lifestyle and stressful situations?
- What remedies have you tried for the symptoms? What were the results?
- Do you have a history of acute or chronic diseases, surgery or weight problems? For example, obesity, eating disorders, diabetes mellitus, heart disease, cancer, ulcers, gallstones, intestinal disorders?
- Are you taking any prescriptions or over-the-counter medications? If so, which drugs and what dosages?

Health Promotion and Health Protection Patterns

- Do you drink products containing caffeine (coffee, tea, cola), salt, or sugar? If so, how much and how often?
- Do you drink alcohol? If so, how much? How often?
- Do you smoke? If so, how much? For how many years?
- Do you have an active or sedentary lifestyle? What are your usual daily activities? Work-related? Recreation-related? Do you exercise regularly? If so, what kind? How often? How long?
- How do you care for your teeth and gums?
- Are you aware of Canada's Food Guide? Do you try to follow it?

---

* An effective method of obtaining information about nutritional patterns and eating habits is the 24-hour dietary recall. This may be obtained by interview or by asking the patient to prepare a written record of all foods and fluids taken in the previous day or on a typical day. Some agencies also use a self-administered questionnaire.

cardiovascular disease, diabetes and some cancers. It is believed that every individual has a *desirable weight* for optimal health and fitness and that this weight can be estimated on the basis of certain measurements and by comparing these measurements to selected standards.

A person's weight depends on his or her height, frame size, and body composition. Measurements of the size and proportions of the body are called **anthropometric measurements**. These include height and weight, circumferences of various body parts and measurements of skinfold (fatfold) thickness. The measurements are used to estimate the patient's body frame, body mass index and the amount of subcutaneous fat, all of which are needed to determine whether a person's weight is desirable or whether he or she is underweight or overweight.

Tables of Desirable Weights for Height

Tables of desirable weights for height, such as those used by the Metropolitan Life Insurance Company (1983 revision), provide a general guide for establishing a person's desirable weight or determining whether someone is over- or underweight. These tables have recently been criticized as a standard of measure because they are based on weights associated with the lowest mortality rate in insured people and, therefore, do not apply to the entire population. In addition, they provide no information on the distribution of body fat or degree of obesity and they fail to account for the usual weight changes associated with aging. Therefore, these tables should be used only as general guidelines in the evaluation of relative weights and should be used in conjunction with other indices (BCDNA, 1992). The 1983 Metropolitan Life Insurance values of desirable weights for height for adults may be found Table 19.7.

Frame Size

Body weight is influenced by frame size or body build. Understandably, a person with a large frame size will weigh more than a person of the same height but with a smaller body build. Body frame is usually divided into three categories — small, medium and large. One can assess the general type of body frame by looking at the person. However, a more accurate measure of a person's frame size may be determined by calculating the ratio of the individual's height to wrist circumference and then comparing that value to standard values for the different frame sizes. The wrist is measured at its smallest circumference (see Figure 19.7) and a height to wrist circumference ratio is computed as follows:

Ratio = height (cm) ÷ wrist circumference (cm)

The patient's frame size is established by comparing the patient's ratio value to standard values as outlined in Table 19.8.

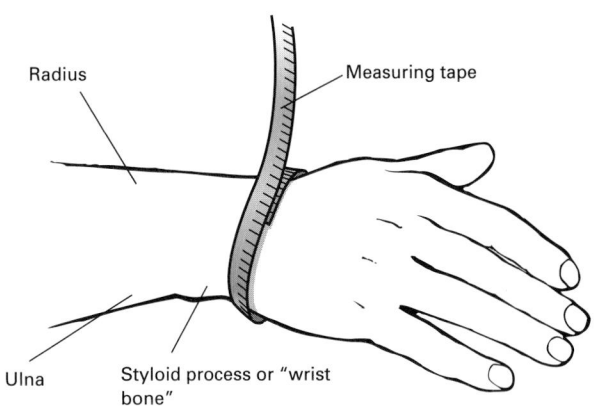

FIGURE 19.7 Measuring wrist circumference: Place the tape around the smallest circumference distal to the styloid process.

Body Mass Index (BMI)

The body mass index is a measure of a person's weight in relation to height. It is computed by dividing the weight (in kilograms) by the height (in metres) squared. Thus:

BMI = weight (kg) ÷ height (m)²

Because the body mass index was found to correlate best with the risk of diseases, an Expert Group on Weight Standards for Health and Welfare Canada recommended the use of BMI as a measure of body weight (1988). "The BMI provides an estimate of healthy weights and identifies individuals at risk for complications associated with being overweight or underweight" (BCDNA, 1992). Its use is limited to men and nonpregnant women between 20 and 65 years of age. In addition, BMI does not account for weight differences due to frame size or fat distribution. Thus, an assessment of fat distribution is recommended for assessing body weight (BCDNA, 1992).

Standards for Interpreting Body Mass Index

- BMI <20   May be associated with health problems for some people
- BMI 20-25   Healthy weight for most people
- BMI 25-27   May lead to health problems in some people
- BMI >27   Increased risk of developing health problems

SOURCE: Health and Welfare Canada (Health Services and Promotion Branch). (1988). *Promoting healthy weights: A discussion paper.* Ottawa: Author.

TABLE 19.7   1983 Metropolitan Life Insurance Values for Desirable Weights for Height for Adults

Weights are for the lowest mortality in ages 25-59 years. Individuals were weighed wearing clothing weighing 1.4 kg (3lb) and shoes with 2.5 cm (1 in) heels.

MALES

7A. Desirable Weight (kg)

Height cms	Small Frame	Medium Frame	Large Frame
158	58.3–61.0	59.6–64.2	62.8–68.3
159	58.6–61.3	59.9–64.5	63.1–68.8
160	59.0–61.7	60.3–64.9	63.5–69.4
161	59.3–62.0	60.6–65.2	63.8–69.9
162	59.7–62.4	61.0–65.6	64.2–70.5
163	60.0–62.7	61.3–66.0	64.5–71.1
164	60.4–63.1	61.7–66.5	64.9–71.8
165	60.8–63.5	62.1–67.0	65.3–72.5
166	61.1–63.8	62.4–67.5	65.6–73.2
167	61.5–64.2	62.8–68.2	66.0–74.0
168	61.8–64.6	63.2–68.7	66.4–74.7
169	62.2–65.2	63.8–69.3	67.0–75.4
170	62.5–65.7	64.3–69.8	67.5–76.1
171	62.9–66.2	64.9–70.3	68.0–76.2
172	63.2–66.7	65.4–70.8	68.7–77.5
173	63.6–67.3	65.9–71.4	69.1–78.2
174	63.9–67.8	66.4–71.9	69.5–78.9
175	64.3–68.3	66.9–72.4	70.1–79.5
176	64.7–68.9	67.5–73.0	70.7–80.3
177	65.0–69.5	68.1–73.5	71.3–81.0
178	65.4–70.0	69.6–74.0	71.9–81.2
179	65.7–70.5	69.2–74.6	72.3–82.5
180	66.1–71.1	69.7–75.1	72.8–83.3
181	66.6–71.6	70.2–75.8	73.4–84.0
182	67.1–72.1	70.7–76.5	73.9–84.7
183	67.7–72.7	71.3–77.2	74.5–85.4
184	68.2–73.4	71.8–77.9	75.2–86.1
185	68.7–74.1	72.4–78.6	75.9–86.3
186	69.2–74.8	73.0–79.3	76.6–87.6
187	69.8–75.5	73.7–80.0	77.3–88.5
188	70.3–76.2	74.4–80.7	78.0–89.4
189	70.9–76.9	74.9–81.5	78.7–90.3
190	71.4–77.6	75.4–82.2	79.4–91.2
191	72.1–78.4	76.1–83.0	80.3–92.1
192	72.8–79.1	76.8–83.9	81.2–93.0
193	73.5–79.8	77.6–84.8	82.1–93.9

SOURCE: Ontario Dietetic Association and the Ontario Hospital Association. (1989). *Nutrition Care Manual* (6th ed.). Ontario: Author.

TABLE 19.7   *continued*

FEMALES

7A. Desirable Weight (kg)

Height cms	Small Frame	Medium Frame	Large Frame
148	46.4–50.6	49.6–55.1	53.7–59.8
149	46.6–51.0	50.0–55.5	54.1–60.3
150	46.7–51.3	50.3–55.9	54.4–60.9
151	46.9–51.7	50.7–56.4	54.8–61.4
152	47.1–52.1	51.1–57.0	55.2–61.9
153	47.4–52.5	51.5–57.5	55.6–62.4
154	47.8–53.0	51.9–58.0	56.2–63.0
155	48.1–53.6	52.2–58.6	56.8–63.6
156	48.5–54.1	52.7–59.1	57.3–64.1
157	48.8–54.6	53.2–59.6	57.8–64.6
158	49.3–55.2	53.8–60.2	58.4–65.3
159	49.8–55.7	54.3–60.7	58.9–66.0
160	50.3–55.2	54.9–61.2	59.4–66.7
161	50.8–56.7	55.4–61.7	59.9–67.4
162	51.4–57.3	55.9–62.3	60.5–68.1
163	51.9–57.8	56.4–63.3	61.0–68.8
164	52.5–58.4	57.0–63.4	61.5–69.5
165	53.0–58.9	57.5–63.9	62.0–70.2
166	53.6–59.5	58.1–64.5	62.6–70.9
167	54.1–60.0	58.7–65.0	63.2–71.7
168	54.6–60.5	59.2–65.5	63.7–72.4
169	55.2–61.1	59.7–65.1	64.3–73.1
170	55.7–61.6	60.2–66.6	64.8–73.8
171	56.2–62.1	60.7–67.1	65.3–74.5
172	56.8–62.6	61.0–67.6	65.8–75.2
173	57.3–63.2	67.8–68.2	66.4–75.9
174	57.8–63.7	62.3–68.7	66.9–76.4
175	58.3–64.2	62.8–69.2	67.4–76.9
176	58.9–64.8	63.4–69.8	68.0–77.5
177	59.5–65.4	64.0–70.4	68.5–78.1
178	60.0–65.9	64.5–70.9	69.0–78.6
179	60.5–66.4	65.1–71.4	69.5–79.1
180	61.0–66.9	65.6–71.9	70.1–79.5
181	61.6–67.5	66.1–72.5	70.7–80.2
182	62.1–68.0	66.6–73.0	71.2–80.7

TABLE 19.8	Frame Size According to Height-Wrist Circumference Ratio	
FRAME SIZE	**MALE RATIO VALUES**	**FEMALE RATIO VALUES**
Small	>10.4	>10.9
Medium	10.4-9.6	10.9-9.9
Large	<9.6	<9.9

SOURCE: British Columbia Dieticians' and Nurses' Association (1992), 80.

Fat Distribution

An indirect estimate of the body's fat deposits can be obtained by measuring the thickness of skin folds using calipers. This is referred to as a *fatfold* or *skinfold* test. The measurement is usually taken from the back of the arm — the triceps skinfold thickness (see Figure 19.8). The fat under the skin in this region, and in other regions such as the back, represents about half of the body's total fat tissue, and in most people, it is roughly proportional to total body fat (Whitney, Cataldo and Rolfes, 1991). The fatfold test can yield reliable information providing it is done by trained professionals using reliable calipers. Skinfold thickness measurements must be interpreted with caution. Their main use is in monitoring body composition and fat deposits over a long period of time. "Depletion of stores can reflect chronic inadequate intake and, therefore, these measurements provide an estimate of the duration and severity of inadequate intake" (BCDNA, 1992, 76).

PHYSICAL ASSESSMENT

There are many outward signs of both good nutrition and malnutrition that are readily observable to the trained eye. Characteristics that the nurse can observe in people with good nutrition and those with poor nutrition (a comparison) are shown in Table 19.9. Particularly important aspects to note are the eyes, the mouth (especially the teeth and mucous membranes), the skin and its underlying fat and muscle tissues and the limbs. The general appearance, the pace and vigor with which they carry out activities, and general emotional tone should be noted. Do they look overweight or underweight? Do they look emaciated? Do they appear listless and apathetic or do they tackle things with enthusiasm? Are they good-natured, irritable or depressed?

In severe cases of malnutrition, the heartbeat may be accelerated and its rhythm altered. The blood pressure may be elevated and they may lose their sense of position — it may be difficult to sit up or stand erect. The lips and tongue may be red and swollen; the gums may be spongy and may bleed easily; and the nails may become spoon-shaped, brittle and ridged. The face may look drawn, with hollow cheeks and dark circles under the eyes and on the cheeks. The parotid glands and the thyroid glands often become swollen. The person may become confused, and may have a burning or tingling sensation in the hands and feet. Muscles may appear wasted and the joints swollen (Keithley, 1979).

The nurse can supplement subjective data by noting the person's reactions to foods. Do reports of heartburn, indigestion or flatulence occur after the patient eats certain foods? Is food pushed away at mealtime without being touched? Does the patient simply toy with food, and actually eat very little? Such behaviour can indicate that a person is anorectic and perhaps nauseated. The nurse may note that the patient expresses no interest in food and appears apathetic and listless.

The person who has indigestion is usually obviously uncomfortable, as is the one who is nauseated. The nauseated person, and the one about to vomit, usually show pallor and

FIGURE 19.8   Measuring triceps skinfold thickness

TABLE 19.9 Clinical Signs of Nutritional Status

FEATURES	GOOD	POOR
General appearance	Alert, responsive	Listless, apathetic; cachexia
Hair	Shiny, lustrous, healthy scalp	Stringy, dull, brittle, dry, depigmented
Neck glands	No enlargement	Thyroid enlarged
Skin, face and neck	Smooth, slightly moist; good colour, reddish pink mucous membranes	Greasy, discolored, scaly
Eyes	Bright, clear; no fatigue circles	Dryness, signs of infection, increased vascularity, glassiness, thickened conjunctivae
Lips	Good colour, moist	Dry, scaly, swollen, angular lesions (stomatitis)
Tongue	Good pink colour; surface papillae present; no lesions	Papillary atrophy, smooth appearance; swollen, red, beefy (glossitis)
Gums	Good pink colour; no swelling or bleeding; firm	Marginal redness or swelling; receding, spongy
Teeth	Straight, no crowding; well-shaped jaw; clean, no discoloration	Unfilled cavities, absent teeth, worn surfaces; mottled, malpositioned
Skin, general	Smooth, slightly moist; good colour	Rough, dry, scaly, pale, pigmented, irritated; petechiae, bruises
Abdomen	Flat	Swollen
Legs, feet	No tenderness, weakness, swelling; good colour	Edema, tender calf; tingling, weakness
Skeleton	No malformations	Bowlegs, knock-knees, chest deformity at diaphragm, beaded ribs, prominent scapulae
Weight	Normal for height, age, body build	Overweight or underweight
Posture	Erect, arms and legs straight, abdomen in, chest out	Sagging shoulders, sunken chest, humped back
Muscles	Well developed, firm	Flaccid, poor tone; undeveloped, tender
Nervous control	Good attention span for age; does not cry easily; not irritable or restless	Inattentive, irritable
Gastrointestinal function	Good appetite and digestion; normal, regular elimination	Anorexia, indigestion, constipation or diarrhea
General vitality	Endurance; energetic; sleeps well at night; vigorous	Easily fatigued, no energy, falls asleep in school, looks tired, apathetic

SOURCE: Williams, S.R. (1989). *Nutrition and diet therapy* (6th ed.). St. Louis: Mosby, p. 6. Reproduced with permission.

increased perspiration. Beads of perspiration may be evident on the person's forehead or upper lip. Pulse and respiratory rates taken at this time may be markedly increased. The pulse rate may increase at first, but it usually then drops to below normal. Blood pressure usually drops as well.

In projectile vomiting, the impulse to vomit is very sudden, occurring with little or no warning (that is, with no symptoms of nausea beforehand). Moreover, the ejection of the stomach's contents is more forceful than in ordinary vomiting. This type of vomiting is often seen in infants with disorders of the gastrointestinal tract and in patients with head injuries.

Vomiting should be assessed in terms of both the nature of the vomiting and the characteristics of the vomitus (material vomited). In relation to vomiting, the nurse should determine its type — that is, whether it is projectile or re-gurgitated (ordinary vomiting); whether it is preceded by feelings of nausea; its frequency; and its occurrence in re-lation to intake of food, the administration of drugs and the individual's emotional state. Characteristics of the vom-itus that should be noted are amount; colour; consistency (watery, liquid or solid); the presence of undigested food, blood or other foreign substances; and odour.

Gastrointestinal disturbances quickly result in deteri-oration of the patient's nutritional status. Food and fluids, especially the chloride ions, are lost as a result of vomiting of gastric juices. Prolonged deficiency in nourishment and in fluid intake results in malnutrition and dehydration; de-hydration, in turn, can cause constipation. The patient can be expected to be constipated because of the fluid with-drawn from the feces in an effort by the body to compensate for the lowered fluid intake or excessive fluid loss. There will probably also be a decrease in the amount of urine ex-creted, and the urine will be more concentrated.

A person who suffers from anorexia or nausea over a pe-riod of time will lose weight and, in addition to showing signs of dehydration and malnutrition, will become weak and listless owing to inadequate intake of nutrients. The individual who has experienced prolonged vomiting will show more pronounced effects due not only to the lack of intake but also to the loss of food and fluids through vom-iting. This individual may show a marked weight loss and rapidly progressive signs of weakness and prostration, as well as signs of fluid and electrolyte imbalance (see Chapter 22). Prolonged vomiting in children is more serious than in adults because of the relatively greater loss of fluids and electrolytes in proportion to body weight.

DIAGNOSTIC TESTS

Blood and urine tests are considered the most reliable means of assessing nutritional status.

Blood Tests

Blood tests for hemoglobin and hematocrit indicate iron as well as protein deficiencies. Laboratory tests which reflect protein adequacy include total protein and serum albumin, prealbumin, and transferrin (total iron-binding capacity). A total lymphocyte count (TLC) is taken to assess the per-son's immune status. Because the TLC is depressed when nu-trient deficiency problems exist, the TLC can be used as gauge of nutritional status. For example, "moderate nutri-tional problems are characterized by a TLC between 800 and 1200 mm^3" (Davis and Sherer, 1994). Blood levels of sodium and potassium, glucose, and cholesterol and triglyc-eride are used to assess electrolyte balance, carbohydrate metabolism and lipid metabolism respectively.

Urine Tests

A 24-hour sample of urine may be ordered for creatinine levels to assess protein metabolism. Creatinine is a by-product of muscle metabolism and is used as an indicator of muscle protein breakdown and malnutrition. Similarly, a 24-hour urinary urea nitrogen test is used to determine protein catabolism and nitrogen balance. Urea nitrogen refers to nitrogen in the form of urea. Urea is formed in the liver as a by-product of protein metabolism. It is ex-creted from the body through the kidneys and so levels in the urine can be used to evaluate protein (nitrogen) balance in the body. When protein intake equals protein output, the body is in a state of nitrogen equilibrium. Often, during illness or starvation, the body loses more protein than it takes in. The body is then in a state of negative nitrogen balance. In practice, the assessment of nitrogen balance requires a battery of tests which you will learn more about in your advanced-level courses.

DIAGNOSING NUTRITIONAL PROBLEMS

Nutritional problems that fall within the domain of inde-pendent nursing intervention are generally labelled *Altered nutrition*. In cases where the intake of nutrients is actually or potentially insufficient to meet metabolic demands, the nursing diagnosis is stated as *Altered nutrition: Less than body requirements*. This can include any number of situations in which the person can ingest food but the quantity and/or quality of intake is inadequate. For example, people who eat less than required amounts of food because of anorexia, nausea, fatigue, pain, chewing or swallowing difficulties, inadequate family budgets for procuring food, personal lifestyles and food habits or lack of knowledge of required nutrient intake may experience or be at risk for insufficient intake. Furthermore, because metabolic needs increase dur-ing illness, trauma and healing, a person who is ill necessarily faces the risk of inadequate intake even when eating patterns remain unchanged. For instance, someone who sustained a fractured wrist in a skiing accident might notice a loss in weight even if food and fluid intake is not affected during the course of healing. Defining characteristics of insuffi-cient nutrient intake might include reported or observed food intake below daily nutrient requirements, weight loss, BMI below 20, presence of hypermetabolic disease states (such as fever, trauma, infection, cancer), decreased energy level and muscular weakness and tenderness.

The diagnostic statement, *Altered nutrition: Less than body requirements* should not be used for patients who are NPO (nothing per mouth) or unable to ingest food because there are no interventions nurses can prescribe to improve the nutritional status of these patients. Instead, the nursing diagnoses should focus on the resulting problems that nurses can treat, such as *Altered comfort* or *Altered oral mucous membrane integrity*. In addition, potential problems that may result from the patient's NPO status and the medical treatment regimen, which nurses have a collaborative responsibility to monitor, manage and minimize, should be stated as collaborative problems. For example, a person on NPO might be at risk for hypoglycemia and a negative nitrogen balance.

Altered nutrition: More than body requirements is the diagnosis used for individuals who are experiencing or are at risk of experiencing weight gain because their food intake is greater than their metabolic needs. This diagnosis might apply to patients who gain or are at risk for gaining weight because of pregnancy, changes in taste or smell or medications, such as corticosteroids (Carpenito, 1993). Carpenito advises that the nurse should be careful using this diagnostic statement with patients who are overweight or obese because of the multiplicity of factors usually involved in obesity. Furthermore, a successful weight loss program includes more than limiting food intake; behaviour modification and lifestyle changes are also necessary. Thus, for these persons, a better diagnosis would be *Altered Health Maintenance related to intake in excess of metabolic requirements* (1993).

Some examples of nursing diagnoses for patients with nutritional problems are:

- *Altered nutrition: Less than body requirement related to chewing difficulty secondary to wired jaw*
- *Altered nutrition: Less than body requirement related to difficulty procuring food secondary to lack of transportation to supermarket*
- *High risk for altered nutrition: Less than body requirement related to anorexia secondary to pain and chemotherapy*
- *PC: Hypoglycemia*

PLANNING NUTRITIONAL INTERVENTIONS

A plan of care for people with nutritional problems is based on the nursing diagnoses, and focusses on maintaining adequate nutrition and hydration during illness, restoring a satisfactory nutritional status if their nutritional balance has been disturbed and promoting optimal nutrition in daily living.

As we discussed previously, dietary habits and food intake are greatly influenced by personal preferences and lifestyle practices, cultural and religious beliefs and practices, psychological and emotional factors and socioeconomic determinants. A plan of care must take these factors into consideration and, furthermore, must involve the patient (and family as necessary). The patient's participation is mandatory when setting goals and planning strategies to change dietary habits and food intake, if successful outcomes are to be achieved. Unless the goals reflect outcomes the patient is willing or able to achieve, the plan of care

KEY PRINCIPLES

Principles Relevant to Nutrition

1. An adequate intake of essential nutrients and energy-giving foods is required for optimal health.
2. An individual's nutritional status is determined by the adequacy of the specific nutrients and energy-giving foods taken into the body, absorbed and utilized.
3. Nutritional needs depend on an individual's age, sex, body composition, amount and kind of daily activity, the secretions of endocrine glands and health status.
4. Nutritional needs are usually altered in illness.
5. Food has psychological meaning for people.
6. Food habits are learned.
7. Food habits are related to cultural, religious and moral beliefs.

will likely be ineffective. Goals and expected outcomes should be stated as short-term steps towards long-term achievement. For example, a long-term goal of reducing weight by 25 kg in 12 weeks may be overwhelming to the patient, whereas a short-term goal of reducing weight by 1 kg per week may be easier to deal with.

Examples of goals or expected outcomes pertaining to nutritional problems include:

- The patient will show adequate nutrition by eating all foods on the meal tray.
- The patient will list high-fibre foods and the amounts he or she will add to the daily diet.
- The patient will describe how to select restaurant foods to avoid high-fat and high-salt intake.
- The patient (family) will explain how he or she will buy and prepare nutritious meals and snacks according to Canada's Food Guide.

IMPLEMENTING NUTRITIONAL INTERVENTIONS

HEALTH PROMOTING STRATEGIES

A proper intake of food is essential for optimal health. "Eating the right kinds and amounts of food and following good dietary habits throughout one's entire life means a healthier body and mind, greater vitality, greater resistance to disease, efficiency, happiness, and longevity" (Poleman and Peckenpaugh, 1991, 9). Inadequate food intake and poor eating habits affect one's physical fitness, decrease strength and endurance, and interfere with the capacity to think, work and cope with the stresses of everyday living. Nurses can assist individuals, families and groups to promote optimal nutrition in three ways:

1. They can encourage and help people to examine lifestyle factors and personal, cultural, and religious values and practices that affect their dietary patterns and eating habits.

2. They can provide information that will enable individuals, families and groups to determine whether their usual patterns and habits need changing.

3. They can provide teaching about healthy eating and other health practices, such as regular exercise and dental care, that are intended to promote optimal nutrition and wellness.

PROMOTING HEALTHY FOOD INTAKE

The wise selection of foods can significantly affect an individual's health and well-being. A well-balanced diet will supply the amounts of essential nutrients that are needed to sustain life and health. In addition, while epidemiological and experimental studies linking nutrition and disease have not been conclusive, available evidence suggests that a diet containing the recommended essential nutrients has the potential for reducing the risk of chronic diseases such as cardiovascular diseases, diabetes and cancer.

Guidelines for Healthier Nutrition

A resource used by nurses, nutritionists and physicians in teaching and counselling individuals, families and groups about nutrition is *Canada's Food Guide to Healthy Eating*. Issued by the Department of Health and Welfare Canada, this *Food Guide* is based on the nutrition recommendations, including recommended nutrient intakes. It specifies amounts to be included in a daily diet from each of four basic food groups: grain products, vegetables and fruit, milk products and meat and alternatives. It also includes guidelines for intake of other foods, such as fats and oils, sugars, beverages, herbs, spices, alcohol, and caffeine, as well as vitamin and mineral supplements. *Canada's Food Guide to Healthy Eating* is outlined in Figure 19.9. The key nutrients in the *Food Guide* are listed in Figure 19.10. In addition to the *Food Guide*, there are a number of other guidelines which individuals and families may use to make food choices for healthier nutrition. These are outlined in the box, Promoting Healthy Nutrition.

The Vegetarian Diet

Vegetarian diets exclude or limit the intake of meat, poultry and fish and, in some instances, eggs and dairy products. There are four basic types of vegetarian diets:

1. *lacto-ovo-vegetarian*, which avoids meat, fish and poultry
2. *lacto-vegetarian*, which avoids meat, poultry, fish, and eggs
3. *ovo-vegetarian*, which avoids meat, poultry, fish, milk, and milk products
4. *vegan*, also referred to as strict vegetarian, which avoids all foods of animal origin.

In practice, there are many individual variations of vegetarian diets. For example, some people call themselves vegetarians because they exclude only red meat, such as beef and pork, from their diet. Others allow only poultry and fish, while excluding all other animal products including milk and eggs.

When foods are selected carefully, vegetarian diets are healthy and nutritionally adequate. If they are not properly planned, the person may suffer from nutritional deficiencies of protein, iron, calcium and riboflavin. A vital concern for people on a vegan diet is that they obtain the right amounts of protein. You will recall from our previous discussion that plant products are incomplete proteins. While certain vegetable products, such as grains (wheat, rice and corn), legumes (fruit or pod of vegetables including soybeans, peas, beans, lentils), nuts and seeds, are good sources of protein, they lack one or more essential amino acids in sufficient quantity. If eaten individually, they are not generally adequate in maintaining proper nutrition. However, if eaten in proper combinations or complementary patterns, they can supply all of the amino acids essential to life. In what is termed protein complementation, a vegetable food low in a particular amino acid is eaten with a food high in that particular amino acid to provide the equivalent of a complete protein. For example, grains complemented by nuts or seeds, such as noodles with sesame seeds, will provide a complete protein. It is important to note that complementary patterns of amino acids are not necessary within each meal but should be included within the intake for a given day (BCDNA, 1992). A Vegetarian Food Guide is shown in Table 19.10.

CHANGING DIETARY PATTERNS

It is sometimes necessary for people to change dietary patterns and food habits because of illness. They may be told by a physician that they can no longer use salt to flavour their food, or they may have to give up eating a favourite dish. Patients may be put on low-fat diets, or any one of a number of special diets. In these situations, people react differently. Some accept the restrictions of a special diet fairly easily; others are less amenable to change.

One of the most common reasons a person fails to adhere to a diet is lack of understanding of why it is necessary.

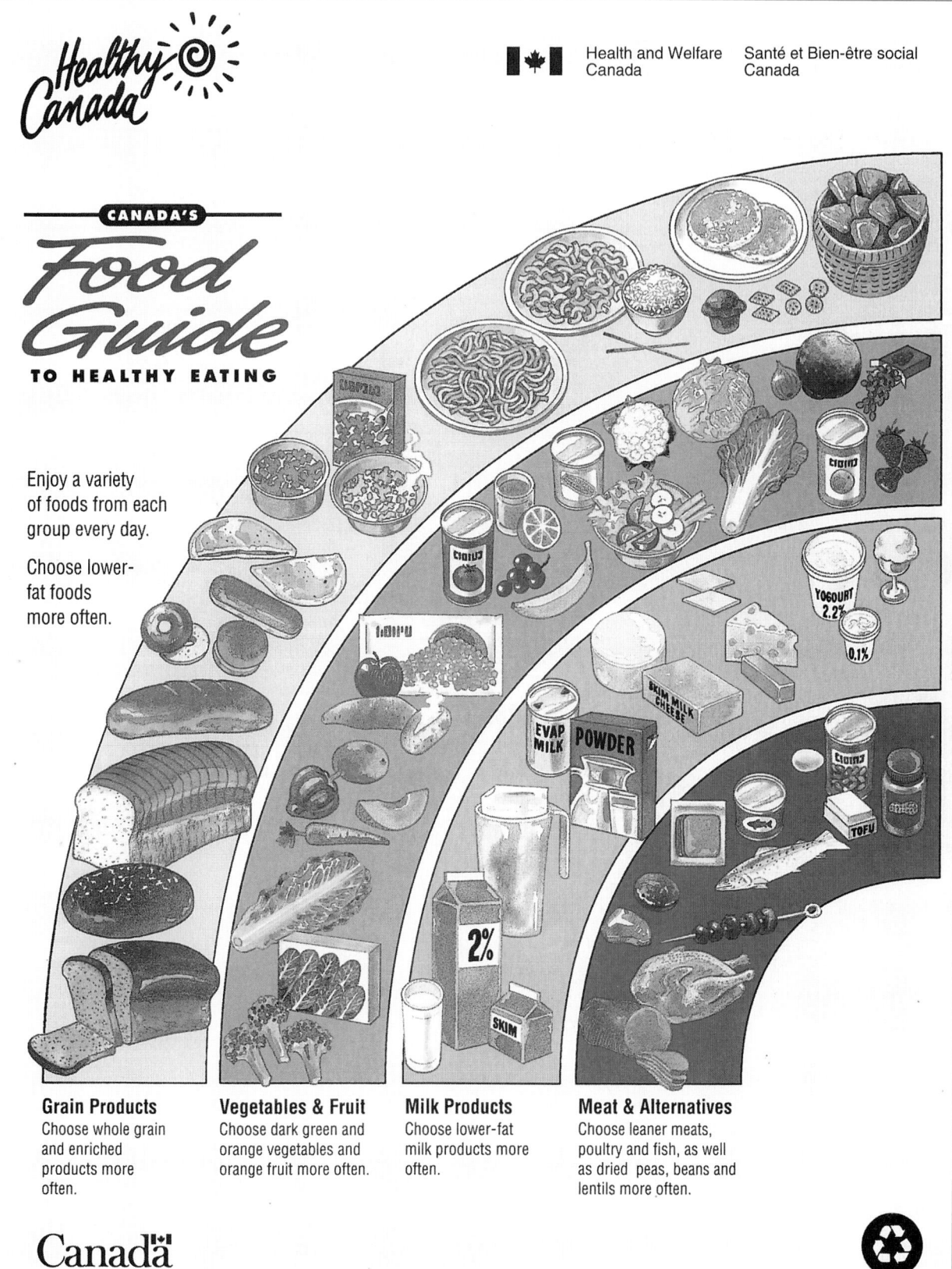

Health and Welfare Canada   Santé et Bien-être social Canada

CANADA'S
Food Guide
TO HEALTHY EATING

Enjoy a variety of foods from each group every day.

Choose lower-fat foods more often.

Grain Products
Choose whole grain and enriched products more often.

Vegetables & Fruit
Choose dark green and orange vegetables and orange fruit more often.

Milk Products
Choose lower-fat milk products more often.

Meat & Alternatives
Choose leaner meats, poultry and fish, as well as dried peas, beans and lentils more often.

Canada

FIGURE 19.9   Canada's Food Guide to Healthy Eating

continued on the next page

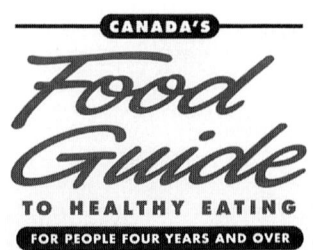

Different People Need Different Amounts of Food

The amount of food you need every day from the 4 food groups and other foods depends on your age, body size, activity level, whether you are male or female and if you are pregnant or breast-feeding. That's why the Food Guide gives a lower and higher number of servings for each food group. For example, young children can choose the lower number of servings, while male teenagers can go to the higher number. Most other people can choose servings somewhere in between.

Grain Products
5–12
SERVINGS PER DAY

Vegetables & Fruit
5–10
SERVINGS PER DAY

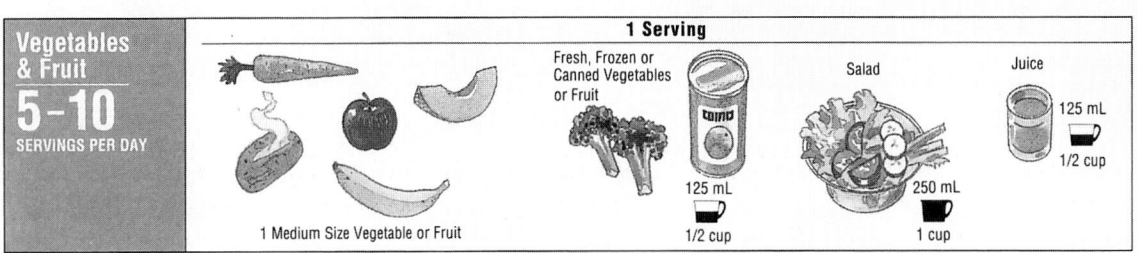

Milk Products
SERVINGS PER DAY
Children 4–9 years: 2–3
Youth 10–16 years: 3–4
Adults: 2–4
Pregnant & Breast-feeding
Women: 3–4

Meat & Alternatives
2–3
SERVINGS PER DAY

Other Foods

Taste and enjoyment can also come from other foods and beverages that are not part of the 4 food groups. Some of these foods are higher in fat or Calories, so use these foods in moderation.

Enjoy eating well, being active and feeling good about yourself. That's VITALITÉ

© Minister of Supply and Services Canada 1992 Cat. No. H39-252/1992E No changes permitted. Reprint permission not required.
ISBN 0-662-19648-1

FIGURE 19.9

continued

SOURCE: Health and Welfare Canada. (1992). Ottawa: Minister of Supply and Services. (Catalogue H39–252/1992E)

Promoting Healthy Nutrition

- Eat a variety of foods from the four food groups. Eating a wide variety will ensure a balanced and adequate intake of all essential nutrients.

- Eat foods rich in calcium and iron (especially women and children). For calcium choose skim or low-fat milk and dairy products; dark green leafy vegetables, such as spinach and broccoli; dried peas and beans; cauliflower; fish with bones, such as canned salmon. For iron choose lean meats, shellfish, dried peas and beans; dark green leafy vegetables, such as spinach and broccoli; and dried fruits, such as raisins, apricots, dates.

- Eat moderate amounts of protein, balancing intake of plant and animal sources. Choose leaner meats, poultry, and fish, as well as dried peas, beans, and lentils.

- Eat more complex carbohydrates, fibre, and natural sugars. Choose whole grain and enriched products, legumes (peas and beans), and fruits and vegetables. Choose dark green and orange vegetables and orange fruits (high sources of vitamin A, vitamin C, and folacin). As well, choose cruciferous vegetables, such as cabbage, Brussels sprouts, broccoli, and cauliflower, since they appear to provide protection against lung, stomach, colon, and rectal cancer.

- Choose lower-fat foods more often since diets high in fat have been associated with heart disease and certain types of cancer.

- Eat less meat with high fat content. Avoid hot dogs, processed luncheon meats, sausage, and bacon.

- Use skim, partly-skim, and reduced-fat dairy products.

- Use less butter or margarine on bread, buns, or bagels.

- Avoid butter, margarine, or rich sauces on vegetables.

- Limit consumption of fast and deep-fried foods.

- Eat more fish and select meat, poultry, or fish that are baked, broiled, or microwaved.

- Use less dressing on salads or use lower-fat dressings.

- Limit snacks such as chips and chocolate bars.

- Limit intake of salt and sodium.

- Avoid highly salted foods.

- When shopping check labels; select unsalted foods or foods low in salt or sodium.

- Use less salt at the table.

- Taste foods before adding salt.

- Use herbs, spices, and lemon juice instead of salt in cooking.

- Avoid taking dietary supplements in excess of the daily RNI.

- Eat fresh, natural foods as much as possible and avoid foods with questionable additives such as dyes, saccharin, sodium nitrate, and sulfites.

- Use alcohol and caffeine in moderation. For adults, this means no more than 1 alcoholic drink a day and no more than 7 drinks a week. Limit caffeine intake from all sources to no more than the equivalent of 4 cups of coffee a day.

SOURCES: Health and Welfare Canada, (1990, 1992); Williams, (1993).

Another underlying cause may be fear resulting from the loss of a familiar food. The person who has been used to eating pasta all the time, and for whom this represents a basic security food, will find it difficult to adjust to a diet on which this is banned. An individual may rebel against being told what to eat or may resent the loss of personal choice in the matter.

There are other factors that must be taken into consideration also. These include socioeconomic factors; the cultural, religious and moral values of the patient; and the matter of control over the purchase and preparation of food in the home. The most influential member of a household in regard to purchasing and preparing food is, in most instances, the mother. Young, well-educated homemakers usually have good nutritional knowledge and are fairly adaptable, but it is often necessary to work with others who may be more resistant to change.

Many older people find it hard to alter the eating patterns they have been used to all their lives; yet often they are the ones on whom dietary restrictions are imposed. In addition, it has been recognized that in new Canadian families, food habits from the homeland are retained long after language, clothing and other aspects of daily living are altered. Often, strong resistance may be encountered to suggested changes involving the removal or alteration of familiar foods.

When helping people to change their dietary patterns, it is often better to work within the framework of the individuals' existing food habits, and to suggest modifications wherever possible rather than complete change. The

Each food group is essential. That's because it provides its own set of nutrients.

Grain Products	+	Vegetables & Fruit	+	Milk Products	+	Meat & Alternatives	=	The Food Guide
protein				protein		protein		protein
				fat		fat		fat
carbohydrate		carbohydrate						carbohydrate
fibre		fibre						fibre
thiamin		thiamin				thiamin		thiamin
riboflavin				riboflavin		riboflavin		riboflavin
niacin						niacin		niacin
folacin		folacin				folacin		folacin
				vitamin B_{12}		vitamin B_{12}		vitamin B_{12}
		vitamin C						vitamin C
		vitamin A		vitamin A				vitamin A
				vitamin D				vitamin D
				calcium				calcium
iron		iron				iron		iron
zinc				zinc		zinc		zinc
magnesium		magnesium		magnesium		magnesium		magnesium

FIGURE 19.10   Key nutrients in *Canada's Food Guide to Healthy Eating*

SOURCE: Health and Welfare Canada. (1992). *Using the food guide*. Ottawa: Minister of Supply and Services, 5. (Catalogue No. H39–253/1922E)

elderly person's protein intake may be increased, for example, by the addition of cheese to his or her usual lunch of tea and toast. Supplementing a familiar diet of beans and rice by the addition of meat and milk may be accepted more readily by a Puerto Rican family than the suggestion of a completely different way of eating.

Another important factor to consider is the effect of the patient's diet on other members of the family. Can the family afford to buy the special foods that are required for the patient? What problems may develop as a result of the need to prepare a different meal for one individual?

PROVIDING NOURISHMENT FOR THE ILL

Food for the sick person should be both therapeutic and a source of pleasure and nourishment. Most patients, if they are not too ill, look forward to mealtimes; meals provide diversions in a sometimes otherwise monotonous day and a pleasant change from the necessary treatments that many people must undergo when they are ill.

Usually other personnel are employed in a health agency to prepare and, often, serve food to the patient. The nurse, however, has important responsibilities with regard to the patient's nourishment.

Illness, as we have mentioned, has a very great bearing upon a person's acceptance of food. Those who are nauseated, dyspeptic or in pain or who have a fever are less desirous of food than are healthy people. The nurse has a responsibility to modify these factors as much as possible so that the patient will accept nourishment. Small, frequent meals are often more acceptable to the sick person than larger servings at regular mealtime hours. Also, finding out about particu-

lar likes and dislikes, and offering foods the patient likes, will increase the likelihood of nourishment intake.

A sedentary person is less likely to have a big appetite than one who exercises regularly. If a patient is able to perform some activity he or she should be encouraged to do so, for it will stimulate appetite. It is important, however, that this activity be carried out well before meals, not directly afterward, and that the amount of exercise is not exhausting.

Anxiety may affect a patient's desire for food, as well as the ability to digest it. Sometimes anxiety is manifested in complaints about the food. Often these complaints are a vocalization of a deeper anxiety. Understanding and acceptance on the part of the nurse can do much to help the patient to accept the illness as well as the new diet.

The amount of food that patients eat and the amount of fluids they drink are sometimes very important therapeutically. It is the nurse who observes how much they eat and drink and who has the responsibility for communicating this knowledge to other members of the health team. Many health agencies have a standard intake and output (I & O) form that is kept at the patient's bedside so that fluid consumption can be recorded. Often the patient can help to keep the bedside record. Once the record is completed, the information is transferred to the fluid balance record in the patient's chart (fluid balance records are discussed more fully in Chapter 22).

The nurse is also responsible for helping the patient to get ready for meals. The patient is offered a bedpan or urinal and is provided with facilities for washing his or her hands prior to eating. Often patients who have unpleasant tastes in their mouths will find their appetites improved if they brush their teeth before eating.

Another factor which affects a person's appetite is the environment in which he or she eats. If a patient is served

TABLE 19.10 Vegetarian Food Guide

A variety of foods from each of the following groups should be eaten daily:

Breads and Cereals: 6 servings daily

Whole grain products are recommended.

Examples of one serving:

Bread, 1 slice
Bagel, 1/2
Bannock, 60 g (2 oz)
Cereal, ready-to-eat, 200 mL (3/4 cup)
Cereal, cooked, 125 mL (1/2 cup)
Chapati or roti, 1
Crackers, 4-6
Hamburger or hot dog bun, 1/2
Muffin, 1 small or 1/2 large
Pancake or waffle, 1
Pita bread, 1/2
Popcorn, 375 mL (1 1/2 cups)
Rice, cooked, 125 mL (1/2 cup)
Roll, 1 small
Rye cracker, 2
Spaghetti, macaroni or other pasta, cooked,
   125 mL (1/2 cup)
Tortilla, 1

Vegetables and Fruits: 6 servings daily

Include 1-2 servings of dark green vegetables daily and at least one other vegetable.

Examples of one serving:

Vegetable or fruit, fresh, frozen or canned,
   125 mL (1/2 cup)
Vegetable or fruit juice, 125 mL (1/2 cup)
Medium sized potato, carrot, tomato, apple,
   banana, orange or peach, 1
Small fruit, apricot or plum, 2

Iron and Protein Foods: 2 servings daily

Eat these plant sources of iron at the same meal with a vitamin C source (a vegetable or fruit) to increase iron absorption.

Examples of one serving:

Legumes, cooked, 250 mL (1 cup)
Firm tofu, 125 mL (1/2 cup)
Nuts or seeds, 125 mL (1/2 cup)
Nut or seed butter, 75 mL (1/3 cup)
Soy yogurt (cultured soy), 125 mL (1/2 cup)
Soybean milk, 500 mL (2 cups)

In addition, for ovo-vegetarian diets:

Eggs, 2

Calcium Foods: 6 servings daily

Each serving provides approximately 100 mg calcium. Some foods can be counted as Fruit and Vegetable servings *as well as* Calcium Foods servings (for example, dark green leafy vegetables and broccoli).

Some foods can be counted as Iron and Protein Foods *as well as* Calcium Foods (for example, moderately firm and firm tofu that is made with calcium, legumes, nuts and seeds).

The serving sizes for some foods are small when counted as calcium servings. Soy milk does not serve as a calcium source.

Examples of one serving:

Firm tofu made with calcium, 50 mL (1/4 cup)
Legumes, cooked, 250 mL (1 cup)
Unhulled sesame seeds or butter, 15 mL (1 Tbsp)
Sesame tahini, 30 mL (2 Tbsp)
Almonds, 30 g (1 oz)
Seaweeds, (hijiki, kelp, wakame) dried, 4-7 g
Dark green vegetables (beet greens, bok choy,
   broccoli, collards, kale, mustard greens, okra,
   turnip greens) cooked 125 mL (1/2 cup)

In addition, for lacto-vegetarian diets:

Milk, 75 mL (1/3 cup)
Yogurt, 75 mL (1/3 cup)
Cheddar cheeses, 14 g (1/2 oz)

Also Include

For vitamin B_{12}:

5 mL (1 tsp) nutritional yeast grown on a vitamin B_{12} enriched medium

For vitamin D:

15 mL (3 tsp) vitamin D-fortified margarine

For additional energy:

Add energy-rich roods such as nuts, seeds, nut and seed butters, and oils. Servings of breads, cereals, legumes, fruits and vegetables may also be increased.

SOURCE: British Columbia Dietitians' and Nutritionists' Association (BCDNA). (1992). *Manual of nutritional care* (4th ed.). Vancouver: Author, 17. Reproduced with permission.

in the hospital room, the air should be fresh and free from unpleasant odours. In addition, the patient's unit should be free of unpleasant sights. Bedside treatment trays should be neatly covered and any unnecessary equipment removed.

The nurse can also see that the patient is free from pain at mealtimes and that he or she is not subjected to unpleasant treatments immediately before or after meals. Enemas and

dressing changes should be carried out at a time when they will have little effect on the patient's appetite.

Some patients like to get out of bed to eat their meals. If this is allowed, the nurse can help the patient to get up a few minutes before the tray arrives. Patients find it very difficult to eat and to swallow when they are flat in bed. If a patient cannot be raised to a sitting position, he or she

Complementary Plant Protein

Combination	Examples
Grains plus Legumes	Whole grain bread and baked beans
	Whole grain crackers and lentil or split pea soup
	Brown rice and tofu
	Cornmeal tortillas and vegetarian chili beans
	Chapatis and dahl
	Felafel (pita bread and garbanzo beans)
	Peanut butter sandwich
	Pita bread and humus
	Toast and scrambled tofu
	Muffins and soy milk
	Cereal with soy milk or tofu yogurt
	Bun with tofu patty
Grains plus Nuts or Seeds	Whole grain bread and nut butter
	Whole grain bread and sesame tahini
	Granola or muesli with nuts
	Noodles with sesame seeds

SOURCE: British Columbia Dietitians' and Nutritionists' Association (BCDNA). (1992). *Manual of nutritional care* (4th ed.). Vancouver: Author, 15. Reproduced with permission.

will be more comfortable lying on the side to eat. A comfortable position with adequate support helps make meals more enjoyable experiences.

Some patients prefer company at mealtime. Pleasant conversation with visitors or members of the nursing staff often relaxes the patient, so that the meal is more pleasurable and appetite and digestion are improved. If the nurse stops to talk with a patient, he or she should be guided by the patient's wishes in regard to mealtime conversations.

TRAY SERVICE

Although dining-room service for patients is becoming popular, most patients in hospitals still receive their food on trays in their rooms. Patients are not always physically able to go to a dining room, and not all hospitals have such facilities for their patients.

The nurse may need to work with the dietary department or aides to help promote good standards for tray service. The following standards should be adhered to:

1. The tray should be large enough to hold the dishes and utensils needed for the patient's meal and, at the same time, small enough to fit on the patient's over-bed or bedside table.

2. Food must be served at the proper temperature; that is, hot food should not be allowed to cool and cold food should not be allowed to become warm.

3. Food should always be covered when it is being carried to the patient's bedside. Covering food helps not only to maintain the proper temperature but also to prevent drying out which affects the flavour, texture and appearance of food.

4. Food should be served as attractively as possible, in arranged portions, with garnishes to give colour appeal. Small portions are more stimulating to the appetite than large portions.

5. The napkins, dishes, utensils and the tray itself should be spotlessly clean.

6. The arrangement on the tray should be neat and organized. Any spilled food should be replaced.

7. China and utensils should be attractive and in good condition.

8. The patient should always get the right tray with the right diet. Each tray has a card with the patient's name, bed number and type of diet. If the nurse has any doubts as to the correctness of a patient's tray, he or she should check the diet orders before the patient is served.

FEEDING THE PATIENT

If it is necessary for the nurse to feed the patient, a few simple rules will enhance the patient's comfort:

1. Whenever possible, use the utensils that are normally used for the food being served.

2. Never hurry the patient. Sit down to feed him or her whenever possible.

3. Offer the patient small rather than large amounts of food.

4. Offer the food in the order that the patient prefers.

5. Note whether any food or liquid is hot and if it is, warn the patient to take only small portions or sips.

6. Provide a straw or drinking cup if possible — these will often help a patient to take liquids.

7. If the patient can hold bread or toast, let the patient do so.

8. Be careful not to spill food. Wipe the patient's mouth and chin whenever necessary. Always protect the patient with a napkin.

After the patient has finished the meal, the tray is removed promptly. Patients are never hurried with their meals. If a patient's fluid intake is to be recorded, the amounts are noted on the I & O form. The nurse should be familiar with the amount of fluid contained in the commonly used containers. Many agencies have printed materials defining volumes of specified cups, bowls and containers.

Patients should be provided with facilities for washing their hands and brushing their teeth after meals. This offers a good opportunity for the nurse to teach oral hygiene and the correct method for brushing teeth.

HEALTH PROTECTING STRATEGIES

In caring for people with nutritional problems, health protecting strategies are implemented to prevent or minimize indigestion, anorexia, nausea and vomiting and to ensure safety, comfort and hygiene for patients who are unable to swallow, who are experiencing anorexia and nausea or who are vomiting. Nurses can also help protect individuals and families from food poisoning by providing information and instruction on preventive measures in the home.

PREVENTING INDIGESTION, ANOREXIA, NAUSEA AND VOMITING

Indigestion

There are a number of things people can do to prevent indigestion. These include:

1. Eating small meals rather than large ones. Dividing the total daily food intake into five small meals — breakfast, lunch, a mid-afternoon snack (the British afternoon tea), a light supper and a snack before bedtime — is often helpful for older people. Children, with their smaller stomach capacities, often do better with smaller meals and snacks at mid-morning and

A relaxed, unhurried atmosphere and an attractively arranged tray contribute to the patient's enjoyment of a meal.

FIGURE 19.11 Special utensils for people who are ill

mid-afternoon and before bedtime than with three large meals. Pregnant women also benefit from having smaller, more frequent meals, because the growing fetus presses on the abdominal organs to effectively lessen stomach capacity.

2. Avoiding coffee, tea, cola drinks and other drinks containing caffeine.

3. Avoiding fried foods and those high in fat content.

4. Avoiding highly spiced foods.

5. Avoiding any foods that the person has found to give him or her indigestion.

6. Having some mild exercise, such as walking, after meals.

Anorexia, Nausea and Vomiting

The prevention of anorexia, nausea and vomiting always involves a consideration of both the patient and his or her environment. Nursing measures that are effective in preventing these problems are often specific to the causes that have been discussed. The nurse can often help the patient to identify situations and stimuli that are causing the problem. They can then help to modify or eliminate these. Frequently the patient is aware of events or subjective experiences, such as pain, which cause nausea and vomiting.

An environment that is clean and pleasant will help to stimulate the appetite and prevent nausea and vomiting. If the patient eats while in bed, the nurse can provide a clean table that is free of equipment. The emesis basin should be kept out of sight. If the patient feels more secure with it nearby, it can be kept within easy reach.

Unpleasant odours, sights and sounds are noxious stimuli that may contribute to anorexia, nausea or vomiting. To dissipate unpleasant odours, a well-ventilated room is important, and the use of deodorants may be necessary at times. Vomitus is always removed immediately and treatment trays are covered and placed as inconspicuously as possible. Personal cleanliness is particularly important in the case of the person who has anorexia or a tendency to become nauseated. Other preventive measures include those described in the section earlier in this chapter on provision of nourishment for the sick.

Collaborative measures to prevent nausea and vomiting involve the use of antiemetic drugs. Antiemetic drugs have a specific action on the vomiting centre, and they may be given 20 to 30 minutes before mealtimes or otherwise as ordered. Many people who are susceptible to motion sickness travel much more comfortably if they take an antiemetic medicine shortly before embarking on a plane trip or other journey. It is important to remember that these drugs usually produce some drowsiness as a side effect.

PREVENTING FOOD POISONING

The prevention of food poisoning involves teaching people about selecting, preparing and storing foodstuffs and cooked foods to prevent unsafe quantities of disease-carrying bacteria (or their toxins) from being consumed. Specifically, people should do the following:

1. Buy from reputable dealers. Patronize only clean stores.
2. Keep hot foods hot (60° C or higher) and cold foods cold (4° C or lower).
3. After marketing, place frozen foods in the freezer compartment of the refrigerator or in a deep-freeze until ready for use.
4. Do not buy foods that are supposed to be frozen but are actually thawed. Frozen foods that have been completely thawed or have been held at refrigerator-temperature more than one or two days should not be refrozen.
5. Heat pre-cooked frozen foods, such as TV dinners and meat pies, for the time and temperature recommended on the labels. Read the labels.

6. Refrigerate left-overs from prepared dishes within an hour and keep refrigerated until re-serving or reheating. Store left-over poultry and stuffing separately.
7. After preparing foods containing eggs, meat, milk, gravy or salads with dressing, such as sandwiches, picnic or buffet dishes, serve them within two hours or refrigerate.
8. If canning foods at home
   a) always follow professional directions carefully
   b) never can non-acid foods such as meat, fish, meat-vegetable mixtures, soups or non-acid vegetables (beans, peas, asparagus, corn) unless a properly attended pressure-cooker is used.
9. Do not taste foods from bulging and leaking cans, or cans whose contents spurt out or are bubbly, off-colour or off-odour.
10. Do not eat foods that have an "off" flavour.
11. Keep everything in the kitchen clean.*

SAFETY, COMFORT AND HYGIENE MEASURES

In caring for seriously ill patients, who may not be fully conscious, the nurse should make sure that they are able to swallow before attempting to give them fluids or food. In assessing the swallowing reflex, the presence of the gagging reflex should be established first. A standard method of testing for the gagging reflex is to touch the back of the throat with an applicator or tongue depressor. If the gagging reflex is present, the person may be given small sips of water first, while the nurse watches for the swallowing movements in the neck. It is helpful to support the person's shoulders and head to make swallowing easier.

With most patients who are anorectic or nauseated, the immediate problem is usually to prevent aggravation of the symptoms. The nauseated individual usually feels better lying down in a cool and quiet room with adequate ventilation. If this is not possible, the person should be encouraged to sit quietly and take a few deep breaths. This helps to relax the diaphragm. Measures to take the person's mind off his or her gastrointestinal problems may also help.

The patient who is vomiting needs prompt attention, directed first of all at making sure that the patient does not aspirate the vomitus. A person who is lying down and starts to vomit should be helped to a sitting position if this is possible and not contraindicated. Otherwise, the head should be turned to the side and the person positioned so that the vomitus will drain from the mouth. It is particularly important to watch helpless patients, such as those who are unconscious, semiconscious or paralyzed, to make sure that the airway is not blocked. Other priorities in nursing care of the vomiting patient are to relieve the symptom and to provide comfort and support to the patient.

---

* Selected nutrition teaching aids (1976).

The nurse can assist the vomiting patient by holding a curved basin (emesis basin) under the chin to catch the vomitus, and supporting the head and shoulders. The nurse should provide tissues and help to wipe the patient's mouth. Vomiting is an unpleasant experience. Not only is it physically distressing but there is a loss of control and dignity which most people find embarrassing. The nurse can do much to reassure the patient by a calm acceptance of the situation and sympathetic yet efficient care. For the patient's own feelings of dignity, and because most people find it distressing to watch someone vomiting, the patient should be screened from the view of others. Curtains can be quickly drawn around the patient's bed, or the door of their room closed, to ensure privacy.

After the patient has stopped vomiting, mouth care and a hand and face wash will promote patient comfort. Any linen that has been soiled should be changed promptly. The room should be aired and the patient allowed to rest. If the patient is unable to tolerate food or fluids, frequent mouth care is essential to prevent complications.

HEALTH RESTORING STRATEGIES

Helping a person to restore hydration and nutritional status is an important nursing function. Some strategies are implemented as independent nursing measures, while others are performed in collaboration with the physician. This section will focus on measures to stimulate appetite and relieve nausea and vomiting, on how to insert and manage gastrointestinal tubes and on how to provide enteral and total parenteral nutrition.

STIMULATING APPETITE AND RELIEVING NAUSEA AND VOMITING

People who are experiencing anorexia may become even more anorectic when confronted with large servings of food. Small portions, attractively served, are usually more appealing. Patients are also more likely to eat if they are given foods that they particularly like. Assisting persons who cannot manage their meals alone may help as well.

Antiemetic drugs are often given as prescribed by the physician to control nausea and vomiting. However, there are a number of non-pharmacologic measures that may also be effective and should be attempted. Weak tea, flattened carbonated beverages (such as ginger ale) or Gatorade are frequently tolerated much better than other fluids when the stomach is upset. Dry crackers and toast may help as well. When people have difficulty retaining fluids, offering small amounts of fluid at frequent intervals may help them to achieve adequate fluid intake. Small amounts taken regularly are more likely to be retained than a large volume taken all at once. Patients must be monitored carefully and if signs of dehydration become evident, the physician should be notified. When dehydration becomes severe, intravenous fluid therapy will be necessary to restore fluid balance. The nursing responsibilities regarding intravenous therapy are outlined in Chapter 22.

Patients who have been vomiting are usually permitted only clear fluids until vomiting subsides. When other fluids are introduced into the patient's diet, those that are high in carbohydrate and protein are preferable because of the body's need for energy and tissue-building nutrients. For infants and small children, half-strength apple juice (diluted with water) is often easily tolerated. High carbohydrate fluids containing needed electrolytes, such as Lytren or Pedialyte, are also available on the market specifically for infants and small children. Lytren also comes in a grape flavour which makes it more palatable and easier for children to ingest.

GASTROINTESTINAL INTUBATION

Many patients with gastrointestinal problems require gastrointestinal intubation. Intubation refers to the placement of a tube into the stomach or intestine through the mouth (orogastric) or nasopharynx (nasogastric or nasointestinal) or through an artificial opening made in the abdominal wall to the stomach (gastrostomy) or jejunum (jejunostomy). The nasal route is preferred over the mouth for gastric and intestinal intubation because it evades the effects of the gag reflex at the base of the oropharynx and is more comfortable on a long-term basis. Orogastric tubes are often used in premature infants whose gag reflex is nonfunctional. Tubes are inserted into the digestive tract for a number of reasons. They are commonly used to prevent distention following surgery or intestinal blockage by removing fluids and gas from the intestinal cavity (gastric decompression) and to provide nutrition to individuals who are not able to ingest foods orally but retain adequate bowel function (enteral nutrition). Nurses are responsible for inserting some tubes and for managing associated patient care, such as irrigating decompression tubes, administering tube feedings, monitoring patient status, providing patient comfort and removing nasogastric tubes.

INSERTING A NASOGASTRIC DECOMPRESSION OR FEEDING TUBE

Nurses may insert nasogastric tubes for abdominal decompression and enteral feedings. The procedure is performed only with a physician's order. Extra care must be taken during the procedure to avoid trauma to the nasal passages and the esophagus, and to ensure correct placement of the tube

Purposes of Gastrointestinal Intubation

Decompression	To establish a means of draining the stomach by suction following surgery or blockage of the intestinal tract.
Nutrition	To establish a route for feeding the patient who is unable to take nourishment by mouth but whose digestive functions are intact.
Lavage	To aspirate or wash out the stomach contents, as when a person has taken poisonous materials or an overdose of medication.
Diagnostic	To aspirate contents for laboratory analysis.

in the stomach. Because of the proximity of the esophagus to the trachea, the tube can easily enter the lungs and result in severe complications. Procedure 19.1 outlines the steps for inserting a nasogastric tube.

Preparing the Patient

Before the insertion of a gastric tube, the procedure is explained to the patient. Not only do most patients want to know how they can help, but explanations frequently allay fear and anxiety. The passage of a tube is not painful but it may be uncomfortable. The patient may feel some irritation as the tube is passed through the nose and may gag or shed tears. Explain that mouth-breathing, panting and swallowing will alleviate some of the discomfort and make it easier to advance the tube. Inform the patient that he or she will be instructed to sip on some water as the tube is passed down. A hand signal is established, permitting the patient to alert the nurse of the need to pause during the procedure.

Assembling Equipment

The nurse must know the purpose of intubation in order to select the appropriate gastric tube. Usually the physician will order the size of tube to be inserted. In some cases of enteral nutrition, the size of tube is recommended by the manufacturer of the solution (formula) to be administered. Nasal tubes differ in size, length and composition. The size, or outside diameter of a tube, is gauged by use of the French scale and is indicated with a number followed by the sym-

bol *Fr*. Each number on the French scale is approximately equal to 0.33 millimetres. The larger the number, the larger the diameter of the tube. Large-sized nasogastric (NG) tubes, referred to as *large-bore* tubes, are used for gastric decompression. They are usually 12 Fr or larger in diameter. *Small-bore* tubes are less than 12 Fr in diameter; these are preferred for enteral feeding. Nasogastric tubes are usually shorter than nasoenteric feeding tubes since they terminate in the stomach. Nasoenteric feeding tubes vary in length. Many are designed so that they can be placed in the stomach, duodenum or jejunum. Enteral feedings are generally administered into the stomach. In some institutions, patients who are at risk for pulmonary aspiration, for instance, those with altered pharyngeal reflexes or those who are unconscious, are fed into the upper small intestine (Metheney, 1988). However, a recent study indicated that these complications did not decrease with postpylorus feedings (Strong, et al., 1992, cited in Davis and Sherer, 1994).

Two basic types of tubes are used for gastric decompression: the single-lumen Levin tube and the double-lumen sump tube (Salem sump tube). The Levin tube is a straight non-vented tube with holes near the tip. It is used less commonly nowadays because it does not have the venting capability of the Salem sump tube. The Levin tube works effectively as long as flow is maintained and the tube openings do not adhere to the gastric mucosa. If flow stops and the tube adheres to the stomach lining, a vacuum forms producing suction levels that can cause trauma to the mucosa. The Salem sump tube overcomes this problem by providing a constant flow of atmospheric air through a venting lumen which prevents the tube from adhering to the stomach lining. The blue "pigtail" on the Salem sump tube connects the venting lumen to the outside air. Both of these types of tubes are made of a stiff polyvinyl chloride which can cause erosion of the nose and oropharynx along with other discomforts such as difficulty swallowing. They should not be used for enteral nutrition. These stiff plastic tubes may be placed in some warm water to make them more flexible for insertion.

Nasoenteric feeding tubes are made of soft silicone rubber or polyurethane, which reduce oropharyngeal irritation, cause less trauma to the tracheoesophageal wall and increase patient comfort and tolerance. Because of their flexibility and softness, these tubes are weighted with tungsten and contain a wire guide or stylet which facilitates their passage through the nose and esophagus into the stomach or upper intestine. The guide is removed once the feeding tube is in place. The weight also helps to keep the tube in its proper place once inserted. Both polyvinyl chloride NG and enteric feeding tubes have a radiopaque strip or marker at the distal end which allows visualization of the tube's placement on X-ray.

A. To tape the nasogastric tube to the nose: (1) Split one half of the tape into two tails. (2) Place the broad tab on the patient's nose and wrap one tail around the feeding tube. (3) Wrap the other tail around the tube in the opposite direction. **B.** Small-bore nasoenteric tubes may be taped to the forehead to allow access to the mouth and to keep tube out of patient's line of vision.

A   B

FIGURE 19.12   Nasogastric tube placement

SOURCE: Flynn J.M. and Kackel, R. (1990) *Technological foundations in nursing.* Norwalk, CT: Appleton & Lange, p.575 with permission.

PROCEDURE 19.1

Inserting A Nasogastric and Nasointestinal Tube

ACTION	RATIONALE
1. Prepare the patient for what to expect and what he or she can do to aid in the procedure.	Reduces anxiety and enables patient participation. Insertion is easier if the patient is relaxed.
2. Gather: • NG tube or feeding tube • Water-soluble lubricant • 50 ml catheter-tip syringe • Glass of water with a straw • Water-proof pad or towel • Emesis basin • Hypoallergenic adhesive tape 2.5 cm wide • Clean gloves • Penlight • Elastic band and safety pin • pH test strip.	Facilitates efficiency and economy of time.
3. Wash hands thoroughly.	Limits the spread of microorganisms.
4. Help the patient into a sitting position unless contraindicated. Cover the patient with a water-proof pad or towel and place the emesis basin, some tissues and the glass of water with a straw on the bedside table in easy reach. Have the patient remove dentures if they don't fit well.	Facilitates passage of the tube by the pull of gravity. Stimulation of the throat may cause gagging and vomiting. Passage of the tube also causes tearing. Readies the water for later use. Prevents choking on the dentures if they should become dislodged.

Continued on the next page

ACTION	RATIONALE
5. If right-handed, stand at the patient's right side; if left-handed, stand at the left side.	Facilitates ease of insertion and prevents unnecessary strain on the nurse's body.
6. Apply gloves. Ask the patient to blow nose. Then ask the patient to breathe while alternately blocking each nostril. Using the penlight examine the patient's nostrils for deformities or obstructions.	Clears the nostrils and determines which side has better air flow. Using the nostril that is larger and has better air flow will facilitate easier passage of the tube.
7. Measure the length of tube to be inserted by holding the distal end of the tube at the tip of the patient's nose, and then extending the tube to the earlobe and down to the xiphoid process. Mark the distance with a piece of adhesive tape.	Approximates the distance from the nose to the gastric cavity, thereby ensuring that the distal end of the tube reaches the stomach.

ACTION	RATIONALE
8. Prepare a small-bore feeding tube according to the manufacturer's directions.	Manufacturers differ in the treatment of tubes. Some require the insertion of the wire guide; in others the guides are preinserted but a specified amount of water must be instilled into the tube to activate a self-lubricating coating which eases removal of the guide. Be sure the guide is properly secured in the tube.
9. If inserting a large-bore polyvinyl tube, coil the distal end around the fingers for a few seconds.	Reduces stiffness, making insertion easier.
10. Lubricate the first 12 to 15 cm of the tube with water-soluble jelly. If using a self-lubricating tube, immerse the tip in water. **Do Not** use mineral oil or petroleum jelly.	Reduces mucosal irritation and facilitates passage of the tube. Some tubes are coated with a water-activated lubricant. Avoids respiratory complications should the tube enter the trachea since oil-based lubricants do not dissolve as water-soluble preparations do.
11. Have the patient hyperextend his or her neck. Hold the tube with its natural curve pointing downward. Carefully insert the tube into the nostril, directing it towards the patient's ear and downward. Advance the tube along the floor of the nostril into the nasopharynx.	Decreases the curvature of the nasopharyngeal junction. Follows the natural contour of the nasal passage and avoids injury to the turbinates (projections) along the lateral wall.

ACTION

RATIONALE

Turbinates

---

12. Slight pressure may be needed to advance the tube. If resistance is met, withdraw the tube a bit, rotate it, and readvance it to the nasopharynx. **Do Not** force the tube against resistance. If the obstruction persists, withdraw the tube, relubricate it, and try the other nostril.

Alters the direction of the tube which may better follow the curvature of the nasal canal.

Avoids the risk of trauma.

13. When the tube reaches the nasopharynx, a resistance will be felt. Ask the patient to lower his or her head slightly and rotate the tube 180° inward towards the other nostril.

Closes the trachea and opens the esophagus. Rotating the tube directs it away from the mouth and into the posterior pharynx.

14. Unless contraindicated, hand the patient the glass of water and instruct him or her to sip and swallow, while slowly advancing the tube. Do not push the tube faster than the patient can swallow.

Swallowing closes the epiglottis and aids passage of the tube.
May cause the tube to kink at the epiglottis and come out of the mouth (Camp and Otten, 1990).

15. Watch the patient carefully as the tube is being advanced. If gagging occurs, instruct the patient to pant and swallow. If gagging continues, check the oropharynx. If the tube is coiled in the throat, withdraw it until it is straightened and continue the procedure.

Suppresses the gag reflex.
Determines whether the tube has coiled in the throat.

If respiratory distress occurs (e.g., patient coughs, gasps for air, becomes cyanotic) immediately withdraw the tube back into the nasopharynx. Give the patient a few moments to readjust breathing pattern, then continue the procedure.

Indicates the tube has entered the trachea and is obstructing breathing.

16. Should the guide of a small-bore tube slip out during insertion, **Do Not** reinsert it while the tube is in the patient.

Prevents potential trauma to surrounding tissue should the guide puncture the tubing as it is being pushed back into the tube.

Instead, withdraw the entire tube, explain to the patient what has happened, and reinsert the guide, making sure it correctly joins to the weighted tip and that all necessary connections are secure. Then, relubricate and reinsert the tube.

Continued on the next page

ACTION	RATIONALE
17. Once the tube is inserted to the premeasured position, tape it lightly to the nose.	Prevents displacement while proper placement is confirmed.
18. Confirm proper tube placement.	
Large-bore tube and small-bore feeding tube with guide removed:	
a) Aspirate stomach contents and measure the acidity with pH test strip.	Provides a reliable indication of proper placement. The mean pH of gastric aspirate is 3.02 compared to 6.57 for intestinal and 7 or more for lung aspirates (Metheney, McSweeney, Wehrle and Wiersema, 1990).
b) If there is any doubt about proper tube placement, obtain an X-ray.	Provides the most reliable means of verifying tube placement.
Small-bore feeding tube with guide in lumen: Obtain an X-ray.	Confirms placement of the tube. (The tube cannot be aspirated because the lumen is occluded by the guide.)
19. Once placement of a small-bore feeding tube is confirmed, remove the guide according to the manufacturer's directions. Store it in a place designated by agency policy (e.g., taped to the head of the patient's bed).	Keeps the guide available for use in case the tube is accidentally removed and must be reinserted. (These tubes are expensive.)
20. Secure the tube with hypoallergenic tape as in Figure 19.12 on page 509. Loop a rubber band around the tube and fasten it to the patient's gown using a safety pin.	Prevents pressure against the nostrils causing irritation and excoriation, reduces the risk of displacement, and promotes comfort.
21. Plug the tube with a catheter plug or connect it to a suction source or feeding apparatus as required.	Initiates treatment as ordered.
22. Discard supplies and wash hands.	Maintains cleanliness and safety in the workplace.
23. Document the procedure, note the type and size of tube, the means by which placement was confirmed, and how the patient responded.	Fulfills requirement for nurse accountability. Promotes continuity of care.

PROVIDING NASOGASTRIC SUCTION AND TUBE CARE

Gastric decompression refers to the drainage of fluid and gaseous contents from the stomach by use of negative pressure or suction. It is indicated as a measure to prevent or relieve distention and vomiting following surgery with general anesthesia and to remove the stomach contents of patients who have gastrointestinal obstructions. A large-bore NG tube, commonly the Salem sump or the Levin tube, is used for gastric decompression. The external end of the tube is connected to a suction device which drains and collects the gastric contents. Effective decompression depends on equipment that functions properly and an NG tube that is patent and placed correctly in the stomach. Thus, care involves monitoring the equipment for proper functioning as well as ensuring patency and correct placement of the tube. Patency is maintained by irrigating the tube at regular intervals to keep it free of blockage from accumulated tissue debris or blood.

Nurses must be aware that the constant presence of the large, inflexible tube in the nasopharynx is a source of discomfort and potential trauma to the patient. Prolonged pressure from the tube on the mucous membrane lining of the nose can cause irritation and painful excoriation. Because one of the nostrils is occluded by the tube, the patient tends to breathe more through the mouth. This, combined with the lessened flow of saliva (due to NPO), leads to a dry mouth and throat. Special care is needed to prevent local excoriation

FROM RESEARCH TO PRACTICE

Metheney, N., McSweeney, M., Wehrle, M.A. and Wiersema, L. (1990). Effectiveness of the auscultatory method of predicting feeding tube location. *Nursing Research, 37*, 324–329.

To ensure patient safety, nurses must verify the placement of nasogastric or nasointestinal feeding tubes when they are inserted and before each feeding. One technique that has traditionally been used for this purpose is the auscultatory method. It consists of injecting air through the tube (insufflation) while listening over the epigastrum or left upper quadrant with a stethoscope. A "whooshing" or "gurgling" sound should indicate that the tube is in the stomach or correct position.

The efficacy of this method came into question as a reliable technique for confirming that the tube was placed in the stomach rather than in the lungs or esophagus. Gurgling sounds have been reported when tubes inadvertently placed in the respiratory tract were insufflated. A clinical study was conducted to determine the extent to which sounds generated by air insufflations through feeding tubes can be used to predict placement of the tubes' port end in the gastrointestinal tract (esophagus, stomach or proximal small intestine) and to differentiate between gastric and respiratory placement.

Sounds generated by air insufflations through the tubes of 85 acutely ill adult subjects were simultaneously transmitted to a tape recorder as they were heard by the investigators. A total of 115 usable tape recordings of sound sequences were obtained. A research team of skilled clinicians listened to the tapes and recorded their impressions of the sounds. The results were collated and compared against the exact tube location as identified by x-ray. Overall, the average percentage of correct classifications of each tape was 34.4 percent. Descriptive data provided by members of the research team present when three tubes were inadvertently placed in the respiratory tract indicated that air insufflations were clearly audible in two out of three cases. Thus, this study found the auscultatory method to be ineffective in distinguishing the location of feeding tubes in the gastrointestinal tract or in differentiating gastric from respiratory placement of tubes.

The authors recommend the use of pH determinations of feeding tube aspirates in differentiating between gastric and intestinal placement, and gastric and respiratory placement. They reported recent clinical studies which indicated the mean gastric pH was 3.02, compared to 6.57 for intestinal pH; in most instances respiratory aspirates have pH values of seven or more.

and discomfort in the nose and to keep the lips and mucous membranes moist and clean. To ease irritation by the tube on the patient's throat, the patient is often allowed to have throat lozenges or to chew gum. Techniques for establishing and maintaining gastric suction, for irrigating the NG tube, and for providing hygiene and comfort to the nose and mouth are detailed in Procedure 19.2.

Since gastric suction returns are an important part of the patient's fluid output, the amount of drainage is measured and the clarity, colour, and consistency of the drainage are noted. These observations are reported on the patient's record. Any untoward changes in the patient's suction returns, such as bright red returns, or in the patient's condition, such as an accelerated pulse, are reported promptly so that the physician can be notified.

Preparing the Patient

The techniques for managing suction, maintaining tube patency, and providing hygiene to the nose and mouth are painless. Telling patients what to expect and how they can help will enable them to better participate in the procedure.

Assembling Equipment

Decompression is established by connecting the NG tube to a suction device. There are a variety of suction devices available. Some are wall-mounted units that generate continuous or intermittent negative suction; others are portable machines that create an intermittent negative pressure by use of an electric pump. Figure 19.13 presents examples of two common types of suction units. The type and amount of suction to be maintained are dictated by the physician's order and the type of NG tube in place. When a single-lumen Levin tube is used, the suction is usually set at "intermittent low" to avoid the risk of mucosal trauma as discussed previously. A continuous high or low setting may be ordered for the double-lumen Salem sump. For wall-mounted suction devices, a high setting is established by adjusting the regulator between 80 and 100 mm Hg; a low setting means 40 to 80 mm Hg. Connecting tubing and a connector will be needed to attach the NG tube to the suction apparatus. Some tubes, for example, the Salem sump, come packaged with a connector. If available in the agency, an antireflux valve can also be used on the venting lumen (pigtail) to prevent spills and soiling of bed linen due to reflux of gastric contents (see Procedure 19.2–B, step 3).

Nasogastric tubes are usually irrigated with normal saline; however, a particular irrigant may be ordered by the physician. Water should not be used as an irrigant because it may cause electrolyte imbalances (Earnest, 1993; Flynn and Hackel, 1990). Disposable irrigating sets are available which contain a basin and a 50 ml catheter-tip syringe; some may also contain a water-proof pad. Since NG tube irrigation is a clean procedure, the irrigation set is kept at the bedside and reused. The set is changed every 24 hours.

FIGURE 19.13 Gastric suction units. A. Portable suction machine B. Wall-mounted unit

PROCEDURE 19.2

Providing Nasogastric Suction and Tube Care

ACTION	RATIONALE
A. ESTABLISHING GASTRIC SUCTION	
1. Check the physician's order for type and amount of suction.	Ensures accuracy and reduces the risk of error.
2. Prepare the patient.	Promotes the patient's well-being and enables participation in care.
3. Gather: • Suction device • Connecting tubing • Connector if one is not supplied with NG tube.	Facilitates efficiency and economy of time.
4. Wash hands thoroughly.	Limits the spread of microorganisms.
5. At the bedside, set up the suction device according to agency protocol. Attach the connecting tubing to the suction container. Check that all connections are tight. Turn on a portable machine to check that it is working. A continuously flashing red light indicates proper functioning. To check a wall unit, squeeze the connecting tubing, turn on the regulator, and watch the gauge for movement of the dial.	Prepares the device for effective functioning.

ACTION	RATIONALE
6. Set the type and amount of suction. **Single-lumen Levin**: set the suction on "intermittent" and "low." **Salem sump tube**: set the suction on "continuous" and "low" unless otherwise ordered. Turn off the suction unit.	Reduces mucosal trauma should the tube adhere to the stomach lining. Air vent prevents suction pressures that would traumatize tissue.
7. Attach the NG tube to the connecting tubing using a connector and turn the suction on. With a Salem sump, connect the primary (larger) lumen to the suction device.	
8. Check for proper functioning of the system: a) Gastric contents in the tubing are moving towards the collecting container. b) Red light on a portable unit is continuously flashing. c) There is no leakage of air or fluid at connection points and no fluid leakage from the air vent (pigtail) of a Salem sump. A Salem sump makes a soft, hissing sound. d) For intermittent suction, the portable suction pump turns on and off in cycles lasting several seconds. Or, the pressure gauge of a wall suction moves up and down at regular intervals.	Indicates that suction is effective and that tube is patent. Indicates machine is working. Indicates that connections are tight and that the tubing and collection container are placed correctly. Indicates effective suction.
9. Anchor the tubing to the patient's gown and place it on the bed so that it lies above the collection container. Keep a Salem sump pigtail higher than the level of the stomach.	Promotes effective suction and prevents reflux of gastric contents through a Salem sump pigtail. Negative pressure decreases when tubing lies below the collection container because the suction device must work against the force of gravity to draw fluids from the stomach. When the pigtail is placed below the level of the stomach, the venting mechanism, aided by the pull of gravity, acts like a siphon, drawing gastric contents into its lumen.

B. MAINTAINING GASTRIC SUCTION

ACTION	RATIONALE
1. Monitor the patient and the suction system regularly.	Indicates tube blockage or ineffective system function.
Patient: Note abdominal distention, stated discomfort, nausea, and feeling of fullness in stomach. Assess bowel sounds and look for electrolyte imbalances if gastric output is excessive.	Bowel sounds indicate gastric function. Electrolytes are lost in gastric drainage.
System: As in A, step 7 and 8. Also inspect the tubing for kinks or blockages.	As above.
Drainage: Note the amount, colour, consistency, and odour. Normal secretions may appear colourless or yellow-green if bile is present and have a mucoid consistency. Note a coffee-ground colour and consistency. Test for pH and blood according to agency protocol.	Provides data for ongoing assessment of patient status and evaluation of care. May indicate bleeding.

Continued on the next page

ACTION	RATIONALE
2. Irrigate the NG tube at regular intervals according to the physician's preference or to agency protocol, or, as necessary, if a blockage occurs. Section C below details the procedure.	Prevents or corrects tube blockage.
3. If available, insert the blue end of an antireflux valve into the pigtail of a Salem sump.	Prevents soiling of patient's gown and bed linen from inadvertent reflux through the venting lumen.

ACTION	RATIONALE
4. To ambulate the patient, turn off the suction. Disconnect the NG tube from the suction source. Close the lumen of the NG tube with a catheter plug. If using an antireflux valve on a Salem sump pigtail, close the primary lumen by inserting the white end of the antireflux valve into it.	Prevents gastric contents from draining out of the tube when the patient is ambulating.
5. Empty and measure gastric drainage from the collection container when the container is three-quarters full or at least q.8h. Disconnect the tube from the suction device as in B, step 4 above. Remove the container from the suction unit. Inspect the drainage, discard, and then rinse the container with warm water. Replace the container and reestablish suction. Record the amount of drainage on the Fluid Balance Record (see Chapter 22) and the characteristics of drainage in the nurses' notes.	Maintains cleanliness and provides data for assessment and evaluation of care. A full collection container may reduce the effectiveness of suction.

C. IRRIGATING THE NG TUBE

ACTION	RATIONALE
1. Check the physician's order or agency protocol for the frequency, type, and amount of irrigant.	Promotes accuracy and avoids risk of error.
2. Gather: • Irrigation set • Irrigating solution • Water-proof pad • Gloves	NG irrigation is a clean procedure. Thus, to conserve equipment and supplies, the materials are kept at the bedside and reused.

ACTION	RATIONALE
3. Place a water-proof pad on the bed under the NG tube-tubing connection.	Prevents soiling bed linen.
4. Apply gloves and check tube placement as in Procedure 19.1, step 18.	Prevents accidental instillation of irrigant into lungs.
5. Draw up 30 to 50 ml of irrigant, or amount as ordered into the syringe.	
6. Disconnect the Ng tube from the connector and attach the catheter-tip syringe. Instill the irrigant gently and slowly. **Do Not** force solution.	The mucosal lining of the stomach is easily damaged. Excessive suction may cause trauma.
7. Gently aspirate the solution or reattach to gastric suction. If fluid returns freely, reestablish gastric suction. Check the system for proper functioning as in A, step 8.	Prevents excessive pressure on a suture line or gastric mucosa.
8. If there is no gastric return, repeat the irrigation and aspirate. If no fluid returns, inject 20 to 30 ml of air and aspirate, reposition the patient, or reposition the tube slightly. If using a Salem sump, instill 10 to 20 ml of air into the venting lumen.	Injecting air or altering the position of the patient and the tube may shift the tube away from the stomach wall and, thereby, promote drainage.
If there are still no fluid returns, set the suction on "low" and notify the charge nurse or physician.	Maintains and verifies patency of the venting lumen.

D. PROVIDING PATIENT COMFORT AND HYGIENE

ACTION	RATIONALE
1. Provide mouth care at least q.4h. or as needed (see Procedure 30.1, Chapter 30)	Promotes comfort and prevents dryness of mucous membranes and lips.
2. Clean the nose and remove secretions with moistened cotton-tip applicators as necessary. Apply water-soluble lubricant to inside of nares.	Prevents irritation from dried secretions. Soothes the tissues and provides a cushion against friction caused by movement of the tube.
3. Remove tape anchoring the tube if it loosens. While holding the tube in place, wash the skin, remove adhesive residue from the skin with a solvent. Slightly reposition the tube, and retape as in Procedure 19.1, step 20.	Skin oils cause the tape to loosen and may produce a gummy residue that is not water-soluble (Berger and Williams, 1992).
	Changes the point of contact in the nose and throat, thereby reducing the risk of irritation and excoriation.

E. DOCUMENTATION

ACTION	RATIONALE
1. Document the procedures in the nurses' notes as per agency protocol. Record nursing assessments, date and time suction was established, suction pressure and any equipment malfunctions. Note tube placement, any blockages, irrigations, and gastric return characteristics. Record hygiene and comfort measures as well as the patient's physical and emotional responses to NG intubation and continuing suction. Record the amounts of drainage in the Fluid Balance Record.	Fulfills requirements for nurse accountability and promotes continuity of care.

PROVIDING ENTERAL NUTRITION

Enteral nutrition is the provision of nourishment in liquid form directly into the stomach or upper intestine through a feeding tube. The tube may be inserted nasally or surgically through an incision in the abdominal wall. A tube surgically inserted into the stomach is called a gastrostomy; one inserted into the small intestine is a jejunostomy. A feeding delivered into the stomach through a nasogastric feeding tube is called a *gastric gavage*. Enteral nutrition is indicated for persons who are unable to take food orally but who retain their gastrointestinal functions. This may include, for instance, a person with impaired swallowing because of cancer or neuromuscular dysfunction, or one with oral or esophageal trauma or obstruction. Gastric and intestinal feedings are also given to unconscious patients and to persons who cannot ingest food because of extensive gastrointestinal surgery.

Tube feedings can be given for an indefinite period of time. The nasogastric route is most commonly used for short-term feeding. It is not recommended for long-term use because the presence of the tube interferes with the functioning of the lower esophageal sphincter — reflux esophagitis, regurgitation and aspiration are high risks, particularly in unconscious patients. Similarly, a nasointestinal tube inserted into the duodenum or jejunum does not lessen the risk of regurgitation and aspiration. Furthermore, the need for radiographic verification of placement and the ease of displacement from coughing, sneezing or vomiting make nasogastric and nasointestinal tubes less desirable for long-term use. Thus, permanent feeding tubes, surgically inserted through a gastrostomy or jejunostomy, are indicated for long-term feedings (Davis and Sherer, 1994). Patients may be sent home with feeding tubes in place after they or their family caregivers have been provided with education for home management.

Enteral feedings are given on an intermittent schedule (for example, every four hours) or by a continuous slow drip over a 24-hour period. The frequency, type and amount of feedings, as well as the rate of infusing continuous feedings, are ordered by the physician in collaboration with the dietitian and the nurse. The dietitian monitors the patient's weight, electrolyte balance, and hydration status to avoid electrolyte imbalances and fluid overload and to ensure the nutritional adequacy of the feedings. In addition to administering the tube feedings, the nurse monitors the patient for common problems and provides protective or therapeutic measures as necessary — some independent and some collaborative. Table 19.11 shows common problems associated with tube feedings, as well as the possible causes and preventive or treatment measures.

Procedures 19.3 and 19.4 outline the steps for administering enteral feedings via the nasogastric, nasointestinal, gastrostomy and jejunostomy routes. Finally, the steps for removing a nasogastric tube are outlined in Procedure 19.5.

Preparing the Patient

As for all procedures, explain to the person what is to be done. A tube feeding is not painful, but the patient may expect a feeling of fullness following an intermittent feeding. Any discomforts such as nausea, vomiting, cramps, bloating or diarrhea must be reported. Intermittent feedings generally take about 20 to 30 minutes; some may take up to an hour. A continuous feeding is administered with a pump and it carries on day and night. The feeding will be stopped periodically so that assessments can be made and the tube flushed. The patient does not have to remain in bed because of the feeding. He or she may be up in a wheelchair or walking around as the condition permits. Before preparing the feeding, the patient is assessed for abdominal distention and bowel sounds. Feedings are withheld if bowel sounds are absent or if the abdomen is distended.

Enteral Formula

Enteral formulas consist of pureed foods or commercially prepared solutions containing carbohydrate, fat, amino acids, vitamins, minerals and other nutrients. There are numerous commercial formulas on the market made to suit the differing clinical needs and permit feeding with small-bore tubes (see Table 19.12). The formulas vary in their composition of carbohydrates, fats, proteins, and residues and in their osmolality (the osmotic pressure of a solution that results from the concentration of particles in a given volume of fluid). It is the responsibility of the dietitian to determine the formula most suited to the patient's needs. If a person's gastrointestinal tract is functioning normally (allowing for the digestion and absorption of nutrients), a pureed or polymeric formula made from intact nutrient sources may be prescribed. If a person's gastrointestinal tract is not fully functional, an elemental formula made from predigested nutrients may be administered. Elemental formulas require minimal digestion because basic nutrients are ready to absorb and do not overly stimulate the pancreatic, biliary and intestinal secretions (Davis and Sherer, 1994). They are absorbed readily from the upper intestinal tract. A modular formula consists of one essential nutrient — either protein, carbohydrate or fat. Modular formulas may be mixed together or added to a basic formula to meet the specific needs of patients. There are also formulas designed for special problems and specific disease states, such as a hepatic formula especially planned for the decreased functional abilities of the liver.

Formulas are provided in ready-to-use or powdered forms. Powdered preparations are reconstituted with water or milk according to manufacturers' directions. Once opened or mixed, formulas must be refrigerated to avoid bacterial contamination. Unused quantities must be discarded after 24 hours. Expiry dates on commercial formulas must be checked; outdated formulas are discarded.

TABLE 19.11 Common Problems Associated with Tube Feedings

PROBLEM	POSSIBLE CAUSE	PREVENTION/TREATMENT
Nausea, vomiting, abdominal distension	Administration too rapid, delayed gastric emptying	Avoid bolus feedings, administer by slow continuous drip Dilute formula, gradually increase concentration
Diarrhea, abdominal cramps	Intolerance to hypertonic formula	Dilute formula, gradually increase concentration
	Bacterial contamination	Refrigerate open containers of formula Use medical sepsis when handling formula and equipment. Change bag and tubing at least q24h, rinse equipment used for intermittent feeding with each use
	Rapid administration of formula	Use slow continuous drip administration
	Lactose intolerance	Use lactose-free formula in high-risk patients
Clogged feeding tube	Medications not adequately flushed through tubing	Use liquid forms of drugs when available Finely crush tablets and mix with water Flush tube with water before and after medications
Dehydration	Diarrhea	See above
	Insufficient fluid intake	Calculate fluid needs, administer supplementary fluids to match needs
	Osmotic diuresis related to high carbohydrate concentration	See hyperglycemia
Hyperglycemia	High carbohydrate concentration	Assess blood and urine glucose, change to lower carbohydrate formula, dilute formula or slow rate of administration. Physician may consider giving insulin

Cans and bottles must be shaken well to thoroughly mix the contents. Refrigerated solutions must be warmed to room temperature. This may be done by pouring the measured amount of formula into a container and then placing the container in a pan of warm water. Never warm formula over direct heat because heat may cause the solution to curdle or change its chemical composition. In addition, hot formula may injure the patient (Shollenberger, 1993).

Assembling Equipment

There are many types of tube feeding equipment. Feeding sets are available which consist of a plastic bag attached to tubing complete with a drip chamber and a roller clamp for regulating the rate of infusion and an adapter to connect the tubing to the feeding tube. A feeding pump or infusion controller is used for all continuous feeds and, in

TABLE 19.12   Classification of Enteral Formulas

TYPE	COMMERCIAL PREPARATIONS	COMMENTS
Pureed	Compleat B (Sandoz) Formula 2 (Cutter) Vitaneed (Sherwood)	Blended natural foods; ready-to-use
Polymeric milk-based	Meritene (Sandoz) Instant Breakfast (Carnation) Sustacal Powder (Mead Johnson)	Pleasant-tasting oral supplements; provide intact nutrients
Polymeric lactose-free	Ensure, Jevity, Osmolite (Ross) Sustacal liquid, Isocal, Ultracal (Mead Johnson) Fibersource, Resource (Sandoz) Entrition, Nutren (Clintec) Attain, Comply (Sherwood)	May be used as tube feeding, or oral supplement; made with intact protein isolates, oligosaccharides and starches, and fats; provide 1 kcal/ml (others available providing up to 2 kcal); in adequate quantities meet RDIs for vitamins and minerals; ready-to-use; isotonic (except Ensure and Sustacal)
Elemental or monomeric formulas	Vital HN (Ross) Vivonex T.E.N. (Sandoz) Criticare HN (Mead Johnson) Travasorb (Clintec) Peptamen (Clintec) Reabilan (O'Brien)	Partially digested nutrients for feeding; hypertonic (except for Reabilan and Peptamen); require reconstitution (except for Peptamen, Reabilan, and Criticare)

SOURCE: Davis, J.R. and Sherer, K. (1994). *Applied nutrition and diet therapy for nurses.* Philadelphia: Saunders, 349. Reproduced with permission.

some agencies, for selected intermittent feedings which require careful control of the infusion rate. A feeding set and an enteral feeding pump are illustrated in Figure 19.14. When a continuous feeding is set up, a four- to six-hour supply of formula should be hung to limit the chance for bacterial growth. A 50 or 60 ml catheter-tip syringe will also be necessary for checking tube placement, measuring gastric residuals (amounts of feeding remaining in the stomach), and flushing the tube after the feeding. Tubes are flushed with tap water.

FIGURE 19.14   Feeding set attached to an enteral feeding pump

Administering Enteral Feedings Through Nasogastric and Nasointestinal Tubes

ACTION	RATIONALE
1. Check the physician's order for frequency, type, amount, and rate of infusion.	Ensures accuracy and reduces the risk of error.
2. Prepare the patient. Auscultate for bowel sounds and observe for distention. Withhold feeding if bowel sounds are absent and/or distention is present. Report to charge nurse or physician.	Promotes the patient's well-being and enables participation in care. Bowel sounds indicate gastrointestinal function. Abdominal distention may indicate delayed gastric emptying and increases the risk of regurgitation and pulmonary aspiration (Petrosino, Christian and Becker, 1989).
3. Gather: • Prescribed formula • Tube feeding administration set • Adapter if one not supplied • Feeding pump as necessary • Large catheter-tip syringe • IV pole • Basin • 10 X 10 cm gauze pad and elastic band (optional).	Facilitates efficiency and economy of time.
4. Wash hands thoroughly.	Limits the spread of microorganisms.
5. At the bedside, set up the feeding. Clamp the tubing on the administration set and pour the formula into the bag. Hang the feeding set on the IV pole. Open the clamp and slowly run formula through the tubing (referred to as priming the tubing). Close the clamp. For a **continuous** feed, attach the tubing to the pump according to the manufacturer's directions. Set the infusion rate.	Prepares the equipment for the feeding. Prevents infusion of air which may cause discomfort.
6. Help the patient into a semi or high Fowler's sitting position.	Aids gastric emptying, prevents regurgitation, and reduces risk of pulmonary aspiration.
7. Attach the syringe to the feeding tube and **gently** aspirate contents. a. Check the pH as in Procedure 19.1, step 18 a). b. **Intermittent feeding**: Measure the amount of gastric residual and reinstill immediately. If gastric residual is more than a specified amount (by physician or agency protocol), withhold the feeding. c. If placement of the feeding tube is in doubt, obtain X-ray confirmation.	Excessive or vigorous suction will collapse small-bore tubes. Confirms correct placement of tube. Prevents overfilling which can lead to vomiting and aspiration. Residuals contain gastric secretions; returning residuals prevents electrolyte imbalance. The small-bore feeding tubes are prone to displacement even if they are weighted. Coughing, sneezing, retching, or vomiting, for example, can displace a gastric tube into the esophagus or the lungs.

Continued on the next page

ACTION	RATIONALE
8. Administer the feeding.	
Intermittent: Connect the feeding tube to the administration tubing. Slowly open the roller clamp and adjust the rate of infusion, allowing the formula to infuse over 20 to 30 minutes. Ensure that the formula container is about one metre above the patient's head.	A large volume introduced into the stomach quickly can cause diarrhea, nausea, cramping and vomiting. Flow depends on the force of gravity.
Continuous: Connect the feeding tube to the administration tubing. Open the roller clamp and start the feeding pump. Check the infusion rate.	A slow, continuous rate of infusion is better tolerated and reduces the likelihood of diarrhea. Promotes safety and accuracy of infusion.
9. **Intermittent feeding:**	
a. Monitor the feeding.	
b. When the infusion is finished, flush the feeding tube with 50 ml of water.	Helps to prevent clogging of the tube and decreases the risk of bacterial growth.
c. Pinch the tube while disconnecting it from the administration set. Then insert a catheter plug or bend the end of the tube onto itself, cover it with gauze, and secure the gauze with an elastic band.	Prevents air from entering the stomach and gastric contents from draining out.
d. Flush the bag and tubing with warm water. Hang it upside down to drain and dry. Store it for reuse. Replace the set every 24 hours.	Removes residual formula, thereby reducing the risk of bacterial growth.
10. Leave the patient comfortable. Ask him or her to stay in a sitting position for at least 30 minutes, if able.	Facilitates gastric emptying.
11. **Continuous feeding:**	
a. Monitor the patient and the feeding every one to two hours. Check the flow rate and assess for diarrhea, abdominal distention, nausea, and cramping. Precise rates of flow are crucial for tolerance of the formula.	Indicates the patient's tolerance of the feeding. The rate of infusion is generally set to lessen complications such as diarrhea and abdominal cramping. An antidiarrheal, like diphenoxylate (Lomotil), may also be ordered to control diarrhea.
b. Interrupt the feeding q.4h. or as ordered to:	
1) Flush the feeding tube with at least 50 ml water.	Prevents clogging of the tubes.
2) Add formula to the container. Rinse the set with warm water before adding new formula.	Prevents buildup of residue which may invite bacterial growth.
3) Administer supplemental water if ordered.	Patient may require water to prevent dehydration.
4) Replace the feeding set every 24 hours.	
12. Document the feedings. Note the frequency, type, amount, and rate of infusion. Include patient responses and associated assessments. Enter volume of feedings and water delivered into the Fluid Balance Record.	Fulfills requirement for nurse accountability and promotes continuity of care.

PROCEDURE 19.4

Administering Gastrostomy or Jejunostomy Tube Feedings

ACTION	RATIONALE
1. Follow steps 1 to 6 of Procedure 19.3.	
2. Flush the tube with 25 to 30 ml of water.	Establishes patency of the tube.
3. Administer the feeding as in Procedure 19.3, steps 8 to 11.	
4. Provide care to the gastrostomy or jejunostomy site according to the physician's order or agency protocol. Use principles of wound care outlined in Chapter 32.	Leakage of gastric and jejunal contents can cause irritation and skin breakdown.
5. Document as in Procedure 19.3.	

PROCEDURE 19.5

Removing a Nasogastric Tube

ACTION	RATIONALE
1. Check the physician's order to remove the tube.	Ensures accuracy and reduces the risk of error.
2. Prepare the patient: a) Some irritation of the nose and throat may occur and the eyes may water as the tube is removed. b) Breathing out as the tube is removed will reduce irritation and ease removal.	Promotes well-being and enables patient participation in the procedure.
3. Gather: • Water-proof pad • Clean gloves • Moisture-proof bag • Tissues	Facilitates efficiency and economy of time.
4. Help the patient into a sitting position if able. Place the pad over the patient's chest. Give the patient some tissues.	Protects patient's gown from secretions and drainage in tube.
5. Disconnect the tube from the suction device or feeding pump, detach the tubing from the patient's gown, and remove the tape anchoring the tube. Apply clean gloves.	Prepares tube for removal. Protects the nurse from contact with patient's secretions.
6. Instruct the patient to take a deep breath and blow out. Pinch the tube and withdraw it smoothly and rapidly as the patient exhales.	Creates a distraction for the patient and relaxes the pharynx which eases removal, decreases irritation, and prevents aspiration.
7. Wrap the tube in the water-proof pad, remove gloves and place into moisture-proof bag.	Maintains cleanliness and prevents transfer of microorganisms to environment.

Continued on the next page

ACTION	RATIONALE
8. Provide mouth care and hygiene as needed (see Chapter 30).	Promotes patient comfort.
9. Provide fluids as ordered. Instruct the patient to sip fluids at first and gradually increase intake.	Rapid, large intake of fluid may cause nausea and vomiting, especially if the patient was on NPO and gastric suction.
10. Measure drainage in collecting container if gastric suction was used. Dispose of equipment and discard supplies according to agency policy. Wash hands.	Maintains cleanliness and safety in the workplace.
11. Document the procedure and the patient's response. Record the amount of drainage in suction container in the Fluid Balance Record.	Fulfills legal requirements for nurse accountability and promotes continuity of care.

TOTAL PARENTERAL NUTRITION

When the body is seriously depleted of nutrients, when the rate of metabolism places excessive demands on the body's resources or when the body is unable to absorb nutrients through its digestive tract, a person's nutritional status can be improved and maintained over extended periods solely through intravenous feeding. This method of providing nutrients directly into the bloodstream is called total parenteral nutrition (TPN).

Indications for TPN therapy   There are three basic indications for use of TPN:

1) Availability of the digestive tract. If the gastrointestinal tract has been rendered totally unavailable for use, an alternative method of nutrition is an obvious necessity. This may include, for example, conditions in which feeding by means of the gastrointestinal tract is impossible, hazardous or inadequate (as for major abdominal injury, obstruction, fistulae, malignant disease, coma) or conditions in which the bowel must rest (such as pancreatitis or inflammatory bowel disease).

2) Malnutrition. In the presence of malnutrition, the chances of successful medical intervention are greatly diminished. Patients with conditions such as severe anorexia nervosa, chronic vomiting or diarrhea, or malabsorption states, and with poor pre- or postoperative nutritional status benefit from the nutrient support provided by TPN.

3) The degree of hypermetabolism or catabolism. In the presence of severe illness, the increased nutritional requirements can place extensive demands on the body's reserves as, for instance, in people with sepsis or burns,

those with extensive trauma or surgery, and those with malignant diseases requiring radiation and/or chemotherapy (Williams, 1989).

The goal of TPN   In a healthy individual, the function of protein is to support the growth and maintenance of body tissues. Adequate protein function is reflected as a state of nitrogen equilibrium. In illness, protein breakdown (catabolism) can exceed protein synthesis (anabolism) and is reflected as a negative nitrogen balance (more nitrogen loss than intake). The goal of TPN is to maintain a state of positive nitrogen balance in an effort to counter catabolic deterioration.

Nutritional Assessment

Prior to the initiation of TPN, it is important to gather a broad assessment of the individual's nutritional and metabolic status to provide a baseline by which to measure progress. Then, at regular intervals throughout TPN therapy, certain tests are repeated to measure the patient's response to therapy. These assessments are presented in the box below.

Administering Parenteral Nutrition

The administration of parenteral nutrition can be approached in two ways: peripheral parenteral nutrition (PPN) and total parenteral nutrition (TPN). The advantages of peripheral parenteral nutrition are the ease of access to the peripheral veins and the much lower rate of infection and catheter-related complications. However, PPN is also subject to complications. For instance, phlebitis and thrombus occur with the administration of hyperosmolar solutions (those containing increased concentration of particles per kilogram of solution) into peripheral veins owing to the slower flow rates within these vessels. As well, peripheral vein access is prone to problems of infiltration. PPN is therefore limited to short-term administration as a supplement (amino acid solutions and lipid emulsions) for patients who are able to consume some oral nutrients or as a means of providing total parenteral nutrition on a very short-term basis (amino acid solutions, lipid emulsions and 10 percent dextrose solutions).

Long-term administration of TPN therapy requires a large central vein such as the subclavian vein. TPN solutions commonly contain 25 percent to 35 percent dextrose in

Assessment of an Individual during TPN Therapy

1. **Dietary adequacy**: Dietary adequacy is determined by comparing the person's caloric intake (diet history) with the estimated caloric expenditure. Basal energy expenditure (BEE) is calculated (by the physician or dietitian) using the parameters of weight, height and age.

2. **Protein status**: To establish the body's need for protein intake, an assessment of the individual's nitrogen balance is essential. Nitrogen balance is determined from 24-hour urine specimen. Protein status is also determined on measurements of lean body mass, body fat stores, skeletal muscle mass, and immune function.

3. **Possible sources of infection**: The high concentrations of dextrose solutions used in TPN and the person's compromised immune status pose a serious risk for infection. Any existing infection must be cultured and treated prior to initiation of therapy. Patients must be monitored carefully throughout therapy for signs of infection.

4. **Liver function**: Laboratory tests include total protein, albumin, AST (aspartate amino transferase), alkaline phosphatase, LDH (lactic acid dehydrogenase).

5. **Kidney function**: Laboratory tests include BUN (blood urea nitrogen), serum creatinine and 24-hour urine collection for Na, K, and Urea.

6. **Biochemistry evaluation**: Studies include electrolytes and fasting glucose.

7. **Hematology evaluation**: Studies include CBC and differential.

SOURCE: Hunt, P. (1988). *Total parenteral nutrition: A learning package*. Vancouver, B.C.: University Hospital, Shaughnessy Site.

addition to amino acids, vitamins, minerals, trace elements, and electrolytes. The brisk blood flow through the large central veins allows for rapid dilution of these hypertonic solutions. While the administration of TPN via central lines provides the secure access essential for long-term therapy, it is not without complications (in Chapter 22 we discuss the care for patients with central venous lines). The nurse needs to be aware of potential complications arising from the infusion of the TPN solution, primarily sepsis and metabolic disturbances, namely hyperglycemia (the most common), rebound hypoglycemia, osmotic diuresis, fluid excess or deficit and electrolyte imbalances. A plan of care that focusses on monitoring for complications and implementing health protecting strategies is critical in TPN therapy. As with all care, the plan should be made in collaboration with the patient. The nurse should assess the patient's learning needs and provide instruction and information accordingly. Patients should be advised, when possible, to watch for potential complications with their therapy and to notify the nursing personnel as necessary.

Sepsis   The individual receiving TPN therapy is in an already compromised state and his or her ability to fight infection is limited. The amino acid-dextrose solution is a potential growth medium for yeast organisms, and bacteria thrive in lipid solutions. The nurse needs to be aware of signs and symptoms that would indicate the presence of any superimposed infection. The nurse should monitor for local (erythema, tenderness and drainage at insertion site) and systemic (sudden glycosuria in a previously glucose tolerant patient as the body mobilizes extra glucose to fight the infection, fever, chills, nausea and vomiting and hypotension) signs of infection. Other nursing interventions should include monitoring vital signs, daily assessment of capillary blood glucose levels and of urine for ketones. If drainage were present at the site of insertion, a swab would be taken for culture and sensitivity.

Hyperglycemia   Monitor the patient for signs and symptoms such as glycosuria, polyuria, increased thirst, weakness, nausea and vomiting, flushed skin, acetone breath and abdominal pain. The TPN solution should be initiated gradually to allow the patient time to adapt to the increased glucose concentration. Use of an infusion pump will ensure the infusion at the prescribed rate (+ or – 10 percent, DO NOT play "catch up"). Insulin may be administered or added to the solution for individuals with persistent hyperglycemia. The patient is also monitored for signs of fluid volume deficit.

Hypoglycemia   TPN therapy should be discontinued gradually in order to prevent hypoglycemia. If concentrated dextrose solutions are discontinued suddenly, an imbalance between pancreatic insulin production and available glucose will occur, resulting in hypoglycemia. The patient is monitored for diaphoresis, tachycardia, confusion, tremors, anxiety and altered levels of consciousness. If any of these symptoms are present, an infusion of 10 percent dextrose (as per doctor's order) is given to maintain glucose levels.

Osmotic diuresis Hyperglycemia increases serum osmolarity, which causes fluid to shift from the intracellular compartment into the plasma, where it is subsequently lost in the urine. A sudden increase in urinary output and signs of dehydration (dry mucous membranes, reduced skin turgor) may indicate osmotic diuresis. Nursing interventions include notifying the physician and infusing additional fluids and electrolytes as prescribed.

Fluid excess Fluid excess results from an infusion that is too rapid or from electrolyte imbalances. The patient is monitored for edema (facial, sacral or peripheral), rapid weight gain and pulmonary edema. Daily weights are taken and intake and output levels are maintained to monitor for fluid excess. The use of an infusion pump for administering solutions should help to prevent this complication. If fluid excess occurs, the rate of infusion is decreased as ordered by the physician.

Fluid deficit An inadequate rate of infusion, hyperglycemia, electrolyte imbalance, diarrhea and loss from other sites (for example, fistula) result in fluid deficit. The patient is monitored for signs of dehydration and imbalances between intake and output. Nursing interventions include increasing the rate of the infusion or changing the composition of the infusion as per the doctor's order.

Electrolyte imbalance The composition of the TPN solution is based on each patient's individual requirements. Throughout the course of therapy, alterations may need to be made to adjust to changes in the patient's response to therapy. The nurse should monitor the patient for signs of hypokalemia (such as lethargy, muscle cramps, nausea and vomiting, arrythmias, glycosuria), hypocalcemia (abdominal muscle cramps, tetany, tingling of fingers and toes, circumoral tingling, positive Chvostek's and Trousseau's signs and convulsions) and hypophosphatemia (progressive weakness of muscles in extremities, pain in long bones). Nurses should be aware of the need for blood work to be done daily or several times weekly. They should monitor the results and notify the physician of any abnormalities.

EVALUATING NUTRITIONAL INTERVENTIONS

The patient goals, or expected outcomes, provide directions for nursing care. An example of a patient goal for a man who is reluctant to eat might be "eats all of his meals each day." Evaluation of the goals depends on the outcome criteria set by the nurse and the patient cooperatively. These should be specifically stated. Some questions for the nurse to keep in mind when evaluating nutritional interventions are:

1. Is the individual eating meals? Has he or she adopted better eating habits, including an adequate, nutritious diet?
2. If on a special diet, is the person adhering to it? If in hospital, does the person select foods that are compatible with his or her prescribed diet from the diet menu?
3. Have the symptoms of digestive disorders been alleviated? That is, has vomiting stopped? Is nausea less troublesome? Is the patient beginning to regain appetite? Is the patient free from indigestion?
4. Is the patient comfortable?
5. Is the patient able to retain fluids for gradually extended periods of time?
6. Is the patient able to take and retain adequate food and fluids for his or her nutritional needs?
7. Do results of laboratory tests reflect adequate nutrition?

The nurse also observes the patient to assess nutritional status and the progress made towards achieving the goals. Comparison of the nurse's observations of the patient with the characteristics of good nutrition and poor nutrition (see Table 19.9) are helpful in this regard.

KEY TERMS

nutrient p. 465
digestion p. 465
peristalsis p. 465
hydrolysis p. 465
mucosal folds p. 466
villi p. 466

metabolism p. 466
catabolism p. 466
anabolism p. 466
carbohydrates p. 466
fats p. 467
triglycerides p. 468

saturated p. 468
unsaturated p. 468
cholesterol p. 469
proteins p. 469
amino acids p. 469
complete proteins p. 469

IN REVIEW

Food is vital to all aspects of health. Physiologically, the body needs a constant supply of nutrients to sustain life. Food provides the fuel for human metabolism; for growth, maintenance and repair of tissues; for the synthesis of enzymes and hormones; and for regulating all body processes. Food also plays a significant role in psychological, social, cultural and spiritual health and well-being. It is used to promote feelings of security and comfort, for social acceptance and prestige value, for traditional customs and religious ceremonies, and to promote family solidarity and relaxation.

Nutrients are ingested, digested and absorbed into the blood stream for delivery to the cells. Metabolism refers to all physical and chemical changes that nutrients undergo after being absorbed from the gastrointestinal tract and their use by body cells. Nutrients may be oxidized for energy (catabolism) or they may be used in the synthesis of hormones, enzymes and proteins needed by the body (anabolism).

The essential nutrients are carbohydrates, fats, proteins, vitamins, minerals and water. Carbohydrates are starches and sugars used primarily for energy. They vary in complexity from simple sugars to complex carbohydrates and fibre. Dietary carbohydrates, except for fibre, are converted to glucose, the major sugar found in the bloodstream. Glucose may be metabolized directly by tissues for energy, stored in the liver or muscles as glycogen, converted into fat and stored in adipose tissue or excreted in urine.

Fats are compounds that are insoluble in water. They function as a source of heat and energy, provide essential fatty acids, spare the burning of proteins for energy, promote the absorption of fat-soluble vitamins and insulate vital organs. They add flavour to food and enhance satiety by slowing digestive processes and retarding hunger.

Proteins are nutrients made up of amino acids. They provide the major source of building material for the maintenance and repair of tissues. They are necessary in the formation of hormones, enzymes, antibodies and blood proteins and in the regulation of water balance, nitrogen balance and nutrient transport. They may also be used for energy. Of the 22 amino acids needed by the body, nine must be supplied by food; these are the essential amino acids. The others are synthesized in the body; they are the nonessential amino acids. Complete proteins are foods that contain all of the essential amino acids. Animal sources are generally complete proteins. Plant sources must be eaten in proper combinations to provide a complete protein.

Vitamins are necessary constituents in the chemical processes involved in converting food to energy, building and repairing tissues and protecting cells. Minerals function in the building and maintenance of bones, teeth and various body systems. Water is essential for the transportation of all nutrients and is part of all body secretions and excretions.

The body uses energy for basal metabolism, physical activity and the thermic effect of food. Daily energy requirements vary greatly depending on lean body mass, body fat, age, sex and physical activity. Nutritional guidelines have been established for Canadians to provide advice in the selection of foods that will ensure an adequate supply of essential nutrients in their daily diets.

Nutritional needs vary considerably during the life cycle. Nutrient requirements increase during pregnancy and lactation. Infants' nutrient requirements change in accordance with growth and the maturation of their gastrointestinal and neuromuscular systems. Growth is rapid during the first year of life. It slows in the second year, as toddlers move to table foods and begin drinking from a cup. Physical and social skills related to eating develop rapidly during the toddler and preschool years. Good eating habits can be established during this time. Children need the same types of foods as adults but the quantities vary according to their growth and energy requirements. Adolescents' nutritional needs increase greatly as they undergo growth spurts. Needs for calories and protein usually decline as people reach full adulthood. As the years pass, there is a gradual slowing down of activity and the need for calories decreases. At the same time, however, intake usually does not drop, and people may put on weight. The nutritional problems of older adults often stem from inadequate intake. Factors such as insufficient funds, lack of information, physical inability to shop and prepare food, as well as feelings of loneliness or depression, and physical changes such as loss of appetite, may contribute to inadequate intake in older adults.

A person's nutritional status reflects the balance between the body's requirements for nutrients and energy and the intake of food. Many factors affect food intake including socioeconomic status, family composition, level of education, physical difficulties, emotional status, culture and religion, personal preferences and health problems.

Nutritional needs are affected by illness. Demands for proteins increase and, if patients are unable to tolerate food, the body's stored sources of energy are used up quickly.

A state of protein-calorie malnutrition rapidly ensues. Therapeutic diets, designed to suit the individual needs of patients, may be prescribed during illness.

Malnutrition, starvation, and obesity are the most common nutrition problems in the world. Malnutrition can be caused by an inadequate food supply and overpopulation in underdeveloped countries, or by inadequate intake from lack of knowledge, time, or money in developed countries. In industrialized nations many people experience inadequate nutrition, often in the form of obesity. Malnutrition and starvation can also occur in hospitalized patients because of inadequate food intake owing to periods of fasting for tests and procedures or alterations in diet due to therapeutic regimens. Careful assessment of patients' nutritional status is important so that problems can be prevented or remedied.

In assessing nutritional status the nurse considers all of the factors that affect a person's nutrition. Assessments include the nursing health history, physical examination, anthropometric measurements, and laboratory tests.

Nursing diagnoses for patients with nutritional problems are generally stated as *Altered nutrition*. There are many causes of nutritional problems. Etiologies must be stated in specific terms so that the diagnoses are described clearly.

A plan of care must take all factors affecting the person's nutrition into account, for example, their socioeconomic status, cultural and religious practices, and personal preferences and lifestyle. The patient's (and family's) participation in setting goals is mandatory if successful outcomes are to be achieved. Goals and expected outcomes should be stated as short-term steps towards long-term achievement.

Nurses can assist patients to promote optimal nutrition by encouraging them to examine their dietary patterns and eating habits and by providing information and teaching about healthy eating and regular exercise. Failure to adhere to a special diet is often due to a lack of understanding of why the diet is important to health. Factors that must be considered in assisting patients to change dietary patterns are comfort foods, socioeconomic level, cultural, religious, and moral values, and who controls the purchase and cooking of food in the home.

When modifications can be made to the individual's existing food habits rather than complete change, success is more likely.

People who are ill may need help maintaining adequate nourishment. Health protecting strategies may include preventing or minimizing problems such as indigestion, anorexia, nausea, and vomiting, and providing safety, comfort, and hygiene measures. Nurses can also help protect individuals and families from food poisoning by providing information and instruction on preventive measures in the home.

Enteral feedings and total parenteral nutrition may be prescribed by the physician to restore hydration and nutritional health in persons unable to ingest or absorb nutrients through the digestive tract. In addition to administering the methods of feeding safely, the nurse monitors patients for potential complications and implements preventive and therapeutic measures accordingly.

LEARNING ACTIVITIES

1. Record all of the food and beverages you consume in a typical day (24-hour period). Compare your intake to *Canada's Food Guide for Healthy Eating*.

   a) What is healthy about your diet? What is not?

   b) What changes should you make to eat a more nutritious diet?

2. Select an ethnic or religious diet and identify the characteristics and main dishes. Examine the diet in terms of the four food groups.

   a) What are the diet's strengths?

   b) How could the diet be improved?

3. Janice, age 7 years, has iron-deficiency anemia. In an interview, her mother tells you that the family is vegetarian and that Janice has a very poor appetite.

   a) What questions are important in a nutritional assessment for Janice?

   b) Plan a strategy for counselling the mother about nutrition.

   c) What advice could you give the mother to help increase Janice's appetite?

4. You are a home care nurse assigned to a 71-year-old woman who speaks little English. She is in need of teaching to improve her eating habits. What are some of the things you could implement in an attempt to change her food habits?

5. Susan Jones, aged 20, works at a day-care centre and lives with five other people on a communal farm at the edge of town. Susan has not been feeling well for the past few days. She was admitted to hospital this morning suffering from severe abdominal pains, vomiting and bloody diarrhea. She looks thin and pale and she has a fever. Susan weighs 43.1 kg. She is 157 cm tall. Her wrist measurement is 15.24 cm. Laboratory test results show that her blood levels of hemoglobin, hematocrit, and serum protein are below normal. The physician establishes a medical diagnosis of regional enteritis (Crohn's Disease) and prescribes TPN.

   a) What are some of the factors contributing to Susan's nutritional problem?

   b) What assumptions might you make about actual or potential problems for Susan?

   c) What assessments would you make regarding Susan's nutritional status?

   d) What signs and symptoms of malnourishment might you observe in Susan?

   e) How much is she below the average weight for her height and body frame?

   f) What should be monitored while Susan is receiving TPN?

   g) What specific nursing interventions would you consider in Susan's care?

   h) How would you evaluate the effectiveness of these interventions?

REFERENCES AND READINGS

ASIAN DIET FACT SHEET: CULTURAL AND RELIGIOUS BACKGROUNDS. (1977). *Nursing Times, 73*, 108–110.

BERGER, K.J. and WILLIAMS, M.B. (1992). *Fundamentals of nursing: Collaborating for optimal health*. Norwalk, CT: Appleton & Lange.

BRITISH COLUMBIA DIETITIANS' AND NUTRITIONISTS' ASSOCIATION (BCDNA). (1992). *Manual of nutritional care* (4th ed.). Vancouver: Author.

CAMP, D. and OTTEN, N. (1990). How to insert and remove nasogastric tubes quickly and easily. *Nursing 90, 20*(10), 59–63.

CAMPBELL, C.C. and HORTON, S.E. (1991). Apparent nutrient intakes of Canadians: Continuing nutritional challenges for public health professionals. *Canadian Journal of Public Health, 82*, 374–380.

CARPENITO, L.J. (1993). *Nursing diagnosis: Application to clinical practice* (5th ed.). Philadelphia: Lippincott.

CHAPPELLE, M.L. (1972). The language of food. *American Journal of Nursing, 72*, 1294–1295.

CHEZ, R.A. (1991). Advising pregnant women about nutrition. *Contemporary Obstetrics and Gynecology, 36*, 80.

DAVIS, J.R. and SHERER, K. (1994). *Applied nutrition and diet therapy for nurses*. Phildelphia: Saunders.

EARNEST, V.V. (1993). *Clinical skills in nursing practice* (2nd ed.). Philadelphia: Lippincott.

FLYNN, J.M. and HACKEL, R. (1990). *Technological foundations in nursing*. Norwalk, CT: Appleton & Lange.

GILLIS, D. (1981). Adapting foodstyle: Counselling tips. *Canadian Nurse, 77*(3), 19.

HEALTH AND WELFARE CANADA. (1988). Canadian guidelines for healthy weights. *Report of an expert group convened by Health Promotion Directorate, Health Services and Promotion Branch*. Ottawa: Author.

HEALTH AND WELFARE CANADA. (1992). *Canada's food guide to healthy eating*. Ottawa: Minister of Supply and Services. (Catalogue No. H39–252/1992E)

HEALTH AND WELFARE CANADA. (1989). *Nutrition recommendations... A call for action*. Ottawa: Minister of Supply and Services. (Catalogue No. H39–162/1990E)

HEALTH AND WELFARE CANADA. (1990). *Nutrition recommendations: The report of the Scientific Review Committee*. Ottawa: Minister of Supply and Services. (Catalogue No. H49–41/1990E)

HEALTH AND WELFARE CANADA. (1992). *Using the food guide*. Ottawa: Minister of Supply and Services. (Catalogue No. H39–253/1992E)

HEALTH AND WELFARE CANADA (Health Services and Promotion Branch). (1988). *Promoting healthy weights: A discussion paper*. Ottawa: Author.

HEALTH PROMOTION DIRECTORATE, HEALTH AND WELFARE CANADA AND CANADIAN PEDIATRIC SOCIETY. (1988). *Feeding babies*. Ottawa: Minister of Supply and Services.

HEWAT, R.J. (1987). Nutritional assessment and infant feeding. In E.R. Knor (Ed.). *Decision making in obstetrical nursing*. Toronto: B.C. Decker.

HUNT, P. (1988). *Total parenteral nutrition: A learning package*. Vancouver, B.C.: University Hospital, Shaughnessy Site.

KATCH, F.I. and MCARDLE, W.D. (1988). *Nutrition, weight control and exercise* (3rd ed.). Philadelphia: Lea and Febiger.

KEITHLEY, J. (1979). Proper nutritional assessment can prevent hospital malnutrition. *Nursing '79, 9*(2), 68–72.

KENNER, C.A. and MACLAREN, A. (1993). *Essentials of maternal and neonatal nursing*. Springhouse, PA: Springhouse.

KINNEY, J.M., JEEJEEBHOY, K.N., HILL, G.L. and OWEN, O.E. (1988). *Nutrition and metabolism in patient care*. Philadelphia: Saunders.

LAQUATRA, I. and GERLACH, M.J. (1990). *Nutrition in clinical nursing*. New York: Delmar.

METHENEY, N. (1988). Measures to test placement of nasogastric and nasointestinal feeding tubes: A review. *Nursing Research, 37*, 324–329.

METHENEY, N., EISENBERG, P. and MCSWEENEY, M. (1988). Effect of feeding tube properties and three irrigants on clogging rates. *Nursing Research, 37*, 165–169.

METHENEY, N., MCSWEENEY M., WEHRLE M.A. and WIERSEMA, L. (1990). Effectiveness of the auscultatory method in predicting feeding tube location. *Nursing Research, 39*, 262–267.

METHENEY, N. SPIES, N.A. and EISENBERG, P. (1988). Measures to test placement of nasoenteral feeding tubes. *Western Journal of Nursing Research, 10*(4), 367–383.

METHENEY, N, WILLIAMS, P., WIERSEMA, L., WEHRLE, M.A., EISENBERG, P. AND MCSWEENEY, M. (1989). Effectiveness of pH measurements in predicting feeding tube placement. *Nursing Research, 38*, 280–285.

OVERFIELD, T. (1977). Biological variation concepts from physical anthropology. *Nursing Clinics of North America, 12*(3), 19–26.

PETROSINO, B.M., CHRISTIAN B.J. and BECKER, H. (1989). Implications of selected problems with nasoenteral tube feedings. *Critical Care Nursing Quarterly, 12*(3), 1.

PILLITTERI, A. (1992). *Maternal and child health nursing: Care of the childbearing and childrearing family*. Philadelphia: Lippincott.

POLEMAN, C.M., and PECKENPAUGH N.J. (1991). *Nutrition: Essentials and diet therapy* (6th ed.). Philadelphia: Saunders.

SELECTED NUTRITION TEACHING AIDS. (1976). Ottawa: Department of National Health and Welfare.

SHOLLENBERGER, D. (1993). Physical treatments. In Springhouse. *Nursing procedures: Student version*. Springhouse, PA: Springhouse.

SHUBIN, S. (1980). Nursing patients from other cultures. *Nursing 80, 10*(6), 78–81.

SPECK, P. (1976). East Comes West. *Nursing Times, 72*, 662–664.

WARDLAW, G.M., INSEL, P.M. and SEYLER, M.F. (1992). *Contemporary nutrition: Issues and insights*. St. Louis: Mosby.

WHITNEY, E.N., CATALDO, C.B. and ROLFES, S.R. (1991). *Understanding normal and clinical nutrition*. St. Paul, MN: West Publishing.

WILLIAMS, E.J. (1980). Food for thought: Meeting the nutritional needs of the elderly. *Nursing 80, 10*(9), 60–63.

WILLIAMS, M.W. (1993). *Lifetime: Fitness and wellness* (3rd ed.). Madison, WI: Brown and Benchmark.

WILLIAMS, S.R. (1989). *Nutrition and diet therapy* (6th ed.). St. Louis: Mosby.

CHAPTER 20

Urinary Elimination Needs

CENTRAL QUESTIONS

1. In what way is adequate urinary elimination important to the health and well-being of the individual?

2. What are the structures and functions involved in urinary elimination?

3. How does normal urinary functioning vary throughout the life cycle?

4. What are the main determinants of urinary functioning?

5. What are some common urinary elimination problems?

6. What basic principles would the nurse apply when assisting individuals to meet their urinary elimination needs?

7. How does the nurse assess an individual's urinary elimination status?

8. What are the common nursing diagnostic statements for individuals with urinary elimination problems?

9. How would the nurse develop a plan of care for individuals with urinary elimination problems?

10. What strategies might the nurse implement in helping individuals, families or groups to promote optimal urinary functioning and prevent potential urinary problems?

11. What health restoring and supportive strategies might the nurse implement when caring for individuals with urinary elimination problems?

12. How would the nurse evaluate the individual's response to nursing interventions?

INTRODUCTION

In order to maintain healthy functioning, the body must rid itself of wastes. There are four principal mechanisms for the removal of wastes: from the urinary tract as urine, from the gastrointestinal tract as feces, through the skin as perspiration and through the lungs as expired air. Each mechanism has its specific function in clearing the body of wastes that result from the processing of nutrients and their subsequent utilization in the cells.

The focus of this chapter is on urinary elimination. Urinary elimination primarily functions in removing nitrogenous waste products of cellular metabolism and in regulating fluid and electrolyte balance. Both of these functions are essential to the maintenance of chemical homeostasis of the blood. When urinary elimination is impaired all body systems may be affected and the individual may become very ill.

In addition, the act of voiding is an important area of independent functioning for an individual. Control over voiding is learned early in childhood and actual or potential loss of independence in this vital function constitutes a serious threat to an individual's social and emotional well-being. Such a loss can lead to fear of a return to the dependent state of infancy, as well as feelings of reduced self-esteem. This chapter provides the basis for understanding urinary elimination, common urinary elimination problems and the management of these common problems. The assessment of urinary elimination and measures by which nurses can help individuals to promote optimal urinary elimination or to maintain or restore their usual patterns of functioning when urinary dysfunction has occurred are also outlined.

ANATOMY AND PHYSIOLOGY OF URINARY ELIMINATION

Normally, the urinary tract consists of two kidneys, two ureters, a bladder and a urethra (see Figure 20.1). The elimination of urine from the body depends on effective functioning of these structures.

Kidneys   The kidneys are situated in the back of the abdominal cavity, behind the peritoneum and just below the diaphragm, one on either side of the spinal column. They are attached to the dorsal wall by connective tissue and an extensive cushion of fat. The kidneys primarily function to control the composition and volume of body fluids, including blood; and to excrete excess fluids, electrolytes, nitrogenous wastes, as well as toxic substances and drugs. These functions are accomplished through the complex processes of filtration, selective reabsorption and secretion

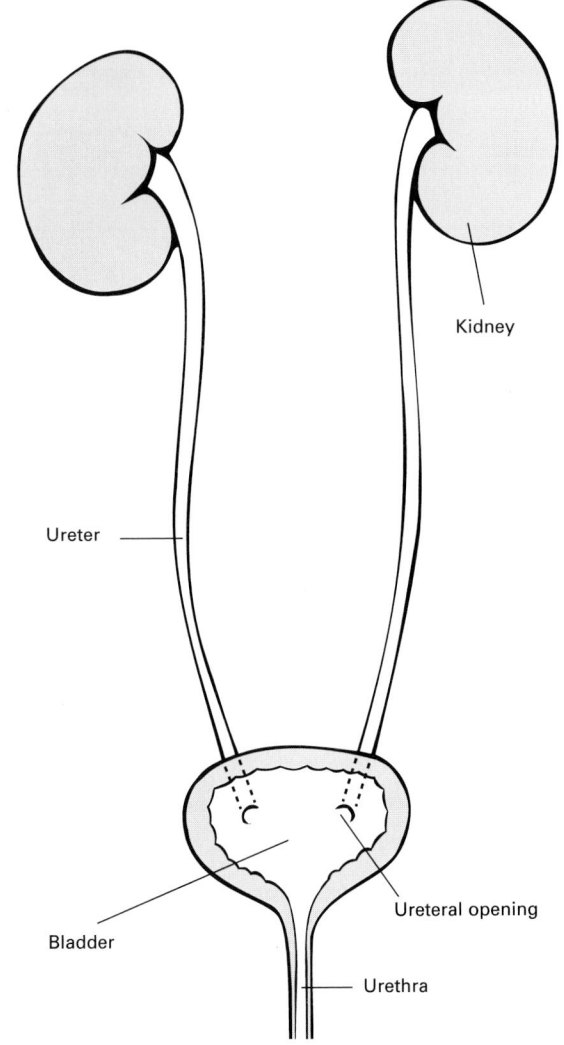

FIGURE 20.1   The urinary system

in which essential elements needed by the body are retained and waste products are removed in the form of urine.

The functional unit of the kidney is the **nephron** (see Figure 20.2). Each kidney contains about one million nephrons. Urine is formed in the nephrons through the processes of filtration, reabsorption and secretion. A single nephron consists of the glomerulus (a cluster of capillaries) which filters fluid from the blood and a renal tubule in which the glomerular filtrate is transformed into urine. The renal tubule begins as a sac (Bowman's capsule) which encases the capillary cluster. It winds through the kidney tissue and opens into a collecting tubule. Each collecting tubule joins other collecting tubules at a collecting duct. The collecting duct carries urine to the pelvis of each kidney.

Blood is brought to the kidneys by way of the renal arteries. About 20 to 25 percent of the resting cardiac

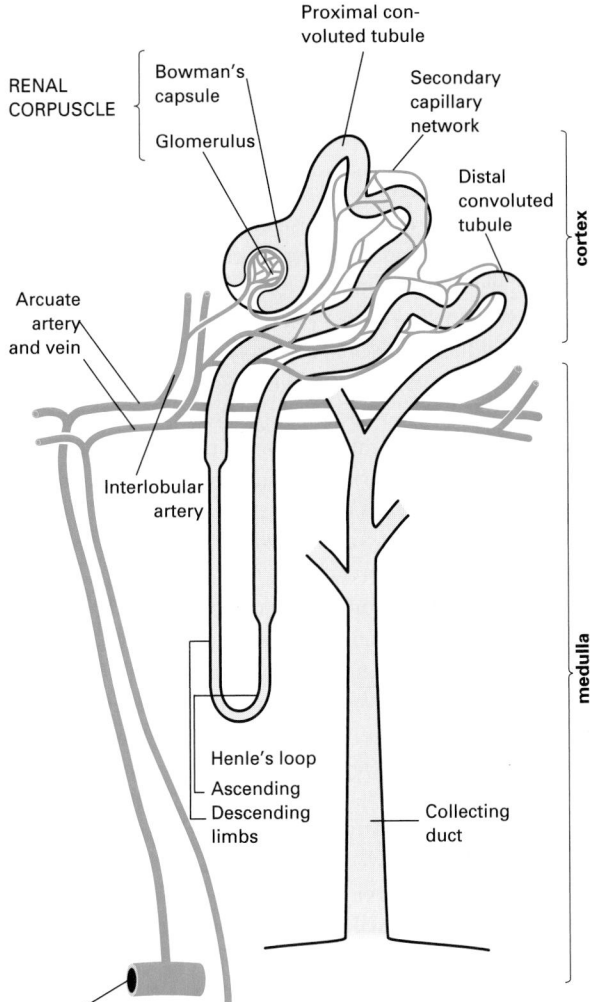

FIGURE 20.2 Cross-section of the kidney, illustrating a nephron

output (approximately 1200 ml per minute) passes through the kidneys. As the blood circulates through the kidneys, water-soluble waste products and excess water are filtered into the renal tubules. The nephrons process this filtrate by reabsorbing the essential constituents back into the blood stream, ignoring the unwanted constituents, and secreting other constituents (hydrogen ions, potassium ions, ammonia) to the filtrate. Waste products are concentrated in the tubule, converting the filtrate into urine.

Ureters   Urine produced in the nephron empties into the pelvis of the kidney. From the kidney, urine is transported at a rate of one to five ml per minute by means of peristalsis along long muscular tubes called the **ureters** to the urinary bladder. The ureters enter the bladder at an oblique angle and the entrances are covered by a fold of mucous

membrane, so that urine is not forced back up the ureters when pressure exists within the bladder.

Bladder   The **urinary bladder** is a distensible muscular sac which lies on the pelvic floor behind the symphysis pubis. The bladder wall contains three layers of smooth muscle and a special mucosal lining (transitional epithelium) which allow the bladder to collapse when empty and then expand as it fills with urine. Normally, the bladder holds about 200 to 500 ml of urine but it is capable of holding more than double that amount. The smooth muscle layers form the *detrusor muscle* of the bladder. Contraction of this muscle compresses the bladder and expels urine into the urethra. At the base of the bladder, where it joins the urethra, smooth muscle fibres form the involuntary *internal sphincter* which controls the release of urine from the bladder. The bladder wall contains sensory receptors which respond to distention from the accumulation of urine and relay information to the central nervous system, activating the mechanism for urination. The bladder is innervated by the autonomic nervous system. Sympathetic impulses cause relaxation of the detrusor muscle and contraction of the internal sphincter, thus inhibiting urination. Parasympathetic impulses, on the other hand, cause contraction of the detrusor muscle and relaxation of the internal sphincter, which activate urination.

Urethra   The **urethra** is a short, muscular tube which carries the urine from the bladder to its exit point from the body. The female urethra is approximately three to five cm long and opens just above the vagina. The urethra of the male serves both the urinary and reproductive systems. It is about 20 cm long from its origin in the bladder to its external opening in the glans penis. Three distinct regions can be identified in the male urethra: the prostatic urethra, the membranous urethra (where the external sphincter is located) and the penile urethra. In both males and females, the urethra contains a circular band of skeletal muscle which forms the *external sphincter*. This sphincter is under voluntary control; thus the individual is able to exert control over the act of voiding. **Meatus** is the term used for the external opening of the urethra in both men and women.

The entire urinary tract is lined with a continuous layer of mucous membrane that stretches from the meatus to the pelvis of the kidney. The mucous membrane of the bladder has a phagocytic ability which, combined with the unidirectional flow of urine, guards against ascending infections of the urinary tract (Lewis and Collier, 1992).

Micturition   **Micturition** refers to the act of emptying the bladder. Two terms more frequently used for this act are *voiding* and *urination*. When a sufficient amount of urine accumulates in the bladder (200 to 300 ml for most people), stretch receptors are stimulated. These receptors relay information via the pelvic nerve to the micturition reflex centre in the sacral (S1, S2, S3) region of the spinal cord and to the voluntary control centre in the cerebral cortex. The pelvic nerves also carry parasympathetic motor impulses to the detrusor muscle in the bladder wall and to the internal sphincter.

At the same time that the sensation of the need to void is perceived in the brain, impulses sent to the spinal cord activate the micturition reflex. This reflex produces parasympathetic stimulation which causes contraction of the detrusor muscle and relaxation of the internal sphincter. If the person responds by voluntarily relaxing the external sphincter, micturition will ensue. If the individual does not cooperate voluntarily, the internal sphincter will remain closed and the bladder wall will gradually relax. As the bladder continues to fill, however, the micturition reflex returns with a more powerful urge to void. Voluntary control of micturition is a learned response which involves the development of an inhibitory mechanism within the cerebral cortex and the maturation of various portions of the spinal cord. Voluntary control of micturition is usually developed by three or four years of age.

URINARY FUNCTIONING IN HEALTH

The average adult usually excretes between 1000 and 1500 ml of urine in a 24-hour period. The total volume varies with the amount of fluid intake, as well as with the amount of fluids lost through other routes, such as perspiration, vomiting or diarrhea.

The number of times a person voids during the day and the amount eliminated each time is highly individual. It is dependent, among other things, upon such factors as early childhood training, habitual response to the urge to urinate, amount of fluids consumed and the capacity of the individual's bladder. Most individuals void first thing in the morning, possibly four to six times throughout the day, and again before retiring. Due to hormonal influences, the volume of urine produced at night is usually less than half that produced during the day. Therefore, it is not usually necessary to void during the night, unless the individual has consumed a large amount of fluids prior to bedtime.

Normal urine is clear and straw-coloured or light amber in appearance. Darker coloured urine generally indicates increased concentration. Usually, the first urine voided in the morning is more concentrated than that excreted at other times of the day. Freshly voided urine is generally slightly acidic with a faintly aromatic odour. When urine is left standing, it develops a stronger odour, it becomes alkaline (owing to the disintegration of its constituents) and a cloudy sediment develops.

URINARY FUNCTIONING THROUGHOUT THE LIFE CYCLE

Infancy   Most newborns void within the first 24 hours of life. The first voiding is usually cloudy and may be pink in colour due to uric acid crystals and mucus. Babies who do not void within this time are examined for problems such as obstruction in the urinary tract, urethral stenosis or absence of kidneys or ureters. Because their glomerular filtration rate is low, newborns have limited capacity to excrete excess solutes and regulate body fluid composition. The glomerular filtration rate reaches 30 percent of adult values within the first two days of extrauterine life and gradually attains full adult value by the age of two years (Kenner and MacLaren, 1993). Urine is usually dilute and odourless and voiding may occur frequently. The frequency of voiding decreases gradually during infancy, although this is highly dependent on the amount of fluids consumed and on the surrounding temperature. The infant's body temperature is more readily affected by environmental temperatures than is an adult's and more fluids are needed for internal body processes when body temperature is high.

Childhood   By early childhood, the specific gravity and other urine findings are similar to those in adults. Children usually have to void more frequently than do adults, due to the smaller size of their bladders. The urge to void is usually more intensely felt in children, although in many instances it is ignored if they are busy, resulting in a race to the bathroom. The neurophysiological pathways necessary for voluntary control of the bladder mature later than do those for bowel control. Most children become physiologically ready for voluntary bladder control by the age of two to three years. In general, readiness can be assessed by children's ability to hold their urine for one to two hours, communicate their need to void, and hold their urine until seated on the toilet. As well, willingness to participate in the process must be considered. Children sometimes learn faster if they have a slightly older sibling whose activities they like to imitate. Night-time control is sometimes accomplished at the same time as the child learns to stay dry during the day. However, control at night occurs later in some children. Most children have achieved night-time control by the age of three to four years.

The school-aged child has generally mastered bladder control. It is not uncommon, however, for accidents to still occur, particularly if the child is under stress or gets too busy, particularly with outdoor activities, to get to a bathroom in time. As growth continues, the bladder also grows and its capacity increases. Urinary elimination usually settles into an adult pattern well before adolescence and, unless problems develop, the pattern continues through adulthood, with variations as noted below.

Pregnancy Pregnant women usually experience the need to void more often and with greater urgency, particularly during the early and late stages of pregnancy. There is a dilation of the urinary system, partly due to pressure on the bladder by the enlarging uterus, but there is also a relaxation of smooth muscle due to hormonal changes. This dilation may lead to stasis or slowing down of urine flow, with a resultant increased vulnerability to urinary tract infections.

Adulthood Many women in the middle years of adulthood experience difficulty in retaining urine within the bladder as the muscles of the pelvic floor, weakened by childbirth, begin to lose their tone. A small amount of urine may leak out of the bladder if a woman in this stage of life laughs heartily, coughs or sneezes. This is known as stress incontinence. Men also may experience some age-related changes in their urinary pattern. As the male ages, there is a likelihood that the **prostate gland** (located below the bladder neck, surrounding the urethra) will become enlarged resulting in such difficulties as increased frequency and nocturia (excessive urination at night). As both men and women age, they may experience a generalized loss of muscle tone, decreased bladder capacity, incomplete bladder emptying and increased residual urine. The lessened efficiency of the kidneys, coupled with a delayed sensation to void, contributes to the need to void more frequently and with increased feelings of urgency.

DETERMINANTS OF URINARY FUNCTIONING

A number of factors may affect the volume of urinary output and the pattern of voiding, as well as the characteristics of the urine excreted. These factors should be taken into consideration in the nurse's assessment of an individual's urinary elimination status.

Individual differences In addition to those changes in urinary function that occur throughout the life cycle, there are also inborn differences in anatomical structure and physiological functioning. Some individuals have a larger bladder capacity than others or a seemingly more efficient urinary system. They may not need to void as often as others. Early childhood training also plays its part in an individual's response to the urge to urinate. Since voiding is under voluntary control, however, individuals may alter their voiding patterns in response to situational factors such as the availability of toilet facilities, mealtimes, and the pressures of work.

Fluid and food intake One of the kidney's functions is to remove excess water from the body; therefore, both fluid intake and the amount of fluids lost through other routes will affect the volume and frequency of urinary output.

When large amounts of liquids are consumed, the kidneys will excrete more urine. Conversely, when fluid intake is decreased or the body is dehydrated, the kidneys will retain fluid, resulting in decreased amounts of concentrated urine.

Urine output is influenced by fluids and foods which contain alcohol and caffeine. Alcohol and caffeine inhibit the release of the antidiuretic hormone (ADH) which, in turn, inhibits the reabsorption of water from the renal tubules, causing a diuretic effect. Cola, cocoa, coffee and tea all have a diuretic effect on the kidney. Fruits and vegetables which have a high water content, for example, celery, may also increase urine output. Conversely, foods that are high in sodium, such as processed cheese and meats, may cause water reabsorption and decreased urine production. Certain foods may also affect the acidity of urine. For example, vegetarian diets may cause alkaline urine.

Psychological states Psychological factors such as stress, anxiety and pain may also cause urinary disturbances. Anxiety, for example, often stimulates the urge to void more frequently, strong fear may cause a person to void involuntarily and pain may inhibit voiding.

Disease and illness Urinary elimination patterns are often altered by disease and illness states and associated medical treatments. Infection is one of the most common causes of urinary disturbances. The urinary tract is lined with a continuous mucous membrane; therefore, an infection that begins in one part of the system can progress rapidly to all parts of the tract. It is not unusual for bacteria commonly found in the large intestine (for example, *Escherichia coli*) to be the cause of urinary tract infection. The proximity of the outlets of the gastrointestinal and urinary tracts contributes to this transfer.

In infants and children, urinary tract infections (UTIs) are treated vigorously to prevent possible spread to the kidneys. UTIs continue to be a problem in adolescence and young adulthood, especially in women. Frequency of occurrence is thought to increase with sexual activity. A bladder infection sometimes called "honeymoon cystitis" identified as an irritation of the urethral mucosa often occurs after initial sexual activity in girls. The shortness of the urethra and proximity of the meatus to the vagina and rectum in women makes them particularly prone to bladder infections.

Stasis of urine in the bladder, as a result of retention, is another factor predisposing people to infections, as well as to the formation of bladder stones. In hospitalized individuals, UTIs are most commonly associated with invasive diagnostic and therapeutic procedures of the urinary tract.

Obstructions may occur in almost any part of the urinary tract. Most commonly, they are seen in the pelvis of the kidney, in the ureter and, in the male, in the prostatic section of the urethra. Blockage of the urinary tract, whether by a malignancy, stones or stricture, hinders the excretion of urine.

Congenital structural anomalies may cause blockage of the urinary tract or give rise to other functional problems. Many congenital problems are discovered in infancy and early childhood and are surgically corrected at that time. Some anomalies, however, may go undetected until later in life or not at all. An individual with a solitary kidney, for example, may not discover this fact until an x-ray of the abdomen is taken during examination for reasons other than urinary tract dysfunction.

Generalized trauma to the body, such as hemorrhage, burns or shock, or systemic infection can also affect the kidneys. In severe dehydration, for example, there is a depletion in the amount of fluid within the body, which can severely disturb kidney function, to the point of failure.

Interference with or injury to the nervous supply of the bladder and urethra can interfere with normal urinary function. Drugs that depress the central nervous system can cause a loss of voluntary control over micturition as can damage to the spinal cord, the pathways that transmit impulses from the spinal cord to the brain, or to the brain itself.

COMMON PROBLEMS

Disturbances in urinary functioning may cause localized alterations in voiding patterns or generalized problems resulting from impairment of elimination of waste products from the body.

LOCALIZED PROBLEMS

Urinary incontinence   *Urinary incontinence*, or the inability to voluntarily control voiding, may result from infection, damage to the nerve supply of the bladder, lesions of the spinal cord or brain or cerebral clouding of the aged. Urinary incontinence sometimes occurs temporarily after an operation. *Stress incontinence*, the excretion of small amounts of urine involuntarily with exertions such as coughing or laughing, occurs in many middle-aged women.

The inability to control urination is often very demoralizing and individuals feel embarrassed when it happens. Incontinence may also result in irritation of the skin in the perineal area.

Dysuria   The term *dysuria* refers to difficult, painful voiding. It is generally associated with urinary tract infections as well as a number of other pathophysiological conditions, such as blockage, trauma or muscular abnormalities of the bladder or urethra. In men, hypertrophy of the prostate gland, which surrounds the urethra, is a common cause of dysuria. Dysuria may also be caused by the excretion of a more highly concentrated urine than normal.

Frequency   *Frequency*, or voiding more often than usual, may simply result from an increased intake of fluids. Anxiety can stimulate voiding and cause distressing frequency, at times with loss of control. However, frequency, particularly combined with urgency, is also commonly seen in individuals with infections of the urinary tract.

Urgency   The need to void in a hurry is known as *urgency*. Its most common cause is urinary tract infection although it may also be due to the same causes that produce frequency.

Nocturia   *Nocturia* is the need to get up during the night to void. While nocturia may simply be the result of drinking a large amount of fluids prior to bedtime, particularly those containing caffeine or alcohol, it may also be the symptom of urinary dysfunction. Nocturia should not be confused with *enuresis* (the involuntary loss of urine, or bedwetting), the causes of which can range from psychosomatic sources to actual physical impairment.

Polyuria   The passage of an increased amount of urine is called *polyuria* or *diuresis*. Excessive fluid intake, particularly fluids containing alcohol and caffeine, and disease states such as diabetes mellitus and diabetes insipidus are among the common causes. Polyuria can also be caused by the use of *diuretics*, drugs given to increase urine output in people who suffer from hypertension and fluid retention.

Urinary retention   *Urinary retention* refers to the inability to pass urine despite bladder distention. It is generally the result of an obstruction to the flow of urine. Anesthetics and certain drugs such as opiates and anticholinergics may also cause urinary retention. Occasionally an individual will void small amounts of urine which minimally relieves feelings of pressure within the bladder but does not empty the bladder completely. This "voiding with overflow" predisposes the individual to bladder infection (*cystitis*).

Oliguria and anuria   *Oliguria* is the term used for urine production that is less than 30 ml per hour. *Renal anuria* is the cessation of urine production and clinically means a urine output of less than 100 ml per day. It usually indicates serious kidney impairment and, if prolonged, toxic substances will build up within the body resulting in death. Kidney disease, heart failure, severe dehydration and shock may cause oliguria and anuria.

GENERALIZED PROBLEMS

The impairment of renal function can result in generalized problems affecting most systems of the body. A reduction in the ability of the kidney to excrete the nonprotein nitrogenous waste products of metabolism results in an accumulation of these wastes within the blood. This condition is called **uremia**. It may result from infection or trauma, for example, or from chronic renal disease.

The impairment in renal functioning has several effects on the body in addition to oliguria and anuria. Fluid retention results in the formation of edema (accumulation of fluid in the tissues) and possible development of hypertension. Retention of the acidic products of metabolism causes disturbance of the acid-base balance leading to development of metabolic acidosis. Potassium (normally excreted by the kidney) is retained, which may result in neuromuscular irritability and cardiac dysrhythmias. There are significant changes in blood chemistry. The blood urea nitrogen (BUN) and creatinine levels rise. The extent of the increase in blood levels of these substances provides an indication of the severity of the kidney impairment.

In an attempt to rid itself of wastes normally excreted in the urine, the body will use other channels, which lead to additional problems for the individual. Perspiration is increased and deposits of salts may accumulate on the skin (*urea frost*). The skin becomes pale and powdery, and the patient may have problems such as itching (*pruritus*). An offensive odour develops on the skin due to the urea deposits. When metabolic acidosis occurs, the lungs compensate through changes in respiration. Respirations become rapid and deep (*Kussmaul's respirations*) in an attempt to increase the excretion of carbon dioxide. Occasionally the individual's breath has the odour of urine.

URINARY DIVERSIONS

When the urinary bladder is removed because of trauma, disease or congenital anomalies, a new route for urinary elimination must be created. An artificial opening or **stoma** is made to divert urine from the kidneys to the abdominal wall. This opening is called a urinary ostomy or **urostomy**. There are a variety of urinary diversion procedures; however, the most common are the ileal conduit and the continent urostomy. The **ileal conduit** consists of a reservoir, constructed from a portion of the ileum, and a stoma (see Figure 20.3). The ureters are attached to the reservoir. Urine drains continuously from the ileal conduit; thus it is an *incontinent* diversion. The individual must wear an external collection bag or appliance to collect the urine.

The **continent urostomy** is a type of ileal conduit that functions similarly to a real bladder. In addition to the formation of an internal pouch, two nipple valves are constructed by intussuscepting sections of bowel. One valve (inlet valve) prevents urine from flowing back into the ureters, thus reducing the risk of ascending infection. The second valve (outlet valve) prevents urine from flowing out of the stoma, thus maintaining continence. Urine is stored in the pouch until it is emptied by means of a catheter passed through the stoma. An external collection appli-

ance is not necessary. Two common types of continent urostomies are the Kock's pouch and the Indiana pouch. In a Kock's pouch, both reservoir and stoma are created from ileum. In an Indiana pouch, the stoma is made from ileum and a larger reservoir is constructed from ileum, ascending colon, and cecum (see Figure 20.3).

Living with a urostomy is a life-long challenge. Individuals must deal with alterations in body image and learn to manage a stoma. Those with incontinent diversions have to care for an external appliance and those with continent diversions have to pass a catheter regularly to drain the internal pouch. Nurses in the community and in inpatient facilities may need to assist individuals with urinary diversions to meet their elimination needs.

ASSESSING URINARY ELIMINATION NEEDS

The assessment of an individual's urinary status involves the collection of data from all sources. The nursing health history and physical assessment provide the basis for planning individualized care. Information about the nature of the patient's health problem, past and current medical history, and the physician's diagnostic and therapeutic plans of care for the patient will be found in the medical record. Data from diagnostic tests or examinations such as blood work, urinalysis, x-rays, scans, biopsies or cystoscopy will add valuable information to the data base.

THE NURSING HEALTH HISTORY

In taking a nursing health history pertaining to urinary elimination the nurse questions patients (or a family member) about their usual patterns of voiding, their ability to toilet themselves, urinary control and any aids required in elimination (urinals, bedpans, commodes). The nurse asks about recent changes in patterns of elimination and the nature, onset and severity of symptoms. The presence of urinary diversions, and, if present, the patient's usual routines, are determined at this time. Factors which may influence the elimination pattern are also considered. This includes, for instance, the patient's age, usual food and fluid intake, and any disturbances currently being experienced with regard to sufficient intake of food and fluids to maintain optimal urinary functioning (such as nausea and vomiting).

In many cultures, the subject of elimination is surrounded by social taboos. Once toilet trained, children are taught that this is not a topic for general conversation. The act of urinary elimination, for the most part, takes place in private. Additionally, the intimate anatomical relationship between the urinary and the reproductive tracts contributes to making urinary functioning a sensitive topic. As a

A

B

FIGURE 20.3 A. Ileal conduit. B. Indiana pouch.

result, individuals often have difficulty in discussing urinary functions and any related problems. The nurse can set the patient at ease with a sensitive but matter-of-fact approach. A private, quiet area for discussion may minimize the individual's feelings of embarrassment. A guide for obtaining a urinary elimination health history follows.

PHYSICAL ASSESSMENT

The nurse uses physical assessment skills to obtain objective data. Observation of the characteristics of the patient's urine (colour, odour, consistency, amount and the presence of abnormal constituents) should be compared against normal values. Careful notation of the patient's fluid intake and output should be related to observations of the patient's voiding pattern and the characteristics of the urine.

Examination of the patient's abdomen may reveal kidney tenderness, bladder distention or the presence of a urinary ostomy. For this, the patient is placed in the dorsal recumbent position and draped appropriately. The nurse begins by inspecting the abdomen for skin colour, contour, symmetry and the presence of scars or urinary stomas. Light palpation or percussion over the costovertebral angle (area which lies

where the 12th rib joins the spine) or flank region may reveal kidney tenderness. Palpation just above the symphysis pubis is used to determine the presence of bladder distention. If the bladder is distended, the nurse will feel a firm roundness and the patient may express the desire to void when pressure is applied. As well, percussion with the fingers over this area will cause a dull sound when the bladder is full.

In addition, the nurse should be alert to manifestations of the localized and generalized problems in relation to urinary dysfunction as described in the preceding section. Assessment and recording of pertinent observations is a primary responsibility of the nurse in caring for patients with urinary tract dysfunction. The early detection of edema, changes in the pigmentation of the skin and signs of central nervous system or neuromuscular dysfunction can contribute significantly to the total plan of care for the patient.

MEASUREMENTS

Exact measurement of fluid intake and output is necessary in monitoring patients with urinary dysfunction. Detailed guidelines for measuring fluid intake and output will be found in Chapter 22. Measurements are recorded in milli-

Urinary Elimination

Health and Illness Patterns

USUAL PATTERN OF URINARY ELIMINATION

- How often do you urinate? How many times in a day?
- Describe the usual amount, colour and odour of your urine.
- Do you often awaken in the night to void? How many times a night?
- Do you have any difficulties with toileting? If so, describe them.
- What assistance will you require while in hospital? Assistance walking to the bathroom? Commode? Bedpan? Urinal?

For patients with urinary diversions:
- What type of urostomy do you have?
- What is your usual urostomy routine?
- Have you had any problems with your urostomy, e.g., skin irritation?
- What assistance will you need managing your urostomy?

For patients with long-term catheters:
- What is your usual catheter routine?
- Do you have any problems with your catheter?
- What assistance will you need managing your catheter?

RECENT CHANGES IN PATTERN OF URINARY ELIMINATION

- Have you noticed any change in your normal pattern of elimination or urine characteristics? If so, describe the changes.
- Have there been any recent changes in your life that may be affecting your normal pattern? Recent illness? Medication use? Surgery? Stressful events?

PRESENTING HEALTH PROBLEM

- Describe the symptoms you are experiencing now. Frequent small amounts of urine? Large amounts of urine? Urgency? Painful voiding? Bleeding? Dribbling of urine? Passing urine when you cough, sneeze or laugh? Trouble starting or maintaining a urinary stream?
- How long have you had these symptoms?
- What remedies have you tried, if any, for the symptoms? What were the results?
- Do you have a history of acute or chronic conditions that might disrupt urinary elimination? For example, heart disease, high blood pressure, diabetes, multiple sclerosis?
- Have you had urinary tract problems in the past? Infections? Kidney stones? Surgery to the urinary or reproductive tracts?
- Are you taking any medications (prescription and over-the-counter) that could affect urinary function, for example, diuretics, antihistamines, anticholinergics, antihypertensives? Dosage of medications?

Health Promotion and Protection Patterns

- How much and what type of fluid do you drink in a day?
- Do you drink alcohol and products containing caffeine? How much and how often?
- Do you smoke? If so, how much and for how many years?

litres and documented on a Fluid Balance Record on the patient's chart. In extreme cases, it may also be necessary to record the amount of fluid ingested as a part of the patient's food and the amount lost in perspiration and feces.

For accurate measurement of fluids, the nurse should drain larger collecting containers into a smaller, calibrated container. Placement of this smaller container on a flat surface and at eye level allows the nurse to accurately visualize the amount within the container. Care must be taken at all times when handling urine and other body fluids. Gloves must be worn and care taken to avoid splashing.

DIAGNOSTIC EXAMINATIONS

In order to diagnose and evaluate urinary function, patients may undergo a variety of tests and examinations. These include urine tests such as urinalysis, dipstick examination, and culture and sensitivity, as well as diagnostic procedures such as cystoscopy and x-ray examination.

URINE TESTS

Urinalysis   The routine **urinalysis** is probably the most common test available. For this examination, a sterile specimen of urine is not required. The patient is asked to void into a clean container, bedpan or urinal. A small amount of urine (five to ten ml is considered sufficient) is then transferred into a clean test tube, labelled and sent to the laboratory with its accompanying requisition. Normal urinalysis values are outlined in Table 20.1.

Dipstick examinations   In some cases, the nurse may be asked to perform a test on urine by means of a dipstick. This procedure provides a quick method of determining such aspects as pH, sugar, protein, ketones and the presence of blood in urine. Dipsticks or reagent strips are impregnated with chemicals which react with specific substances in the urine producing colour changes. Results are obtained by matching colour changes on the dipstick to colour charts usually on the container. A dipstick test is performed on a clean, fresh urine specimen. The tip of the reagent stick is placed into the specimen and after a period of specified time, the colour changes are compared to the colour chart. Table 20.1 gives the normal values for these tests.

Urine cultures   Normally urine is sterile; it does, however, provide an excellent growth medium for those bacteria which invade the urinary tract. Urine cultures are done to determine the presence of pathogenic organisms. Whenever possible, specimens for culture should be ob-

A dipstick is dipped in urine and then held against a colour chart to obtain test results.

tained from the first urine voided in the morning, as bacterial counts will be highest at that time. A clean voided midstream specimen of three to five ml is generally sufficient; however, specimens may also be collected by catheterization or from an indwelling catheter. Due to the risk of introducing bacteria into the urinary tract, collection of urine for culture by catheterization should be avoided if at all possible.

To obtain a midstream specimen from a male patient, it is necessary to cleanse the urinary meatus with an antiseptic solution. The patient next voids some urine (which is discarded), stops the stream, and then voids into a sterile container. Obtaining a midstream specimen from a female patient is somewhat more difficult. The labia and vestibule should be thoroughly cleansed with soap and water or antiseptic solution. If soap is used, it must be rinsed off thoroughly. Holding the labia apart, the patient then voids. The first part of the stream is discarded, the midstream specimen is caught in a sterile container, and the remainder of the urine discarded. The specimen should be sent to the laboratory for immediate processing; otherwise it must be stored at 4°C until processing is possible.

When possible, most patients prefer to do this procedure themselves. A thorough explanation of the procedure will ensure proper collection of the specimen. The nurse can assist in collecting the midstream specimen by positioning the patient on a bedpan or the bedside commode. In this instance, the nurse dons disposable gloves, cleanses the patient as above and collects the middle of the stream as the patient voids.

24-hour specimens   For some tests a *24-hour* sample of urine is required. The first urine voided in the morning is usually discarded and collection begins with the next voiding.

Common reagent dipsticks for urine testing.

TABLE 20.1   Normal Urinalysis Values

GENERAL CHARACTERISTICS AND MEASUREMENTS	CHEMICAL DETERMINATIONS	MICROSCOPIC EXAMINATION OF SEDIMENT
Colour: pale yellow to amber	Glucose: negative	Casts negative: occasional hyaline casts
Turbidity: clear to slightly hazy	Ketones: negative	Red blood cells: negative or rare
Specific gravity: 1.015-1.025 with a normal fluid intake	Blood: negative	Crystals: negative
pH: 4.5-8.0 average person has a pH of about 5 to 6	Protein: negative	White blood cells: negative or rare
	Bilirubin: negative	Epithelial cells: few
	Urobilinogen: 0.1-1.0	
	Nitrate for bacteria: negative	
	Leukocyte esterase: negative	

SOURCE: Fischbach, F. A. (1992). *Manual of laboratory and diagnostic tests* (4th ed.). Philadelphia: Lippincott, 148. Reproduced with permission.

All urine voided during the subsequent 24 hours is collected, including the first urine of the following morning. The urine is collected in one large container. Urine must be stored according to agency protocol for the test being performed. Occasionally, this requires that the urine be kept cool. This can be achieved by placing the collection container on ice in a large basin or tub in the patient's bathroom. With proper preparation, ambulatory patients are often responsible for collecting their own urine. If necessary, a sign may be posted above the patient's bed or in the bathroom as a reminder to staff, family and the patient that a 24-hour urine collection is in progress.

DIAGNOSTIC PROCEDURES

There are many examinations of the urinary tract which facilitate diagnosis of urinary tract dysfunction. A **cystoscopy** is the examination of a patient's bladder with a lighted instrument inserted through the urethra. The physician can visualize the interior of the bladder, obtain a biopsy specimen, and perform therapeutic treatments as well. This procedure is done under a local or general anesthetic in the operating room or day-care surgery department. The *intravenous* **pyelogram** (IVP) and *retrograde pyelogram* are radiological procedures which outline the pelvis, calices, ureters and urinary bladder by means of a contrast medium. As well, patients may undergo more definitive radiological testing such as ultrasonography and computerized tomography (CT) scanning. These procedures are described in Chapter 15.

The nurse is responsible for preparing the patient for any diagnostic procedure. This can involve physical preparation of the patient, such as evacuation of the bowels. It also involves the psychological preparation by thorough explanation of the procedure to be performed and admin-

istration of any pre-procedure medication. By doing so, patient anxiety is diminished and patient participation throughout the procedure is achieved.

DIAGNOSING URINARY ELIMINATION PROBLEMS

Urinary elimination problems that can be treated by independent nursing intervention may be generally stated as: *Altered pattern of urinary elimination.* According to Carpenito, this diagnostic statement is too broad for use in clinical practice and should be applied when the etiologic or contributing factors for incontinence have not been identified (1993). When the etiology of incontinence is known, the diagnostic statement should identify the specific nature of the problem. For example, in a woman who has recently had a baby and is now experiencing leakage of small amounts of urine whenever she sneezes, coughs or laughs, the nursing diagnosis would be: *Stress incontinence related to weakened pelvic floor muscles secondary to childbirth.* NANDA categorizes the types of incontinence as functional, reflex, stress, total and urge incontinence:

- *Functional incontinence:* The state in which an individual experiences a difficulty or inability to reach the toilet in time due to urgency, environmental barriers, decreased attention to the urge to void or physical limitations. Example: An elderly person who cannot get to the bathroom in time because of side rails on the bed and because the bathroom is too far away.

- *Reflex incontinence:* The state in which an individual experiences an involuntary loss of urine caused by damage to the spinal cord between the cortical and sacral

(S1, S2, S3) bladder centres. Example: A person with a spinal cord injury who has lost voluntary control of micturition.

- *Stress incontinence*: The state in which an individual experiences an immediate involuntary loss of urine upon an increase in intra-abdominal pressure. Example: As above.

- *Total incontinence*: The state in which an individual experiences continuous, unpredictable loss of urine. Example: A confused individual who is not aware of the urge to void.

- *Urge Incontinence*: The state in which an individual experiences an involuntary loss of urine associated with a strong sudden desire to void. Example: A person who experiences urgency with incontinence following a cystoscopy*

Urinary retention is a diagnostic label used to identify problems in which the individual experiences an inability to void, followed by involuntary voiding. Bladder distention will be present and the individual may dribble or void small frequent amounts, and may verbalize the feeling that the bladder is not empty after voiding. This problem occurs frequently following surgery due to the effect of anesthesia or surgical manipulation of tissues proximal to the bladder, as, for example, in prostate surgery. It may also result from drug therapy with antihistamines, such as cyclizine (used for motion sickness); adrenergics (sympathetic stimulants) such as epinephrine or isoproterenol; or anticholinergics (parasympathetic depressants), such as Atropine or propantheline.

Problems with urinary elimination often cause difficulties in other areas of functioning. For example, urinary incontinence may lead to impaired skin integrity. Urinary incontinence may also cause a disturbance in self-esteem. A perceived loss of independence and control over the act of micturition may be demoralizing to the individual and, in addition, may lead to ineffective individual coping capacity. Individuals with urinary ostomy diversions may experience a body image disturbance and will likely have a knowledge deficit in self-management of the urinary diversion ostomy. Following are examples of common nursing diagnoses pertaining to urinary elimination problems:

- *Altered pattern of urinary elimination related to unknown etiology as evidenced by incontinence.*

- *Functional incontinence related to avoidance of the urge to void and mobility deficit secondary to arthritis.*

- *High risk for urinary retention related to spinal anaesthesia and bladder trauma secondary to pelvic surgery.*

- *Low self-esteem related to incontinence.*

---

* Carpenito, 1993.

PLANNING URINARY ELIMINATION INTERVENTIONS

A plan of care for individuals with urinary elimination problems is based on the nursing diagnoses and takes into account each person's elimination patterns and toileting practices. Patient goals focus on understanding normal urinary elimination, maintaining or restoring normal urinary elimination patterns, preventing associated problems such as skin breakdown and infection and promoting healthy urinary functioning in daily living. Specific goals or expected outcomes are established for each nursing diagnosis. Some examples of expected outcomes include:

- The patient will explain the cause of incontinence and the measures to promote continence.

- The patient will remain continent during the night.

- The patient will remain free of infection from the indwelling catheter.

- The patient will describe the exercises to strengthen pelvic floor muscles.

- The patient will demonstrate self-care for an indwelling catheter.

The successful achievement of patient goals depends on the patient's state of health, his or her ability to participate in care, and the resources available to the patient. Regaining continence, for example, is a learning process which requires maximum participation of the individual and full support of the family and all health personnel. The process takes time — often weeks and even months — and frustration from lapses of incontinence is not unusual. Goals should be stated as short-term steps towards long-term achievement. They should be set mutually with the patient (and family) and reflect levels of performance the patient is realistically capable of achieving. Learning begins in hospital but continues once the person is at home. Thus, planning should also include referrals to appropriate home care services.

IMPLEMENTING URINARY ELIMINATION INTERVENTIONS

HEALTH PROMOTING STRATEGIES

The urinary tract provides an effective mechanism for eliminating nitrogenous wastes of cellular metabolism and maintaining fluid, electrolyte and acid-base balance in the body.

KEY PRINCIPLES

Principles Relevant to Urinary Elimination

1. Most of the nitrogenous wastes of cellular metabolism are eliminated by the kidneys.
2. The kidneys play an important role in maintaining the fluid and electrolyte balance of the body.
3. The suppression of urine formation in the kidneys threatens the life of an individual.
4. The kidneys normally mature to full functioning ability by two years of age.
5. The necessary neuromuscular structures for voluntary control of voiding are not usually sufficiently developed until the age of two to three years.
6. Loss of voluntary control over voiding can be a serious threat to an individual's self-esteem.
7. The average adult voids 1000 to 1500 ml of urine in a 24-hour period; the average school-age child voids up to 1000 ml in 24 hours.
8. Awareness of the need to void normally occurs in the adult when the bladder contains 200 to 300 ml of urine.
9. The lining of the urinary tract consists of a continuous layer of mucous membrane.
10. The intimate anatomical relationship between the urinary and reproductive tracts makes urinary functioning a sensitive topic for most people.
11. The location of the urinary meatus in close proximity to the anus and to the external sex organs makes the urinary tract vulnerable to infection from these sources.
12. Urinary output of less than 30 ml per hour (720 ml in a 24-hour period) is considered inadequate for adults.

An adequate fluid intake, emptying the bladder when the urge arises, proper hygiene practices and strong perineal muscle tone will foster healthy urinary functioning in daily living. Nurses can help individuals promote optimal urinary elimination by providing information and encouraging them to examine their urinary patterns and toileting practices.

PELVIC-FLOOR STRENGTHENING EXERCISES

Pelvic floor exercises, also called **Kegel exercises**, are beneficial for strengthening perineal muscle tone and pre-

venting stress incontinence in both men and women. These exercises consist of repetitive contraction and relaxation of the perineal muscles. The individual is instructed to squeeze the perineal muscles as if trying to stop the flow of urine and tighten the muscles around the anus, then hold to the count of five and release. The person will feel the pelvic floor rise during tightening of the muscles. At least five contraction-relaxation cycles should be performed during a set and the sets repeated several times a day. Pelvic floor exercises can be performed while lying down, sitting or standing, anywhere and anytime during the day. They should also be performed several times while voiding.

HEALTH PROTECTING STRATEGIES

Maintenance of adequate urinary elimination is important to physiological functioning. When people are ill or in hospital their voiding habits may be disrupted and they may need assistance maintaining normal patterns.

MAINTAINING NORMAL URINARY ELIMINATION

The best way to maintain normal urinary patterns is to void at regular times and when the urge is felt. An adequate fluid intake will help to maintain regularity. Patients who are ambulatory can generally attend to their elimination needs by using bathroom facilities. This is most desirable both physiologically and psychologically — psychologically, because the patient can void in private and physiologically, because the patient can assume the natural positions for micturition. For women, voiding is facilitated in a sitting or squatting position. Men void more effectively in the standing position. If they cannot ambulate to the bathroom, women may find it easier to void using a bedside commode than a bedpan. Male patients find it easier to stand at the side of the bed when using a urinal. When patients need assistance with urinary elimination, prompt attention to their call for help is essential to avoid delaying the micturition reflex. In addition, teaching and encouraging patients to perform Kegel exercises will promote bladder emptying.

ASSISTING THE PATIENT WITH A BEDPAN OR URINAL

Patients who are confined to bed must use the bedpan or the urinal for elimination purposes. Female patients use the bedpan for both urination and defecation; the male patient needs the bedpan for defecation and the urinal for voiding. Having to use these utensils for elimination is embarrassing for many people. Thus, the nurse must ensure the patient's privacy, avoid unnecessary exposure of body parts considered private by most individuals, and make the

HEALTH PROMOTING STRATEGY

Promoting Healthy Urinary Elimination

* Urinate as soon as the urge is felt. Ignoring the urge to void will lead to urinary stasis and bladder distention which may cause infection, and, in older persons may lead to urgency and possibly incontinence.
* Drink about 2 litres of fluid daily.
* Limit foods containing sodium, caffeine and alcohol.

For people who tend to wake up in the night to void:
  * Limit the intake of fluids in the evening.
  * Limit foods containing caffeine and alcohol.
  * Void before retiring.

For women:
  * Wipe the perineum from front to back. This prevents the transfer of organisms from the anus to the urethra.
  * Void soon after intercourse. This helps to flush organisms from the urinary meatus and reduce opportunities for bacterial growth.

* Wash hands before and after urinating.
* Practise pelvic-floor strengthening exercises (Kegel exercises) regularly.

procedure as safe and as comfortable as possible for the patient, both physically and psychologically.

To ensure privacy, the curtains are drawn around the patient's unit, or the door of a private room closed. The nurse assesses the patient's need for assistance. If the patient can use the bedpan or urinal independently, the nurse ensures these utensils and the call bell are within easy reach. The patient who needs help is assisted onto the bedpan as described in Chapter 21. Assisting the male patient with a urinal will be described later in this section. The nurse remains available just outside the patient's unit or room to provide help as necessary.

Generally, men do not require cleansing following urination, other than provision of the means for washing their hands. Assistance in cleansing the perineal area following urination for the female patient may be required. Using a bedpan can be an extremely uncomfortable experience. Prompt response to a patient's call light and competent and proper use of equipment can ensure that the procedure is made as comfortable as possible.

As in all other contact with patients, the nurse must remember to use principles of body substance precautions (these are described in more detail in Chapter 31). Hands must be washed before and after assisting patients, and disposable gloves worn when handling urine and feces or when providing perineal care following urination.

The nurse assesses the amount and characteristics of the urine prior to disposal in the toilet or hopper. Cleaning of the bedpan is outlined in Chapter 31. If the patient is on intake and output measurements, the amount is documented on the patient's intake and output record.

In most institutions, separate bedpans and urinals are available for each patient. These are usually stored in the bedside locker. Once the patient is discharged from the hospital, these utensils are returned to the central supply department for sterilization.

A

B

FIGURE 20.4   A. Male urinal. B. Female urinal.

Using a urinal The male urinal is designed to fit over the patient's penis so that urine could be excreted without spillage. It has a handle for convenience (specially designed urinals are available for patients who have the use of only one hand) and is usually flat on either one side or the bottom so that it can be set down on a flat surface after use without spilling the contents. Some agencies provide a bag for storing the urinal at the patient's bedside.

The patient can use a urinal in the supine position, the lateral position (either side) or Fowler's position or when standing at the side of the bed. Most patients prefer to use the urinal without help. If help is needed, however, the nurse separates the patient's legs sufficiently to allow placement of the urinal between them. Then, holding the urinal with one hand, the nurse inserts the penis into the urinal far enough to prevent urine from spilling onto the bedclothes or the patient's skin. If necessary, the nurse holds the urinal in place until the patient has finished voiding.

Although not common, urinals for use by female patients are available. These are similar in design to the male urinal, but with a long, wide top, shaped like a spout (Figure 20.4). In order to use the urinal, the patient stands at the side of the bed, sits on the edge of the bed or sits in bed. If necessary, the urinal may also be used in the side-lying position. To use the urinal correctly, the spout must be positioned towards the rectum and must be in contact with the patient's skin. Otherwise, urine will leak out.

HEALTH RESTORING STRATEGIES

Restorative care for urinary elimination problems includes measures to reestablish normal voiding patterns (bladder retraining programs) and facilitate bladder emptying. Measures to stimulate micturition, urinary catheterization, indwelling catheter care, bladder irrigation, external drainage (condom catheter) and urostomy care will be outlined here.

RETRAINING FOR BLADDER CONTROL

Individuals with urinary dysfunction may experience urinary retention or incontinence. For instance, a patient who has had a catheter in place over a period of time may experience a phase of urinary incontinence before regaining bladder control. Neuromuscular conditions which interfere with sensory and motor impulses involved in voluntary control of voiding; psychological changes such as anxiety, fear or disorientation; and the use of medications affecting urine output can also result in urinary incontinence.

Incontinence can affect all age groups; however, older individuals are more likely to experience this problem. Urinary incontinence can cause psychological and physiological problems for individuals and their families. People

with urinary incontinence may suffer lowered self-esteem, depression, and apathy, all of which can lead to a pattern of social isolation (MacLeod and MacTavish 1988). Nurses can help patients to train their bladders to function at regular and predictable times. To achieve success, the patient must be willing and physically able to undertake a training program.

A program to reestablish bladder control begins with an assessment of the patient's normal pattern of voiding and usual times for toileting. A program is then established to comply with these usual habits. It is important that all nursing and support personnel adhere to the planned schedule for the patient. Consistency is the key to an effective retraining program.

All of the measures for promoting normal urinary elimination are used in implementing a bladder retraining program. The patient is encouraged to void at regular intervals or as soon as the urge to void is felt. Individuals who require toileting assistance from nursing personnel should not be kept waiting or allowed to become incontinent because their call for assistance has been ignored. If incontinence does occur, bed linen should be changed at once, thus preventing skin irritation and promoting psychological well-being.

In a bladder retraining program it is essential that the micturition reflex be activated at regular intervals. Therefore, an adequate intake of fluids is necessary so that sufficient urine is produced to distend the bladder and stimulate the micturition reflex. Withholding fluids in a mistaken attempt to control incontinence can lead to fluid and electrolyte imbalances, as well as constipation and cystitis. The provision of fluids at regular intervals helps to ensure an adequate intake; that is, under normal circumstances, a minimum of 2000 ml per day, although 3000 ml or more is preferred if tolerated by the patient. Patients are encouraged to avoid caffeine-containing beverages, which stimulate the urge to void. Water, milk and fruit juices are recommended (Powers and Williams, 1992).

Bladder retraining is a learned behaviour much like toilet training in children. Achievement of continence can take time for many individuals when voluntary control has been lost for a period of time. In some instances, it may take months, but success when it comes can be very rewarding for both the patient and the nursing staff.

Patients require both physical and psychosocial support during a bladder retraining program. Dependence on others and the lack of control over a basic function such as voiding can be very distressing. It is important that the nurse and other personnel have a good working relationship with the patient, as this will help to lessen any anxiety the patient may experience, as well as any embarrassment due to any incontinence that should occur. A sensitive, caring approach and patience are required of the nurse in helping individuals with urinary problems. Every effort should be made to provide only positive reinforcement during the program. The individual can be very sensitive to signs of displeasure on the part of staff.

In some individuals, however, voluntary bladder control cannot be achieved. For these people, the plan of care may include a schedule of regular toileting (either on the toilet, commode chair, urinal or bedpan) and the use of absorbent pads or waterproof garments. The male patient may benefit from the use of an external urine collecting device such as a Texas catheter. As a last resort, intervention may involve the long-term use of an indwelling catheter.

FACILITATING MICTURITION

There are a number of measures the nurse can implement to stimulate micturition in patients who are having difficulty in initiating voiding. These include:

1. Providing privacy and helping the patient to assume a natural position for voiding

2. Providing a commode or, preferably, assisting the patient to the bathroom if this is possible (male patients frequently find it easier to void when standing rather than sitting or lying down)

3. Running water within the patient's hearing

4. Providing warm water in which to dangle their fingers

5. Pouring warm water over the perineum (The water must be measured if the patient is on intake and output measurements.)

6. Gently stroking the inner thighs or applying pressure over the symphysis pubis

7. Providing relief of pain.

The application of warmth to the bladder and perineal areas helps to relax the muscles used in voiding and therefore facilitate this process. If possible, having the patient sit in a Sitz bath or bathtub with warm water is also very helpful. When conservative measures have been unsuccessful in stimulating micturition and the patient is very uncomfortable, a urinary catheterization may be ordered.

URINARY CATHETERIZATION

Catheterization of the urinary bladder is the introduction of a narrow tube, called a catheter, through the urethra into the bladder. It provides a means of emptying the bladder for individuals unable to control micturition and those with urinary obstructions. It is inserted prior to operative procedures in which there is a high risk of bladder trauma or urinary complications. It is also used as a means of monitoring urinary output when frequent, accurate measurements are essential to the patient's care. The insertion of a urinary catheter carries a very high risk of nosocomial infections. If at all possible, catheterization should be avoided. However, when it is required, careful attention to meticulous aseptic technique is absolutely essential during every phase of catheter care from insertion to removal. Surgical aseptic technique is described in Chapter 31. The steps for inserting a catheter in a female and a male patient are outlined in Procedures 20.1 and 20.2 respectively.

Preparing the Patient

Before carrying out a catheterization, the nurse explains the procedure and the reasons for it to the patient. It is important to emphasize that insertion of a catheter should not be a painful experience; however, a sensation of pressure may be felt as the catheter is inserted. The patient will be asked to assume a dorsal recumbent or lithotomy position during the procedure. A side-lying or Sims' position may also be used for a female patient who cannot abduct her legs at the hip joint. Drapes will be used to minimize exposure. Every effort should be made to alleviate anxiety and put the patient at ease. Catheter insertion is easier for the nurse, and discomfort is minimized, when the patient relaxes.

In most cases, the patient should be encouraged to thoroughly wash the perineal area with warm soapy water immediately prior to the procedure. If the patient is unable to perform this procedure independently the nurse can carry out this function. This can provide the nurse with the opportunity to identify the urinary meatus in the female patient and retract the foreskin in the uncircumcised male patient. As well, this expedites the cleaning process during the catheterization.

Assembling Equipment

There are many types of catheters available and the choice of the catheter is determined by the reason for the catheterization. A straight, single-lumen catheter is used to collect a sterile specimen, measure a residual urine (amount of urine left in the bladder after voiding), or intermittently drain the bladder. If the catheter is to remain in place for a period of time, an indwelling or retention catheter (often called a Foley catheter) is used.

Retention catheters are kept in place by a balloon which is inflated once the catheter has been inserted. These catheters have two or three lumens. In the double-lumen catheter, one lumen is connected to the balloon which holds the catheter in place while the second lumen drains the urine from the bladder. The triple-lumen catheter has an additional lumen that is used for instilling solution during bladder irrigation. Figure 20.5 provides an illustration of the types of catheters.

In most institutions, sterile, prepackaged catheterization sets are available for catheter insertion. Each kit contains a pair of sterile gloves, sterile drapes, one of which is fenestrated (has an opening in the middle), cleansing solution, lubricant, cotton balls, a specimen container, forceps, a pre-filled syringe and a basin to collect urine. Some kits may contain a standard-size catheter and all kits can be used for both male and female patients. The kits are discarded after

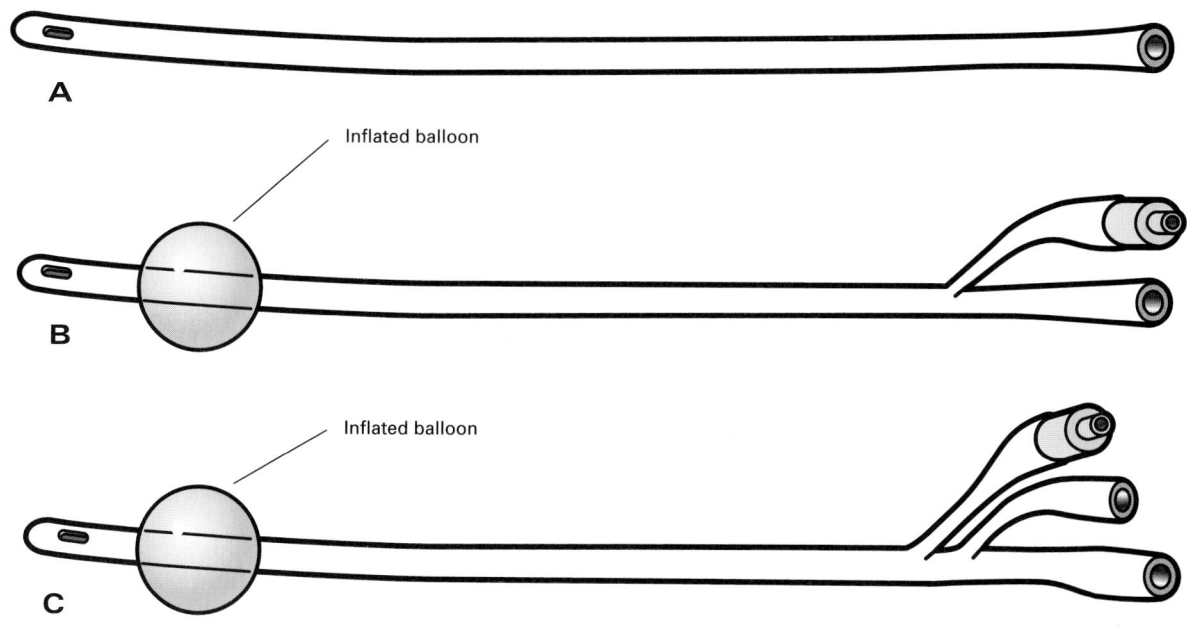

FIGURE 20.5   A. Straight catheter. B. Double-lumen indwelling catheter. C. Triple-lumen indwelling catheter.

use. Catheters are graded in size according to the French scale; 14 Fr and 16 Fr catheters are commonly used for the catheterization of the adult patient. The larger the number, the larger the lumen of the catheter. Smaller lumen catheters are generally not necessary and the smaller lumen results in an increased length of time required to empty the bladder. However, if there is any chance of injury to the urethral mucosa or if the patient experiences discomfort during the procedure, smaller sized catheters can be used. It is always wise to take an extra catheter and an extra pair of sterile gloves along in case of contamination during the procedure.

When an indwelling catheter is being inserted, a urine drainage bag and tubing will also be needed (Figure 20.6). The tubing connects the catheter to the collecting bag, forming a closed drainage system which should not be entered unless absolutely necessary. The drainage bag and tubing are sterile and must be attached to the catheter using aseptic technique to prevent the introduction of microorganisms into the system.

In order to visualize the urinary meatus and prevent contamination of the catheter as it is inserted, the nurse requires a good light source. Either an extension lamp or an extendible goose-neck lamp can be used to illuminate the perineal area. If necessary, the nurse can enlist the aid of an assistant with a flashlight.

FIGURE 20.6   Urinary drainage system

Inserting a Straight or Indwelling Catheter in a Female Patient

ACTION	RATIONALE
1. Prepare the patient.	Reduces anxiety and enables patient participation.
2. Wash hands thoroughly for one minute with antiseptic agent.	Prepares for sterile technique and use of sterile gloves (see Chapter 31).
3. Gather: • Catheter kit • Two catheters, size and type as appropriate • Extra pair of sterile gloves • Light • Urine collection bag and tubing • Tape, elastic band and safety pin • Moisture-proof bag • Water-proof protective pad • Bath blanket (optional)	Facilitates efficiency and economy of time.
4. Ensure adequate lighting. If necessary enlist the aid of an assistant to hold a flashlight.	Facilitates visualization of the urinary meatus.
5. Close the door (if private room) and pull bed curtains.	Provides privacy and may lessen feelings of embarrassment.
6. Place a protective pad under the patient and position her.	Prevents soiling of bed linen. Enables access to urinary meatus.
• Assist the patient to a dorsal recumbent position. Knees should be flexed and thighs externally rotated. Pillows can be used to support the knees and to elevate the buttocks.	Reduces muscle tension and promotes comfort.
• If unable to lie supine or abduct the thighs, assist the patient to a side-lying position with the upper leg flexed at the hip and knee. Position the buttocks close to the edge of the bed.	Promotes comfort, and, for some women, lessens feelings of exposure.

ACTION	RATIONALE
7. Drape the patient. Cover her upper body with a bath blanket, pull the gown up over her hips. Cover her legs and feet with the bed sheet.	Lessens feelings of exposure and keeps the patient warm.
8. If not done by the patient, don clean gloves and wash the genital area with warm soap and water. Rinse well and dry. Discard gloves and wash hands again.	Reduces microorganisms near the urethral meatus and enables the nurse to see the meatus in women with increased vaginal secretions.
9. If inserting an indwelling catheter, attach the urine drainage set to the bed according to the manufacturer's specifications. Leave the cover on the connector end of the tubing.	Prepares equipment for connection to the catheter after insertion. Maintains sterility.
10. Attach the moisture-proof bag to the side of bed placed to ensure minimal reaching over the sterile field.	Provides a receptacle for wrappings and used equipment. Prevents spread of microorganisms.
11. Position the light to illuminate the perineal area.	Provides sufficient light to view the urinary meatus.
12. Set up a sterile field on the overbed table using the inner wrapper of the catheterization kit and don sterile gloves (see Procedure 31.3). Open catheter package, if not included in kit.	Allows for easy access to equipment. Aseptic technique prevents contamination of sterile supplies by microorganisms.
13. Don sterile gloves (see Procedure 31.2).	Allows the nurse to handle sterile equipment without contamination.
14. Organize the equipment on the sterile field. • Add the catheter.	Readies equipment for the insertion while both gloves are sterile.
• If the catheter is indwelling, attach the pre-filled syringe to the valve of the balloon lumen and inject the fluid until the balloon inflates. Then withdraw all fluid from the balloon and leave the syringe attached to the valve port.	Tests for intactness of the catheter balloon and allows replacement of faulty equipment.
• Open and add cleansing solution to cotton balls.	Cleanses the urinary meatus and reduces the possibility of introducing microorganisms into the bladder.
• Open the specimen container if a specimen is to be obtained.	
• Lubricate 2.5 to 5 cm of the catheter tip.	Aids in catheter insertion and reduces trauma to the tissues.
15. Drape the patient. • Pick up the plain drape and open it away from any unsterile surfaces. Wrap the drape around gloved hands and place it between the patient's legs under the buttocks, without allowing the gloves to come in contact with the patient's skin.	Provides a sterile surface close to the perineal area. Protects the hands from contact with unsterile surfaces and maintains sterility of work area.
• Open the fenestrated drape in the same manner and wrap it around gloved hands. Place the drape over the patient's perineal area taking care not to touch any unsterile surfaces.	*Continued on the next page*

ACTION	RATIONALE

16. Place the sterile collecting basin containing the necessary supplies on the drape between the patient's thighs.	Maintains asepsis and allows access to supplies during the procedure.
17. Using the nondominant hand gently open the labia to expose the urethral meatus. Keep the labia separated and maintain this hand position throughout the procedure.	Allows the nurse to see the meatus and prevents contamination of the area around the meatus as well as the catheter. *This hand is no longer sterile and cannot be used to touch sterile items.*

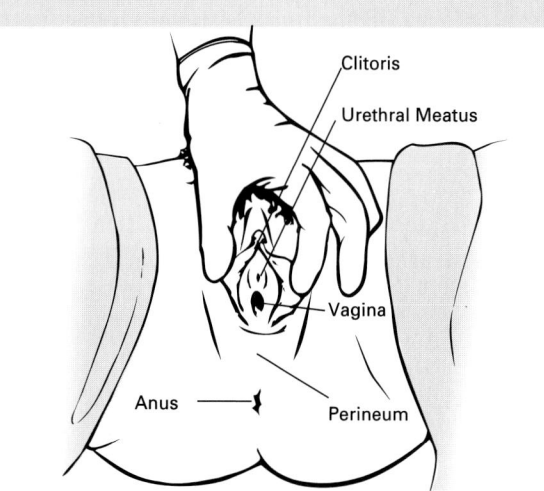

Clitoris
Urethral Meatus
Vagina
Anus
Perineum

18. Using forceps to hold the cotton balls, cleanse between the labial folds and over the urinary meatus. Use each swab just once and discard after use. Clean from the cleanest area (near the symphysis pubis) towards the most contaminated area (near the rectum). A minimum of five cotton balls is needed. Discard the cotton ball container and forceps.	Prevents the spread of microorganisms from dirtier to cleaner areas. Cleaning over the urinary meatus last helps to prevent the introduction of microorganisms into the bladder during insertion of the catheter.

ACTION	RATIONALE

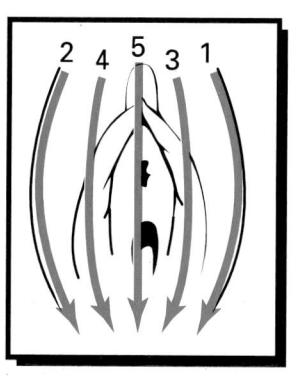

19. Pick up the lubricated catheter approximately 7.5 to 10 cm from the tip and ensure the distal end is in the collecting basin. Ask the patient to bear down as if to void or take a deep breath. Insert the catheter gently into the urethra to a distance of 5 to 7.5 cm or until urine begins to flow. If inserting an indwelling catheter, advance catheter a further 1 to 2.5 cm. Do not force the catheter if any resistance is felt.

Facilitates control of catheter. Prevents drainage onto the bed when the catheter is inserted.
Allows the sphincter to relax, making passage of the catheter easier.
The female urethra is about 3.7 to 6.2 cm in length.
Ensures placement of the catheter and allows inflation of the balloon without traumatizing urethral mucosa.

20. Straight catheter: Hold the catheter in place with thumb and forefinger of the nondominant hand until the bladder empties. Collect a specimen if required.

Prevents dislodgement.

Indwelling catheter: Hold the catheter in place with thumb and forefinger of the nondominant hand. Gently inflate the balloon according to the manufacturer's directions, while watching for any signs of patient discomfort. If discomfort is evident, aspirate the fluid back into the syringe, advance the catheter further into the bladder and attempt to inflate the balloon again. Detach the syringe without allowing any of the fluid to flow back into the syringe. Gently tug on the catheter. Collect a specimen if required.

Prevents dislodgement.

Holds the catheter in place in the bladder. If the balloon is not fully inflated the catheter may slip out of the bladder.

If resistance is felt when the catheter is tugged, the nurse can presume the balloon is inflated.

21. Straight catheter: Once the urine has stopped flowing, the catheter is pinched and withdrawn slowly.

Indwelling catheter: Attach the catheter to the urinary drainage system and secure the tubing to the patient's thigh using tape. Anchor the tubing to the drawsheet using the safety pin and elastic band.

Establishes a closed urinary drainage system.

Prevents trauma to the urethral meatus during movement.

Continued on the next page

ACTION	RATIONALE

22. Dry the perineal area and assist the patient to assume a comfortable position.

Promotes patient comfort and well-being.

23. Discard used equipment as per agency protocol. Send the specimen to the laboratory and wash hands.

Maintains cleanliness and safety in the workplace.

24. Document the procedure on the patient's record. Include the size and type of catheter used, a description of the urine obtained (amount, colour, clarity and odour), the patient's tolerance of the procedure, and that a specimen has been sent to the laboratory.

Fulfills legal requirements for nurse accountability and promotes continuity of care.

PROCEDURE 20.2

Inserting a Straight or Indwelling Catheter in a Male Patient

ACTION	RATIONALE

1. Follow steps 1 to 5 of Procedure 20.1.

2. Assist the patient to a supine position with thighs slightly abducted.

Prevents tensing of abdominal and pelvic muscles.

3. Follow steps 7 to 13 of Procedure 20.1.

4. Organize the equipment on the sterile field.
  • Add the catheter.

Readies equipment for the insertion while both gloves are sterile.

  • If the catheter is indwelling, attach the pre-filled syringe to the valve of the balloon lumen and inject the fluid until the balloon inflates. Then withdraw all fluid from the balloon and leave the syringe attached to the valve port.

Tests for intactness of the catheter balloon and allows replacement of faulty equipment.

PROCEDURE 20.2
continued

ACTION	RATIONALE
• Open and add cleansing solution to cotton balls.	Cleanses the urinary meatus and reduces the possibility of introducing microorganisms into the bladder.
• Open the specimen container if a specimen is to be obtained.	
• Lubricate the catheter generously for a length of 15 to 17.5 cm.	Aids in catheter insertion and reduces trauma to the tissues.
5. Drape patient.	
• Pick up the plain drape and open it away from any unsterile surfaces. Wrap the drape around gloved hands and place it over the patient's thighs below the penis.	Provides for a sterile surface close to the perineal area. Protects gloves from contact with unsterile surfaces and maintains sterility of the work area.
• Open the fenestrated drape in the same manner and wrap it around gloved hands. Place the opening of drape over the patient's penis.	
6. Place the sterile collecting basin containing the necessary supplies on the drape between patient's thighs.	Maintains asepsis and allows access to supplies during procedure.
7. If the patient is not circumcised and the foreskin is not already retracted, gently retract it. With the nondominant hand, grasp the penis just below the glans. Keep the hand in this position throughout the procedure.	If the foreskin is released, the area becomes contaminated and cleansing has to be repeated. *This hand is no longer sterile and cannot be used to touch sterile items.*
8. Using forceps to hold the cotton balls, cleanse the tip of the penis, using a circular motion. Proceed outwards from meatus to the base of the glans. Repeat the procedure at least three times, using a clean cotton ball each time. A final cotton ball may be held for a few moments over the urinary meatus.	Reduces the number of microorganisms in the area of the meatus. Cleansing from an area of least contamination to an area of greater contamination helps to prevent the spread of microorganisms. Cleansing over the urinary meatus last helps to prevent the introduction of microorganisms into the bladder during insertion of the catheter.

Continued on the next page

ACTION	RATIONALE
9. Lift the penis to a position perpendicular to the patient's body and apply slight traction. Pick up the lubricated catheter approximately 7.5 to 10 cm from the tip and ensure the distal end is in the collecting basin. Ask the patient to bear down as if to void and insert the catheter gently into the urethra to a distance of 15 to 20 cm or until urine begins to flow. It is not unusual to feel some resistance when the catheter reaches the area of the external sphincter. The nurse may also keep a gentle forward pressure on the catheter while the patient takes a few deep breaths.	Straightens the downward curvature of the prepubic urethra. Facilitates control of the catheter. The male urethra is approximately 20 cm in length. Allows the sphincter to relax, allowing the catheter to pass more readily.
If inserting an indwelling catheter, advance 1 to 2.5 cm more. Do not force the catheter if any significant resistance is felt.	Ensures placement of the catheter and allows inflation of the balloon without traumatizing urethral mucosa.
10. Follow steps 21 to 24 of Procedure 20.1. Before leaving the patient who is uncircumcised, ensure that his foreskin has been pulled forward over the glans.	If the foreskin is left retracted, circulation of blood to the glans can be impeded.

PROVIDING INDWELLING CATHETER CARE

Care for the patient with an indwelling catheter primarily includes monitoring for problems, preventing infection and maintaining unobstructed flow of urine through the drainage system. Many patients can participate in the care for their catheter once they know how the system functions and what care is required.

Immediately after a catheter insertion, some patients may experience irritation of the urethral mucosa. The nurse can reassure the patient that such discomfort is usually of short duration and it should soon pass. The patient is encouraged to drink adequate fluids (3000 ml per day if the patient's condition permits) to aid the urinary tract in flushing out unwanted microorganisms and to keep the tubing free of sediment.

Hand-washing and basic hygiene are essential for preventing infection. Hands must be washed before and after caring for a patient with an indwelling catheter. In addition, gloves should be worn to protect the nurse from exposure to blood and body substances. Patients should have perineal care administered at least twice a day to remove secretions and encrustations on the catheter which may cause infection (perineal care is outlined in Chapter 30; Procedures 30.3 and 30.4). Tub baths or showers should be taken as the patient's condition permits.

The correct positioning and maintenance of the urinary drainage system is an essential aspect of care. Urine drains from the bladder into the drainage bag by the force of gravity. The bag must be kept lower than the level of the patient's bladder for urine to drain freely. When the drainage bag is positioned higher than the bladder, urine will flow back into the bladder (backflow) bringing with it unwanted microorganisms. If the catheter bag is positioned above the level of the bladder (for example, for a tub bath), the tubing must be clamped to prevent urine backflow. The tubing should not loop below the receptacle because a kink may form, occluding the lumen. The tubing should be kept secured, with excess loops coiled on the bed, allowing the urine to drain into the drainage bag in a straight drop from the bed. Care must be taken to ensure that tubing does not become trapped under the patient's leg causing occlusion of the lumen.

When a continuous drainage system is in place, the drainage bag should be emptied as it fills, or at regular intervals. The amount, colour, clarity and odour of the urine are noted at that time. Urine meters are often used when the measurement of hourly urine outputs is required. The meters are rigid plastic containers attached to a drainage bag. The meters are calibrated to measure small amounts (300 ml or less) of urine (see Figure 20.7).

A closed drainage system should never be opened to measure urine or to obtain a specimen. Doing so would allow bacteria to enter the system and cause infection. The drainage bag is emptied through a drainage port at the bottom of the bag into a graduated container. This provides a means of measuring the amount of urine and then disposing of it, usually into a hopper in the soiled utility room (the technique for obtaining a urine specimen from an indwelling catheter is outlined in Procedure 20.3). If it is necessary for the catheter to be disconnected from the tubing for a period of time, for example, during a bladder irrigation, it is important that the sterility of both the catheter and the tubing be maintained. Small disposable devices are available which provide a sterile cover for the tubing and a plug for the catheter.

Patients with indwelling catheters are not confined to bed. In fact, such patients should be up and about as much as possible. The benefits of exercise to well-being are discussed in Chapter 28. Some agencies have cardboard receptacles designed to hold the drainage bag which

the patient then can carry, much like a shopping bag. Ambulatory patients may also use drainage bags which strap to the leg. These leg bags are equipped with a drainage port which can be opened to drain out the urine into the toilet or other receptacle as the bag fills. Leg bags are easily concealed under clothing and allow patients to participate in public without the embarrassment of displaying the catheter.

On occasion, it is necessary to change a retention or indwelling catheter. This is usually done according to the physician's order or agency protocol. Due to the risk of introducing microorganisms into the patient's bladder, catheters are never changed without good reason. Any obstruction to urine flow which is not cleared by irrigation would indicate a need for catheter replacement. Other signs that a catheter may need changing are insufficient urine in the collection bag relative to the fluid intake of the patient and abdominal distention just above the symphysis pubis. When a catheter is changed, the catheter *in situ* is removed as per Procedure 20.4, perineal care is completed and a new catheter is inserted as per Procedure 20.1 or 20.2.

FIGURE 20.7   Urinary drainage bag with urine meter attached

Patient Teaching for Indwelling Catheter Care

1. It is common to feel the need to void while the catheter is in place.

2. Increased amounts of fluid (approximately 3000 ml per day) are needed to flush the bladder and keep the tubing free of sediment.

3. Move freely in bed and, if allowed, be up and about with catheter in place.

4. Avoid lying on the catheter tubing.

5. Keep the drainage bag below the level of the bladder.

6. If able, wash the perineal area (and the urinary meatus, for male patients) and catheter with soap and water at least twice daily. If unable, this will be done by the nurse. When taking tub baths or showers, clamp the tubing if the drainage bag must be suspended above the level of the bladder.

7. Watch for and report untoward signs such as strong odours, burning sensations, or discharge at the meatus.

Obtaining a Urine Sample from an Indwelling Catheter

ACTION	RATIONALE
1. Wash hands and gather: • Alcohol swab • Sterile syringe with 25 gauge needle attached • Sterile container for specimen • Clamp • Clean gloves	Reduces transfer of microorganisms and facilitates efficiency and economy of time.
2. Tell the patient what you are going to do.	Promotes patient well-being and participation in care.
3. Check that the drainage tube has urine in it. If necessary, apply a clamp to the tubing below the puncture port and wait until urine collects in the tubing.	
4. Cleanse the puncture port with an alcohol swab.	Prevents contamination of the specimen and introduction of surface microorganisms into the system.
5. Insert the needle into the port and withdraw the sample of urine. Usually 3 to 5 ml of urine provides a sufficient sample. If used, be sure that the clamp is removed from the tubing.	
6. Put the specimen into the sterile container. Dispose of syringe into a Sharps container, remove gloves and wash hands.	Ensures safe handling of used equipment.
7. Send the specimen to the laboratory with its appropriate requisition.	
8. Document the procedure. Record the time that the specimen has been sent to the laboratory for culture and sensitivities.	Fulfills requirement for nurse accountability.

Note: Urine collected for culture and sensitivity needs to be clean and as recently produced as possible; therefore, it is never obtained from the urine in the collecting bag.

REMOVING AN INDWELLING CATHETER

Following the doctor's order for removal of an indwelling catheter, the nurse first needs to assess the patient's understanding of the procedure to be performed. If appropriate, the reason for the removal and the procedure is explained. If this is a first-time experience for the patient, he or she will likely be concerned about pain on withdrawal of the catheter. The nurse can assure the patient that at most there may be a slight burning sensation. This will be more pronounced for the male patient than for the female.

Prior to the procedure, thorough cleansing of the perineal area must be performed. Most patients will prefer to do this independently; however, on occasion it will be the responsibility of the nurse. This is a good time for the nurse to assess the size of the balloon holding the catheter in place so that the appropriate size of syringe can be collected later. The technique for removing an indwelling catheter is detailed in Procedure 20.4. Once the catheter is removed, the nurse discusses measures to promote return of the patient's normal urinary elimination pattern. These are summarized in the box on page 558.

Removing an Indwelling Catheter

ACTION	RATIONALE

1. Wash hands and gather:
  • Clean gloves
  • Syringe (without needle)
  • Moisture-proof bag
  • Water-proof protective pad
  • Graduated container
	Prevents the transfer of microorganisms and facilitates efficiency and economy of time.

2. Assist the patient to a dorsal recumbent position, with legs slightly apart. Place the protective pad under the patient's buttocks.	Promotes patient comfort. Protects bed linens.
3. Apply clean gloves.	Protects the nurse from exposure to body secretions.
4. Empty the urinary drainage bag into the graduated container and measure the output.	Readies the bag for removal.
5. Remove the tape securing the tubing to the patient's thigh.	Readies the tube for removal.
6. Insert the tip of the syringe into the valve of the balloon lumen and withdraw the fluid until negative pressure is felt.	Readies the catheter for removal.
7. Ask the patient to take several deep breaths and then while the patient is relaxed wrap the catheter in a protective pad and gently withdraw it from the urethra. Observe the patient for signs of discomfort. If discomfort occurs, stop the procedure and again attempt to withdraw fluid from balloon port.	Promotes relaxation. If the balloon has not been emptied completely, the patient may experience discomfort.
8. Place used equipment into the moisture-proof bag, remove gloves and discard appropriately. Wash hands.	Promotes cleanliness and safety in the workplace.
9. Ask the patient to perform, or, if necessary, help the patient to perform, perineal care.	Cleanses area of any spilled urine.
10. Document the procedure. Record the time, patient tolerance and any teaching done.	Fulfills requirements for nurse accountability and promotes continuity of care.

Note: In some agencies, a sample of urine for culture and sensitivity is obtained prior to removal of the catheter.

BLADDER IRRIGATION

A bladder irrigation is performed to maintain or restore patency of a catheter when drainage is obstructed with blood or sediment. It is also done to flush a bladder or instill medications. For example, the physician may order an irrigation to flush the bladder for extensive bleeding with clots in a patient with cancer, or to instill an antibiotic agent in a patient with infection. If the patient does not have an indwelling catheter in place, one has to be inserted first.

Patient Teaching Following Removal of an Indwelling Catheter

1. Void into a urinal or bedpan until otherwise directed so that output can be measured.

2. Continue increased fluid intake.

3. A burning sensation during the first couple of voidings is a normal occurrence.

4. Report any untoward signs such as continued burning on voiding, bleeding, unusual odours or indications of fever.

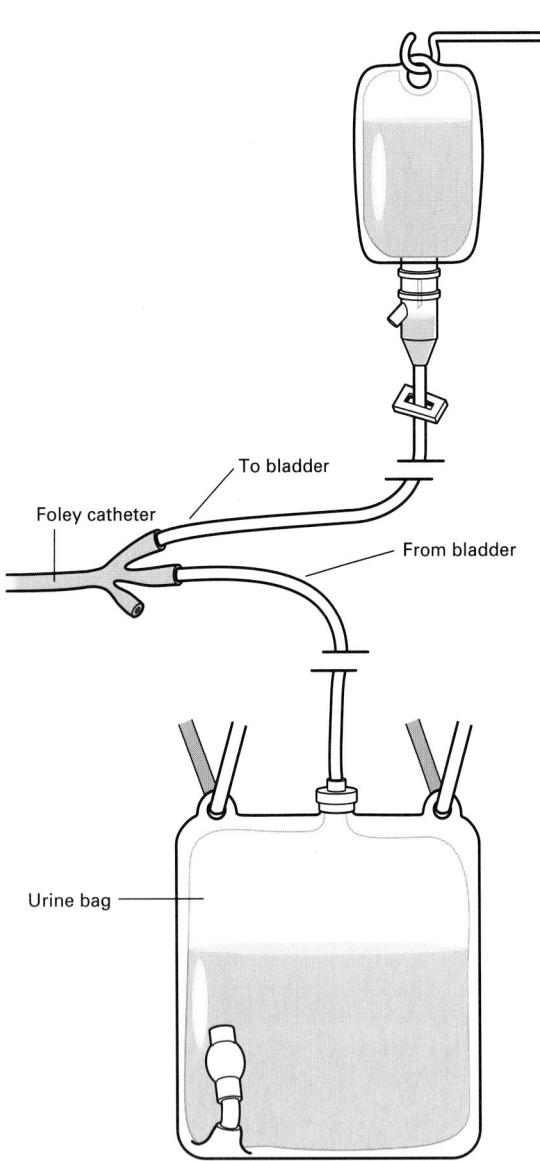

To bladder

Foley catheter

From bladder

Urine bag

FIGURE 20.8 Continuous bladder irrigation using a closed system via a triple-lumen catheter

Bladder irrigations are performed on the physician's order. They may be carried out on an intermittent or continuous basis. There are two methods for bladder irrigation: open and closed. The *open method* is used for intermittent irrigation when the patient has a double lumen indwelling catheter in place. It involves separating the catheter from the drainage tubing and flushing the catheter with a syringe. The *closed method* uses a triple-lumen catheter. The irrigating solution (irrigant) is instilled through the third (irrigating) lumen while the return solution is drained through the catheter drainage system (see Figure 20.8). This method permits frequent intermittent or continuous irrigation without disruption of the sterile drainage system. The steps for performing a bladder irrigation using the open method are outlined in Procedure 20.5. The closed method for continuous bladder irrigation is detailed in Procedure 20.6. Meticulous aseptic technique is required throughout the procedure.

Preparing the Patient

Explain the procedure to the patient. Patients may experience a feeling of fullness in the bladder. They should inform the nurse of any discomfort.

Assembling Equipment

Normal saline is most commonly used for bladder irrigations. Irrigating solutions (irrigants) are administered at room temperature. Disposable irrigation kits are available for open bladder irrigations. A kit includes a container for the irrigating solution, a receptacle for the irrigation return (outflow) and an Asepto syringe. An Asepto syringe is a large bulb-type syringe with a tip that fits into the urinary catheter (see Figure 20.9). In cases where there are large blood clots occluding urinary drainage, the nurse might choose to use a 50 to 60 ml piston type syringe, called a Toomey syringe, which permits greater forward pressure and return suction than does the Asepto syringe.

A continuous bladder irrigation is set up much like an intravenous infusion (see Procedure 22.1 in Chapter 22). Sterile irrigating solution is usually supplied in three-litre bags of normal saline. The irrigation administration set consists of straight or Y-type tubing which connects to the solution container, a roller clamp for adjusting the rate of irrigant entering the bladder and an adapter end that attaches to the catheter. The Y-type tubing is used when it is necessary to hang two solution bags at once. The solution container is suspended on an IV pole and the tubing is primed in the same manner as intravenous tubing.

A

B

FIGURE 20.9   A. Asepto syringe. B. Toomey syringe.

PROCEDURE 20.5

Open Bladder Irrigation

ACTION	RATIONALE
1. Prepare the patient.	Promotes patient well-being and enables participation in care.
2. Wash hands thoroughly.	Prevents the spread of microorganisms.
3. Gather: • Disposable irrigation kit • Sterile irrigation solution • Toomey syringe (optional) • Sterile gloves • Sterile tip to protect end of drainage tubing • Water-proof protective pad • Bath blanket (optional)	Facilitates efficiency and economy of time.
4. Close the door to the room, and pull bed curtains.	Promotes privacy.
5. Help the patient into a dorsal recumbent position, with legs slightly separated. Pull down the bed covers to expose the catheter where it joins the drainage tubing and place a protective pad under the patient's buttocks. Cover the patient's upper body with a bath blanket.	Promotes patient comfort, facilitates access to the catheter, and aids flow of irrigant into the bladder. Protects bed linen from soiling. Provides warmth.
6. Open the irrigation kit on the overbed table, creating a sterile field. Add solution.	Maintains sterility of equipment.

Continued on the next page

PROCEDURE 20.5
continued

ACTION	RATIONALE
7. Put on gloves.	Maintains asepsis and protects the nurse from exposure to body substances.
8. Place the sterile drape between the patient's thighs, under the catheter-tubing junction, and put the irrigating equipment on it.	Creates a sterile field. Readies equipment for the procedure.
9. Disconnect the catheter from the tubing, place a cap over the end of the drainage tube and secure it to the bed linen. Position the end of the catheter in the collecting basin, holding the catheter about 2.5 cm from its open end. Cleanse the end of the catheter with an antiseptic swab.	Keeps the end of the drainage tube sterile. Protects the bed linen from spillage of urine. Prevents entry of microorganisms into the system.
10. Aspirate 30 ml to 50 ml of irrigant into the syringe.	Prepares the syringe for irrigation and ensures a record of the amount of irrigant instilled.
11. Insert the syringe into the catheter lumen, compress the bulb and gently instill the solution.	Minimizes the potential for discomfort and damage to delicate bladder tissues.
12. Keeping the bulb of the syringe compressed, remove the syringe from the catheter and allow the solution to drain by gravity into the collecting basin. If there is no fluid return, gently aspirate solution from the bladder. Repeat the procedure as indicated by the effect of irrigation or as per physician's order.	Repetition may be required to dislodge obstructions and establish urine flow.
13. Reattach the catheter to the drainage tube, ensuring that the ends remain sterile. Secure the catheter to patient's thigh.	Reestablishes closed drainage system.
14. Remove gloves and assist the patient into a comfortable position.	Promotes patient well-being.
15. Discard equipment and wash hands.	Promotes cleanliness and safety.
16. Document the procedure. Note how the patient tolerated the procedure as well as the characteristics and amount of drainage obtained.	Fulfills requirements for nurse accountability.

PROCEDURE 20.6

Continuous Bladder Irrigation

ACTION	RATIONALE
1. Prepare the patient.	
2. Wash hands thoroughly.	Prevents the spread of microorganisms.

ACTION	RATIONALE
3. Gather: • Sterile irrigation solution • Irrigation administration set • IV pole • Water-proof protective pad • Catheter clamp • Large-size graduated container • Clean gloves • Alcohol swab • Moisture-proof bag	Facilitates efficiency and economy of time.
4. Prepare the irrigant. • Remove the solution bag from its outer wrapper and hang it on the IV pole. • Attach and prime the tubing as in Procedure 22.1 maintaining sterility of equipment.	Readies equipment.
5. Close the door to the room, or pull bed curtains. Put on gloves, expose the catheter and place a protective pad under the catheter where it joins the drainage tubing.	Promotes privacy. Gloves protect the nurse from exposure to body substances. Protects bed linen.
6. Cleanse the irrigation lumen of the catheter with an alcohol swab.	Reduces the risk of introducing microorganisms into the system.
7. Connect the tubing to the irrigation lumen.	
8. Slowly open the roller clamp and establish flow of irrigant. Adjust the flow rate according to the amount ordered over time or by the character of the irrigation returns.	Provides for a continuous flushing of the bladder. The amount is regulated to irrigate the bladder without distending it.
9. Remove gloves and leave the patient in a comfortable position. Discard unnecessary equipment and wash hands.	Promotes cleanliness and safety.
10. Monitor the patient and the irrigation regularly. It will be necessary to empty the bag more frequently.	Promotes safety and establishes need for care. For patients with hematuria and clot formation which blocks bladder drainage, the rate of the irrigation may have to be changed frequently. This does not require a specific physician's order, but changes in the character of returns must be recorded.
11. Document the procedure. Note the time irrigation was established, the type of solution used, changes in the character of urinary returns and the patient's tolerance of the procedure. In some agencies, the amount of fluid instilled into the bladder is subtracted from the amount of returns obtained, giving a record of urinary output.	Fulfills requirements for nurse accountability and facilitates continuity of care.

FIGURE 20.10   An external urinary appliance. The urine is collected in a bag that can be attached to the calf or thigh.

EXTERNAL URINARY DRAINAGE

Alternative methods are sometimes used instead of a retention catheter for individuals who are unable to control urination. For women, protective pants made of a nonabsorbent plastic or rubberized material are worn over an absorbent pad. An external urinary appliance, called a condom catheter, is often used by men. This appliance consists of a latex condom with a short tube which can be connected to a drainage bag. Known by various names, such as urosheath, "Texas condom" or condom catheter, it provides a convenient method of collecting urine from pa-

tients who are incontinent, and reduces the risk of infection from an indwelling catheter. The psychological impact of being able to empty the bladder in a more "normal" fashion cannot be overemphasized. The condom is disposable, relatively inexpensive and easily applied, all of which make frequent changes possible. It comes with a self-adhesive or velcro tape which is used to secure the condom in position at the base of the penis (see Figure 20.10). The technique for applying a condom drainage device in outlined in Procedure 20.7.

PROCEDURE 20.7

Applying a Condom Drainage Device

ACTION	RATIONALE
1. Explain the procedure to the patient.	Promotes well-being and enables participation in care.
2. Wash hands and gather: • Basin with warm water, soap, washcloth and towel • Condom catheter with velcro or adhesive strap • Urinary drainage tube and collecting bag or urinary leg bag and straps • Clean gloves • Bath blanket	Lessens transfer of microorganisms and promotes efficiency and economy of time.
3. Close the door to the room or draw bed curtains. Assist the patient into a dorsal recumbent position, cover him with a bath blanket and expose the genitals.	Promotes privacy and lessens feelings of embarrassment. Keeps the patient warm.
4. Apply gloves and thoroughly wash and dry the penis and perineal area.	Removes urine and other secretions which may be harmful to skin integrity.
5. Unroll the condom over the the penis so that the narrow tube opening at the end is over the urinary meatus. Leave approximately 2.5 cm to 5 cm space between the end of the penis and the end of the condom.	Permits proper application of condom. Decreases the chance of skin irritation and allows urine to drain more freely.

ACTION	RATIONALE
6. Wrap the tape or velcro strap snugly (but not too tightly) over the condom around the shaft of the penis and secure in place.	Wrapping too tightly may impede circulation to the penis.
7. Connect the tube opening of the condom to the urinary drainage set (or leg bag).	Establishes a route for collecting urine.
8. Remove gloves and assist the patient to a position of comfort. Remove used equipment and wash hands.	Promotes patient well-being. Promotes cleanliness and safety in the workplace.
9. Document procedure. Record the patient's response to the procedure. Record urinary drainage as necessary.	Fulfills requirements for nurse accountability and facilitates continuity of care.

Care for a condom drainage device Once condom drainage has been established, it is important to assess the patient from time to time to ensure that the condom has not become twisted at the point where it joins the drainage tubing and that tubing has not become kinked, thus blocking drainage. Removal and reapplication of the condom device is dependent upon the integrity of the skin on the patient's penis and the patient's ability to be continent for any length of time.

UROSTOMY CARE

Individuals with urostomies generally have achieved a measure of independence in dealing with their unique method of urinary elimination. When they are ill or hospitalized they may need assistance in carrying out their usual routines.

The nurse should assess the individual's ability to care for the urostomy independently. As well, the condition of the stoma, fluid intake and output and changes that would indicate urinary tract dysfunction should be monitored. If the agency has access to an enterostomal therapist, the nurse can enlist his or her aid in formulating the most effective plan of care for the patient.

Incontinent urinary diversions Individuals with incontinent urinary diversions (for example, ileal conduit)

wear an external collecting appliance. This is a one- or two-piece appliance consisting of a collecting bag with an adhesive wafer that sticks to the skin surrounding the urinary stoma. The appliance can be kept in place for three to seven days, but generally, it is changed twice a week. If it is a two-piece appliance, the collecting bag can be changed more frequently and the wafer can stay in place up to ten days. The collecting bag is fitted with a valve at the bottom through which it is emptied into a toilet or other receptacle. For most individuals, the collecting bag is attached by means of a connector to a closed urinary drainage system (as is used for catheter drainage) for drainage during the night. This reduces the risk of leakage or rupture of the bag and ensures peace of mind while the individual sleeps. The technique for changing an external collecting appliance in outlined in Procedure 20.8.

Throughout the procedure, the nurse should observe the condition of the peristomal skin, condition of the stoma and characteristics of the urine. One of the normal functions of the bowel is to produce mucous to facilitate passage of fecal matter. For individuals with urinary reservoirs created from portions of their intestine, it is normal for the urine to be somewhat cloudy and to contain mucous shreds. However, the nurse must remain alert for any signs of urinary tract dysfunction such as foul-smelling urine, hematuria and increased body temperature.

PROCEDURE 20.8

Changing an External Two-Piece Urostomy Appliance

ACTION	RATIONALE
1. Wash hands and gather: • Type and size of appliance used by the patient • Clean gloves • Water-proof protective pad • Basin with warm water, soap, washcloth and towels (or cotton gauze wipes) • Urine collection container • Scissors • Moisture-proof bag	Reduces the spread of microorganisms. Promotes efficiency and economy of time.
2. Provide for privacy, position the patient, place the protective pad under the patient on stoma side.	Individuals with incontinent diversions have no control over urinary elimination. Protects bed linens.
3. Don clean gloves.	Protects nurse from exposure to body fluids and substances.
4. Position the urine collection container under the valve and open it. Drain any urine collected in the bag into the container. Measure and discard urine.	Provides accurate measurement of urinary output. Allows for appropriate disposal of urine.

PROCEDURE 20.8
continued

ACTION	RATIONALE
5. Prepare the new wafer. If necessary, cut an opening on the wafer large enough to accommodate the size of stoma. Some patients may have a guide to gauge the size of the opening.	Allows the barrier to be fitted over the stoma.

ACTION	RATIONALE
6. Remove the old appliance by carefully lifting one corner of the wafer from the skin using one hand while pressing down with the other. Discard into garbage bag.	Protects the patient's skin from damage. Maintains a clean environment.
7. Gently cleanse area around the stoma with warm soapy water, rinse clean and dry well.	Provides for skin protection from urine. The stoma is fragile and will bleed readily if handled in a rough manner.

Continued on the next page

ACTION	RATIONALE
8. Apply the new wafer quickly, pressing the wafer firmly to the skin around the stoma.	A urinary stoma drips urine constantly. If the appliance is applied quickly, the skin will remain dry and the wafer will stick.

9. Attach the collecting bag to the wafer. Ensure that the valve is closed and positioned at the bottom.	Allows for effective drainage and proper filling of collecting bag.

SOURCE: Figures from ConvaTec (1986). *For a better way of living with a urostomy — every day.* Princeton, NJ: E.R. Squibb & Sons, Inc., Pamphlet 567-042CE. Reproduced with permission.

Collecting a sample of urine from urinary diversions To collect a urine sample for urinalysis from a patient with a urinary diversion, the nurse first empties the collecting bag, waits for more urine to collect and then takes the sample from the fresh supply. If a urine for culture and sensitivity is required, the nurse will need to remove the collecting bag, insert a sterile, straight catheter into the stoma, position the other end of the catheter into the sterile specimen container and, once the specimen is collected, withdraw the catheter and reapply the collecting bag.

Continent urinary diversions Individuals with continent urinary diversions meet their need for urinary elimination by catheterizing their urinary reservoirs on a regular basis throughout the day. If assistance is required, the nurse needs to know the size of catheter used and the frequency of catheterization.

ASSISTING WITH MEASURES TO REDUCE THE WORKLOAD ON THE KIDNEYS

The primary function of the kidneys is to maintain the composition and volume of the body fluids in homeostasis. In cases of renal failure, the kidneys are unable to excrete the waste products of metabolism, chiefly the nitrogenous wastes of cellular metabolism. This may be an acute, potentially reversible state resulting from major trauma, metabolic disturbances or surgery, for example. It may also, however, be a chronic condition requiring long-term management.

Careful monitoring of the patient's fluid intake and output, electrolyte balance and response to therapy and medications can identify those individuals who are at risk for development of acute renal failure. Individuals with acute renal failure require comprehensive medical and nursing intervention.

The nurse can implement various measures to relieve some of the workload of the kidney. The patient is generally put on bed rest in an effort to minimize activity and lessen cellular metabolism. Diet therapy for the renal patient is highly individualized. Protein metabolism results in the formation of nitrogenous waste products. Therefore, unless the patient is losing large amounts of protein in the urine (which occurs in some conditions), the patient is placed on a low protein diet in an attempt to minimize the amounts of nitrogenous wastes produced.

In renal failure, the kidney does not excrete or retain sodium and potassium appropriately. Higher levels of sodium cause fluid retention, while accumulation of potassium can result in serious neuromuscular disturbances. Fluid intake may be restricted in an effort to prevent or lessen edema. Meticulous monitoring of the fluid intake and output is critical to the patient's therapeutic management. Patients with renal disorders often suffer from anorexia and may need encouragement to eat their meals. The nurse needs to ensure that the patient is made aware of the importance of adhering to the ordered diet and fluid intake. Many patients are able to keep track of their fluid intake, and gains in their fluid management can often be achieved by encouraging patient participation in their own care.

Edematous tissue is more prone to breakdown than is normal tissue; therefore, if edema is present, the nurse must be alert for any sign of impaired skin integrity. Patients who are confined to bed require particular attention to prevent the development of pressure areas. Fluid tends to collect in the dependent parts of the body such as the lower limbs and the sacral area in bed patients. These areas particularly should be monitored for signs of impending tissue breakdown, and measures should be taken to prevent this. See Chapter 25 for further discussion of pressure ulcers.

Meticulous skin care is important in the care of patients with renal impairment, not only as a factor in maintaining skin integrity, but also to cleanse the skin of perspiration and rid the patient of any unpleasant odours arising from the accumulation of nitrogenous wastes being eliminated by this route. Bathing is particularly important for the patient's cleanliness and comfort.

In an effort to compensate for the decreased ability of the kidneys to excrete excess acid, an increased amount of carbonic acid is eliminated through the respiratory tract. Measures to facilitate breathing are therefore important. The position of the patient when in bed should be such that maximum expansion of the chest is possible. The room should be well ventilated, and an adequate supply of oxygen ensured.

Accumulated nitrogenous wastes may cause disturbances in neuromuscular functioning. Headaches and lethargy are not uncommon, and in severe cases of renal impairment, the patient may become disoriented and subsequently comatose. In these cases, it is especially important to consider the safety needs of the patient. Although the sensorium can remain clear even in patients with considerable kidney damage, the nurse must be alert to any signs of mental confusion. Measures such as side rails to protect the confused patient from injury and the application of mitts to prevent pulling at catheters or other tubing are frequently needed.

Muscle weakness may result from the retention of potassium, and the renal patient is usually easily fatigued. The heart is particularly susceptible to changes in potassium levels. Therefore, the apical heartbeat provides a more accurate assessment of the patient's cardiac status.

At times, if the kidneys have ceased to function adequately or if the kidneys need to be put at complete rest in an effort to promote recovery, the patient will be put on *renal dialysis*. This can be accomplished by means of *hemodialysis* or *peritoneal dialysis*.

Hemodialysis removes waste products and excess water by circulating blood from an artery through an external dialyzer (sometimes referred to as an artificial kidney). Waste products are removed by the process of diffusion across a semipermeable membrane which mimics the processes of filtration, reabsorption and secretion normally carried out by the kidney. The composition of the *dialysis fluid* on one side of the membrane is the same as the blood with the exception of urea and other waste products. Thus, movement of the waste products across the membrane occurs by diffusion and filtration. The cleansed blood is then returned to the patient through a vein. Several types of machines for renal dialysis are now available, including units for home use. Some patients require renal dialysis for a short period of time, until recovery from the acute episode has been achieved. However, many individuals with nonfunctioning kidneys and no hope of recovery have been maintained on dialysis over a period of years. For those patients without access to home dialysis, outpatient departments or renal clinics provide dialysis on a scheduled basis, usually three times a week.

In place of hemodialysis, patients may be treated by **peritoneal dialysis**. This technique requires large amounts of *dialyzing fluid* to be instilled into the peritoneal cavity and later removed. Dialysis occurs in this method by the circulation of waste products through the peritoneal capillaries diffusing across the peritoneal membrane into the dialysis fluid. This procedure has been refined to the extent that the patients no longer need be hospitalized and are taught to do dialysis at home.

The initial experience of undergoing renal dialysis can be very frightening for the patient. Often the individual is very ill, and the exposure to highly technical machinery, the numerous personnel involved and the attendant tests required can provoke anxiety. Many large acute-care hospitals are equipped with renal units staffed by specially trained personnel who can provide the thorough explanations required to allay patient anxiety. However, the nurse in the general patient areas or in the community should be aware of patients' (and families') need for continuing encouragement and supportive care. It is important for the nurse to consider the patient ability to adjust to the effects of renal failure as a chronic condition. Stress, such as that caused by the inability of the individual to work, may be a significant factor to be addressed in the nursing care plan.

Once the patient's condition is stabilized, the patient is usually treated on an outpatient basis. For some, dialysis may be done in the home environment. On occasion, however, these individuals may require hospitalization. Usually all that is required is notifying the renal unit of the patient's admission and noting the scheduled times for dialysis on the patient's kardex. However, the nurse in the general patient areas should also be aware of the need to assess the patient's access site for dialysis. Normally, a thrill can be felt by palpation over the vascular access site or a bruit can be heard by use of a stethoscope. This would indicate patency of the site used for individuals on hemodialysis. A sign indicating that no venipunctures or blood pressures be done on this arm should be posted above the patient's bed.

For the patient on peritoneal dialysis, the nurse should assess the peritoneal catheter insertion site. Usually the patient can be provided with the necessary supplies and is able to change the dressing independently. If assistance from the nurse is required, the dressing around the catheter should be changed daily and whenever necessary.

EVALUATING URINARY ELIMINATION INTERVENTIONS

The expected outcomes established in the planning phase of the nursing process provide the basis for evaluating the effectiveness of nursing interventions. Changes in the patient's plan for care are made accordingly. Examples of questions the nurse might ask in evaluating care for urinary elimination problems are given below.

1. Is the patient voiding an adequate amount in relation to fluid intake?
2. Are the laboratory test results showing improvement in the patient's condition?
3. Does the patient maintain voluntary control of micturition?
4. Can the patient state or identify factors that interfere with his or her normal voiding pattern?
5. Can the patient describe measures to promote or maintain normal urinary elimination.
6. Is the patient's skin in good condition?
7. Is the patient comfortable — free from pain, restlessness and anxiety?

KEY TERMS

nephron p. 532

ureters p. 533

urinary bladder p. 533

urethra p. 533

meatus p. 533

micturition p. 533

prostate gland p. 535

urinary incontinence p. 536

stress incontinence p. 536

dysuria p. 536

frequency p. 536

urgency p. 536

nocturia p. 536

enuresis p. 536

polyuria p. 536

IN REVIEW

The primary functions of urinary elimination are to remove nitrogenous waste products and to regulate fluid and electrolyte balance. Both of these functions are essential in the maintenance of chemical homeostasis of the blood. When urinary elimination is impaired, all body systems may be affected and the individual may become very ill.

For most people, the act of voiding is a private matter and an important area of independent functioning. Control over voiding is learned early in childhood. Actual or potential loss of this control can lead to fear of a return to the dependent state of infancy and feelings of reduced self-esteem.

The urinary tract consists of two kidneys, two ureters, a bladder and a urethra. The kidneys primarily function to control the composition and volume of body fluids (including blood), and to excrete excess fluids, electrolytes and nitrogenous wastes, as well as toxic substances and drugs. These functions are accomplished through the complex processes of filtration, selective reabsorption and secretion in which essential elements needed by the body are retained and waste products are removed in the form of urine. Urine is transported from the kidneys to the urinary bladder by way of the ureters. The urinary bladder is a distensible muscular sac which holds the urine and the urethra is a short, muscular tube which carries the urine from the bladder to its exit point from the body. Normal urine is clear and straw-coloured or light amber in appearance.

Micturition (urination) is both voluntary and involuntary. The average adult usually excretes between 1000 and 1500 ml of urine in a 24-hour period. The total volume varies with the amount of fluid intake as well as with the amount of fluids lost through other routes, such as perspiration, vomiting or diarrhea.

Urinary functioning changes throughout the life cycle and is affected by individual differences, fluid and food intake, psychological states (such as stress, anxiety and pain), states of disease and illness and associated medical treatments. For example, medications that depress the central nervous system can inhibit voluntary control of micturition. Common urinary problems include localized disturbances such as incontinence, dysuria, frequency, urgency, nocturia, polyuria, oliguria, anuria and retention. The impairment of renal function can cause generalized problems affecting most systems of the body. Renal dialysis may be used when the kidneys have ceased to function adequately or when they need to rest in an effort to promote healing. Some medical problems of the urinary tract such as trauma, dis-ease or congenital anomalies of the bladder may require urinary diversion. Urine is eliminated from the body through a urostomy, an artificial opening which is created to divert urine from the kidneys to the abdominal wall.

A urinary status assessment includes the nursing health history, physical assessment and review of laboratory data. Notable areas of assessment include usual patterns of urination and toileting, urinary control, the presence of urinary diversions, characteristics of urine output (colour, odour, consistency, amount and the presence of abnormal constituents), kidney tenderness, bladder distention and dysuria. Intake and output measurements are necessary in monitoring patients with urinary dysfunction. Nurses are responsible for collecting urine specimens, performing dipstick examinations, and preparing patients for diagnostic procedures.

Common nursing diagnoses for patients with urinary elimination problems are: *Incontinence* and *Urinary retention*. When the etiologic or contributing factors for incontinence are known, the diagnostic statement should identify the specific nature of the problem. For example, for a woman who experiences leakage of small amounts of urine whenever she sneezes, coughs, or laughs, the diagnostic label would be: *Stress incontinence*.

Nursing care (planning and implementing) for individuals with urinary elimination problems is based on the nursing diagnoses and focusses on promoting optimal urinary elimination, maintaining or restoring normal patterns and preventing associated problems such as skin breakdown and infection.

Restorative care includes measures to reestablish normal voiding patterns (bladder retraining programs), measures to stimulate micturition, urinary catheterization, external urinary drainage and measures to reduce the workload on the kidneys. Urinary catheterization carries a high risk of infection. Meticulous aseptic technique is essential during every phase of catheter care from insertion to removal.

Methods of external urinary drainage are sometimes used instead of catheterization for patients unable to control urination. Protective pants made of a nonabsorbent plastic or rubberized material are worn over an absorbent pad. An external urinary appliance, called a condom catheter, is often used by men.

Individuals with urostomies may need assistance in carrying out their usual routines when they are ill or hospitalized. This can include changing an external urostomy appliance or assisting with a urostomy catheterization.

LEARNING ACTIVITIES

1. Mrs. Smith needs an indwelling catheter prior to her surgery tomorrow afternoon. Mrs. Smith is an intelligent person; she understands the purpose of her surgery, but she has never had a urinary catheterization. The catheter is to be inserted tomorrow morning.

   This afternoon Mrs. Smith's husband comes to the nursing unit desk greatly disturbed. His wife has told him that she has to have a tube inserted and he does not understand why. In talking with Mr. Smith, you learn that his mother had a tube inserted and she died two days later.

   a) What factors should you consider in your explanation?

   b) What should you include in your explanation to Mr. Smith? Why?

   c) What principles would guide you in carrying out a urinary catheterization?

   d) Why is a urinary catheterization a distressing measure?

   e) What nursing interventions would be essential for Mrs. Smith, as a result of the indwelling catheter?

   f) How can you evaluate the effectiveness of your nursing care after the catheterization?

   g) What problems could Mrs. Smith encounter following removal of the indwelling catheter?

   h) What would you teach Mrs. Smith following removal of the indwelling catheter?

2. With the aid of your instructor, arrange to spend a day with an enterostomal therapist in your agency. How does the enterostomal therapist establish a teaching plan for a patient with a urinary diversion? What techniques does he or she use in helping individuals learn how to manage their urostomies?

REFERENCES AND READINGS

ALLEN, P. (1992). Nursing care: Kock pouch continent urinary diversion — the Hamilton experience. *Canadian Association for Enterostomal Therapy, 11*(4), 17–19.

BERGER, K.J. and WILLIAMS, M.B. (1992). *Fundamentals of nursing: Collaborating for optimal health*. Norwalk, CT: Appleton & Lange.

BRINK, C. (1980). Promoting urine control in older adults: Assessing the problem. *Geriatric Nursing, 1*, 241–245.

BRISTOLL, S., FADDEN, T., FEHRING, R., ROHDE, L., SMITH, P. and WOHLITZ, B. (1989). The mythical danger of rapid urinary drainage. *American Journal of Nursing, 89*(3), 344–345.

BROWN, J., MEIKLE, J. and WEBB, C. (1991). Collecting midstream specimens of urine — the research base. *Nursing Times, 87*(13), 49–52.

CARPENITO, L.J. (1993). *Nursing diagnosis: Application to clinical practice* (5th ed.). Philadelphia: Lippincott.

EARNEST, V.V.(1993). *Clinical skills in nursing practice* (2nd ed.). Philadelphia: Lippincott.

FARRELL, J. (1990). *Nursing care of the older person*. Philadelphia: Lippincott.

FISCHBACH, F.A. (1992). *Manual of laboratory and diagnostic tests* (4th ed.). Philadelphia: Lippincott.

KENNER, C.A. and MACLAREN, A. (1993). *Essentials of maternal and neonatal nursing*. Springhouse, PA: Springhouse.

KOHLER-OCKMON, J. (1993). Catheter concerns. *Nursing Times, 89*(2), 34–36.

KUMAR, K.T. (1991, Spring). Surgery for cancer of the bladder. *Ostomy Quarterly*. 71–73.

LEWIS, S.M. and COLLIER, I.C. (1992). *Medical-surgical nursing: Assessment and management of clinical problems* (3rd ed.). St. Louis: Mosby.

MACLEOD, F. and MACTAVISH, M. (1988). Adult incontinence. *Canadian Nurse, 84*(8), 45–47.

MARTINI, F. (1989). *Fundamentals of anatomy and physiology*. Englewood Cliffs, NJ: Prentice-Hall.

MCCORMICK, K.A., NEWMAN, D.K., COLLING, J. and PEARSON, B.D. (1992). Urinary incontinence in adults. *American Journal of Nursing, 92*(10), 75–88.

MILNE, A. (1993). Men only: Male catheterisation procedures. *Nursing Times, 89*(8), 55–58.

MOORE, K. (1992). Indwelling catheters: problems and management. *The Canadian Nurse, 88*(6), 33–35.

MURRAY, R.B. and ZENTNER, J.P. (1993). *Nursing assessment and health promotion: Strategies through the life span* (5th ed.). Norwalk, CT: Appleton & Lange.

NESKY, K. and LOEHNER, D. (1994). Urinary diversion with an Indiana pouch. *Nursing 94, 24*(1), 32c–32h.

NEWMAN, D.K., LYNCH, K., SMITH, D. and CELL, P. (1991). Restoring urinary continence. *American Journal of Nursing, 91*(1), 28–36.

OROVAN, W.L. (1992). Kock pouch continent urinary diversion: The Hamilton experience. *Canadian Association for Enterostomal Therapy, 11*(4), 11–16.

PEARSON, B. (1993). Liquidate a myth: Reducing liquid intake is not advisable for elderly with urine control problems. *Urologic Nursing, 13*(3), 86–87.

PILLITTERI, A. (1992). *Maternal and child healthy nursing: Care of the childbearing and childrearing family*. Philadelphia: Lippincott.

ROBERTS, A. and GARDINER, P. (1991). Systems of life: The urinary system. *Nursing Times, 87*(28), 51–54.

SMITH, S. and DUELL, D. (1992). *Clinical nursing skills: Nursing process model, basic to advanced skills*. Norwalk, CT: Appleton & Lange.

TAYLOR, C., LILLIS, C. and LEMONE, P. (1993). *Fundamentals of nursing: The art and science of nursing care* (2nd ed.). Philadelphia: Lippincott.

TOOTLA, J. and EASTERLING, A.D. (1992). Current options in bladder cancer management. *RN, 55*(4), 42–49.

WEBBER-JONES, J. (1991). Performing clean, intermittent self-catheterization. *Nursing 91, 21*(8), 56–59.

WOZNIAK-PETROFSKY, J. (1993). Fundamental urodynamics (part one): Normal bladder function and patient assessment. *Urologic Nursing, 13*(3), 88–92.

CHAPTER 21

Bowel Elimination Needs

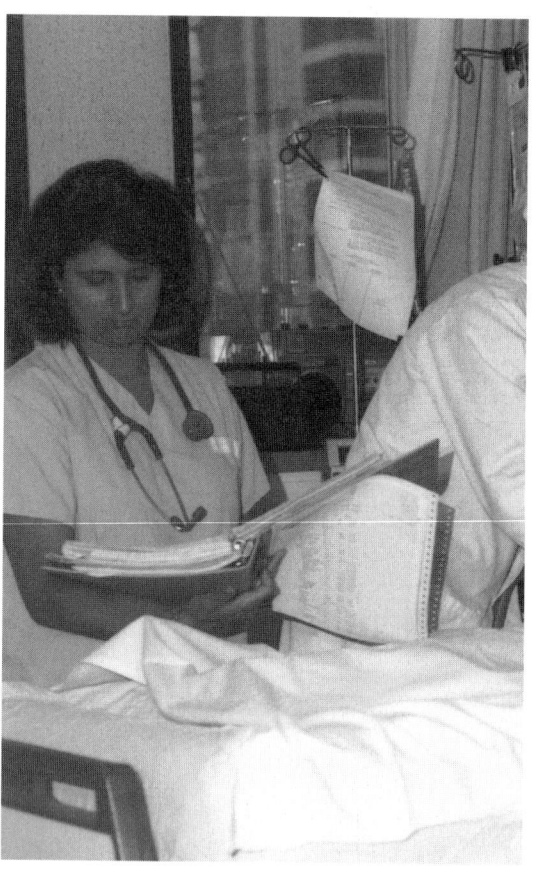

1. In what way is bowel elimination important to health and well-being?

2. What are the structures and functions involved in bowel elimination?

3. How does bowel elimination vary throughout the life cycle?

4. What are the main determinants of bowel functioning?

5. What are some common bowel elimination problems?

6. What basic principles would the nurse apply in assisting individuals to meet bowel elimination needs?

7. How does the nurse assess an individual's bowel elimination status?

8. What are the common nursing diagnostic statements for individuals with bowel elimination problems?

9. How would the nurse develop a plan of care for individuals with bowel elimination problems?

10. What strategies might the nurse implement in helping individuals, families or groups to promote optimal bowel functioning and prevent potential bowel elimination problems?

11. What health restoring and supportive strategies might the nurse implement in the care of individuals with bowel elimination problems?

12. How would the nurse evaluate the individual's response to nursing interventions?

INTRODUCTION

Bowel elimination is the excretion of gastrointestinal waste products. The maintenance of normal bowel elimination is an essential part of health. A proper diet, adequate intake of fluids, exercise and regular bowel habits contribute to healthy bowel elimination patterns. Anyone can encounter difficulty maintaining bowel elimination at one time or another. For example, a person may develop mild constipation or diarrhea after eating certain foods or may suffer severe diarrhea from a bout of gastrointestinal flu. Illness, travel, medications, surgery or a change in activity and eating patterns can disrupt normal patterns of elimination.

While most bowel elimination problems are not serious, individuals usually feel uncomfortable and are often distressed. If a disruption in bowel elimination is not restored, the functioning of all other body systems may be affected. For instance, prolonged and severe diarrhea can lead to such problems as nutritional deficits, water and electrolyte imbalances, alterations in comfort, and impaired skin integrity. In developing countries, infectious diarrhea is the most significant cause of infant and early childhood mortality. Individuals may need assistance to maintain or promote normal bowel elimination patterns or to restore their usual pattern of elimination when a disturbance has occurred.

This chapter provides basic knowledge of the physiology of bowel elimination, the factors that affect bowel function and common bowel elimination problems. This knowledge will enable the nurse to assess a person's bowel elimination needs and plan individualized care. Nursing interventions for helping people to promote normal bowel patterns in daily living; to prevent bowel disruption during illness, diagnostic testing and medical treatment; and to restore bowel function following illness are also outlined.

ANATOMY AND PHYSIOLOGY OF BOWEL ELIMINATION

During digestion, food and fluids taken into the body are mixed and processed, nutrients are selected and absorbed for utilization by body tissues and the waste products of digestion are excreted. The principal structures of the gastrointestinal tract concerned with elimination are the small and large intestine.

The *small intestine* is a narrow muscular tube approximately 2.5 cm in diameter and 6.4 m in length. It consists of three sections: the duodenum, jejunum and ileum (see Figure 21.1). Food in the stomach is propelled into the small intestine by stimulation of the gastrocolic reflex. The duodenum receives food, in the form of chyme (viscous, liquid contents of the stomach), from the stomach about half an hour after ingestion. Chyme moves through the small intestine slowly via wave-like contraction and relaxation of

smooth muscles (peristalsis). It mixes with digestive enzymes from the gallbladder and pancreas, further breaking down food for digestion. This mixing action is called segmenting. The duodenum is the primary site for iron and calcium absorption; the jejunum absorbs fats, proteins and carbohydrates; and the ileum absorbs specific vitamins and bile salts (Society of Gastroenterology Nurses and Associates, 1993). By the time chyme reaches the large bowel, it consists mostly of nondigestible substances.

When chyme has moved through the small intestine, the duodenocolic reflex is initiated and pushes the digestive content into the large intestine.

The large intestine is larger in diameter than the small intestine (5 cm), but is shorter in length (5.5 m). Divisions of the large intestine include the cecum; the ascending, transverse, descending and sigmoid colon; and the rectum (see Figure 21.1). The large intestine's primary functions are the absorption of water, electrolytes and remaining nutrients; the synthesis of vitamins; and the storage and elimination of feces.

The cecum receives unabsorbed chyme from the small intestine and, through peristalsis, moves it forward through the colon. Most absorption of water, nutrients and electrolytes, such as sodium and chloride, occurs in the cecum, ascending and transverse colons. The amount of water that is absorbed is dependent on the speed of peristaltic action. If propelled too rapidly, the resultant stool will be loose and watery. If peristalsis is too slow, water will continue to

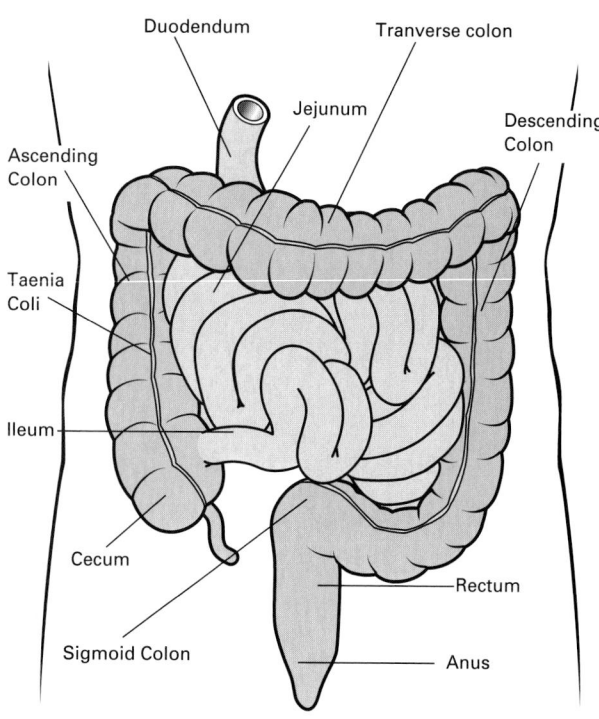

FIGURE 21.1 The small and large intestines

be absorbed and the stool will become dry and hard. The synthesis of certain vitamins, including folic acid, riboflavin and vitamin K, occurs in the large bowel aided by the activity of intestinal bacteria. Bacteria are typically found in the intestinal cavity and are often referred to as normal intestinal flora. If bowel function is impaired, serious nutritional and electrolyte imbalances can develop.

Finally, the distal colon (descending and sigmoid colons) stores and removes waste products and gas (flatus). To protect itself from injury as the waste moves towards the rectum and becomes drier, the distal colon releases mucus. Waste products are stored in the sigmoid colon and are called *feces*. Normal feces consist of digestive residues and water, with water making up approximately 75 percent of the total. Digestive residues include those from undigested and unabsorbed foods and from digestive secretions. The feces also contain cells and mucus sloughed off the lining of the gastrointestinal tract, as well as bacteria. Added to the resident bacteria are those that have been ingested through food and fluids, from fingers or in swallowed air.

When feces and flatus accumulate in the sigmoid colon, the muscle layers are stimulated to contract. Mass peristaltic movements force the feces into the rectum. These movements are strong and occur only a few times a day. The rectum is normally empty of stool. In the adult, the rectum is approximately 12 to 15 cm in length and 2.5 to 4 cm in width at the anal opening. The walls of the rectum consist of transverse and vertical folds. The transverse folds assist in keeping the feces in the rectum until defecation (the act of emptying stool from the anus and rectum) is initiated. The vertical folds each contain an artery and veins. Hemorrhoids occur when the veins become engorged due to pressure from straining during defecation.

The anal canal forms approximately the last 2.5 cm of the rectum. Two muscular sphincters control the discharge of feces from the anus. The internal sphincter is composed of smooth muscle and its control is involuntary, responding to distention of the rectum; the external sphincter is composed of striated muscle and is under voluntary control.

The rectal reflex is initiated when the rectum is full. Parasympathetic nerve endings transmit impulses to the brain to initiate the rectal reflex. The internal sphincter of the anus relaxes and the colon contracts. The urge to have a bowel movement is felt. However, the external sphincter can be controlled voluntarily so if the time is not suitable for defecation, the act of defecation can be delayed and the urge to defecate will disappear.

During the act of defecation, the external sphincter relaxes and a number of accessory muscles are brought into play. Contraction of the muscles of the abdominal wall and fixing of the diaphragm increase pressure within the abdominal cavity which aids expulsion of feces. Closing of the glottis by holding the breath while bearing down also increases intra-abdominal pressure. This is called a Valsalva manoeuvre. Finally, defecation can be assisted by assuming the sitting position.

BOWEL FUNCTIONING IN HEALTH

Normal stools are brown in colour (due to the presence of urobilinogen), soft and solid in consistency and cylindrical in shape. The amount of fecal matter excreted is highly dependent on the coarseness of the foodstuffs consumed. It may vary from 100 to 200 gm per day in a person whose diet contains a large proportion of refined food to 300 to 400 gm per day in the person who eats a diet high in fibre. The number of bowel movements a person has also varies from one individual to another, with the average being between one or two bowel movements every day to one movement every two to three days. Fecal odour is caused by the by-products of bacterial activity. Flatus (air or gas in the intestine) is formed by bacterial action on the digestive products, diffusion of gas from the blood stream and from swallowing air while eating or talking. It is estimated that 400 to 700 ml of flatus is produced daily (Guyton, 1991).

BOWEL ELIMINATION THROUGHOUT THE LIFE CYCLE

Bowel elimination patterns are affected by growth and development throughout the life cycle. Knowledge of the variations in bowel function and stool characteristics will assist the nurse in assessing patients and determining their elimination needs.

The first bowel movement of the newborn infant is called **meconium**; it is a greenish black, tarry substance that is present in the gastrointestinal tract of the full-term fetus. During the first week of life, stools gradually change from greenish black to yellow. Because the infant's stomach is small and peristalsis is rapid, food moves quickly through the digestive tract. Breast-fed infants may have four to six bowel movements a day, and bottle-fed babies one to three a day. In breast-fed babies the stools are usually looser and lighter yellow in colour and do not have as strong a fecal odour as those of bottle-fed babies. Breast-fed babies also rarely develop constipation, although they may do so when they are weaned, if their fluid intake is not sufficient. With the addition of solids to the diet, the stools become fewer in number, darker brown in colour and firmer in consistency.

Infants and young toddlers normally have a bowel movement whenever the rectum is full. The necessary neuromuscular development for voluntary control is usually not present until the age of two to three years (Guyton, 1991). By four years, most children have fairly good control over defecation, although accidents may still happen if the child is in a stressful situation, is too busy to go to the bathroom or has diarrhea.

The elimination patterns of school-age children and adolescents tend to remain fairly constant. However, there is rapid growth of the large intestine during the teenage years and an increase in the amount of food consumed.

Among adults variations in bowel patterns occur in pregnant women and in older people. During pregnancy, the entire gastrointestinal tract becomes more sluggish owing to the relaxing effect of hormones on smooth muscle. This, combined with the pressure of the growing uterus on the abdominal organs, causes constipation. Hemorrhoids also frequently occur in pregnant women and add to the discomfort of bowel elimination.

In the older adult, many changes occur that influence elimination. Appetite decreases and the ability to chew food thoroughly may be reduced by the loss of teeth or poorly fitting dentures. Partially chewed food enters the digestive tract and is processed less efficiently because of the decrease in digestive enzyme secretions. Also, peristaltic action slows down and the absorptive ability of the intestinal mucosa changes. There is weakening of the muscle tone in the perineal floor and the anal sphincter, as well as slowing of the rectal reflex nerve impulses. The older adult is more likely to experience constipation and may have difficulty controlling bowel elimination.

DETERMINANTS OF BOWEL FUNCTIONING

In addition to the variations that occur at different stages in the life cycle, many other factors affect bowel functioning. These include health practices such as dietary and fluid intake patterns, personal habits, activity and exercise. Illness, pain, emotions, surgery and anesthesia, and medications also influence bowel elimination.

Dietary pattern and fluid intake   The type of food and the amount of fluids a person consumes influence both the nature and frequency of bowel movements. An adequate amount of fibre in the diet is important in providing sufficient bulk to stimulate peristaltic action of the intestines. Fibre is the undigestible residue in food. It absorbs water which increases stool mass and keeps the stool soft. Raw fruits and vegetables, greens and whole grains contain high amounts of fibre. Natural bran has the highest fibre content of any food and is the most satisfactory bulking agent (Jensen, 1990). People whose diet consists mostly of highly refined foods usually have fewer bowel movements and their stools are likely to be firmer and darker in colour than those who ensure that they include high-fibre foods in their daily diet.

Certain foods cause flatus in some individuals. Flatus stimulates peristalsis by distending the bowel wall and it can cause abdominal discomfort. Some notoriously gas-forming foods are cabbage, turnips, onions and beans. Fried and spicy foods can cause peristalsis and watery stools. Food-borne infection may also cause gastrointestinal upsets.

An adequate daily intake of water and other fluids (1900 to 2400 ml) is necessary to maintain the soft consistency of feces (Basch and Jenson, 1991). Reduced fluid intake slows the passage of food through the bowel and makes stool harder. In some individuals, hot liquids stimulate peristalsis and milk causes constipation.

Personal habits   Elimination habits affect bowel function. Most people have established a habit of emptying their bowels at a certain time of the day or ingesting certain foods to stimulate peristalsis. A glass of hot water with lemon juice or a cup of coffee before breakfast often promotes regularity. Many people benefit from eating prunes at breakfast or eating a bowl of bran flakes before going to bed at night. Others habitually take laxatives, or use suppositories to clear their bowels.

Bathroom facilities play an important role in maintaining a regular pattern of elimination. People enjoy the convenience and privacy of their own toilet facilities and are often uncomfortable in situations such as the hospital where bathrooms may be shared. The odours and sounds associated with using the toilet in a shared environment are often embarrassing and can encourage an individual to ignore the urge to defecate. This can lead to constipation.

Activity and exercise   Daily exercise helps to improve muscle tone, stimulate peristaltic action and promote digestion. Inactivity contributes to constipation, and prolonged sitting is conducive to hemorrhoids. People who are bedridden lose tone in their abdominal and pelvic floor muscles very rapidly, and constipation can become a serious problem. Therefore, early ambulation is important after illness or injury to maintain normal bowel function.

Medications   Medications may also affect bowel functioning. Laxatives act by softening stool, lubricating stool or stimulating peristalsis. They are a safe aid to defecation if used properly. However, misuse can cause the intestine to lose muscle tone and, over time, the bowel will become less responsive to the medication. Constipation or diarrhea may result from laxative misuse.

Drugs that depress the nervous system lessen the motility of the intestines and have constipating side effects. Narcotic analgesics, such as morphine, and anticholinergics, such as atropine, are examples. Iron preparations cause constipation in many individuals. Antibiotics, on the other hand, may cause diarrhea by changing the normal bacterial flora in the gastrointestinal tract.

Anesthesia and surgery   Agents used for general anesthesia impair bowel motility temporarily by blocking the nerve impulses to the intestinal muscles. Peristalsis slows or stops entirely. In addition, surgery that involves direct handling of the intestine stops peristalsis. According to Erwin-Toth and Doughty, it is normal for peristalsis to be affected for a period of 24 to 48 hours after surgery (1992).

This condition is known as paralytic ileus. Further delay in the return of bowel motility occurs if the surgical patient does not ambulate quickly.

Pain   Defecation is normally painless; however, certain conditions may cause discomfort. These include hemorrhoids, anorectal surgery and perianal skin irritation. People who experience pain on defecation may suppress the urge to defecate, and this results in constipation.

Emotions   The effect of emotions on bowel functioning is not to be underestimated. Stress and anxiety stimulate the parasympathetic nervous system to speed up digestive and peristaltic action so that nutrients may be utilized for defence. Diarrhea and gaseous distention often result. Sadness or depression can have the opposite effect on the digestive tract as these emotions tend to slow peristalsis.

Other illnesses   There are many congenital abnormalities, injuries and disease processes that affect bowel functioning. For example, some infants are born with Hirschprung's disease, a condition in which the intestinal ganglia are absent. This results in failure of the internal sphincter to relax, resulting in severe constipation. Persons with spinal cord injuries may lose control of defecation because of damage to the parasympathetic nerves in the sacral area which normally transmit the rectal reflex. Incontinence of feces may result. And persons with ulcerative colitis may experience diarrhea as a symptom of the disease.

COMMON PROBLEMS

Because of the multitude of factors that affect bowel function, the nurse is likely to encounter patients with bowel problems in all age groups and practice settings. Common bowel problems include constipation, fecal impaction, diarrhea, incontinence and hemorrhoids.

Constipation   **Constipation** refers to the passage of infrequent, hard, dry stools. Feces become hard and dry when peristalsis is slowed or delayed and water content is absorbed.

There are many causes of constipation. The most frequent causes are the self-induced failure to respond to the urge to defecate because of the pressures of time, inconvenient bathrooms or lack of privacy; insufficient dietary fibre and fluid; and lack of daily exercise. Immobility and extended bedrest can contribute to constipation. Constipation can be induced by medications such as opiates, anticholinergics and iron which slow the motility of the intestine. Strong emotions are believed to be responsible for constipation through the increased production of epinephrine, with resulting inhibition of peristalsis. The physical changes of aging, including decreased peristalsis, weakness in abdominal and pelvic floor muscles, and reduced intestinal mucus secretion make the older adult prone to constipation. Gastrointestinal abnormalities can also cause constipation. These include congenital defects, bowel obstruction from tumours, neurological injury to the spine and paralytic ileus, to name but a few. Finally, pain from hemorrhoids or anal fissures can contribute to constipation (Jensen, 1990).

The person who is constipated usually complains of a "bloated" feeling. This is caused by abdominal distention, which results from the accumulation of gas when waste products remain too long in the gastrointestinal tract. Swallowed air makes up over 75 percent of intestinal gas. Other sources of intestinal gas include the consumption of gas-forming foods and the methane and carbon dioxide gases produced in the colon by bacterial action on food (Guyton, 1991). If not expelled, the gas can lead to crampy abdominal pain. Headache, anorexia and nausea are additional symptoms a constipated person may experience. These usually disappear upon defecation and the establishment of a healthier bowel pattern.

Painful straining in unproductive attempts at defecation is called **tenesmus**. Constipation and tenesmus are serious health hazards and efforts should be made to avoid these, particularly for people who have had recent rectal surgery or who have heart disease, glaucoma or increased intracranial pressure from a head injury.

Fecal impaction   Untreated constipation can lead to a large, hardened mass of stool that cannot be expelled. This condition is known as **fecal impaction**. The causes of fecal impaction include dehydration, immobility, medications, neurologic diseases and barium retention. The nurse should be alert to seepage of small amounts of liquid stool from the anus with accompanying symptoms of abdominal distention, cramping and inability to defecate despite the urge. These are indicators of fecal impaction. The seepage, caused by feces higher up in the bowel moving around the mass, can easily be mistaken as a bowel movement leaving the constipation problem overlooked.

Diarrhea   **Diarrhea** is the frequent discharge of loose, watery stools. There are many possible causes of diarrhea. Pre-examination diarrhea, resulting from emotional tension, is a fairly common occurrence among students. Medications, such as antacids, cathartics and antibiotics, may cause diarrhea. Diarrhea may result from dietary indiscretions such as eating coarse foods or an excessive amount of seasonings, alcohol or caffeine. It may occur as an allergic reaction to certain foods. Inflammation of the intestinal mucosa due to pathogenic organisms is a very common cause of diarrhea. Patients with inflammatory bowel diseases such as Crohn's and ulcerative colitis have diarrhea as a symptom of the disease because of anatomical defects in the bowel mucosa which interfere with the absorption of water and nutrients. Surgical operations in which significant portions of the bowel are removed, thus reducing the size of absorptive surface, can also lead to diarrhea.

Patients with diarrhea often complain of generalized abdominal pain. This is usually caused by flatus which distends the colon. As well, pains of a piercing, gripping nature are not uncommon. They are usually spasmodic in nature and are caused by the strong peristaltic contractions of the intestinal musculature as the waste products are propelled precipitously through the gastrointestinal tract. These pains are frequently accompanied by a feeling of urgency in the need to defecate. Although an increase in the number of stools is not always an indication of diarrhea, it often occurs with diarrhea. The frequency and the irritating nature of diarrheal stools often causes redness and *itchiness* around the anal area. Care must be taken to cleanse the area well after each movement.

If diarrhea is prolonged, fatigue, weakness and general malaise are experienced. In addition, the individual is in danger of fluid and electrolyte imbalance (see Chapter 22). Nausea and vomiting frequently accompany diarrhea and further aggravate the loss of fluids and electrolytes.

Incontinence   Incontinence of feces is lack of control over bowel evacuation and may vary from infrequent, minor soiling to the inability to control stool of normal consistency. The highest incidence of **fecal incontinence** is in the older population, most often caused by undetected fecal impaction or simply by degenerative changes in the muscles controlling defecation (Rothenberger and Orrom, 1991).

Diarrhea is another common cause of incontinence because some individuals cannot control the precipitous delivery of liquid stool to the rectum. Incontinence may also occur as a result of direct injury to the rectal sphincters from childbirth or surgery. Illnesses that impair the neural pathways transmitting impulses from the sacral area to the brain, for instance, stroke, spinal cord injury, tumour or multiple sclerosis, can also induce incontinence. Finally, incontinence may also occur in people with mental disorders in which awareness of the need to defecate is altered or awareness of what is socially acceptable behaviour is lost; dementia, confusion or severe depression are some examples (Basch and Jensen, 1991).

Fecal incontinence is a distressing problem which can cause great embarrassment and affect self-esteem. Defecation is very much a private matter, so soiling clothes in a social situation can be demoralizing. Fear of having an "accident" can lead to social isolation and this can be particularly harmful to the patient's psychological well-being. Incontinent patients may become extremely anxious and preoccupied with their bowels. The nurse must provide reassurance and support. In many cases, continence can be restored with a good bowel retraining program. This will be discussed in more detail later in the chapter. Scrupulous attention to personal hygiene is necessary since incontinence can cause severe perianal skin breakdown.

Hemorrhoids   **Hemorrhoids** are swollen veins of the anus or rectum. There are two types: internal or external.

Internal hemorrhoids cannot be seen as they develop above the anal sphincter. External hemorrhoids protrude through the anal opening and can be visualized. Increased pressure on the rectum and anus secondary to straining with constipation, pregnancy, obesity and abdominal tumours are the most common causes of hemorrhoids.

Hemorrhoids can cause bleeding, pain and itchiness. Usually they disappear with conservative treatment, such as warm baths, and preparations containing astringent or anesthetic agents, or a combination of both. A common astringent is witch-hazel, supplied in compresses known as Tucks. Anusol or Preparation H are examples of preparations containing astringent and local anesthetic properties. Surgery may be required for unresolved hemorrhoidal pain. Prevention of hemorrhoids can be achieved by proper diet, exercise and the use of stool softeners.

BOWEL DIVERSIONS

Some bowel diseases are so life-threatening or their symptoms are so severe that feces must be diverted from passing through the colon. A temporary or permanent artificial opening from the colon to the surface of the abdomen may be created surgically. The opening is called a **stoma**. An **ileostomy** (see Figure 21.2) is an opening from the ileum of the

FIGURE 21.2   Ileostomy. The shaded portion, namely the colon and rectum, is usually removed. The surgeon creates a stoma in the lower right hand quadrant of the abdomen.

small intestine to the abdominal wall, whereas a **colostomy** is an opening from the large intestine. A plastic pouch or bag must be worn over the stoma to collect the stool.

The nature and consistency of the fecal matter that flows from these ostomies are different. Since an ileostomy bypasses the large intestine, fecal discharge or effluent from an ileostomy is frequent and more liquid in consistency. The presence of digestive enzymes in the effluent causes irritation to the skin of the abdomen. Feces from a colostomy is generally formed and soft, more like normal stool.

There are three types of colostomies: end, loop and double-barrelled (see Figure 21.3). The type of colostomy the surgeon creates depends on the patient's medical problem. An *end colostomy* is usually constructed in the treatment of sigmoid or rectal colon cancer. This type of colostomy is usually permanent. The diseased portion of the bowel is removed and the proximal functioning portion is brought to the abdominal wall and sutured in place. Thus, one stoma is created.

A *loop colostomy* is usually created as a medical emergency when the bowel cannot be prepared for surgery, for example, in repairing a gunshot wound to the abdomen or a ruptured diverticulum. This type of colostomy is often performed on the transverse colon and is temporary. In other words, the physician expects to be able to reconnect the bowel at a later date once the bowel has healed. A loop of bowel is pulled up to the surface of the abdomen and a plastic rod is placed under the loop to prevent it from falling back into the abdominal cavity. The loop is sutured to the skin of the abdomen and is opened to create a stoma. This stoma has two openings: a proximal one that emits feces and a distal one that drains mucus. The rod is removed from beneath the stoma in approximately seven to ten days.

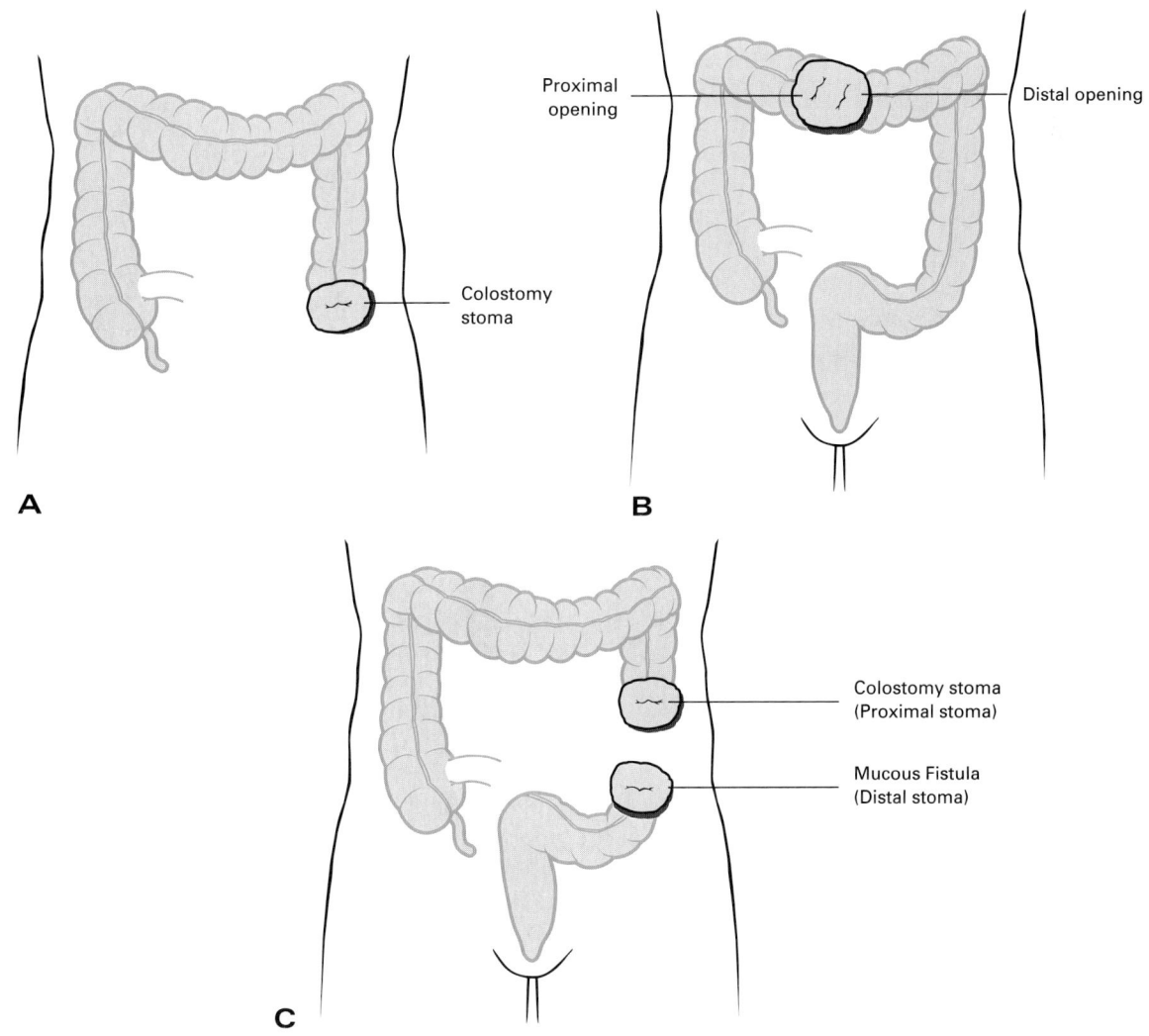

Proximal opening — Distal opening

Colostomy stoma

A

B

Colostomy stoma (Proximal stoma)

Mucous Fistula (Distal stoma)

C

FIGURE 21.3 Types of colostomies. A. End colostomy. B. Loop colostomy. C. Double-barrelled colostomy.

KEY PRINCIPLES

Principles Relevant to Bowel Functioning

1. The function of the bowels is to eliminate the waste products of digestion.
2. Normal bowel elimination is essential to efficient body functioning.
3. The body's fluid and electrolyte balance can be seriously affected by disturbances in bowel functioning.
4. Obstruction of the bowel poses a serious threat to life.
5. The oral intake of food or fluids stimulates a mass peristaltic action in the gastrointestinal tract.
6. The urge to defecate results from stimulation of the rectal reflex by distention of the lower colon and rectum.
7. The act of defecation is normally under voluntary control after the age of two to three years.
8. The necessary neuromuscular structures are not sufficiently developed for voluntary control over bowel elimination until the age of 15 to 18 months.
9. Once achieved, control over defecation is an important area of independent functioning for the individual.
10. The normal pattern of bowel elimination in individuals after infancy varies from one or two bowel movements every day to one bowel movement every two to three days.
11. Patterns of bowel elimination and consistency of feces are highly dependent on an individual's food and fluid intake.
12. Stress, anxiety, and other strong emotions may interfere with bowel functioning.

A *double-barrelled colostomy* has two separate stomas. Again, typically a temporary diversion, it is located most often in the descending colon. The affected part of the bowel is excised and both proximal and distal ends of the large intestine are brought to the abdominal surface. Like the loop colostomy, feces drains from the proximal stoma and mucus from the distal stoma. The term, double-barrelled, is sometimes confusing and this procedure is now often referred to as an *end stoma with a mucous fistula*. The mucous fistula is the distal stoma.

A pouch or ostomy appliance must always be worn for continence because the anal sphincter is removed or by-passed in diversional procedures. For ileostomy patients, the pouch must be emptied and cleaned frequently because the stool is so liquid. Management of the bag for the patient with a colostomy is less concerning as the stool is more solid and less frequent. Some people with colostomies can regulate their bowel movements by the food they eat, just as they would do if their bowel were intact. Others establish bowel regularity by irrigating their stoma every morning, although this procedure is not as highly recommended as it once was. Irrigations will be covered later in this chapter.

A great deal of sensitivity is needed by the nurse when caring for the patient with an ileostomy or colostomy. The operation itself is extensive and the alteration in bowel elimination patterns causes body image changes. Many people are repulsed by the stoma and are overwhelmed by the presence of the pouch and the care it requires. The inability to control defecation and the management of odour, gas and leakage of stool are major concerns to these patients.

ASSESSING BOWEL ELIMINATION NEEDS

To assess bowel elimination status, the nurse needs information about all of the factors that affect a patient's bowel functioning. This includes subjective data obtained in a health history and objective data gathered through physical assessment, observation of fecal characteristics and review of diagnostic test results. Information about the patient's illness or any diagnostic or treatment measures that may affect bowel functioning will be found in the chart.

THE NURSING HEALTH HISTORY

The nursing health history provides the nurse and other members of the health care team with baseline information about the patient's usual bowel habits and patterns of defecation. People vary in bowel elimination patterns so it is important to determine what the patient describes as "normal." The nurse can then ascertain whether bowel dysfunction exists, since what the patient considers to be normal may differ from the nurse's knowledge of the parameters of healthy elimination and the factors that influence it.

Knowledge of the normal process and the factors that affect elimination can assist the nurse in structuring the health history. Many people are embarrassed to talk about their bowel functioning. The nurse should take care to ask questions in simple, nontechnical language that allows the patient to provide pertinent information yet maintain feelings of dignity. Privacy during the interview helps to alleviate embarrassment. A guide for taking a health history pertaining to bowel elimination is outlined below.

Bowel Elimination
Health and Illness Patterns

USUAL PATTERN OF BOWEL ELIMINATION

* How often do you have bowel movements? What time of day?
* Describe a typical stool. Colour? Texture? Shape? Odour?
* Describe your usual routine for bowel elimination.
* Do you use any natural aids for defecation? A glass of warm water? A cup of coffee?
* Do you use any specific foods or fluids, laxatives, suppositories or enemas to aid elimination? If so, what type? How frequently?

For patients with bowel diversions:

* What type of ostomy do you have?
* What is your usual routine?
* Have you had any problems with your ostomy, for example, protrusion, retraction, or irritation?
* What assistance will you need in managing your ostomy?

RECENT CHANGES IN PATTERN OF BOWEL ELIMINATION

* Have you noticed any change in your normal pattern of elimination or stool characteristics? If so, describe the changes?
* Have there been any recent changes in your life that may be affecting your normal bowel pattern? Recent illness? Surgery? Stressful event? Travel? Change in diet or activity?

PRESENTING HEALTH PROBLEM

* Describe the symptoms you are experiencing now.

Constipation? Diarrhea? Bleeding? Excessive flatulence? Incontinence? Pain in the abdomen or rectum?

* Have you recently had any unintentional weight loss, appetite loss, unexplained fatigue or fever?
* How long have you had these symptoms?
* What remedies have you tried for the symptoms? What were the results?
* Do you have an acute or chronic condition that might be causing your bowel problem? For example, gastroenteritis, inflammatory bowel disease, polyps? Have you had surgery lately?
* Are you taking any medications (prescription and over-the-counter) or treatments for other health problems? If so, what are they? Dosage of medications?
* Has anyone in your family ever had cancer of the colon or rectum, or polyps?

Health Promotion and Protection Patterns

* Do you eat a regular, well-balanced diet high in fibre? Whole grain cereals and breads? Fresh fruit? Raw vegetables such as carrots and celery?
* Are you aware of certain foods that tend to cause bowel problems? If so, do you try to avoid them in your diet?
* How much and what type of fluid do you drink in a day?
* Do you participate in a regular exercise program?
* Do you smoke? If so, how much and for how many years?
* Do you drink products containing caffeine? How much and how often?

PHYSICAL ASSESSMENT

The physical assessment of bowel elimination status involves an examination of the abdomen, rectum and anus. The skills used for this assessment are inspection, auscultation and light palpation. Palpation is performed last because palpation stimulates peristalsis which may alter auscultation. Deep palpation and percussion are advanced nursing skills and, therefore, will not be discussed in this book.

THE ABDOMEN

Prior to beginning the abdominal assessment, the nurse should ensure that the patient has an empty bladder. The patient is then assisted into a supine position with hands by the side. The abdomen is exposed and the chest and pubic area are appropriately draped. The examiner's hands and the stethoscope should be warmed before touching the patient to prevent muscular contraction which can alter the findings.

Inspection The nurse inspects all four quadrants of the abdomen, noting contour, symmetry, skin colour and appearance, abdominal girth and abdominal movements. The presence of masses, scars or stomas should also be noted. Normally the contour of the abdomen is slightly rounded or flat. A concave abdomen might indicate weight loss and a protuberant abdomen may be caused by intestinal gas, a tumour, hernia or fluid in the peritoneal cavity from cirrhosis of the liver, for example. The abdomen is normally symmetrical; asymmetrical areas may be the result of previous surgery, weak muscles or a mass.

The skin on the healthy abdomen should look smooth and intact, and feel soft and supple. It should be free of abnormal colour, rashes, lesions or scars. For instance, if the individual has liver or biliary tract disease, the abdominal skin may appear jaundiced or yellow. If abdominal distention is severe, the nurse may see tense, glistening skin. In the case of a distended abdomen, the nurse should measure the abdomen's girth daily to determine if the distention is increasing. To measure abdominal girth, a measuring tape is placed around the abdomen at the widest point, usually the umbilicus. For accuracy, measures at this same anatomical landmark should be taken each day. Finally, the abdomen should be free of observable movements. Visible peristaltic waves may mean impending bowel obstruction.

Auscultation The abdomen is auscultated to evaluate bowel motility via bowel sounds. This is done by placing the diaphragm of the stethoscope over each of the four quadrants starting with the right lower quadrant (RLQ). The RLQ is the point at which the cecum and ileum join, so if bowel sounds are heard here it may not be necessary to listen further. Proceeding in a clockwise manner, the nurse listens to each quadrant for one full minute. Bowel sounds are caused by air and fluid moving through the intestine and usually occur every five to fifteen seconds. They are described as soft, bubbling or gurgling sounds. Hypoactive (infrequent or absent) bowel sounds occur normally after surgery or they may be related to advanced bowel obstruction. Hyperactive bowel sounds may be heard with early intestinal obstruction, diarrhea and hypermotility of the intestine related to hunger.

Light palpation Light palpation is used to identify abdominal distention, masses and areas of tenderness. The abdomen is normally soft and nontender. The nurse should ask the patient to identify any tender areas first and palpate that area last. If not contraindicated, the nurse begins at the RLQ and moves around the abdomen in a clockwise pattern. Using the dominant hand and with fingers close together, the nurse depresses the skin one to two centimetres, palpating in a dipping, rotating motion. The nurse then lifts the hands to the next site. It is important for the individual to breathe slowly during the examination to aid in the relaxation of the abdominal muscles. The nurse must distinguish between voluntary muscle guarding from coldness or ticklishness, and involuntary muscle rigidity from tissue inflammation or injury. Deep palpation of masses or specific body organs is not usually part of the nurse's routine physical abdominal assessment.

THE RECTUM AND ANUS

Usually, a rectal exam is performed only on a person over the age of 40; however, it may be performed on individuals of any age if they have a history of bowel elimination problems. Digital examination of the rectum is not routinely done by the nurse as a component of the physical assessment. However, when fecal impaction is suspected, the nurse may perform a rectal exam if institutional policy permits. To examine the anus, the nurse instructs the patient to assume a side-lying position on the bed or examination table. The upper leg is flexed towards the chest. Wearing a disposable glove, the nurse gently raises the buttock to view the anus. The anus and surrounding skin are inspected for external hemorrhoids, inflammation, scars, fissures, rectal prolapse or discharge. In addition, the tissue around the anus may be palpated for tenderness or nodules.

The nurse uses the physical findings of the abdominal and rectal assessment to supplement the information collected from the nursing history and records normal and abnormal findings in the patient's chart. The nurse can continue the assessment of bowel elimination by focussing on the characteristics of stool and diagnostic test results.

FECAL CHARACTERISTICS

Assessment of fecal characteristics is the nurse's responsibility. Knowledge of what normal stool is like assists the nurse in determining whether alterations in elimination exist. These characteristics are described in the box below. Stool may also be examined for other constituents, such as fat and pathogenic organisms. Stools that are clay-coloured indicate the absence of bile and the presence of fat. In this case, obstruction in the biliary tract might be suspected.

DIAGNOSTIC TESTS

Diagnostic examinations of the intestinal tract can reveal helpful information about elimination problems. Common procedures include direct and indirect visualization techniques and laboratory tests of feces. They are usually performed when there are changes in bowel habits, chronic constipation and blood or mucus in the stool (Kee, 1991).

VISUALIZATION STUDIES

Direct visualization techniques Direct visualization of the inner cavity of the anal canal, the rectum

Characteristics of Normal Feces

Colour	Brown
Consistency	Soft-formed
Shape	Cylindrical
Amount	Adult: 100–400 gm/day depending on coarseness
Frequency	Once or twice a day to 3 times a week
Odour	Pungent
Constituents	Undigested food, bacteria, cells lining the intestinal mucosa, water, fat and bile pigment

and the lower colon permits examination of the intestinal mucosa for disease, tumours, fissures or hemorrhoids and allows for the collection of tissue specimens. A tubular instrument or scope with an attached light source is inserted into the anal canal (anoscopy), the rectum (proctoscopy) or the sigmoid colon (sigmoidoscopy).

Prior to the test, the nurse ensures that the patient signs a consent form. An enema or suppository is usually given the evening before the examination and the morning of the test to clear the gastrointestinal tract of fecal material. The patient may be allowed a light breakfast. The nurse should explain that pressure or discomfort may be experienced as the instrument is introduced into the bowel and as air is injected to distend the bowel for better visualization.

For the examination, the patient is asked to assume a knee–chest position. If unable to do so, the Sims' position on the left side may be used. The patient should be draped carefully for comfort, privacy and to reduce embarrassment. Assisting the patient with relaxation breathing techniques, ensuring unnecessary exposure during the procedure, and offering reassurance that the discomfort is of short duration are helpful nursing measures during the procedure. The examination usually takes about 30 minutes. After the exam, the nurse observes the patient for rectal bleeding, abdominal pain and fever. The patient is also encouraged to rest for several hours.

Indirect visualization techniques

Indirect visualization of the bowel is achieved by x-ray examination and fluoroscopic examination. The small intestine is examined by an upper gastrointestinal (UGI) and small bowel follow-through test; the lower colon by a barium enema. Both tests use barium, a white chalky radiopaque substance, which is usually flavoured to enhance taste and facilitate ingestion. In the UGI series, meglumine diatrizoate (Gastrographin), a water-soluble contrast agent, may also be ingested. The UGI and small bowel follow-through study al-

lows the radiologist to observe for ulcerations of the intestinal mucosa, tumours or diverticula.

Again the nurse must have the patient sign a consent form. In preparation for the test, the patient must follow a low residue diet for two days prior to the examination and an enema may be ordered the evening before. The patient is permitted nothing by mouth after midnight. In the x-ray department, the patient will be given a barium meal or Gastrographin drink to swallow and the agent will be observed as it passes through the digestive tract. The patient is positioned supine on a tilting x-ray table which moves to various positions as x-rays are taken. The test can take four to six hours if the bowel series is included. After the examination the patient may resume eating. The patient should be instructed to increase fluid intake as barium is constipating. The doctor may order a laxative to aid excretion of the barium. Stools are light in colour for up to three days until the barium is expelled.

The barium enema permits observation of the large bowel for abnormalities. Nursing care prior to the procedure is similar to that for the UGI and small-bowel series except that a more extensive bowel preparation is required. The patient is restricted to clear fluids the day before the test and permitted nothing by mouth after midnight. A laxative and enemas to clear the bowel are given that same evening. Another enema or suppository is given the morning of the examination. It is the nurse's responsibility to ensure that the patient's bowel is clear of feces. During the examination, the patient lies on the tilt table and barium is administered slowly via a rectal tube. As different positions are assumed, bowel filling is monitored by spot x-rays. The procedure takes approximately one hour to complete. Posttest observations and instructions to the patient are the same as for the UGI series.

FECAL EXAMINATIONS

Collection of stool specimens   The collection of stool specimens for laboratory analysis is the responsibility of the nurse. The nurse must know why the stool specimen is required so that an appropriate container is used and the correct method for obtaining the specimen is carried out. For example, some specimen jars have preservative solution in them whereas others do not. Some tests require a single stool sample; others require a series of timed specimens. Agencies usually have a laboratory resource manual available which details the requirements for specific fecal examinations.

Gloves are always worn when handling stool specimens. A wooden tongue depressor is useful for transferring the stool from the bedpan or other receptacle to the specimen container. Care must be taken not to contaminate the outside of the container. These practices are necessary to lessen the chance of spreading microorganisms, since feces is largely composed of bacteria. The purpose of specimen collection determines the amount of stool needed. Generally about 2.5 cm or 15 to 30 ml of liquid stool is sufficient (Kee, 1991). Specimens must be labelled carefully and sent to the laboratory as quickly as possible along with the appropriate requisitions. If stool specimens are left at room temperature for a period of time, bacteriological changes can occur which could affect the accuracy of the test results.

In most cases, patients can obtain their own specimens. Instructions they will need in order to do this include the following:

- Defecate in a special receptacle that fits under the toilet seat or in a clean bedpan or commode.
- Avoid mixing the stool with urine or blood from menstruation (may alter test results).
- Avoid placing toilet paper in with the stool (may affect test results).
- Alert the nurse as soon after defecation as possible.

Test for occult blood **Occult blood** refers to microscopic amounts of blood in stool that are hidden to the naked eye on gross examination. A simple fecal test can detect occult bleeding in the intestinal tract. It is used as a screening test for colon cancer and in diagnosing conditions known to cause bleeding such as inflammatory bowel disease. The test can be carried out on the ward of an inpatient facility or in the home. There are several test products available; common ones are Hematest and Hemoccult slide. The testing instructions are given on the product packages and are easy to follow.

- For **Hematest**, apply a thin layer of stool on filter paper, add a tablet to the centre of the specimen and apply two drops of water. Time as directed and note colour changes.

- For **Hemoccult slide**, apply a thin smear of stool to both boxes of filter paper inside the slide package, add two drops of reagent solution to the paper and time. Note colour changes.

With both products, a blue colour change indicates a positive test for occult blood. Sometimes blood can be seen on a stool specimen quite easily. This may simply be indicative of bleeding hemorrhoids. More serious bleeding from the upper gastrointestinal tract usually results in black stools. This is called *melena*.

DIAGNOSING BOWEL ELIMINATION PROBLEMS

Problems with bowel elimination which are amenable to nursing intervention include constipation, diarrhea and incontinence. *Constipation* is the diagnosis used for problems in which elimination is infrequent and stools are hard and dry. These problems are often related to inadequate fibre in the diet, inadequate fluid intake, immobility, the use of constipating medications, pain on defecation or a change in routine. When patients pass three or more loose, liquid stools in a day, the diagnosis *Diarrhea* is appropriate. Diarrhea may be caused by stress, the side-effect of medications, an allergy, excessive spices in food or inflammation of the bowel. Diagnoses for problems in which people experience involuntary passage of stool because of such factors as fecal impaction, confusion or neuromuscular impairment from stroke or spinal cord injury are stated as *Bowel incontinence*.

Bowel elimination disturbances often cause other related problems that require nursing attention. For instance, bowel incontinence or prolonged diarrhea may lead to anal skin breakdown, and fecal seepage from a poorly fitting ileostomy pouch may cause skin breakdown around the stoma. In such cases the diagnoses *High risk for* or *Impaired skin integrity* would be used. Prolonged diarrhea is a very common cause of fluid volume deficit. When diarrhea is present, the nurse should always consider the problem *High risk for fluid volume deficit* in the plan of care.

People who have difficulty with bowel elimination often experience a disturbance in their body image, self-esteem, and coping capacity. Examples of nursing diagnoses for such problems might include: *Body image disturbance related to a colostomy or fecal incontinence*; *Self-esteem disturbance related to the need for digital removal of stool*; and *Ineffective individual coping related difficulty adapting to an ileostomy*. In addition, the diagnosis *Altered health maintenance* may be used for patients who need to learn how to live with and care for a bowel diversion, or those who require bowel retraining.

Following are two examples of nursing diagnoses made from assessment data:

Normal Constituents of Feces

Bulk	100-200 gm/24 hours (may be up to 300-400 depending on coarseness of diet)
Dry matter	32-64 gm/24 hours
Water	Approximately 75%
Total fat	Less than 6.0 gm/24 hours
Total nitrogen	Less than 2.0 gm/24 hours
Urobilinogen	50-300 mg/24 hours
Blood	Negative
Ova and Parasites	Negative

SOURCE: Springhouse Corporation, 1991, 437.

A. Data: Mrs. S, age 83, is bedridden because of arthritis. Her abdomen is distended and her bowel sounds have decreased. She says she feels full and has not eaten much food in the last few days. Her last bowel movement was four days ago.

Nursing Diagnosis:

- *Constipation related to inactivity from disability and insufficient fibre and fluid in the diet.*

B. Data: Mr. B reports having loose, watery brown stools with some blood for the last week. He has crampy abdominal pain when defecating. He is weak and has lost weight. He recently returned from a vacation in Peru where sanitary conditions were poor. He was not always able to drink bottled water and he ate some unfamiliar food.

Nursing Diagnosis:

- *Diarrhea related to possible bacterial invasion from contaminated water and food.*

PLANNING BOWEL ELIMINATION INTERVENTIONS

When planning care for the patient with elimination problems, the nurse includes the patient and family as much as possible. Because bowel habits are learned early in childhood and each individual's pattern of elimination is different, the plan of care must take into account previously established patterns. Previous healthy bowel habits should be maintained with an emphasis on incorporating new ones. Goals are generally directed towards understanding normal defecation; achieving a regular elimination pattern; understanding the influence of dietary fibre, fluids and exercise on bowel elimination; achieving comfort; and maintaining self-esteem.

Patient goals or expected outcomes are set for specific nursing diagnoses. Following are some examples of expected outcomes for bowel elimination problems.

Constipation:

- The patient will report soft, brown bowel movements every two days.
- The patient will report absence of pain or straining during defecation.
- The patient will verbalize ways to promote regular bowel habits, respond to the urge to defecate when it arises, eat high-fibre foods, increase fluid intake and exercise regularly.
- The patient will describe foods high in fibre.
- The patient will describe the hazards of laxative use and relate intent to avoid their use on a regular basis.

Diarrhea:

- The patient will report no more than two bowel movements per day.
- The patient will defecate brown, solid stool.
- The patient will relate intent to modify known factors which cause diarrhea: avoid intake of spicy foods, participate in relaxation techniques.

Bowel incontinence:

- The patient will pass a soft, formed stool in the bedpan, in the bathroom or on the commode every second or third day.

IMPLEMENTING BOWEL ELIMINATION INTERVENTIONS

HEALTH PROMOTING STRATEGIES

Bowel elimination is a very basic physiological need. Regular bowel evacuation helps to maintain physiological functioning by eliminating wastes from the body and promotes physical comfort and emotional well-being. Many people experience some degree of disruption in bowel elimination from time to time. Nurses can assist individuals to promote regular bowel evacuation in the course of daily living by providing information and encouraging them to examine their health habits and practices which affect elimination. The Health Promoting Strategy box gives a summary of guidelines to assist individuals in promoting healthy bowel elimination patterns. The major points are discussed more fully here.

Regularity Regularity of defecation is the key to maintaining healthy bowel habits. To establish regularity, one must defecate when the urge arises and take the time for elimination. People should select a convenient time in the day when they will not be rushed or disrupted by busy or changing work schedules. Since the urge to defecate is usually strongest after breakfast, this is a good time for a bowel elimination routine. Eliminating after breakfast is also beneficial because it allows for the act of defecation in the privacy of one's home. Many people suppress the urge to defecate when they are in a strange environment or when others are present.

Dietary pattern Normal elimination is influenced by diet. The type of foods and the amount of fluids consumed may impair or promote elimination. Foods high in fibre and a daily fluid intake of 1900 to 2400 ml is considered sufficient to maintain soft stool (Basch and Jensen, 1991). Eating a variety of foodstuffs containing complex carbohydrates with emphasis on cereals, breads and other whole grain products will ensure adequate fibre in the diet (Health and Welfare Canada, 1990). Fresh fruits, raw root vegetables such as carrots and celery and cooked fruits such as apricots and prunes are other good sources of fibre. A regular mealtime schedule will also help to maintain bowel regularity.

Certain foods cause gastrointestinal upsets such as flatulence, distention or cramping in some individuals. For example, cabbage, turnips, onions and beans often cause gas distention; fried, spicy foods tend to cause watery stools. Gum chewing and drinking alcohol and carbonated beverages may contribute to flatulence (BCDNA, 1992). People who experience such upsets should avoid foods and drinks they find troublesome and "in some cases, yogurt and buttermilk may reduce flatus" (BCDNA, 1992).

Exercise   Regular exercise helps to establish a regular bowel pattern and prevent elimination problems. Walking, running, swimming and biking are all excellent exercises for stimulating intestinal motility.

Positioning   A sitting or squatting position is the natural one assumed to evacuate the bowels. In this position, it is easier to increase abdominal pressure which is needed to expel stool. People who have difficulty squatting because of weakness or disability may find regular toilet seats too low. Raised toilet seats can be purchased so that less effort is needed to sit down or stand up from the toilet.

Toileting hygiene practices   All people should be reminded to wash their hands thoroughly after using the toilet. Female patients should be told of the need to wipe their perineal area from front to back in order to prevent the

introduction of microorganisms from the rectum and vagina to the urinary meatus.

HEALTH PROTECTING STRATEGIES

Illness and hospitalization often interfere with a person's usual pattern of bowel elimination. Change in food and fluid intake, decreased activity and exercise, medications, diagnostic procedures, surgery, being in a strange environment and lack of privacy all contribute to altered elimination patterns. This section focusses on strategies a nurse may use in assisting patients to maintain their usual bowel habits, prevent disruptions in bowel functioning and maintain comfort and hygiene.

MAINTAINING USUAL BOWEL ELIMINATION PATTERNS

When people are ill or in hospital (or long-term care facility) every effort should be made to maintain their usual pattern of functioning. Established routines to aid defecation, for example, drinking hot water at meals, should become part of the individual's plan of care. Sufficient time must be allowed for defecation and the nurse should ensure that other treatments or nursing activities do not interfere with these routines. In addition, when the patient calls for assistance, the nurse should be prompt in providing help before the urge to defecate passes.

Bowel evacuation is enhanced when people use the natural position for defecation in the privacy of a bathroom. Therefore, unless ambulation is contraindicated, the

HEALTH PROMOTING STRATEGY

Promoting Healthy Bowel Elimination

- Defecate when the urge arises and take the time to defecate. If needed, establish a routine around the time the urge to defecate often occurs. Ignoring the urge to defecate will cause constipation.

- Drink eight to ten glasses of fluid daily.

- Eat a well-balanced diet including high-fibre foods such as whole wheat cereals, breads and other grain products. Fresh fruits, raw root vegetables and cooked fruits such as apricots and prunes are good sources of fibre.

- Avoid foods which cause troublesome gas distention, cramping or diarrhea, for example, cabbage, turnips, onions, carbonated beverages or fried, spicy foods.

- Participate in a regular exercise program three to four times a week.

- *Female patients*: Always wipe the perineal area from front to back to prevent the introduction of microorganisms from the rectum or vagina into the urinary tract.

- Always wash hands after using the toilet.

FIGURE 21.4   Bedside commode

FIGURE 21.5   Bedpans. A. Regular bedpan
B. Slipper bedpan

patient should be assisted to the bathroom or to use the bedside commode (see Figure 21.4). Patients who are restricted to bed will need assistance in using the bedpan. When assisting patients with defecation, the nurse must ensure as much privacy as possible, since the urge to defecate may be suppressed in the presence of others.

Ambulation and exercise are essential for maintaining bowel function and preventing elimination problems such as constipation and fecal impaction. Patients who are ill or who have had surgery are ambulated as early as possible to encourage the return of peristalsis and normal defecation patterns. Bedridden patients can be assisted with exercises to strengthen weak abdominal and pelvic floor muscles. Two simple exercises which will help bowel evacuation are as follows:

- Lying supine, pull the abdominal muscles inward, hold for a count of five, and release. Repeat the sequence at least five times, several times a day.
- Again lying supine, contract the thigh muscle, hold for a count of five, and relax. Repeating the sequence five times, several times a day helps to improve leg strength and thereby facilitate the use of a bedpan.

ASSISTING THE PATIENT WITH A BEDPAN

Patients who are not ambulatory must use a bedpan for elimination. The nurse should do all that is possible to en-

sure the privacy, safety and comfort of the patient using a bedpan.

There are two types of bedpans: the regular bedpan and the slipper pan (see Figure 21.5). The slipper pan is designed with a low back to facilitate ease of placement for patients who are unable to raise their buttocks or who are restricted from such movements. Bedpans are made of metal or plastic. Metal bedpans can become cold when they are stored; they should be rinsed with warm water and dried before use to lessen the patient's discomfort. Bedpans are usually stored in the patient's bedside table, in an adjoining bathroom or in a utility room on the nursing unit. Female patients use the bedpan for feces and urine, whereas male patients use it for feces only.

When assisting a patient with a bedpan, it is important that proper technique is used to avoid muscle strain for both the patient and the nurse. For patients who can lift their buttocks, the nurse first elevates the head of the bed about 30 degrees to avoid hyperextension of the back. The patient is then asked to bend the knees and push into the mattress with the heels or raise the buttocks. If the patient needs help raising their buttocks, the nurse places a hand under the patient's lower back and rests the elbow on the bed, using the forearm as a lever to help lift the buttocks. The nurse then slides the bedpan under the patient so that the rounded, smooth end is under the buttocks. A slipper pan should be placed with the flat end under the buttocks.

For the patient who cannot raise the buttocks on and off a bedpan, the bedpan can be given by first placing the bed flat, with the side rail up on the far side of the bed from the nurse. The patient is assisted to a side-lying position, backside towards the nurse, and is asked to grasp the side rail. The bedpan is placed in position under the buttocks (see Figure 21.6), and supported there while the patient is rolled to the back-lying position. The head of the bed should then be elevated, if permissible, to bring the patient into a sitting position. Raising or bending the knees may also help support the patient on the pan. The position of the bedpan may need some adjusting for the patient's comfort and to prevent spillage.

The patient's privacy is maintained while on the bedpan. The bed covers are replaced and the nurse leaves the room unless the patient is weak or requests help. Toilet paper and the call bell are placed within easy reach. The nurse must respond to the call bell as soon as possible to avoid undue discomfort. To remove the pan, the patient should raise the buttocks while the nurse holds the pan steady to avoid spillage when removing it. If the patient cannot raise the buttocks, the nurse can assist the patient to roll off to the side. If assistance is needed cleaning the perineal area, the nurse must wear gloves and wipe from the pubic area back to the anus to reduce the spread of microorganisms. Care to wash and dry the perianal area thoroughly is essential to prevent skin breakdown. The patient should be offered a wet face cloth to wash the hands after defecating.

MAINTAINING COMFORT AND HYGIENE

Meeting the comfort and hygiene needs of patients with elimination problems is very important to their safety and well-being. In the patient with diarrhea, for example, the frequency and enzymatic content of liquid stool together with repeated wiping with toilet paper poses the risk of perianal skin breakdown. The same potential problem exists for the incontinent patient as well, particularly if the incontinence is frequent and stool remains in contact with the skin for a period of time.

Cleanliness is essential in bowel elimination. The sight and odour of fecal material is unpleasant and the high bacteria count in feces makes it a possible source of contamination. Basic hand washing prevents the spread of microorganisms. The patient who cannot get to the bathroom for defecation must be provided the opportunity to wash the hands afterwards. The rectal area should be cleaned with soap and water and dried thoroughly after each evacuation. Products, such as zinc oxide, can be applied to protect the perianal skin from breakdown. Soiled linen should be removed immediately.

After defecation, the environment may require ventilating and freshening to eliminate unpleasant odours. The nurse should take the initiative to use a room deodorizer or open a window.

FIGURE 21.6   Assisting the patient on to the bedpan from a side-lying position

HEALTH RESTORING STRATEGIES

Measures to restore bowel elimination involve activities related to specific problems. Often, diet alterations are enough to relieve constipation. If not, a laxative, rectal suppository, enema or colonic irrigation may be needed to produce a satisfactory bowel movement. At times, manual extraction of feces is necessary. Diet and medications are also used to bring relief from diarrhea. Individuals with incontinence may require a bowel training program while those with bowel diversions may need extensive education in ostomy self-care. Some measures, such as diet therapy, may be implemented independently by the nurse; others, such as use of rectal suppositories and enemas, are dependent upon the physician's order.

DIET THERAPY

The patient who experiences constipation needs additional high-fibre foods and fluids to activate peristalsis and achieve soft, bulky stools. Bran, fruit and whole-grain cereals and breads are excellent high-fibre foods. The usual dose of bran is 15 to 30 ml daily to establish regularity. Hot liquids stimulate peristalsis and prune juice has a natural cathartic effect. It is important for people to know that diet is a life-long measure for healthy bowel patterns and may not provide immediate relief from elimination problems.

When diarrhea is the problem, the patient may try bland foods that are less stimulating to the gastrointestinal tract, such as tea, toast and custards. Foods that are binding, such as rice, cheese, bananas and applesauce, may also be helpful. Extra fluid intake to compensate for the fluid lost through the gastrointestinal tract is important. Foods high in potassium, for example, chicken broth, are encouraged because diarrhea can lead to potassium loss. Hot and cold foods should be avoided because they stimulate peristalsis. If the patient cannot tolerate food or fluids, medical help should be sought; hospitalization may be required so that intravenous therapy and potassium replacement can be initiated.

DRUG THERAPY

Laxatives and cathartics   **Laxatives** and **cathartics** are agents that promote evacuation of the bowel. "Laxatives promote a soft stool and cathartics result in a soft to watery stool with some cramping" (Kee and Hayes, 1993, 440). Some laxatives, such as bisacodyl (Dulcolax), act by increasing intestinal peristalsis while others, such as psyllium hydrophilic mucilloid (Metamucil), act by absorbing water into the intestine and increasing fecal bulk. Still others, including ducosate sodium (Colace), act as emollients which soften stool and decrease straining during

defecation. These agents are available in oral and suppository form. How to administer oral medications and suppositories is outlined in Chapter 33.

Laxatives and cathartics are useful on a short-term basis in patients whose activity is restricted and whose food intake is limited. They are also used to evacuate the bowel in preparation for diagnostic tests and abdominal surgery.

Because laxatives are readily available over-the-counter, many people use them to promote regular bowel function. Long-term use of these agents can lead to fluid and electrolyte imbalances and dependence. The nurse should caution individuals against frequent use of laxatives and cathartics, especially if they are capable of promoting normal bowel function through diet, exercise and regular habits.

Antidiarrheal medications   **Antidiarrheal agents** are drugs which counteract diarrhea. They act by decreasing intestinal motility or immobilizing toxic substances, for example bacteria, that cause diarrhea. Diphenoxylate (Lomotil) is an example of an opiate-related agent which decreases peristalsis and kaolin-pectin (Kaopectate) is an adsorbent which binds substances to its surface. It is important to note that antidiarrheal medications do not treat the underlying cause of diarrhea and, therefore, should not be used until the etiology has been identified. Until this is known, non-pharmacologic measures, such as the dietary interventions described above, should be implemented.

ENEMAS

An **enema** is the instillation of fluid into the rectum to stimulate peristalsis and remove feces or flatus from the colon. Enemas act by distending or irritating the bowel or by providing lubrication to make evacuation easier. They are usually administered to relieve constipation, remove fecal impaction, administer medication and cleanse the rectum and colon prior to diagnostic tests or as a safety measure to prevent possible infection in patients who are undergoing surgery. They may also be used to reduce fever or cerebral edema. As with laxative overuse, normal defecation is impaired with frequent use of enemas.

The nurse must check the doctor's order before administering an enema to determine the type and amount of enema and time it is to be given. In some institutions, enemas are given at the nurse's discretion. In this case, it is essential that the nurse be knowledgeable about the types and purposes of enemas so that the enema selected is the best one for the patient's needs and physical condition. Because the bowel contains bacteria, the enema requires clean technique only. The nurse wears gloves to ensure that cross-contamination of microorganisms is prevented. The steps for administering an enema are outlined in Procedure 21.1.

Types of Enemas

There are several different kinds of enemas. These include cleansing, oil retention, carminative and medicated enemas.

Cleansing enemas

Cleansing enemas are given chiefly to remove feces from the colon. Preparations commonly used for cleansing enemas include normal saline, tap water, soapsuds and hypertonic solution.

The *normal saline enema* is an isotonic solution given in large volume to distend the bowel and thereby stimulate peristalsis and evacuation. Since normal saline is isotonic — that is, most like the fluid in tissue cells — it minimizes the danger of fluid shifts in the bowel and makes it a very safe solution. For this reason, it is the safest enema for adults with preexisting fluid and electrolyte imbalances, and for infants and children who tolerate fluid and electrolyte imbalances poorly. A saline enema is prepared by adding 10 ml of salt to 1000 ml of tap water.

The *tap water enema*, on the other hand, is hypotonic. When introduced into the bowel lumen, the difference in osmotic pressure causes the water to move from the bowel lumen into the blood stream. However, before large amounts of water are actually absorbed, the sheer volume stimulates peristalsis and the complete mass is eliminated within minutes. Caution is necessary when administering tap water enemas because the volume of water absorbed can lead to fluid and electrolyte imbalance such as circulatory overload. The nurse is advised to check with the physician or agency policy regarding the number of tap water enemas that can be repeated consecutively.

The *soapsuds enema* acts by irritating the bowel mucosa. Only pure castile soap should be used since harsh soaps and detergents can cause serious intestinal inflammation. Approximately 5 to 15 ml of castile soap is added to 1000 ml of water or normal saline to make a soapsuds enema.

The *hypertonic enema* is a low-volume, concentrated solution, which pulls fluid from the surrounding tissues into the bowel lumen, thus distending the bowel and promoting defecation. The most commonly used preparation is sodium phosphate (the Fleet enema). Commercially prepared and disposable, this type of enema is easy to use and comfortable for the patient because of its small volume (100 ml).

Oil retention enema

An oil retention enema may be given in cases in which there is severe constipation or the patient has a painful anal condition. The oil not only lubricates the rectal mucosa but also softens the stool, easing its passage. Oil enemas are small-volume (90 to 120 ml) preparations made with mineral, olive or cottonseed oil. The effectiveness of the oil enema is enhanced if the individual can retain the enema for one to two hours. A cleansing enema may be ordered following an oil retention enema.

Carminative enema

A carminative enema is given to relieve the discomfort from gas distention. These enemas are usually low-volume solutions which help to move gas by stimulating peristalsis. The 1-2-3 enema (30 g magnesium, 60 ml glycerin, 90 ml water) and the Mayo enema (240 ml water, 60 ml brown sugar, 30 ml sodium bicarbonate) are two common examples.

Medicated enema

A medicated enema is given to administer medications that are absorbed by the rectal mucosa. For example, the antibiotic neomycin can be administered by enema to cleanse the bowel of microorganisms prior to surgery.

Preparing the Patient

An explanation of the enema procedure for the patient should include the purpose, the position to be assumed, breathing instructions to reduce abdominal cramping and the length of time to retain the enema. A feeling of fullness or abdominal cramping may be experienced when the enema is administered. In general, enemas are retained for about 10 minutes, but this is really dependent upon the patient's ability to contract the anal sphincter. In older patients, holding an enema is often problematic so bed linen should be well protected and a commode readily available at the bedside. If the doctor orders "enemas to clear," the nurse must explain what this means: the enemas are repeated until the results are free of stool. However, it is generally advised that not more than three consecutive enemas be given. The nurse should notify the physician if the third enema fails to produce clear returns.

Assembling Equipment

Disposable, plastic enema kits are available with an attached rectal-tip tubing and sliding clamp. The rectal tip is often prelubricated. Reusable equipment may still be used in some agencies. This includes a metal or plastic solution container, tubing, a rubber or plastic rectal tube and a clamp. Rectal tubes come in sizes 12-30 Fr; the sizes of tubes that should be used for the various age groups are listed in Table 21.1. Small-volume enemas, for example Fleet or oil retention, are contained in prepackaged disposable units consisting of a squeezable bottle and a nozzle tip. The nozzle tip is prelubricated and covered with a protective cap. Figure 21.7 illustrates the various types of enema equipment.

Prepackaged, disposable enemas come with their own instructions for use. To prepare enema solutions using a disposable enema kit or reusable equipment, first assemble the equipment and clamp off the tubing. Lubricant will be needed for a reusable rectal tube and an IV pole to suspend a soft disposable container. The volume of solution that may be administered varies according to age (see Table 21.1) and should be indicated in the doctor's order. The solutions should be warmed to 40.5° to 43.3° C for adults and 37.7° to 40.5° C for children (Earnest 1993; Flynn and Hackel, 1990).

FIGURE 21.7 Enema equipment and supplies. A. Metal reusable container with attached tubing and a clamp. B. Rectal tube. C. Disposable enema kit. D. Prepackaged disposable enema.

SOURCE: Norton, B. A. and Miller, A. M. (1986). *Skills for professional nursing practice*. Norwalk, CT: Appleton-Century-Crofts, 610. Redrawn with permission.

TABLE 21.1   Enema Volumes and Tube Sizes

AGE	CLEANSING VOLUME (ML)	RETENTION VOLUME (ML)	TUBE SIZE (F)
Adult	500–1000	15–200	22–30
School age/adolescent	350–750	100–150*	18–22
Toddler/preschooler*	250–350	75–150*	14–18
Infant*	Under 250	Under 75*	12

* Should be stipulated in physician's order.

SOURCE: Flynn, J.M. and Hackel, R. (1990). *Technological foundations in nursing*. Norwalk, CT: Appleton & Lange, 620. Reproduced with permission.

An enema that is too cold lowers the body temperature and causes cramping; one that is too warm may cause thermal injury. Once the solution is in the container, rid the tubing and rectal tube of air by opening the clamp and running solution through it; then clamp the tubing. If the patient cannot ambulate, a bedpan or commode should be readied.

Administering an Enema

ACTION	RATIONALE
1. Confirm doctor's order for the type of enema and number to be given.	Prevents error and promotes accuracy.
2. Prepare the patient.	Promotes patient well-being and facilitates participation in care.
3. Gather equipment: • Enema kit or reusable container, tubing, rectal tube, and clamp; or prepackaged enema. • Enema solution • Water-soluble lubricant • Water-proof protective pad • Clean gloves • Bedpan or commode if required • Toilet tissue • Towel and washcloth • Paper bag for equipment disposal	Facilitates efficiency and economy of time.
4. Pull the bed curtains and help the patient into a left-lateral position with the right leg flexed. However, this position may be varied according to the patient's condition. Place a protective pad under the patient's buttocks, then drape the patient appropriately.	Provides privacy. Facilitates the flow of fluid since the rectum and sigmoid colon are on the left side of the body. Flexion of the leg provides access to the anus. Provides warmth and comfort.
5. Apply clean gloves.	Protects the nurse from exposure to blood, body substances and microorganisms.
6. Administer the enema.	
For small-volume prepackaged enemas:	
• Remove the rectal tip covering and inspect for lubricant. Add lubricant if necessary.	Facilitates insertion into the rectum and lessens irritation of the mucous membrane.
• Raise the upper buttock.	Exposes the anus.
• Ask the patient to breathe deeply and insert the rectal nozzle into the anus. Advance the tip 7 to 10 cm in adults or 5 to 7.5 cm in children.	Relaxes the internal sphincter and makes insertion easier.
• Squeeze the enema bottle until all of the solution has entered the rectum.	
For large-volume enemas:	
• Lubricate the rectal tube if not already lubricated.	As above.
• Insert the rectal tube as above.	
• Hold the tubing in the rectum with one hand.	
• Raise the enema container on the IV pole 30 to 45 cm above the rectum, open the clamp and slowly instill the solution. A litre of solution should take about 10 minutes, but this can vary depending on the patient's tolerance.	Decreases the force exerted by the solution on the rectal tissue and thereby lessens the risk of injury.

ACTION	RATIONALE

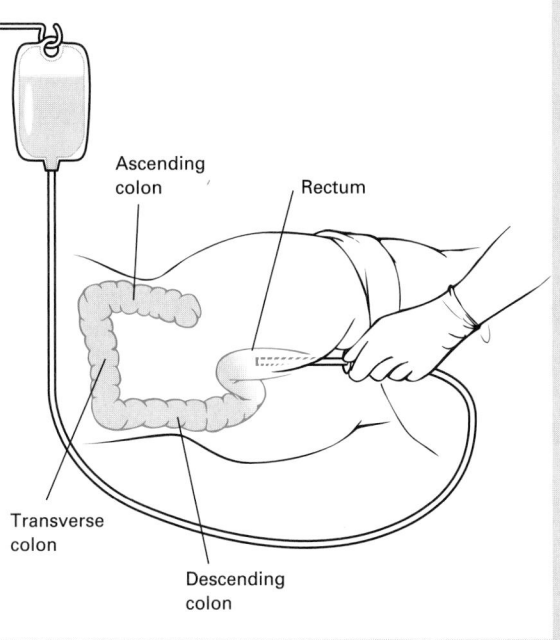

- Allow the solution to infuse slowly.

  Prevents cramping and pain from rapid distention of the rectum.

- Instruct the patient to signal if the instillation is painful or if it is becoming difficult to hold the solution. If the patient experiences cramping, lower the enema container or clamp the tubing.

  Gives the patient some control over the procedure and directs the nurse's activities.

  Allows the patient to rest.

  Instruct the patient to breathe slowly through the mouth.

  Promotes relaxation and enhances tolerance of the solution.

- When all of the solution is instilled or the patient is unable to tolerate any more, clamp and remove the tube.

  Intolerance is indicated when cramping continues or solution seeps out around the rectal tube.

7. Instruct the patient to remain in the side-lying position and hold the enema for the required time.

   Helps to retain the enema.

8. Assist the patient to the bathroom, commode, or with the use of a bedpan.

9. If the patient is using the toilet, ask them not to flush it.

   Permits the nurse to observe the enema results.

10. Dispose of equipment according to agency policy. Wash hands.

    Maintains cleanliness and safety in the workplace.

11. Record relevant information. Note the type of enema, amount of solution given or tolerated; the amount, colour and consistency of the returns; and relief of gas or abdominal distention.

    Fulfills requirements for nurse accountability and facilitates continuity of care.

FECAL DISIMPACTION

If laxatives and enemas administered over a course of days are ineffective in removing feces, a manual extraction of stool from the rectum is necessary. This is done with the finger and can be painful for the patient. Digital removal of feces can be dangerous for some people because rectal stimulation causes a vagal response which may in turn result in a slowing of the heart rate. For this reason, the nurse should check agency policy regarding who can perform a disimpaction.

Digital removal of stool requires a rectal glove, paper bag for glove disposal, lubricant, protective bed covering and a bedpan. Once the procedure has been explained, the nurse proceeds to assist the patient into a lateral position with the knees flexed. Waterproof protective pads are placed under the buttocks and the bedpan is placed nearby. With donned gloves, a lubricated index finger is gently inserted into the rectum. The rectum is massaged along its wall and at the same time the finger works the hard stool mass. The nurse must work the feces down towards the anus and piece by piece remove the stool, discarding it into the bedpan. It is important to assess the patient for fatigue, pallor, sweating and pain, and to allow rest periods. After the procedure, the patient should be encouraged to use the toilet, commode or bedpan as rectal stimulation can induce the need to defecate.

Meticulous observations of bowel patterns and fecal characteristics by the nurse is necessary to prevent further impaction. Attention to diet, mobility, bathroom facilities and drug regimens are important aspects of nursing care for the person with fecal impaction.

MANAGING INCONTINENCE

Some people with fecal incontinence, particularly those who have retained some sensory awareness and sphincter control, may be able to achieve normal elimination with a bowel retraining program. A thorough assessment of the cause of the patient's incontinence, physical readiness and ability to gain from bowel training must be completed first. The patient is then put on a daily routine using interventions that promote defecation. Patience, consistency and time are necessary for a successful bowel training program. Success may not be achieved for several weeks.

The program usually involves establishing a time for bowel training that fits with the patient's normal elimination pattern or incontinence. The best times are 20 to 40 minutes after meals when the gastrocolic reflex is stimulated. Attempts at evacuation are made daily within 15 minutes of the scheduled time. Bulking agents, such as natural bran or Metamucil, are administered daily. As well, hot liquids may be offered each day as a stimulant to defecation 30 minutes before the scheduled time. At the selected time, the patient should be assisted to the bathroom to defecate and given a time limit of 20 minutes. Teaching the patient to lean for-ward when sitting on the toilet, to bear down and to massage the abdomen are useful measures to aid defecation. Of course, regular meals with adequate amounts of fibre foods and fluids, and exercise are important ingredients of a successful bowel training program (Basch and Jensen, 1991).

For patients with incontinence related to sensory or motor deficits of the rectum and anus, digital stimulation is a commonly used approach to bowel training. Using a gloved, lubricated finger, the anal wall is massaged in a circular motion until the sphincter relaxes. Usually bowel evacuation quickly follows. If not, digital stimulation may be repeated. Again, timing defecation by rectal stimulation after meals, ensuring a sitting position and encouraging abdominal massage help establish a regular defecation pattern.

Other bowel training therapies may include sphincter training with biofeedback and pelvic floor exercises. Surgery may be indicated for people with incontinence that cannot be treated by these other methods (Basch and Jensen, 1991).

For those with incontinence, a variety of absorbent pads are available, or fecal collection devices can be worn. Prompt disposal of feces, management of odour and skin protection must be provided to restore the comfort and dignity of the patient with incontinence.

OSTOMY CARE

An individual with an ostomy no longer eliminates in the same way as a person with an intact bowel. In most cases, a pouch to collect the feces must be worn on the abdomen at all times. Successful adjustment of the person to the ostomy requires well planned nursing care. To live independently with an ostomy, the individual must learn about normal stoma characteristics, how to change and empty the pouch and how to care for peristomal skin. In addition, the person needs information about diet and fluid modifications, control of gas and odour and management of many unique health care problems associated with ostomies.

In addition to the practical management of the ostomy, the person must also adjust emotionally to the surgery. Many people find the idea of feces emptying onto the abdomen repugnant and are acutely aware of the reactions of others. They may feel a loss of health and fear that major changes in lifestyle will be necessary. Others may also be coping with a poor prognosis if the ostomy is a palliative measure. It is not unusual for patients and families to go through a period of grieving. It is important for the nurse to communicate understanding of the emotions and reactions of the patient and family. Acceptance and care aimed at protecting the patient's dignity and need for privacy can do much to assist the patient in his or her recovery. Enterostomal therapists are nurses with specialized knowledge and skills in the management of ostomies. Some institutions have enterostomal therapists on staff to assist patients in their recovery and to consult with other nurses in developing and implementing a patient care plan.

Stoma Characteristics

Assessment of the condition of the stoma after surgery is an essential nursing intervention. Stoma characteristics must also be included in the patient's teaching plan and can be addressed preoperatively or in the immediate post-operative phase. Stoma assessment should include stoma colour, size and shape, condition of peristomal skin, stoma bleeding and stoma functioning.

The stoma is normally red or deep pink in colour and appears moist. A pale or dark, bluish-coloured stoma indicates poor circulation and should be brought to the attention of the physician. Loop colostomies are larger in size than end colostomies or ileostomies. Most stomas are round in shape and protrude from the abdomen approximately 1.5 to 2.5 cm. It generally takes 4 to 8 weeks for a new stoma to shrink to its final size (Erwin-Toth and Doughty, 1992). The peristomal skin (5 to 13 cm of skin around the stoma) should appear intact and free of redness. The stoma will often bleed when cleaned as it contains many small blood vessels. When bleeding occurs, the patient should be reassured that this is normal.

Assessment of stoma functioning includes the characteristics of the drainage as well as the presence of flatus. Stoma output from an ileostomy in the first few weeks is likely to be liquid and of high volume — up to 1500 ml per day (Erwin-Toth and Doughty, 1992). This volume will decrease over time and should thicken slightly. Colostomy drainage, on the other hand, will be like the preoperative bowel pattern in terms of frequency and consistency. Flatus occurs when bowel peristalsis returns after an operation. Large amounts of flatus and noise are commonly experienced by the patient and are usually of concern. It should be explained that flatus can be modified by the diet and that the pouches are odour-proof.

Changing an Ostomy Appliance

In the first few days after surgery, changing an ostomy appliance (also referred to as *pouching the stoma*) is the responsibility of the nurse or enterostomal therapist. During this time the patient is usually emotionally and physically unprepared to learn this skill. Once patient readiness is determined, the instruction process can begin. First the patient is encouraged to watch the nurse change the pouch while explanations are given with each step. Thereafter, the patient takes on more of the pouch changing procedure until the patient can demonstrate the ability to change the pouch independently. Procedure 21.2 outlines the steps in changing an ostomy pouch.

Types of appliances   Many types of ostomy appliances are available. The nurse should be familiar with the available products so that a suitable one can be chosen for the patient. Most have the following common features: a plastic pouch, an adhesive skin barrier and a drainable end. Skin barriers come in various forms: wafers, rings, pastes and powders. They are used to protect the peristomal skin from drainage, build a flat pouching surface on the abdomen or to treat peristomal skin breakdown. Fecal pouches are classified as one-piece or two-piece, disposable or reusable and closed-end or drainable. Figure 21.8 illustrates the ostomy appliance.

Faceplate

Stoma opening

Pouch

Pouch clip

Drainable end

FIGURE 21.8   The ostomy appliance

FIGURE 21.9 A two-piece appliance. A. A Stomadhesive wafer with flange is applied directly to the peristomal area. B. A pouch is positioned over the stoma and snapped into place. C. and D. The pouch may be removed and the stoma assessed without removing the wafer.

SOURCE: Rosdahl, C. (1991). *Textbook of basic nursing* (5th ed.). Philadelphia: Lippincott, 858. Redrawn with permission from the J. B. Lippincott Company and ConvaTec, a Division of E.R. Squibb and Sons, Inc., Princeton, N. J.

In the one-piece system, the pouch is attached to an adhesive back or ring which affixes to the abdomen. The two-piece appliance has a wafer skin barrier with flange separate from the attachable snap-on pouch (see Figure 21.9). The two-piece appliance provides some benefits over the one-piece system, including ease in centring the skin barrier over the stoma, greater visualization of the stoma for assessment and the ability to empty or replace the pouch without disturbing the adhesive wafer. Another advantage of the two-piece system is the type of flange. The floating flange permits the nurse to slide fingers under the flange for pouch application thereby easing the potential discomfort caused by pressure on the sensitive abdomen of the post-surgical patient.

Another feature of pouches is the size of the stomal opening. Some ringed pouches have this opening already cut in premeasured sizes, others have starter holes. Starter holes are small openings in the centre of the skin barrier that can be cut to fit the exact size and shape of the stoma. While these pouches provide a custom fit, they also demand good eyesight and more dexterity on the part of the patient to apply.

Pouches come in disposable or reusable form. Most agencies stock the disposable pouch. Disposable pouches are made of a lightweight plastic and come in one- or two-piece systems. They are simply discarded after use. The reusable pouch is made of heavier plastic or rubber, comes pre-sized, and in one- or two-piece systems. They may benefit the patient who has a limited budget and needs frequent pouch changes. On the other hand, reusable pouches require more maintenance. The patient must learn how to clean the pouch and how to use and remove the cements that are necessary for adhering the appliance to the skin.

Finally, pouches can be drainable or closed-end. Drainable pouches have an open end that must be tied with an elastic band or closed with a pouch clip until emptying is desired. A closed-end pouch does not permit emptying. They are generally used by colostomates who are well regulated by irrigation.

Guiding principles for pouching   Protection of the peristomal skin and stoma from damage as a result of effluent or repetitive removal of the appliance serves as the guiding principle for pouching. The degree of skin damage from fecal matter depends on the effluent's enzymatic content, volume and consistency. For example, the effluent from an ileostomy is liquid, and high in enzymes. If allowed to pool on the skin, rapid skin breakdown results. Colostomy drainage contains few if any enzymes, and is therefore less corrosive to the skin. The nurse must ensure the appliance is sized snugly to the stoma so little skin is exposed to the effluent. If the pouch is sized larger than the stoma, a barrier paste must be applied to protect the skin. If leakage occurs around the appliance, it must be changed immediately. Otherwise, disposable ostomy appliances can remain secure for up to seven days. Unnecessary and frequent removal of the pouch can result in skin trauma. Irritated skin requires prompt treatment and more frequent pouch changes so that the appropriate healing products can be applied.

Preparing the Patient

Explain the procedure to the patient and determine, with the patient, an optimum time to change the pouch. It is best to select a time when the ostomy is least likely to function. Avoid meal times and visiting hours. Effluent odour may affect appetite and make an unpleasant environment for guests. The patient's comfort should be ensured before beginning the procedure since pain will interfere with learning. The patient should observe or participate in the procedure to the extent that he or she is able.

Assessing the Need for a Pouch Change

The following criteria will assist the nurse in determining when a pouch change is required:

- Note the condition of the existing bag for leakage or melt down of the skin barrier. Effluent on the skin causes skin irritation. Melting of the skin barrier predisposes the patient to a poor seal and leakage.

- Determine if the patient experiences any discomfort around the stoma. A burning sensation may indicate skin irritation from deterioration of the skin barrier of the pouch.

- Assess the amount of drainage in the pouch. Pouches should be emptied when they are no more than half full as the weight of the drainage may separate the pouch from the skin.

- Change the pouch if any of the above conditions are seen.

Assembling Equipment

The nurse selects the type of pouch and skin barrier by considering the type of effluent or drainage, stoma size and shape, abdominal contours, visual acuity and manual dexterity of the patient, the patient's preferences in terms of equipment and the cost and availability of supplies. After surgery, as the patient's stoma size decreases, abdominal contours change or activity level improves, pouching needs may require adjustment (Erwin-Toth and Doughty, 1992). When applying a skin barrier, a stoma measuring guide is used to determine the size of the stoma so as to ensure that the hole cut into the skin barrier will fit around the stoma exactly. Tissues, water and a towel will be needed to cleanse the stoma and peristomal skin of effluent or wastes. A mild, non-oily and non-perfumed soap or skin cleanser such as Sween or Bard may also be used if needed, to cleanse the peristomal skin.

PROCEDURE 21.2

Changing an Ostomy Pouch

ACTION	RATIONALE
1. Prepare the patient.	Promotes well-being and enables participation in care.

Continued on the next page

ACTION	RATIONALE
2. Gather equipment: • Pouch • Pouch clip • Clean gloves • Moisture-proof bag • Cleaning materials such as tissues, washcloth, basin of warm water, towel • Mild, non-oily, and non-perfumed soap, if required • Peristomal skin paste or powder, if required • Measuring guide and pen • Scissors • Micropore tape	Promotes efficiency and economy of time.
3. Provide privacy.	Promotes dignity and comfort.
4. Ideally the pouch should be changed in the bathroom with the patient sitting or standing. If unable to ambulate, help the person into a lying or sitting position in bed.	Lying or standing positions are preferred. In these positions there is less wrinkling of the skin which makes application of the pouch easier.
5. Apply clean gloves.	Protects the nurse from exposure to blood, body substances and microorganisms.
6. Remove the old appliance. • Empty the pouch of drainage and measure. • Remove the appliance by gently pressing the skin away from the appliance starting at the top and working to the bottom. • Discard the appliance into the moisture-proof bag.	This prevents spillage during the change. Minimizes peristomal skin damage and patient discomfort.
7. Prepare the peristomal skin. • Remove remaining stool with toilet tissue. Slight stomal bleeding may occur during cleaning and is normal. • Clean the skin with warm water and mild soap or skin cleanser. • Dry the skin thoroughly. • Remove hair from around the stoma if required. An electric or safety razor may be used.	Prevents drying or irritation of the skin. Ensures solid bonding of barrier to the skin. Allowing the hair to grow and then be pulled out during pouch change may cause infection of the hair follicle.
8. Inspect the stoma and skin. • Assess the skin for redness, broken areas or rash. Note the condition of peristomal sutures, if applicable. • Note the size, shape, and colour of the stoma.	Provides data for ongoing evaluation of care.

ACTION	RATIONALE
9. Prepare for pouch application.	
For a two-piece pouch system with a wafer skin barrier and flange:	
• Measure the size of the stoma with the measuring guide. For the first four to eight weeks, the stoma size should be measured with each pouch change.	Ensures a correct fit of the skin barrier. Allows for stomal shrinkage during this time.
• Draw the measured size of the stoma opening on the back of the wafer.	
• Using scissors, cut out the traced pattern.	Makes an opening in the skin barrier.
• Remove the paper backing of the skin barrier to expose the adhesive side. Save the paper backing.	Readies the barrier for application. Serves as a template for sizing the skin barrier on the next pouch change.
• Apply skin barrier paste to the inner diameter of the cut wafer, if necessary.	Smoothes out creases in the skin and provides extra protection from effluent.
• Permit the paste to dry for one to two minutes.	
10. Apply the pouch.	
• Centre the wafer over the stoma and press down. Work in a circular fashion, pressing the skin barrier from the stoma to the outside. Remove any air bubbles.	Ensures a good seal and prevents leakage.
• Snap the pouch onto the flange. Position the end of the pouch towards the feet if the patient is ambulatory or slightly to the side if the patient is not active.	Facilitates emptying.
• Give the pouch a slight tug.	Makes sure it is on.
• Remove any air in the pouch.	
• Secure the end of the pouch with a tail-closure clip or elastic band. If a clip is used, ensure it snaps into place by giving a slight tug on the closure.	Provides extra reinforcement.
• Apply micropore tape in a window-framing manner around the wafer edges.	
11. Attach the belt to the pouch if the patient prefers. Otherwise the wings to which the belt attaches may be cut off.	Facilitates patient comfort and provides extra security. May be useful for the patient with a large abdomen.
12. Dispose of or clean reusable equipment.	
• Wash reusable pouches with warm water and soap, dry and store.	Promotes cleanliness and prevents the spread of microorganisms.
• Remove and dispose of gloves into the moisture-proof bag and discard into the appropriate garbage receptacle.	

Continued on the next page

PROCEDURE 21.2
continued

ACTION	RATIONALE
13. Record pertinent information. Note the characteristics of the stoma, the condition of the peristomal skin, the amount and type of drainage, the type and size of appliance used, any significant patient behaviours during the change and any skills learned.	Fulfills requirements for nurse accountability and promotes continuity of care.
14. Modify the teaching and nursing care plan as needed.	Promotes continuity of care.

POUCH EMPTYING

Most types of pouches are closed with a pouch clip (tail closure) or elastic band. To empty the pouch, the clip or band must be removed. Pouch emptying is easiest if the patient can sit on the toilet seat, allowing the fecal effluent to drain into the toilet. At the bedside, a bedpan or other receptacle may be used to collect the output. The patient is taught to cuff the bottom of the pouch after the clip is removed. This helps to keep the end of the pouch clean which further prevents odour. The cuff also helps to keep the patient's hands clean during the procedure. Squeezing the pouch facilitates emptying and toilet paper or a damp paper towel is useful in cleaning the bottom of the pouch. The patient may wish to rinse the pouch to remove all the stool, although this is unnecessary as the pouch is odour-proof. A squeeze bottle can be used to direct the water into the pouch, but the patient should be instructed not to be too rigorous with cleaning as the water may disturb the pouch seal. After the pouch is cleaned, the cuff is uncurled and the clip is reapplied.

If the patient is wearing a two-piece pouch system, the pouch may be snapped off and a new one applied. The old one may be rinsed to be used again later. The patient should be taught to empty the pouch when it is no more than half full. The weight of a full pouch risks the integrity of the pouch seal and may cause leakage.

IRRIGATING A COLOSTOMY

The patient with a colostomy may use colonic irrigation as a means of regulating bowel function. However, the individual must understand that irrigation is a management option, and is not essential to maintain healthy bowel patterns. While the choice to irrigate is the individual's, not all people are suitable candidates and thoughtful assessment and counsel by the nurse is required. For instance, the patient who has a descending or sigmoid colostomy only, who has a history of regular, formed bowel movements and who is capable of learning the procedure is likely a good candidate. Irrigation is ill-advised for the patient with a stoma higher in the intestinal tract, who is very young, has a temporary colostomy, has had pelvis irradiation or has a prolapsed stoma (Erwin-Toth and Doughty, 1992).

Irrigation acts by stimulating the bowel through bowel distention. Routine irrigation trains the bowel to evacuate at the time of irrigation which is usually performed every second day. The benefit of irrigation is that the patient can avoid wearing the pouch. The disadvantages are that irrigations can take up to an hour to complete and bowel dependency can occur over time. Irrigation does not provide effective bowel regulation at all times; careful attention to the diet is also required so that unexpected evacuation is avoided. The technique for performing an ostomy irrigation is outlined in Procedure 21.3. Universal or body substance precautions are necessary when performing this procedure.

Preparing the Patient

At the beginning, the irrigation procedure should be simply explained. The patient needs to understand that the stoma has no sphincter and therefore he or she has no voluntary control over evacuation. The most convenient location for the colostomy irrigation is in the bathroom. The patient can sit on the toilet and the end of the sleeve can be placed directly in the toilet. If the patient is unable to tolerate sitting, the irrigation can be performed in bed. The patient should lie on the side of the colostomy stoma. The end of the sleeve can be closed and drained into a bedpan placed at a lower level when full.

Assembling Equipment

The supplies for the irrigation include an irrigating bag with tubing and a clamp, water-soluble lubricant, a stoma cone and an irrigation sleeve with belt. A stoma cone (see Figure 21.10) is a colon catheter with a seal or cone that prevents backflow of irrigating fluid. A catheter or rectal tube is not recommended for colostomy irrigation due to the risk of bowel perforation. Because the stoma does not have nerve endings, the patient cannot report injury. Using a stoma cone reduces the risk that the bowel will be perforated during the procedure. The irrigation sleeve is a disposable, plastic appliance that fits over the stoma to contain the irrigant and evacuated stool as it flows out of the stoma. If a two-piece ostomy appliance is used, the irrigation sleeve will attach to the system.

Tap water is the most commonly used irrigating solution. Patients who are severely debilitated or for whom fluid balance is disrupted may need a saline solution. A normal saline solution may be made by adding 10 ml of salt to 1000 ml of warm water. As with enemas, lukewarm water is most appropriate. Water that is too cold may cause cramping, and water that is too warm may cause mucosal injury and slow the return of feces.

The amount of irrigating solution varies among individuals (500 to 1500 ml), with 1000 ml generally producing the best results. Too much water can tire the patient and contribute to fluid and electrolyte imbalance. Initially a small amount of solution (500 ml or less) will stimulate the bowel. Pour warm tap water into the irrigation bag to the desired volume. Allow the solution to flow through the tubing to clear the air and clamp the tubing. Suspend the bag on the IV pole. Attach the cone catheter to the tubing and remove any air. Figure 21.10 illustrates a colostomy irrigation.

FIGURE 21.10   Colostomy irrigation. The patient sits on the toilet. The irrigating solution is suspended 30 to 45 cm above the stoma. The plastic irrigation sleeve is applied over the stoma and the distal end is lowered into the toilet. The stoma cone and colon catheter are inserted through the top of the irrigating sleeve.

PROCEDURE 21.3

Irrigating a Colostomy

ACTION	RATIONALE
1. Prepare the patient.	Promotes well-being and enables patient participation.
2. Gather equipment:	Promotes efficiency and economy of time.
• Irrigation set (solution bag with tubing, clamp; stoma cone; stoma -irrigation sleeve with belt)	
• Irrigating solution	
• A clean ostomy appliance	
• Moisture-proof bag	
• Clean gloves	
• Lubricant	
• IV pole	
• Protective pad	
• Bedpan or commode	
3. Provide for privacy.	Promotes patient's dignity and comfort.
4. Assist the patient to a side-lying position if unable to get out of bed, or on to a commode at the bedside, to the bathroom on a toilet. If performed in bed, place a protective pad under the stoma and the bedpan on a chair beside the bed. Move the patient's clothing out of the way.	Allows the irrigant to flow into the stoma through the force of gravity. Protects the bed linen from soiling. Exposes the colostomy.
5. Put on clean gloves.	Protects the nurse from contaminants.
6. Attach the irrigation sleeve. A sleeve for a two-piece system will snap onto the flange. A reusable sleeve is belted into place; a disposable adhesive-backed sleeve sticks to the peristomal skin; both require the removal of the old pouch. Place the sleeve bottom into the toilet, commode, or bedpan.	Collects the irrigant and evacuated stool. Directs the returns.
7. Adjust the height of the IV pole so that the solution bag hangs about 30 to 45 cm above the stoma.	Ensures adequate pressure to allow irrigant to flow into stoma.
8. Administer the irrigation.	
• Lubricate the cone catheter and insert it into the stoma through the top of the sleeve.	Makes insertion easier.
• Hold the cone firmly against the stoma.	Prevents backflow of irrigant.
• Open the clamp and begin the flow of solution. Expect the irrigation to take 10 minutes to infuse. If cramping occurs, stop the flow until it subsides, then resume the flow.	Alleviates discomfort.
• Close the clamp and remove the cone when the solution has been instilled or when the patient senses bowel distention.	

ACTION

- Expect initial returns to be complete in 15 minutes. Instruct the patient to massage the abdomen. After this the patient has the option to close the bottom of the bag and move around. Allow about 45 minutes for completion of returns.

9. When bowel evacuation is complete, remove and rinse the sleeve.

10. Clean the peristomal skin, and apply a new pouch.

11. Assist the patient to a comfortable position if required.

12. Prepare the equipment for repeat use and discard disposable supplies. Remove gloves and wash hands.

13. Record pertinent information. Note the type and amount of irrigant used, the characteristics of fecal returns, the patient's response and abilities during the procedure.

RATIONALE

Encourages emptying by stimulating peristalsis.

Movement stimulates peristalsis.

Maintains cleanliness and prevents transfer of contaminants.

Promotes skin integrity.

Maintains cleanliness and safety in the workplace.

Fulfills requirements for nurse accountability and promotes continuity of care.

PROMOTING OPTIMAL OSTOMY ELIMINATION

Diet management is important for the individual with an ostomy. For most ostomates there are few diet restrictions. Control of odour and gas can be achieved by monitoring the intake of foods which produce gas and may cause odour. The individual may choose to omit these foods, but it should be stressed that the most important odour-control measures are the odour-proof pouch and the practice of keeping the pouch bottom clean and dry. In some cases, buttermilk and yogurt may reduce flatus and eating parsley, yogurt and buttermilk may also help to reduce odour (BCDNA, 1992). Management of constipation and diarrhea is the same as for the person whose bowel is intact.

The person with an ileostomy must be more cautious about diet because of the location of the ostomy and the nature of the output. Bowel obstruction, for example, is a significant concern. The ileostomate is at risk for food blockage because the ileum, from which the ileostomy is created, has a narrow lumen. Further narrowing may occur at the fascia-muscle or where the intestine comes through the abdominal wall. Consequently, intestinal waste can collect at this point and cause a partial or complete blockage. The nurse describes the types of high-fibre foods that can contribute to blockage (see box) and explains preventive measures to the patient: avoid high-fibre foods in the first six to eight weeks after surgery, add high-fibre foods one at a time

Gas and Odour Producing Foods

GAS PRODUCING FOODS	ODOUR CAUSING FOODS
broccoli	asparagus
Brussels sprouts	broccoli
cabbage	Brussels sprouts
cauliflower	cabbage
corn	cauliflower
cucumber	cheese
legumes (dried peas, beans and lentils)	eggs
	fish
melon	garlic
peppers (green and red)	legumes (dried peas, beans, lentils)
pickles	onion
radishes	spices
sauerkraut	turnip
turnip	

SOURCE: BCDNA. (1992). *Manual of nutritional care* (4th ed.). Vancouver: Author, 216, 218.

in small amounts, and chew food well and drink plenty of fluid (Erwin-Toth and Doughty, 1992).

The nurse must also inform the patient of the signs and symptoms of bowel obstruction and discuss home management strategies. The signs and symptoms of partial bowel obstruction usually initiate with cramping abdominal pain and diarrhea. Abdominal distention, stomal swelling and nausea may occur, with progression to absence of fecal output as indicative of complete bowel obstruction. To manage these signs and symptoms at home, the patient should sit in a warm bath and massage the abdomen to relax the muscles. Solid food should be avoided and fluids increased. If no stool is passed and vomiting occurs despite these measures, the physician should be contacted.

EVALUATING BOWEL ELIMINATION INTERVENTIONS

The effectiveness of nursing care is determined on an ongoing basis by collecting data pertinent to the expected outcomes established by the nurse and patient. Optimally, the desired outcomes might be that the individual will defecate a soft, formed stool every day or every other day; that defecation will be pain free; that the patient will demonstrate knowledge of the factors that influence defecation, such as diet and exercise, and apply this knowledge over an extended period of time until the modifications are expressed as a normal pattern of living; that aids to defecation will be used minimally or cautiously to avoid overuse; that the individual with an ostomy will adjust to the ostomy, incorporating it as part of daily life; or that the patient will achieve independence with the technical management of ostomy care and demonstrate an understanding of factors that affect ostomy functioning.

Following is a sample guide for evaluating the effectiveness of interventions to aid bowel elimination:

1. If the patient has been constipated, has the patient had a soft stool and has a regular bowel pattern been reestablished?
2. If the patient has had diarrhea, have the stools returned to normal consistency and frequency?
3. If the patient has had abdominal distention, does the abdomen feel soft? Have flatulence and abdominal pain been relieved? Is the patient comfortable and free from distressing symptoms?
4. If the patient has had hemorrhoids, have they disappeared? Has pain on defecation been relieved?
5. Is the patient aware of dietary and fluid needs to ensure adequate fecal elimination? Does the selection of foods and fluid intake indicate this?
6. Is exercise part of the patient's daily routine?
7. Does the patient practise good hygiene? For example, does the patient wash hands after a bowel movement?

KEY TERMS

small intestine p. 574

feces p. 575

meconium p. 575

constipation p. 577

tenesmus p. 577

fecal impaction p. 577

diarrhea p. 577

fecal incontinence p. 578

hemorrhoids p. 578

stoma p. 578

ileostomy p. 578

colostomy p. 579

occult blood p. 584

Hematest p. 584

Hemoccult slide p. 584

laxatives p. 589

cathartics p. 589

antidiarrheal agents p. 589

enema p. 589

cleansing enema p. 590

IN REVIEW

Bowel elimination is the excretion of the gastrointestinal waste products of digestion. In health, bowel elimination is usually maintained with proper diet and fluids, exercise and regular bowel habits. Normal patterns can be disrupted by certain foods, gastrointestinal flu, illness, travel, medications, surgery and change of activity. Prolonged diarrhea can lead to imbalances in nutrition, water and electrolytes, impaired skin integrity and discomfort.

The principal structures involved in bowel elimination are the small and large intestines. The small bowel (intestine) consists of the duodenum, jejunum and ileum. The duodenum receives chyme from the stomach. Chyme moves along the small intestine by peristalsis and mixes with digestive enzymes, further breaking down the food substances. The duodenum is the primary site for absorption of iron and calcium; the jejunum absorbs fats, proteins and carbohydrates and the ileum absorbs some vitamins and bile salts. When chyme enters the large bowel it is mostly in the form of nondigestible substances. The primary functions of the large bowel are the absorption of water, electrolytes and remaining nutrients; the synthesis of vitamins; and the storage and elimination of feces.

The average person defecates from once or twice a day to every two to three days. The amount of feces varies with the coarseness of foodstuffs in the diet. Normal stools are brown in colour, soft and solid in consistency and cylindrical in shape. Fecal odour is caused by byproducts of bacterial activity. Flatus is the result of bacterial action on the digestive products, diffusion of gas from the blood stream and swallowing of air while eating or talking.

Bowel elimination patterns are affected by growth and development. In newborns, stools change over the first week from the initial greenish-black, tarry meconium to a yellow colour. As solids are introduced into the infant's diet, stools become darker brown and firmer in consistency. Bowel control is not usually gained until two to three years of age. Elimination patterns are fairly constant in school-age children and adolescents. There is rapid growth of the large intestine during adolescence as the amount of food consumed increases. Among adults, variations in bowel patterns occur in pregnant women and older adults. Pregnancy often produces constipation from the pressure of the uterus on the abdominal organs and the relaxing effect of hormones on smooth muscles. In older adults, bowel elimination is affected by such influences as poor appetite, inability to chew properly, decreased digestive enzyme secretion, slowed peristaltic action, less efficient absorptive ability of the intestinal mucosa, weakening muscle tone of the perineal floor and anal sphincter and a slowing of the rectal reflex nerve impulses. Constipation or loss of control are common.

Many factors affect bowel functioning. These include diet and fluid intake, personal habits, activity, exercise and emotions. Illness, pain, anesthesia and surgery and medications also influence elimination patterns.

Common bowel problems are constipation, fecal impaction, diarrhea, incontinence and hemorrhoids. Constipation often results from poor habits, lack of time, lack of privacy, low intake of fibre and fluid, immobility, medications, aging, abnormalities and pain. Fecal impaction results from dehydration, immobility, medications and neurological disease. The patient with fecal impaction may have small liquid stools, abdominal distention, cramping and inability to defecate despite the urge. Diarrhea may be caused by emotions, medications, foods, alcohol, caffeine, inflammation and infectious processes and allergies. Individuals often experience abdominal pain accompanied by urgency in the need to defecate. Prolonged diarrhea leads to skin irritation, fatigue, weakness, malaise and fluid and electrolyte imbalance. Incontinence may result from lack of control in the aged, diarrhea, injury to the rectal sphincters, neural disorders, confusion or depression. It is a distressing problem affecting self-esteem and causing great embarrassment. Hemorrhoids are the cause of increased pressure on the rectum and anus secondary to straining from constipation, childbirth, obesity and abdominal tumours. They cause bleeding, pain and itchiness.

A bowel diversion is an artificial opening, created surgically, from the colon to the surface of the abdomen. The opening is called a stoma. An ileostomy is created from the ileum and a colostomy from the large intestine. An ostomy appliance or pouch is worn over the stoma to collect the stool.

In assessing bowel elimination needs, the nurse uses subjective information obtained from the nursing health history. Objective data are gathered through physical observations and review of the chart for diagnostic test results and information about the patient's illness or diagnostic or treatment measures that may affect bowel functioning. Physical examination of the abdomen is done for skin colour, contour, symmetry, girth, abdominal distention, tenderness, masses and bowel sounds. The anus is examined for hemorrhoids, skin irritation, scars, and rectal discharge or prolapse.

Diagnostic tests include direct visualization studies in which the inner cavity of the anal canal, the rectum and the lower colon are examined using a scope. Indirect visualization is achieved by x-ray examination and fluoroscopy, both of which use barium or meglumine diatrizoate (Gastrographin) to outline the gastrointestinal tract. The collection of stool specimens for laboratory examination is the responsibility of the nurse. Stool specimens must go to the laboratory promptly because bacterial changes can occur which could affect the accuracy of the test results.

Common nursing diagnoses for bowel elimination problems are *Constipation*, *Diarrhea* and *Bowel incontinence*. Interventions for bowel elimination should be established in collaboration with the patient and family and should take into account previous healthy habits. Goals are generally directed towards understanding normal defecation and achieving a normal elimination pattern.

Health promotion strategies are aimed at helping individuals promote regular bowel elimination in daily living. Health protection strategies focus on assisting individuals who are ill or hospitalized to maintain their normal bowel habits, prevent disruptions in bowel functioning and maintain comfort and hygiene. When assisting a patient with a bedpan, the nurse should do all that is possible to ensure privacy, safety and comfort. If the patient needs help with cleansing the perineal or anal area the nurse wears gloves and wipes from front to back. The perineal area should be washed and dried thoroughly to prevent skin breakdown. The patient should be provided with a wet cloth to wash the hands after defecating.

Measures to restore healthy bowel patterns involve diet and drug therapy and bowel training programs. A high-fibre diet and fluids are often enough to relieve constipation. If not, a laxative, cathartic, rectal suppository or enema may be needed to produce satisfactory bowel elimination. Manual extraction of feces may sometimes be necessary. Foods that are binding or less stimulating and antidiarrheal medications are used for relief of diarrhea. Individuals with incontinence may require bowel training; those with bowel diversions may need help with ostomy self-care.

Evaluation of expected outcomes involves determining whether the patient's problem has been resolved or a regular elimination pattern has been maintained. This may be demonstrated by regular soft feces with no expressed pain during defecation, expressed knowledge of the factors influencing regularity or independent management of ostomy care by ostomates.

LEARNING ACTIVITIES

1. Mr. S. Norris is a 70-year-old man who has abdominal pain. He has been retired for five years after an active life as a house painter, and he now spends most of his time watching television. Mr. Norris lives alone in a small house just outside the city. He has three grandchildren who live a few miles away and he visits them on Sundays.

   Mr. Norris has been increasingly uncomfortable because of constipation during the past few years. He says he never took medicines when he worked but now has to take a laxative every day. Because he does not like to cook, he generally eats frozen TV dinners, sandwiches and cookies, and occasionally eggs. His doctor has referred Mr. Norris to home health care services for assistance in regulating his bowel habits. You have been assigned to his case.

   a) What factors should you take into consideration before assisting Mr. Norris?

   b) What questions would you ask Mr. Norris about his bowel habits?

   c) For what reasons might Mr. Norris be constipated? What associated problems might he have?

   d) What interventions would you think best to try? Outline the expected outcomes of nursing interventions for Mr. Norris.

   e) What would you include in your teaching program for this patient? How would you evaluate the effectiveness of your teaching?

   f) Mr. Norris's physician has ordered an enema for the patient. How would you explain this measure to him?

   g) Describe the best position for the administration of an enema and why it is desirable.

   h) What observations should you record regarding the enema?

REFERENCES AND READINGS

BARISONEK, K., NEWMAN, E. and LOGIO, T. (1984). Assessment under pressure: When your patient says "My stomach hurts." *Nursing 84, 14,* 34–41.

BASCH, A. and JENSEN, L. (1991). Management of fecal incontinence. In D. Doughty. *Urinary and fecal incontinence: Nursing maintenance,* St. Louis: Mosby, 235–268.

BERGER, K.J. and WILLIAMS, M.B. (1992). *Fundamentals of nursing: Collaborating for optimal health.* Norwalk, CT: Appleton & Lange.

BRITISH COLUMBIA DIETITIANS' AND NUTRITIONISTS' ASSOCIATION (BCDNA). (1992). *Manual of nutritional care* (4th ed.). Vancouver: Author.

CARPENITO, L.J. (1993). *Nursing diagnosis: Application to clinical practice* (5th ed.). Philadelphia: Lippincott.

EARNEST, V.V. (1993). *Clinical skills in nursing practice* (2nd ed.). Philadelphia: Lippincott.

ERICKSON, P. (1987). Ostomies: The art of pouching. *Nursing Clinics of North America, 22,* 311.

ERWIN-TOTH, P. and DOUGHTY, D. (1992). Principles and procedures of stomal management. In B. Hampton and R. Bryant. *Ostomies and continent diversions: Nursing management.* St. Louis: Mosby, 29–103.

EWING, G. (1989). The nursing preparations of stoma patients for self-care. *Journal of Advanced Nursing, 14,* 411.

FLYNN, J.M. and HACKEL, R. (1990). *Technological foundations in nursing.* Norwalk, CT: Appleton & Lange.

GUYTON, A. (1991). *Textbook of medical physiology* (8th ed.). Philadelphia: Saunders.

HEALTH AND WELFARE CANADA. (1990). *Nutrition recommendations: The report of the Scientific Review Committee.* Ottawa: Minister of Supply and Services. (Catalogue No. H49–41/1990E)

JENSEN, L. (1990). Fecal incontinence. In K. Jeter, N. Faller and C. Norton. *Nursing for continence.* Philadelphia: Saunders, 223–240.

KEE, J.L. (1991). *Laboratory and diagnostic tests with nursing implications* (3rd ed.). Norwalk, CT: Appleton & Lange.

KEE, J.L. and HAYES E.R. (1993). *Pharmacology: A nursing process approach.* Philadelphia: Saunders.

KOZIER, B., ERB, G. and OLIVIERI, R. (1991). *Fundamentals of nursing, concepts, process and practice* (4th ed.). Redwood City, CA: Addison-Wesley.

MARTINI, F. (1989). *Fundamentals of anatomy and physiology.* Englewood Cliffs, NJ: Prentice-Hall.

MCGARITY, W. Gastrointestinal surgical procedures. In B. Hampton and R. Bryant. *Ostomies and continent diversions: Nursing management.* St. Louis: Mosby, 349–373.

MORTON, P. (1989). *Health assessment in nursing.* Springhouse, PA: Springhouse.

NORTON, B.A. and MILLER, A.M. (1986). *Skills for professional nursing practice.* Norwalk, CT: Appleton-Century-Crofts, 610.

POTTER, B. (1986). *Pocket guide to physical assessment.* St. Louis: Mosby.

POTTER, P. and PERRY, A. (1993). *Fundamentals of nursing: Concepts, process and practice* (3rd ed.). St. Louis: Mosby.

RIDEOUT, B. (1987). The patient with an ileostomy: Nursing management and patient education. *Nursing Clinics of North America, 22,* 253.

ROSDAHL, C. (1991). *Textbook of basic nursing* (5th ed.). Philadelphia: Lippincott, 858.

ROTHENBERGER, D. and ORROM, W. (1991). Anatomy and physiology of defecation. In D. Doughty. *Urinary and fecal incontinence: Nursing maintenance.* St. Louis: Mosby.

SMITH, C. (1988). Assessing bowel sounds: More than just listening. *Nursing 88, 18,* 42–43.

SMITH, C. (1985). Detecting acute abdominal distention. *Nursing 85, 15,* 34–39.

SOCIETY OF GASTROENTEROLOGY NURSES AND ASSOCIATES. (1993). *Gastroenterology nursing: A core curriculum*. St. Louis: Mosby.

SPRINGHOUSE CORPORATION. (1991). *Diagnostic tests*. Springhouse, PA: Author.

WARDLAW, G.M., INSEL, P.M. and SEYLER, M.F. (1992). *Contemporary nutrition: Issues and insights*. St. Louis: Mosby.

WILLIAMS, M.W. (1993). *Lifetime: Fitness and wellness* (3rd ed.). Madison, WI: Brown and Benchmark.

CHAPTER 22

Fluid, Electrolyte and Acid–Base Balance

CENTRAL QUESTIONS

1. In what way is fluid, electrolyte and acid–base balance important to the health and well-being of the individual?

2. How are water and electrolytes distributed in the body?

3. What mechanisms regulate fluid and electrolyte balance?

4. What are the functions of the major electrolytes?

5. Why is acid–base regulation important?

6. What mechanisms maintain the normal pH range of body fluids?

7. What are the main determinants of fluid, electrolyte and acid–base balance?

8. How does fluid, electrolyte and acid–base balance vary throughout the life cycle?

9. What are the common fluid, electrolyte and acid-base balance problems?

10. What basic principles might the nurse apply in assisting patients in meeting fluid, electrolyte and acid–base balance needs?

11. How does the nurse assess a patient's fluid, electrolyte and acid–base balance status?

12. What are the common nursing diagnostic statements for patients with fluid, electrolyte and acid–base balance problems?

13. How might the nurse develop a plan of care for patients with fluid, electrolyte and acid–base balance problems?

14. What strategies might the nurse implement in helping individuals, families or groups promote optimal fluid, electrolyte and acid–base balance and prevent potential problems?

15. What health restoring and supportive strategies might the nurse implement in the care of patients with fluid, electrolyte and acid–base balance problems?

16. How might the nurse evaluate the patient's response to nursing interventions?

INTRODUCTION

Water has been called the indispensable nutrient. Approximately 60 percent of the total body weight of an average adult is made up of water and its dissolved constituents; 70 to 80 percent of the total body weight of the full-term infant is in a fluid state. The fluid system plays an essential role in the body. Its principal functions are (1) the transportation of nutrients to the cells and the removal of waste products from them, and (2) the maintenance of a stable physical and chemical environment within the body. Important in this latter function are the electrolytes. *Electrolytes* are substances which, when dissolved in solution, split into electrically charged ions of atoms or molecules that conduct an electrical current. Atoms or molecules that carry a positive charge are called *cations*, while those carrying a negative charge are called *anions*— for example, sodium (Na^+) is a cation and chloride (Cl^-) is an anion. The electrolytes in body fluids are important in the chemical reactions that occur within cells. They help regulate the distribution of water and are vital in the maintenance of acid-base balance. They are also essential in the transmission of electrical energy within the body. Without the calcium ion, for example, muscle contraction could not occur.

Healthy bodies maintain a very precise fluid, electrolyte and acid-base balance. Both the volume and constituents of body fluids vary little from day to day, and they usually return to a state of equilibrium within a few days following any minor disturbance.

Serious fluid and electrolyte imbalance may occur as a result of many health problems. The nature of the imbalance may be either a deficit or an excess. An individual may retain an excess amount of fluid in the tissues, or he or she may lose an inordinate amount of fluids (through persistent vomiting, for example). Whenever fluids are lost or retained in excessive amounts, there is an accompanying loss or retention of electrolytes, so that both fluid and electrolyte balances are disturbed. Disturbances in fluid and electrolytes can cause serious repercussions within the body. Both the transportation and regulatory functions of the fluid system are likely to be affected. The cells may not get enough nourishment, for instance, or there may be an accumulation of waste products owing to the inefficient removal. The body's acid-base balance may be upset and temperature regulation impaired. There may also be interference with the transfer of materials across the cell membrane so that a shift occurs in the distribution of fluids and electrolytes. Activities within the body that depend on the transmission of electrical energy, such as muscle contraction and the relay of nerve impulses, may be impaired.

This chapter provides an introduction to the physiology of fluid, electrolyte and acid-base balance in the body; the common fluid, electrolyte and acid-base imbalances; and the management of these problems. Assessment of fluid, electrolyte and acid-base status and nursing interventions for assisting individuals to promote, protect and restore fluid, electrolyte and acid-base balance during health and illness are also detailed.

THE PHYSIOLOGY OF FLUID, ELECTROLYTE AND ACID–BASE BALANCE

In order to understand the physiological processes involved, it is perhaps easier to consider different aspects of fluid, electrolyte and acid–base balance under separate headings:

1. The distribution of body fluids
2. The composition of body fluids
3. The transport of body fluids
4. Fluid and electrolyte balance
5. Principal electrolytes
6. Acid–base balance.

THE DISTRIBUTION OF BODY FLUIDS

Fluid within the body is generally distributed in two basic compartments. First, body fluids are found within the cells of the body. This type, termed *intracellular fluid* (ICF), accounts for approximately 40 percent of the total body weight. Second, fluid occurs outside the cells of the body;

FIGURE 22.1 Percentage of total body weight composed of water and dissolved constituents

50% to 70% water

70% to 80% water

Extracellular fluid

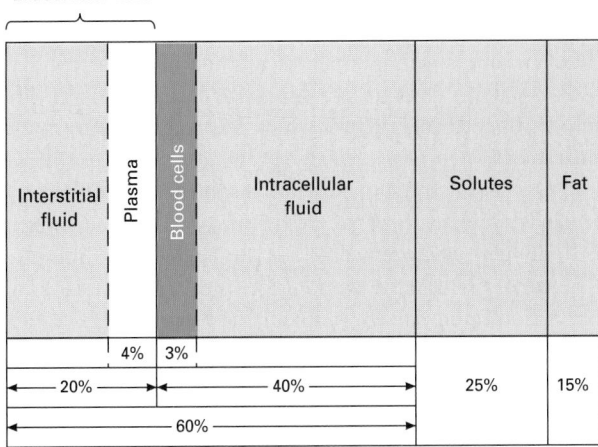

Body weight

FIGURE 22.2 Distribution of fluid between ICF and ECF in relation to body weight

SOURCE: Martini, F. (1989). *Fundamentals of anatomy and physiology.* Englewood Cliffs, NJ: Prentice-Hall, 780. Reproduced with permission.

TABLE 22.1 Approximate Values of Total Body Fluids as a Percentage of Body Weight in Relation to Age and Sex

AGE	TOTAL BODY FLUID (% BODY WEIGHT)
Full-term newborn	70%–80%
1 year	65%
Puberty to 39 years	Men: 60% Women: 52%
40 to 60 years	Men: 55% Women: 47%
More than 60 years	Men: 52% Women: 46%

SOURCE: Metheny, N.M. (1992). *Fluid and electrolyte balance.* Philadelphia: Lippincott, 5. Reproduced with permission.

this is ***extracellular fluid*** (ECF). There are two kinds of extracellular fluid. One is the fluid in the spaces between the cells; called ***interstitial fluid*** (ISF), this component accounts for about 16 percent of the body weight in an adult. The other component, the plasma or ***intravascular fluid,*** is the fluid in the blood and lymph vessels; it makes up about four percent of total body weight in an adult. A minor component of ECF is *transcellular fluid,* which includes cerebrospinal, synovial and pleural fluid as well as aqueous humor. A comparison of the distribution of intracellular and extracellular fluid as related to body weight is depicted in Figure 22.2.

Water, or fluid, from both the ICF and ECF compartments combined is referred to as total body water or fluid. The content of total body water depends on such factors as age, body fat to lean mass ratio and sex. Infants have proportionately more ECF than adults. Over half of the total body fluid in infants is extracellular as compared to about one third ECF in adults. Since ECF is more easily lost from the body than is ICF, infants are especially vulnerable to fluid volume deficits. The infant's percentage of total body fluid gradually decreases over the first two years, reaching about 64 percent of body weight by one year of age and 60 percent by the end of the second year. However, ECF is proportionately higher (24%) than ICF (36%), and remains so until puberty.

After puberty, the proportions of ECF and ICF reach adult levels but the total body fluid content varies according to body fat and sex. Lean tissue contains more water than adipose tissue. Thus, the leaner the person, the greater the percentage of total body fluid to body weight. Conversely, the

more obese the person, the lesser the percentage of body weight that is fluid. Since females have more fat tissue than males, their total body fluid is less than that of males. Correspondingly, as people get older, the percentage of total body fluid to body weight decreases as lean body mass lessens and body fat increases. See Table 22.1 for a comparison of total body fluid in relation to sex and age.

THE COMPOSITION OF BODY FLUIDS

Body fluids consist of water and dissolved substances. Water is considered to be the major constituent of the body and the ***solvent*** in which substances are either dissolved or suspended. Substances that dissolve in a solution are called ***solutes.*** These include electrolytes, minerals and substances such as glucose, urea and creatinine. The primary solutes in body fluid are the electrolytes.

The principal electrolytes and their concentrations in ECF (plasma) and ICF are given in Table 22.2. In studying this table it can be readily seen that the electrolyte composition of ECF and ICF is quite different. The fluid contained within cells is essentially a potassium and phosphate solution, whereas extracellular fluid is high in sodium and chloride.

The electrolyte composition of the two types of extracellular fluid (interstitial and plasma) is essentially the same insofar as principal electrolytes are concerned. The fluid within the blood vessels does, however, contain a much greater concentration of protein than is found in interstitial fluid.

TABLE 22.2 Electrolyte Composition in Plasma and Intracellular Fluid

PLASMA ELECTROLYTES	mmol/L	ICF ELECTROLYTES	mmol/L
Cations:			
Sodium (Na^+)	142	Potassium (K^+)	150
Potassium (K^+)	5	Magnesium (Mg^{2+})	40
Calcium (Ca^{2+})	5	Sodium (Na^+)	10
Magnesium (Mg^{2+})	2		
TOTAL CATIONS	154		200
Anions:			
Chloride (Cl^-)	103	Phosphates &	
Bicarbonate (HCO_3^-)	26	Sulfates	150
Phosphate (HPO_4^{2-})	2	Bicarbonate (HCO_3^-)	10
Proteinate	17	Proteinate	40
Sulfate (SO_4^{2-})	1		
Organic acids	5		
TOTAL ANIONS	154		200

Clinically, plasma is used to measure concentrations of extracellular electrolytes because this component best represents the electrolyte levels in the body as a whole. It is also easily accessible and samples can be obtained with minimal risk and discomfort to the patient. Usually, electrolyte concentrations are measured on serum, the portion of plasma remaining after clotted blood is removed. Thus the term **serum electrolytes** is used.

THE TRANSPORT OF BODY FLUIDS

There is a constant shift or transfer of body fluids and dissolved substances from one compartment to another as nutrients and oxygen are transported to the cells and wastes and manufactured products are removed from cells. This transfer is accomplished by several different means, the four most common being diffusion, osmosis, active transport and filtration.

Diffusion is the process whereby dissolved particles (ions and molecules) distribute themselves equally within a given space. Diffusion occurs as a result of the constant motion of molecules. The particles move from an area of higher concentration to an area of lower concentration until equilibrium is reached. In the human body, diffusion usually takes place across a **selectively permeable membrane**. A selectively permeable (or semipermeable) membrane allows some substances to pass freely through it but not others. The exchange of oxygen and carbon dioxide both in the lungs between the alveoli and the blood and in the tissues between the cells and the blood occurs by diffusion across semipermeable membranes. Electrolytes such as sodium, chloride, potassium and calcium can also diffuse across cell membranes which are permeable to these substances.

Osmosis is the movement of a solvent, such as water, through a selectively permeable membrane. The membrane is freely permeable to water but not to all of the solutes. The water passes from the solution with a low solute concentration (more solvent to solute) to the one with a higher solute concentration (less solvent to solute) until the concentrations of solutes in both solutions are equalized.

A common example of osmosis is the movement of water between two salt solutions separated by a semipermeable membrane. The water goes from the weaker salt solution to the stronger salt solution until both solutions contain the same concentrations of salt. The water is drawn across the membrane by the force of the particles in the more concentrated solution. The force which moves fluid from an area of low solute concentration to an area of high solute concentration is called **osmotic pressure**. The degree of osmotic pressure is dependent on the solute concentration, or the number of osmotically active particles per unit of volume of solvent. The more active the particles are, the greater the osmotic pressure. **Osmolality** is a term used to indicate osmotic pressure. Measured in millimoles, it refers to the number of osmotically active particles per kilogram of water (mmol/kg).

Some substances dissolved in body fluid — electrolytes, for instance — do not move across membranes as readily as water. Therefore, when it is necessary for the body to transfer electrolytes from within the cells to the extracellular fluid to achieve a balance, an **active transport** is brought into play. Active transport is the movement of solute particles from an area of lower concentration to an area of higher concentration with the use of a carrier molecule. Although the mechanism is not completely understood, it is believed that a substance known as *adenosine triphosphate (ATP)* is released from the cell. This substance appears to give the electrolytes the energy required to pass through the semipermeable membrane. The transfer of sodium, potassium and a number of other ions, including amino acids, takes place via this mechanism.

Filtration is the process whereby water and dissolved substances are forced from an area of high pressure to an area of low pressure. In the body, the pressure involved is hydrostatic or fluid pressure. Hydrostatic pressure is generated by something pushing against fluid contained within a wall. The pumping action of the heart as it propels blood through the circulatory system creates hydrostatic pressure. Filtration occurs across arterial capillary walls where water and dissolved nutrients are driven into the tissues. It also occurs in specialized tissues of the kidney in the production of urine.

FLUID AND ELECTROLYTE BALANCE

The mechanisms that maintain fluid and electrolyte balance are closely connected. That is, there are no separate receptors that monitor fluid balance or specific ion concentrations. Instead, fluid and electrolyte adjustments are made in response to osmotic pressure (osmolality) or volume of extracellular fluid. In the healthy adult, body fluid volume remains fairly constant, despite intake variations. This is due to the regulatory mechanisms that balance intake (gains) and output (losses).

FLUID INTAKE AND OUTPUT

People derive fluid and electrolytes from three main sources: the fluid that is ingested in liquid form, the fluid content of the various foods that are eaten and water that is formed as a by-product of the body's oxidation of foods and body substances. The total daily intake of water under normal circumstances is approximately 2100 to 2900 ml. Water is lost from the body through the skin by perspiration, through the lungs during expiration and from the kidneys in the urine. In addition, a small amount of fluid is excreted in the feces. The total daily loss of water from the body in normal circumstances is approximately 2100 to 2900 ml, depending largely upon the amount of fluid intake. The average amounts of daily fluid gains and losses are listed in the accompanying box.

MECHANISMS REGULATING FLUID INTAKE AND OUTPUT

Although individual water molecules move from one fluid compartment to another, the volume of fluid in each compartment remains relatively stable. The main forces at work in holding water within the various compartments of the fluid system of the body (hydrostatic pressure and osmotic pressure) are generated by proteins and electrolytes. In the intravascular compartment (blood vessels) the force is generated largely by the serum albumin; in the interstitial fluid by the sodium ion; and within the cells by protoplasm. Water passes freely through the capillary walls and membranes, but the protein molecules and the sodium ions do not move as freely. These substances exert an osmotic pressure that tends to hold water in their respective compartments. A patient who has lost a great deal of serum albumin through malnutrition tends to become edematous, as fluid is drawn from the blood plasma into the interstitial spaces. This happens because the osmotic pressure holding the water in the blood vessels has been reduced.

By far the most important regulatory mechanism operating to maintain the body's fluid balance is the kidneys. When the intake of fluid is insufficient or when there is an

Average Daily Fluid Gains and Losses		
GAINS		
Ingested fluids	1000	to 1500 ml
Ingested foods	900	to 1000 ml
Metabolic oxidation	200	to 400 ml
TOTAL GAINS	2100	to 2900 ml
LOSSES		
In urine	1000	to 1500 ml
In feces	100	to 200 ml
Through skin	600	to 700 ml
Through lungs	400	to 500 ml
TOTAL LOSSES	2100	to 2900 ml

excessive loss of fluid from the body, the amount of urine that is excreted is decreased. Conversely, when an excess amount of fluid is ingested, urine output increases. This is accomplished through the selective reabsorption of water in the tubules of the kidney.

The kidney also exerts the main control over the sodium and potassium balance of the body through the selective reabsorption of these ions in the tubules. When sodium and potassium levels are low in the body, increasing amounts are reabsorbed into the blood stream. When sodium and potassium levels are high in the body, the excess is excreted in the urine. If there is an acute shortage of sodium in the body, the excretion of this ion through the urine may be cut to almost zero. In the case of potassium, however, there appears to be an obligatory excretion of a certain amount in the urine (MacBryde and Backlow, 1970). Thus, there is always some potassium in the daily urine output, even though the body reserves may be dangerously low. This factor is taken into account by physicians in planning replacement therapy.

The control of fluid by the kidneys is influenced by two sets of hormones. The *antidiuretic hormone* (ADH), which is produced primarily in the anterior hypothalamus and stored in the posterior pituitary gland, is a major factor in controlling water reabsorption. When the osmotic pressure of the ECF is greater than that of the cells because of insufficient water intake, deprivation of water from other sources or excessive sodium intake, for instance, the secretion of ADH is stimulated. This in turn causes increased reabsorption of water in the kidney tubules and a lessened volume of urinary output. *Aldosterone*, one of several steroid hormones produced in the adrenal cortex, exerts a major influence in promoting the retention of sodium and the excretion of potassium. Aldosterone secretion appears to be stimulated by such factors as lessened sodium intake, an excess of potassium, muscular activity, trauma and emotional tension (MacBryde and Backlow, 1970).

The gastrointestinal tract also helps to regulate fluid and electrolyte balance. Selective reabsorption of water and solutes takes place principally in the small intestine. Although the volume of digestive juices secreted into the intestinal tract each day is considerable (approximately 8200 ml), all but about 100 to 200 ml of fluid is reabsorbed. Under normal circumstances, only a small amount of the body's daily fluid loss is from the gastrointestinal tract in the feces, and the loss of electrolytes by this route is normally negligible. Both fluid and electrolytes may be lost in considerable quantity, however, in such conditions as vomiting and diarrhea.

Thirst is another of the regulatory mechanisms working to maintain fluid balance. Thirst is the desire for more fluids. It usually indicates a basic physiological need for water, although it may sometimes occur as a result of dryness of the mucous membranes of the mouth and throat from other causes, such as mouth breathing. *True thirst*, due to a basic lack of water, usually occurs when body cells are dehydrated, extracellular volume is lessened (by hemorrhage, for example), or certain centres in the hypothalamus are stimulated. The thirst mechanism is related to the control of water balance by the antidiuretic hormone (ADH). When the body is suffering from a lack of water, the thirst mechanism operates to increase the desire for intake of water, while ADH acts on the distal convoluted tubules of the kidney to increase reabsorption of water (Woodtli, 1990).

The lungs are also important in the regulation of fluid and electrolyte balance. Ordinarily, the amount of water lost from respiration is quite small. Whenever respirations are increased in rate and depth, however, the amount of water lost via this route is also increased and may become a significant factor to consider. This may occur, for example, with strenuous muscular exercise, in fevers or any condition in which respirations are considerably increased or when the air that is breathed is very dry. The loss of electrolytes through respiration is normally minimal, although the lungs play an important role in maintaining acid–base balance of the body as will be discussed later.

PRINCIPAL ELECTROLYTES

As we mentioned previously, electrolytes are the primary solutes of body fluid and are necessary for maintaining homeostasis within the body. In this respect they primarily function in three physiological processes: body fluid distribution and osmolality; nerve and muscle irritability and contractility; and acid–base balance. There are many electrolytes in the body; each has its distinct functions and regulating mechanisms. Only the principal cations and anions will be outlined here.

Sodium

Sodium is the major cation within extracellular fluid. In fact, more than 90 percent of osmolality of the ECF comes from sodium salts, namely sodium chloride (NaCl) and sodium bicarbonate ($NaHCO_3$). Because of its abundance in quantity and the fact that it does not move across cell membranes with ease, sodium is largely responsible for maintaining water balance. Indeed, its primary functions are to control the distribution of water throughout the body and to regulate the extracellular fluid volume.

A basic assumption behind sodium's role in water balance is that where sodium goes, water goes with it. If sodium is retained or excreted, water will be retained or excreted, too. Because extracellular volume is exceptionally stable in health, sodium balance must be maintained within normal limits. Furthermore, the regulation of sodium balance is interrelated with the regulation of other electrolytes and with acid–base balance, owing to its ability to combine readily with chloride and bicarbonate. Therefore, sodium imbalances are often accompanied by electrolyte and acid–base disturbances as well (Keys, 1985).

Sodium plays an important role in neuromuscular activity and the transmission of nerve impulses. As part of the cellular sodium–potassium exchange, sodium moves into nerve cells that have been stimulated and generates action potentials. An **action potential** is a change in electrical charge on the cell membrane that activates nerves to transmit impulses to muscles, causing muscles to contract.

The average daily requirement for sodium is two to four grams. Sodium is taken into the body from food and fluid sources. A list of foods rich in sodium is presented in Table 22.3. A very common dietary source is table salt used in cooking. It is also abundant in most processed foods. Sodium ions enter the ECF through the digestive epithelium, mainly in the small intestine, by the processes of diffusion and active transport. The normal serum concentration of sodium is 135 to 150 mmol/litre. The amount that enters the ECF is directly proportional to the amount of sodium in the diet. To maintain a stable extracellular volume, the intake of sodium must equal its output. Sodium balance is regulated within narrow limits by the kidneys, which are influenced primarily by the action of aldosterone, the glomerular filtration rate and the physical condition of the kidneys themselves. Excess sodium is excreted in the urine. Small amounts are also lost through perspiration and feces.

Potassium

Potassium is the main cation of intracellular fluid. About 98 percent of the body's content of potassium lies inside the cells; the remaining two percent is extracellular. It is this two percent of extracellular potassium that represents serum potassium levels. Since it is the major intracellular electrolyte, potassium accounts for a large portion of osmotic

TABLE 22.3 Functions and Food Sources of Principal Electrolytes

ELECTROLYTE	FUNCTIONS	FOOD SOURCE
Sodium	Regulates body fluid volume Generates and transmits nerve impulses Aids in acid–base balance Involved in enzyme activities	Table salt Baking soda Soy sauce Processed dairy products: cheese, butter, margarine Eggs Processed, canned or smoked meats Celery, spinach Canned vegetables Processed cereals Condiments such as mayonnaise, ketchup, mustard, pickles, salad dressings
Potassium	Helps maintain the intercellular osmotic pressure Regulates body fluids (primarily within the cell) Transmits and conducts nerve impulses Involved in muscle fibre contraction Maintains regular cardiac rhythm Activates cellular enzymes	Fresh apricots, bananas, citrus fruits and juices Dried fruits such as figs, dates, peaches, raisins Avocados, fresh tomato, mushrooms, broccoli, Brussels sprouts, spinach Cooked kidney beans, baked potato Chicken, salmon, sardines, scallops Whole milk, yogurt
Calcium	Forms and maintains healthy bones and teeth Aids in transmission of nerve impulses, muscle contraction, and blood clotting Maintains cell membrane permeability	Milk, cheese, yogurt Green, leafy vegetables such as kale, turnip and mustard greens, broccoli Sardines and salmon Tofu
Magnesium	Aids in transmission of impulses in nerves and muscles Activates enzymes Aids in bone formation	Green vegetables Roasted peanuts Bananas Milk, yogurt Soybeans Grains, bran
Chloride	Transports CO_2 (chloride shift) Maintains osmotic pressure Aids in acid–base balance Component of hydrochloric acid in stomach	Table salt Seafood Meats Eggs Milk
Phosphorus	Provides strength and rigidity to bones and teeth Buffer in acid–base balance Participates in fat, carbohydrate and protein metabolism	Beef, pork, poultry, fish and fish eggs Milk and milk products, especially cheddar cheese Peanuts Cooked dry beans Carbonated beverages Whole grains, fruits and vegetables are fair sources

FOOD SOURCES FROM: Stanfield, P. (1986), 81–93; Holman, S.R. (1987), 48–50; 58–59.

pressure within the intracellular fluid compartment and in this way is involved in the distribution of body water.

Potassium is necessary for the transmission of nerve impulses and the contraction of skeletal, smooth and cardiac muscles. Once a nerve impulse has been generated by the influx of sodium ions, potassium shifts out of the cell and in so doing restores the resting state of the cell membrane. Until the neuron is restored to a resting state, it cannot conduct another impulse. In this way potassium regulates the excitability of nerve and muscle cells and controls neuromuscular activity in the body.

Potassium plays a major role in activating specific cellular enzymes necessary for carbohydrate metabolism and it participates in protein synthesis. It is involved in normal kidney function and promotes acid–base balance through its cellular exchange with the hydrogen ion.

The average daily requirement for potassium is three to four grams. Food sources high in potassium are listed in Table 22.3. Most vegetables, when eaten raw, are rich in potassium. Bananas, citrus fruits and juices and dried fruits are also good sources of potassium, as are chicken and seafood. Virtually all potassium that is ingested is absorbed through the small intestine. The normal serum concentration of potassium is 3.5 to 5.0 mmol/litre. In health, potassium ions are conserved; potassium balance is maintained when the rate of urinary excretion equals the amount absorbed from the digestive tract. Potassium balance in the body is regulated by the kidneys in response to alterations in the potassium ion concentration or pH of the interstitial fluid and through the influence of aldosterone (Martini, 1989). Small amounts of potassium are eliminated in the feces and sweat.

Calcium

Calcium, which is a cation, is the major element involved in maintaining the structure and function of bones and teeth. Only about one percent of the total body calcium is part of extracellular fluid. Of this, over half is bound to proteins such as albumin and globulin or combined with ions such as citrate, sulfate or phosphate. Less than half of the extracellular calcium is freely ionized and available for use in chemical and biological functions in the body. Calcium is needed for the transmission of nerve impulses and for the contraction and relaxation of muscles. It is necessary for maintaining the permeability of cell membranes and is an essential element in blood coagulation.

The average adult requires about 800 mg of calcium daily. Large-bodied people, children and pregnant and lactating women require more. Calcium is primarily absorbed from the small intestine. It is important to note that not all of the calcium that is ingested is absorbed. The average adult absorbs 30 to 60 percent of daily ingested calcium; about 15 percent is considered nonabsorbable (Stroot, Lee and Barrett, 1984). Intestinal absorption is prevented by low vitamin D intake and by binding agents which are present in certain vegetables.

The normal serum calcium level is 2.12–2.62 mmol/litre. This value includes the ionized, *complexed* (combined with citrate, for example) and protein-bound calcium. The normal concentration of calcium in plasma is regulated by a fairly complex set of organ and hormonal factors. The primary hormones include parathyroid hormone (PTH), calcitonin (secreted by the thyroid gland) and Vitamin D. When plasma levels of ionized calcium drop, PTH is secreted. PTH stimulates the release of calcium from bones and teeth and increases the reabsorption of calcium from the kidney. Calcitonin, on the other hand, has the effect of lowering extracellular calcium concentrations. It decreases plasma calcium levels by inhibiting the release of PTH, facilitating the transfer of calcium from plasma to bone, and increasing renal excretion of calcium. Vitamin D promotes the absorption of calcium from the intestine and assists PTH in the reabsorption of calcium from the bone. The bulk of excess calcium is excreted in the urine. Smaller amounts are also lost in feces, digestive secretions and perspiration.

Magnesium

Magnesium is the second most abundant cation found in intracellular fluid. However, it must be noted that 60 percent of magnesium in the body is located in bone, muscle and soft tissues. In addition, as with calcium, it is only the ionized fraction of serum magnesium that is free for chemical activity and physiological processes.

Magnesium plays a role in neuromuscular activity. It is thought to mediate the release of acetylcholine by motor nerve impulses, creating a sedative effect, and in so doing helps to regulate the transmission of activating impulses in nerves and muscles.

Magnesium is also an important activator of enzymes involved in protein and carbohydrate metabolism. It is necessary for energy production (that is, the formation of ATP) and it works with calcium, phosphorus and vitamin D in the formation of bone. The average daily nutrient requirement for magnesium is 300 mg. The principal sources of dietary magnesium are listed in Table 22.3. The normal serum concentration of magnesium is 0.69- 1.07 mmol/litre. The regulation of magnesium balance in the body is not completely known (Keyes, 1985). The kidneys play a large role in conserving and excreting magnesium.

Chloride

Chloride is the principal anion of the ECF. A very small quantity of chloride is present in the ICF, where it plays a significant role in the functioning of specialized cells such as neurons. In the ECF, this electrolyte parallels that of sodium and is generally considered to have a passive relationship with sodium. That is, when serum sodium increases, chloride also increases and when serum levels of sodium drop, chloride levels usually drop, too. Sodium and chloride dissolved in water constitute the saline solution of the ECF compartment; both tend to hold water. Thus, like sodium, chloride functions in maintaining fluid balance and osmotic pressure of the ECF. Chloride also plays a passive role in acid–base balance where the kidneys excrete chloride or bicarbonate ions, and sodium conserves chloride or bicarbonate ions along with it to maintain acid–base balance. In cases where bicarbonate ions are retained, as in metabolic alkalosis, for example, chloride will be excreted while sodium is reabsorbed with bicarbonate. When this happens, chloride losses will not be in proportion to sodium losses, which is a deviation from the parallel, passive nature of chloride's relationship with sodium. Thus, while increases in serum chloride levels follow those of serum sodium, losses in serum sodium and chloride can differ.

Chloride plays a part in the chloride shift, which is the chloride-bicarbonate buffer system that functions to maintain the pH balance of the blood. It is also a necessary component of hydrochloric acid in gastric juice.

The average daily requirement for chloride is three to five grams. Substantial amounts of chloride are found in table salt, dairy products and meats. It is often ingested in combination with sodium or potassium, as a sodium or potassium salt. Normal serum levels of chloride are 98–109 mmol/litre. Chloride is absorbed readily from the small intestine along with sodium and potassium. It is chiefly excreted from the body by the kidneys; however, it is also lost in sweat and gastrointestinal secretions.

Bicarbonate

The bicarbonate molecule is the second most abundant anion of extracellular fluid; it is found in intracellular fluid as well. It is an essential component of the bicarbonate–carbonic acid buffer system which functions to maintain normal hydrogen ion concentration and acid–base balance of the body fluids. Bicarbonate differs from the other principal electrolytes in that it is not ingested through food and fluid sources, but is synthesized in the body as the end product of fat metabolism. Base bicarbonate (pertaining to the buffer bicarbonate) is produced when sodium, potassium, calcium or magnesium combine with bicarbonate. Normal serum levels of bicarbonate are 23–33 mmols/litre. Since it is a principal base buffer within the body, the regulation and excretion of bicarbonate is discussed in the section on acid–base balance.

Phosphorus and Phosphate

Phosphorus is found in the body in the form of organic and inorganic compounds. Most of it is located in the ICF, mainly as organic phosphate. In fact, 80 percent of the total body phosphorus is comprised of cellular organic phosphate located in bone. Another 10 percent of cellular phosphate is

found in muscles and one percent is located in nerve tissues. The remaining nine percent of the total body phosphorus is located in the ECF (Stroot, Lee and Barrett, 1984).

The phosphate ion is the major intracellular anion. Phosphate plays a role in many body functions. In conjunction with calcium, it provides strength and rigidity to bones and teeth. It acts as a buffer in maintaining acid–base balance and participates in carbohydrate, protein and lipid metabolism. Phosphate is required for normal nerve and muscle activity, and is important for many cellular activities such as the formation of high energy compounds (for example, ATP), the utilization of B vitamins and the transmission of hereditary traits.

The average daily requirement for phosphorus is 800 mg. Growing children and pregnant and lactating women need more. Dietary sources rich in this electrolyte are listed in Table 22.3. The normal serum phosphorus level is 0.81–1.58 mmol/litre. Phosphorus is absorbed easily from the small intestine, especially when vitamin D_3 (activated vitamin D) is present. When dietary intake of calcium is excessively high, however, absorption of phosphorus is inhibited. In the presence of too much calcium, phosphorus binds with the calcium forming insoluble compounds that are excreted in the feces. Phosphorous, like calcium, is regulated by the parathyroid hormone and calcitonin. It is excreted primarily in the urine and is, in fact, the major urine buffer.

ACID–BASE BALANCE

BODY PH BALANCE

Intimately connected with the fluid and electrolyte balance of the body is the maintenance of acid–base (H^+) balance. **Acids** ionize in water and release hydrogen ions (H+). **Bases** combine with the hydrogen ions released by acids to neutralize their effects. Bases make a solution more alkaline. The relative acidity or alkalinity of body fluids is expressed in terms of pH, which refers to the concentration of hydrogen ions in the fluid. The pH is measured on a negative logarthimic scale of 1 to 14. Water, which is considered a neutral substance (being neither acid nor alkaline), has a pH of 7.0. The pH scale is based on a negative logarithm. Acid solutions have a pH lower than 7.0 and alkaline solutions a pH higher than 7.0. Body fluids are not as neutral as water; they tend towards the basic side of the scale.

When large amounts of fluids are lost or retained in the body, the acid–base balance can swing in the direction of a higher concentration of either acid or base. The term *acidosis* refers to a swing towards the acid side through either a retention of excess acid (H^+ concentration) in the body or a depletion of the body's base reserves. The normally basic state of body fluids becomes more acidic. A pH below 7.35, the lowest point on the normal range for blood, is generally considered to indicate acidosis.

Alkalosis is the opposite of acidosis; there is either a lessening of the acid (H⁺ concentration) of body fluids or an excess of base reserves. When the pH of blood exceeds 7.45, the highest point in the normal range, the condition is called alkalosis. When acidosis or alkalosis results from disturbances in metabolism, the term *metabolic acidosis* or *metabolic alkalosis* is used; when it results from disturbed respiratory functioning, it is called *respiratory acidosis* or *respiratory alkalosis*.

REGULATING MECHANISMS

In order for the body to function normally, the pH of body fluids must be maintained within the normal range, that is, between 7.35 and 7.45. Any deviation from this range poses a threat to homeostasis because changes in hydrogen ion concentration disrupt the stability of cell membranes, alter protein structure, and change the activities of important enzymes. The nervous system is particularly sensitive to fluctuations in pH, becoming depressed in acidosis and hyperexcitable in alkalosis (Martini, 1989). Therefore, the control of pH is essential for normal physiological functioning in the body. The acid–base balance of body fluids is maintained by four mechanisms: dilution, buffer systems, respiratory regulation and renal regulation.

Dilution

A local small buildup of extra acid or base may be corrected by the simple process of *dilution* — the circulating fluid picks up the extra ions and takes them away from the trouble spot; they become diluted in the total volume of fluid circulating. The excess acid accumulated in a muscle after exercise, for example, may be removed in this way.

Buffer Systems

The body also has a system of *buffers*, which function within the fluid system to correct the tendency towards either acidity or alkalinity. Buffers are pairs of substances consisting of a weak acid and its salt, which act as sponges to absorb extra hydrogen or base ions as required. The principal buffering agents in body fluids are the carbonic acid-bicarbonate system, which operates mainly in the extracellular fluid; the phosphate buffer system, which operates predominantly in the intracellular fluid; and the protein buffer system, which operates in both (proteins can act as acids or bases as needed). The primary buffer in the body is the bicarbonate–carbonic acid system.

Buffers act immediately to correct changes in the body's pH balance. However, their ability to function on a long-term basis is limited, because as soon as they react, they are used up and eventually have to be replaced. Therefore, the body brings two other mechanisms into play — the *lungs* and the *kidneys*.

Respiratory Regulation

The lungs aid in maintaining acid–base balance through their control of carbonic acid. They can eliminate either more or less carbonic acid (in the form of carbon dioxide and water), thus either ridding the body of excess acid or conserving it. When you have engaged in strenuous exercise, for example, you may find that you are breathing more quickly and more deeply than usual, as the body attempts to rid itself of the extra acid from the waste products of muscle cell metabolism.

Renal Regulation

The kidneys can vary the acidity of the urine in response to the body's need to throw off excess acid or base. They act principally by controlling base bicarbonate. See the accompanying box on mechanisms for maintaining normal hydrogen ion concentration.

DETERMINANTS OF FLUID, ELECTROLYTE AND ACID–BASE BALANCE

Many factors will disturb the body's fluid and electrolyte balance. These factors fall under the following general headings: Insufficient Intake, Disturbances of Gastrointestinal Function, Disturbances of Kidney Function, Excessive Perspiration or Evaporation and Volume Losses.

INSUFFICIENT INTAKE

The sources of water and electrolytes for the body are the food and fluids ingested. Any disturbance in the source of nourishment is reflected in the body. People who do not take in a sufficient amount of food and fluids, either because these are not available or because of lifestyle, fad dieting or illness, will usually show a disturbed fluid and electrolyte balance, particularly if the insufficient intake is prolonged.

DISTURBANCES OF GASTROINTESTINAL FUNCTION

A very large volume of fluid in the form of digestive juices is secreted into the gastrointestinal tract each day. Almost all of this fluid is reabsorbed during the process of digestion. Interference with the normal processes of secretion and reabsorption can result in serious fluid and electrolyte imbalance. The nature of the imbalance depends to a large extent on the portion of the gastrointestinal tract affected.

Mechanisms for maintaining normal hydrogen ion concentration

The buffer system

Bicarbonate–carbonic acid (primary buffer system)

Carbonic acid (weak acid)
$$H_2CO_3 \rightleftharpoons H_2O + CO_2$$
Sodium bicarbonate (weak base)
$$NaHCO_3$$

In the presence of a buffer system
the pH shifts only slightly

$$NaHCO_3 + HCl \rightarrow H_2CO_3 + NaCl$$
(strong   (weak
acid)   acid)

$$H_2CO_3 + NaOH \rightarrow NaHCO_3 + H_2O$$
(strong   (weak
base)   base)

The respiratory system

The respiratory system acts as a feedback system for
controlling hydrogen ion concentration

H^+ concentration increases
pH $7.4 \rightarrow 7$
Respirations $\rightarrow$ rapid and deep
More CO_2 exhaled
Less CO_2 to combine
Therefore, less H_2CO_3

50% to 75% efficient

pH from 7 to 7.2 or 7.3 within minutes
OR
H^+ concentration decreases
pH $7.4 \rightarrow 7.8$
Respirations $\rightarrow$ slow and shallow
Less CO_2 exhaled
More CO_2 to combine
Therefore, more H_2CO_3

pH from 7.8 to 7.6 or 7.7 within minutes

The renal system

This complex mechanism continues to act
until the pH reaches normal; requires more time

Can excrete more or less H^+ to achieve balance
Can excrete more or less bicarbonate to achieve balance

SOURCE: Weldy, N.J. (1992). *Body fluids and electrolytes* (5th ed.). St. Louis: Mosby, 54. Reproduced with permission.

In order to appreciate the significance of this point, it is helpful to keep in mind the volume, the pH and the electrolyte composition of the various digestive juices. The approximate volumes and pH of the principal digestive juices secreted per day are given in Table 22.4

The major components involved in electrolyte and acid–base balance are found in the gastric and intestinal secretions. Gastric juice contains large quantities of hydrochloric acid and a significant amount of sodium. Gastric mucus contains a high proportion of sodium and chloride, small but significant amounts of potassium, and a relatively small amount of carbonate. Thus, when fluids are lost from the stomach through vomiting, there may be a significant loss of acid as well. Prolonged vomiting may cause severe

TABLE 22.4 Approximate Daily Volumes and pH of Principal Digestive Juices

SECRETION	DAILY VOLUME	USUAL PH
Saliva	1000 ml	6.7
Gastric juice	2500 ml	1.0–3.5
Small bowel fluid	3500 ml	7.5–8.0
Pancreatic juice	700 ml	8.0–8.3
Bile	500 ml	7.8

SOURCE: Metheney, 1992, 223.

sodium depletion and loss of chloride ions. The body's reserves of potassium may also be decreased. Gastric suctioning removes hydrochloric acid and fluids; gastric washings can severely deplete the store of chloride ions, particularly if these washings are done with water rather than saline. All gastric tube irrigations as well as gastric washings should therefore be done with isotonic saline to prevent the depletion of these electrolytes.

Pancreatic juice, bile and the intestinal secretions are predominantly basic and contain relatively large amounts of bicarbonate, as well as sodium and chloride. In addition, a portion of the total volume of potassium excreted from the body daily is via the gastrointestinal tract in the feces. Thus, diarrhea generally results in the loss of fluids, and of sodium and chloride ions, as well as of the base secreted in the intestine. Severe diarrhea also depletes the body's potassium levels.

DISTURBANCES OF KIDNEY FUNCTION

Because the kidney is so intimately connected with the regulation of fluid, electrolyte and acid–base balance, any impairment in renal function may disturb this balance. Damage to the kidney itself may interfere with its ability to reabsorb water and electrolytes in the tubules. An imbalance in the antidiuretic hormone (caused by pituitary gland dysfunction, for example) affects kidney functioning, particularly the reabsorption of water. Similarly, an imbalance in aldosterone (which may result from steroid therapy) affects sodium retention and potassium excretion by the kidneys.

The kidneys are also affected by disturbance in cardiovascular functioning. For example, a poorly functioning heart may cause an insufficient flow of blood through the kidneys to produce an adequate amount of glomerular filtrate. As a result, body tissues may retain fluid. This is evidenced by edema, which is a frequent accompaniment of many cardiac conditions.

EXCESSIVE PERSPIRATION OR EVAPORATION

One of the most significant variables in the amount of water lost from the body daily is the volume of perspiration. This may range from zero to several litres per day, depending on such factors as the amount of physical activity engaged in, the temperature of the environment and the presence of fever. When there is excessive perspiration, two protective mechanisms are brought into play: thirst, which increases the amount of fluid intake; and adjustment of the water output by the kidneys (MacBryde and Backlow, 1970).

When fluids are lost through sweating, there is a loss of sodium chloride as well. Hence, people who live in hot climates, and those who must work in temperatures above normal, often find they need more salt in their food to replace that lost through perspiration. As a person becomes acclimatized to higher environmental temperatures, however, the body usually adjusts by lessening the salt content of sweat so that the loss of sodium and chloride ions by this route is minimized.

VOLUME LOSSES

Conditions which cause a loss of fluid volume may cause severe disturbances in fluid, electrolyte and acid–base balance. Hemorrhage causes not only a loss of fluid but also a percentage of all the blood elements. The total circulatory volume is decreased and, in a large hemorrhage, the body's adaptive mechanisms may collapse and shock may ensue.

In burns, as well as in some trauma to the body (including surgical trauma), fluid and electrolytes are lost from the general circulation, as these tend to accumulate in the interstitial spaces. Fluids are removed from the plasma, sodium is depleted throughout the body generally, and potassium is released in excessive amounts from the damaged cells. Proteins are also depleted. Therefore, there is a need to replace not only fluids but also sodium, potassium and proteins in order to restore a balance.

FLUID AND ELECTROLYTE NEEDS THROUGHOUT THE LIFE CYCLE

The pregnant woman's circulatory system must take care of the fluid and electrolyte and oxygen needs of the fetus, as well as her own. To cope with these demands, her total blood volume is increased by approximately 50 percent, the production of red blood cells in her body is stepped up by almost one third, and total cardiac volume is increased by approximately 10 percent. The pregnant woman's heart must also beat faster (her resting pulse rate increases) with the extra demands on her circulatory system. There is also a marked increase in the body's water content. An average of 6.5 to 7 litres is gained, including 3.5 litres for the needs of the fetus and the balance for the mother's needs.

Many pregnant women experience fluid retention, which may be caused by such factors as a decrease in blood protein, hypervolemia (in which fluid readily leaves the intravascular spaces to equalize osmotic pressure), an increase in capillary permeability, and a tendency to retain sodium. Some edema is common, particularly in the late stages of pregnancy. Some women develop a pregnancy-induced hypertension (a complication that can cause problems for both fetus and mother). This hypertension is related to sodium and water retention.

As mentioned at the beginning of the chapter, 70 to 80 percent of a newborn's body weight is water. Until around the age of two years, fluids continue to make up a greater proportion of total body weight than they do in older children and adults. Much of the additional fluid is extracellular, and is rapidly lost in the event of illness, a factor that makes the infant very vulnerable to fluid and electrolyte and acid–base imbalances.

The infant also has a high metabolic rate, because of his or her greater proportional body surface area, growth needs, and relatively large body organs. The high metabolic rate means that there is more rapid turnover of water in the body of children than in adults, and that children need a larger amount of fluid proportional to body weight. Another factor contributing to the infant's vulnerability to fluid and electrolyte imbalances is the immaturity of the homeostatic mechanisms. For example, the infant's kidneys have a limited ability to concentrate and dilute urine, a mechanism that is important in maintaining fluid balance.

By the time the child is two years of age, fluid volume as a percentage of total body weight, as well as its distribution in the body, is similar to that in an adult. The basal metabolic rate gradually decreases through childhood until maturity, and the water turnover gradually slows down to adult levels. Children, however, continue to need a greater volume of fluids proportionate to body weight than adults do and also lose a proportionately greater volume in urine.

In children there is also a greater exchange of fluids in the gastrointestinal tract than there is in adults. This factor is important because it is through this exchange that water and sodium are absorbed. Thus, problems interfering with the reabsorption of fluids in the gastrointestinal tract can cause major fluid losses in children. Children can become dehydrated quickly with even minor gastrointestinal upsets. Edema is often seen in refugee children who are starving. In this case the fluid flows from the blood vessels into the tissues because lowered levels of plasma protein are insufficient to hold the fluid in the intravascular compartment.

With adolescence, there is a maturing of all body systems and the homeostatic mechanisms for regulating fluid and electrolyte balance begin to function as they do in adults. In fluid and electrolyte balance, as in so many other aspects of physiological functioning, there is a difference between males and females; women have a tendency to retain fluids during the two or three days immediately prior to the menstrual period. Just before the menstrual period, there is an increase in the level of the hormone progesterone. This hormone is related in chemical composition to aldosterone and has a similar effect in promoting the retention of sodium, which, in turn, leads to the retention of water in the body.

Throughout adulthood, there is a gradual decrease in the functional capacity of the cardiovascular system as blood pressure increases and the individual becomes more vulnerable to cardiovascular diseases. A gradual lessening in efficiency of the fluid and electrolyte regulating mechanisms contributes to making the older adult slower to recover from imbalances than the younger adult.

During menopause many women have a problem with fluid retention. Although a number of theories have been postulated, no single definitive cause has been isolated.

TABLE 22.5 Range of Average Water Requirement of Children at Different Ages under Ordinary Conditions

AGE	AVERAGE BODY WEIGHT IN KG	TOTAL WATER IN 24 HOURS, ML	WATER PER KG BODY WT. IN 24 HOURS, ML
3 days	3.0	250–300	80–100
10 days	3.2	400–500	125–150
3 months	5.4	750–850	140–160
6 months	7.3	950–1100	130–155
9 months	8.6	1100–1250	125–145
1 year	9.5	1150–1300	120–135
2 years	11.8	1350–1500	115–125
4 years	16.2	1600–1800	100–110
6 years	20.0	1800–2000	90–100
10 years	28.7	2000–2500	70–85
14 years	45.0	2200–2700	50–60
18 years	54.0	2200–2700	40–50

SOURCE: Vaughan, V.C. III., McKay, R.J. and Behrman, R.E. (1993) *Nelson textbook of pediatrics* (11th ed.). Philadelphia: Saunders, 107. Reproduced with permission.

Generally it is usually considered to be *idiopathic*, that is, due to no known cause.

In the older adult, the prevalence of hypertension and the incidence of cardiovascular disease increase. The arteries thicken and become less elastic. Many older people have a problem with varicose veins. If the varicosities occur in the deep veins, there will be reduced venous return and edema of the ankles. Older adults have a blunted thirst mechanism which makes it difficult to get them to drink a sufficient amount of fluids to meet their bodily needs, particularly when they are ill. It is important to make a point of offering extra fluids between meal times and encouraging them to drink more water, milk and juices.

COMMON PROBLEMS

Disturbances in fluid, electrolytes and acid–base balance are often not disease entities themselves, but complications of other disorders or trauma. The underlying pathophysiology of many disease processes cause either gains or losses of body water and/or solutes. The resulting fluid, electrolyte and acid–base disturbances can cause many problems to the body's internal environment. As we already discussed, all other systems in the body depend on the effective functioning of the fluid system. It serves not only as the transport mechanism for moving nutrients and removing wastes, but also provides an optimal environment for the efficient functioning of body cells.

As a result of fluid, electrolyte and acid–base imbalance, problems may arise in any of the body's functional areas. These problems often require medical or nursing intervention. The type of problem and the intervention required depend to a large extent on the specific nature of the imbalance and the degree of disturbance. The most common problems that the nurse will encounter are those associated with fluid and electrolyte excesses or deficits, and the accompanying disturbances in acid–base balance.

FLUID VOLUME IMBALANCES

FLUID VOLUME DEFICIT

Fluid volume deficit (FVD) is a general term used to designate a condition in which the body or tissues are deprived of water. It may result from a number of causes, such as insufficient intake of fluids, or disease conditions causing excess fluid loss, as outlined in Table 22.6.

There are three types of fluid volume deficit. The first, called **isotonic** or extracellular *fluid deficit*, occurs when water and electrolytes are both lost in approximately the same proportions, and the osmolality of the remaining fluids are normal. In this type of disturbance, the loss of fluid comes primarily from the ECF; that is, intravascular fluid and interstitial fluid which lead to hypovolemia (decreased volume of circulating blood) and dehydration. Since there is no change in osmolality, there is very little movement from other compartments. Therefore, loss of fluid from the ICF does not occur.

Extracellular fluid deficit occurs when fluid is lost from the body as with hemorrhage and diarrhea or when it becomes trapped in a third space. A *third space* is an area such as a body cavity in which fluid accumulates and cannot be drawn back into the circulatory system. An example of third space fluid loss is the accumulation of fluid in the bowel due to obstruction. With hemorrhage, in addition to intravascular fluid loss, there is a loss of ICF because the fluid within the red blood cells belongs to the intracellular compartment. Hemorrhage can lead to volume deficit from both the ECF and ICF compartments (Keyes, 1985).

The second type of fluid volume deficit is a **hypotonic dehydration**. In this case, solutes are lost from the ECF without a proportionate loss of water. As a result, the remaining ECF is hypotonic; it has less solute than water. This causes water to move from the extracellular compartment into the cells (ICF) by osmosis until osmotic equilibrium is reached. The ECF volume decreases while the ICF volume increases, and the osmolality of both compartments is lowered. Hypotonic fluid volume deficit can occur after sweating if water is ingested without an adequate intake of salt. It also can occur when diuretic therapy is used in conjunction with a salt restricted diet (Keyes, 1985). The signs and symptoms (see Table 22.6) tend to be more severe with hypotonic dehydration (Weldy, 1992). In addition, it must be noted that weight loss does not provide a good estimate of hypotonic dehydration because some of the ECF shifts into the ICF compartment resulting in minimal loss of weight (Keyes, 1985).

Hypertonic dehydration is the third type of fluid volume deficit. It occurs when more water than solute is lost and the remaining body fluids become hypertonic (concentrated). At first the water loss comes from the ECF compartment. This causes water to shift from the ICF compartment until osmotic equilibrium is reached. The end result is that fluid volume is lost from both compartments and the osmolality of both ICF and ECF is increased. Hypertonic dehydration occurs when **insensible water losses** (losses of fluid from the lungs and the skin through respiration and perspiration) are not replaced. This may result from sweating with no intake of water or inability to ingest adequate amounts of water. Since the fluid shifts from the ICF to the ECF compartment, the signs and symptoms of fluid volume deficit are not readily apparent; however, the neurological manifestations become evident (Weldy, 1992). Table 22.6 outlines fluid volume deficit, including the common causes, signs and symptoms and nursing interventions.

FLUID VOLUME EXCESS

Fluid volume excess (FVE) is a condition in which excessive fluid is retained in the interstitial fluid space (tissues), causing generalized or localized edema. Fluid is first retained in the peripheral tissues and then in the lungs; in severe cases edema becomes more generalized and fluid passes into body cavities, such as the peritoneal cavity. Fluid volume excess may result from disturbances in kidney function, disturbances in circulatory function (as, for example, in people with heart conditions), inflammation, increased permeability of the cell membranes or a number of other health problems. This condition is outlined further in Table 22.6.

ELECTROLYTE IMBALANCES

SODIUM DEFICIT

Sodium deficit is called **hyponatremia**. Specifically, it refers to a condition in which the concentration of sodium in the ECF (serum sodium) is below normal levels, that is, less than 135 mmol/litre. It is a hypotonic (hypo-osmolar) state that can result from an excessive loss in sodium without a proportionate loss in water or an excessive gain in water without a proportionate gain in sodium. When there is a deficit in sodium, the extracellular fluid becomes less concentrated; in other words, more dilute. Thus, water is pulled, by osmosis, from the ECF space into the cells, causing an intracellular water excess. While edema is not present *per se*, the tissues swell because of the increased cellular water content. In fact, the signs and symptoms of hyponatremia are probably due to cellular swelling — in particular, the neurological manifestations are the result of cerebral edema (Metheney, 1992). The increased content of intracellular water makes the tissues "plastic," allowing for a phenomenon known as sternal fingerprinting. When a finger is pressed firmly over the sternum (or another bony prominence) for 15 to 30 seconds, a fingerprint remains. Sternal fingerprinting indicates excessive intracellular fluid and is a positive sign of sodium deficit.

Hyponatremia can occur alone — that is, a loss of sodium within a normal ECF volume — or it can occur in conjunction with a fluid volume excess or deficit. It is associated with fluid volume excess (edema) in conditions such as congestive heart failure or renal disease where total body water increases to a greater extent than does sodium. It occurs with hypotonic dehydration when the deficit of sodium is relatively greater than that of total body water; when, for example, a loss of secretions from the gastrointestinal tract is due to vomiting and/or diarrhea.

The treatment for hyponatremia is sodium replacement or restriction of fluid. When the signs and symptoms indicate a hyponatremia with a water deficit, treatment is to replace sodium and fluid through oral intake of food and fluids high in sodium or intravenous infusion for those patients unable to eat or drink. Hyponatremia with signs and symptoms of water retention is corrected by restricting fluid intake. The causes, signs and symptoms, and nursing interventions for hyponatremia are presented in Table 22.7.

SODIUM EXCESS

Sodium excess, in which the concentration of sodium in the ECF (serum sodium) is above normal levels (more than 145 mmol/litre), is called **hypernatremia**. It is a hypertonic (hyperosmolar) state in which there are greater gains in sodium than in water or conversely there are greater losses in water than in sodium. Excesses in sodium cause the ECF to become more concentrated and as a result water is pulled from the cells by osmosis, causing a cellular dehydration. Consequently, cells shrink and their function is impaired. Indeed, the neurological manifestations of hypernatremia are attributed to cellular dehydration, and in particular to the water loss from brain tissues.

As with hyponatremia, hypernatremia can occur in patients whose fluid volume is normal or in those with fluid volume deficits or excesses. People who experience increased insensible water loss, through hyperventilation for instance, can lose water but not sodium, which leads to a mild hypernatremia. The amount of water loss, however, is not large enough to deplete the extracellular space; thus the ECF volume remains nearly normal. This type of hypernatremia often goes unnoticed because the body corrects itself by triggering the thirst centre, which induces the person to drink water.

More severe hypernatremia is often associated with hypertonic dehydration where loss of water exceeds loss of sodium. This can occur with more severe insensible water loss, for instance, from sweating profusely because of high environmental temperature, fever or strenuous muscular exercise. Hypernatremia associated with a volume deficit also occurs in people who are deprived of water because they cannot perceive thirst (for example, unconscious patients or very young children) or because they cannot ingest water (for example, paralyzed individuals). Hypernatremia can also be related to fluid volume excess; for example, when hypertonic saline solutions are administered intravenously there can be a greater gain of sodium in relation to water (Metheney, 1992).

Hypernatremia in conjunction with a water deficit is corrected by replacing water orally or by intravenous infusion of five percent dextrose in water. Sodium excess combined with ECF excess is treated with diuretic drugs, which remove both sodium and water from the body, and by restricting the intake of sodium and fluids. The causes, signs and symptoms and nursing interventions for hypernatremia are outlined in Table 22.7 starting on page 628.

TABLE 22.6 Fluid Volume Imbalances

COMMON CAUSES	SIGNS AND SYMPTOMS

Fluid Volume Deficit

Insufficient intake	Thirst (earliest sign)
Vomiting	Dry mucous membranes
Diarrhea	Dry, fissured tongue
Gastric suction	Decreased skin turgor
Fistulas	Weight loss (rapid change)
Excessive laxative use or tap water enemas	2% (mild deficit, such as 1 kg in a 50 kg person)
Polyuria	5% (moderate deficit, such as 2.5 kg in a 50 kg person)
Excessive use of diuretics	8% (severe deficit, such as 4 kg in a 50 kg person)
Fever	Systolic blood pressure drops 10 mm Hg or more when
Excessive diaphoresis	position changes from supine to standing or sitting
Muscular exercise	Slow filling of peripheral veins
Third space fluid shifts	Pulse weak and rapid
Hemorrhage	Respirations rapid
Burns	Temperature subnormal (i.e., 35°–36.7°C) or low-grade
	elevation (e.g., 37.2°C) unless infection is present
	Urine output <30 ml/hr (in an adult) and concentrated
	Dizziness, vertigo, syncope
	Behavioural changes (in severe FVD), e.g., lethargy, irritability,
	disorientation
	Laboratory results:
	Urine specific gravity>1.030
	Hematocrit (Hct) is elevated in isotonic and hypotonic
	dehydration, and decreased in hypovolemia secondary
	to bleeding
	Blood urea nitrogen (BUN) and creatinine are increased

Fluid Volume Excess

Conditions which cause a decreased renal perfusion or blood flow, e.g., renal disease, cardiac insufficiency, cirrhosis	Pitting edema in upper and lower extremities, and periorbital and presacral areas
Intravascular protein depletion	Weight gain (rapid change)
Rapid intravenous infusion of sodium containing fluids	2% (mild excess, such as 1 kg in a 50 kg person)
	5% (moderate excess, such as 2.5 kg in a 50 kg person)
Excessive intake of table salt or other sodium salts	8% (severe excess, such as 4 kg in a 50 kg person)
Release or administration of aldosterone as occurs with stress or steroid therapy	Distended neck and peripheral veins
	Bounding pulse
	Irritating cough, difficulty in breathing (due to fluid in the lungs)
	Moist crackles in lungs
	Laboratory results:
	BUN, hemoglobin and hematocrit decreased (due to hemodilution)

NURSING INTERVENTIONS

Fluid Volume Deficit

1. Assess the status of FVD.
   - Observe signs and symptoms
   - Measure and record intake and output from all sources
   - Obtain accurate daily weights (1 kg loss in weight represents 1 litre of fluid lost)

2. Provide oral fluids if indicated.
   - Select fluids containing lost electrolytes and adequate calories
   - Establish patient likes and dislikes
   - Ensure patient comfort:
     provide frequent mouth care
     choose non-irritating fluids
     give antiemetics as ordered for nausea

3. Fluids may be administered to patients who are unable to eat or drink through tube feedings (i.e., nasogastric, gastrostomy or jejunostomy tubes) as ordered by the physician. Nursing care for tube feedings is discussed in Chapter 19.

4. Fluids will be replaced intravenously if the patient is vomiting, FVD is prolonged or large volumes of fluid are required.
   - Careful monitoring of intake and output and serum electrolytes is necessary for intravenous therapy because the type and amount of fluid prescribed is determined by the type and amount of fluid lost. Nursing interventions for intravenous therapy are discussed later in this chapter.

5. Evaluate the patient's response to fluid therapy. Indicators of effective therapy:
   - increasing urine output (40–60 ml/hour)
   - decreasing urine concentration and specific gravity
   - blood pressure returns to normal baseline
   - pulse and respiratory rates return to baseline
   - return to baseline weight
   - return of skin and tongue turgor
   - increasing moisture in skin and mucous membranes
   - improved behaviour and sense of well-being
   - laboratory values return to normal

Fluid Volume Excess

1. Assess the status of FVE.
   - Observe signs and symptoms
   - Measure and record intake and output
   - Obtain accurate daily weights (1 kg gain in weight represents 1 litre of fluid)

2. Restrict sodium and fluid intake as ordered.

3. Administer diuretics as ordered.

4. Monitor response to diuretics; observe for potassium depletion and replace as necessary.

5. Regulate intravenous fluids as ordered.

6. If breathing difficulty occurs, position the patient in semi-Fowler's position to facilitate lung expansion.

7. Frequently turn and position the patient on bed rest (edematous tissue is prone to skin breakdown).

8. Provide instruction for self-care:
   - sodium-restricted diet
   - avoidance of over-the-counter drugs containing sodium
   - rest (side-lying positions promote diuresis)
   - monitoring of weight, intake and output, diuretic therapy and potassium replacement

9. Evaluate the patient's response to treatment and care. Indicators of effective care:
   - laboratory values return to normal
   - absence of dependent and pitting edema
   - return to baseline weight
   - pulse returns to baseline
   - clear lungs; easy breathing

SOURCES: Metheney, 1992, 40–45; 48–54; Stroot, Lee and Barrett, 1984, 17–23; Kee, 1986, 259–260; 263–264; 281.

POTASSIUM DEFICIT

Potassium deficit, or **hypokalemia**, occurs when the extracellular concentration of potassium is less than 3.5 mmol/litre. Hypokalemia is quite a common condition because the kidneys do not conserve potassium. Even when intake is decreased, the kidneys continue to excrete potassium. In addition to decreased intake, hypokalemia is caused by excessive renal excretion which may result from treatment with potassium-wasting diuretics or steroid hormones which promote excretion of potassium.

Hypokalemia is also caused by stress and disease of the adrenal cortex in which excess aldosterone is secreted, since aldosterone causes sodium and water retention and potassium loss from the kidney. Gastrointestinal secretions are rich in potassium. Therefore, fluid loss from the gastrointestinal tract will cause significant loss of potassium and hence hypokalemia.

The signs and symptoms of hypokalemia (see Table 22.7) stem primarily from its effect on neuromuscular function. Potassium plays a large role in the transmission and conduction of nerve impulses, and in the contraction of skeletal, smooth and cardiac muscles. Potassium deficit results in decreased neuromuscular excitability and subsequent diminished muscular contractility, thus muscle weakness.

Early detection and treatment of hypokalemia is important because potassium deficit can be life-threatening. The primary objective in treating hypokalemia is prevention. Patients at risk for hypokalemia require increased potassium through diet and supplements. Individuals who cannot ingest food and fluid receive a maintenance dose of potassium by the intravenous route. Actual potassium losses must be replaced either orally through liquid or tablet forms or intravenously if hypokalemia is severe or oral intake is not possible. See Table 22.7 for an outline of nursing interventions pertaining to hypokalemia.

POTASSIUM EXCESS

Extracellular potassium excess or **hyperkalemia** is an increased accumulation of potassium in the blood stream and results when the serum potassium level is above 5.5 mmol/litre. Hyperkalemia is not common in people with normal kidney function; however, it can occur in renal dysfunction associated with decreased urinary output. Probably the most common cause of hyperkalemia is excessive or very rapid oral or intravenous fluid intake combined with renal failure.

Like hypokalemia, hyperkalemia affects the excitability of nerve and muscle cell membranes. In the case of potassium excess, the excitability of the cell membrane increases while the resting potential decreases. As a result, the spread of stimuli along nerves and muscle fibres are blocked. Muscle weakness and paralysis follow. The most dangerous effect of hyperkalemia is its influence on the heart. The increased excitability of cell membranes can lead to disturbances in cardiac conduction causing cardiac arrhythmias, bradycardia, heart block and cardiac arrest.

The signs and symptoms of potassium excess are outlined in Table 22.7. It cannot be overemphasized that hyperkalemia is life-threatening; early detection and treatment is imperative. Muscle weakness progressing to flaccid paralysis is the most common sign of hyperkalemia. Paresthesias and tingling sensations are also common. Respiratory paralysis and involvement of the facial muscles are late manifestations.

As with hypokalemia, prevention is the best treatment of hyperkalemia. For instance, eliminating the use of salt substitutes in a patient taking potassium-sparing diuretics may be required to prevent an accumulation of extracellular potassium. Treatment of hyperkalemia depends on the cause and severity of potassium excess. In mild cases restriction of oral or intravenous potassium may be all that is necessary. For more severe forms and especially when cardiac manifestations are present, treatment may include intravenous administration of hypertonic glucose and insulin to pull potassium back into the cells. Once the potassium moves back into the cells it is no longer toxic. Calcium gluconate will be given intravenously to stimulate the heart when life-threatening cardiac manifestations are present. Calcium works by antagonizing the effect of excessive potassium on conductivity of cardiac tissue.

Hyperkalemia, particularly when associated with acidosis, may be corrected with intravenous sodium bicarbonate. By buffering the hydrogen ions in the plasma, bicarbonate helps shift potassium back into the cells. Hypertonic glucose and insulin, calcium and sodium bicarbonate are temporary measures for controlling hyperkalemia and are, therefore, used in emergency and transient hyperkalemic states. Acute, nontransient forms of hyperkalemia are treated with cation-exchange resins, such as Kayexalate, that absorb potassium from the intestinal tract; or peritoneal- and hemo-dialysis which filter potassium along with other waste products from the extracellular fluid.

CALCIUM DEFICIT

Hypocalcemia refers to a deficit in the serum concentration of calcium and is reflected in total serum values below 2.12 mmol/litre. It is caused by dietary deficiency of calcium or vitamin D, or by diseases which limit intestinal absorption, as in acute pancreatitis or diarrhea. Diseases of the parathyroid gland resulting in an inadequate secretion of parathyroid hormone lead to calcium deficits. Hypocalcemia is also associated with excesses of serum phosphates (hyperphosphatemia), through a mechanism that is not clearly understood (Keyes, 1985) and with renal failure, in which phosphorus is retained while calcium is excreted.

A calcium deficit can also occur when the body is in an alkalotic state because calcium will not ionize when alkalosis is present. The signs and symptoms of hypocalcemia are related primarily to its effect on neuromuscular irritability. Calcium exerts a sedative effect on the nerve cell membranes. A lack of calcium leads to increased neuro-muscular irritability and results in tonic muscle spasms (tetany) and cramps. It decreases the contractility of heart muscle and reduces blood clotting. The signs and symptoms of calcium deficit are listed in Table 22.7. Chronic hypocalcemia is treated with oral calcium supplements. Vitamin D may also be given to enhance absorption from the intestinal tract. Acute hypocalcemia in which severe tetany or convulsions have set in is a medical emergency which requires immediate administration of intravenous calcium.

CALCIUM EXCESS

The condition in which there is an excess of extracellular calcium is called *hypercalcemia*. A total serum calcium reading above 2.62 mmol/litre indicates hypercalcemia. Extracellular calcium excess is caused by conditions which release calcium from the bones into the extracellular fluid. The most common of these are malignant tumours (cancers) followed by hyperparathyroidism. In hyperparathyroidism, calcium is not only reabsorbed from the bones and teeth but also absorbed in greater quantities from the intestines and the kidneys.

Excessive intake of calcium and vitamin D can result in hypercalcemia. People who take large doses of pharmacologic vitamin D and people who ingest excessive milk and alkaline antacids, particularly calcium carbonate, (for example, those with peptic ulcer), may develop hypercalcemia. The signs and symptoms of hypercalcemia (Table 22.7) are related to the increased sedative effect on the nerve cell membranes and the decreased tone of skeletal and smooth muscle. The increased urinary excretion of excess calcium may lead to kidney stones and the loss of calcium from bones may cause deep bone pain and pathological fractures. Increased serum calcium may also be demonstrated through mental and behaviour changes, notably depression, lethargy and apathy.

Treatment for hypercalcemia must be directed towards the cause; for instance, removal of tumours by surgery, chemotherapy or radiation. However, general measures are also instituted to eliminate serum calcium excesses. A diet low in calcium may be used. Fluids are forced to dilute serum levels and promote diuresis and renal excretion of calcium. Intravenous solutions of normal saline are administered for this purpose as well. Serum calcium concentrations can also be lowered by administering organic phosphorus through oral, nasogastric, enema or intravenous routes.

MAGNESIUM DEFICIT

A magnesium deficit or *hypomagnesemia* is present when the serum magnesium is less than 0.69 mmol/litre. Hypomagnesemia is a relatively rare state, which can be caused by a number of diseases. It can occur in conditions which result in an inadequate intake of magnesium, for instance, prolonged malnutrition or starvation associated with alcoholism. Hypomagnesemia is also caused by the administration of magnesium-free intravenous or total parenteral nutrition solutions, particularly when there is no oral intake or when magnesium is also being lost through nasogastric suctioning.

Diseases of the small bowel causing impaired absorption lead to hypomagnesemia, as does hypercalcemia. Calcium and magnesium share a common site for absorption in the distal small bowel. They have a mutually suppressive effect on one another so that excesses in one will inhibit absorption of the other. Thus, excessive calcium intake inhibits magnesium absorption and vice versa. Diuretic therapy and conditions resulting in increased renal excretion and fluid loss, such as renal disease, diabetic ketoacidosis and primary hyperaldosteronism, can also cause magnesium deficits.

The signs and symptoms of hypomagnesemia are primarily associated with its effects on neuromuscular function and on potassium and calcium balance. Since magnesium exerts a sedative effect on the neuromuscular system, deficits in magnesium will lead to hyperactive neuromuscular manifestations. Magnesium facilitates the transport of potassium across cell membranes. When there is a deficit in magnesium the kidneys excrete more potassium; thus a deficit in magnesium leads to a deficit in potassium. With regard to calcium balance, low levels of magnesium inhibit the action of parathyroid hormone causing a hypocalcemia. Mild hypomagnesemia may be treated with diet alone. More severe forms may require oral or parenteral replacement of magnesium salts.

MAGNESIUM EXCESS

Hypermagnesemia occurs when the serum concentration of magnesium is above 1.07 mmol/litre. The most common cause of magnesium excess is renal failure in which excretion of the mineral is inadequate. The risk of hypermagnesemia is even greater in these cases if excessive antacids or laxatives containing magnesium salts are being used over prolonged periods of time. Excessive administration of magnesium for other reasons, such as controlling convulsions in pregnancy-induced hypertension, can lead to hypermagnesemia. People suffering from severe extracellular volume depletion with oliguria may also develop a magnesium excess.

The signs and symptoms vary according to serum concentration levels as outlined in Table 22.7. Mild hypermagnesemia is asymptomatic. As the serum levels increase, manifestations beginning with vasodilating effects — hypotension, flushing and diaphoresis — advance to the neuromuscular blocking effects at the myoneural junction — lethargy, drowsiness, hypoactive reflexes, respiratory depression, coma and death. The effects on the heart lead to bradycardia and eventually cardiac arrest. Thus, although hypermagnesia is quite rare, when it occurs it can be fatal.

TABLE 22.7   Electrolyte Imbalances

COMMON CAUSES	SIGNS AND SYMPTOMS
Hyponatremia	
Vomiting	Headache
Diarrhea	Faintness
Gastric suction	Weakness
Renal disease	Muscle cramps
Potent diuretics	Anorexia
Lack of sodium intake	Nausea
Adrenal insufficiency	Vomiting
Profuse perspiration followed by a large intake of water	Abdominal cramping
	Sternal fingerprinting
Wound drainage and weeping skin lesions	Vertigo
Mental confusion	Muscle twitching
Burns	Seizures
Excessive intake of water or electrolyte-free solutions (e.g., 5% dextrose in water)	Coma
	Serum sodium <135 mmol/L
	Serum osmolality <285 mmol/kg
	Urine S.G. <1.010
Hypernatremia	
Increased insensible loss:	Mild to moderate:
Fever	•Intense thirst
High environmental temperature	• Dry, sticky mucous membranes
Strenuous exercise	• Swollen, dry tongue
Water deprivation	• Flushed skin
Watery diarrhea	• Decreased urine output
Renal failure with sodium retention	• Temperature may rise
Increased sodium intake:	Severe:
Hypertonic tube feedings without water supplement	• Restlessness and agitation
	• Disorientation
Excessive ingestion of salt	• Hallucinations
Excessive parenteral infusion of sodium-containing solutions	• Lethargy when undisturbed
	• Seizures
	• Coma
	Serum Sodium >145 mmol/L
	Serum osmolality >295 mmol/kg
	Urine S.G. >1.015
Hypokalemia	
Diarrhea	Muscle weakness
Vomiting	Malaise
Gastric suction	Decreased muscle tone
Potassium-losing diuretics	Hyporeflexia
Corticosteroid use	Paresthesias and muscle cramps
Diseases leading to increased adrenal cortical hormone release	Hypotension
	Cardiac arrhythmias due to increased irritability of the heart muscle
Metabolic alkalosis	Anorexia
Poor intake	Nausea and vomiting
	Abdominal distention
	Decreased peristalsis
	Polyuria
	Serum potassium <3.5 mmol/L

NURSING INTERVENTIONS

Hyponatremia

1. Identify patients at risk for hyponatremia, for example, those with gastrointestinal fluid losses, diuretic therapy in conjunction with a low-salt diet, or patients with adrenal insufficiency who are exposed to stress such as surgery.
2. Assess the status of hyponatremia.
   - Observe signs and symptoms. Be aware of their significance in the presence of sodium-containing fluid losses, low sodium intake and excessive intake of water and electrolyte-free solutions.
   - Measure and record intake and output from all sources
   - Obtain accurate daily weights
3. Administer fluid and foods high in sodium as ordered.
4. Know the sodium content of commonly used parenteral fluids and monitor patients with cardiovascular disease for fluid overload (signs of fluid volume excess).
5. In cases of severe hyponatremia, hypertonic saline solutions (3% or 5% NaCl) are administered, using extreme caution. These patients are cared for in an intensive care unit where their status and response to therapy can be closely monitored.
6. Evaluate the patient's response to treatment and care. Indicators of effective care:
   - absence of sternal fingerprinting
   - resolution of the gastrointestinal and neurological signs and symptoms
   - return of normal laboratory values

Hypernatremia

1. Identify patients at risk for hypernatremia, for example, debilitated patients who are not able to perceive or respond to thirst, or stroke patients who are unable to communicate thirst.
2. Assess the status of hypernatremia.
   - Observe signs and symptoms. Be aware of their significance in the presence of risk for water deprivation and insensible water loss, high sodium intake, and excessive intake of salt-containing solutions.
   - Observe for fluid volume deficit and excess
   - Measure and record intake and output
   - Obtain accurate daily weights
3. Restrict sodium intake as ordered.
4. Provide fluids at regular intervals to patients who are debilitated or cannot communicate. If intake is inadequate, collaborate with the physician for alternative method of administering fluids.
5. Evaluate the patient's response to treatment and care. Indicators of effective care:
   - absence of thirst
   - moist, shiny mucous membranes
   - normal body temperature
   - resolution of neurological signs and symptoms
   - gradual return of serum sodium to normal value

Hypokalemia

1. Identify patients at risk for hypokalemia, for example, patients on potent diuretics or corticosteroids, those who are allowed nothing by mouth (NPO), or those who are chronic laxative users.
2. Assess the status of hypokalemia.
   - Observe signs and symptoms
   - Observe for signs of metabolic alkalosis
   - Measure and record intake and output from all sources
   - Check serum potassium reports and notify physician of results
3. Implement preventive care for hypokalemia in patients at risk.
   - Encourage increased intake of potassium, providing there are no dietary restrictions. Patients who use salt substitutes may not need extra potassium because these substances contain significant amounts of potassium.
4. Administer oral potassium supplements as ordered.
5. Intravenous potassium must be administered carefully following strict guidelines because excessive or rapid intake of this mineral can be lethal. Even a transient excess in potassium is dangerous because it can lead to a cardiac arrest.
6. Evaluate the patient's response to treatment and care. Indicators of effective care:
   - resolution of neuromuscular signs and symptoms
   - return of gastrointestinal function
   - normal pulse rate and rhythm
   - gradual return of serum potassium to normal value

continued on next page

TABLE 22.7   Electrolyte Imbalances

COMMON CAUSES	SIGNS AND SYMPTOMS
Hyperkalemia	
Renal failure with decreased urinary output	Vague muscle weakness
Excessive or rapid oral or intravenous intake	Cardiac arrhythmias, tachycardia followed by bradycardia,
Crush injuries, burns	heart block and cardiac arrest
Adrenal insufficiency	Oliguria or anuria
Respiratory and metabolic acidosis	Paresthesias of face, tongue, hands and feet
Rapid infusion of old blood (potassium released	Flaccid paralysis which begins in legs and spreads to trunk and
from deteriorated red blood cells)	arms; facial and respiratory muscles become involved later
	Abdominal cramps
	Nausea and diarrhea
	Serum potassium >5.5 mmol/L
Hypocalcemia	
Dietary deficiency of calcium or vitamin D	Numbness and tingling in the fingers, around the mouth,
Pancreatitis	in toes
Diarrhea	Spasms in the hands, feet and face
Excessive laxative use	Hyperactive reflexes
Hypoparathyroidism	Trousseau's sign
Hyperphosphatemia	Chvostek's sign
Renal failure	Skeletal muscle cramps
	Abdominal spasms and cramps
	Laryngospasm
	Convulsions
	Mental changes such as anxiety, confusion, impaired memory
	Serum calcium <2.12 mmol/litre
Hypercalcemia	
Malignant tumours	Muscle weakness
Hyperparathyroidism	Hypotonic muscles
Hyperthyroidism	Constipation, anorexia, nausea, vomiting
Excessive vitamin D intake	Polyuria
Excessive calcium intake	Thirst
	Kidney stones
	Deep bone pain
	Depression, lethargy
	Behaviour changes

NURSING INTERVENTIONS

Hyperkalemia

1. Identify patients at risk for hyperkalemia, for example, those on potassium-sparing diuretics, potassium supplements or salt substitutes, or those with poor kidney function who are experiencing metabolic acidosis.
2. Assess the status of hyperkalemia.
   - Observe signs and symptoms
   - Observe for signs of metabolic or respiratory acidosis
   - Measure and record intake and output from all sources
   - Check serum potassium reports and notify physician of results
3. Implement preventive care for hyperkalemia in patients at risk.
   - Administer oral and intravenous potassium safely
   - Administer fresh blood transfusions if possible
   - Provide self-care teaching. Advise patients to:
      take potassium supplements as prescribed and avoid over-use
      use salt substitutes sparingly if taking diuretics in conjunction with potassium supplements
      avoid potassium-sparing diuretics, potassium supplements or salt substitutes if renal function is impaired
      know the signs and symptoms of hyperkalemia and report any adverse effects immediately
      avoid foods high in potassium if chronically prone to hyperkalemia
4. Implement treatment measures for hyperkalemia as ordered. Use established procedures and guidelines to ensure safety.
5. Evaluate the patient's response to treatment and care. Indicators of effective care:
   - resolution of neuromuscular signs and symptoms
   - gastrointestinal comfort, absence of diarrhea
   - normal pulse rate and rhythm
   - return of serum potassium to normal value

Hypocalcemia

1. Identify patients at risk for hypocalcemia, for example, those who have had surgery to thyroid gland or parathyroid glands, patients with malabsorption syndromes or conditions causing increased gastrointestinal motility with diarrhea.
2. Assess the status of hypocalcemia.
   - Observe signs and symptoms
   - Observe breathing, noting airway status
   - Monitor serum calcium levels for 24 to 48 hours postoperatively following thyroid surgery or radical neck dissection
   - Observe for prolonged bleeding and clot formation
   - Monitor acid–base status
3. Implement preventive care for hypocalcemia in patients at risk.
   - Institute seizure precaution care
   - Have a tracheotomy tray at the bedside
   - Reduce environmental stimuli
   - Teach individuals with inadequate calcium intake about diets high in calcium or self-administration of calcium supplements as necessary. An adequate intake of Vitamin D is necessary to aid intestinal absorption of calcium.
4. Administer oral calcium supplements as ordered.
5. Know parenteral calcium solutions and administer according to established procedure.
6. Evaluate the patient's response to treatment and care. Indicators of effective care:
   - resolution of neuromuscular irritability
   - return of patient's usual pattern of behaviour, mental alertness
   - return of total serum calcium to normal level

Hypercalcemia

1. Identify patients at risk for hypercalcemia, for example, women with breast cancer or patients using thiazide diuretics.
2. Assess the status of hypercalcemia.
   - Observe signs and symptoms
   - Strain urine to monitor for kidney stones
3. Encourage a fluid intake of three to four litres per day. Unless contraindicated, fluids containing sodium are recommended because sodium enhances calcium excretion.
4. Restrict dietary intake of calcium and vitamin D supplements as ordered. Provide instruction on foods the patient should avoid, that is, those rich in calcium.

continued on next page

TABLE 22.7 Electrolyte Imbalances

COMMON CAUSES	SIGNS AND SYMPTOMS

Hypomagnesemia

Prolonged inadequate intake
Malnutrition
Alcoholism
Prolonged IV or TPN without magnesium
  replacement
Nasogastric suction
Severe diarrhea
Malabsorption syndrome
Severe renal disease
Diabetic ketoacidosis
Hyperaldosteronism
Hyperparathyroidism
Diuretics
Excessive calcium or vitamin D intake

Neuromuscular irritability
Increased reflexes
Coarse tremors
Facial twitching
Positive Chvostek's and Trousseau's signs
Painful paresthesias of hands and feet
Muscle cramps
Cardiac tachyarrhythmias
Disorientation, confusion
Behaviour changes
Convulsions
Serum magnesium <0.8 mmol/L
Signs of hypocalcemia and hypokalemia when
  hypomagnesemia is severe

Hypermagnesemia

Renal failure
Excessive, prolonged use of magnesium-containing
  antacids and laxatives
Excessive administration of magnesium salts
Severe extracellular fluid volume deficit with
  oliguria

Serum magnesium 1.5-2.5 mmol/L:
- Hypotension
- Facial flushing, warmth
- Diaphoresis

Serum magnesium 2.5-3.5 mmol/L:
- Lethargy, drowsiness
- Loss of deep tendon reflexes
- Muscular weakness

Serum magnesium 5 mmol/L:
- Respiratory depression

Serum magnesium 6-7.5 mmol/L:
- Coma

Serum magnesium >7.5 mmol/L:
- Cardiac arrest

NURSING INTERVENTIONS

Hypercalcemia cont'd

5. Ambulate patients as soon as possible. Assist with active and passive exercises for patients on bed rest. Mobility prevents loss of calcium from the bones and promotes the transfer of calcium from the bloodstream back into the bones.
6. Implement preventive care for complications in patients with hypercalcemia.
   - Position and transfer patients carefully to prevent pathological fractures
   - Force fluids to dilute the urine and prevent kidney stones. Ensure an intake of fluids that will produce an acid urine, such as cranberry juice and prune juice. An acid urine will increase the solubility of calcium in the urine.
   - Teach patients about and encourage a diet high in bulk to counteract the propensity for constipation
7. Evaluate the patient's response to treatment and care. Indicators of effective care:
   - resolution of neuromuscular weakness and cramps
   - return to normal gastrointestinal function and comfort
   - absence of pathological fractures or kidney stones
   - return of patient's usual pattern of behaviour, mental alertness
   - return of total serum calcium to normal level

Hypomagnesemia

1. Identify patients at risk for hypomagnesemia, for example, people who abuse alcohol chronically and do not eat adequately, postoperative patients receiving magnesium-free intravenous solutions and on nasogastric suction and people taking calcium and vitamin D supplements.
2. Assess the status of hypomagnesemia.
   - Observe signs and symptoms
   - Monitor vital signs and observe for cardiac arrhythmias
   - Observe breathing, noting airway status (laryngospasm can occur)
3. Implement preventive care for hypomagnesemia in patients at risk.
   - Institute seizure precaution care in severe cases
   - Know the commonly used intravenous solutions that do not contain magnesium, for example, 5% Dextrose in water, lactated Ringer's solution, and collaborate with physician regarding replacement if necessary
   - Implement safety precautions in patients with behaviour changes
   - Because patients with hypomagnesemia may suffer difficulty with swallowing, check swallowing ability before giving food, fluids or oral medications
4. Teach patients who are able to ingest food and fluid about foods high in magnesium.
5. Administer oral and parenteral magnesium salts as ordered and according to established procedure to ensure safety.
6. Evaluate the patient's response to treatment and care. Indicators of effective care:
   - resolution of neuromuscular irritability
   - normal vital signs and cardiac function
   - return of patient's usual pattern of behaviour, mental alertness
   - return of serum magnesium to normal level

Hypermagnesemia

1. Identify patients at risk for hypermagnesemia, for example, patients with renal failure who use antacids and laxatives containing magnesium salts or obstetrical patients who are being treated with magnesium sulfate.
2. Assess the status of hypermagnesemia.
   - Observe signs and symptoms
   - Monitor vital signs and observe for hypotension, bradycardia and cardiac arrhythmias
   - Observe breathing, noting shallow respirations with periods of apnea
3. Implement preventive care for hypermagnesemia in patients at risk.
   - Teach patients with poor renal function to avoid antacids and laxatives containing magnesium salts
   - Provide sufficient fluids to ill patients to ensure adequate urinary output. When patients are receiving parenteral magnesium, always have intravenous calcium gluconate available for emergency use.
4. Evaluate the patient's response to treatment and care. Indicators of effective care:
   - resolution of neuromuscular depression
   - normal vital signs and cardiac function
   - return of serum magnesium to normal level

continued on next page

TABLE 22.7 Electrolyte Imbalances

COMMON CAUSES	SIGNS AND SYMPTOMS
Hypophosphatemia	
Inadequate intake	Anorexia
Malnutrition	Muscle weakness
Vitamin D deficiency	Paresthesias
Hyperparathyroidism	Skeletal muscle pain and aches
Vomiting, chronic diarrhea	Behavioural changes such as apprehension, confusion
Diabetic ketoacidosis	Hemolytic anemia
Glucose administration	Decreased tissue oxygenation
Respiratory alkalosis	Serum phosphorus <0.8 mmol/L
Phosphate-binding antacids	
Thiazide diuretics	
Hyperphosphatemia	
Chronic renal failure	Symptoms of hypocalcemia such as tetany, hyperreflexia, flaccid paralysis, muscular weakness and cramps
Antineoplastic drugs	Symptoms of soft-tissue calcification in such sites as the kidney, joints, cornea and arteries
Excessive use of phosphate containing laxatives	
Excessive intake of oral or intravenous phosphate supplements	
Hypoparathyroidism	

Prevention is the best treatment for hypermagnesemia. Antacids and laxatives containing magnesium should not be given to patients with renal failure or poor urinary output. In milder forms, magnesium excess may be corrected by discontinuing use of magnesium salts. Severe forms with respiratory and cardiac involvement are controlled with intravenous calcium gluconate. Since calcium has a direct antagonistic effect on magnesium it is an effective temporary measure. Ventilatory support may be required. Hemodialysis with a magnesium-free dialysate may also be used.

PHOSPHORUS DEFICIT

A decrease in the serum concentration of inorganic phosphorus is known as **hypophosphatemia**. Concentrations less than 0.81 mmol/litre constitute hypophosphatemia.

While this serum value generally indicates a deficiency in phosphorus, hypophosphatemia can occur in a wide variety of situations in which the total body stores of phosphate may be normal, increased or decreased.

Hypophosphatemia is associated with low intake, poor absorption from the small bowel (often due to a lack of vitamin D), loss from vomiting and diarrhea and increased renal excretion. Increased renal excretion may be due to hyperparathyroidism (since PTH secretion causes phosphorus excretion) and altered carbohydrate metabolism such as diabetic ketoacidosis (glycosuria and polyuria promote renal excretion while parenteral insulin therapy causes phosphorus to shift into the cells, thus lowering serum phosphorus levels). The intake of nonabsorbable antacids containing aluminum or magnesium hydroxides may also decrease phosphate levels by binding with phosphorus in the bowel and preventing absorption.

continued

NURSING INTERVENTIONS

Hypophosphatemia

1. Identify patients at risk for hypophosphatemia, for example, older, debilitated patients who are being re-fed after malnourishment; chronic alcoholic patients being treated with intravenous glucose; or patients in diabetic ketoacidosis being treated with intravenous glucose and insulin.
2. Assess the status of hypophosphatemia.
   - Observe signs and symptoms
   - Observe urinary output
   - Observe for signs of hypercalcemia (calcium excess is often associated with phosphorus deficit)
3. Implement preventive care for hypophosphatemia in patients at risk.
   - Monitor serum phosphorus values in patients at risk and report to the physician
   - Teach patients about foods high in phosphorus
   - Monitor closely patients taking phosphorus-binding antacids in conjunction with thiazide diuretics or if they have other associated conditions such as hyperparathyroidism or hypercalcemia
5. Administer oral phosphorus as ordered.
6. Evaluate the patient's response to treatment and care. Indicators of effective care:
   - resolution of neuromuscular weakness and pain
   - return of patient's usual pattern of behaviour, mental alertness
   - return of serum phosphorus to normal level

Hyperphosphatemia

1. Identify patients at risk for hyperphosphatemia, for, example patients with renal insufficiency being treated for peptic ulcer with large quantities of milk or children receiving large quantities of phosphate-containing enema solution.
2. Assess the status of hyperphosphatemia.
   - Observe signs and symptoms
3. Implement preventive care for hyperphosphatemia in patients at risk.
   - Teach patients about the dangers of excessive use of phosphate laxatives and enemas
   - Administer oral and intravenous supplements cautiously, frequently monitoring serum phosphorus levels
4. Teach patients on a low-phosphorus diet about foods that should be avoided.
5. Evaluate the patient's response to treatment and care. Indicators of effective care:
   - resolution of neuromuscular irritability
   - absence of signs of soft-tissue calcifications
   - return of serum phosphorus to normal level

SOURCES: Metheney, 1992, 56–130; Stroot, Lee and Barrett, 1984, 54–90; Kee, 1986, 43–155; Keyes, 1985, 13–164; Weldy, 1992, 11—176.

The signs and symptoms of hypophosphatemia (Table 22.7) are related to central nervous system (CNS), muscular and hematologic abnormalities. Treatment of phosphorus deficit includes replacement therapy, usually by the oral route, and correction of the underlying pathology.

PHOSPHORUS EXCESS

Hyperphosphatemia is an excess of phosphorus in the ECF and is indicated by serum concentrations above 1.58 mmol/litre. The incidence of hyperphosphatemia is relatively rare because normally functioning kidneys excrete excess phosphorus. It is associated with an intake of large amounts of phosphate-containing enemas or oral laxatives, with chronic renal insufficiency when the glomerular filtration rate falls below 30 ml per minute (Schrier, 1986) and with the administration of antineoplastic agents for cancer which cause tumour cells to break down and release phosphate into the ECF.

Hypocalcemia usually occurs in conjunction with hyperphosphatemia. While the mechanism by which this occurs is not completely known, it is thought the increased phosphate concentration stimulates an increase in bone formation which requires more calcium (Keyes, 1985). The symptoms of hyperphosphatemia are often seen as those of hypocalcemia. Phosphate excess itself causes little symptomatology; the most significant is soft tissue calcification, seen most commonly in patients with renal failure. Treatment is directed towards correcting the underlying cause. If excessive intake is the cause, discontinuing dietary ingestion and use of substances containing phosphorus may be all that is necessary. Phosphate-binding antacids may also be used to precipitate and consequently excrete excess phosphate through the gastrointestinal tract.

ACID–BASE IMBALANCES

The acid–base balance of body fluids is kept within a very narrow range by the chemical blood buffers, the lungs and the kidneys. Any condition that interferes with the function of any one of these regulating mechanisms or that either increases or decreases the concentration of hydrogen ions (acid) or bicarbonate (base) will cause an acid–base imbalance in the body. Acidosis will result when there are more hydrogen ions circulating in the blood than there are bicarbonate ions to absorb and buffer them. Alkalosis results when there is too much bicarbonate and not enough acid in the extracellular fluid.

Whenever an acid–base imbalance occurs in the body, a set of processes are put into motion by the lungs and the kidneys to minimize the change in pH and return it to normal. These processes are referred to as *compensation*. *Compensation*, as it refers to acid–base imbalance, must not be confused with the terms buffering and correcting. **Buffering** is the immediate chemical response to changes in the hydrogen ion concentration of body fluids, whereas **correction** implies the return of all acid–base components to normal.

Compensation is the result of the physiologic mechanisms that attempt to maintain the ratio of one carbonic acid molecule to 20 bicarbonate ions. For example, in compensated respiratory acidosis, the plasma pH values are normal even though carbonic acid is elevated, because the kidneys excrete hydrogen ions and retain bicarbonate ions. When the kidneys are no longer able to help restore balance, the condition is termed *uncompensated*. These compensating mechanisms actually accentuate the abnormal levels of carbon dioxide and bicarbonate in the blood; and they are "expensive" because when compensation occurs, some other regulatory process is compromised and normal body function is altered (Keyes, 1985).

There are two primary types of acid–base imbalance: respiratory and metabolic. Each can result in acidosis or alkalosis. These imbalances are depicted in Figure 22.3. The manifestations of acid–base imbalances in the body vary depending on the cause, the amount of cellular injury and the success of the compensatory mechanisms (that is, the retention or release of carbon dioxide by the lungs and the retention or release of bicarbonate or hydrogen ions by the kidneys) that are mobilized to return body pH to normal.

In addition, the signs and symptoms are not always specific to the acid–base imbalance; for instance, in metabolic alkalosis many of the manifestations are attributed to the concomitant deficits in potassium and chloride. Therefore, the best method for assessing and evaluating acid–base status is arterial blood gas analysis. The components of blood gas analysis and their significance in diagnosing acid–base imbalances are presented in Table 22.8. The common types of acid–base imbalance, along with their causes, compensatory mechanisms, signs and symp-

toms, treatment and nursing interventions, are outlined in Table 22.9 starting on page 640 and supplement the following discussion.

Respiratory Acidosis

Respiratory acidosis is caused by conditions which prevent the lungs from exhaling carbon dioxide. Excessive amounts of carbon dioxide are retained in the blood which combine with water to form carbonic acid. The increased carbonic acid causes the blood pH to decrease. The kidneys attempt to compensate for this imbalance by retaining base bicarbonate and eliminating hydrogen ions. However, renal compensation is very slow, taking from a few hours to several days to occur. Therefore, in acute cases, renal compensation may not be effective in shifting the pH back to normal. Very low respiratory rates, as in hypoventilation, or any disease that obstructs the exchange of oxygen and carbon dioxide in the lungs will result in respiratory acidosis.

Respiratory Alkalosis

Respiratory alkalosis occurs when respirations are very rapid. Excessive carbon dioxide is exhaled; as a result, carbonic acid decreases and blood pH rises. Attempting to correct this imbalance, the kidneys save hydrogen ions and excrete bicarbonate ions. Hyperventilation, fever or stimulation of the respiratory centre can cause respiratory alkalosis.

Metabolic Acidosis

Metabolic acidosis is characterized by a deficit of base bicarbonate (alkali) in the extracellular fluid. It is caused by an excessive loss of bicarbonate from the gastrointestinal tract or the kidneys, or by an excessive accumulation of acids from faulty nutrient metabolism or renal inability to excrete acid products of metabolism. In either case, the ratio of bicarbonate to carbonic acid is decreased, and without enough base the blood pH rises. The lungs try to compensate by getting rid of carbon dioxide; thus, breathing becomes rapid and deep. The kidneys respond by excreting more hydrogen ions and retaining bicarbonate ions; therefore, the urine becomes acidic. Metabolic acidosis is due primarily to altered nutrient metabolism. Some causative conditions include uncontrolled diabetes mellitus, severe diarrhea, excessive exercise, severe infection, starvation and a high fat diet.

Metabolic Alkalosis

In metabolic alkalosis there is either an excess of base bicarbonate or a loss of hydrogen ions in the blood. Vomiting or gastric suction result in a loss of hydrochloric acid from the

FIGURE 22.3   Acid–Base Balance and Imbalance

SOURCE: Kee, J.L. (1986). *Fluids and electrolytes with clinical applications* (4th ed.). Albany NY: Delmar Publishers Inc., 175. Reproduced with permission.

TABLE 22.8   Arterial Blood Gases

TERM	NORMAL VALUE	DEFINITION–IMPLICATIONS
pH	7.35–7.45	Reflects H+ concentration; acidity increases as H+ concentration increases (pH value decreases as acidity increases) • pH < 7.35 (acidosis) • pH > 7.45 (alkalosis)
P_aCO_2	34–46 mmHg	Partial pressure of CO_2 in arterial blood • When <34 mmHg, hypocapnia is said to be present (respiratory alkalosis) • When >46 mmHg, hypercapnia is said to be present (respiratory acidosis)
PaO_2	>70 mmHg (decreases with age)	Partial pressure of O_2 in arterial blood • Any reading above 70 mmHg (on room air) is considered acceptable • In adults younger than 60 years (on room air) <70 mmHg indicates mild hypoxemia <60 mmHg indicates moderate hypoxemia <40 mmHg indicates severe hypoxemia • Somewhat lower levels are accepted as normal in aged persons because there is some loss of ventilatory function with advanced age
Standard HCO_3	23–33 mmol/L	HCO_3 concentration in plasma of blood that has been equilibrated at a $PaCO_2$ of 40 mmHg, and with O_2 to fully saturate the hemoglobin
Base excess (BE)	–3 – +3 mmol/L	Reflects metabolic (nonrespiratory) body disturbances, which may be primary or compensatory in nature Always negative in metabolic acidosis (deficit or alkali or excess of fixed acids) Always positive in metabolic alkalosis (excess of alkali or deficit of fixed acids) Arrived at by multiplying the deviation of standard HCO_3 from normal by a factor of 1.2, which represents the buffer action of red blood cells

SOURCE: Metheney, N.M. (1992). *Fluid and electrolyte balance*. Philadelphia: Lippincott, 134. Adapted with permission.

stomach. The sodium that is left behind when chloride is lost combines with bicarbonate to form a base bicarbonate excess. Excessive ingestion of bicarbonate-containing antacids (for example, Alka-Seltzer) can cause metabolic alkalosis as well. In any case, the blood pH is elevated and the lungs retain carbon dioxide, causing slow shallow breathing. The kidneys also respond by conserving hydrogen ions and excreting bicarbonate; as a result, the urine becomes alkaline.

Combined and Mixed Imbalances

Acid–base imbalances can occur as separate entities or as combinations or mixtures of disturbances. That is, a patient can have respiratory acidosis or alkalosis or metabolic acidosis or alkalosis alone, or two of the types can occur at the same time. In *combined acid–base* disturbances, respiratory and metabolic acidosis or respiratory and metabolic alkalosis occur together. For instance, an anxious patient who is hyperventilating and vomiting will experience both respiratory and metabolic alkalosis simultaneously.

Mixed acid–base imbalances occur as respiratory acidosis and metabolic alkalosis or respiratory alkalosis and metabolic acidosis. A common example of the latter mixed imbalance is salicylate (aspirin) poisoning. At first, the respiratory centre in the medulla is stimulated causing hyperventilation and thus respiratory alkalosis. Later, the salicylates cause a metabolic disturbance which leads to an accumulation of acids in the body, resulting in metabolic acidosis.

In both the combined and mixed imbalances, the body's compensatory mechanisms are impaired and compensation cannot occur. Medical treatment is necessary to reverse the imbalances and prevent death.

ASSESSING FLUID, ELECTROLYTE AND ACID–BASE BALANCE

In order to assess a patient's fluid, electrolyte and acid–base needs, the nurse has to identify factors in the patient's history which would contribute to health or illness. The nurse should also be alert to signs and symptoms as well as significant laboratory findings in the patient that might be indicative of fluid, electrolyte and acid–base imbalances.

In addition, the nurse should know the physician's plan of therapy for the patient and understand the rationale on which this plan is based.

The patient's medical history provides the nurse with information about actual or potential fluid, electrolyte and acid–base problems. The person who has had a history of nausea and vomiting over several days, for example, is likely to show disturbances from the loss of fluids generally, the loss of acid from gastric secretions and possibly a depletion of the sodium ions as well. The patient who is admitted for surgery may develop fluid, electrolyte and acid–base imbalance

HEALTH HISTORY GUIDE

Fluid, Electrolyte and Acid–Base Balance

Health and Illness Patterns

USUAL PATTERN OF FLUID INTAKE AND OUTPUT

- What types of fluid do you usually drink in a day?
- How much water do you drink in a day?
- What foods do you usually eat? (Focus on proteins and foods rich in minerals such as sodium and potassium.)
- What is your usual frequency and amount of urination? How often do you void in a 24-hour period? Is urine concentrated or dilute?

RECENT CHANGES IN PATTERN OF INTAKE AND OUTPUT

- Have there been any recent changes in your usual patterns of intake and output? Have you noticed that you are drinking more or less than usual?
- Have you noticed that you have been voiding more or less often than usual?
- Have you noticed any loss or gain in weight?
- Have you had a recent illness that affected your fluid intake and output?
- Have you experienced nausea, vomiting, diarrhea or excessive perspiration?
- Have you noticed any signs of too much or too little hydration in your body? (Too much — swollen fingers and ankles, difficulty breathing, weight gain. Too little — dry mouth and skin, thirst, concentrated urine.)
- Have you noticed any change in your muscle strength, or signs of muscular irritability, such as tremors or twitching of the muscles?

PRESENTING HEALTH PROBLEM

- Describe the symptoms you are experiencing now. (Use questioning techniques as necessary to explore the symptoms.)
- When did the symptoms begin?
- What remedies have you tried for the symptoms? What were the results?
- Do you have a history of any acute or chronic diseases that might disrupt fluid, electrolyte and acid–base balance? For example, diabetes mellitus, high blood pressure, heart disease, kidney disease?
- Are you taking any medications or treatments that might disrupt fluid, electrolyte and acid–base balance? For example, diuretics, laxatives or enemas, steroids, potassium supplements, tube feedings, total parenteral nutrition, dialysis?
- Have you had any dietary restrictions? If so, what kind? Do you need help to plan a diet to meet these restrictions?

Health Promotion and Protection Patterns

- Do you drink products containing caffeine (for example, coffee, tea and cola), salt or sugar? If so, how much and how frequently?
- Do you drink alcohol? If so, how much and how often?
- Do you exercise regularly? If so, what is the nature of your program? What do you do to maintain hydration during strenuous exercise? What precautions do you take when exercising in hot weather?
- Do you work in a hot, humid environment? Does your work require strenuous activity? For example, using tools in a vigorous way, moving and carrying furniture or engaging in rigorous sporting activity?

TABLE 22.9 Acid–Base Imbalances, Causes, Compensation, Signs and Symptoms, Treatment and Nursing Intervention

CAUSES	COMPENSATION	SIGNS AND SYMPTOMS
Respiratory Acidosis (Carbonic acid excess) Hypoventilation, e.g., Airway obstruction Pulmonary edema Infection Atelectasis Paralysis of respiratory muscles Overdose of sedatives or anesthetics Postoperative pain Tight abdominal binders or dressings Severe abdominal distention	Kidneys excrete hydrogen ions but the process is slow (takes from a few hours to several days to develop)	Dyspnea Anxiety Disorientation Mental confusion Feeling of fullness in head (due to high $PaCO_2$ which causes cerebral vasodilation and increased blood flow) Dizziness Decreasing level of consciousness Tachycardia Cardiac arrhythmia, e.g., ventricular fibrillation Blood Gases: pH <7.35 $PaCO_2$ >46 mm Hg HCO_3 normal or slightly elevated (uncompensated) HCO_3 >33 mmol/L (compensated) Serum K elevated
Respiratory Alkalosis (Carbonic acid deficit) Hyperventilation, e.g., Severe anxiety of hysteria (most common) High fever Brain lesions involving respiratory centre Hypoxemia Early salicylate poisoning Excessive ventilation with mechanical ventilator	Kidneys excrete bicarbonate but the process is slow	Rapid breathing Signs related to a decrease in calcium ionization, e.g., dizziness, numbness and tingling of fingers and toes, circumoral paresthesias tetany Lightheadedness (a low $PaCO_2$ causes cerebral vasoconstriction and decreased blood flow) Headache Vertigo Palpitations Blood Gases: pH >7.45 $PaCO_2$ <34 mm Hg HCO_3 normal (uncompensated) HCO_3 <23 mmol/L (compensated) Serum K decreased
Metabolic Acidosis (base bicarbonate deficit) Diabetic ketoacidosis Renal failure (uremic acidosis) Severe diarrhea Excessive exercise (lactic acidosis) Starvation	Lungs "blow off" carbon dioxide, respirations rapid and deep Kidneys excrete hydrogen ion and retain bicarbonate ion	Lethargy Headache Drowsiness Nausea and vomiting Fruity, acetone breath Increased respiratory rate and depth

TREATMENT	NURSING INTERVENTIONS

Respiratory acidosis

Treat underlying cause,e.g., antibiotics for infection
Improve ventilation, e.g.,
• Clear airway by suction, postural drainage
• Deep breathing exercises
• Intermittent positive pressure breathing (IPPB)
Oxygen therapy for hypoxia
Severe cases:
• Ventilation via endotracheal tube, tracheostomy and mechanical
• Intravenous lactate or bicarbonate to help restore balance

Maintain a patent airway:
• Assist patient to turn and change position frequently
• Use semi-Fowler's positionunless contraindicated
• Assist patient to deep breathe frequently, cough as necessary
• Suction the nose and throat as necessary
Maintain hydration (2–3 litres per day), unless contra-indicated to keep secretions thin and facilitate removal
Administer oxygen as ordered
Monitor the patient's status as per signs and symptoms
Report signs of difficult breathing promptly, especially respiratory rates of 12 or less per minute or 24 or above per minute

Respiratory Alkalosis

Treat underlying cause, e.g., tranquilizer for hysteria
Increase level of carbon dioxide:
• Rebreathe exhaled air from a paper bag or a rebreathing mask
• Voluntary breath-holding
• Intermittent inhalations of carbon dioxide

Provide reassurance and emotional support to anxious and hysterical patients
Teach and encourage slower breathing, breath-holding, or rebreathing techniques

Metabolic Acidosis

Treat underlying cause, e.g., correct diabetic ketoacidosis with glucose and insulin
Replace water, electrolytes, and nutrients

Monitor the patient's status as per signs and symptoms
Report signs of worsening condition immediately, e.g., restlessness, confusion, Kussmaul respirations, tetany bradycardia, unconsciousness

continued on next page

TABLE 22.9 Acid–Base Imbalances, Causes, Compensation, Signs and Symptoms, Treatment and Nursing Intervention

CAUSES	COMPENSATION	SIGNS AND SYMPTOMS
Metabolic Acidosis continued (base bicarbonate deficit) Salicylate poisoning High fat diet		Kussmaul breathing (when HCO_3 is very low) Warm, flushed skin Dehydration Restlessness Confusion Unconsciousness Convulsions Blood Gases: pH < 7.35 HCO_3 <23 mmol/L $PaCO_2$ <34 mm Hg (compensated) Base excess negative Serum K is often elevated
Metabolic Alkalosis (base bicarbonate excess) Excessive intake of sodium bicarbonate Excessive vomiting orgastric suction Use of potent diuretics	Lungs retain carbon dioxide, respirations slow and shallow Kidneys retain hydrogen ion, excrete more bicarbonate	Shallow breathing Nausea, vomiting, diarrhea May be signs of hypokalemia May be signs related to decreased calcium ionization, such as muscle cramps, tremors, muscle twitching Irritability Unconsciousness Possible convulsions Blood Gases: pH >7.45 HCO_3 >33 mmol/L $PaCO_2$ normal (uncompensated) $PaCO_2$ >46 mm Hg (compensated) Base excess positive Serum K often decreased Serum Cl disproportionately lower than Na

postoperatively and will need careful observation to detect impending imbalances. The baseline data entered on the patient's record by the physician, other nurses and other members of the health care team can alert the nurse to the presence of health problems.

NURSING HEALTH HISTORY

The health history for fluid, electrolyte and acid–base balance focusses on obtaining information about the patient's usual patterns of fluid intake and output, determining changes in these patterns and exploring symptoms relating to the presenting health problem. The patient's health-promoting and -protecting patterns are also scrutinized to help identify potential problems and opportunities for health teaching.

MEASUREMENTS

FLUID INTAKE AND OUTPUT

Accurate measurement and recording of fluid intake and output is essential for identifying fluid balance problems and for planning and evaluating patient care. Abnormal

TREATMENT	NURSING INTERVENTIONS
Metabolic Acidosis continued	
Alkaline solutions, such as sodium bicarbonate or lactated Ringer's, may be given parenterally	Measure and record intake and output (required for calculating fluid replacement) Administer alkaline solutions according to established procedure to ensure safety Have sodium bicarbonate available for emergency use Implement safety precautions for restless, confused, unconscious or convulsing patients
Metabolic Alkalosis	
Treat underlying cause, e.g., stop use of sodium bicarbonate antacids for relief of indigestion Acidifying solutions, such as ammonium chloride, may be used intravenously or orally Oral or intravenous sodium chloride is administered Potassium deficits are replaced intravenously or orally	Monitor the patient's status as per signs and symptoms Report signs of worsening condition immediately, e.g., confusion, irritability, twitching, tremor, unconsciousness, convulsions Measure and record intake and output Monitor potassium, chloride and hydrogen ion losses (necessary to determine replacement) Instruct patients on foods high in potassium Administer oral sodium chloride and potassium supplements as ordered Administer intravenous sodium chloride and potassium as per established procedure to ensure safety Implement safety precautions for confused, agitated, irritable, unconscious or convulsing patients

SOURCES: Metheney, 1992, 133–142; Stroot, Lee, and Barrett, 1984, 99–123; Kee, 1986, 174–202; Weldy, 1992, 66–73.

gains or losses of fluids are valuable signs of fluid and electrolyte imbalances. Accurate recording of intake and output is especially important for correctly estimating fluid replacement therapy. When patients have existing or potential fluid and electrolyte problems, the nurse should implement fluid intake and output recording as an independent nursing function, even though this may sometimes be ordered by the physician.

All fluids the patient takes into and eliminates out of the body must be measured. Intake consists of fluids given orally, intravenously, interstitially and rectally, as well as fluids administered through tubes (tube feedings) or fluids used for tube irrigations. Fluid output includes urine, emesis and any drainage such as bile and suction returns. Significant amounts of fluid lost in the feces (with diarrhea), from wounds, during hyperventilation or through perspiration are estimated and recorded.

Fluid intake and output is recorded on a form commonly referred to as an I & O record or a Fluid Balance Record (see Figure 22.4) that is kept at the bedside or on the patient's chart. In most agencies, printed materials defining volumes of cups, glasses, bowls and containers enable accurate measurement of fluid intake. Graduated containers are also available for measuring output. Patients and their families can help to keep their own records, particularly if they understand the need for documentation and have been

LIONS GATE HOSPITAL

FLUID BALANCE / IV THERAPY RECORD

INTAKE ☐　　**OUTPUT** ☐

DATE: From 0700 _____ to 0700 _____

INTAKE											OUTPUT						
INTRAVENOUS							ORAL			URINE			OTHER FLUID LOSS				
													GASRIC			TUBE (Specify)	
START TIME	STOP TIME	SOLUTION VOLUME	RATE	INITIAL	TOTAL IV IN	TOTAL BLOOD IN	TIME	ORAL	TUBE	TIME	VOID	CATH.	EMESIS	N/G	BOWEL		
SUBTOTALS																	

12 HOUR TOTAL:　　IN:　　　　　　　　　　OUT:

START TIME	STOP TIME	SOLUTION VOLUME	RATE	INITIAL	TOTAL IV IN	TOTAL BLOOD IN	TIME	ORAL	TUBE	TIME	VOID	CATH.	EMESIS	N/G	BOWEL		
SUBTOTALS																	

12 HOUR TOTAL:　　IN:　　　　　　　　　　OUT:

24 HOUR TOTAL:　　IN:　　　　　　OUT:　　　　24 HOUR BALANCE + or –

A601 10M-S-TS
Rev. (03/91)

FIGURE 22.4　　Fluid Balance Record

SOURCE: Courtesy of Lions Gate Hospital, North Vancouver, BC.

Guidelines for Measuring and Recording Fluid Intake and Output

ESTABLISH INTAKE AND OUTPUT PROTOCOL

- Post an "Intake and Output" sign on the patient's bed or on the door of the room.
- Place an I & O sheet at the bedside and a fluid balance record on the chart. In some agencies only the fluid balance record is used. It is kept at the bedside and entries are made directly on it, eliminating the need to transfer amounts from one sheet to another at the end of the shift.
- Note fluid intake and output recording on the patient's nursing care plan or Kardex.

INSTRUCT THE PATIENT AND/OR FAMILY

- Explain why intake and output measurement is necessary.
- If patients are able to participate, explain how to measure and record intake and output.
  - Oral intake may be recorded in millilitres, using the agency list of fluid content in glasses, cups, soup bowls and other containers. Alternatively, the number of glasses, cups, bowls or containers of fluid ingested may be recorded, leaving the computation into millilitres to be done by the nurse.
  - The patient should void into a bedpan or urinal, pour the urine into a graduated container, measure the amount and then discard the urine. Demonstrate how to read amounts using the graduated container.
  - Record the time and amounts of intake or output on the I & O sheet.

MEASURE AND RECORD INTAKE

- Record the time, amount and type of intake on the I & O sheet.
- Water ingested from the bedside pitcher
  - Note the amount in the pitcher at the beginning of the shift.
  - Record the amount taken in when the pitcher is refilled or at the end of the shift.
  - Determine the amount of fluid ingested by subtracting the volume remaining in the pitcher from the volume it originally held, that is, the amount at the beginning of the shift or in the refilled pitcher.
- Ice chips
  - Determine the amount consumed by multiplying the volume of ice by 0.5 (for example, 240 ml of ice equals 120 ml of water).

- Oral fluids taken during or between meals
  - Record the time and amounts immediately after meals and intakes throughout the day.
  - Indicate the type of liquids ingested, (juice, carbonated beverages, coffee, tea, broth, milk, jello, ice cream, sherbet, hot cereals, etc.). Pureed foods are not included.
  - Measure the amount ingested using standard volumes of measurement specified for the agency.
- Enteric fluids or feedings (nasogastric, gastrostomy, jejunostomy)
  - Note the amount in the bag or bottle at the beginning of the shift.
  - Record the type, amount and time when the feeding is completed.
  - For feedings in progress at the end of a shift, measure and record type and amount taken in, and note the amount remaining.
  - Record the time, type and amount of fluid (water or normal saline) used to clear or irrigate the tube that was not withdrawn during the irrigation.
- Parenteral fluids
  - Record the time, type and amount to be absorbed (TBA) when the bag or bottle is hung or note the amount TBA at the beginning of the shift.
  - Record the time and amount when the bag has infused.
  - Record the time, type and amount of fluid infused with intravenous medications.
  - At the end of the shift, record the time and amount infused and indicate the amount TBA for the next shift.

MEASURE AND RECORD OUTPUT

- Record the time, amount and source of output on the I & O sheet.
- Urine
  - Measure amount using a graduated container, and record the time and amount following each voiding.
  - For urinary incontinence, estimate the amount or note the amount of clothing or bed linen saturated with urine.
  - For newborn babies or infants, measure output by weighing wet diapers.

- For indwelling urinary catheters, record the time and amount of urine when the drainage bag is emptied and at the end of the shift. Always empty the drainage bag at the end of the shift, regardless of how full it is. If measuring output hourly, drain the catheter tubing into the collection apparatus before measuring the amount to ensure an accurate measurement.
- Diarrhea, Emesis
  - Measure amounts using a graduated container and record, time, type and amount.
  - Estimate amounts that cannot be measured, for example, indicate the area (in cm) of vomitus or liquid stool on clothing or bed linen.
- Drainage tubes (wound drains, chest tubes, nasogastric tubes)
  - At the end of each shift or as frequently as ordered, empty drainage from the collecting container into a measuring device.
  - If the collecting container is graduated, an alternative method is to place a tape on the container and mark the drainage level with the date and time. Determine the amount of drainage by subtracting the previous level from the latest level.
  - Note amount of fluid taken out during tube irrigation if more fluid was withdrawn than was instilled.
- Blood and wound exudate
  - Describe the amount by measuring the size of the stained area and the thickness of the dressing or by weighing soaked dressings and subtracting the dry weight.
- Perspiration
  - Describe the amount of clothing or bed linen saturated with sweat.
  - An alternative method is to estimate perspiration as +, ++, +++, or ++++. The value + depicts sweating that is just visible, whereas ++++ depicts extreme sweating.

TOTAL INTAKE AND OUTPUT

- At the end of each 8- or 12-hour shift, or more frequently if ordered, calculate the total intake and output, and enter these amounts into the appropriate columns of the I&O Record.

---

taught how to do it. Guidelines for measuring and recording fluid intake and output are outlined in the box on p. 645.

The nurse totals the patient's intake and output at the end of each shift and also computes a 24-hour total. Fluid loss should equal fluid intake over a 48- to 72-hour period. The urine output of the average adult is between one and two litres in a 24-hour period. A general rule is that the kidneys produce approximately one millilitre of urine per kilogram of body weight per hour (1ml/kg/hr), regardless of age. Urine output that is less than 30 ml or more than 500 ml per hour is generally abnormal. Abnormalities of either excess or inadequate output must be reported to the patient's physician so that appropriate therapy can be instituted.

DAILY BODY WEIGHT

When patients have fluid and electrolyte disturbances, it is important to measure body weight on a daily basis — rapid changes in fluid volume are reflected in body weight. A loss or gain of one kg of body weight is almost equal to the loss or gain of one litre of fluid. To ensure accuracy of measurement, weights should be taken at the same time each day — before breakfast and after voiding. The same scale should be used each time and the patient should wear similar clothing.

VITAL SIGNS

Many disturbances in fluid, electrolyte and acid–base balance may be indicated by changes in vital signs. For example, an elevated body temperature in a patient who experienced profuse sweating without water replacement may indicate hypernatremia or hypertonic dehydration. Tachycardia is often one of the earliest signs of fluid volume deficit. A full bounding pulse is commonly associated with fluid volume excess. Deep rapid respirations may accompany metabolic acidosis as a compensatory mechanism. Blood pressure is a sensitive indicator of hypovolemia. Vital signs are important measures of the occurrence or worsening severity of fluid, electrolyte and acid–base problems and should be monitored carefully.

PHYSICAL ASSESSMENT

Because many organs and body functions are involved in the maintenance of fluid, electrolyte and acid–base balance, a variety of parameters must be examined. In order to make astute observations, the nurse must have knowledge of the normal characteristics of fluid, electrolyte and acid–base balance as well as the common defining signs and symptoms of imbalances. The parameters that should be appraised in assessing fluid, electrolyte and acid–base status are outlined here. These have been adapted from Metheney (1992).

Skin and Tongue Turgor

Skin turgor, which refers to the elasticity of skin, provides an indication of interstitial fluid volume or hydration. It is assessed by pinching a fold of skin on the sternum or forehead, under the clavicle, or on the inner aspect of the thigh and then observing how quickly it returns to its normal position. In a well-hydrated person, the skin returns to position immediately. If a fluid volume deficit is present, the pinched skin returns to position slowly and may stay elevated for a few seconds. Skin turgor can vary with age, nutritional state and even complexion and race. It may not be an effective indicator of hydration status in people older than 55 to 60 years because the loss of elasticity associated with aging reduces turgor.

Tongue turgor is an effective indicator of hydration for all age groups, because it does not change with age. The tongue of a hydrated person has one longitudinal furrow. The tongue of a patient with fluid volume deficit will have additional longitudinal furrows and will appear smaller. In a patient with sodium excess, the tongue will look red and swollen.

Moisture in Oral Cavity

A dry mouth can be the result of fluid volume deficit or mouth breathing. In fluid volume deficit, all tissues in the oral cavity will be dry. Conversely, if dryness is caused by mouth breathing, the areas where the gums meet the cheek membranes will be moist. Dry, sticky mucous membranes are indicative of hypernatremia (sodium excess).

Tearing and Salivation

Tearing and salivation are reduced in patients with fluid volume deficit. In infants and very small children, tears may be absent (Trucker and Sussman-Karten, 1987).

Appearance and Temperature of Skin

The skin takes on a pale appearance and feels cool to touch in patients with severe fluid volume deficit. This is due to peripheral vasoconstriction that occurs as a compensatory response to hypovolemia. Metabolic acidosis can cause warm, flushed skin due to peripheral vasodilation. Skin temperature is best palpated using the back of the hand or fingers because the skin over these areas is thin, permitting better perception of subtle changes.

Facial Appearance

The patient with a severe fluid volume deficit may have a pinched, drawn expression. The eyeballs may appear sunken and feel soft to the touch because the fluid deficit causes decreased intraocular pressure.

Edema

"*Edema* is defined as an excessive accumulation of interstitial fluid (the body fluid that bathes the cells)" (Metheney, 1992, 22). The formation of edema may be localized in one area of the body, such as the swelling in an ankle that sustained trauma, or it may be generalized and spread throughout the body. An accumulation of interstitial fluid predominantly in the lower extremities of ambulatory patients and over the sacral area in bedridden patients is known as *dependent edema*. Edema related to salt retention is described as *pitting* and can be appraised by pressing one's finger into soft tissues over a bony prominence such as the ankle or tibia and then removing it. If pitting edema is present, an indentation will remain (see Figure 22.5).

Gauging edema by appearance is a subjective measure. Peripheral edema may be described using plus signs to indicate the amount, ranging from +1 to +4. The value +1 indicates barely perceptible, +2 and +3 moderate, and +4 severe edema. A more exact method is to measure the same extremity or body part every day using a millimetre tape measure. Pitting edema may be described by measuring the degree of pitting with a tape measure. If pitting is 0 to 0.6 cm, edema is described as mild; if it is 0.6 to 1.3 cm, edema is moderate; and if it is 1.3 to 2.5 cm, edema is severe (Bowers and Thompson, 1984).

FIGURE 22.5   Pitting Edema

Neck and Hand Veins

Intravascular fluid volume can be indirectly assessed by observing the filling and emptying of veins in the neck and the hands. Normally, the external jugular veins distend and become visible when a person lies flat in bed or when the head is lower than the heart. The veins should empty easily when the person is brought back to a sitting position. If fluid volume excess is present, the veins may remain distended when the patient's position is changed. In fluid volume deficit, the veins will remain flat even in the supine position, or they will fill slowly.

Normally, the veins on the back of the hand will empty or flatten in three to five minutes when hands are elevated. Likewise, they will fill or expand in three to five minutes when hands are held in a dependent position. Increases or decreases in fluid volume are exhibited by vein-emptying or -filling times that are longer than three to five minutes. A prolonged vein-filling time indicates fluid volume deficit. In fluid volume excess, vein-emptying time is prolonged; the veins will remain distended and clearly visible.

Neuromuscular Irritability

Electrolyte changes, in particular changes in levels of calcium, magnesium, potassium and sodium, can cause notable neuromuscular responses. Tests for increased or decreased muscular irritability should be made when imbalances in these electrolytes are suspected.

Chvostek's sign   Chvostek's sign is checked by tapping the facial nerve about two cm anterior to the earlobe. A positive Chvostek's sign is shown by a unilateral twitching and contraction of the facial muscles — the upper lip, side of the face, nose and eyelid (Figure 22.6). It is indicative of hypocalcemia and hypomagnesemia.

Trousseau's sign   Trousseau's sign can also occur with calcium and magnesium deficits. It is tested by applying a blood pressure cuff on the upper arm and inflating it above systolic pressure for three minutes. A positive response will elicit a carpal spasm (adducted thumb with fingers extended), as shown in Figure 22.6.

Deep tendon reflexes   Electrolyte and acid–base imbalances can cause hyperactive or diminished reflexes. Deep tendon reflexes often become hyperactive in states of hypocalcemia, hypomagnesemia, hyperkalemia, hypernatremia and alkalosis. Conversely, they are diminished in hypercalcemia, hypermagnesemia, hypokalemia, hyponatremia and acidosis.

Other Signs

Changes in behaviour, for instance, changes in level of consciousness, restlessness or confusion and varying levels of fatigue, may accompany the signs and symptoms of fluid, electrolyte and acid–base balance. Their significance must

A **B**

FIGURE 22.6   A. Chvostek's sign B. Trousseau's sign

TABLE 22.10 Laboratory Tests for Fluid, Electrolyte and Acid–Base Balance

TEST	NORMAL VALUES	IMBALANCES INDICATED
Serum electrolytes: Measures the concentration of electrolytes in blood serum.		
Sodium (Na^+)	135–150 mmol/L	Hyponatremia and hypernatremia
Potassium (K^+)	3.5–5.0 mmol/L	Falling trend (0.1–0.2 mmol per day) indicative of a developing deficiency Hypokalemia and hyperkalemia
Calcium (Ca^{2+})	2.12–2.62 mmol/L	Hypocalcemia and hypercalcemia
Chloride (Cl^-)	98–108 mmol/L	Hypochloremia and hyperchloremia
Magnesium (Mg^{2+})	0.70–1.10 mmol/L	Hypomagnesemia and hypermagnesemia
Phosphate (PO_4)	0.81–1.58 mmol/L	Hypophosphatemia and hyperphosphatemia
Serum Osmolality: Measures the concentration of dissolved particles (electrolytes, sugar, urea) in the serum.	M 275–295 mmol/kg F 280–290 mmol/kg	Elevated levels indicate hemoconcentration, dehydration and hypernatremia Decreased levels indicate hemodilution, overhydration and hyponatremia
Hematocrit (Hct): Measures the red blood cell mass in a volume of whole blood.	M 0.40–0.51 F 0.35–0.45	Elevated levels indicate hypovolemia and dehydration
Urine Specific Gravity: Measures the kidney's ability to concentrate urine.	1.003–1.035	Low values indicate fluid excess and overhydration. High values indicate fluid deficit and dehydration.
Arterial Blood Gases: Give information on acid–base status and the adequacy of ventilation and oxygen-carbon dioxide exchange.	pH: 7.35–7.45 PO_2: >70 mm Hg PCO_2: 34–46 mm Hg Bicarbonate: 23–33 mmol/L Base excess: –3.0-+3.0 mmol/L	A pH <7.35 indicates acidosis; >7.45 alkalosis. An elevated PCO_2 indicates respiratory acidosis; decreased PCO_2 indicates respiratory alkalosis. Decreased bicarbonate and base excess indicate metabolic acidosis; elevated values indicate metabolic alkalosis.

SOURCE: *Laboratory Ward Manual.* (1992). North Vancouver, BC: Lions Gate Hospital.

be considered in the context of the specific imbalances (Metheney, 1992).

DIAGNOSTIC TESTS

There are a large number of diagnostic tests for fluid, electrolyte and acid–base disturbances. You will learn about many of them in the more advanced levels of your program. In this section, we will focus on the common laboratory tests performed on blood and urine specimens. These are outlined in Table 22.10.

DIAGNOSING FLUID, ELECTROLYTE AND ACID–BASE BALANCE PROBLEMS

Fluid and electrolyte problems that are amenable to nursing therapy are related to deficits or excesses in fluid volume. *Fluid volume deficit* occurs in situations where oral intake is insufficient or large amounts of fluids are lost from the body. People who feel too ill to eat, who are nauseated, tired, weak or in pain or those who are fasting may experience or be at risk for fluid volume deficits as a result of insufficient intake. Similarly, individuals experiencing vomiting, diarrhea, excessive perspiration, gastric suction and wound drainage may develop fluid deficits from abnormal losses. Defining characteristics of *Fluid volume deficit* might include insufficient oral fluid intake, less fluid intake than output, thirst, dry skin with decreased turgor and a decreased volume of concentrated urine.

Fluid volume excess problems may occur when there is excessive intake of sodium or water, high salt intake, low protein intake or excessive intravenous fluids. Defining characteristics of these problems may include peripheral and sacral edema, taut shiny skin, greater intake than output and weight gain. Many problems associated with fluid volume excess, however, are not within the realm of independent nursing intervention and should be viewed as collaborative problems. These might include pulmonary edema, ascites (accumulation of fluid within the abdominal cavity) or massive generalized edema. Electrolyte and acid–base problems should also be regarded as collaborative problems because physicians' orders are necessary for initiation of treatment measures; and many aspects of care, such as initiation and maintenance of intravenous therapy, are directed by hospital policy.

Common examples of nursing diagnoses and collaborative problems for fluid, electrolyte and acid–base problems as taken from the list of NANDA diagnoses include:

- *Fluid volume deficit related to vomiting, diarrhea and decreased intake*
- *High risk for fluid volume deficit related to nausea and poor fluid intake*
- *Fluid volume excess related to high salt intake*
- *PC: electrolyte imbalance*
- *PC: acidosis (metabolic, respiratory)*
- *PC: alkalosis(metabolic, respiratory).**

PLANNING FLUID, ELECTROLYTE AND ACID–BASE BALANCE INTERVENTIONS

Once diagnosis is complete, the nurse formulates a plan for care. Planning must be done in conjunction with the patient, taking into account individual and family beliefs, preferences, lifestyle practices and socioeconomic considerations. In addition to therapeutic interventions for the particular problems, emphasis should be placed on self-care and strategies that enable patients to achieve optimum fluid, electrolyte and acid–base balance in their daily lives.

_____
* Carpenito, 1993.

Goals or expected outcomes direct the selection of nursing interventions. Common expected outcomes related to fluid, electrolyte and acid–base balance might be as follows:

- Patient will maintain a balanced fluid intake and output, averaging 2500 ml per day for 2 days
- Patient will show signs of hydration
- Patient will verbalize how to maintain increased fluid intake during strenuous exercise
- Patient will exhibit arterial blood gases within normal range.

IMPLEMENTING FLUID, ELECTROLYTE AND ACID–BASE BALANCE INTERVENTIONS

HEALTH PROMOTING STRATEGIES

The human body possesses a very effective system for maintaining and regulating fluid, electrolyte and acid–base balance. An adequate fluid intake and a well-balanced diet containing the essential minerals are necessary to maintain optimal fluid, electrolyte and acid–base balance on a day-to-day basis. Difficulties arise when water intake is not adequate or when water losses greatly exceed intake, as can happen during strenuous exercise or manual labour, for example.

Deficiencies or excesses in the intake of minerals may also cause problems. Nurses can help individuals and families maintain optimum fluid, electrolyte and acid–base balance in three basic ways. First, they can encourage and assist individuals and families to explore lifestyle factors, values and health practices that may affect their fluid, electrolyte and acid–base needs. Second, nurses can provide information that will enable people to decide whether or not they need to change their usual patterns and practices. Third, nurses can provide teaching about healthy living practices aimed at promoting optimum fluid, electrolyte and acid–base balance.

HEALTH PROTECTING STRATEGIES

Disturbances in fluid, electrolyte and acid–base balance can have serious effects on body functioning. The nurse must be particularly alert in noting early indications of imbalance. These should be reported promptly so that appropriate therapy can be instituted before the condition

HEALTH PROMOTING STRATEGY

Promoting Healthy Fluid, Electrolyte and Acid–Base Balance

- Drink about two litres of fluid daily
- Eat a well-balanced diet from all four food groups
- Minimize consumption of salt, sugar, caffeine and alcohol
- Keep body weight within normal limits
- Maintain a regular exercise program
- Note early signs of dehydration
  - Thirst, dry mouth, dry skin, decreased urine output
- Note early signs of fluid retention
  - Puffy fingers, ankle edema, sharp weight gain
- When undertaking strenuous activity:
  - Wear minimal clothing. Clothes worn should be loose and porous to permit circulation of air and evaporation of heat.
  - Drink fluids frequently. Consume about 240 ml every 25 minutes. Pour water over head and chest to cool down.

- Replenish lost electrolytes. Add extra salt to meals except if high blood pressure is a problem; eat foods high in potassium, such as bananas, dried fruits (figs, peaches) and oranges.
- In hot climates, work or exercise in the morning or evening, if possible, to avoid the heat of the day. Stay in the shade, if possible, to avoid the sun's radiation and wear white clothing to reflect the radiant heat.
- Hyperhydrate if planning to exercise or work in the heat. To do this, drink half to one litre of fluid within an hour of commencing the activity.
- Note signs of heat exhaustion: fatigue, weakness, nausea, cramps and headache. If these should occur, stop exercising, rest in a cool place and drink cool fluids.
- In cold climates, cover head, hands and wrists. Wear several layers of clothing with a windbreaker on the outside. Heat must be allowed to dissipate without getting clothes wet.

becomes too advanced. The consequences of marked imbalances of fluids and the major electrolytes in the body have been documented throughout this chapter. It should be stressed, therefore, that all measures to maintain and restore fluid, electrolyte and acid–base balance are nursing priorities.

Patients with elevated temperatures are especially vulnerable to disturbances in fluid and electrolyte balance. In fever states between 38.3° and 39.4° C, an adult's fluid need increases by 500 ml over the basic 24-hour requirement. When body temperatures exceed 39.4° C, an adult requires an additional litre of fluid (Condon and Nyhus, 1988).

HEALTH RESTORING STRATEGIES

Whenever a disturbance in fluid, electrolyte and acid–base balance occurs, steps must be taken to restore homeostasis. Since the principal sources of fluids and electrolytes are the foods and fluids consumed, adjustments in diet or fluid intake or both may be sufficient to rectify a mild disturbance. In the case of deficiencies of specific electrolytes, supplements may be given in the form of medications. Often, however, fluid loss is too extensive and the accompanying loss of electrolytes too great to be corrected by

oral intake alone; or this method of replacement may be contraindicated. Fluids and electrolytes may then be administered by other routes, namely intravenous infusion, blood transfusion, enteral tube feeding, or total parenteral nutrition. The physician orders the route and the type of solutions to be administered based on knowledge of the patient's condition and the particular factors causing the imbalance. Enteral tube feedings and total parenteral nutrition are discussed in Chapter 19.

ORAL FLUID AND ELECTROLYTE THERAPY

Of primary importance in the care of the patient with fluid and electrolyte problems is the maintenance of a therapeutic fluid intake. In many instances the physician orders the exact amount of oral fluid for the patient. Sometimes, however, it is a nursing function to judge the oral needs and prescribe fluid intake. For example, the nurse may determine that a patient with a fever or an infection requires larger amounts of fluid per day.

Generally speaking, patients who are dehydrated or have lost excessive amounts of fluid should be encouraged to take in extra fluids, unless contraindicated by other conditions. If patients are nauseated or vomiting, for example, it is not reasonable to expect that they will tolerate oral fluids. Patients with kidney or heart conditions may require restriction of their fluid intake. The nurse should be aware of the physician's objectives in medical therapy and never push or force fluids beyond the limit prescribed.

People normally obtain electrolytes from the foods and fluids they ingest. Therefore, to maintain good electrolyte balance, adequate nutrition is essential. When a patient is deficient in certain electrolytes or more are needed in the body, these may be replaced by medication. For example, calcium supplements may be ordered for older individuals because they absorb calcium poorly and ingest less in their diets.

In addition, restricted electrolyte intake may be prescribed; for example, the physician might order a salt-free or low-salt diet for the patient. The usual purpose here is to restrict the oral intake of sodium (Na^+). It is frequently the nurse's responsibility to help patients understand the necessity for the restriction and help them plan meals accordingly. Most people are able to assume responsibility for restricting their diets. Nevertheless, in hospitals it is not unknown for a "helpful" roommate to lend his or her salt shaker to a person on a restricted diet.

INTRAVENOUS THERAPY

The infusion of fluids directly into a vein is often indicated for patients who are unable to ingest fluids orally. Intravenous infusion provides a safe, rapid and controlled route for administering a variety of fluids, electrolytes, nutrients, medications and blood or blood products. It is a vital treatment measure in the care of most surgical and a large number of medical patients. Patients no longer have to be in hospital to receive intravenous infusion. An increasing number of people today are being sent home on intravenous therapy after they or their caregivers in the family are taught the necessary skills for home care. Home care nurses also supervise home intravenous therapy.

Intravenous fluids are delivered into both peripheral and central veins through what are referred to as *peripheral* and *central venous lines*. In peripheral intravenous therapy, solutions are administered through a catheter or inserted into a vein in the hand, the arm or, occasionally, the leg or foot, and into a scalp vein in infants. This method is commonly used for short-term or intermittent fluid therapy.

In central venous therapy, a catheter is inserted into the right or left subclavian vein or the internal or external jugular veins. This route is preferred for patients who require large volumes of solution, those who need more than one infusion at the same time and those who receive hypertonic or irritating solutions such as total parenteral nutrition (discussed in Chapter 19). Central venous lines are also used in patients whose peripheral veins are inaccessible or collapsed because of prolonged therapy or the disease process. A mod-

ification of the central venous line is the *implanted vascular access device*. Consisting of a port connected to a catheter, the device is surgically implanted into a pocket of subcutaneous tissue adjacent to a central vein, into which the catheter is inserted. Intravascular access devices are favoured for prolonged, intermittent intravenous therapy (months or even years) because patients are able to maintain activities of daily living with complete freedom when solutions are not being infused.

The decision to administer intravenous fluids rests with the physician. The route of administration, the type and amount of solution, the rate of flow and the duration of infusion is ordered by the doctor according to the patient's age, condition and need for fluid, electrolytes and nutrients. Although nurses may not be required to insert all types of intravenous lines, they are responsible for preparing, maintaining and discontinuing the infusions as well as teaching patients and their families about intravenous therapy and relevant aspects of self-care. Nurses are also responsible for assisting physicians with the insertion of central venous lines.

TYPES OF INTRAVENOUS SOLUTIONS

The most common intravenous solutions contain water with additives, usually nutrients and electrolytes. Nutrient solutions contain water or saline with carbohydrates. They supply fluid and calories for energy needs. Electrolyte solutions are made up of saline alone or saline with electrolytes. They are used to correct electrolyte imbalances as well as acidosis and alkalosis. Blood volume expanders are solutions that are used to restore blood volume following losses from hemorrhage and to prevent or treat shock.

Intravenous solutions are classified according to their tonicity or osmotic pressure equivalents to concentrations within cells. A solution that has approximately the same osmolarity as blood plasma is called *isotonic*. One with a lower osmolarity than blood plasma is called *hypotonic* and one with a higher osmolarity is called *hypertonic*. Isotonic solutions produce no change in the osmotic pressure of plasma. They increase circulating fluid volume without altering the interstitial and intracellular compartments. Iostonic solutions are infused to treat hypotension caused by hypovolemia. Hypotonic solutions lower serum osmolarity and cause water to move out of the blood vessels into the interstitial spaces and the cells. Hypotonic solutions are administered to correct cellular dehydration. When hypertonic solutions are administered, serum osmolarity increases. Fluid is pulled from the cells and interstitial spaces into the blood vessels. Hypertonic solutions are commonly used in postoperative patients to maintain circulating fluid volume and prevent edema.

TABLE 22.11 Common Intravenous Solutions

TYPE	COMPOSITION	PURPOSE
Nutrient Solutions		
Dextrose in water D_5W (isotonic) $D_{10}W$ (hypertonic)	Water with carbohydrate	Provide water and calories
Dextrose and saline $D_5W/0.9$ NaCl (hypertonic) $D_5W/0.45$ NaCl (hypertonic)	NaCl with carbohydrate	Provide calories and electrolytes
Electrolyte Solutions		
Saline solution 0.45 NaCl (hypotonic) 0.9 NaCl (isotonic)	NaCl and water	Provide salt and water
Multiple electrolyte solutions Ringer's solution (hypertonic) Lactated Ringer's (RL)(isotonic)	Varying electrolytes: Na, K, Ca, Cl	Maintenance therapy; correct electrolyte and acid–base imbalances
Electrolyte solutions with dextrose D_5W/RL (hypertonic)	Electrolytes and dextrose	Provide electrolytes and calories
Blood Volume Expanders		
Serum albumin		Restores normal blood volume
Dextran	Large carbohydrate molecules in water	Temporarily increases blood volume; used to treat shock

PERIPHERAL INTRAVENOUS THERAPY

Starting a Peripheral Infusion

When intravenous therapy is ordered, nurses must complete a number of tasks. Namely, they have to check the doctor's order, prepare the patient, collect and assemble the equipment and solution, perform the venipuncture and establish the infusion. In some agencies, graduate nurses perform venipuncture; in others this is done by a specialized team of nurses, called the *IV Team*. When the venipuncture is performed by an IV Team, the nurse caring for the patient is responsible for preparing the patient and assembling the equipment.

Preparing the Patient

It is important to explain the procedure and make the patient feel relaxed. Tension and anxiety can cause vasoconstriction which makes insertion of the catheter or needle more difficult and uncomfortable for the patient. Patients will also feel more relaxed when the nurse is organized. Begin your teaching by asking patients if they have had an IV before. Allow them time to express experiences and understanding. Try to dispel any misconceptions or apprehensions by providing clear explanations.

Information you give might include why the patient needs intravenous therapy, how the venipuncture will be performed, sensations that might be felt, how long the infusion will last, how the patient can help maintain the infusion, when to call the nurse and any limits the intravenous may put on activity. Explain that slight transient pain may be felt during the insertion of the needle or catheter, but the discomfort will stop once the device is in place. Initially, the IV fluid can feel cool but this too will subside in a few minutes. Emphasize that any discomfort or change in the rate of flow should be reported to the nurse. Reassurance that showering and bathing are usually possible is comforting to many patients. If available and if time permits, pamphlets, demonstrations and audiovisual aids may be used to enhance the patient's understanding and comfort. Play therapy is frequently used with children. Encourage patients to ask questions and provide clarification as necessary.

One last detail in preparing the patient for intravenous therapy is to ensure that clothing can be removed over the IV apparatus. Some agencies have special hospital gowns with openings at the shoulder for this purpose.

Assembling Equipment

The basic equipment for intravenous infusion includes a bag or bottle containing the solution, an intravenous administration set (tubing), a label for the tubing and an IV pole.

Intravenous bags and bottles. Intravenous containers are either plastic bags or glass bottles that are vacuum-sealed (see Figure 22.7). Currently, most solutions come in plastic bags; however, glass bottles are sometimes necessary for solutions containing substances that are incompatible with plastic, for example, lipid emulsions. Plastic bags are advantageous because they do not require an air vent to enable the flow of solution into the vein. Aided by the pull of gravity and atmospheric pressure, these bags simply collapse as solution flows out. Because of their ability to collapse, plastic containers provide a closed system which reduces the possibility of contamination by microorganisms.

Glass bottles, on the other hand, cannot collapse because they are rigid. Therefore, an air vent is needed to draw air into the bottle as fluid flows out. This mechanism is necessary to prevent the creation of a vacuum within the container which stops the flow of fluid. The air vent can be a plastic tube placed in the bottle or it can be an attachment on the IV administration set. Due to the air vent, glass containers are open to room air and more likely to become contaminated, thereby posing an increased risk for infection in patients. At the neck end of both plastic and glass containers there is a port or a rubber stopper into which the IV administration set is inserted. Plastic bags also have a resealable port for instilling medication into the container. Solutions for infusion are commonly supplied in 500 or 1000 ml containers, whereas those for medications come in 50 or 100 ml capacities.

Intravenous administration set. The IV administration set is a closed system of connective tubing that delivers the solution from the container to the needle or catheter situated in the patient's vein. Figure 22.8 shows the parts of the IV administration set. Commonly referred to as the IV line, the administration set consists of an insertion spike, a drip chamber, tubing, a movable roller or screw clamp, one or more Y-type injection ports, an antireflux or backcheck valve, and a

FIGURE 22.7 IV Solution Containers   A. Glass Bottle   B. Plastic Bag

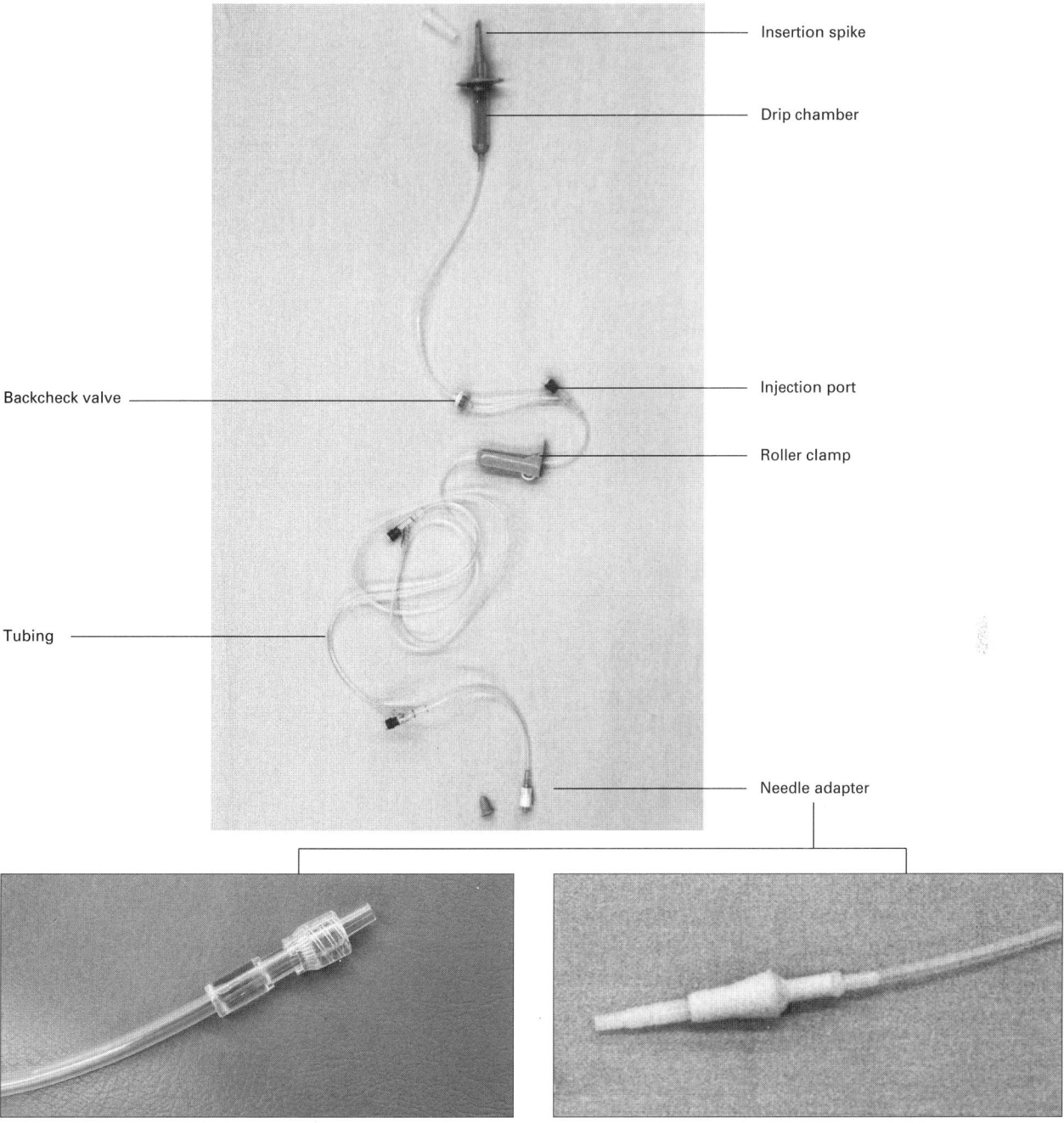

Insertion spike

Drip chamber

Backcheck valve

Injection port

Roller clamp

Tubing

Needle adapter

Luer–lock needle adapter

Flashball with friction-type needle adapter

FIGURE 22.8 Parts of the IV administration set

needle adapter. Protective caps over the insertion spike and the needle adapter ensure sterility before use.

The *insertion spike* is a sharply pointed plastic cannula that is pushed into the port of the solution container. Below the insertion spike is an enlarged, clear plastic tube called the *drip chamber*. Fluid passes from the spike to the drip chamber through a drip tube in the form of drops. Administration sets are calibrated to deliver a specified number of drops per millilitre of solution. This is called the *drop factor*. The drop factor, indicated as drops per millilitre, is indicated on the package. The drip chamber allows one to observe the drops of solution leaving the container and entering the tubing. The rate of infusion over time can be established by counting the number of drops per minute.

Clear tubing connects the drip chamber and the needle adapter. Situated on the tubing is the *roller clamp*, which is a movable apparatus used to control the amount of fluid passing through the tubing. Also along the tubing, there

Macrodrop Set

Definition: Refers to the size or diameter of the drip tube that forms the drops entering the drip chamber. The macrodrop delivers 10, 12, 15 or 20 drops per millilitre of solution.

Uses: To deliver large quantities of solution or when rapid infusion is necessary.

Microdrop Set

Definition: The microdrop delivers 50 to 60 drops per millilitre of solution.

Uses: To deliver small quantities of solution or when a very slow, precise rate of infusion is necessary, for example, in infants and small children, or in older patients to prevent circulatory overload.

Nonvented Set

Definition: Refers to tubing without an air vent.

Uses: With plastic bags or vented bottles.

Vented Set

Definition: Refers to tubing that contains an air vent allowing air to replace solution as it flows out of the bottle. Vented sets usually have filters to remove contaminants from the air that enters the bottle.

Uses: With nonvented bottles, for example, for albumin and fat emulsions.

In-Line Filter

Definition: A filter within the IV line that removes particles and microbes from the solution, helping to decrease the risk of contamination and complications such as infusion phlebitis.

Uses: For total parenteral nutrition; when administering solutions to immunodeficient patients; or for administering solutions containing several additives.

Add-On Filter

Definition: A filter added on to the tubing serving the same purposes as in-line filters.

Uses: For total parenteral nutrition and infusion of plasma, blood and blood products.

Volume-Control Container

Definition: Small calibrated container situated between the solution container and the drip chamber. Examples: Soluset® and Buretrol®

Uses: To deliver small doses of fluids or medications over extended periods. Often used in pediatrics and critical care areas.

Secondary Set

Definition: Tubing that connects a secondary solution to the primary line. This can be a tandem set-up as pictured here or a piggyback set-up as described in Chapter 33.

Uses: For intermittent or simultaneous infusion of medications with the primary solution.

FIGURE 22.9   Types of administration sets and devices

are one or two *Y-type injection ports* which permit simultaneous or intermittent infusion of a secondary solution. Many sets also contain backcheck valves which prevent the flow of solution from a secondary line into the main solution. At the end of the tubing is the *needle adapter*, a plastic connector to which the needle or cannula is connected. Many adapters contain a lock apparatus, known as a *luer lock*, which secures the tubing to the needle or cannula with a twisting motion. Others are slip adapters which simply fit into the needle or cannula hub by friction. Some administration sets have a resealable injection port, called a *flashball*, between the tubing and the needle adapter. However, this type of tubing is being used less frequently.

There are a number of variations to the basic IV administration set. In most situations that require fluid maintenance or replacement in adult patients, a regular administration set is used. The regular set, called the *macrodrop*, can deliver large quantities of solution at rapid rates because the drops contain a larger volume of solution. In pediatrics, on the other hand, where smaller volumes of solution are to be infused, *microdrop* sets are preferred.

Sometimes, particularly when medications are being administered, two solutions may be put up at the same time. This requires a primary administration set with a secondary injection port or a piggyback port and a *secondary set* which connects the second solution to the primary line (we talk about this in Chapter 33 in the section on medication administration). In some cases, when administering total parenteral nutrition or blood products, for instance, an administration set with a *filter* is required. Other times, such as in the need to deliver very small, precise amounts of fluid to infants, a *special volume control device* is attached to the administration set.

In order to assemble the correct administration set, the nurse must know the type of solution that has been ordered, the rate of flow and the type of container that will be used. Many of the variations are built into basic administration sets or they are available as separate devices that can be added as necessary. It is important to note at this point that IV administration sets and related devices vary according to the different manufacturers. To ensure correct use of equipment nurses should read and follow the manufacturer's instructions carefully. The most common types of IV administration sets and devices are illustrated in Figure 22.9.

Needleless systems. Nurses working with intravenous equipment are at risk for needlestick (sharps) injuries. Needles, including those used for injecting solution into IV tubing, and the IV tubing spike are examples of sharps used in IV therapy. Needlestick injuries have the potential to transmit blood borne pathogens (microorganisms that are present in human blood and can cause disease). Contaminated, as well as clean, needlestick injuries expose health care workers to infection. Nurses are accountable for the safe handling of IV equipment to prevent injury to themselves and other health team members. This aspect will be discussed later in the chapter. In addition, some agencies use needleless intravenous devices to protect health care workers. Examples of needleless devices are illustrated in Figure 22.10. Shields are also available to protect the opposing hand from a needlestick injury.

IV pole. An adjustable rod or pole, called the *IV pole*, is necessary to hold the IV container above the level of the patient. In order for solution to flow from the container into the patient's vein, the force of gravity is required to overcome venous pressure. This is accomplished by hanging the container upside down on the pole and adjusting the height to approximately one metre above the needle insertion site. Flow rates can be adjusted by raising or lowering the IV pole. The more distance between the container and the patient, the greater the force of gravity; thus the faster the solution flows into the vein. IV poles can be attached to the bed or they can hang from the ceiling. They are also mounted on wheels so that patients can get out of bed and ambulate freely.

Performing the Peripheral Venipuncture and Establishing the Infusion

The process of inserting a needle or a catheter into a vein is called **venipuncture**. This procedure is done to establish intravenous infusion of fluids, to administer medications and to obtain venous blood samples. Agencies have their own guidelines as to who will be responsible for performing venipunctures. In some this is done by the nurses on the ward after they have successfully completed an in-service education program. In others this task is left to specialized nurses on the IV team. Whether or not you will learn the skill of venipuncture as a student will depend on your school's curriculum. Not all schools regard venipuncture as a skill required for graduation.

Venipuncture is considered a relatively simple procedure by those who are skilled in doing it. It involves, however, a number of tasks that require proper knowledge, skill and dexterity for safe performance. These tasks include selecting an appropriate venipuncture device (needle or catheter) and site for insertion, inserting the device into the patient and establishing the infusion.

Selecting a venipuncture device
Several factors have to be considered in selecting a venipuncture device. The duration and purpose of intravenous therapy; the type of solution; and the patients age, condition of veins and activity level will influence the type of device to be used. A variety of venipuncture devices are available for intravenous therapy. Two of the most common devices are the over-the-needle catheter and the wing-tipped (butterfly) needle (see Figure 22.11).

FIGURE 22.10 Needleless intravenous devices. A, B and G are prepierced, self-sealing ports. The blunt cannula in F is inserted into the prepierced port. Use of this system replaces the sharp needle and avoids the risk of injury. C is an adapter which is attached to IV tubing. Secondary IV tubing and syringes can be attached directly to this adapter without a needle. D is a connector used to attach a secondary IV set to a primary line. This adapter shields against injury by having the needle permanently retracted. E is a prepierced vial adapter, designed to permit the withdrawal of solution from a vial with the blunt cannula in F.

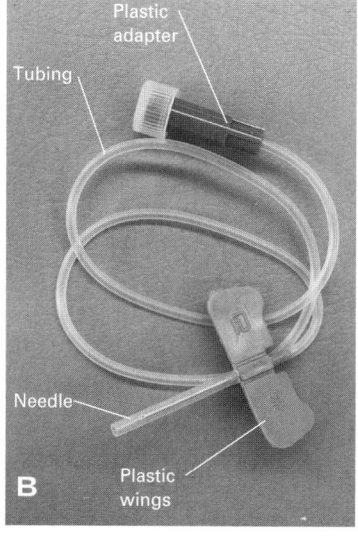

FIGURE 22.11 Common venipuncture devices A. Over-the-needle catheter B. Wing-tipped needle

The over-the-needle catheter consists of a plastic tube mounted over a needle, the bevel of which protrudes out of the end of the catheter. The needle functions to stabilize the catheter during insertion and is withdrawn once the catheter is inside the vein. This type of catheter is used for long-term therapy (more than 24 hours) and for administering all solutions including blood. It is also used in emergency situations because large volumes of solution can be administered quickly. Since the catheter is a flexible tube, it is less likely to puncture the vein, thus reducing the risk of infiltration. Also, once in place, the catheter is more comfortable and permits the patient to move normally. One disadvantage is that over-the-needle catheters are more difficult to insert.

The butterfly needle consists of a thin-walled stainless steel stem with plastic flaps attached to the shaft. The flaps are used to hold the needle during insertion.

Preparing the Intravenous Infusion

ACTION	RATIONALE
A. PREPARING THE SOLUTION CONTAINER	
1. Check physician's order for type of solution and rate of flow.	Ensures accurate delivery and reduces risk of error.
2. Gather equipment: • Correct solution • Administration set • Label for the tubing • IV filter as per agency policy • IV pole	Safe, effective infusion depends on correct solution and proper equipment.
3. Wash hands thoroughly and maintain sterile technique throughout the procedure.	Aseptic technique is required to prevent contamination which can lead to local or systemic infection.
4. Inspect the container for leaks, cracks or tears; the solution for expiry date, clarity and foreign particles; and the tubing for cracks, holes or missing clamps.	Ensures sterility and freshness of solution and sterility of the tubing.
5. Place a bag on a flat surface or hang it on an IV pole; place a bottle upright on a stable surface.	Facilitates ease of inserting spike.
6. Slide the roller clamp below the drip chamber and close the clamp.	Facilitate easy access of clamp and prevents escape of fluid through the tubing.
7. **Bag:** Remove the protective cover from the tubing port by pulling downward, uncap the spike, and, while holding the port with one hand, insert the spike with the other hand using a firm twisting motion.	Pulling downward quickly removes the cover and maintains sterility of the port. A twisting motion is needed to puncture the seal on the bag.
Nonvented Bottle: Remove the metal cap and inner disk, uncap the spike, and push the spike straight down, through the centre of the rubber stopper .	Twisting or angling the spike during insertion can cause pieces of the rubber stopper to break off and fall into the solution.

8. Hang the container on an IV pole (if not already done) and squeeze the flexible drip chamber until it is half full. Note: firm drip chambers will fill automatically.	Squeezing the drip chamber pushes air into the container causing fluid to flow into the chamber. It also prevents air from moving downward into the tubing. When the chamber is partially filled, drops can be easily seen and counted.

Continued on the next page

ACTION

B. PRIMING THE INTRAVENOUS TUBING

1. Hold the capped needle adapter end of the tubing over a sink or clean container.

2. Partially open the roller clamp and allow solution to flow slowly through the entire tubing. Invert injection ports and backcheck valve before the solution flows through them.

3. Close the roller clamp.

4. Remove air bubbles from the tubing by holding the tubing vertically while lightly tapping the area with fingers.

5. Loop the tubing over the IV pole or attach it to the roller clamp.

6. Label the container and the tubing as required by agency policy.

RATIONALE

To catch solution. Most protective coverings over the needle adapter permit the flow of solution.

Forces air out of the tubing, fills ports and backcheck valves with solution, and prevents air bubbles. A large collection of air can act as an embolus in the patient's bloodstream.

Bubbles will rise into the drip chamber.

Prevents contamination of tubing.

Labelling the tubing with date and time permits regular replacement according to agency policy.

They are flattened and taped to the skin once the needle is inside the vein. The butterfly needle may be chosen for intravenous therapy lasting less than 24 hours and for therapy of any duration in infants, children, older patients or patients with fragile veins. The current design of small, over-the-needle catheters, however, has resulted in a decrease in the use of butterfly needles. As well, butterfly needles can easily dislodge, causing fluid infiltration into tissues.

Catheters and needles vary in length and in the size or diameter of the lumen (the gauge). Lengths vary from 1.5 to 3 cm whereas lumen sizes range from 16 to 27 gauge. The gauge number relates inversely to the size of the lumen, so that the smaller the number, the larger the diameter of the lumen. It is generally recommended that the shortest length and the smallest gauge of a device possible should be used for infusion. Smaller devices cause less trauma to veins and more blood flow around their tips which results in less risk of clotting. Short needle lengths and large lumens permit more rapid infusion of solution.

Choosing the infusion site The selection of an infusion site is based on a consideration of the duration and type of solution to be infused and on the patient's age, hand dominance, preference, comfort and need for mobility. It is also important to consider the condition, size and location of the vein. In adults, the superficial veins of the arm or hand can be used for most IV fluids. However, the most common sites are the basilic or cephalic veins in the arm and the metacarpal or dorsal networks in the hand (see Figure 22.12). The most distal veins in the forearm or hand should be used first. This keeps the more proximal sites in good condition for future use. If a vein has been traumatized, sites below the trauma cannot be used until the vein has had a chance to heal.

Sites on the dominant arm or over joints, such as the wrist or elbow, should be avoided because infusions into these areas interfere with the patient's mobility and comfort and can result in phlebitis. In addition, frequent flexion of the joint can alter the rate of flow or cause the device to become dislodged. The insertion of venipuncture devices into the feet should be avoided because circulation to these extremities may be compromised, especially in older patients. The risk of thrombophlebitis is higher with infusions into feet. Also, a limb that suffers circulatory or neurological impairment (for example, the affected arm of a patient with a mastectomy or an arm with an arteriovenous shunt) should not be used for venipuncture. Additionally, an extremity that is edematous, reddened, infected or contused should be avoided. The smallest vein to accommodate the needle or catheter needed for the infusion should be selected. Ideally, the vein should be straight, smooth, firm, resilient and large enough to permit sufficient circulation around the needle or catheter.

Protection for the nurse The safe handling of IV equipment is mandatory in order to prevent injury to self and others in the workplace. Body substance precautions

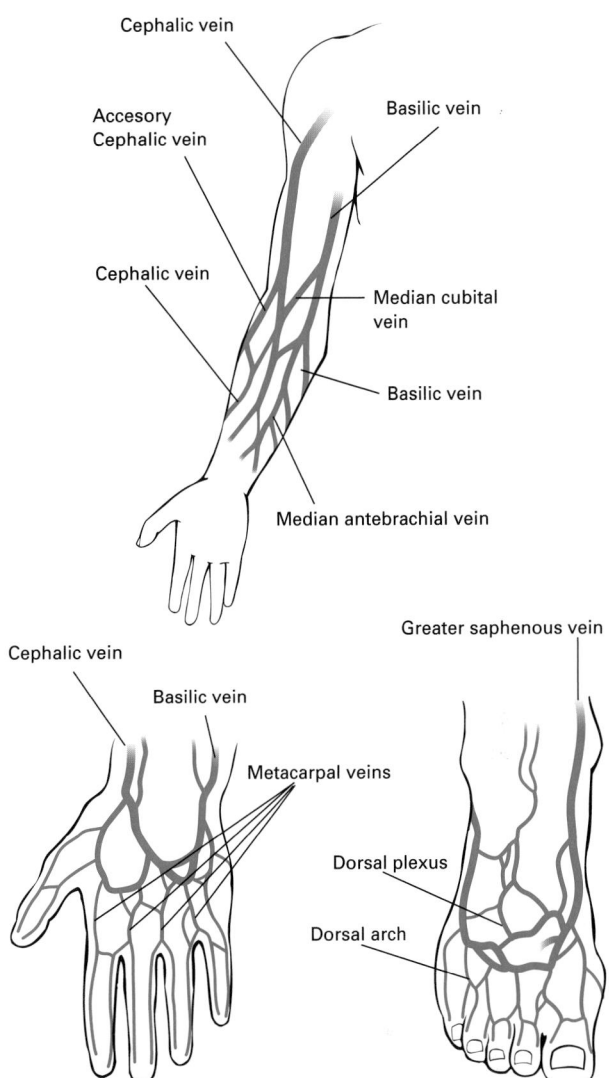

FIGURE 22.12 Peripheral venipuncture sites

for blood and body fluids must be used when performing the venipuncture or at any time during intravenous therapy that contact with patients' blood is likely. Body substance precautions warn that blood and body fluids from *all* patients be treated as potentially infected with Hepatitis or HIV, both of which are blood borne pathogens. Gloves must be worn whenever working with IV infusions and IV equipment. After each use, gloves must be discarded into appropriate waste containers, and the hands washed thoroughly. If the possibility of blood splashing is anticipated, additional protection must be worn, such as a gown, a mask or eye goggles or coverings. Special attention must be paid to the handling of needles and catheters. Do not bend, break, recap, separate from syringe or in any way manipulate needles or catheters by hand. Place these devices into puncture-resistant containers called sharps containers promptly after use.

PROCEDURE 22.2

Establishing the Infusion (Peripheral Venipuncture)

ACTION	RATIONALE
1. Gather equipment: • Venipuncture device • Tourniquet • Alcohol or antiseptic swab • Gauze sponges, transparent semipermeable dressing, non-allergenic tape • Sharps container, protective underpad, disposable gloves • Primed IV solution on IV pole	Facilitates efficiency and economy of time.
2. Identify the patient.	Avoids error.
3. Prepare the patient for what to expect during each stage of the procedure.	Knowing what to expect reduces anxiety and tension which enhances the patient's comfort and makes it easier to insert the venipuncture device.
4. Wash hands thoroughly and maintain sterile technique.	Prevents introducing contaminants during preparation.
5. Ready all equipment. Open packages maintaining aseptic technique. Cut tape and store it on the inside cover or a sterile package.	Facilitates efficiency. Starting an IV infusion is a sterile procedure. Sticking cut tape on hospital surfaces results in the transfer of microorganisms.
6. Place the extremity in a dependent position (below level of heart), apply a tourniquet 15 to 20 cm above the possible site, ask the patient to clench and unclench the fist, lightly pat the area with fingertips. Warm packs can also be applied. Check for a distal pulse. If one is not present, reapply the tourniquet less tightly. Do not use a tourniquet if the veins are fragile or rolling.	These measures distend the vein making it easier to visualize the vein and insert the needle or catheter. The tourniquet should be applied tightly enough to dilate the vein but it should not occlude the artery. A palpable radial pulse indicates adequate arterial blood flow. Fragile veins can rupture or "blow" when distended.

ACTION	RATIONALE
7. Select a veinpuncture site by inspecting and palpating the veins. Choose a vein that is visible, feels firm, and has a straight section. Avoid areas of flexion. If necessary, shave excessive hair over venipuncture area as per agency policy and with permission from the patient.	Makes insertion easier. Prevents the risk of phlebitis. Makes tape removal more comfortable and decreases risk of bacterial contamination.

ACTION

RATIONALE

8. Place a protective pad under the site. Put on gloves and cleanse the site with an antiseptic swab using a firm circular motion working from the centre of the site outwards. Let dry.

Protects bed linen if bleeding occurs. Reduces skin bacteria which would be introduced into the patient's vascular system during the venipuncture.

9. Using the nondominant hand, hold the extremity so that the thumb is placed below and slightly lateral to the site and the forefinger placed above and lateral to the site. Hold the skin taut by gently pulling downward with the thumb while pushing upward with the forefinger.

Stabilizes the skin and anchors the vein.

10. Insert the needle or the catheter.

   a. Grasp the catheter by the hub, leaving the flashback chamber visible.

   Enables the nurse to see the blood return.

   b. Holding bevel side up and pointing in the direction of blood flow, pierce the skin at a 30° angle.

   Decreases injury to the skin and is more comfortable for the patent.

   c. Decrease the angle of the device so that it is almost flush with the skin, then pierce the vein. Watch for a backflow of blood into the needle tubing or the catheter. A sensation of released resistance can sometimes be felt when the device enters the vein.

   Reducing the angle of entry decreases the chance of puncturing both walls of the vein. The backflow of blood confirms placement of the device in the vein.

Continued on the next page

ACTION

RATIONALE

d. Advance the catheter up to the hub or until resistance is felt, then release the tourniquet.

e. Remove the stylet (needle) from inside the catheter and discard into a sharps container. Attach the administration set to the catheter and open the roller clamp to start the flow of solution.

A

B

C

D

E

F

ACTION	RATIONALE
f. **Do Not** reinsert the stylet into the catheter at any time.	The needle may cut the catheter and cause embolus.
g. If using a needle, advance it into the vein up to the hub. While holding the needle in place with one hand, release the tourniquet with the other, attach the administration set, and open the roller clamp to start the flow of solution.	Ensures the device is curently in the vein. The flow of solution is necessary to prevent blood from clotting in the needle.
11. Tape the needle or catheter in place and dress the site using adhesive tape, transparent tape, antiseptic creams and gauze dressing as per agency policy. Secure the device so that the insertion site and the hub–tubing connection is free of tape. See Figure 22.13.	The device must be stabilized to prevent dislodgement. Antiseptic ointment and dresings prevent infection by keeping bacteria from the site. Facilitates inspection of the site and tubing changes later on.
12. Loop the IV tubing on the patient's limb near the venipuncture site and secure with tape.	Prevents the weight of the tubing from pulling on the needle or catheter thereby dislodging it.

ACTION	RATIONALE
13. Regulate the flow rate as ordered.	Maintain accurate infusion.
14. Remove gloves, wash hands.	
15. Apply an armboard if necessary.	Stabilizes the needle or catheter situated near a joint.
16. Document the procedure noting the time, site, size and type of device, the type of solution and rate of infusion, any problems with the procedure and nursing actions as per agency protocol.	Fulfills legal requirements for nurse accountability.

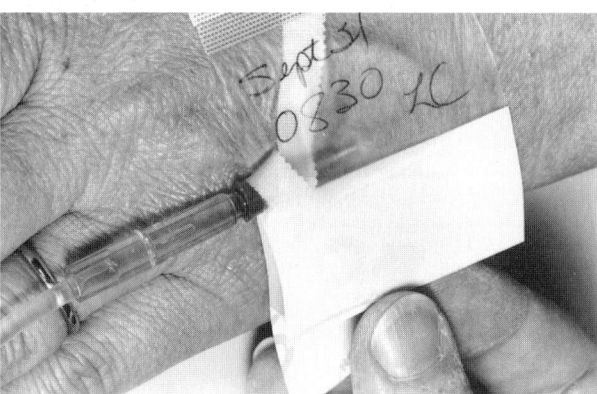

FIGURE 22.13   Securing an infusion needle or catheter with tape and transparent dressing. A. Tape the catheter securely using Chevron technique (or as per hospital procedure), pinching tightly to secure the catheter. B. DO NOT apply tape over the sterile entry point. C. Apply a sterile transparent dressing or a sterile bandaid. Document with date, time, catheter size and your initial.

SOURCE: Chase, L. (1993). Venipuncture for initiating peripheral intravenous therapy. *Parenteral Therapy Manual.* Vancouver, BC: Vancouver General Hospital. Reproduced with permission.

Maintaining the Peripheral Infusion

Intravenous therapy carries the risk of many complications. Some of these, such as infiltration and phlebitis, are local-ized and cause discomfort for the patient. Others, such as fluid overload or sepsis, are systemic and can lead to life-threatening problems. The risk of complications can be reduced through careful assessment and meticulous care. An intravenous infusion must be regulated, assessed and maintained on a regular basis to ensure a constant rate of flow, to identify and correct problems and to reduce the risk of complications. Table 22.12 outlines common complications of intravenous therapy.

Regulating and Monitoring the Infusion Rate of Flow

The intravenous flow rate is routinely expressed as the total volume of solution to be infused over a specified period of time or as the amount in millilitres per hour (ml/hr). For example, the physician's order may be written as *D5W 1 litre every 8 hours* or *D5W 100 ml/hr*. The nurse must ensure that the infusion flows at the specified rate. A rate of flow that is too slow can deprive the patient of needed fluids, electrolytes and nutrients. Conversely, an infusion that is too rapid can cause complications such as circulatory overload. Various devices are used to regulate the rate of infusion. The roller clamp on the IV administration set which is adjusted manually is the most basic device used. There are also controllers, flow regulators and infusion pumps that are set to adjust the rate of flow electronically.

When the infusion is regulated with a *roller clamp* on the IV administration set, the flow rate is measured in drops per minute. In order to calculate the *rate of flow*, also referred to as *the drip rate*, the nurse has to know the amount of solution to be infused, the duration of infusion, and the drop factor (the number of drops per millilitre of solution). The most common method of calculating the rate of flow determines first, the number of millilitres per hour (ml/hr) and second, the drops per minute (gtt/min).

Step 1. $\dfrac{\text{Total volume of solution}}{\text{Number of hours}} = \text{millilitres/hour}$

Step 2. $\dfrac{\text{Number of ml/hr} \times \text{drop factor}}{\text{Time in minutes}} = \text{drops/minute}$

Suppose, for example, 1000 ml of solution are to be infused over 8 hours. With a drop factor of 10, the drip rate would be calculated as follows:

Step 1. $1000 \div 8 = 125 \text{ ml/hr}$
Step 2. $125 \times 10 \div 60 = 20.8 \text{ or } 21 \text{ drops/min}$

Once the drip rate is determined, the infusion is regulated by adjusting the roller clamp on the administration set and counting drops until the desired rate of flow is achieved. Holding a watch next to the drip chamber expedites the counting of drops. It is recommended that the drops be counted for one minute to account for irregularities in flow (Krozek, 1992).

FIGURE 22.14   Time tapes

A *time tape* placed on the solution container is commonly used as a quick guide for monitoring the rate of flow and checking that the correct amount of solution has infused over an hourly period. Commercially prepared time tapes are available; however, a piece of tape placed vertically on the container adjacent to the millimetre calibrations is a common alternative. Based on the calculated flow rate, the time tape is marked at intervals showing the expected volume to be infused per hour (see Figure 22.14). The flow rate is monitored by comparing the level of solution in the container to the expected fluid level on the time tape. Necessary adjustments are made to the flow rate using the roller clamp and validated by counting drops per minute.

One of the biggest challenges in managing intravenous therapy is maintaining a consistent rate of infusion. Several factors alter the flow of solution into the vein causing the rate to speed up or slow down over time. These include:

1. *The distance of the solution container from the venipuncture site.* The higher the container, the greater the force of gravity overcoming venous pressure, therefore, the more rapidly the solution flows into the vein.

2. *The position of the extremity.* The flow rate may increase or decrease when the limb is moved, flexed, or held above (increases) or below (decreases) the level of the heart.

3. *The patency of the venipuncture site and the tubing.* Taping of the IV site too tightly may restrict flow. An infusion can also slow down if the tubing becomes kinked, crimped, looped, compressed, or if it is allowed to dangle below the insertion site.

4. *The viscosity of the solution.* Thicker fluid such as blood forms fewer and smaller drops than less viscous solutions, therefore flows more slowly.

5. *The condition of the vein.* Hard, sclerosed veins impede the flow of solution.

6. *The size of the vein and the venipuncture device.* The smaller the vein and the size of the device, the slower the infusion of solution. Conversely, solution flows more rapidly into large veins when large gauge venipuncture devices are in place.

Infusions must be monitored frequently in order to ensure consistent flow rates. How often this is done varies according to agency policy, the patient's age and condition, the type of solution and how well it is infusing. Generally, the drip rate is checked and readjusted as necessary at least every hour. Some nurses do this every time they are in the patient's room. If the infusion has been too slow, an increase in the drip rate may be necessary to "catch up," that is, reestablish the infusion at the specified rate. When this happens, the drip rate should not be increased more than 30 percent without consulting the physician first (Krozek, 1992).

Intravenous infusions are also regulated with electric or battery-operated infusion control devices, namely pumps and controllers. These devices maintain flow rates more accurately than the standard gravity flow and clamp systems. Although infusion pumps and controllers work on different principles, both devices can be used to administer a wide range of fluids, electrolytes, medications and nutrients. They are necessary for all central venous infusions and for administering total parenteral nutrition (see Chapter 19). Infusion pumps and controllers are used for peripheral infusions when a precise rate of flow is necessary, as, for example, in an older patient at risk for developing circulatory overload.

An *infusion pump* (Figure 22.15) maintains a preset flow rate by applying variable positive pressure on the fluid or the administration set. Solutions are propelled into the vein at a constant rate by a slight change in the pressure

FIGURE 22.15   Infusion Control Devices A. Infusion controller with photoelectric sensor on the drip chamber. B. Infusion pump

exerted on the fluid. For example, if flow is restricted because the patient flexes an arm and increases pressure in the vein, the pump responds by increasing pressure on the administration set to overcome the resistance and thereby maintain a constant rate of flow. An *infusion controller* is a device that regulates the rate of flow by using a photoelectric sensor attached to the drip chamber. The sensor recognizes whether the solution is flowing into the drip chamber at the preset flow rate and keeps this rate constant by speeding up or slowing down the drops of fluid. The controller depends on the force of gravity to propel solution into the vein; therefore, height is an important factor in its effectiveness. To work correctly a controller must be located at least 76 cm above the insertion site.

Infusion devices ensure safe, accurate infusion of fluids. They also save time because nurses do not have to constantly check and readjust flow rates. Most devices are equipped with alarms that sound if the flow rate is not being maintained or if there are infusion difficulties, such as occlusions or air in the tubing. However, these devices do not always detect inflammation at the venipuncture site or dislodgement of the device, nor do they detect patients' responses to IV therapy. Therefore, it is important to complete the regular assessments required for intravenous infusions. Checks of the pump or controller should also be routinely made to ensure that it is programmed correctly and that it is working properly. A time tape on the solution container is recommended as a gauge for accuracy.

Assessing the Infusion

Systematic assessment is made of the venipuncture site, the administration set, the accuracy of therapy and the patient's response to therapy. First, the *venipuncture site* is thoroughly inspected for tenderness, redness, swelling or coolness at or just above the site of insertion. These findings indicate that the needle or catheter may have slipped out of the vein allowing fluid to flow into the surrounding tissues (infiltration) or that the vein has been irritated by the venipuncture device or solution (phlebitis). When signs of infiltration or phlebitis occur, the infusion should be discontinued and restarted on the other limb. A warm compress may be applied to the site for patient comfort.

The site is also assessed for leakage or bleeding which can be caused by a loose connection between the venipuncture device and the tubing, faulty equipment or movement of an improperly secured needle or catheter. A loose connection between the venipuncture device and the tubing is corrected by simply tightening the connection. Faulty equipment must be replaced promptly. When leakage or bleeding occurs from the site because the needle or catheter was not securely taped in place, the site must be cleansed with an antimicrobial agent and retaped. The area should be carefully inspected for signs of irritation and infection caused by the movement of the device in the vein and skin. An armboard

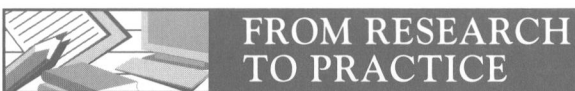

FROM RESEARCH TO PRACTICE

Pelletier, D. S. (1992). Patients' experience of technology at the bedside: Intravenous infusion control devices. *Journal of Advanced Nursing, 17,* 1274–1282.

This exploratory study was undertaken to determine patients' perceptions of their experience with infusion control devices (ICD) used in intravenous therapy. Insights into patients' experiences with clinical equipment at the bedside will allow nurses to incorporate such devices into their care more optimally. The objectives of the study were to explore patients' understanding of the ICD; their fears, concerns and degree of comfort with the ICD; their perception of the focus of nursing attention; the relationship of the ICD to their feelings of safety and level of illness; and their feelings in response to alarms and other mechanical noises. A 22-item questionnaire of single-response multiple-option closed questions was developed for the study. A sample of 150 patients on general medical surgical wards were surveyed over a nine-month period. All participants were over 18 years of age, had over 12 hours experience with the device and were willing to participate. Generally, the study found a positive patient response to the use of the ICD and its management. The majority of participants understood the reasons for the use of the ICD and were not greatly disturbed by the alarms and mechanical noises. Nearly 25 percent of the sample indicated they had not received an explanation for the ICD or its purpose even though explanations were given to all. A majority of respondents were willing to use the device again and most perceived the patient to be the focus of nursing attention, not the device. These insights into patients' experiences with clinical technology provide valuable knowledge which nurses can use to enhance patient care.

may be applied to further stabilize the insertion site. The site is also checked to ensure that it is free from pressure. Lying on the venipuncture site or keeping the limb tightly flexed increases the blood pressure in the extremity and can cause the infusion to slow or stop completely.

Next, the *venipuncture device* is assessed to ensure that it is patent and securely positioned in the vein. There are several ways of doing this. The most common way is to lower the solution container below the insertion site and pinch the tubing several centimetres away from the venipuncture device. When the tubing is released blood should be pulled into the tubing by the force of gravity. Another way of establishing patency of the needle or catheter is to apply a tourniquet above the insertion site tight enough to restrict venous flow and open the roller clamp. If the device is correctly positioned in the vein, the flow of solution should stop.

Patency of the device can also be assessed by inserting a syringe into the port nearest to the insertion site, and while pinching the tubing, slowly withdrawing some fluid from the tubing and the device. Blood will return if the device is properly situated and in a large enough vein. Lastly, the patency of the venipuncture device can be determined by gently palpating the vein two to three cm beyond the end of the device. Palpation will cause a mechanical compression of the vein. If the device is patent, blood flow will slow or stop.

The *administration set*, namely the tubing, should be assessed for patency. Checks are made to ensure the tubing is filled with solution and free from air bubbles, particulate matter, kinks, obstructions and disconnections. Excess tubing should be looped and placed on the bed next to the patient. Inspections are also made to determine that the roller clamp is open, the drip chamber is half-full of solution, the spike is securely inserted into the container and the container holds enough fluid for the next hour.

It is also important to assess the *accuracy of intravenous therapy*. At the beginning of each shift, the nurse should check the physician's order for IV therapy and then examine the existing administration set, flow rate, type of solution, amount of solution to be absorbed and the height of the container. If an electronic infusion device is being used, the flow rate and machine should be checked for proper functioning. Labels on the tubing and the solution containers should be examined for expiry dates. Necessary changes must be made promptly in order to prevent infection.

The *patient's response to intravenous therapy* is often manifested through his or her vital signs. An elevated temperature, pulse, respirations or blood pressure may indicate a complication such as infection, pulmonary edema or circulatory overload. Another response is demonstrated by the patient's fluid balance. If IV therapy is effective, urinary output should be proportionate to fluid intake, assuming there are no renal problems. When patients are receiving electrolyte solutions, blood work results should be monitored for excessive levels and the patient examined for untoward effects. For example, when potassium solutions are being infused, laboratory results should be monitored for increased potassium levels and the patient observed for signs of hyperkalemia. High levels of potassium can cause cardiac arrhythmias or, in some instances, even cardiac arrest. Finally, the nurse should examine the patient's emotional response to therapy. Does he or she have any questions or concerns about the therapy?

Care of the Infusion Site and System

Routine maintenance of a peripheral infusion site and system includes changing solution containers and administration sets, rotating the infusion sites and in some agencies changing the IV site dressings. Agencies differ in how frequently administration sets are replaced or IV sites rotated and in the type of dressings and antibacterial preparations that are used. Therefore, agency policies should be followed for all routine maintenance procedures.

Solution containers are ordinarily changed when they become empty, when the physician writes a new order, or if they have been hanging for 24 hours. Bags and bottles should be changed once every 24 hours because the sterility of the solution cannot be guaranteed for more than one day. In addition, solution containers must be replaced immediately if signs of contamination, such as discolouration, leaks or foreign particles become evident. Administration sets are generally replaced every 48 to 72 hours as a precaution against bacterial growth. These are most simply and efficiently changed when new containers of solution are put up. Sometimes, however, the administration set may have to be changed before the solution container is empty, for example, if there are leaks, incompatibilities or occlusions in the line, when the tubing becomes contaminated, or if a different calibration of tubing (drop factor) is required to facilitate regulation of flow rate.

Venipuncture sites are redressed when administration sets are replaced or whenever they become damp, soiled or loosened. Changing an opaque gauze dressing allows the

Regular, systematic assessment of the infusion ensures safe, accurate intravenous therapy.

nurse to inspect the infusion site and helps to prevent infection. Transparent semipermeable dressings allow easy assessment of the site; therefore, they are not changed routinely. These dressings are waterproof and impervious to microorganisms, so that the chances of infection from airborne bacteria are decreased. Venipuncture sites should be rotated every 48 to 72 hours as a precaution against infection and phlebitis. However, this may not be realistic in some cases. For example, frequent changes of venipuncture devices in people who are receiving long-term therapy or in those with poor veins would soon leave few accessible veins.

Therefore, in circumstances such as these, the sites are carefully assessed by the nurse and changed only when necessary. When an infusion site is changed, a vein that is proximal to the old site or in the opposite limb should be used in order to promote patient comfort and prevent complications. When rotating an infusion site, the nurse follows the procedure for establishing a peripheral venipuncture (Procedure 22.2). Procedures for maintaining the infusion system — that is changing the solution container, replacing the tubing and redressing the infusion site — are outlined in Procedure 22.3 below.

PROCEDURE 22.3

Maintaining the Infusion System

ACTION	RATIONALE
A. GENERAL ACTIONS	
1. Gather equipment as outlined in each section below.	Ensures efficiency and economy of time.
2. Wash hands thoroughly and maintain sterile technique.	Reduces the risk of contamination during the procedure.
3. Explain the procedure to the patient.	Allays anxiety and enhances emotional well-being.
4. Assess the site and IV system.	Ensures the system is working properly and enables early detection and intervention for complications.
B. CHANGING THE SOLUTION CONTAINER	
1. Collect the prescribed solution, check the container as outlined in Procedure 22.1, apply a time tape, and obtain an alcohol swab.	Ensures accurate delivery and reduces the risk of error.
2. At the bedside, hang a bag on the IV pole; place a bottle on the overbed table.	Readies the equipment for the change-over.
3. Close the roller clamp on the administration set or turn off the infusion control device.	Keeps fluid in the drip chamber and prevents air from entering the tubing.
4. **Bag:** Remove the protective cap from the administration port. **Bottle:** Remove the cap and seal.	Maintains sterility of the port or stopper.
5. Remove the old container from the IV pole, invert it and remove the spike. Insert the spike into the new container as in Procedure 22.1. Hang container on IV pole.	Prevents the escape of left-over fluid from the container.
6. Open the roller clamp and adjust the rate of flow, or restart the infusion control device.	Maintains the patency of the system and the desired rate of flow.
7. Discard used equipment.	Maintains cleanliness and safety in workplace.

ACTION

C. CHANGING THE SOLUTION CONTAINER AND THE ADMINISTRATION SET

1. Gather equipment:
   - Administration set
   - Correct IV solution
   - Time tape, label for tubing
   - Sterile gauze sponges, adhesive tape
   - Two pair of clean gloves
   - Optional: hemostat

2. Prepare the solution container and prime and label the tubing as per Procedure 22.1.

3. At the bedside hang the new solution container and primed set on the IV pole and lay the needle adapter end of the tubing near the infusion site. Loosen protective cap on new tubing.

4. Put on gloves.

5. Remove tape and dressing from the infusion site to expose the connection, taking care not to displace the needle or catheter. Remove tape anchoring tubing to limb.

6. Place a sterile gauze under the needle or catheter.

7. Close off the roller clamp of the old tubing.

8. Hold the hub of the needle or catheter with the nondominant hand and gently disconnect the old tubing using a twisting, pulling motion.

Option: a hemostat may be used to stabilize the device; however, the hemostat must not be clamped shut on the device as doing so will crack the hub.

RATIONALE

Promotes efficiency and economy of time.

Readies the equipment for the change-over.

Maintains body substance precautions.

Promotes access to the venipuncture device.

Provides a sterile working area and absorbs leakage when the tubing is disconnected.

Avoids undue leakage of solution.

Ensures the device is kept securely in the vein.

Continued on the next page

ACTION	RATIONALE
9. Quickly remove the cap from the new tubing and insert the adapter into the device.	Facilitates exchange with minimal blood loss and minimal risk of infection.
10. Open the roller clamp.	Prevents clotting of the device.
11. Clean the site of any leakage, working from the site outward.	Maintains sterility of the site.
12. If gloves are soiled, remove them and apply new ones.	Prevents contamination of the site.
13. Apply antibacterial ointment according to agency policy and redress the site as necessary. Loop and tape the new tubing securely onto the patient's limb.	Prevents airborne bacteria from entering the site. Prevents strain on the venipuncture device .
14. Regulate the IV flow rate as prescribed. Label the tubing with date and time.	Maintains accurate infusion. Promotes continuity of care.
15. Discard the used administration set and equipment. Remove gloves and wash hands.	Maintains cleanliness and safety in the workplace.

D. REPLACING THE ADMINISTRATION SET ONLY

1. Gather equipment:
   - Administration set
   - Label for tubing, sterile gauze sponges, antiseptic swab, adhesive tape
   - Two pair of clean gloves
   - Hemostat

2. Reduce the infusion rate of flow.

Ensures patency of the venipuncture device and prevents air from entering the tubing.

3. Clamp off the port of a bag with a hemostat. Remove a bottle from the IV pole and invert it.

Prevents fluid spilling from the container.

4. Remove the spike from the container and keep it upright above the level of the patient's heart. Remove the protective cap from the new spike and place it over the old spike. Tape the old spike to the IV pole or place it on a pillow, next to the patient.

Maintains the infusion during the change-over.

5. Insert the new spike into the solution container and prime the tubing as in Procedure 22.1.

6. Put on gloves and continue as in section C, numbers 4 to 15.

E. CHANGING THE SITE DRESSING

1. Gather equipment:
   - Sterile gauze sponges or transparent semipermeable dressing, adhesive tape

ACTION	RATIONALE
• Povidone-iodine or antiseptic solution, alcohol swabs, povidone-iodine ointment or antibacterial ointment as per agency policy	
• Clean gloves	
2. Put on gloves.	Maintains body substance precautions.
3. Stabilize the venipuncture device with the non-dominant hand. Gently remove the old tape and dressing.	Prevents displacement of the device.
4. Clean the insertion site with povidone-iodine or alcohol, using a circular motion and working from the site outward.	Avoids contaminating the site. An antiseptic solution decreases the risk of infection by reducing the number of microorganisms.
5. Allow the area to dry. Apply antiseptic ointment as per protocol.	Drying area maximizes effect of antiseptic solution. Ointment protects against infection.
6. Retape the device and cover with sterile gauze or transparent semipermeable dressing.	Prevents displacement of the device. Decreases contamination of the site.
7. Remove gloves and wash hands.	Prevents spread of microorganisms.
8. Label the dressing with date.	Promotes continuity of care.
F. DOCUMENTATION.	
Document the procedure in the Nurses' Notes or Fluid Balance Record as per agency protocol. **Changing solution container:** Note the type and amount of solution infused; the time, type, and amount of solution added; the flow rate; and the assessment findings. **Changing administration set:** Note the date and time of replacement. **Changing IV site dressing:** Note the date and time the site was redressed. Indicate the cleansing solution and antiseptic ointment used, the type of dressing applied, assessment findings, and the patient's response to the procedure.	Maintains a record of intake and fulfills requirements for nurse accountability.

Discontinuing the Peripheral Intravenous Infusion

Intravenous therapy is discontinued when ordered by the physician or when complications such as infiltration or phlebitis develop. An infusion is also discontinued and restarted in another area for routine site rotation. Procedure 22.4 details the nursing actions for discontinuing an infusion.

Preparing the Patient

Before gathering the equipment, the nurse should inform the patient of the procedure. Even though this is a procedure patients look forward to, they often want to know if it will hurt. Discontinuing an infusion is usually a painless procedure. The dressing and tape are removed from the site, the device is withdrawn slowly and pressure is applied to the site for a few minutes. Pressure is necessary to stop bleeding. A bandaid is placed over the site. It should be kept in place for at least eight hours. Normal activities can be resumed immediately.

Discontinuing the Peripheral Infusion

ACTION	RATIONALE
1. Gather equipment: sterile gauze, bandaid, gloves.	Ensures efficiency and economy of time.
2. Wash hands thoroughly and maintain sterile technique.	Reduces the risk of contamination during the procedure.
3. Close the roller clamp.	Prevents escape of fluid.
4. Loosen the tape and dressing by pulling towards the site while applying countertraction to the skin with the nondominant hand.	Countertraction helps to prevent pulling of the skin thereby lessening patient discomfort.
5. Put on gloves.	Maintains body substance precautions.
6. Place gauze over the site and apply gentle pressure with the nondominant hand. Withdraw the device in line with the vein, using a steady pulling motion.	Prevents trauma to the vein and breaking/binding of the device.
7. Apply direct, firm pressure over the site for one or two minutes or until bleeding stops. If the patient is on heparin or an anticoagulant, maintain pressure for a longer period and elevate the limb slightly.	Prevents bleeding and hematoma formation.
8. When bleeding has stopped apply a bandaid. Leave the bandaid in place for at least eight hours.	Prevents microorganisms from entering the site and slight pressure prevents further oozing.
9. Discard used equipment appropriately. Remove gloves and wash hands.	Ensures cleanliness and safety in the workplace.
10. Document the procedure in the Nurses' Notes or on the Fluid Balance Record as per agency policy. Note date and time; reason for discontinuing infusion; condition and intactness of the device; condition of the infusion site; patient's response; any complications and nursing interventions; and the amount and type of infusion infused.	Fulfills requirements for nurse accountability.

Special Considerations for Peripheral Intravenous Therapy

Intravenous equipment taken to the bedside too early may cause undue anxiety for some patients. Therefore, equipment should be assembled in the utility room and brought to the patient's unit for immediate use. When patients are confused, the roller clamp should be positioned high enough on the tubing so that they cannot reach up and adjust the flow rate. Additionally, restraints may be necessary with confused or aggressive patients to prevent them from pulling out the infusion device.

Some patients may not accept intravenous infusions due to religious beliefs. Jehovah's Witnesses, for instance, will accept blood substitutes but not whole blood. Christian Scientists avoid use of medications or infusions. Patients who choose to refuse intravenous infusions are required to sign a "refusal of treatment" form which is attached to their record.

The inspection of a site for redness or streaking may be difficult to do for dark-skinned patients. In such cases, other techniques, such as palpation of the area for tenderness and warmth, can be used.

Older and very young patients are more susceptible to circulatory overload; therefore, infusion rates must be monitored very carefully. Use of microdrop administration sets or pumps/controllers is recommended for these patients.

Troubleshooting Peripheral Intravenous Infusion Problems

Begin assessment at the infusion site and work upward to the solution container.
Look for obvious problems and then correct them.

ASSESSMENT

INTERVENTION

1. **IV site**

   Check for possible complications:

   • infiltration

   • phlebitis

   • thrombophlebitis

   • infection

   See Table 22.12 for signs and symptoms and interventions.

2. **IV device**

   Check for:

   • placement in the vein. Is the device in line with the vein or is it pressed against the vein wall, restricting flow?

   If pressed against the vein wall, gently pull back on the device. Gently rotate an over-the needle catheter. Never rotate a butterfly, as it will puncture the vein wall. Slightly raise or lower the angle of the device in the vein by adjusting the gauze pad under the hub.

   • restriction by tape or pressure from the patient's limb.

   If restricted, retape the device or reposition the limb. Apply an armboard if necessary.

   • positional flow (rate is affected by joint movement).

   Apply a splint or armboard. Instruct the patient to keep the limb below the level of the heart and avoid direct pressure on the site.

   • patency.

   Follow the techniques outlined under "Assessing the infusion." If the device is patent but the flow is sluggish, pinch and release the tubing near the site several times. This increases the pressure within the tubing, which may clear the device. Do not compress the flashball. Doing so creates pressure which may rupture the vein. Never irrigate a device. Doing so may dislodge a clot into the bloodstream, resulting in an embolism. If the device is obstructed, remove it and relocate the infusion.

3. **Tubing**

   Check for:

   • kinks, crimps, or pressure (other equipment or patient lying on tubing).

   Straighten the tubing or reposition the patient or other equipment.

   • sections dangling below the level of the infusion site (prevents gravity from propelling fluid into the patient).

   Coil excessive tubing and reposition it on the bed.

ASSESSMENT	INTERVENTION
3. Tubing *(continued)*	
• patency and large air bubbles.	If there are large air spaces or if there is precipitate, replace the tubing. For air bubbles high in the tubing, turn off the flow and while stretching the tubing downward, tap or flick the tubing with a finger. The air will rise into the drip chamber. Regulate the flow rate. For air low in the tubing, slow the rate of flow. Insert a sterile needle into the port nearest to the IV site. Hold the hub of the needle above the port. When the air reaches the port it will rise and flow out through the needle because air is lighter than fluid. Regulate the flow rate.
4. Clamps	
Check that all clamps are open.	Open the roller clamp completely, change it to a new position, regulate the flow rate.
5. Air vent	
Check that the air vent is: • present • patent	Glass containers require air vents. If absent, replace the administration set with one containing an air vent or insert a vent into the rubber stopper. If obstructed, replace administration set or vent.
6. Filter	
Check that the filter is: • present • patent	Filters are required for solutions with some additives and when administering blood. If obstructed, replace the filter. A blocked filter will interrupt flow.
7. Drip chamber	
Check fluid level (should be able to count drops).	If the drip chamber is full, pinch off the tubing, invert the container and squeeze the drip chamber. The fluid squeezed into the container will be replaced by air from the container. Rehang the container and release the tubing. Regulate flow.
8. Spike	
Check placement in port of container.	If the spike is not placed securely into the port, push it further upward with a twisting motion.
9. Solution container	
Check: • level of fluid • temperature of solution	If fluid level is low (50–100 ml), replace the container. If the solution is cold, which happens when blood is administered, the vein may go into spasm, thereby decreasing flow. Apply a warm compress to the infusion site. Never warm blood unless ordered by the physician. Adjust the height of the IV pole.
• height of the container (should be one metre above the infusion site).	
10. The system has been systematically assessed, there are no obvious problems, but the infusion has stopped.	Discontinue the infusion and reestablish in another site.

TABLE 22.12 Complications of Peripheral Intravenous Therapy

COMPLICATION	POSSIBLE CAUSES	SIGNS & SYMPTOMS	INTERVENTIONS
Infiltration: The escape of solution into interstitial tissues	Venipuncture device dislodged from vein Perforated vein wall	Blanching of skin at the site Coolness Swelling at or above the site Feeling of fullness or tightness at the site Pain or burning at the site but may also be painless Infusion continues when the vein is occluded	**Restorative:** Reassure patient there is no permanent harm. Discontinue the infusion. Restart the IV in an other site above infiltrated area or preferably in other limb. Apply warm compresses to the site to aid absorption and for comfort. Elevate the limb to encourage venous return. **Protective:** Use an over-the-needle catheter, if possible. Select the most appropriate device. Avoid sites in areas of flexion or excessive movement. Anchor the device securely. Check the infusion frequently. Instruct the patient to report any discomfort or swelling.
Phlebitis: Inflammation of the vein wall	Mechanical trauma during insertion of infusion device or from sliding movement of the device Needle or catheter too large for size of vein Device left in vein too long Infection due to contamination Weakened veins from repeated infusions Chemical irritation from IV solutions, medications, or incompatible additives Infusion rate too rapid	Local tenderness, pain along the vein Redness, warmth, and induration (hardness) along the course of the vein Swelling at or above the site Burning sensation along the vein Slight temperature elevation	**Restorative:** Discontinue the infusion. Apply warm compresses to stimulate circulation and for comfort. Restart the IV in other limb. Report to physician if temperature is elevated. **Protective:** Use the smallest device possible. Use an over-the-needle catheter if possible. Stabilize the device securely to prevent sliding movement. Change the IV site every 48 to 72 hours. Use intermittent rather than prolonged continuous infusions. Use large veins if infusing irritating solutions. Dilute solutions or additives sufficiently. Infuse solutions at the prescribed rate. Use pumps or controllers for irritating solutions.

continued on next page

TABLE 22.12 *continued*

COMPLICATION	POSSIBLE CAUSES	SIGNS & SYMPTOMS	INTERVENTIONS
Thrombophlebitis: A blood clot at the tip of the needle or catheter or along the inner wall of the vein. Can be a potential source of bacterial growth	IV inserted in an area of flexion. Infusion rate too slow. Inflammation leading to damage of the tunica intima (platelets adhere to roughened surface). Incompatible drug additives resulting in obstruction	Tenderness. Redness. Swollen, hardened vein. Slow or stopped infusion	**Restorative**: Discontinue the infusion. Apply warm compresses. Restart the IV in other limb. DO NOT massage or rub of the affected limb. Report to physician. Watch for signs of infection. **Protective**: Maintain the prescribed rate of flow. Use a microdrop set or an infusion pump or controller for slow infusion rates. Check the infusion frequently. Dilute additives. Check drug incompatibilities carefully.
Infection: Invasion of pathogenic organisms into the body. May be local or systemic	Entry of microorganisms during insertion or with breaks in techniques during site care. Movement of device allowing organisms into the vein. Break in aseptic technique. Use of contaminated equipment. Leaking in the system. Opening the system, thus exposing the patient to airborne bacteria. Patient's own bacteria. Device left in vein too long. Weakened immune system	Redness, warmth, and swelling at site. Tenderness. Purulent drainage from site. Possible chills, malaise, elevated temperature	**Restorative**: Assess for all possible causes. If local, discontinue the infusion. Send a sample of the solution and needle or catheter tip for bacterial analysis. Report to physician. Monitor vital signs. Restart the IV in the other limb. **Protective**: Wash hands and use meticulous aseptic technique during all IV procedures. Use sterile equipment. Check equipment for contamination and leaks. Replace contaminated equipment promptly. Change equipment as per agency policy or as recommended by the CDC. Ensure that venipuncture device is securely anchored. Avoid using sites near joints or immobilize the joint with an armboard as necessary.

TABLE 22.12
continued

COMPLICATION	POSSIBLE CAUSES	SIGNS & SYMPTOMS	INTERVENTIONS
Circulatory overload: An increase in circulating fluid volume above normal	Infusion rate overly rapid Excessive volume of infused fluid in patients with impaired cardiac and renal function	Headache Discomfort Flushed skin Engorged neck veins Tachycardia Tachypnea Increased blood pressure Shortness of breath Cough and crackles heard in lung bases on auscultation Cyanosis Chest pain	**Restorative:** Slow the infusion rate and keep the vein open. Place the patient in semi-Fowler's position. Report to physician. Monitor vital signs and intake and output. Administer oxygen as ordered. **Protective:** Maintain prescribed flow rate. Question IV orders which call for excessive amounts of fluids to be infused. Monitor the infusion and patient's response frequently.

CENTRAL VENOUS THERAPY

Increasingly, in modern-day health care, patients are receiving intravenous solutions containing medications (for example, anticancer agents) or nutrients (for example, additives in total parental nutrition) that are irritating to small peripheral veins. These solutions, however, are well tolerated by large veins because the high volume of blood flowing through them permits rapid dilution of the irritating substances. In addition, there are many people for whom peripheral intravenous therapy is no longer possible because their veins are inaccessible due to scarring or sclerosing that resulted from prior repeated infusions of irritating solutions. An effective alternative for these patients is central venous therapy.

In central venous therapy a large-gauge catheter, made of polyurethane, polyvinylchloride (PVC) or silicone rubber, is inserted into a major vein in the body. The vessels most commonly used are the right and left subclavian veins, but the right cephalic vein, the right or left internal jugular veins and the femoral veins in the groin may be used as well. A sterile catheter is inserted into a central vein through an incision made in the skin or through a tunnel made in the subcutaneous tissue. The catheter is threaded through the vein until its tip rests in either the superior vena cava, the inferior vena cava or the right atrium of the heart. A central catheter may also be inserted through a peripheral vein and advanced into the central venous circulation. Referred to as a *peripherally inserted central catheter* (PICC), the catheter is usually inserted into the basilic vein in the antecubital fossa of the arm and threaded into the axillary vein, the subclavian vein or the superior vena cava.

There are several benefits to central venous therapy. As we mentioned above, central venous infusion provides a safe, effective way of administering solutions that must be diluted, such as irritating medications or hypertonic fluids. It allows rapid delivery of large amounts of fluids in emergency situations or in cases where peripheral veins have collapsed due to decreased peripheral circulation. A central venous line also permits monitoring of central venous pressure, which is an indicator of the patient's circulatory functioning, blood volume and pumping efficiency of the heart. By providing a long-term (six months to two years or more) venous access, this route eliminates the frequent venipunctures needed to establish peripheral lines or to withdraw blood samples for diagnostic testing. Patient anxieties and discomforts associated with venipunctures are thereby decreased while peripheral veins are preserved and, in some cases, restored.

Central venous therapy also provides a benefit to patients who require the infusion of two or more solutions at the same time. For example, a patient with cancer may need to receive analgesics, antibiotics and chemotherapy along with parenteral nutrition. A multi-lumen catheter in which two or three lumens function separately permits uninterrupted infusion of parenteral nutrition while medications are being administered and also provides a port for drawing blood. When used intermittently, the lumens are capped and flushed with a heparin solution to keep them patent. Finally, long-term central venous catheters are less likely to become obstructed with blood clots and are less prone to infection than are short-term devices. For these reasons, patients are better able to maintain central venous therapy at home.

The illustrations below show several common pathways for central venous (CV) catheter insertion. Typically, a CV catheter is inserted into the subclavian vein or the internal jugular vein. The catheter may terminate in the superior vena cava or in the right atrium.

Insertion: Subclavian vein
Termination: Superior vena cava

Insertion: Subclavian vein
Termination: Right atrium

Insertion: Internal jugular vein
Termination: Superior vena cava

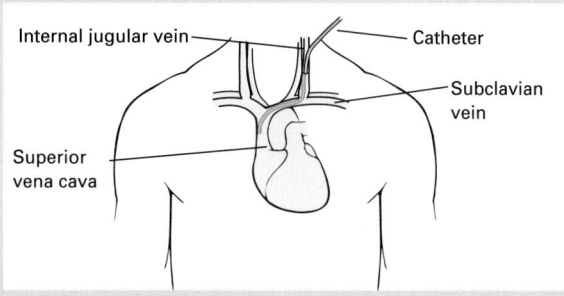

Insertion: Basilic vein (peripheral)
Termination: Superior vena cava

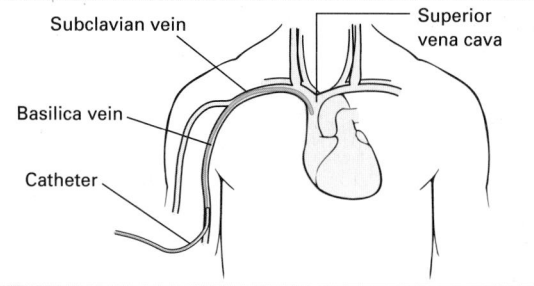

Insertion: Through a subcutaneous tunnel to the subclavian vein (Dacron cuff helps hold catheter in place)
Termination: Superior vena cava

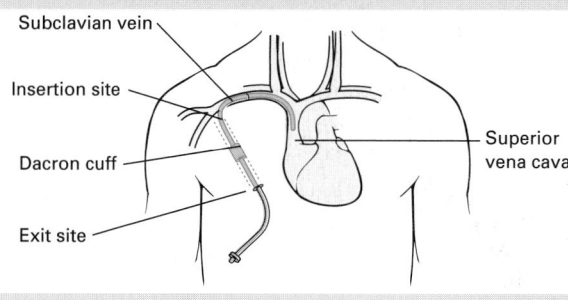

FIGURE 22.16   Central venous catheter pathways

SOURCE: Krozek, C. *Nursing procedures* (1993). Student Version. Springhouse, Pennsylvania: Springhouse Corporation, 1993, 292. Reproduced with permission.

Central venous therapy, however, also has a number of disadvantages. More skill and time is required to insert central venous lines: some of the catheters have to be inserted surgically in an operating room. Because of the location of the catheters, there is an increased risk of life-threatening complications such as pneumothorax, sepsis, thrombus formation and perforation of the vessel and adjacent organs. Central venous lines require specialized, meticulous nursing care to maintain the infusion(s) and prevent complications.

Insertion of a Central Venous Line at the Bedside

Central venous lines are inserted at the bedside using strict aseptic technique. In Canada, nurses do not insert central venous catheters but assist physicians in the procedure.

Preparing the Patient

Ensure that the patient understands the purpose and benefits of central venous therapy, the insertion procedure and possible risks involved. In addition, answer any questions or concerns that he or she might have. Tell patients that, for their safety and well-being, it is important that they lie still during the procedure and stay in the position in which they are placed. When the jugular vein is used, a sterile cloth or drape is placed over the head and the patient may be asked to wear a face mask covering the mouth and nose. Reassure patients that although it may feel dark and warm under the drapes, they will be able to breathe normally. Reassure them, too, that while the procedure may feel uncomfortable because of positioning and draping, it is not painful. A stinging sensation might be felt at the insertion site when the local anesthetic is given and the patient may feel pressure when the catheter is inserted. Any pain should be reported to the doctor immediately.

During insertion of the catheter, the patient will be instructed to perform the Valsalva manoeuvre. The Valsalva manoeuvre prevents air from entering the catheter by raising intrathoracic pressure. It also slows the heart rate, decreases the return of blood to the heart and increases venous pressure. Therefore, you should not teach this procedure to patients who have increased intracranial pressure or patients who are not alert and not able to comply with instruction. To perform the Valsalva manoeuvre, instruct the patient to take a deep breath, hold it, and then bear down for 10 seconds. After this, the patient can exhale and breathe normally.

Once inserted, the catheter will be sutured in place to prevent dislodgement. After the insertion, any feelings of pain or pressure at the site, shortness of breath or lightheadedness should be reported to the nurse. The patient should also call the nurse if the dressing becomes wet or loose, or if the tubing has air in it or becomes disconnected.

Assembling Equipment

Many agencies have specially prepared carts which hold the supplies and equipment for central venous catheter insertions. A typical cart would include:

1. reusable CV catheter insertion bundles or sets containing a sterile gown for the physician, drapes, containers for solutions, forceps and kelly clamps, a needle driver and gauze sponges
2. disposable CV catheterization kits containing a CV catheter, an inducer needle and vessel dilator, a 5 ml syringe, a scalpel and blade, straight silk suture material, prep sponges and gauze pads
3. dressing trays
4. IV administration sets, extension tubing, vented tubing, pump sets and solutions
5. masks and sterile gloves
6. shave preparation kits and razors
7. local anesthetic solutions and 25 gauge needles

8. skin cleansing solutions such as untinted chlorhexidine, povidone–iodine solution and ointment and 70% alcohol
9. adhesive tape, transparent semipermeable dressing and extra sponges
10. intermittent injection caps. An IV pole and infusion pump are also needed.

The cart is taken to the bedside, where the nurse assists the physician by opening packages and readying the equipment. The choice of catheter type and size depends on the purpose of therapy. For example, a multi-lumen catheter would be selected for the patient who needs multiple infusions over a short period of time. Catheters vary in length, number of lumens, purposes, duration of use and method of insertion. Table 22.13 illustrates some of the more commonly used central venous catheters. Agency policies vary with respect to priming the administration set. Sometimes this is done by the nurse; other times the physician will prime the tubing immediately before establishing the infusion as a means of ensuring that the connector end is completely sterile.

An extension tubing is attached to the administration set. On this tubing is a *slider clamp* (Figure 22.17) which is used as a safety device to guard against entry of air into the system. It is kept open when an infusion is running but must be closed if an infusion has stopped.

FIGURE 22.17   Slider Clamp

TABLE 22.13   Types of Central Venous Lines

TYPE	CHARACTERISTICS	INDICATIONS FOR USE	ADVANTAGES AND DISADVANTAGES	NURSING IMPLICATIONS
Single-lumen catheter	• Polyvinylchloride (PVC) or polyurethane • 20 cm long • Lumen gauge varies • Inserted percutaneously • Sutured in place	• Short-term CV access • Emergency access • Patient requires one type of infusion solution	**Advantages** • Easy to insert at bedside • Easy to remove **Disadvantages** • Limits infusion to one solution • Short-term therapy • PVC is thrombogenic and irritates inner lumen and vessel	• Minimize patient movement • Assess frequently for signs of infection or clot formation

Multi-lumen catheter	• PVC or polyurethane • Two, three or four lumens exiting at 2 cm intervals • Lumen gauges vary • Inserted percutaneously • Sutured in place	• Short-term CV access • Patient requires multiple types of infusion solutions	**Advantages** • As for single-lumen catheter • Allows simultaneous infusion of multiple purpose (even incompatible) solutions **Disadvantages** • As for single-lumen catheter	• Know gauge and purpose of each lumen • Use the same lumen for the same purpose

TYPE	CHARACTERISTICS	INDICATIONS FOR USE	ADVANTAGES AND DISADVANTAGES	NURSING IMPLICATIONS
Hickman catheter	• Silicone rubber • 90 cm long • Dacron cuff • Single- or multi-lumen • Tunnelled	• Long-term CV access • Home therapy	**Advantages** • Less thrombogenic • Dacron cuff prevents excessive motion and migration of bacteria **Disadvantages** • Requires surgical insertion • Requires doctor for removal • Tears and kinks easily	• Sterile dressings required • Handle catheter gently • Observe for kinks or tears • Have repair kit available

| ***Hickman/ Broviac catheter*** | • Hickman catheter combined with a Broviac (like a Hickman but with a smaller lumen) | • Long-term CV access
• Patient requires multiple infusions | **Advantages**
• Allows blood sampling without interrupting infusions
Disadvantages
• As for Hickman | • Know the purpose of each lumen
• Label lumens to avoid confusion |

SOURCE: Krozek, 1993, 294-295.

PROCEDURE 22.5

Assisting With a Bedside Central Venous Catheter Insertion

ACTION	RATIONALE
1. Gather equipment and supplies: • CV catheter insertion set • CV catheterization kit • Dressing tray • IV administration set, tubings and solutions as per agency policy • Masks and sterile gloves • Shave preparation kit and razor • Skin cleansing solutions, povidone–iodine solution and ointment, and 70% alcohol • Local anesthetic solutions and 25 gauge needle • Intermittent injection caps for multi-lumen catheters • Sterile gauze pads • Non-allergenic tape and transparent semipermeable dressing • IV pole and infusion pump	Facilitates efficiency and economy of time.
2. Identify the patient.	Avoids error.
3. Prepare the patient for what to expect and provide support during each stage of the procedure.	Helps to reduce anxiety and tension which enhances the patient's well-being and comfort.
4. Apply a mask and wash hands thoroughly.	Prevents introducing contaminants during procedure.
5. Set up a sterile field on the overbed table and ready the equipment for insertion.	
6. Shave (as necessary) and cleanse the site as per agency protocol.	Decreases microorganisms on the skin.
7. When using the subclavian or jugular vein, place the patient in the Trendelenburg position, with a towel between the scapulae.	Dilates the vein and decreases risk of air embolism.
8. Turn the patient's head away from the insertion site.	Makes the site more accessible and prevents possible contamination from airborne bacteria in the patient's breath.
9. After masking, gowning and gloving the physician will cover the site with sterile drapes.	Creates a sterile field.
10. Assist with injection of local anesthetic as required.	Promotes patient comfort.
11. Support the patient while the catheter is inserted through the skin and threaded through the vein to the vena cava or right atrium.	Promotes physical and emotional well-being.

PROCEDURE 22.5
continued

ACTION	RATIONALE
12. Assist with attaching the catheter to the primed administration set. Instruct the patient to perform the Valsalva manoeuvre while the physician attaches the tubing to the catheter hub.	Keeps the vein patent and closes the catheter to air. Due to the forces of fluid flow and pressure changes in the thoracic cavity, a negative pressure develops at the tip of the catheter if it is not filled with fluid or if it is open to air. This negative pressure draws air into the catheter, creating an air embolism. The Valsalva manoeuvre prevents air from being drawn into the catheter by increasing intrathoracic pressure.
13. Set the infusion flow at a keep-the-vein open rate.	Keeps the vein patent. D_5W or NS is used until placement of the catheter is confirmed. Infusing an isotonic solution avoids the risk of vessel wall thrombosis.
14. After the catheter is sutured in place, cleanse the insertion site and apply a sterile dresing according to agency protocol.	Stabilizes the catheter and prevents entry of microorganisms.
15. Assist the patient to a comfortable, Fowler's position.	Makes it easier to breathe and decreases the chance of hematoma formation.
16. Monitor the patient's response to the catheter insertion. Observe patient's breathing and note any chest pain.	Indicates possible complications of pneumothorax and arrythmias.
17. Complete requisition for x-ray as ordered.	Since the catheter is radiopaque, its placement is easily seen on x-ray or fluoroscopy.
18. Document the procedure noting the date and time of insertion; length, type, and location of catheter; name of physician; type of solution and rate of infusion; blood samples drawn; type of dresing applied; condition of the site; and patient's response to the procedure. Once the x-ray has been completed and placement is confirmed, document where the catheter is situated and that the physician has been notified.	Fulfills requirements for nurse accountability.

Surgical Insertion of a Central Venous Line

Some central venous catheters, for example, Hickman and Broviac, are surgically inserted in the operating room. A tunnel is created in the subcutaneous tissue of the chest wall so that the insertion site in the vein is away from the exit site in the skin (Figure 22.16). In the subcutaneous tunnel, the catheter is encircled with a Dacron cuff. Tissue growth into the material of the cuff anchors the catheter and forms a seal against microorganisms.

Preoperative Preparation

Preoperative care for a patient having a surgical insertion of a central venous catheter is similar to that for any operative procedure. A preoperative checklist is completed and a consent form is signed. As with any invasive procedure, the patient must be informed about and have an understanding of the procedure and the possible risks involved. Blood work and a chest x-ray are done prior to the procedure. If a general anesthetic is to be used, the patient may be required to fast after midnight. Frequently, the insertion is completed under local anesthetic, in which case fasting is not required. The morning of or a few hours before the procedure, the patient should have a bed bath or take a shower with an antibacterial soap as per agency protocol. The anterior chest wall is cleansed thoroughly and the appropriate area is shaved.

During the procedure, a small incision is made in the chest wall above the chosen vein and another incision is made between the nipple and the sternum. An instrument is inserted through the subcutaneous tissue to create a tunnel. The catheter is pulled through the tunnel and out the exit incision. The catheter is threaded through the vein under fluoroscopic examination to verify that the tip is positioned correctly in the superior vena cava or the right atrium of the heart. The procedure is not painful. The patient may feel a stinging sensation when the local anesthetic is injected and pressure when the catheter is inserted. Sutures are used to close the incisions and sterile opaque dressings are applied.

Postoperative Care

When the patient returns to the ward the nurse will assess the patient's comfort level, vital signs and dressings on a frequent basis for a few hours. The patient is asked to stay in bed for a few hours to ensure that there is no bleeding from the sites. The dressing over the insertion site may be removed after 48 hours. Patients may shower or bathe once the dressing is off but the incision must be kept dry for at least seven days. The exit site must be dressed and cared for as long as the catheter remains in place.

Maintaining a Central Line Infusion

After a central line has been inserted, the primary responsibility of *all* nurses is to maintain the infusion accurately and safely and to prevent complications. Each agency has its own specific policies stating who is certified to care for central lines and what care is necessary, but, with minor variations, care is generally the same.

Regulating the Infusion Rate of Flow

Infusion pumps are used for all central lines to ensure accurate flow and patient safety. The nurse must program the pump correctly and monitor it frequently to ensure proper functioning.

Assessing the Infusion

Frequent careful and systematic assessments of the central venous line are necessary to ensure safe and accurate infusion. The assessment of a central venous infusion is similar to that of a peripheral intravenous infusion. Beginning at the insertion site, the nurse checks for any tenderness, redness, warmth, swelling or discharge. The catheter is also checked for kinks, obstructions or leakage. The sutures should be clean and firmly securing the catheter in place. There should be no redness in adjacent tissues. The transparent dressing should be dry and intact; all edges should be well secured to prevent entry of microorganisms. The date and time of last dressing change is noted. In some agencies the external length of the catheter is also noted so that a measurement can be made to determine whether the catheter may have become displaced.

Next, the administration set is inspected to ensure that all connections are secure. Because accidental disconnections can be life-threatening, a number of steps are taken to ensure patient safety. First, only tubing with luer locks and Y connectors are used in central venous therapy. All tubing connection sites are joined firmly and then luer locked. In addition, the connections are tab-taped with waterproof tape. The tape is tabbed to facilitate ease of removal and to avoid trauma to the connection. The tubing is also pinned onto the patient's gown to prevent strain on the connection sites. The threads of the locking connectors are inspected daily for wear, tear and cracks. Tubings are checked for kinks, leaks, obstructions, air bubbles or precipitate matter and the date of the last tubing change is noted. Finally, the safety slider clamp is inspected. The clamp should be open when solution is infusing. However, if the infusion has stopped or the catheter is not in use, the clamp should be closed to prevent air from entering the catheter.

The infusion pump is watched to make sure the infusion is set at the prescribed rate and that it is functioning properly. An inspection is then made of the solution container, noting the type of solution, the amount and type of additives, the amount that has infused and the amount remaining, as well as the date and time the solution began.

The patient's response to the infusion is also monitored. The nurse must be especially alert for signs of infection including increased temperature, chills and malaise. It is important to monitor the patient's respiratory status. Is the patient experiencing any dyspnea or shortness of breath and are there unusual sounds on auscultation? The pulse or apical beat should be taken to determine arrhythmias, increases in rate or decreases in strength. Finally, the fluid record is examined to determine imbalances in intake and output.

Routine Interventions for Central Venous Lines

In most agencies, routine interventions for central venous lines, with the exception of solution container changes, are carried out by nurses who are certified in the necessary skills. These skills include changing dressings, tubings and intermittent injection caps, as well as flushing and heparinizing the lumens to maintain patency of the catheters. Central venous dressings are routinely changed every 48 to 72 hours or when they become loose, soiled or wet. Occlusive dressings must be changed more frequently so that the site may be assessed. Administration sets are replaced when dressings are changed in order to limit interruptions in the infusion. Every time a connection in the system is opened, there is a risk that air and microorganisms will enter the catheter. In addition, frequent interruptions of the infusion can cause the formation of clots and occlusions.

When the central venous line or a lumen of a multiple catheter is not kept open with continuous infusion, it may be capped with an intermittent injection cap. An injection cap is a short luer-lock device placed at the distal end of the line or lumen of the catheter. The cap keeps the line sterile and ready for access when necessary. Central venous catheters must be flushed regularly to keep them patent. Agency policies vary on the flushing procedure, the frequency and the amount and type of flushing solution that is used.

While most of the skills needed for central venous therapy are carried out by specialized nurses, the nurse assigned to care for the patient is responsible for regulating the infusion, making assessments and alerting a certified nurse immediately should problems arise. The nurse caring for the patient (and this includes the nursing student as well) is also required to change the solution container. In central venous therapy, solution containers are changed in much the same way as they are for peripheral infusions. Meticulous aseptic technique must be used to prevent the entry of microorganisms into the venous system and care must be taken to ensure that no air bubbles enter the tubing during a container change. Should air enter the tubing at this time, the infusion must be slowed and the assistance of a certified nurse must be obtained immediately. If the air in the tubing is near to the patient, the infusion must be stopped by closing the slider clamp on the administration set. Prompt help from a certified nurse is imperative in this instance.

Preventing Complications

Complications may occur at any time during central venous therapy. It is essential for nurses to have knowledge of the common complications so that preventive measures are implemented rigorously. Restorative actions must be enacted promptly.

Infection

The threat of infection is always present; therefore, when providing any care to a central venous catheter, meticulous aseptic technique is mandatory. Once contaminated, the catheter becomes a haven for the growth of microorganisms. Furthermore, bacteria and fungi are readily transported to the heart, the great blood vessels and the intracardiac valves.

The chief cause of infection in central venous therapy is a break in sterile technique. Frequent interruptions of the system, wet or soiled dressings that remain in place, contaminated equipment and immunosuppression also contribute to infection. The importance of strict, thorough hand washing as a preventive measure before each procedure cannot be overemphasized. In fact, meticulous hand washing has been recognized as the most important action against infection.

A number of measures can be implemented to prevent infection in central venous therapy. Ideally, all medications given into central venous catheters should be prepared in the Pharmacy Department under a laminar flow hood. Blood work, tubing changes, flushings and other procedures should be coordinated to reduce the number of times the system is opened. Intravenous push medications should be avoided, except in emergency situations, to decrease the number of times the injection cap is punctured. When the cap is used, a small needle such as a 22 gauge is recommended.

When signs and symptoms of infection such as fever, chills, tenderness along the insertion site or shoulder, redness, swelling or purulent drainage from the site become evident, blood cultures are taken from the central catheter and from peripheral veins. Antibiotic therapy is instituted. If the source of infection is indeed the central venous catheter and the medications are ineffective, the catheter must be removed.

Air Embolism

Although **air embolism** — the presence of a large amount of air in the circulatory system — is a rare complication, its consequences are life-threatening. An air embolism can disrupt the blood supply to parts of the body and cause serious trauma. Death can ensue if the air embolism obstructs the pulmonary circulation. The exact amount of intravenous air that can cause death is not known; therefore, the entry of any amount of air into the venous system should be prevented.

As we discussed earlier, because central veins have a negative venous pressure, air can enter the circulatory system whenever a catheter is open to air or it is not filled with fluid. This can occur when a catheter is inserted or during procedures in which the line is opened, for example, when changing containers, tubings and injection caps. Air can also enter the system when a connection becomes disconnected, a solution container runs dry or a clamp remains open after a continuous infusion has stopped.

The signs and symptoms of air embolism will depend on the rate and amount of air taken into the venous system. The patient may display a sudden onset of chest pain, difficulty breathing, cyanosis, anxiety and confusion. On examination, the nurse may find an increasing respiratory rate, a rapid thready pulse, churning heart sounds over the precordium and hypotension. The patient may also experience nausea, restlessness, possible loss of consciousness, faintness, convulsions, diaphoresis and possibly cardiac arrest.

The entry of air into the patient's venous system is an emergency situation that must be dealt with immediately. The nurse must remain calm because his or her behaviour will have an impact on the patient's response. The central line must be clamped immediately using the slider clamp. If available, a padded or non-toothed hemostat may also be used. The patient is turned onto the left side in a Trendelenburg (head down) position. This position is necessary because it causes air to collect in the upper portion of the right atrium, and thereby prevents the air from moving through the tricuspid valve into the right ventricle and on into the pulmonary artery. The physician must be notified promptly. Oxygen is administered and the patient's vital signs are monitored. The physician may attempt to aspirate the air.

Occlusion and Dislodgement of the Catheter

A central venous catheter can become partially or completely occluded when an infusion flows too slowly or stops for a long period of time, or when it has not been irrigated frequently enough. When an infusion has stopped or is *positional* (will infuse only when the patient assumes a certain position), or will infuse only at a reduced rate, a certified nurse should be notified immediately. Like peripheral infusions, central catheters can become dislodged and cause infiltration. Thrombus formation can occur but it is rare because rapid blood flow in central veins and the slippery nature of silicone materials in the catheter inhibit clot formation.

Implanted Vascular Access Device

An implanted vascular access device (IVAD) consists of a small port or reservoir with a self-sealing rubber disc (septum) and a radiopaque silicone catheter (see Figure 22.18). The device is surgically implanted into a subcutaneous pocket adjacent to the central vein (commonly the subclavian or internal jugular) into which the catheter is inserted. A special type of needle, called the Huber Point needle, is used to access the catheter. This needle has a curved tip that slices the septum rather than coring it; as a result, the septum reseals itself more effectively. The needle is then taped to the skin and attached to intravenous equipment.

An IVAD is aesthetically more appealing to patients than a central venous catheter because there are no external parts and it allows complete freedom in daily activities when not in use. There is less chance of infection because

FIGURE 22.18 Implanted vascular access device. A. Port design B. Common sites C. Huber needle

A. SOURCE: Camp-Sorrell, D. (1992) Implantable ports: Everything you always wanted to know. *Journal of Intravenous Nursing, 15,* 264. Redrawn with permission.

the catheter does not exit the skin and there are no exposed parts to be subjected to damage or dislodgement.

The purpose and functions of an IVAD are like those of long-term central venous catheters, that is, to deliver intravenous fluids, parenteral nutrition, medications and blood and blood products and to obtain blood samples. IVADs are inserted into patients who require intermittent or continuous venous access for periods of months to years. This includes individuals of any age with terminal illnesses such as cancer, cystic fibrosis and AIDS as well as people with sickle cell anemia, inflammatory bowel disease and congestive heart failure. The IVAD is not recommended for patients with inadequate body tissue (for example, those who are malnourished) to support the device. It is also not recommended for patients who are extremely obese and those who have had mastectomies and radiation to the chest.

Care for an IVAD is the same as for a central venous catheter. Preoperative and postoperative care for implanting an IVAD is like that for a surgical insertion of a central venous catheter. In the first 24 hours postoperative, the head of the patient's bed should be raised 30–40° to decrease pressure on the area and promote comfort. The tissue surrounding an IVAD is very tender and may be bruised from the creation of the pocket. Patients may require analgesia for the control of discomfort. The pressure dressing over the insertion site is usually removed in 24 to 48 hours. It is not uncommon to have a scant amount of serosanguineous drainage on the dressing. The site is assessed for tenderness, redness and swelling. After the dressing is removed, the patient may shower or bathe. However, the site should remain dry. The sutures are usually removed seven to 14 days postoperatively.

The care for an accessed IVAD (that is, one being used for intravenous therapy) is similar to the care for a central venous line. In addition to the standard assessment for a central venous catheter, the Huber needle must be checked to ensure that it is firmly secured in the skin at a 90° angle. The covering dressing should be dry and intact. As with central venous lines, the nurse caring for the patient may change solution containers. All other interventions — tubing and injection cap changes as well as flushing and heparinizing the device — are carried out by certified nurses.

Although the incidence is low, the risk of complications with implanted venous access devices is always present. Infection, the most common complication, can be prevented with strict aseptic technique. Thrombosis, occlusions, infiltration and air embolism have occurred occasionally. One unique complication with an IVAD is *Twiddler's Syndrome*. In this syndrome the catheter becomes disconnected from the port as a result of frequent manipulation of the device by the patient. The signs and symptoms include tenderness, redness and edema at the insertion site. Should such a disconnection be suspected, the nurse must stop the infusion and notify the physician promptly.

Comfort measures such as cold compresses to the site may be implemented. The patient is also prepared for an x-ray.

Implanted venous access devices require minimal care when they are not being used for intravenous therapy. Any type of clothing may be worn but care should be taken to avoid clothes that rub or apply pressure to the site. Car seat belts, especially shoulder straps, may have to be adjusted. Individuals may bathe, shower or swim as they normally would. There are no restrictions on activities, although aggressive contact sports such as football should be avoided. The patient should manipulate the device as little as possible to decrease the potential for infection and Twiddler's syndrome.

Daily inspection for swelling, redness, tenderness and discharge should be carried out. Any abnormal findings should be reported immediately. IVADs require monthly flushing with normal saline or a heparin solution to maintain their patency. Patients may go to an agency to have the device flushed or they may be taught how to do this procedure at home. The patient should wear a medical alert bracelet or necklace and carry a medical information card stating the type of IVAD that is in place and who should be contacted in the case of emergency.

BLOOD TRANSFUSION THERAPY

The administration of whole blood or blood components, such as plasma, red blood cells or platelets, into the venous circulation is called a *blood transfusion*. Blood transfusions are given to restore circulating blood volume following hemorrhage, trauma, surgery, shock and burns; to correct red blood cell deficiency and improve oxygen-carrying capacity of the blood in cases of severe anemia; and to maintain the blood's clotting ability when clotting factors are deficient, for example, in patients with bone marrow suppression or hemophilia. While blood transfusion is often a life-sustaining therapy, it is a procedure that is accompanied by the risk of serious and even life-threatening reactions.

One of the major risks associated with blood transfusion is due to the fact that the blood is taken from one individual, the *donor*, and infused into another individual, the *recipient*. Blood is collected from a donor, processed and stored under controlled conditions and then infused into a recipient. Known as a *homologous* or *indirect transfusion*, this method carries the potential for incompatibility between the donor's blood and the recipient's blood, and for exposure to blood borne diseases such as hepatitis and AIDS.

A method that is becoming more popular is the *autologous transfusion* in which blood is collected from a person, stored and then transfused back into the same person at a later time. This method is safer than the homologous transfusion because it significantly decreases the risk of blood incompatibility and avoids exposure to blood borne diseases. Autologous transfusion is discussed further in a later section.

Blood and Blood Components

Blood is made up of formed elements and a fluid called plasma. Erythrocytes (red blood cells), leukocytes (white blood cells) and thrombocytes (platelets) comprise the formed elements. The plasma contains largely water (serum) and protein (albumin, globulin and fibrinogen) as well as various substances (for example, electrolytes, carbohydrates, lipids and vitamins).

Each component of the blood has its own distinctive function. For example, erythrocytes carry oxygen from the lungs to the cells and carbon dioxide from the cells to the lungs for elimination from the body. Leukocytes guard the body against infection while thrombocytes aid in blood clotting. The plasma carries the formed elements and other substances. Table 22.14 outlines the most common blood components along with indications for their use in blood transfusion therapy. Whole blood is rarely transfused today because the components can be separated out and used for the specific needs of patients.

TABLE 22.14   Blood and Blood Components

TYPE	DESCRIPTION	USES AND SPECIAL CONSIDERATIONS
Whole blood	Contains all blood components	To replace blood loss from hemorrhage, surgical intervention, trauma or extensive burns. Shelf-life of 21 days when stored at 5°C. Crossmatch is necessary.
Packed red blood cells	Whole blood with 80% of the plasma removed	To restore or maintain oxygen-carrying capacity in patients with anemia. To increase red blood cell mass and maintain hemoglobin levels following surgical blood loss or gastrointestinal bleeding. Shelf-life of 21 days for stored fresh packed cells. Frozen cells may be stored for three years. Must be used within 24 hours after opening or thawing. Crossmatch is necessary.
Platelets	Platelet sediment from platelet-rich blood re-suspended in 30 to 50 ml plasma	To control or prevent bleeding associated with deficiencies in the number or function of platelets. Must be administered within 72 hours after whole blood is collected. Crossmatch is not necessary for red-cell-free products.
Plasma (fresh, freshfrozen)	Serous component separated from whole blood. Contains clotting factors	To increase clotting factors and plasma protein levels and to expand plasma volume. Fresh plasma must be administered within six hours of collection. Fresh frozen plasma may be stored for 12 months and must be given within two hours of thawing. Crossmatch is not necessary.
Cryoprecipitate	Factor VIII (antihemophilic factor) and fibrinogen recovered from frozen plasma	To control bleeding in patients with classical hemophilia or Factor VIII deficiency and replace fibrinogen. Frozen cryoprecipitate may be stored for 12 months. Must be given within six hours of thawing. Crossmatch is not necessary.
Albumin 5% or 25%	Heat treated, chemically processed fraction of pooled plasma	To expand blood volume in patients with hypovolemia, replace plasma albumin and maintain electrolyte balance. May be stored for three years at room temperature. Crossmatch is not necessary.

SOURCES: *Nursing PhotoBook: Managing IV therapy.* (1980), 114–115; Earnest (1993), 558; Flynn and Hackel (1990), 760–761.

Blood Group and Rh (Rhesus) Factor

Human blood is classified according to **blood group** (type) and Rh (Rhesus) factor. Successful transfusion therapy depends on blood group and Rh compatibility between recipient and donor blood.

Blood type depends on the presence of specific antigens on the red cell surfaces and corresponding antibodies in the plasma. *Antigens* initiate an immune response and stimulate the formation of *antibodies* to destroy the foreign invaders. In blood, the antibodies inactivate antigens by agglutination (clumping together of red blood cells) and hemolysis (disintegration of red blood cells with the release of hemoglobin into the plasma). Tests for blood type and compatibility are based on these antigen-antibody reactions.

A person's blood type (A, B, AB, or O) is genetically determined by two antigens, A and B, which are present on the surface of the red blood cells. People with A antigens have type-A blood and those with B antigens have type-B blood. Some people have both A and B antigens; their blood group is type-AB. Still others carry neither A nor B antigens on their red cell surfaces. These people have type-O blood.

Correspondingly, plasma contains genetically determined antibodies which act against any A or B antigens that are naturally not present in the blood. For example, type-B blood, which does not normally contain A antigens, has naturally occurring anti-A antibodies present in the serum. Giving type-A blood to a person with type-B blood would result in a blood incompatibility because the anti-A antibodies in the recipient's plasma would act against the A antigen in the donor blood.

Therefore, in homologous transfusion therapy, the blood of the donor must be matched to the blood type of the recipient, since the recipient's plasma contains the incompatible antibodies. Table 22.15 lists ABO compatibilities and incompatibilities. Note that type-O blood has neither A nor B antigens. It, therefore, can be donated to individuals with any of the four blood groups. A person with type-O blood is referred to as a *universal donor*. On the other hand, people with type-AB blood have neither anti-A nor anti-B antibodies in their plasma. These people are called universal recipients because they can receive all blood types.

Another constituent of blood that can cause a hemolytic reaction is the Rh factor. The **Rh factor** is also an inherited antigen, referred to as antigen D, present on the surface of red blood cells. People with antigen D in their blood are classified as Rh positive (Rh+); those without it are Rh negative (Rh−). Unlike the ABO system in which anti-A and anti-B antibodies occur naturally, exposure to the D antigen is necessary for production of Rh antibodies. If a person with Rh negative blood receives Rh positive blood, that person's body will begin to produce anti-D antibodies. These antibodies stay in the system; a subsequent transfusion with Rh positive blood would result in a reaction causing hemolysis and agglutination of red blood cells.

Blood Typing and Crossmatching

In order to administer blood safely, the recipient's blood must be typed and compared with donor blood to ensure that the two are compatible. The blood test that is done to determine a patient's blood group is called *typing*. **Crossmatching** is a procedure performed to establish compatibility between donor and recipient blood.

Administering Blood and Blood Components

Blood transfusions can result in life-threatening complications, the most common resulting from incorrect identification of patients or the administration of incompatible blood (LaRocca and Otto, 1989). When administering blood transfusions, nurses must judiciously follow the agency protocol and guidelines for identifying the patient and blood product, initiating and maintaining the infusion and monitoring the patient for adverse reactions. Procedure 22.6 outlines the nursing actions for administering, maintaining and discontinuing a blood transfusion.

TABLE 22.15   ABO Blood Compatibilities and Incompatibilities

BLOOD TYPE	ANTIGEN	ANTIBODY	COMPATIBLE DONOR	INCOMPATIBLE DONOR
A	A	Anti-B	A, O	B, AB
B	B	Anti-A	B, O	A, AB
AB	A, B	None	A, B, AB, O	None
O	None	Anti-A, Anti-B	O	A, B, AB

Preparing the Patient

The nurse explains the need for a blood transfusion, the component the patient will be getting and the possibility of adverse reactions. Sometimes patients refuse blood transfusion for religious or personal reasons. When this happens, the patient is asked to sign a "refusal of treatment" form and the physician is notified of the patient's decision. Once verbal agreement for the transfusion is given, the nurse obtains information about allergies and previous experiences with blood transfusions. In addition, the patient is instructed to report chills, nausea, itching, rash, headache, shortness of breath or any other unusual symptoms.

The patient's vital signs are taken within 30 minutes prior to starting the transfusion for later assessment and evaluation. If the patient has a peripheral or central venous line or an IVAD, the nurse should assess the site and the infusion for patency and signs of complications. With peripheral lines, the needle or catheter gauge must be large enough for blood infusion, that is, at least a 19 gauge butterfly needle and an 18 gauge or 20 gauge catheter. Smaller gauge needles can cause damage to the red blood cells and significantly slow the transfusion. Larger gauge catheters (16 gauge or 14 gauge) may be necessary in emergency situations where blood must infuse rapidly. A smaller gauge needle (21 gauge or smaller) may be used for children because the rate of infusion is slower owing to the smaller body size and the smaller amount that has to be infused.

When a peripheral line is already in place, the solution that is infusing must be replaced with normal saline. A 0.9% saline solution is preferred in transfusion therapy because it simulates plasma's isotonicity. Other solutions may cause problems. Dextrose solutions, for example, cause hemolysis and clumping of red blood cells while solutions containing calcium, such as Ringer's lactate, cause blood to clot in the bag and tubing.

Assembling Equipment

The equipment needed for blood transfusion includes a straight or Y-type blood administration set (see Figure 22.19), normal saline solution (500 ml bag) and the blood or blood product. A standard filter is incorporated into all straight and Y-type administration sets to remove small clots, degenerated platelets, leukocytes and large fibrin strands that accumulate during storage. The Y-type set has two branches with spikes; one branch attaches to the blood and the other to the normal saline.

When a straight blood administration set is used, a primary IV line is established using normal saline. If the patient does not have an existing IV line or if the venipuncture device is too small for blood transfusion, equipment is assembled for a peripheral venipuncture using an 18 or 20 gauge catheter. Infusion pumps may be used to administer and regulate the infusion of blood and blood components.

FIGURE 22.19 Y-type blood administration set

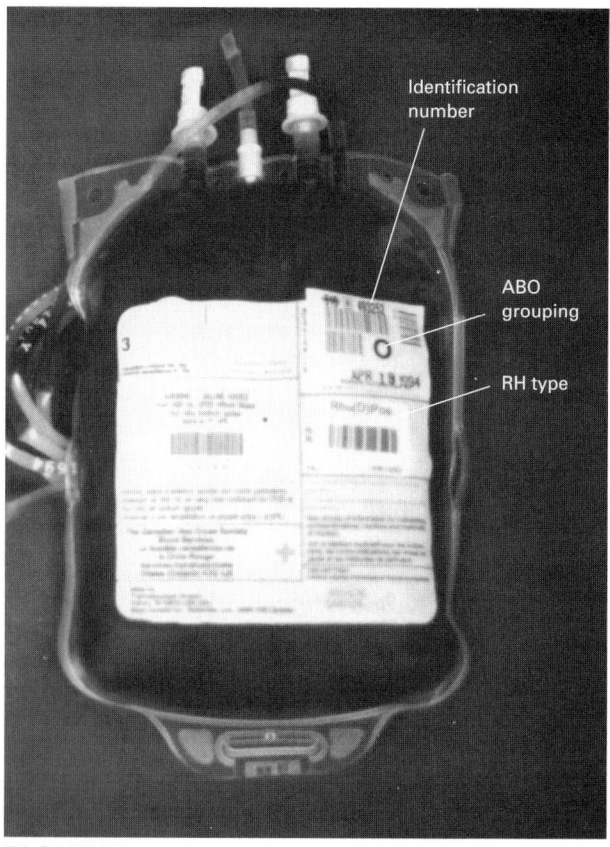

FIGURE 22.20 Blood product label

Before using a pump, the nurse must check the manufacturer's instructions to make sure the pump will not cause hemolysis of the red blood cells.

The blood product is obtained from the blood bank according to established agency policy and procedure. Some practitioners consider identification of the patient and the proper blood component as the most important measure in transfusion therapy (LaRocca and Otto, 1989). The transfusion process begins with confirmation of the physician's order. The blood is then obtained from the blood bank. The blood bag will have a blood identification label put on by the Canadian Red Cross containing donor or unit number, the donor's ABO blood group and Rh factor and the expiration date (Figure 22.20). There will also be a recipient identification tag attached to the bag with a rubber band. This tag is put on by blood bank personnel in the agency. It includes the recipient's name and hospital number, the donor's ABO blood group and Rh factor and the unit number.

All information on the label and tag must be matched and compared with the blood requisition form. If there are any discrepancies in the information, the blood must be returned to the blood bank. As a safeguard, the identification procedure is conducted by two health care professionals, first in the blood bank and then at the nursing station. This double check is documented on the blood requisition form and noted in the patient's chart. In addition, the nurse who administers the blood checks the patient's name, birth date and hospital number against that on the recipient identification tag to ensure the correct patient is receiving the blood. The product's unit number and the time that the transfusion was commenced is entered onto the patient's chart.

PROCEDURE 22.6

Administering Blood and Blood Components

ACTION	RATIONALE
1. Prepare the patient. Assess an existing IV line for patency and note the gauge of the venipuncture device. Take the patient's TPR and BP.	Keeps the patient informed and reduces anxiety. Facilitates decision-making and organization of care. Provides baseline values.
2. Gather equipment and supplies: • Straight or Y-type blood administration set with filter • Primary IV administration set if using a straight blood set • 500 ml normal saline solution • Supplies for venipuncture if required (see Procedure 22.2). Use an 18 or 20 gauge catheter or larger • Alcohol swabs, adhesive tape • Clean gloves	Facilitates efficiency and economy of time.
3. Wash hands.	Reduces risk of contamination.
4. Establish normal saline infusion. **When using a straight blood set with an existing IV:** replace the solution bag with normal saline. **When using a Y-type blood set with an existing IV:** don gloves, discontinue the existing solution and tubing and connect the primed Y-type set to the venipuncture device. **When establishing a peripheral line for use of a straight blood set:** initiate the IV using a primed primary administration set. **When establishing a peripheral line for use of a Y-type administration set:** initiate the IV using the primed Y-type tubing. Make sure the branch of the tubing that will be attached to the blood bag is clamped off.	Prepares the line and keeps the vein open until the blood transfusion is commenced. Blood and blood components must be commenced within 30 minutes of leaving the fridge in the blood bank. Therefore, the infusion should be established before the blood product is obtained from the blood bank.

Continued on the next page

ACTION	RATIONALE
5. Obtain and, with a second registered nurse, identify the blood product.	Ensures safety. Avoids error and possible reactions.
A. Verify doctor's order.	
B. Compare the information on the blood bag identification label and recipient identification tag to that on the blood requisition form:	
• the patient's first and last name, birth date and hospital number.	
• the unit number, the blood group, Rh factor and expiration date.	
C. Verify that the unit number on the blood identification label is the same as on the recipient identification tag.	
D. Check the blood for abnormal colour, clumping or bubbles.	Indicates contamination.
E. Enter signatures as indicated on the blood requisition form.	
6. At the bedside, identify the patient. Compare the first and last name, birth date and hospital number on the patient's identification bracelet to that on the recipient identification tag. Blood must **NEVER** be administered to a patient who is not wearing an identification bracelet.	Ensures that the correct patient will receive the blood product.
7. Gently invert the blood bag several times.	Mixes the plasma and cells.
8. Prime the blood administration set and start the infusion.	
When using a Y-type set: Insert the spike of the remaining branch into the blood bag and hang the bag on the IV pole. Open the clamp on the tubing which connects the spike to the filter and squeeze the drip chamber until the filter is entirely covered with blood. Clamp off the normal saline to begin the infusion of blood.	To function optimally, the filter should be entirely covered with blood.
When using a straight set: Prime the tubing using established procedure. Don gloves, disconnect the primary tubing with normal saline and connect the blood tubing to the venipuncture device. To begin infusion, open the roller clamp on the blood administration set. Put a sterile cap on the connector end of the primary tubing and attach it to the roller clamp.	Keeps the primary IV line with normal saline ready for hook-up should blood reaction occur.
9. Regulate the infusion rate of flow to no more than 3 ml/minute for the first 15 minutes.	Transfusion reactions of flow frequently occur within the first 15 minutes.
10. Check vital signs and monitor the patient as per agency protocol. Observe for signs of transfusion reaction. See Table 22.16.	Enables early detection of and prompt intervention for transfusion reactions.

ACTION	RATIONALE
11. If signs of reactions appear, stop the blood immediately. Reestablish the primary IV and keep the vein open with normal saline. Take vital signs and notify the doctor.	Minimizes the severity of the reaction.
12. If there are no reactions after 15 minutes, regulate the flow at the prescribed rate. A unit of blood should be infused within four hours. Blood that has not infused within the time allowance must be stopped and returned to the blood bank.	Red blood cells start to deteriorate after 30 minutes out of the fridge and lose their effectiveness after two hours. The longer the blood remains at room temperature the higher the risk of bacterial growth.
13. Document the procedure on the appropriate forms, including date and time infusion commenced, size of needle or catheter, venipuncture site, type of blood component, serial number, sequence number if more than one unit, infusion rate of flow, vital signs, patient responses, and any adverse reactions.	Maintains requirements for nurse accountability.
14. Continue to monitor the patient and the infusion according to agency protocol.	Reactions can occur throughout the transfusion.
15. When the infusion is completed, flush the blood tubing with normal saline.	Ensures infusion of the small amounts of blood that remain in the tubing.
16. If the patient is to receive a subsequent unit of blood, keep the vein open with normal saline.	Maintains patency of the IV until the subsequent unit is established.
17. If the transfusion is completed, reestablish an existing IV or discontinue the infusion and document the procedure and time the transfusion was finished.	
18. Return blood bag to the blood bank as per agency policy.	
19. Take vital signs and continue to monitor the patient for signs of adverse reactions as per agency protocol.	Delayed reactions can occur for two to three hours following an infusion.

What Not to Do When Transfusing Blood

- Do not store any blood component on a nursing unit or in an unmonitored refrigerator.
- Do not keep blood out of the transfusion service's refrigerator for longer than 30 minutes before starting the transfusion.
- Do not warm blood for transfusion in a microwave oven, in an unmonitored water bath, under running water or in a sink.
- Do not heat blood components to a temperature higher than 38°C.
- Do not transfuse any blood component without using the appropriate blood filter.

- Do not use the same blood filter longer than four hours.
- Do not transfuse a unit of blood over a period longer than four hours.
- Do not add drugs to blood components or infuse drugs and blood through the same blood-administration set.
- Do not use any solution other than 0.9% (normal) saline to prime a blood-administration set, to flush the IV line or to dilute the blood product.

SOURCE: National Blood Resource Education Program's Nursing Education Working Group. (1991). Choosing blood components and equipment. *AJN*, June, 45. Reproduced with permission.

TABLE 22.16   Common Transfusion Reactions

TYPE	CAUSES	SIGNS & SYMPTOMS	INTERVENTIONS
Hemolytic	Antibodies in the recipient's plasma react with antigens in donor blood	Chills, shakiness, flushed skin, fever, nausea, vomiting, headache, backache, dyspnea, cyanosis, chest pain, tachycardia, hypotension, oliguria, flank pain and bleeding abnormalities	Stop the transfusion immediately. Keep the vein open with normal saline. Notify the physician immediately. Return blood container and administration set to the blood bank along with a sample of patient's blood for repeat typing and crossmatch. Monitor vital signs, intake and output, and observe for signs of bleeding. Administer oxygen and medications as ordered.
Febrile (Bacterial)	Blood contaminated with bacteria	Mild chills, fever, warm flushed skin, headache, malaise, nausea, vomiting, diarrhea. Symptoms may be mild to extreme resembling a hemolytic reaction	Stop the transfusion immediately. Keep the vein open with normal saline. Notify the physician immediately. Treat mild symptoms with antipyretics and antihistamines as ordered. Severe cases are cared for like hemolytic reactions.
Allergic	Sensitivity to substances in donor blood	*Mild:* itching, urticaria, mild facial edema, nasal congestion, bronchial wheeze, chills, fever, nausea, vomiting. *Severe:* Increasing severity of signs above, tightness in chest, substernal chest pain, difficulty swallowing, progression to shock and death	*Mild:* Slow the infusion. Notify the physician. Administer antihistamines as ordered. *Severe:* Stop the infusion. Keep the vein open with normal saline. Notify the physician immediately. Monitor vital signs. Administer oxygen and medications as ordered.
Hypervolemia (Circulatory overload)	Transfusion too large or too rapid	Dry cough, dyspnea, tightness in chest, pulmonary congestion, distended peripheral and neck veins, full bounding pulse	Stop the transfusion immediately. Keep the vein open with normal saline. Notify the physician immediately. Administer oxygen and medications as ordered.

TRANSFUSION REACTIONS

Even when all of the safety checks have been completed, transfusion reactions can still occur during, immediately after or within 96 hours of the blood transfusion. The primary types of blood reactions are hemolytic, febrile, hypervolemic or allergic. The most serious and potentially dangerous type is the hemolytic reaction, which occurs from incompatibilities between donor and recipient blood. Antibodies in the recipient's plasma react with antigens on the donor's red blood cell surfaces, causing hemolysis and agglutination. Table 22.16 provides an outline of the common transfusion reactions, detailing the causes, signs and symptoms and nursing interventions.

AUTOLOGOUS BLOOD TRANSFUSION

An autologous transfusion is the collection and reinfusion of a person's own blood or blood components at a later time. Autologous transfusion is a desirable alternative for individuals whose religious beliefs prohibit homologous blood transfusion and for those concerned about the risk of contracting blood borne diseases such as hepatitis and AIDS. In addition, receiving one's own blood significantly decreases the risk of febrile, allergic and hemolytic reactions. Another advantage of autologous transfusion is that it reduces the demands for donor blood and, thus, helps to conserve blood supply. However, the risk of bacterial contamination is always

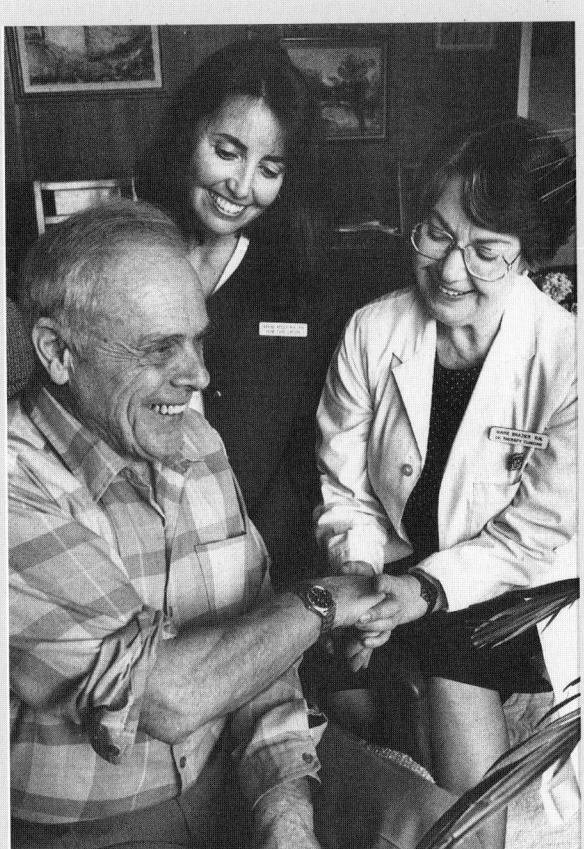

A home IV program allows patients to receive intravenous medications and/or fluids in the comfort and privacy of their home.

creased demands for hospital beds. The benefits for patients are many. Their well-being is enhanced because they feel more comfortable in their own surroundings and they are able to perform many of their normal activities. They feel a sense of control and independence because they are caring for themselves.

The types of intravenous care that are currently undertaken in the home include the administration of fluids and medications such as antibiotics, antifungal agents, analgesics, chemotherapeutic (anticancer) agents and total parenteral nutrition. Some programs also administer blood transfusions in the home. Intravenous therapy may be given via a central venous line, an intermittent injection cap or an IVAD.

Safe and successful home intravenous therapy is dependent on two important factors. The first is a comprehensive assessment of the patient and his or her home environment; the second is thorough patient teaching. Candidates are selected carefully for the program.

Candidates must demonstrate a specific level of self-care and have the mental ability to understand the basis of treatment and asepsis, as well as the physical abilities and coordination to perform the procedures safely. They must also be able to recognize complications and deal with potential emergency situations. In addition, the candidates must have a care-giver, a relative or a friend in the home who can provide the necessary care for them. The home environment is also evaluated. Obvious essentials such as running hot and cold water, adequate lighting, telephone service and transportation must be present. An area for clean, safe storage of supplies and equipment as well as an area for performing the procedures must be available. Finally, the accessibility of a hospital or 24-hour health care support service is considered.

Once a candidate is recommended for the program, thorough patient teaching begins. Patients and their care-givers are taught about the following:

- therapy-related procedures
- care of the infusion site
- daily assessments
- restrictions in activities
- trouble-shooting problems
- prevention of complications
- when to call for the assistance of a physician or a nurse
- actions to be taken in case of emergencies
- safe methods of discarding used equipment
- where to obtain supplies and equipment
- arrangements for blood sampling or testing.

Patients and their care-givers should feel secure with their knowledge base and the physical skills required before discharge.

present, as is the chance of transfusing the wrong unit of blood into the patient. Therefore, the same stringent procedures for collecting, processing, storing, and transfusing homologous blood must be used for autologous transfusion.

Unfortunately, not all patients can qualify for autologous transfusion. Those with malignant cancer, blood clotting disorders or hemolytic conditions involving excessive destruction of red blood cells are not eligible. Patients with active infections are also not eligible for autologous transfusion because the bacteria may proliferate while the blood is stored. Autologous transfusion is most appropriate for healthy patients who are undergoing planned surgery such as a hip replacement. The individual must have a hemoglobin of at least 110 and be free of active infection or enteric contamination. Blood may be collected four to six weeks prior to the surgery. Blood lost during and after surgery or trauma can also be salvaged and re-infused (Drago, 1992).

INTRAVENOUS HOME CARE

One of the trends of the 1990s is the administration of intravenous therapy in the home. Intravenous home care is beneficial for both health care agencies and patients. For the health care system there are reduced costs for care and de-

INTERSTITIAL INFUSION

Interstitial infusion, hypodermoclysis and subcutaneous infusion are synonymous terms referring to the administration

KEY PRINCIPLES

Principles Relevant To Fluid, Electrolyte and Acid–Base Balance

1. The average adult requires 2100 to 2900 ml of fluid in a 24-hour period.
2. Children require a greater volume of fluids, proportional to body weight, than adults.
3. Normally, fluid intake is balanced against fluid loss.
4. When fluids are lost or retained in excessive amounts, there is an accompanying loss or gain of electrolytes.
5. The signs and symptoms accompanying electrolyte imbalance vary according to the excess or deficiency of the specific electrolyte.
6. The specific electrolytes lost from the body in any fluid loss depend on the route of the loss.

of large amounts of fluid into subcutaneous tissue. This measure is not used often: it is utilized when a person is unable to take fluids orally, rectally or intravenously. Its purpose is to supply the patient with fluids, electrolytes and occasionally nourishment. Hyaluronidase (Wydase) is often added to the fluid to hasten its absorption. The enzyme breaks down the hyaluronic acid in the connective tissue.

Whether the initiation of an interstitial infusion is the responsibility of the nurse or the physician depends on the policy of the specific agency. The common sites for the administration of an interstitial infusion are just below the scapula, the abdominal wall above the crest of the ilium, the lower aspect of the breast and the anterior aspect of the thigh. The equipment that is used is similar to that used in intravenous infusions. A 19 gauge to 22 gauge needle is used. Often, two sites are used simultaneously.

After the equipment has been set up, the needle is inserted into the skin at a 20° angle. It is then taped in place and the flow of the fluid is adjusted in accordance with the physician's order. The usual rate of flow for an interstitial infusion is 60 to 120 drops per minute. The rate is dependent upon the ability of the individual to absorb the fluid. Thin people usually absorb fluid more easily than obese people, because they have fewer fat cells.

The nurse assists the patient in assuming a comfortable position, since this treatment is often lengthy. Observations are indicated to detect untoward signs, particularly those related to circulatory collapse (for example, an accelerated, weak pulse). The patient should be watched for signs of respiratory difficulty that could indicate overhydration, such as dyspnea or moist and noisy breathing. Sometimes, the infusion is poorly absorbed and the nurse may notice the tissues at the site of the injection are becoming edematous. If untoward symptoms develop, the infusion should be stopped and the physician notified promptly.

At the termination of an infusion the needle is removed. A small antiseptic dressing is taped over the wound with slight pressure to prevent leakage of the fluid. The nurse records the time of initiation and termination of the infusion, as well as the type of fluid, the amount of fluid absorbed, the addition of any medications, the rate of flow and the patient's response to the treatment. Again it is wise to record site of the infusion so that the injection sites can be rotated.

EVALUATING FLUID, ELECTROLYTE AND ACID–BASE BALANCE INTERVENTIONS

The evaluation of a care plan for fluid, electrolyte and acid–base balance is based on the expected outcomes or goals outlined in the planning phase of the nursing process. Following is a guide for evaluating the effectiveness of nursing intervention.

1. Is the patient taking adequate food and fluids to meet his or her fluid and electrolyte needs?
2. Is the patient's urine output compatible with fluid intake?
3. If there are restrictions on the patient's fluid or electrolyte intake, are these being followed?
4. If parenteral fluids have been prescribed, have they been given at the correct time? Have sterile precautions been observed in their administration? Is the infusion flowing at the proper rate?
5. Is the patient's skin in good condition? Is the mouth?
6. Do the patient and family have all the information they need to enable them to maintain and restore the patient's fluid, electrolyte and acid–base balance?

KEY TERMS

electrolyte p. 610

cation p. 610

anion p. 610

intracellular fluid p. 610

extracellular fluid p. 611

interstitial fluid p. 611

intravascular fluid p. 611

solvent p. 611

solute p. 611

serum electrolyte p. 612

diffusion p. 612

selectively permeable
 membrane p. 612

osmosis p. 612

osmotic pressure p. 612

osmolality p. 612

active transport p. 612

filtration p. 612

action potential p. 614

acid p. 617

base p. 617

acidosis p. 617

alkalosis p. 618

fluid volume deficit p. 622

isotonic fluid deficit p. 622

hypotonic dehydration p. 622

hypertonic dehydration p. 622

insensible water loss p. 622

hyponatremia p. 623

hypernatremia p. 623

hypokalemia p. 626

hyperkalemia p. 626

hypocalcemia p. 626

hypercalcemia p. 627

hypomagnesemia p. 627

hypermagnesemia p. 627

hypophosphatemia p. 634

hyperphosphatemia p. 635

buffering p. 636

correction p. 636

compensation p. 636

skin turgor p. 647

edema p. 647

venipuncture p. 657

air embolism p. 687

blood transfusion p. 689

donor p. 689

recipient p. 689

homologous or indirect
 transfusion p. 689

autologous transfusion p. 689

blood group p. 691

Rh factor p. 691

typing p. 691

crossmatching p. 691

IN REVIEW

Water is an indispensable nutrient. Body fluids make up approximately 60 percent of the total body weight of an adult and 70 to 80 percent of the total body weight of a full-term infant. The fluid system transports nutrients to the cells, removes waste products and maintains a stable physical and chemical environment in the body.

Body fluids are distributed in the intracellular compartment and extracellular compartment, the latter being interstitial and intravascular. The proportions of ICF and ECF vary with age, sex and body fat.

Body fluid is made up of water (solvent) and dissolved substances (solutes) such as electrolytes, minerals, glucose and urea. Electrolytes are the primary solutes in body fluid. Body fluid and dissolved substances constantly shift from one compartment to another. Water moves by osmosis and filtration; electrolytes by diffusion and active transport.

Fluids and electrolytes are derived from the ingestion of fluids and food and from metabolic oxidation. They are lost through urine and feces, expiration and perspiration. Fluid and electrolyte balance is regulated by osmotic pressure and kidney function. The gastrointestinal tract and thirst also play a role in maintaining this balance.

The acid-base or pH balance of the body is upset with large losses or gains of fluid or with a depletion or excess of essential acid or base reserves, resulting in acidosis or alkalosis. The pH of body fluids is maintained within a narrow range of 7.35 and 7.45 for normal body function. It is regulated by four mechanisms: dilution, buffer systems (bicarbonate, phosphate and protein) and respiratory and kidney regulating systems.

Insufficient intake, disturbances in the gastrointestinal tract or the kidneys, excess perspiration or volume losses from hemorrhage, burns and trauma can all lead to fluid, electrolyte and acid-base imbalances. Severe electrolyte deficits or excesses can be life-threatening and require medical intervention. Many are associated with a disease condition which inhibits absorption or excretion of one or more electrolytes. Imbalances must be watched for in patients who have been vomiting for several days or are postoperative. Acid-base imbalances can be respiratory or metabolic and are diagnosed by arterial blood gas analysis.

Fluid and electrolyte needs vary through the life cycle. In pregnancy, total blood volume is increased by approximately 50 percent and many pregnant women experience fluid retention. Until the age of two, a large proportion of a child's total body weight is made up of water. Infants are vulnerable to fluid and electrolyte imbalances because of this and because their homeostatic mechanisms are still immature. Children continue to need a greater volume of fluids in proportion to their body weight. They become dehydrated quickly with even minor gastrointestinal disturbances. With adolescence, all body systems mature and the homeostatic mechanisms for regulating fluid and electrolyte balance begin to function as they do in adults.

Women tend to retain fluids two to three days immediately prior to the menstrual period. Many women also experience difficulty with fluid retention during menopause. A gradual lessening in the efficiency of the fluid and electrolyte regulating mechanisms throughout adulthood makes it harder for older adults to recover from imbalances. Also older adults often drink insufficient amounts to meet their bodily needs, particularly when they are ill.

Assessment of a patient's fluid, electrolyte and acid-base balance includes the nursing health history and the measurement of body weight, vital signs and intake and output. Accurate recording and measurement of fluid intake and output is essential in suspected imbalance situations. These should be about the same in any 48-hour period. Physical assessments are related to the signs and symptoms of imbalances. The parameters of physical assessment include skin and tongue turgor, moisture in the oral cavity, tearing and salivation, appearance and temperature of the skin, facial appearance, edema, distention of neck and hand veins, and neuromuscular irritability. Laboratory tests are valuable in confirming findings.

The two common nursing diagnostic labels for fluid volume problems are *fluid volume deficit* and *fluid volume excess*. Problems associated with fluid volume excess, like pulmonary edema, and electrolyte and acid-base imbalances fall out of the realm of independent nursing intervention. Such problems are regarded as collaborative problems since physicians' orders are usually needed to initiate treatment.

Nursing interventions include health teaching, the maintenance of therapeutic fluid intake and the administration of electrolyte supplements. Fluid and electrolyte therapy is ordered by the physician. Fluids are provided orally and intravenously (for those unable to tolerate oral intake). Patients with fluid retention may be placed on fluid and dietary restrictions.

Intravenous fluids are delivered into peripheral and central veins. Meticulous care and careful assessment is mandatory throughout intravenous fluid therapy to prevent complications. Body substance precautions must be used to protect not only the nurse but also other members of the health care team from blood borne infections. Blood transfusion therapy is prescribed to restore circulating blood volume, to correct red blood cell deficiency or to maintain clotting ability. While blood transfusion is often a life-sustaining intervention, it is accompanied by the risk of serious reactions, most notable blood incompatibility. Strict agency protocol and guidelines must be followed in identifying the patient and the blood product, initiating and maintaining the infusion, and monitoring the patient for reactions.

LEARNING ACTIVITY

Case Study: Mr. Miller is admitted to an active treatment hospital in a large city. His diagnosis was tentatively given as dehydration and emaciation. The physician, Dr. Shirley Black, has ordered food and fluids as tolerated and various laboratory tests. She has also ordered an intravenous of $D_5W/0.45$ NaCl to infuse at 100 ml/hr.

Mr. Miller is 70 years old and lives on Social Security. He has no family and lives alone in a rooming house where he cooks on a small hot plate. A friend accompanied him to the hospital. Mr. Miller is very thin and says he has not eaten well in months. He appears frightened; this is his first admission to hospital.

a.   What is dehydration?

b.   What subjective and objective observations might you anticipate? Why?

c.   What factors should be taken into consideration in explaining the intravenous infusion to Mr. Miller?

d.   The intravenous infusion has been established using a macrodrop administration set with a drop factor of 10. Calculate the intravenous rate of flow in drops/minute.

e.   What observations could you make regarding Mr. Miller's intravenous infusion?

f.   Outline a nursing plan of care for this patient, including nursing diagnoses, expected outcomes, and interventions.

g.   How can you evaluate the results of your planned nursing interventions for this patient?

REFERENCES AND READINGS

BOWERS, A.C. and THOMPSON, J.M. (1984). *Health assessment* (2nd ed.). St. Louis: Mosby.

BULLOCK, B.L. and ROSENDAHL, P.P. (1988). *Pathophysiology: Adaptations and alterations in function* (2nd ed.). Glenview, IL: Scott, Foresman.

CAMP-SORRELL, D. (1992) Implantable ports: Everything you always wanted to know. *Journal of Intravenous Nursing, 15*, 262.

CAPKA, M.B., CAREY, S., MARKS, D., WILSON, M. and BENARD, J. (1991). Nursing observations of central venous catheters. *Journal of Intravenous Nursing, 14*, 243.

CHASE, L. (1993) Venipuncture for initiating peripheral intravenous therapy. *Parenteral Therapy Manual.* Vancouver, B.C.: Vancouver General Hospital.

CONDON, R. and NYHUS, L. (1988). *Manual of surgical therapeutics* (7th ed.). Boston: Little, Brown.

COULTER, K. (1992). Intravenous therapy for the elder patient: Implications for the intravenous nurse. *Journal of Intravenous Nursing, 15*(Supplement), S18.

DRAGO, S. S. (1992). Banking on your own blood. *AJN. 92*(3), 61.

EARNEST V.V. (1992). *Clinical skills in nursing practice* (2nd ed.). Philadelphia: Lippincott.

FISCHBACH, F.A. (1992). *Manual of laboratory and diagnostic tests* (4th ed.). Philadelphia: Lippincott.

FLYNN, J.M. and HACKEL, R. (1990) *Technological foundations in nursing.* Norwalk, CT: Appleton & Lange.

GILLIS, A. (1983). Hazards and complications of IV therapy. *Dimensions in Health Services, 60*(5), 9.

GROER, M.W. and SHEKLETON, M.E. (1989). Basic pathophysiology. St. Louis: Mosby.

HEALTH AND WELFARE CANADA. (1991). Intravenous therapy guidelines. Ottawa: Minister of Supply and Services. (Catalogue H39-49/3-1989E).

HOLDER, C. and ALEXANDER, J. (1990). Guide to IV therapy. *AJN. 90*(2), 43.

HOLMAN, S.R. (1987). *Essentials of nutrition.* Philadelphia: Lippincott.

INTRAVENOUS NURSES SOCIETY (1990). Intravenous nursing standards of practice. *Journal of Intravenous Nursing.*

IV THERAPY: CLINICAL SKILLBUILDERS. (1990). Springhouse, PA: Springhouse.

JOSEPHSON, A. (1985). The relationship between IV fluid contamination and the frequency of tubing replacement. *Infection Control, 6,* 367.

KEE, J.L. (1986). *Fluids and electrolytes with clinical applications* (4th ed.). New York: Wiley.

KEE, J.L. (1990). *Handbook of laboratory and diagnostic tests with nursing implications.* Norwalk, CT: Appleton & Lange.

KEYES, J.L. (1985). *Fluid, electrolyte, and acid–base regulation.* Monterey, CA: Wadsworth.

KROZEK, C. (1993). Intravascular therapy. In *Nursing procedures: Student version.* Springhouse, PA: Springhouse.

LABORATORY WARD MANUAL. (1992). North Vancouver, BC: Lions Gate Hospital.

LaROCCA, J.C. and OTTO, S.E. (1989). *Pocket guide to intravenous therapy.* St. Louis: Mosby.

LESLIE, L. (1991). Intravenous therapy and direct IV medication. *Acute Care Nursing Orientation Manual.* Vancouver, BC: University Hospital, Shaughnessy Site.

MACBRYDE, C.M. and BACKLOW, R.S. (Eds). (1970). *Signs and symptoms: Applied pathologic physiology and clinical interpretation* (5th ed.). Philadelphia: Lippincott.

MARTINI, F. (1989). *Fundamentals of anatomy and physiology.* Englewood Cliffs, NJ: Prentice-Hall.

MESSNER, R. and PINKERMAN M.L. (1992). Preventing a peripheral IV infection. *Nursing, 22*(6), 34.

METHENEY, N.M. (1992). *Fluid and electrolyte balance* (2nd ed.). Philadelphia: Lippincott.

MILLIAM, D.A. (1988). Managing complications of IV therapy. *Nursing, 18*(3), 34.

NATIONAL BLOOD RESOURCE EDUCATION PROGRAM'S NURSING EDUCATION WORKING GROUP. (1991). Choosing blood components and equipment. *AJN. 91*(6), 42.

NORTON, B.A. and MILLER, A.M. (1986). *Skills for professional nursing practice.* Norwalk, CT: Appleton & Lange.

NURSING PHOTOBOOK: MANAGING IV THERAPY. (1980). Horsham, PA: Intermed Communications.

OLINGER, M. (1989). Disorders of calcium and magnesium. *Emergency medical clinics of North America, 7*(4), 796.

PILLITTERI, A. (1992). *Maternal and child heath nursing.* Philadelphia: Lippincott.

RITTER, H.T.M. (1990). Evaluating and selecting general purpose infusion pumps. *Journal of Intravenous Nursing, 13,* 156.

SCHRIER, R. (1986). *Renal and electrolyte disorders* (3rd ed.). Boston: Little, Brown.

SHERIDAN, E., PATTERSON, H.R. and GUSTAFSON, E.A. (1982). *Falconer's the drug, the nurse, the patient* (7th ed.). Philadelphia: Saunders.

SMITH, A.J. and JOHNSON, J.Y. (1990) *Nurses' guide to clinical procedures.* Philadelphia: Lippincott.

SOMMERS, M. (1990). Rapid fluid resuscitation: How to correct dangerous deficits. *Nursing, 20*(1), 52.

SPEER, E.W. (1990). Central venous catheterization: Issues associated with the use of single- and multiple-lumen catheters. *Journal of Intravenous Nursing, 13,* 30.

STANFIELD, P. (1986). *Nutrition and diet therapy.* Boston: Jones and Bartlett.

STROOT, V.R, LEE, C.A. and BARRETT, C.A. (1984). *Fluids and electrolytes* (3rd ed.). Philadelphia: F.A. Davis.

TACKETT, J.J. and HUNSBERGER, M. (1981). *Family centered care of children and adolescents.* Philadelphia: Saunders.

TRUCKER, J.A. and SUSSMAN-KARTEN, K. (1987). Treating acute diarrhea and dehydration with oral rehydration solutions. *Pediatric Nurse, 13,* 169.

VAUGHAN, V.C. III, McKAY, R.J. and BEHRMAN, R.E. (1979). *Nelson textbook of pediatrics* (11th ed.). Philadelphia: Saunders.

WELDY, N.J. (1992). *Body fluids and electrolytes.* St. Louis: Mosby.

WILLIAM, M.H. (1993). *Lifetime: Fitness and wellness* (3rd ed.). Madison, WI: Brown and Benchmark.

WOODTLI, A.O. (1990) Thirst: A critical care nursing challenge. *Dimensions of Critical Care Nursing, 9*(1), 6.

CHAPTER 23

Oxygen Needs

CENTRAL QUESTIONS

1. In what way is oxygen essential to life?

2. What are the structures and functions of the respiratory and cardiovascular systems?

3. How do the processes of ventilation, diffusion and transportation supply oxygen to body cells?

4. What are the body's lung clearance mechanisms and how do they function to ensure clean air intake?

5. What are the main determinants of adequate oxygen supply to tissues?

6. How do oxygen needs vary throughout the life cycle?

7. What are the common oxygenation problems?

8. What basic principles does the nurse apply in assisting individuals to meet their oxygenation needs?

9. How does the nurse assess an individual's oxygenation status?

10. What are the common nursing diagnostic statements for individuals with oxygenation problems?

11. How might the nurse develop a plan of care for individuals with oxygenation problems?

12. What strategies might the nurse implement in helping individuals, families or groups to promote optimum oxygenation?

13. What health protecting strategies might the nurse implement to maintain respiratory function, oxygen transport and tissue perfusion in individuals who are ill?

14. What health restoring and supportive strategies might the nurse implement in the care of individuals with oxygenation problems?

15. How might the nurse evaluate the individual's response to nursing interventions?

INTRODUCTION

Oxygen is an essential nutrient for life. Body cells need a continuous supply of oxygen for all metabolic processes and for the production of energy. As the physiologist Haldane noted, "oxygen lack not only stops the motor but wrecks the human machine" (cited in Lacey, 1988, 17). Deprived of oxygen, cells malfunction, become damaged and eventually die. Cells of the brain and the heart are particularly sensitive to a lack of oxygen. Within only a few minutes of oxygen deprivation, these cells suffer irreversible damage and death quickly follows.

The supply of oxygen to body cells, referred to as **oxygenation**, is a complex process involving the respiratory and cardiovascular systems. Normally, oxygen is taken into the body by the respiratory system through the air we breathe. It is carried to all body cells within seconds by the cardiovascular system. The cells use the oxygen to produce energy and then release quantities of a metabolic waste product, carbon dioxide. Carbon dioxide is taken up by the blood and carried to the lungs for immediate elimination from the body.

The term **respiration** is used to describe the exchange of oxygen and carbon dioxide between the atmosphere and the cells of the body. The body cannot store oxygen and excessive amounts of carbon dioxide are poisonous to cells. Therefore, it is essential that both the respiratory and cardiovascular systems are functioning optimally. Problems in either system or insufficient oxygen in the atmosphere will interfere with the ability to meet our need for oxygen.

This chapter will provide the nurse with basic knowledge of oxygenation, factors affecting oxygenation and common oxygenation problems. Methods of assessing oxygen health status and measures to protect and restore the health of individuals experiencing problems meeting their oxygen needs are outlined. In addition, ways of assisting people to promote healthy oxygenation in daily living are also presented.

PHYSIOLOGY OF OXYGENATION

The respiratory and cardiovascular systems work together to supply oxygen to the cells and eliminate carbon dioxide from the body. The respiratory system consists of the upper and lower **airways** and the lungs (see Figure 23.1). The upper airways consist of the nose, pharynx, larynx and trachea. Their primary functions are to provide a passageway for air entering and leaving the body and to warm, filter and moisturize it on entry. The lower airways are the two bronchi and their branches which deliver oxygen to the functional areas of the lungs and return unused air and carbon dioxide to the atmosphere. The lungs are tissues made up of clusters of tiny airways (bronchioles), blood vessels

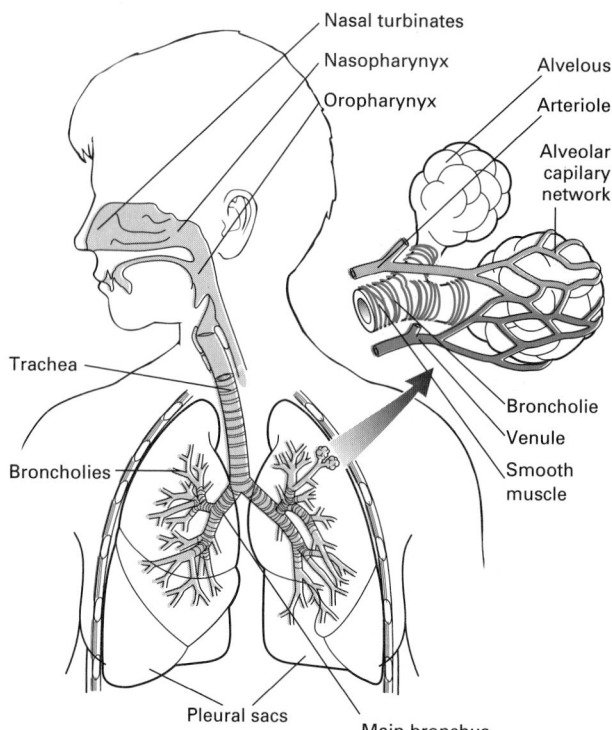

FIGURE 23.1   The respiratory tract

SOURCE: Berger, K.J. and Williams, M.B. (1992). *Fundamentals of nursing: Collaborating for optimal health*. Norwalk, CT: Appleton & Lange, 1218. Reproduced with permission.

and the alveolar membrane. The exchange of gases occurs in the alveolar sacs of the lungs. The upper and lower airways and the bronchioles are lined with mucous membrane, part of which contains cilia and secretes mucus to trap organisms and other foreign material.

The cardiovascular system includes the heart; the network of arteries, veins and capillaries; and blood. It provides the mechanism for transporting oxygen and carbon dioxide. The heart supplies the force or pumping action that circulates blood throughout the body. Oxygen is carried from the lungs via the arteries to the tissues and carbon dioxide is carried from the tissues via the veins back to the lungs. There are three major processes involved in oxygenation. These are ventilation, diffusion and transport.

VENTILATION

Ventilation is the mechanical movement of air in and out of the lungs. It is achieved by a pressure gradient in which gases flow from an area of higher pressures to one of lower pressures. Air is taken into the lungs when the pressure inside the lungs (intrapulmonic) is less than air pressure in the atmosphere. Inhalation ceases when atmospheric air pressure and intrapulmonary pressures are equal. When the pressure inside the lungs is greater than atmospheric pressure, air is moved out. Intrapulmonic pressures are generated by changes in the size of the thoracic cavity through the work of breathing.

Breathing   Breathing has two phases: *inhalation* (inspiration) when air is taken into the lungs, and *exhalation* (expiration) when air is passed out of the lungs. During inhalation, the inspiratory muscles, namely the diaphragm and the external intercostals, contract increasing the size of the thoracic cavity. The diaphragm flattens and descends, the ribs lift upward and outward and the sternum moves outward to lengthen the thorax and expand its lateral and anteroposterior dimensions. The lungs, which adhere to the walls of the thoracic cavity by the attraction of the pleural membranes for each other, expand as the thorax enlarges. Intrapulmonic pressure decreases and air enters the lungs. Air ceases to enter when the intrapulmonic and atmospheric pressures are equal.

Exhalation is a more passive process. The diaphragm relaxes (recoils) and moves upward, the ribs move downward and inward and the sternum moves inward, all of which cause the thoracic cavity to decrease in size. This, combined with the upward push of the abdominal organs against the diaphragm, compresses the lungs and increases intrapulmonic pressure. Air is expelled from the lungs until intrapulmonic and atmospheric pressures are equal. Inhalation normally lasts 1 to 1.5 seconds and exhalation 2 to 3 seconds.

When the effort involved in breathing increases, as, for example, during exercise or with disease, accessory muscles become involved in ventilation. The scalene, sternocleidomastoid and internal intercostal muscles help to increase the size of the thoracic cavity so that more air will enter the lungs. The internal intercostal muscles are activated in forced exhalation to help decrease the size of the rib cage and squeeze air out of the lungs.

Compliance and recoil   Compliance and recoil refer to properties of muscles and tissues which allow them to stretch or expand and then to contract or return to their original position. As the rib cage expands and the lungs enlarge during inhalation, the elastic components of the chest wall and the lungs — skeletal muscle fibres, elastin fibres of the lungs, surrounding connective tissues and the parietal pleura — stretch accordingly. When the inspiratory muscles relax, these elastic components are able to contract, thus returning the rib cage and the lungs to their original positions. This phenomenon is called *elastic recoil*. The ease with which the chest wall and the lungs can expand to fill with air and contract to empty the air is called *compliance*. When compliance is low, greater force is needed to fill and empty the lungs. People with emphysema, for example, have reduced compliance because they have neither the elasticity to expand the lungs fully, nor the elastic recoil to return them to their normal position on exhalation.

Pulmonary volumes and capacities   Pulmonary (or respiratory) volumes and capacities represent the amount of air contained within the lungs, the amount of air that moves in and out of the lungs during quiet breathing and the amount that can be moved in and out with forceful breathing. The terms for the various volumes and capacities are described in Table 23.1. Combinations of pulmonary volumes make up the pulmonary capacities. For example, total lung capacity is the sum of the tidal volume, the inspiratory reserve volume, the expiratory reserve volume and the residual volume. Pulmonary volumes and capacities vary among individuals depending on such factors as body size and build, sex, age and physical condition. Average adult values are given in Table 23.1.

Control mechanisms   The principal mechanism controlling respiration is the respiratory centre in the medulla and pons. The respiratory centre functions as the "control central" for ventilations. It receives chemical and mechanical impulses from the body, coordinates the information to determine respiratory need, and forwards nerve impulses to the muscles that control breathing. The nervous system adjusts the rate, depth and pattern of ventilations so that oxygen and carbon dioxide levels remain relatively constant.

Normally, our breathing patterns change without our awareness in response to fluctuations in the chemical composition of blood and body fluids. This involuntary control of respiration is possible because of chemical receptors (chemoreceptors) located in the respiratory centre, aorta and carotid sinuses. These chemoreceptors are groups of nerves cells that sense changes in oxygen, carbon dioxide and hydrogen ion concentrations. Chemoreceptors in the aorta and carotid sinuses are sensitive to concentrations of oxygen and carbon dioxide in arterial blood. Central chemoreceptors respond only to concentrations of carbon dioxide in the cerebral spinal fluid. The chemoreceptors monitoring carbon dioxide levels are sensitive to hydrogen ions released from the dissociation of carbonic acid. Thus, other conditions altering the pH of body fluids can affect respiratory performance (Martini, 1989). Under normal conditions, the level of carbon dioxide in the blood is the primary regulator of ventilation. For most individuals, an increase in carbon dioxide concentration (hypercapnia) or a decrease in pH causes an immediate increase in respiratory rate.

Mechanical stretch receptors are important in regulating respiratory activity. Stretch receptors located in the visceral pleura around the lungs initiate the Hering-Breuer reflex, which prevents overexpansion of the lungs, particularly during forced ventilations such as those accompanying strenuous exercise. At a specific point in inspiration, these receptors transmit impulses to the respiratory centre, which inhibits inspiration and triggers the expiratory phase of respiration. The reverse takes place during expiration. Other stretch receptors, for example, baroreceptors in the

TABLE 23.1 Summary of Respiratory Volumes and Capacities

	MEASURMENT	ADULT MALE AVERAGE VALUE	DESCRIPTION
Respiratory volumes	Tidal volume (TV)	500 ml	Amount of air inhaled or exhaled with each breath under resting conditions
	Inspiratory reserve volume (IRV)	3100 ml	Amount of air that can be forcefully inhaled after a normal tidal volume inhalation
	Expiratory reserve volume (ERV)	1200 ml	Amount of air that can be forcefully exhaled after a normal tidal volume exhalation
	Residual volume (RV)	1200 ml	Amount of air remaining in the lungs after a forced exhalation
Respiratory capacities	Total lung capacity (TLC)	6000 ml	Maximum amount of air contained in lungs after a maximum inspiratory effort: TLC = TV + IRV + ERV + RV
	Vital capacity (VC)	4800 ml	Maximum amount of air that can be expired after a maximum inspiratory effort: VC = TV + IRV + ERV (should be 80% TLC)
	Inspiratory capacity (IC)	3600 ml	Maximum amount of air that can be inspired after a normal expiration: IC = TV + IRV
	Functional residual capacity (FRC)	2400 ml	Volume of air remaining in the lungs after a normal tidal volume expiration: FRC = ERV + RV

SOURCE: Marieb, E.N. (1992). *Human anatomy and physiology,* 2nd ed. Redwood City, CA: Benjamin/Cummings, 727. Reproduced with permission.

aorta and carotid sinuses, also have an effect on respirations. When blood pressure rises, the respiratory rate increases; it decreases when blood pressure falls.

Breathing can be consciously controlled by activating or restricting muscles of the chest and diaphragm. For instance, breathing is controlled while eating, drinking, singing or speaking. People might hold their breath for short periods while swimming under water, or while trying to avoid inhaling a noxious fume in the air. However, people cannot hold their breath to the detriment of their health. When oxygen levels become too low and carbon dioxide levels too high, we loose consciousness. At this point the nervous system regains control and the individual begins to breathe again.

DIFFUSION

Diffusion is the process by which oxygen and carbon dioxide are exchanged between the air and the blood (external respiration) and between the tissue cells and the blood (internal respiration). External respiration takes place in the lungs, more specifically, in the alveoli across the alveolar–capillary membrane. The alveolar–capillary membrane is a very thin layer of cells that separates each alveolus from its surrounding capillaries. Each lung contains about 150 million alveoli and it has been estimated that the total surface for gas exchange provided by the alveoli equals the area of a tennis court (Martini, 1989; Marieb, 1989).

All gases exert pressure. When gases are mixed together, each gas contributes to the total pressure in proportion to its relative amount in the mixture (Dalton's Law). The pressure exerted by a single gas in a mixture is called the **partial pressure** and it is indicated by a capital P before the chemical abbreviation for the gas (for example, PO_2, PCO_2). The diffusion of a particular gas from the air into a solution (blood) is dependent on its partial pressure alone. Thus, the amount of force exerted by oxygen molecules will affect how much oxygen enters the solution but it will not affect rates of carbon dioxide or nitrogen diffusion. Each gas behaves on its own.

Gases are exchanged in the lungs according to the laws of diffusion. That is, the gases move across a membrane towards the area of lower concentration. On inhalation, oxygen pressure is higher in the alveoli than in the capillary blood; thus oxygen passes from the alveoli into the blood. The same principle holds true for the passage of carbon dioxide from the blood to the alveoli. The pressure of carbon dioxide is higher in the pulmonary capillaries than in the alveoli; thus carbon dioxide diffuses into the alveoli for excretion.

The rate of gas exchange is influenced by the thickness of the alveolar–capillary membrane and the gas exchange surface provided by the alveolar walls. In health, diffusion is rapid because the alveolar–capillary membrane is very thin and the alveolar surface is expansive. Conditions that increase the thickness of the membrane or decrease the size of the alveolar surface reduce gas exchange. For example, edema present in lung tissue increases the thickness of the membrane and slows diffusion. Chronic diseases, such as emphysema or silicosis, damage the alveolar epithelium. As a result, less surface area is available for diffusion to take place.

TRANSPORT

The third process involved in oxygenation is the transport of oxygen and carbon dioxide between the capillaries in the lungs and the cells of the body. This process depends upon an adequate blood volume, an adequate amount of hemoglobin and an effective heart action to pump blood throughout the body.

When oxygen enters the blood it is transported in two forms — a small percentage (about 3%) is dissolved in the plasma and the remaining amount is carried by erythrocytes (red blood cells). Hemoglobin (Hgb) molecules make up the major portion of erythrocyte protein and are responsible for transporting oxygen and carbon dioxide.

Heme is the oxygen-carrying component of hemoglobin. Heme units hold iron ions which combine with oxygen to form oxyhemoglobin. The iron–oxygen interaction is such that oxygen can easily separate from hemoglobin, allowing it to leave the blood and enter the body cells. Oxygen that diffuses from the hemoglobin molecules into plasma is carried via interstitial fluid to the cells.

Carbon dioxide, the end product of cellular metabolism, is transported in several forms. About 5 percent is attached to hemoglobin (carbaminohemoglobin), 5 percent is dissolved in plasma, and the remaining 90 percent is carried in the form of bicarbonate (HCO_3).

LUNG CLEARANCE MECHANISMS

The body has an effective set of mechanisms for ensuring clean air intake and for removing unwanted debris and contaminants. These include filtration, mucociliary action, coughing and sneezing.

Filtration   The body's first clearance mechanism is nasal hair. As air is inhaled, large particles such as sand or dust are trapped in the hairs and thus prevented from entering the nasal cavity.

Mucociliary action   Mucous-secreting glands and tiny hair-like projections called *cilia* line the respiratory passageways. The mucus traps small particles while cilia move the collected particles towards the pharynx, where it is swallowed. It is estimated that a normal adult swallows about 10 ml of transported mucus daily (Traver, Mitchell and Flodquist-Priestley, 1991).

Coughing   Coughing is a defense mechanism the body uses for clearing the airways of secretions and debris. It is triggered by irritants such as smoke, smog, dust or toxic gases; by the infectious process; or by obstructions in the pharynx, larynx, trachea and bronchi. In the act of coughing, the glottis is forcibly closed while the lungs are relatively full. The abdominal and intercostal muscles contract suddenly, pushing the diaphragm upward and creating pressures which force air from the lower respiratory tract upward against the glottis. The glottis reopens and a blast of air passes upward carrying mucus, foreign particles and irritants out of the respiratory system.

Sneezing   A sneeze clears the upper respiratory passages. It is much like a cough except that air is expelled into the nasal cavity instead of the mouth. When someone sneezes, the uvula becomes depressed, closing the oral cavity off from the pharynx and directing the air upward through the nose.

DETERMINANTS OF OXYGENATION

Adequate oxygenation of body tissues is affected by a multitude of factors. We have categorized some of the more basic ones under the headings Environment, Physiological Factors and Health Status, and Health Practices and Lifestyle. Age related influences on oxygenation are discussed in the next section.

ENVIRONMENT

The presence of atmospheric oxygen in adequate concentrations is vital to optimal respiratory functioning. Normally, the atmosphere supplies all the oxygen an individual requires. At sea level, air contains approximately 21 percent oxygen and 0.04 percent carbon dioxide. These concentrations appear to be the most conducive for normal breathing. At higher altitudes, however, the situation is different. As altitude increases, atmospheric pressure decreases. The alveolar pressure correspondingly goes down and less oxygen diffuses into the blood. The body responds by increasing the rate and depth of respirations. Visitors to high altitude areas may experience fatigue until they become acclimatized to the rarefied atmosphere.

Air pollutants such as smoke, industrial gaseous wastes and automobile exhaust fumes may alter the availability of oxygen and have detrimental effects on respiratory functioning. Noxious or toxic gases in the air displace the oxygen normally present and decrease the amount of oxygen available for diffusion.

The respiratory rate is also affected by climate. In hot weather, the peripheral blood vessels dilate. The resistance of blood flow decreases and, consequently, blood pressure drops. The heart responds by increasing cardiac output to maintain blood pressure. With the increase in cardiac output, there is a need for more oxygen. Thus, the rate and depth of respirations increase. In cold weather blood vessels constrict. Blood pressure increases, cardiac action decreases and the need for oxygen is reduced. As a result, respirations become slower.

PHYSIOLOGICAL FACTORS AND HEALTH STATUS

In addition to an adequate supply of oxygen in the atmosphere, our ability to meet our need for oxygen depends on the patency of airways, proper muscular functioning, pulmonary compliance and an adequate mechanism for transporting oxygen and carbon dioxide. Both physiological factors and health status can influence the effectiveness of these processes in oxygenation.

Patent airways   In ventilation, oxygen passes through the nose, pharynx, larynx, trachea, bronchi and bronchioles to the alveoli and then carbon dioxide passes back. Obstructions (partial or complete) in any of the passageways will interfere with the efficiency of ventilation and cause considerable breathing difficulty. Airways can be obstructed by food and fluids. Children often put small objects such as toys and coins into their mouths and subsequently aspirate them. Airway obstruction is always a danger in unconscious individuals, since the tongue can fall back into the oropharynx and block it.

The airway may also be obstructed by excessive or thickened secretions, tumours or tissue growths and edema in the respiratory tract. Diseases such as emphysema, asthma or bronchitis affect ventilation because they obstruct the airway or increase the resistance to the normal flow of air during inhalation and exhalation. Normally, a certain amount of resistance is present in the airways owing to the slight expansion and contraction of the relatively rigid airway structures. When the airways become less elastic because of tissue changes, or obstructed by thickened secretions, the effort involved in breathing increases in an attempt to move air through the narrowed passageways.

Some patients have difficulty clearing secretions for various reasons — because it is painful to cough, because of unconsciousness or because of lack of muscle strength. During the aging process, the pressure an individual can achieve during a maximum inspiration or expiration decreases so that the ability to generate the high air flows re-

quired for effective coughing is reduced. Also, there is decreased ciliary movement in lower airways which slows the cough reflex. Whatever the cause, secretions can accumulate and the patient may require assistance for their removal.

Muscle functioning   The condition of the body's musculature affects breathing. If the chest is unable to expand because of trauma or thoracic or abdominal surgery, ventilation will be impaired. Disease processes that weaken or paralyze the muscles that move the rib cage, such as Guillain-Barré syndrome or poliomyelitis, affect the ability to breath normally.

Continual bed rest and immobility alter ventilation of the lungs. Pressure of the bed against the body limits chest expansion and alveolar ventilations. In the supine or dorsal recumbent position, abdominal organs push against the diaphragm restricting its movement and thus the movement of air through the lungs. Limited or inadequate chest expansion leads to stasis and pooling of respiratory secretions which harbour microorganisms and may cause infection (hypostatic pneumonia).

Pulmonary compliance   Lungs that have the elastic properties to expand and recoil with ease during the act of breathing are said to be compliant. Lungs with low compliance (lungs that are stiff) require greater than normal energy expenditure to achieve adequate levels of ventilation. When extra energy is used routinely for breathing, there is less available for other needs and body functions are compromised. Low or inadequate compliance results from restrictive lung diseases, for example, fibrosis, emphysema, tumour, paralysis, kyphosis or scoliosis (curvature of the spine).

Transport of oxygen and carbon dioxide   Many factors can affect the transport of oxygen and carbon dioxide to and from the cells. There may be an inadequate force from the heart to pump blood through the lungs, or there may be an impediment in the return flow of blood from the lungs to the heart causing a slowing up (stasis) of blood in the small vessels that surround the alveoli. Such conditions will interfere with oxygenation by disturbing the balance of partial pressures of oxygen and carbon dioxide circulating through the lungs.

Similarly, any condition affecting the blood volume and the circulation of blood to the tissues can interfere with the transportation of oxygen from the lungs to the cells. This would include all types of heart diseases, bleeding disorders and arterial or venous disorders, as well as blood dyscrasias. In anemia, for example, the blood lacks adequate hemoglobin to carry oxygen to the cells of the body.

Among the major diseases affecting the cardiovascular system are those which cause the blood vessels to narrow and deteriorate, resulting in inadequate oxygenation and subsequent damage of tissues in vital organs, such as the heart, the brain, the kidneys or other parts of the body.

Most of the damage is caused by three major types of heart disease — atherosclerosis (hardening of the arteries), hypertension (high blood pressure) and congenital defects. These diseases may lead to congestive heart failure, myocardial infarction and stroke.

HEALTH PRACTICES AND LIFESTYLE

There are many health practices and lifestyle factors that can affect the ability to meet one's oxygen needs. The positive influence of exercise and fitness as well as the negative effects of cigarette smoking and occupational hazards will be discussed here.

Exercise increases the efficiency of all body functions and processes. Regular exercise, particularly aerobic exercise, such as sustained speed walking, running or swimming, enhances respiratory and cardiovascular endurance, as well as muscular strength and tone. During exercise, the metabolic rate goes up and demands for oxygen increase. The person breathes more deeply and rapidly to take in extra oxygen, and the heart beats more rapidly and forcefully to supply the needed oxygen to the cells. Over time, the lungs increase their capacity to take up oxygen, the blood increases its capacity to pick up and carry more oxygen and the heart strengthens in its capacity to supply the oxygenated blood to the muscles. Furthermore, the muscles become very effective in using oxygen to generate the energy needed for their activity. The more conditioned the muscles become, the less

Regular exercise, particularly aerobic exercise such as swimming, enhances respiratory and cardiovascular functioning.

oxygen they need to accomplish their work. In short, with regular exercise, cardiopulmonary effort and oxygen use in the body become very efficient, bringing significant benefits to the health and well-being of the individual.

Cigarette smoking is a hazard to health and a major factor associated with lung cancer, chronic obstructive pulmonary disease (COPD) and coronary artery disease. In the lungs, cigarette smoke induces a variety of inflammatory changes which lead to disease. Small airways become ulcerated, narrowed and fibrosed. Mucous secretion in the bronchi produces sputum and a characteristic smoker's cough. Cilia are damaged and ciliary movement is impaired, thereby interfering with effective ciliary clearance. The alveoli themselves may suffer from inflammation and structural abnormalities which result in disease. While a direct cause-and-effect relationship between smoking and coronary artery disease has not been determined, the relationship is thought to be due to the physiologic effect of nicotine and other chemicals that increase the risk of atherosclerosis. Cigarette smoking "has been shown to cause changes in blood lipid levels, increasing triglycerides and total cholesterol while decreasing high density lipoprotein cholesterol, a lipid profile more prone to atherosclerosis" (Williams, 1993, 180).

Not only is smoking detrimental to the health of those who smoke, it is also harmful to those exposed to the passive or sidestream smoke given off by burning cigarettes. Epidemiological studies have found that lung cancer is more prevalent in people exposed to passive smoke than those living in a smoke-free environment. Similarly, children of parents who smoke suffer more episodes of respiratory illness such as chronic coughing, bronchitis and laryngitis than do children of non-smoking parents (Williams, 1993; Ellis and Nowlis, 1994).

Certain occupations expose workers to irritants that may cause lung disease. People working at construction sites, mines, shipyards and chemical plants are exposed to dusts and hazardous materials that pervade the atmosphere, for example, coal dust, asbestos fibres, silica dust or toxic fumes. Irritants infiltrate the lining of the air passageways and lung tissues, causing inflammation and damage. Scar tissue forms which reduces lung elasticity and restricts air flow along the passageways. "Chronic irritation and stimulation of the epithelium and its defences cause changes in the epithelium that increase the likelihood of lung cancer" (Martini, 1989, 651).

MEDICATIONS

Drugs and anesthetics that act as depressants on the central nervous system decrease the rate and depth of respirations and may, when administered in large dosages, cause respiratory arrest. Morphine and meperidine are common examples of drugs that depress respirations.

OXYGEN NEEDS THROUGHOUT THE LIFE CYCLE

During pregnancy, the diaphragm is pushed upward as the fetus grows and the uterus expands in the abdominal cavity. The lungs of the mother are gradually squeezed as space in the chest cavity decreases. Pregnant women usually find that they breathe more rapidly than usual and may experience shortness of breath and dyspnea (difficult breathing) after mild exertion.

The fetus receives its needed oxygen from the mother, the supply being transferred from the mother's circulation to the placenta and, then, via the umbilical cord to the fetus. Readers interested in the fetal circulation and the changes that take place in cardiovascular and pulmonary function after birth are referred to an obstetrical nursing book.

Infants are obligatory nose-breathers during the first year of life. Therefore, congestion in the nasal passages can create problems, especially during feeding. Infants breathe much more rapidly than adults; 30 to 50 breaths per minute is the normal range. The rate remains high through the first months of life, slowing down gradually to about 20 to 40 breaths per minute at 12 months. The higher rate is due to the smaller lung capacity. A normal full-term infant has a total lung capacity of only 300 ml and a tidal volume of 25 ml.

Respiratory infections are common in infants and children. Newborns are usually immune, because of antibodies received from the mother, until they are two to three months old. During the first two to three years of life, respiratory infection is not uncommon as children gradually build up active immunity to the organisms normally prevalent in their environment. Immunization (which confers passive immunity) to whooping cough is routinely started in infancy to protect the child from this disease.

During childhood, the diameter of the upper respiratory tract is small, and obstruction caused by the accumulation of secretions from an infection, an allergy or the inhalation of a foreign body can be serious. Coins and toys are common sources of obstruction in young children.

With adolescence, there is a rapid increase in lung capacity as the chest expands. Boys show a greater increase than girls do, the chest cavity of the male becoming larger and the shoulders broader than those of his female counterpart. Adolescence can be a time of respiratory health risk, as many smokers begin their habit in the teenage years, exposing themselves to serious future health problems.

Respiratory infections, in the form of colds, bronchitis and pneumonia, are a common cause of short-term illness in adults. Most people appear to be most resistant to these infections in the late middle years. However, this is also the time that chronic respiratory ailments become more prevalent. The term *chronic obstructive pulmonary disease* (COPD) is used to refer to a group of disorders associated with chronic obstruction of air flow into and out of the lungs. COPD includes such conditions as emphysema, chronic bronchitis and asthma. These are irreversible conditions commonly associated with cigarette smoking, air pollution and exposure to hazardous substances.

The efficiency of an individual's cardiorespiratory system gradually declines with age. The effects may not be evident at rest but become noticeable when effort is required. Adults who remain physically active, however, maintain higher aerobic capacities than do sedentary individuals. In the normal aging process, the chest wall stiffens and the lungs lose their elasticity. As a result, the ability to ventilate the lungs slowly decreases. According to Marieb, "vital capacity decreases by about one-third by the age of 70" (1984, 258). In addition, as people age, their ciliary activity and cough efficiency decrease making them more vulnerable to respiratory infections. The cardiovascular system also undergoes gradual change during aging. Usually maximum cardiac output decreases so that by the age of 65 years it is typically 20 to 30 percent less than that of a young adult. In middle age, blood pressure increases owing to the diminishing elasticity of blood vessel walls but stabilizes, by about the age of 65 years (Bell, 1983).

COMMON PROBLEMS

Disturbances in oxygenation may cause a number of health problems. These commonly include hypoxia and hypoxemia, dyspnea, cough and chest pain.

Hypoxemia and hypoxia   **Hypoxemia** refers to a decrease in the oxygen content of the blood and is frequently associated with **hypoxia**, which is an insufficient supply of oxygen to the tissues. The body's responses to hypoxemia and hypoxia depend on how suddenly these states develop. With rapidly developing hypoxia there are changes in CNS functioning because the higher centres are more sensitive to oxygen depletion. The patient may exhibit motor incoordination and impaired judgement, increased (rapid) pulse, rapid, shallow respirations, dyspnea, increased restlessness and flaring of nares. Patients with long-standing conditions (for example, COPD) may show signs of fatigue, drowsiness, apathy, inattentiveness or delayed reaction time, altered thought process, headache, chest pain, enlarged heart, anorexia, decreased urinary output, weakness of extremity muscles or muscle pain.

Dyspnea   People whose oxygen needs are not being met often experience **dyspnea**, defined as difficult or laboured breathing. An individual with dyspnea may not be able to climb a flight of stairs or walk a block to the corner store without finding it hard to breathe. Often, it is more difficult to breathe when lying flat (orthopnea). Asthmatic patients, those with chronic obstructive lung disorders and those with heart conditions frequently use numerous pillows to raise themselves to a sitting position for more comfortable sleeping. The sitting position promotes maximum expansion of the chest and also prevents the pooling of blood in the large abdominal vessels. Excessive fatigue is commonly experienced, as even normal daily activities can be exhausting to the person who does not have enough oxygen to supply bodily needs.

Cough　　Coughing is the body's mechanism for ridding the respiratory tract of irritations and obstructions. It is also a troublesome symptom associated with respiratory disease. The characteristics of the cough and the nature of sputum produced are often indicative of specific diseases. For instance, a harsh productive cough of yellow–green sputum is indicative of bacterial infection. Clear, white sputum can be characteristic of asthma and pink froth sputum indicative of pulmonary edema. A brassy, *nonproductive cough* (a cough without the production of mucus) is associated with pressure on the trachea. *Hemoptysis* is the coughing up of sputum containing varying amounts of blood. It may be associated with cancer of the lung or chronic conditions such as bronchiectasis.

Chest pain　　Many patients with respiratory problems experience pain in the chest. The pain may or may not be associated with the act of breathing. Pain may be caused by a number of different factors, such as inflammation, the presence of space-occupying lesions or increased muscular activity as the patient works harder to breathe. The presence or absence of chest pain should be noted. A description of the pain (for example, sharp, dull, intermittent or steady) should be reported, as should the location of the pain and its relationship to breathing.

ASSESSING OXYGEN NEEDS

The assessment of a patient's ability to meet his or her oxygen needs is a critical nursing activity. Using interviewing techniques and physical assessment skills, the nurse gathers subjective and objective data about the patient's oxygenation status. In determining oxygen needs and developing a plan of individualized care, the nurse also draws information from the medical history, from laboratory and diagnostic test results and from the physician's plan of care.

NURSING HEALTH HISTORY

The health history provides the basis for planning individualized patient care. The nurse gathers information about the patient's usual pattern of oxygenation, including information about home environment, activity level, and whether or not the patient smokes. Recent changes or deviations from the patient's usual breathing pattern, any recent or past related health problems (for example, respiratory and cardiovascular diseases) and symptoms relating to the presenting problem are explored. The patient's family history is also pertinent. Problems such as allergies, asthma, chronic bronchitis or frequent bouts of pneumonia tend to be genetically predisposed. Many people with chronic respiratory problems use oxygen at home (portable units), and they often use humidifiers, nebulizers and other aids as well. These should be noted on the patient's record. Finally, the individual's health-promoting and health-protecting patterns are examined to determine opportunities for health teaching.

Patients who are admitted with oxygen problems may be in severe distress. They may be hypoxic, or have difficulty breathing or severe chest pain. They may not have the energy to speak and they may be anxious and confused. A quick visual assessment before undertaking the health history will determine the degree of distress a patient is in. When patients are in distress, the health history interview is deferred until their immediate needs are met and they are more comfortable. The nurse may need to collect data during several visits or allow for periods of rest for patients who become short of breath or experience chest pain during the interviews. The history may also be obtained from a family member. A guide for taking an oxygen health history follows.

MEASUREMENTS

VITAL SIGNS

The assessment of oxygenation status includes measurement of the vital signs — temperature, pulse, respirations and blood pressure. The techniques for obtaining these measurements are described in Chapter 15.

PULSE OXIMETRY

Pulse oximetry is a simple, painless and non-invasive method of measuring a patient's arterial blood oxygen saturation levels. Oxygen saturation is the amount of oxygen being carried by hemoglobin, expressed as a percentage of the maximum oxygen-carrying capacity of the hemoglobin. Measurements are made with an oximeter that uses a light-sensitive probe attached to cutaneous tissue with a pulsating vascular bed, such as the fingertip, ear lobe, toe or bridge of the nose. Oximetry is used in a wide variety of situations to monitor responses to treatment or to observe patients who are at risk for developing hypoxemia. For instance, it may be implemented for patients recovering from anesthesia in the immediate postoperative period. Monitoring can be intermittent or continuous. The steps involved in conducting pulse oximetry are outlined in Procedure 23.1.

Oxygenation

Health and Illness Patterns

USUAL PATTERN OF OXYGENATION

- Describe your usual pattern of breathing. Is it effortless? Difficult?

- Does activity affect your breathing?

- Do you tire easily?

- Does your breathing pattern affect your activities of daily living?

- Do you have allergies in different seasons?

- Do you smoke? If so, what type of tobacco (cigarette, cigar, pipe)? For how many years? How many cigarettes per day?

- Does anyone in your home smoke? Are you exposed to smoke at work?

- Are you exposed to respiratory irritants at home or at work? For example, glue, paints, silica, asbestos, pesticides, grain dust, pets, plants?

- Do you use any aids for breathing such as oxygen, humidifiers or nebulizers?

- Do you routinely use over-the-counter nasal sprays or inhalers?

- How many pillows do you sleep with?

RECENT CHANGES IN PATTERN OF OXYGENATION

- Have there been any recent changes in your usual pattern of oxygenation? Shortness of breath? Difficulty breathing? Wheezing? Troublesome cough? Excessive sputum? Fatigue? Chest pain?

- Have you had a recent illness that affected breathing? A cold? Respiratory infection (for example, strep throat, tonsillitis)?

- Any recent injuries to the thoracic cage (ribs) or surgeries?

PRESENTING HEALTH PROBLEM

- Describe the symptoms you are experiencing now. Do you have wheezing? Tightness in the chest? Shortness of breath? Do you have a cough? How did it begin (sudden or gradual)? Is it dry or accompanied by sputum? Does it cause fatigue? Does it affect your sleep?

- Do you have sputum? If so, describe it. What is the amount? Appearance (clear, mucoid, yellowish, greenish, purulent, blood-tinged, bloody)?

- Do you have pain associated with breathing? If so, describe it. Onset (gradual or sudden)? Intensity? Frequency? Location? Any radiation?

- Do your lips or nail beds turn blue?

- Do you feel dizzy when you change positions?

- Do your shoes or rings feel tight?

- Does your heart sometimes feel as though it is pounding?

- Do you feel tired or fatigued?

- Have you experienced anorexia and weight loss?

- When did the symptoms begin? Duration? Are they constant or intermittent?

- Are the symptoms associated with an activity, time of event or environmental factors? For example, asthma attack brought on by exposure to cats?

- What remedies have you tried for the symptoms? Have you tried sitting up? Sleeping with pillows? Over-the-counter drugs such as decongestants, nasal sprays? What were the results?

- Do you have a history of any acute or chronic diseases that disrupt oxygenation? For example, colds, allergies, asthma, bronchitis, pneumonia, emphysema, high blood pressure, heart disease, anemia?

- Are you on any medications for respiratory problems, high blood pressure or heart disease? If so what kind? Dosage? Frequency?

- Have you had rheumatic fever, a heart murmur or tuberculosis?

- Has any member of your family had emphysema, asthma, respiratory allergies, tuberculosis, heart disease or high blood pressure?

- Have you had past occupations that exposed you to respiratory irritants?

Health Promotion and Protection Patterns

- Do you drink alcohol? If so, how much and how often?

- Do you exercise regularly? If so, what is the nature of your program?

- When was your last chest x-ray?

- When was your last tuberculin test?
- Are your immunizations up to date?
- What home remedies do you use for respiratory problems?
- Do you use an air conditioner, air purifier or humidifier in your home?

- If smoking, do you have any feelings about or interest in quitting?
- Would you like to know about ways to protect yourself from respiratory irritants and pollution?

Pulse oximetry carried out by a respiratory therapist.

Preparing the Patient

Explain the purpose and procedure for the test. Pulse oximetry requires little time and is painless.

Assembling Equipment

The pulse oximeter is a small device with a spectrophotometer probe that contains two sensors. One sensor emits red and infrared light beams through the tissues and the other receives wavelengths of light reflected from capillary hemoglobin. Hemoglobin that is saturated (red) absorbs light differently than does hemoglobin that is desaturated (blue) and reflects light in accordance with the amount it absorbs. The probe measures the amount of light reflected from the hemoglobin and sends the information to a computer which calculates the oxygen saturation and displays the value on a digital screen. The pulse rate is displayed as well.

PHYSICAL ASSESSMENT

Physical assessment of oxygen status involves an examination of the patient's cardiovascular and respiratory functioning. The nurse uses inspection, palpation, auscultation and percussion techniques as outlined in Chapter 15.

Before starting the physical examination it is important to ensure the room is well lit, quiet, warm and private. Natural lighting is necessary to examine subtle colour changes and breathing patterns. Minimal noise facilitates detection of respiratory sounds. Every effort should be made to ensure patient privacy and no interruptions. This enables the patient to relax and helps ensure a comprehensive assessment. Each step of the examination should be carefully explained and clear directions given when needed, for example, "Please breathe in deeply and hold it," so the patient knows what to expect. A calm matter-of-fact manner can often allay anxiety, even for patients who are in distress.

For examination of the chest and lungs, the patient should wear a gown that can be dropped to the waist. Bras and undershirts should be removed to provide maximum view of the chest. The patient should sit upright, lean slightly forward, and have the arms rest comfortably across the lap; shoulders should be brought forward to abduct the scapula so that a greater lung surface can be examined. Assessments should be made in an organized manner. The posterior and lateral aspects of the chest are examined first and then the nurse moves to face the patient for the anterior examination. One side is compared to the other for variations, proceeding from the top downward.

INSPECTION

The nurse begins inspection by exposing the chest and observing the patient's posture and the contour or shape of the thorax. Normally, the transverse diameter should be greater than the anteroposterior (AP) diameter. The normal chest is symmetric with bilateral muscular development although slightly greater muscle development may be present on the patient's dominant side. The rib cartilages should curve slightly out from the sternum. The spinal processes of C7, T1 to T7 should be straight and the scapulae should be symmetrical. The intercostal spaces should

Performing Pulse Oximetry

ACTION	RATIONALE
1. Prepare the patient	Promotes well-being and enables patient participation.
2. Wash hands and gather pulse oximeter and sensor probe.	Reduces transmission of microorganisms.
3. Select a site with adequate peripheral circulation, for example, finger, ear, toe or bridge of nose. If using a finger or toe, check the proximal pulse and capillary refill closest to the site.	Test requires an adequate vascular area for transmission of light.
4. Cleanse the site with water and dry well. If using a finger probe, remove nail polish or false nails.	Body oils, artificial nails or nail polish interfere with transmission of light.
5. Attach the probe to the site according to manufacturer's directions.	Incorrect placement gives an inaccurately low reading or no reading at all.
6. Ask the patient to remain still. If the patient is restless, the probe may be taped **lightly**.	Saturation reading may be inaccurate if circulation is restricted.
7. Turn the machine on.	
8. When the oxygen saturation reading has stabilized, wait 30 seconds and note reading.	Readings can be affected by motion, low perfusion, vasoconstriction, impaired tissue perfusion, intravenous fluids, nail polish and direct excessive lighting.
9. Remove the probe, turn off the machine, and clean the probe with alcohol.	Prevents the spread of microorganisms.
10. Document the date, time, oxygen saturation, observations and nursing continuity of care.	Fulfills requirements for nurse accountability and facilitates interventions.

be flat or depressed. Normal and abnormal configurations of the thorax are illustrated in Table 23.2.

The patient's respiratory movements and breathing pattern are examined next. At this time, the nurse also listens for audible breath sounds (sounds heard without the use of a stethoscope). During breathing, the chest should expand symmetrically and without obvious use of accessory muscles. There should be no retractions or bulging of the intercostal spaces on inspiration. The normal adult breathing pattern is smooth and regular with 12 to 20 breaths per minute. The ratio of respirations to pulse rate is 1:4. Breathing should be quiet and effortless. Audible breath sounds are usually the result of extra breathing effort combined with obstruction. **Stridor** is a harsh high-pitched "crowing" sound heard on inspiration when there is a narrowing of the upper airway, that is, the larynx or trachea. Infants and young children with croup often manifest stridor. **Stertor** is a snoring sound made when secretions are present in the trachea or large bronchi. **Wheezing** is a high-

pitched "whistling" sound often made on inspiration when the airway is partially obstructed. People with asthma make wheezing sounds. Table 23.3 describes and illustrates normal and abnormal breathing patterns.

Sputum, if produced, must be inspected. Sputum is not saliva. It is a mucous secretion from the lungs, bronchi and trachea composed of mucus, dust particles and microbial debris, saliva, nasal and sinus secretions, normal oral bacteria and epithelial cells. Normal sputum is clear, white and slightly frothy because it contains air bubbles. Abnormal sputum is produced as a pulmonary reaction to any constant recurring irritant including nasal discharge. The characteristics and amounts of sputum reflect the patient's overall condition and the particular pulmonary dysfunction. In assessing sputum, the nurse notes the amount (in millilitres), consistency (thin, watery, thick, sticky, tenacious, mucoid), odour (musty, foul), colour (clear, cloudy, white, yellow, greenish, pink or rusty) and the presence of blood (hemoptysis).

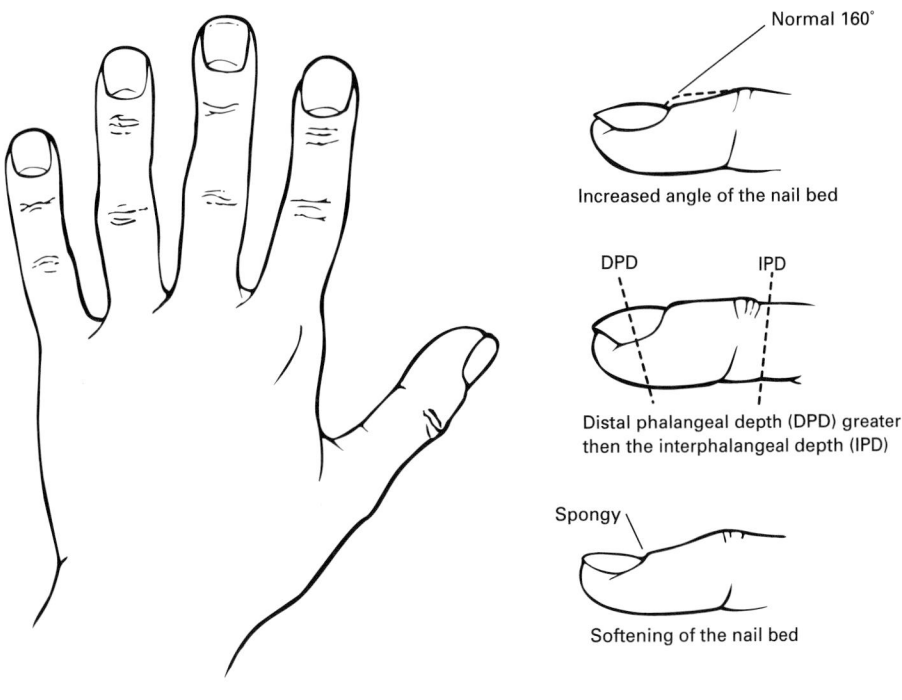

Normal 160°

Increased angle of the nail bed

DPD   IPD

Distal phalangeal depth (DPD) greater then the interphalangeal depth (IPD)

Spongy

Softening of the nail bed

FIGURE 23.2   Clubbing of the fingers

SOURCE: Brill, E.L., and Kilts, D.F. (1986). *Foundations for nursing* (2nd ed.). Norwalk, CT: Appleton-Century-Crofts. Redrawn with permission.

The colour of skin and mucous membranes are also assessed. The patient's skin colour should be consistent with his or her genetic background. If well oxygenated, the skin, nail beds and mucous membranes should be pink in colour. People with darker skin colour should have rosy undertones. There should be no pallor or cyanosis in highly vascular areas. In light-skinned people, cyanosis can be detected in the lips, nail beds, tip of the nose, top of the ear and underside of the tongue. Colour changes can be more subtle in dark-skinned individuals. A bluish hue in the nail beds, lips and gums is normal in people with very dark skin so the buccal mucosa or conjunctivae are the most reliable areas for detection of cyanosis. The facial skin may also be pale grey in a dark-skinned person with central cyanosis.

Finally, the fingers are examined for signs of clubbing. **Clubbing** is an increase in the angle between the base of the nail and fingernail from the normal angle of 160°–180° (Figure 23.2). Clubbing is also manifested by an increase in the depth of the nails; they feel bulky and spongy compared to a normal firm nail base. Clubbing is best seen in the fourth and fifth fingers. It indicates signs of lung disease found in patients with chronic hypoxic conditions, for example, cystic fibrosis, chronic lung infections or cancers of the lung.

PALPATION

Palpation is performed to evaluate thoracic expansion, spasticity or rigidity, chest symmetry during respiration, areas of sensitivity, masses, edema and depressions, unusual movements with respiration, vibrations or pulsations. Skin temperature, turgor or moisture are also assessed. The nurse's hands should be clean and warm before proceeding with the examination.

Palpation of the posterior chest   To palpate the posterior chest, place the hands flat against the chest on the lower third of the rib cage (level of tenth rib), with thumbs pointing towards each other almost touching, and fingers pointing laterally (see Figure 23.3). Ask the patient to inhale deeply. Note the movement of the area between thumbs. It should move upward and outward equally during inspiration. The space between the thumbs on inspiration is a rough measure of expansion and equality of movement. Normal expansion is two to five centimetres; both sides should move equally.

Next, palpate the chest wall for fremitus. **Fremitus** is a vibration that can be felt on the exterior chest wall when a person speaks. Sounds produced in the larynx are transmitted through patent airways and lung tissue to the chest wall where they are felt as vibrations. To palpate for fremitus, place the palmar base of the fingers of one hand over the chest wall and ask the patient to say "ninety-nine" or "one, two, three" or "how now brown cow." These words are effective in examining fremitus because they are resonant and thus produce strong vibrations. Begin at the lung apices and palpate from one side to the other as shown in Figure 23.4. Normally, all people have fremitus. It is loudest

FIGURE 23.3   Palpating the chest for respiratory expansion. A. Posterior. B. Anterior.

TABLE 23.2   Configurations of the Thorax

Normal Adult (for Comparison)

The thorax has an elliptical shape with an anteroposterior: transverse diameter of 1:2 or 5:7

Barrel Chest

Note anteroposterior = transverse diameter and that ribs are horizontal instead of the normal downward slope. This is associated with normal aging and also with chronic emphysema and asthma due to hyperinflation of lungs.

TABLE 23.2 *continued*

Pectus Excavatum

A markedly sunken sternum and adjacent cartilages (also called funnel breast). Depression begins at second intercostal space, becoming depressed most at junction of xiphoid with body of sternum. More noticeable on inspiration. Congenital, usually not symptomatic. When severe, sternal depression may cause embarrassment and a negative self-concept. Surgery may be indicated for cosmetic purposes.

Pectus Carinatum

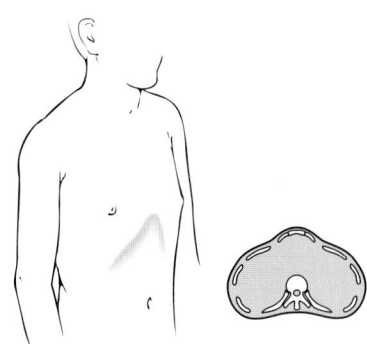

A forward protrusion of the sternum, with ribs sloping back at either side and vertical depressions along costochondral junctions (pigeon breast). Less common than pectus excavatum, this minor deformity requires no treatment. If severe, surgery may be indicated for cosmetic purposes.

Scoliosis

A lateral S-shaped curvature of the thoracic and lumbar spine, usually with involved vertebrae rotation. Note unequal shoulder and scapular height and unequal hip levels, rib interspaces flared on convex site. More prevalent in adolescent age groups, especially girls. Mild deformities are asymptomatic. If severe (> 45 degrees) deviation is present, scoliosis may reduce lung volume, then person is at risk for impaired cardiopulmonary function. Primary impairment is cosmetic deformity, negatively affecting self-image. Refer early for treatment, often surgery.

Kyphosis

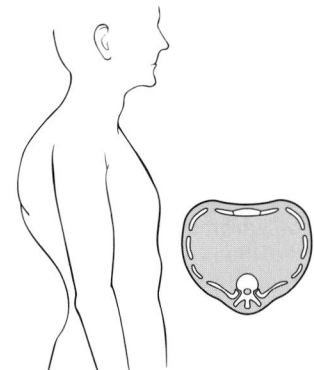

An exaggerated posterior curvature of the thoracic spine (humpback). Mild deformities are asymptomatic. Severe deformities impair cardiopulmonary function. Also associated with aging. Compensation may occur by hyperextension of head to maintain level of vision.

SOURCE: Jarvis, C. (1992). *Physical examination and health assessment*. Philadelphia: Saunders, 514-515. Reproduced with permission.

TABLE 23.3   Breathing Patterns or Rhythm

Normal Adult

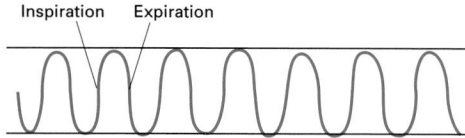

Rate: 10 to 20 breaths per minute
Depth: deep
Pattern: easy, smooth, quiet, even, effortless, occasional sigh, automatic
The ratio of pulse to respirations is constant, about 4:1.

Sigh

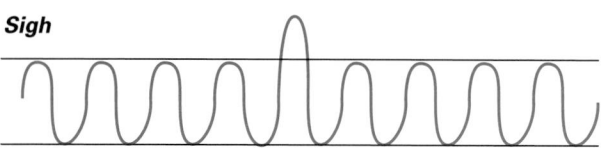

Occasional sighs are normal; their purpose is to expand alveoli. Frequent sighing may indicate emotional dysfunction and may lead to hyperventilation and dizziness.

Tachypnea or Polypnea

Rapid, shallow breathing
Rate: increased over 24 breaths per minute. This is a normal response to fever, fear, or exercise. Also occurs with respiratory insufficiency, pneumonia, alkalosis, pleurisy.

Bradypnea

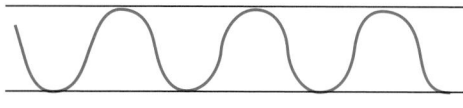

Slow breathing — less than 10 breaths per minute
Regular rate
Occurs in protective response to pain, depression of medulla (respiratory centre), increased intracranial pressure, diabetic coma.

Hyperventilation

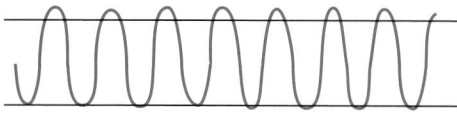

Increase in rate and depth. Normal with extreme exertion, fear or anxiety or when amphetamines are given. Also occurs when blood gas concentrations are altered (either an increase in carbon dioxide or decrease in oxygen). Hyperventilation blows off carbon dioxide causing a decreased level in the blood (alkalosis).
Amount of air in alveoli exceeds the body's metabolic requirements.

Hypoventilation

An irregular shallow slow pattern of inadequate alveolar ventilation which does not meet the body's requirements. Carbon dioxide is retained in the blood (hypercapnia). May be caused by prolonged bed rest, conscious splinting of the chest to avoid respiratory pain, side effect of some medications. Occurs in respiratory diseases such as pneumonia, asthma, emphysema, airway obstructions.

TABLE 23.3 *continued*

Cheyne-Stokes Respiration

A regular cycle in which there is a gradual increase (wax) followed by a gradual decrease (wane) in the depth of respiration and then a period of apnea (temporary cessation of breathing).

Breathing periods last 30–45 seconds with periods of apnea lasting 20 seconds.

Most common causes are congestive heart failure, renal failure, increased intracranial pressure or drug overdose. Occurs normally in infants and aging persons during sleep.

Ataxic

Irregular breathing pattern with both deep and shallow breaths occurring randomly.

Seen in patients with lesions of the medulla.

Biot's Respiration

Disorganized pattern of shallow breaths with irregular periods of apnea. The cycle length is variable, lasting anywhere from 10 seconds to one minute. Usually seen in patients with CNS disturbances, for example, meningitis, encephalitis, head trauma or brain abscess.

Kussmaul

Also called air hunger. Characterized by increased rate (greater than 20 breaths per minute) and increased depth, that is, deep sighing breaths without pauses, laboured breathing. Body attempts to give off excess hydrogen ions by blowing off carbon dioxide. Seen in patients with metabolic acidosis and renal failure.

SOURCES: Jarvis 1992, 515-516; Wilson and Thompson, 1990, 25.

at the level of the tracheal bifurcation and should be equal bilaterally. Fremitus is increased in conditions that increase lung density, for example, consolidated lobar pneumonia. It is decreased or absent in airway obstruction or in any condition that blocks the transmission of vibrations such as emphysema or thickening (fibrosis) of the pleura. Fremitus is assessed on the posterior thorax since there is less muscle tissue and no breast tissue to interfere with the transmission of vibrations.

Finally, palpate the entire posterior surface noting the presence and location of tenderness, masses, depressions or unusual movements with respiration. Palpations that produce audible crackling sounds, called *crepitations*, indicate subcutaneous emphysema in which fine beads of air are trapped under the skin (Malasanos, Barkauskas and Stoltenberg-Allen, 1990). A course crackling sensation may also be felt over the skin surface. This is called *crepitus* (Jarvis, 1992). The skin surface should feel warm, smooth and dry, and have elastic turgor. The spinal processes should be straight and nontender. The rib cage should feel somewhat elastic, but the sternum and xiphoid should be relatively inflexible.

FIGURE 23.4 Palpating fremitus

Palpation of the anterior chest Standing directly in front of the patient, palpate the sternal notch. This aids in identifying the location of the internal organs. Palpate the intercostal spaces noting the presence, location and characteristics of tender or painful areas or masses. To identify the extent of chest expansion with respirations, place the hands on patient's lateral rib cage with thumbs placed along the costal margins. The thumbs are placed together (see Figure 23.3). Ask the patient to take a deep breath and, again, note the movement of the areas between the thumbs; this represents the chest expansions. Movement should be symmetrical.

PERCUSSION

Percussion is used in the chest examination to determine the presence of air, fluid or solid material in the underlying lung tissue and to help identify the location and boundaries of underlying organs such as the diaphragm, lungs, heart and liver. Both the posterior and anterior thoracic cage should be percussed. Percussion techniques are discussed in Chapter 15. If the patient is too ill or is unable to sit up, percussion of the posterior thorax is performed with the patient positioned on the side. Start at the top of the shoulder to identify the apices of the lung. Then progress downward and side to side at five to six centimetre intervals. Compare the sounds of each area with the sound of the opposite side as percussion proceeds. Normally, the entire thorax to the level of the diaphragm elicits a resonant sound: that is, a loud, hollow, low-pitched sound of long duration. A dull, flat sound is heard over the heart and liver, or in the presence of a mass, pneumonia or atelectasis.

AUSCULTATION

The nurse listens to the patient's chest using a stethoscope to determine the presence of normal and abnormal breath sounds. The breath sounds are created by air passing through the tracheobronchial tree (trachea, bronchi and branching bronchial tubes). Before starting, explain the procedure and ask the patient to take slow deep breaths through the mouth, a little deeper than normal. Nasal breathing tends to produce false abnormal sounds. Hyperventilations can develop quickly, so the patient should not breath too fast. If the patient feels lightheaded or dizzy, he or she should inform the examiner so that auscultation can be stopped and time allowed for the patient to rest and breath normally.

The diaphragm of the stethoscope is used to auscultate the chest because it transmits the higher pitched sounds more common in respirations. Hold the diaphragm firmly on the patient's chest to eliminate outside extraneous sounds. Beginning posteriorly at the apices, proceed downward towards the lung bases at four to five centimetre intervals comparing the right and left sides (see Figure 23.5). Ask the patient to raise his or her arms when auscultating the lateral chest walls.

Take time to evaluate and correlate what is being heard; listen for at least one full respiration in each location. The examiner's ear must be trained to differentiate the various sounds. Listen for the pitch (high/low), intensity and duration of breath sounds. These will vary over different parts of the lung. If abnormal breath sounds are heard the nurse should ask the patient to cough and should then auscultate again for at least two breaths to note any change. Note the location of the sound and the phase (inspiration or expiration) in which it occurs.

A nurse listens to the patient's breath sounds.

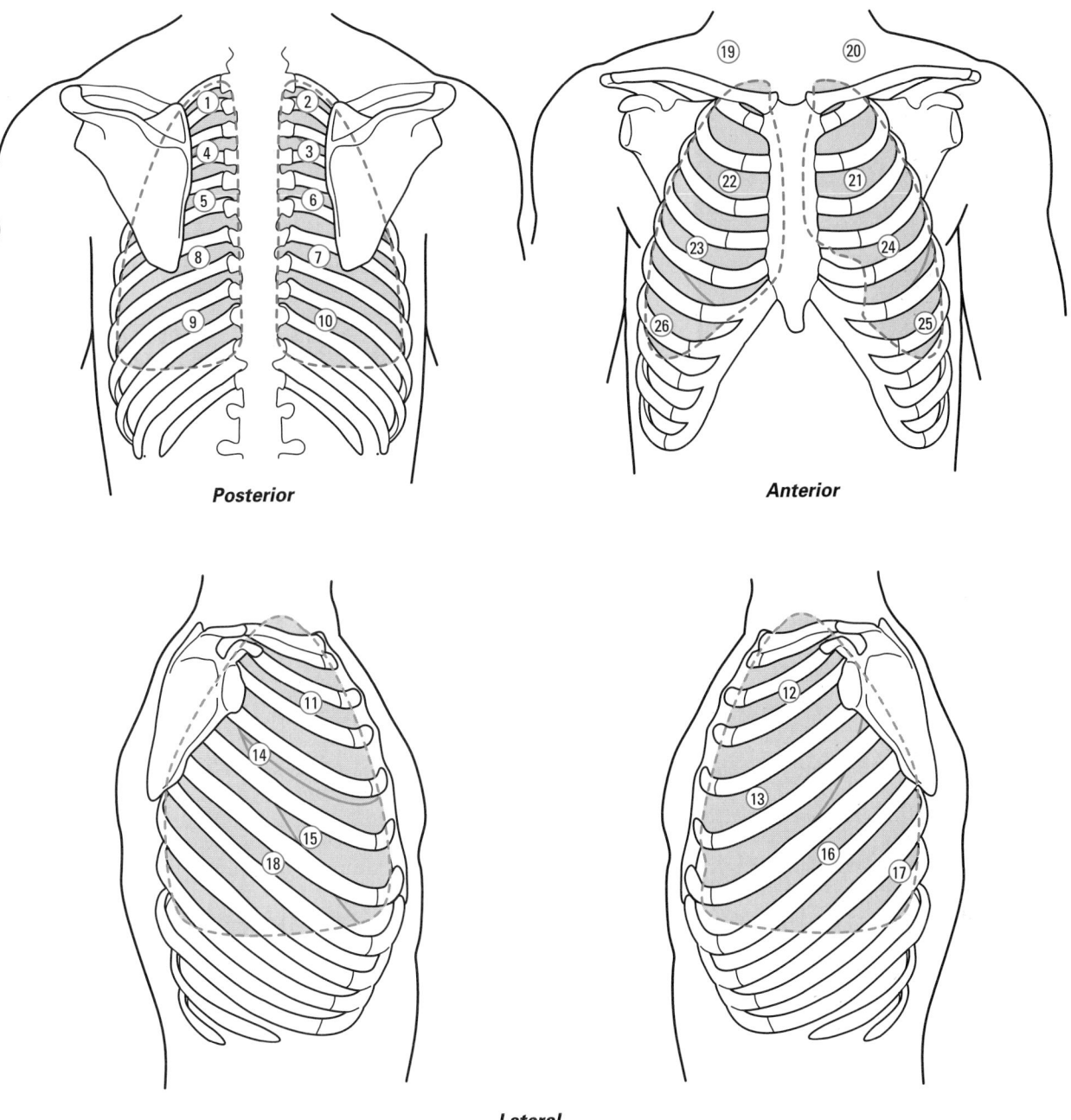

Posterior

Anterior

Lateral

FIGURE 23.5   Locations and sequence for percussing and auscultating the chest.

The characteristics of normal breath sounds are depicted in Table 23.4. Abnormal breath sounds include two categories: 1) absent or diminished sounds and 2) superimposed sounds not normally heard in the lungs. Absent or diminished sounds occur when air does not enter a portion of the lung due to obstruction of the air passages or from the accumulation of pleural fluids or air between the chest wall and the adjacent lung. Superimposed sounds include **crackles** (formerly called rales), **gurgles** (formerly called rhonchi), wheezes and **pleural friction rubs**. These are caused by air colliding with secretions in the tracheobronchial passageways or by the reopening of previously deflated airways. These abnormal breath sounds are described in Table 23.5.

TABLE 23.4 Characteristics of Normal Breath Sounds

	PITCH	AMPLITUDE	DURATION	QUALITY	NORMAL LOCATION
Bronchial (Tracheal)	High	Loud	Inspiration < expiration	Harsh, hollow, tubular	Trachea and larynx
Bronchovesicular	Moderate	Moderate	Inspiration = expiration	Mixed	Over major bronchi where fewer alveoli are located: posterior, between scapulae especially on right; anterior, around upper sternum in first and second intercostal spaces
Vesicular	Low	Soft	Inspiration > expiration	Rustling, like the sound of the wind in the trees	Over peripheral lung fields where air flows through smaller bronchioles and alveoli

SOURCE: Jarvis, C. (1992). *Physical examination and health assessment.* Philadelphia: Saunders, 496. Reproduced with permission.

DIAGNOSTIC TESTS

A number of laboratory and diagnostic tests are used to evaluate oxygenation status. Testing includes blood, sputum and pleural fluid analysis, direct and indirect visualization techniques and pulmonary function studies. Nurses must be knowledgeable about these procedures so that they can prepare patients for the tests and provide care afterwards. The nurse may also assist in some procedures performed at the bedside, such as a thoracentesis.

BLOOD STUDIES

Complete Blood Count (CBC)

A complete blood count is a routine screening test that provides general information about overall state of health and respiratory function. The elements that most directly relate to respiratory status are the red blood cell (RBC) count, hematocrit (Hct), hemoglobin (Hgb) and white blood cell

(WBC) count and differential. Table 23.6 outlines the purpose and clinical significance of these tests along with the normal values of the elements being measured.

Arterial Blood Gases

Arterial blood gas analysis is essential in diagnosing and monitoring patients with respiratory disorders. The tests measure the partial pressures of oxygen and carbon dioxide dissolved in the arterial blood. They also reveal the acid–base status and how well the oxygen is being carried in the blood.

The blood sample is taken by a specially trained nurse, doctor or respiratory therapist. The nurse on the unit provides care before and after the procedure and, in addition, may be asked to assist the health team member who is drawing the sample.

In preparing the patient, the nurse explains the purpose and the procedure for collecting the blood sample. Because the sample is taken from an artery, the procedure

TABLE 23.5 Abnormal Breath Sounds

SOUND	CHARACTERISTICS	COMMENTS
Crackles	Described as fine, medium or coarse, discontinuous sounds. **Fine**: high pitched, soft, crackling, short. Sound like several hairs rubbing together between fingertips, air-filled rice breakfast cereal in milk or crinkling of cellophane. Crackling, popping sound. **Medium**: lower pitched, moist. Sound like bubbling or a fizzing carbonated drink. **Coarse**: low pitched, loud, short. Sound like bubbling or gurgling, or like opening a Velcro fastener; heard on inspiration; can only be cleared somewhat with a cough.	Produced in the small airways by air passing through fluid or mucous. Can also be found in alveoli. Patients with pneumonia, heart failure, asthma, or pulmonary edema may have these sounds.
Gurgles	Continuous sound, coarse. Prominent on expiration. **Low pitched**: sounds are sonorous, rumbling and originate in the larger airways. **High pitched**: musical quality, rattling; may be changed or cleared with coughing.	Produced by air flowing through large passages narrowed by secretions, mucosal swelling, edema, tumour or obstruction. Occurs in patients with lung disease e.g., asthma, emphysema, COPD.
Wheeze	High pitched, continuous. More apparent on expiration. Sounds like musical whistling, squeaky; may clear somewhat with coughing.	Occurs with constriction of large or small airways; in patients with broncho-spasms, fluid, mucus, inflammation or obstructive lesion. Caused by rapid vibrations of bronchial walls.
Pleural Friction Rub	Loud, low-pitched, coarse, dry. Jerky sound, rubbing, grating. Sounds like two pieces of leather being rubbed together. Loudest over lower lateral anterior surface. Heard during inspiration and expiration. May get louder with coughing. Variable duration.	May be confined to a small area of the chest. Originates in inflamed pleura that has lost its normal lubricating fluid. Opposing roughened pleural surfaces rub together during respiration. Pain with breathing; patient may splint the chest when breathing.

may be uncomfortable for a few minutes. In order to obtain the most accurate reading, the patient should rest for approximately 20 to 30 minutes before the test. If the patient is on oxygen therapy, the rate of flow should not be changed, nor should interventions such as suctioning or positioning be performed for 20 minutes before obtaining the sample unless absolutely necessary.

The sample may be taken from the radial, brachial or femoral arteries. During the procedure, the nurse provides support and reassurance, and assists the patient to maintain proper positioning. Because the pressure from these arter-

ies is quite high, direct pressure must be applied to the site for five to ten minutes after the needle is withdrawn to prevent hemorrhage. The site is then covered with a firm dressing. The blood sample must be placed in a basin of ice and taken to the lab immediately. Specimens stored at room temperature will yield lower pH and PO_2 levels. Further, if the sample is not analyzed straight-away, continuing blood cell metabolism could alter the results of the test.

If the patient is on oxygen therapy, the laboratory requisition should include the amount and method of oxygen administered over the last 20 to 30 minutes. Following the

TABLE 23.6 Common Blood Studies For Assessing Oxygenation

TEST	NORMAL VALUES	PURPOSE	CLINICAL SIGNIFICANCE
RBC **(erythrocytes)**	M: $4.4–6.5 \times 10^{12}$/L F: $3.8–5.6 \times 10^{12}$/L	Determines oxygen-carrying capacity	Increased in chronic lung disease. Decreased in anemia. Results from insufficient dietary intake of iron or folic acid, RBC destruction, blood loss, or bone marrow suppression
Hemoglobin	M: 136–168 g/L F: 115–151 g/L	Determines amount of Hgb available for combining with oxygen	Same as RBC
Hematocrit	M: 0.40–0.51 F: 0.35–0.45	Determines the percentage of RBCs to plasma	Increased in severe dehydration (when blood plasma is lost, concentration of RBCs increases), disease, and high altitude. Decreased in over-hydration disease, and reaction to blood transfusions.
WBC	$4.0–10.0 \times 10^9$/L	Determines immune system response to antigen	Increased in acute bacterial infections, carcinoma, diabetes mellitus, acute hemorrhage. Decreased in acute viral infections, bone marrow depletion.

SOURCE: Values taken from *Laboratory Ward Manual*. (1992). North Vancouver, BC: Lions Gate Hospital.

procedure, the nurse assesses the patient's vital signs and response to the procedure, and examines the puncture site for bleeding, arterial thrombosis (common occurrence) and signs of infection or ulnar nerve trauma. Documentation includes the date and time the blood sample was drawn, the puncture site, the name of the health team member who drew the sample, the oxygen concentration and flow rate (if applicable), the patient's response to the test, and any relevant observations (for example, patient's vital signs, colour, condition of site). The purpose and significance of arterial blood gases tests along with normal values are given in Table 23.7.

SPUTUM STUDIES

Sputum analysis is valuable in identifying the cause of pulmonary dysfunction, diagnosing bacterial infections and determining and evaluating treatment regimens. Periodic sputum exams may be necessary for patients receiving antibiotics, steroids and immunosuppressive drugs for prolonged periods, as these agents give rise to opportunistic infections. The most common tests performed on sputum are culture and sensitivity (C&S) to determine the organisms causing bacterial infection and their sensitivities to antibiotics; acid-fast stain (AFB) to detect the acid-fast bacilli

when tuberculosis is suspected; and cytology to identify cancer including the specific cell type.

Because the results of a C&S may take 24 to 48 hours, a gram stain is performed to determine whether the organisms are gram-negative or gram-positive. The gram stain report is available within a few hours, and, therefore, is useful in selecting immediate antibiotic therapy until the C&S results are obtained. C&S and gram staining examinations require one specimen collected in a sterile container. The specimen should be collected before antibiotic treatment is started. Specimens for AFB are collected in a special glass container for three consecutive days. The results are usually available in three to eight weeks. A single specimen is needed for cytology. It is collected in a special container with a fixative solution. The specimen must be sent to lab promptly to ensure accuracy of the examination.

Collection of Sputum Specimens

Sputum is best collected in the morning because secretions pool in the bronchi during the night and require only a few deep coughs to bring them to the back of the throat. The patient should be supplied with the correct wide-mouthed specimen container and taught how to collect the specimen. If the sight of a specimen is objectionable to the

TABLE 23.7 Arterial Blood Gases (ABGs)

TEST	VALUES	PURPOSE AND SIGNIFICANCE
pH	7.35–7.45	Assesses acid–base status. It is the free H+ ion concentration in circulating blood. The pH must remain constant for health. Values <7.35 indicates acidosis; >7.45 indicates alkalosis. Values <7.2 or >7.6 (panic values) can be life-threatening.
$PaCO_2$	34–45 mm Hg	Assesses the amount of carbon dioxide in blood and indicates the effectiveness of alveolar ventilation. High values indicate impaired respiratory function, e.g., airway obstruction, lung damage. Low values indicate hyperventilation. Panic values: <20 or >70.
PaO_2	1–60 years: 75–100 mm Hg >60 years: >63 mm Hg	Assesses the amount of oxygen dissolved in plasma and represents the status of alveolar gas exchange with inspired air. PO_2 values decrease with age.
SaO_2	95–98%	Is the percentage of available Hgb that is saturated with oxygen and available for transport throughout the body.
HCO_3	23–33 mmol/L	Bicarbonate is a component of the body's acid–base system that influences pH; tells how the kidneys are able to absorb or excrete bicarbonate ions to maintain normal pH.
BE	–3.0 – +3.0 mmol/L	Base excess is taken to determine acid–base balance.

SOURCE: Values taken from *Laboratory Ward Manual*. (1992). North Vancouver, BC: Lions Gate Hospital.

NOTE: PaO_2 and $PaCO_2$ refer to partial pressures of oxygen and carbon dioxide in arterial blood. SaO_2 refers to oxygen saturation of arterial blood.

patient or others in the room, the outside of the container may be covered. To produce a suitable specimen, the patient must know the difference between saliva (the clear liquid secreted by the salivary glands in the mouth) and sputum, and that it is necessary to cough to bring up sputum. The patient can be taught how to cough, if necessary. The patient should brush the teeth, clear the throat and rinse the mouth so that saliva and oral debris do not contaminate the specimen. Mouthwash and toothpaste should be avoided because these substances affect the mobility of organisms. The patient then takes a deep breath to full capacity and exhales with an expulsive deep cough directly into the sterile sputum container without touching the edges. Usually 5 to 30 ml of sputum is enough for examination.

Once the specimen is produced, the container is labelled and the specimen sent to the laboratory. If the specimen is a series specimen, the number of the specimen is included on both the requisition and label. When patients are on antibiotics, this should be indicated on the requisition. In addition, specimens obtained by suctioning should also be noted on the requisition because these specimens commonly appear watery and may resemble saliva. The specimen should be taken to the laboratory immediately, because results are most accurate when analysis is completed within one hour of collection. Some specimens may

be refrigerated; consult the laboratory for specific directives. Mouthwash or water should be offered to the patient after producing a specimen to remove any unpleasant taste.

The specimen collection is documented in the patient's record. The date and time of collection, number of the specimen if serial, method used to obtain the specimen, how the patient tolerated the procedure, the characteristics of the sputum and its proper delivery to the laboratory are recorded.

THORACENTESIS

Thoracentesis (also called a thoracocentesis) is the aspiration of fluid or air from the pleural cavity (the cavity within the thorax that contains the lungs). It involves the insertion of a needle through the chest wall and into the pleural space to remove fluid for diagnostic or therapeutic purposes or to obtain a needle biopsy of the pleura. Medication can also be instilled in the pleural space.

The procedure is performed at the bedside using aseptic technique. The nurse assists by preparing the patient and providing support during the procedure.

Patient preparation includes an explanation of the reasons for the procedure, what is going to happen and how the patient can help. Normally, thoracentesis is not painful;

some pressure will be felt when the needle is inserted. A local anesthetic is given to promote comfort. When the needle is inserted, the patient must avoid movement and refrain from talking or coughing to avoid puncturing of the lung. An informed consent is obtained per hospital policy and allergies to local anesthetics are determined. Preprocedure sedation or analgesia may be ordered.

The patient is helped into a comfortable position for the procedure. This may be a sitting position, as illustrated in Figure 23.6, or a side-lying position with the patient lying on the unaffected side. The nurse offers support and reassurance and monitors the patient's response during the procedure. After the needle is withdrawn, pressure and a small sterile dressing are applied to the puncture site. The patient is placed on bed rest on the unaffected side to permit the pleural site to seal itself and to prevent fluid seepage from gravity or coughing.

Specimens, if any, are sent to the laboratory and a chest x-ray is requisitioned. A chest x-ray is taken to verify the absence of pneumothorax and to evaluate the result of the procedure (if the purpose was to remove excessive fluid or air). Vital signs are taken and the patient is monitored for signs of respiratory problems (dyspnea, coughing, hemoptysis (blood tinged sputum) chest pain, wheezing, cyanosis, hypoxia, headache and lightheadedness). A check of the puncture site is made for bleeding or seepage of fluid. The documentation of the procedure should include the total amount of fluid withdrawn, the characteristics of the fluid (colour, viscosity), specimens sent, thoracentesis site, response of the patient and whether or not a chest x-ray was taken.

VISUALIZATION STUDIES

Bronchoscopy

The larynx, trachea and bronchi may be examined with a fibreoptic bronchoscope, a tubular instrument with an attached light source (see Figure 23.7). **Bronchoscopy** permits direct examination of tissues for abscesses, tumours or localized bleeding. It is also used to obtain tissue biopsies, remove foreign objects or mucus plugs and aspirate secretions for laboratory analysis.

An informed consent is obtained prior to the test as per agency policy and allergies to local anesthetics are determined. The purpose and procedure must be carefully explained to the patient to reduce anxiety and correct misinformation. Patient participation during the test is very important. The patient will be asked to assume a sitting or lying position with the neck hyperextended. The throat is sprayed with a local anesthetic to reduce the cough reflex and promote the patient's comfort. A flexible fibreoptic scope is passed through the mouth or nose into the larynx and trachea. This may create a feeling of being unable to breathe. The patient must be reassured that the airway remains open, and that the procedure will be more comfortable if the patient concentrates on breathing normally. The procedure takes approximately 45 to 60 minutes. Test results (except secretion analysis) are available within one to two days. The patient may experience hoarseness, a sore throat or blood-tinged sputum after the procedure.

The patient must fast for a minimum of six to twelve hours before the test. In some agencies fasting begins at

FIGURE 23.6   Positioning the patient for thoracentesis. The nurse assists the patient to one of three positions, and offers comfort and support throughout the procedure. A. Sitting on the edge of the bed with head and arms on and over the bed table. B. Straddling a chair with arms and head resting on the back of the chair. C. Lying on unaffected side with the bed elevated 30 to 40 degrees.

Source: Suddarth, D.S. (1991). *The Lippincott Manual of nursing practice* (5th ed.). Philadelphia: Lippincott, 168. Reproduced with permission.

Fibreoptic bronchoscope
smaller bronchus

FIGURE 23.7   Fibreoptic bronchoscopy

SOURCE: Smeltzer, S. and Bare, B. (1992). *Brunner and Suddarth's textbook of medical-surgical nursing.* Philadelphia: Lippincott, 516. Redrawn with permission.

midnight. Contact lenses, eye glasses and dentures are removed. Loose or capped teeth are noted on the chart. A pre-procedure medication is administered as prescribed. This may be atropine (to inhibit vagal stimulation and guard against bradycardia, dysrhythmias and hypotension), a sedative or tranquilizer (to sedate the patient and relieve anxiety) or an analgesic (to promote pain tolerance).

After the procedure the patient is placed in a semi-Fowler's position to prevent aspiration; the patient is permitted to turn from side to side. Vital signs are monitored q15 minutes or as ordered until stable. The physician is notified immediately if complications develop or the patient's condition deteriorates. An emesis basin is provided and the patient is instructed to spit out saliva rather than swallow it because the anesthetic impairs the protective laryngeal reflex and interferes with correct swallowing. Sputum is observed for bleeding, especially if a biopsy has been taken. Patients who have had a biopsy are instructed to refrain from clearing the throat and coughing so as not to dislodge the clot at the biopsy site and cause bleeding.

The patient is advised to avoid smoking for the rest of the day because smoking irritates the tissues and may cause coughing and clot displacement. Fluids or food are restricted until the gag and swallowing reflexes return (approximately two hours). The return of reflexes may be tested by touching the back of the throat with a tongue depressor. The patient is started with ice chips, sips of water and then a normal diet (soft if throat is sore) within a few hours.

Medicated lozenges or warm saline gargles may be provided to ease throat discomfort. Patients are encouraged to avoid straining the voice and, if necessary, an alternative means of communicating may be used such as a magic slate, letter board or pad and pencil.

Indirect Visualization Studies

A number of indirect visualization techniques are used to examine respiratory function. These include the standard chest x-ray, fluoroscopy, computerized tomography (CT scan) and lung scans. X-ray, fluoroscopy and CT scanning are discussed in Chapter 15. Lung scans are performed to assess pulmonary blood flow and ventilatory function when pathology is suspected. Abnormalities such as pulmonary embolism, tumours, lung cancer, bronchitis and emphysema may be detected.

Usually two tests are involved in lung scanning: the perfusion scan and the ventilation scan. A perfusion scan is obtained by injecting a radioactive agent labelled with technetium into a peripheral vein. The isotope particles pass through the right side of the heart and are distributed throughout the lungs in proportion to the active blood flow. The radioactive emissions are traced with a scanner and the image is recorded with a camera. Areas in which radioactive uptake is absent or low indicate vascular obstruction or poor perfusion. In the ventilation scan, the patient inhales a radioactive gas (xenon or krypton) through a mask. The gas diffuses through the lung but does not cross the alveolar–capillary membrane (the radioactive particles are too large). Scanning shows the air spaces in the lung and can detect abnormalities in ventilation such as pneumonia, emphysema or infarction.

In preparation for lung scanning, the nurse explains the purpose and procedure of the tests. The tests usually cause minimal discomfort. When the radioactive agent is injected into a vein for the perfusion scan, the patient may feel a flushed sensation or nausea. This is normal and only lasts a very short time. The scanning time lasts 20 to 40 minutes; the patient will be asked to lie very still under the camera so as to ensure the most accurate results. A mask may be placed over the nose and mouth during the test. The patient should breathe normally.

For the ventilation scan the patient will be asked to inhale a gas and hold the breath for a short period of time. The gas is not harmful and will not cause any distressing symptoms. The scanning process will take approximately five minutes. Both tests are completed in approximately two hours. The radioactive isotope disintegrates and is excreted within six to twenty-four hours. It will cause no harm to the patient or visitors. An informed consent is obtained and any previous reactions to diagnostic dyes or allergic reactions to shellfish or iodine are determined. Jewellery and metal objects are removed so the results of the test will not be distorted. Following the tests, the patient is watched for allergic reactions to the radioactive materials. The patient is encouraged to drink fluids to help flush the contrast materials from the kidneys.

PULMONARY FUNCTION TESTS

Pulmonary function tests are performed to assess lung function and to identify the presence and severity of respiratory disease. A number of tests are carried out because no single measurement provides a complete picture of pulmonary functioning. These include measurements of ventilation function, lung volumes, diffusion capacity and gas exchange.

Pulmonary function tests are usually performed by a respiratory therapist. As with all procedures, the nurse prepares the patient for the testing. The tests are painless but patient participation is essential. Testing involves breathing as deeply as possible and blowing as hard, as fast and as long as possible into a machine. The tests take approximately 20 to 30 minutes. They are tiring, so resting prior to and following the tests will be helpful. A nose clip is applied for the testing. Patients often report feeling as though they can't catch their breath or that they are "going to suffocate." Reassure the patient that this will not happen but that it is essential to breathe through the mouth. Practising mouth breathing prior to the test helps to alleviate distress. A consent is not required for pulmonary function studies.

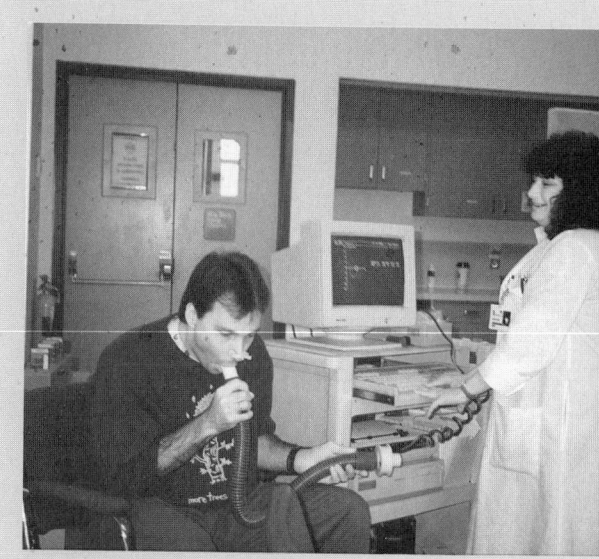

A pulmonary function test underway.

The patient is advised not to smoke prior to the tests. Eating is permitted but a heavy meal is discouraged four to six hours before testing to prevent gastric distention which may alter test results. Dentures can remain in the mouth. The patient is advised to avoid restrictive clothing and to void before leaving the ward.

DIAGNOSING OXYGENATION PROBLEMS

Actual or potential problems with oxygenation that are treated by independent nursing interventions may relate to respiratory dysfunction itself or to the effects of respiratory dysfunction on other facets of functioning. Alterations in respiratory function may include difficulties with airway clearance and ineffective breathing patterns. When patients experience a threat to their respiratory status because they cannot cough effectively, the diagnosis *Ineffective airway clearance* is useful. This diagnosis applies to cases where a suppressed cough reflex (for example, due to medications or anesthesia), pain, weakness, fatigue or improper positioning interfere with effective coughing. It may also be used for patients who are able to cough but for whom the tenacity of secretions prevents effective airway clearance.

The diagnosis *Ineffective breathing patterns* may be used when a patient's breathing pattern fails to provide adequate ventilation. In this situation the patient will be either hyperventilating or hypoventilating. He or she will display changes in the respiratory rate or pattern from the baseline measure, as well as changes in pulse rate and rhythm.

According to Carpenito, the diagnosis *High risk for altered respiratory function* may be used to describe potential problems which may affect both the passage of air through the respiratory tract and the exchange of gases between the lungs and the vascular system. She identifies smoking, immobility and environmental allergy as etiologies for this diagnosis (Carpenito, 1993). Nursing interventions are directed towards health protective measures, such as teaching deep breathing exercises and ways to maintain an allergen-free environment and providing education about the effects of smoking on respiratory health.

The diagnoses *Ineffective airway clearance* and *Ineffective breathing patterns* should only be used when the nurse can initiate treatment measures independently. For instance, in a patient with *High risk for ineffective airway clearance related to postoperative incisional pain*, the nurse may intervene by providing pain relief measures and teaching the patient how to cough effectively. Many oxygenation problems, however, are medical problems for which the nurse collaborates with the physician in monitoring the patient's status and implementing therapeutic interventions. Hypoxemia in a patient with emphysema; impaired gas exchange due to pulmonary embolus or destruction of lung tissue; and decreased tissue perfusion secondary to anemia are but a few examples. These problems are best identified as collaborative problems, in which case the label *Potential Complication* is used.

Insufficient oxygenation often interferes with the ability to function effectively in daily living. A major problem is activity intolerance. The diagnostic label *Activity intolerance* is appropriate for individuals with respiratory and cardiovascular disorders who experience dyspnea or shortness of breath when attempting physical activity. This diagnosis is outlined more fully in Chapter 28. *Anxiety* almost always accompanies breathing difficulty and a lack of oxygen. To be unable to breathe normally is a frightening experience. People with chronic respiratory problems may live in constant fear that the next breath will be their last. In addition, the demands of living with a chronic illness often require adjustments in lifestyle and compliance with therapeutic regimens that individuals may find difficult. Diagnoses such as *Alteration in health maintenance* and *Ineffective coping capacity* may be used to describe such problems. Some examples of nursing diagnoses and collaborative problems follow.

- *Ineffective airway clearance related to inadequate coughing secondary to chest pain, positioning in bed and thick secretions*
- *Ineffective breathing pattern: Hyperventilation related to anxiety and extreme pain*
- *High risk for altered respiratory function related to immobility*
- *PC: Hypoxemia*
- *Altered health maintenance related to dyspnea with exertion, confusion, and difficulty remembering therapeutic regimen.*

PLANNING OXYGENATION INTERVENTIONS

A nursing plan of care for individuals with oxygenation problems is based on the established nursing diagnoses and is generally directed towards maintaining and restoring airway patency, pulmonary ventilation and oxygen/carbon dioxide transport; preventing deterioration of respiratory function; and promoting optimal functioning in daily living. Expected outcomes are set and interventions are selected jointly by the nurse and patient, to the extent that the condition allows. When patients are very ill, the nurse may collaborate with the patient's family and other health care

 KEY PRINCIPLES

Principles Relevant to Oxygen Needs

1. Oxygen is essential to life.
2. A person can survive only a few minutes without oxygen.
3. An insufficient supply of oxygen impairs functioning of all body systems.
4. Irreparable brain damage may result from prolonged periods of inadequate oxygen.
5. Cells of the cerebral cortex begin to die as soon as they are deprived of oxygen.
6. Air at sea level containing approximately 20 percent oxygen and 0.04 percent carbon dioxide is normally adequate to meet human oxygen needs.
7. Carbon dioxide concentrations between 3 and 10 percent increase the rate and depth of respirations.
8. The body's ability to meet its oxygen needs depends on the adequacy of functioning of the cardiovascular and the respiratory systems.
9. A patent airway is essential to normal respiratory functioning.
10. The respiratory tract is lined with mucus-secreting epithelium.
11. Coughing, swallowing and sneezing are mechanisms by which the body attempts to rid itself of foreign materials in the respiratory tract.
12. Difficulty in breathing provokes anxiety.

members in establishing the plan of care. Care is provided through a multidisciplinary team approach involving physicians, respiratory therapists, physiotherapists and nurses. The nurse must take into account treatments prescribed by the physician as well as interventions implemented by the respiratory therapist and the physiotherapist.

As with all care planning, expected outcomes are developed from the nursing diagnoses and reflect the changes in behaviours or health status anticipated as a result of care. Some expected outcomes might be:

- The patient will show an effective breathing pattern as evidenced by rate, depth and rhythm in normal range.
- The patient will describe the allergens causing asthmatic attacks and the methods of avoiding contact with them.
- The patient will demonstrate how to correctly use an inhaler.
- The patient will walk to the bathroom and back to bed without dyspnea.

IMPLEMENTING OXYGENATION INTERVENTIONS

HEALTH PROMOTING STRATEGIES

A constant supply of oxygen to the body is fundamental to life. Most people take oxygenation for granted until they experience a serious problem. There are many ways to preserve and promote optimal oxygenation. Nurses can assist individuals by providing information and encouraging an exploration of lifestyle factors and health practices which may ultimately affect optimal oxygenation.

HEALTH PROTECTING STRATEGIES

Patients who are ill, especially those who are immobilized or who have undergone major surgery, often need help in maintaining optimal respiratory function, oxygen transport and tissue perfusion. The nurse assists by implementing measures to enhance these processes and prevent complications.

Techniques include positioning to ensure a clear airway and to promote ventilation; breathing exercises to facilitate maximum lung expansion; effective coughing to clear the airway; use of an incentive spirometer to enhance deep breathing and coughing; and leg exercises to strengthen circulation and venous return. Leg exercises are discussed in Chapter 28. Here we will focus on positioning, breathing exercises, effective coughing and use of an incentive spirometer.

POSITIONING

Airway patency and ventilation are affected by body positioning. Patients who are unconscious or partially conscious (for example, those recovering from anesthesia) or those with swallowing difficulty should never be positioned on their back. In the supine position, the lower jaw and tongue fall backward and occlude the airway. Also, secretions pool at the back of the throat, making aspiration likely. These individuals should be placed in a semi-prone position with the lower jaw (mandible) extended forward and upward. This prevents the tongue from falling back and also permits drainage of fluids from the mouth. For the conscious patient, an upright position (Fowler's or semi-Fowler's) is best because the abdominal contents move downward and away from the diaphragm, allowing maximum expansion of the thorax. Expectoration of sputum is also easier in a sitting position. Patients are encouraged and helped to change position (that is, from side to side) frequently while in bed to aid expansion of all lung areas and prevent stasis and pooling of pulmonary secretions.

Individuals experiencing dyspnea will be most comfortable in an orthopneic position, which promotes use of the accessory muscles to help obtain maximum expansion. In this position, the patient sits in bed or on the side of the bed and leans on the overbed table (raised a suitable height). The patient can also press the lower part of the chest against the table to help in exhalation.

BREATHING EXERCISES

Breathing exercises are performed to improve ventilation and blood oxygenation, decrease the work of breathing by coordinating patterns of respiratory muscle action and relieve anxiety due to dyspnea. Three basic breathing techniques are deep breathing, diaphragmatic or abdominal breathing and pursed-lip breathing. Procedure 23.2 outlines how to teach these exercises to patients.

Deep Breathing

Patients who are at risk for respiratory impairment should be taught this technique. This includes people who are immobile, obese, elderly and those receiving medications (narcotics) that depress the rate and depth of respiration. Patients undergoing surgery are taught deep breathing and coughing (discussed later) in the preoperative period. Teaching should begin upon admission and practice should be encouraged hourly while awake. Even while semi-conscious, a person who has been instructed in these techniques will respond to a verbal reminder. Postoperatively, deep breathing helps to clear general anesthetic (given by inhalation) agents from the body and hastens recovery, thereby preventing stasis of secretions and the tendency to hypoventilate.

HEALTH PROMOTING STRATEGY

Promoting Healthy Oxygenation

- Engage in a regular exercise program, preferably aerobic, three to four times a week for at least 30 minutes of continuous activity.
- Eat a nutritious, well-balanced diet, low in fat. Avoid excessive intake of salt and maintain normal body weight.
- If you are a smoker, consider quitting.
- If you are not a smoker, do not start.
- Avoid passive or sidestream smoke.
- Use protective masks, gloves and clothing when exposed to hazardous materials or gases.
- Avoid occupational hazards by adhering to safety regulations of the industry.
- Avoid going outside when the air is severely polluted.

- Support public programs aimed at promoting a pollution-free environment.
- Maintain a pollution-free environment in the home.
- Avoid stagnation of air. Open windows and allow fresh, clean air into the house. Sleep with a window opened but avoid a direct draft.
- Keep dust to a minimum by damp dusting and vacuuming at least once a week.
- Use an air purifier, if possible, and have carpets cleaned to remove animal hair, dust and smoke.
- Maintain a clean air filter in the furnace.
- Visit the physician regularly for health screening examinations.

Diaphragmatic or abdominal breathing

Diaphragmatic breathing uses the diaphragm instead of the accessory muscles to achieve maximum inhalation. During inspiration, the diaphragm moves downward and outward resulting in an enlargement of the upper abdomen which allows air to flow in. During exhalation, the abdominal muscles contract, pushing air out. Diaphragmatic breathing helps to expand and ventilate the bases of the lungs. It slows respirations, opens more alveoli and permits better gas exchange. It also helps to relax the entire body and is, therefore, useful as a sleep aid. This technique is useful for patients with COPD.

Pursed-lip breathing The goal of pursed-lip breathing is to prolong exhalation by increasing airway pressure and preventing bronchiolar collapse and air trapping. It provides a way of controlling respirations when a patient is experiencing dyspnea or anxiety.

PROCEDURE 23.2

Teaching Breathing Exercises

ACTION	RATIONALE
1. Explain the purpose of the breathing exercise.	Understanding the benefits of the exercise facilitates learning and promotes active participation.
A. Deep Breathing	
1. Assist the patient to a comfortable sitting or Fowler's position. Make sure there are no constricting clothing or restraints.	Permits full chest expansion.
2. Instruct and demonstrate how to:	
• Take a slow, deep breath in through the nose (unless prevented by a nasal condition), raising the rib cage and making the bottom ribs move outward.	Allows maximum inspiration, decreases work of respiration, and relaxes the patient.

Continued on the next page

ACTION	RATIONALE
• Exhale slowly through the mouth.	Facilitates maximum expiration.
3. Repeat the exercise, slowly inhaling and exhaling a few times every hour while awake.	Repetition reinforces learning. Regular deep breathing promotes ventilation and prevents complications.

B. Diaphragmatic or Abdominal Breathing

ACTION	RATIONALE
1. Assist patient to a comfortable semi-Fowler's or supine position.	Enables full contraction and relaxation of the diaphragm.
2. Instruct and demonstrate how to:	
• Place one hand on the stomach and one on the mid-chest area.	Enables awareness of the diaphragm and its movement in breathing.
• Slowly, take a deep breath in through the nose, letting the lungs fill. The chest should not move.	
• Hold breath for a count of three.	Slows down the respiratory rate.
• Purse the lips and slowly exhale, while tightening the abdominal muscles. Press inward and upward on the abdomen with the hand while breathing out.	Increases pressure within the bronchi which minimizes collapse of the small airways and allows more complete exhalation.
3. Repeat the technique for one minute or 15 times, with a short rest after each group of five.	Promotes maximum benefit of the exercise without causing undue fatigue.
4. Practise the exercise several times during the day. If you become short of breath, concentrate on breathing slowly and rhythmically.	Regular exercise is needed to improve pulmonary function.

C. Pursed-Lip Breathing

ACTION	RATIONALE
1. Help the patient to a comfortable upright position.	Decreases pressure of the abdominal organs on the diaphragm, thus creating space for lung expansion.
2. Instruct and demonstrate how to:	
• Inhale slowly through the nose while counting one, two, three or "one one hundred," "two one hundred," "three one hundred."	Facilitates a deep inhalation.
• Purse the lips as if about to whistle, or as if blowing through a straw. Then exhale slowly and evenly through the pursed lips for six seconds. The sound made will be like a small soft whistle.	Prevents collapse of the small airways and promotes more complete exhalation. Exhalation takes twice as long because expiratory airflow is slowed due to collapse of airways.
3. Practise the technique eight to ten times per interval, three to four times a day until it becomes automatic. Practise the technique in other positions, for example, lying flat in bed, standing, or walking. While walking, the patient should inhale for two steps and then exhale through pursed lips for the next four steps.	Prepares for use of the exercise in daily living.
4. Document the teaching, patient response, and effectiveness of teaching.	Fulfills requirement for nurse accountability and promotes continuity of care.

COUGHING

Coughing is used to force collected and consolidated secretions from the lungs and to maintain a clear airway. Postoperatively, patients are often reluctant to cough because of pain. Secretions can pool in the lungs causing airway obstruction, decreased alveolar gas exchange and lung complications such as hypostatic pneumonia. Because deep breathing tends to stimulate the cough reflex, deep breathing and coughing were formerly taught together in preoperative teaching. This is not recommended, however, in current practice. "Routine coughing in the absence of secretions has been found to cause atelectasis and, because of associated pain, to decrease motivation for effective deep breathing" (Berger and Williams, 1992, 1261). Thus, postoperative coughing should be done only when secretions are present. The steps for teaching effective coughing are given in Procedure 23.3.

Because incisional pain limits the effectiveness of deep breathing and coughing for the postoperative patient, the nurse also teaches the patient how to splint the incision, so that the patient can obtain maximum benefit from the exercises. *Splinting*, which provides support to the incision during coughing, involves applying external pressure against the abdominal muscles. This limits pain and strengthens the force of the muscular contraction. To splint an incision, the patient can put his or her hands across the incisional site with fingers interlaced or place a pillow or bath blanket against the abdomen (Figure 23.8). Splinting can be done by the nurse for patients who need help.

Patients with lung secretions may need to be reminded to cough. Coughing is advised upon awakening, because secretions consolidate through the night; and before meals to aid oxygenation, promote ease of respirations, and allow more energy for eating (in addition, the removal of foul secretions along with mouth care may increase the taste of food).

INCENTIVE SPIROMETRY

Incentive spirometers are used to increase lung functioning and improve pulmonary ventilation. They are effective in counteracting the effects of anesthetic agents and/or hypoventilation, loosening respiratory secretions, facilitating gaseous exchange, preventing atelectasis and expanding collapsed alveoli. Patients on prolonged bed rest, postoperative patients at risk for pulmonary complications (those who have had abdominal or thoracic surgery, older people, those who are obese, smokers and people with decreased ability to cough effectively and expel lung secretions) benefit from incentive spirometry.

The incentive spirometer is designed to increase the depth and duration of lung inflation beyond normal deep breathing in what is called a *sustained maximal inspiration*. The device measures the flow of air through the mouthpiece during inhalation and gives visual feedback to the patient which provides an incentive to improve deep breathing. If spirometry is to be used postoperatively, teaching takes place preoperatively along with deep breathing. Teaching a patient to use an incentive spirometer is outlined in Procedure 23.4. There are two general types of spirometers: the flow-oriented spirometer and the volume-oriented spirometer.

FIGURE 23.8   Splinting incisions to aid effective coughing

Teaching Effective Coughing

ACTION	RATIONALE
1. Explain the purpose of the breathing exercise.	Understanding the benefits of the exercise facilitates learning and promotes active participation.
2. Auscultate lungs.	Establishes a baseline for evaluating effectiveness of coughing.
3. Help the patient to a comfortable sitting or well-supported Fowler's position.	Aids full expansion of the lungs, permitting maximum ventilation and removal of retained secretions.
4. Provide tissues and/or an emesis basin.	Prepares for collection of secretions.
5. Splint the incision, if necessary.	Decreases pain and promotes lung expansion.
6. Instruct the patient to:	Prevents secretions from being taken deeper into the lungs. Deep inhalations stimulate the cough reflex and build up air within the airways behind the secretions which will aid in moving them upward.
• Take a slow, deep breath and exhale. Repeat two or three times.	
• Lean forward, take another deep breath, hold it for a second, and then exhale, with the throat closed, by contracting the diaphragm and abdominal muscles.	Builds up intrathoracic pressure. Maximal air volume combined with pressure creates a bolus of air, which moves secretions (Berger and Williams, 1992).
• Open the mouth and cough forcefully, without inhaling, until nearly out of breath. Expectorate into tissues or basin.	Clears trachea and bronchi and moves secretions out of the smaller airways.
• Pause and breathe normally for about 10 to 15 seconds. Repeat coughing technique until secretions are expectorated.	Relaxes the muscles, provides rest, and permits normal ventilation between coughing episodes.
7. Auscultate the lungs.	Evaluates the effectiveness of coughing.
8. Assist the patient with mouth care.	Removes secretions retained in the mouth and refreshes the patient.
9. Encourage fluids, if not contraindicated.	Liquefies secretions making expectoration easier.
10. Leave the patient in a comfortable position. Encourage rest.	Restores energy used up in coughing.
11. With gloves on, dispose of tissues or basin.	Eliminates microorganisms from contaminated secretions; gloves prevent contact with blood and body secretions.
12. Document the procedure, the patient's response, effectiveness of treatment, characteristics of the secretions, chest auscultation findings.	Fulfills requirements for nurse accountability and promotes continuity of care.

Flow-oriented device This device consists of one or more clear plastic chambers containing freely movable coloured balls or disks which move up and down as the patient breathes (see Figure 23.9). It does not measure the specific volume of inhaled air. The patient's task is to elevate the balls and keep them elevated for as long as possible before exhaling. This device is low-cost, disposable and can be used independently by patients.

Volume-oriented device The volume-oriented device measures the inhalation volume maintained by the patient. It contains pistons or bellows that are raised by inhalation to a predetermined volume (see Figure 23.9).

A   **B**

FIGURE 23.9   Incentive spirometers. A. Flow-oriented devices. B. Volume-oriented devices.

SOURCE: Traver, G. A., Mitchell, J. T. and Flodquist-Priestly, G. (1991). *Respiratory care: A clinical approach.* Gaithersburg, MA: Aspen, 112. Reproduced with permission.

PROCEDURE 23.4

Teaching Use of an Incentive Spirometer

ACTION	RATIONALE
1. Explain the purpose of the incentive spirometer.	Understanding the benefits of exercise facilitates learning and promotes active participation.
2. Teach the patient how to use the spirometer. For a volume device, set the volume level pointer at a predetermined level.	Enables independent use of the spirometer.
3. Assess the patient's breath sounds and comfort level. Administer pain medication if necessary.	Establishes a baseline for evaluation of treatment. Pain control allows maximum effort and chest expansion.
4. Help the patient into a comfortable sitting or semi-Fowler's position. If the patient can't assume or maintain an upright position, the procedure can be performed in any position as long as the device remains upright.	Promotes optimal lung expansion.
5. Instruct the patient to: • Exhale normally. • Seal the lips tightly around the mouthpiece. • Hold the spirometer in an upright position.	 A weak seal may alter flow or volume readings. A tilted flow device requires less effort to raise the ball and a volume device will not function correctly unless upright.

Continued on the next page

ACTION	RATIONALE
• Take a slow deep breath in to elevate the balls or cylinder while watching the balls or gauge rise in the spirometer.	Achieves maximum lung expansion. Indicates when the preset goal is achieved.
• Hold the breath for two seconds initially and increase to six seconds as tolerance increases. Try to keep the balls or cylinder elevated during this time.	Facilitates maximum ventilation of the alveoli.
• Remove the mouthpiece and exhale normally.	Spirometers are not designed for exhalation through the chambers.
• Relax and take several normal breaths before repeating the exercise.	
• Try to cough; splint the incision as necessary.	Deep ventilations may loosen secretions that can be expectorated.
• Repeat the procedure several times (that is, 10 per hour while awake).	Repetition increases inspiratory volume, maintains alveolar ventilation and prevents atelectasis.
• Avoid exercising at meal times.	Prevents nausea.
6. Auscultate the breath sounds.	Determines effectiveness of treatment.
7. Clean the mouthpiece with water and shake dry. Do not immerse the spirometer. Change disposal mouth pieces every 24 hours.	Moisture enhances bacterial growth and impairs effectiveness of the internal filter.
8. Label the spirometer with the patient's name and store at the bedside within easy reach.	Limits transmission of microorganisms and reminds the patient to use it.
9. Document the procedure, type of spirometer, volume or flow levels achieved, number of breaths taken, the patient's tolerance and results of auscultation.	Fulfills requirements for nurse accountability and promotes continuity of care.

HEALTH RESTORING STRATEGIES

Restorative care for individuals experiencing interferences with oxygenation involves a variety of measures to establish airway patency, increase ventilatory efficiency, ensure adequate oxygen intake and decrease bodily needs for oxygen. Nurses work in collaboration with health professionals such as physicians, respiratory therapists and physiotherapists in administering necessary interventions. Some measures, for example, managing chest tubes and tracheostomies, require knowledge and skill beyond the level of the beginning student and, therefore, will not be considered in this text.

MEASURES TO DECREASE DEMANDS FOR OXYGEN

The need for oxygen by the body is related to the rate of metabolism of the tissue cells. Factors affecting metabolic rate include physical activity, disease processes and emotional reactions. Although a certain amount of activity is essential to promote optimum ventilation of the lungs, excessive activity should be avoided. The patient's level of tolerance must be carefully assessed and care must be taken to avoid overexertion. Patients who experience dyspnea on exertion will need assistance from the nurse in completing activities of daily living until activity tolerance improves.

Uninterrupted periods of rest are essential to restore energy and support optimal oxygenation.

Because an elevated body temperature increases the basal metabolic rate, oxygen requirements will increase accordingly. Patients with oxygenation problems may not be able to meet these extra demands for oxygen. Measures to keep body temperatures within normal limits are essential. Care must be taken to prevent infection; when infections develop the causative organism(s) must be identified and treatment instituted promptly.

Emotional tension is also a factor to be considered in patients with respiratory problems. Anxiety, for example, may stimulate the parasympathetic nervous system and result in constriction of the smooth muscles of the bronchioles. The expression of other emotions, such as fear, anger and grief, is also closely related to respiration. Strong emotions initiate responses to prepare the body for action, and respirations become faster and deeper.

The patient's anxiety contributes to respiratory problems, and a vicious circle may develop. The patient becomes dyspneic; the dyspnea produces anxiety; the anxiety results in more dyspnea. It is essential that this circle be broken.

Helping to establish the patient's confidence in the care being given is an important factor in alleviating anxiety. Prompt attention to the patient's needs, such as answering the call-bell immediately and attending to needs without delay, can often prevent or minimize an attack of dyspnea. It is important in this regard to remember that anxiety is not always expressed openly. Patients may not necessarily say "I am frightened," but often their actions convey this meaning to the astute and observant nurse; the patient may make a seemingly excessive number of requests, or attempt to keep the nurse engaged in conversation. The physical presence of someone competent who can help if needed is reassuring to the patient.

Efficient handling of equipment and skillful execution of procedures contribute to the patient's feeling of security and well-being. The nurse should be familiar with the equipment used in the care of patients with respiratory problems and should feel confident about performing the necessary procedures.

Caring for a patient who has difficulty breathing can also be an anxiety-provoking experience for the nurse. Knowing what measures to take and how to use equipment contribute to feelings of confidence in giving care.

NUTRITION AND FLUID THERAPY

Patients with dyspnea often have little energy for eating and may have difficulty holding their breath while swallowing. In addition, eating large amounts of food creates difficulty in breathing because a full stomach pushes upward on the diaphragm limiting its movement. A well-balanced diet, taken in small frequent meals over the day, is recommended. Activities should be scheduled so that meals are eaten one to two hours after treatments or exercises, when respirations are easier, airways are clear, and the patient has had some rest.

Adequate hydration is essential for people with respiratory secretions. Water depletion increases the viscosity of secretions and impairs clearance of the lungs. A fluid intake of one to two litres daily is necessary to keep secretions thin and easy to expectorate. People who are mouth-breathers need extra fluids because they are also losing fluids through respiration.

HUMIDITY THERAPY

The provision of air with a high water content is a form of therapy that has been used for people with respiratory problems for many generations. Traditionally this has taken the form of steam inhalations, but there are now other devices available for humidification. The purpose of humidity therapy is to provide extra moisture to the mucous membranes lining the respiratory tract. The moisture prevents drying and irritation of the mucous membranes, and helps to dilute thick secretions.

Humidifiers are devices that add moisture to inspired air. Vapour is produced by passing air or oxygen through water in a process referred to as *bubbling*. One of the most common humidifiers in use is the bubble humidifier for humidifying oxygen in oxygen therapy. It consists of a bottle filled with sterile distilled water that is attached to an oxygen source by means of a flowmeter. Moisture is picked up as the gas bubbles through the bottle before moving through the tubing to the patient. Room humidifiers are also used at the bedside to humidify the atmosphere immediately surrounding the patient.

AEROSOL-NEBULIZATION THERAPY

Aerosol-nebulization therapy involves the delivery of medications into the tracheobronchial tree by inhalation. Medication is nebulized or reduced to a fine spray (aerosol) that is inhaled deeply into the respiratory tract where absorption occurs. Two commonly used *nebulizers* for medication therapy are the small volume jet nebulizer (mini-nebulizer) and the hand nebulizer. A mini-nebulizer is a hand-held device which uses oxygen or air under pressure to create a suspension of microscopic particles in the form of a mist which the patient inhales (see Figure 23.10).

A hand nebulizer or inhaler consists of a plastic outer shell holding a pressurized canister designed to release a controlled dose of medication through a nosepiece or mouthpiece (see Figure 23.10). The canister contains the medication and a gas propellant. When the inhaler is activated by pressing down on the canister, a dose of medication, suspended in the propellant gas, is released from the inhaler (Traver, Mitchell and Flodquist-Priestly, 1991).

A

B

FIGURE 23.10   A. Small volume jet nebulizer. B. Hand nebulizers or inhalers.

SOURCE: A. Traver, G. A., Mitchell, J. T. and Flodquist-Priestly, G. (1991). *Respiratory care: A clinical approach*. Gaithersburg, MA: Aspen, 87. Reproduced with permission.

Patients use inhalers independently once instructed in the correct technique.

Medications commonly delivered by aerosols include bronchodilators and mucokinetics. Mucokinetics are drugs that alter the consistency and clearance of tracheobronchial secretions. They include diluents (water and saline); mucolytics, which liquefy and loosen thick secretions; and expectorants, which loosen bronchial secretions so they can be removed with coughing. The steps in administering aerosol therapy using a mini-nebulizer are outlined in Procedure 23.5. Treatment should be given before meals to increase lung ventilation and therefore decrease the fatigue that accompanies eating.

Preparing the Patient

The nurse explains the purpose and procedure to the patient. To maximize the benefit of the treatment, the patient should sit upright and breathe in slowly and deeply through the mouth, hold the inspiration for two to three seconds, and then exhale normally. The procedure is painless and not tiring; it usually lasts 15 to 20 minutes.

Assembling Equipment

A mini-nebulizer is a small device that is attached to a gas source. In a hospital, wall oxygen or compressed air is used for this purpose; at home the patient may have an air-powered compressor. The nebulizer has a small reservoir (nebulizer cup) into which the medication and diluent are added. The medication is prepared in a syringe (according to the procedure outlined in Chapter 33) and added to the nebulizer cup. If necessary, water or saline may also be added to dilute the medication. The nebulizer cup and tubing are changed according to agency policy to maintain cleanliness and prevent respiratory infections.

CHEST PHYSIOTHERAPY

Chest physiotherapy, also referred to as *postural drainage*, is used to loosen and move secretions into the large airways so they can be expectorated with greater ease. It is usually performed by a physiotherapist or respiratory therapist, and in some situations by a specially trained nurse. The procedure uses positioning to aid in drainage of secretions by the

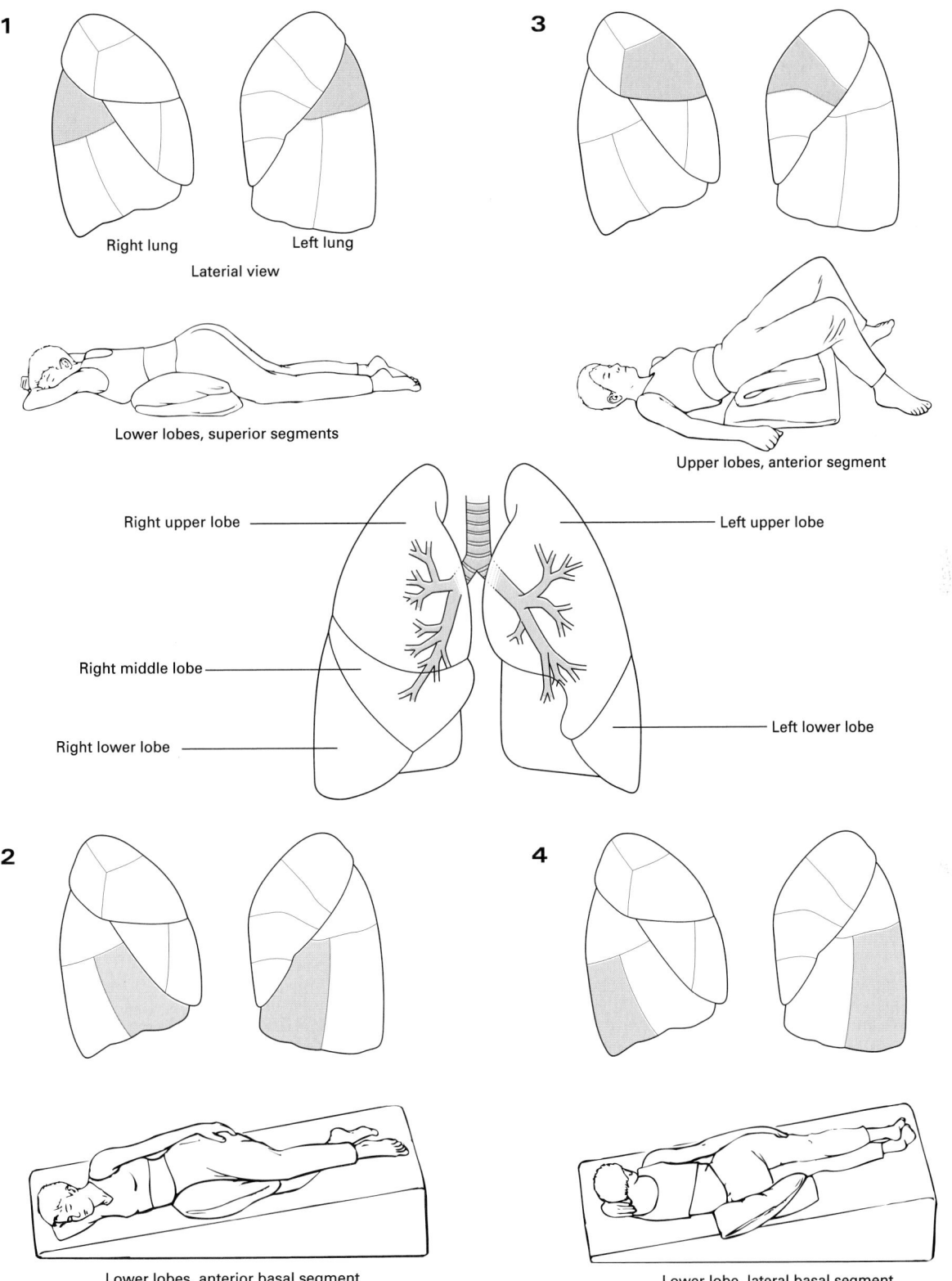

FIGURE 23.11   Anatomic segments of the lungs with four postural drainage positions. The numbers relate the position to the corresponding anatomic segment of the lung.

SOURCE: Smeltzer, S. and Bare, B. (1992). *Brunner and Suddarth's textbook of medical-surgical nursing.* Philadelphia: Lippincott, 528. Reproduced with permission.

PROCEDURE 23.5

Administering Nebulization Using a Mini-Nebulizer

ACTION	RATIONALE
1. Prepare the patient.	Promotes patient well-being.
2. Wash hands and gather: • Mini-nebulizer • Air or oxygen flowmeter • Medication	Reduces transfer of microorganisms, promotes efficiency and economy of time.
3. Prepare the equipment at the bedside. • Attach the flowmeter to the air or oxygen outlet. • Attach the nebulizer to the gas source. • Inject the medication into the medication cup. • Adjust the flowmeter to about 6 L/min.	Usually 5 to 7 L/min are adequate to create a fine mist.
4. Help the patient to an upright position.	Facilitates maximum chest expansion and aerosol dispersion.
5. Auscultate the chest for breath sounds.	Establishes a baseline for evaluation of care.
6. Instruct the patient to breathe in slowly and deeply through the mouth, hold the breath for two to three seconds, and then exhale normally.	Ensures maximum benefit of aerosol therapy.
7. After the treatment, encourage the patient to cough and expectorate the secretions. Provide suction if necessary.	Removes liquefied and loosened secretions.
8. Auscultate the chest.	Determines the effectiveness of treatment.
9. Document the treatment including the date and time, type and amount of medication, breath sounds, and patient's response to treatment.	Fulfills requirements for nurse accountability and promotes continuity of care.

flow of gravity, and deep breathing (see Figure 23. 11), coughing, percussion and vibration techniques to mobilize secretions. Percussion is carried out by lightly and rhythmically striking the chest wall with cupped hands (see Figure 23.12). Vibration is achieved by a rapidly repetitive shaking and a gentle compression of the chest wall during exhalation. Figure 23.12 shows the proper placement of hands for vibration. Effective coughing is necessary to help raise the secretions. It may take several hours following therapy before secretions are expectorated.

Chest physiotherapy is usually performed at least two hours after meals to prevent nausea, and before bed. Bronchodilators are sometimes ordered before the procedure to dilate the bronchial tubes and reduce spasm of the bronchial walls. These should be administered 20 minutes prior to the procedure. Chest physiotherapy is very tiring. A rest period beforehand will conserve energy for the procedure and improve the patient's tolerance.

OROPHARYNGEAL AND NASOPHARYNGEAL SUCTIONING

Oropharyngeal and nasopharyngeal suctioning refers to the removal of secretions from the pharynx by means of a catheter inserted through the mouth or nose (as shown in Procedure 23.6). It is used to maintain a patent airway in patients who have difficulty swallowing or expectorating secretions. Suction is provided by a suction machine or wall outlet.

Guidelines for Using Inhalers

- Clear the chest of secretions as completely as possible before using the inhaler. *Maximizes inhalation and absorption of the medication.*

- Make sure the canister is firmly and fully inserted into the outer shell of the inhaler. *Ensures correct delivery of the prescribed medication.*

- Remove the cap from the mouthpiece. Hold the inhaler in the upright position and shake well five to six times. *Ensures even suspension of the medication.*

- Exhale slowly and fully, then administer the medication using either open- or closed-mouth technique.

Open-Mouth Technique:

- Place the mouthpiece three to five cm in front of open mouth. Keep the tongue and teeth from blocking the mouthpiece of the inhaler.

- Take a slow deep inhalation through open mouth while firmly pressing down on the canister.

Closed-Mouth Technique:

- Place the mouthpiece over the tongue and well into mouth. Keep the teeth from blocking the mouthpiece of the inhaler.

- Close lips tightly around the mouthpiece of the inhaler.

- Press down firmly on the canister once while breathing in slowly and deeply.

- Hold the breath for 10 seconds or as long as comfortable. *Creates a resistance against airflow from the lungs and increases pressure within the bronchi forcing full expansion of the airway.*

- Release pressure on the canister, remove the inhaler from the mouth, purse the lips and breathe out slowly. *Permits greater expansion of the airway.*

- Wait one to two minutes to deliver a second puff (if prescribed).

- Rinse mouth with water after using the inhaler. *Prevents dryness of the mouth and throat.*

- If two inhalers are prescribed, that is, a bronchodilator and a corticosteroid, use the bronchodilator first. This opens the airways and allows the corticosteroid to get into the airways more effectively. It will take a few minutes for the medication to be effective.

- Clean the inhaler once a week. Remove the canister and wash the outer shell in warm soapy water, rinse it well, and let it air dry overnight.

A

B

FIGURE 23.12   A. Hand position for cupping. B. Hand position for vibration.

Because the suction catheter may inadvertently slip into the lower airway or esophagus, sterile technique (discussed in Chapter 31) is used throughout the procedure. When both nasal and oral suctioning are required at the same time, the nose is suctioned first. This limits the introduction of microorganisms from the mouth to the nasal passages. Normally, the mouth harbours more organisms than does the nose.

The mucous membrane of the respiratory tract can easily be injured during suctioning. Therefore, suctioning should only be used when secretions have accumulated and abnormal breath sounds are audible. These are indicated by noisy, wet respirations or rattling, bubbling breath sounds. Signs of respiratory distress caused by obstruction (restlessness, cyanosis), drooling or the obvious presence of secretions alert the nurse to the need for suctioning.

Preparing the Patient

The patient is reassured that the procedure will make him or her more comfortable by relieving the breathing difficulty. Suctioning of the throat is usually a painless procedure but it can cause the patient to gag, cough or sneeze. If the patient can cough during the procedure, it will facilitate removal of mucus.

Assembling Equipment

Suction is established by a device which creates a negative pressure that draws liquids and solid materials towards the source of pressure (much like a vacuum cleaner). A suction unit consists of a collection container, a regulator with a gauge that registers the degree of negative pressure during suctioning and a control knob for setting the pressure (see Figure 23.13). Tubing connects the suction unit to the catheter. Wall-mounted and portable suction units will be found in agencies. Wall-mounted units are attached to a piped-in source of negative pressure. The negative pressure is measured in millimetres of mercury (mm Hg). In some portable units the negative pressure can only be set as "low," "medium," or "high."

Suction catheters are made of soft plastic material and are available in different sizes ranging from 5 Fr to 18 Fr. Recall from previous chapters that the smaller the French number, the smaller the diameter of the catheter. Sizes 12 Fr to 18 Fr are used for adults. The size of catheter selected for a patient should be large enough to remove secretions but not so large as to occlude the airway. Most catheters have a suction control port on the distal end, called a thumb port, which is used to establish suction once the catheter is inserted. This permits insertion of the catheter without causing trauma to tissues along the way.

Sterile suction kits are available which are used once and then discarded. These kits contain a catheter with a thumb port, one or two gloves, water-soluble lubricant and a container for the irrigant. Sterile water or saline is used to flush the catheter during the procedure. If the catheter in the kit is not the correct size for the patient, a separately packaged catheter is obtained. A clean glove will also be necessary when using a suction kit that provides only one glove. When a patient is in distress, the airway must be cleared promptly. For this reason, a suction unit and a supply of necessary equipment is usually kept at the bedside of patients who require suctioning.

Suctioning the oropharynx with a tonsillar tip catheter   The mouth can also be cleared with a *tonsillar or Yankauer suction tip*. It is a rigid catheter which can be easily directed to all parts of the mouth. Patients can be taught to use this type of catheter themselves. Once connected to the suction source, the suction is continuous (the catheter has no suction control mechanism). Clean technique is used with a tonsillar tip device because it is used only to remove secretions from the mouth. The procedure is the same as for oropharyngeal suctioning. All areas of the mouth are cleared: along the top of the tongue, under the tongue and along the sides of the mouth to the pharynx. The catheter is reusable. After use, it is cleaned with water and hydrogen peroxide to remove secretions, rinsed with water and air dried.

FIGURE 23.13   Suction unit

PROCEDURE 23.6

Performing Oropharyngeal and Nasopharyngeal Suctioning

ACTION	RATIONALE
1. Prepare the patient.	Reduces anxiety and fear, and enables patient participation.
2. Wash hands and gather: • Portable or wall suction unit with tubing • Sterile suction kit and appropriate-sized catheter, if necessary or • Sterile suction catheter • Sterile gloves • Sterile water or saline • Sterile disposable container • Towel or water-proof pad • Clean glove, if suction kit used	Reduces transfer of microorganisms and facilitates efficiency and economy of time.
3. Draw the bed curtains.	Promotes privacy.
4. Help the patient to a semi-Fowler's position, if conscious. In unconscious, place the patient in a lateral recumbent position, facing the nurse.	Catheter insertion aided by gravity. Promotes drainage of secretions and lessons the risk of aspiration.
5. Place a towel or waterproof pad across the patient's chest.	Protects patient's clothing from secretions.
6. Turn suction to appropriate pressure. **Wall unit:** Adult: 100-120 mm Hg Child: 80-110 mm Hg Infant: 50-95 mm Hg **Portable:** Adult: 10-15 mm Hg Child: 5-10 mm Hg Infant: 2-5 mm Hg	Negative pressure must be at a safe level to minimize injury to mucosa.
7. Prepare the sterile equipment using sterile technique (see Procedure 31.3). Add sterile saline or water to the container and open the sterile suction (if appropriate).	Reduces the risk of infection. Patients with pulmonary dysfunction are very vulnerable to infection.
8. Don sterile gloves (Procedure 31.2). Or, apply a clean glove on the nondominant hand and a sterile glove on the dominant hand.	The dominant hand will be used to handle the catheter; it must be kept sterile. The nondominant hand will be used to manipulate unsterile equipment. The glove protects the nurse from contact with body secretions.
9. Using the dominant hand, pick up the catheter and coil it around the hand. Grasp the connecting tube with the nondominant hand and attach the catheter to the tubing.	Prevents inadvertent contamination of the catheter.

Continued on the next page

ACTION	RATIONALE

10. Moisten the catheter by dipping it into the container of sterile irrigant and occlude the thumb port. Fluid should move through the tube.

Lubricates the lumen of the catheter which aids movement of secretions and checks that equipment is functioning.

11. Coil the catheter around the dominant hand so the tip is between the thumb and forefinger.

As in Step 9.

12. Insert the catheter.

Nasopharynegeal suction:

• Estimate the distance from the earlobe to the patient's nose and hold at that point between thumb and forefinger.

Determines the length of catheter needed to reach the pharynx.

ACTION

- With the thumb port open, gently insert the catheter into one nostril as the patient inhales.
- Direct the catheter along the floor of the nasal cavity (medially and inferiorly).

Oropharyngeal suction:

- With the thumb port open, insert the catheter along the side of the mouth towards the oropharynx.

13. Apply suction by placing the thumb of the non-dominant hand over the thumb port for five to 15 seconds at a time. Gently rotate the catheter while suctioning and when it is removed.

14. Flush the catheter with sterile irrigant and wipe it with sterile gauze if it is thickly coated with secretions.

15. Repeat suctioning until the air passage is clear. Allow at least 20 to 30 seconds of rest between suction passes. Apply oxygen and encourage coughing and deep breathing between suctionings.

16. If the patient shows signs of increasing hypoxia, or the heart rate becomes excessively slow or rapid, or if there are sudden frank bloody secretions, stop suctioning and have someone notify the doctor.

RATIONALE

Absence of negative pressure lessens injury to the mucosa and reduces oxygen depletion.

Prevents injury to the nasal turbinates or coiling in the nasal cavity.

Minimizes gagging.

Reduces mucosal trauma and clears mucus from all the walls of the airway.

Cleans and clears the catheter and lubricates it for the next insertion.

Helps to compensate for hypoxia caused by suctioning. Helps to eliminate secretions naturally and reduces the need for further suctioning, or moves the secretions from the trachea and bronchi into the pharynx so they can be removed.

Continued on the next page

ACTION	RATIONALE
17. When suctioning is complete, disconnect the catheter from the tubing, coil the catheter in the palm of the sterile hand and remove the glove so that it turns inside out over the catheter.	Prevents the transfer of microorganisms.

ACTION	RATIONALE
18. Turn off the suction, dispose of equipment in the proper receptacle and wash hands.	Maintains cleanliness and safety in the workplace.
19. Auscultate the breath sounds, note the patient's colour and respiratory status. Take pulse and respirations.	Determines effectiveness of suctioning.
20. Assist the patient with oral or nasal hygiene and leave the patient comfortable.	Enhances patient well-being.
21. Document the procedure, including the frequency and method of suctioning, patient's colour, respiratory status and characteristics of secretions.	Fulfills requirements for nurse accountability.

OXYGEN THERAPY

Oxygen therapy is a method of supplying supplemental oxygen in concentrations greater than that of environmental air. It improves cellular oxygenation, decreases the work of breathing and reduces stress on the heart. In clinical use, oxygen is considered a drug. Therefore, the principles of medication therapy (as discussed in Chapter 33) apply when oxygen is being administered. A physician's order is needed to administer oxygen. The physician specifies the method of oxygen delivery and the rate of flow or the concentration, expressed as a percentage of oxygen in inspired air. Sometimes the physician orders the level of oxygen (hemoglobin) saturation to be maintained, as determined by pulse oximetry. For example, the order might read: *Administer oxygen by nasal cannula and keep O_2 saturation at 96%.* In this case the nurse adjusts the flow rate to maintain the necessary oxygen saturation level.

Oxygen must be administered carefully because excessive oxygen is not only harmful, but is also potentially fatal in some people. It can produce toxic effects in the lungs and central nervous system, and cause depression of ventilation. High concentrations of oxygen are especially dangerous in people with chronic hypoxia, for example, a patient with COPD. Such patients become accustomed to abnormally high $PaCO_2$ levels in the blood, and, for them, the stimulus to breathe is a lack of oxygen. Administering high levels of oxygen to these patients would take away their respiratory stimulus and they may stop breathing completely. In general, patients with respiratory conditions are given oxygen at the lowest flow rate or concentration that will maintain the arterial oxygen pressure at their normal baseline. This can vary from 63 to 100 mm Hg.

Oxygen is an odourless, colourless and tasteless gas. People may not be aware of its presence. In addition, while oxygen by itself does not burn, it does support combustion.

Therefore, safety measures must be taken by everyone, including visitors, when oxygen therapy is in progress. Precautions to be taken during oxygen therapy are outlined in the box below.

PREPARING OXYGEN EQUIPMENT

In order to administer oxygen safely the nurse must have an understanding of oxygen equipment and know how to use it. Procedure 23.7 outlines the steps involved in setting up oxygen equipment.

Assembling Equipment

Therapeutic oxygen is supplied from central storage reservoirs piped to wall outlets or from portable tanks or cylinders. Most hospitals today use a piped-in oxygen system; however, portable units are necessary for transporting patients (for example, to the x-ray department) or in case of emergencies in designated areas. Portable tanks are also used for home care.

Oxygen tanks are steel cylinders containing oxygen under high pressure. A pressure regulator with a pressure-reducing valve is used to control the release of oxygen from the tank. The regulator normally has two gauges: a content gauge and a flowmeter. The content gauge, calibrated in pounds per square inch (psi), indicates the amount of

oxygen in the tank. A flowmeter controls the release of oxygen to the patient. This is measured in litres per minute (L/min). Figure 23.14 shows an oxygen tank with an attached regulator, content gauge and flowmeter.

The oxygen gauges are generally attached to the tank before it is brought to the patient. In most hospitals, respiratory technologists supply and service the oxygen equipment. Because of the extreme pressure within the cylinder, oxygen tanks must be handled with caution and care. The force of gas escaping from a damaged regulator or outlet could cause the tank to behave like a rocket. Cylinders are held in wheeled carriers or stands and secured with metal straps to prevent them from falling and damaging the regulator and outlet. They should be placed away from high traffic areas and heat registers when in use. Tanks in storage have a protective cap to avoid accidental damage to the cylinder outlet.

Piped-in oxygen is stored in reservoirs under low pressure between 50 to 60 psi. A flowmeter is used to regulate the amount of oxygen released from the wall outlet (see Figure 23.14).

Oxygen is a dry gas (has no moisture content). Continuous administration of oxygen above 4 L/min dries respiratory tissues and mucous secretions, both of which can lead to airway obstruction and the risk of infection. Thus, oxygen delivered at high flow rates (>4 L/min) should be humidified. In some agencies, it is standard practice to humidify all oxygen delivered to patients, regardless of the flow rate. The nurse should consult agency policy in this regard. Oxygen is humidified with a humidifier attached to the oxygen flowmeter. Pre-filled disposable humidifiers are commonly used. Reusable humidifiers are packaged in sterile wrappers and must be filled with sterile distilled water before use. An adapter is needed to connect the humidifier to the flowmeter. Adapters may be packaged separately or with the humidifier. Tubing is needed to connect the oxygen source to the delivery device, for example, an oxygen mask.

Establishing Oxygen Therapy

Oxygen is administered by a delivery device, such as a nasal cannula or a mask, in an amount prescribed by the physician. The amount is ordered as a rate of oxygen flow, indicated in litres per minute, or a concentration, expressed as a percentage of oxygen in inspired air. For example, the physician may order *O₂ per nasal cannula at 4 L/min* or *O₂ by venturi mask at 36%.*

Oxygen delivery devices are categorized as either low-flow or high-flow systems. In a low-flow system, the device delivers a set flow of 100 percent oxygen which is then mixed with room air as the patient inhales. The amount of room air that is entrained (pulled in and trapped like air in a vacuum) varies according to the person's rate and depth of respirations and consequently influences the final

---

Safety Measures During Oxygen Therapy

- Place "Oxygen in Use" and "No Smoking" signs in conspicuous places: at the patient's door, foot or head of bed and on oxygen equipment.

- Instruct patients and visitors regarding safety precautions.

- Avoid smoking, open flames, matches and lighters. For the confused patient, remove cigarettes and lighters from the bedside.

- Eliminate sparks by ensuring electrical equipment (electric call bells, razors, radios, television sets) are in good working order. Ground electrical equipment.

- Avoid materials that generate static electricity (woolen blankets, synthetic fabrics).

- Avoid volatile, flammable materials, for example, alcohol, petroleum-based lip agents (Vaseline, for example), nail polish remover. Oil can ignite spontaneously in the presence of oxygen. Use water-soluble lubricants.

FIGURE 23.14 A. Oxygen tank B. Close-up of regulator, content gauge and flowmeter C. Flowmeter used with a piped-in oxygen source

concentration of oxygen delivered. For instance, when respirations are shallow, little room air is drawn in (entrained) to dilute the supplemental oxygen. Therefore, the percentage of oxygen in the inspired air increases. On the other hand, when a person takes a deep or rapid respiration, more room air is drawn in. As a result, the room air–oxygen mixture is more diluted and the inspired oxygen concentration decreases. "Low flow refers to this variable mixing with room air, not the oxygen flow rate set on the flow meter" (Traver, Mitchell, and Flodquist-Priestly, 1991, 96). The nasal cannula and simple face mask are the two most common low-flow delivery devices. They are indicated for people who require supplemental oxygen but not in precise concentrations.

High-flow delivery systems are able to control the percentage of oxygen in the inspired more precisely. This is achieved primarily with masks designed to regulate the amount of room air that is entrained to mix with supplemental oxygen. The mask's ability to deliver a precise percentage of oxygen is not affected by the patient's respiratory pattern, but it does require a properly fitting mask that is consistently kept in place. The most common high-flow

device in use is the venturi mask. The techniques for establishing oxygen therapy by nasal cannula and face mask are outlined in Procedure 23.8.

Preparing the Patient

The administration of oxygen is often a frightening experience for the patient and family. To many people, it denotes a serious illness; some may remember a relative or a friend who died while receiving oxygen. Oxygen is essential to life and to have to depend upon equipment in order to live is in itself anxiety-producing. It is a situation over which patients often have little control, and, because they are dependent upon others for the air they breathe, they may feel helpless.

Such fears can often be allayed with knowledge and an opportunity for the patient to become familiar with the equipment. Information about oxygen equipment should be geared to the patient's needs. Some people want to understand in great detail; others are satisfied with a simple explanation. When possible, patients should hold the device, put it on their face, and get used to the sensation of the

Preparing Oxygen Equipment

ACTION	RATIONALE
1. Gather equipment:	
• Oxygen flowmeter	
or	
• Portable tank and regulator with flowmeter	
• Humidifier, as appropriate	
• Oxygen connecting tubing	
A. Wall-Outlet System	
1. Make sure the flowmeter control is in the off position. Push the flowmeter into the wall outlet using firm pressure.	Prevents escape of oxygen when the flowmeter is attached to the wall outlet.
2. If appropriate, attach a humidifier to the flowmeter. Attach the adapter to the top of the humidifier bottle. Then connect the humidifier to the flowmeter and turn the adapter clockwise until it is tight.	Prevents oxygen from leaking around the connection and causing a fire hazard. Indicates that oxygen is flowing freely.
Open the flowmeter to establish oxygen flow and look for bubbles in the container. Turn the flowmeter off.	
3. Connect one end of the oxygen tubing to the flowmeter if a humidifier is not used, or to the outlet port of the humidifier, if used.	Readies the equipment for connection to the oxygen delivery device.
B. Portable Oxygen Tank	
1. If necessary, set up a new cylinder.	When cylinders drop to about 500 psi, they should be replaced.
• Remove the protective cap from the cylinder outlet.	
• Open the hand wheel at the top of the cylinder slightly by turning it clockwise and then closing it quickly. A loud hissing sound will be made.	Called "cracking the cylinder," this removes dust from the outlet.
• Connect the pressure regulator with flowmeter to the cylinder outlet and tighten it with the wrench, supplied with the tank.	Oxygen is stored under pressure. The connections must be tight to ensure safety during use.
2. Open the cylinder valve by slowly turning the hand wheel until it is fully open and then turn it back a quarter turn.	Readies the tank for the flow of oxygen.
3. Follow steps 2 and 3 of section A.	
4. To turn off the flow of oxygen, close the hand wheel by turning it clockwise. Wait until both gauges indicate empty. Then, turn the flowmeter control off.	Clears oxygen from the regulator during storage.
5. Store the unit in a safe location away from high traffic areas and heat.	Promotes safety in the environment. Heat causes gases to expand.

device on their face. When patients are well enough to help with the therapy, the nurse can teach them to administer the oxygen themselves and thus help them to feel that they have some control over the situation. The nurse must also review the safety precautions for oxygen therapy and ensure that patients have a good understanding of them.

Assembling the Oxygen Delivery Device

There are many different devices for delivering oxygen. Some, like the oxygen hood and oxygen tent (croupette), are used primarily in pediatrics. The nasal cannula, oxygen masks and the face tent will be described here.

Nasal cannula. The nasal cannula, also referred to as *nasal prongs*, is the most commonly used aid to breathing. It is an inexpensive, disposable, plastic tube with two protruding curved hollow prongs that fit into the nostrils and is placed around the patient's head with an elastic band (see Procedure 23.8). A nasal cannula has several advantages. It is easy to apply, relatively comfortable for the patient and does not cause feelings of claustrophobia, or interfere with eating, talking or coughing. It permits some freedom of movement without interrupting oxygen flow. To use a cannula effectively, the patient must have clear nasal passages and must be alert and able to keep the device in place. Nasal obstruction from a deviated septum, mucosal edema, polyps or excessive secretions, for example, prevents effective use of a cannula and it can be easily dislodged. Because of the limited area of the nasal cavity to act as a reservoir, the nasal cannula delivers a low range of oxygen concentration. Flow rates of one to six L/min are recommended.

Simple face mask. The simple face mask is a dome-shaped, clear plastic mask that can be molded to fit over the nose and mouth (see Procedure 23.8). It has a metal clip that is bent over the bridge of the nose to ensure a snug fit and prevent leakage of oxygen. It is held in place by an elastic strap around the head that can be adjusted to the patient's comfort. There are several holes (or ports) on each side of the mask through which room air is taken in and mixed with oxygen, and carbon dioxide is exhaled. A flow rate of at least five L/min is necessary to flush exhaled carbon dioxide from the mask. The simple face mask delivers a moderate range of oxygen concentrations at five to eight L/min. It is indicated when a patient requires an increased delivery of oxygen for a short period, for instance less than 12 hours.

Face masks have several disadvantages. First, they are very uncomfortable to wear. Because of the snug fit, masks are warm, confining and cause a closed-in feeling. Pressure can also cause irritation of the face and tops of the nose and ears. Masks must be taken off to eat, speak or cough and for care of the face, thus interrupting the continuity of treatment. If the patient is vomiting, there is a danger of aspiration because the mask inhibits clearance of the vomitus from around the mouth; the danger increases with unconscious or comatose patients. Close observation is mandatory.

Venturi mask. The venturi mask can deliver precise concentrations of oxygen providing the mask fits snugly and remains in place. The venturi system (see Figure 23.15) is designed to limit the amount of room air that is blended with a fixed flow of oxygen. The mask has a specific setting for the desired oxygen concentration. Therapeutic oxygen is delivered at the flow rate (L/min) indicated on the mask, to a small jet (Venturi device) in the centre of a side base cone. A specific amount of room air is entrained in the cone through an opening, called an entrainment port, which mixes with the oxygen. The size of the entrainment opening can be adjusted to control the amount of room air entrained and the percentage of oxygen delivered to the patient. The mask also has large vents through which exhaled air can escape.

When using the venturi mask it is very important to prevent occlusion of the air entrainment ports by bed linen

FIGURE 23.15 Venturi mask. Two views of the mask are shown. In the upper panel, the mask is set to deliver 24% oxygen; note that the litre flow is indicated as 3 L/min and the entrainment opening is wide. In the lower panel, the mask is set to deliver 30% oxygen; the litre flow is now to be set at 6 L/min and the air entrainment opening is much smaller.

SOURCE: Traver, G. A., Mitchell, J. T., and Flodquist-Priestly, G. *Respiratory care: A clinical approach*. Gaithersburg, MA: Aspen, 99. Reproduced with permission.

or clothing. If the jets are occluded the efficiency of the venturi mask is reduced to that of a simple mask and the concentration of oxygen delivered will vary. The venturi mask is used for individuals with COPD because it can provide precise low levels of supplemental oxygen, while avoiding the risk of suppressing the hypoxic drive. The disadvantages of using a venturi mask are the same as for simple masks.

Face tent. The face tent is an enclosure that covers the lower half of the face and fits snugly under the chin (see Figure 23.16). It is open at the top at about the level of the eyes. It is beneficial for patients who cannot tolerate the simple mask or who have facial burns. A large-bore tubing connection at the base of the shield supplies the oxygen. The concentration of oxygen delivered by a face tent is unpredictable. Therefore, it is often used in conjunction with a venturi system. When using a face tent, the nurse should frequently inspect the patient's face for dampness, chafing or irritation and provide care as necessary.

FIGURE 23.16   Face tent

PROCEDURE 23.8

Establishing Oxygen by Nasal Cannula and Face Mask

ACTION	RATIONALE
1. Check the physician's order for the amount and route of administration.	Protects the patient from injury and promotes accuracy.
2. Prepare the patient. Review safety precautions and place "No Smoking, Oxygen in Use" signs in appropriate areas.	Reduces fear and anxiety and enables patient participation. Alerts staff and visitors that oxygen is in use, thereby promoting safety.
3. Gather: • Oxygen source • Flowmeter and tubing • Humidifier bottle containing sterile distilled water • Oxygen delivery device	Facilitates efficiency and economy of time.
4. Set up the equipment as in Procedure 23.7 and connect the delivery device. Adjust the flowmeter control to the prescribed rate.	
5. Apply the delivery device. **Nasal Cannula:** • Position the prongs so they follow the natural curve of the nostril and are directed into the nasal passages. Adjust the strap and tubing according to the type of equipment:	Ensures proper oxygen flow.
a) slip the elastic band around the patient's head.	Secures the cannula in place.

Continued on the next page

ACTION	RATIONALE
b) adjust the tubing around the patient's ears and slide the plastic holder to secure the tubing under the chin.	
• Ensure that adjustments are not too tight.	Avoids pressure areas and patient discomfort.
• Pin or tape the tubing to the patient's gown leaving slack for movement.	Prevents displacement of the prongs and undue stress against the nasal tissues when the patient moves.

a)

b)

Mask

Simple Mask:

• Position the mask so that it covers the nose and mouth, and fits the contours of the patient's face. — Ensures maximum benefit from the oxygen being delivered by preventing its escape around the edges of the mask.

• Fasten the elastic band over the patient's ears and adjust it so the mask fits snugly against the face.

• Mold the nose clip to fit snugly but avoid excessive pressure. — Avoids skin irritation, breakdown or necrosis.

• Attach the oxygen tubing to the patient's clothing. — Prevents unnecessary strain against the mask and potential displacement.

Venturi Mask:

• Adjust the control device on the mask to the prescribed concentration. — Ensures delivery of specified concentration oxygen.

• Apply the mask using the same steps as for the simple mask above.

6. Monitor the patient's status frequently. Note the patient's colour, respiratory status and activity tolerance. Take the pulse and respirations. — Determines effectiveness of oxygen therapy.

7. Document the procedure. Note the device applied, the flow rate, assessments of the patient's oxygenation and respiratory status and the patient's response to therapy. — Fulfills requirements for nurse accountability.

MAINTAINING OXYGEN THERAPY

When oxygen is being administered, frequent monitoring of the patient and the equipment is important. The nurse assesses the patient's vital signs, oxygenation status, colour, level of consciousness, activity tolerance and respiratory pattern. Pulse oximetry for oxygen saturation levels may also be taken at specified intervals. In addition, blood gas analysis may be performed. Oxygen therapy is considered completely effective if it improves a patient's oxygen status and acid–base balance. Equipment must be checked at frequent intervals to ensure proper functioning. The nurse notes, for example, the oxygen flow rate, water level in the humidity bottle (if appropriate) and position of the device on the patient's face. If a venturi mask is in use, the ports are examined for obstructions to ensure delivery of the correct percentage of oxygen.

Therapy will be most effective if the delivery of oxygen is maintained at a constant level. Oxygen flow should only be interrupted to provide necessary care to the face, or the nose in the case of a cannula. Patients who are receiving oxygen via a face mask are provided with nasal prongs for ambulating and eating meals. If the patient is able to sit in a chair or ambulate to the bathroom, tubing long enough to allow for the accomplishment of these activities will be required. A portable tank may offer the patient more mobility and freedom, if the condition allows. The patient can maintain the health of mucous membranes and keep secretions thin by drinking as much fluid as the condition allows.

Care must be taken to promote patient comfort and protect the skin around the delivery device. With a cannula, the patient's nostrils are inspected q2h for dryness, irritation or bleeding. The nares are cleansed and then lubricated with a water-soluble lubricant as necessary to prevent skin breakdown. Petroleum-based agents, such as Vaseline, should not be used because they can ignite spontaneously in the presence of oxygen and cause a fire. Gauze pads are placed under the tubing around the patient's ears or along the cheekbones, if necessary, to reduce irritation and pressure, thereby preventing skin breakdown. The cannula is removed and cleaned as frequently as recommended by the manufacturer to maintain patency of the openings and, as specified by the agency infection control policy, to limit the spread of microorganisms. The patient with a mask is monitored q2–4h for moisture build-up. The mask is removed temporarily and the skin dried as necessary to prevent skin breakdown.

Oxygen therapy equipment is a potential source of bacterial cross-infection. The delivery devices and tubing must be changed frequently according to manufacturer's recommendations and hospital infection control policies to reduce the spread of microorganisms.

OXYGEN HOME CARE

For some patients, oxygen therapy becomes a life-long need. Individuals learn to manage oxygen therapy at home as a part of daily living. The doctor determines the choice of delivery system according to the patient's problem. The systems available for home use are oxygen concentrators, compressed oxygen and liquid oxygen in portable devices. These allow the patient the convenience of being able to leave the home while receiving oxygen therapy.

Patients and family members require support and teaching to manage oxygen therapy efficiently and safely. The nurse can help the patient and family by providing information and coordinating the efforts of the health-care team. This may include, for instance, the respiratory therapist, the home-care nurse and the oxygen supplier in the community.

The patient and family members are taught the reason for the treatment, the importance of using the oxygen only as prescribed by the doctor, the correct administration, safety precautions and maintenance of the equipment. Safety issues are extremely important. Oxygen therapy must be avoided around open flames, for example, lit cigarettes, a gas cooking flame, a fireplace or a wood-burning stove. Tanks or cylinders should be secured on a cart or stand to prevent accidental falls and punctures. Lengthy tubing is useful for mobility, but creates many physical hazards. The patient must be very careful to avoid tripping over the tubing or draping it over the cooking stove. Pets or small children must be kept away from tubing so they cannot chew it.

Cleanliness is very important. Oxygen tubing must be cleaned weekly with gentle soap and water to prevent the growth of microorganisms. Extra long tubing must be replaced monthly. Distilled water used for humidification is always capped and stored in the refrigerator. Hand-held nebulizers (inhalers) should be washed daily in soap and water, rinsed with water, soaked for 20 to 30 minutes in a 1:1 white vinegar–water solution, rinsed with water and finally air-dried. Commercial respirator cleaning agents may also be used if instructions are followed. Cleaning the inhaler in the top shelf of an automatic dishwasher saves time and the hot water destroys most organisms.

ARTIFICIAL AIRWAYS

An **artificial airway** is a tube inserted into the airway by way of the mouth or nose, or through a surgical opening in the trachea called a *tracheostomy*. It is used to maintain airway patency, to provide a route for administering mechanical ventilation and to facilitate suctioning of secretions. The insertion of a tube is called *intubation*; removing it is *extubation*.

An **oral** *(oropharyngeal)* **airway** is a curved, plastic device which slides over the tongue to hold it down and forward (see Figure 23.17). Its main purpose is to prevent the tongue from falling back into the pharynx of the unconscious or semiconscious patient. It also facilitates easy removal of secretions. An oral airway may be used in emergency situations such as respiratory or cardiac arrest when bag-mask ventilation (Ambu bag and mask) is employed during cardiopulmonary resuscitation. The airway facilitates adequate ventilation by keeping the tongue out of the way.

An oral airway is often inserted by the nurse. To be effective, the artificial airway must not be too long and it must be positioned correctly. If an airway is too long or positioned incorrectly, it can stimulate the gag and cough reflexes, causing gagging, vomiting and aspiration. A properly sized airway for a patient is equal in length to the distance from the corner of the patient's mouth to the angle of the jaw below the ear. The steps for inserting an airway are listed in the box below. An airway is *never* inserted if the patient is alert or conscious enough to resist or to push it out . Similarly, an airway is removed as soon as the patient has regained consciousness and the gag and cough reflexes have returned. Keeping airways in conscious patients could stimulate the gag reflex and cause them to aspirate their secretions.

An *endotracheal tube* is passed via the nose or mouth, through the larynx and into the trachea when short-term airway assistance is needed. It is a soft rubber tube used to

FIGURE 23.17   An oral airway in place

provide mechanical ventilation in unconscious or semiconscious patients and to administer anesthetic gases and then mechanically ventilate individuals undergoing surgery. Endotracheal tubes also permit the removal of pulmonary secretions and the administration of medications such as epinephrine hydrochloride in emergency situations (Springhouse, 1989). The procedure is performed by physicians, anesthetists, respiratory therapists and specially trained nurses. Care for a patient with an endotracheal tube requires advanced nursing skills learned in higher levels of nursing programs.

A *tracheostomy* is performed when long-term airway management and mechanical ventilation are anticipated. The major advantages of tracheostomy tubes over endotracheal tubes are that they avoid laryngeal damage and enable patients to take fluid and food orally, if their condition permits (Traver, Mitchell and Flodquist-Priestly, 1991). Like endotracheal care, tracheostomy care is an advanced clinical skill and, therefore, will not be addressed in this book.

EMERGENCY MEASURES

The Heimlich manoeuvre and cardiopulmonary resuscitation (CPR) should be familiar to the reader and thus will not be considered in this text. Nursing students are required to complete a course in basic life support before entering their program of studies and then maintain their skills through yearly recertification. As well, health care providers working in facilities across Canada must maintain certification in basic life support or advanced life support by taking yearly courses set by the Heart and Stroke Foundation of Canada.

Inserting an Oral Airway

- Select the proper size of airway.
- Don clean gloves.
- Rinse the airway in cold water. *Lubricant effect aids insertion.*
- Place the patient in a supine position with the neck hyperextended. *Prevents the tongue from falling back into the pharynx.*
- Open the mouth and place a tongue blade on the front half of the tongue. *Flattens the tongue and facilitates insertion.*
- With the airway sideways, insert it into the mouth and once it is over the tongue, rotate it over and down to the correct position. *Promotes insertion without stimulating the gag reflex.*
- Suction the mouth if needed.
- Position the patient on the side. *Decreases risk of aspirating secretions.*

FIGURE 23.18 Using an Ambu bag and mask. Note the basic position of the hands in holding a bag mask in place. A tight seal should be maintained between the mask and the patient's face with one hand while the bag is squeezed with the other hand. The patient's airway must be kept open by keeping the neck extended as shown.

In the health care setting, a compressible bag, called an Ambu bag, and a mask are used to assist ventilations in the patient who has suffered a respiratory or cardiac arrest (see Figure 23.18). To use the Ambu bag, position the patient with head tilted back and jaw pulled forward to open the airway. An oral airway may be inserted to prevent airway obstruction, which could interfere with adequate ventilation. Hold the mask tightly over the patient's nose and mouth with one hand and, with the other hand, squeeze the bag at a rate of approximately 16 to 20 breaths per minute. The bag will inflate automatically; a one-way valve in the mask allows exhaled air to escape. Continue artificial ventilations, or "bagging," until spontaneous breathing is established, until another mechanical assistance is established or until death is confirmed by a doctor. Oxygen tubing can usually be attached to the bag to increase the oxygen supply to the patient. Many devices also have an adapter that can be directly connected to a tracheostomy or endotracheal tube for manual ventilations of a patient who is intubated.

EVALUATING OXYGENATION INTERVENTIONS

Evaluation of the effectiveness of measures to improve oxygenation are based on the expected outcomes. Following is a list of criteria which the nurse may generally find useful in evaluating care.

1. Is the patient breathing more easily?
2. Has the patient's anxiety been relieved?
3. Is the patient's airway patent?
4. Has ventilatory efficiency been improved?
5. Have distressing symptoms such as coughing been relieved?
6. Has cyanosis been lessened?
7. Is the patient able to bring up sputum sufficiently to clear the bronchial tree?
8. Has activity tolerance increased?
9. Has the patient or the patient's family gained the knowledge and skills necessary to continue treatment at home?

KEY TERMS

IN REVIEW

Oxygen is an essential nutrient for life. Without oxygen, cells malfunction, become damaged and die. Tissues of the brain and heart are particularly sensitive as they can die within a few minutes of oxygen deprivation.

Oxygenation is a complex process carried out by the respiratory and cardiovascular systems. The upper respiratory tract provides a passageway which warms, filters and moisturizes the inhaled air. The lower respiratory tract delivers oxygen to the alveoli and returns carbon dioxide to the atmosphere. The exchange of oxygen and carbon dioxide between the lungs and the circulation occurs in the alveoli. The cardiovascular system includes the heart, blood vessels and blood. It transports oxygen from the lungs to the tissues and carbon dioxide from the tissues back to the lungs. The three major processes involved in oxygenation are ventilation, diffusion and transportation.

The body has an effective set of lung clearance mechanisms to ensure intake of clean air and remove harmful debris. These are filtration, mucociliary action, sneezing and coughing.

An adequate supply of oxygen to the body is affected by numerous factors. In addition to an adequate supply of clean air and oxygen in the atmosphere, effective oxygenation depends on patent airways, proper muscle functioning, pulmonary compliance and adequate oxygen/carbon dioxide transport. Health practices, such as regular aerobic exercises and avoidance of exposure to cigarette smoke and hazardous occupational materials, have a positive influence on oxygenation and on one's health and well-being.

Assessment of oxygenation status is a critical nursing activity. The nursing health history collects subjective data about the patient's usual pattern of oxygenation, smoking history, recent changes in the pattern of oxygenation, symptoms of the presenting health problem, recent or past related health problems and family history. Review of the patient's chart and physical observations supply objective data. The chart shows diagnostic test results and also provides information about the patient's illness and diagnostic or treatment measures that may affect oxygenation. Physical examination includes inspection of the chest, respiratory movements and breathing pattern. The nurse also measures pulse, respirations and blood pressure and examines sputum, colour of skin and mucous membranes. Fingers are inspected for clubbing and the chest wall is palpated for expiratory expansion and fremitus. Auscultation is carried out to determine the presence of normal and abnormal breath sounds. Pulse oximetry, laboratory tests of CBC and arterial blood gases, sputum studies and diagnostic tests (such as bronchoscopy, lung scans, and pulmonary function tests) provide valuable information.

Nursing diagnoses pertaining to oxygenation problems include *Ineffective airway clearance* and *Ineffective breathing patterns*. *High risk for altered respiratory function* may be used to describe potential problems caused by smoking, immobility and environmental allergies. The diagnostic label *Activity intolerance* is appropriate when insufficient oxygenation interferes with the ability to move and function effectively in daily living.

Nursing interventions are planned to maintain and restore airway patency, pulmonary ventilation and oxygen/carbon dioxide transport; prevent deterioration of pulmonary function; and promote optimal functioning in daily living.

Health promoting strategies are those for general good health. Health protecting strategies include positioning, breathing exercises, effective coughing, use of an incentive spirometer and leg exercises. Unconscious patients should be placed in a semi-prone position to prevent aspiration and blockage of the airway by the tongue. Upright positions — Fowler's or semi-Fowler's — should be used for conscious patients. Breathing exercises include deep breathing, abdominal breathing and pursed-lip breathing. Coughing helps to clear secretions and debris from the lungs. It should be done only when there are secretions. Splinting a surgical incision aids with coughing and deep breathing. Incentive spirometry increases lung functioning and improves pulmonary ventilation.

Health restoring strategies establish airway patency, increase ventilatory efficiency, ensure adequate oxygen intake and decrease bodily needs for oxygen. Patients who experience dyspnea need assistance in completing activities of daily living. Uninterrupted rest periods, a well-balanced diet taken in small frequent meals and measures to alleviate emotional tension and anxiety are essential for restoring energy and supporting oxygenation.

Patients with respiratory secretions need adequate hydration and humidity therapy. Medications to dilate the tracheobronchial tree and liquefy secretions may be administered using aerosol-nebulization therapy. Chest physiotherapy (postural drainage) loosens and moves secretions into the large airways so they can be expectorated. Suctioning of the oropharynx and nasopharynx is necessary in patients who have difficulty swallowing or expectorating secretions.

Oxygen therapy supplies supplemental oxygen which improves cellular oxygenation, decreases the work of breathing and reduces stress on the heart. Clinically, oxygen is considered a drug, so it must be administered according to principles of medication therapy. Oxygen must be administered carefully because excessive amounts produce harmful effects. Because oxygen supports combustion, safety measures are very important.

LEARNING ACTIVITIES

1. **Case Study**: Mr. Rowlands is a 38-year-old patient who has been in the hospital for three weeks. His medical diagnosis is acute bronchial asthma. When he was admitted his breathing was dyspneic, he appeared cyanotic, and his respiratory rate varied from 28 to 34 respirations per minute.

   Mr. Rowlands did not want his bed to be flat; he demanded five pillows from the nurse and spent most of his time bent forward in bed. He was thin and appeared anxious. In addition to intravenous corticosteroids and bronchodilators administered by a mini-nebulizer, the physician ordered oxygen by nasal cannula. Mr. Rowlands liked to use the oxygen and preferred to turn it on and off himself.

   a. What factors should be taken into consideration in explaining to this patient how to use the oxygen equipment?

b. By what means can the patient's need for oxygen be assessed?

c. For what reason might the patient demand five pillows, and why would he like to handle the oxygen himself?

d. Identify the nursing diagnoses in this situation. Outline expected outcomes and interventions to resolve the identified problems.

e. How can the effectiveness of these measures be evaluated?

2. With the aid of your instructor, arrange to spend a day with a respiratory therapist in your agency. What types of care does the respiratory therapist provide? In what ways do nurses and respiratory therapists collaborate to provide care in this agency?

REFERENCES AND READINGS

BELL, R. (1983). The body works...Physiology of aging and exercise. In *Fitness for seniors: A handbook for leaders*. Ottawa: Minister of State, Fitness and Amateur Sport, Government of Canada.

BERGER, K.J. and WILLIAMS, M.B. (1992). *Fundamentals of nursing: Collaborating for optimal health*. Norwalk, CT: Appleton & Lange.

BJORNDAHL, S. (1990). *Pulse oximeter: Module*. Vancouver: Vancouver Hospital.

BRILL, E. L., and KILTS, D. F. (1986). *Foundations for nursing* (2nd ed.). Norwalk, CT: Appleton-Century-Crofts.

CAMPBELL, E., BAKER, M. and CRITES-SILVER, P. (1988). Subjective effects of humidification of oxygen for delivery by nasal cannula. *Chest, 93*(2), 289–293.

CARPENITO, L.J. (1993). *Nursing diagnosis: Application to clinical practice* (5th ed.). Philadelphia: Lippincott.

CARPENTER, K.D. (1993, August). A comprehensive review of cyanosis. *Critical Care Nurse*. 66–71.

EARNEST, V.V. (1993). *Clinical skills in nursing practice* (2nd ed.). Philadelphia: Lippincott.

ELLIS, J.R. and NOWLIS, E.A. (1994). *Nursing: A human needs approach*. Philadelphia: Lippincott.

FISCHBACH, F. (1992). *A manual of laboratory and diagnostic tests* (4th ed.). Philadelphia: Lippincott.

FLYNN, J.M. and HACKEL, R. (1990). *Technological foundations in nursing*. Norwalk, CT: Appleton & Lange.

JARVIS, C. (1992). *Physical examination and health assessment*. Philadelphia: Saunders.

LABORATORY WARD MANUAL. (1992). North Vancouver, BC: Lions Gate Hospital.

LACEY, G. (1988). Physiology of oxygenation. *Emergency Prehospital Medicine, 2*(4), 17–22.

LEWIS, S.M. and COLLIER, I.C. (1992). *Medical-surgical nursing: Assessment and management of clinical problems* (3rd ed.). St. Louis: Mosby.

MALASANOS, L., BARKAUSKAS, V. and STOLTENBERG-ALLEN, K. (1990). *Health assessment* (4th ed.). St. Louis: Mosby.

MARIEB, E.N. (1984). *Essentials of human anatomy and physiology*. Menlo Park, CA: Addison-Wesley.

MARIEB, E.N. (1989). *Human anatomy and physiology*. Redwood City, CA: Benjamin/Cummings.

MARTINI, F. (1989). *Fundamentals of anatomy and physiology*. Englewood Cliffs, NJ: Prentice-Hall.

PATIENT INSTRUCTIONS FOR INHALER USE (Patient Information Pamphlet #343 10/92). (1992). Department of Pharmacy and Education Services, Vancouver: University Hospital.

PATRICK, M.L., WOODS, S.L., CRAVEN, R.F., ROKOSKY, J.S. and BRUNO, P. M. (1991). *Medical-surgical nursing: Pathophysiological approach* (2nd ed.). Philadelphia: Lippincott.

SMELTZER, S. and BARE, B. (1992). *Brunner and Suddarth's textbook of medical-surgical nursing*. Philadelphia: Lippincott.

SMITH-TEMPLE, J. and YOUNG-JOHNSON, J. (1994). *Nurses' guide to clinical procedures* (2nd ed.). Philadelphia: Lippincott.

SPRINGHOUSE CORPORATION. (1989). *Respiratory care: Handbook*. Springhouse, PA: Author.

STIESMEYER, J.K. (1993, August). A four-step approach to pulmonary assessment. *American Journal of Nursing*. 22–28.

SUDDARTH D.S. (1991). *The Lippincott Manual of nursing practice* (5th ed.). Philadelphia: Lippincott.

TRAVER, G.A., MITCHELL, J.T. and FLODQUIST-PRIESTLY, G. (1991). *Respiratory care: A clinical approach*. Gaithersburg, MA: Aspen.

WEILITZ, P.B. (1991). *Pocket guide to respiratory care*. St. Louis: Mosby.

WILLIAMS, M.W. (1993). *Lifetime: Fitness and wellness* (3rd ed.). Madison, WI: Brown and Benchmark.

WILSON, S.F. and THOMPSON, J.M. (1990). *Respiratory disorders*. St. Louis: Mosby.

YEAW, E.M.J. (1992, March). How position affects oxygenation: Good lung down? *American Journal of Nursing*. 27–29.

CHAPTER 24

Temperature Regulation Needs

CENTRAL QUESTIONS

1. What are the heat-regulating mechanisms of the body and how do they maintain a stable temperature within the body?

2. What are the main determinants of body temperature regulation?

3. How does temperature regulation vary throughout the life cycle?

4. What are the common problems of disturbed temperature regulation?

5. How does the nurse assess temperature regulation status?

6. What are the common nursing diagnostic statements for patients with temperature regulation problems?

7. How does the nurse develop a plan of care for patients with temperature regulation problems?

8. What information might the nurse give to individuals, families, or groups in helping them to promote optimum temperature regulation?

9. What health protecting measures can the nurse implement for a patient with a fever?

10. What health restoring and supportive strategies can the nurse implement in the care of patients with temperature regulation problems?

11. How does the nurse evaluate the patient's response to nursing interventions?

12. How does the nurse implement therapeutic heat and cold measures?

13. What basic principles does the nurse apply when administering heat and cold treatments?

INTRODUCTION

The surface temperature of the body varies with environmental changes, and human beings have had to learn to dress appropriately to protect themselves from both the hot tropical sun and the cold northern winds. Over the centuries, humans also have developed the ability to modify their immediate surroundings to provide an environmental temperature most comfortable for them.

With regard to the *core temperature* (or internal temperature) of the body, humans are **homeothermic**, or warm-blooded, with inborn mechanisms for maintaining a stable temperature within the body.

Heat regulation, or *thermoregulation*, involves not only those mechanisms concerned with the production of heat within the body, but also those involved in its dissipation. These mechanisms of the body maintain a precise balance between heat production and heat loss. In this way, the internal body temperature is kept within a very narrow range, usually varying not more than 0.5 to 1°C within a 24-hour period (Cooper, 1969; Ganong, 1989). The heat-regulating system is one of the body's most important homeostatic mechanisms.

Every once in a while, however, the balance is upset and deviations outside the normal range of body temperature occur. Many people who are ill have an elevated temperature. It is, indeed, one of the cardinal signs of illness, often being one of the first observable indications that there is a disturbance of body function. The maintenance of a higher-than-normal temperature puts considerable stress on the body's adaptive mechanisms, and is very debilitating.

The balance also may be upset in the opposite direction. Mild degrees of lowered body temperature (1 to 2°C) apparently do not do as much harm to the body as fever does. At lower temperatures, all body processes slow down and when the body warms up, they commence to function at normal levels again. However, the problem of *hypothermia* (excessively low body temperatures) both in accidental and clinical situations due, in most cases, to prolonged exposure to cold environmental temperatures continues to be a concern. It appears to be more common than was once thought. *Frostbite*, which involves freezing of the skin tissues in one area of the body, such as exposed earlobes, the tip of the nose, fingers, or toes, has always been a problem in cold climates. *Chilblains*, a mild form of frostbite, also are a common source of discomfort, particularly to older people who live in cold, damp climates and whose homes are not equipped with central heating.

Applications of both heat and cold have been used for centuries to treat various disorders of the human body. Both have systemic and localized effects on body tissues and are still frequently used in therapy. This chapter describes the mechanisms underlying body temperature regulation and the therapies employed to maintain thermal health.

THE BODY'S MECHANISMS FOR TEMPERATURE REGULATION

Human beings are in a state of thermal health when their central body temperature is about 37°C. Body temperature is a measure of the body's heat; it reflects the ability to maintain a balance between heat gain and loss. Human beings produce heat continuously through the process of cellular metabolism. The body heat produced through metabolism must be lost to the environment so that a constant body temperature can be maintained. Heat is lost from the body through a variety of means as outlined in the accompanying box.

To maintain thermal health, it is necessary to adapt to changing conditions in the immediate (ambient) environment and to internal metabolic processes. Humans have various adaptive mechanisms to promote heat if body temperature falls too low, or to lose excess heat if the temperature goes too high. Figure 24.1 illustrates thermal health and adaptation. According to Erickson (1982), thermal health exists when environmental challenges (ambient and metabolic) are balanced by the individual's adaptive capabilities, which include biological, behavioural and social modes. When the environmental demands exceed the individual's adaptive capacities, body temperature rises or falls below normal range, and thermal dysfunction occurs. The goal of nursing is to tip the balance towards thermal reserve and wellness by enhancing the patient's adaptive potentials.

Biological Adaptive Modes

The regulatory mechanisms controlling body temperature are located in the preoptic area of the hypothalamus which acts as the body's thermostat. Neurons in this area respond to changes in the temperature of the blood circulating through it by sending impulses either to the anterior heat-losing centre (in the hypothalamus) or to the posterior heat-gaining centre. These centres have a reciprocal effect on each other; when one is activated, the other is depressed. Both peripheral (skin) and core temperature receptors play a role in the control of thermoregulation.

It is generally believed that body temperature is regulated around a narrowly defined temperature or *setpoint* (Benzinger, 1969; Bruck, 1983). Although individuals vary somewhat in the temperature at which their body is maintained, (Ganong, 1989) temperature homeostasis results in a relatively constant central temperature. When body temperature deviates from the setpoint, the heat-losing or heat-gaining centre is stimulated.

Mechanisms of Body Heat Loss

MECHANISM	EXAMPLE
Conduction: The direct transfer of heat from the body to cooler objects in the immediate environment.	Lying on a cold stretcher
Convection: Body heat is transferred to air currents circulating around the body.	The cooling effect of a fan
Evaporation: Body heat is used up to convert moisture on the surface of the skin to vapour.	The effect of sweating
Radiation: The transfer of heat, in the form of electromagnetic waves, from the body to cooler objects in the environment. Over half of body heat loss occurs through this process.	Lying next to a cold window

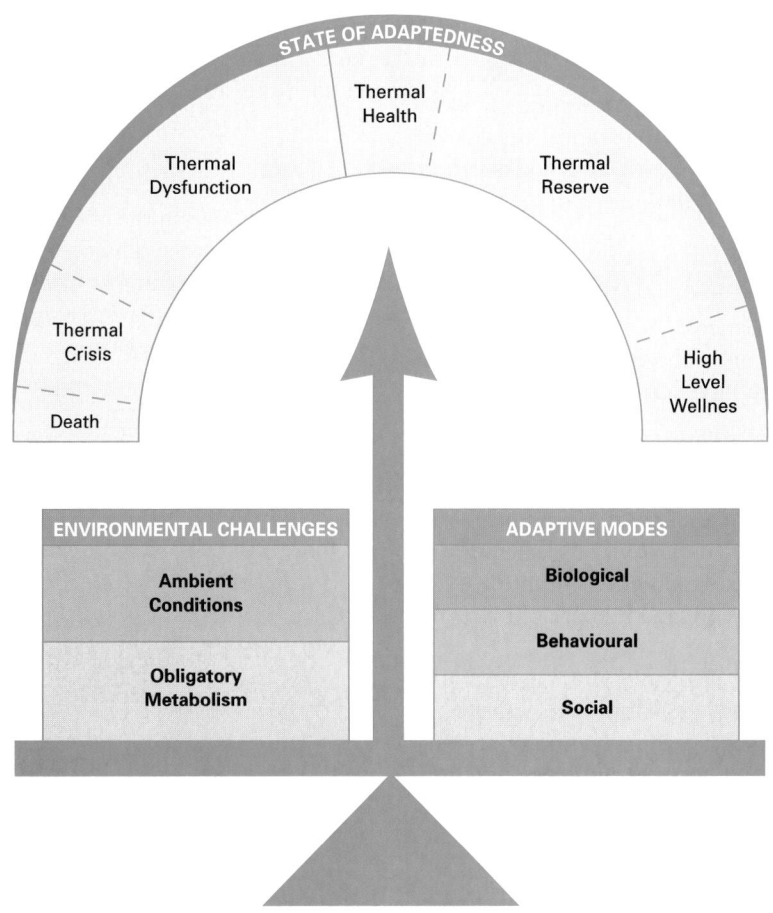

FIGURE 24.1   A model of adaptation to the thermal environment

SOURCE: Erickson, R. (1982). A model of adaptation to the thermal environment. *Advances in Nursing Science, 14*(4), 1-12. Reproduced with permission of Aspen Publishers Inc.

When the temperature at the preoptic nucleus drops below the setpoint, the heat-gaining centre is activated. Stimulation of the heat-gaining centre initially increases wakefulness and stimulates muscular activity. If the individual does not engage in some form of exercise in response to this, the body will initiate its own muscular activity involuntarily in the form of shivering, which can produce a considerable amount of heat within the body — as much as 400 percent (Martini, 1989).

At the same time, stimulation of the sympathetic nervous system facilitates the release of both epinephrine and norepinephrine into the blood stream. As a result, glucose stores in the liver are released for energy. Cellular metabolism is accelerated and heat is produced.

Stimulation of the sympathetic nervous system also results in the phenomenon of *piloerection*, in which hairs stand on end. In human beings, this mechanism is usually manifested in the milder reaction of a "goose flesh" appearance of the skin. In animals with long hair, this mechanism serves to entrap a layer of warm air next to the skin. In human beings, the mechanism is not as effective in providing insulation, but it occurs nonetheless. Cessation of sweating usually occurs as well, to reduce the amount of heat lost through evaporation of water from the body surface.

Concomitantly, vasoconstriction takes place and blood is drawn away from surface vessels to minimize the amount of heat lost through conduction, convection and radiation. Individuals become pale and their skin is cold to the touch. They also feel cold.

With prolonged exposure to colder temperatures than normal, the thyroid gland is stimulated to increase production of the hormone thyroxine. This results in an increased metabolic rate and subsequent increased heat production. However, this process is slower, occurring over a period of weeks.

Conversely, stimulation of the heat-losing centre when the temperature setpoint is exceeded has an inhibitory effect on the mechanisms for heat production, and the reverse effects are seen. Muscular activity is decreased and metabolism is slowed; vasodilation occurs resulting in increased circulation to the skin; and the rate of thyroxine production gradually decreases.

The body also has two mechanisms unique to the facilitation of heat loss; these are panting and sweating. In other animals, rapid shallow breathing (panting) increases the amount of heat lost by evaporation of moisture from the respiratory tract or tongue. Rapid deep breathing (hyperventilation) in humans has the same effect. In our case, however, the principal mechanism for cooling the body is by increasing perspiration. This greatly facilitates the loss of heat from the body through the process of evaporation of moisture from the skin. If the environmental temperature is higher than body temperature, perspiration is the only mechanism available to us for heat loss.

Behavioural Adaptive Modes

Our ability to modify the surrounding environment is the most powerful mode of adaptation to extremes in environmental conditions. This behavioural adaptation is motivated by the conscious appraisal of the thermal environment. Thermal comfort is the subjective feeling of satisfaction with the temperature of the surrounding environment, desiring it to be neither warmer nor cooler (ASHRAE, 1982). Thermal comfort is said to indirectly reflect the heat balance in the body. It is related to an individual's level of activity and clothing, and to ambient conditions (Mount, 1979). Individuals at rest, wearing light clothing, usually feel comfortable in an ambient environment of 24 to 25°C and, when unclothed, are comfortable in an environment of about 28 to 30°C (Erickson, 1982).

Adaptive behaviours to maintain thermal comfort include altering posture to change the amount of exposed body surface (by curling or stretching out), ingesting hot or cold foods or beverages, creating a favourable environment by using artificial heating or cooling devices and donning clothing appropriate to the ambient temperature. Clothing, of course, decreases the effects of environmental temperatures on body heat. The insulation of the body by adequate, warm clothing lessens the impact of cold temperatures. In warm climates, cottons are more comfortable to wear because they absorb moisture. Synthetic fibres and wool do not absorb as well; hence, they inhibit the removal of perspiration from the body.

Several factors influence the ability to behaviourally adapt to the environment. Conscious perception and voluntary movement is essential for all behavioural responses (Erickson, 1982). The unconscious or immobilized patient

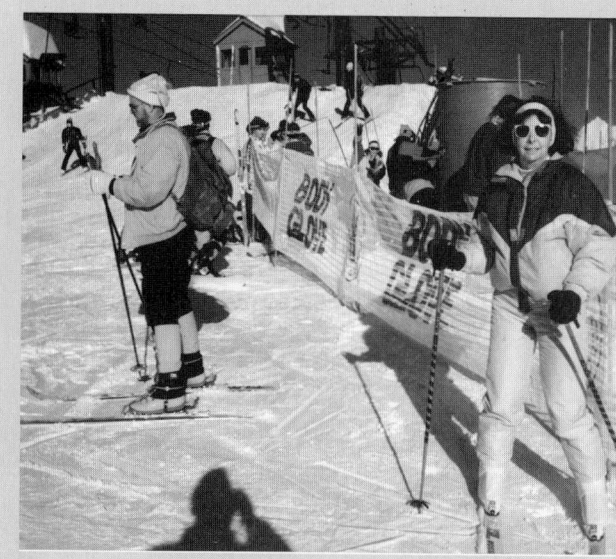

Wearing warm clothing insulates the body from cold temperature.

is therefore at risk for thermal dysfunction. Furthermore, the individual's knowledge of risk factors and available resources will affect behaviour.

Social Adaptation

Individuals with impaired ability to biologically or behaviourally adapt to thermal challenges in their environment can achieve thermal comfort and health through social adaptation. Direct practical assistance through physical care, material resources and education can help individuals to achieve comfort (Erickson, 1982). For example, nurses can provide a warming blanket and warm intravenous solutions to the hypothermic patient.

DETERMINANTS OF BODY TEMPERATURE

Body temperature may be affected by a number of factors. These include conditions that increase metabolic rate, emotions, body size and mass, illness and disease states and environment.

Conditions that Increase Basal Metabolic Rate

Any factor that increases the metabolic rate will raise the temperature of the body; conversely, a decreased metabolic rate will lower body temperature. In exercise, muscular activity increases body temperature as a result of heat production by body muscles. With heavy muscular exercise rectal temperature may rise as high as 40°C (Guyton, 1981). When the temperature begins to rise, the body's heat-regulating mechanisms start to function. Blood is drawn to the surface for cooling and the person starts to perspire. Usually an elevated temperature due to exercise quickly returns to normal with the cessation of activity.

Disturbances in the production of thyroxine by the thyroid gland also affect body temperature. An excess production of thyroxine (due to an overactive thyroid gland) increases the basal metabolic rate, thereby stimulating heat production. People with a thyroid deficiency, on the other hand, have a lower metabolic rate, and consequently a body temperature that is usually at the low end of the normal range.

An increase in body temperature itself will stimulate the cells to increase the rate of cellular metabolism and heat production. For each 1°C rise in temperature, the rate of heat production increases 13 percent and the metabolic rate may be 40 times as high as normal (Dubois, 1921). As a result, an increased temperature tends to heighten a fever. A lowered body temperature for a prolonged period has the

reverse effect of decreasing metabolism, which will in turn lessen body temperature still further.

The specific dynamic action of foods also affects body temperature. The body's metabolic rate is stimulated by the intake of food and remains elevated for several hours after a meal. Underfeeding, on the other hand, decreases the metabolic rate, reducing internal heat production. Foods differ in their specific dynamic qualities. Proteins increase the metabolic rate (up to 30 percent) more than fats and carbohydrates do, and the increase remains high over a longer period of time (three to twelve hours after the meal) (Martini, 1989).

There is a circadian rhythm to metabolism and body temperature. In humans, core temperature may fluctuate between 0.5°C and 1.0°C over a 24-hour period. It is generally lowest in early morning between midnight and 6 AM and peaks between 4 and 8 PM (Britten, 1986).

Emotions

Strong emotions, such as anger, can also raise body temperature because of stimulation of the sympathetic nervous system. It is thought that this may be the result of muscle tensing (Ganong, 1989). "The heat of anger" and "feverish with excitement" are common expressions that represent genuine physical conditions. One notices the relationship between emotional and physical states particularly with children, whose body temperatures are more labile (that is, they fluctuate more easily) than those of adults.

Body Size and Mass

Other factors such as body size and mass influence an individual's capacity to maintain thermal health. Subcutaneous fat is an efficient insulator, conducting heat at a slower rate than other tissues (Martini, 1989). This is how long distance swimmers (who generally have a thicker layer of adipose tissue) maintain their body temperatures even in relatively cold water. Conversely, older people are more vulnerable to cold because they generally have a thinner layer of subcutaneous tissue. Obese individuals have a tendency to retain heat and have difficulty tolerating hot environmental conditions.

When the body surface area is large in proportion to weight, there is less muscle mass to produce metabolic heat. This is why infants lose heat rapidly and therefore require warmer environments than adults.

Illness and Disease States

Disease states affect the efficiency of the body's temperature-regulating mechanisms. Poor circulation related to cardiac or vascular disease impairs the body's ability to dissipate heat. Disorders that affect the nervous system can interfere with the reflexive responses to changes in body temperature.

Environment

The surrounding environment has a pronounced effect upon body temperature. Not only permanent changes, such as those encountered when moving to a hot or cold climate, but also temporary changes, such as a brief hot spell, affect the body by raising or lowering its temperature. The body's ability to withstand high environmental temperatures is dependent on the humidity of the atmosphere. When the air is dry and there are sufficient air currents to carry heat away from the body by convection, an individual can stand very high temperatures with little or no increase in body temperature. If, on the other hand, the humidity is high, then the amount of heat lost through evaporation from the surface of the body is decreased and body temperature begins to rise quickly. This explains why one feels so uncomfortable on hot, "muggy" days.

Similarly, a cold environment decreases body temperature. Cold, damp weather is much more chilling than cold dry weather, and when there is considerable amount of air movement, increasing amounts of heat are carried away from the body. The "wind chill" factor can produce the effect of a temperature much lower than that which is registered on the outdoor thermometer.

There is a range of ambient temperatures within which normal body temperature is maintained with minimal metabolic work or evaporative losses. This temperature range, called the thermoneutral zone, is between 27 and 33°C for the naked adult (Mitchell and Laburn, 1985).

TEMPERATURE REGULATION THROUGHOUT THE LIFE CYCLE

Early in pregnancy, there is a slight rise in the body temperature of most women, which continues until about the fourth month. Body temperature generally returns to normal levels at about this time and stays within the normal range the remainder of pregnancy.

Maternal fever in early pregnancy (four to six weeks) can be *teratogenic*, that is, it can cause the development of physical defects in the fetus, particularly in the brain. Pregnant women should take precautions to avoid developing a fever during this time.

Normally the fetus is maintained for nine months in the warm, protected environment of the uterus. Immediately after birth, the newborn's temperature usually falls 1 to 2°C

Premature infants are cared for in a unit with a neutral thermal environment.

because of the evaporation of amniotic fluid from the skin as the infant's total body surface is exposed to the cooler environment outside the mother's body. Further heat loss is prevented in the birthing room by drying and placing the newborn under radiant heat. The newborn may also be placed on the mother's abdomen. By maintaining skin-to-skin contact, the newborn is kept warm by the mother's body heat. A newborn's temperature is quite unstable because the heat regulating system is not yet fully developed. Hence, it is important to maintain a stable environmental temperature. A *neutral thermal environment* (32°C) is considered best because it requires minimum oxygen consumption at rest. This point is particularly important in the care of premature infants, whose heat-regulating mechanisms are even less mature than those of full-term infants.

During the first year of life, infants continue to be highly dependent on environmental temperature to maintain their own internal temperature because of immaturity of the heat-regulating system. The shivering mechanism does not usually begin to function until after the first year. Heat must be produced through the use of specialized adipose tissue known as *brown fat* which can quickly accelerate the infant's metabolic rate (Martini, 1989). This mechanism, although short-lived, plays an important role in temperature maintenance during infancy (McCance and Huether, 1990). Because their body surface area is relatively large, it is important that infants be protected from becoming too cold, or too warm, with changes in the environmental temperature. Appropriate clothing for the climate is essential (warm wool clothing for winter weather and cool cottons for summer or in the tropics).

Infants can develop a high fever very rapidly, and this frequently occurs with the acute respiratory infections that are common in early childhood. The high fever may produce convulsions — a very frightening experience for the new parent. Another concern is that seizures, as a result of fever, may cause brain damage. Although many children have seizures at relatively low temperatures (38.3°C) on the first day of illness, these seizures do not recur on subsequent days when the fever reaches its peak (Fruthaler, 1985). Unless they are due to brain injury or tumour, seizures accompanying fever rarely result in permanent damage to neurologic tissue (Fruthaler, 1985).

During childhood, the body temperature averages approximately 37°C. A child can run a fever as a result of excitement, for example; however, fever in children is usually secondary to infection, and is often the first indication that they are ill. It is not until adolescence that sweating in the axilla occurs; younger children do not have this mechanism to assist in cooling the body.

With onset of the menses, girls experience a cyclical rise and fall of body temperature which continues through the childbearing years. There is a fall in the early morning temperature of most women just after the onset of menstruation. The temperature remains at this lower level until ovulation takes place. There is then an abrupt rise of 0.5 to 1.0°C that occurs with ovulation (Kemp, Pillitteri and Brown, 1989). The body temperature remains at this increased level until the beginning of the next menstrual period. This pattern in body temperature can be used by women to determine ovulation and is therefore helpful in family planning (Kemp, Pillitteri and Brown, 1989).

Women also experience variations of body temperature during the menopause. Once ovulation has ceased, secretion of the female hormones, the estrogens, declines rapidly. One of the distressing side effects is a disturbance in temperature regulation that gives rise to the characteristic "hot flushes" (or "hot flashes") experienced by many women in middle-age. During these episodes, the woman suddenly feels very warm, her skin becomes extremely flushed, and she often finds herself drenched with perspiration. These episodes usually last for only a few minutes. Irregular intervals of hot flashes may be experienced by women for a number of years.

Hot flashes can be triggered by things such as stress, alcohol, caffeine, spicy foods and monosodium glutamate (Manitoba Health, 1990). Interestingly, hot flashes are reported less frequently by women from non-Western cultures (Manitoba Health, 1990). The reason for this cultural difference remains unknown.

Many women have been relieved of this and other symptoms of menopause by taking a low dosage of estrogen replacement therapy (ERT). There is concern, however, that the long-term use of estrogen increases the risks of endometrial cancer (cancer of the lining of the uterus) and gall bladder disease (Manitoba Health, 1990). Many physicians advise women not to take estrogen therapy for too long a period. There are other measures that have been found helpful in relieving hot flashes. Among these are non-hormonal medications (Clonidine and Bellargal) and self-care strategies (such as wearing cotton undergarments, keeping a diary of episodes and triggering agents) (Manitoba Health, 1990).

The basal metabolic rate gradually decreases with age, so that older men and women usually have a body temperature lower than that of young adults. The decreasing efficiency of most body systems that accompanies the aging process also renders the older person more vulnerable to the effects of changing environmental temperatures. Older people often do not cope very well with heat. Sweat glands atrophy and circulation becomes sluggish, limiting their ability to dissipate heat through perspiration (Caruso and Posey, 1985). Hypothermia also can be a problem because the older person tends to be undernourished, and has a slower metabolic rate, which limits heat production. The vasoconstrictor response and shivering reflex also become delayed and less effective (McCance and Huether, 1990).

Medications such as diuretics ("water pills") and anticholinergics (used to treat neuromuscular symptoms) inhibit the normal thermoregulatory processes of vasodilation and sweating. The physiological changes associated with aging, combined with underlying disease states and medications, place older people at high risk for heat-related illnesses and hypothermia.

COMMON PROBLEMS

Although normal processes can cause mild fluctuations in body temperature, many illnesses also cause deviations from the normal. Most frequently, the fluctuations are in the direction of an elevated temperature, giving rise to a fever. The most common of these illnesses are infections, diseases of the central nervous system, neoplasms and metabolic disorders. These heat-related illnesses continue to be a common problem. Fluctuations in the opposite direction, resulting in hypothermia (in both accidental and clinical situations), can also create challenges for the practitioner. Figure 24.2 provides a summary of normal and abnormal variations in body temperature.

FEVER

The physiological mechanisms responsible for fever are not known for all disease processes. It is generally felt that fever may be caused by abnormalities in the brain itself or by toxic substances that affect the heat-regulating mechanisms.

A number of stimuli may activate the hypothalamic centres. Important among these are the substances called *pyrogens*, which are secreted by toxic bacteria or released by degenerating tissue. It is believed that these substances stimulate the release of a second substance, *endogenous*

Major Physiological Effects	Thermoregulatory Capabilities	F°	C°	Associated Condition
Death		114		
Proteins denature, tissue damage accelerates	Severely impaired	110	44	Heat Stroke
Convulsions Cell damage	Impaired	106	42	CNS damage
Disorientation	Effective	102	40	Disease-related fevers Severe exercise Active children
			38	
Systems normal		98	36	Normal range (oral)
Disorientation	Impaired	94	34	Early mornings in cold weather Severe exposure
Loss of muscle control		90	32	
Loss of consciousness		86	30	
Cardiac arrest	Severely impaired	82	28	Hypothermia for open heart surgery
		78	26	
Skin turns blue	Lost		24	
		74		
Death				

FIGURE 24.2   Normal and abnormal variations in body temperature

SOURCE: Martini, F. (1989). *Fundamentals of anatomy and physiology.* Englewood Cliffs, NJ: Prentice-Hall, 736. Reproduced with permission.

pyrogen, from the leukocytes that have been drawn to the diseased area. The endogenous pyrogens then act on the thermoregulatory centres (Guyton, 1981).

There is evidence to suggest that fever caused by pyrogens has some beneficial effects in helping the body to combat infection. It is felt that the fever acts in two ways: (1) it creates an undesirable temperature for the survival of bacteria; and (2) the increased rate of metabolism in the cells increases their production of immune bodies and also their ability to phagocytize foreign bodies, thus impeding bacterial invasion.

Dehydration can also affect the hypothalamic centres directly so that the temperature rises to febrile levels. Part of the elevation is due to lack of fluids for sweating, which deprives the body of one of its principal mechanisms for losing excess heat.

Fever may occur postoperatively owing to a number of causes. It may be due to excessive heat production, as in the case of pathogenic infection, or due to inadequate heat elimination as a result of peripheral vasoconstriction. Fever may occur secondary to the surgical stress response, to respiratory atelectasis or to lung congestion.

Fever frequently accompanies a head injury and is often seen in patients with spinal cord injuries. In the case of head injury, it is felt to be caused by pressure on, or injury to, the hypothalamus or the tracts leading to and from the heat-regulating centres (MacBryde and Blacklow, 1970). In the spinal cord-injured patient, vasoconstriction, piloerection and sweating mechanisms are impaired below the level of the injury in the spinal cord (Lewis and Collier, 1992).

A term that is frequently used synonymously with fever is **pyrexia**. *Hyperpyrexia* and *hyperthermia* are used interchangeably to designate an abnormally high fever, that is, 40.5°C or higher.

Although prolonged fevers are not seen as commonly today as in the years before the use of antibiotics, it is well for the nurse to know the technical terms used for different types of fevers. The terms are descriptive and explain the nature of the fever.

An *intermittent* or *quotidian* fever is one in which the temperature rises each day but falls to normal sometime during the 24-hour period, most often during the early morning hours. A *remittent* fever is one which shows marked variations in the temperature readings during a 24-hour period, the lowest reading, however, always being above the patient's normal level. In a *relapsing* fever, the patient's temperature may be normal for one or two days, then elevated for varying periods. These periods of normalcy are interspersed irregularly throughout the course of a relapsing fever. The term *hectic* or *septic* may be used to describe an intermittent fever in which there are wide fluctuations in daily temperature readings. It is not unusual for the temperature to vary as much as 2.2°C within a 24-hour period with this type of fever. Another type of fever is called a *sustained* or *continuous* fever. In this type, the patient's temperature remains at essentially the same level over a period of days or weeks.

Fever also may be classified as being either low-grade, above 37.1°C but below 38.2°C, or high-grade, above 38.2. A fever of undetermined origin is one in which there is no identifiable cause (Britten, 1986).

THE STAGES OF A FEVER

The typical stages of fever occur in response to the physiological processes taking place within the body. There are three distinct stages to a fever: (1) the *chill* phase, or period of rising temperature; (2) the *course* of the fever, when the temperature is maintained at an elevated level; and (3) the *termination*, or period when the temperature falls to normal. During the three stages, different sets of mechanisms are operating, giving rise to the signs and symptoms characteristic of each stage.

The Chill Phase

During the onset of a fever, it is thought that there is a resetting of the body's internal "thermostat" at a higher level (Guyton, 1981; Martini, 1989). This may be a response to the presence of pyrogenic substances, or to any one of the other causes listed in the section on the etiology of fever.

The resetting of the internal thermostat brings the body's heat-producing mechanisms into play as an attempt is made to bring the temperature up to the "desired" level. Until this level is reached, the patient experiences what is known as a **chill**. Muscular activity, in the form of shivering, is increased, and may vary in severity from merely a feeling of being cold, with slight shivering, to violent muscular contractions (shaking chills).

At the same time as the shivering mechanism is induced, the rate of cellular metabolism increases, and the waste products of metabolism — carbon dioxide and water — are formed in greater quantities. The increased carbon dioxide level in the blood stimulates the respiratory centre and breathing becomes faster and deeper. This leads to extra fluid loss and the patient often feels thirsty. Also, as metabolism is accelerated, there is an increased demand by the cells for more oxygen and glucose. The heart beats more rapidly in response to this demand, and the nurse will note that the patient's pulse rate is higher than normal.

Concomitantly, heat-conserving mechanisms are instituted. Vasoconstriction occurs, the patient becomes pale, and the skin is cold to the touch. As a result of feeling cold, the patient may ask for extra blankets. Often, there is a "goose flesh" appearance to the skin as piloerection takes place. Sweating also may cease.

During the chill phase, body temperature rises steadily and may be increased by as much as 1.1 to 4°C (MacBryde and Blacklow, 1971). A chill may last for a few minutes or as long as an hour. In mild cases of fever, such as one sees with the common cold or in mild cases of influenza, the chill phase is usually brief. It is important that temperature be assessed at the completion of the chill phase in order to determine its upper limit.

The Course of a Fever

During the second stage of a fever, when the fever is "running its course," the temperature has reached the preset level and there is a balance between heat production and heat loss. Because of the increased body temperature, there is usually a generalized flushing of the skin and it feels warm to the touch. The increased metabolic rate required to maintain the elevated temperature puts heightened demands on the body for more oxygen and glucose. The heart and respiratory rates remain high, and water loss through respiration increases the patient's feeling of thirst. The elevated temperature also increases nervous irritability. Headache, photophobia (sensitivity to light) and restlessness or drowsiness (or both) are not uncommon symptoms. An abnormally high fever is often accompanied by a state of mental confusion, which may progress to delirium. Patients may become disoriented as to time and place and may not know what day it is or where they are. Sometimes patients have hallucinations. They may become quite irrational and combative. Finally, prostration (collapse) may ensue. In young children, a convulsion not infrequently accompanies fever, usually at the outset.

The maintenance of an elevated temperature is very debilitating to the patient. During the first week or so of a fever, there is always some destruction of body protein and *albuminuria* (protein in the urine) is usually noted in the laboratory findings (Guyton, 1981). The patient often complains of a generalized weakness and is not inclined to much activity. Aching of the muscles and joints is also frequently present. In addition to the destruction of tissue protein, it is believed that the parenchyma (the tissue of an organ, not of the supporting or connective tissue) begins to be damaged when the body temperature rises above 40°C (Guyton, 1981).

Most authorities concur that children and adults can tolerate temperatures up to 41°C (Fruthaler, 1985; McCance and Huether, 1990). In sustained high fevers above 41.7°C, there may be permanent damage to brain and nervous tissue which do not regenerate (Fruthaler, 1985; McCance and Huether, 1990). The upper limit for survival of vital organs is at a body temperature of 43°C (McCance and Huether, 1990; Mitchell and Laburn, 1985; Porth, 1990).

Febrile patients usually lose weight. Although the increased metabolic rate maintained during the course of a fever increases the body's need for nourishment, most patients have little interest in food. The combination of increased need for food and loss of appetite (anorexia) leads to a loss of weight.

Usually during the course of a fever, the temperature does not remain at a constant level but fluctuates. Thus, periods when body temperature is rising are usually interspersed with periods when it is falling, even though the lowest temperature reached may always be above normal. When the heat-loss centre is stimulated, temperature falls and mechanisms for heat loss are dominant. Vasodilation occurs and the skin becomes flushed and warm. **Diaphoresis** (sweating) is usually present to maximize heat loss through evaporation. The body thus loses more fluids, and the possibility of dehydration becomes a problem.

When fever is prolonged, the problem of dehydration is more likely to occur. This is due to a number of factors, including the greater loss of water through increased respiration and the further loss of fluids from sweating during periods when the elevated body temperature is falling. There is often a lessening in the output of urine as more than the usual amount of fluid is lost through the skin and lungs. Other evidences of dehydration may be noted. The skin and mucous membranes may appear parched and dry. The patient's lips may become cracked and sore, and lesions may occur at the corners of the mouth. These lesions are termed *herpes simplex*, but are often referred to as "fever blisters" because they are so frequently seen in patients with high fever. The nurse may note other signs and symptoms of dehydration, such as those discussed in Chapter 22. It is well to remember that young children in particular become dehydrated very quickly if there is a sustained fever.

The Termination of a Fever

When the cause of the elevated temperature has been removed, for example, when antibiotics have eliminated the cause of infection, the body's thermostat is reset at its original level. The mechanisms for increased heat production cease to operate, and mechanisms for increased heat loss are instituted. These are the same mechanisms that have already been described as operating when there is a temporary drop during the course of a fever. The patient's temperature may drop to normal quickly, over a period of hours (by crisis), or gradually over a period of days or weeks (by lysis).

OTHER HEAT DISTURBANCES

Other disturbances in the body's homeostatic heat balance that require prompt intervention include heat cramps, heat exhaustion, heat stroke and malignant hyperthermia.

Heat Cramps

Heat cramps may occur in hot climates or hot weather as a result of prolonged, excessive sweating. This depletes the sodium chloride in body fluids and results in pallor, extreme thirst, nausea and dizziness. The muscle cramps that characterize this condition result from micro-circulatory failure that may be caused by dehydration (Mitchell and Laburn, 1985). The body temperature may be normal or slightly elevated. Putting the patient with heat cramps in a cool room and giving fluids with salt added (as, for example, lemonade with salt in it) will relieve mild cases. Salt tablets are not recommended because they are absorbed slowly and may result in gastric irritation, vomiting and cerebral edema (Porth, 1989).

Heat Exhaustion

Also known as *heat prostration*, heat exhaustion may result from lengthy exposure to heat, especially if combined with high humidity. The patient usually becomes very pale, and has cold, clammy skin, lowered blood pressure and generalized weakness. These are signs of shock. The individual may experience profuse sweating, and nausea and vomiting, culminating in dehydration. Generally, moving the patient to cooler and less humid surroundings and giving fluids will relieve this condition.

Heat Stroke

A condition of severe prostration, heat stroke may be caused by prolonged exposure to high environmental temperatures, and is potentially lethal. It is most frequently seen in the elderly and is believed to be due to predisposing factors such as atrophy of sweat glands, decreased circulation, underlying disease conditions and the side effects of drug therapy (Caruso and Posey, 1985). Other factors that increase the risk for heat stroke include dehydration, obesity, lack of acclimatization, lack of sleep, chronic illness, alcoholism and restrictive clothing (Khogali and Mustafa, 1984; Mitchell and Laburn, 1985).

Heat stroke is characterized by a very high rectal temperature (above 40°C), coma and the absence of sweating (Mitchell and Laburn, 1985). It is generally accepted that temperatures above 43°C are incompatible with life (McCance and Huether, 1990; Mitchell and Laburn, 1985). The physiological effects of a dangerously high body temperature include damage to the brain and central nervous system tissues, increased blood clotting, metabolic acidosis, tissue hypoxia and severe potassium imbalance which leads to cardiac arrest (Khogali and Mustafa, 1984). Heat stroke requires immediate action to lower the body temperature as quickly as possible. Some authorities recommend the optimum rate of cooling to be a decrease of 0.3°C every five minutes (Khogali and Mustafa, 1984). Prompt medical intervention is needed and the patient should be hospitalized (Cain, 1980).

Malignant Hyperthermia

Malignant **hyperthermia** (hyperpyrexia) is a sudden and potentially lethal hypermetabolic crisis state triggered by certain volatile anesthetic or neuromuscular blocking agents in persons genetically prone to this. A rapid elevation in temperature at a rate of 1°C every five minutes may result unless appropriate treatment is initiated rapidly. Careful family history assessment preoperatively is necessary to screen patients for this genetic defect.

HYPOTHERMIA

On the other side of the temperature spectrum, the most common problem from lack of heat is accidental hypothermia.

Hypothermia is a chilling of the whole body from exposure to cold such that the core temperature drops below 35°C (Mitchell and Laburn, 1985). This state can occur in accidental situations (such as from exposure to cold weather or from immersion in cold water); it can be induced clinically during specific types of surgery (such as in cardiac and neurosurgery) (Clark and Edholm, 1985); or it can occur as a secondary clinical problem resulting from a predisposing disease condition (such as hypothyroidism, hypoglycemia, alcoholism, hypopituitarism or severe burns) (Mitchell and Laburn, 1985).

Although older patients account for the majority of victims of hypothermia, children and young adults can also be exposed to environmental conditions leading to life-threatening drops in body temperature. Nor does accidental hypothermia only occur in cold, northern climates or in people who have been caught in a snowstorm in the mountains. People vary considerably in their ability to withstand cold temperatures. Persons with darkly pigmented skin, older people and those in poor physical condition are more affected by the cold than others. The amount and type of clothing worn for insulating the body is also important. Multiple layers of lightweight clothing serve to entrap warm air close to the skin and have been found to be more effective than fewer layers of bulky, heavy clothing for keeping the body warm. Water acts as a heat conductor, and damp clothing therefore conducts heat away from the body. The "wind chill" factor, as we mentioned, considerably increases the effect of cold environmental temperatures on the body. Rarefied atmospheres, as experienced by mountain climbers, also magnify the effect of cold on the body.

Regardless of the underlying cause or the victim's age, treatment of hypothermia takes precedence over any accompanying problems because of the threat to life. In cases of *accidental hypothermia,* (in which the victim survived) the body temperature has been known to go down as low as 14.2 °C rectally (personal communication, Dr. John Burgess, Plains Hospital, Regina, Saskatchewan, May 12, 1994). In this instance, a two-year-old was exposed to several hours of extreme winter conditions on the Canadian prairies. The body is well preserved at low temperatures because metabolism is suppressed and oxygen stores to the vital tissues are maintained (Mitchell and Laburn, 1985). For this reason, it is generally accepted that even profoundly hypothermic patients should be resuscitated and warmed to normal body temperature regardless of their apparent unresponsiveness on admission to hospital.

If the patient is in the early stages of mild hypothermia (34°C to 35°C) (Potter, 1990), he or she should be protected from the elements and from the cold and possibly wet ground. If possible, wet garments should be removed, the individual should be wrapped in dry clothing and put into a sleeping bag for gradual rewarming. Other acceptable forms of warming the mildly hypothermic patient include direct body contact with a normothermic individual, immersion in a warm bath (Mitchell and Laburn, 1985) or consumption of hot liquids.

If the patient has become stuporous or unconscious, it is probable that moderate to severe hypothermia (body temperature lower than 34°C) has occurred (Potter, 1990). This condition requires prompt medical intervention because of the possibility of lethal complications such as myocardial irritability and "afterdrop" (in which the core temperature drops further at the onset of rewarming) (Mitchell and Laburn, 1985). It is necessary to transport such a patient to medical facilities where intensive rewarming techniques and monitoring are available. The victim should be placed between blankets and protected from

further cold en route. For this condition, there has been no agreement on the merits of surface warming (such as the application of external heating measures) versus core warming techniques (such as peritoneal dialysis or extracorporeal blood warming) (Mitchell and Laburn, 1985).

The basic physiological mechanism operating in hypothermia is a constriction of the blood vessels in the peripheral tissues of the body. With the vasoconstriction, there is a decreased flow of blood to the area and consequently a decreased supply of oxygen to the tissues. The decreased blood flow results in diminished local sensation (a numbness is perceived) and weakness of the muscles. The skin feels cold and becomes pale. The walls of blood vessels in the area may be directly damaged by the cold, with the result that plasma fluid leaks into interstitial spaces and the area becomes swollen. The blood in the vessel then becomes more concentrated and small clots begin to appear, giving a typically mottled look to the tissues. Eventually, the clots will close off the vessel completely and the area becomes avascular (without blood supply). A pulse can no longer be felt. If there is a quick freezing of the tissues, as sometimes happens in very cold climates to exposed noses, cheeks or ears, the affected part becomes white and shiny, sometimes with a blue tinge.

The skin is the first tissue to be cooled and the most likely to be damaged. Blood vessels, nerves and muscles are also very vulnerable and easily damaged. Bones, connective tissue and tendons are more resistant to damage from cold exposure. The areas of the body that are most vulnerable to damage from the cold are those that are most exposed, such as the hands, the face (especially the cheeks and the nose), the ears and the feet.

In addition to the localized reactions to cold, the patient who has suffered from exposure under conditions of extreme cold may develop cold exhaustion. This usually begins with mild hypothermia, characterized by intense shivering, profound vasoconstriction and accelerated heart rate which help to resist lowering of temperature (Potter, 1990). Urinary flow is increased (cold diuresis) and the patient will hyperventilate — a reaction which could culminate in dehydration during early hypothermia (Potter, 1990).

In response to the prolonged cold exposure, physical and mental responses slow down. At a body temperature of 34°C, the patient becomes clumsy and muscle control is impaired as the temperature of the muscles becomes lower. Speech is slurred and the patient becomes amnesic and irrational (Martini, 1989; McCance and Huether, 1990; Mitchell and Laburn, 1985). The thermoregulatory mechanisms of shivering and vasoconstriction are lost when body temperature drops below 33°C (McCance and Huether, 1990; Mitchell and Laburn, 1985). If body temperature drops further, the individual will become drowsy, and will usually fall asleep. Loss of consciousness and cardiac arrest ensues at a body temperature of 28°C. The lowest limit for survival is considered to be a body temperature of 23°C (except in the unusual situations described earlier in the chapter).

ASSESSING TEMPERATURE REGULATION NEEDS

Usually the first thing nurses do on admission of patients to a health care agency is take their temperature. Indeed, fever is such a universal sign of illness that it is important to interview and observe all patients for the signs and symptoms of disturbed body temperature. In order to know what to look for and the relevant questions to ask the patient (or family or significant other), the nurse needs to understand the mechanism of fever — the types of fever commonly encountered and the stages of fever. The nurse should also understand the effect of cold on body tissues and be able to make pertinent observations. The nursing health history, temperature measurements and observations made during physical assessment of the patient that are recorded on the patient's chart furnish data which aid the nurse in determining patient problems and needs for care.

In addition, the patient's record will provide information about actual or potential problems with temperature regulation. The nurse will want to check for conditions that place the patient at risk for temperature disturbances. These may include:

- open wounds
- recent surgery
- recent invasive diagnostic procedures (colonoscopy, catheterization)
- drug therapy that causes immunosuppression (steroids, chemotherapy)
- malnutrition
- burn injury

THE NURSING HEALTH HISTORY

If the patient is admitted to the health agency running a fever, it is important to find out how long he or she has had it, how high the temperature has been and whether the patient has had any other signs and symptoms of illness. In the case of children, it is particularly important to ask if they have been exposed to a communicable disease, so that they may be isolated to protect other children on the unit. Some agencies have a policy of putting all children with an elevated temperature on isolation precautions for 24 hours to observe them for development of a rash or other indication of one of the childhood diseases.

When a patient is admitted with a cold-weather injury, the nurse should find out the circumstances of the accident. How long was the exposure? Under what conditions? What parts of the body are affected? What first aid measures were used before admission? It is also helpful to know

how old the patient is, the general physical condition and any existing health problems.

As with all needs, the nurse will also question the patient or family about usual health promoting and protecting patterns to help identify potential problems and opportunities for promoting optimal thermal well-being. A health history guide follows.

MEASUREMENTS

TEMPERATURE, PULSE AND RESPIRATIONS

Body temperature, taken with a clinical thermometer, is an objective measure of the body's temperature-regulating status. The methods of taking a body temperature are given in Chapter 14. In order to have a baseline on which to judge whether a patient's temperature is above, or below, his or her normal range, it is helpful to take the temperature over a period of several successive days at different times of the day and to plot the readings on a temperature graph (flowsheet).

Many inpatient agencies have specific policies for the taking of temperatures. Some require that all patients have their temperature taken once, or sometimes twice, a day to screen for fever. If once a day, it is usually considered that early evening is the best time, since in many patients with a fever, this is the time when the temperature is most elevated. If temperatures are taken in the morning, this should be done an hour or so after the patient wakens, when the body temperature is stabilized.

When a patient has a fever, the temperature should be monitored at more frequent intervals. All newly admitted patients have their temperature taken, as do all preoperative and postoperative patients. Postoperatively, the temperature is usually taken every four hours for the first 48 hours. In addition to these general guidelines, when signs and symptoms indicating fever are present, the nurse should monitor the patient's temperature. The temperature should be evaluated in relation to such factors as the patient's usual normal temperature, the time of day, the environmental temperature and the normal physiological processes that may affect body temperature. Pulse and respiratory rates are elevated in hyperthermic disturbances while in hypothermia these are decreased.

PHYSICAL ASSESSMENT

Physical assessment of a patient with a disturbance in thermoregulation is very basic. The appearance and temperature of the skin are appraised and the patient is observed for physiological and behavioural manifestations of the disturbance. The skin is appraised for characteristic features

Temperature Regulation

Health and Illness Patterns

USUAL TEMPERATURE PATTERN

- Do you know your normal temperature range? If so, what is it?
- Do you usually feel cold and need an extra sweater or blanket even in warm weather?
- Are you usually too warm when others are comfortable indoors or outdoors?

RECENT CHANGES IN TEMPERATURE PATTERN

- Have there been any recent changes in your usual temperature pattern? Are you feeling warmer or colder than usual? What has been your recent temperature range?
- How long have you noticed this temperature disturbance?
- Have you had prolonged exposure to excessively hot or cold environmental temperatures?

PRESENTING HEALTH PROBLEM

If admitted with a fever:

- How long have you had this fever?
- How high has the temperature been?
- Describe any symptoms you are experiencing now. Chills? Headache? Fatigue or malaise? Pain or absence of sensation in a body part? Anorexia, nausea, or vomiting? Thirst?
- Do you have a history of acute or chronic disease that may cause a fever? Flu? Chronic bronchitis? Bladder infection?
- Are you taking any medications at present (including over-the-counter medications)? If so, what?

If admitted with a cold-weather injury:

- What was the nature of your accident?
- How long were you exposed to the cold? What were the weather conditions?
- What parts of your body are affected?
- Were any first aid measures used to treat the injury? If so, what?

Health Promotion and Protection Patterns

- Do you spend a lot of time in a hot environment or in the sun? Examples: Working on road maintenance, at construction sites, or in steel mills? Spending time on the beach?
- What precautions do you take in very hot weather or in a hot environment?
- Do you spend a lot of time in a cold, windy environment? Examples: Skiing or working outdoors in the winter?
- What precautions do you take in very cold weather?

---

of fever and hypothermia. What is the colour of the patient's skin? Is it pale, white or flushed? Does it feel warm, cool or cold to the touch? Does it have a goose flesh appearance or is it smooth and shiny? Is it dry, clammy or wet with moisture? What is the appearance of the parts of the body affected by thermal injury?

The patient is examined for physiological manifestations of temperature disturbances. Does the patient show signs of having a chill, namely shivering and muscular tremors? Are there signs of dehydration (poor skin turgor, a dry and furrowed tongue, rapid weight loss, absence of tearing and salivation)? Does the patient's urine appear normal in colour and amount? The behavioural manifestations accompanying fever and hypothermia are also noted. Is the patient restless, irritable, drowsy, clumsy, stuporous? Are there signs of mental confusion?

DIAGNOSING TEMPERATURE REGULATION PROBLEMS

Clinical problems in temperature regulation amenable to nursing intervention are related to an imbalance between heat losses and heat gains, leading to an excessive rise or fall in core body temperature. Common nursing diagnoses related to temperature regulation are: *Hyperthermia, Hypothermia* and *High risk for altered body temperature* (Carpenito, 1993).

Trauma, illness, increased metabolic rate, exposure to a hot environment, inability to perspire, dehydration and the side effects of certain medications on thermoregulatory responses are situations that could lead to increased heat

Subjective and Objective Data in Patients with Disturbances of Body Temperature

SUBJECTIVE DATA	OBJECTIVE DATA
Fever	
Chill Phase	
Feeling of being cold	Skin cool to touch
Intermittent chills	Pale goose flesh appearance
Apprehension	Observable shivering or shaking
	Increased pulse rate
	Increased respiratory rate
	Increased rectal temperature
Course of the Fever	
Feeling of being warm	Skin flushed
Thirst	Hot to touch
Lips sore	Perspiration (may be profuse)
Feeling of generalized weakness	Elevated temperature (may fluctuate)
Restlessness, drowsiness	Dry mouth and lips
Headache	Fever blisters
Sensitivity to light	Tongue coated, "furry"
Aching muscles and joints	Scanty urine
Anorexia, nausea, vomiting	Lethargy
	With high fever, may show disorientation
	Delirium, with hallucinations
	Irrational combative behaviour
	Convulsions (in children)
	Loss of weight
	Dehydration
Termination of Fever	
Feels improved	Bodily functions return to normal
	Skin flushed
	Sweating (diaphoresis) often profuse
	Increased respiration
	Increased pulse
	Dropping temperature
	Clearing sensorium
	Return to normal functioning
Hypothermia	
Exposed area feels cold	Skin cold to touch
Diminished local sensation	Pale — becoming white or blue-tinged
(feeling of numbness)	Sometimes mottled appearance of skin
Weakness of muscles	Absence of pulse
Inability to flex joints	Swelling
Tiredness	Slow, often stumbling movements
Drowsiness	Sometimes irrational behaviour
	Vision impaired
	Breathing slow and shallow
	Pulse rate slow

production and a nursing diagnosis of *Hyperthermia*. Along with a body temperature above normal range, the patient who is hyperthermic will exhibit warm, flushed skin, increased pulse rate (tachycardia) and an increased respiratory rate (tachypnea). This person may report headache and may appear lethargic or restless. Complete blood count results may reveal an elevated white blood cell count, if infection or inflammation is present. An elevated hematocrit and hemoglobin may be suggestive of dehydration.

Hypothermia is the nursing diagnosis applicable to the patient who is exposed to a cold environment for a prolonged period, or whose thermoregulatory responses are affected by alcohol, disease, trauma, medications or anesthetics. Other related factors include aging, inadequate clothing, inactivity, malnutrition and inability or decreased ability to shiver (McFarland and McFarlane, 1989). Defining characteristics of a hypothermic individual may include a reduction in body temperature below normal range; cool, pale, blanched or reddened skin; piloerection; decreased heart rate (bradycardia); decreased respiratory rate (bradypnea); decreased blood pressure (hypotension); and decreased level of consciousness (drowsiness, confusion or coma).

The nursing diagnosis, *High risk for altered body temperature*, may be applied to individuals who are identified to be at risk. Risk factors may include extremes in age or weight, exposure to extremes in environmental temperature, inappropriate clothing, disease or trauma affecting temperature regulation, dehydration or intake of alcohol or medications affecting temperature control (McFarland and McFarlane, 1989).

The management of severe hyperthermia and profound hypothermia requires collaboration between nursing and medical disciplines. These and other problems associated with these potentially lethal conditions, such as compartmental syndrome from thermal injury, fluid volume deficit and decreased cardiac output, should be labelled as collaborative problems. Examples of nursing diagnoses and collaborative problems are *High risk for altered body temperature related to surgery and sedation, Hyperthermia related to dehydration, Hypothermia related to exposure to a cold environment, PC: Hyperthermia, and PC: Compartmental syndromes thermal injury*.

PLANNING TEMPERATURE REGULATION INTERVENTIONS

The plan of care for patients with thermoregulation problems is based on the severity of the problems and on the appropriate treatment modalities to restore body temperature. In cases of fever, nursing interventions are selected to reduce the amount of heat produced within the body,

to facilitate the elimination of heat from the body, to minimize the effects of fever on vital functions of the body (circulation, respiration, nutrition and fluid balance) and to collaborate with other health professionals in identifying and eliminating the cause of the fever. Nursing actions for patients with excessive lowering of surface or core body temperature focus on rewarming the patient, preventing tissue damage and, in severe hypothermia, preventing and treating complications such as acid–base imbalance, fluid and electrolyte imbalance, hypoxemia and cardiac arrythmias. As with all needs, the plan of care incorporates patient preferences and beliefs, usual lifestyle practices and socioeconomic status. Strategies that enable self-care and achievement of optimal thermal regulation in the course of daily functioning are essential.

In determining priorities for nursing action, the nurse must assess the severity of the patient's condition. If the patient's temperature is extremely high (above 40°C) or profoundly low (below 32°C), the situation is considered a medical emergency and requires immediate intervention (McFarland and McFarlane, 1989).

Common expected outcomes of interventions for the patient with a body temperature problem include the following:

- Oral temperature will be within normal limits (35.8–37.3°C).
- Blood pressure, pulse and respirations will be within the normal limits.
- Patient's skin will be of normal warmth.
- Patient will be alert and oriented.
- Patient will verbalize environmental risk factors for hyperthermia or hypothermia.
- Patient will verbalize how to maintain body temperature regulation during temperature extremes.

IMPLEMENTING TEMPERATURE REGULATION INTERVENTIONS

HEALTH PROMOTING STRATEGIES

Human beings are equipped with an efficient heat-regulating mechanism for maintaining a stable body temperature. The body's adaptive mechanisms produce heat when temperature falls and lose excess heat when temperature rises. Thermal dysfunction occurs when environmental challenges (ambient temperature and metabolic processes) exceed the individual's adaptive capacity. People can promote optimal thermal health in the course of daily living by modifying

HEALTH PROMOTING STRATEGY

Promoting Healthy Temperature Regulation

- Keep a comfortable temperature in the home. An ambient temperature of 21–23°C is considered comfortable for day-time; lower levels are recommended for sleeping.
- Avoid extremes of environmental temperature whenever possible.
- In hot climates, stay out of the sun as much as possible. Wear loose, light-weight, and light-coloured clothing to allow air circulation and dissipation of heat. White is best for reflecting radiant heat. Wear a large hat to shade your eyes and deflect the radiant heat from the head and back of the neck.
- In cold climates, wear multiple layers of light-weight clothing to entrap warm air close to the skin. Cover the head, hands and wrists. The head and neck can lose up to 40 percent of body heat (Williams, 1993).
- If planning strenuous work or exercise in hot weather, drink ample fluids within an hour of commencing activity. It takes more energy to work in a hot climate. Pace yourself and work slowly.

environmental conditions and doing certain things to conserve or dissipate body heat.

HEALTH PROTECTING STRATEGIES

MANAGING FEVER

The presence of a temperature above the normal level puts stresses on the body's adaptive mechanisms. Patients are usually uncomfortable; they are losing more than the normal amount of fluids and using more energy than usual to maintain the elevated body temperature. Nursing action should be directed towards minimizing these stresses and enhancing the body's coping capabilities.

Maintaining rest   The patient who has an elevated temperature needs rest. It is essential to minimize the patient's energy requirements. Rest and inactivity decrease the rate of the metabolic process and muscular activity and thereby decrease the amount of heat produced in the body. Usually, patients are restricted to bed in order to curtail their activities. Physical activity should be kept to a minimum. During the convalescent stage, activity should be increased gradually to prevent tiring the patient unduly.

Rest, however, involves more than restrictions on physical activity; it also means mental rest. Sometimes the simple act of taking a patient's temperature may cause anxiety. An elevated temperature may result in having surgery postponed, or in delaying a much anticipated return to home and family. Febrile patients need to be assured that all is being done for their welfare and that they are in competent hands. Anticipating the needs of patients helps them to relax. Very often, a simple explanation of procedures and treatments can alleviate many anxieties.

The patient with a fever needs a cool, quiet environment. He or she may be irritable and may be hypersensitive to stimuli. An effort should be made to minimize noise and to provide the opportunity for rest. A cool, comfortable room increases heat elimination and helps the patient to rest more easily. Sometimes a fan is used to increase the circulation of air in the room and facilitate the removal of heat from the body through conduction and convection. Care should be taken, however, to ensure that the patient does not become chilled. The bedclothes of the patient with a fever should be light and comfortable, since heavy coverings inhibit heat elimination.

Maintaining comfort and hygiene   Good hygiene is important to the patient's health and comfort. Diaphoresis, which frequently accompanies fever, is uncomfortable. Bathing, and a change of gown and bedding, may be required to ensure that the patient remains clean and dry. Because sweat glands are more numerous in the axilla and around the genitalia, these areas need particular care when the patient is bathed. Flannelette sheets, because of their greater absorbency, are often used in place of ordinary cotton ones on the beds of patients who are perspiring profusely.

Maintaining hydration   The hydration of the febrile patient is of primary importance. Diaphoresis and the loss of additional fluids through increased respirations increase the amount of fluid eliminated from the body, and this fluid needs to be replaced. In addition, during a fever, there is increased production of metabolic waste products, which must be eliminated. The necessity for removing these products from the body, together with any toxic substances that may be present, emphasizes the importance of fluids. If the patient is unable to take fluids orally or in sufficient amounts, parenteral fluids may be ordered.

An accurate record of the patient's fluid intake and output must be maintained. Intake records should include all fluids taken orally and those given parenterally. In computing output, urine should be measured accurately and a note made of the extent of sweating and the loss of any fluids through vomiting or diarrhea. Suction returns also should be included in the output calculations.

The patient should be observed carefully for signs of dehydration. When a patient becomes dehydrated during the course of a fever, the skin often becomes dry and scaly. The application of creams helps to keep the skin in good condition. Dehydration frequently results in cracks in the patient's lips, tongue or mucous membrane lining of the mouth. Good oral hygiene is imperative to prevent infection from developing and also to contribute to the patient's comfort. There is a need to cleanse, hydrate and lubricate the mouth and lips.

Frequent intake of fluids helps to maintain hydration of the oral cavity. Rinsing the mouth with water (or mouthwash) and chewing gum also help to preserve hydration. If patients are unable to take fluids orally, rinse their mouth, or chew gum, the nurse can help them by cleaning the mouth with swabs. Commercially prepared swabs or swabs dipped in mouthwash are used in many places for this purpose.

Lubrication may be accomplished by the application of creams or petrolatum to the lips. Patients unable to apply lubricating cream themselves may require the assistance of the nurse. Sterile petrolatum should be used because of frequent splits or cracks in the lips due to the fever, which provide a portal of entry for infection.

Maintaining nutritional status   As a result of the body's increased metabolic rate and the increased destruction of tissues that are so often a concomitant of fever, there is a need for proteins and carbohydrates in the diet of the febrile patient. Proteins aid in the formation of body tissue; carbohydrates supply the body with much-needed energy. Frequently these products are supplied in the liquids taken orally or given parenterally. The patient's weight should be checked at frequent intervals, and the physician should be kept informed of the patient's nutritional status so that appropriate therapy may be instituted.

An important function of the nurse is the communication of observations to other members of the health team. The nutritional status of the patient with a fever must be carefully monitored and accurately reported and recorded. See Chapter 19 for the signs of good and poor nutritional status in patients.

RESTORATIVE STRATEGIES

MEASURES TO REDUCE HEAT PRODUCTION AND FACILITATE HEAT LOSS

Since fever may be a useful defence mechanism, it is not always advisable to treat it. However, in situations where it has been deemed necessary to treat fever, a number of measures may be used to bring about a rapid reduction in body temperature. These include the use of antipyretic drugs, which have a systemic action, as well as various techniques for *surface cooling* of the body.

ANTIPYRETIC AND ANTIBIOTIC DRUG THERAPY

Antipyretic drugs, such as acetylsalicylic acid (Aspirin) or acetaminophen, are often ordered to reduce a patient's fever. These drugs have a specific action on the heat-regulating centres but do not eliminate the cause of the fever. Their administration may be designated at specific times, when the patient's temperature reaches certain levels or according to the nurse's judgement. Antibiotics, when prescribed, are usually administered at regular intervals in order to maintain a therapeutic drug level in the patient's body. The use of antibiotics for patients with infections reduces the fever by eliminating the cause of it — that is, the infection within the body.

TEPID SPONGE BATH

A tepid sponge bath is a temporary measure to lower a patient's temperature. This simple nursing measure can be employed either in a home situation or in the hospital. It is carried out on the order of a physician because decreasing the temperature below the setpoint may trigger the shivering response and consequently increase heat production (Donahue, 1983). When fever is the result of imbalances in the heat loss–heat production mechanism, tepid sponge baths are particularly beneficial. The technique is based on the principle that the body loses heat through the mechanisms of conduction to a cooler substance (in this case the tepid water), evaporation of water from the surface of the body and convection of the heat away from exposed body surfaces during the bathing process. The procedure for tepid sponge bath is outlined in Procedure 24.1. The bath is usually repeated until the patient's temperature has reached the level designated by the physician. If the physician's order does not include the temperature at which treatment is to be discontinued, the bath should be stopped before the normal temperature is reached. A further drop in temperature may occur after it is discontinued.

Preparing the Patient

Prior to the bath explain the procedure to the patient and take temperature, pulse and respirations as a baseline for subsequent evaluation. Ensure that the patient's room is warm and free of drafts.

Assembling Equipment

The equipment and supplies are the same as for a basic sponge bath. Use a bath thermometer to ensure the bath water is between 32 and 38°C. The use of isopropyl (rubbing) alcohol with the bath is controversial. Alcohol, alone or added to tepid water, causes the most rapid reduction in temperature because it evaporates faster. However, alcohol is very drying and irritating to the skin. In addition, the rapid reduction in heat due to the use of alcohol may cause chilling and a rebound rise in temperature (Malloch, 1993). Therefore, some agencies have eliminated the use of alcohol in the tepid bath.

USING A FAN

A nursing intervention that is somewhat similar to the tepid sponge bath is the use of a fan to increase heat elimination from the body. The patient is covered only by a sheet and a fan is positioned so that there is constant movement of air over the sheet. This measure promotes evaporation and convection and thereby increases heat loss from the body.

PROCEDURE 24.1

Tepid Sponge Bath

ACTION	RATIONALE
1. Prepare the patient and take TPR.	Promotes patient well-being and provides a baseline for evaluation.
2. Gather: • Basin of water 32 to 38°C • Towels • Washcloth • Bath blanket	Promotes efficiency and economy of time.
3. Close the door (if private room) or pull bed curtains. Fan-fold the top bedclothes to the foot of the bed, drape the patient with the bath blanket, and then remove the gown.	Protects the patient's privacy and prevents undue shivering from exposure.
4. Apply wet cloths to the axillae, wrists and groin. Change the cloths as they warm.	Enhances the cooling effect because the blood vessels in these areas are close to the body surface, thus allow heat to dissipate.
5. Sponge large areas at a time, for example, one side of the leg, one side of the arm, the chest and the abdomen. Long strokes are used on the legs and on the back.	Heat is lost from the body as water is sponged onto the body surface and some of the water is permitted to evaporate.
6. Use a gentle patting motion to dry each area.	Brisk rubbing increases the activity of the cells and therefore the rate of heat production.
7. Take the patient's TPR 20 minutes after the sponge bath.	Determines effectiveness and need to repeat the procedure.
8. Document the procedure. Note the patient's TPR and condition before and after the procedure.	Fulfills legal requirements for nurse accountability.

HYPOTHERMIA MACHINES

Many hospitals have a hypothermia machine (cooling blanket) that is used for rapid surface cooling of the body. This machine may be used when it is deemed essential to bring the body temperature down quickly (for example, in a case of malignant hyperthermia) or when there has been brain damage to the heat-regulating centres of the brain and it is necessary to maintain artificial cooling of the body over a prolonged period of time.

This technique uses the mechanisms of radiation and conduction. The patient is placed on or between cooling blankets, which are attached to a refrigerating machine. The blankets contain coils in which a liquid, often water, circulates. The machine is set to operate according to either the desired body temperature or to the desired water blanket temperature. The temperature of the patient is continuously monitored with an attached temperature probe, which is lubricated and inserted into the rectum. A considerable amount of heat is lost from the body through direct conduction to the cooling substance and through the radiation of heat waves from the body to the cooler blankets. Because some people shiver in response to the application of the hypothermia blanket, drugs are sometimes given to minimize shivering. Patients receiving hypothermia treatment frequently need a great deal of reassurance and explanation about the treatment. It is an uncomfortable procedure, according to people who have experienced it.

THERAPEUTIC MEASURES TO FACILITATE HEAT PRODUCTION AND PROMOTE HEAT GAIN

Patients with lowered body temperature require generalized warmth in order to maintain or regain normal body temperature. In addition to the simple application of additional blankets, particularly flannelette sheets, which help to conserve heat, other measures are available. In some health care facilities, warming cupboards in which sheets or blankets are heated may be useful, particularly in post-anesthetic (recovery room) areas. As a result of cool temperatures in the operating room, patients frequently exit these areas with lowered body temperature.

For patients requiring additional warmth, commercial warming devices are available. One such device (Bair Hugger®) injects warmed air into disposable light-weight plastic/paper blankets. Small openings on the patient side of the blanket allow the air to circulate over the patient. This simple but effective device is user-friendly and is especially useful in the emergency department and post-anesthetic areas where patients with varying degrees of hypothermia may be admitted. Temperature settings of low, medium or high may be selected.

Home Care: Managing Fever in a Child at Home

Fever in children is commonly treated at home by parents who may need guidance and reassurance. Nurses can teach parents how to care for their child during a febrile episode. The following guidelines should be included in parent teaching.

1. Children are considered febrile when their temperature is greater than:
   - 37.3°C (axilla)
   - 37.8°C (oral)
   - 38.3°C (rectal)

2. The child's doctor should be consulted if the febrile child:
   - is under 6 months of age.
   - has persistent diarrhea, vomiting or difficulty breathing.
   - is very lethargic.

3. The child whose fever persists beyond 24 hours should be brought to the attention of a doctor.

Treatment of fever:

1. Unwrap the child into light clothing (for example, vest and diaper). Keep the room comfortably warm.

2. Give the child acetaminophen according to instructions on the bottle.

3. Encourage the child to drink plenty of fluids.

4. Give the child a warm sponge bath for 10 to 20 minutes. The water temperature should be 1°C lower than the child's body temperature. Rationale: Research has revealed that warm sponging has an additive effect and reduces fever more quickly than giving an antipyretic alone. Most children enjoy the warm sponging and parents are most receptive to this treatment.

(Victoria General Hospital, 1993; Kinmouth, Fulton, Cambell, 1992.)

Another device, the hyperthermia blanket (warming blanket), may also be used. This apparatus is similar to the hypothermia blanket described earlier, with the exception that warmed, instead of cooled, liquid circulates through the coils in the blanket. The hyperthermia machine is particularly useful for patients with extreme hypothermia. Again, rectal temperature is continuously monitored throughout the procedure and the physician orders the desired patient or blanket temperature to be achieved.

FIGURE 24.3 Warming blanket

SOURCE: Augustine Medical, Inc. Reproduced with permission.

EVALUATING TEMPERATURE REGULATION INTERVENTIONS

The evaluation of care for patients experiencing disturbances in temperature regulation is based on the expected outcomes for identified problems. The following guidelines may assist the nurse in determining effectiveness of care.

1. Has the patient's temperature come down? gone up? Is it within safe limits?
2. Is the fluid intake adequate for the patient's needs?
3. Is the diet adequate?
4. Is the patient comfortable?
5. Is the patient obtaining sufficient rest?
6. Are the skin and oral cavity in good condition?

THERAPEUTIC USE OF HEAT AND COLD

Applications of heat and cold as therapeutic measures are well known to most people. Applying a hot water bottle or a heating pad to cold feet is a comfort familiar to many, particularly to those who live in cold climates. The application of ice as a means of stopping nosebleed (epistaxis) is a common therapeutic measure carried out in the

FROM RESEARCH TO PRACTICE

Kinmouth, A., Fulton, Y. and Cambell, M. J. (1992). Management of feverish children at home. *British Medical Journal*. 305, 1134–1136.

This study compared the acceptability and effects on body temperature of the addition of the antipyretic agent paracetamol (acetaminophen) or warm sponging to unwrapping and encouraging cool drinks among feverish children at home. The sample comprised 52 children aged from 3 months to 5 years with axillary temperatures before treatment ranging between 37.8°C and 40°C. The children were randomized within blocks stratified by age into four treatment groups: unwrapping, warm sponging plus unwrapping, paracetamol plus unwrapping, and paracetamol and warm sponging plus unwrapping. The children were treated at home by parents. A research nurse studied each child over four hours after treatment and followed the children until they were well. The nurse advised parents on the treatment measures as follows:

Unwrapping—Dress your child in light clothing (shirt and diaper) in a room warm enough for an adult to feel comfortable naked. Encourage frequent cool drinks.

Warm sponging—In a warm room (as above) sit your child in a tub or basin containing a few inches of warm water (at a temperature just below that of your child). Wet the child all over for 10 to 20 minutes or as long as the child is comfortable. Do not leave the child unattended. Then unwrap the child (as above).

Paracetamol—Give amounts as prescribed according to age. Then unwrap as above.

Paracetamol and warm sponging—The advice given above was combined.

The response to advice was assessed over four hours. Temperature was measured by continuous logging from an axillary thermometer. Acceptability of treatment to child and parent were scored on Likert scales immediately after treatment and on return to health. The response to treatment advice varied. Unwrapping alone had little effect on temperature. Paracetamol increased the time spent below 37.2°C by 109 minutes compared with unwrapping. Warm sponging caused the fastest reduction in temperature and almost half of the children enjoyed warm sponging. Parents, however, were happiest with treatments that included paracetamol. The researchers concluded that giving an antipyretic is more effective and is more acceptable to parents than sponging or unwrapping alone. Warm sponging has an additive effect and reduces fever more quickly than does the antipyretic.

home. The student has probably already had firsthand experience with many of these therapeutic measures.

Applications of heat and cold are used in health care agencies and in the home as therapeutic measures. These measures are often used to relieve inflammation and aid healing. Because perceptions of temperature sensations vary (as described in the following section), applications of heat and cold pose hazards to skin integrity. Therefore, they must be carried out with caution. In many agencies, these measures require a written order from a physician. Occasionally heat and cold also serve as comfort measures in the home setting. If patient comfort is the sole reason for their use, it is often left to the judgement of the nurse and patient whether and how to apply them. Nurses therefore need a knowledge of the physiological reactions resulting from these measures and of the untoward reactions that may occur. If nurses are ever in doubt about the use of heat or cold, they should consult the physician before applying these measures.

Applications of heat and cold also are used in the course of physical medicine as part of certain rehabilitation programs. In these instances physical therapists use measures such as paraffin baths and whirlpool baths.

TEMPERATURE SENSATION

Heat and cold are relative degrees of warmth dependent to some extent upon the perception of the individual. The temperature at the surface of the skin of the torso is generally 33.9°C. Local skin tolerance to cold and hot is thought to range between 4.4°C and 43.3°C. Generally any application that is outside of this range can cause tissue damage.

Temperature is perceived in gradations: cold to cool, tepid, indifferent, warm and finally to very, very hot. Different areas of the body have varying sensitivity to changes in heat and cold. People perceive temperature more acutely when the temperature of the skin is changing. Eventually the skin's heat and cold receptors that relay sensation become conditioned to the given temperature. That is why a hot bath feels hotter at first than it does after the skin becomes adjusted to it. This mechanism can be dangerous as it allows people to be burned or frost-bitten without their realization. Extremes in temperatures, both hot and cold, are perceived as painful.

TYPES OF APPLICATIONS

Many different types of hot and cold applications can be used as therapeutic measures. Both heat and cold can be applied as dry treatments or as moist treatments, and the source can be varied according to the purpose. Hot and cold applications must be applied with good nursing judgement. Good judgement is based on knowledge of the reasons for the therapeutic heat and cold measures, as well as on the patient's health status.

REASONS FOR THE APPLICATION OF HEAT

Heat is applied to the body for any of several reasons. It can be applied to produce a local or a systemic effect or both. A *local effect* is one that is specific to a defined area of the body, for example, one which relieves a local muscle spasm. A *systemic effect* is one that is reflected in the body as a whole — for example, general warmth felt throughout the body.

The effect of local application of heat involves several responses: peripheral vasodilation which increases blood supply to the area and increased cellular metabolism and oxygen demand by the local tissues. The maximum effect of heat is reached after 20 to 30 minutes of the application. After an hour, a secondary vasoconstriction occurs which could result in detrimental rather than beneficial effects (Kemp, Pillitteri and Brown, 1989). To avoid this secondary effect, 20 minutes to an hour should be allowed to elapse between heat treatments.

Heat is known to relieve pain in two ways: by relaxing muscle tone and by increasing blood flow where circulation is poor. Pain caused by the contraction of muscle fibres is relieved when the muscle spasm is reduced by heat. Heat can relieve pain related to ischemia (decreased blood supply) by increasing circulation to an area. Similarly, the pain and swelling caused by increased pressure accompanying the collection of fluid in an area can be reduced by the application of heat. As blood circulation improves, fluid is more easily absorbed from the tissues and consequently swelling or edema is reduced. Toxins and waste products are also thought to be causes of discomfort which can be relieved by an increase in blood circulation to the irritated tissues.

Heat helps the healing process by bringing leukocytes and lymph to the area. The suppurative process (pus formation) is increased and wound healing is enhanced. Heat can be applied to improve the oxygenation and nourishment of tissues, thus aiding tissue metabolism and subsequent healing. For example, heat applied to an infected surgical incision not only hastens suppuration but also increases the nourishment of the tissue cells and the healing process.

Another purpose of applying heat locally is to soften exudates. An exudate is a discharge produced by body tissues. Sometimes the discharge from an open wound forms hardened crusts over the area. Hot moist compresses are often used to soften these crusts so they can be easily removed.

The fact that heat helps to alleviate many types of pain does not mean that it is indicated for all instances of pain. Since heat can hasten the suppuration process, it could aggravate an underlying inflammatory process. In the case of an inflamed appendix, heat applied to the abdomen can cause the appendix to rupture. Although the physician supplies the directions regarding the application of heat, the nurse must always be aware of the purpose of the treatment and alert to possible untoward actions. There is, for instance, always a danger that a burn may result from the local application of heat, or that deeper-lying tissues may be affected and an inflammatory process aggravated.

If a systemic effect is desired, a hyperthermia blanket is applied. A heated liquid or air is circulated through the blanket, providing various degrees of heat as required. A physician's order is usually required in order to apply this treatment.

REASONS FOR THE APPLICATION OF COLD

Cold is applied to the body for both local and systemic effects. The local response to cold includes vasoconstriction and decreased blood flow to the area, and decreased cell perfusion and slowed cellular metabolism. Cold can be applied to stop hemorrhage, since it constricts the peripheral arterioles and increases the viscosity of the blood, in addition to contracting the muscles and depressing cardiac action. Ice bags are applied routinely to patients after a tonsillectomy as a prophylactic measure against hemorrhage.

Cold applications slow the suppurative process and the absorption of tissue fluids. Cold applied immediately after an injury such as a sprained ankle helps reduce swelling by de-

creasing blood flow to area. Once edema has formed, cold prevents its absorption. For this reason, cold application is recommended only within the initial 24 hours after an injury and heat is applied thereafter (Kemp, Pillitteri and Brown, 1989).

Pain can also be relieved through the use of cold applications. Intense cold reduces nerve impulse conduction and decreases the perception of pain. As a result, cold is used as a local anesthetic. There is, however, a danger in the prolonged use of intense cold; it interferes with the supply of oxygen and nourishment to the tissues and may result in tissue death. As with heat, a secondary vasodilation effect occurs after an hour of cold application. The maximum therapeutic effect of cold applications is reached in 30 minutes, and it is recommended that at least 20 minutes be allowed between treatments (Kemp, Pillitteri and Brown, 1989).

For systemic purposes, cold is used to slow the basal metabolic rate. This is indicated in certain kinds of heart surgery, because a low basal metabolic rate results in a lessened demand of the body tissues for oxygen and nourishment, and thus decreases the work of the heart. Cold also slows the blood circulation. For this reason a patient's limb may be packed in ice prior to amputation. The effect of the cold enables the surgeon to control bleeding more easily during the operation.

ASSESSMENTS FOR THERAPEUTIC APPLICATIONS OF HEAT AND COLD

Prior to implementing heat and cold treatments, nurses must assess their patients for age and condition of the skin, general physical health and area of the body that is affected. The choice of the kind of application to be used will depend on the purpose of the application, the duration of the treatment and the availability of the equipment.

The age of the patient and the condition of the skin   Infants and older adults tend to have thinner and more fragile skin. Because older adults have decreased perception of pain, and infants are not able to describe these sensations, both groups require special consideration when applying heat and cold treatments.

The general physical health of the patient Patients with circulatory problems or heart disease are particularly sensitive to applications of heat and cold (Kemp, Pillitteri and Brown, 1989). Heat applied to a large area of the body draws a significant volume of blood supply to that area and away from other areas. This could result in an inadequate amount of blood within the central circulation and compromise kidney function. Alternatively, cold application to an area with poor circulation could result in cell damage.

Guide for Assessing Therapeutic Applications of Heat or Cold

1. Does the patient understand the purpose of the treatment?
2. What precautions need to be taken to protect the patient from harm?
3. Is the patient aware of the dangers?
4. Are added safety precautions required because of age, general physical condition, the skin condition or the mental state of the patient?
5. Is the patient able to participate in the treatment? Is this desirable?
6. Are there specific skills that the patient (or family) needs to learn or knowledge that must be gained in order to carry out the treatment at home?
7. Is the patient safe during the application?
8. Is the patient comfortable?
9. Is the hot or cold application producing the desired physiological effect, for example, increased circulation to the part, or relief of pain?

People who are sedated (by analgesics, anesthetics or sedatives), and those who have decreased neurological sensation (for example, diabetics, paraplegics), are less able to detect heat or cold. They may sustain tissue injury without realizing its severity.

The area of the body that is affected   Certain body areas, depending on the condition of the skin, are better able to tolerate heat and cold. The hands, for example, can withstand greater warmth or cold than can the abdomen or the neck. Newly formed tissues (such as a fresh surgical incision) are more tender than surrounding tissue. Thus, applications of heat or cold to the new tissue may not be tolerated very well (Kemp, Pillitteri and Brown, 1989).

LOCAL APPLICATIONS OF HEAT

Heat can be applied as radiant heat, conductive heat or conversive heat. *Radiant heat* is heat with a wavelength in the infrared portion of the electromagnetic spectrum. A commonly used example is the infrared lamp. *Conductive heat* is heat transferred by direct application, for example, by a hot water bottle or hot compress. Radiant and conductive heat provide heat to the superficial tissues only. *Conversive heat* is heat converted from primary sources of energy, for example, from short wave or ultrasound wave energy. The application of this latter type of heat is classified as medical diathermy; it is used to provide heat to deep tissues. Use of this type of heat treatment requires consultation with the physical therapist or physician because the increased temperature in the deep tissues may accelerate underlying inflammatory processes, such as cartilage inflammation in arthritis (Burrell, 1992).

Both moist and dry forms of heat can be applied to the skin or mucous membranes. All patients receiving dry and moist heat should be observed closely for any untoward reactions to heat applications, such as a prolonged erythema (redness), blister formation or discomfort.

DRY HEAT APPLICATIONS

The advantages of dry heat applications are that they can be directed to the local site without macerating surrounding tissues, and they help prevent contamination from microorganisms. Dry heat does have disadvantages though. These include fluid loss from evaporation at the site and less penetration than moist heat.

HOT WATER BOTTLES

The hot water bottle has long been used as a vehicle for applying dry heat to the body. It is used as both a therapeutic and a comfort measure, although therapeutically its

KEY PRINCIPLES

Principles Relevant to the Therapeutic Use of Heat and Cold

1. Heat is distributed throughout the body by the circulating blood and by direct conduction throughout the tissues.

2. Heat is lost from the body chiefly through conduction, convection and evaporation at the surface of the skin.

3. The amount of heat that is lost from the body is directly proportional to the amount of blood that is circulating close to the surface of the skin.

4. The amount of blood that circulates close to the surface of the skin is influenced by the dilatation and constriction of peripheral arterioles.

5. Applications of heat and cold influence the dilatation and constriction of peripheral blood vessels.

6. Moisture conducts heat better than air does.

7. People vary in their ability to tolerate heat and cold applications. People at both extremes of the age spectrum — that is, the very old and the very young — are particularly at risk for tissue damage from heat and cold treatments.

8. The length of time of exposure to extremes in temperature affects the body's tolerance of the temperature.

9. A decreased sensitivity to heat and cold occurs with prolonged applications.

10. Prolonged applications of heat and cold result in secondary (vasoconstriction/vasodilation) effects which may reduce the benefits of the treatment.

11. The maximum therapeutic effect of heat and cold applications is reached after 30 minutes of the application.

use is being surpassed by the electric heating pad. Some hospitals and other inpatient health agencies have prohibited the use of hot water bottles because of the ever-present danger of burns to patients. Procedure 24.2 outlines how to administer a hot water bottle.

Preparing the Patient

Explain the purpose and duration of the procedure to the patient. Since patients become accustomed to heat after

PROCEDURE 24.2

Applying a Hot Water Bottle

ACTION	RATIONALE
1. Prepare the patient.	Promotes patient well-being.
2. Gather:	Facilitates efficiency and economy of time.
• Hot water bottle	
• Protective cover	
• Thermometer	
3. Fill the hot water bottle and let it remain full for a few minutes, then empty it.	Allows the rubber to warm.
4. Fill the hot water bottle one-half to two-thirds full, then squeeze the sides together before putting on the top.	Expels air from the remainder of the bottle making it light and easy to mold to the body.
5. Dry the outside of the hot water bottle, test it for leakage, then place it in its entirety in a cloth cover before taking it to the patient.	The cover slows the transmission of heat, absorbs perspiration, and thereby lessens the danger of burning the patient.
6. Place the hot water bottle on the desired area and mold it to the patient's body. If the patient is a person who burns easily, place a sheet or blanket between the patient and the bottle.	Facilitates the effectiveness of heat. Protects the patient from thermal injury.
7. Caution the patient against refilling the bottle without checking the temperature.	Protects the patient from thermal injury.
8. Document the procedure and any responses to the treatment.	Fulfills requirements for nurse accountability.
9. When a hot water bottle is not in use, hang it upside-down with the top unscrewed.	This allows the bottle to dry inside and prevents the sides of the bottle from sticking together.

prolonged applications, they should be cautioned not to refill a hot water bottle without checking the temperature. Any pain or discomfort should be reported immediately. The TPR is taken prior to commencing the application as a baseline for evaluating the patient's response to treatment.

Assembling Equipment

Because the rubber of the hot water bottle readily heats up to the temperature of the inside water, it can cause a burn. Therefore, the water for a hot water bottle must be tested for its exact temperature. Maintaining water temperature between 38 and 43°C is generally considered to be a safe guideline. A temperature at the lowest end of this range is considered safe for children (Whaley and Wong, 1992) and for adults who are unconscious or debilitated or who have

impaired circulation. The water for a hot water bottle can be obtained from the hot water tap; its temperature is checked by the thermometers that most hospitals provide for measuring the temperature of unsterile solutions. As a general guide, the temperature of the water should be comfortable when tested on the nurse's inner wrist.

HEATING PADS

Electric heating pads and electric blankets are frequently used as a means of providing dry heat. They have the advantages of being light, of being easily molded to the patient's body and of providing constant heat at a constant temperature. Their disadvantages are related to their cleaning and to the danger of short circuits. Guidelines for applying heating pads pad are outlined in Procedure 24.3.

Preparing the Patient

Patient preparation is the same as that for applying a hot water bottle. The patient should be cautioned against turning up the temperature setting on the heating pad to avoid the risk of thermal injury.

Assembling Equipment

There are two basic types of heating pads. The first, called an *electric heating pad*, is a flat waterproof pad made up of a coiled element that converts electric current to dry heat and a control switch. The temperature should be set at the lowest setting unless otherwise prescribed by the physician. Settings at the highest and medium temperatures place the patient at risk for burn injury; this is of particular concern with children, older people and patients whose perception of pain and warmth may be dulled by analgesics or other medications. The temperature control switch should be secured so that is cannot be changed. This can be done by putting adhesive tape on both sides of the control switch, and placing it out of reach of the patient. It is recommended that this be done routinely for children under 12 years of age, and for those patients who may be tempted to increase the temperature setting.

The second type of heating pad is the *aquamatic* or **aquathermia pad**. It is a vinyl pad consisting of channels through which heated water circulates, transmitting dry

FIGURE 24.4   The Aquathermia pad and unit

SOURCE: Norton, B.A. and Miller, A.M. (1989). *Skills for professional nursing practice.* Norwalk, CT: Appleton–Century–Crofts, 438. Reproduced with permission.

heat of a constant temperature. The pad is attached to an electrically operated unit which stores, heats and circulates warmed distilled water(see Figure 24.4). Distilled water is used because tap water leaves mineral deposits in the unit. The temperature is preset with a plastic key and thermostatically controlled. This adds a safety feature in that the temperature setting cannot be changed without the use of a key. Aquathermia pads come in various sizes.

Both types of heating pads are made of a plastic material. If this covering comes in contact with perspiring skin, maceration can occur. Therefore, these electric pads must be covered before use on patients.

PROCEDURE 24.3

Applying the Heating Pad

ACTION	RATIONALE
1. Prepare the patient.	Promotes the patient's well-being.
2. Gather: • Electric heating pad or aquathermia pad and unit • Towel or flannel cloth • Distilled water for aquathermia unit	Promotes efficiency and economy of time.
3. Wrap a thin towel or flannel cloth around the heating pad.	Avoids direct contact with the patient's skin.
4. **Electric heating pad:** Set the temperature at its lowest setting, or as ordered. **Aquathermia pad:** Set the temperature at 40.5°C or as ordered.	Prevents burn injury.
5. At bedside, plug unit into an electrical outlet and allow pad to warm for a few minutes. Place aquathermia unit on a stable surface and slightly higher than the patient.	Force of gravity assists the flow of water through the pad.

Continued on the next page

PROCEDURE 24.3
continued

ACTION	RATIONALE
6. Check the temperature of the pad by pressing it against the inner aspect of the forearm.	Alerts the nurse to mechanical dysfunction and prevents accidental burning.
7. Apply the pad to the designated area.	
8. Monitor the patient for untoward reactions.	Ensures patient safety.
9. Remove the pad after treatment is completed. Store unit as per agency policy.	
10. Document the procedure and any responses to the treatment.	Fulfills requirements for nurse accountability.

CHEMICAL HEAT PACKS

These packs are made of heavy-duty plastic with separate compartments filled with chemicals that produce heat when they react with each other. To activate the chemical reaction, the nurse strikes the pack against the countertop or kneads it between the hands. The temperature of the pack reaches between 40.5 and 46°C and may vary according to the manufacturer (Kemp, Pillitteri and Brown, 1989).

The principles for applying chemical heat packs are similar to those used for a hot water bottle and electric pad. Specific to heat packs, safety pins should not be used to secure the pack because a puncture could precipitate leakage and a chemical burn.

MOIST HEAT APPLICATIONS

Moist heat applications have the advantage of providing more penetrating warmth than dry heat because moisture is conducive to heat transfer. By the same token, moist heat applications tend to cool more quickly (through evaporation) and they need to be reapplied to maintain the therapeutic effect. Moisture on the skin makes it prone to maceration; nurses must carefully assess the site of application and the surrounding skin for breakdown.

HOT COMPRESSES

Hot compresses are moist applications of sterile or unsterile gauze sponges. Sterile precautions are indicated when the compress is to be applied to an open wound or to an organ such as the eye. Hot compresses are often indicated to hasten the suppurative process and to improve the circulation of blood to the tissues. Normal saline and antiseptic solutions are frequently ordered by the physician. Procedure 24.4 outlines how to apply hot compresses.

Preparing the Patient

Explain the purpose, duration and sensations the patient may feel during the procedure. The compresses will feel warm but should not be painful. Pain should be reported immediately.

Assembling Equipment

Hot compresses may be applied by clean or sterile techniques. When clean technique is used, a basin with hot tap water is assembled along with clean forceps, gauze sponges, towels, plastic wrap, dressing supplies and a waterproof protective pad. When the compress is to be applied with sterile technique, the solution, basin, gauze sponges, forceps and dressing supplies must be sterile. Sterile gloves may also be used. Sterile solution is heated by placing the solution container in a sink or large basin of hot water. The temperature of the solution should be 55°C for adults and 40.6°C for children, older people and for eye compresses (Malloch, 1993). The temperature can be tested by pouring a small amount of solution into a container, checking it with a thermometer and then discarding the solution. Clean tap water can be tested directly.

Some agencies use commercially prepared compresses. These eliminate the need for a basin of solution. The compresses (contained in sealed packages) are heated in a special heater and then taken to the bedside. A sterile absorbent pad or towel and plastic wrap are placed over the compress to retain heat and moisture during the procedure. If the patient's skin is prone to maceration, petroleum jelly is applied to the area (sterile jelly is used on the edges of an open wound if present). Petroleum jelly acts as a water barrier and protects the skin from maceration. It also protects the area from burns because it decreases the rate of heat penetration (Malloch, 1993).

PROCEDURE 24.4

Applying Hot Compresses

ACTION	RATIONALE
1. Prepare the patient.	Promotes patient's well-being.
2. Gather clean or sterile: • Basin • Tap water or solution • Gauze sponges or prepared compresses • Forceps • Gloves • Sterile absorbent pad or towel • Plastic wrap • Petroleum jelly and applicator • Water-proof protective pad • Dressing supplies	Promotes efficiency and economy of time.
3. Expose the area to be treated. Place a water-proof pad under the treatment site.	Protects the bed linen from moisture.
4. Prepare solution and compresses. Open a sterile basin, add sterile gauze sponges, and pour in hot solution. Add gauze sponges and hot tap water to a clean basin. Test temperature. Have commercially prepared packs in easy reach.	Readies supplies for the procedure.
5. Using gloves, remove old dressing, if present, and discard. Remove and discard gloves. Apply petroleum jelly to area if necessary. Use sterile gloves or applicator for a sterile procedure.	Acts as a water barrier and protects the skin from maceration.
6. Using clean or sterile technique, wring out excess fluid from the compresses.	Prevents rapid evaporation and cooling of compresses.
7. Apply the gauze to the area. Check for skin reaction. If no excessive redness, blistering or pain, mold the compress to the site.	Protects the patient from thermal injury. Molding the compress facilitates heat retention.
8. Cover the moist dressing with plastic wrap and then a dry towel. For sterile procedures, place a sterile abdominal pad over the compress before applying the plastic wrap. If ordered, apply a hot water bottle or aquathermia pad over the compress. Never use an electric heating pad for this purpose.	Facilitates heat retention by slowing evaporation and the cooling process. Holds the heat of the compress more uniformly. Moisture may cause an electric shock.
9. Leave the compress on for 15 to 20 minutes. Monitor the site and the patient's response during the procedure.	Maximum therapeutic effect is reached in this time.
10. Remove the compress, assess the condition of the site, and dress it as necessary.	Provides data for evaluating the effectiveness of treatment.

Continued on the next page

ACTION	RATIONALE
11. Discard supplies, and clean and store equipment as per agency protocol.	Promotes cleanliness and safety in the workplace.
12. Document the procedure, the condition of the site and the patient's response to treatment.	Fulfills requirements for nurse accountability.

HOT PACKS

A hot pack is sometimes referred to as a *hot fomentation* or *foment*. It is a piece of heated moist flannel or similar material that is applied to a patient's skin in order to supply superficial moist heat. It is used for a larger area than the hot compress is. Hot packs are frequently indicated to relieve muscle spasm. They are also applied to hasten the suppurative process and to decrease muscle soreness.

A hot pack can be prepared by boiling or steaming pieces of flannel or by heating commercially prepared packs. If the flannel is boiled it is necessary to wring it out before applying it. There are hot pack machines available which steam the flannel to prepare it for application. Because intense heat can be applied in this manner, there is a danger that the patient may be burned. This danger is minimized if the hot pack is sufficiently dry that water does not drip from it.

The procedure for applying a hot pack is similar to that for a hot compress. The patient is prepared by explaining the procedure. Sometimes petrolatum is applied to the skin beforehand to serve as a protective coating and to slow the transfer of heat. Once the foment has been heated, it is shaken slightly before it is applied. This step distributes the heat evenly, and reduces the danger of burning the patient. The hot foment is covered with an insulating water-proof material and then secured to the patient with a towel or binder. As with hot compresses, a hot water bottle or aquathermia pad may be applied over a hot pack to maintain its heat.

A hot pack usually keeps hot for 10 to 15 minutes. Once it has cooled it is removed and, if a longer treatment is required, it is replaced with another pack. If the patient does not need another application for some time, the skin is dried.

Erythema (redness) of the skin is expected with the application of hot packs because the heat causes dilatation of the local blood capillaries. If blistering of the skin occurs, it should be reported and the treatment withheld until the physician is consulted.

HYDROTHERAPY

Hydrotherapy, also known as "tubbing" or "tanking" (from Hubbard tanks), is used in burn therapy for wound cleansing, range of motion exercises and total body bathing. Whirlpool baths are units that are small enough to accommodate a leg or an arm for these same purposes. Special portable containers, such as arm and foot baths, also are available commercially for use at home. Water agitation in whirlpools and Hubbard tanks is created by air bubbled into the water. This swirling motion stimulates circulation, promotes relaxation and helps to clean wounds. When the body is totally submerged in water, the limbs become weightless, thus facilitating active and passive range of motion exercises. Hydrotherapy is often carried out in the physiotherapy department or in specialized burn units.

Whirlpool bath.

SITZ BATHS

The *sitz bath* is a special bath, the purposes of which are chiefly to provide warmth, to cleanse and to provide comfort to the patient's perineal area. It is often indicated after rectal or perineal surgery and is used routinely after child-birth for promoting perineal healing and comfort. Procedure 24.5 outlines how to administer a sitz bath.

Preparing the Patient

Explain the purpose and the procedure, as well as sensations the patient may feel. Comfort is an important concern for patients who have experienced perineal trauma. Tell patients that initially they may experience some discomfort because the tissues are tender. However, this should subside within a few minutes. Some patients may require analgesia prior to the procedure. The bath takes about 20 minutes. The patient may want to take some reading material to help pass the time. Because of the localized vasodilation that occurs in response to the heat, dizziness and faintness may occur when getting out of or off the sitz bath. The patient should be warned about this and instructed to stand up and change position very slowly.

Assembling Equipment

There are several commercially manufactured sitz baths available. Some models are portable and disposable. These models can fit over toilets, on commode chairs or on beds. There are also comfort seats and inflatable rings that can be placed in bathtubs, as well as separate sitz bath units. The sitz bath is generally ordered with saline solution or tap water. The temperature should be 38.9 to 40.6°C.

FIGURE 24.5   Portable sitz bath

PROCEDURE 24.5

Administering a Sitz Bath

ACTION	RATIONALE
1. Prepare the patient.	Promotes patient participation and well-being.
2. Gather: • Portable sitz bath or inflatable ring • Towels • Bath blanket • Patient's clean clothing	Facilitates efficiency and economy of time.
3. Fill the basin or bathtub with water or ordered solution until it is two-thirds (basin) or one-third (tub) full.	Ensures the perineal area will be adequately immersed.
4. Check the temperature of the water with thermometer or the inner aspect of the wrist.	Protects the patient from thermal injury.

Continued on the next page

PROCEDURE 24.5
continued

ACTION	RATIONALE
5. **Bathtub:** Place an inflatable ring on tub bottom. **Portable basin:** Place the basin on the toilet or commode.	
6. Assist the patient into a comfortable position in the sitz bath, ensuring that the perineal area is immersed in water. Provide adequate support with towels, particularly if there is doubt about the patient's ability to tolerate the procedure.	Promotes patient comfort and effectiveness of therapy.
7. Cover the patient with a towel or bath blanket.	Promotes privacy and avoids chilling.
8. Stay with the patient if an analgesia was given; otherwise show the patient how to use the call bell and assess condition at regular intervals.	Protects the patient from injury. Analgesia may cause lightheadedness.
9. After 20 minutes assist the patient to get off of the bath or out of the tub. The patient should stand up slowly and hold onto a safety rail if one is available.	Protects the patient from accidentally falling.
10. Dry the area and dress the wound as necessary. Assist patient to dress and to return to bed.	
11. Dispose of supplies and clean the sitz bath as per agency protocol.	Ensures safety and cleanliness in the workplace.
12. Document the procedure, the condition of the site, and the patient's response to treatment.	Fulfills requirements for nurse accountability.

ULTRAVIOLET LAMPS

Ultraviolet radiation is used clinically to treat wounds and skin diseases. The sun is a natural source of ultraviolet light, but artificial sources are used therapeutically. The hot quartz mercury lamp, the carbon arc lamp and, of course, the sun lamp are all used.

Generally, ultraviolet radiation treatment is carried out in a special department, such as the physiotherapy department. The normal skin reaction produces an erythema, tanning and a proliferation of the cells of the epidermis. The physician generally orders ultraviolet treatments every other day for maximum effect. Fair-skinned people are more sensitive to ultraviolet radiation than dark-skinned people are. Sulfanilamide medications also increase sensitivity.

DIATHERMY

Medical diathermy is the provision of heat to the deep tissues of the body by transforming certain kinds of physical energy into heat. It is usually done in a physical therapy department under the direction of a physician.

Various high frequency currents are used: short wave, microwave and ultrasound. The treatment is painless; the patient's chief perception is one of warmth. Diathermy is used for much the same reasons as superficial heat is. Although this therapy may not affect all models, it is generally not administered to individuals with cardiac pacemakers because the currents may interfere with the function of the pacemaker.

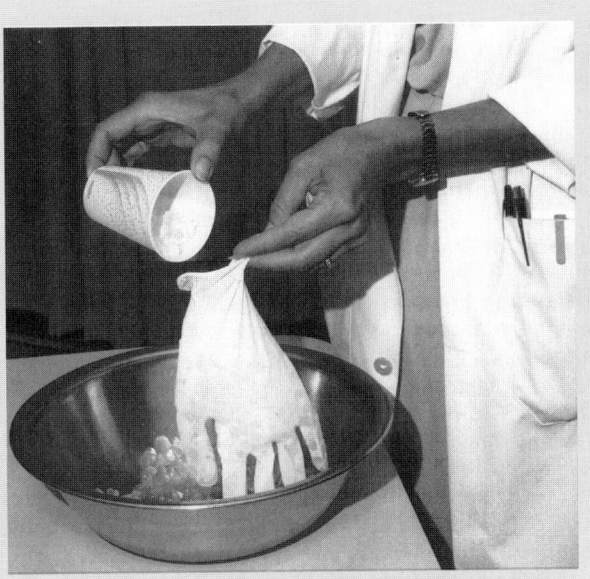

Nurse prepares an ice bag by filling a disposable glove with crushed ice.

LOCAL APPLICATIONS OF COLD

Cold applications are available in dry or wet forms. Tissue damage can ensue from intense and prolonged cold applications. Signs of tissue damage include mottling, purplish or bluish colour of the skin surface, blisters and numbness.

DRY COLD APPLICATIONS

The ice bag, ice cap, ice collar and ice pack are commonly used means of applying dry cold to the body. An ice collar is a long narrow rubber or plastic bag that fits around the neck. Commercial plastic packs that can be frozen and reused are frequently used in lieu of the ice bag. Care should be taken to avoid puncturing these packs because the chemicals in the coolant liquid can cause tissue injury. An ice bag can also be made by filling a disposable glove with crushed ice.

Ice bags are usually made with an opening through which small pieces of ice are inserted. The procedure for applying an ice bag is similar to that for a hot water bottle. Once the ice bag is filled to two-thirds of its capacity, the air is expelled before the top of the ice bag is secured. As with the hot water bottle, the air in the ice bag is removed so that it can be molded to the patient's body.

Ice applications should never be in direct contact with the skin; a cold injury could result from the intense cold. Therefore, a flannel cover should be put over an ice bag once it is dried. The cover retains cold for more gradual application and it absorbs the water formed by atmospheric condensation. The bag is placed on the area of the body to be cooled.

When an ice bag is in place, it is important to ensure that the pressure of the bag does not cut off circulation. At the first sign of tissue numbness and a mottled bluish appearance, the bag should be removed and the physician notified. These signs could be the result of either the cold or pressure upon the tissues.

Ice bags that are not in use are stored with the tops removed so that the air will dry the inside and prevent the sides from sticking together. An economic alternative to an ice bag, which can be used at home, is a small bag of frozen peas which can be easily molded and applied. The bag of peas can be refrozen for future use. It should be labelled "for external use only" since defrosted and refrozen foods should not be eaten.

MOIST COLD APPLICATIONS

Moist cold can be applied by means of ice compresses. These are frequently used to terminate a nosebleed (epistaxis) or to supply moist cold to the eye.

An ice compress is usually made of gauze or other cloth material. Moistened gauze is cooled over ice chips, wrung out and then applied. The compress is covered with a waterproof pad to keep it cool longer and for patient comfort, as this prevents moisture from dripping on the patient. It is replaced as it becomes warm.

KEY TERMS

core temperature p. 760

homeothermic p. 760

thermoregulation p. 760

neutral thermal
   environment p. 764

pyrexia p. 766

chill p. 767

diaphoresis p. 767

hyperthermia p. 768

hypothermia p. 768

aquathermia pad p. 783

hot compress p. 784

hydrotherapy p. 786

sitz bath p. 786

IN REVIEW

Human beings are in a state of thermal health when their central body temperature is about 37°C. This temperature is a measure of body heat, reflecting a balance between heat gain and heat loss. For a constant body temperature to be maintained, heat produced by cellular metabolism must be lost to the environment. This is accomplished by the mechanisms of conduction, convection, evaporation and radiation. To maintain thermal health, individuals must adapt to changing conditions in the ambient environment and to internal metabolic processes. According to Erickson (1982) individuals' adaptive capabilities include biological, behavioural and social modes. Thermal dysfunction occurs when the body temperature rises or falls outside the narrow range of normal.

The regulatory mechanisms controlling body temperature are located in the preoptic area of the hypothalamus, which acts as the body's thermostat. Neurons which respond to the temperature of circulating blood trigger the heat-gaining or the heat-losing centre. Stimulation of the heat-gaining centre elicits activities to produce more heat and to prevent its loss from the body. Conversely, stimulation of the heat-losing centre inhibits the heat-producing and heat-conserving mechanisms and activates heat loss through panting and sweating. Humans can also maintain thermal comfort through adaptive behaviours such as altering posture, ingesting hot or cold foods or beverages, adding or removing clothing and using artificial heating or cooling devices. Individuals with impaired ability to adapt biologically and behaviourally can achieve thermal comfort through the education and the assistance of others.

Body temperature is affected by any condition which increases the basal metabolic rate, such as activity, thyroxine production, the dynamic action of food and circadian rhythm. Strong emotions, body size and mass and the surrounding environment also affect temperature. Temperatures are normally lowest in the early morning and highest in late afternoon. Illness and disease states, poor circulation and disorders of the nervous system affect the efficiency of the temperature-regulating mechanisms and interfere with an individual's ability to respond to changes in body temperature.

Temperature regulation varies throughout the life cycle. High fever during early pregnancy is teratogenic; thus pregnant women should try to avoid developing a fever during this time. At birth and during the first year of life, an infant's body temperature is unstable because the heat-regulating mechanisms are immature. In addition, because their body surface is large in relation to their body size, infants can become too cool or too warm very rapidly. Infants are dependent on a stable environmental temperature to maintain their own internal temperature.

High fevers occur with the common acute respiratory infections of infancy and early childhood and may precipitate seizures. Fever is often the first indication of these infections.

Sweating begins in the teen years; this cooling mechanism is not functional in younger children. Girls have a cyclic rise and fall of temperature with the onset of menses and this continues throughout the childbearing years.

Women often experience variations in body temperature during menopause; the characteristic "hot flushes" occur in many middle-aged women. Older people tend to have a lower body temperature than young adults and they tend not to cope well with heat or cold.

Fever is thought to be caused by abnormalities in the brain or by toxic substances that affect the temperature regulating mechanisms. Pyrogens produced by toxic bacteria or degenerating tissue stimulate the release of endogenous pyrogens which act on the thermoregulatory centres. Fever creates an unfavourable temperature for the survival of bacteria and it increases the cellular metabolic rate which increases the production of immune bodies and phagocytic action.

The stages of a fever are the chill phase, the course of the fever and the termination. During the chill and fever phases, the rate of cellular metabolism increases and bodily demands for fluid, oxygen and glucose rise. Respiratory and pulse rates become elevated and remain high. As the cause of the fever is controlled, the process reverses and mechanisms for heat dissipation are instituted.

The body's homeostatic heat balance can be upset by heat cramps, heat exhaustion, heat stroke, malignant hyperthermia and accidental hypothermia. These conditions, especially hypothermia, require prompt care.

The nurse assesses a patient's temperature-regulating status by measuring body temperature with a clinical thermometer, taking a health history and observing the individual for signs of disturbed thermoregulation. Because fever is a universal sign of illness, temperatures are taken routinely in most inpatient agencies.

Problems in temperature regulation that nurses may treat independently are related to an imbalance between heat losses and heat gains leading to an excessive rise or fall in core body temperature. The common nursing diagnostic labels are *Hyperthermia* (fever), *Hypothermia* and *High risk for altered body temperature*. The management of severe hyperthermia and profound hypothermia requires collaboration between nursing and medical disciplines. These and other associated problems are identified as collaborative problems.

In planning care for patients with thermoregulation problems, the nurse considers the severity of the problems and the appropriate treatment modalities to restore body temperature. Collaboration with other health care professionals is often necessary.

Nurses can assist individuals to achieve optimal thermal health by providing information about environmental challenges and suggesting ways to conserve or dissipate heat in the course of daily living. Interventions for patients with a fever are directed towards minimizing the stresses of an elevated temperature on the body's adaptive mechanisms. Rest, comfort, hygiene measures and an adequate fluid and food intake are important protective strategies.

In implementing restorative interventions for fever, the nurse might administer antipyretic and/or antibiotic medications, give tepid sponge baths and use fans. Hypothermia machines (cooling blankets) may also be employed. Health restoring strategies for a hypothermic patient include the use of extra blankets, flannelette sheets, warmed bedding and commercial warming devices.

Applications of heat and cold are used as therapeutic measures in health care agencies and in the home. Because perceptions of temperature sensations vary, therapeutic heat and cold measures pose hazards to skin integrity and therefore must be carried out with caution. Usually a physician's order is required in hospital.

Heat applied locally causes an increase in circulation to an area. It provides warmth and comfort, reduces muscle tension and swelling, increases suppuration, hastens healing and softens exudates. Conversely, cold applied locally causes a decrease in circulation and blood flow. It stops hemorrhage, slows suppuration, reduces swelling immediately after an injury and relieves pain. Systemic cold is sometimes used to slow basal metabolic rate in certain types of heart surgery.

Both moist and dry forms of heat can be applied to skin or mucous membranes. Dry heat can be applied to a local area but causes evaporation and has less penetration than moist heat. Hot water bottles, electric heating pads, aquathermia pads and chemical heat packs are means of providing dry heat. Moist heat applications provide more penetrating warmth than dry heat because moisture conducts heat. However, they cool quickly and can cause maceration of the skin. Moist heat is applied by hot compresses, hot packs, hydrotherapy and Sitz baths.

Cold can be applied in dry or moist forms but it can cause tissue damage if prolonged. Dry cold is applied by ice bags and moist cold by ice compresses.

LEARNING ACTIVITIES

1. **Case Study:** Mrs. S. James is a 34-year-old woman who works as an aide in one of the city hospitals. She is married and has a 5-year-old son. Mrs. James was admitted to the hospital with an elevated temperature of unknown etiology. Her temperature at admission was 39.1° C, her pulse 100 and her respirations 24. The patient had a chill during her first evening in the hospital, when her fever rose to 40° C. The following morning she felt improved, but she still perspired profusely and in the evening appeared restless and flushed.

   The doctor left orders that Mrs. James was to have a tepid sponge bath and acetaminophen if her temperature rose above 39° C. He also asked the patient to drink at least one glass of fluid hourly.

   a. What factors are relevant to your explanation of a tepid sponge bath to this patient?

   b. How can the patient's production of body heat be minimized?

   c. How can the loss of body heat be facilitated?

   d. What is the action of acetaminophen?

   e. How should you evaluate the effectiveness of the nursing care?

   f. Why did the doctor want Mrs. James to drink at least one glass of fluid every hour?

   g. What observations would indicate that the patient is taking insufficient fluid?

   j. Describe an environment which would be therapeutic for this patient.

2. **Case Study:** Mrs. J. Watson has an infected cut on her right hand. She is at home and the physician has ordered hot compresses for her hand. As the home care nurse you have been asked to assist Mrs. Watson. This patient is 75 years old and has poor blood circulation.

   a. What are the specific problems of this patient in relation to her infected cut?

   b. What factors should you take into consideration in helping to plan this patient's care?

   c. What physiological reactions are to be expected as a result of the hot compresses?

   d. How could the effectiveness of the compresses be evaluated?

   e. What specific precautions should be taken? Why?

   f. Outline the nursing diagnoses, expected outcomes and a plan of care for this patient.

REFERENCES AND READINGS

AMERICAN SOCIETY OF HEATING, REFRIGERATION AND AIR CONDITIONING (ASHRAE). (1982). Health Facilities. In *ASHRAE handbook: Applications* (sections 7.1–7.12). Atlanta: Author.

BATES, B. (1991). *A guide to physical examination and history taking*. Philadelphia: Lippincott.

BENZINGER, T. H. (1969). Heat regulation: Homeostasis of central temperature in man. *Physiological Review, 49*(4), 671–759.

BRITTEN, M. (1986). Monitoring body temperature and understanding its significance. In J. Luckman and K. C. Sorenson (Eds). *Basic nursing: A psychophysiologic approach*. Philadelphia: Saunders, 551–571.

BRUCK, K. (1983). Heat balance and the regulation of body temperature. In R. F. Schmidt and G. Thews (Eds). *Human physiology*. Berlin: Springer Verlag, 531–547.

BURRELL, L. O. (1992). *Adult nursing in hospital and community settings*. Norwalk, CT: Appleton & Lange.

CAIN, H. D. (1980). *Flint's emergency treatment and management* (6th ed.). Philadelphia: Saunders.

CARPENITO, L. J. (1993). *Nursing diagnosis: Application to clinical practice* (5th ed.). Philadelphia: Lippincott.

CARUSO, C. and POSEY, V. (1985, July/August). Heat waves threaten the old. *Geriatric Nursing*. 209–212.

CLARK, R. P. and EDHOLM, O. G. (1985). *Man and his thermal environment*. London: Edward Arnold.

COOPER, K. E. (1969, June). Regulation of body temperature. *British Journal of Hospital Medicine*. 1065–1067.

CUNHA, B. A., DIGAMON-BELTRAN, M. and GOBBO, P.N. (1984). Implications of fever in the critical care setting. *Heart and Lung, 13*(5), 460–465.

DONAHUE, A.M. (1983). Tepid sponging. *Journal of Emergency Nursing, 9*(2).

DUBOIS, E. F. (1921). The basal metabolism in fever. *JAMA, 77*(5), 352–355.

EARNEST, V.V. (1993). *Clinical skills in nursing practice* (2nd ed.). Philadelphia: Lippincott.

ERICKSON, R. (1982, July). A model of adaptation to the thermal environment. *Advances in Nursing Science*, 15(2), 1–12.

FLYNN, J. M. and HACKEL, R. (1990). *Technological foundations in nursing.* Norwalk, CT: Appleton & Lange.

FRUTHALER, G. J. (1985, November). Fever in children: Phobia vs. facts. *Hospital Practice.* 49–53.

GANONG, W. (1989). *Review of medical physiology.* Norwalk, CT: Appleton & Lange.

GUYTON, A. C. (1981). *Textbook of medical physiology* (6th ed.). Philadelphia: Saunders.

HOLTZLAW, B. J. (1992). The febrile response in critical care: State of the science. *Heart and Lung*, 21(5), 482–501.

KEMP, B., PILLITTERI, A. and BROWN, P. (1989). *Fundamentals of nursing* (2nd ed.). Glenview, IL: Scott, Foresman.

KHOGALI, M. and MUSTAFA, M. K. Y. (1984). Physiology of heat stroke: A review. In Hales, J. R. S. (Ed), *Thermal Physiology.* New York: Raven Press, 503–510.

KINMOUTH, A., FULTON, Y. and CAMBELL, M. J. (1992). Management of feverish children at home. *British Medical Journal, 305*, 1134–1136.

LEWIS, S. and COLLIER, I. (1992). *Medical-surgical nursing: Assessment and management of clinical problems* (3rd ed.). St. Louis: Mosby.

MACBRYDE, C. M. and BLACKLOW, R. S. (Eds). (1970). *Signs and symptoms: Applied pathologic physiology and clinical interpretation* (5th ed.). Philadelphia: Lippincott.

MALLOCH, K. (1993). Physical treatments. In Springhouse. *Nursing procedures: Student version.* Springhouse, PA: Springhouse.

MANITOBA HEALTH. (1990). *Menopause and midlife health for women.* Winnipeg: Author.

MARTINI, F. (1989). *Fundamentals of anatomy and physiology.* Englewood Cliffs, NJ: Prentice-Hall.

McCANCE, K. and HUETHER, S. (1990). *Pathophysiology: The biologic basis for disease in adults and children.* St. Louis: Mosby.

McFARLAND, G. K. and McFARLANE, E. A. (1989). *Nursing diagnosis and intervention: Planning for patient care.* St. Louis: Mosby.

MITCHELL, D. and LABURN, H. P (1985). Pathophysiology of temperature regulation. *The Physiologist*, 28(6), 507–517.

MOUNT, L. E. (1979). *Adaptation to thermal environment: Man and his productive animals.* Baltimore: University Park Press.

NORTON, B. A. and MILLER, A.M. (1986). *Skills for professional nursing practice.* Norwalk, CT: Appleton-Century-Crofts.

PORTH, C. (1990). *Pathophysiology: Concepts of altered health states* (3rd ed.). Philadelphia: Lippincott.

POTTER, P.A. (1990). *Clinical nursing skills and techniques* (2nd ed.). St. Louis: Mosby.

TROFINO, R. B. (1991). *Nursing care of the burn-injured patient.* Philadelphia: F. A. Davis.

VICTORIA GENERAL HOSPITAL. (1993). *Fever in a child* (Teaching pamphlet). Winnipeg: Victoria General Hospital Education Department.

WHALEY, L. and WONG, D. (1992). *Nursing care of infants and children* (4th ed.). St. Louis: Mosby.

WILLIAMS, M. H. (1993). *Lifetime: Fitness and wellness* (3rd ed.). Madison, WI: Brown and Benchmark.

INTRODUCTION

Comfort is a multi-faceted concept indicating a sense of physical, psychological, social, spiritual and environmental ease. It is a subjective experience. Health care professionals rely on subjective reports and on observable behaviour to determine a patient's comfort. The patient, however, remains the authority on his or her experience of feeling comfortable.

Discomfort may result from myriad psychosocial, spiritual or physical stimuli. A person who is afraid or worried may be as uncomfortable as one who is cold or in pain. For example, newly hospitalized patients are subject to the stresses that accompany entering any unfamiliar environment. Unwell individuals often fear pain, disability or death, and worry about their ability to cope with impending stresses. Nurses perform a crucial role in alleviating the psychosocial and spiritual discomfort that occurs when patients enter the hospital environment.

Physical discomforts may also cause distress. Pain, nausea, heat and even an untidy environment are stimuli patients may find uncomfortable. Nurses, therefore, need to be alert for observable signs of physical discomfort and implement interventions to alleviate or diminish it, such as anticipating analgesic needs.

Nursing actions which promote comfort often centre around dialogue and touch. For instance, taking time to listen and talk as well as explaining procedures and the function of equipment may help patients to feel less anxious, and thereby, more comfortable (Gropper, 1992).

Rest is synonymous with repose or relaxation, and implies freedom from emotional tension and physical discomfort. Rest does not necessarily mean inactivity. People often find a change of activity as relaxing as sitting or lying down to rest. The person who has a sedentary job, for example, may find that physical activity in the form of walking, skating or swimming is relaxing and restful. The person who has been physically active all day may feel rested by watching television, reading, playing cards or just sitting down and talking with family or friends. People who are ill may also find these activities more restful than lying in bed.

Sleep is a period of decreased mental alertness and physical activity which is part of the normal pattern of daily living. Sleep is a necessary part of life and takes up approximately one third of our time. All body cells need a period of inactivity to restore themselves. Sleep is essential for growth and healing.

THE PHYSIOLOGY OF SLEEP AND REST

Sleep is a cyclical phenomenon affecting all body functions. Stages of sleep have been identified through the use of sophisticated methods of measurement such as the elec-troencephalogram (EEG). The EEG provides a graphic representation of the electrical waves emanating from the brain. Using instruments such as the EEG it has been possible to identify the changes occurring in the brain during sleep. Cardiovascular and muscular activity and changes have also been recorded and used to identify the sequence of sleep stages.

CIRCADIAN RHYTHMS

Human beings, like plants and animals, possess biological clocks which regulate body functions in regular cyclical fashion. Some cycles, such as the female menstrual cycle, occur monthly; others occur at approximately 24-hour intervals. *Circadian rhythms*, from the Latin words *circa* (about) and *dies* (day), refer to physiologic events that follow a 24-hour cycle. Sleep–wake cycles, changes in body temperature, heart rate and blood pressure and fluctuations in metabolism and hormonal secretions are influenced by circadian rhythms.

The sleep–wake cycle follows a sequential pattern of awareness (wakefulness) and unawareness (sleep) which constitutes circadian rhythm. These patterns vary among individuals. Some people are early risers, performing their best in the morning. They prefer to go to bed early and sleep throughout the night. Others perform their best late in the evening and into the night; they prefer to sleep in the morning. Generally, however, "morning is a time of peak alertness in most people" (Dotto, 1990). This is because the sleep–wake cycle coincides with other biological rhythms such as body temperature, heart muscle contraction and hormone secretions that decline during sleep and rise during the day. A disruption in the sleep–wake cycle may affect other physiological functions and interfere with general health and well-being.

STAGES OF SLEEP

Normally, the adult sleep cycle recurs every 90 minutes. There are usually four to six 90-minute cycles in a person's sleep time. There are five stages in each 90-minute sleep cycle.

Stage 1 sleep is the lightest and shortest sleep phase. A person is easily aroused from this stage and may be unaware of having been asleep. This is a transitional state during which vital signs begin to slow, muscles become relaxed and body temperature begins to decrease. The EEG reading flattens. A sudden involuntary muscle jerk may be experienced at this point in the cycle.

It is more difficult to wake someone who has entered *Stage 2 sleep*. Some activity appears on the EEG and the individual, although in a more relaxed state, may still be aroused. A person in *Stage 3 sleep* is difficult to rouse. Blood pressure, pulse and body temperature decrease. EEG waves are larger and slower. The individual in *Stage 4 sleep* is

CENTRAL QUESTIONS

1. How are comfort, rest and sleep important to health and well-being?

2. What are the characteristics of the five stages of sleep?

3. How do normal sleep patterns vary throughout the life cycle?

4. What is the relationship between illness and sleep disturbances?

5. What are the main factors which interfere with a patient's comfort, rest and sleep?

6. What are the common sleep problems?

7. What basic principles does the nurse apply in assisting patients meet their comfort, rest and sleep needs?

8. How does the nurse assess comfort, rest and sleep needs?

9. What are the common nursing diagnostic statements for patients with comfort, rest and sleep problems?

10. What is a sleep plan and why is it important in patient care?

11. What information might the nurse give to individuals, families, or groups in helping them to promote optimum comfort, rest and sleep?

12. What health protecting measures does the nurse implement to maintain normal rest and sleep patterns and to prevent the development of sleep problems in hospitalized patients?

13. What strategies does the nurse implement to restore normal patterns for patients with rest and sleep problems?

14. How does the nurse evaluate the patient's response to nursing interventions?

CHAPTER 25

Comfort, Rest and Sleep Needs

completely relaxed and may not move. It is extremely difficult to wake a person in this stage of sleep. It is believed that bedwetting and sleepwalking are most likely to occur at this time, due to incomplete arousal. During this phase of the sleep cycle there is an increase in the release of hormones regulating growth and promoting tissue healing.

Stage 3 and Stage 4 sleep are commonly referred to as slow wave sleep (SWS) due to the large, slow brain waves depicted on EEG tracings. This state is the phase of physically restorative sleep (Dotto, 1990; Edwards and Schuring, 1993; Hayter, 1980).

Upon completion of Stage 4 sleep, the individual retraces the cycle back to Stage 2 and then enters **REM (rapid eye movement)** sleep (see Figure 25.1). It is during REM sleep that dreaming occurs. Dreams are believed to promote the psychological integration of daily activities. This stage is considered the psychologically restorative stage of sleep (Dotto, 1990; Edwards and Schuring, 1993; Knapp, 1993). During this stage, there is also a great deal of autonomic activity — vital signs fluctuate widely, the eyes move rapidly back and forth and muscular relaxation increases. The EEG reading is similar to that of a person who is awake.

With the completion of the REM stage, approximately 90 minutes after falling asleep, the individual recommences the cycle at Stage 2, proceeds through to Stage 4, returns to Stage 2 and again experiences REM sleep. During the first few hours of sleep, the individual will spend more time in Stage 3 and Stage 4 than in later cycles. The length of the REM stage increases towards morning and may last as long as 60 minutes. Most adults will experience four to six complete sleep cycles during the night. In the final cycle, the individual continues beyond REM to Stage 1, and wakens.

Anytime an individual is awakened, sleep is regained by starting again at Stage 1 and proceeding directly to REM sleep. Consequently, patients disturbed frequently by nursing care may suffer deprivation of the other sleep stages (Dotto, 1990; Hayter, 1980). The importance of REM sleep suggests that dreaming is a very necessary part of our lives.

SLEEP DEPRIVATION

Sleep deprivation refers to a decrease in the amount, quality or consistency of sleep. Lack of sleep has a profound effect on an individual's abilities, particularly their physical endurance, mental alertness and social relationships. A person deprived of sleep is likely to appear tired, irritable, depressed, anxious or apathetic. Thought processes may be impaired; the ability to concentrate is reduced, forgetfulness occurs and response to stimuli may be inappropriate. Minor troubles may become major problems. Sensory perception may be distorted, causing increased sensitivity to pain. Delusions or hallucinations may occur. When a person experiences gross deprivation of sleep, the body will try to catch up and REM stage sleep may be entered almost immediately. Sleep deprivation is common

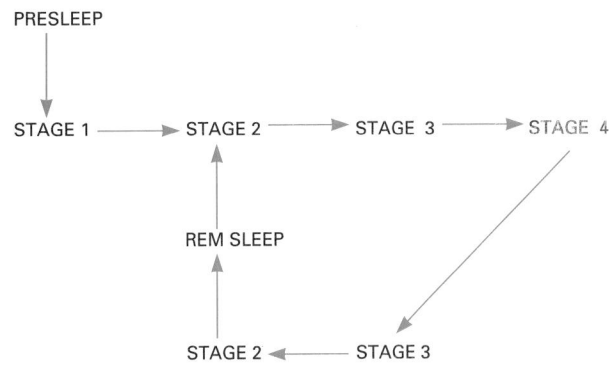

FIGURE 25.1   The adult sleep cycle

among hospitalized patients owing to the frequent interruptions for assessments and care. Nurses can do much to help patients satisfy their rest and sleep needs by thoughtful planning and implementing of care so as to prevent sleep deprivation.

DETERMINANTS OF SLEEP AND REST

There are a multitude of factors, both physical and psychological, that may affect a patient's ability to rest and sleep. Age, personal habits, illness, medications, emotional stress, nutrition and exercise are common determinants. As well, environmental factors and feelings of comfort or discomfort affect one's ability to rest and sleep.

Frequent interruptions for assessments and care can cause sleep deprivation.

Sleep Habits

Most people have a bedtime ritual that forms part of their sleep habits. For example, many adult Canadians like to watch the late news on television as one of their nightly rituals. Many people enjoy a light snack before going to bed. Some like a cup of coffee or tea and find that, for them, it does not interfere with getting to sleep. For many people, a warm bath or shower is part of their nightly ritual. Each person has particular habits related to going to bed and getting ready for sleep. Most people also have a particular position they find most comfortable for sleeping. Some like to curl up in a ball, some are "tummy" sleepers and others prefer a back-lying position.

Interferences with these bedtime habits are likely to cause disturbances in sleep patterns. In unfamiliar environments people often find it hard to get to sleep the first night or so. A major change in habit patterns can result in stress that disturbs all body functions. Nurses, because they frequently have to work evening or night shifts, often experience disturbances in their normal circadian rhythm. It usually takes a few days to become accustomed to sleeping in the daytime and having one's first meal late in the day. Other people who work shifts have the same problems.

Physical

Excessive stimulation will often make it harder for people to get to sleep, unless they are exhausted by the stimulation. A lack of sufficient exercise may be another reason some people find it difficult to sleep; the muscles are not tired enough. A person who is hungry often cannot rest. On the other hand, an excessive intake of food, particularly highly seasoned food that may cause problems in digestion, may also interfere with sleep. A larger than usual amount of fluid intake before retiring usually means having to get up during the night to relieve a distended bladder. Things that often disturb rest patterns of hospitalized people are medications that must be taken at night and the early morning awakening (often followed by a long delay before breakfast is served) that is still part of the routine in many agencies.

Psychological

Emotional stress and anxiety are common causes of an inability to rest. And, as a person lies awake and worries, the worries magnify and sleep becomes increasingly elusive. In addition, once sleep comes, the sleep cycle is disturbed. REM sleep, in particular, is decreased, which leads to more stress and anxiety.

Environment

Excessive sensory stimulation can disturb the comfort, rest and sleep of hospital patients (see Chapter 27). Noise and other disturbances to a sleeping patient may disturb the cyclical pattern of sleep. Other environmental factors which may be a problem include the warm temperatures of most hospital rooms, the hardness of most hospital pillows, lights that are turned (or left) on, the noise of nurses at the nursing station and the sudden stillness after patients have been awakened by some noise.

Discomfort and Illness

Discomfort of any kind interferes with the ability to rest and to sleep. A number of causes of discomfort were discussed in the introduction to this chapter. Pain is, of course, always a deterrent to rest and sleep. Often, however, it is the minor irritations and discomforts that are most troublesome to patients.

Illness and sleep problems go hand in hand. People who are ill require more sleep because of their need for increased growth hormone to promote tissue repair, and yet this increased need is often thwarted by the fact that illness disturbs the normal rhythm of sleep and wakefulness. Sleep deprivation, as we mentioned, can itself be a cause of illness.

Medications

Drugs will also distort sleep patterns. The reticular formation in the brain is thought to control sleep. Cerebral depressant drugs that induce sleep work in one or more of several ways. First, they may depress the reticular formation so it no longer responds to stimuli. Second, they may depress the response of the cerebral cortex to stimuli from the reticular formation. Third, they may cause a specific reduction in the response to stimuli producing wakefulness (for example, anxiety, depression or pain). Alcohol, for instance, has this effect, as do many of the tranquilizing drugs.

Hypnotics and barbiturates have a tendency to depress REM sleep, resulting in an abnormal sleep cycle. Amphetamines and antidepressant drugs also reduce REM sleep. A patient who is taken off these drugs after having taken them for several days, or who fails to take them, usually has a considerable increase in dream activity, and may be convinced that he or she never slept at all. Barbiturates also depress the parts of the brain that are responsible for inhibitory activity. Hence, they often have an excitatory effect, somewhat like alcohol. Older people are particularly susceptible to this reaction and may become confused and excited instead of going to sleep when they are given barbiturate sedatives.

SLEEP AND REST THROUGHOUT THE LIFE CYCLE

Growth and development are crucial factors in the sleep–wake cycle. Our need for sleep and certain stages of sleep change as we mature. As well, the manner in which we meet our sleep and rest needs alters with maturation.

The developing infant is said to sleep in *utero* or, at least, to have rest periods. Newborns fall into a deep sleep shortly after birth. Most newborns sleep for an average of 16 hours a day, with the longest uninterrupted sleep being a little more than four hours. Approximately half of newborns' sleep corresponds to REM stage sleep.

The infant proceeds to quickly establish a diurnal pattern and sleep cycle. By about six weeks of age, most infants are sleeping for longer periods during the night than during the day, and by four months most are sleeping through the night, with the longest sleep period averaging around eight-and-a-half hours. The pattern of the sleep cycle in the three-month-old infant begins to resemble that of the adult. Approximately two thirds of the infant's total sleep is quiet sleep by this time.

Toddlers generally sleep 10 to 14 hours a day in total, and usually require daily naps until they are approximately three years old. During the toddler stage bedtime rituals become important. Bedtime rituals such as story time, or engaging in some other quiet activity, help establish good sleep habits. A quiet period and consistent bedtime routines are important for all children. Preschool-age children are often apprehensive about being left in the dark and may need a night light. Nightmares and bedwetting (*enuresis)* are common problems which usually disappear as the child matures. A school-aged child usually sleeps 11 to 12 hours a night. The amount of sleep required gradually diminishes to around nine to ten hours by age 12. Teenagers require longer periods of sleep once again, a fact which may be related to their growth needs.

Healthy adults generally sleep six to eight hours a night. During pregnancy, however, women require extra sleep, particularly during the first and third trimesters. Their sleep is frequently interrupted because of the need to void, caused by pressure of the enlarging uterus on the bladder. Additional rest is important throughout pregnancy and a short nap or rest period during the day is advocated.

As adults mature the amount of sleep required remains the same, though the quality of sleep seems to degenerate. Older adults tend to have difficulty falling asleep and staying asleep. Many older adults experience frequent periods of wakefulness during the night as well as early morning awakenings. Some of the difficulty may be due to aging brain cells and a concomitant decrease in Stage 3 and Stage 4 sleep (Dotto, 1990). Lost nighttime sleep results in the need for daily rest periods.

COMMON PROBLEMS

Sleep problems may be divided into two broad categories — *dyssomnias* and *parasomnias*. **Dyssomnias** are characterized by difficulties with the quantity and quality of sleep and include problems such as insomnia (inability to fall asleep or excessive wakefulness), hypersomnia (excessive sleeping, especially during the day) and narcolepsy (sudden, irresistible sleep attacks). **Parasomnias** refer to disruptions of the sleep cycle and include problems such as somnambulism (sleepwalking), enuresis (bedwetting) and night terrors (Dotto, 1990). Sleep apnea is a physiological difficulty affecting the sleep–wake cycle which doesn't fall into either of the principal categories.

DYSSOMNIAS

Insomnia

Insomnia is the most common of all sleep disturbances and may be described as difficulty falling asleep or staying asleep. Most people, at some time, have problems falling asleep, usually during periods of stress and anxiety. This type of insomnia is termed *situational* or *temporary insomnia* and, over the short term, does not significantly affect waking performance. Individuals who experience *chronic insomnia*, however, often feel continuously fatigued due to difficulty falling asleep or frequent awakenings. These people may also suffer from depression and anxiety. Their work or school performance may be severely affected. Insomnia is usually treated symptomatically with the use of various relaxation techniques and by encouraging the development of appropriate sleep habits.

Hypersomnia

One explanation for sleeping excessively (**hypersomnia**) is that sleep is being used as a defence mechanism to escape anxieties or frustrations in the fulfilment of basic needs. This, of course, is not always the case; a person who seems to require more than a usual amount of sleep requires referral to a physician for a complete medical examination. Patients exhibiting signs of hypersomnia are generally investigated for possible causes such as insufficient sleep, drugs, tumours or other medical conditions. Oftentimes the cause is related to sleep apnea or narcolepsy (Dotto, 1990).

Narcolepsy

Narcolepsy is a disorder characterized by brief episodes of sleep that are uncontrollable. The sleep attacks, which may occur frequently, may or may not be preceded by drowsiness. Sleep attacks may last from 30 seconds to 20 minutes. Narcoleptic individuals often have vivid dreams and may be unable to move on waking. They experience hypersomnia during the day and yet during the night often experience insomnia. Many of these people also experience *cataplexy* (profound loss of muscle tone) often brought on by strong emotions (Dotto, 1990; Rogers and Aldrich, 1993).

Accidents are more common among narcoleptics than the general population. People with this condition are usually prohibited from working with machinery or at occupations where falling asleep without warning would be a safety hazard. Treatment generally involves taking stimulants and naps.

PARASOMNIAS

Somnambulism

Somnambulism (sleepwalking) is more common among children than adults. It tends to occur during Stages 3 and 4 of the sleep cycle; hence people who are sleepwalking are usually confused and disoriented. It is not wise to wake them; rather they should be gently guided back to bed.

Nightmares and Night Terrors

While nightmares may occur occasionally among adults, nightmares and night terrors are common sleep problems in children. These disturbances reach their peak in the preschool years. **Nightmares** occur during REM sleep. The child wakes completely following the frightening dream. He or she will be reassured by the presence of someone else and will return to sleep once calm. **Night terrors** often occur during Stage 4 sleep. The child may sit bolt upright in bed, or assume bizarre postures and scream, or cry. The child is terrified. Pulse and respirations are rapid, and diaphoresis occurs. The child is usually disoriented, and may not recognize the person attempting to offer reassurance. It is often difficult to wake the child from this state (Waley and Wong, 1991).

Enuresis

Enuresis, or bedwetting, generally occurs in Stage 4 sleep and is a common problem in children. Some adults may experience this difficulty as well. It generally occurs more frequently in males and in emotionally disturbed children. Some reports indicate that enuresis is more prevalent among children in low socioeconomic groups. It is believed to be caused in many cases by immaturity of the bladder and many children "grow out of it." Enuresis may, however, be a sign of health problems and sufferers should be referred for medical attention (Waley and Wong, 1991).

SLEEP APNEA

Sleep apnea is characterized by "repetitive pauses in breathing lasting from 10 seconds to 2 minutes" during sleep (Dotto, 1990, 106). This disorder most commonly occurs in men over the age of 50 and in postmenopausal women. Individuals with this disorder often experience hypersomnia, insomnia and loud snoring. Severe morning headaches, impotence, depression and confusion, daytime lethargy and poor performance are common symptoms. High blood pressure and heartbeat irregularities also occur; these cardiovascular problems usually get progressively worse unless the sleep disorder is treated (Dotto, 1990). These secondary symptoms are the result of periods of decreased blood oxygenation during the night.

The pathology of sleep apnea is classified as obstructive, central or mixed. The most common form, obstructive sleep apnea, is characterized by complete occlusion of the upper airway despite continued respiratory effort by the diaphragm. Loud snoring signals the resumption of breathing. The usual treatment of obstructive sleep apnea is continuous positive airway pressure (CPAP). The patient wears a face mask connected to a device that forces air through the upper airway. The force of the air maintains the airway in an open position. Many patients do not like the device, however, because of the noise it creates. Weight loss can often lessen the severity of sleep apnea and is suggested for many patients. Surgery, specifically a uvulopalatopharyngoplasty (UPP) may be an option for less serious obstructive apnea. In this procedure, the tonsils, uvula and posterior portion of the soft palate are excised and the posterior pharyngeal wall is tightened (Weaver and Millman, 1986).

Central sleep apnea is often associated with infections such as encephalitis or bulbar poliomyelitis. Spinal cord surgery or brainstem infarction may also be causes. These patients do not have the characteristic snoring of obstructive apnea and often require sophisticated ventilatory support. Mixed sleep apnea involves episodes of central apnea (no respiratory effort), followed by obstructive apnea (respiratory effort) and finally by airflow (Weaver and Millman, 1986).

ASSESSING COMFORT, REST AND SLEEP NEEDS

Making sure that patients are comfortable and that they receive sufficient rest and sleep are essential nursing responsibilities. In order to assess a patient's health status with regard to comfort, rest and sleep, the nurse needs information about usual rest and sleep patterns, specific problems the patient may have and the nature of any health problems that may be affecting his or her sleep patterns. Much of this information is collected during the health history; however, focussed enquiries about rest and sleep status are made on a day-to-day basis.

Anxiety is a common cause of emotional discomfort as well as of sleep and rest problems. Therefore, the nurse needs to be aware of any particular health-related worries the patient has. Knowing the nature of the patient's current health problem and the physician's plan of care — that is, the medications the patient is receiving, the nature of planned diagnostic and therapeutic measures and the results of diagnostic tests — will enhance the nurse's sensitivity to the patient's needs. This information is contained in the patient's record. It is also helpful to know of any other stresses that may be causing the patient anxiety. Many people are aware of the sources of their anxiety, and when given the opportunity, will make them known. The nurse who takes the time to listen can frequently identify specific sources of worry and discomfort.

NURSING HEALTH HISTORY

In hospitals there is a tendency to treat all patients in a similar fashion. Often, it is expected that everyone will go to sleep between 2200 and 2300 and sleep until 0600. This assumption does not respect differences in patients' circadian rhythms, nor does it acknowledge individual habits and preferences. It is essential that nurses identify and note each patient's unique routines and find the measure or combination of measures which will effectively promote comfort, rest and sleep for each individual patient. Data about a patient's usual rest and sleep pattern and bedtime habits are collected in the nursing health history. This information is also recorded on the Kardex to ensure effective communication among the health care team members. In addition, as is the case with other needs, the patient is questioned about recent changes in rest and sleep patterns; if a problem becomes evident, a more detailed exploration of the problem ensues.

PHYSICAL ASSESSMENT

Patients may communicate their inability to sleep to the nurse. However, nurses must also look for behaviours that indicate sleep disturbances. During the night, nurses make frequent rounds of patients noting those having difficulty falling asleep or who are wakeful. Nurses on the day shift check the night report to determine how well patients slept. Nurses also observe patients during the day and evening to see if they appear to be getting sufficient rest and sleep.

In assessing a patient's physical comfort, the nurse must be attentive to both verbal and behavioural cues. The patient who is uncomfortable may appear restless, or tense, perspire profusely or lie rigidly in bed. Nurses also need to be aware of any restrictions on the patient's level of activity. Is the patient confined to bed, or restricted to a certain position for therapeutic reasons? Individuals with cardiac or respiratory problems may be most comfortable sleeping with the head of the bed elevated — this is also the best position for them therapeutically. The patient with a fracture may have to lie flat, or have an injured extremity main-

tained in a specific position. The nature of the surgical intervention a patient has undergone often determines the position taken in bed. Even an intravenous infusion affects the patient's position in bed.

DIAGNOSING COMFORT, REST AND SLEEP PROBLEMS

Problems associated with the quantity and quality of sleep that the nurse can independently treat are labelled as *Sleep pattern disturbance*. Carpenito defines a *Sleep pattern disturbance* as "the state in which the individual experiences or is at risk of experiencing a change in the quantity or quality of [his or her] rest pattern that causes discomfort or interferes with desired life-style" (1993, 723). The defining characteristics can include difficulty falling or remaining asleep, fatigue on awakening or during the day, mood alterations and dark circles under the eyes (Carpenito, 1993). It is important to determine the precise etiology of the problem, so that proper interventions can be implemented. For instance, the diagnosis, *Sleep pattern disturbance related to hospitalization* does not indicate the treatment measures that should be instituted. However, saying *Sleep pattern disturbance related to a noisy environment or a stuffy overheated room* gives direction to the care that may be implemented, in this case eliminating the noise or cooling down and ventilating the room.

Problems with rest and sleep that fall under the diagnosis of *Sleep pattern disturbance* must be differentiated from sleep disorders such as narcolepsy or sleep apnea. These are chronic conditions treated by the physician which nurses care for as collaborative functions. Thus, a problem such as sleep apnea is better identified as *Potential complication: Sleep apnea* (Carpenito, 1993).

The body needs sufficient rest and sleep for optimal health. A deficit in the quantity and quality of sleep affects daily functioning and causes difficulties in other facets of life. For instance, an individual's performance at work and coping capabilities may be decreased by a prolonged lack of sleep. Thus, the sleep disturbance itself becomes the etiology of other problems. Using the example above, the diagnosis might be stated as *Ineffective individual coping related to prolonged lack of sleep*.

Examples of nursing diagnoses and collaborative problems related to comfort, rest and sleep problems are:

- *Sleep pattern disturbance related to uncomfortable position and pain associated with fractured elbow*

- *Sleep pattern disturbance related to the changes in usual bedtime routine and noisy hospital environment*

- *Fatigue related to sleep deprivation*

- *PC: Dependency on sedatives prescribed for sleep*

Rest and Sleep

Health and Illness Patterns

USUAL PATTERN OF REST AND SLEEP

- What are your usual hours of sleeping (including naps)?
- Describe a typical night's sleep. Do you sleep through? wake up? If so, how many times a night? Why do you wake up? thirst? to use the bathroom?
- Describe your usual routine before bedtime. Do you have a snack or warm beverage? What are your hygiene practices? Do you read? listen to music?
- Do you usually take medicine to help you sleep at night? If so, what?
- What are your usual sleeping habits? Describe the placement and number of pillows, your position. Do you use other aids for sleeping?
- Describe your usual sleep environment. Is your room warm or cool? Is it dark ? quiet or noisy? Do you use a night light?
- Do you feel sufficiently rested in the morning?

RECENT CHANGES IN PATTERN OF REST AND SLEEP

- Have there been any recent changes in your pattern of rest and sleep? If so, describe the changes. Do you find you sleep more? sleep less?
- Are you having difficulty falling asleep? staying asleep?
- Can you identify any recent changes in your life that may be upsetting your sleep pattern?

PRESENTING HEALTH PROBLEM

- Describe the difficulty you are having with rest and sleep, falling asleep, staying asleep? Are you sleeping more or less than usual? snoring?
- Have you been having bad dreams? nightmares?
- Do you have difficulty waking up in the morning?
- How do you feel when you awaken in the morning? tired? depressed? irritated? Do you often have a headache? How has this sleep difficulty affected your daily functioning? Have you noticed changes in your behaviour? Do you always feel tired? have trouble concentrating? feel irritable?
- When did this sleep disturbance begin? What remedies have you tried for the sleep disturbance? What were the results?
- Do you have an acute or chronic condition that may be causing your sleep disturbance? any medications?
- Do you have a history of long-standing problems with sleeping and resting?

Health Promotion and Protection Patterns

- Do you try to maintain a consistent pattern for sleep and rest?
- Do you exercise regularly? If so, at what time of the day?
- Do you drink products containing caffeine? If so, how much and at what times during the day?
- Do you usually drink alcohol after dinner?

PLANNING COMFORT, REST AND SLEEP INTERVENTIONS

Interventions to promote comfort, rest and sleep are an integral part of nursing care for all patients. Particularly with ill patients, in whom rest and sleep are essential for healing, the nurse must ensure that factors causing the patient discomfort or interfering with their rest and sleep are eliminated or, at least, minimized. This aspect of nursing care is considered so important that, in some agencies, the nurses have developed "sleep care plans" for patients (Grant and Klell, 1974).

A specific sleep care plan, or a sleep and rest plan, is helpful in focussing attention on these important aspects of patient care and in facilitating communication about individual needs, preferences and problems with regard to comfort, rest and sleep. Sleep care plans ensure that a definite series of nursing activities is planned to help each patient obtain adequate sleep. Interventions that nurses have found helpful for a particular patient are communicated to others so there is consistency in the approach used by all nursing personnel. The same holds true for interventions related to the patient's level of comfort. The selection, implementation and communication of interventions is a significant nursing action which permits all health team members to assist patients to maintain a satisfactory level of comfort.

KEY PRINCIPLES

Principles Relevant to Comfort, Rest and Sleep

1. Definite periods of sleep are an essential component of the circadian rhythm in human beings.

2. Adequate amounts of sleep are needed for optimal physical and psychosocial functioning.

3. Growing people require more sleep.

4. Individual needs for sleep vary with age, growth patterns, health status and individual differences.

5. Lack of sufficient sleep impairs physical functioning, mental alertness and social relationships.

6. Individual habits vary with regard to bedtime rituals.

7. Sleep patterns may be disturbed by changes in normal daily living patterns, by social and emotional problems, by physical problems and by minor irritations or discomforts, as well as by pain.

8. Sleep patterns are almost invariably disturbed by illness.

As with all care planning, a sleep and rest plan is based on the patient goals which are derived from the nursing diagnoses. Examples of patient goals or expected outcomes may include the following:

- The patient will have six hours of uninterrupted sleep.
- The patient will describe factors that prevent or inhibit sleep.

- The patient will report feeling refreshed and energetic after awakening.
- The patient will fall asleep within 15 minutes of using relaxation techniques to induce sleep.

IMPLEMENTING COMFORT, REST AND SLEEP INTERVENTIONS

HEALTH PROMOTING STRATEGIES

People usually fall asleep more easily when their lifestyle permits regular habits for mealtimes, work or school hours, periods of relaxation and bedtime. Adequate nutrition and exercise are important in promoting restful sleep. Generally it is suggested that strenuous exercise not occur within two hours of bedtime. Restful and relaxing activities should be encouraged prior to sleep. Many find specific relaxation techniques helpful (some of these are discussed in Chapter 35). Tea, coffee and alcohol are best avoided prior to bedtime. A bedtime snack which includes milk is considered by some to be an aid to sleep. Warm milk is particularly effective. Milk contains a potentially sleep-inducing amino acid (L-tryptophan) which is activated when milk is warmed. The development of effective sleep habits needs to begin early in childhood. An especially effective habit is the use of the bedroom for no other activity but sleep.

It is important for individuals who work rotating schedules, such as nurses, to be especially aware of sleep habits. Circadian rhythms may be disturbed and individuals may experience sleep deprivation when continually shifting from a day to a night routine. Shift workers generally require more sleep than usual when they begin working

HEALTH PROMOTING STRATEGY

Promoting Healthy Rest and Sleep

1. Get up at the same time of day, every day, regardless of the amount of sleep obtained during the night.

2. Exercise as vigorously as possible in the afternoon or early evening.

3. Reduce caffeine intake.

4. Avoid alcohol after supper.

5. Set aside some quiet time before sleep to relax and unwind.

6. Go to bed only when feeling sleepy.

7. Use the bedroom for sleeping only.

8. Control the sleep environment. Keep the bedroom dark, cool and quiet.

9. If you have difficulty falling asleep, focus on something monotonous. If sleep does not come within a reasonable length of time, get up and do something boring until you feel sleepy. Also, drink a glass of warm milk.

SOURCES: Dotto, 1990; Knapp, 1993; Walgenbach, 1990; Webster, 1986.

through their usual sleep time. Therefore, it is important to have a quiet, comfortable place to sleep uninterrupted during the day.

Almost everyone has an occasional sleepless night. If the sleeplessness continues, however, for more than two or three nights, a physician should be consulted for a thorough investigation of the problem.

HEALTH PROTECTING STRATEGIES

Rest and sleep are crucial for restoring health. Yet, many patients in hospital fail to obtain sufficient rest and sleep. There are a number of health protecting strategies that nurses can implement to foster adequate rest and sleep in their patients. These include measures to prevent disruption in a patient's sleep–wake cycle, maintaining a comfortable bed and administering a back massage.

PREVENTING SLEEP–WAKE CYCLE DISRUPTION

Normal patterns of daily living, including the sleep–wake cycle, are disrupted during illness. There are a number of measures that can be implemented to avoid or lessen the disruption in a patient's sleep–wake cycle. Diversional activities, if these are not ruled out by health problems, will keep patients from sleeping so much during the day that sleep at night becomes difficult. Morning naps are considered more beneficial than afternoon ones, because they are a continuation of light REM sleep; whereas afternoon sleep is often slow wave sleep, which can result in the patient waking up feeling groggy.

Maintaining some of the patient's usual bedtime rituals facilitates a sense of security and promotes comfort, rest and sleep. The dietary department needs to be alerted to usual bedtime snacks and, if the patient is accustomed to having a bath or shower before retiring, the opportunity to continue this practice will be beneficial to sleep.

Most bedtime rituals involve some type of personal hygiene. In hospital, patients require an opportunity to wash their hands and face and clean their teeth prior to sleep. As well, patients need to be assisted to the bathroom or offered the use of a bedpan or a urinal.

Some people are fond of their own pillow, and may find hospital pillows uncomfortable. Patients may have their own pillow if desired. Familiar objects or routines also help promote a sense of security. A patient may like the pillows arranged in a certain way, the head of the bed elevated to a certain angle, position just so, or a clock turned to facilitate viewing. Small things like these contribute to a patient's comfort and effective rest and sleep. The nurse will find that it is worthwhile to spend a few extra minutes "settling" patients by attending to these small but important

FROM RESEARCH TO PRACTICE

Johnson, F. E. (1993). Progressive relaxation and sleep in older men and women. *Journal of Community Nursing, 10*(1), 31-38.

Prior research has shown that older adults experience changes in their sleep patterns. They often have difficulty getting to sleep, wake up frequently and rouse early in the morning. Non-pharmacological methods are considered the safest approach to promote sleep in older adults. The purpose of this study was to determine the effects of one non-pharmacological method — progressive relaxation — on the self-reported sleep patterns of healthy, non-institutionalized men and women over the age of 65 years. The population used was a volunteer sample of 156 men and women over 65 years of age, all of whom were living in their own homes. Measures were taken to ensure that all subjects were clear of drugs or medications that might affect the study findings. The study consisted of three stages: pretest (nights 1, 2 and 3), instruction and practice (nights 4, 5, 6 and 7) and post-test (nights 8, 9 and 10). The Baekeland and Hoy Sleep Pattern Questionnaire (SPQ) was administered to all subjects during both the pretest and post-test stages. Subjects were taught a standard method of progressive relaxation and practised it on going to bed. The study found that self-reported sleep patterns improved with use of the technique, both for men and women, with more success reported in those 65 to 84 years than in those over 85 years. The subjects were more calm at bedtime, took less time getting to sleep, were more refreshed in the morning and were more satisfied with their sleep. The study draws attention to the changes that occur in sleep patterns with age, which all nurses should be aware of, and emphasizes the importance of non-pharmacological methods to improve sleep patterns.

details. Patients' comfort, rest and sleep is facilitated by these actions.

Most patients find a back massage soothing and an aid to sleep. For some, relaxation techniques are beneficial. Besides relaxing exercises, a number of techniques for learning to control tension in the muscles and induce relaxation have been developed. The use of progressive relaxation techniques is especially useful with older adults (Johnson, 1993).

When the patient is settled, and all details attended to, the lights are dimmed. Noise is kept to a minimum, and the patient not disturbed unless absolutely necessary.

MAINTAINING A COMFORTABLE BED

The bed is particularly important to most people who are ill. Much of a patient's comfort depends on the condition of the bed, particularly if the patient is in it for long periods of time. When a patient appears unduly particular about the bed, remember that the patient may spend 24 hours a day in it. A neat, clean and wrinkle-free bed is necessary for comfort. Often patients who are exacting in regard to their beds and bed units may be clinging to a position from which they can control some aspect of their environment at a time when they believe that many decisions and activities are beyond their control. The ill patient's horizons often narrow, and matters about which he or she normally would have no concern become important.

There are two types of bed making: *occupied* (with the patient in it) and *unoccupied* (with the patient out of it). Whether the nurse makes an occupied or unoccupied bed depends on the patient's condition and the physician's order. An occupied bed is often made as part of the patient's daily hygiene care, after the bath. The nurse should try to schedule the making of an unoccupied bed when the patient is in the bath or shower, taking a walk or off the unit for tests and treatments. Linen is also changed whenever it becomes damp or soiled. Soiled or wet linen predisposes a patient to skin breakdown and infections.

When the bed is made, soiled linen is changed and the bed is aired and remade. Making an occupied bed is similar to making an unoccupied bed, except that in the former case the nurse is also concerned about maintaining the pa-

Infection Control and Bed Making

1. Microorganisms are present on the skin and in the general environment.
2. Some microorganisms are opportunists; that is, they can cause infections when conditions are favourable. For example, a break in the skin or mucous membrane of the patient may become a site of infection.
3. Patients are often less resistant to infections because of the stress resulting from an existing disease process.
4. Microorganisms may be transferred from one person to another or from one place to another by air, by inanimate objects or by direct contact among people. Therefore:
   - avoid holding soiled linen against the uniform
   - never shake linen
   - always wash your hands before going to another patient.

Effective Body Mechanics and Bed Making

1. *Maintain good body alignment.* For example, stand facing the direction in which you are working and move so as not to twist your body.
2. *Use the large muscles of the body rather than the small muscles.* For example, flexing the knees and bringing the body to a comfortable working level is preferable to bending at the waist. The former uses the large abdominal and gluteus muscles, whereas the latter puts strain upon the back muscles and shifts the centre of gravity outside the base of support.
3. *Work smoothly and rhythmically.* This is less fatiguing because the muscles are alternately contracted and relaxed.
4. *Push or pull rather than lift* because it requires less effort.
5. *Use your own weight to counteract the weight of an object.* This decreases the effort and strain involved. Shifting your own weight when pulling a mattress requires less effort than pulling the mattress with your arms. In addition, back and arm strain is reduced.

tient's body alignment, safety and comfort. Some patients are unable to assume a supine position because of their condition; for example, they may have difficulty breathing. In such cases, the nurse makes a comfortable, neat bed while the head of the bed is elevated.

When changing bed linen, the nurse must remember that microorganisms are present in the environment and be aware of the methods by which they spread. The use of good body mechanics is also important when making a bed. The principles that underlie body movements in helping the patient to move (see Chapter 28) are equally applicable to bed making. The accompanying boxes outline principles of infection control and the effective use of body mechanics with respect to making.

The method used for stripping and making beds differs among agencies. Basically, however, every health agency wants the end product to be neat, clean, comfortable and durable, and the bed-changing process to be an economical use of time, equipment and the patient's and nurse's energies. Procedure 25.1 details the steps involved in stripping and making an unoccupied or an occupied bed.

Assembling Linen and Equipment

The linen required for the basic hospital bed includes two sheets (a fitted or flat bottom sheet and a flat top sheet), two pillowcases, one plastic or rubber drawsheet (optional), one cotton drawsheet (optional), one or two blankets (also optional) and one spread.

Cotton and rubber drawsheets have traditionally been used on the sick person's bed for two reasons: they are easier to change than bottom sheets are, and they protect the mattress. With the availability of plastic-covered mattresses, however, and increasing use of cotton mattress pads (similar to the ones that are commonly used in the home), the routine use of drawsheets, both rubber (or plastic) and cotton, is disappearing. In many agencies the use of drawsheets is now reserved for the beds of patients who need them; they are no longer put on every bed.

When a plastic or rubber drawsheet is used, it is placed under a cotton drawsheet since the rubber (or plastic) retains heat and is uncomfortable. The drawsheet usually extends from above the patient's waist to the mid-thigh. Thus it can serve to absorb secretions in cases of urinary or fecal incontinence.

The cotton that is used for sheets, pillowcases and drawsheets must be of a heavy weight that wears well in spite of strong pulling and frequent washing. Moreover, because linen is often washed in disinfectant solutions in order to kill microorganisms, a heavy weight is necessary to withstand the laundering.

The blankets that are used in hospitals and most other health agencies are frequently made of a loose cotton weave or a mixture of flannel and cotton. The blankets should be able to withstand frequent washings without damage or shrinkage. In many hospitals, patients' rooms are warm enough that no blankets are needed. However, blankets are sometimes necessary for warmth. Usually one or two blankets suffice. An extra blanket is sometimes used as a throw blanket over the spread. The extra blanket can be rolled and stored at the foot of the bed, fan-folded down to the bottom of the bed, or put in the patient's closet until it is needed. Blankets should never be used by more than one patient because of the danger of transferring microorganisms from one patient to another. Elderly patients are often more sensitive to the cold than younger patients are and require more covers for warmth.

A complete linen change is not made every day. This is unnecessary and would only serve to increase already costly health care expenditures. It is customary practice to change a pillow and the drawsheet on a daily basis and other linen only when it becomes soiled. A receptacle is needed for soiled linen. In some agencies hampers are provided that may be taken right into the patient's room. If such a hamper is not available, the corners of the bedspread may be tied to the foot of the bed to collect soiled linen. Clean gloves are necessary if the linen is soiled with body substances and fluids.

PROCEDURE 25.1

Making an Unoccupied and an Occupied Bed

ACTION	RATIONALE
A. General Actions	
1. Gather equipment:	Ensures efficiency and economy of time.
• Receptacle for soiled linen	
• Clean linen as needed:	
• top and bottom (fitted) sheet	
• drawsheet	
• bedspread	
• blanket	
• pillowcases	
• Clean gloves as necessary	
2. Wash hands thoroughly.	Reduces the risk of contamination.
3. Explain procedure to the patient.	Enhances emotional well-being and enables patient participation.
B. Stripping the Bed	
1. Remove equipment from the bed. Detach the call light and garbage bag, and place them on the bedside table.	Provides a clear working space.

ACTION	RATIONALE
2. Lower the head of the bed and raise the bed to a comfortable working height.	Promotes the nurse's use of good body mechanics.
3. Place a chair beside the bed. An overbed table may be used in place of a chair.	Provides a clean area to place linen.
4. Remove pillowcases and place them in the laundry bag. Place the pillows on the seat of the chair or on top of the table.	Promotes organization of work space.
5. Starting at the head of the bed loosen the top and bottom sheets from the mattress while walking around the bed.	
6. Remove the blanket by grasping it at the centre and near side and folding it to the bottom of the bed. Pick the blanket up at the centre and lay it, folded in quarters, across the back of the bedside chair. Remove the bedspread and top sheet in the same way, if they are to be reused.	Prevents linen from touching the floor. Folding the linen in such a manner permits efficient replacement on the bed.
7. Linen not to be reused is rolled into itself and discarded into the laundry hamper.	Prevents contact with the nurse's uniform, thereby preventing transmission of microorganisms.
8. If necessary, turn the mattress side to side, or push to the head of the bed.	Adjusting the mattress after bed making loosens the linens.
9. Wash hands thoroughly when finished stripping the bed and before putting on the clean linen.	Avoids transferring microorganisms.

C. Making the Unoccupied Bed

ACTION	RATIONALE
1. Place the bottom sheet on the lower half of the mattress with its centre fold on the centre of the mattress. Align the end of the sheet with the lower edge of the mattress. Open the sheet to the head of the bed. If using a fitted sheet, secure the nearest top and bottom corners. If using a flat sheet, tuck the top under the mattress at the head of the bed and mitre or square the corners on one side (see Figure 25.2 following this procedure). Tuck the sheet in smoothly along the sides so that it is free of wrinkles.	Prevents wrinkles which are a source of irritation against the patient's skin.
2. Place and tuck in the drawsheet.	
3. Place the top sheet on the lower half of the mattress as with the bottom linen. Unfold the sheet towards the top of the bed. Align the top edge of the sheet to the top edge of the mattress. The blankets and bedspread are applied in the same manner but are brought to within about 23 cm of the edge of the mattress. Fold the top sheet down to make a cuff over the blankets and bedspread.	

Continued on the next page

ACTION

RATIONALE

4. Make a toe pleat in the top covers. To do this, raise the upper sheet and blankets and make a 5 cm vertical fold, perpendicular to the bed. Tuck the linen under the mattress. As an alternative, the top covers may be loosened at the foot of the bed.

Allows room for the patient's feet and prevents pressure that can cause discomfort, skin breakdown and foot drop.

5. Tuck the remaining top linen under the mattress and make a modified mitred corner. This is done as in Figure 25.2, except that the top edge is left to hang down at the side of the bed.

ACTION

6. When the bed has been made completely on one side, make the other side in the same way.

7. To replace a pillowcase, grasp the closed end of the pillowcase in one hand. With the other hand gather up the sides of the pillow case and rest them over the forearm of the hand holding the case. Then, with the hand holding the pillowcase, grasp the pillow and slide the sides of the case over the pillow. Align the corners of the case and the pillow.

8. Replace any equipment the patient requires. Attach the call light to the bed, place the bedside chair beside the bed, and place the bedside table within the patient's reach. Remove all unnecessary equipment, and place small articles in the bedside table. Ask the patient's permission before discarding any belongings, including flowers.

D. Making the Occupied Bed

1. Check the physician's orders regarding the patient's position and activity.

2. Draw privacy curtain around bed.

3. Raise the bed to a comfortable working position. Lower the side rail on the near side and remove the call bell.

4. When stripping the bed, leave a pillow under the patient's head.

5. Remove the spread and blankets, then place a bath blanket over the top sheet. Remove the top sheet by drawing it down from under the bath blanket. If the patient is to be washed, it is done at this time, before the foundation of the bed is changed.

RATIONALE

Promotes efficiency and economy of time.

Promotes patient's well-being, comfort and safety.

A neat environment promotes a sense of comfort.

Ensures safety and avoids errors.

Maintains privacy, promoting comfort and security.

Promotes the nurse's use of good body mechanics.

Promotes comfort.

Prevents the clean sheet from becoming dampened or soiled during the bath.

Continued on the next page

PROCEDURE 25.1
continued

ACTION	RATIONALE
6. Help the patient move to the far side of the bed. Loosen the foundation on the near side. Fold the linen to be removed into the centre of the bed. Place clean linen on the near side of the bed and tuck it in. Raise the side rail on the near side. Help patient to roll over the folded linen to the near side of the bed.	Promotes patient safety and security.
7. Move to the other side of bed. Lower the side rail. Remove the soiled linen and pull the clean linen tightly across the bed and tuck it in.	
8. Assist the patient to the centre of the bed and re-place the second pillow.	
9. Remove the bath blanket and replace the top covers as for an open bed.	
10. Replace the patient's call bell and lower the bed. Return all equipment to proper position. Tidy the bedside unit.	Promotes patient safety and comfort.

FIGURE 25.2   Mitring a corner. To mitre a corner, tuck the bottom edge of the sheet securely under the mattress. Lift the side edge of the sheet about 30 cm from the corner, and hold it at a right angle to the mattress. Tuck in the part of the sheet that hangs below the mattress. Drop the triangular edge down and firmly tuck it under the mattress.

ADMINISTERING THE BACK MASSAGE (BACK RUB)

Many patients have trouble sleeping because they feel anxious about being in a hospital. A back massage can be a very effective way of increasing a patient's comfort and alleviating stress, allowing the patient to sleep more soundly.

To administer a massage in preparation for sleeping, after a bath and at other times as indicated, the nurse rubs the patient's back with an emollient lotion or cream. In addition to promoting relaxation, the back rub also increases circulation to the skin, thereby reducing the risk of skin breakdown. The technique of administering the back rub is outlined in Procedure 25.2

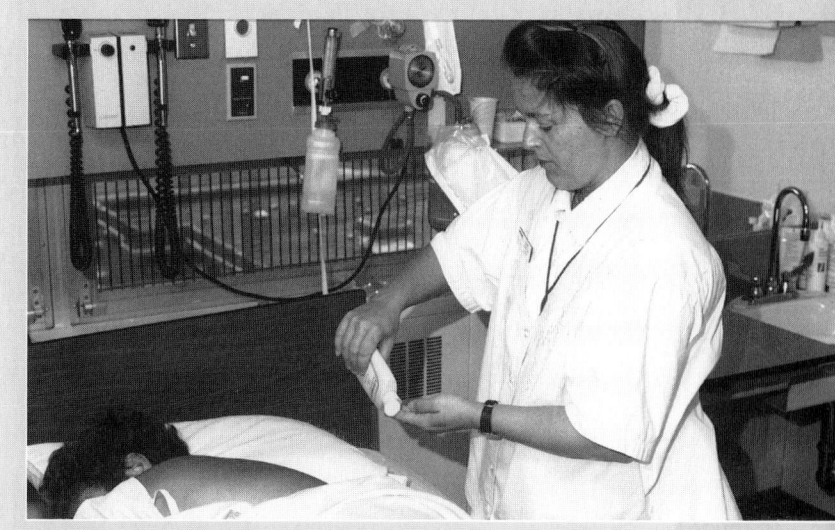

A soothing back rub helps to relax the patient and promotes comfort and rest.

PROCEDURE 25.2

Administering a Back Massage

ACTION	RATIONALE
1. Wash hands thoroughly.	Reduces the risk of contamination.
2. Explain the procedure to the patient.	Enhances emotional well-being and enables patient participation.
3. Help the patient to lie in the prone or side-lying position.	Permits use of long, firm strokes, which are both soothing to the patient and stimulating to the blood circulation.
4. Expose the patient's back from shoulders to sacrum.	
5. Warm the lotion by holding a small amount in the palms of your hands for a minute. The bottle of solution may also be placed in warm water.	Warm solutions feel more comfortable.
6. Starting at the shoulders and using the palms and fingertips, rub the patient's neck with circular motions extending to the hairline.	Helps to relax the shoulder and neck muscles, which so often are tense.

Continued on the next page

ACTION	RATIONALE
7. Move the hands to the sacral area and repeat the circular motions with palms and fingertips.	
8. Move to sacrum and rub up the centre of the back to the hairline, using long smooth strokes, then over to the shoulders, and down the sides of the back, using broad circular motions.	The circular motions are designed to increase circulation to bony prominences. The pressure of the nurse's motions should be sufficiently firm to stimulate the muscle tissue.
9. Now, move to lower edge of the patient's buttocks and sacrum, continuing with the broad circular motions.	
10. Massage the patient's knees, elbows, heels and any other reddened areas or bony prominences.	Increases blood circulation to the area, thereby reducing the risk of skin breakdown.

HEALTH RESTORING STRATEGIES

THERAPEUTIC BEDS, MATTRESSES AND DEVICES

Mattresses

There are many different kinds of mattresses available for both therapeutic and comfort purposes. The regular hospital mattress is firm and often covered with a plasticized material. Patients allergic to these mattresses have a foam pad placed on top of the usual mattress. This pad also has an advantage in that it places less pressure upon the patient's bony prominences. Because of this it is often used in the prevention and treatment of pressure ulcers for patients who must remain in bed for long periods of time.

Another type of mattress is the alternating pressure mattress. An air pump alternately deflates and inflates areas of the mattress, with the result that there is a continual change in the pressure upon the various parts of the patient's body. These alternations of pressure stimulate circulation to the skin which facilitates tissue nourishment and waste product removal. This mattress is most effective with only a single layer of linen between the mattress and the patient. Care must be taken not to prick the mattress with safety pins or sharp instruments, or pinch or shut off the tubing to the motor.

There are a variety of other therapeutic mattresses available to assist in making patients feel comfortable. Air-fluidized beds use the flotation principle to provide uni-

form support to the body. The mattress portion of the bed consists of fine glass beads. Air is blown through these spheres to keep them constantly moving, and the patient experiences a sensation of floating. Other types of mattress available include low-air-loss, oscillating low-air-loss, oscillating support surfaces, static air mattresses and water mattresses. Each of these mattresses has specific indications for use, often related to pain management or wound healing. An increased sense of comfort is the outcome experienced by the patient.

It should be noted that the use of these special mattresses is not a substitute for nursing care. Patients continue to require turning, skin care and proper positioning.

The Fracture Board

The **fracture board** (bed board) is placed under the patient's mattress to increase support. It is usually made of wood or Plexiglas. Some fracture boards have hinges so that the head and knee gatches (adjustable joints) of the bed can be used with the board in position. The fracture board is used in situations where patients require additional support such as following a spinal injury or surgery.

The Bed Cradle

The **bed cradle** is a device used to keep the weight of the top bed covers off the patient. Patients who have burns, uncovered wounds or wet casts often need to keep the top bedclothes away from the injured area. When applying a cradle to the patient's bed it is securely fastened to, or under, the mattress. Some bed cradles are hoop arrangements which extend from one side of the bed to the other; others extend only to the midline of the bed. The cradle is carefully positioned so that the area of the patient's body that is to be free from the weight of the top bed covers is directly under the cradle. The top bedclothes must be pulled up higher than usual to cover the patient's shoulders. Bed cradles are made of metal or plastic.

The Footboard

The *footboard* is placed at the foot of the patient's bed to serve as a support for the feet. Footboards are usually made out of plastic or wood and fit onto the bed frame across the foot of the bed.

Normally the feet of the patient lying in the dorsal position will be bent into plantar flexion (see Chapter 28). In time, if the patient's feet are not exercised or supported, they may become fixed in plantar flexion. This condition, known as *footdrop*, is the result of contractures of the gastrocnemius or soleus muscles and prevents the patient from standing with heels flat on the floor. Footdrop is usually treated by physiotherapy, but sometimes can only be modified by surgery.

The Balkan Frame

The **Balkan frame** is a metal frame that extends lengthwise above the bed supported at either end by a pole attached to the bed frame (see Figure 25.3). A trapeze may be attached to the frame just above the patient's head as a mobility aid. This simple measure provides patients with the ability to move themselves in bed, thus increasing their sense of independence and ultimately their comfort. The Balkan frame may also be used as an attachment for the pulleys and weights of traction equipment used for patients who have fractures of the lower limbs, particularly the femur.

FIGURE 25.3 Balkan frame

Specialized Beds

A number of specialized beds have been devised for patients who will be immobilized for long periods of time and for those with specific health problems. Examples include the Stryker Frame, the CircOlectric bed, the HighLow Tilt bed, the Rocking bed and the Chair bed. The use of these beds is generally confined to a specific area and nurses will be educated about their use when working in the area.

POSITIONING THE PATIENT IN BED

Generally patients assume the positions that are most comfortable for them. For the patient who is able to move easily and freely in bed without therapeutic considerations, the nurse's chief responsibility in regard to position is comfort. The astute use of pillows and the provision of a firm foundation assist in achieving a comfortable position for the patient.

Patients must sometimes assume positions for therapeutic reasons. Some of the reasons are to maintain good body alignment, to prevent contractures, to promote drainage, to facilitate breathing and to prevent the development of skin breakdown over bony prominences.

The physician may prescribe the appropriate therapeutic position for a patient, but usually the nurse decides which position is best. Intelligent assessment of a patient's problems and a knowledge of anatomy and physiology are important bases for such judgements. Also, the nurse needs to be aware of the variety of positions possible and the supportive measures available to promote comfort in these positions.

COMMON BED POSITIONS

Dorsal Recumbent and Supine Position

In the **dorsal recumbent position** (see Figure 25.4) the patient lies on the back with the head and shoulders slightly elevated. Usually one pillow suffices for this purpose. A small pillow is placed under the lower legs to slightly flex the limbs and prevent hyperextension of the knees. It also keeps the patient's heels off the bed and helps to reduce lumbar lordosis.

If the patient does not have support for the thighs, they will tend to rotate outward. Two rolled towels or a rolled bath blanket tucked in at the lateral aspects of the thighs under the trochanter of the femur will maintain the patient's legs in alignment. In the dorsal recumbent position, the patient's feet will normally assume a plantar flexion position. Prolonged positioning in plantar flexion, however, can result in footdrop. Preventive measures for

FIGURE 25.4   Dorsal recumbent position

this complication include the use of the footboard, which helps the patient to maintain the feet in dorsal flexion and removes the weight of the bedclothes from the toes; and the heel protector, which supports the foot's position as well as providing protection for the heel. Flexion, extension and circumduction of the patient's ankles help maintain muscle tone and ankle joint mobility.

In some cases, the patient's head and shoulders are not elevated by pillows and rolls. The patient lies on the back with the head and shoulders on the flat surface. This is called the *supine position*. It is frequently prescribed for patients who have had spinal anesthetics. Supports similar to those just described are used when indicated.

Prone Position

The *prone position* is one in which the patient lies on the abdomen with the head turned to one side. Many people are relaxed and sleep well in this position; some find it most comfortable to flex their arms over their heads (see Figure 25.5).

Supportive measures for the patient in this position include a small pillow or pad, as needed, under the abdomen at the level of the diaphragm in order to give support to the lumbar curvature and, in the case of the female patient, to take weight off the breasts. A small pillow or towel

roll under each shoulder helps to maintain the anatomical position. In addition, a pillow under the lower legs elevates the toes off the bed and permits slight flexion of the knees. Alternatively, the patient can extend the toes over the end of the mattress to take the weight off the toes. Plantar flexion is minimized if the patient's lower legs are also supported. When the patient is in a prone position, there is pressure on the knees. A small pad under the thighs can be used to relieve this pressure. Sheepskin or sponge rubber pads may also be used under the knees.

The patient may want a pillow for his or her head. Unless the physician wishes the patient's head to lie on a flat surface, in order to promote drainage of mucus, for example, a small pillow may be provided to make the patient more comfortable; however, the pillow should not be so thick as to hyperextend the patient's head.

Lateral (Side-lying) Position

In the *lateral position*, the patient lies on the side with both arms forward and knees and hips flexed (see Figure 25.6). The upper leg is flexed more than the lower leg. Weight is borne by the lateral aspects of the patient's ilium and by the scapula.

The upper knee and hip should be at the same level; the upper elbow and wrist should be at the same level as

FIGURE 25.5   Prone position

FIGURE 25.6   Lateral (side-lying) position

the upper shoulder to prevent the limbs from being in a dependent position. The heels and ankles may be protected by using small pads (sheepskin or sponge rubber) to keep them from rubbing against the bedclothes.

If the upper arm falls across the chest, the patient's lung capacity may be restricted; a pillow to support the patient's arm permits greater chest expansion and enables the nurse to readily observe the character and rate of respirations.

The patient who lies laterally will probably want a pillow for the head. A pillow of proper depth should prevent lateral flexion of the head. Frequently the patient will also require the support of a pillow placed lengthwise behind the back.

The lateral position is prescribed in situations where it is necessary to take weight off the sacrum of the patient. The patient can also eat more easily in this position than in the supine position. It also facilitates some kinds of drainage. Finally, many people find it a relaxing position.

Fowler's Position

Fowler's position is one of the most frequently assumed positions. It is a sitting position in which the patient's head and trunk are raised between 45° and 90° (see Figure 25.7). There are two variations of Fowler's position: the *semi-Fowler* (or *low Fowler*) and *high Fowler* positions. In the semi-Fowler position the head and trunk are elevated 15° to 45°. This is a comfortable position for the patient who must keep the head and chest slightly elevated. The high Fowler position refers to the full sitting position, that is, with the head of the bed elevated 90°; the knees may or may not be flexed.

In Fowler's position the patient usually needs at least two pillows for support and comfort. The first pillow is best placed far enough down the patient's back to provide support for the lumbar curvature. A second pillow supports

the head and shoulders. An emaciated patient will probably need three pillows. For patients who are very weak, pillows placed laterally will support the arms and help to maintain good body alignment.

Small pillows or a pad under the patient's thighs permits slight flexion of the knees and a footboard permits dorsal flexion and prevents the patient from sliding towards the foot of the bed. Occasionally the knee gatch of the bed is used to support flexion of the knee. If the knee gatch is used, the knees should not be flexed too much because of the danger of putting pressure on the popliteal nerve and major blood vessels that are close to the skin surface in the popliteal area. Prolonged pressure can cause serious interference with both nerve supply and circulation to the lower limbs. Hence, the knee gatch is seldom used for patients now.

In Fowler's position the main weight-bearing areas of the patient are the heels, sacrum and posterior aspects of the ilium. The nurse should pay particular attention to these areas when giving skin care.

FIGURE 25.7   Fowler's position

Fowler's position is indicated for patients who suffer either cardiac or respiratory distress, since it permits maximal chest expansion. A position somewhat similar to the high Fowler is the sitting position in which the patient leans over an overbed table upon which several pillows have been placed for comfort. Some patients with respiratory problems find this position makes breathing easier for them. Patients who have difficulty exhaling tend to lean forward to compress the chest for additional force on expiration. The pillows on the overbed table provide support for the arms and help to maintain the individual in as erect a position as possible to increase total lung capacity.

Sims' (Semiprone) Position

Sims' position is similar to the lateral position except that the patient's weight is on the anterior aspects of the shoulder girdle and hip (see Figure 25.8). The patient's lower arm is behind the back, and the upper arm is flexed at the shoulder and elbow. The upper leg is acutely flexed at the hip and knee and the lower leg is slightly flexed at the hip and knee.

A rolled pillow placed laterally and in front of the patient's abdomen will support the patient in this position. Pillows for the upper arm and upper leg will prevent adduction of these limbs, and a small pillow for the patient's head will prevent lateral flexion. If, however, the patient is unconscious and the nurse wants to promote mucus drainage from the mouth, a pillow under the head is contraindicated.

In Sims' position the patient's feet naturally assume the plantar flexion position. If the patient is to maintain Sims' position for some time, supports should be provided in order that the feet assume the dorsal flexion position. A footboard or sandbag can be used for this purpose.

Sims' position can be established on both the left side and the right side. The patient's position should be changed frequently; if he or she is unable to move unaided, the nurse can help the patient turn every two hours, or more often if needed. When turning the patient who is unconscious, the nurse should be sure that the patient's eyelids are closed to prevent the possibility of the cornea's being scratched by the bedclothes. Good skin care, particularly to the anterior aspects of the patient's ilium and shoulder girdle, is also indicated.

This position is prescribed for patients who are either unconscious or unable to swallow. It permits the free drainage of mucus. Sims' position also allows maximal relaxation and is therefore a comfortable sleeping position for many people.

POSITIONING THE PATIENT

When patients are confined to bed and cannot move, improper positioning and support of joints can lead to contractures and skin breakdown. Regardless of the position of the patient, certain principles must be applied. The body parts must be properly aligned and the joints adequately supported. The patient's position must be changed frequently. Adequate exercise (to the extent the patient's condition allows), good skin care and supportive measures must always be carried out. A general guide for positioning patients as well as the principles of anatomical position and body alignment are listed in the boxes below. Although there are situations in which positions that do not follow the therapeutically anatomical position fully may be required, the basic principles should be kept in mind and applied insofar as is possible. The steps for helping patients assume the various positions are detailed in Procedure 25.3.

When patients cannot move, care must be taken to maintain the fingers in a functioning position, that is, with fingers flexed and thumb in opposition. A small hand roll may be placed in the palm of the hand and the fingers curved

FIGURE 25.8   Sims' position. A small pillow may or may not be placed under the patient's head.

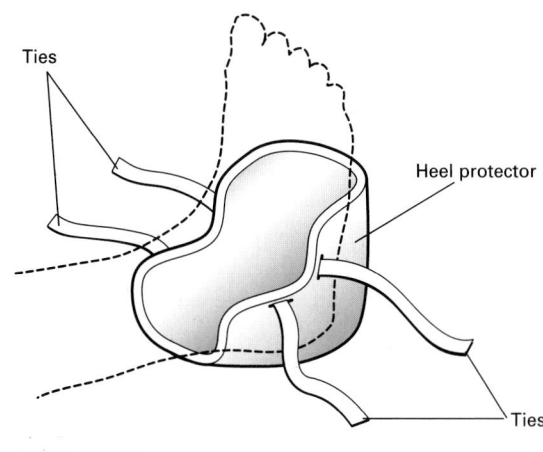

FIGURE 25.9 Heel protector

Guide for Positioning Patients

1. Positions that are as close as possible to the basic anatomical position provide good body alignment.
2. Joints should be maintained in a slightly flexed position. Prolonged extension creates undue muscle tension and strain.
3. Positions should be changed at least every two hours. Prolonged pressure on one area may cause the skin to break down, with resultant pressure sores (decubitus ulcers).
4. All patients require daily exercise unless medically contraindicated.
5. When a patient changes position, joints should be manipulated through the full range of motion unless medically contraindicated.

Principles of Anatomical Position

1. Good alignment of all body parts
2. Equal weight distribution of body parts
3. Maximal space in body cavities for internal organs
4. Joints in functional position (for walking, grasping objects, etc.)

Assembling Aids for Positioning and Comfort

Pillows are used to maintain proper position and provide support to joints. There are also a number of aids and supportive devices that may be used to ensure comfort and safety.

Sheepskin pads and small pillows Sheepskin pads and small pillows serve as supportive devices. Placed under bony prominences, they relieve pressure; placed in the lumbar curve or under a limb, they support or elevate an extremity. Figure 25.9 shows a heel protector which supports the foot in dorsal flexion and protects the skin from friction against the bed linen.

Sponge pad A small sponge pad placed in the patient's hand can be used as an exercise aid. It can also be used to prevent flexion of the hand and to separate skin

around it. This is particularly important for unconscious patients and for those who have limited movement in one or both hands. Wristdrop must also be prevented. The hand should never be left in a dependent position. It should be supported so that it is in a straight line with the lower arm.

FIGURE 25.10 A trochanter roll can be used to prevent external rotation of the hip. The safety pins used to secure the roll are placed so that they face away from the patient.

surfaces in conditions of spastic contraction. The size of the pad allows slight flexion of the hand and fingers, with the thumb comfortably placed in its normal anatomical position, that is, in opposition.

Trochanter rolls   **Trochanter rolls** are used to prevent external hip rotation. They may be made from bath towels or bath blankets. The towel is folded lengthwise once and then rolled to within six inches of one end. The roll may be secured with safety pins fastened between the body and the tail of the roll. To support the patient's thigh and prevent

external rotation the tail of the roll is placed under the patient's thigh, with the safety pins away from the patient. The roll is then firmly secured along the patient's thigh until the patient's toes point directly upward. Figure 25.10 on page 817 illustrates a trochanter roll.

Sandbags   Sandbags also serve as a means of providing support to the patient. They are firmer than trochanter rolls and, because of their weight, are less easily moved. For this reason, sandbags are desirable when body alignment must be maintained — for example, in the case of fractures.

PROCEDURE 25.3

Positioning Patients

ACTION	RATIONALE
A. General Actions	
1. Assess the patient's alignment and comfort level.	Determines equipment that will be needed.
2. Gather equipment and supplies as necessary: • Pillows • Aids for positioning and comfort • Sheepskin pads • Sponge pads • Heel or elbow protector • Trochanter roll • Footboard	Ensures efficiency and economy of time.
3. Obtain assistance as necessary.	Ensures safety for patient and nurse.
4. Explain procedure to the patient.	Enhances emotional well-being and, where possible, facilitates patient's participation in care.
5. Wash hands.	Prevents transmission of microorganisms.
6. Provide privacy.	Promotes patient comfort.
B. Dorsal Recumbent Position	
1. Position the patient on the back with one pillow under the head and shoulders.	Prevents hyperextension of the neck.
2. Place a small pillow or folded towel under the lumbar curvature of the back.	Supports the lumbar curvature.
3. Place rolled towels or a rolled bath blanket at the lateral aspects of the thighs.	Supports the thighs, prevents outward rotation, and maintains the patient's legs in alignment.
4. Place a small pillow under the lower legs, below the popliteal area.	Slightly flexes the limb and prevents hyperextension of the knees. Placing the pillow below the popliteal area avoids possible interference with circulation to the extremities and injury to the popliteal nerve.

ACTION	RATIONALE
5. Place a footboard at end of the bed.	Helps to maintain the feet in flexion and removes the weight of the bedclothes from the toes.

C. Prone Position

ACTION	RATIONALE
1. Assist the patient to lie on the abdomen with the head turned to one side. The head may or may not be supported with a small pillow. If a pillow is used it should not be so thick as to hyperextend the patient's head.	
2. Position a small pillow or pad under the abdomen below the level of the diaphragm.	Provides support to the lumbar curvature and, in the case of the female patient, takes weight off the breasts. A pillow placed at or above the level of the diaphragm will impede respiration.
3. Place a pillow under the patient's lower legs. Alternatively, the patient can extend the toes over the end of the mattress.	Takes the weight off the toes. Lifts the patient's toes off the bed and permits slight flexion of the knees. Plantar flexion is minimized.

D. Lateral (Side-lying) Position

ACTION	RATIONALE
1. Position the patient on the side with both arms forward and the knees and hips flexed. The upper leg is flexed more than the lower leg. Weight is borne by the lateral aspects of the patient's ilium and scapula.	
2. Place a pillow under the patient's head.	Maintains alignment of the head to trunk.
3. Place a pillow under the patient's upper arm.	Support of the patient's arm permits greater chest expansion and enables the nurse to observe respirations.
4. Place one or two pillows under the upper leg.	Promotes correct alignment and decreases pressure of top leg resting on bottom leg.
5. Place a pillow lengthwise behind patient's back.	Increases support and promotes sense of comfort.

E. Fowler's Position

ACTION	RATIONALE
1. Place a pillow behind the patient's back. A second pillow supports the head and shoulders.	Provides support for the lumbar curvature.
2. Place a small pillow or a pad under the patient's thighs.	Permits slight flexion of the knees.
3. Place a footboard at the end of the bed.	Permits dorsal flexion and prevents the patient from sliding towards the foot of the bed.

F. Sims' Position

ACTION	RATIONALE
1. Position patient laterally but lying partially on abdomen. The lower arm is placed behind the body and the upper arm is flexed at the shoulder and elbow. The upper leg is acutely flexed at the hip and knee, and the lower leg is slightly flexed at the hip and knee.	

Continued on the next page

ACTION	RATIONALE
2. Place a rolled pillow laterally and in front of the patient's abdomen.	Supports the patient in this position.
3. Place pillows under the patient's upper arm and upper leg.	Prevents adduction of these limbs.
4. Place a small pillow under the patient's head.	Prevents lateral flexion. However, if the patient is unconscious and the nurse wants to promote mucus drainage from the mouth, a pillow under the head is contraindicated.

EVALUATING COMFORT, REST AND SLEEP INTERVENTIONS

All interventions must be evaluated for effectiveness. This is especially important when considering the patient's level of comfort and the quantity and quality of rest and sleep.

When an intervention related to comfort is implemented, the patient's comfort level is assessed every two to four hours. The following questions can help in evaluating the effectiveness of care.

1. Does the patient verbally indicate increased comfort?
2. Does the patient appear more comfortable, that is, more relaxed or less restless?
3. Has the frequency of the patient's requests for analgesics decreased?

Expected outcomes of interventions regarding rest and sleep relate to the amount of rest and undisturbed sleep the patient achieves, as well as the ease with which he or she falls asleep. Questions which may assist evaluation of rest and sleep interventions might include the following.

1. Has the patient been able to fall asleep without difficulty?
2. Has the patient been able to rest quietly?
3. Does the patient feel refreshed following sleep?

Sedatives or hypnotics may be prescribed for patients having difficulty sleeping. These drugs tend to decrease the length of time spent in REM sleep. There is also a rebound effect when these drugs are discontinued. That is, once the drug is discontinued the patient may encounter a significant increase in REM sleep and may experience considerable dreaming and possibly nightmares (Knapp, 1993).

KEY TERMS

comfort p. 796

rest p. 796

sleep p. 796

circadian rhythm p. 796

REM (rapid eye movement) p. 797

sleep deprivation p. 797

dyssomnias p. 799

parasomnias p. 799

insomnia p. 799

hypersomnia p. 799

narcolepsy p. 799

somnambulism p. 800

nightmare p. 800

night terror p. 800

enuresis p. 800

sleep apnea p. 800

fracture board p. 812

bed cradle p. 812

footboard p. 813

Balkan frame p. 813

dorsal recumbent position p. 813

supine position p. 814

prone position p. 814

lateral position p. 814

Fowler's position p. 815

Sims' position p. 816

trochanter roll p. 818

IN REVIEW

Comfort is the subjective experience of physical, psychological, social, spiritual and environmental ease. Discomfort may be caused by myriad psychosocial, spiritual or physical stimuli. Nurses perform a crucial role in preventing and alleviating patients' discomforts. Nursing actions which promote comfort often centre on dialogue and touch. Rest is synonymous with repose or relaxation and implies freedom from emotional tension and physical discomfort. It does not necessarily mean inactivity, since people often find a change of activity as relaxing as sitting or lying. Sleep is a period of decreased mental alertness and physical activity which is a part of the normal pattern of daily living. It is a necessary part of life and is essential for growth and healing.

Sleep is a cyclical phenomenon affecting all body functions. Each individual has a sleep–wake cycle which follows a sequential pattern (a circadian rhythm) which is intricately involved with other body rhythms. Most adults have a 90-minute sleep cycle and pass through four to six cycles in their sleep time. Each cycle has five stages. People must progress through the stages in sequential fashion in order to obtain the physiological and psychological benefits of sleep. People who are awakened frequently may not progress through all of the stages and suffer sleep deprivation as a result.

Sleep deprivation is a decrease in the amount, quality or consistency of sleep. If prolonged, it can have a profound adverse effect on physical and psychological functioning.

Many factors affect a person's ability to rest and sleep. Among these are age, sleep habits, discomfort, emotional stress, environment, illness and medications.

Sleep patterns change through the life cycle. Newborns need the most sleep and approximately half of their sleep is REM sleep. By three months of age the infant's sleep-cycle pattern begins to resemble that of the adult. By this time, about two thirds of the infant's total sleep is quiet sleep. The amount of sleep required throughout childhood gradually diminishes. Adolescents need longer periods of sleep once again, a fact which may be related to their growth needs. Sleep requirements remain the same throughout adulthood; however, the quality of sleep seems to degenerate. Frequent periods of wakefulness and early morning awakenings result in the need for daily rest periods.

Common sleep disturbances include the dyssomnias (insomnia, hypersomnia and narcolepsy) and the parasomnias (sleepwalking, nightmares, night terrors and enuresis). Sleep apnea is a physiological difficulty affecting the sleep–wake cycle.

The nursing health history should include information about the patient's usual sleep and rest patterns, any sleep problems and present worries or anxieties. It is essential that nurses identify and note each patient's unique routines, and find the measure or combination of measures which will effectively promote comfort, rest and sleep for each patient.

Nursing diagnoses associated with the quantity and quality of sleep are labelled *Sleep pattern disturbance*. Sleep disorders such as narcolepsy or sleep apnea are conditions which nurses care for in collaboration with the physician; these are identified as collaborative problems.

A sleep care plan facilitates communication about the patient's rest and sleep needs, as well as individual preferences and problems. It arranges a definite series of activities to help each patient obtain adequate sleep.

Nurses can help individuals, families and groups promote optimal rest and sleep in daily living through information sharing and teaching. Health protecting interventions include encouraging daytime diversional activities and morning naps, fostering usual bedtime rituals, providing back massages, teaching and encouraging the use of relaxation techniques and ensuring a quiet environment and a comfortable bed. A therapeutic mattress, fracture board, bed cradle, footboard or Balkan frame may be used for comfort and therapeutic purposes. Proper positioning of the patient in bed is important for comfort, relaxation and healing. Therapeutically, patients are positioned to maintain good body alignment, prevent contractures, promote drainage, facilitate breathing and prevent skin breakdown. Positions include dorsal recumbent, supine, prone, lateral, Fowler's and Sims'. Pillows of various sizes, sheepskin or sponge pads, rolled towels and sandbags are used for comfort and proper positioning.

LEARNING ACTIVITIES

1. Keep a record of your hours of sleep (including naps) for a typical week. Note factors in your lifestyle that may affect your sleep. Analyse your sleep pattern and determine whether or not it is adequate. If not, what changes should you make to promote optimum rest and sleep?

2. **Case Study**: Mrs. R. Rogers is a 56-year-old woman who was admitted to the hospital with acute rheumatoid arthritis involving her back, knees and feet. Mrs. Rogers is an obese woman and she finds it difficult to breathe when the head of her bed is flat. She experiences pain in her joints continually. Mrs. Rogers has a limited income and lives by herself in a small apartment. Her husband died four years ago, and her one daughter lives out of town and finds it difficult to visit frequently.

    The physician has ordered a low calorie diet. Her medications include enteric-coated acetylsalicylic acid (650 mg four times a day) and secobarbital (50 mg at bedtime).

    a. What factors might cause Mrs. Rogers to have problems with regard to comfort, rest and sleep?

    b. How would you assess Mrs. Rogers' present comfort, rest and sleep status?

    c. What objective data (signs) would indicate to you that Mrs. Rogers is uncomfortable or is not resting or sleeping well?

d. What subjective data (symptoms) of Mrs. Rogers might you note?

e. What other members of the health team are, or might be, involved in helping Mrs. Rogers? For what purpose?

f. What positions do you think might be most comfortable for Mrs. Rogers?

g. What supportive devices might make Mrs. Rogers more comfortable? How should you use them?

h. Outline a nursing care plan for Mrs. Rogers.

REFERENCES AND READINGS

ALWARD, R.R. (1988). Are you a lark or an owl on the night shift? *American Journal of Nursing, 88,* 1337–1339.

CAMERON, B.L. (1993). The nature of comfort to hospitalized medical surgical patients. *Journal of Advanced Nursing, 18,* 424–436.

CLOSS, S.J. (1988). Assessment of sleep in hospitalized patients: A review of methods. *Journal of Advanced Nursing, 13,* 501–510.

DOTTO, L. (1990). *Asleep in the fast lane: The impact of sleep on work.* Toronto: Stoddard.

EDWARDS, G.E. and SCHURING, L.M. (1993). Sleep protocol: A research-based practice change. *Critical Care Nurse, 13*(2), 84–88.

GRANT, D.A., and KLELL, C. (1974). For goodness sake, let your patients sleep. *Nursing '74, 4,* 54–57.

GROPPER, E.I. (1992). Promoting health by promoting comfort. *Nursing Forum, 27*(2), 5–8.

HAYTER, J. (1980). The rhythm of sleep. *American Journal of Nursing, 30*(3), 457–461.

JOHNSON, J.E. (1993). Progressive relaxation and the sleep of older men and women. *Journal of Community Health Nursing, 10*(1), 31–38.

KNAPP, M. (1993). Night shift: The restorative sleep specialists. *Journal of Gerontological Nursing, 19*(5), 38–42.

KOLCABA, K.Y. (1992). Holistic comfort: Operationalizing the construct as a nurse-sensitive outcome. *Advanced Nursing Science, 15*(1), 1–10.

KOZIER, B. and ERB, G. (1989). *Techniques in clinical nursing* (3rd ed.). Redwood City, CA: Addison-Wesley.

POTTER, P. and PERRY, A.G. (1991). *Basic nursing theory and practice* (2nd ed.). St. Louis: Mosby.

ROGERS, A. and ALDRICH, M.S. (1993). The effect of regularly scheduled naps on sleep attacks and excessive daytime sleepiness associated with narcolepsy. *Nursing Research, 42*(2), 111–117.

WALGENBACH, J.C. (1990). Lullabye and not a good night? *Geriatric Nursing, 11,* 278–279.

WHALEY, L.F. and WONG, D.L. (1991). *Nursing care of infants and children* (4th ed.). St. Louis: Mosby.

WEAVER, R. and MILLMAN, R.P. (1986). Broken sleep. *American Journal of Nursing, 86*(2), 146–150.

WEBSTER, R.A. and THOMPSON, D.R. (1986). Sleep in hospital. *Journal of Advanced Nursing, 11,* 447–457.

CHAPTER 26

Pain
Management

CENTRAL QUESTIONS

1. How is pain important as a protective mechanism for the body?

2. How do the mechanisms of pain reception, transmission and perception function in the physiology of pain?

3. What is the gate-control theory of pain?

4. What are the various types of pain stimuli and how do they cause pain?

5. What are the types of pain and the determinants of the personal experience of pain?

6. How do pain experiences vary throughout the life cycle?

7. How does the nurse assess a patient's pain experience?

8. What are the common nursing diagnostic statements for patients with pain?

9. How can the nurse apply principles relevant to pain and pain management in planning and implementing nursing interventions
   a. to prevent or minimize pain
   b. to help patients cope with their pain
   c. to modify the patient's perception of pain?

10. How does the nurse evaluate the patient's response to nursing interventions?

INTRODUCTION

Pain is a universal experience. It is a difficult experience to describe and a phenomenon not yet completely understood. Clinically, pain is difficult to measure. Though sophisticated equipment and methods of diagnosis exist for most other disease symptoms, pain measurement remains almost completely subjective. Health care professionals rely on subjective reports and on observable behaviour. The individual experiencing pain is the authority and the only person able to describe the experience. According to McCaffery, pain is "whatever the experiencing person says it is, existing whenever he[she] says it does" (1979, 11).

In most circumstances, the sensation of pain is due to **noxious** (harmful, injurious) stimuli, and is a protective mechanism that warns the individual of actual or potential damage to body tissues. This type of acute experience is familiar to most people. However, pain can become chronic. Prolonged or intractable pain lasting longer than six months is considered to be chronic pain. We will discuss acute and chronic pain in more detail later on in the chapter.

Published research indicates that pain is often undertreated. There are some common misconceptions about pain and pain management which may account for this lack of treatment. Many health care professionals are concerned that use of pain medications will promote drug abuse. It is often assumed that individuals with chronic pain grow accustomed to the pain and therefore require less attention to pain management. Another common misconception concerns children and pain. There is an assumption that children may not feel pain, and that if they do, they quickly forget the experience. Older adults are assumed to be less sensitive to pain and therefore not to require pain management. These common fallacies have led to the discomfort and anxiety of many individuals of all ages.

Pain is a major factor affecting the functional capacity to cope with the activities of daily living. Healing can be interrupted or prolonged if pain is unmanaged. Untreated pain may cause a number of negative responses, including blood pressure, pulse and respiratory changes, as well as anxiety, fear and feelings of helplessness. Therefore, a significant nursing function is assisting patients to achieve relief from pain. Appropriate assessment and analysis of data enables nurses to develop and implement a plan of care which will assist patients to alleviate or manage their pain. In order to do this, nurses must have an understanding of the physiology of pain and the interventions available for pain management.

THE PHYSIOLOGY OF PAIN

The experience of pain is a complex process involving both the nervous and the endocrine systems. Though the physiology of pain is not completely understood, the physiological mechanisms of pain may be characterized by three components: reception, transmission and perception.

PAIN RECEPTION

Free sensory nerve endings (**nociceptors**) are responsible for the reception of noxious stimuli and for beginning the transmission of pain impulses along afferent nerve fibres. Nociceptors are not found in all areas of the body. The skin, arterial walls, joints, periosteum and some internal organs such as the gallbladder and bile duct are richly supplied with nociceptors, while other areas, such as the brain and alveoli of the lung, lack these free nerve endings.

It is generally assumed that acute cellular damage stimulates the production of *endogenous pain producing substances*, such as bradykinin. Other neuropeptides which may be released at the site of injury and which produce pain impulses include acetylcholine, histamine, prostaglandins, potassium, serotonin and substance P. Not all noxious stimuli generate pain impulses. A stimulus must reach a sufficient level of intensity to create a nerve impulse. The point at which a stimulus reaches sufficient intensity to create a nerve impulse is called the **pain threshold**. This is the point at which the pain is first felt. Normally the pain threshold is the same for all individuals, and does not differ between cultures or races. In controlled laboratory experiments individuals subjected to increasingly painful stimuli reported feeling pain at almost the same point of intensity. The pain threshold, however, may be altered by **pain tolerance**, which is the amount of pain an individual is willing to endure. Pain tolerance is influenced by the physical and emotional condition of the individual, as well as cultural conditioning.

PAIN TRANSMISSION

The transmission of pain occurs via complex neural pathways. Once the nociceptor receives a stimulus of sufficient strength, an electrical impulse is generated along peripheral afferent nerve fibres to the spinal cord. Pain impulses are primarily transmitted by two types of peripheral nerve fibres: larger, myelinated A delta fibres and smaller, unmyelinated C fibres.

Myelinated A delta fibres rapidly transmit impulses. These fibres permit information to be localized and degrees of intensity to be differentiated. The type of impulses transmitted are usually sharp or pricking. Pain transmitted by A delta fibres generally subsides quickly.

Persistent, diffuse, burning sensations are conducted slowly by unmyelinated or poorly myelinated C fibres. Approximately two thirds of the fibres in the peripheral nerves are C fibres. The abundance of C fibres permits the transmission of large amounts of information despite slow conduction (Meinhart and McCaffery, 1983).

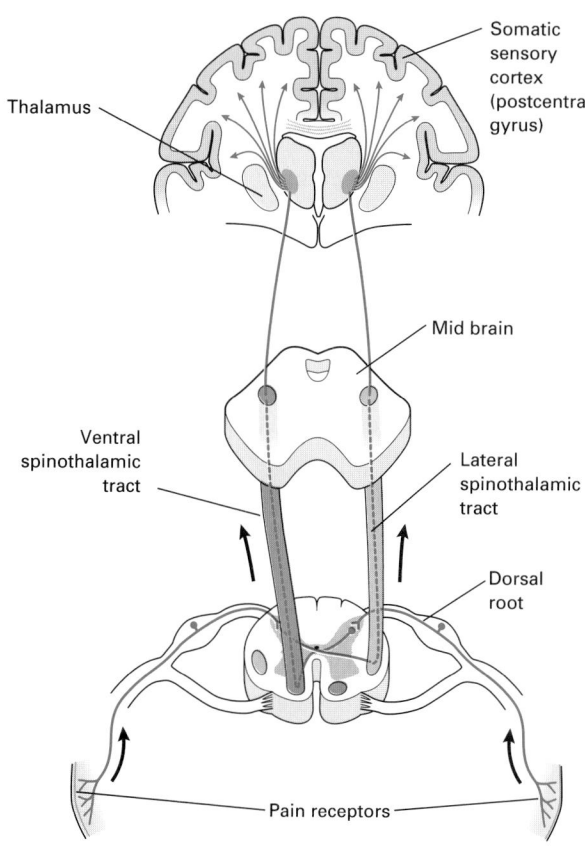

FIGURE 26.1   Pain transmission via ventral and lateral spinothalamic pathways

The difference between the experiences of A delta and C fibre pain is easily exemplified. Catching the tip of a finger in a door initially produces sharp, intense and well-localized pain — A delta pain. Several moments later, aching and diffuse C fibre pain is experienced.

Both A delta and C fibres enter the spinal cord through the dorsal roots of a spinal nerve and terminate in the grey matter (*substantia gelatinosa*) of the dorsal horns. From here the impulses ascend to brain centres including the thalamus, reticular formation, limbic system and somatosensory cortex.

Impulses ascend to the reticular formation and thalamus by neurons that form the spinothalamic pathway. The spinothalamic pathway may be divided into ventral, lateral and spinoreticular tracts. The lateral spinothalamic or neospinothalamic tract is composed of both A delta and C fibres and transmits sharp, localized pain sensations. It is believed that this tract conveys information regarding the location, duration and intensity of pain. Innervation of this tract may also be responsible for initiating autonomic reactions, such as the fight or flight response.

The spinoreticular or paleospinal tract is composed primarily of C fibres. This tract conducts impulses slowly and is associated with burning and diffuse sensations. Visceral sensations may also be transmitted along this tract. It is further hypothesized that this system affects brain structures that regulate memory and recall, and consequently, influence the emotional component of pain.

PAIN PERCEPTION

Perception begins the moment an individual experiences pain. The ability to perceive pain is dependent upon the integrity of the nerve fibres and structures that receive, transmit and interpret pain impulses. Injury to sensory nerves, sensory tracts in the spinal cord, the thalamus or sensory areas in the cerebral cortex will interfere with pain perception. For example, patients with paralysis due to spinal cord injury will not feel pain below the level of the injury. Pain perception is also altered by an individual's level of consciousness. The unconscious patient or the patient under general anesthetic, for example, is presumed to not feel pain.

In some circumstances, individuals become hypersensitive to painful stimuli. Unlike other receptors, nociceptors adapt poorly, or not at all, to continuous stimulation. Pain is triggered as the receptors increasingly respond to any type of stimulation. The pain threshold is lowered, and individuals experience increased sensitivity to pain. This is often true for individuals with continuous or chronic pain syndromes.

In contrast, intense pain in one part of the body may raise the pain threshold in other areas. An individual suffering considerable pain from a broken leg may be unaware of pain from an elbow abrasion. This is due to selective perception, whereby the stimulus of greater priority (or intensity) assumes precedence in attention over the less intense, or less significant stimulus.

Areas of the body adjacent to injured areas are usually more sensitive to pain. The skin adjacent to a wound, for example, is generally tender. Also, damaged tissues react to additional painful stimuli, even of minimal intensity, more readily than intact tissue. The sensitivity of sunburned skin attests to this phenomenon.

Several factors within the central nervous system moderate pain perception. In some instances, the stimulus is of sufficient intensity for a protective response to be initiated in the spinal cord before the impulse reaches the somatosensory cortex and conscious perception. For example, touching a hot stove will generate a reflex action, causing an individual to immediately withdraw his or her hand.

Pain impulses travelling via the spinothalamic tract, reaching the thalamus and finally the cortex, may also be modified by *endogenous opiates* such as the *enkephalins, endorphins* and *dynorphins*. Enkephalin-containing fibres are prevalent throughout the nervous system. Enkephalins produce a weak analgesic effect by binding to opiate receptors on nociceptive fibres and inhibiting the release of excitatory neurotransmitters, such as substance P. This decreases the intensity of the pain impulse being transmitted.

Endorphins are large polypeptides with an opioid-like pharmacological action. Endorphins are believed to be synthesized and stored by the pituitary gland. These molecules, like enkephalins, alter pain impulse transmission by binding to opiate receptor sites throughout the nervous system and inhibiting the release of neurotransmitters. Several endorphins have been isolated. The most powerful is Beta-endorphin.

Dynorphins are the most powerful of the identified endogenous opiates. These substances have an analgesic effect 50 times more powerful than beta-endorphin (Meinhart and McCaffery, 1983).

Enkephalins, endorphins and dynorphins are triggered by pain and stress. Stimulation of this internal system of endogenous opiates activates descending nerve fibres which transmit inhibitory impulses to cells in the dorsal horns of the spinal column. The result is an alteration of the intensity of the pain impulse and analgesia. However, the degree, or amount, of pain necessary to trigger the system is unknown.

PAIN THEORIES

Despite rigorous research, the mechanisms of pain are not completely understood. Several theories of pain, such as the specificity theory, pattern theories, and the gate-control theory, have been proposed. The gate-control theory, however, dominates present thinking about pain.

GATE-CONTROL THEORY

The gate-control theory proposed by Melzak and Wall (Melzak, 1973) is presently the most popular theory of pain. This theory proposes that a neural mechanism located in the substantia gelatinosa of the spinal cord dorsal horns acts as a gate which controls the flow of pain impulses to higher centres in the brain. Typically, the gate is partially closed. Stimulation of the substantia gelatinosa further closes the gate, thereby blocking the transmission of impulses. Inhibition of the substantia gelatinosa, on the other hand, opens the gate and allows impulses to flow through it. Beyond the gating mechanism are T (transmission) cells. When the degree of stimulation passing through the gate to the T cells reaches a critical (threshold) level, these cells fire, activating areas within the central nervous system that are responsible for pain perception and response.

Activity in both the peripheral and the central nervous systems may alter the position of the gate and either increase or decrease the transmission of pain impulses from the peripheral fibres to the somatosensory cortex and conscious awareness. Pain impulses carried by A delta and C fibres enter the spinal column at the level of the dorsal root and terminate in the substantia gelatinosa. Input from C fibres has an inhibiting effect on the gating mechanism, causing the gate to remain open, or to open further. This action permits the transmission of pain impulses. A delta fibres, which have a larger diameter than C fibres, conduct impulses which stimulate the substantia gelatinosa, causing the gate to close. Thus, impulses from A delta fibres may be halted at the level of the spinal cord and prevented from reaching the brain, that is, conscious awareness (Meinhart and McCaffery, 1983).

In addition to the A delta fibres, larger diameter A-beta (touch) fibres have been identified. These large afferent fibres also enter the spinal cord at the level of the dorsal root. Stimulation of A-beta fibres opposes the activity of the smaller diameter fibres, thereby closing the gate and inhibiting the transmission of pain impulses. Stimulation of the A-beta fibres also facilitates the release of enkephalins in the dorsal horn which further modifies pain impulse transmission along the spinothalamic tracts.

The majority of the larger diameter A fibres lie close to the skin surface. Cutaneous stimulation of these fibres by massage, heat, cold or TENS (transcutaneous electrical nerve stimulation) provides effective modalities for decreasing pain impulse transmission and contributing to pain relief.

The gating mechanism is also affected by motivational and cognitive influences from the higher brain centres. These influences, which include such factors as attention, anxiety, expectations, suggestion and memories of previous experiences (including cultural and social background), send messages from the brain which modulate pain impulses travelling upward from peripheral sites. Through a process of input comparison from the sensory systems, the thalamus and the cerebral cortex, the spinal-gating mechanism will be excited and close, or will be inhibited and open.

There are a number of pain-relief measures which stimulate the activity of the thalamus and cerebral cortex to close the gating mechanism. These include relaxation strategies, distraction techniques, guided imagery and hypnosis. It is believed that these methods may also activate the endogenous opiate system. The gate-control theory provides plausible explanations for some of the observations about pain, such as why stimulating a painful area, by rubbing it, for example, may result in pain reduction. This theory also recognizes the potency of cognitive activities, particularly distraction, in decreasing the perception of pain.

COMMON CAUSES OF PAIN

Pain begins with stimulation of free sensory nerve endings located near the skin surface or within deeper structures. Stimulation of nociceptors may be generated by a number of different stimuli including chemical substances, mechanical trauma and thermal extremes.

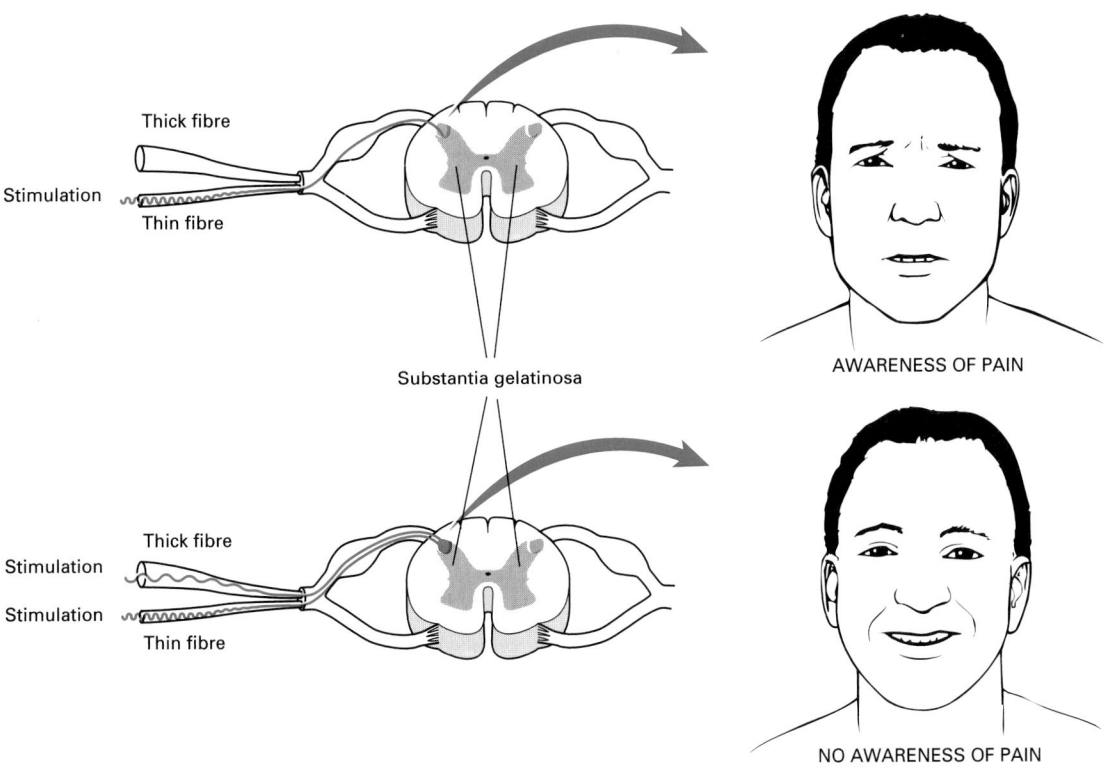

FIGURE 26.2   Stimulation of thick nerve fibres, which may be done by nursing measures such as massage, may stimulate the release of endorphins so that pain impulses from thin nerve fibres are blocked in the substantia gelatinosa.

CHEMICAL STIMULI

Direct stimulation of nociceptors by irritating chemical substances is the most common cause of pain. Chemical stimulation may occur both internally and externally. Any contact lens wearer who replaces a lens, having forgotten to first rinse the lens with normal saline, can attest to the pain of external chemical stimulation caused by the hydrogen peroxide.

Internal (*endogenous*) chemical stimulation occurs when there is a disruption in the usual body chemistry. An example of this is the lactic acid accumulation in the gastrocnemius muscle experienced by runners. When the acidic waste products of cellular metabolism collect, pain results from the irritating effect of these substances on nociceptors.

Ischemic pain is an example of the effect of endogenous chemicals. An insufficient blood supply results in tissue death. The decaying cells liberate endogenous chemical substances which irritate the nociceptors and generate pain impulses. Ischemic pain is further intensified by the inability of the blood supply to remove the accumulated metabolic waste products.

MECHANICAL TRAUMA

Mechanical stimulation usually involves trauma to body tissue, such as spraining an ankle or accidentally hitting the thumb instead of the nailhead when hammering a nail. The pain felt initially is due to pressure on the free nerve endings.

Pain may also result from over-stretching or contraction of tissues. Distention of a hollow organ such as the stomach is an example of over-stretching the tissues. An individual who eats a large meal may feel considerable discomfort in the region of the stomach. This feeling of pain is related to two factors: stretched nerve endings in the sensory receptors and occlusion of small blood vessels in the stretched tissue, producing localized ischemia.

Muscle spasm is an example of pain occurring during contraction. Intramuscular blood vessels are compressed, producing localized ischemia. In addition, prolonged muscular contraction increases the cellular metabolic rate, resulting in an accumulation of metabolic waste products, which constricted blood vessels cannot remove. These metabolic waste products are chemically irritating to sensory nerve endings and contribute to the sensation of pain.

THERMAL STIMULATION

Extreme heat or cold causes pain and damage to body tissues. Pain due to a sunburn or small burn on the tip of the finger is a common experience. The initial burning pain probably results from the intensity of the thermal stimulus. The lingering after-pain is due to the chemical substances released following tissue destruction.

Extreme cold, particularly if there is freezing of body tissues, as in frostbite, causes tissue damage and pain. Cold constricts the blood vessels in the affected tissue and may completely obliterate the blood supply. The pain in a frostbitten nose or finger is most severe when the blood flow is returning and the constricted vessels are being dilated.

THE EXPERIENCE OF PAIN

The personal experience of pain is mediated by the type of pain perceived and by the influence of a variety of determinants.

TYPES OF PAIN

Pain may be divided into two categories: acute and chronic. *Acute pain* is a protective mechanism that warns of potential or actual tissue damage. This type of pain has a rapid onset, varies in intensity and generally lasts less than six months. Acute pain usually has an identifiable pathology, and tends to resolve as healing occurs. This type of pain is usually responsive to treatment modalities. Pain lasting longer than six months, that may or may not be connected to a pathological process, is chronic pain. *Chronic pain* varies in intensity and is often unresponsive to treatment.

Both acute and chronic pain may arise from two sources: somatic and visceral. *Somatic pain* originates from the skin, muscles or joints and it may be superficial or deep. *Superficial somatic pain* is usually described as having a sharp, burning or pricking quality. It arises from stimulation of receptors in the skin or the mucous membranes of the body. As a rule, an individual is able to localize surface pain fairly accurately because of the large number of free sensory nerve endings on the surface of the body. *Deep somatic pain* comes from the deeper structures of the body, such as the muscles, tendons, joints and fasciae. Pain originating from these areas is easily localized. It is frequently described as dull, aching, cramping, gnawing or boring. Muscles and tendons are particularly sensitive to pain and may give rise to pain of considerable intensity.

Visceral pain arises from sources in the abdominal cavity or thorax. It is more difficult to localize the source of visceral pain because there are fewer sensory nerve endings in the viscera than in the skin and mucous membranes.

Visceral pain is similar to deep somatic pain and frequently includes gripping, cramping, dull aching and burning sensations, as well as a feeling of pressure. In the case of a peptic ulcer, the patient may describe the pain as having a gnawing, burning or sometimes knifelike quality.

Acute pain   There are two categories of acute pain: intermittent pain and referred pain. **Intermittent pain** is characterized by exacerbations and remissions of acute episodes of pain. The patient is generally free of pain between these episodes. This type of pain syndrome is common in conditions such as sickle cell anemia or migraine headaches.

Pain that is felt in one region of the body from a stimulus in another area is called **referred pain**. This type of pain most commonly occurs with visceral pain. The pain originates in an organ but the sensation is felt in a somatic area, often, superficial areas in the skin. In referred pain, the afferent fibres carrying impulses from the viscera and those from cutaneous tissues enter the spinal cord and converge onto the same spinothalamic tract. The brain is unable to distinguish between the two sources of painful stimuli and the pain sensation is referred to the most superficial structures innervated by the converging neurons (Seeley, Stephens and Tate, 1992). The individual may experience the sensation of pain coming from the skin alone or from both viscera and skin.

The nature of the referred pain is typically specific to the organ involved and the pathological process that is occurring. For example, a person with myocardial infarction (ischemia of the heart muscle) often describes the pain as constricting, viselike or compressing and radiating to the left shoulder and down the left arm. Pain may or may not be felt in the region of the heart.

Chronic pain   Chronic pain is pain that is experienced continuously and is often resistant to relief measures (intractable). There is no predictable end point in chronic pain. Consequently, people with chronic pain often encounter significant disruption in their personal and professional life. They may become overwhelmed by the pain and lose their ability to cope with the activities of daily living. Feelings of frustration, helplessness and hopelessness in managing the pain frequently lead to anxiety and depression.

Phantom limb pain and central pain syndromes are examples of chronic pain. **Phantom limb pain** occurs following amputation of a limb. Individuals with this syndrome usually experience pain prior to the amputation and feel pain as though the affected limb had not been amputated. The pain tends to be severe and may be described as burning, crushing or cramping. Individuals may also feel that the limb is edematous, or lying in a distorted position. Phantom limb pain may be triggered by touch, illness, fatigue or stress (Meinhart and McCaffery, 1983). The physiology of phantom pain is not well understood, but it is suggested that a pattern of impulses may be generated between the brain and the sensory receptors, even though the receptors are not present. Also, the lack of usual neural mediating mechanisms, due to the amputation, tends to result in sensations of increased intensity.

Central pain syndromes usually arise from injury to sensory nerves, neural pathways or areas in the brain concerned with pain perception. The pain is severe, occurs spontaneously and is often continuous. It may be described as gnawing, burning or crushing. Trigeminal neuralgia (*tic douloureux*) is an example of a central pain syndrome.

RESPONSES TO PAIN

An individual's response to pain is characterized by physiological and behavioural manifestations. Pain activates both the sympathetic and parasympathetic divisions of the autonomic nervous system. The physiological manifestations of low- to moderate-intensity acute pain, or superficial pain, are generally the result of sympathetic nervous system stimulation. Commonly referred to as the "fight or flight" reaction, observable signs and symptoms include an elevated blood pressure, pulse and respiratory rate. Pallor, diaphoresis, dilation of the pupils and the bronchial tubes, increased skeletal muscle tension and decreased gastric motility are also evidence of autonomic nervous system response. Restlessness and irritability are frequently observed.

When an individual experiences severe or deep pain, the parasympathetic nervous system is activated and the individual exhibits pallor, a decrease in blood pressure and heart rate, as well as muscle tension and rapid irregular breathing. Nausea and vomiting often occur and the body's defenses may collapse. In such an event, there are observable signs of exhaustion and prostration. The patient might appear "as white as a ghost." Collapse and loss of consciousness may ensue.

An individual with chronic pain does not usually demonstrate the same overt signs and symptoms of pain. The exact mechanism of the compensatory response of the body to chronic pain is not well understood, but, over time, there is a decrease in the sympathetic nervous system response. As a result, the individual may display fewer physiological pain indicators.

DETERMINANTS OF THE PAIN EXPERIENCE

The behavioural responses to pain differ much more widely from one individual to another than do the physiological manifestations. Everyone has observed individuals who "never flinch" even though the pain they experience is intense. On the other hand, some people react to pain with loud groans, weeping, screaming or attempts to remove themselves from the source of pain. An individual's re-sponse to pain is influenced by several factors. We have categorized these according to the individual's physical condition, emotional state and cultural conditioning.

Physical condition   When tired or physically weak, an individual's usual resistance and control over reactions diminishes. In such circumstances the individual may react to a minimal stimulus with an exaggerated response. When tired, even a small cut may seem too much to endure. Therefore, a busy parent attempting to cook dinner and at the same time look after small children may find the pain of a slight burn at the stove to be intense.

However, in cases of extreme exhaustion, an individual's attention span is reduced and concentration on any one stimulus for a long time is unlikely. Therefore, an extremely exhausted individual may be unable to focus on the location or intensity of the pain, and thus feels it less.

Emotional state   The emotional state of the individual also modifies the reaction to pain. Pleasurable emotions tend to nullify pain perception. A contented or happy individual often does not feel pain to the same extent as someone who is worried.

Anxiety and fear aggravate pain. Anxiety, fear and pain all provoke the same physiological "fight or flight" reaction. If anxiety is relieved, the patient's reaction to pain is lessened. It is suggested that anxiety-relieving measures are associated with the release of endorphins that block or moderate the transmission of pain impulses.

Strong emotional responses to stimuli other than the pain stimuli may block out the awareness of pain. A football player injured during a game may not notice an injury until the game is over. Excitement and the desire to win may be so intense that the sensory impressions of pain from the injury are of less priority and, therefore, are not perceived. A similar explanation may account for the numerous reports of wounded soldiers who stated they did not feel pain despite significant injuries. The overriding fear during battle and the necessity for self preservation at all costs took precedence over impressions from other sensory stimulation, so that pain perception was inhibited.

Cultural conditioning   Cultural values and beliefs influence behavioural responses to painful stimuli. Culture is a complex and multi-faceted influence involving ethnicity, age, sex, religion and socioeconomic status. Many sociologists have investigated the differing reactions of various cultural groups to pain. People of the First Nations are often cited as examples of members of a cultural group in which stoic indifference to pain is a highly valued characteristic. Among people of Latin or Mediterranean origin, on the other hand, an open display of suffering is considered a socially acceptable response to pain.

It is important for nurses to be aware of their own cultural biases with respect to pain. Cultural influences, though subtle, may affect the manner in which a nurse may perceive and react to another's pain. Nurses who have been raised with the belief that "only babies cry" may find themselves reacting negatively to patients who do not handle their pain in the "approved" manner. Similarly, nurses raised to expect open displays of suffering must not assume that a patient is not in pain simply because he or she does not cry. If nurses realize that their reactions are a reflection of their own social values, which may be different from those of the patient, they will be better able to understand that these feelings should not interfere with judgements about the patient's pain experience.

THE PAIN EXPERIENCE THROUGHOUT THE LIFE CYCLE

Individuals of all ages experience pain as a reaction to noxious stimuli. Response to pain and pain tolerance, however, are unique to each individual. As we age, responses and tolerance to pain may change due to physiological maturity and to the acquisition of a greater number of cognitive responses.

Neonates exhibit a reflex withdrawal response to harmful or potentially harmful stimuli. Other signs of pain in neonates include intense crying, restlessness or lethargy. Neonates in pain have also been observed to lie very quietly, as though sleeping. Poor sucking and decreased appetite are also indicators of pain in an infant. Infants, like older people, may try to protect the painful area by positioning themselves in a particular way. For example, infants with abdominal pain will draw their legs up to the abdomen.

All children experience pain, but their ability to describe the pain they are experiencing is affected by their limited cognitive understanding, insufficient verbal skills and fear of the consequences. Toddlers, in particular, have limited cognitive ability to describe pain. Nurses must rely on behavioural manifestations of pain in these children. Abnormal gait, guarding a part of the body, persistent crying or consoling behaviours such as rocking or sucking are a few examples of pain manifestations in young children. Older children (those over three years of age) have ample cognitive ability to describe their pain but they may be reluctant to do so because they fear painful diagnostic or treatment measures. Nurses must be sensitive to the pain management needs of children. They require the same attention to their pain as do adults. With respect to pain-relief measures, children are able to tolerate opioid analgesics and effectively use many behavioural and cognitive strategies for pain relief.

Older adults frequently suffer from chronic diseases which may cause pain. It is important to note that pain is not a symptom of aging. Some older adults, however, may believe pain to be related to aging and may hesitate to ver-

FROM RESEARCH TO PRACTICE

Holm, K., Cohen, F., Dudas, S., Medema, P.G. and Allen, B.L.(1989). Effect of personal pain experience on pain assessment. *Image* 21(2), 72-75.

This study was undertaken to determine the impact of nurses' personal experience with pain on their assessment of patients' pain. A sample of 134 registered nurses employed in three U.S. Midwestern hospitals participated in the study. Participants were asked to provide sociodemographic data, to complete a personal pain history questionnaire and to assess the degree of physical pain and psychological distress in hypothetical patients described in a series of vignettes. The nurses rated each situation on a standard "measure of inference of suffering" scale. Pain with headache, menstrual distress and dental events were the types of pain most frequently experienced personally by respondents. Most also had family members who had experienced pain in their presence. A major finding of the study was that the intensity of pain experienced by nurses significantly affected their assessment of a patient's pain. Those experiencing more severe pain were generally more sympathetic to the patient in pain. The intensity of personal pain experience also influenced the nurses' assessment of psychological distress, with those having personal experience with severe pain appearing more empathetic. Nurses with a religious preference tended to infer less pain than those claiming no religious preference. Findings of this study indicate that it is important for nurses to be aware of possible biases that may affect their assessment of patients' pain and their subsequent decisions about interventions.

balize what they think is a normal process. Therefore, any statement of pain or behaviour that may indicate pain must be investigated.

Older adults often experience sensory-related age changes. Perception of information and information processing is slower, but the intensity of the pain experience is *not* reduced. Cardiovascular disease, diabetes, arthritis, osteoporosis and cancer are some common pathologies which may cause pain for older adults. The usual presentation of pain in these pathologies may not occur due to age-related physiological changes. For example, in older patients, headache may be an indication of cardiovascular disease or cervical osteoarthritis. Chest pain may indicate herpes zoster or disease of the upper spine (Saxon, 1991). It is important to assess the older adult as a unique individual, whose pain experience is also unique.

KEY PRINCIPLES

Principles Relevant to Pain

1. Pain has a protective function in warning of present or potential damage to body tissues.
2. Pain may be caused by a number of different kinds of stimuli.
3. Tissues of the body differ in their sensitivity to painful stimuli.
4. Severe pain can cause collapse of the body's adaptive mechanisms.
5. The ability to perceive pain is dependent upon integrity of the neural structures which receive, transmit and interpret pain impulses.
6. Pain perception may be altered by physical and emotional factors.
7. Reactions to pain are highly individualized and depend on a number of physical, emotional and cultural factors.

ASSESSING PAIN

Pain is one of the most personal and distressing of all disease symptoms. Only the individual experiencing the pain really knows what it is like. Therefore, the primary source of information about pain is always the patient. When patients are unable to provide adequate descriptions of their pain by themselves, their family or significant others become essential sources of information. The nurse also makes observations about the patient's physiological and behavioural responses to pain and consults with other members of the health care team for observations they may have made.

NURSING HEALTH HISTORY

Because pain is a highly subjective experience, the majority of data about a patient's pain is collected through an interview. Many agencies supplement the standard nursing history form with a special pain assessment tool. When gathering information about an individual's pain experience, the nurse needs to ascertain, whenever possible, the following aspects of the pain:

1. quality
2. location
3. intensity
4. time and duration
5. precipitating factors

6. aggravating factors
7. effect on activities of daily living
8. personal meaning
9. usual coping strategies and pain-relief measures
10. affective responses.

Quality   Graphic terms are frequently used when describing pain. Patients generally characterize pain in terms of something familiar to them. For example, sharp pain may be compared to the cutting action of a knife. When recording and reporting pain, it is best to use the patient's exact words, in order to convey an accurate description of the patient's perceptions of pain. If the patient is having difficulty describing the pain, it may be necessary to provide some prompting. One way to do this is to ask the patient to describe what would be necessary to make you feel the same pain.

Location   The patient is usually able to identify fairly accurately superficial pain and pain originating from bones, muscles, joints and blood vessels. It is more difficult to identify the source of visceral pain. The patient may complain of pain in the general epigastric region, the lower abdomen, the chest or the lower back when a visceral organ is affected. Pain from the viscera may also be referred to a surface area, such as the referral of myocardial pain to the left shoulder.

When assessing the location of pain, ask patients to point to the area of discomfort on their own body and also any area where the pain radiates. If patients have difficulty doing this, it sometimes helps to ask them to show you the area of discomfort by pointing to that area on your body. This is a useful technique with both adults and children.

Intensity   The intensity of pain is completely subjective and it is sometimes difficult for a patient to quantify the severity of the experience. There are many tools available to assist with this area of assessment. The simplest technique is to ask the patient to numerically indicate the severity of the pain on a scale of one to ten. One represents no pain, and ten indicates the most severe pain. Similar tools may be used with children three years of age and older. These are discussed further in the section on Measurement of Pain.

For children younger than three years, and for cognitively impaired adults, it is necessary to rely on behavioural cues to determine the intensity of pain. Restlessness, lethargy, decreased appetite or increased irritability may indicate increasing intensity of pain. Often, it is only by 24-hour monitoring of all activities that a picture of the individual's response to pain can be determined.

When the intensity of a patient's pain changes abruptly, it is usually an indication of a change in the patient's condition. For example, when an inflamed appendix ruptures, or a peptic ulcer perforates, the patient usually experiences persistent sharp and severe pain, different both in quality and intensity from the pain felt previously.

Time and duration   An accurate description of a patient's pain includes when it begins, how long it lasts and whether it is intermittent or persistent. Does the pain come and go, or does it remain constant? Does the pain become more severe at night? Does it wake the individual at night? Pain sometimes seems more severe at night, when a person is alone and unoccupied. It is suggested that, in the absence of other people or distracting activities, the patient's full attention becomes focussed on the pain.

Precipitating factors   Pain is often precipitated by certain physical or emotional activities. In some cardiac conditions, chest pain may be caused by exertion. Patients with musculoskeletal problems frequently have pain associated with movement of the affected limb. Pain in the gastrointestinal tract may be precipitated by eating certain foods, or pain may be related to an intolerance to factors in the environment. Noise, for example, may induce a headache. Often, the patient is able to identify the specific factor or factors that cause pain, and these should be recorded and reported, again using the patient's own words. If the patient cannot identify precipitating factors, it is often helpful to ask him or her about activities engaged in prior to noticing the pain. The answer may provide a clue to the precipitating cause. Arguing with a teenager, for example, may raise a parent's blood pressure and precipitate a headache. Similarly, waiting for a job interview may activate stomach ulcers.

Aggravating factors   A variety of factors may worsen the patient's pain. Secondary symptoms such as nausea, constipation or dyspnea may exacerbate pain. Patients with peripheral vascular disease or a herniated disk often find the physical exertion of walking heightens their pain. It is important to ask patients about activities that worsen the pain.

Effect on activities of daily living   Sometimes pain can be so overriding that it interferes with a patient's ability to carry out the usual functions of daily living. For example, the severe pain associated with rheumatoid arthritis may prevent patients from washing, dressing and feeding themselves as well as getting to and from the bathroom. Pain interferes with rest and sleep, decreases appetite and reduces concentration. Severe pain may keep a person away from work or school and curb usual leisure and social activities. Knowing the extent of disruption in daily functioning gives clues about the severity of pain and provides information needed to determine the assistance patients may require in coping with the activities of daily living.

Personal meaning of the pain   How people interpret their pain depends on the significance of the pain, on their past experiences with pain and on social and cultural influences. Individuals withstand pain extremely well if they identify the painful experience with a positive outcome. For example, a woman giving birth or an individual undergoing cosmetic surgery often tolerates pain very well. Conversely, pain with no benefit is viewed as a threat to well-being. People with chronic, unabating pain experience fear, anxiety and depression which further act to exacerbate the pain experience.

Usual coping strategies and pain-relief measures   People in pain often use the same coping strategies they do with any illness. Some people do not allow the pain to disrupt their functioning; they implement pain-relief measures and continue the activity at hand. Other people allow the pain to take precedence over everything else. They stop what they are doing and attempt to relieve the pain. For example, someone with acute abdominal pain may take a warm drink and lie down until the pain has subsided. Still other people turn to others for help and comfort. This is perhaps a vestige of a coping strategy learned in childhood when they found that their mother saying, "I'll kiss it better" worked. Knowing something about a patient's coping strategies helps the nurse better understand the patient in pain. In addition, identifying pain-relief measures the patient has tried and noting the effectiveness of these measures provides valuable information when developing a pain management plan. For example, does rest relieve pain brought on by exertion? Does holding the limb in a certain way prevent pain? Does medication relieve the pain?

Affective responses   Many feelings accompany pain depending on the severity and duration of discomfort and the degree of disruption in a person's life. Feelings of fear, anxiety, depression and exhaustion are common with long-standing pain. Furthermore, individuals may feel powerless to control their pain and consequently lose hope. Expressions like "I can't take this anymore," "I feel like I don't have a life" or "I don't know what else to do" indicate feelings of hopelessness. Information about affective responses to pain are necessary in determining the supportive care patients will need.

A health history guide for assessing a patient's pain experience follows. It will draw the nurse's attention to the presenting pain pattern as well as the patient's usual health patterns that promote and protect pain-free healthy living. The nurse is cautioned, however, to use this guide in a sensitive manner. For example, if the patient is in severe, acute pain, the nurse would logically focus on determining the location and intensity of pain and administering pain-relief measures first. Then, when the pain has subsided, a more detailed assessment of the pain experience may continue.

Pain Experience

Presenting Pain Pattern

- Describe the quality of pain you are experiencing. (Is it sharp, burning?)
- Where do you feel the pain?
- Does the pain radiate anywhere? Can you point to the pain on yourself? on me?
- On a scale of one to ten, if ten is the worst pain, how would you rate your pain?
- Have you noticed any patterns to the pain? Is it worse at certain times of the day? in the morning or during the night? Does the pain wake you at night?
- Do you have a history of any disease that might bring on pain?
- What were you doing when the pain started?
- Does anything bring the pain on?
- Does anything make the pain worse?
- Have you had difficulty with nausea, vomiting, constipation, diarrhea or shortness of breath?
- How does the pain affect your usual daily functioning? Are you able to perform hygiene activities, continue to work (or go to school), exercise, socialize with friends? Are you able to rest?
- What does this pain mean to you? Do you have any fears about the pain?
- How do you usually cope with pain?

- Is there anything that makes the pain better or go away?
- What have you tried to make the pain go away?
- Have you taken any drugs to relieve the pain? If so, have the drugs helped?
- How does the pain makes you feel? anxious? depressed? helpless? hopeless?
- What do you expect from health care professionals in regard to treating the pain?

Health Promotion and Protection Patterns

- What is your usual outlook on life? optimistic? positive? happy? sad? depressed? unhappy?
- Describe your usual mood. Do you tend to be relaxed? calm? tense?
- Do you eat a well-balanced diet and avoid foods and beverages that cause gastric upset, abdominal pain or headache?
- Do you keep fit, exercise regularly but avoid excessive, overzealous workouts?
- Do you wear a seat belt when riding in a car?
- Do you practise proper body mechanics when moving or lifting heavy objects?
- Do you practise safety in the workplace?

MEASUREMENTS
PAIN RATING SCALES

Pain rating scales are objective measurement tools used to help patients describe the intensity of their pain. These scales use numbers, words and faces to describe pain of varying intensity. Patients are asked to rate their pain by selecting the word, number or face that describes the intensity of the pain they are feeling. Figure 26.3 gives an example of a word scale. There are similar scales that use numbers instead of words.

A "faces" rating scale is depicted in Figure 26.4. It consists of a range of faces, from happy to grimacing. Patients point to the face that best represents how they feel. Faces

scales are commonly used with children. Another tool used to rate pain intensity is the visual analogue scale (VAS), also depicted in Figure 26.4. This scale consists of a ten-centimetre line which represents a continuum of pain intensity. One end of the line represents *no pain* and the other end *unbearable pain*. The patient places a mark on the line that represents the intensity of pain experienced. The distance from the zero point of the line to the patient's mark signifies the intensity of pain. Pain rating scales provide a valuable tool for evaluating pain-relief measures because the patient's descriptions before and after treatment can be compared. These techniques require that patients be alert and cognitively aware.

UNIVERSITY OF OTTAWA   SCHOOL OF NURSING   FACULTY OF HEALTH SCIENCES

PAIN ASSESSMENT

Name _____ Ward _____ Room _____

Age _____ Diagnosis _____

Doctor _____ Nurse Assessing _____ Date _____

Medications for pain_____

LOCATION

Mark drawings with an X where pain is felt. Indicate sites of pain with an I (internal), E (external), EI (if both). Use arrow to indicate direction and spread.

SEVERITY

Rate pain on a 0-5 scale:

0. no pain
1. mild
2. discomforting
3. distressing
4. horrible
5. excruciating

At present_____

Worst it gets_____

Best it gets _____

1 hour after meds_____

FIGURE 26.3   Pain assessment tool

SOURCE: Logan, M. and Fothergill-Bourbonnais, F. (1991). *Continuous subcutaneous infusion of narcotics: Patient care and family support.* Markham: Knoll Pharmaceuticals Canada, 25-26. Reproduced with permission.

QUALITY

Have patient describe pain in own words (e.g. dull, sharp, throbbing, burning, aching)

_____

_____

Note non-verbal observations _____

_____

TIMING

When did the pain start? _____

How long have you had it? _____

How often does it appear? _____

How long does it last? _____

AGGRAVATING/RELIEVING FACTORS

What brings on the pain?_____

What makes it worse? _____

What makes it better? _____

IMPACT ON PATIENT

Does pain affect your sleep? _____

Does pain affect your mood? _____

How is pain affecting your activities? _____

What is pain preventing you from doing that you would like to do?_____

Describe your food intake (appetite)_____

Are you experiencing other symptoms? _____

PREVIOUS THERAPY   (drugs and other therapies that have helped or failed to relieve pain)

_____

FAMILY INFORMATION

Patient's personality/coping prior to cancer _____

_____

View on the impact of pain to the patient _____

_____

Strengths, weaknesses and dynamics of family _____

_____

FIGURE 26.3   Continued

VITAL SIGNS

Pain is accompanied by autonomic nervous system responses that are reflected in the patient's vital signs. Acute or superficial pain of low to moderate intensity will cause stimulation of the sympathetic nervous system resulting in elevations of heart rate, blood pressure and respirations. Severe, prolonged and deep pain cause parasympathetic stimulation and a concomitant decrease in blood pressure and heart rate.

Pain Scale/Description	Instructions	Recommended Age
A Faces Scale* (Wong and Baker, 1988). Consists of six cartoon faces ranging from very happy, smiling face for "no pain" to increasingly less happy faces to final sad, tearful face for "worst pain"	Explain to the child that each face is for a person who feels happy because there is no pain (hurt) or sad because there is some or a lot of pain. Face 0 is very happy because there is no hurt. Face 1 hurts just a little bit. Face 2 hurts a little more. Face 3 hurts even more. Face 4 hurts a whole lot, but Face 5 hurts as much as you can imagine, although you don't have to be crying to feel this bad. Ask child to choose face that best describes own pain.	Children as young as 3 years

No Pain   Worst Pain

B Visual Analogue Scale consists of a 10-centimeter line ranging from "no pain" to "unbearable pain"	Explain to the patient that one end of the line represents "no pain" and the other end represents "unbearable pain"—"the worst pain imaginable." Ask the patient to place a mark on the line that shows the intensity of pain he or she is feeling.	Adults

No Pain   Unbearable Pain

FIGURE 26.4   A. Faces Scale*   B. Visual Analogue Scale

*SOURCE: Wong and Baker, 1988, cited in Whaley and Wong, 1991, 1148. Reproduced with permission.

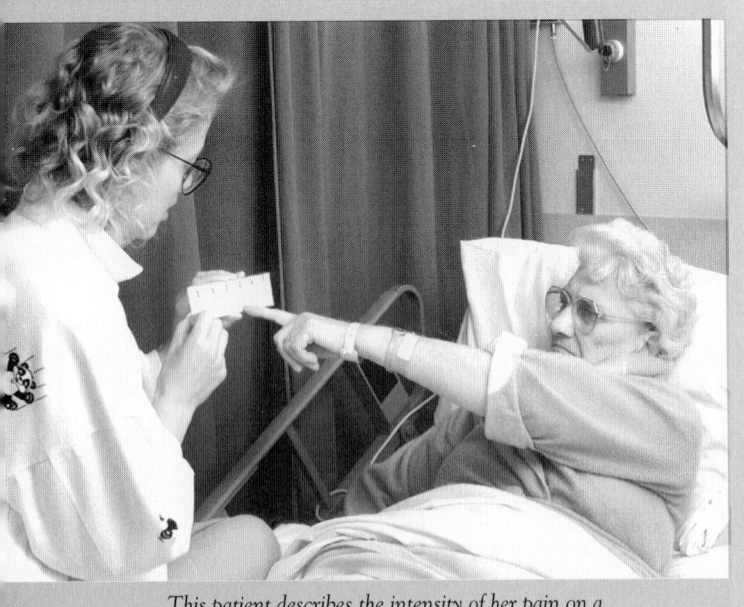

This patient describes the intensity of her pain on a rating scale.

PHYSICAL ASSESSMENT

When assessing a patient in pain, it is important to supplement information obtained from the patient with observations of physiological and behavioural manifestations of pain. An individual's facial expression, posture and body movement will indicate pain. Patients in pain often appear tense and drawn. In addition, they may assume a particular position to minimize the discomfort. For example, individuals with abdominal pain often draw their knees up and curl into a ball. Patients in severe pain sometimes lie rigidly because the discomfort is intensified by any movement.

Some patients do not like to complain of pain. As a result, they may not verbally acknowledge the existence of pain. Pallor, muscle tension (demonstrated by drawn facial muscles or clenched fists), posture, inactivity and diaphoresis may be the only outward evidence of pain in these individuals.

Other individuals may respond to pain with restlessness and increased sensitivity to stimuli in the environment, such as noise and bright lights. Some patients may demonstrate increased emotional tension, reacting irritably

Facial expression and body posture are behavioural manifestations of pain.

to people or events. They may also exhibit a change in common routines and a decrease in social interactions. When working with individuals in pain, these are all important observations which provide cues in the diagnosis and management of pain.

INFORMATION FROM OTHER HEALTH CARE TEAM MEMBERS

Pain is frequently the principal symptom that prompts people to seek medical help. A physician may have investigated the nature of the patient's pain, and the nurse can often obtain much information from the patient's physician or from notes made on the patient's record. Of particular importance are notations regarding factors that precipitate pain, since the nurse may be able to institute measures to eliminate or minimize these factors.

Sharing observations made by all members of the nursing team contributes to the completeness of the patient's pain assessment and intervention plan. All observations should be accurately reported and recorded so that all nursing personnel are aware of measures that prevent, minimize or alleviate the patient's pain, as well as factors that aggravate it.

In addition, other members of the health care team, such as the physiotherapist, often contribute information regarding a patient's pain. The physiotherapist usually assists in assessing the patient's mobility and functional ability and may be able to provide insight to nursing team members regarding activities and schedules that the patient can tolerate.

The patient's family may also be helpful in establishing the nature of the patient's pain, precipitating factors and effective relief measures. Some people minimize the severity of pain when talking to medical personnel; yet may have confided the extent of their discomfort to their spouse. Additionally, a spouse may be aware of the patient's inability to sleep or restlessness and increased irritability. Therefore, it is important to include information given by family members as part of the assessment data.

DIAGNOSING PAIN

Diagnosing pain problems presents a challenge to nurses. Pain may be a response that nurses identify and treat independently (nursing diagnosis) or a problem that nurses treat in collaboration with the physician (collaborative problem). Furthermore, pain may be an etiology of many other problems for which nurses prescribe treatment.

The nursing diagnoses for patients manifesting pain are *Pain* and *Chronic pain*. The diagnosis should include an accurate description of the type, intensity and nature of the pain as well as its cause (if known). These aspects are necessary for planning interventions to relieve pain and to minimize the effects of pain on the patient's lifestyle and daily functioning. To identify a specific pain, for example, as *Headache*, without a statement of etiology, gives no direction for selecting measures to eliminate the cause of headache. However, the diagnosis *Headache related to stressful daily living and skipping meals* tells us what interventions are necessary to alleviate the problem.

Chronic or acute pain related to medical conditions which involve nurse-prescribed and physician-prescribed interventions should be stated as collaborative problems. For example, in treating pain related to cancer, the nurse would be responsible for evaluating the pain, administering pain-relief medications, monitoring for adverse reactions to the medications, teaching patients how to self-administer pain-relief measures and assisting them in coping with necessary lifestyle modifications. The problem statement for patients such as these would be written as *Potential Complication: cancer*.

Pain is a powerful etiological factor affecting many aspects of a person's life. For example, in a postoperative patient, pain can cause impaired mobility, ineffective breathing patterns, self-care deficits, fear and anxiety, just to name a few. Patients with prolonged chronic pain may experience hopelessness, powerlessness, ineffective individual coping or altered health maintenance, all of which may be caused by the pain itself, fear of the consequences of pain or a lack of knowledge of effective relief modalities.

Thus pain is not a simple problem to diagnose. A correct diagnosis requires complete and accurate information about a patient's pain and the effects of the pain on his or her lifestyle and daily functioning. It requires collaboration with the patient and family as well as other members of the health care team.

Examples of nursing diagnoses and collabortive problems related to pain are:

- *Pain in legs related to improper positioning and use of pillows when in bed*
- *Impaired mobility related to postoperative incisional pain*
- *Altered health maintenance and hopelessness related to lack of knowledge of pain-relief measures for arthritis*
- *PC: Angina*

PLANNING PAIN-RELIEF INTERVENTIONS

Nursing actions for patients who are or may be experiencing pain are primarily directed towards protective strategies that assist patients to prevent, minimize and cope with pain. Restorative strategies focus on modifying the perception of pain by decreasing or eliminating painful stimuli. When determining appropriate pain-relief measures, the nurse uses knowledge about the patient's condition and unique reaction to pain.

Common patient goals or outcomes expected from pain-relief interventions might include:

- Patient will describe relief of pain as evidenced by a rating of 5 on a pain scale of 0 to 10.
- Patient will perform selected pain-relief measures.
- Patient will show improvement in pain as evidenced by walking to the bathroom without guarding incision.

IMPLEMENTING PAIN-RELIEF INTERVENTIONS

HEALTH PROMOTING STRATEGIES

Because pain is a protective mechanism that alerts us to potential injury or trauma in the body, no one can always be pain-free. However, there are a number of things people can do to maintain most freedom from pain in the course of daily living. For example, we know that fatigue, lack of physical fitness and a poor mental outlook will increase one's perception of pain. We also know that eating certain foods brings on headaches and stomach and bowel ailments in certain people. People can promote a pain-free existence by limiting or avoiding potential sources of pain and by maintaining a healthy lifestyle.

HEALTH PROTECTING STRATEGIES

People recover from illness better and faster when their pain is controlled and they are able to get up, move around and perform the activities of daily living for themselves. Health protecting strategies in pain management focus on measures to prevent or minimize pain and to help patients cope with their pain. For example, in some cardiac conditions, chest pain may be caused by exertion. Therefore, the nurse should know how much activity a cardiac patient can tolerate in order to avoid causing undue discomfort. It may be necessary to space nursing interventions to permit the patient to rest between activities. In some cases it may be wise to leave a patient's bath until an hour or so after breakfast, so that the patient may rest after the exertion of eating a meal.

Measures to Help Patients Tolerate and Cope with Pain

One of the most important nursing functions is the provision of psychological support for the patient in pain. Discussing the meaning of pain for the patient is one way to provide support. The nurse may find that it is not really pain that is bothering the patient but something else. The patient may be concerned about the results of surgery or about his or her ability to tolerate pain.

Knowing what to expect in the way of pain often enables a person to cope with an upcoming situation; it also removes the fear of the unknown so that anxiety is lessened. Many diagnostic and therapeutic procedures are uncomfortable or painful. It is wise to explain to the patient exactly

HEALTH PROMOTING STRATEGY

Promoting Pain-Free Health

- Obtain adequate rest and avoid fatigue.
- Avoid foods and beverages you associate with pain.
- Keep physically fit and in good condition.
- Exercise in moderation.
- Avoid sporadic episodes of strenuous exercising.

- Practise safety in the home and workplace.
- Use proper body mechanics for lifting and moving heavy objects.
- Wear a car seat belt at all times.
- Avoid stress and keep a positive, happy outlook on life.

what is going to be done, the nature of the pain that may be experienced and what the patient can do to assist. Explanation of this sort often helps change the individual's attitude towards the experience.

It is important to be honest with children. Telling them that a procedure is going to hurt a little and what the hurt will be like is preferable to telling them that it will not hurt and then inflicting pain. The latter course of action can destroy a child's sense of trust. A factual explanation of exactly what is going to happen usually eliminates fear and anxiety for both adults and children.

Reassuring patients that pain will not be beyond their level of tolerance is advisable. Assure patients that something will be done to relieve their pain. During a painful procedure, placing a hand on the patient's arm is often considered supportive. Care needs to be taken with touch, however, as some patients dislike it, particularly if they are striving to maintain their independence.

Enabling the patient to retain a measure of control over the situation can also help minimize the reaction to pain. "Tell me when it hurts and we will stop for a minute" is one way of doing this. The nurse can also involve patients in some part of the activity. Holding a piece of the equipment, for example, is an effective way to allow children to feel involved. Distraction can sometimes be used effectively in these situations. The patient is less focussed on pain when concentrating on taking deep breaths.

Be sure that the patient is settled comfortably following a painful experience. Evidence of the procedure, such as the dressing tray, should be removed as quickly as possible. Some nurses have found that encouraging the patient to talk about the experience helps put it into perspective.

HEALTH RESTORING STRATEGIES

The management of pain is based on several principles of therapy which guide all health care professionals in the development of health restoring interventions for pain. These principles were formulated in 1984 by the Expert Advisory Committee on the Management of Severe Pain in Cancer Patients, charged with preparing a Monograph on the management of cancer pain to the Minister of National Health and Welfare (1984). Nurses can also use both non-invasive and non-pharmacologic pain-relief measures as well as pharmacological measures to help patients manage pain.

ALLOW THE PATIENT TO BE IN CONTROL

The foundation of effective pain management is to allow patients to be in control. Participation and commitment to therapeutic regimens increase when patients are involved in discussions regarding treatment options.

KEY PRINCIPLES

Principles of Pain Management

1. Allow the patient to be in control.
2. Involve the whole family.
3. Utilize a team approach.
4. Use multiple modalities.
5. Acknowledge and treat secondary symptoms.

Allowing patients to be in control also requires prompt attention to requests for pain relief. Many treatment modalities are more effective when administered before pain intensity peaks. Early intervention, at the beginning of pain, often prevents a serious attack. This is important in conditions such as myocardial infarction or biliary or renal colic (stones in the bile duct or the ureter of the kidney), in which the pain can reach agonizing proportions.

INVOLVE THE WHOLE FAMILY

When any member of a family experiences pain there is disruption to the usual structure and roles and functions of the family. As well, the meaning and the expression of pain within the family is a significant variable. Therefore, it is important to involve the whole family in the treatment plan. Acute pain is often quickly relieved, allowing family functioning to return to normal. Chronic pain, however, generally has a significant and long-term effect on family behaviours.

It is important that family members be viewed as active participants in the therapeutic process. They often are able to contribute valuable information needed to complete the picture of the patient's pain experience. As well, families often develop unique methods of coping with pain, which, when shared with health care professionals, may provide insight into treatment modalities most suited to the patient. It is also important to provide family members with practical advice, aid and emotional support so that they, in turn, can support the family member in pain.

UTILIZE A TEAM APPROACH

Pain, particularly unrelenting chronic pain, is a complex experience which involves physiological and psychosocial dimensions. Consequently, pain is best managed by a comprehensive multidisciplinary team of professionals.

Pain teams may function within acute-care hospitals, ambulatory care departments or free-standing pain clinics. The team is directed by the needs of the patient in pain,

---

Members of the Pain Team

- patient and family
- family physician
- specialist/internist
- surgeon
- psychiatrist
- psychologist
- acute care nurse
- home care nurse
- palliative care nurse
- social worker
- pharmacist
- chaplain
- physiotherapist
- occupational therapist
- dietitian
- volunteers

Methods of Pain Relief

MODIFY THE DISEASE PROCESS

- Chemotherapy
- Medical Treatment
- Radiation
- Surgery

MODIFY PAIN PERCEPTION

- Application of Cold/Heat
- Distraction
- Guided Imagery/Visualization
- Hypnosis
- Massage
- Pharmacological Treatment
- Relaxation Techniques
- Therapeutic Touch

INTERRUPT PAIN TRANSMISSION

- Acupuncture
- Acupressure
- TENS (transcutaneous electrical nerve stimulation)
- Nerve Blocks
- Surgery

---

and generally concentrates on long-term methods to completely relieve or control pain. Usually these teams develop individualized programs integrating physical, cognitive and psychosocial strategies for alleviating pain. Working collaboratively, multidisciplinary pain teams ensure practical, integrated and consistent therapy for individuals in pain.

USE MULTIPLE MODALITIES

According to the gate-control theory of pain, there are several points along the nervous system where pain impulses may be modified. Therefore, effective pain management involves employing a combination of pain-relief measures. These are presented in the accompanying box.

ACKNOWLEDGE AND TREAT SECONDARY SYMPTOMS

There are a variety of secondary symptoms which, independently, may cause significant discomfort. When these symptoms are combined with another painful process, patients may have a perception of increased pain.

Control of secondary symptoms can decrease the perception of pain. For example, food can prevent or relieve the uncomfortable muscular contractions of an empty stomach. Ensuring that patients are taking sufficient fluids helps prevent the distressing effects of dehydration. The pain caused by a distended bladder and the discomfort of constipation are both preventable by specific nursing techniques (see Chapter 20 and 21). Ensuring that patients obtain sufficient rest and sleep is another important consideration.

Secondary Symptoms of Pain

- Anorexia
- Constipation
- Cough
- Dehydration
- Diarrhea
- Dyspnea
- Hiccups
- Hunger
- Incontinence
- Insomnia
- Nausea
- Vomiting
- Weakness

NON-INVASIVE AND NON-PHARMACOLOGIC PAIN-RELIEF MEASURES

The experience of pain can be lessened or relieved by modifying the perception of the pain impulse. Many strategies are available to alter the perception of pain. Nurses may independently implement a variety of non-invasive and non-pharmacologic strategies to assist patients in achieving pain relief. Some of these nursing measures are easily accomplished. For example, changing patients' position to ensure proper body alignment aids in preventing painful contractures and muscle spasm, relieves muscle strain and prevents pressure sores from developing. Consequently, patients may perceive less pain. A back rub often assists patients to relax by easing muscular tension. Removing external sources of irritation, such as loud noises or bright lights, also aids in the elimination of painful stimuli. All the comfort measures identified in Chapter 25 are useful for eliminating sources of pain.

There are many other non-invasive pain management modalities which nurses may independently employ with patients. These include cognitive strategies such as visualization, distraction, hypnosis and many relaxation techniques. According to the gate theory, these measures stimulate the activity of the thalamus and cerebral cortex to close the gating mechanism and thereby decrease the perception of pain. Massage, the application of heat or cold and therapeutic touch are physical therapies which the nurse may implement. The effective use of modalities such as hypnosis and therapeutic touch generally requires the completion of formal post-graduate education in the specific area.

APPLICATION OF HEAT OR COLD

The application of heat or cold to modify the perception of pain is a familiar strategy (see Chapter 24), and may be used with both acute and chronic pain. Muscular aches and pain are often effectively relieved by heat. Heat increases the circulation in the part of the body where it is applied. The increased circulation transports metabolic waste products (a factor in causing muscular pain) away from the painful area. Consequently, a warm bath may help to relieve aching muscles following strenuous exercise.

Cold has the opposite effect — it decreases circulation. In doing so, edema and pressure on sensory nerve endings may be reduced. Ice is frequently used to relieve edema and pain for many joint-related problems. Most athletes and arthritis sufferers are aware of the benefits of ice applied to sore and inflamed joints. Cold may also be used as a local anesthetic agent. The cold numbs the sensory nerve endings, decreasing the transmission of pain impulses. Prior to administering an injection, ice may be briefly applied to the site. The patient will experience less puncture pain due to the numbness. This technique is useful both with children and with adults who have difficulty accepting an intramuscular injection.

DISTRACTION

Distraction is a useful tool for helping alleviate both acute and chronic pain. Distraction techniques work equally well with adults and children. It simply involves diverting the patient's attention away from the sensation of pain towards other thoughts. The number of sensory impressions competing for attention produces a decreased perception of pain. Because the effectiveness of this technique is based on competing sensory impressions, it is important to involve as many of the senses as possible in these strategies. Some examples of specific techniques include the following:

1. Encourage the patient to recount a recent exciting or pleasant experience. Narrating the action of a sports event, the plot of a movie or a story may all function as distracters. Encourage the patient to relate information from all the senses: touch, taste, smell, hearing and sight. Children can be encouraged to recite rhymes, or participate in a game. The key component is active participation by the patient.

2. Music is an excellent distracter and relaxant. The type of music selected is crucial to the effectiveness of this method. Therefore, the patient needs to select music based on personal preference. For example, older adults may prefer music from the time when they were growing up, or music that reminds the patient of a happy time (McCaffery and Beebe, 1989).

    Encourage the patient to actively listen. Have the patient close the eyes, concentrate on the music, and tap out the rhythm of the music.

3. Participating in rhythmic singing is also an effective distracter. Chants, hymns or simple songs with a strong beat are good to use with both adults and children. Adults are usually more self-conscious than children, however, and often prefer to mouth the words silently. Tapping the foot or fingers for emphasis is an additional distracter that can be used with this technique.

4. Teach the patient rhythmic breathing exercises. The patient may do these exercise with eyes closed, or by focussing intently on an object. Breathing is to be deep and slow, preferably from the abdomen. The patient focusses on the breath and silently repeats "In, 2, 3, 4 — Out, 2, 3, 4."

    Another rhythmic breathing technique is a form of Yoga breathing known as the Alternate Nostril Breath (see box on page 845). Frequent practice of this technique promotes the patient's ability to use the technique beneficially. This method of breathing may not be useful with patients experiencing severe or acute pain.

Another technique, especially useful with children, is blowing bubbles using, for example, a straw in a glass of water.

5. Encourage the patient to reminisce. This is an especially useful technique with older adults. Encourage the patient to remember and articulate a happy or pleasant time. Or have the patient imagine that he or she is standing at the front door of a childhood home. Have the patient describe everything that can be seen while standing in front of the door. Encourage use of all senses. Ask the patient to imagine opening the door and walking down the street. Again, have the patient tell you everything that is seen, heard or felt.

VISUALIZATION

Visualization is a form of distraction that uses images to modify the perception of pain and decrease the intensity of the pain experience. This technique is a useful strategy with all age groups; practising it for approximately 20 minutes, two to three times a day, will improve the effectiveness of the images. One common method of visualization is guided imagery.

The following steps provide a guideline for implementing imagery. Until the technique is learned by the patient, it is necessary for the nurse to spend time guiding the patient through the process.

1. Identify the focus of the imagery. The patient needs to be clear about the problem that will be the focus of attention. Is it a headache, stomach pain or a backache?

2. Create a relaxed environment. It is advantageous to darken the room and remove any sources of distraction.

3. Encourage the patient to relax using rhythmic breathing. Spend a few minutes simply relaxing. It is helpful at this point to have the patient visualize a safe and comfortable place.

The Alternate Nostril Breath

I. BENEFITS:

The Alternate Nostril Breath

- has a marvellously calming effect on the nervous system
- helps overcome insomnia
- relaxes and refreshes the body
- purifies the bloodstream and aerates the lungs
- soothes headaches
- improves digestion and appetite
- helps free the mind of anxiety and depression.

II. TECHNIQUE:

1. Sit in a comfortable position, back straight.
2. Raise your *right* hand and place your ring finger against your *left* nostril, closing it off (Figure 26.5 A).
3. Inhale deeply and slowly through the *right* nostril to the count of 4.
4. Close off the *right* nostril with your thumb and retain the breath for a count of 1–4 seconds (Figure 26.5 B).
5. Open the *left* nostril and exhale for a count of 4–8 seconds. The longer you make the exhalation, the better. Concentrate on completely emptying the lungs.
6. Breathe in through the same nostril (the *left*) to the count of 4.

7. Close off the nostril with the ring finger again and hold to the count of 1–4 seconds.
8. Exhale through the *right* nostril to the count of 4–8 seconds. This makes one cycle.
9. Repeat five cycles of alternate nostril breathing, or up to ten minutes if you are concerned about insomnia.
10. Practise a ratio of 4:4:8, if at all possible. Increase this to 8:4:8 eventually, then 8:8:8, after some months.

III. DO'S AND DON'TS:

- *Do not* push yourself by maintaining the holding position too long, or by increasing the ratio until you are comfortable doing so.
- *Do* make the breathing rhythmic, smooth and slow. You can work on making it inaudible slowly.
- *Do* practise the Alternate Nostril Breath whenever you need calming — if you are nervous, upset or irritable.

  The importance of this particular breath cannot be overemphasized. The body and mind are closely interrelated and one influences the other to a much greater extent than Western medicine acknowledged for many years. As an all-round "soother" the Alternate Nostril Breath is incomparable.

SOURCE: Zebroff, K. (1971). *The ABC of Yoga*. Vancouver, BC: Fforbez Enterprises, Ltd. Reproduced with permission.

FIGURE 26.5   The alternate nostril breath
A. Step 2 B. Step 4

4. Ask the patient to visualize an image that represents the pain. A tight headband around the forehead for a headache. Knotted ropes may indicate muscular pain. A mound of cold and rough cement may indicate back pain. It is important that this image is identified by the patient. Try not to suggest images, but allow the patient to find an image that represents his or her pain.

5. Have the patient visualize an image that represents relieving the pain. The headband loosening, the ropes untangling, the cement being smoothed out like glass. Once the headband is loose and the ropes are untangled, the patient should focus on this image for a few minutes.

6. Have the patient imagine the positive effects of less pain. The patient visualizes him- or herself as being dynamic, energetic and in good health (Dossey, 1991; Saxon, 1991).

Guided imagery is also an effective technique with children. An imaginary "magic glove" or "magic blanket" may be put in place before a painful procedure such as an intravenous injection (Kachoyeanos and Friedhoff, 1993). The child's perception of pain is lessened by imagining that the magic glove or blanket is protecting him or her during the procedure.

HYPNOSIS

The clinical application of hypnosis is usually executed by a registered hypnotherapist. This technique works with all age groups. Hypnosis is an altered state of consciousness during which the patient is sensitive to suggestion. Even though the patient may be in a suggestible state, the patient remains in control, and will not perform any action that is incompatible with personal beliefs or values. Many patients with chronic pain use self-hypnosis as one method of achieving pain relief.

A hypnosis-like technique that may be used with some patients is conscious suggestion. This technique involves achieving deep relaxation, and then listening to or giving oneself positive suggestions. When patients are first learning this technique, suggestions may be given by the nurse. Begin by having the patient perform rhythmic breathing. It is helpful for the patient to visualize a safe place at home or in natural surroundings. Allow the patient a few minutes to simply relax; then in a calm, soothing voice offer the patient positive suggestions of well-being or of decreased sensations of pain.

MASSAGE

Massage has had a long history of use in the treatment of muscular pain. The effect of massage is similar to heat in that circulation and removal of cellular waste products is enhanced. The gate control theory of pain suggests that massage stimulates the large A-beta and A delta fibres which cause closure of the gating mechanism to pain impulses.

When it is impossible to reach a painful area — a limb in a cast, for example, or an area covered by a dressing that cannot be removed — the skin in an opposite area can be stimulated (contralateral stimulation). This may provide some relief in the painful area.

Massage is a valuable technique for reducing anxiety and promoting relaxation. The muscular relaxation generated by massage may promote decreased sensations of pain for many hours. This technique is also an excellent modality for promoting family involvement. Family members may actively participate in care by massaging a patient's back, hands or feet.

RELAXATION TECHNIQUES

As we discussed earlier in the chapter, anxiety and fear are contributing factors in pain and may intensify an individual's reaction to pain. Successful reduction of anxiety and fear will assist the individual to feel more comfortable and experience a decreased perception of pain. Some techniques that may be used for relaxation include biofeedback techniques, meditation, rhythmic breathing exercise and yoga.

Biofeedback techniques   Biofeedback is useful for individuals with chronic pain. In biofeedback, individuals learn to control nonconscious physiological responses such as blood pressure and muscle tension through the use of mental images and thought processes. Biofeedback techniques require training with the use of special monitoring equipment that measures nonconscious events and feeds information back to the person in the form of varying tones or meter readings. With practice, people develop mental strategies to control the nonconscious processes enough to promote relaxation and relieve problems such as high blood pressure and tension headaches.

Meditation   Meditation is also a useful relaxation technique for patients with acute or chronic pain. Prior to beginning the meditation, the patient selects a soothing word, such as *relax* or *calm*. The patient begins by performing slow rhythmic breathing and imagining a safe place. The patient may wish to close the eyes or leave them open and focus on an object. With every breath in, the patient silently says the word that was chosen. Frequent practice facilitates the effectiveness of this technique.

Rhythmic breathing exercises   Rhythmic breathing, which we discussed in the section on distraction, can also be used on its own for relaxation. Slow deep breathing is a powerful technique for promoting relaxation. Patients can participate in this method of relaxation whenever they are feeling uncomfortable and anxious.

Therapeutic touch   Therapeutic touch is a method of directing energy through the hands. The technique of therapeutic touch involves internally centring yourself and consciously focussing on the intent to assist a person in pain. Practitioners assess the patient's energy field by passing their hands over the individual, just above the body. Areas that feel warm or cool, or stimulate pins and needle sensations in the practitioner, are areas of energy congestion, blockage or depletion. Through a technique known as *unruffling the field*, the practitioner smoothes the patient's energy field (Brown, 1993; Krieger, 1979).

The technique of unruffling produces a relaxation response and a perception of pain relief. Therapeutic touch has been used effectively with acute and chronic pain. This technique is easy to learn, but requires some formal education to be completed by the nurse.

PHARMACOLOGICAL PAIN-RELIEF MEASURES

The administration of medication continues to be a major focus in pain management. There are various categories of

KEY PRINCIPLES

Principles of Analgesic Administration

- Use the oral route whenever possible.
- Use only one medication for pain relief.
- Administer the medication regularly (around the clock).
- Individualize the dose.
- Use adjuvant medications to enhance analgesia.
- Treat tolerance appropriately.
- Use modalities other than just opioids.
- Do not use placebos.

drugs available for pain relief including opioids, such as morphine and codeine, and agonists/antagonists, such as pentazocine. Opioids and agonists/antagonists are commonly referred to as narcotic analgesics. Other categories of medication include non-narcotic pain relievers, of which aspirin is the most common agent; nonsteroidal anti-inflammatory drugs (NSAID); and some tranquilizers. Pain-relief medications are given by oral, subcutaneous, intramuscular, intravenous, rectal, epidural and intrathecal routes. The administration of medication and the observation of patients' responses to medication are within the purview of the nurse. As members of health care and pain teams, nurses need to be aware of the principles that guide decision making regarding analgesic administration.

Nurses have a crucial responsibility in the administration of analgesics. They must understand the actions and effects of the drugs being administered in order to ensure that patients are achieving maximum pain relief. They must also understand how the different routes of delivery may alter or enhance the outcome of medications administered. The timing of administration is very important. Prescriptions may be written for analgesics to be given every four hours or at other specified times (as is frequently the case with patients who have arthritic and rheumatic disorders). In most instances, however, the orders are written *prn* (an abbreviation for *pro re nata*, the Latin phrase meaning "as needed"). Nurses must judge the most suitable time of administration and the interval between doses. Medications for pain relief are most effective when given regularly, around the clock, because it is easier to prevent pain than to control pain. This is true even for the postoperative patient receiving intramuscular analgesics. The different categories of pharmacological agents used for pain relief are summarized in Table 26.1 and outlined in the text below.

TABLE 26.1 Categories of Drugs for Pain Management

MEDICATION	ACTION	USES	ROUTE	SIDE EFFECTS	TOXIC EFFECTS
Opioids	Alter pain perception by binding to opiate receptors within the CNS	Treatment of moderate to severe pain Used for acute and / or chronic pain Primarily used to treat visceral pain	PO SC IM IV *PR *epi *inth	nausea vomiting constipation pruritis sedation or drowsiness hypotension urinary retention	Respiratory depression (usually relieved with Narcan)
Agonist/ Antagonists	Produce a narcotic effect, but in the presence of a true narcotic will counteract the effect of the narcotic	Used for patients unable to tolerate true narcotic analgesics	PO IM IV	drowsiness nausea psychotomimetic effects such as hallucinations or euphoria	
Non-narcotics	Act at the peripheral level by inhibiting the release of prostaglandins	Used alone for mild to moderate pain May be used as an adjuvant for severe and persistent pain	PO *top	hepatotoxicity gastric irritation ASA use inhibits platelet formation	tinnitus with ASA
NSAIDs	Act at the peripheral level by inhibiting the release of prostaglandins Have a ceiling effect—reach a point where increasing the dose does not have an effect Have analgesic, antipyretic, antiplatelet and anti-inflammatory effects	Used alone for pain due to inflammation May be used as an adjuvant for severe and persistent pain Especially effective for metastatic bone pain	PO IM PR	GI upset and irritation May prolong coagulation time Hepatotoxicity	GI bleeding

*PR = per rectum
*epi = epidural
*top = topical
*inth = intrathecal

Indications for Using Opioids

- Moderate to severe acute pain
- Moderate to severe chronic pain
- When immediate pain relief is required

Opioids

Opioids are drugs which bind to opiate receptors in the central nervous system and inhibit or alter the transmission of pain impulses. Codeine, hydromorphone, levorphanol, methadone and morphine are examples of opioids. These medications all produce similar outcomes. All are effective analgesics, and may produce side effects such as sedation, nausea and vomiting, and constipation (see the accompanying box on coping with the side effects of opioids). There is also a possibility of toxicity which usually manifests as respiratory depression. Morphine tends to be the most frequently used of the opioids, likely because it is effective for both acute and chronic pain, and because it can be administered in any form.

While opioids are effective analgesics there is often a reluctance to use these drugs. The concern generally expressed by physicians and nurses relates to addiction and toxicity. Physicians are reluctant to prescribe opioids in adequate dosages and nurses are hesitant to administer these drugs in adequate amounts regularly, fearing that patients will experience toxic reactions or become dependent on the drugs. To use these drugs effectively, then, the health care professional must have an understanding of the effects of therapeutic opioid drug use. This understanding begins with knowing the meanings of the terms *addiction*, *dependence*, and *tolerance*.

Addiction refers to the psychological need to use drugs for other than medical reasons such as pain relief. The addicted individual exhibits compulsive drug use and craving for the opioid. **Dependence** is the state in which the individual experiences symptoms of withdrawal which occur when the drug is abruptly discontinued. Signs of physical withdrawal may include anxiety, irritability, chills, diaphoresis, nausea, vomiting, abdominal cramps and occasionally seizures. **Tolerance** occurs when there is a need to increase the dose of the drug in order to achieve the same effect that a smaller dose originally gave. Tolerance does not suggest psychological dependence (American Pain Society, 1988).

Any individual receiving opioids for a week or more may develop physical dependence and tolerance. However, this does not imply addiction. Behaviours such as clock-watching and frequently requesting medication may be interpreted as addictive behaviours, but it is more likely that such a patient is experiencing inadequate pain relief due to tolerance. A patient experiencing tolerance requires an increased medication dose in order to maintain an effec-

Coping with the Side Effects of Opioids*

CONSTIPATION

- Stool softeners are a must with opioid therapy. Patients using opioids tend to become constipated.
- Monitor and record bowel movements.
- Encourage fluids — at least eight glasses of water a day.
- Include high-fibre foods in the diet.

SEDATION

- All patients will experience sedation during the initial three to five days. This is normal, and the patient will develop tolerance to this effect.
- If the patient remains persistently sedated, drowsy or confused, the dose may have to be decreased, or another opioid tried.

NAUSEA AND VOMITING

- This is often the most distressing side effect for patients. If it persists the opioid dose may need to be reduced. An antiemetic may also be necessary.
- Encourage the patient to eat cold foods and avoid foods with strong smells.

---

*Remember that not only analgesics cause these symptoms. Assess all patients carefully and thoroughly.

---

tive state of analgesia. Any symptoms of physical withdrawal can be minimized by decreasing the dosage slowly when the medication is no longer required.

Children can safely be administered opioids. Those twelve years of age and older are often able to tolerate an adult dose of medication. Children between the ages of seven and twelve usually require about half an adult dose. Youngsters between the ages of two and six years need about a quarter of an adult dose for effective pain relief. Children younger than two years generally require the medication dosage to be adjusted according to body weight (American Pain Society, 1988). Older adults may also safely use opioids, but due to slower excretion of the drug, may require a reduced dose.

Agonists/Antagonists

Examples of these drugs include pentazocine, buprenorphine and butorphanol. These narcotic analgesics also interact with the opiate receptor sites within the central nervous system to alter the perception of pain. It is important to note that agonists/antagonists, such as pentazocine, may inhibit the effectiveness of pure agonists or opiates, causing ineffective analgesia.

Non-narcotic Pain Relievers

Analgesic–antipyretic medications are the primary non-narcotic pain relievers. These agents block the transmission of pain impulses at the peripheral level, by interfering with the production of prostaglandin. Aspirin is used extensively for the relief of mild to moderate pain and is an example of a non-narcotic analgesic. Non-narcotics are often used in conjunction with narcotics. Because one group of drugs acts on the central nervous system and the other acts peripherally, the combination strikes the pain at two levels. When this type of combination is effective, analgesia is often achieved using less narcotic.

Nonsteroidal Anti-inflammatory Drugs (NSAIDs)

Medication in this category acts similarly to non-narcotic analgesics. The action occurs peripherally through inhibition of the prostaglandin system. Generally, the effects of NSAIDs include analgesic, anti-inflammatory, antipyretic and anticoagulant properties. Ibuprofen, indomethacin and naproxen are examples of drugs in this group. While all medication within this classification may have similar properties, each drug has a unique monograph. That is, not all NSAIDs affect the same degree of each property. Consequently, patients may need to try several drugs in this group before finding one that is effective. It may also be necessary to carefully titrate the medication dose for each individual. NSAIDs may be used in conjunction with opioids and antagonists to facilitate analgesia.

METHODS OF MEDICATION ADMINISTRATION

There are numerous methods for administering medications. The preferred route for the administration of analgesic medication is oral. The oral route is considered to be effective and the least invasive of all routes. However, there are a variety of conditions, such as nausea and vomiting or gastrointestinal obstruction, which prevent patients from swallowing or absorbing medication taken orally. The conventional alternative method for the delivery of analgesia is via intramuscular or intravenous routes.

Intramuscular Injections

The administration of medication via the intramuscular injection is a familiar strategy. It is often the route of choice for patients unable to swallow. However, some difficulties

do exist with this method. There is frequently a significant lapse of time between the administration of an analgesic and the initial request for it. After the analgesic has been requested, the patient must wait for the nurse to obtain the narcotic keys, sign for the medication and prepare the injection. During this time, the patient's pain and anxiety are likely to increase.

The actual administration of the medication may also create some difficulties. Many patients dislike the puncture pain of injections. Also, many nurses attempt to reduce puncture pain by using shorter needles, with the result that, in effect, the medication is delivered subcutaneously. Because subcutaneous tissue has less blood supply than muscle, the rate of medication absorption may be slowed, thus prolonging the onset of relief from pain. Even when medications are delivered quickly and into the appropriate muscle, absorption may be erratic, depending on the age and weight of the individual and on previous use of analgesics.

It is difficult to maintain pain control using the intramuscular route. The time lapse between the request for and the administration of an analgesic promotes the development

When giving an analgesic by intramuscular injection...

- When giving an IM analgesic, identify the site carefully and insert the needle quickly and smoothly. The faster the needle is inserted the less puncture pain.
- Inject the analgesic slowly to avoid creating pressure in the muscle.
- Withdraw the needle rapidly and smoothly.
- Gently massage the muscle once the needle has been removed. This brings blood to the area and aids in dispersing the analgesic and in increasing absorption. Gentle exercise will produce a similar effect. So wiggling the toes after an injection in the gluteal muscle is a good idea.

Does size really matter?

- Many analgesics are administered via intramuscular injection, and needle size *does* make a difference.
- Most adult patients require intramuscular analgesic administration with a $1\frac{1}{2}$-inch needle. Using a 1-inch needle frequently results in the analgesic being injected into subcutaneous fat rather than muscle. Because there is less blood supply in subcutaneous fat, the analgesic is absorbed slowly and often incompletely. Therefore, patients do not experience effective pain relief.

of peaks and troughs. The patient is likely to be feeling uncomfortable at the time of the initial request. By the time the medication is administered and absorbed, the degree of pain control will have probably decreased significantly. The sudden rise in the blood level of the narcotic analgesic is likely to precipitate observable side or toxic effects. Sedation and possibly respiratory depression are more likely to occur because of the sudden peak of medication in the patient's system.

Attempts to overcome inadequate pain control with intramuscular injections for both acute and chronic pain have led to the development of innovative methods for delivering analgesics. These methods include subcutaneous infusions, sophisticated methods of intravenous injection and epidural and intrathecal medication administration.

Continuous Subcutaneous Infusion (CSCI)

Continuous subcutaneous infusions provide an effective means of achieving pain control for patients who may not be able to tolerate oral analgesics, or for whom oral analgesics are ineffective. However, CSCI is not an acceptable means of analgesic administration for all patients. Patients experiencing pain due to nerve damage, or patients with intermittent acute pain, do not achieve effective analgesia with this method. This modality is also not as effective for severe pain. The other important consideration when selecting patients for this therapy is the amount of subcutaneous tissue. Emaciated patients have too little subcutaneous tissue for satisfactory absorption of the medication.

This therapy does, however, have some significant advantages. The frequency of injections is decreased, and the lightweight portable pumps do not affect mobility. The system is easy to maintain in a home environment. As well, side effects are less frequent and severe because a smaller dose of opioid is administered. This method also avoids the peak and trough levels observed with intramuscular injections (Poniatowski, 1991).

To begin treatment with CSCI, the 24-hour dose is calculated and the correct concentration of narcotic is diluted and added to the pump reservoir. The pump is then programmed to infuse the medication at a rate of 1 to 2 ml/hour. A rate greater than this tends to cause irritation at the site. A 25 or 27 gauge needle is inserted into subcutaneous tissue usually in the anterior chest, abdomen or thighs. The site is covered with a transparent occlusive dressing. The infusion is begun and peak effect is usually achieved within 30 to 120 minutes (Poniatowski, 1991).

Assessment and evaluation of the effectiveness of this technique proceeds as with any other pain treatment. The site requires routine monitoring every four to six hours for pain, redness, edema and leakage. Sites require changing every three to seven days (Logan and Fothergill-Bourbonnais, 1991). The pump is checked routinely to en-

---

Rescue Orders

- Any patient receiving opioids for pain, using any method other than IM injections, requires a rescue order.
- A rescue order is a medication order of the same drug that the patient is receiving.
- The rescue order is used when the patient begins to experience breakthrough pain.

---

sure accurate medication delivery. Evaluation of the effectiveness of treatment occurs by assessing the patient's level of pain and reaction to the opioid being administered. Side effects are noted and treated appropriately.

Patients and families discharged home with this modality require teaching about the type of medication and what to expect regarding side effects. Information about assessing the site and pump is also necessary. As well, the patient and family need to know how to contact resources for problem-solving assistance at any time during a 24-hour period. Patients and families are encouraged to maintain a comfort record so that the effectiveness of the medication dose can be assessed.

Intravenous Delivery Systems

Traditionally, the intravenous method of delivering analgesics was reserved for terminally ill patients. Continuous morphine infusions were only for the dying. However, continuous opioid infusions often require as long as 15 hours to reach a therapeutic level of analgesia (Lubenow and Ivankovich, 1991). To combat the ineffectiveness of this route an innovative intravenous technique known as *patient-controlled analgesia* (PCA) has been developed. Patient-controlled analgesia may not completely relieve pain but it allows the patient to remain in control of his or her pain-relief needs. Published research indicates that patients on the PCA system use less narcotic and experience fewer side effects than do patients who receive conventional intermittent intramuscular injections of narcotics (Fleming and Coombs, 1992; Ryder, 1991; St. Marie, 1991).

Patient-controlled analgesia is administered intravenously through an indwelling catheter by use of a special electronically controlled infusion pump which contains a timing device. Many of the pumps are small and portable allowing the patient freedom of movement. The PCA pump permits patients to self-administer, on a demand basis, predetermined doses of narcotic analgesics within prescribed time intervals to maintain a more stable serum level of analgesia.

There are two types of PCA administration: continuous narcotic infustion with bolus injections or bolus injec-

Patient-controlled analgesia allows patients to self-administer doses of analgesia as needed.

doses are administered within a prescribed time interval and prevents the patient from administering a second dose before the first has had time to take effect.

The continuous narcotic infusion with bolus injections is a method of PCA which delivers a maintenance dose of narcotic continuously, yet allows patients to self-administer bolus doses as patients feel they are needed. This method is beneficial for postoperative patients and for patients with chronic pain. It has "the advantage of maintaining analgesia while a patient is sleeping and minimizes the problem of patients being awakened by sharp, unrelenting pain" (Lubenow and Ivankovich, 1991, 38). When a continuous infusion with bolus injections is used, the rate of infusion (called the basal rate) is set to deliver a low dose of medication continuously. This is similar to any IV infusion controlled by a pump. However, the patient may also self-administer bolus doses as described previously.

There are a number of safety features within the PCA system. The amount of medication that the patient can administer, as prescribed by the physician, is set and locked into the pump controls. All pumps have a "lock-out" feature which prevents overdosage. The patient presses the button to administer the medication but the pump will only administer the programmed amount. Once the programmed amount is used up, the patient must wait a set amount of time before the next bolus can be administered. Also, many pumps have a four-hour maximum that prevents the patient from administering more than a preset total during a four-hour period.

Effective use of PCA requires that patients be cognitively aware, physically able and psychologically willing to participate in their treatment. This modality is feasible with all age groups, though it is generally suggested that children be at least seven years of age (St. Marie, 1991). PCA is a valuable therapy for patients with acute intermittent pain, acute constant pain or chronic pain. PCA may be effectively used for chemically dependent patients but the amount of medication may have to be increased in order to achieve pain control.

Patient teaching is critical for this group. The patient must understand the reason for the type of medication being administered. It is important that the patient feel comfortable with this modality. All questions need to be honestly answered. A working knowledge of the pump, the control button and safety features is essential. The patient needs to be confident that inadvertent overdosage cannot occur.

Assessment and evaluation of the patient's response to patient-controlled analgesia are crucial for safe care. A flowsheet indicating sedation level, pain control and respiratory rate is usually maintained. If the agency does not use a flowsheet, the nurse enters these assessment parameters in the nurses' notes. Any side effects that are noted and treated are recorded.

tions only. In patient-controlled analgesia, a *bolus injection* refers to an intermittent small dose of narcotic that the patient self-administers on demand. Solitary bolus injections, without continuous narcotic infusion, are generally used for acute intermittent pain such as the pain related to passing a kidney stone. The nurse programs the pump to deliver the prescribed analgesic dose. When pain is felt, the patient administers a bolus injection, for example, 1 to 2 mg of morphine sulfate, into the intravenous catheter by pressing a control button. The timer ensures that repeat

---

Patient-Controlled Analgesia Terms and Definitions

- *On-demand dose*: a predetermined amount of narcotic delivered with the system is activated as necessary.
- *Lockout interval*: the delay time during which no additional medication can be administered.
- *Basal rate*: the rate of low-dose continuous infusion.
- *Attempts*: the number of times the patient attempts an on-demand dose. The difference between successful attempts and the number of attempts before pain relief is achieved is an indication of pain control. Frequent unsuccessful attempts may indicate that pain is out of control.

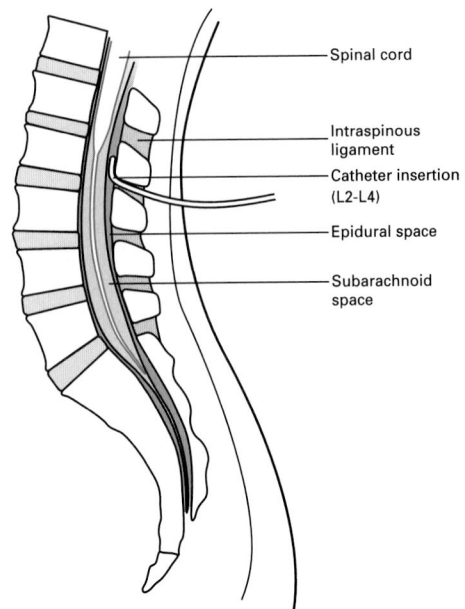

- Spinal cord
- Intraspinous ligament
- Catheter insertion (L2-L4)
- Epidural space
- Subarachnoid space

FIGURE 26.6   Epidural analgesia

Epidural and Intrathecal Medication Administration

Epidural analgesia has become an accepted method of analgesic delivery for postoperative patients. An external catheter with a bacterial filter attached to the distal end is inserted by an anesthesiologist, into the potential space between the dura mater and the spinal cord (see Figure 26.6). This space is composed of fat, connective tissue and a network of thin-walled veins (St. Marie, 1991). Opioids, administered by a physician into the epidural space, bind to opiate receptor sites on the dorsal horns of the spinal cord. Generally patients who receive analgesics in this manner require less opioid and experience fewer side and toxic effects (Faut-Callahan, 1991; Paice and Magolan, 1991; Woodin, 1993).

The effect of an epidural injection may last from 8 to 24 hours. Patients often experience fewer side effects than they do with IM injections. Consequently, they are able to perform deep breathing and coughing exercises and to mobilize with ease. There are some disadvantages to this method of medication delivery, however. The medication must be administered by a physician, and the catheter may kink or migrate into the subarachnoid space, resulting in a loss of effective pain control.

Nurses caring for patients receiving epidural analgesia must check the insertion site frequently, at least every four hours. The site is assessed for redness, warmth, edema and leakage. The patient's level of pain is assessed to determine the effectiveness of the analgesic. Agency policy usually dictates the frequency of monitoring respirations. Generally respirations are monitored hourly for at least the first 24

hours. All vital signs are assessed every four hours. An increased temperature may indicate the beginning of infection and hypotension may occur due to vasodilation. Patients should be encouraged to move from a lying to a sitting or standing position slowly and with assistance. The effect of the opioid on nerves innervating the bladder may lead to retention, so patients need to be assessed for urinary retention at least every four hours. The physician must be informed of side effects such as nausea and vomiting or pruritis so that appropriate action may be taken.

Opioids may be administered by bolus or pump-controlled continuous infusion. Continuous infusions may be used for postoperative patients with severe pain or for patients experiencing chronic pain. In long-term management, a port and catheter may be implanted to decrease the risk of infection. Because epidural analgesics may not totally alleviate patients' pain, the use of systemic opioids and/or adjuvant drugs may still be necessary.

Implanted ports are generally used for the administration of **intrathecal analgesia** (medication injected into the subarachnoid space). A small reservoir is implanted and a catheter is tunnelled directly to the intrathecal space (see Figure 26.7). The intrathecal space contains circulating CSF and is located between the subarachnoid and pia membranes (Paice and Magolan, 1991). Accessing the implanted port in home use is often difficult. Because the reservoirs tend to be implanted in the back, the assistance of a willing family member is necessary for the patient to be maintained at home with this treatment.

Intrathecal opioids behave is a manner similar to opioids administered epidurally. The drug binds to opiate receptors within the central nervous system and alters the transmission of the pain impulse. With intrathecal opioids, as with epidural opioids, patients experience fewer side effects. Patients are, therefore, able to mobilize and perform pulmonary hygiene exercises comfortably.

The monitoring of patients receiving intrathecal opioids is similar to that for patients receiving epidural medication. However, temperature must be observed more

---

SAFETY MEASURES WHEN GIVING OPIOIDS

- ANY PATIENT RECEIVING AN OPIOID MUST HAVE RESPIRATIONS MONITORED FREQUENTLY
- A RESPIRATORY RATE OF LESS THAN 10/MINUTE REQUIRES IMMEDIATE ACTION
  - NOTIFY THE APPROPRIATE PHYSICIAN
  - BE SURE THAT NALOXONE IS AVAILABLE

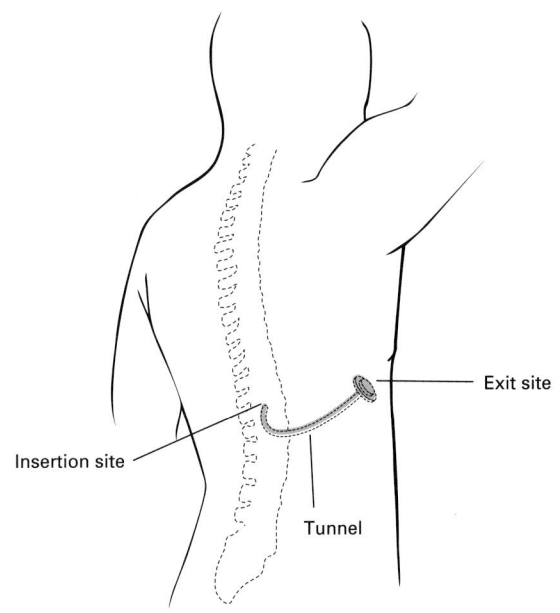

FIGURE 26.7 Implanted port for intrathecal medication

frequently with these patients, due to the possibility of developing meningitis. Table 26.2 gives a summary of care for patients receiving intrathecal analgesics.

EVALUATING PAIN-RELIEF INTERVENTIONS

All therapeutic modalities must be evaluated for effectiveness. A key nursing responsibility is to evaluate the effectiveness of any intervention. This is especially important when evaluating pain management regimes. The patient's level of comfort requires continual monitoring. Initially the patient's comfort level is assessed every two to four hours when a new modality, or a change in pain management, is implemented. The following questions suggest some of the ways pain management interventions might be evaluated.

1. Does the patient verbally indicate increased comfort? Has the pain disappeared or lessened in intensity?

2. Does the patient appear more comfortable; that is, is the patient more relaxed or less restless and irritable?

TABLE 26.2 Nursing Care Guidelines for Patients Receiving Intrathecal Analgesics

PROBLEM	NURSING INTERVENTION
Incomplete Pain Management	• Assess pain level every 4 hours • Notify appropriate physician if patient experiencing pain
Hypotension	• Monitor and assess BP at least every 4 hours • Notify appropriate physician if systolic BP < 100 • Hypotensive patient to remain flat in bed with head elevated on one pillow • If physician approves patient may be up with assistance
Nausea and Vomiting	• Notify appropriate physician and administer antiemetic if ordered
Pruritis	• Keep patient cool and dry • Notify appropriate physician and administer antihistamine or naloxone if ordered
Urinary Retention	• Assess bladder and voiding every 4 hours • Catheterize if necessary
Fever	• Monitor temperature at least every 4 hours • Assess insertion site for redness, swelling, edema and leakage • Notify appropriate physician if dressing non-occlusive or wet • Assess for signs of meningitis
Respiratory Depression	• Monitor respirations hourly for first 24 hours • A respiratory rate of < 10/minute requires prompt attention • Notify appropriate physician and have naloxone available

*Many agencies have developed assessment parameters for patients receiving intrathecal analgesics.

3. Has the patient been able to get to sleep without difficulty, or to rest quietly?
4. Is the patient able to enjoy his or her usual activities?

OTHER PAIN-RELIEF INTERVENTIONS

Methods to alter the disease process or interrupt the transmission of the pain impulse tend to involve specialized techniques. These procedures are often performed by specialized practitioners. They include modalities such as surgery, chemotherapy, radiation, acupressure, acupuncture, transcutaneous electrical nerve stimulation (TENS) and nerve blocks.

Surgery, chemotherapy and radiation therapy are within the realm of the physician. The physician attempts to decrease pain by interfering with the disease process. Surgery may also be performed to interrupt pain impulse transmission. For example, rhizotomy (resection of dorsal nerve root) may be performed to relieve intractable pain. Physicians may also try to interrupt the pain impulse using a nerve block, in which a small amount of anesthetic is injected along the course of the nerve innervating the painful area.

Acupressure, acupuncture and TENS are effective adjuvant modalities, usually performed by practitioners skilled in the specific areas. Acupuncture has, for centuries, been used in China for the treatment of various disorders, for the relief of pain and for surgical anesthesia. During the past few years it has attracted the attention of Western medicine and is now being used as an alternative method of treating pain.

Acupuncture

The acupuncture technique consists of inserting long, fine needles into particular areas of the body. The peripheral needle placement sites are associated with specific internal organs of the body. The needles are inserted with a continuous twirling motion. Additional heat in the area may be generated by applying moxa to the skin or to the needle.

The physiological mechanisms involved in the relief of pain by acupuncture are not fully understood. However, the gate-control theory suggests that stimulation of particular nerves or tissues by acupuncture needles results in increased input to the gate-control mechanism, causing the gate to close and interrupt the pain impulses from selected areas of the body.

Acupressure Acupressure works on the same principles as acupuncture. However, in this case, pressure is applied to specific peripheral points, without the use of needles. Pressure is applied with the hands, elbows and knees, depending on the point to be stimulated. These techniques may be used effectively for both acute and chronic pain.

Transcutaneous Electrical Nerve Stimulation (TENS)

Transcutaneous electrical nerve stimulation is an effective adjuvant therapy for pain relief that can be used with all age groups. There are two common types of TENS — CTENS (conventional TENS) and ALTENS (acupuncture-like TENS). CTENS interrupts the transmission of pain impulses by stimulating peripheral nerve fibres with low-voltage electrical impulses, causing the gating mechanism to close. It is suggested that stimulation of peripheral fibres by ALTENS initiates the release of endorphins (Finlay, 1992).

Transcutaneous electrical nerve stimulation is usually applied by physiotherapists, but nurses may need to assist patients with therapy during the evening and night. CTENS involves the placement of two to four small electrodes around the painful area. The electrical impulse is adjusted for comfort. Stimulation of the area needs to be strong enough to induce numbness, but not so intense as to induce spasm. The effect of CTENS may decrease over time as peripheral fibres accommodate. The unit may be turned off, or the intensity increased for a few minutes to promote neural excitability (Finlay, 1992).

Acupuncture-like TENS electrodes are positioned over muscle motor points. The objective is to produce nonpainful, rhythmic, muscular contractions. ALTENS treatments are usually administered twice a day for 20 to 45 minutes (Finlay, 1992).

Most patients are able to monitor TENS independently. Children may require more supervision. Nursing care for individuals using TENS involves assessing the skin for reactions to the conductive jelly or to the electrodes. Dermatitis requires that electrode positions be altered. Patients cannot shower or bath with the units (Finlay, 1992).

SPECIAL SITUATIONS

While the general principles of pain management apply to all situations, there are some circumstances which deserve special consideration. Caring for the surgical patient, the drug dependent patient and the cognitively impaired adult in pain are three such situations.

CARING FOR THE SURGICAL PATIENT

Postoperative pain may be the result of more than just the surgical incision or wound itself. There may also be pain due to the effect of the anesthetic drugs and to the position of the patient during surgery. It is therefore important that all the patient's statements about pain be acknowledged and considered when developing and implementing

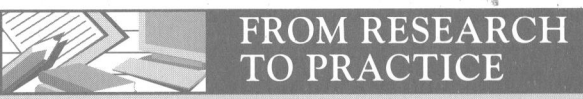

FROM RESEARCH TO PRACTICE

Puntillo, K. and Weiss, S. J. (1994). Pain: Its mediators and associated morbidity in critically ill cardiovascular surgical patients. *Nursing Research, 43*(1), 31-35.

This study explored the effects of age, sex, personality adjustment and analgesic administration on the extent of pain experienced by patients during the first few days following cardiac and abdominal vascular surgery. It also examined the relationship between pain magnitude and postoperative complications. The sample consisted of 60 cardiac patients (44 male, 16 female) and 14 abdominal vascular patients (13 male, 1 female). The mean age was 64 with a range of 34 to 83. Pain intensity was measured by a 10-cm horizontal numerical rating scale (NRS); sensory and affective pain were measured using word descriptors derived from the McGill Pain Questionnaire–Short Form (MPQ–SF). Personality adjustment was measured by the California Q-Set, a 100-item Q-Sort procedure. The amount of analgesia was computed by summing all dosages of opiates administered by IV and by mouth during the course of the study. Dosages were converted to morphine sulfate equivalents. Once a day, beginning no sooner than 12 hours after admission to the unit and at least two hours after the last opiate administration, patients rated their pain using the NRS and MPQ–SF tools. Sometimes during their recovery a family member or significant other completed the personality Q-Set in order to minimize patients' stress because of the critical nature of their condition.

The study found that pain intensity was moderate and did not diminish over the first few postoperative days; physical sensations and emotional tension associated with pain caused minimal distress. The primary consistent mediator of pain magnitude after surgery was the amount of analgesics received, although small amounts were administered. The findings indicated that the analgesics administered were not effective in reducing pain. The researchers suggest that less conservative use of analgesics may be warranted, as well as increased use of non-pharmacologic interventions. Age and personality adjustment did not influence the extent of pain experienced. However, women and patients having abdominal vascular surgery reported more disturbing physical sensations associated with their pain. Finally, patients with greater pain intensity were found to have a significantly greater incidence of atelectasis (collapse of lung tissue) as a postoperative complication. Sixty-seven percent of patients in this study experienced atelectasis. The implications of this finding cannot be ignored. More aggressive pain reduction strategies are necessary to support patients' abilities to deep breathe, cough and ambulate. These aggressive measures should minimize the development of atelectasis.

a pain management plan. Pain may also be the result of misconceptions about the effect and duration of narcotics, tolerance levels and drug addiction. Physicians and nurses concerned about oversedation or respiratory and other complications have been reluctant to administer narcotic analgesics. Consequently, many postoperative patients are undermedicated.

Strategies for alleviating postoperative pain begin preoperatively. Decreasing anxiety can reduce later complications and aid in reducing pain. Informing the patient during the preoperative teaching session about what to expect regarding the surgery and afterward may ease feelings of fear and anxiety. Developing and explaining the plan for pain relief preoperatively will also enable the patient to participate in pain management strategies postoperatively.

When the patient returns from the post-anesthetic area, the nurse should complete a thorough assessment. The type of anesthetic the patient received and any analgesics that were administered during the operation or in the post-anesthetic room should be noted. Following the initial assessment, the patient should be assessed for pain every two to four hours. During the first 24 to 48 hours postoperatively it is wise to administer analgesics regularly and round-the-clock.

Postoperative patients in pain tend to guard their surgical area. The resultant muscle tension decreases circulation to the injured area, thereby decreasing the transport of nutrients and waste products to and from the healing area. A patient in pain is generally reluctant to move or ambulate, and respirations also tend to become shallow. Effective analgesia permits the patient to breathe deeply and to relax tense muscles, facilitating circulation and healing and decreasing the possibility of complications. It is helpful to explain this to the patient preoperatively.

It is a good idea to assure the patient that the use of narcotics for 24 to 48 hours will not encourage addiction. While the administration of analgesics provides the patient with effective pain relief, the need for other comfort measures remains paramount. Nursing actions such as supporting the incision with a pillow during pulmonary hygiene exercises and ensuring proper positioning also assist in achieving pain relief.

Other modalities should also be used with surgical patients. Relaxation techniques, imagery and massage may all be effective adjuncts for the surgical patient feeling pain.

Postoperatively, patients often experience muscle pain and backache. Muscle aches — the "hit by a truck" feeling — may be due to the relaxants used during surgery. Some relaxants, such as succinylcholine, cause muscle fasciculations which may leave the patient tired and sore. These aches usually resolve spontaneously but oral analgesics may also be beneficial (Rowland, 1990).

Many patients experience low back pain postoperatively. Muscle relaxation during anesthesia and the resultant stretching of the ligaments in the lower spine is generally the cause. Patients who received spinal or epidural anesthesia may have a sensation of bruising at the injection site. The application of heat to the lower back provides many patients with comfort for this type of pain (Rowland, 1990).

CARING FOR THE CHEMICALLY DEPENDENT PATIENT

Caring for patients with chemical addictions, whether to alcohol or drugs, is complex and challenging. Misconceptions regarding addiction and tolerance often precipitate inadequate pain management practices for these patients.

Individuals with chemical addictions often have a higher tolerance to opioids and require larger doses of narcotic analgesics to experience pain relief. Consequently, the first challenge is to identify chemically addicted patients so that appropriate analgesic treatment may be instituted. Many times, these patients do not overtly identify their addiction and the first suspicion of addiction is raised when patient behaviours become a concern. Constant "clock-watching," expressions of anger or withdrawal or refusal to participate in care are often behaviours indicating inadequate pain relief. In most instances, the solution is to raise the dose of the prescribed analgesic.

There is, however, often a hesitancy to increase the narcotic dose for chemically dependent patients. There seems to be a fear that increasing the dose will contribute to the addiction. There may also be concerns that the patient is feigning pain to obtain more drug. It is of paramount importance in these situations to remember that pain is a subjective experience. Only the patient truly knows the severity and intensity of the pain. It is the professional responsibility of the nurse to assist the patient to achieve pain relief. If the patient is not genuinely experiencing pain and is attempting to obtain more drug, it is the patient who is irresponsible, not the nurse who administers medication based on an assessment of the situation. It is also important to remember that rehabilitation is not possible when the patient is experiencing acute pain. Furthermore, rehabilitation needs to occur in a specialized setting. Most acute care units are not organized to provide the intense counselling and physical care required (McCaffery and Vourakis, 1992).

Therefore, chemically dependent patients deserve the same respect and sensitivity to their needs as other patients. All statements of pain must be assessed and appropriate treatment implemented.

CARING FOR THE COGNITIVELY IMPAIRED OLDER ADULT IN PAIN

Assessment and evaluation of pain management techniques for the cognitively impaired older adult are often frustrating. Older adults may suffer from a variety of conditions which affect cognition, including aphasia, confusion, dementia, depression, memory loss and sensory deficits. Unable to articulate the experience of pain, the cognitively impaired older adult often expresses pain behaviourally.

Assessment of these individuals must occur over a 24-hour period with input from all health care personnel who have contact with the patient during that time period. Expressions such as frowning or widely opening the eyes; aggressive behaviour, such as biting or hitting; rocking movements; sudden onset of confusion; and the guarding of a body part may all be behavioural indicators of pain. Remember that, though this patient may not be able to communicate the experience verbally, the pain experience is as intense as it would be for a younger person. Older adults who suffer from memory loss or certain types of aphasia may be able to communicate the experience if the nurse speaks slowly and uses short sentences or even just a few words. Terms such as *sore* or *hurt* accompanied by pointing to a body area may be all that is required to obtain a response (Parke, 1992).

Once pain has been identified for an older adult, it is necessary to implement an appropriate plan of care. Careful documentation of all attempted strategies for pain management and the patient's response is critical. Because the patient cannot verbally indicate the effectiveness, it is necessary to observe for behaviour cues. Watch for evidence of increased relaxation, willingness to participate in daily care and decreased irritability.

KEY TERMS

noxious p. 826
nociceptor p. 826
pain threshold p. 826
pain tolerance p. 826
acute pain p. 830
chronic pain p. 830

somatic pain p. 830
visceral pain p. 830
intermittent pain p. 830
referred pain p. 830
phantom limb pain p. 830
central pain syndrome p. 831

addiction p. 848
dependence p. 848
tolerance p. 848
patient-controlled analgesia p. 850
epidural analgesia p. 852
intrathecal analgesia p. 852

IN REVIEW

Pain is a personal experience and can only be described by the person experiencing it. It is a protective mechanism that warns the person of actual or potential damage to body tissues.

Pain is often undertreated because health care professionals hold the misconceptions that pain medication will produce drug abuse, that people with chronic pain get used to it, that children don't feel pain or will soon forget the experience and that older adults are less sensitive to pain. These misconceptions are wrong. Pain can cause physiological and psychological changes in individuals and interfere with the capacity to cope with the activities of daily living.

The physiology of pain is not completely understood but it involves three components: reception, transmission and perception. Nociceptors are free sensory nerves which receive noxious stimuli in the tissues and begin the transmission of pain impulses. Pain impulses are transmitted along peripheral afferent nerve fibres to the spinal cord. From here the impulses ascend through the spinothalamic pathways to the reticular formation, the thalamus and the cortex where pain is perceived and interpreted. Pain perception can be modified by endogenous opiates, namely enkephalins, endorphins and dynorphins.

The gate-control theory proposes an explanation of how pain is transmitted and perceived. A neural mechanism in the spinal cord acts as a gate to control the flow of pain impulses from the peripheral afferent nerves to the brain. The gate is opened or closed depending on input from small and large nerve fibres. Input from the small C fibres causes the gate to open, allowing the transmission of pain inpulses. Input from large A delta and A-beta fibres closes the gate, preventing pain impulses from reaching the brain. Pain is perceived when stimuli passing through the gate have reached threshold levels and activate areas within the brain that are responsible for pain perception and response. The gating mechanism is also affected by motivational and cognitive influences from the higher brain centres. These include such factors as attention, anxiety, expectations and memories of past pain experiences. A number of pain-relief measures, such as relaxation techniques, distraction and hypnosis, work by stimulating the activity of the thalamus and the cerebral cortex to close the gating mechanism.

Pain is caused by chemical substances, mechanical trauma or thermal extremes. Pain may be acute or chronic. Acute pain lasts less than six months, has a rapid onset, usually an identifiable pathology, and usually subsides as healing occurs. Chronic pain lasts more than six months, may or may not be connected to a pathological process and is often unresponsive to treatment (intractable). Pain has two sources: somatic and visceral. Somatic pain may be superficial (if arising from the skin or mucous membranes) or deep (if arising from muscles, joints, tendons or fascia). Visceral pain originates in the abdomen or thorax.

Responses to pain are both physiological and behavioural. The physiological responses are due to activation of the sympathetic and parasympathetic divisions of the autonomic nervous system. People react differently to pain depending upon their physical condition, emotional state and cultural conditioning.

Pain is experienced throughout the life cycle although it is manifested differently at different ages. It is important to watch for pain behaviours in those who do not verbalize well, such as children, elderly people and those with little command of the English language.

The primary source of information about pain is the patient. Many agencies supplement the standard nursing history form with a special pain assessment tool. The assessment of pain should include the quality, location, intensity, time and duration, precipitating and aggravating factors, effects on activities of daily living, the personal meaning of pain, usual coping strategies and affective responses. Sometimes a pain rating scale with words, faces or a visual analogue is used with the patient. Physical and behavioural manifestations of pain are also noted. In addition, other health team members such physicians, nurses and physiotherapists, as well as family members, contribute information about a patient's pain.

The nursing diagnoses for patients experiencing pain are *Pain* and *Chronic pain*. Pain is also a powerful etiological factor for other diagnoses such as *Ineffective individual coping*, *Hopelessness* or *Self-care deficits*. The diagostic statements should be specific about the pain, its cause, and the effect it has on ADL and the patient's emotional state (where possible) to enable effective care planning.

Nursing interventions are directed primarily towards protective strategies that assist patients to prevent, minimize and cope with pain. Restorative strategies focus on modifying the perception of pain by decreasing or eliminating stimuli.

The principles of pain management include allowing the patient to be in control, involving the family, using a team approach, using multiple modalities and acknowledging and treating secondary symptoms. Many of the noninvasive techiques may be implemented to ease pain, such as heat and cold, distraction, visualization, hypnosis, massage, relaxation and therapeutic touch. Relaxation techniques may help to lessen the anxiety and fear contributing to acute or chronic pain and lessen the dosage or frequency of the analgesics.

The administration of medication continues to be a major focus in pain management. The categories of drugs available for pain relief include the opioids, agonists/antagonists and non-narcotic pain relievers such as aspirin and NSAIDs. Pain-relief drugs are given by oral, intramuscular, subcutaneous, intravenous, epidural and intrathecal routes. With any of these medications, the patient must be watched for side effects. Respiratory depression requires immediate attention.

Evaluation of the effectiveness of any therapy is part of nursing intervention, and is especially important in pain management. Continual monitoring of the patient's comfort level is required.

LEARNING ACTIVITIES

1. Explore at least three cultural groups with respect to the values and beliefs that influence behavioural responses to pain. What are the similarities and differences among the various groups in their reactions to pain? How do your own values and beliefs about pain compare to those of the cultural groups studied? What have you learned from this exercise that will help you understand the personal experiences of pain and implement individualized pain-relief measures?

2. **Case Study:** Mrs. Roberts is admitted to the hospital after an automobile accident in which she has possibly fractured her ribs. Mrs. Roberts' husband was also injured at the same time, and he is admitted to a nearby nursing unit. He has a fractured pelvis. Mrs. Roberts is 33 years old, has three small children at home and is in a great deal of pain upon admission. Her orders include meperidine 100 mg IM q.4h prn; secobarbital 50 mg q.hs; up and about as desired; food and fluids as desired; chest x-ray.

a. Describe the physiology of this patient's pain.

b. What factors might enter into this patient's perception of and reaction to pain?

c. How might this patient describe her pain?

d. What observations would indicate to the nurse that the patient has pain?

e. What should the nurse include when recording this patient's pain? Give an example of the recording, including subjective data, objective data and assessment.

f. What are the goals of nursing care of this patient?

g. What specific measures might help alleviate this person's pain?

h. By what criteria can the nurse evaluate the success of the nursing care?

3. Find out about the services that are available in your community for people who have pain.

REFERENCES AND READINGS

ABRAM, S.E. (Ed.) (1990). *The pain clinic manual.* Philadelphia: Lippincott.

AMERICAN PAIN SOCIETY (1988). Relieving pain: An analgesic guide. *AJN, 88,* 816–825.

BERGER, K.J. and WILLIAMS, M.B. (1992). *Fundamentals of nursing: Collaborating for optimal health.* Norwalk, CT: Appleton & Lange.

BERNE, R.M. and LEVY, M.N. (1988). *Physiology* (2nd ed.). St. Louis: Mosby.

BROWN, J. (1993). When words can't take the pain away. *Nursing BC, 25*(4), 16–19.

CAHILL-WRIGHT, C. (1991). Managing postoperative pain. *Nursing 91, 21*(12), 42–45.

COPP, L.A. (1993). An ethical responsibility for pain management. *Journal of Advanced Nursing, 18,* 1–3.

DOLAN, M.B. (1993). Pain empowerment for patients and families. *Caring, 12*(2), 34–37.

DOSSEY, B. (1991). Awakening the inner healer. *American Journal of Nursing, 91*(8), 30–34.

EXPERT ADVISORY COMMITTEE ON THE MANAGEMENT OF SEVERE CHRONIC PAIN IN CANCER PATIENTS. (1984). *Cancer pain: A monograph on the management of cancer pain.* Ottawa: Minister of Supply and Services. (Catalogue No. H42-2/5–1984E)

FAUT-CALLAHAN, M. (1991). Update on drug interventions. *Nursing Clinics of North America, 26*(2), 463–475.

FERRELL, B.R. (1991). Managing pain with long-acting morphine. *Nursing 91, 21*(10), 34–39.

FERRELL, B.R., NASH, C.C. and WARFIELD, C. (1992). The role of patient controlled analgesia in the management of cancer pain. *Journal of Pain and Symptom Management, 7*(3), 149–154.

FINLAY, C. (1992). TENS: An adjunct to analgesia. *The Canadian Nurse, 88*(8), 24–26.

FLEMING, B.M. and COOMBS, D.W. (1992). A survey of complication documented in a quality-control analysis of patient-controlled anal-gesia in the postoperative patient. *Journal of Pain and Symptom Management, 7*(8), 463–469.

FULTON, J.S. and JOHNSON, G.B. (1993). Using high-dose morphine to relieve cancer pain. *Nursing 93, 23*(2), 35–39.

HESTER, N., JACOX, A., MIASKOWSKI, C., and FERRELL, B. (1992). Excerpts from guidelines for the management of pain in infants, children, and adolescents undergoing operative and medical procedures. *MCN, 17,* 146–152.

HOLM, K., COHEN, F., DUDAS, S., MEDEMA, P.G. and ALLEN, B.L. (1989). Effect of personal pain experience on pain assessment. *Image, 21,* 72–75.

KACHOYEANOS, M.K. and FRIEDHOFF, M. (1993). Cognitive and behavioural strategies to reduce children's pain. *MCN, 18,* 14–19.

KOZIER, B., ERB, G. and OLIVIERI, R. (1991). *Fundamentals of nursing: Concepts, processes, and practice.* Redwood City, CA: Addison-Wesley.

KRIEGER, D. (1979). *The therapeutic touch: How to use your hands to help or heal.* Englewood Cliffs, NJ: Prentice-Hall.

LEA, P. (1992). Pain and the chemically dependent patient. *The Canadian Nurse, 88*(6), 24–25.

LEWIS, S.M. and COLLIER, I. C. (1992). *Medical-surgical nursing: Assessment and management of clinical problems* (3rd ed.). St. Louis: Mosby.

LOGAN, M. and FOTHERGILL-BOURBONNAIS, F. (1991). *Continuous subcutaneous infusion of narcotics: Patient care and family support.* Markham: Knoll Pharmaceuticals Canada.

LUBENOW, T.R. and IVANKOVICH, A.D. (1991). Patient-controlled analgesia for postoperative pain. *Critical Care Nursing Clinics of North America, 3*(1), 35–41.

MARIEB, E.N. (1989). *Human anatomy and physiology.* Redwood City, CA: Benjamin Cummings.

McCAFFERY, M. (1979). *Nursing management of the patient with pain* (2nd ed.). Philadelphia: Lippincott.

McCAFFERY, M. and BEEBE, A. (1989). *Pain clinical manual for nursing practice*. St. Louis: Mosby.

McCAFFERY, M. and BEEBE, A. (1992). Do you know the value of a non-narcotic. *Nursing 92, 22*(10), 48–49.

McCAFFERY, M. and FERRELL, B. (1990). Do you know a narcotic when you see one. *Nursing 90, 20*(6), 62–63.

McCAFFERY, M. and VOURAKIS, C. (1992). Assessment and relief of pain in chemically dependent patients. *Orthopaedic Nursing, 11*(2), 13–27.

McCONNAN, L. (1992). Measuring a child's pain. *The Canadian Nurse, 88*(6), 20–22.

McCONNELL, E.A. (1993). Myths and facts about pain in the elderly. *Nursing 93, 23*(6), 83.

McSHANE, F.J. (1992). Epidural narcotics: Mechanism of action and nursing implications. *Journal of Post Anaesthesia Nursing, 7*(3), 155–162.

MEINHART, N.T. and MCCAFFERY, M. (1983). Pain: A nursing approach to assessment and analysis. Norwalk, CT: Appleton-Century-Crofts.

MELZAK, R. (1973). *The puzzle of pain*. New York: Basic Books.

MELZAK, R. (1990, February). The tragedy of needless pain. *Medicine*, 45–51.

NEWTON, M., NEWTON, D. and FUDIN, J. (1992). Reviewing the "Big Three" injection routes. *Nursing 92, 22*(2), 34–41.

NICHOLS, B.S. (1986). Pain. In *Nurse Review Neurologic Problems*. Springhouse, PA: Springhouse, 143–157.

NOBACK, C.R. and DEMAREST, R.J. (1981). *The human nervous system: Basic principles of neurobiology*. New York: McGraw-Hill.

NOLTE, J. (1993). *The human brain: An introduction to its functional anatomy* (3rd ed.). St. Louis: Mosby.

PAICE, J.A. and MAGOLAN, J.M. (1991). Intraspinal drug therapy. *Nursing Clinics of North America, 26*(2), 477–497.

PARKE, B. (1992). Pain in the cognitively impaired elderly. *The Canadian Nurse, 88*(7), 17–20.

PONIATOWSKI, B.C. (1991). Continuous subcutaneous infusions for pain control. *Journal of Intravenous Nursing, 14*(1), 30–35.

POTTER, P.A. and PERRY, A.G. (1991). *Basic nursing theory and practice* (2nd ed.). St. Louis: Mosby.

PUNTILLO, K. and WEISS, S.J. (1994). Pain: Its mediators and associated morbidity in critically ill cardiovascular surgical patients. *Nursing Research, 43*(1), 31–35.

RYDER, E. (1991). All about patient-controlled analgesia. *Journal of Intravenous Nursing, 14*(6), 372–380.

ROMYN, D. (1992). Pain management: Know the facts. *The Canadian Nurse, 88*(6), 26–27.

ROWLAND, M.A. (1990, May). Myths and facts about postop discomfort. *American Journal of Nursing*, 60–64.

ST. MARIE, B. (1991). Narcotic infusions: A changing scene. *Journal of Intravenous Nursing, 14*(5), 334–343.

SAWAKI, Y., PARKER, R.K. and WHITE, P.F. (1992). Patient and nurse evaluation of patient-controlled analgesia delivery systems for postoperative pain management. *Journal of Pain and Symptom Management, 7*(8), 443–453.

SEELEY, R.R., STEPHENS, T.D. and TATE, P. (1992). *Anatomy and physiology* (2nd ed.). St. Louis: Mosby.

SHEPHERD, G.M. (1988). *Neurobiology* (2nd ed.). New York: Oxford University Press.

SIMMONDS, M., WESSEL, J. and SCUDDS, R. (1992). The effect of pain quality on the efficacy of conventional TENS. *Physiotherapy Canada, 44*(3), 35–40.

SKIDMORE-ROTH, L. (1993). *Nursing drug reference*. St. Louis: Mosby.

SOFAER, B. (1984). *Pain: A handbook for nurses*. London: Harper and Row.

WALKER, M. and WONG, D. (1991, June). A battle plan for patients in pain. *American Journal of Nursing*, 32–36.

WHALEY, L. and WONG, D.L. (1991). *Nursing care of infants and children* (4th ed.). St. Louis: Mosby.

WILD, L. and COYNE, C. (1992, April). The basics and beyond: Epidural analgesia. *American Journal of Nursing*, 26–34.

WOODIN, L.M. (1993). Cutting postop pain. *RN, 56*(8), 26–33.

ZEBROFF, K. (1971). *The ABC of Yoga*. Vancouver, BC: Fforbez Enterprises, Ltd.

UNIT 5

Activity Needs

C H A P T E R 27

Sensory Needs

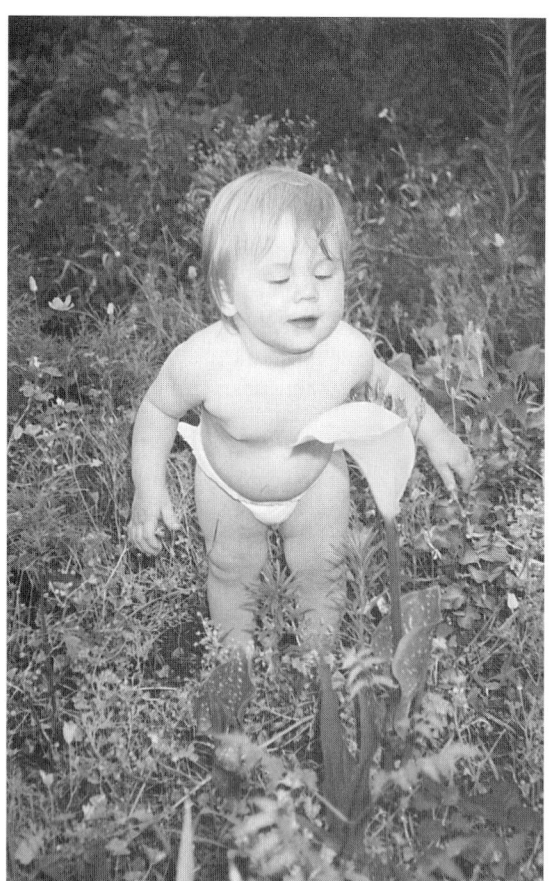

CENTRAL QUESTIONS

1. *In what way is sensory stimulation a basic human need?*

2. *What are the main determinants of sensory functioning and how do they affect sensory perception?*

3. *How does sensory perception vary throughout the life cycle?*

4. *What are some of the common problems in sensory functioning?*

5. *What basic principles would the nurse apply in assisting individuals to meet their sensory needs?*

6. *How does the nurse assess the patient's sensory abilities?*

7. *How would the nurse identify nursing diagnoses pertaining to sensory functioning?*

8. *How would the nurse develop a plan of care for patients with sensory disturbances and deficits?*

9. *What strategies might the nurse use to promote and protect the patient's sensory functioning?*

10. *What strategies would the nurse use to help the patient to cope with a partial or complete sensory deficit?*

11. *How would the nurse evaluate the patient's response to nursing interventions?*

INTRODUCTION

Sensory stimulation is a basic human need. Psychologists and educators have long been aware of the need for adequate sensory stimulation to promote the optimal growth and development of children, but only in recent years has the subject received much attention in other areas of the health field, and only recently has its importance to adults been acknowledged.

Sensory stimulation is a vital component of our lives. Our sensory faculties of sight, hearing, smell, taste and touch are the antennae that enable us to pick up signals that give us information about our environment. Without these abilities, we would not know what is going on in the world around us. Nor would we be able to communicate with other people, since communication involves both visual and auditory abilities, as well as the abilities to symbolize, to write and to make sounds. The ability to communicate is usually included in discussions of sensory functioning because of the interrelationship between sensory functioning and communication.

Receiving and accurately interpreting *sensory input* (stimuli from the external environment) is essential for survival. Losing the use of one of the senses is considered a handicap; it means that one of the antennae is missing and that stimuli must be picked up from other sources to compensate.

The person who is blind, for example, learns to distinguish sound with much more discrimination than does the person whose sense of sight is intact. Such a person also develops the sensitivity of the fingers in learning to read Braille. But he or she may still require the help of another person or of a seeing-eye dog to offer protection from hazards in the environment.

Similarly, the person who is deaf learns to "listen" to other people by reading their lips. People who are deaf may learn to talk in sign language. They also develop their sense of sight more keenly to interpret the meaning of nonverbal communications. Limitations in the ability to communicate, either in speech or in writing, can reduce one's ability to make contact with other human beings and, hence, these limitations cut off a major area of sensory stimulation. If speech is affected, the individual must either write messages or depend on nonverbal means of communication.

Appetite is aroused by the sight and smell of food, but it is also dependent on direct stimulation of the taste buds. Thus, if the ability to taste is lost, appetite diminishes, and the nourishment taken in may be insufficient to meet bodily requirements. Loss of the sense of smell lessens the pleasure of many foods, since aroma contributes a great deal to the enjoyment of eating and drinking. The loss of the sense of smell also entails other handicaps. People without the sense of smell may not be able to detect important odours, such as fumes. They may not, for example, smell the smoke of a fire, and may have to depend on their senses of sight and hearing to alert them to the danger.

The loss of the sense of touch in a part of the body, for example, through the paralysis of an arm or leg as a result of stroke, can also leave an individual vulnerable to danger. He or she will be unable to tell if tissues in the affected extremities are being damaged (by burning from a hot water bottle, for instance). Loss of the sense of touch affects the ability to perceive pain, heat and cold and pressure. It also affects balance, since we use touch to align our bodies with objects or persons in the immediate environment. A person without the sense of touch is cut off from contact with other objects or human beings so far as the affected area is concerned.

We have talked mainly of sensory deficit; but, of course, people can also suffer from too much sensory input. The excessive noise and constant barrage of stimuli from a variety of sources that are a part of contemporary life can overload sensory receiving mechanisms and result in problems in sensory functioning.

SENSORY PERCEPTION

The perception of sensory stimuli is a complex process which has its origin in the five sense organs: the eyes (visual), the ears (auditory), the skin (*tactile*), the nose (*olfactory*) and the mouth (*gustatory*). Receptors in the sense organs pick up sensory input and send this information along to the brain via channels in the nervous system. The sensory information passes through several levels of increasing complexity in the brain, where it is modified, refined and interpreted. This interpretation depends on a number of factors, including the individual's state of well-being, past experiences with stimuli of this sort and the interrelationship of stimuli coming in from various sources. The result of this process, which takes less than a second to occur, is known as *perception*.

In order to process sensory perception, the brain (in particular, the reticular activating system of the reticular formation) depends on a constant and varied input of stimuli from the environment. If the receptors are not picking up enough stimuli or are getting too much of the same stimuli, *adaptation* occurs, and the brain will no longer perceive the available stimuli. To illustrate this effect, try sitting in a quiet, darkened room and staring at a luminous object. Gradually the object will seem to disappear until it can no longer be seen. Extreme concentration on any object or person will produce the same effect. This phenomenon has been known to be used by some cult leaders as a demonstration of their power over their followers.

A lack of environmental stimulation will likewise result in a form of sensory adaptation. It is believed that, in such a case, the brain will focus on higher thought processes and disregard the small amount of external stimulation that is available. Either situation — too much of one stimulus or not enough stimuli altogether — results in sensory deprivation.

In addition to the sense organs, which receive information from the outside world, the body also possesses *proprioceptors* (sensory nerve endings) which provide information about movement and the position of the body in space. Proprioceptive senses allow us to move about effectively and to orient ourselves to the environment. *Kinesthesia* is the sense that tells us where our body parts are in relation to one another. Kinesthetic information, which comes primarily from joint receptors, enables smooth, coordinated movement of the body. We would not be able to develop any motor skill, from walking to complex athletic movements, without kinesthetic information. The *vestibular system* in the inner ear is another proprioceptive sense. It conveys information about the position of the body in space and is often thought of as the sense of balance. We are usually not aware of the vestibular sense unless we overstimulate it, by spinning around, for example, and become dizzy (Bernstein, Roy, Srull and Wickens, 1988).

DETERMINANTS OF SENSORY FUNCTIONING

Two major sets of factors affect sensory functioning: environmental and biological. Environmental determinants involve either inadequate or excessive sensory stimuli in the environment. Besides the physiological changes that occur throughout the life cycle, biological determinants include the impairment of the sensory receptors themselves or the neural structures transmitting sensory impulses, and the impairment of the centres for processing sensory stimuli.

ENVIRONMENTAL FACTORS

Inadequate Stimuli

People who have all of their sensory abilities intact are just as likely to suffer from a lack of sensory stimuli as are people with impairment of these abilities. The lack of stimulation may come from the physical environment, the psychosocial environment or both. People with limited mobility, such as those confined to a wheelchair or bed or those whose ability to get around is limited in any way, are particularly vulnerable. Their opportunities for varying their surroundings and for meeting and talking with other people are seriously hampered. The potential for inadequate sensory stimulation is therefore greatly increased. People whose work or home environments are monotonous and lacking in stimulation may also suffer from sensory deprivation. The person who works on an assembly line, for example, and has few hobbies or after-work activities, and the parent who stays home day after day with the same monotonous round of housework and who has

no interests outside the home, are both likely to suffer from sensory deprivation.

Lack of stimulation is a very common problem in people who are ill, particularly in the hospital setting. Whether at home or in hospital, sick individuals fail to receive adequate sensory input because of monotony from meaningless stimuli or restrictions imposed by therapeutic interventions. Having to remain in the same room, look at the same walls, be exposed to dim lighting and a quiet environment, undergo a repetitive, unchanging routine and have limited contact with others are common examples of factors which lead to sensory deprivation. Disturbances caused by this form of sensory deprivation have been documented on patients in isolation, in intensive care units and in coronary care units, all of whom have minimal contact with the outside world (Halm and Alpen, 1993; MacKellaig, 1986).

Excessive Stimuli

It is also possible to experience an overload of sensory stimulation. This can even occur in the hospital setting. Although the atmosphere of the hospital is traditionally quiet and conducive to rest, this is not always the case. Many humorous articles have been written by patients about the disturbances in a hospital, but the situation is not always amusing. The patient may be subjected to bright lights or disruptive noises, for example, those produced by a respirator or a renal dialysis (artificial kidney) machine. The patient's rest may be constantly interrupted by members of the health team checking his or her vital signs or those of a roommate. Adequate rest and sleep are important to physical and psychological well-being, as well as to sensory

Sensory overload is possible in the hospital, especially in an Intensive Care Unit.

perception; the specific effects of sleep deprivation are discussed more fully in Chapter 25.

BIOLOGICAL FACTORS

Impairment of the Sense Organs

The sense organs and their accessory muscles, nerves and blood supply must be intact for optimal sensory stimulation to occur. Disease, injury or a congenital defect can interfere with the ability to receive adequate sensory input. The impairment may be temporary, or it may be permanent. A patient recovering from eye surgery who has both eyes bandaged may be suffering only a temporary loss of vision, but it is nonetheless a very distressing experience. While the patient's eyes are bandaged, he or she must adjust to life as a blind person. The person with a permanent sensory deficit must learn to adapt by making greater use of remaining sensory abilities and learning to live with the deficit.

Sensory impairment may be either partial or total. Partial loss of any of the senses can be almost as disturbing as total impairment. The individual who has some hearing loss often becomes very anxious and frustrated trying to hear what other people are saying. Social relationships may be impaired and sensory stimulation may be lost because of the difficulties in receiving spoken messages.

Distorted sensory perception can be equally distressing and potentially harmful. A person with distorted vision, for example, may stumble and fall while trying to find where to put his or her foot next. If you have ever walked through a "fun house" in an amusement park, you may remember how it feels to have your vision distorted in one of the convex or concave mirrors. This experience helps to give you some idea of the feelings of a person with distorted vision.

Impairment of the Centres for Processing Sensory Stimuli

Any factors that impair the functioning of centres in the brain that refine, modify and interpret sensory input interfere with sensory abilities. Diseases or injury affecting mental processes or causing damage to the brain may cause disturbances in sensory functioning. Fever, for example, often distorts sensory perception — a very high fever may cause hallucinations. Hallucinations may be visual or auditory. Other senses, such as smell and touch, may also be involved, and sometimes several sensations may be experienced at the same time. When this occurs, the feeling that this is real, and not a hallucination, may be overpowering (Gregory, 1973).

A stroke (cerebrovascular accident) is a common cause of temporary or permanent impairment to brain tissues that interferes with sensory functioning. Paralysis and interference with speech and hearing often result from a stroke. Because the speech area in the brain is located in the dominant hemisphere, a stroke affecting this side of the brain may cause difficulties in speaking or *aphasia* (the loss of the ability to speak). In patients with existing heart problems, general circulation is impaired and there may be interference with the blood supply to the brain. These patients may also experience disturbances in sensory functioning because of inadequate oxygenation of brain tissues.

One's level of consciousness affects both the ability to receive sensory input and the ability to process it. The ability to receive sensory stimuli and the complicated mechanisms in the brain that process the input function at less than optimal efficiency when the level of consciousness is decreased.

Drugs that depress the central nervous system can decrease sensory functioning, since this system carries information from the sensory receptors and processes it. Many drugs are known to cause distortions in sensory perception. Hallucinogenic drugs, such as marijuana and LSD, cause hallucinations. Other drugs commonly used in the treatment of illness may have side-effects which cause disturbances in sensory functioning, such as blurring of vision, ringing in the ears or distorted taste. When caring for patients on any type of medication therapy, the nurse should be aware of potential side-effects and be alert for their appearance in the patient.

Emotional state can also affect sensory abilities. When people are happy they tend to see everything in a different light than when they are worried or depressed. The flowers have more colour; other people look different, perhaps more friendly. The depressed individual, on the other hand, may be unaware of things in their immediate environment — their eyes just do not see them.

SENSORY FUNCTIONING THROUGHOUT THE LIFE CYCLE

Newborn babies possess amazing sensory capabilities. Even before birth, sensory antennae are beginning to function. The fetus responds to sound starting in the fifth month of gestation (Caplan and Caplan, 1979). At birth, most of the essential sensory organs are fairly well developed and ready to function. From birth, infants are very sensitive to touch and pressure. Newborn babies will respond to cutaneous stimulation (soothing touch) with quiet, relaxed behaviour and they will withdraw from painful stimuli, such as a pinprick. Skin contact and warmth are the most powerful stimuli in the first few months.

Newborn babies can see to a distance of approximately 22 cm to 30 cm and can detect visual patterns; black and white geometric shapes are especially stimulating (Ludington-Hoe, 1983). Their sense of smell is functional and they respond to noxious odours by averting their head (Kenner and MacLaren, 1993). By the time infants are three weeks old, they can imitate the mouth movements of an adult. Because infants have taste buds all over the mouth, they tend to stuff their mouth as full as they can once they start to feed themselves.

People often remark on the fact that babies have very large eyes. The eye of a newborn is three fourths the size of an adult's. During the first 12 months of life, the eyes grow rapidly. This growth gradually slows down until the third year, when the eyes reach anatomical maturity. Visual maturity is reached in the sixth year. Newborns do not shed tears — the tear glands are usually not functional until the infant is two weeks old. Infants are aware of the relationship between sight and sound at a very early age, and by the time children are ready to crawl, they are able to perceive depth.

If the mother was not sedated during the birth process, the baby is likely to be very responsive and alert. If the baby is tired and hungry, however, he or she is capable of shutting out excessive stimulation. During infancy, it is important for the child to have a variety of sensory inputs. A lack of stimulation, as might exist in institutional care, for example, can result in depression and developmental delays. Screening for hearing defects can be done by the time an infant is six to twelve months old.

The major change in sensory perception during the early years of childhood is the maturation of vision. The young child's eye is normally *hyperopic*; that is, a distant image will fall behind the retina. However, because children's eyes have malleable lenses, they accommodate for this easily. Sometimes hyperopia persists into adulthood. If the eye becomes too long during growth, the child will become *myopic*, that is, nearsighted. Children with myopia do not usually complain of poor vision, however, since they do not know anything else. With most children, vision usually improves up to the age of five, when most have 20/20 vision. An annual vision screening is done in most school systems from kindergarten through the high school years. Periodic auditory screening is also done in most schools. This is important because a significant hearing loss is one of the most commonly overlooked serious handicaps in children.

By the time the individual reaches adolescence, there is a cessation of growth and a stabilization of sensory powers. As people grow older, their sensory functioning decreases. It takes more stimulation to whet the appetite, for example, because there are fewer taste buds functioning in the mouth.

Vision also deteriorates as people grow older. As people approach middle age, they generally find that they need to wear glasses, even if they have never needed them before. In old age, vision is often impaired by cataracts or retinal degeneration. Most elderly people are farsighted, because the lens of the eye loses elasticity. The pupils are often small, and there may be white, ringlike deposits of cholesterol just inside the edge of the cornea. Eyeglasses are an important part of the older person's sensory equipment. Nurses should be especially careful to handle them gently and to make sure that the lenses are clean.

Hearing also becomes less acute as a person gets older. Men tend to lose the ability to hear high tones, while women tend to lose the ability to hear low tones. The older person usually needs the radio or television volume set much louder than a younger person does. It is often necessary to speak more loudly and to enunciate words distinctly when talking with an older patient.

Depth perception and position sense are two other sensory abilities that deteriorate with age. This makes older people more susceptible to falls for two reasons. First, an increased length of time is required for sensory impulses to travel to the brain and for motor impulses to travel from the brain to the periphery. Hence, reaction time is increased. Second, there are degenerative changes in the sensory organs themselves, which cause decreased vestibular functioning and lessened visual acuity.

Older people are more susceptible to burning themselves. One of the reasons for this is that an older adult's response to temperature is decreased. It is usually the middle ranges of temperature that are not perceived accurately, and the older person can be easily burned by water that is just a little too hot, or a heating pad that has been turned up too high.

Stronger impulses are needed to stimulate the senses as a person gets older. The ability to perceive light touch and vibration is often lost, and even deep pressure sensitivity is diminished. An example of the loss of deep pressure sense is the lessened response to the rectal reflex for evacuation of the bowel. As you will recall from Chapter 21, this reflex is activated by the perception of a feeling of fullness in the rectum.

COMMON PROBLEMS

The most common sensory disturbances the nurse will encounter are sensory deprivation, sensory overload and sensory deficit (partial or complete). **Sensory deprivation** may be defined as "a prolonged reduction in exposure to sensory stimuli" (Bernstein, Roy, Srull and Wickens, 1988, 156). It may result from inadequate or monotonous stimuli, poorly functioning sense receptors, an inability to perceive environmental data, physical or social isolation, immobilization or restricted movement or sensory overload. Humans rely on constant and varied sensory experiences in order to function. A lack of or alterations in sensory input may result in symptoms such as boredom, impaired consciousness, lack of coherent thinking, anxiety, fear, depression and hallucinations (Moore, 1991).

Sensory overload simply means the bombardment of an individual by too many stimuli at the same time. Sensory deprivation and sensory overload are relative terms. What might be sensory deprivation for one person may be peace and tranquillity for another. People who come from large families may enjoy a quiet time by themselves. They may, on the other hand, not find noise as disturbing as those who are used to a quiet household. They may even miss the stimulation of an active, busy home.

A ***sensory deficit*** is a lack or a deficiency in one of the sensory abilities. It may be partial, as for example impaired vision, or complete, as in total blindness.

ASSESSING SENSORY NEEDS

In order to assess a patient's sensory needs, the nurse obtains a health history and examines the patient for sensory deficits and manifestations of sensory deprivation or overload. Tests done on specific sensory abilities, such as a hearing test or an eye examination, will be included in the patient's record, and the nurse can supplement the nursing data with this information. Similarly, information about the patient's health problems and the plan of therapy for these should also be available to the nurse from the physician's notations and orders on the record.

NURSING HEALTH HISTORY

The health history helps to identify patients' sensory capabilities and to determine the type of assistance they will need. Patients are the most reliable source of information about the condition of their senses. However, the family is a valuable source when the patient cannot communicate adequately. The nurse can add to subjective data by making observations of behaviours that indicate sensory disturbances.

In the health history, the nurse obtains information about the patient's usual and current status with regard to sensory abilities. Long-standing sensory deficits or problems the patient has, and any that have occurred recently, are identified. Information about corrective devices that the patient uses, such as eyeglasses or hearing aids, is also obtained. In assessing sensory functioning it is also helpful to gather information about the individual's personality, usual lifestyle and environment. This will help to determine whether the patient's lifestyle and environment are providing adequate sensory stimulation for health. Through talking with the patient and with the family or friends, the nurse can usually learn something about the patient's basic personality. Is this individual usually quiet or talkative? Is the patient gregarious and does he or she enjoy the company of other people? What are usual activities during the day?

What is the environment like? Does the patient live alone or with family? How easily can he or she get out and around? What are some leisure interests?

PHYSICAL ASSESSMENT

Physical examinations of the sensory organs are outlined in Chapter 15. In this section we will focus on assessments of sensory deprivation, sensory overload and sensory deficits.

OBSERVING FOR SENSORY DEPRIVATION

It is important for nurses to recognize signs that may indicate possible sensory deprivation in their patients. Once these are recognized, the nurse can take steps to prevent deprivation from occurring or to remedy the situation if it does occur.

Below is a list of the continuum of behaviours manifested by the patient suffering from sensory deprivation.

- boredom
- inactivity
- slowness of thought
- daydreaming
- increased sleeping
- thought disorganization
- anxiety
- panic
- hallucinations*

Patients who are *bored* may be overactive, usually doing trivial or inappropriate things. They may annoy other patients or continually push their call button to summon staff members, usually for small requests that they could handle themselves. Often they are irritable. Alternatively, people who are *bored* may also be *inactive*. If they are *inactive*, they may appear apathetic and just lie or sit in one place without seeming to respond to any form of stimulation.

A person experiencing *slowness of thought* may take considerable time to grasp even simple concepts, and there may be great lapses in conversation as the patient tries to think of what to say. Reaction time will be reduced and the patient may appear clumsy and awkward.

Daydreaming individuals may sit for seemingly endless periods of time, happily absorbed in their thoughts and fantasies, ignoring what else is going on in the room. It may be difficult to rouse these people, and they may not know when they have taken a medication or when someone is talking to them. They may confuse reality with fantasy.

The person who *sleeps* for longer than usual periods of time may be bored and consider this an effective way to

*Cameron, Kessler, Kramer and Warren (1972).

Sensory Functioning

Health and Illness Patterns

USUAL PATTERN OF SENSORY FUNCTIONING

- How would you describe your ability to:
  - hear sounds and voices?
  - see near or far objects?
  - differentiate among a variety of tastes?
  - distinguish smells and pick up odours?
  - sense heat, cold and different textures?
  - know where body parts are without looking at them?
  - maintain a sense of body position and balance?
- Do you use any assistive devices such as a hearing aid or eyeglasses?
- What kind of assistance would you require in caring for these devices?
- Do you live alone or with family? Describe where you live.
- Describe what you do in a typical day.
- What do you usually do for recreation and leisure?
- Do you spend time with other people or do you prefer to do things alone?

RECENT CHANGES IN PATTERN OF SENSORY FUNCTIONING

- Have you noticed any recent changes in your sensory functioning? If so, describe the changes.
- Can you identify any recent changes in your life that may be upsetting your sensory functioning, for instance, loss of companionship through death of a spouse, relocating from a quiet environment to one that is noisy?
- How have these changes affected your daily living?

PRESENTING HEALTH PROBLEM

- Describe the difficulty you are having with your sensory functioning.

- Do you have difficulty hearing? unusual sensations, such as ringing or humming in the ears? pain in the ear?
- Are you having blurred vision, double vision, or other visual disturbances such as sensitivity to light or blind spots?
- Do you have pain in or around the eyes?
- Have you noticed an inability to taste foods or distinguish odours?
- Have you noticed any unusual sensations, such as a bitter or metallic taste in the mouth?
- Do you have difficulty feeling hot and cold temperatures, or distinguishing different textures?
- Do you have numbness, tingling, or unusual tactile sensations? altered sense of body position? dizziness or loss of balance?
- How long have you experienced these disturbances? Do you have an acute or chronic condition (such as multiple sclerosis, diabetes, an old head injury or chronic eye or ear infections) that may be causing your sensory disturbance?
- Are you taking any medications or treatments? If, so what are they?
- Do you have a family history of eye disease or deafness?

Health Promotion and Protection Patterns

- Do you visit an optometrist or ophthalmologist periodically?
- Do you vary your recreation and leisure activities?
- Do you need rest during the day?
- How would you describe an emotionally stressful situation? How would you handle such a situation?
- Do you use alcohol or other mood-altering drugs?

---

pass the time. Such a person may find it difficult to stay awake with no stimuli to arouse the nervous system.

Individuals suffering from *thought disorganization* may find it difficult to remember what they were saying, or may experience space and time disorientation. They may not know what time of day it is, which meal they have just eaten or where they are. They may make inappropriate responses both in conversation and in action. For example, a person may intend to put on eyeglasses, and instead remove shoes or put on a dressing gown. *Thought disorganization* may cause distortions in sensory perception and, for instance, cause people to think they are eating fish when in fact they are eating fruit.

People experiencing *anxiety* may feel that they are losing all faculties one by one or that they have a terrible brain disease affecting sensory perception. These people may become frightened and resort to the use of the defence mechanisms (Chapter 8).

Panic, which we discuss in Chapter 35, is a severe state of anxiety. When people reach the stage of panic where sensory functioning is disturbed , they may feel that they will be permanently blind, deaf or paralyzed or that they are going mad.

A person suffering from hallucinations has lost all contact with reality. An explanation of the reason for hallucinations appearing in people who have experienced sensory deprivation is found in the following quotation.

> *It seems that the brain is always spontaneously active, and that the activity is normally under the control of sensory signals. When these are cut off [as in an isolation chamber] the brain activity can run wild and instead of perception of the world, we become dominated by hallucinations which may be terrifying and dangerous, or merely irritating and amusing.*

(Gregory, 1973)

OBSERVING FOR SENSORY OVERLOAD

The nurse should be alert to factors in the patient's environment that may cause sensory overload and to signs of this in the patient. Ambulatory patients may suffer from an excess of sensory stimulation in their work or home environment, or in the sum of their daily activities. Everyone needs a quiet place in which to relax, to be free from the constant ringing of the telephone and from all the other noises and activities that form a part of the lifestyle of many active, busy people.

The busy parent with a house full of noisy children may show signs and symptoms of stress, as may the harried executive whose phone is constantly ringing, and who goes immediately from one meeting to another. The noise of machines in a factory constitutes a real health hazard to employees, as does the constant noise of planes for people who work in airports. Both the physical and psychological effects of excessive sensory stimulation are significant stress factors contributing to illness.

People who are ill are particularly vulnerable to the effects of excessive stimulation. Rest and quiet are still considered the best therapy for many illnesses. The body will often heal itself if it is not overwhelmed with the exigencies of the usual everyday activities. Indeed, illness is frequently the body's way of telling us that rest is needed.

We have already mentioned some of the sources of excessive sensory stimulation in people who are ill. The nurse should be alert to the factors that have been discussed as well as to excessive noise, interruptions of the patient's rest, too many people attending to the patient or too many visitors, particularly for the patient who is acutely ill.

The primary effect of overstimulation is fatigue. Patients may express weariness verbally but often it is the nurse's responsibility to note if the patient's face looks tired and drawn, if reactions are slowing down and every movement seems an effort, or if the patient is lying quietly in bed, trying to ignore the noise and activity in the surrounding area.

OBSERVING FOR SENSORY DEFICITS

There are a number of basic techniques a nurse can use to assess sensory deficits. These are not usually conducted during the initial patient assessment; however, the techniques are very useful if a sensory deficit is suspected.

Visual

Visual acuity refers to the ability to see objects or persons clearly. The simplest way to test visual acuity is to ask the patient to read printed material. If the patient normally wears glasses, the nurse should also check to see if these are still suitable. Many times, people find that illness affects their sight, and the glasses they used to wear no longer help them. This may be one reason that some ill patients do not read.

Visual acuity may also be measured with a Snellen eye chart (Figure 27.1). It is commonly used as a screening test for vision. The tool measures the ability to read letters or symbols on a chart from a distance of six metres (20 feet). Each eye is tested separately. The patient is asked to read through the chart beginning at the top line and continuing to the smallest line of letters possible. The lines on the chart have standardized numbers representing degrees of visual acuity. Normal visual acuity is 20/20. The first number represents the distance the patient is positioned from the chart. The second number is the visual acuity. It represents the distance at which the normal eye can read a particular line. Thus a reading of 20/20 means the patient can read at 20 feet (6 m) what the normal eye can read at 20 feet. The greater the second number is, the poorer the visual acuity. A score of 20/60 means that a person standing at a distance of 20 feet from the chart can read a line that a normal eye reads from 60 feet (18 m).

The assessment of visual acuity yields information about a person's central vision. Peripheral vision is tested with a visual fields test (also called a confrontation test). A **visual field** is the entire area an eye sees when it is fixed on a central point. In a visual fields test, the examiner compares the patient's peripheral vision to his or her own, assuming it is normal. To conduct a visual fields test, the patient is positioned at eye level about 60 cm away from the examiner. The patient is asked to cover one eye and look directly at the examiner. The examiner also covers the eye opposite to the patient's covered eye and looks at the patient so that the visual fields mirror one another (see Figure 27.2). Holding

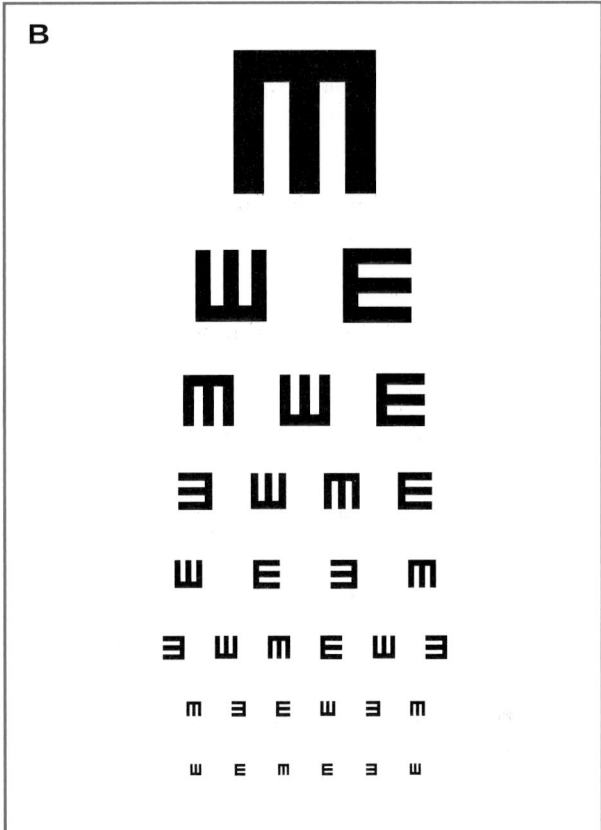

FIGURE 27.1 Snellen charts use letters (A) or symbols (B) to measure visual acuity

SOURCE: Burns, K.R. and Johnson, P.J. (1980). *Health assessment in clinical practice.* Englewood Cliffs, NJ: Prentice-Hall, 98. Reproduced with permission.

a pen or other testing object midway between the examiner and the patient, the examiner moves the object from the periphery into the field of vision. The patient is directed to say "Now" as soon as the object comes into view. The object is moved in from several different directions: above, below and laterally. The steps are repeated with the other eye. If the patient is unable to see the object when the examiner does, a peripheral field deficit is suggested.

Auditory

Auditory acuity is best tested with an audiometer which gives a precise quantitative measure of the ability to hear sounds of varying frequencies. This test is conducted by audiologists and other professionals with specialized training in the field. The nurse may conduct a simple voice test to help detect the presence of a hearing loss. One ear is tested at a time. While the patient covers one ear, the examiner positions his or her lips 30 to 60 cm away from the patient's unoccluded ear in such a way that the patient cannot read the examiner's lips. The examiner exhales and, beginning with a low whisper, slowly says two-syllable words that the patient repeats. If necessary the examiner may increase the intensity of the voice to a medium whisper, a loud whisper and then a soft,

FIGURE 27.2. Position of the examiner and the patient for a visual fields test

medium and loud voice (Bates, 1991). The inability to correctly repeat whispered words indicates a hearing loss.

Olfactory

The sense of smell is tested by presenting the patient with familiar and non-irritating odours. Substances such as coffee, vanilla, soap, chocolate or oils of wintergreen, oranges or lemons may be used. Patients are asked to close their eyes, occlude one nostril, and identify the smell of the substance held under the open nostril.

Gustatory

The taste sensation is tested by applying selected solutions to the tongue with an applicator and asking the patient to discriminate sweet, sour, salty and bitter tastes. A different applicator is used for each substance and the patient takes sips of water between substances to avoid confusing tastes. A simple method is to ask the patient to identify sweet, sour, salty or bitter flavours of foods on the meal tray. While the patient keeps his or her eyes closed, the nurse offers the various foods with a spoon.

Tactile

In testing for touch the patient is asked to discriminate sharp, dull, light and firm touch, as well as heat, cold and pain. The nurse can use a cotton ball for applying light touch and a safety pin for inducing pain. The safety pin should be discarded after use to avoid the possibility of transmitting blood-borne pathogens to other patients.

Speech

While interacting with patients the nurse should always observe the patient's formation and perception of speech. Problems in phonation (the ability to articulate words), and in the ability to understand and initiate speech, will be evident if there is a deficit.

DIAGNOSING SENSORY PROBLEMS

Sensory-perceptual alterations is a diagnostic label that may be used to describe problems with sensory functioning that are amenable to independent nursing intervention. *Sensory-perceptual alteration* is defined as "a state in which the individual/group experiences or is at risk of experiencing a change in the amount, pattern, or interpretation of incoming stimuli" (Carpenito, 1993, 695). This may include, for example, the patient who is responding to decreased stimulation from social isolation or excessive stimulation from a noisy environment, or to physiological influences such as pain, immobility or sleep deprivation. Such problems are evidenced by signs and symptoms of sensory deprivation or overload. With respect to sensory deficits (for example, visual loss), nurses independently treat patients' responses to the deficit rather than the deficit itself. In

these situations, the nursing diagnosis should describe the response, not the deficit; the sensory deficit becomes the etiology of the problem. Examples of these nursing diagnoses are below:

- VISUAL: *High risk for injury related to blurred vision*
  - *Self-care deficit related to visual disorder*
  - *Diversional activity deficit related to impaired vision*
- AUDITORY: *Impaired communication related to hearing loss*
  - *Impaired social interactions related to hearing deficit*
- KINESTHETIC: *High risk for injury related to dizziness and loss of balance*
  - *Impaired physical mobility related to altered balance*
- OLFACTORY: *Altered nutrition related to reduced sense of smell*
- GUSTATORY: *Altered nutrition related to impaired taste buds*
- TACTILE: *High risk for injury related to inability to perceive heat and cold*
  - *Impaired tissue integrity related to decreased tactile sensation**

PLANNING SENSORY INTERVENTIONS

Once the nursing diagnoses are established, the nurse develops a plan of care to suit the patient's individual needs. The goals or expected outcomes depend on the nature of the problem. In people with actual or potential problems of sensory deprivation or overload, goals are directed towards preventing the problems or restoring adequate sensory input and normal perception. For people with temporary or permanent sensory deficits, the goals focus on adjusting to the deficit and on maintaining or restoring self-care.

The patient and family should be involved in setting goals and selecting interventions as much as possible. This is especially important for permanent sensory losses, such as those of vision and hearing. In such situations, successful achievement of the goals will depend on the patient's emotional adjustment to the loss and on the support provided by family, health care professionals and community organizations. When establishing the plan of care, the nurse may collaborate with physical, occupational and speech therapists, audiologists and professionals providing specialized services (for example, representatives of the Canadian National Institute for the Blind).

If sensory disturbances are temporary, goals are usually short-term. For instance, the patient with *Diversional*

*Carpenito (1993)

KEY PRINCIPLES

Principles Relevant to Sensory Functioning

1. Psychosocial equilibrium requires that individuals have adequate sensory stimulation.
2. Stimuli picked up by the sense organs provide the body with information about the external environment.
3. Integrity of the sense organs is essential for sensory perception.
4. Sensory perception can be distorted in persons who are ill.
5. Damage to brain tissues caused by disease processes or by injury can interfere with sensory perception.
6. Communication provides an important means of sensory stimulation.
7. All sensory receptors adapt, either partially or totally, to their various stimuli over a period of time.
8. The brain is active even in the absence of stimuli from the external environment.
9. Sensory perception diminishes as a person get older.
10. The length of time an impulse takes to travel to the brain increases with age.
11. Reaction time to environmental stimuli increases with age.

HEALTH PROMOTING STRATEGY

Promoting Healthy Sensory Functioning

- See an optometrist or ophthalmologist regularly for eye examinations.
- Watch the ultraviolet index. Wear proper sunglasses or a brimmed hat to avoid direct sunlight.
- Wear protective goggles when handling dangerous chemicals or materials that may fragment.
- Use proper, nonglare lighting for reading, doing close work and in the workplace. Avoid extreme lighting conditions that may be caused by high intensity light sources.
- Avoid eye strain from excessive use of computers. Rest the eyes about 20 minutes every two hours.
- Avoid persistent loud noise. Wear protective ear covers if exposure is continuous.
- Maintain regular oral hygiene and drink ample fluids to keep the taste buds hydrated. A well-balanced diet with a variety of seasonings and textures will heighten taste perception.
- Keep the environment clean and fresh. Provide pleasant fragrances with deodorizers or flowers.
- Establish a variety of leisure activities to stimulate the senses.
- Balance activities with ample rest.
- Visit with friends and relatives frequently.

activity deficit related to impaired vision secondary to eye patches will need intervention only as long as the eye patches are in place. Adjustment to a permanent sensory loss often requires major changes in a patient's life. This may be a long process for some people. It is important to set short-term goals when striving towards long-term accomplishment. Success with short-term goals will help to provide the motivation needed to continue the long-term efforts.

The nurse should ensure that goals are realistic, attainable and measurable for each patient. For example, for a patient who remains in his or her room, sitting in a wheelchair most of the day, the expected outcome might be to increase the number of hours spent outside the room each day. It is helpful to set definite criteria, starting perhaps with two hours, and eventually increasing to eight hours per day. Or for the patient who takes no initiative in going to arts and crafts or other activities, possible goals might be that the patient will participate in these activities and take increasing responsibility for getting to the arts and

crafts room. For the patient who is depressed or apathetic, even the initiation of conversation would be a major achievement.

IMPLEMENTING SENSORY INTERVENTIONS

HEALTH PROMOTING STRATEGIES

The sensory organs enable individuals to relate to and function effectively and safely in their environment. Health practices, lifestyle and occupation can alter sensory functioning and place individuals at risk for sensory loss. Individuals can do much to preserve and promote sensory capabilities in everyday living. Guidelines for promoting optimal sensory functioning are given in the box above.

HEALTH PROTECTING STRATEGIES

People who are ill often experience alterations in sensory functioning which may affect psychosocial well-being and interfere with the ability to communicate with others and function safely in their environment. A change in normal environment, exposure to unfamiliar sights and sounds, restricted mobility, medications, treatment measures and a lack of diversional activity and meaningful social interactions all contribute to altered sensory patterns. In addition, sensory impairments such as a loss of vision or hearing affect the ability to protect against hazards in the environment and to perform activities of daily living. Measures to promote patient safety and to enable self-protection are outlined in Chapter 29. This section will consider strategies the nurse can use in assisting patients to maintain their sensory functioning, prevent sensory deprivation or overload, maintain communication and perform activities of daily living.

PREVENTING SENSORY DEPRIVATION

Sensory deprivation has long been thought to be a problem requiring nursing intervention. Florence Nightingale was evidently concerned about this when she wrote:

> It is an ever recurring wonder to see educated people who call themselves nurses, acting thus. They vary their own objects, their own employments, many times a day; and while nursing some bedridden sufferer, they let him be there staring at a dead wall, without any change of object to enable him to vary his thoughts; and it never occurs to them at least to move his bed so that he can look out of the window.

(Nightingale, 1946)

The logical approach to nursing action for the patient at risk for sensory deprivation is to ensure that the environment contains adequate meaningful stimuli. This implies a certain amount of environmental management on the nurse's part.

People in a home situation should be encouraged to vary both their physical and their psychosocial environment. The nurse may be able to make some suggestions in this regard, or to involve family and friends or community organizations to assist individuals if they are unable to do this for themselves. Radio and television are great comforts to people who are unable to get out of their everyday environment; these comforts help to keep individuals in touch with the outside world. Radio and television can

be supplemented with active participation in games, crafts and other activities that keep individuals in contact with their environment. For the person who is fond of reading, mobile libraries are available in many communities. A visit by a library staff member not only provides new books and magazines to read, but also provides the stimulation of a new face and some conversation to relieve the monotony of the day.

Volunteers who deliver "Meals on Wheels" find that their patients often look forward to the social aspects of the service as much as the actual meal. A number of service clubs, lodges and other community groups visit people unable to leave their home, and arrange outings for senior citizens and handicapped persons. The nurse should be familiar with services available in the community. Community centres and organizations also provide activities for those who are ambulatory. Bridge clubs, arts and crafts classes and a variety of courses, including academic subjects as well as gardening, swimming and exercise classes, are among the many activities offered in a number of these centres.

For the person who is ill and in an institutional setting, approaches similar to those in the community setting may be used. Volunteers and community resources can help to provide the individual with sufficient change in both physical and psychosocial environment to ensure an adequate amount of sensory input. Varying the patient's surroundings, even if it only involves moving the bed near the window, as Florence Nightingale suggested, provides a different perspective.

For the resident in an extended care facility, or one who is low-functioning disabled and confined to home, it is important to maintain contact with reality. It is helpful to provide some devices to enable this contact. The use of clocks, calendars, fixed time schedules, regular television or radio programs, and similar means helps to keep the person oriented to time and place. Newspapers and magazines provide a contact with what is going on in the world outside the agency setting.

The nurse may find brief explanations to the patient of nursing functions and treatments helpful too, even if the activities are routine ones. These explanations help to keep patients aware of where they are and what is being done for and to them. The nurse should not think that just because the patient does not respond that he or she does not hear. It is important to maintain auditory stimuli for the person who is seriously deprived of sensory input.

Therapeutic touch is an effective way of increasing stimulation to the brain and communicating with the patient. The use of touch that is so much a part of nursing has been shown to have definite therapeutic healing properties, from both a physical and a psychological point of view. The nurse's presence also means the patient has someone to talk to, and the different nurses coming on for different shifts help to provide a variety of people, which patients often find stimulating.

Active participation in games or crafts with other people provides a variety of sensory input and helps to keep an individual in touch with his or her environment.

The nurse functions both as a source of sensory input to the patient, and as a resource person who can enlist the assistance of family, friends, visitors and volunteers from community organizations to help the patient to receive adequate sensory stimulation. The nurse is frequently called upon to use imagination to think of ways of getting people involved and to provide the type of stimulation needed for a particular individual.

PREVENTING SENSORY OVERLOAD

For the patient at risk for sensory overload, interventions that help to reduce the number of stimuli in the environment are indicated. In the community, the nurse may be able to help the individual to plan periods of rest in a busy day or to engage in relaxing activities. Physical exercise is often a good antidote for people whose work keeps them in an office, a factory or other enclosed surroundings. Some people need assistance in order to be able to rest and relax. Other people enjoy music or reading or a game of bridge. A change of stimuli is often as relaxing as a cessation of stimuli.

Some people need help in learning how to relax and clear their minds of stimuli. Relaxation techniques are discussed in Chapters 26 and 35.

Some of the ways the nurse can help to reduce environmental stimuli for the ill person, at home or in hospital,

have already been discussed. In addition, it helps to explain the reasons for the tubes and machines that are surrounding the patient, the purposes of treatments and the reasons why other personnel come in to see the patient. Putting a structure to the sensory input helps people to interpret stimuli meaningfully; they are not so apt to feel disoriented, and anxiety is reduced.

MAINTAINING COMMUNICATION

Individuals with sensory deficits, such as visual and hearing losses, require alternate methods of communicating with others. People with loss of vision rely on their sense of sound and touch and are very sensitive to spatial perception. Those with hearing loss make maximum use of their sight. Individuals with hearing loss may communicate in a number of different ways. They may use sign language, read lips, listen with the help of a hearing aid or use a note pad.

MAINTAINING ACTIVITIES OF DAILY LIVING

Individuals with sensory deficits may need assistance in handling their physical environment and maintaining daily activities. The nurse should be sensitive to the patient's

Communicating with People with Vision Loss

- Always announce your presence when entering the room.
- Speak in a normal tone of voice.
- Inform the patient when you are going to touch him or her, explain all procedures, and explain what will happen next.
- Describe the patient's environment in detail and allow the patient to touch objects in the surroundings.
- Inform the patient when changes have been made in the placement of items in their environment.
- Tell the patient when you are going to leave the room.
- Make sure the call bell is within easy reach.

Communicating with People with Hearing Loss

- Encourage the patient to use a hearing aid. Make sure the aid is in place and working
- Make your presence known, but avoid startling the patient. Do not approach or do anything unexpectedly from behind.
- Stand where your face can be easily seen and maintain eye contact when speaking. Make sure the lighting is adequate so that the patient can see you.
- Speak clearly and a little more slowly than usual. Do not exaggerate lip movement because this interferes with lip reading. Refrain from speaking with anything in your mouth. Keep your voice at a normal volume.
- Use visible aids. Speak with your hands, your voice, your face and your eyes.
- If the patient does not understand what you have said, rephrase words or sentences rather than repeating the whole conversation. Use pictures or written information to supplement the spoken word.
- Eliminate background noise; for instance, turn off the radio or television, or close windows to control noise from outside.
- Be sensitive. An ill or fatigued patient may not hear as well as usual.

SOURCE: Chovaz, C. (1989). Nursing the hearing impaired patient. *Canadian Nurse*, 85(3), 34–36.

needs and offer help before the patient has to ask for it. For example, the nurse can tell the patient who is having problems with vision what foods are on the meal tray and help to locate the food and silverware. Cutting up food for a patient who has the use of only one hand, anticipating the need for help in putting on a dressing gown or helping a patient to the bathroom are other ways the nurse can assist individuals with sensory impairments to meet daily needs.

The nurse should be aware of tools that have been developed to assist people to maintain physical independence.

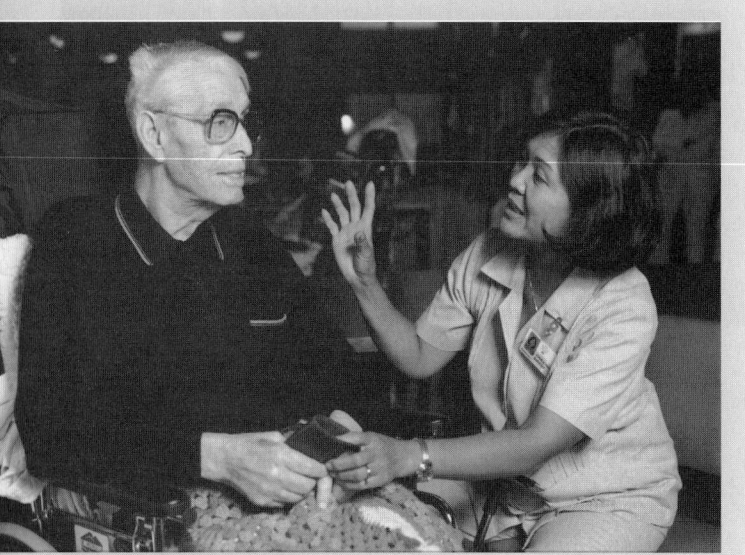

This nurse is speaking with her hands, her face and her eyes.

Many utensils and mechanical devices are now available commercially. It is also possible to adapt ordinary utensils to assist with such activities as eating, reading, getting in and out of bed and moving about. These items eliminate problems for people who are blind, paralyzed or otherwise handicapped in performing both necessary and leisure activities. The nurse can call upon physical and occupational therapists for help in suggesting ways of increasing an individual's independence when one of the sensory abilities has been lost.

HEALTH RESTORING STRATEGIES

The strategies for restoring sensory functioning when a patient is experiencing sensory deprivation and overload are the same as the health protecting strategies discussed above.

In helping a person to cope with either a temporary or permanent sensory deficit, the nurse must first of all be aware of the individual's reaction to it. Loss of sensory functioning has both physical and psychosocial ramifications. Some of the psychosocial effects have already been discussed. If a permanent and total disability of one of the senses has occurred, the patient feels an acute sense of loss and grief. If the nurse is caring for someone who has recently experienced such a loss, it may be helpful at this point to read Chapter 36.

With a partial or a temporary loss of sensory functioning, people may be anxious and worried. Will they regain total functioning? What if they become totally blind or deaf or remain permanently paralyzed? What if their speech never comes back? How are they going to cope with partial impairment? These are some of the spoken and unspoken questions these patients ask.

Often people with sensory losses need the help of specialized health professionals or specialized agencies to enable them to learn to live with a sensory deficit. The nurse supports the work of specialists such as the physical, occupational and speech therapists by following through on activities suggested by them. The patient's increased independence is ensured when all nursing personnel are aware of the goals for the patient, and are consistent in their approach to the patient.

Rehabilitation centres offer tremendous help for people who are learning to live with a sensory deficit, such as blindness, deafness, and paralysis, and also for patients who have lost the ability to speak. The nurse should, if possible, visit one of these centres early in his or her career to become aware of things that are available to help individuals with sensory deficits cope with the daily activities of living.

EVALUATING SENSORY INTERVENTIONS

When expected outcomes have been explicitly stated, the nurse is able to evaluate the effectiveness of various interventions or to try other alternatives if these have not been successful. It also helps the nurse and the patient to feel a sense of accomplishment when progress towards goal achievement has been made. This aspect of nursing care is important for the nurse as well as for the patient and family.

FROM RESEARCH TO PRACTICE

Allen, M.N.(1989). The meaning of visual impairment to visually impaired adults. *Journal of Advanced Nursing.* 14, 640-646.

Nurses who understand the personal meaning attached to an illness or life event are better able to help people cope with the adaptive demands involved. This study was undertaken to explore the subjective meanings of visual impairment to adults as it concerns them in their daily lives. Using phenomenological methodology, data were gathered through observations and interviews of a convenience sample of 25 men and women who had been visually impaired for one to more than 20 of their adult years. Data were analyzed to identify the social and symbolic context of visual impairment in order to better understand the world of visually impaired individuals.

The study found that adjustment to visual impairment was a gradual process with five distinct and identifiable stages:(1) pre-impact/early loss, (2)impact/realization of loss, (3) implications of the loss, (4) decision to live with the visual impairment and (5) adjustment and readjustment. The most difficult aspect of being visually impaired was needing to ask for help. The respondents felt obligated or indebted to the person(s) helping them and therefore they were unable to maintain a balance of give and take in the relationship. The most helpful aid to adjustment was contact with other visually impaired people whereas lack of social support — someone to talk and share mutual experiences with — was a major hindrance. People often coped by learning to do things. Reactions to blindness included not only the shock, disbelief, anger and depression noted in the literature, but also a fear of going out alone, learning new skills and coping with the future. Understanding the personal meaning of visual impairment can help the nurse to identify those patients at risk for further health problems such as depression. Nurses can also provide support during the early stages of adjustment as the patients come to terms with their loss and reorganize their lives. Nurses can also help people to establish and maintain social networks to overcome feelings of loneliness and social isolation.

KEY TERMS

sensory input p. 864

tactile p. 864

olfactory p. 864

gustatory p. 864

perception p. 864

adaptation p. 864

proprioceptors p. 865

kinesthesia p. 865

vestibular system p. 865

aphasia p. 866

sensory deprivation p. 867

sensory overload p. 868

sensory deficit p. 868

visual acuity p. 870

visual field p. 870

IN REVIEW

Sensory stimulation is a basic human need and is essential for optimal growth and development. The senses are sight, hearing, smell, taste and touch. Our sensory abilities enable us to know what is going on in the world around us and to communicate with other people.

Sensory perception is a complex process which originates in the five sense organs: the eyes, ears, skin, nose and mouth. Receptors in these organs receive sensory input from the external environment. The information passes along the nerves to the brain where it is modified, refined and interpreted. This interpretation depends on the person's state of well-being and past experiences as well as the interrelationship of stimuli coming in from other sources. The result of this process is known as perception.

In addition to the sense organs, the body also possesses proprioceptive and kinesthetic senses. These senses allow us to move about smoothly and effectively and to orient ourselves to the environment. The vestibular system in the inner ear conveys information about the position of the body in space and is thought of as the sense of balance.

Determinants of sensory functioning include environmental and biological factors. Environmental factors involve either inadequate or excessive stimuli in the environment which cause sensory deprivation or sensory overload. Biological factors include the physiological changes that occur throughout the life cycle, impairment of the sensory receptors or the neural structures transmitting sensory impulses and impairment of the centres for processing sensory stimuli.

Newborn babies possess amazing sensory capabilities. At birth, most of the essential sensory organs are fairly well developed. The major change in sensory perception during the early childhood years is the maturation of vision. With most children vision improves up to the age of five years when most attain 20/20 vision. All of the senses are fully developed by the teen years and gradually diminish in the later years.

The common problems of sensory functioning are sensory deprivation, sensory overload and sensory deficit. Sensory deprivation can occur from a lack of stimulation, monotonous stimuli, poorly functioning receptors, an inability to perceive environmental data, physical or social isolation, immobility or sensory overload. Sensory overload occurs when an individual is bombarded with too many stimuli. A sensory deficit is a deficiency in one of the sensory abilities.

In assessing sensory needs, the nurse obtains a health history and examines the patient for sensory deficits and manifestations of sensory deprivation and sensory overload. The nurse can supplement the data with information from tests done on specific sensory abilities, such as auditory studies or eye examinations. The patient's record provides information about the patient's health problems and the physician's plan of therapy.

Nursing diagnoses describing sensory deprivation or sensory overload may be labelled as *Sensory-perceptual alteration*. With respect to sensory deficits, nurses independently treat patients' responses to the deficits rather than the deficit itself. Thus, the sensory deficit becomes the etiology of the problem — for example, *High risk for injury related to loss of balance*.

Nursing interventions are planned and implemented to suit patients' individual needs. For people with actual or potential problems of sensory deprivation or overload, care is directed towards preventing problems and restoring sensory input and perception. For individuals with temporary or permanent sensory deficits, interventions focus on helping patients to adjust to the sensory loss and on assisting them to maintain or restore their independence. People with sensory losses often need the help of specialized health professionals and agencies in learning how to live with the deficit.

LEARNING ACTIVITIES

1. **Case Study**: Mr. Jones is a 75-year-old retired school principal who had a cerebrovascular accident (stroke) with resultant hemiplegia (left-sided) nine months ago. Following the acute episode, he was admitted to a rehabilitation unit but did not progress as well as expected and was transferred to an extended care facility, where he has been ever since. His mental faculties appear unimpaired and his speech is intact, but his visual and auditory functioning are decreased. He has some movement in the left leg, but the arm is flaccid. He is helped into a wheelchair daily and can propel himself about a little.

Mr. Jones' wife died two years ago; two of his four adult children (a son and a daughter) live in town—the other two sons at a considerable distance—and both visit frequently, as do their children.

Prior to his disability, Mr. Jones was active in the local community centre, played golf regularly and liked to travel. However, on the ward, he spends most of his time in his room, staring out of the window. He does not go to the TV room and has given up reading newspapers because he says he can read nothing but the headlines. He has his radio on most of the time, but keeps the volume low because other patients were complaining about it. He can never remember if visitors have been in or not.

As his nurse, what can you do to help Mr. Jones?

2. Visit an agency or rehabilitation centre in your community that offers assistance to people learning to live with sensory deficits such as vision or hearing loss. What types of services do these agencies provide?

REFERENCES AND READINGS

ALLEN, M.N. (1989). The meaning of visual impairment to visually impaired adults. *Journal of Advanced Nursing, 14,* 640–646.

BATES, B. (1991). *A guide to physical examination and history taking* (5th ed.). Philadelphia: Lippincott.

BERNSTEIN, D.A., ROY, E.J., SRULL, T.K. and WICKENS, C.D. (1988). *Psychology.* Boston: Houghton Mifflin.

BURGENER, S.C. and BARTON, D. (1991). Nursing care of cognitively impaired institutionalized elderly. *Journal of Gerontological Nursing, 17*(4), 37–43.

BURNS, K.R. and JOHNSON, P.J. (1980). *Health assessment in clinical practice.* Englewood Cliffs, NJ: Prentice-Hall, 98.

CAMERON, C.F. KESSLER, J.C., KRAMER, W. and WARREN, K.E. (1972). When sensory deprivation occurs. *Canadian Nurse, 68*(11), 32–34.

CAPLAN, F. and CAPLAN, T. (1979). *The second twelve months of life.* New York: Grosset and Dunlap.

CARPENITO, L.J. (1993). *Nursing diagnosis: Application to clinical practice* (5th ed.). Philadelphia: Lippincott.

CHOVAZ, C. (1989). Nursing the hearing impaired patient. *Canadian Nurse, 85*(3), 34–36.

DOOTSON, S. (1990) Sensory imbalance and sleep loss. *Nursing Times, 86*(35), 26–29.

GREGORY, R.L. (1973). *Eye and brain* (2nd ed.). New York: McGraw-Hill.

HAHN, K. (1989). About sensory loss. *Nursing 89*(2), 97–99.

HALM, M.A. and ALPEN, M.A. (1993). The impact of technology on patients and families. *Nursing Clinics of North America, 28,* 443–457.

JARVIS, C. (1992). *Physical examination and health assessment.* Philadelphia: Saunders.

KEE, C.C. (1990). Sensory impairment: Factor X in providing nursing care to the older adult. *Journal of Community Health Nursing, 7*(1), 45–52.

KENNER, C.A., and MACLAREN, A. (1993). *Essentials of maternal and neonatal nursing.* Springhouse, PA: Springhouse.

KRIEGER, D. (1975). Therapeutic touch: The imprimatur of nursing. *American Journal of Nursing, 75,* 784.

LEVINE, M.W. and SHEFNER, J.M. (1991). *Fundamentals of sensation and perception* (2nd ed.). Pacific Grove, CA: Brooks/Cole.

LUDINGTON-HOE, S. M. (1983). What can newborns really see? *American Journal of Nursing, 9,* 1286–1289.

MACKELLAIG, J. (1986). A study of psychological effects of intensive care with particular emphasis on patients in isolation. *Intensive Care Nursing, 2,* 176–185.

MALASANOS, L., BARKAUSKAS, V. and STOLTENBERG-ALLEN, K. (1990). *Health assessment* (4th ed.). St Louis: Mosby.

MOORE, T. (1991). Making sense of...Sensory deprivation. *Nursing Times, 87*(6), 36–38.

NEY, D.F. (1993). Cerumen impaction, ear hygiene practices, and hearing acuity. *Geriatric Nursing, 14*(2), 70–73.

NIGHTINGALE, F. (1946). *Notes on nursing.* New York: Appleton & Lange.

SCHIFFMAN, H.R. (1990). *Sensation and perception: An integrated approach* (3rd ed.). New York: Wiley.

WILSON, L.D. (1993). Sensory perceptual alteration: Diagnosis, prediction, and intervention in the hospitalized adult. *Nursing Clinics of North America, 28,* 747.

CHAPTER 28

Movement and Exercise Needs

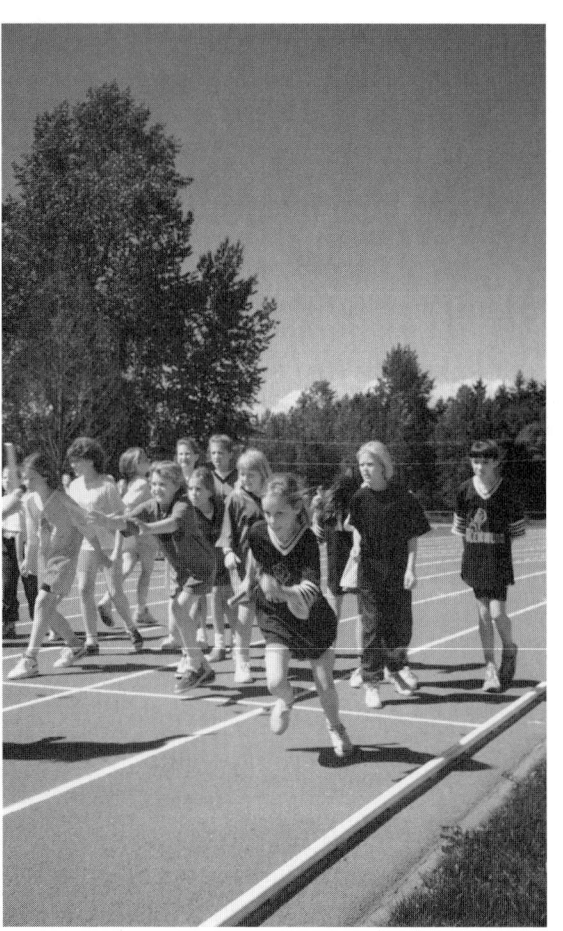

CENTRAL QUESTIONS

1. How are movement and exercise important to health and well-being?

2. What are the major functions of bones, muscles, joints, nerves and their blood supply in body movement?

3. How does the capacity for coordinated movement and exercise vary throughout the life cycle?

4. What are the main determinants of movement and exercise?

5. What are some common mobility problems?

6. What basic principles does the nurse apply in assisting patients meet movement and exercise needs?

7. How does the nurse assess movement and exercise needs?

8. What are the common nursing diagnostic statements for patients with movement and exercise problems?

9. How does the nurse develop a plan of care for patients with movement and exercise problems?

10. What strategies does the nurse implement in helping individuals, families or groups promote optimum physical fitness and prevent potential mobility problems?

11. What health restoring and supportive strategies does the nurse implement in the care of patients with mobility problems?

12. How does the nurse evaluate the patient's response to nursing interventions?

INTRODUCTION

Most people take for granted the ability to move around freely. We rely on free movement to carry out activities of daily living (ADL), such as getting out of bed, washing, dressing and eating. We also rely on movement for work, for play, for defending ourselves from danger and for communicating with others. We give little thought to how our skeletal system functions, or how our muscles and joints work, until illness or trauma impairs our capacity to move. Indeed, movement is such a vital part of our lives that we consider permanent loss of the ability to move any part of the body to be one of the major tragedies that can occur.

A loss of mobility lessens self-concept and affects body image. Such a loss tends to make people think less of themselves. Independence is threatened and if the immobility affects one or more of the principal locomotor parts of the body, the threat may assume major proportions. Opportunities for communication are also jeopardized if mobility is impaired, and sensory deprivation becomes a real possibility. Communication depends on motor abilities for speaking, writing and using nonverbal "body language" to send messages to other people.

Just as movement is necessary for fulfilling basic human needs, exercise is essential for promoting physical and psychological health. People who exercise regularly not only have higher energy levels, they look better and feel better about themselves. There is growing evidence that exercise, in conjunction with other healthy behaviours such as eating healthily and quitting smoking, offers some protection against health problems and chronic diseases (Williams, 1993).

When people are ill or become immobilized, the muscles and the nerves that regulate movement become inactive. Disuse of the neuromuscular system quickly leads to degeneration and subsequent loss of functioning. If muscles are immobilized, the process of degeneration begins almost immediately. The restoration of muscle strength and tone, on the other hand, is a very slow process that may take months or years to accomplish. With this in mind, prevention is the better part of care. Nurses caring for patients whose movement is restricted have a responsibility to prevent the degeneration of unused muscles and the development of complications that might limit mobility or prolong the recovery and restoration to health.

PHYSIOLOGY RELATED TO MOVEMENT

The principal systems involved in body movements are the skeletal system, the muscular system and the nervous system. The circulatory system is also involved in that it provides nourishment to the tissues of these other systems. If circulation to any part of the body is impaired, degeneration of the tissues in the area begins, since body cells cannot live without ade-

Children find many ways to exercise.

quate nourishment. However, it is the bones, the nerves and the muscles, working together, that make movement possible.

INTEGRATION OF THE BONES, MUSCLES AND NERVES IN MOVEMENT

The bones of the skeletal system have two functions in movement: they provide an attachment for muscles and ligaments, and they act as levers. The *proximal* end of a muscle is attached to a less movable bone, such as the scapula in the shoulder. This point of attachment is called the *origin of the muscle*. The *distal* end of the muscle is attached to a freely movable bone, such as the humerus in the upper arm. This point is called the *insertion of the muscle*.

The muscles contract to produce motion. Muscles that are used for movement are always in pairs, one on either side of a bone or joint, and have opposing functions; as one contracts, the other extends (stretches) to cause the bone to move in a certain direction. This action is similar to that involved in the manipulation of a puppet by strings; you shorten one string and lengthen another to make the puppet move in the direction you want it to go.

Muscles tend to work in groups, though, rather than in single pairs. Breathing, for example, requires the coordinated activity of a number of muscles, including the intercostals, the diaphragm and the sternocleidomastoid muscles, the scalenes, the thoracohumeral and the thoracoscapular muscles. Just to move the thigh involves all of the gluteus muscles, as well as the hip adductor and flexor muscles.

The spinal nerves are directly involved in trunk and limb movements. Each spinal nerve has an anterior and a posterior root in the spinal column. The anterior root conducts impulses to the muscles from the central nervous system. The posterior root conducts messages from the peripheral sensory receptors to the central nervous system.

Almost all patterns of movement can be initiated by the spinal cord alone. Balance and the progression, coordination and purposefulness of movement, however, require the participation of progressively higher levels of the brain. Motor areas located in the frontal lobes of the cerebral cortex control the voluntary movements of all muscles of the body (Jacob and Francone, 1989).

TYPES OF JOINTS

The various types of body movements are made possible by the *joints*, which connect one bone to another. Each movable joint is constructed to make possible a certain type of movement and each has a circumscribed range of motion. These joint movements are defined in Table 28.1 and illustrated in Figure 28.1.

The body does have some joints that are immovable, such as those connecting the bones in the skull, but the major purpose of joints is to serve as fulcrums to enable the body to move. The body has six types of movable joints (see Table 28.2).

TABLE 28.1   Types of Body Movement

TYPE OF MOVEMENT	EXPLANATION
Abduction	Movement away from the central axis (midline) of the body.
Adduction	Movement towards the central axis (midline) of the body.
Flexion	The act of bending; the angle between the two moving parts is decreased.
Extension	The act of straightening; the angle between the two moving parts is increased.
Hyperextension	Extension beyond the normal range of motion, for example, bending the head back towards the spine.
Gliding	Movement in one plane, as in sliding.
Rotation	Turning in a circular motion around a fixed axis.
Circumduction	Circular motion of a limb or part when the limb or part forms part of a cone, as in swinging the arm in a circular motion. It is a combination of abduction, adduction, flexion and extension.
Pronation	Turning down towards the ground.
Supination	Turning upward (the opposite of pronation).
Inversion	Turning inward towards the body.
Eversion	Turning outward away from the body.

TABLE 28.2   The Six Types of Movable Joints

TYPE OF JOINT	EXPLANATION
Hinge	This is a uniaxial joint that permits flexion and extension. An example of a hinge joint is the knee.
Pivot	This is also a uniaxial joint. It permits rotation. An example is the atlantoaxial joint (between the first cervical vertebra and the base of the skull).
Condyloid	This is a biaxial joint. It permits flexion, extension, abduction and adduction. The wrist is a condyloid joint.
Saddle	This is another biaxial joint. It permits flexion, extension, abduction, adduction and circumduction. An example is the thumb.
Ball and socket	This type of joint is polyaxial. Movements permitted include flexion, extension, abduction, adduction, circumduction, and rotation. The hip joint is a ball and socket joint.
Gliding	This is a *plane* joint and permits gliding movements. An example is the acromioclavicular joint of the shoulder.

FIGURE 28.1 Types of joint movements

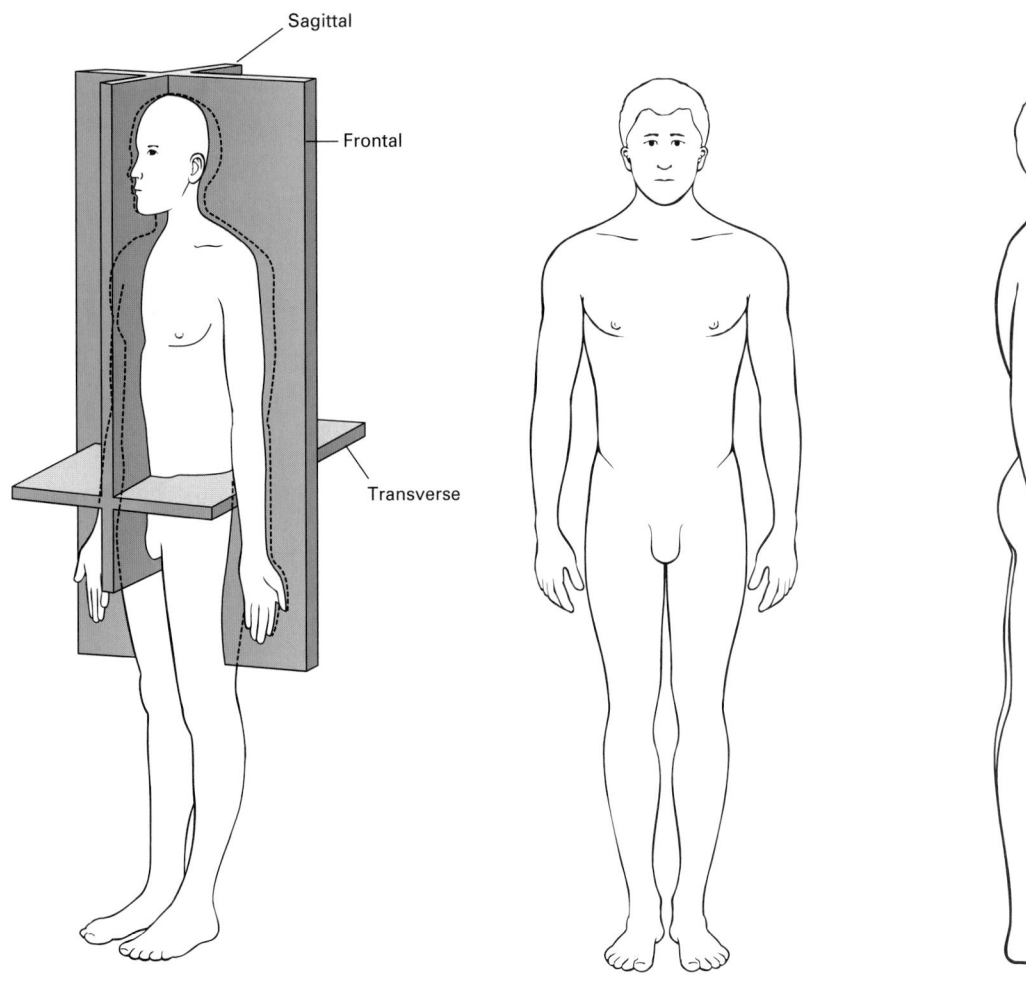

FIGURE 28.2 Sagittal, frontal and transverse planes of the body

FIGURE 28.3 Normal anatomic position

BODY PLANES AND ANATOMIC POSITION

Body movements are often described in relation to *planes*, another term from the physical sciences. When the body is in a standing position, as shown in the Figure 28.2, the *sagittal plane* divides it into right and left sections, the *frontal plane* into dorsal and ventral sections, and the *transverse plane* into upper and lower sections.

Anatomic position refers to the **body alignment** or relationship of body parts to the midline of the body. In anatomic position (see Figure 28.3), the body is erect; the head, pelvis, legs and feet are balanced and their weight is evenly distributed. The arms hang down at the sides with the palms facing forward. The feet are slightly apart and pointed forward; the knees and fingers are slightly flexed.

Movement of the body is much easier when the body parts are well aligned, when the weight of the body is evenly balanced, and when the feet are set a little farther apart (about 30 cm) than in the anatomic position. Setting the feet this far apart provides the body with a wider foundation or **base of support** for its weight than the normal standing posture does.

The **centre of gravity** (also called centre of mass or centre of weight) of the body is located in the pelvis at approximately the level of the second sacral vertebra. The **line of gravity** is an imaginary straight line that passes from the top of an object through its centre of gravity to form a right angle with the ground.

When the body is in anatomic position, the line of gravity falls in the frontal plane downward behind the ear, through the centre of gravity in the pelvis, and slightly in front of the knee and ankle joints, to the middle of the body's base of support, so that the line is perpendicular to the ground, as shown in Figure 28.3. The body is more stable in this position because its line of gravity is in direct line with the gravitational pull of the earth.

THE ROLE OF EXERCISE IN HEALTH AND WELLNESS

Exercise increases the efficiency of all body processes. The physiological, psychological and social benefits of exercise have been receiving increasing attention in recent years. The predominantly sedentary way of life of so many North Americans has been a major factor contributing to many illnesses, such as heart disease and stroke, hypertension, diabetes and obesity.

Many studies have been undertaken in the United States, Canada and a number of other countries to determine the exact physiological changes that result from a regular exercise program. Some of the changes indicated by these studies are listed below.

- Increased muscle strength, tone and size
- Increased efficiency of the heart
- Increased pulmonary efficiency
- Improved digestion
- Increased work tolerance
- Better mental alertness
- Improved sleep patterns
- Increased hemoglobin levels in the blood
- Decreased blood pressure
- Decreased deposits of fatty tissue
- Decreased cholesterol levels in the blood*

Numerous research studies have also demonstrated that proper exercise can help to slow the aging process. For example, regular exercise has been shown to maintain cardiovascular functioning and pulmonary reserve, glucose tolerance, bone density and physical strength and endurance. It has also been shown to reduce serum lipids and cholesterol and systolic blood pressure (Williams, 1993).

MOVEMENT AND EXERCISE THROUGHOUT THE LIFE CYCLE

Our capacity for movement and exercise is influenced by our age and our current phase of the life cycle. The development of coordinated movement begins in infancy and continues throughout childhood and adolescence. Strength, endurance and motor coordination reach maximum potential in late adolescence and early adulthood, and then gradually decline through middle and late adulthood.

Pregnancy

During late pregnancy, there is a general relaxation of all body ligaments, particularly those involving the pelvic bones and the back. A woman's centre of gravity is moved backwards by the enlarging uterus, tending to upset her balance. She usually feels awkward in her movements, being hindered by her increasing bulk as well as her protruding abdomen. A woman needs exercise throughout pregnancy to keep herself in overall good physical condition. Specifically, being in good physical condition aids circulation, strengthens the muscles used in delivery of the baby, and makes it easier to learn relaxation techniques. The relaxation techniques are helpful in making labour and delivery easier for the woman. Learning to relax specific muscles used in delivery, such as the pelvic and perineal diaphragms, is essential to further ease labour and delivery.

After delivery, exercises are needed to strengthen the abdominal muscles and the muscles of the pelvic floor, which have been stretched during labour and delivery. Most prenatal programs teach both pre- and postnatal exercises, as well as relaxation techniques.

Expectant parents are usually excited when the mother first feels the baby kick in her womb. This event is called "quickening" and usually occurs during the fourth or fifth month of gestation. The infant continues to move until just before birth, when the head becomes engaged in the birth canal.

Infancy

The newborn's movements are mainly random. Babies have poor motor control at first, because most of their movements are reflex actions. Some infants are much more active than others and some acquire motor skills at an earlier age than others do. It can be very traumatic to a new parent when a one-year-old child is still not walking while the neighbour's child has been running around since nine months of age. It helps if the nurse can reassure parents that their child is just as normal as the neighbour's. A chart of development for the first year of life (see Figure 28.4) identifies the *average* age in months when specific achievements are attained by 95 percent of normal infants. The chart is helpful in reassuring parents and is also useful in identifying children who are not developing at a normal rate.

During the first year of life, the major accomplishments in motor skills are learning to walk and learning to use the

---

*Greenberg and Dintiman (1992).

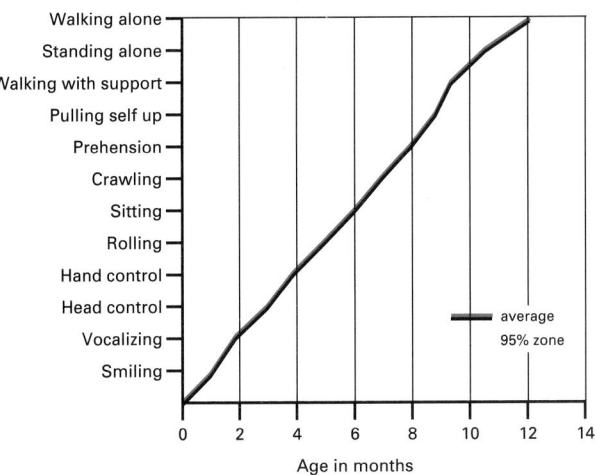

FIGURE 28.4 Average age for the achievements selected and the zone in which 95 percent of observations fell in a group of 215 normal infants

SOURCE: Johnson, T.R. and Moore, W.M. (1978). *Children are different: Developmental physiology.* Columbus, OH: Ross Laboratories, 33.

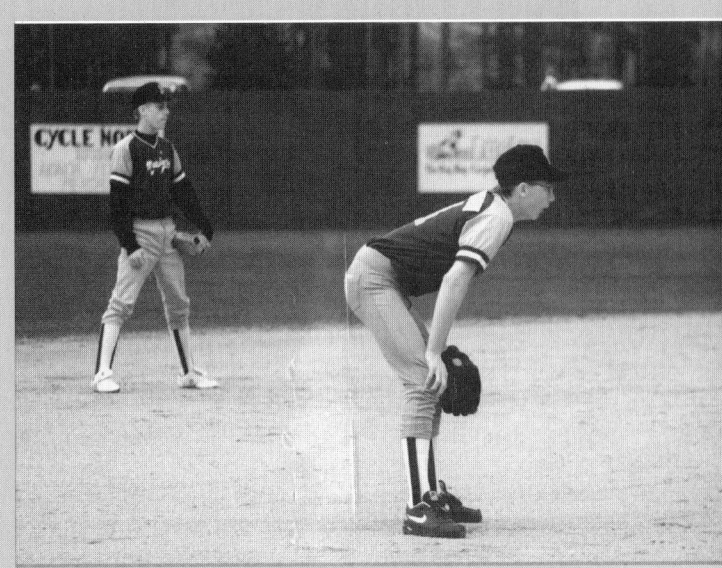

Adolescents enjoy outdoor sports and active physical exercise.

hands as tools (prehensile skill). These skills depend on physical maturation, although it is generally believed that a stimulating environment can accelerate motor development. A musical mobile, or brightly coloured objects suspended above the crib within the infant's reach, can stimulate a child's interest for movement, grasping and hand–eye coordination.

During infancy, the bones are soft and pliant and the pelvis is usually tilted forward. The back is rounded when the baby is sitting. Because the head is large in comparison with the body, balance is difficult. This is why babies often fall over when first learning to sit and totter in first attempts at walking.

Childhood

During childhood, the extremities grow faster than the trunk of the body, the pelvis straightens, and a pronounced spinal curvature develops. The toddler usually "toes out," and the older preschooler may "toe in" when walking. Children delight in activities that use their large muscles, such as running, hopping or jumping. By the time children are six years of age, they have usually acquired rudimentary motor skills that enable them to get about on skates, to ride a two-wheel bicycle and to swim. By the time they are 11, children have gained control of their motor skills to the extent that they appear graceful and coordinated in their movements. The development of fine motor skills usually lags behind that of gross motor skills. Girls as a general rule develop dexterity with their fingers and hands much earlier than boys do. Hence, girls' writing is generally better in school, and their drawings are usually neater.

Adolescence

Adolescence is characterized by a rapid growth spurt, and for a while, adolescents look as if they are all arms and legs. Hands and feet grow rapidly in length, pelvic and shoulder diameters increase and head circumference gets larger. They also attain an adult posture. With all of this growth going on, adolescents often look and feel awkward as they learn to adjust to their new body size. The adolescent usually has a lot of excess energy, which needs to be channelled constructively. This is the time for outdoor sports and active physical exercise to wear off the tremendous amount of energy that adolescents seem to have. It is during the late teens that an individual's strength, endurance and coordination reach the maximum potential.

Adulthood

The maximum potential for movement continues through early adulthood and begins to decline as people approach the middle years. Muscle strength peaks at the age of 30 and begins to decline after that (Timaris, 1988). If the individual continues to put excessive demands on the musculoskeletal system to reach the same levels as before, injury and inflammatory conditions are likely to occur. Because of this, traumatic injuries, such as fractures caused by skiing accidents, are common.

During the middle years, bone density and mass progressively decrease. Accidents that previously would have caused only minor injuries may now result in fractures. As people get older, they gradually lose height because of a gradual compression of the vertebrae bodies and the dehydration of vertebral discs. The regenerative capacity of articular cartilage is also diminished, and the cumulative effect of injuries to the joints may lead to arthritis. The frequency of joint disease increases with age. Most people do not participate in active sports to the same extent they did in their youth, and the more sedentary lifestyle of many adults often leads to "middle-age spread." Functional aerobic capacity also diminishes with age because the heart and lung function are not as efficient. Regular exercise is important for several reasons.

- It improves functional aerobic capacity
- It reduces the risk factors that can lead to coronary artery disease (such as being overweight and developing cholesterol accumulation in the blood stream)
- It maintains joint flexibility and it produces a general sense of well-being

People over the age of 65 are usually an inch or so shorter than they were in their youth. This is because of the thinning and, sometimes, anterior wedging and collapse of the intervertebral discs, in addition to the previously mentioned compression of the vertebral bodies themselves. There is also a loss of cartilage in the large joints and a proliferation of adjacent bone. Women in particular are vulnerable to osteoporosis. The reflexes that minimize sway in the erect posture become sluggish and blunted and deep tendon reflexes are often diminished or absent. There is a gradual, progressive loss of muscle bulk and strength. Often, there is a limited range of motion in the neck. The changes taking place in the musculoskeletal system and the changes taking place in the nervous system combine to make walking and other coordinated movements more difficult. Exercises that promote joint flexibility and improve circulation are particularly important for the older person.

DETERMINANTS OF MOVEMENT AND EXERCISE

A multitude of factors may affect movement and exercise. Many of these factors are related to alterations in health status. Others are the result of heredity, immobility and environmental and lifestyle factors.

ALTERATIONS IN HEALTH STATUS

The ability of the body to move its various parts and to control these movements and perform them in a coordinated fashion depends on the integrity of the muscles, the bones, the joints, the nerves innervating these structures and the circulation nourishing them. Injury, disease or congenital problems affecting the bones, muscles, joints, or

their collateral nerve or blood supply may cause impairment of motor functioning.

Even a minor injury, such as a sprained ankle (which damages muscles and ligaments), will limit the ability to walk until the muscle fibres and ligaments have healed. A bone fracture limits the ability to move the part of the body in which the fracture is located. People injured in car accidents, severe falls or other types of accidents may sustain injury to the spinal cord. Because the spinal cord is essential in the transmission of nerve impulses to and from the area in the brain controlling motor function, all movements below the site of the injury may be cut off. The person may be paralyzed from the waist down (*paraplegic*), if the injury is located at that level, or from the neck down (*quadriplegic*), if the injury is in the cervical region.

A *stroke* is the result of a cerebrovascular accident. This problem frequently impairs the blood supply to motor areas in the frontal lobe of one hemisphere of the brain, with resultant loss of motor functioning on one side of the body (*hemiplegia*). The motor abilities needed for speech may also be impaired if the accident occurs in the dominant half of the brain.

Serious illness of any kind lessens an individual's muscular strength and tone. Ill people may be completely dependent and unable to lift appendages or move around in bed, or they may have some limitations; they may require assistance to be able to do some of these activities. Inactivity of muscles leads to **contractures** — the abnormal flexion and fixation of joints caused by the shortening and atrophy of muscles fibers. Contractures at the wrist or ankle, for example, will cause limitations in mobility. These contractures frequently result from a hand or foot not being supported in good anatomical position and not being exercised when the patient is immobilized for another reason. Correcting these contractures requires intensive therapy over a prolonged period of time.

Movement is usually restricted in surgical patients because of pain in the operative area. Restrictions are put on patients' movement as soon as they are placed on bedrest for any reason in any type of illness. Limitations may be placed on mobility for therapeutic reasons, even if patients are not confined to bed, for example, in the case of a sprained ankle or a "wry neck" (*torticollis*).

Mobility may also be restricted because of nonmotor-related disabilities that limit the ability to get around without help, for example, vision or hearing loss.

HEREDITY

Congenital abnormalities are common troubles that often cause hospitalization in infants and small children. Many children the nurse will encounter on the pediatric units of hospitals are there for the correction of congenital malformations that interfere with the ability to walk, for example, "club-foot" or "congenital hip dislocation."

IMMOBILITY

The dangers of immobility have been well documented in numerous studies, books and articles in both nursing and medical literature over the past 30 or 40 years. Some of the adverse effects of lengthy bedrest are noted below.

- A slowing down of the basal metabolic rate
- A decrease in muscle strength, tone and size
- Postural changes
- Constipation
- Increased vulnerability to pulmonary and urinary tract infections
- Circulatory problems, such as thrombosis (the development of a clot in the blood stream) and embolus (the detachment of a clot and subsequent travelling through the blood stream until it becomes lodged in a vessel too small for it to pass through)

The degenerative process associated with immobility affects bone and skin tissues as well.

When the body is in a horizontal position, an extra amount of blood is "dumped" from the legs into the general circulation. When this happens, the pulse rate increases as the heart works harder in an attempt to cope with this extra blood. There is increased excretion of calcium, nitrogen and phosphorus, and the patient may suffer severe depletion of these elements. Patients who are subjected to lengthy bedrest usually develop feelings of anxiety and, frequently, hostility as a result of disturbed functioning of physical and mental activity. Sleep patterns can also be disrupted (Olsen, 1990).

ENVIRONMENT

The environment may significantly restrict mobility. People in nursing homes, for example, may have limited opportunities to move about and usually have physical mobility problems as well. Mobility is restricted in patients who are isolated because of communicable disease precautions since they cannot leave the immediate surroundings. The movements of some patients may be curtailed by the use of restraints if it is in their best interests to do so, for example, confused patients who may hurt themselves trying to get out of bed.

Air quality may greatly affect outdoor activity such as walking, jogging or participating in sports. Air pollution can interfere with respiratory function. Weather is another part of the environment that needs to be considered in relation to mobility. Air temperature can be too cold or too hot for many activities, and rain or snow can be a deterrent.

LIFESTYLE

The growth of technology has contributed to sedentary lifestyles for many people in developed countries. Jobs are often less physically demanding. Computers and electronic information transfer systems (e-mail and fax) have reduced the mobility required for many jobs, while electronic lifts and mechanical devices have eliminated the physical challenge of many others. Highly developed transportation systems and the extensive use of automobiles coupled with more conveniently placed public services and commercial enterprises also contribute to reduced physical activity, creating a more sedentary lifestyle. For example, mail is delivered to the door, the bus stop is located nearby, the corner mall contains most of the goods and services necessary for living and, in the extreme, nearly all of the essentials of life can be obtained without even leaving the home. In this technological age, individuals must plan for and include physical activity in their daily lives in order to keep fit and healthy.

Over-eating, drinking alcohol and smoking are all lifestyle factors that affect the ability to exercise. Financial concerns may also come into play, as some individuals cannot afford to participate in activities that are costly, such as skiing or belonging to a fitness centre.

COMMON PROBLEMS

The ability to make parts of the body move and to control these movements enables us to develop the motor skills (a series of coordinated movements) needed for the functions of daily living. It also permits the development of more highly refined motor skills, such as playing the piano, playing tennis or dancing. Common problems with movement include impaired motor function, limited range of motion, decreased muscle strength, lack of balance and coordination and pain and discomfort.

Impaired motor function   People whose motor abilities are impaired because of illness or injury often need help to perform the activities of daily living (ADL). Among the common problems for which the nurse's help may be needed is the inability or limited ability to raise the head, to grasp objects, to move around in bed, to turn on the side or to turn over, to raise the buttocks when lying flat or when sitting up (necessary for use of the bedpan), to sit up, to stand, to transfer (as from the bed to a chair or the reverse) or to walk. Such limitations make it difficult to be independent with respect to dressing, grooming, toileting, bathing, hygiene and feeding. Difficulties in performing these activities of daily living are called self-care deficits, (Carpenito, 1993).

Limited range of motion (ROM)   In expressing how much ROM a person has in all joints, the terms *full*, *partial* and *limited* ROM can be used. Individuals who have no difficulty with ADL are considered to have full range of motion with all joints. Impairment in either the upper or lower extremities or weakness on one side of the body may give patients partial ROM in an affected joint. The patient may only need assistance with some aspects of ADL, such as putting on socks and shoes or fastening snaps or buttons. When several joints are impaired, the patient may have very limited ROM, causing even more difficulty in maintaining ADL without assistance.

Decreased muscle strength   A decrease in muscle tone and strength accompanies many illnesses. A common example is the patient who has had a stroke. Patients are usually affected on one side of the body, and are left with weakness or no movement at all. As a result, they are unable to perform the activities of daily living by themselves. Large motor control may be compromised, denying independence in walking, standing or even sitting in a chair without using assistive devices. A lack of fine motor control may interfere with activities such as handling utensils for eating, combing hair, doing up buttons or holding a pencil.

Lack of balance and coordination   Falls are common problems that have to do with movement or exercise. They may be due to the type of activity or to a physical impairment, such as one-sided weakness associated with a stroke or an abnormal gait related to ataxia (compromised muscle coordination). Neurological disorders will also impair muscle coordination causing instability when ambulating or when transferring from one place to another (for example, moving from a bed to a chair). All age groups are at a certain risk of falling which is dependent upon the developmental stage and the activities in which people participate. Toddlers are prone to falling because they are learning to walk and have unsteady gaits due to balance reactions and undeveloped coordination. Older adults may be at higher risk than other age groups because of slower response time, degenerative disease or disorientation.

Pain and discomfort   The ability to move freely may be compromised by pain which occurs with movement. This pain can be related to traumatic injury such as sprains, strains or fractures, or to degenerative disease such as arthritis or osteoporosis. Post-surgical patients may be reluctant to move because of incisional pain.

ASSESSING MOVEMENT AND EXERCISE NEEDS

In assessing the need for movement and exercise, the nurse uses data from a variety of sources, namely the health history, the physical examination, the patient's chart and other health team members. The family is a primary source of information when a patient is unable to communicate. The nurse will find the patient's chart a particularly useful source. The medical examination and physician's diagnostic and

therapeutic plan for care, along with reports from the physiotherapist, the occupational therapist and other allied health team members, are contained in the chart. Radiology reports and results from laboratory and other diagnostic tests will also be found in the chart. The Kardex is another valuable source as it contains current information about the patient's functional abilities, level of activity, aids to ambulation, ability to transfer and exercise programs.

NURSING HEALTH HISTORY

The nursing history provides subjective data about how a patient meets the need for movement and exercise in daily living. This includes information about the patient's usual level of activity and exercise, ease of movement and motor function. Recent changes in mobility, any related health problems and current difficulties with ambulation or activities of daily living are explored. In patients with self-care deficits, the nature of assistance they will need is also determined. The patient's lifestyle, current physical fitness patterns and attitudes and knowledge about the benefits of exercise in health promotion are examined to help identify opportunities for health teaching.

PHYSICAL ASSESSMENT

Physical assessment is performed to gather objective data about a patient's mobility status. The examination is primarily carried out through the use of inspection and palpation techniques.

General observation   By observing the patient as a whole, the nurse can get a sense of the uniformity of the skeletal system, muscle structure, symmetry and posture. Body alignment can be assessed when the patient is standing, sitting and lying. Balance, coordination, weakness, lethargy and fatigue can also be assessed and validated through interviewing. The nurse can then move to more specific areas of the body. It is logical to start at the head of the body and work down systematically to the feet when collecting data. Since there may be great differences in strength, flexibility and ROM in the upper and lower extremities, these areas should be assessed separately.

Muscles   Muscles are assessed for symmetry, size, tone, strength and endurance. Assessment of the strength and equality of the upper extremities can be done using hand grips. The patient is asked to squeeze both of the examiner's hands as firmly as possible. To assess the lower extremities, foot presses can be done. Foot presses involve asking the patient to push the foot as hard as possible against the force exerted by the palm of the examiner's hand. This helps to establish whether a weakness exists in one side or

Movement and Exercise

Health and Illness Patterns

USUAL PATTERN OF MOVEMENT AND EXERCISE

- What are the activities you carry out in a typical day? (activities of daily living, work-related, home management, cooking, cleaning, gardening, recreation, leisure and social?)
- Do you usually get around by car? by bus? on foot?
- Do you exercise regularly? If so, what type of exercise do you do? how often? for how long?
- Do you use any assistive devices such as a cane, walker or brace?
- What kind of assistance would you require in hospital for ambulating and performing activities of daily living?

RECENT CHANGES IN PATTERN OF MOVEMENT AND EXERCISE

- Have any of your usual activities become difficult or impossible for you? Do you have any problems caring for yourself? working? getting around? exercising? Describe any changes.
- How long have you been experiencing these changes?
- Do you know the cause of these changes? Are the changes due to lifestyle? environmental factors? financial resources?
- Have you had a recent illness or health problem that has affected your ability to perform the activities of daily living and to exercise (for example, activity intolerance following a heart attack)?
- Are you taking any medications or treatments that may affect your daily motor activities and exercise?
- Do you think you would be helped by an assistive device such as a cane, walker or brace?

PRESENTING HEALTH PROBLEM

- Describe the symptoms you are experiencing now. Is there any pain? muscle weakness? joint stiffness? swelling?
- Can you point to the area where you feel pain?
- How would you describe the pain? Is it an aching, a burning, a stabbing, or a throbbing pain?
- When you have this pain, do you also have pain in another location?

- When did this pain begin? What were you doing at the time?
- What activities seem to decrease or increase the pain?
- Do you have any other unusual sensations, such as tingling, with the pain?
- Describe your weakness. When did you first notice muscle weakness? Did it begin in the same muscles where you notice it now?
- When did you first notice swelling? Did you injure this area?
- When did the stiffness begin? Has the stiffness increased or has it been constant?
- Do you ever hear a grating sound?
- Do weather changes seem to affect the problem? For example, does the pain increase in cold or damp weather?
- What methods have you tried to reduce the stiffness?
- Are you taking any prescription or over-the-counter drugs or using home remedies to treat the problem? If so, which ones, at what strengths and for how long have you been using them?
- Have you ever had any injury to a bone, muscle, ligament, cartilage, joint or tendon?
- Have you ever had surgery or other treatment involving bone, muscle, ligament, cartilage, joint or tendon?

Health Promotion and Protection Patterns

- What are your beliefs about exercise and physical fitness?
- Are you aware of the benefits of a regular fitness program to health and the prevention of illness? If not, would you like to learn about physical fitness and exercise?
- Do you follow a regular fitness schedule? If so, describe it. How has your current problem affected your usual exercise routine?
- Are you experiencing any difficulties with your exercise and fitness activities? Are you experiencing any fatigue? decreased endurance? pain? dyspnea? dizziness?
- Do you supplement your diet with vitamins, calcium, protein or other products?

another. Normally, muscle strength should be equal on either side of the body and should fully resist the examiner's opposing force.

Bones and joints   Bones and joints are also assessed through observation and palpation. Contour, prominence and symmetry are observed. Each joint must be examined individually. For the upper extremities, the shoulder, elbow, wrist and finger joints are examined for range of motion. In the lower extremities, the hip, knee, ankle and toes are all assessed separately. Normally, a person should be able to move joints independently through the full range of motion without pain. The nurse notes the degree to which each joint can move, its flexibility or any resistance felt when attempting to passively move the joint. The nurse should never attempt to force a joint if resistance is felt or if the patient expresses pain.

Body alignment   It is important to note whether a patient has good body alignment while standing, sitting and lying. In order to assess body alignment, the nurse must be aware of the body's normal anatomic position and know how to determine the body's centre of gravity. The centre of gravity may be explained as an imaginary line that runs through the centre of the body from head to toe vertically, and horizontally through the pelvis (see Figure 28.3).

Body balance   To determine body balance related to large motor control, the individual is observed in a standing (walking) or sitting position. The patient should be able to maintain balance whether walking independently or with assistive devices, such as walkers or canes. When sitting, a patient should be able to maintain an upright position without leaning to one side or another. Assessing balance is an important factor in determining the risk for injury.

Coordination   To assess fine motor control, the nurse observes the patient carrying out activities of daily living that involve dexterity, such as handling eating utensils, buttoning buttons, tying shoe laces, combing hair or writing with a pencil. These activities allow an individual to function independently and are an important part of daily living.

Assistive devices   It is important to note whether patients walk independently or whether they need the help of devices to maintain independence. Do they require the use of a cane, walker, crutches or wheelchair for mobility? How well do they use these devices?

Ability to transfer   A person who requires no assistance transferring from bed to chair, or from chair to toilet is considered to be independent. It is essential to assess the type of help an individual requires to move from one place to another. Some individuals may only require supervision for safety; others may need the assistance of one

or two nurses for a transfer. If the patient is too heavy or too incapacitated, a mechanical lift will be needed.

DIAGNOSTIC TESTS

The most common diagnostic tests used to assess mobility involve radiographic examination. Fractures, dislocations and other abnormalities can be detected with x-ray. Specific radiographic tests that may be done to assess joints, bones and muscles include the arthogram (visualization of a joint), myelogram (visualization of the spinal canal) and arthroscopy (examination of a joint through the use of fibreoptic technology).

DIAGNOSING MOVEMENT AND EXERCISE PROBLEMS

Movement and exercise problems pertain not only to difficulties or limitations in physical mobility and motor function but also to the effects of these difficulties on other facets of regular functioning. *Impaired physical mobility* is the nursing diagnosis often used for problems in which "the individual experiences or is at risk for experiencing limitation of physical movement but is not immobile" (Carpenito, 1993, 488). This can occur in patients with neuromuscular or musculoskeletal conditions such as multiple sclerosis or arthritis; in those who have undergone surgical procedures; or in those undergoing treatment with such measures as casts, traction devices or drainage tubes connected to suction units. Impaired physical mobility may be characterized by the inability to move purposefully within the environment (including bed mobility, transferring and ambulation), limitations in ROM, limited muscle strength and control, impaired coordination and imposed restriction on movement (Carpenito, 1993).

When a patient is unable to endure physical movement and exercise at the usual or desired level, the nursing diagnosis *Activity intolerance* applies. Many factors can cause activity intolerance. Cardiac, pulmonary, circulatory or chronic diseases, nutritional disorders, treatments such as surgery or chemotherapy, prolonged bedrest, medications and a sedentary lifestyle are a few of the possible related factors. Activity intolerance is defined by altered physiological responses to activity, in particular respiratory and cardiovascular function. These may include shortness of breath, dyspnea, change in rhythm, blood pressure and heart rate. Weakness, fatigue, pallor or confusion are other defining characteristics (Carpenito, 1993).

Impairments in motor function which lead to difficulties in performing the self-care activities of daily living (the ADLs) are stated as *Self-care deficits*. NANDA has identified five categories of self-care deficits, listed below.

- Feeding
- Bathing and hygiene
- Dressing and grooming
- Toileting
- Instrumental

The inability to cut food, open packages or bring food to the mouth define self-feeding deficits. In the self-bathing deficit, the patient may be unable to wash body parts or attend to personal care. Self-dressing deficits include difficulties with dressing, undressing and grooming. Patients requiring assistance to use the toilet, carry out adequate hygiene, transfer to and from the toilet, handle clothes and flush the toilet have a self-toileting deficit. Instrumental self-care deficits describe problems in which people experience an impaired ability to perform certain activities or access services essential to managing a household, such as using a telephone, accessing transportation, shopping or preparing meals (Carpenito, 1993).

Because the ability to move freely is so vital to human functioning, mobility impairments can become the etiology of other nursing diagnoses. For example, a patient with mobility impairment following extensive surgery might experience a self-care deficit. This can lead to a sense of powerlessness if the patient is confined to bed for a prolonged period of time and feels that personal control of the situation has been lost. Mobility impairments may also lead to deficits in diversional activity, alterations in health maintenance, impairments in management at home, fear of falling and difficulties in meeting safety needs. Indeed, when patients cannot move freely, they are at risk for injury because of the limited capacity to protect themselves from harm.

Many people today seek to enhance their level of wellness through lifestyle changes that centre around exercise and fitness. Physical fitness and exercise are key components of health practices which help to improve the quality of life and prevent such health problems as heart disease and stroke. When individuals and families indicate a desire to achieve a higher level of physical fitness and exercise, the diagnostic statement *Potential for enhanced physical fitness and exercise* may be used (Carpenito, 1993).

Following are some examples of nursing diagnoses that may apply to patients with movement and exercise problems.

- *Impaired physical mobility related to insufficient knowledge of managing a lower limb prosthesis*
- *Activity intolerance related to a sedentary lifestyle and inadequate diet*
- *Diversional activity deficit related to prolonged bedrest and inability to perform favourite activities*
- *Altered health maintenance related to decreased flexibility and muscle strength secondary to aging*
- *High risk for injury related to unsteady gait secondary to weakness and uncoordinated use of crutches*

PLANNING MOVEMENT AND EXERCISE INTERVENTIONS

A plan of care for patients with mobility and exercise problems is based on the nursing diagnoses and is designed to suit each individual's needs. Goals are generally aimed at maintaining, strengthening and restoring mobility and motor function, preventing further deterioration in function and promoting optimal functioning in daily living. The patient and family should be involved in establishing expected outcomes and selecting interventions as much as possible. The nurse works closely with the physiotherapist and the occupational therapist to plan exercises that are consistent with the physician's plan of care for the patient. The prevention of muscle deterioration and the maintenance and improvement of muscle strength and tone in patients whose mobility is limited requires the intensive effort of all concerned.

The process of recovery for patients who have partially or completely lost one or more of their motor abilities is often a long one. Short-term goals are therefore very important. The achievement of each small step of progress is something to strive for and provides the nurse, the patient and the family with motivation to work towards further goals. In setting goals, the nurse must ensure that the expected outcomes reflect levels of performance that are realistic and attainable in terms of the patient's capabilities.

According to Dr. Sidney Katz (cited in Meissner, 1980), who developed the index of independence in ADL, there is a natural order of progression in regaining independence. Functions such as feeding, continence, transfer, toileting, dressing and bathing follow a definite hierarchy, beginning with feeding and moving up towards bathing. It is important to note that, in establishing goals, a person who has had a fracture, for instance, will not regain full independence in dressing or toileting until the ability to transfer has been achieved. Similarly, a patient who has had a stroke will be able to achieve independence in feeding and continence before achieving independence in dressing and bathing (Meissner, 1980).

The following is a list of some examples of expected outcomes.

- The patient will demonstrate correct body alignment when standing, sitting or lying.
- The patient will show progressive activity tolerance as evidenced by maintaining pulse, respirations and blood pressure within predetermined ranges.
- The patient will feed him- or herself independently using special feeding utensils.
- The patient will walk with crutches, unassisted.
- The patient will demonstrate ways of preventing injury when transferring to and ambulating in a wheelchair.

In establishing priorities of care for patients with limited mobility, the nurse considers two sets of problems. For the patient whose mobility is curtailed, the foremost priority is the promotion of optimal strength and tone in unused muscles and the prevention of muscle degeneration and joint contractures. Patients who cannot move by themselves and need the nurse's help in turning and performing the activities of daily living should rank high on the nurse's list of priorities. Patients who cannot feed themselves should be helped while their food is still hot. Patients who need help in turning must be turned at scheduled times or serious skin problems may result. When patients need assistance to use the bedpan or a urinal, the nurse should ensure they receive help immediately. The patient who needs assistance in getting up, getting in or out of bed or getting in or out of the wheelchair likewise should not be left waiting too long.

Priorities of care may change from day to day depending on the patient's status. The nurse must use judgement in scheduling activities to ensure that patients who have problems in meeting basic physiological needs are given the needed assistance at the time they need it. The nurse must also be sufficiently flexible to interrupt other activities that can be deferred in order to assist patients who need immediate assistance with the basic needs. Recording, for example, can be interrupted when the nurse sees a patient's call light go on. Ignoring or responding slowly to signals for help devalues the patient-centred approach to treatment and is one of the most common complaints patients have when they are in hospital.

IMPLEMENTING MOVEMENT AND EXERCISE INTERVENTIONS

HEALTH PROMOTING STRATEGIES

Since the Lalonde Report (1974) and the fitness revolution that followed, as evidenced by such programs as "Participaction," *fitness* has become a key buzzword. Physical fitness, exercise, and other health promotion practices such as proper nutrition, a positive mental outlook and the avoidance of stress enable individuals to increase control over their lives and to function at maximum potential. By definition, physical fitness means "a set of abilities individuals possess in order to perform specific types of physical activity" (Williams, 1993, 13). Physical fitness related to health refers to the development of cardiovascular–respiratory vitality, maintenance of an optimal body weight and the development of joint flexibility and muscular strength and endurance. To maintain or improve physical fitness, it is important to participate in some form of regular physical activity and exercise.

TYPES OF PHYSICAL ACTIVITY AND EXERCISE

Physical activity generally involves bodily movement caused by muscular contraction that results in the expenditure of energy. There are two types of physical activity that promote health-related physical fitness—unstructured physical activity and structured physical activity.

Unstructured Physical Activity

Usual activities of daily living, such as walking, climbing stairs, cycling, gardening and home maintenance, domestic activities (house cleaning, changing bed linen, doing laundry), occupational activities and recreational activities fall into the category of unstructured physical activity. Unstructured activity, because of its low intensity, generally does not improve physical fitness, but it does maintain health and provide some protection against the development of certain chronic diseases, particularly if carried out for longer periods of time (Williams, 1993).

Structured Physical Activity

Structured physical activity refers to exercise programs designed to improve physical fitness. These include aerobic exercise, muscle strengthening exercises and flexibility or stretching exercises.

Aerobic exercise Of all of the different exercise programs available, those that involve aerobic activity possess the greatest potential for improving health. ***Aerobic exercise*** refers to sustained physical activity which increases heart rate, blood circulation and metabolic demands for oxygen. Aerobic exercises strengthen cardio–respiratory function and endurance and enhance the capacity of muscle tissues to extract oxygen from the blood and use it to generate energy via the oxygen system (Williams, 1993). Aerobic exercises involve the use of large muscle groups in a rhythmical manner. Aerobic exercises include speed walking, jogging, stationary bicycling, swimming, cross-country skiing, aerobic dancing, rowing and active games and sports, such as basketball, soccer or squash.

Muscular strengthening exercise Muscular strength and endurance are developed through physical activity in which force is exerted against resistance, thus the name resistance (weight) training. There are three basic types of exercises in resistance training: isotonic, isometric and isokenetic. ***Isotonic exercises*** are those in which the tension in the muscle remains constant while its length changes to move the resistance (weight) through a range of motion. The biceps curl is an example of an isotonic routine. In ***isometric exercise*** the tension of the muscles is increased, but there is neither movement of the joint nor

Potential Benefits of Aerobic Exercise

- Reduces risk of heart attack by
  - increasing blood serum HDL cholesterol, the "good" cholesterol
  - decreasing blood serum triglyceride levels
  - reducing high blood pressure
  - reducing the desire to smoke
  - improving the efficiency of the heart
- Reduces risk of developing certain forms of cancer
- Reduces risk of developing noninsulin-dependent diabetes
- Reduces excess body weight and helps maintain optimal weight
- Reduces risk of developing osteoporosis
- Increases resistance to stress, anxiety and fatigue; enhances mood and lowers depression
- Increases stamina, strength and working ability
- Improves self-esteem

SOURCE: Williams, M.H. (1993). *Lifetime fitness and wellness* (3rd ed.). Dubuque, IA: Wm C. Brown Communications Inc., 49. Reproduced with permission. All rights reserved.

Everybody should be encouraged to participate in a regular exercise program, unless health reasons preclude this. Exercises are planned to suit individual needs, interests and motor abilities, taking into consideration age, sex, degree of mobility and limitations imposed by chronic or current health problems and interests. The individual who starts on an exercise program should always have a complete physical examination first to make sure there are no contraindications to exercise, and to find out if there are any limitations on the type or amount of exercise planned.

Exercise programs may be carried out at home or outside the home. Exercise programs can be designed to accommodate all age groups and to cater to virtually all interests, from hiking, swimming and other active sports to simple calisthenics. Many community organizations offer a graded series of exercise classes to assist people in maintaining or regaining optimal physical fitness. Exercises for older people have become a regular feature of many of these programs.

A regular program of aerobic exercise is recommended. Regular aerobic exercise three to four times weekly, for thirty minutes of continuous activity, has been shown to produce a number of health benefits in all ages (Greenberg and Dintiman, 1992). All exercise sessions should start with a *warm-up* period of exercises that gradually increase respiration, circulation and body temperature and stretch muscles. A proper warm-up helps to prevent excessive strain on the heart as well as muscular soreness and injury. The warm-up is followed by a *stimulus* period of more vigorous activity designed to challenge the cardiovascular system by significantly increasing blood flow to the working muscles over an extended period of time. It is important that the intensity of the activity is moderate, not exhaustive. Exercise tolerance should be built up gradually, through regular sessions of gradually increasing intensity, rather than in intermittent spurts. Sessions should never be carried to the point of exhaustion.

change in the length of the muscle. This occurs when the muscular force generated to move an object is inadequate to overcome the resistance. Attempting to push or pull against an immovable object is an example of an isometric exercise. *Isokinetic exercise* involves activity in which the speed of muscle shortening is controlled by a machine or electronic device. Rehabilitative exercises for knee injuries, for example, use devices to regulate resistance through a complete range of motion.

Stretching exercise Flexibility is enhanced when muscles and joints are gently moved through their full range of motion. Stretching, yoga and calisthenics (systematic exercises for attaining strength and gracefulness) increase range of motion, improve circulation and also promote relaxation.

PROMOTING PHYSICAL FITNESS AND EXERCISE

Nurses can help to promote physical fitness by providing education and information to patients. Knowledge of physical fitness and of the benefits and risks of exercise will enable individuals to explore fitness practices and determine exercise needs. Patients may want to know how to go about establishing and maintaining an exercise program and the nurse should be prepared to provide this information.

Exercise classes assist people in maintaining physical fitness.

HEALTH PROMOTING STRATEGY

Promoting Fitness and Healthy Exercising

- Make exercise part of your daily routine.
- Use every opportunity for unstructured exercise, for example, take stairs instead of the elevator, walk instead of drive and walk at a brisk, fast pace.
- Plan a personal fitness program suited to you. If you have any health concerns, consult your physician before planning the program.
- Select activities that are rhythmic, repetitive and which challenge the circulatory system, at an intensity appropriate for you.
- Select a variety of modes of aerobic exercise that you enjoy, that are suited your needs and that can be done year-round.
- Wear comfortable clothes and shoes with proper support.
- Follow your program regularly, at least three times a week and not more than six, preferably on alternate days.

- Remember to warm up and cool down.
- Begin your sessions with less vigorous activities and gradually build the intensity as your body adapts to the exercise routine and your physical fitness improves.
- Avoid exercising to the point of exhaustion and never force a joint beyond its range of motion.
- If you experience muscle pain, burning or tingling, stop and rest for a few minutes.
- Stop exercising and consult the physician if you experience
  - pain in the chest, in the arm, or any other unexplained pain.
  - irregular pulse rate — too fast or too slow, flutters, rapid rate changes.
  - palpitations in the chest or throat.
  - dizziness, light-headedness, fainting or confusion.

(Williams, 1993; Corbin and Lindsey, 1994)

Following the exercise period, a gradual cooling-down is advised. This should involve slower movements, such as relaxing exercises or simply walking around for a few minutes, to allow the body time to adjust to lessened physical demand and return the heart rate to near normal. Stretching at this time may help to improve flexibility and prevent muscle stiffness.

HEALTH PROTECTING STRATEGIES

Patients who remain in bed for prolonged periods are prone to develop complications as a result of inactivity. Exercise helps to create and maintain good muscle tone and to prevent atrophy. Exercise also helps in the elimination of waste products from the muscles. The contraction of muscles increases circulation and the metabolism of wastes from the body. Increased circulation is particularly important for the person who remains in bed. Stasis of blood is a predisposing factor in the formation of clots, which can lead to serious complications. The increased basal metabolic rate that results from exercise increases the body's need for oxygen. This in turn results in an increase in both the rate and depth of respirations, which improves lung aeration and helps to prevent infectious processes in the lungs — these can occur as a result of inactive lung areas and stagnant secretions. Improved blood circulation also increases the delivery of oxygen and nutrients to tissues, maintaining their health and preventing deterioration and ulcer formation.

Contractures and stiffening of the joints are other unfortunate side effects of prolonged inactivity. By putting joints through their full range of motion, these complications can often be avoided.

MUSCLE STRENGTHENING EXERCISE

Patients who are inactive because they are confined to bed or a wheelchair or because they are recuperating from illness can maintain strength and flexibility of muscles and joints and prevent muscle wasting and joint stiffness or contractures through regular exercise. The patient is encouraged to exercise actively those muscles that can be used. Patients can learn how to do isometric exercises while they are otherwise inactive. For example, the patient who is confined to bed can perform isometric exercises of the lower limbs by periodically contracting the quadriceps and gluteal muscles for 10 to 15 seconds, or by pushing the back of the knee against the bed while the leg is extended. Clenching the fist or squeezing a ball are isometric exercises for increasing hand strength. Isometric contraction, sometimes referred to as "muscle setting" exercise, can help considerably in maintaining or improving muscle strength and tone.

Principles Relevant to Exercise Programs for Patients

1. The process of degeneration starts almost immediately when muscles are unused.

2. The process of degeneration involves bone and skin tissues as well as muscle tissue.

3. All joints have a circumscribed range of motion.

4. Passive exercise of the body's movable parts through their full range of motion prevents the development of contracture that can interfere with joint mobility.

5. Active contraction of muscles is required to maintain and improve their strength and tone.

6. Active contraction of muscles on one side of the body causes the corresponding muscles on the other side of the body to contract.

7. Exercise has beneficial effects on all body systems.

Isotonic exercise is often prescribed as part of the patient's therapy but it may also be used for preventive care. In isotonic exercise, the muscle actively contracts or shortens, causing the limb to move. Active range of motion exercises, which we discuss in the next section, are isotonic activities. This type of exercise is beneficial for preventing joint stiffness and weakness, as well as for promoting muscle strength and tone. Patients may go to the physiotherapy department for this, or the physiotherapist may come to the nursing unit.

If a program of regular exercise is not undertaken by another health care worker for a patient, the nurse institutes one. This is done for all patients for whom active exercise is not contraindicated. Both individual and group exercises are used. Group exercises are helpful from a psychosocial point of view (increasing sensory stimulation), and for their physically therapeutic benefits. There is greater motivation for patients to put forth more effort in a group when everyone is doing the same thing. In many agencies, group therapy classes are organized by the physiotherapy department, but there is no reason why a nurse cannot organize these on a nursing unit. This is frequently done in some obstetrical units to assist patients to regain lost muscle tone resulting from pregnancy and childbirth, or on an extended care unit to reactivate residents.

Occupational therapy also assists people to maintain or regain muscular strength and to prevent loss of joint mobility. The focus of occupational therapy is to assess activities of daily living and to help the patient become as functionally independent as possible.

RANGE OF MOTION EXERCISE

Range of motion exercises (ROM), in which a body part is moved through a range of motion, are carried out to promote circulation, maintain muscle tone and promote flexibility. In doing this, joint stiffness and debilitating contractures are prevented. **Active ROM** is range of motion carried out by the patient. It is a form of isotonic exercise and as such, it maintains strength, tone and flexibility. In patients unable to move body parts due to paralysis or extreme illness, ROM is performed by someone else. This is called **passive ROM** exercise. Passive exercise helps to maintain joint flexibility and prevent stiffness and contractures. Because this type of exercise involves no active movement on the part of the muscles, it does not contribute to muscle tone or strength.

ROM exercises are planned as a regular part of nursing activities. During a bath, for example, the nurse has an excellent opportunity to move the patient's limbs through their full range of motion. The patient is encouraged to exercise actively those muscles that can be used. However, in certain cases, the nurse may need to assist the patient in performing ROM (active assisted ROM), or to perform passive ROM.

Performing ROM Exercises

The body has six large movable parts: the head, the trunk, two arms and two legs. It also has smaller movable parts, such as the hand, fingers, feet and toes, which form parts of larger parts but may move independently All of these body parts are capable of the various kinds of movements defined previously. You can move your hand without moving the rest of your arm, for example, or your finger independently of any other part of your body.

The degree to which people can tolerate exercise varies considerably. A patient should avoid fatigue and pain while exercising. Joints need to be exercised to the full range of motion. In active assisted and passive exercises, the nurse should not force movement when it is painful to the patient or when resistance is met. When passive range of motion is performed, the joint must be properly supported to prevent muscle strain or injury. The nurse does this by placing the hands directly above or below the joint to be moved. Table 28.3 illustrates and provides instructions for performing both active and passive range of motion exercises.

When a patient is exercising, the joints should go through their full range of motion. For example, the normal shoulder and upper arm movements are flexion, extension, hyperextension, abduction, adduction, circumduction, inward rotation and outward rotation. The chief muscles involved in these movements are the deltoid (abducts the upper arm), pectoralis major (flexes and adducts the upper arm), trapezius (raises and lowers the shoulders), latissimus dorsi (extends and adducts the upper arm) and serratus anterior (pulls the shoulder forward).

Hand and finger exercises are very important. Flexing, extending, abducting and adducting the hand, as well as flexing and extending the joints of the fingers, are exercises commonly carried out by patients who have some functional impairment as a result of a stroke. It is particularly important to exercise the thumb. The ability to bring the thumb in opposition to the tip and base of the fingers is a key factor in the use of the hands.

The elbows and the knees can be flexed and extended. The biceps, triceps, quadriceps and hamstring muscles are active when these movements are performed. The forearm can be supinated and pronated. The four principal muscles that move the forearm are the biceps brachii (flexes and supinates), the brachialis (flexes and pronates), the triceps brachii (extends) and the pronator quadratus (pronates).

Thigh movement involves the glutei muscles and the adductor and flexor muscles. The glutei muscles (maximus, medius and minimus) extend, rotate and abduct the thigh. The adductor muscles adduct the thigh and adduct and flex the leg. Flexion, extension, abduction, adduction and inward and outward rotation from the hip are usually possible. Most hip movements involve movement of the pelvis as well.

Movement of the feet and toes is also important. The ankle is a hinged joint that permits *plantar flexion* (pointing the foot down) and *dorsiflexion* (bending the foot backwards). Inversion and eversion of the feet take place in the gliding joints. The joints of the toes permit flexion, extension, abduction and adduction.

Normally the vertebral joints permit flexion, extension, lateral flexion and rotation of the cervical spine and trunk. The rectus abdominis, the external and internal oblique muscles and the sacrospinal muscle are involved in these movements.

TABLE 28.3   Assisting with Range of Motion

| MOVEMENT | ACTIVE | | PASSIVE | |
	ILLUSTRATION	INSTRUCTIONS FOR PATIENT	ILLUSTRATION	DESCRIPTION OF NURSE'S ACTION
HEAD **Rotation**		Tell patient to turn head as far as possible to the left, then to the right.		Cup the palm of your hand under the patient's chin. Pull or push chin in an arc toward each shoulder and return. (Note: no pillow)
Forward Flexion		Move head as if to look at feet, then return to resting position.		Cup hands behind patient's head, pulling head upward toward chest.
Lateral Flexion		Tilt head so left ear moves toward left shoulder. Repeat for right.		Supporting the head as above, tilt the head so left ear moves toward the left shoulder. Repeat for right.
Hyperextension		Tip head back as if looking up.		Seated or side-lying — done after all supine exercises. Place one hand on the patient's forehead, the other under chin. Move the head in an arc toward the back.

	ACTIVE		PASSIVE	
MOVEMENT	**ILLUSTRATION**	**INSTRUCTIONS FOR PATIENT**	**ILLUSTRATION**	**DESCRIPTION OF NURSE'S ACTION**
Circumduction		Roll head as if drawing a large circle with the top of the head, left to right, then right to left.		Support chin and occiput (back part of head) with palms of hands when patient is sitting up. Rotate head in circular motion to right, then to left.
UPPER EXTREMITY *Shoulder Flexion*		Start with arm at side or flexed so forearm is across chest. Move arm above head in a smooth arc. (Hand or elbow will make a half-circle in movement.)		Flex arm across chest. Cup elbow in one hand, grasp wrist joint to support wrist and hand. Move arm above patient's head so elbow makes a 180° arc.
Adduction		Bring arm across chest, moving elbow as close to middle of body as possible.		Bracketed movements are performed together: Grasping elbow and wrist joint as above, move elbow across chest toward midline.
Abduction		After the above, move arm outward, away from the body, then up over head.		Starting in adduction and keeping arm flexed and supported as above, move arm away from the body, then over the head.
Internal rotation		Start with arm straight out to side from shoulder with palm facing front and elbow bent in 90° angle. Move hand downward so fingers point to floor. If lying down, hand should be raised above body. Move hand forward so palm touches bed next to hip. Upper arm remains on the bed.		Move arm straight out from shoulder; flex elbow so hand is raised. Support wrist joint as above and stabilize upper arm. Press gently on shoulder with your other hand. With elbow as fulcrum, move the hand downward so hand makes an arc, touching bed next to patient's hip if possible.

(continued on next page)

	ACTIVE		PASSIVE	
MOVEMENT	**ILLUSTRATION**	**INSTRUCTIONS FOR PATIENT**	**ILLUSTRATION**	**DESCRIPTION OF NURSE'S ACTION**
External rotation		After completing internal rotation, move hand so fingers point up. If lying down, keep upper arm on bed and move hand so back of hand touches bed next to head.		After above, move the hand upward so the back of the hand touches the bed next to patient's head.
Circumduction		Extend arm straight out from body at shoulder. Move hand as if to draw a circle.		After above, extend the elbow so the arm points out from body. Cupping the elbow and supporting the wrist joint, move the arm in a circular motion.
Hyperextension		When standing or sitting with arm at side, swing arm backwards as far as possible without turning hand. May also be done lying on side.		(Done at the completion of all exercises in the supine position.) With patient prone or side-lying, arm at side, cradle arm to support elbow and wrist joint. Move arm toward the back as far as possible, so that hand makes an arc.
ELBOW **Pronation**		Starting with arms at sides, bend arm with palm facing upward, then turn palm toward floor.		Hold patient's hand as if to shake hands; elbow may rest on bed or be cupped by other hand. Turn your hand so patient's hand faces the floor.
Supination		Starting in elbow pronation position, turn palm up toward ceiling.		When above is completed, turn palm up toward ceiling.

MOVEMENT	ACTIVE		PASSIVE	
	ILLUSTRATION	INSTRUCTIONS FOR PATIENT	ILLUSTRATION	DESCRIPTION OF NURSE'S ACTION
Flexion		Starting with arm at side, bend elbow, moving hand toward shoulder.		
Extension		Return to starting position.		Place patient's arm at the side, palm up or facing thigh. Grasp patient's hand and wrist. With patient's elbow resting on bed, move patient's fingers toward the shoulder and return to straight position.
Circumduction		Place elbow out so it is level with shoulder. Move hand in a circle.		Rest elbow on bed. Grasp wrist and describe circle with hand while stabilizing upper arm with your other hand.
WRIST *Adduction (ulnar deviation)*		Tell the patient to: With arm at side, bend wrist as if to touch side of arm with little finger.		Place patient's palm in yours. Grasp wrist with your other hand. Move patient's hand from side to side as if to touch thumb (abduction) and little finger (adduction) alternately on either side of arm.
Abduction (radial deviation)		With arm at side, bend wrist as if to touch thumb on side of arm.		

(continued on next page)

	ACTIVE		PASSIVE	
MOVEMENT	**ILLUSTRATION**	**INSTRUCTIONS FOR PATIENT**	**ILLUSTRATION**	**DESCRIPTION OF NURSE'S ACTION**
Flexion		Bend wrist so palm moves toward it.		Rest elbow on bed, grasp wrist. Hold patient's hand so yours and patient's fingers are perpendicular. Flex palm toward wrist.
Hyperextension		Bend wrist so back of hand moves toward it.		When wrist flexion completed, extend wrist, then move back of hand toward wrist.
Circumduction		Move hand as if stirring — make a circle with hand.		Supporting patient's hand as above, move hand in circular motion.
FINGERS ***Adduction/ abduction***		Spread fingers and thumb as far as possible, then bring together.		With arm resting on bed or across chest, move the thumb and each finger away from the adjacent finger and return.
Opposition		Touch each finger to thumb.		With hand still resting on bed, touch each finger to thumb.

MOVEMENT	ACTIVE			PASSIVE	
	ILLUSTRATION	INSTRUCTIONS FOR PATIENT		ILLUSTRATION	DESCRIPTION OF NURSE'S ACTION
Circumduction		Make a circle with each finger and thumb.			Move each finger and thumb in a circle while supporting wrist.
Flexion/extension		Make a fist, straighten and repeat.			Flex elbow, grasp wrist. Place the palm of your other hand on the back of the patient's hand and flex all fingers and thumb with yours. Hook your fingertips under the patient's flexed fingers and thumb and pull them to extension, *or* slide your palm under the patient's flexed fingers, extending the fingers and thumb as you do.
Hyperextension		Stretch fingers and thumb toward the back of hand.			Continue to apply pressure on fingers and thumb to hyperextend them.
LOWER EXTREMITY **Hip** **Internal rotation**		Keeping knee straight and foot perpendicular to leg, turn foot toward center of body.			With leg resting on bed, rotate leg toward midline.
External rotation		In same position as above, turn foot outward.			With leg resting on bed, rotate leg outward.

(continued on next page)

MOVEMENT	ACTIVE		PASSIVE	
	ILLUSTRATION	INSTRUCTIONS FOR PATIENT	ILLUSTRATION	DESCRIPTION OF NURSE'S ACTION
Adduction		Bring one leg across and in front of the other leg.		Support leg behind ankle and knee. Move leg toward midline.
Abduction		Move leg out to the side as far as possible.		Support as above, move leg outward away from midline. Step away from side of bed to fully abduct hip.
Circumduction		With leg straight, move foot in circular motion.		Supporting leg as above, move it in a circular motion, keeping leg straight.
Flexion		Bend hip and knee bringing knee close to chest. Can assist by grasping knee with arms (see knee flexion below).		Support ankle and calf to flex knee and hip, pushing thigh toward abdomen.
Hyperextension		Point toe, move leg backward with knee straight.		(Done after all leg exercises in supine position have been completed.) Place patient on side or prone. Cradle lower leg with arm. Applying counterpressure on buttocks, raise leg off bed. (Move leg backward if lying on side.)
KNEE Flexion		Lying on back, bend knee to chest and grasp with arms.		Done with hip flexion.

MOVEMENT	ACTIVE		PASSIVE	
	ILLUSTRATION	INSTRUCTIONS FOR PATIENT	ILLUSTRATION	DESCRIPTION OF NURSE'S ACTION
Circumduction		With knee flexed, move foot in circular motion.		Support back of knee, ankle. With knee flexed, move lower leg in circular motion.
Hyperextension		Sitting with leg extended, push back of knee against surface below.		Cradle knee joint. Apply counterpressure above knee, gently raise lower leg until you feel resistance.
ANKLE **Inversion**		Tell the patient to: Turn the sole of the foot toward the other leg.		With leg resting on bed, stabilize ankle, grasp forefoot with fingers on sole. Turn sole of the foot toward midline.
Eversion		Turn the sole of the foot to the outside.		Holding forefoot as above, turn the sole away from the midline.
Dorsiflexion		Bend the foot toward the shin.		Holding foot as above, flex the foot toward the shin. (May also cup heel with hand and use forearm to flex foot.)
Plantar flexion		Point the toe.		Holding foot as above, straighten foot as if to point toe.

(continued on next page)

	ACTIVE		PASSIVE	
MOVEMENT	**ILLUSTRATION**	**INSTRUCTIONS FOR PATIENT**	**ILLUSTRATION**	**DESCRIPTION OF NURSE'S ACTION**
Circumduction		Move foot in circular motion at ankle without moving the knee.		With foot in plantar flexion, rotate forefoot in circular motion.
TOES *Flexion*		Curl toes.		Flex toes toward sole of foot by applying pressure with fingers.
Hyperextension		Raise toes off floor without raising foot. Spread toes.		Move one hand behind toes and the other hand to forefoot, apply hand pressure to move toes toward ankle.
Adduction / abduction				With leg resting on bed, separate each toe from the one adjacent.
Circumduction				Move each toe in a circular motion.

SOURCE: Berger, K.J. and Williams, M.B. (1992). *Fundamentals of nursing: Collaborating for optimal health.* Norwalk, CT: Appleton & Lange, 1440–1449. Reproduced with permission.

BODY MECHANICS

The practice of good body mechanics is integral to healthy living for all people. In health and in illness, good posture and efficient body movement are essential both therapeutically and aesthetically. The proper use of body mechanics is especially important for nurses who do a lot of moving and lifting of patients in the course of their work. Improper body mechanics can lead to injury for both the nurse and the patient. Using principles of body mechanics not only prevents injury but also promotes efficient use of energy.

Once people have knowledge of the principles underlying body mechanics, they should put them into practice in order to establish good patterns of body movement. As these patterns are established, movements become smooth and place a minimum of strain upon the muscles. The nurse will find that good patterns of body movement will be beneficial when helping patients to move more easily and be more comfortable.

Understanding the following principles of body movement and their application in the correct use of the nurse's muscular energy and weight will contribute greatly to ease nurse–patient physical interactions and reduce the likelihood of injury to either party.

Large muscles fatigue less quickly than small muscles. Using a group of large muscles places less strain on the body than does using a group of smaller muscles or a single muscle. For example, less strain results when a heavy object is raised by bending the knees rather than by bending from the waist. The former movement uses the large gluteal and femoral muscles, whereas the latter utilizes smaller muscles such as the sacrospinal muscle of the back.

Muscles are always in slight contraction. This condition is called *resting muscle tone.* If the nurse prepares the muscles for action prior to activity, ligaments and muscles will be protected from strain and injury. For example, the nurse will be better prepared to lift a heavy object if the muscles of the abdomen and pelvis and the gluteal muscles of the buttocks are first contracted.

The stability of an object is greater when there is a wide base of support and a low centre of gravity, and when the line of gravity is perpendicular to the ground and falls within the base of support. In nursing action movements, the nurse can assume a broad stance and bend the knees rather than bend at the waist. This practice keeps the vertical line of the centre of gravity within the base of support, thus providing greater stability. For example, when standing with feet apart and bending at the knees rather than at the waist, the nurse maintains better balance when helping a patient move.

The amount of effort required to move a body depends on the resistance of the body as well as on the gravitational pull. By using the pull of gravity rather than working against it, the nurse can reduce the amount of effort required in movement. For example, it is easier to move a patient up in bed

KEY PRINCIPLES

Principles Relevant to Body Mechanics

1. Large muscles fatigue less quickly than small muscles.
2. Muscles are always in slight contraction.
3. The stability of an object is always greater when there is a wide base of support and a low centre of gravity, and when the line of gravity is perpendicular to the ground and falls within the base of support.
4. The amount of effort required to move a body depends upon the resistance of the body as well as on the gravitational pull.
5. The force required to maintain body balance is greatest when the line of gravity is farthest from the centre of the base of support.
6. Changes in activity and position help to maintain muscle tone and avoid fatigue.
7. The friction between an object and the surface on which the object is moved affects the amount of work needed to move the object.
8. Pulling or sliding an object requires less effort than lifting it, because lifting necessitates moving against the force of gravity.
9. Using one's own weight to counteract another patient's weight requires less energy in movement.

when the bed is flat and the centre of gravity has been shifted towards the foot of the bed than when the head of the bed is elevated, in which case the resistance of the body to movement is much greater.

The force required to maintain body balance is greatest when the line of gravity is farthest from the centre of the base of support. Therefore, the person who holds a weight close to the body uses less effort than the person who holds the weight in extended arms. Thus, when moving a patient from a bed to a stretcher, it is easier for the lifters if they hold the patient's body close to their own.

Changes in activity and position help to maintain muscle tone and avoid fatigue. By changing position even slightly while carrying out a task, and by changing the activity from time to time, better muscle tone will be maintained and undue fatigue will be avoided.

The friction between an object and the surface upon which the object is moved affects the amount of work needed to move

---

Back Programs

"In 1990, Canadian hospitals reported 30 487 time-loss injuries. Fifty-three percent were sustained by nurses. Almost half [of the injuries sustained by nurses] were back injuries. Back injury is now recognized as one of the major reasons for ill-health retirement from nursing. Not only is it the most frequent injury sustained by nurses, it is the most debilitating" (Haley, 1994, 57). Many programs are available both in the community and in the workplace to deal with the prevention of back problems. Understanding how the back works and developing knowledge of how to use your back correctly are the keys to promoting and maintaining health. Workers' Compensation Boards have developed pamphlets, books and videos to help educate the work force. Individual hospital programs have developed their own back programs in order to educate staff members about how to use their backs correctly and thereby prevent injury.

---

the object. Friction is a force that opposes motion. The smoothest surfaces create the least friction; consequently less energy is needed to move objects on smooth surfaces. When a patient changes position in bed, the nurse can apply this principle by providing a smooth foundation upon which the patient can move.

Pulling or sliding an object requires less effort than lifting it, because lifting necessitates moving against the force of gravity. If, for example, the nurse lowers the head of a patient's bed before helping to move the patient up in the bed, less effort is required than when the head of the bed is raised.

Using one's own weight to counteract a patient's weight requires less energy in movement. If nurses use their own weight to move or push a patient, the weight increases the force applied to the movement.

MOVEMENT AND POSITION CHANGE

The goal to safe movement and position change is to promote functional mobility in the dependent or semidependent patient while protecting both the patient and the nurse from the risk of injury. The nurse facilitates movement by assisting (as required) the patient to change position using principles of body mechanics and competence in nursing skills. In the following section, various techniques to help patients move and change positions will be outlined. The basic preparation is the same for all of the nurse-assisted patient movements.

Preparing the Patient

Inform the patient of the intent to move, in order to avoid startling him or her and to enlist participation. Approach the patient from a direction in which you can be seen and heard. Ensure the patient's freedom of movement by freeing tubes, leads, cords and restraints, and ensure privacy by closing doors or curtains.

Preparing the Nurse

Remove sharp-edged, dangling jewellery which can cause skin damage. Assess the patient's physical, mental and emotional status. Make sure that you don't do anything that patients are capable of doing for themselves. Imagine the sequence of movement in order to anticipate patient needs. Enlist help if required, and designate a leader when working as a team to coordinate actions. Remember to use the principles of body mechanics.

Assembling Equipment and Preparing the Work Area

Gather necessary equipment (non-skid shoes, clothing, pillows and transfer aids) prior to movement. Check the equipment for safety. Apply brakes to wheelchairs, beds and stretchers, and clear the work area of obstacles, ensuring freedom of movement.

MOVING A PATIENT TO THE SIDE OF THE BED

Procedures 28.1 and 28.2 outline how to help a patient move to the side of the bed using a one-person total and a one-person partial assist. The partial assist procedure is used when a patient has good upper body strength and abdominal muscle tone and can participate in the movement.

MOVING A PATIENT UP IN BED

It is easiest to move dependent patients up in bed with two people rather than one; however, it is possible for one nurse to help a patient using a diagonal motion towards the side of the bed. By moving the patient in sections and by using the nurse's own weight to counteract the patient's weight, the nurse can safely move the dependent patient up in bed. This is most easily done if the head of the bed is lowered; this way the nurse is not working directly against the force of gravity. Procedures 28.3 and 28.4 detail how to move a patient up in bed using a one- and two-person total assist technique.

PROCEDURE 28.1

Moving a Patient to the Side of the Bed: Total Assist (One Person)

ACTION	RATIONALE
1. Stand facing the patient at the side of the bed towards which the patient is moving.	
2. Assume a broad stance with one leg forward of the other and with knees and hips flexed.	A wide base of support facilitates nurse's stability.
3. Move the patient's body in segments: upper, middle, then lower. Place one arm under the patient's shoulder and neck, and the other arm under the rib cage.	Less energy is expended moving parts instead of whole body.
4. Shift body weight from front foot to back foot, and rock backward to a crouched position, pulling the patient to the side of the bed.	Large muscles are less easily fatigued.
5. Repeat the procedure for the middle segment, placing the hands under the patient's buttocks and thighs.	

Assume a broad stance.

Shift body weight and rock backward, pulling the patient to the side of the bed.

ACTION	RATIONALE
6. Align the lower segment by placing arms under knees and ankles.	Maintains body alignment.
7. Avoid excessive friction moving the patient.	Prevents abrasive forces which cause discomfort and skin breakdown.

Patients who have some movement ability may be helped to move up in bed using a partial-assist procedure. This movement is facilitated when the patient can assist by flexing the knees and pushing with the legs. In assisting the patient to make this movement, the nurse should take precautions to ensure that the patient's head does not hit the top of the bed. This is done by lowering the head of the bed and putting a pillow at the head of the bed, where it can act as a pad. Helping the patient move up in bed can be done by one or two nurses; in the latter instance one nurse stands on each side of the patient's bed. Procedure 28.5 describes a one-person partial assist.

Moving a Patient to the Side of the Bed: Partial Assist (One Person)

ACTION	RATIONALE
1. Follow steps 1 and 2 of Procedure 28.1.	
2. Move the middle segment first. Instruct the patient to bend the knees, push down on the bed with the feet, raise the buttocks, and then move over to the edge of the bed, with the aid of the forearms.	Allows the patient to use their femoral muscles for movement.

ACTION	RATIONALE
3. Follow with head and neck, then legs.	Maintains body alignment.

Moving a Patient Up in Bed: Total Assist (One Person)

ACTION	RATIONALE
1. Stand at the side of the patient's bed and face the far corner of the foot of the bed. One foot is placed behind the other, assuming a broad stance.	Increases the base of support which facilitates nurse's stability.
2. Flex the knees so that both forearms are level with the bed. One arm is placed under the patient's head and shoulders, and one arm under the small of the back.	Prevents back injury.

PROCEDURE 28.3
continued

ACTION

RATIONALE

3. Rock forward, then shift weight from the forward foot to the rear foot, hips coming downward. The patient will slide diagonally across the bed towards the head and side of the bed.

Rocking motion develops momentum.

4. Move the patient's trunk and legs as in Procedure 28.1.

Keeps the body in proper alignment.

5. Go to the other side of the bed and repeat the steps. Repeat this process, if required.

PROCEDURE 28.4

Moving a Patient Up in Bed: Total Assist (Two Person)

ACTION

RATIONALE

1. Place the patient in a supine position with the head of the bed flat.

Decreases gravitational pull.

2. Both nurses stand at same side of the bed looking towards the head of the bed.

Movement of the patient is more coordinated.

3. The leader places one arm under the patient's neck and shoulders, supporting the head, and the other arm under shoulder and lower ribs. The second nurse places his or her hands under the patient's buttocks and upper thighs.

Enables equal distribution of body weight.

Continued on the next page

ACTION	RATIONALE

4. At leader's direction, the nurses move the patient up in bed by transferring weight to their forward foot.

Promotes smooth, coordinated effort.

Moving a Patient Up in Bed: Partial Assist (One Person)

ACTION	RATIONALE

1. Help the patient get into position with knees flexed and feet flat on the bed, heels near the buttocks.

Permits the patient to use the femoral muscles for movement.

ACTION	RATIONALE
2. Stand at the side of the bed, facing towards the direction of the movement. One foot is a step in front of the other, the foot that is closer to the bed positioned to the rear.	Prevents twisting of the nurse's body during the movement.
3. Place one arm under the patient's shoulders and one arm under the upper thighs.	Provides support to heaviest parts of the body.
4. Instruct the patient to place the chin on the chest and push with the feet on count of 3. On the count of 3, shift weight from the rear foot to the forward foot and move the patient up as the patient pushes upwards with the feet. The patient may also assist by pulling on an overhead bed bar or by pushing on bent elbows.	Movement is coordinated through a predetermined count of "1-2-3-up." Provides momentum to overcome inertia. Encourages independence.

TURNING AND POSITIONING A PATIENT

Patients may need assistance turning from side to side or changing position in bed. Procedures 28.6 to 28.8 outline the steps in helping a patient turn from a supine to a side-lying position, change from a supine to a semi-prone position and change from a side-lying to a sitting position on the edge of bed.

Turning a Patient from a Supine to Side-Lying Position

ACTION	RATIONALE
1. Assist the patient to the far side of the bed in supine position.	Keeps the patient away from the edge of the bed when the turn is completed.
2. Stand at the side of the bed towards which the patient is to be turned.	Patient will roll towards the nurse; this allows the nurse to control the amount of turn.
3. Place the patient's far arm across the chest and the far leg over the near leg. Check that the patient's near arm is lateral to and away from the body, with palm down.	Uses the patient's weight when rolling. Prevents the patient from rolling on arm during the turn.
4. Stand opposite the patient's waist and face the side of the bed, with one foot a step in front of the other. Slightly flex the knees and put your weight on the leg nearest the bed.	Nurse's body is in the direction of movement, with a wide base of support.

Continued on the next page

PROCEDURE 28.6
continued

ACTION	RATIONALE

5. Place one hand on the patient's far shoulder and the other on the far hip.

Nurse's weight is used to turn patient.

6. While shifting weight from the forward leg to the rear leg, roll the patient towards you as you move.

Shifting weight provides additional turning force by using large muscle groups.

7. The patient is stopped by the nurse's elbows, which come to rest on the mattress at the edge of the bed.

Provides security for patient.

8. Place pillows under the head, along the back, and between the legs.

Provides support and comfort and maintains body alignment.

9. Check for good body alignment and reposition as necessary.

Prevents muscle strain.

PROCEDURE 28.7

Turning a Patient from a Supine to Semi-Prone (Sims' or Recovery) Position

ACTION	RATIONALE
1. Move the patient to far side of the bed in supine position.	Ensures the patient will roll to the centre of the bed.
2. Stand on opposite side of bed.	Patient will roll towards the nurse.
3. Tuck the patient's near arm under the buttock. Place a pillow on bed next to the patient's chest. Cross the patient's far leg over the near leg.	Prepares for the turn. The patient will roll onto the pillow. Uses the patient's weight when turning.

4. Following steps 4 and 5 of Procedure 28.6, turn the patient, rolling over the bottom shoulder so that the arm is behind the patient.

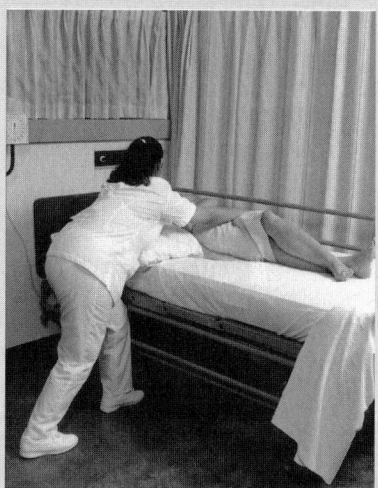

5. Release the patient's arm from under the buttock.	Maintains patient comfort.

Continued on the next page

ACTION	RATIONALE
6. Reposition the patient's head.	Maintains an unobstructed airway.
7. Place pillows under head and chest and between legs.	Maintains comfort and body alignment.

ACTION	RATIONALE
8. Check for good body alignment and reposition as necessary.	Prevents muscle strain.

Assisting a Patient to a Sitting Position on the Edge of the Bed (Dangling)

ACTION	RATIONALE
1. Assist the patient to a side-lying position, with knees bent and lower legs at edge of bed.	Prepares for the change of position.
2. Raise the head of the bed.	Reduces gravitational force.
3. Facing the far bottom corner of the bed, support the patient's shoulders with one arm, while using the other arm to help the patient extend the lower legs over the side of the bed. Assume a broad stance with the foot that is towards the bottom of the bed positioned to the rear of the other foot.	Nurse's body faces the direction of movement. Provides greater stability and balance, and facilitates use of large muscle groups.

PROCEDURE 28.8
continued

ACTION	RATIONALE

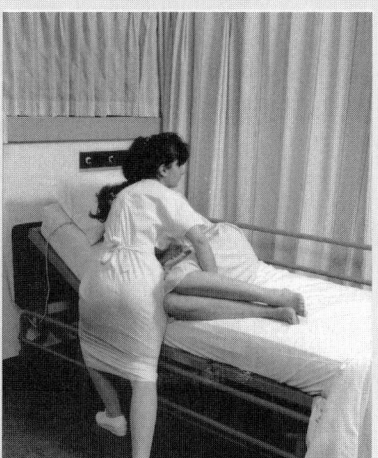

4. While still supporting the patient's shoulders and legs, bring the patient to a natural sitting position on the edge of the bed by pivoting in such a manner that the patient's lower legs are swung downward. The nurse's weight is shifted from the front leg to the rear leg.

Promotes patient safety.

The nurse's weight is used for momentum.

5. The patient assists as able by using the elbow to push up from side-lying position.

Promotes independence.

TRANSFERRING AND LIFTING PATIENTS

Movement from one position to another that involves a change in location, position or equipment is referred to as a transfer or a lift. The distinction between the two terms is that transfers are patient-assisted and lifts are not.

Patients may need assistance moving from the bed to a chair, from a chair to the toilet or commode or from the bed to a stretcher. Procedure 28.9 details the steps involved in moving a patient from the bed to a chair. The variations in transferring from a chair to the toilet or commode are discussed following the procedure.

To move a patient who must remain in the horizontal position — for example, from a bed to a stretcher — three people are usually needed. The tallest person takes the top third of the patient. This person usually has the longest reach and can most easily support the patient's head and shoulders. The shoulders are the heaviest part of the body in men. The second person supports the middle third of the patient, usually the heaviest part in women. The first and third people position their arms beside the second person's. The shortest person supports the patient's legs. To coordinate movements, the three people must work by counting off numbers; the leader who takes the head of the patient calls the numbers. The technique of moving a patient from the bed to a stretcher is outlined in Procedure 28.10.

Transferring a patient from a chair to the toilet or commode is the same as transferring from the bed to a chair, with some modification. In moving from a sitting to standing position from a chair, the patient places both feet on the floor, with the legs angled slightly backward behind knees. This provides a base of support, directly below the patient's centre of gravity. The patient then leans forward and, using the arms of the chair, pushes to a standing position. Assistance may be required to help the patient manage clothing. Grab bars and a raised toilet seat facilitate the patient's independence and safety.

TRANSFERRING AND LIFTING DEVICES

There are a number of devices which nurses can use to make the work of lifting, transferring and moving patients easier and safer. These include transfer belts, lift sheets and mechanical devices such as the hydraulic lift.

Transfer belt   The main objectives of using a transfer belt are to provide security when moving a patient and to minimize the risks of musculoskeletal injury to both the patient and the health care provider. The belt provides a means of guiding a patient's movement from a point close to the patient's centre of gravity while avoiding the use of arms as levers. The belt is positioned securely around the patient's

TABLE 28.4   Characteristics of a Transfer Belt

Dimensions	7.5 cm wide x 122 cm to 137 cm long.
Fabric	Light-weight, soft, supportive, washable, attractive and comfortable.
Fastenings	Simple buckle closure or hook and loop system closure secure when fastened.

waist; the nurse guides movement by grasping the belt. The nurse should ensure that female patients' breasts are not under the transfer belt. Table 28.4 gives the characteristics of a transfer belt. Health care workers who do a lot of patient transfers might consider owning their own transfer belt.

The lift sheet   A lift sheet (or full sheet folded in half) placed under a dependent patient is a useful aid for changing position in many situations. The lift sheet extends from the patient's arm level to the bottom of the buttocks. At least two nurses are needed to move a patient by this means. The nurses stand on opposite sides of the patient, grasp the lift sheet firmly near the patient and move the patient and lift sheet to the desired position — up in the bed or towards the side, for example (Eustace, 1991). Figure 28.5 illustrates the use of a lift sheet to move a patient up in bed.

FIGURE 28.5   The use of a lift sheet to move a patient up in bed

PROCEDURE 28.9

Transferring a Patient from the Bed to a Chair

ACTION	RATIONALE
1. Lower the bed to a height from which the patient can step naturally to the floor.	Facilitates ease of movement and promotes patient safety.
2. Help the patient assume a sitting position on the edge of the bed and put on the patient's shoes and dressing gown. The patient should wear supportive, non-slip footwear.	Prepares for the transfer. Promotes patient dignity and safety.
3. Place a chair at the side of the bed at a right angle to the bed. Position the chair to the stronger side of the patient. If a wheelchair is being used, secure the brakes, and remove the arm and foot rest closest to bed.	Enables the patient to use stronger extremities for support. Provides for safety.
4. Stand facing the patient; the foot that is closer to the chair is a step in front of the other.	Provides a wide base of support.
5. If available, secure a transfer belt around the patient's waist as described in the section on transfer belts. If one is not available, place your hands over patient's posterior iliac crest. Instruct the patient to place his or her hands lightly around your lower waist.	Promotes patient's sense of security and provides support during the transfer. Allows the nurse to guide movement. Enhances the patient's sense of security and ease of movement.
6. As the patient stands, guide the movement by flexing the knees and positioning the forward knee against the patient's knee.	Prevents the patient's knee from bending involuntarily (buckling).

7. Pivot with the patient while maintaining a wide base of support.	Maintains nurse's balance and stability.

Continued on the next page

ACTION	RATIONALE
8. Instruct the patient to move backwards until it is possible to feel the back of the chair on the knees and, at the same time, reach for an arm of the chair with an available hand; then lower gently into a sitting position. Flex your hips and knees while lowering the patient into the chair.	Promotes the patient's sense of space and prevents the patient from sitting down too quickly.
	Prevents back injury.

Transferring a Patient from the Bed to a Stretcher (Three-Person Lift)

ACTION	RATIONALE
1. Place a stretcher at a right angle to the bed, with the head of the stretcher almost touching the foot of the bed. Lock the wheels of the stretcher. Raise the side rails at the far side of the stretcher.	Promotes efficient and safe transfer.
	Prevents the patient from rolling off the stretcher after transfer.
2. The three people who are to move the patient face the side of the patient's bed. Each assumes a broad stance, with the foot that is towards the stretcher placed forward.	Provides balance and stability.
3. At the call of "one," the three bend their knees and place their arms under the patient. The first person places one arm under the neck and shoulders and the other arm under the small of the patient's back.	Distributes weight equally.

ACTION	RATIONALE
The middle person places one arm under the small of the patient's back and the other arm under the hips. The third person places one arm under the patient's hips and the other arm under the legs. Palms are facing the ceiling.	
4. At the call of "two," the patient is turned towards the lifters. This is accompanied by the lifters rolling the patient towards themselves. The patient's arms must not dangle freely. The lifters hold the patient close to their bodies.	Ensures patient safety. Prevents muscle strain.
5. At the call of "three," they rise, step back (with the forward foot), turn and walk in unison to the stretcher.	Facilitates easy, smooth motion, which promotes the patient's sense of security.
6. At the call of "four," they bend their knees and rest their elbows on the stretcher.	Promotes stability and balance and facilitates use of large muscles.
7. At the call of "five," the lifters extend their arms so that the patient rolls to the supine position in the middle of the stretcher.	
8. At the call of "six," the lifters withdraw their arms.	
9. Position the patient, ensuring correct body alignment.	Promotes comfort and avoids muscle strain.

A mechanical lift.

To turn a patient to the side, the arms and legs are first positioned safely. The nurse then reaches over the patient, grasps the lift sheet on the far side, and pulls it forward in such a way that the patient rolls on the side towards the nurse.

Mechanical devices   A wide variety of mechanical devices are available for moving a patient. One is the hydraulic lift, which can raise a person and offers safe, supportive movement. Washable nylon slings fit under the patient's buttocks and back to provide support. These lifts can be used to assist a patient in and out of the bathtub and in and out of bed. The nurse must be taught to use mechanical lifts properly and must have sufficient help to carry out the procedure safely.

HEALTH RESTORING STRATEGIES

Health restoring strategies involve interventions that help individuals to regain mobility following acute illness or traumatic injury or enable independent movement for people with chronic neurological or musculoskeletal conditions. For instance, mobility interventions may allow a patient with multiple sclerosis to move around with the support of a cane or a walker.

PREPARATION FOR WALKING

Everything possible should be done to help individuals maintain strength and tone in the muscles that are needed for walking, or to regain these if they have deteriorated because of illness. Patients who will require a walker, crutches or a cane need to gain additional strength in their hand, arm and shoulder muscles because much of the weight of the body is supported by these muscles when such aids are used. All patients must strengthen the leg and abdominal muscles in preparation for walking. If active exercises are not contraindicated, the patient should be encouraged to do these while in bed.

Active exercises for patients who require additional strength in the arms and shoulders in preparation for crutch or walker-assisted ambulation include push-ups and pull-ups. Push-ups are performed while sitting in a chair. The patient raises the buttocks off the chair seat by pushing down on the fists, while keeping the elbows straight. In pull-ups, the patient pulls him- or herself from a lying to a sitting position. A trapeze supported from a Balkan frame is often used to assist patients to pull themselves up to a sitting position if they are unable to manage it unassisted. Another exercise for strengthening hand, arm and shoulder muscles is to have the patient lie flat in bed, reach up to grasp the head of the bed, and pull him- or herself up in the bed.

AMBULATION

It is often necessary for patients to relearn to walk, often with the aid of crutches, walkers or canes. This is usually the responsibility of the rehabilitation program, but it is beneficial for the nurse to be aware of correct use of these aids to ambulation in order to assist the patient.

The patient may be learning to walk again following an extended period of bedrest. Preparing the patient for this task involves both psychological and physical measures. The nurse can help the patient to gain confidence in the ability to walk again. Often encouragement and faith in the patient's ability can bolster self-confidence. If an appropriate exercise program has been maintained throughout illness, the task is easier. Before attempting to stand, it is important for the patient to learn to maintain good trunk balance first in a sitting position. Then, the patient must achieve good trunk balance in a standing position before attempting to walk. When a standing position can be maintained with confidence and balance, a few steps can be tried. Since good balance is essential and the patient must feel steady, it is important that shoes with good support rather than slippers are worn when standing or walking.

Regaining movement in an injured joint requires gradually increasing exercise.

The patient should not be allowed to become fatigued and should attempt only short distances at first. The nurse can help to promote the patient's feelings of self-confidence by helping to set small goals for each day's activity and acknowledging the accomplishment of these goals.

Most patients who are learning to walk again require physical support when first starting. There are three ways the nurse can provide this support. The nurse can place the arm that is nearer the patient under the arm at the elbow and grasp the patient's hand. The nurse synchronizes walking steps with the patient's, moving the inside foot forward at the same time as the patient's inside foot. A second method is to grasp the patient's left hand in the nurse's left hand, and encircle the patient's waist with the right hand. Again, the walking is synchronized to provide as wide a base of support as possible. The patient can also be supported during walking by being held at the waist from the rear with the use of a transfer belt. This helps the patient maintain balance and keep the centre of gravity within the base of support. If the patient requires more support than this, it is advisable for the nurse to have a second person to assist in the activity.

In some cases, however, the nurse may have to assist a patient with weakness on one side of the body to walk without the help of a second person. To do this, the nurse stands at the patient's weak side. The nurse puts the arm that is nearest to the patient under the patient's arm and grasps the inside of the upper arm. With his or her far arm, the nurse reaches over and takes hold of the patient's lower arm or hand. In this position, the nurse can also provide support with his or her leg to the patient's weakened one if necessary, providing maximum support for the affected side (see Figure 28.6).

FIGURE 28.6 Supporting the patient while walking. A. The nurse supports the patient under the arm at the elbow and grasps the patient's hand. B. The nurse grasps the patient's left hand in the left hand and encircles the patient's waist with the right hand. C. The nurse supports the patient from the rear with the use of a transfer belt. D. The nurse supports the patient with one-sided weakness.

Safety Measures for Crutch Walking

- Check height of crutches
- Check rubber tips
- Assess environment
- Nonslip footwear should be worn

CRUTCH WALKING

It may be necessary for people to use crutches for a period of time. The patient needs to be measured for crutches and taught how to walk with them.

Measuring a Patient for Crutches

Several methods are used to measure a person for an underarm crutch. One method is to measure the distance from the patient's axilla to the heel of the foot while in bed. Five centimetres are then added to this distance. A second method is to measure from the anterior fold of the axilla to a point 15 cm lateral to the heel. When crutches are the correct length, the hand bar permits slight flexion of the elbow, and the weight is borne by the hand and arms rather than at the axilla. The nerves in the axilla are not protected against pressure except by a layer of fat, which is compressible. If weight is borne on the axilla, the pressure may result in nerve damage and possibly paralysis. For this reason the top of the crutch should be 5 cm below the axilla and should not be padded initially.

Teaching Crutch Walking

Patients should be taught more than one gait. The reason for this is twofold: the patient can use a slow or fast gait as necessary and, since each gait requires a different combination of muscles, gaits can be changed when fatigued. There are five basic crutch gaits in crutch walking.

1. **Two point crutch gait** This gait has the following sequence: right crutch and left foot simultaneously; left crutch and right foot simultaneously.
2. **Three point crutch gait** This gait has the following sequence: both crutches and the weaker limb; then the stronger limb.
3. **Four point crutch gait** This gait has the following sequence: right crutch, left foot, left crutch, right foot. This is a particularly safe gait because there are always three points of support on the floor at one time.
4. **Tripod gaits** There are two tripod gaits. A. The patient puts the crutches forward simultaneously and

A walker is often used to assist patients who are relearning to walk following illness.

then drags the body forward. B. The patient puts the crutches forward one at a time, and then drags the body forward.
5. **Swing gaits** There are two swing gaits. A. The patient puts the crutches forward and then swings the body up to the crutches. B. The patient swings the body beyond the crutches.

WALKING WITH A WALKER

There are a variety of walkers available which provide support while walking. When a person uses a walker, much of the weight is carried by the arms and hands as the walker is pushed forward. A safe distance for moving the walker ahead is about 30 cm. The affected leg moves at the same time that the walker is advanced forward. Walker height should be adjusted for maximum efficiency. There should be approximately 15 degrees of flexion of the elbow.

WALKING WITH A CANE

When a patient gradually becomes stronger and has more balance and stability, a cane may be indicated. The patient holds the cane on the strong side of the body. The cane moves forward at the same time that the affected leg moves forward. Stability is increased since there are always two points on the floor as the patient advances (about one foot length at a time). To climb stairs, the patient steps up on the good leg, then follows with the cane and affected leg on the next step. To go down stairs, the procedure is reversed.

ADAPTING TO THE HOME ENVIRONMENT

With the shift in the focus of health care from acute care to community settings, more individuals with mobility problems are returning to home environments. Discharge planning units focus on assisting individuals to be functionally independent by teaching ways to adapt to the environment and to carry out activities of daily living. Occupational therapists assess individual abilities by visiting the home with the patient and seeing what adjustments might have to be made. The occupational therapist may observe the patient cooking a meal or walking up stairs. The therapist will also assess the physical environment in terms of safety and function. The patient may require a homemaker to come in and help with light housekeeping chores, or a community organization such as Meals on Wheels to provide the main meal of the day on a daily basis. Many alternatives are available in the community to assist a patient in making the transition from hospital to home. Through a collaborated effort on the part of the patient (and family) and the health care team, suitable arrangements may be made.

EVALUATING MOVEMENT AND EXERCISE INTERVENTIONS

If the expected outcomes of the nursing interventions have been sufficiently explicit, the process of evaluating the effectiveness of these becomes relatively simple. Have the expected outcomes been achieved? Is the patient's range of motion extended? Can the patient do more of the exercises independently? Does the patient carry out isometric exercises independently, the prescribed number of times as stated in the goals?

The nurse also keeps in mind the long-range goals of nursing action. Have unused muscles for which movement is not contraindicated been maintained in strength and tone? Has the process of degeneration been prevented in these muscles? Have contractures that could interfere with joint mobility been prevented? Has joint mobility been maintained? Have muscular strength and tone been improved? Has the patient regained independence in carrying out activities of daily living or making progress towards this? What progress has been made towards this goal? If the patient requires help in moving to carry out these activities, has help been received when needed, and in such a way as to enable maintenance of other functional abilities? Is there optimal functioning of all other abilities?

KEY TERMS

abduction p. 883

adduction p. 883

flexion p. 883

extension p. 883

hyperextension p. 883

gliding p. 883

rotation p. 883

circumduction p. 883

pronation p. 883

supination p. 883

inversion p. 883

eversion p. 883

body alignment p. 885

base of support p. 885

centre of gravity p. 885

line of gravity p. 885

contracture p. 888

aerobic exercise p. 894

isotonic exercises p. 894

isometric exercises p. 894

isokinetic exercises p. 895

range of motion exercises p. 897

active ROM p. 897

passive ROM p. 897

plantar flexion p. 898

dorsiflexion p. 898

IN REVIEW

Movement and exercise are necessary for fulfilling basic human needs. Free movement allows us to carry out activities of daily living, to work, to play, to protect ourselves from danger and to communicate. Exercise is essential for physical and psychological health and well-being.

Coordinated movement is brought about by the structures and functions of the skeletal system, the muscular system and the nervous system. The circulatory system provides the nourishment tissues need to function. The bones, the muscles and the nerves working together make movement possible.

Movement is easier when the body is in proper alignment, when the weight of the body is evenly distributed and when there is a wide base of support. The body is more stable when its line of gravity runs through the midline of the body and is in direct line with the gravitational pull of the earth.

The capacity for movement and exercise is influenced by age and phase of the life cycle. The development of co-ordinated movement begins in infancy and continues throughout childhood and adolescence. Strength, endurance and motor coordination reach maximum potential in late adolescence and early adulthood, and then gradually decline through middle and late adulthood. Regular exercise slows the aging process and maintains cardiovascular functioning and pulmonary reserve, glucose tolerance, bone density and physical strength and endurance.

Many factors affect movement and exercise. Any condition that interferes with the integrity of the muscles, bones and joints, as well as the nerves innervating these structures, will affect mobility. Injury, disease or congenital anomalies of the bones, muscles, joints or their collateral nerve or blood supply can cause impairment of motor function. Other determinants of movement and exercise are the result of bed rest, immobility and environmental and lifestyle factors.

Common problems with movement include impaired motor function, limited range of motion, decreased muscle strength, lack of balance and coordination and pain and discomfort.

To assess the need for movement and exercise, the nurse uses information from the health history to determine the patient's usual level of activity and exercise, ease of movement and motor function and need for assistive devices. Physical assessment is performed to determine mobility status. This includes a general survey of the patient for uniformity of the skeletal system, muscle structure, symmetry and posture, as well as body alignment, body balance and coordination. Muscles are assessed for symmetry, size, tone, strength and endurance; bones for contour, prominence and symmetry; and joints for range of motion.

Nursing diagnoses pertaining to mobility status include *Impaired physical mobility*, *Activity intolerance* and *Self-care deficits*. Mobility impairments often affect other areas of functioning resulting in such problems as *High risk for injury*, *Powerlessness*, *Altered health maintenance* or *Diversional activity deficit*. A wellness diagnosis — *Potential for enhanced physical fitness and exercise* — may be used when individuals and families express a desire to achieve a higher level of physical fitness and exercise.

Care is generally planned and implemented to maintain, strengthen and restore mobility and motor function, to prevent further deterioration in function and to promote optimal functioning in daily living.

Physical fitness refers to the development of cardiovascular–respiratory vitality, the maintenance of an optimal body weight and the development of joint flexibility and muscular strength and endurance. To maintain physical fitness it is important to participate in some form of regular activity and exercise. Unstructured physical activity such as walking, cycling or climbing stairs is effective for maintaining health. Aerobic exercises, muscular strengthening exercises and flexibility or stretching exercises improve physical fitness. Aerobic exercises have the greatest potential for improving health. Regular aerobic exercise at least three and no more than six times a week, for thirty minutes of continuous activity, is recommended.

Exercise is essential for patients who remain in bed for prolonged periods of time. Muscle strengthening exercises and active or passive ROM promote circulation, maintain muscle tone, promote flexibility and prevent joint stiffness and contractures.

Good posture and efficient use of body mechanics is essential for health. The practice of good body mechanics is particularly important for nurses who do a lot of lifting and moving of patients in the course of their work. The proper use of body mechanics when moving, positioning or transferring patients places a minimum of strain upon muscles, promotes efficient use of energy and prevents injury.

The nurse can use a number of devices to make the work of lifting, moving and transferring patients easier and safer. These include transfer belts, lift sheets and mechanical devices such as the hydraulic lift.

Individuals may need help to regain mobility following acute illness or traumatic injury. It is sometimes necessary for patients to relearn to walk, often with the aid of assistive devices such as walkers, canes or crutches. Muscle strengthening exercises are necessary in preparation for ambulation. Trunk balance in sitting and then standing positions must be achieved before attempting to walk. Shoes with good support as well as support provided by the nurse or assistive devices help the patient maintain balance and feel steady when walking.

LEARNING ACTIVITIES

1. **Case Study**: Mr. George Ellis, age 28, had his foot crushed in a logging accident 3 days ago. He works as a scaler for a large forest products company. Following surgery to repair the soft tissue damage, the physician has encased the foot in a cast. He has ordered that Mr. Ellis remain in bed for an unspecified period of time. He has told Mr. Ellis that when he is allowed up, he must learn to walk with crutches or use a wheelchair to get around in. Mr. Ellis is a healthy, active individual and objects strongly to being confined to bed. He says he is not going to use a wheelchair if he can help it. He wants to know if there is anything he can do while in bed that will help him when he is allowed up from bed.

   a. What information would you need to help you in planning Mr. Ellis's care?

   b. What sources would you use to obtain this information?

   c. What problems might Mr. Ellis have in addition to his impaired mobility?

   d. What other health professionals might be involved in Mr. Ellis's care?

   e. What factors would you take into consideration in planning Mr. Ellis's care?

   f. What exercises might Mr. Ellis do on his own to prevent the deterioration of muscular strength and tone? To prepare himself for using crutches?

   g. What other help would Mr. Ellis require in carrying out daily living activities?

2. With the aid of your instructor, arrange to spend a day with a physiotherapist or an occupational therapist in your agency. What types of care does this health care

professional provide? In what ways do nurses collaborate with physiotherapists and occupational therapists to provide care in this agency?

REFERENCES AND READINGS

ALISON, M. (1991). Aging and exercise: Improving the odds. *Harvard Health Letter, 16*(4), 4–6.

ANDERSON, S. (1990). The health club. *The Canadian Nurse, 86*(6), 34–35.

BERGER, K.J. and WILLIAMS, M.B. (1992). *Fundamentals of nursing: Collaborating for optimal health*. Norwalk, CT: Appleton & Lange.

CARPENITO, L.J. (1993). *Nursing diagnosis: Application to clinical practice* (4th ed.). Philadelphia: Lippincott.

CORBIN, C.B. and LINDSEY, R. (1994). *Concepts of fitness and wellness: With laboratories*. Madison, WI: Brown and Benchmark.

CRAVEN, R.F. and HIRNLE, C.J. (1992). *Fundamentals of nursing: Human health and function*. Philadelphia: Lippincott.

DAWE, D. and CURRAN-SMITH, J. (1994). Going through the motions. *The Canadian Nurse, 90*(1), 31–33.

EUSTACE, C. (1991). Back up and wait. *RN, 54*(6), 49–51.

EXTON-SMITH, N. (1987). The patient's not for turning. *Nursing Times, 83*, 42–44.

GORDON, M. (1976). Assessing activity intolerance. *American Journal of Nursing, 76*(1), 72–75.

GREENBERG, J. and DINTIMAN, G. (1992). *Exploring health: Expanding the boundaries of wellness*. Englewood Cliffs, NJ: Prentice-Hall.

HALEY, E. (1994). One approach to patient lifting. *The Canadian Nurse, 90*(1), 57–58.

HALEY, E. and COLGATE, W. (1990). Standing up for your back. *Canadian Nurse, 86*(11), 26–7.

HEESCHEN, S. (1989). Getting a handle on patient mobility. *Geriatric Nursing, 10*, 146–147.

JACOB, S.W. and FRANCONE, C.A (1989). *Elements of anatomy and physiology* (2nd ed.). Philadelphia: Saunders.

JAMES, B. and PARKER, A.W (1989). Active and passive mobility of lower limb joints in elderly men and women. *American Journal of Physical Medicine and Rehabilitation, 68*(4), 162–166.

JOHNSON, T.R. and MOORE, W.M. (1978). *Children are different: Developmental physiology*. Columbus, OH: Ross Laboratories, 33.

LALONDE, M. (1974) *A new perspective on the health of Canadians*. Ottawa: Information Canada.

MASON, D.J and REDEKER, N. (1993). Measurement of activity. *Nursing Research, 42*, 87–91.

MCCONNELL, E. (1990). Placing your patient in the lateral position. *Nursing 90, 20*(7), 65.

MEISSNER, J.E (1980). Evaluate your patient's level of independence. *Nursing 80, 10*, 72–73.

MILDE, F.K. (1988). Impaired physical mobility. *Journal of Gerontological Nursing, 14*, 20–24.

ODDY, R. and LODGE, L. (1993). Special support... Scheme to change patient handling practices in a continuing care ward. *Nursing Times, 89*(3), 44–46.

OLSEN, E.V, and JOHNSON, B.J. (1990, March). The hazards of immobility. *American Journal of Nursing, 90*, 43–44; 46–48.

OWEN, B. D and GARG, A. (1993). Back stress isn't part of the job. *American Journal of Nursing, 93*(2), 48–51.

RUBIN, M. (1986). The physiology of bed-rest. *American Journal of Nursing, 86*(3),8–50.

TARLING, C. (1992). The right equipment. *Nursing Times, 88* (50), 38–40.

TAYLOR, C., LILLIS, C. and LEMONE, P. (1993). *Fundamentals of nursing: The art and science of nursing care* (2nd ed.). Philadelphia: Lippincott.

TIMARIS, P.S. (1988). Aging of skeleton, joints, and muscle. In P. S. Timaris (Ed). *Physiological Basis of Geriatrics*. New York: Macmillan.

WALTON, J. (1993). Lifting techniques for nurse-aiders. *British Journal of Nursing, 2*(7), 385–386; 388.

WILLIAMS, M. H. (1993). *Lifetime fitness and wellness* (3rd ed.). Madison, WI: Brown and Benchmark.

UNIT 6

Protection and Safety Needs

CENTRAL QUESTIONS

1. What is the nurse's role in protecting against environmental hazards?

2. What are some of the factors affecting a person's capacity for self-protection?

3. How do protection and safety needs vary throughout the life cycle?

4. What are the five principal causes of accidental death in Canada?

5. What are some existing and potential hazards in the home, community, workplace and hospital?

6. How does the nurse assess an individual's safety needs?

7. How does the nurse identify nursing diagnoses pertaining to protection and safety problems?

8. How does the nurse apply relevant principles in selecting, planning and implementing safety interventions?

9. What action does the nurse take to protect the safety of ill persons in case of fire?

10. How does the nurse evaluate the effectiveness of nursing interventions?

INTRODUCTION

As with so many aspects of the nurse's role today, responsibilities regarding environmental safety are rapidly expanding. Nurses, as informed and knowledgeable health professionals, are not only concerned with health hazards in the communities in which they live and work; they are also taking action and making their voices heard, both individually and collectively, to make the environment more conducive to healthy living. Local, provincial and national nursing associations are expressing concerns about air pollution; the pollution of our rivers, lakes and coastal waters; highway safety; the safety of our water, milk and food supplies; drugs and cosmetics; and the presence of disease-carrying animals, insects and other potential sources of infection that adversely affect health. They are issuing statements and lobbying municipal, provincial and federal authorities to take action to eliminate environmental health hazards and they are actively participating in community action to detect, minimize or eliminate these hazards.

The Role of Nurses in Protecting and Improving the Environment

The nurse's role is to:

- Help detect ill effects of the environment on the health of humans, and vice versa.

- Be informed with the available data and apply knowledge in daily work with individuals, families and/or community groups on potentially harmful chemicals, radioactive waste problems, latest health hazards and ways to prevent and/or reduce them.

- Be informed and teach preventive measures about health hazards due to environmental factors as well as about conservation of environmental resources to the individual, families and/or community groups.

- Work with health authorities to point out health care concerns and health hazards in existing human settlements and in the planning of new ones.

- Assist communities in taking action against environmental health problems.

- Participate in research providing data for early warning and prevention of the deleterious effects of the various environmental agents to which we are increasingly exposed. Also participate in research conducive to discovering ways and means of improving living and working conditions.

SOURCE: RNAO News, 1976, 19.

The International Council of Nurses (ICN) has strongly urged nurses to participate in actions to safeguard the human environment. In 1975, the Council of National Representatives (CNR) of the International Council of Nurses adopted a policy statement which outlines the role that nurses can play in protecting and improving the environment and thereby contribute to better health for all people. The ICN Policy Statement reads as follows:

The preservation and improvement of the human environment has become a major goal of man's action for his survival and well-being. The vastness and urgency of the task places on every individual and every professional group the responsibility to participate in the efforts to safeguard man's environment, to conserve the world's resources, to study how their use affects man and how adverse effects can be avoided.

RNAO News, 1976, 19.

In Chapter 11, Health and the Community, a number of environmental health issues were discussed. This chapter on safety is particularly concerned with the protection and safety needs of people with a focus on accident and injury prevention. The factors that influence the capacity for self-protection are described, as well as the specific safety and protection needs of individuals during the various stages of the life cycle. Next, accident prevention and safety in the home, in the community, in the workplace and in hospitals and other inpatient facilities are outlined.

DETERMINANTS OF THE CAPACITY FOR SELF-PROTECTION

A number of factors are involved in the ability to protect ourselves from hazards in the environment. We must, first of all, be aware of things in the environment that are harmful, or potentially harmful, to our health. We must be able to perceive stimuli in the environment and to interpret these stimuli in order to identify what is hazardous and what is not. We also need to know what action is needed to protect ourselves from hazards we have identified and we must be capable of carrying out these actions. For example, a small child may see some pretty red berries on a tree and decide to eat them. The child is able to perceive the visual stimulus but does not know that holly berries are poisonous and is therefore not able to interpret the stimulus as dangerous. For self-protection, then, one needs a knowledge of environmental hazards, an intact sensory system, good mental functioning and reasoning ability, a knowledge of the protective measures to take and adequate motor abilities to take the appropriate action. Age is a factor in all of these requirements.

KNOWLEDGE

Much of what we know about hazards in the environment and how to protect ourselves from these hazards is gained from personal experience (finding out that the tongue sticks to cold metal if you try to lick a wire fence in the winter) and from learning in the home, the school and the workplace as parents, older siblings, teachers and more senior workers share their accumulated experiences. Books and other media also contribute to our knowledge about the environment, its hazards and how to cope with them. A considerable amount of research is currently being undertaken to increase our knowledge about the effects of pollution and other hazards on our health and to discover ways to make our environments more conducive to health.

PERCEPTION AND INTERPRETATION OF STIMULI

In Chapter 27, we discussed the fact that our sensory receptors provide us with information about the surrounding environment. It is through our ability to see, hear, smell, taste and feel that we are alerted to dangers in our environment. Impairment of the sensory receptors, the neural pathways carrying sensory impulses to and through the central nervous system, or the ability to interpret these impulses results in a lessened ability to sense harmful, or potentially harmful, factors in the environment.

A person with limited vision may not see obstacles in the path. The person with some hearing loss may not hear warnings or sirens. Someone without the sense of smell may not be aware of the odour of escaping gas from the kitchen stove. Loss of the ability to taste prevents detection of the slightly "off" flavour of food that has been improperly preserved. A person who cannot feel does not receive warning signals to move from a seat too close to the fire.

The phenomenon of negative adaptation to sensory stimuli can provide hazards. The smell of leaking gas may be so insidious that a person becomes accustomed to it or is never even consciously aware of it. The sense of smell is one that adapts very quickly, it seems. The nurse should keep this in mind when on the nursing unit. It can be helpful for the nurses to make a regular effort to breathe fresh air; this will allow the nose to pick up stimuli again.

If mental faculties are clouded or impaired for any reason, sensory perception is diminished, as is the ability to interpret stimuli. The perceptual abilities of someone suffering from sleep deprivation are usually diminished, or perception may be distorted. Being drowsy is a hazard when driving on the highway because sensory abilities are dulled; you may not see the car approaching on your side of the road. Your own car may veer suddenly because your sense of touch is decreased or you may not perceive the infinitesimal shift in the steering wheel that tells you that you are not on the proper course. It may also take longer than usual to realize that you are dangerously close to the edge of the road or in the wrong lane. Alcohol and drugs, which are central nervous system depressants, have the same dulling effect on the senses as drowsiness does.

In fact, any alteration in the state of consciousness will affect the ability to perceive sensory stimuli, to interpret them and to react appropriately. The confused or disoriented individual may mistake the door leading to the stairs for the door to the bathroom. Believing to be at home, a patient may also try to get out of a hospital bed to go to the bathroom, and climb over the bed rails to do so. Someone who is roused out of a sound sleep is often confused and disoriented. Older people may become excited and confused by medications given to help them get to sleep.

Stress, anxiety and other emotions may also affect the perception of harmful stimuli in the environment, the interpretation of these stimuli, and the ability to react to them. Mild anxiety increases perceptual awareness, but increased levels of anxiety progressively decrease it. We can attend to only so many stimuli at one time, and if other stimuli are of more importance, we may not be alert to potential dangers in our environment. Someone whose thoughts are turned inward or fixed on one object, or who is lost in reverie, may bump into objects because they are not noticed; this person may also step off the curb without looking or do any one of a number of things that could endanger life and limb.

ABILITY TO TAKE PROTECTIVE ACTION

The ability to respond to stimuli must also be considered in looking at self-protection. The brain must be functioning sufficiently well to make decisions and to initiate appropriate action in response to sensory stimuli. Some actions are reflexes that are initiated in the spinal cord, such as the withdrawal of the hand from a hot stove. This reaction becomes an almost instinctive reaction that is a learned cord reflex. Most actions, however—such as moving out of approaching danger— are initiated and controlled by higher centres of the brain. If the ability to initiate, coordinate and carry out motor actions is impaired for any reason, the ability to protect ourselves from environmental hazards is decreased. The sleepy driver may not be sufficiently alert to turn the steering wheel fast enough to get back on course before going over the edge of the road or running into an approaching car. Reaction time is slowed.

Alcohol is well known for its effect of slowing reactions, thus making people who have been drinking a potential hazard both to themselves and to others. The relationship between alcohol consumption and a substantial proportion of motor vehicle accidents, fires and other types of accidents was mentioned in Chapters 2 and 10. Many cities in Canada now set up roadblocks over the Christmas season to check all drivers for the effects of alcohol; police have the power to suspend licences on the spot if drivers are inebriated. The roadblocks have proven to be a good preventive measure.

Injury or illness affecting either the specific areas of the brain that initiate and control movement or the neural pathways that transmit motor impulses will also limit safeguarding abilities. People who have lessened mental faculties because of congenital problems such as cerebral palsy (a motor disorder from non-progressive brain damage) are hampered in their abilities to protect themselves.

People who have impaired motor functioning of any kind or who have had restrictions (such as a cast) placed on mobility are at a disadvantage when it comes to protecting themselves from environmental hazards. People in wheelchairs, for example, cannot move as quickly as able-bodied people, and are hampered by having to manoeuvre the chair around obstacles or out of the way of dangerous objects. People who cannot grasp objects or move an arm or leg with normal agility and speed are disadvantaged as far as protective abilities are concerned.

People who are ill are particularly prone to accidents and injury. They are often physically weak and the ability to carry out normal daily activities is impaired. As a result, they may fall while walking or easily lose their balance on an uneven surface. The protective senses of sick people (for example, sight) may become so impaired that they cannot perceive dangers. Moreover, the anxiety that goes along with illness may interfere with perceptual abilities and with the capacity to concentrate. It may also interfere with the ability to make judgements, and may thus expose sick people to injury. Many people who are ill suffer temporary or prolonged periods of an altered state of consciousness. The preoperative patient who is under sedation, the postoperative patient recovering from anesthesia, the person with a severe head injury and the unconscious patient all have decreased sensory perceptual abilities, as well as decreased abilities to respond to environmental stimuli and to make decisions based on good judgement.

In many illnesses, a patient is rendered helpless or semi-helpless by the nature of the illness. Patients who are paralyzed, for example, must then depend on other people to protect them from environmental hazards. In some instances, it is necessary to restrain mobility to afford protection from the patient's own actions which may cause injury, such as pulling out catheters or intravenous tubing. Restraining a confused or disoriented patient is often distressing, however, and the patient may fight against the restraints, creating additional safety problems.

Sometimes the therapy that is prescribed makes patients more vulnerable to accidents or injuries, or has inherent hazards in itself. Medication therapy carries with it many potential hazards, such as adverse reactions or the possibility that the wrong patient will get the medication. Radiation therapy also has its hazards. The very act of penetrating the skin surface for surgery renders a patient more

vulnerable to infection and causes physiological stress, which makes the patient more susceptible to other disturbances of body functioning, such as fluid and electrolyte imbalance.

> ## *Determinants of the Capacity for Self-Protection*
> - Age
> - Knowledge of environmental hazards
> - Integrity of sensory functioning (vision, hearing, taste, smell, touch)
> - Level of consciousness
> - Mental functioning
> - Emotional state
> - Knowledge of protective measures
> - Motor ability
> - Health status
> - Medications and other therapies

PROTECTION AND SAFETY NEEDS THROUGHOUT THE LIFE CYCLE

REPRODUCTIVE HEALTH

The protection of reproductive health concerns the potential not only of both parents, but also of their children, to have healthy offspring (Zenz, 1988). Particularly in the workplace, many chemical and physical agents are, or could potentially be, *teratogenic* (cause physical defects), *mutagenic* (cause permanent alterations in the genes), or *carcinogenic* (cause cancer). Agents exist which can affect the male reproductive system, as well as the preconception health of the germ cells of both males and females. A classical example is dichlorobromopropane (DCBP), a chemical used in some pesticides. A study found that male factory workers who were chronically exposed to this chemical became sterile (Radike, 1985). Pesticides made with DCBP have now been taken off the market. Exposure to lead compounds has been shown to decrease fertility and cause chromosomal aberrations in males (Roychowdhury, 1990). Organic solvents such as carbon disulfide have been linked with low sperm counts and abnormal genes (Radike, 1985). Radiation is well known for its mutagenic effect on people of both sexes. One study found an association between anesthetic gas and spontaneous abortions in operating room nurses (Chenier, 1982).

Although much is known, more research is needed to investigate reproductive health and to define safe levels of exposure to those chemicals and physical agents that are dangerous to reproductive health. Knowledge of the effects of these substances, and preventing or controlling exposure to them in the workplace, is a key role for the Occupational Health and Safety Team.

PREGNANT WOMEN

The expectant mother must be protected against potential injury, not only for her own sake but also for the sake of the fetus. The fetus is protected, to the extent that nature is able to do so, by its cushion of amniotic fluid within the uterus. However, trauma to the mother, such as a direct blow to the abdomen, may dislodge the placenta from its attachment to the uterine wall, causing a miscarriage or premature labour, depending on the stage of development of the fetus. Pregnant women are generally advised not to participate in sports that cause jolting (such as horseback riding), although swimming and most other sports are not contraindicated. As we mentioned in Chapter 28, exercise in moderation is important to the health of both mother and baby.

Maternal exposure to infectious diseases may pose a particular risk to the fetus. Protection from exposure to rubella, hepatitis B and human immunodeficiency virus (HIV) is very important, and will be discussed more fully in Chapter 31. The effects of smoking and the consumption of alcohol and caffeine (in large quantities) are detrimental to the health of the developing fetus. Because "safe" limits of alcohol or caffeine consumption on the growing fetus have not been determined, it is best for pregnant women to avoid or eliminate taking these substances during pregnancy. During pregnancy and lactation, drugs should be used only under the supervision of a qualified health professional.

INFANTS AND CHILDREN

"Today, injury is the number one killer of children, ahead of cancer, birth defects, diseases of the nervous system and all other causes" (Health and Welfare Canada, 1991, 1). Most of these injuries can be prevented. Newborn infants have very limited abilities to protect themselves and depend on the people who are caring for them to keep them safe. As children grow and develop, they learn to avoid certain hazards in the environment; it is through education and trial and error that they learn to identify harmful and potentially harmful situations and to protect themselves. Accidents often occur because an infant makes a develop-

Neonates are dependent on others to protect them from harm.

mental advance for which the parent is not prepared. Although a baby may appear safe lying on the bed or in a baby carriage, six-month-old infants can achieve a sitting position and, because their balance is still not very good, they may tumble out of the carriage or off the bed.

Infants do not have the ability to push or roll themselves out of water if they fall face down in a pool or bath. Also, the reflex to hold their breath while submerged in water is not fully formed in young children. Therefore, infants and small children need special care around pools and baths. Death rates from drowning are highest in both Canada and the United States in children from one to four years of age (Riley and Paddon, 1989).

Very young children have no sense of danger. It is only as the world they know through experience enlarges that they are able to interpret the meaning of potentially harmful stimuli. Children who play with matches are fascinated by the flame. Until they burn themselves or unless their caretaker is sufficiently impressive in terms of correction, they do not perceive matches as dangerous objects. Indeed, the rate of death from fire in children from one to four years of age is higher than in any other age group except the 75 and up group in both Canada and the United States (Riley and Paddon,1989).

Small children cannot read warning labels, and may ingest poisonous cleaning fluid, or other harmful substances. They may lick chipping lead-based paint on their cribs or on a windowsill and suffer from lead poisoning. Some children suffer from *pica*, the eating of unnatural substances. These children must be supervised especially carefully, and potentially harmful substances must be kept out of reach.

Growing children are most vulnerable to accidents when participating in newly acquired activities and when exercising newly won freedom. A four-year-old may be given permission to visit a friend up the block but, during the visit, may dart out into the street to retrieve a ball that has bounced out of reach. The child just learning to ride a bicycle may not be able to stop and may ride out on the road and into the pathway of an oncoming car.

ADOLESCENTS

By pre-adolescence, prevention has largely become a matter of self-discipline. Some children are accident-prone, however, and always seem to suffer from more cuts, bruises and scrapes than their brothers and sisters. This tendency often persists into adulthood. Some people may drive a car for 20 years without an accident, while others have one accident after another. It is believed that emotional disturbances are often the cause of being accident-prone. Tension of any kind is likely to cause increased susceptibility to accidents by impairing critical abilities and exhausting defenses.

YOUNG AND MIDDLE-AGED ADULTS

Insurance and mortality/morbidity statistics repeatedly point out the disproportionately large number of automobile accidents involving young male drivers (see Figure 29.1). Risk-taking behaviour is common among young adults (especially among males), because they tend to view their bodies as indestructible. Many, though not all, drive at high speeds, take the steepest trail down the mountain when skiing and generally operate under the philosophy that "it can't happen to me." Many young adults also have unrealistic perceptions about their physical capabilities and will push themselves to the limit of endurance. "Shin splints" (periostitis or inflammation of the periosteum) is a common problem that results from excessive demands on the musculoskeletal system. Much of this trauma is related to sports, although the largest percentage of injuries to young adults still results from car and motorcycle accidents.

In adults, most car accidents are related to the use of alcohol. The trauma resulting from motor vehicle accidents usually gives rise to musculoskeletal problems such as fractures, head injuries and torn ligaments. Repetitive trauma may result in painful inflammatory lesions of the periarticular structures. Because bone mass declines in middle age, injuries to the joints that would only affect ligaments in young adults cause fractures in middle-aged adults.

Stress at any age renders an individual more vulnerable to accidents. People who are troubled — children or adults — are much more likely to stumble and fall, or to act hurriedly without too much thought and injure themselves or others. Stress is said to be the disease of the '90s. Tension related to financial, marital, health, alcohol or drug problems can all add to the risk of injury in adulthood. Extra stresses are imposed on the "sandwich generation" who are busy raising children while at the same time helping aging parents with health and housing concerns.

OLDER ADULTS

Falls are the most common type of accident among older people, although the members of the 75 and up age group are more at risk for death or injury from fire than the members of any other age group. The 75 and up age group is also more at risk of death from drowning than any other age group except children aged one to four (Riley and Paddon, 1989).

As people get older, sensory abilities diminish. Vision becomes worse, and hearing may sometimes be considerably decreased. The sensory receptors for smell in the nose are often damaged in accidents when people have any kind of head injury and, in any case, usually diminish with age. Atrophy of the taste buds is one of the unfortunate aspects of getting older, and even the receptors for touch lose acuteness with the changes that occur in aging skin. The older person's skin is less sensitive to heat and cold and is therefore prone to thermal injuries. The older person, like the young child, is very vulnerable to environmental hazards, but for different reasons. Older people's "early warning system" in the sensory receptors is not as efficient, and responses to environmental hazards are slower and not as effective. Vestibular function declines, and there is an increased risk of falling. Absent-mindedness is also a major factor in accidents.

COMMON ACCIDENTS

"An accident is an undesired event that results in physical harm to a person or damage to property. It is usually the result of a contact with a source of energy (i.e., kinetic, electrical, chemical, thermal etc.) above the threshold limit of the body or structure" (American National Standards Institue (ANSI), cited in Bird, 1984). Accidents are among the five leading causes of death each year in Canada and the United States. They are the principal cause of death among children and young adults and a major cause of hospitalization in people of all ages (Riley and Paddon, 1989). Accidents are usually caused by hazards in the environment.

Figure 29.1 contains graphs of age-specific mortality rates for men and women for the five most common types of accidents causing death or hospitalization in Canada and the United States.

The Five Most Common Accidents

- Motor vehicle accidents
- Falls
- Drowning
- Fires
- Poisonings

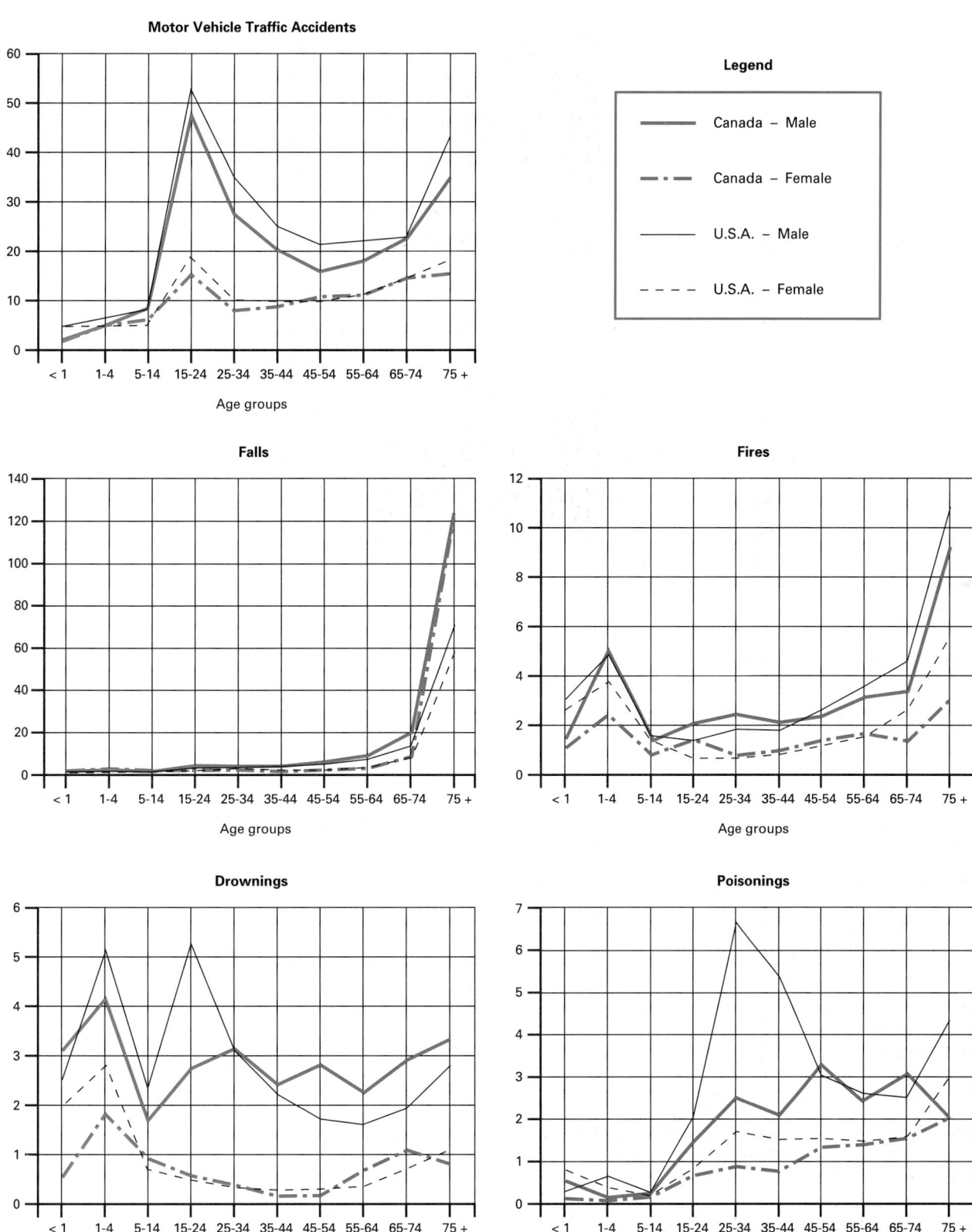

FIGURE 29.1 Accidents, Age-specific Mortality Rates by Sex, Canada and U.S.A. 1985. (Rates per 100 000 population) (Graphs for Motor Vehicle Accidents, Falls, Drownings, Fires and Poisonings.)

SOURCE: Riley, R. and Paddon, P. (1989). Accidents in Canada: Mortality and hospitalization. *Health Reports, 1,* 29. (Statistics Canada Catalogue No. 82-003)

TABLE 29.1	Environmental Hazards		
PHYSICAL	**CHEMICAL**	**BIOLOGICAL**	**PSYCHOLOGICAL**
Noise	Solvents	Bacteria	Shift work
Radiation	Caustics	Viruses	Boredom
Vibration	Fumes	Fungus	Stress
Electricity	Lead	Poisonous plants	Danger
Heat/Cold/Humidity	Dust	Insects, Rodents,	
Repetitive motions	Mercury	Reptiles and	
Lifting	Gases	other disease-	
Slips and Falls		carrying animals	

Environmental Hazards Leading to Accidents

The hazards that can lead to accidents can be divided into four categories: physical hazards, chemical hazards, biological hazards and psychological hazards. Examples of each of the four categories are shown in Table 29.1.

ACCIDENTS IN THE HOME

Although most accidental deaths occur on roads and highways, the majority of other accidents take place in the home (Riley and Paddon, 1989). Home is a place where children and adults should be safe from harm, but the average home contains many hazards. The most common types of accidents in the home involve fire and burns, falls, poisonings, choking and suffocation and drowning.

Fire and Burns

Fire is probably the most common and the most dreaded accident that can happen in a home (Riley and Paddon, 1989). Although no age group is immune to the dangers of fire, the rate of death from fires is higher for the very young and the very old; it is also higher among men than women (see Figure 29.1). A common cause of fire in the home is an overloaded electrical circuit. About 25 percent of house fires are attributed to heating equipment. Wood stoves and wood-burning fireplaces that are poorly installed and/or poorly maintained cause a large number of these fires. Many homes are not equipped with an adequate escape route or with fire detectors. Therefore, many people die in fires because they are trapped or because they are unaware of the fire until it is too late to escape.

Thermal injuries in the home often result from contact with hot water (scalding) or hot pots and pans. Children, in particular, sustain burns when playing with lighters or matches.

Falls

In Canada and the United States, falls are a leading cause of accidental death in people in the 75 and up age group and the leading cause of hospitalization for both men and women (Riley and Paddon, 1989). Children have their share of falls and sustain injuries from these but the death rate from falls is not as high as from other types of accidents. Stairs are a principal cause of home injuries. As well, people often fall in slippery bath tubs or showers.

Poisonings

Deaths due to poisonings appear to be much greater in number for men than for women, with the highest number occurring in the 45–54 age group among Canadian men, and in the 25–34 age group in American men (Riley and Paddon, 1989). Children are also vulnerable to poisoning because of natural curiosity and the tendency to put things into their mouths.

Choking and Suffocation

Choking and suffocation are among the common accidents that occur among infants and small children. Because children like to put many things into their mouths, they may choke on objects that are too big to swallow.

Drowning and Diving Accidents

Deaths from drowning in both Canada and the United States are highest among the one to four age group. Many homes and playgrounds have swimming pools, wading pools, whirlpools or hot tubs to which children are naturally attracted. Drownings unfortunately do occur, even with diligent supervision.

Teenagers and young adults often sustain spinal cord injuries from diving accidents. Diving at night or where visibility is obstructed may cause neck injuries due to hitting the bottom of a lake or pool, or injuries can be sustained by diving into rocks or other submerged objects. Similar to motor vehicle accidents, many drownings are alcohol related.

ACCIDENTS IN THE COMMUNITY

Most of the accidents or injuries that occur in the community are motor vehicle, bicycle or sport- and recreation-related. Motor vehicle accidents are the number one cause of injury and death among children and young people. "Each year in Canada, about 70 children under the age of five die, and 4000 more are injured as passengers in motor vehicle collisions" (Transport Canada, 1990). Motor vehicle accidents are also a major cause of death and permanent disability in adults. Most of these accidents are preventable.

Bicycling, always a popular sport, has become a common mode of transportation in our country. Many cities in Europe and in other parts of the world have separate lanes for bicycle traffic. In most Canadian cities, however, cars, buses and bicycles all compete for road space on clogged city streets. The risk to the lone rider on a bicycle is much greater than to the occupants of a car, should the two collide. In the community, playgrounds for children, playing fields and sports arenas, as well as schools, are places where accidents can happen. Adult supervision in parks and other recreational areas where children play is essential to identify and remedy potential hazards.

ACCIDENTS IN THE WORKPLACE

Despite accident prevention programs, millions of occupational injuries and illnesses are still reported in the industrialized world every year. In Canada, over 520 000 time-loss injuries were accepted for Workers' Compensation in 1991 (Statistics Canada, 1992). The highest number of injuries occurred in the Health and Social Services Industry with service occupations apparently the most hazardous, followed by occupations in medicine and health. Clerical and related workers were third. In British Columbia alone, payments for short-term, long-term and fatality claims were accepted for a total compensation cost of $ 639 951 102. In this province, fatalities in the workplace are most frequent in the logging, construction, heavy manufacturing, trucking and mining industries (Statistics Canada, 1992; WCB of BC, 1993).

Musculoskeletal Injuries

Musculoskeletal injuries affecting the back, neck and shoulders are common in all types of workplaces. Back injuries due to physical hazards, such as lifting and reaching, are common occupational injuries. Safety improvements have decreased certain types of accidents, but new technology creates new types of problems. A group of disorders called **Cumulative Trauma Disorders** (CTD), also known as **Repetitive Strain Injuries**, is the silent epidemic of the '90s. Cumulative Trauma Disorders are usually caused by sustained, unnatural body postures, and repetitive, forceful movements. A common feature of CTDs is overuse of certain joints or muscles groups; therefore, injury is the result of repeated microtrauma leading to a chronic injury. Computer operators and assembly line workers are reporting injuries such as carpal tunnel syndrome, strains, sprains, tendonitis and tenosynovitis. Careful attention to workstation, tool and job task design, training and administrative policies will prevent many CTDs.

Common Occupational Injuries

Other common occupational injuries include slips and falls, lacerations, abrasions, contusions, eye injuries, head injuries, asphyxiation and thermal injuries. Injuries caused from being trapped by or caught in equipment or other heavy material occur especially in the mining, logging and construction industries. Noise-induced hearing loss can occur in any workplace with excessive noise levels, but hearing conservation programs have been in place for many years now.

Occupation-Related Diseases

Pulmonary diseases can be related to occupational exposure to **hazardous substances**. Environmental dust may be inhaled as a solid, fume or a mixture of the two. The type of respiratory injury which could ensue depends on the physical, chemical and toxic properties of the agent involved. Asbestosis (asbestos), Coal Worker's Pneumoconiosis (respirable coal dust), silicosis (silica), Meat Wrapper's Asthma (polyvinylchloride heat process), Occupational Asthma (various causes) and Siderosis (welding fumes, iron oxide) are some of the pulmonary disorders related to occupational exposure.

A number of agents encountered in the workplace have been related to varying types of occupational cancers. These include ethylene oxide, ionizing radiation, coke oven emissions, benzene, radium, asbestos and others (Zenz, 1988). In addition, skin disorders occur from handling or otherwise being in contact with irritating agents in the workplace. Contact dermatitis and various infections may ensue. Causative agents include solvents, resins, detergents, fibreglass, cutting oils, plastics and infectious agents.

The aging workforce, stress and non-occupational factors such as arthritis, diabetes, heart disease and lack of fitness all compound occupational injuries, affecting both the severity of injury and length of recovery.

ACCIDENTS IN THE HOSPITAL

A hospital is generally thought of as a place where the sick and injured come for care; it is seldom thought of as a place where people are injured. Yet the number of accidents that occur in hospitals is extraordinarily high compared with the number that occur in other industries.

Many safety-related problems occur in health agencies. Three groups of people should be considered: the patients, who require additional protection because they are ill; the staff, who because of the nature of the work are vulnerable to many types of accidental injury (such as back strain from lifting heavy patients incorrectly); and the visitors, who are usually anxious and worried about the person they have come to see.

A hospital is a busy place, and is usually fraught with tension and stress. It must function as a hotel, as well as take care of the sick, or, in the case of Long-Term Care facilities, provide health care for residents. Staff members have all the responsibilities of an innkeeper for the safety of the guests.

HAZARDOUS AREAS IN THE HOSPITAL

Many areas of a hospital are particularly dangerous. The nurse should be aware of the dangers of these areas and take extra precautions when working in or around them.

The mechanical plant   A hospital usually has a large mechanical plant with heavy equipment, high voltage areas, hazardous products, boiler rooms, woodworking, ma-

Maintenance personnel ensure a safe mechanical plant.

chining and paint shops. Potentially dangerous activities such as plumbing, carpentry, welding, electrical work, construction and renovation projects are ongoing.

Food and nutrition services   Meal service is part of the daily activities in all inpatient facilities, and safety in food preparation, handling and serving must be considered. Most kitchens have sophisticated food assembly and dish room areas. Many heavy, raw and prepared products are handled. Cooks and chefs are at risk of sustaining serious cuts. Slips and falls are also common in areas where food and water spills occur.

The laundry   Laundry functions involve lifting and moving large, heavy loads. There is always the possibility of exposure to sharps inadvertently left in the laundry, thereby posing a risk of infection for laundry workers. Similar to the hospital kitchen, advances in technology have led to computer-controlled, mechanical devices and equipment which in turn have led to decreased injuries in the laundry facilities.

Diagnostic services   Diagnostic and therapeutic procedures for patients are often hazardous because of the potential for chemical and physical injuries to patients and staff, and because of the potential for infection. Staff could be exposed to ionizing and non-ionizing radiation, laser, radioactive isotopes, antineoplastic agents and others.

HAZARDS FOR HEALTH CARE WORKERS

Accidental injury   Back strains accounted for 34.2 percent of all Short-Term Disability claims in 21 participating acute care community hospitals in 1992 in the province of British Columbia (WCB of BC, 1993). The cost of these claims accounted for 42.6 percent of all costs for the years 1990–1992. Most of the back strains were sustained by practical nurses and nurse's aides and were due to lifting or transferring patients. Registered nurses, housekeepers, maintenance workers and others are also at risk for back injury. Injuries from slips and falls are also common in the hospital, and safe footwear and safe housekeeping signs for wet floors are very important. Cuts, abrasions and contusions can also occur unless proper precautions are taken. Injuries sustained from aggressive patients are being reported more frequently by health care workers.

Exposure to blood and body fluids   Exposure to blood and body fluid can occur through stick injuries from contaminated needles, scalpels or sutures; splashes of blood or body fluid into the eye or mouth; or through contact with non-intact skin. Housekeepers are at a high risk because the source patient is often not known (in the case of a needlestick from a garbage or sharps container) and therefore cannot be tested for hepatitis B antigen to establish infectiousness. Every health care facility should establish first aid and follow-up treatment for blood and body fluid exposure accidents. Chapter 31 discusses infection control programs and body substance precautions in detail.

Stress "Stress is now recognized as being a hazard for those employed in the helping and caring professions" (Bailey, 1985, 1). Nurses and other health professionals generally start their careers with ideal optimism. They become frustrated, however, when time and budget constraints do not permit the type of nurturing care they would like to provide for their patients. Health agencies, like many other employers, are beginning to recognize that stress is an occupational hazard and are endeavouring to provide the necessary support services.

ASSESSING SAFETY NEEDS

There are two distinct yet related components in the assessment of a patient's safety needs. The first component is an appraisal of the factors affecting the patient's (or family's) capacity for self-protection. The second component is the identification of potential hazards in the environment which may affect patients, visitors and staff. This appraisal may be conducted in an inpatient facility or in a patient's home.

ASSESSING THE CAPACITY FOR SELF-PROTECTION

In assessing a patient's capacity for self-protection, the nurse should be aware of both the patient's age and the integrity of the sensory abilities. Does the patient have any sensory deficits, such as a loss of sight, hearing, smell, taste or touch? It is necessary to know any restrictions that have been put on the patient's mobility, such as bedrest, position restrictions, or immobilization of a part (as with a cast or traction apparatus). The use of aids for mobility (a cane, a walker or a wheelchair, for example) may also pose potential hazards for patient safety.

The nurse also needs information about the patient's general state of health, the nature of any health problems, and the physician's plan of diagnostic and therapeutic care. It is important to know if the patient is helpless or semi-helpless or whether the nature of the illness may cause loss of strength, impairment of sensory or motor functioning or short or prolonged periods of altered states of consciousness. Is the patient to have surgery, for example, and experience preoperative and postoperative periods when the patient's mental faculties may be lessened by sedation or anesthesia? The nurse should be aware of diagnostic or therapeutic procedures being performed that may involve the use of potentially hazardous equipment, potentially harmful reactions and the possibility of infection. Information about

medications which the patient is receiving and the nature of other treatments planned for the patient is also essential. Is the patient receiving medications that may diminish the ability to perceive and respond to harmful stimuli? Might the medications cause confusion? Is the patient having treatments, such as oxygen therapy, that require extra safety precautions?

Many patients are anxious, and the nurse should particularly watch for evidence of this in the patient. It is important to note the level of anxiety the patient is showing. An emotionally upset patient, visitor or staff member may rush blindly into danger. Someone who is worried, preoccupied or emotionally distressed is often less able to make judgements that are in the best interests of physical or mental health. These patients require extra vigilance from the nursing staff. The nurse also needs to know if the patient is an accident-prone individual.

Much of the information the nurse requires to assess safety needs may be obtained from the baseline assessment taken at the time of admission. The nursing history and physical assessment will provide data concerning the patient's usual and current patterns of functioning with regard to sensory and motor abilities, state of comfort, rest and sleep and emotional and mental state. The patient's status changes constantly, however, and the nurse must rely on observations and make judgements regarding safety precautions that need to be taken.

The patient's record is, of course, the most reliable source of information about diagnostic procedures, medications and other therapeutic measures in the patient's overall plan of care. Nurses supplement this information by increasing their own knowledge about medications, tests, examinations and treatments by asking knowledgeable people, such as physicians, nursing instructors, nursing team leaders or head nurses, and by reading up on these matters in texts and in the library.

To ensure safety at all times, the nurse should conduct a focus assessment during every nurse–patient encounter. This includes a visual scan of the environment for potential hazards and a quick appraisal of patient-related factors. The nurse will find subjective data very helpful. The patient may say that the things on the bedside table are out of reach, for example, or that sitting, standing or trying to walk causes weakness or dizziness. The patient can alert the nurse to things that are causing pain or discomfort so that appropriate action can be taken to remove the cause. For example, a patient may be lying on an arm and cutting off circulation. The astute and observant nurse should be aware of this, but patients can be very helpful in assisting the nurse to adjust the position to one that is comfortable and safe. The patient is often aware when mental faculties are impaired and may indicate this by expressing an inability to think clearly or by saying that everything "seems to be fuzzy."

The patient's family or significant others often alert the nurse to dangerous situations for the patient. Many agencies permit family members to stay with confused or

Safety Needs Assessment Guide

- How old is the patient?
- Is the patient alert, conscious and in full command of mental faculties?
- Does the patient require additional safety precautions because of age, physical condition or mental state?
- Is the patient receiving medications that impair the senses?
- Does the patient require restraints of any sort?
- Does the patient smoke?
- Is electrical equipment in use in the patient's room? Does the patient have electrical appliances at the bedside?
- Is heat or cold used as a therapeutic agent in the care of this patient?
- Is the patient receiving oxygen therapy?
- Are there any safety practices or information which can help the patient to avoid injury or accident?
- Is the patient comfortable?
- Can the patient reach everything that is needed?
- Is the call signal within easy reach?
- Is the patient safe from mechanical injuries, such as those resulting from falls?
- Is the patient being protected from burns, for example, those from a heating pad or a hot water bottle?
- What precautions are taken to ensure that medications are given safely?

Hospital Hazards Appraisal

- Is all electrical equipment functioning properly? Is it properly grounded (does it have a three-pronged plug)? Are extension cords properly taped to the floor? Look for frayed cords, tangled cords and cords that can be tripped on. Look for loose control knobs, overloaded circuits and placement of appliances near sinks, bath tubs or moisture areas.
- Are "No Smoking" signs clearly displayed in areas where patients are on oxygen therapy?
- Could injury be caused by any obstacles present? Equipment? Misplaced footstools? Chairs? Overbed tables? Bags or suitcases with patient's belongings on the floor?
- Are bathrooms equipped with safety features? Look for hand rails around tubs and toilets, non-slip surfaces, stools or chairs for tubs and showers.
- Is lighting adequate, for instance, can the patient see adequately when getting from bed to bathroom? In the bathroom?
- Are there water spills or wet slippery areas on the floor? Are "Wet Floor" signs clearly displayed by the housekeeping staff when floors are being washed?
- Are hand rails secured properly in bathrooms and hallways?
- Are side rails up for patients who need them?
- Are areas where radiation is in use clearly demarcated?
- Is there a designated smoking area for people who must smoke?

sedated patients and this can be of great assistance to the nurse. However, the nurse must ensure that the family member knows what to do when helping the patient and will call for assistance if it is needed. The patient's safety is the nurse's responsibility at all times, and this should not be neglected when a patient's family member is present.

ASSESSING HAZARDS IN THE ENVIRONMENT

In terms of safety, an astute nurse has a sharp eye for potential hazards in the environment. In the hospital, these hazards could be a dangling electric cord, a misplaced footstool, a side rail that is down or a slippery floor. In the home, hazards might include inadequate lighting, a stairway with loose steps, slip-

pery surfaces in bath tubs or showers or overloaded electrical outlets. Guidelines for appraising hazards in the hospital and the home are given in the boxes above and on the next page.

DIAGNOSING SAFETY PROBLEMS

The patient's safety is an integral component of all facets of the nursing process. Safety needs must be considered when the patient is very young or very old, when perceptual abilities are lessened for any reason, when the ability to react to harmful stimuli is decreased, when potentially harmful equipment is being used in care and when the patient is accident-prone.

Home Hazards Appraisal

1. Are stairs secure both inside and outside? Are the steps the same height and the treads the same width? Are the treads slip-resistant? If carpeted, is the carpet firm and secure?

2. Are handrails present on both sides of the stairs? Do they provide a good handhold? Are they strong enough to support an adult's weight?

3. Are stairways well lit?

4. Are balcony and sundeck railings strong enough to resist the impact of a person falling against them? Are they sturdy and secure? Are exterior guardrails at least 1.07 m high with openings no larger than 100 mm? Can children climb the guardrails without difficulty?

5. Are there decorative decals on glass doors, preventing someone from bumping into or attempting to walk through them?

6. Do floors have non-slip surfaces? Are scatter rugs skid-proof?

7. Are walkways and stairways cluttered with objects that are easily tripped over (such as toys, electrical cords, newspapers, garden hoses)?

8. Do bath tubs and showers have non-slip surfaces or rubber mats?

9. Is a smoke detector located on every level of the home? Is it tested regularly?

10. Is there at least one readily accessible fire extinguisher in the home? Does every family member know how to use it?

11. Are fireplaces, wood-burning stoves and space heaters properly screened? Are portable heaters away from combustible materials?

12. Are electrical outlets overloaded (having too many items on the same outlet)? Is more than one electrical appliance connected to an extension cord? Are electrical cords worn and frayed?

13. Are all electrical wires placed out of reach of children? Are outlets covered with safety plugs?

14. Are all cleaning products, insecticides, medications and other harmful chemicals placed out of reach of children?

15. Are cigarettes, lighters and matches out of reach of children?

16. Is propane or gasoline stored in the home?

17. Are children's toys in good repair? Do they have sharp edges, loose parts or parts small enough for a young child to swallow?

SOURCE: B.C. Ministry of Municipal Affairs, Recreation, and Housing (1991).

The general diagnostic label for patients with problems meeting safety needs is *High risk for injury*. Carpenito defines *High risk for injury* as "the state in which an individual is at risk for harm because of a perceptual or physiologic deficit, a lack of awareness of hazards, or maturational age" (Carpenito, 1993, 446). NANDA has identified four subcategories of potential injury: *High risk for aspiration, poisoning, suffocation* and *trauma* (Carpenito, 1993). These diagnostic statements identify the nature of the problem more specifically and as such, facilitate the selection of appropriate interventions.

The following is a list of some examples of nursing diagnoses for patients who are at risk for injury.

- *High risk for aspiration related to accumulation of secretions secondary to dorsal positioning*
- *High risk for poisoning related to easy accessibility of household cleaners to young children*
- *High risk for injury related to insufficient knowledge of accident prevention in the home*

PLANNING SAFETY INTERVENTIONS

Planning interventions for *High risk for injury* problems involves the selection of strategies to foster a patient's capacity for self-protection or to protect the patient who lacks this capability. Safety needs are among the most basic of all human needs. Safety is important for all people, but especially for those who are ill. The protective aspects of the nurse's role are among the most important of all functions. The nurse must incorporate the patient's safety as the number one priority in all aspects of patient care.

Assuring patient safety in case of fire takes precedence over all other nursing responsibilities. Nurses must know the agency's fire procedure, understand how to use the equipment for controlling fire and know their responsibilities with regard to patient safety. They must be ever alert to potential fire hazards and take action to see that the danger is minimized or eliminated if possible.

KEY PRINCIPLES

Principles Relevant to Patient Safety

1. Normally functioning body senses inform the individual about potential hazards.
2. Age affects both the ability to perceive and interpret sensory stimuli from the environment and the ability to take effective action to provide protection from harmful stimuli.
3. Familiarity with the environment makes it less hazardous.
4. The ability to provide self-protection is affected by sensory status, mental status, emotional status, mobility status and by the status of comfort, rest and sleep.
5. Illness renders a person more vulnerable to accidents and injury.
6. Diagnostic and therapeutic measures have inherent potential for causing a patient harm even while aiding in the resolution of health problems.

IMPLEMENTING SAFETY INTERVENTIONS

The primary goal of nursing action with regard to patient safety is the prevention of accidental injury. A very large aspect of care is educating people to protect themselves from injury in the course of daily living in the home, the workplace and the community. As well, strategies that promote wellness on a personal and occupational level are important because troubled individuals are more prone to accidents. The modelling of safe behaviours is by far the most effective form of teaching safety awareness.

ACCIDENT PREVENTION IN THE HOME

Many accidents such as falls, poisonings, drownings and burns need never happen. A good many of these accidents can be prevented by the careful supervision of children and teenagers and by assessing the home for potential hazards and correcting them. Table 29.2 outlines a number of prevention strategies for protecting children and youth from common accidents.

Fire Prevention

The best fire prevention is to practise home fire safety. Every home should have a fire prevention program. A good home fire prevention program includes the installation of smoke detectors and sprinklers, fire safety education and an evacuation plan. It also includes other measures such as the use of non-flammable materials wherever possible and care and attention to safety precautions in the use of heat-producing equipment (like stoves) and all electrical appliances.

Dwellings should have smoke alarms installed between the bedrooms and the remainder of the house. The batteries should be replaced at least yearly and the alarms should be tested monthly. A sprinkler system is a good idea for homes and it is becoming mandatory for apartments under many municipal building codes. If a family member smokes, particular care should be taken to be sure that smouldering cigarettes are not left unattended and that cigarette butts are cold before being put into the garbage. Clothing and upholstery, window drapes and other articles made of cloth must meet flammability standards. People need to be cautioned about the dangers of overloading electrical circuits. Only one appliance should be connected to an extension cord. As we mentioned earlier, poorly installed and ill-maintained wood stoves cause a large number of fires in the home. People who have wood stoves or wood-burning fireplaces should make sure that the chimney is cleaned regularly. Wood stoves and fireplaces should always be installed in accordance with the local building codes.

Every home should have at least one fire extinguisher and all family members who are old enough should know how to use it. A 5 lb multipurpose ABC dry chemical extinguisher rated 2A is recommended for homes. A 5 lb container is large enough to put out small fires or contain a fire until the fire department arrives, yet it is not so large that it cannot be handled effectively. The ABC type of fire extinguisher is effective against the three basic classes of fires, described in the box below.

It is dangerous to use water or a fire extinguisher labelled Class A only on grease or electrical fires. Class B and C models, however, may be used on Class A fires (National Fire Protection Association, 1992).

Three Basic Classes of Fires
- **Class A** Ordinary combustibles such as wood, paper, cloth, rubber and many plastics
- **Class B** Flammable liquids such as grease, gasoline, oil, oil-based paint
- **Class C** Energized electrical equipment including wiring, fuse boxes, circuit breakers, appliances and machinery.

TABLE 29.2 Injury Prevention Strategies for Children and Youth

INJURY PROBLEM	INTERVENTION	PROVEN EFFECTIVE	PROMISING	MORE STUDY REQUIRED
Motor Vehicle Occupants	Air bags	✓		
	Child restraint loaner programs	✓		
	Child restraints/seat belts	✓		
	Education programs for youth		✓	
	Driver training			✓
Pedestrians	Visibility measures	✓		
	Roadway barriers	✓		
	School zone measures	✓		
	Sidewalks	✓		
	Pedestrian education programs		✓	
Motorcyclists	Helmet use	✓		
	Motorcycle rider training		✓	
Bicyclists	Helmet use	✓		
	Visibility measures	✓		
	Bicycle paths		✓	
	Bicycle selection guidelines		✓	
	Bicycle safety education			✓
Home Accidents	Education programs		✓	
Falls	Window guards	✓		
	Parent education		✓	
	Safety gates		✓	
Fire/Burns	Fire safe cigarettes	✓		
	Flammability standards	✓		
	Reduced tap water temperature	✓		
	Smoke detectors	✓		
	Sprinkler systems	✓		
	Fire safety education		✓	
Poisoning	Poison control centres	✓		
	Prevention packaging	✓		
	First aid training		✓	
	Prevention education programs		✓	
Suffocation/Choking	Heimlich manoeuvre	✓		
	Product safety regulations	✓		
	Education re: choking risks			✓
Drowning	Barriers for pools	✓		
	Personal flotation devices	✓		
	Supervision	✓		
	CPR instruction			✓
	Parent counselling			✓
	Swimming lessons			✓
Sports and Playground Injuries	Protective equipment	✓		
	Surfacing/equipment standards	✓		
	Education programs		✓	
Occupational Injuries	Education programs		✓	
Injuries in Facilities	Safety standards	✓		
	Training programs for workers		✓	

SOURCE: B.C. Ministry of Health, Office for Injury Prevention, Family Health Division. (1993, September). *Injury prevention strategies for children and youth in British Columbia.* Victoria: Queens Printer, 18.

Families are encouraged to prepare an emergency escape plan, which the whole family should periodically review and practise. The local fire department can help families to design this plan. People who live in apartment buildings should make sure that one of the two exit stairs mandatory for apartment buildings under most building codes is always accessible and clear of obstacles. Fire doors should always be kept closed. If the fire alarm rings, people are urged to:

- Proceed outdoors as quickly as possible
- Take the apartment keys
- Walk downstairs, rather than using the elevator

If a person is trapped in an apartment suite, it is important to let the firefighters know and ensure that the trapped person stays near a window or balcony.

Burns from causes other than fire can be prevented by keeping the temperature of the hot water set at or lower than 54° C (130° F) (B.C. Ministry of Municipal Affairs, Recreation and Housing, 1991). Pots and pans that contain hot foods must be kept out of the reach of small children, as should matches and lighters. Propane and gasoline should be stored outdoors or in a garden shed.

Preventing Injuries from Falls

There are a number of ways to prevent injuries from falls in the home. Stairs should be clear of all objects and should be constructed of slip-resistant material. Handrails must be strong enough to support an adult's weight and should be shaped to provide a good handhold. Balcony and sundeck railings must be strong, well secured and meet local building code specifications. Bath tubs and showers should be constructed with slip-resistant materials. Window guards and safety gates should be installed where there is a risk of falling. People should never stand on chairs to reach high places, and all carpets and area rugs should be securely fastened.

Preventing Poisonings

People can do much to protect their families from accidental poisonings. Regulated chemical products are required by law to bear appropriate hazard symbols on the labels and some must be packaged in child-resistant containers. Poisons and medicines should be stored in the original containers and out of reach of children, preferably in a locked cabinet. Parents should never call medicine "candy," nor should they take medicines in front of children. There is a national network of poison control centres in Canada and a poison control centre in every major city in Canada The phone number of the Poison Control Centre should be posted by each telephone and baby sitters and relatives should be made aware of the number. Every household should have at least one person with first aid training. It is helpful to have ipecac syrup on hand at all times to induce vomiting although this measure should only be taken after advice from the Poison Control Centre or a physician. For tips on how to poison-proof your home, see the box below.

Preventing Choking, Suffocation and Drowning

Part of home safety is being prepared for possible accidents such as choking or suffocation. In the home, knowledge of the Heimlich manoeuvre is the most helpful first aid measure. People with swimming pools must take extra precautions in order to ensure water safety. Rules of conduct, safety barriers, personal flotation devices and adequate supervision protect family and visitors from accidents. Swimming lessons for children and knowledge of cardiopulmonary resuscitation are also essential for safe water activity.

General Safety Measures

All home furniture and appliances should meet Canadian Safety Standards specifications. When purchasing clothing, toys, equipment, appliances and furniture, people should give careful consideration to safety features. Parents should be cautious when purchasing or receiving second-hand items such as cribs, playpens, strollers and high chairs, and ensure that these items meet current government safety standard specifications. If parents are uncertain, they should either contact the local health unit which will have the latest information from Consumer and Corporate Affairs Canada (CCAC) or contact the local office of CCAC directly.

Finally, children must be kept away from construction or carpentry areas, and any work area where dangerous machinery or tools (such as chain saws or table saws) are being operated .

ACCIDENT PREVENTION IN THE COMMUNITY

Infant and Child Restraint Systems

Transport Canada publishes regulations governing safety standards for infant and child restraint systems. All provinces require that children be properly restrained when travelling in a motor vehicle. It is imperative that any restraint system meets Canadian Motor Vehicle Safety Standards and is correctly installed according to the manufacturer's instructions. Table 29.3 illustrates the recommended infant and child car restraint systems.

The nurse can assist parents by providing information about current legislation and the suggested types of

How to Poison-Proof Your Home

The average household contains as many as 250 poisons and, each year in Canada, hundreds of fatalities are caused by poisoning. There are two key steps to poison-proofing your home: identification and storage.

Common Household Poisons

- Cleaners and bleaches, including detergents, ammonia, naphtha, oven cleaner, and bleach
- Solvents, including paint remover, kerosene and turpentine
- Polishes and waxes, including paint, car and furniture wax, silver polish
- Herbicides, insecticides and insect repellents
- Mercury from thermometers
- Cosmetics and toiletries, including after-shave, bubble bath, nail polish, hair lotions
- Drugs and medicines, including both prescription and non-prescription drugs such as vitamins, ASA, cough medicines and cold medications
- House plants, ornamental plants and flower and vegetable garden plants

How to Store Them

- Keep products in clearly labelled original containers.

- Store prescription drugs out of the reach of children and in containers with safety lids.
- Store household cleaners in high shelves, not underneath the sink.
- Return medication and cleaning products to a safe place after using them.
- Keep all poisonous liquids and solids out of the reach of children; if possible, install child-proof locking cabinets.
- Never call medicine "candy"; it gives children a distorted idea.
- Warn children at an early age not to eat household plants or wild plants and berries.
- Never keep food and household cleaners next to each other.
- Don't continue to store old products around the house.
- Don't leave a purse or handbag where a child can reach it, since prescription drugs are often inside.
- If poisoning occurs, identify the suspected poison and immediately seek medical help. Many areas have poison information centres. Never attempt to induce vomiting without medical advice.

SOURCE: Colombo, J.R. (1992). *The 1993 Canadian Global Almanac.* Toronto: Macmillan Canada, 684. Reproduced with permission.

---

restraint systems. Children should never be allowed to travel in the cargo area of a van, station wagon or truck. Loose, bulky objects in vehicles should be secured. Travel beds and plastic baby seats should never be used in a vehicle as they are not designed to give crash protection. The infant carrier or seat must be ready for the infant's first ride home from the hospital.

Bicycle Safety

The risk of bicycle-related brain injury can be greatly reduced by the use of bicycle helmets but, as yet, few people actually wear them. Some communities have, however, established mandatory bicycle helmet programs to prevent injuries while cycling.

School and Recreational Safety

In sports arenas and playgrounds, adult supervision is needed to ensure safety for children and youth. Someone skilled in first aid treatment should always be available. Safety is an important area of consideration for school boards, teachers and parents. Both students and teachers need safe working conditions and access to support services (Government of Ontario, 1993).

ACCIDENT PREVENTION IN THE WORKPLACE

Accident prevention should be part of the overall occupational safety and health program in the workplace. Most large companies and hospitals recognize the importance of promoting health and wellness and preventing accidents and are hiring staff and allocating funding for occupational safety and health programs.

THE OCCUPATIONAL SAFETY AND HEALTH TEAM

The Occupational Safety and Health Team may consist of one or more of the following professionals:

TABLE 29.3   Recommended Infant and Child Car Restraint Systems

TYPE OF RESTRAINT	WEIGHT LIMIT	DESCRIPTION	ILLUSTRATION
Infant Carrier	Birth to 9 kg	• Especially designed for children from birth to 9 kg • The seat faces the rear of the car • The baby is securely held in the seat by the harness • The seat itself is fastened by the car seat belt, according to the manufacturer's directions • Attach a locking clip to a continuous lap/shoulder belt, if applicable	
Convertible Seat for Infants and Toddlers	Birth to 9 kg	• The seat faces the rear of the car • The baby is securely held in the seat by the harness • The seat itself is fastened by the car seat belt, according to the manufacturer's directions • Attach a locking clip to a continuous lap/shoulder belt, if applicable	
Convertible Seat for Young Children	9 to 18 kg	• The seat faces forward • The seat is anchored with the lap belt and a tether strap according to the manufacturer's instructions • Attach a locking clip to a continuous lap/shoulder belt, if applicable	
Booster Seat	18 to 27 kg	• Faces forward • Best location — centre back seat • The seat is anchored by placing the lap belt over the shield or low and snug over the hips • Attach a locking clip to a continuous lap/shoulder belt, if applicable	

SOURCE: Insurance Corporation of British Columbia. (1990). *Do it up right* (Pamphlet No. TS244A(0394). Vancouver: Author. Adapted with permission.

- Occupational Safety and Health Manager
- Accident Prevention/Safety Officer
- Occupational Health Nurse
- Full-time, part-time or occasional Occupational Health Physician
- Workers' Compensation Board Claims Manager
- Clerical support

In a large corporation, an expanded department might include:

- Industrial Hygienist
- Physiotherapist
- Occupational Therapist

Other specialists such as ergonomists (specialists in environmental hazards in the workplace), toxicologists (specialists in the field of poisons and toxins), and orthopedic specialists (physicians in the field of the prevention and correction of deformities involving locomotor areas of the body, such as muscles, bones and joints) might be brought in on a consulting basis. The type and number of staff required and their responsibilities will depend on the type and size of the business and on the type of hazards in the workplace.

The occupational health team teaches accident awareness and prevention.

Occupational Safety and Health

An occupational safety and health program usually includes, but is not limited to

- Education and training of employees about
  - Accident prevention and awareness
  - Accident investigation
  - Workplace and job safety audits
  - Workplace Hazardous Materials Information System (WHMIS)
  - Respirator fit testing
  - Programs for specific hazards (such as asbestos, lead or mercury)
  - Back care and lifting education
- Workplace and personal monitoring of physical, chemical, biological or psychological hazards
- Development of safety policies and procedures
- Health assessment and counselling

Workplace Hazardous Materials Information System (WHMIS)

WHMIS is a system designed to communicate information about hazardous materials in the workplace — from the suppliers of controlled products to employers and to workers through the three key elements: **labelling, material safety data sheets*** and **worker education**. The relationships are shown in the diagram.

* to be completed where the employer produces a controlled product.

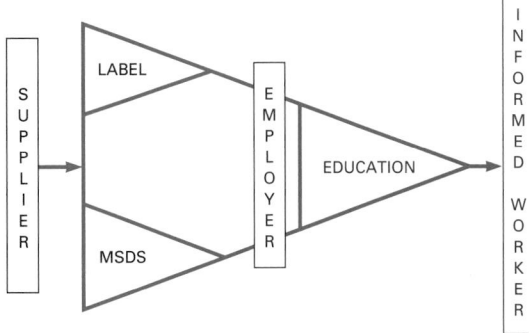

Legislation to implement WHMIS has been enacted at both the federal and the provincial and territorial levels. Federal requirements deal with the importation and sale of controlled products and provincial legislation covers the storage, handling and the use of controlled products in the workplace.

Every province and territory uses a common system of labelling for containers of all controlled products. In addition to this system, WHMIS requires education programs, so that employees will have a thorough understanding of the information on the WHMIS labels (see Figure 29.2) and in the material safety data sheets (MSDS).

SOURCE: Workers' Compensation Board of British Columbia. (1991). *What's WHMIS?* Pamphlet. Richmond, B.C.: Author. Reproduced with permission of the author.

Occupational hazards differ greatly from one workplace to another. The types of equipment, chemicals, machinery, work processes and location of work all affect the focus of the safety program. In general, however, the role of the Occupational Safety and Health Department includes the identification of occupational hazards, the development and implementation of a safety and accident prevention program and the provision of first aid to injured workers. In addition, the Occupational Safety and Health Unit provides health assessment and counselling services for employees of the organization. This is usually one of the responsibilities of the occupational health nurse. The occupational safety and health professional in a health care facility also provides specific expertise regarding infectious diseases.

THE WORKPLACE HAZARDOUS MATERIALS INFORMATION SYSTEM (WHMIS)

The Workplace Hazardous Materials Information System (WHMIS) was developed in response to Canadian workers' request to know — and their right to know — about the hazards of materials used in the workplace to safety and health (WCB of BC, 1991). A brief summary of the program is given in the box above. Figure 29.2 illustrates the labels for various WHMIS hazard classes.

WELLNESS PROGRAMS

At one time, it was believed that occupational accidents happened because workers were not "careful enough." More recently, safety experts suggest that lack of management control is an important factor in causing accidents. Safety programs, policies, accident investigation, safety training and providing a safe environment all fall under management's control. However, supervisors and workers both play key roles in developing and maintaining an accident-free workplace. Joint Occupational Health and Safety

Committees are mandated by law in each province for most workplaces. Management, unionized and non-unionized staff work together on these joint committees to develop and maintain an effective occupational health and safety program.

Programs like the Employee and Family Assistance Program (which offers confidential counselling), Continuous Quality Improvement Programs and Stress Management Programs and other wellness programs aim to alleviate or prevent stress-related problems. It has recently been recognized that accidents are often linked to work-related stress and stress from personal, financial or other worries. People take their worries to work; they do not automatically shed them at the company door. A 1984 Canadian study on work and well-being suggests that "troubled employees tend to make more errors, produce poorer quality material and damage equipment" (Canadian Mental Health Association, 1984, cited in Thomas, 1993).

Corporations have developed wellness programs, realizing that stress is a major factor in absenteeism, work accidents and illnesses, errors of omission or commission and lowered productivity. The wellness program developed in 1986 by Carolyn Mathews and a group of nurses working for

---

A controlled product is a substance or material that meets or exceeds criteria for inclusion in one or more of the following WHMIS hazard classes and divisions.

CLASS A:

COMPRESSED GAS. This class includes compressed gases, dissolved gases and gases liquefied by compression or refrigeration. Examples: gas cylinders for oxyacetylene welding or water disinfection.

CLASS B:

FLAMMABLE AND COMBUSTIBLE MATERIAL. Solids, liquids and gases capable of catching fire or exploding in the presence of a source of ignition. Examples: white phosphorus, acetone and butane. **Flammable** liquids such as acetone are more easily ignited than **combustible** liquids such as kerosene.

CLASS C:

OXIDIZING MATERIAL. Materials which provide oxygen or similar substance and which increase the risk of fire if they come in contact with flammable or combustible materials. Examples: sodium hypochlorite perchloric acid, inorganic peroxides.

CLASS D: POISONOUS AND INFECTIOUS MATERIALS.

DIVISION 1:

Materials Causing Immediate and Serious Toxic Effects. This division covers materials which can cause the death of a person exposed to small amounts. Examples: sodium cyanide, hydrogen sulphide.

DIVISION 2:

Materials Causing Other Toxic Effects. This division covers materials which cause immediate skin or eye irritation as well as those which can cause long-term effects in a person repeatedly exposed to small amounts. Examples: acetone (irritant), asbestos (cancer causing), toluene diisocyanate (a sensitizing agent).

DIVISION 3:

Biohazardous Infectious Material. This division applies to materials which contain harmful microorganisms. Examples: cultures or diagnostic specimens containing salmonella bacteria or the hepatitis B virus.

CLASS E:

CORROSIVE MATERIAL. Caustic or acid materials which can destroy the skin or eat through metals. Examples: muriatic acid, lye.

CLASS F:

DANGEROUSLY REACTIVE MATERIAL. Products which can undergo dangerous reaction if subjected to heat, pressure, shock or allowed to contact water. Examples: plastic monomers such as butadiene and some cyanides.

FIGURE 29.2   What is a controlled product?

SOURCE: Workers' Compensation Board of British Columbia. (1991). *What's WHMIS?* Pamphlet. Richmond, B.C.: Author. Reproduced with permission.

Imperial Oil at various sites across the country exemplifies the trend towards wellness in occupational health. Mathews's program was organized in four parts: increasing health awareness in employees, lifestyles examination/risk management, personal prescription (tailoring a program to meet the needs of the individual employee) and behaviour change.

ACCIDENT PREVENTION IN THE HOSPITAL

In nursing, a knowledge base of safe nursing practices is essential. This involves not only a sound knowledge of the nursing and allied sciences, but also a knowledge of preventive nursing measures. Nurses must recognize circumstances that could result in an accident and intervene.

Enabling Self-Protection

All patients have self-protection learning needs while in the agency. These needs include an orientation to the physical design of the nursing unit and the equipment in the patient's immediate surroundings. Patients must know how to call for assistance if needed (and the call bell must be placed within easy reach). They need to know how to use the equipment in and around the bed, and they must be alerted to safety precautions in the use of this equipment. Each nursing measure, each diagnostic test or examination and each therapeutic measure has important safety precautions that patients need to be aware of to protect themselves from harm. If patients know why the safety measures are being taken, they are more apt to participate.

Environmental Factors

General considerations of environmental factors include arranging everything for the patient's comfort and convenience, as well as that of family members, other visitors and the staff. Equipment used in hospitals is generally portable, so that it can be easily moved to a more convenient position or location. Hospitals try to obtain equipment that is also quiet, durable, simple to operate and easily repaired. In many agencies, equipment is built into the patient's unit so that it is easier to use and always convenient. As a result, fewer hazardous objects are in and around the patient's bed.

The patient's unit and the nursing unit itself should be kept as free of clutter as possible. When giving care to a patient, nurses should always make sure that there is a clear working space, that they can see what they are doing, and that it is possible to practise good body mechanics in any lifting and moving that is involved. It is awkward to work over side rails, for example, or to reach around objects.

Reporting Accidents

All accidents — that is, all events that have resulted or could have resulted in injury to a patient, a visitor or a staff member — are reported so that remedial measures may be instituted. For example, if a patient receives an incorrect medication, notifying the nursing supervisor or the physician initiates measures to prevent a recurrence of this error and to remedy the effects of the incorrect medication. Accidents are ordinarily reported on an Unusual Occurrence Report (see Figure 29.3). Many hospitals require that employees injured at work complete an Accident/Injury On Duty Report (see Figure 29.4) and report to either a designated First Aid Attendant or a physician for care.

Reporting accidents also guides the safety committee of an agency in instituting proper preventive measures. The findings of these committees can be used as the bases for changes in medical and nursing practices and as indications of the need for the education of patients and personnel.

PREVENTING FALLS AND SELF-INFLICTED INJURIES

Among the most frequently occurring types of accidents in hospital are falls. Falling from beds, from chairs, while walking or while getting into or out of a bathtub are not uncommon occurrences but are often preventable. A person who is weakened by illness can lose balance and fall while simply leaning towards a table that is out of reach. Nurses can prevent many accidents of this kind by being alert to potentially dangerous situations and remedying them. For example, adjustable beds can be left in the low position when the nurse is not present. At this level, the patient will be able to get in and out of bed more safely. Also, patients who have been in bed for several days or who are weakened by illness can be helped to recognize their need for assistance in getting about.

Slippery floors can be dangerous to people in any situation, not only to patients. To minimize this danger, non-slippery materials are used on the floor surfaces of hospitals. Also, since anything spilled on a floor may make it slippery, spills should be mopped up before an accident occurs. Floors should be washed and polished at a time when there is little traffic, and signs warning that the floor is wet and slippery should be prominently placed.

Untidiness can also contribute to accidents. People can trip over electric cords, footstools and equipment left on the floor. Walkways, such as areas between a patient's bed and the bathroom, can be particularly hazardous when they are not kept clear. Patients have fallen from beds while reaching for articles on bedside tables or while looking for a misplaced call button. The nurse can help the patient to arrange these items so that they are within easy reach.

SMH   Surrey Memorial Hospital

UNUSUAL OCCURRENCE REPORT

DATE OF INCIDENT: _____   TIME: _____

DEPARTMENT/NURSING UNIT: _____

STATUS: ☐ Patient ☐ Visitor ☐ Staff ☐ Physician ☐ Other _____

LOCATION: ☐ Patient Room ☐ Bathroom ☐ Stairs ☐ Corridor
           ☐ Dining Room ☐ Hospital Grounds ☐ Parking ☐ Other _____

IF NO I.D. PLATE COMPLETE THE FOLLOWING

MR. ☐
MRS. ☐
MISS ☐

NAME _____
     (LAST NAME)   (GIVEN NAMES)

ADDRESS_____

PHONE _____

| DATE OF BIRTH | | | |
| DAY | MO. | YR. | SEX |

TYPE OF INCIDENT: Check the appropriate section below.

☐ Falls - Section A
☐ Medication - Section B
☐ Aggressive Behaviour - Section C

☐ Security/Property - Section D
☐ Equipment Related - Section E
☐ Treatment/Procedure - Section F

☐ Others - Section G
☐ Staff Injury - Complete Form #590
☐ Fire - Complete Form #802F

A. FALL:
(check one)

Ambulation:
1 Independent
2 Req. Asst.
3 Dependent
4 Wheelchair
5 Crutches
6 Walker

Footwear:
1 Shoes
2 Barefoot
3 Slippers / Socks
4 Other
_____

Restraints/Equipment
(circle if yes)
1 Height of Bed in Lowest Position
2 Side Rails Up
3 Red Vest
4 Brakes Applied
5 Call Bell Reachable
6 Security Room
7 Jacket
8 Waist/Leg
9 Lap Belt
10 Other

E. EQUIPMENT RELATED:
(send copy to Biomedical Engineering)
1 Monitor
2 Ventilator
3 IV PUMP
4 Other (Medical Devices)

Equip. Control # _____

COPY TO MAINTENANCE
5 Bed   7 Others (specify)
6 Wheelchair

B. MEDICATION:
1 Omission
2 Wrong Dose
3 Wrong Rate of Infusion
4 Extra Dose Given
5 Unordered Dose Given
6 Wrong Dosage Form

7 Wrong Time
8 Wrong Route/Site
9 Incorrect Dosage Preparation
10 Allergic Patient Given Drug
11 Wrong Drug Given
12 Incorrect Patient
13 Other

ROUTE: ☐ P.O. ☐ I.V. ☐ I.M. ☐ Other _____

F. TREATMENT/PROCEDURE:
1 Missed
2 Incorrect
3 Wrong Patient
4 Blood (product) Problem
5 Specimen Problem
6 Other
_____

C. AGGRESSIVE BEHAVIOUR:
1 Physical
2 Verbal
3 Telephone
4 Other
_____

Injury to:
1 Staff
2 Patient
3 Resident
4 Security
5 Visitor
6 Other
_____

D. SECURITY/PROPERTY:
1 Theft
2 Property Damage
3 Property Loss
4 Patient Property
5 Other
_____

G. OTHERS:
1 Complaints
2 Consent Error
3 Elopement
4 Count Discrepancy
5 Tissue/Damage Loss
6 A.M.A.
2 Other _____

Brief description of incident: _____
_____
_____
_____

Immediate action taken: _____
_____
_____

	Name	Date	Time
REPORTED BY (signature):			
REPORTED TO:			
WITNESSED BY:			
PHYSICIAN NOTIFIED:			
REVIEWED BY (signature):		Title:	
	(Department Manager)		
	(Director Signature)	Title:	

COPIES SENT TO: ☐ Pharmacy ☐ Biomedical Engineering ☐ Security ☐ Occup. H. & S. ☐ Nursing ☐ Maintenance ☐ Other _____

DISTRIBUTION OF COPIES: See reverse side for instructions

FORM 561   REV. 06/93
8415-0740-4

FIGURE 29.3   Unusual Occurrence Report

SOURCE: Surrey Memorial Hospital, Surrey, B.C. Reproduced with permission.

SMH
ACCIDENT/INJURY ON DUTY REPORT

| R E S U L T | ☐ investigation completed _____ D/M/Y hazardous situation | OH & S DEPARTMENT ☐ no treatment ☐ first aid ☐ no time loss ☐ health care (medical aid) ☐ potential loss ☐ lost time |

B. Employee Identification

| Last Name | First Name | Sex | Marital Status | Area Code | Phone No. | Date of Birth day month year |

| Address (no., street, apt.) | City/Town | Province | Postal Code | Department/Unit |

| Date of Employment day month year | Occupation at time of the injury and years of experience in that occupation Years Exp. | Language Spoken if not English | Social Insurance No. |

C. DATE

| D/M/Y OF INCIDENT | TIME OF DAY | ACCIDENT FORM SUBMITTED D/M/Y | TIME OF DAY | OH & S DEPARTMENT CALLED D/M/Y | TIME OF DAY |

D. DESCRIPTION

STATE EXACTLY — WHAT WAS THE SEQUENCE OF EVENTS LEADING UP TO THE INCIDENT, WHERE INCIDENT OCCURRED, WHAT EMPLOYEE WAS DOING, SIZE, WEIGHT AND TYPE OF EQUIPMENT OR MATERIALS INVOLVED, ETC.

_____

_____

_____

_____

_____

_____

SIGNATURE OF PERSON REPORTING INCIDENT   SIGNATURE OF DEPT. HEAD OR SUPERVISOR

E. TYPE OF INCIDENT (√)
SEE DEFINITION ON REVERSE OF WHITE COPY

1. ☐ STRUCK OR CONTACT BY
2. ☐ STRUCK AGAINST / CONTACT WITH
3. ☐ CAUGHT IN, ON, OR BETWEEN
4. ☐ FALL
5. ☐ OVER EXERTION / STRAIN
6. ☐ EXPOSURE
7. ☐ PATIENT ACTION

F. WITNESS

NAMES AND ADDRESSES OF WITNESSES OR PERSONS HAVING KNOWLEDGE OF THE INCIDENT

_____

_____

G. CAUSE

WHAT CONDITIONS CONTRIBUTED TO THE INCIDENT (√)   (Number all contributing causes in order of importance)

1. ☐ OPERATING WITHOUT AUTHORITY
2. ☐ FAILURE TO SECURE OR WARN
3. ☐ WORKING AT UNSAFE SPEED
4. ☐ UNSAFE EQUIPMENT
5. ☐ UNSAFE LOADING, PLACING, MIXING, COMBINING ETC.
6. ☐ UNSAFE POSITION OR POSTURE

7. ☐ WORKING ON MOVING OR DANGEROUS EQUIPMENT
8. ☐ DISTRACTING, TEASING, WILFUL MISCONDUCT
9. ☐ FAILURE TO USE PERSONAL PROTECTIVE DEVICES
10. ☐ WHEELED EQUIPMENT OPERATION
11. ☐ NOT GUARDED OR IMPROPERLY GUARDED
12. ☐ PATIENT ACTION

13. ☐ INADEQUATE ILLUMINATION
14. ☐ FIRE, EXPLOSION, ATMOSPHERIC HAZARD
15. ☐ HAZARDOUS PERSONAL ATTIRE
16. ☐ UNSAFE DESIGN OR ARRANGEMENT
17. ☐ HAZARDOUS METHOD OR PROCEDURE
18. ☐ OUTSIDE HAZARDOUS CONDITION
19. ☐ OTHER (explain)

EXPLANATION OF CAUSES

DETAILS OF PROPERTY DAMAGE

H. CORRECTION

ACTIONS TO PREVENT INCIDENT RECURRENCE   MARK WITH (√) THOSE ACTIONS TAKEN TO PREVENT RECURRENCE, MARK WITH (P) OTHER CORRECTIVE ACTIONS DECIDED UPON OR PLANNED BUT NOT YET CARRIED OUT. MORE THAN ONE ITEM MAY APPLY

1. REINSTRUCTION OF PERSON INVOLVED
2. REASSIGNMENT OF PERSON
3. ORDER JOB SAFETY ANALYSIS DONE
4. IMPROVED PERSONAL PROTECTIVE EQUIPMENT

5. ACTION TO IMPROVE INSPECTION
6. EQUIPMENT REPAIR OR REPLACEMENT
7. CORRECTION OF CONGESTED AREA
8. INSTALLATION OF GUARD OR SAFETY DEVICE

9. ACTIONS TO IMPROVE DESIGN / PROCEDURE
10. CHECK WITH MANUFACTURER
11. INFORM ALL DEPARTMENT SUPERVISION
12. DISCIPLINE OF PERSONS INVOLVED
13. OTHER (explain)

DESCRIBE ACTIONS TAKEN TO PREVENT RECURRENCE _____

SIGNATURE OF DEPT HEAD OR SUPERVISOR

I. INJURY

DESCRIBE INJURY, PART OF BODY INVOLVED AND SPECIFY LEFT OR RIGHT SIDE.

NAME OF: A) ATTENDING PHYSICIAN, AND B) EMPLOYEE'S PHYSICIAN.

TO YOUR KNOWLEDGE, HAS THE EMPLOYEE HAD A PREVIOUS SIMILAR DISABILITY?   YES ☐   NO ☐

J. FIRST AID ATTENDANT - CIRCLE YOUR RESPONSE			K. MEDICAL OFFICER - CIRCLE YOUR RESPONSE		
YES	NO	RETURNED TO WORK	YES	NO	TREATED - RETURNED TO WORK
YES	NO	REFERRED TO PHYSICIAN	YES	NO	TREATED - TO REMAIN OFF WORK
YES	NO	ACCIDENT LOGGED			
YES	NO	FORM 7A COMPLETED			

FORM 590-841509404   WHITE - OH & S DEPARTMENT   CANARY - FIRST AID ATTENDANT   PINK - EMPLOYEES SUPERVISION

FIGURE 29.4   Accident /Injury On Duty Report

SOURCE: Surrey Memorial Hospital, Surrey, B.C. Reproduced with permission.

Other possible causes of falls are movable wheelchairs or stretchers. Often, just as a patient is about to sit in a wheelchair, it moves out of place. Most movable equipment is furnished with locks for the wheels. These locks should be set when the equipment is to be used and released only after the patient is secure.

When a patient first becomes ambulatory after a period of time in bed, some physical support is often required. Many hospitals and other health agencies have rails in the halls to guide and support patients while walking. These and other measures, such as rubber treads on stairs, can help prevent many falls.

Out of concern for a patient's safety, the nurse may employ specific safety devices. There are dangers involved in the use of many of these devices, however. Disoriented patients may become dangerously entangled in restraints, for example, or a safety device may make a patient unable to move in case of a fire. Many safety devices, therefore, should not be used unless absolutely necessary. In most institutions, devices are used either upon the request of the attending physician, or when, in the judgement of the nurse, they become necessary. Policies vary from place to place, however, and the nurse should be familiar with each institution's practices. Students should always check with the primary nurse or with their teacher before using safety devices for patients.

Side Rails

Side rails on beds can stop the patient from rolling off the bed. They do not deter the patient from climbing out. Most hospitals have policies regarding the use of side rails. Frequently side rails are required on the beds of patients who are blind, unconscious or sedated, or who have muscular disabilities or seizures. Some hospitals require that the beds of all patients over the age of 70 have side rails. A number of hospitals have adopted a policy of using side rails on the beds of all patients, particularly at night.

It is important when side rails are in use that both rails be up. For example, even when the patient's bed is against the wall both rails should still be used; the wall does not serve as a good replacement for the rail. When caring for the patient whose bed has side rails, the side rail should be taken down on the side at which the nurse is working. The nurse should go no further than an arm's length away from that side of the bed without returning the side rail to its "up" position.

Many patients dislike the use of side rails; they may find them an embarrassing reminder of childhood cribs. Some people are fearful of them, while to others, side rails signify a loss of independence and control over the situation. An explanation of the purpose for using side rails often helps patients to accept them. Generally, side rails will not keep patients in bed against their will; if patients need restraining, safety jackets should be used.

Jacket and Belt Restraints

Patients who are confused sometimes try to climb over the side rails of the bed. Because they are confused, they are frequently unaware of their surroundings; they just want to leave the bed. These patients can often be restrained comfortably in bed by means of a safety jacket or belt (see Figure 29.5). The jacket is an inconspicuous sleeveless garment which has long cross-over ties either in front or in back that can be attached to the frame on either side of the bed. The ties are secured to the frame out of reach of the patient. Some jacket restraints can also be used to hold patients securely upright in wheelchairs. When applying the jacket, ensure that it is not wrapped so tightly that it restricts breathing. Be sure to check the patient regularly to ensure comfort.

The belt restraint performs the same function as the jacket. It is secured around the patient's body, and ties are attached to the bed frame. Both jacket and belt restraints allow patients to move relatively freely in bed, yet restrain them from climbing over the side rails and possibly falling to the floor. When applying a belt restraint, care must be taken to ensure the belt is not placed too tightly around the patient's chest or abdomen.

Arm and Leg Restraints

Occasionally it is necessary to apply arm or leg restraints to patients in bed. Generally this is an undesirable nursing care measure because it limits a patient's movements, and this in turn often causes anxiety, increasing restlessness and subsequent fatigue. It is particularly dangerous to restrain only one side of the body because this tends to increase restlessness, and patients may injure themselves as they try to move the restrained side of the body. If only two limbs are restrained, they should be opposite limbs. Few patients like to be tied down, regardless of how irrational they are. The reaction is usually to struggle against whatever is hampering movement and patients may become quite agitated. Injury to the tissues of the wrists and ankles may result from the friction engendered by rubbing against the restraints. Occasionally, leather restraints may be used. Many agencies will not permit the use of leather restraints except on a doctor's order. There is a greater possibility of both adverse patient reaction to leather restraints and injury to the patient as a result of them.

An arm restraint may be prescribed during an intravenous infusion. Its chief purpose in this instance is to remind the patient to keep the arm immobilized during the treatment.

Arms and legs should not be restrained any longer than is absolutely necessary, and at least every two hours the restraints should be loosened and the limbs exercised. A patient's circulation may be restricted if a restraint is tight or if a limb is restrained in an abnormal position. Care must be

FIGURE 29.5 A. Hand rails B. Jacket restraint C. Belt restraint

taken to pad the skin and especially bony prominences be-fore restraints are applied. A washcloth or other soft cloth may be used to pad the skin under the restraint. A knot over the pad serves to keep the restraint from being too tight. Absorbent cotton should never be used because it has a tendency to flatten out and form into lumps. At any sign of blueness, pallor or cold or if the patient complains of tingling sensations in the extremity, the restraint is loos-ened and circulation restored by exercise and massage. A limb is best restrained in a slightly flexed position.

Commercially prepared restraints are available; how-ever, a common restraint used in many agencies is the clove hitch. The clove hitch restraint is made of a piece of cloth or tube gauze as illustrated in Figure 29.6. The advantage of this restraint is that it does not tighten as the patient pulls on it. To make a clove hitch, first make a "figure eight" with a strip of material. Then pick up the loops and direct the padded extremity through the loops. Adjust the re-straint so that it is secure but not too tight on the limb.

Mitt Restraints

Mitt restraints are indicated for patients who are confused or semiconscious and may pull at dressings and tubes. The mitts are often used, for example, for a patient with a head injury or for a patient who is confused following a stroke. Mitt restraints have the advantage of not permitting the patient to grasp such objects as dressings, tubing or bed rails, but they do not limit movement. A mitt restraint is like a soft boxing glove that pads the patient's hand. Commercial mitts are available (see Figure 29.7), or mitts may be made using dressing pads, gauze bandage, and adhesive tape. To

A

B

C

FIGURE 29.6 How to make a clove hitch re-straint. A. Make a "figure eight." B. Pick up the loops. C. Put the padded extremity through the loops and adjust the restraint.

FIGURE 29.7 Mitt restraint

make a mitt restraint, the nurse first places the patient's hand in a naturally flexed position. This allows unrestricted circulation and places little strain upon muscles. The patient is asked to grasp a soft rolled dressing so that the thumb approximates their fingers. The soft dressing permits flexion of the hand while the mitt is in place. All skin surfaces are separated to avoid irritation. The patient's wrist is padded with a dressing to avoid rubbing bony prominences. Two dressings are then placed over the patient's hand: one medial to lateral, one dorsal to ventral. Large 20 cm by 40 cm dressings are suggested. These are secured by a gauze bandage applied in figure-eight patterns. A stockinette is then fitted over the hand and secured by adhesive tape just beyond the wrist pad. A double fold of stockinette open at one end is sufficient.

The mitts need to be removed regularly. When they are removed, the patient washes the hands and exercises them, or the nurse may do this. Mitt restraints should not be so tight as to impede circulation, but they must be secure and pad the patient's hands well.

PREVENTING INJURIES FROM FIRE AND OTHER THERMAL ACCIDENTS

Thermal injuries involve the presence of harmful levels of heat or cold. The most common sources of thermal accidents are fire, hot appliances or an improperly functioning electrical circuit. Generally, hospital policy requires electrical appliances to be regularly checked and adequately maintained in order to prevent injury. As an added precaution, patients are often required to have radios, electric razors and other appliances checked by the hospital maintenance staff before they use them in hospital. Hot water bottles, heating pads and heat lamps are also possible sources of thermal injury. Heat that is applied to a patient is generally regulated and is well within the safety limits for that patient.

Fire is a constant threat in institutions. Even though modern construction materials have lessened the danger of the actual building catching fire, many materials within a hospital are highly combustible. Oxygen, for example, supports combustion, and substances such as ether are highly inflammable.

In order for a fire to start, three elements must be present: a combustible material, heat and oxygen. A **combustible material** is anything that will burn. Among the most common materials involved in hospital fires are paper; textiles, such as patient's bedding or oily rags; flammable liquids, such as ether or other liquid gases (for example, those used as anaesthetic agents); and electrical equipment. Heat sufficient to ignite the combustible material may come from such sources as a lighted match, a live cigarette, a spark or friction. There is usually enough oxygen

in the atmosphere to support combustion if the other two elements are present. Fire prevention is usually directed, therefore, towards controlling the combustible materials and heat; fire extinguishing measures are geared towards the reduction of heat (as by water cooling) and the exclusion of oxygen.

Fire Prevention

Most hospitals have active programs in fire prevention. Regular education of the patients, the personnel and the public in safe practices is an essential part of such programs. Some of the areas that are included in the fire control programs of hospitals are discussed in the following paragraphs.

Smoking regulations   Usually smoking is prohibited in most areas of the hospital. Designated smoking areas are well marked and located away from chemical and gas storage areas. Patients who do smoke require ashtrays that do not easily tip and that are constructed so that if a cigarette is left burning it will fall into the ashtray. Some patients (for instance, those who are confused or under the influence of a sedative or hypnotic drug) should not smoke unattended. Matches and cigarettes may be locked in a cupboard if the patient is confused.

Scrupulous housekeeping   Thorough housekeeping and adequate maintenance of equipment lessen the likelihood of accidents and fires. Oily rags, paints and solvents are stored carefully in a special area so as to prevent spontaneous combustion.

Hazardous products   All hazardous products must be labelled, stored, handled and used according to federal and provincial legislation. Workplace Hazardous Materials Information System (WHMIS) training is usually part of both the orientation program for new staff and the annual in-services for all staff.

Volatile gases and liquids (those that are easily turned into vapour) are distributed to the various areas of the agency under strict control and all necessary fire precautions are observed.

Fire prevention and extinguishing   An active fire prevention program requires that all employees receive regular education in fire prevention and fire extinguishing. All agency personnel should be provided with information about specific policy and practice. Demonstrations in the use of fire equipment, practice in moving patients and knowledge of the established practice to be followed upon the discovery of a fire are important. It is only through a continuous in-service educational program in fire prevention and extinguishing methods that everyone's safety is ensured.

Types of Fires and Fire Extinguishers

Fires have been categorized into four major classes, based on the type of material that is burning. Class A fires are those involving paper, cloth, wood and similar solid combustible materials; Class B involves flammable liquids and gases; Class C, electrical equipment; and Class D, metals.

Fire extinguishers are simply containers for an agent, such as water or chemicals, which put out a fire. Many kinds of extinguishers are available for home, institutional and industrial use. They come in dry chemical, carbon dioxide and halogenated types and some contain pressurized water. The right type of extinguisher must be used to fight a fire. Some are dangerous when used on the wrong type of fire, for example, a water extinguisher (for Class A fires) should not be used on a grease (Class B) or an electrical (Class C) fire. The fire extinguisher should be clearly labelled with picture symbols that identify the type(s) of fire it is intended to extinguish (see Figure 29.8).

Nurses need to know the types of fire extinguishers used in their agency and how to operate them. It is important to read the directions on the extinguisher to check for

FIGURE 29.9 Most fire extinguishers are operated by the following four steps. 1. Pull the pin. This may involve releasing a puncture lever, inversion, or other motion. 2. Aim the nozzle at the base of the fire. 3. Squeeze (or press) the handle. 4. Sweep from side to side at the base of the fire until the contents of the extinguisher are discharged. However, some extinguishers are operated slightly differently. Nurses should be familiar with the extinguishers available in the health agency where they work.

any variations. The four basic steps for using most types of extinguishers are illustrated in Figure 29.9.

Fire extinguishers must be accessible to personnel. Generally, they are kept in obvious places in all patient and service areas. The kind of extinguisher that is placed in a specific area depends upon the type of fire most likely to occur there. Part of a safety program is the regular inspection and maintenance of fire extinguishers.

In addition to having fire extinguishers, nursing units and other departments of a hospital are usually equipped with fire hoses, and personnel are trained in their use. In the event of a small fire, it may be easier and quicker to use material near at hand, for example, a blanket or a mattress, to smother the fire.

A	ORDINARY COMBUSTIBLES	TYPE A: ordinary combustibles. Wood, cloth, paper, rubber, many plastics, and other common materials that burn easily.
B	FLAMMABLE LIQUIDS	TYPE B: flammable liquids. Gasoline and other flammable liquids, oil, grease, tar, oil-based paint, lacquer and flammable gas.
C	ELECTRICAL EQUIPMENT	TYPE C: electrical equipment. Energized electrical equipment, including wiring, fuse boxes, circuit beakers, machinery and appliances.
D	COMBUSTIBLE METALS	TYPE D: combustible metals. Metal and metal dust— often used in industry.

FIGURE 29.8 Your extinguisher must fit the fire

SOURCE: National Fire Protection Association. (1988). *Fire extinguishers: Your small fire defense.* (Pamphlet No. BR-3). Quincy, MA: Author. Reproduced with permission.

The Nurse's Responsibilities in the Event of Fire

If a fire does occur in a nursing unit, the nurse should make sure that the following steps are carried out.

1. Remove patients from the immediate danger area.
2. Pull the fire alarm and report the location of the fire according to agency protocol.
3. Shut off the fire area and decrease the ventilation to the area.
4. Employ available extinguishing equipment.

In some health agencies it is accepted practice to telephone the fire department, directly reporting the exact location of the fire. Other agencies have a fire alarm system that when set off causes an alarm to ring in the fire station.

A third method of reporting a fire is to telephone the operator at the central hospital exchange, who then notifies the fire department.

The removal of patients   When a fire occurs, the nurse in charge of the nursing unit assumes responsibility for directing the activities of the hospital personnel until the fire fighters arrive. All fire doors and windows should be closed. Patients in immediate danger must be moved to safety quickly. Generally, ambulatory patients are assisted in walking to safety. In moving immobilized patients, the entire bed is wheeled to a safe area. When it is not feasible to move the entire bed, immobilized patients are moved by stretcher or wheelchair. Occasionally, it is necessary to carry patients in order to remove them from danger. Non-nursing personnel in the agency, for example housekeeping and maintenance staff, may be called upon to assist with evacuation of patients. Patients may be carried from fire areas using either the cradle technique, the pack strap carry, the piggy-back carry, or the two-person swing carry.

HOSPITAL SAFETY PROGRAMS

A safety program is an endeavour to control the physical environment and work procedures in such a manner that accidents can be prevented. In order to be effective, a program must involve all the people who work in the agency. Many hospitals have safety committees whose job it is to plan a safety program for the institution. Nurses are frequently members of these committees.

The safety committee's function is to conduct a continual analysis of the kind of accidents that occur in the hospital and their causes. On the basis of this analysis, an active program is developed. Continual assessment of hospital practices and continual education of employees are important functions of this committee. Another part of a safety program is the regular inspection of agency facilities. To be effective, a safety program must motivate all employees to accomplish the purpose of the program, for it is only through the active cooperation of all the people in an agency that accidents can be prevented.

EVALUATING SAFETY INTERVENTIONS

The risk for injury almost always results from another problem, such as the nature of the diagnostic or therapeutic plans of care for the patient. The patient's safety may be jeopardized, for example, when under sedation for pain relief. Evaluation of the effectiveness of nursing interventions is based on the degree to which accidents and injury are avoided. The patient's condition is subject to constant

---

Techniques for Carrying Patients

CRADLE

This technique is used for people who are not heavy and for children. The nurse lifts the patient by passing one arm beneath the patient's two knees and the other around the back (see Figure 29.10-A).

PACK STRAP CARRY

With the patient in a sitting position in bed, the nurse faces the patient and grasps the patient's wrists, the patient's right wrist in the nurse's left hand and the patient's left wrist in the nurse's right hand. The nurse then pivots, and slips under the patient's arm so that the patient's chest is against the nurse's shoulders and the patient's arms are crossed on the nurse's chest. With one leg forward for balance, the nurse then rolls the patient off the bed and onto the back (see Figure 29.10-B).

PIGGY-BACK CARRY

If the patient is conscious and able to give some help, the familiar *piggy-back* carry can be used (see Figure 29.10-C). The patient sits at the edge of the bed. The nurse stands in front of the patient, back facing the patient. The patient reaches over the nurse's shoulders and clasps hands in front of the nurse. The nurse then grasps the backs of the patient's legs, slightly above the knees. This carry supports the weight of the patient in an easier position for carrying than the pack strap carry.

SWING CARRY BY TWO NURSES

For a swing carry by two nurses, one nurse stands on each side of the patient. The patient's arms are extended around the nurses' shoulders and each nurse grasps one of the patient's wrists with the arm that is farthest from the patient. Each nurse then reaches behind the patient's back with the free arm (nearest the patient) and grasps the other nurse's shoulder. The patient's wrists are then released. Each nurse reaches under the patient's knees and grasps the other's wrist. The patient is then in a sitting position between the nurses. This carry is sometimes called a two-handed seat. A variation of this technique is the four-handed seat, which can be used for patients who are able to sit up without support (see Figure 29.11).

960   UNIT 6: *Protection and Safety Needs*

FIGURE 29.10   A. Position for cradle carry. B. Position for the pack strap carry. C. Position for the piggy-back carry.

A

B

FIGURE 29.11   A. Position for the swing carry. B. Position for the four-handed seat, with a close view of how the hands are held.

change. It is therefore necessary for the nurse both to regularly reassess patients' abilities to protect themselves from environmental hazards and to modify the nursing care plan in accordance with changes in status. The nurse must also be constantly alert to new dangers in the environment that could harm patients, nurses, visitors or other staff.

KEY TERMS

teratogenic p. 934

mutagenic p. 934

carcinogenic p. 934

Cumulative Trauma Disorders p. 939

Repetitive Strain Injuries p. 939

hazardous substances p. 939

thermal injuries p. 957

combustible material p. 957

IN REVIEW

An individual's safety needs include the personal capacity for self-protection and an environment conducive to healthy living. Determinants of a person's capacity for self-protection include age, health status, sensory and mental functioning, motor ability, emotional state, knowledge of environmental hazards and protective measures against these. Environmental hazards may be physical, chemical, biological or psychological.

Safety needs vary at different stages of the life cycle. Of particular concern are the following:

- Reproductive health — agents causing sterility, gene mutation and cancer
- Pregnancy — infectious diseases, jolts, smoking, use of drugs or alcohol, excessive caffeine intake
- Infancy and childhood — traffic accidents, falls, drownings in swimming pools and baths, fire, poisoning
- Adolescence — emotional tension
- Young and middle adulthood — traffic accidents, sports injuries, excessive use of alcohol, stress
- Older adulthood — falls, thermal injuries, environmental hazards.

Most accidental deaths and injuries in Canada result from motor vehicle accidents, falls, drownings, fires or poisonings. Common accidents that occur in the home are burns, falls, poisonings, choking and drownings. In the community, traffic accidents, sports injuries and recreational-related injuries are some of the most common types of accidents. In all types of workplaces musculoskeletal injuries occur. In addition, there are specific occupation-related injuries and diseases. In hospitals and other inpatient facilities, the most frequent hazards for patients, staff and visitors are injuries, infections and stress.

Assessing safety needs includes determining the person's capacity for self-protection and identifying hazards in the environment. People who are unable to judge hazards because of a perceptual or physiologic deficit, a lack of awareness or maturational age are at a high risk for injury. In planning and implementing safety interventions the nurse uses different approaches in the home, in the community and in the workplace. Patient safety is always the top priority in all aspects of care.

LEARNING ACTIVITIES

1. **Case Study**: Mrs. R. Ross is a 73-year-old woman in hospital with a fractured femur. The physician has ordered that she sit in a chair for 15 minutes twice a day. Mrs. Ross walks with considerable difficulty and requires support.

   a. What factors should the nurse be aware of in providing a safe environment for Mrs. Ross?

   b. List six specific measures that the nurse should take to prevent mechanical injury to Mrs. Ross.

   c. If there is a fire in this patient's room, what should the nurse do? How should this patient be moved?

   d. By what criteria can the safety of Mrs. Ross's environment be evaluated?

REFERENCES AND READINGS

BAILEY, R. D. (1985). *Coping with stress in caring.* Oxford: Blackwell Scientific Publications.

BAIRD, P.A. (1992). Reproductive hazards in the workplace, *Canadian Medical Association Journal, 147*, 157–160.

B.C. MINISTRY OF HEALTH (Office for Injury Prevention, Family Health Division). (1993, September). *Injury prevention strategies for children and youth in British Columbia.* Victoria: Queen's Printer.

B.C. MINISTRY OF MUNICIPAL AFFAIRS, RECREATION, AND HOUSING (Office of the Fire Commissioner). (1992). *The British Columbia fire code, 1992.* Victoria: Queen's Printer.

B.C. MINISTRY OF MUNICIPAL AFFAIRS, RECREATION, AND HOUSING. (1991). *Home safety: A guide to common hazards around the home* (Pamphlet). Victoria: Queen's Printer.

BIRD, F.E., Jr. (1984). *The management guide to loss control.* Atlanta: Institute Press.

CARPENITO, L.J. (1993). *Nursing diagnosis: Application to clinical practice.* Philadelphia: Lippincott.

CHENIER, N.M. (1982). *Reproductive hazards at work: Men, women and the fertility gamble.* Ottawa: The Canadian Advisory Council on the Status of Women.

COLOMBO, J.R. (1992). *The 1993 Canadian Global Almanac.* Toronto: Macmillan.

FLETCHER, K. (1990). Restraints should be the last resort. *RN, 53*(1), 52–56.

GOVERNMENT OF ONTARIO (1993). Nurturing health. *Report of the Premier's Council on Health, Well-being and Social Justice (1987–1991).* Toronto: Queen's Printer. (Catalogue 01–93–20M)

HEALTH AND WELFARE CANADA (Health Protection Branch). (1991, October). *Children's hospital injury research and prevention program (CHIRPP).* (Laboratory Centre for Disease Technical Report No. 2). Ottawa: Minister of Supply and Services.

INSURANCE CORPORATION OF BRITISH COLUMBIA. (1990). *Do it up right.* (Pamphlet No. TS244A(0394)). Vancouver: Author.

NATIONAL FIRE PROTECTION ASSOCIATION. (1988). *Fire extinguishers: Your small fire defense.* (Pamphlet No. BR–3). Quincy, MA: Author.

NATIONAL FIRE PROTECTION ASSOCIATION. (1992). *Portable fire extinguishers.* (Pamphlet No. BR–3D). Quincy, MA: Author.

PILLITERI, A. (1992). *Maternal and child health nursing: Care of the childbearing and childrearing family.* Philadelphia: Lippincott.

RADIKE, M. (1985). Reproductive toxicology. In P.L. Williams and J.L. Burson *Industrial toxicology: Safety and health applications in the workplace.* New York: Van Nostrand Reinhold.

REGISTERED NURSES ASSOCIATION OF ONTARIO (1976). ICN Policy Statement. *RNAO News, 32*:19.

RILEY, R. and PADDON, P. (1989). Accidents in Canada: Mortality and hospitalization. *Health Reports, 1,* 23–49. (Statistics Canada Catalogue No. 82 – 003)

ROYCHOWDHURY, M. (1990). Reproductive hazards in the work environment. *Professional Safety, 35*(5), 17–23.

STATISTICS CANADA. (1992). *Work Injuries 1989–1991.* Ottawa: Minister of Supply and Services. (Catalogue No.72–208)

TABER'S CYCLOPEDIC MEDICAL DICTIONARY (16th ed.). (1989). Philadelphia: F.A. Davis.

THOMAS, G. (1993). Working can be harmful for your health. *The Canadian Nurse, 89*(6), 35–38.

TRANSPORT CANADA. (1990). *Keep them safe.* (Pamphlet). Ottawa: Minister of Supply and Services, 1.

WORKERS' COMPENSATION BOARD OF BRITISH COLUMBIA. (1991). *What's WHMIS?* (Pamphlet.) Richmond, BC: Author.

WORKERS' COMPENSATION BOARD OF BRITISH COLUMBIA.(1993). *Annual Report, 1992 (part 2): Statistics.* Richmond, B.C.: Author, 8.

WORKERS' COMPENSATION BOARD OF BRITISH COLUMBIA. (1993). *Short term disability claims by occupation for participating hospitals, 1992, B.C., 1.* Richmond, B.C.: Statistical Services.

ZENZ, C. (1988). *Occupational medicine, principles and practical applications* (2nd ed.). St. Louis: Mosby.

CHAPTER 30

Skin Integrity and Hygiene Needs

CENTRAL QUESTIONS

1. Why is good personal hygiene important for health and well-being?

2. What anatomical structures comprise the skin, the teeth and the mouth?

3. What are the determinants of skin and oral integrity and hygiene needs?

4. How do skin integrity and hygiene needs vary throughout the life cycle?

5. What are some common problems people have in meeting their hygiene needs?

6. How does the nurse assess skin integrity and hygiene needs?

7. What are the common nursing diagnostic statements for patients with hygiene and skin integrity problems?

8. How does the nurse apply relevant principles in planning and implementing nursing interventions
   a. to promote good hygiene practices in patients with respect to bathing and the care of the mouth, nails and hair?
   b. to maintain the skin, hair, nails, teeth and soft tissues in the oral cavity in good condition?
   c. to maintain and restore the integrity of the patient's skin?

9. How does the nurse evaluate the effectiveness of nursing interventions?

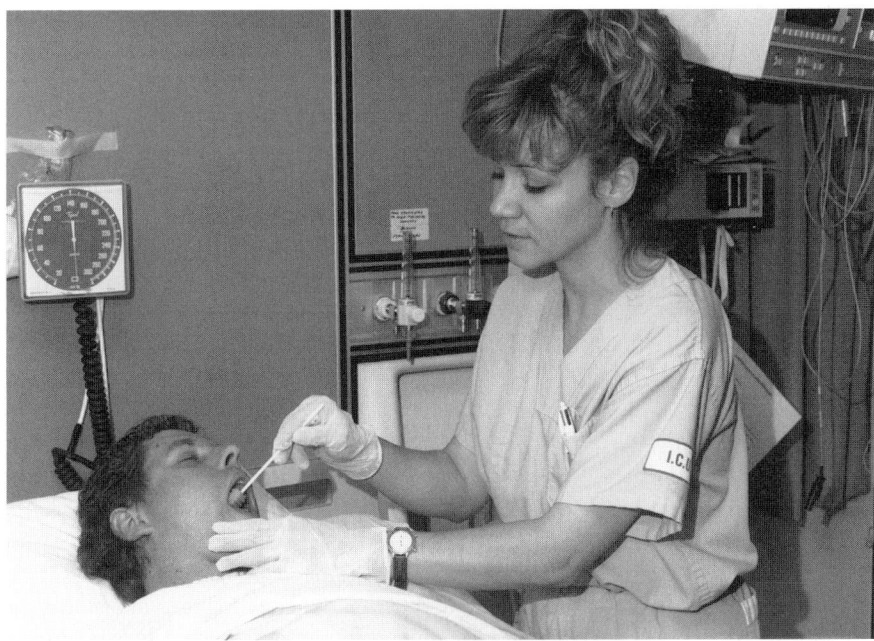

INTRODUCTION

The New Lexicon Webster's Dictionary defines hygiene as "the science of health, its preservation, and the prevention of disease; the practice of measures designed to attain and preserve health." On a personal level, hygiene usually means those measures a person takes to keep the skin, its appendages (hair, fingernails and toenails), and the teeth and mouth clean and in good condition. Hygiene practices have personal meaning that varies according to cultural and social factors and individual values. Hygiene habits are influenced by family practices and values with respect to cleanliness and by knowledge of hygiene needs in health. Nurses must assess each individual's personal bathing and hygiene practices and incorporate these into the plan of care.

Healthy unbroken skin is the body's first line of defence against infection and injury to underlying tissues. The skin is important for the regulation of body temperature and it serves as one means for the excretion of body wastes. Healthy teeth and gums are essential for maintaining nutritional status. Decayed teeth and poor condition of the oral cavity are potential sources of infection and discomfort. Thus, proper hygiene is necessary for healthy bodily functions. The nurse can take a golden opportunity for health promotion by teaching patients about healthy hygiene practices while assisting with daily hygiene needs.

Attending to personal hygiene and grooming needs is an important independent function both for children (once they have learned to do this themselves) and adults. When ill, people often depend on others for help with their hygiene. The loss of the ability to perform these very personal functions independently often impacts self-esteem and contributes to feelings of powerlessness. In addition, having someone else provide very personal aspects of care may be considered demeaning and embarrassing. Both the nurse and the patient feel more comfortable if the nurse can anticipate the patient's needs and provide help in a competent, matter-of-fact manner, and, at the same time, acknowledge the patient's feelings and allow the patient every opportunity for participation in care.

The person who is ill has a lowered resistance to infection. Consequently, the presence of pathogenic bacteria in the environment poses a constant threat. Helping the patient to keep clean by removing dirt, excretory products and secretions eliminates many substances in which these bacteria flourish. In addition to controlling infection, hygienic measures help patients feel more comfortable and relaxed. Most people feel better when they are fresh and clean, and many who have been unable to rest will sleep soundly after a relaxing bath. Unpleasant odours may be distressing and attention to hygiene helps eliminate them. Excessive perspiration and the presence of bacteria in the mouth and on the skin are common causes of such odours. Oral hygiene usually eliminates bad breath (halitosis) which is most frequently caused by bacteria and old food particles in the mouth.

ANATOMY OF THE SKIN, MOUTH AND TEETH

THE SKIN

Skin The skin is composed of two main layers: the outer, thinner layer or *epidermis,* and the inner, thicker layer or *dermis.* Underlying these layers is subcutaneous tissue and adipose tissue. The epidermis itself has four layers on most areas of the body except the palms of the hands and the soles of the feet, where there are five. The outermost, horny layer of epidermis continually flakes off.

Nails The nails of the fingers and toes are composed of epidermal cells that have been converted to *keratin.* Epithelial cells lie under the crescent of each nail, and it is from these cells that the epidermal cells of the nails grow.

Hair Hair is composed of a long, cylindrical shaft and a root that is embedded in a depression, called a hair follicle, which penetrates the epidermis to the subcutaneous tissues. The hair receives its nourishment from the blood supply through the root. **Dandruff** is the term used for the dry, scaly material that is shed from the skin of the scalp.

Skin glands There are three kinds of skin glands in the body. The **sebaceous glands** secrete oil and are present wherever there is hair. The oil (sebum) keeps the hair supple and pliable. The **sweat glands** produce sweat, a mechanism the body uses to cool the skin and reduce body temperature. Waste products are also excreted in sweat. Sweat glands are most numerous in the axilla, on the palms of the hands and the soles of the feet and on the forehead. The action of bacteria on sweat from these glands produces a distinctive odour. The **ceruminous glands,** located in the external ear canal, secrete cerumen (wax). Some people accumulate a large amount of cerumen in their ears which can impair hearing.

THE MOUTH AND TEETH

The *mouth* is the anterior opening of the alimentary canal. It is coated with a mucous membrane, the epithelial tissue layer that lines body cavities and passageways. The mouth contains three important anatomical structures: the tongue, the teeth and the gums. The tongue, a movable muscular organ, is an important sensory receptor. It assists in the acts of chewing (*mastication*), swallowing and sound articulation. Healthy teeth are essential for the chewing of food. Each tooth has a crown and a root or roots. The tooth is solid except for the inner soft pulp cavity. The crown is covered with a hard inorganic substance called *enamel,* which protects the soft structures beneath it. The root is protected by *cementum,* which is true bone. The teeth protrude up through the gums *(gingivae),* which are made up of mucous membrane with supporting fibrous tissue. The hard portion of the gum is firm, dense, pink, stippled and tightly attached to the teeth, the periosteum and the bone of the jaws. A soft portion of the gums protrudes upward in the spaces between the teeth.

DETERMINANTS OF SKIN AND ORAL INTEGRITY AND HYGIENE NEEDS

Nutrition and hydration The skin is nourished by nutrients delivered by the blood. If food and fluid intake is disrupted, the skin will likely show ill effects. If fluid intake is insufficient, a person becomes dehydrated, and the skin appears dry and loose, a condition called *poor tissue turgor.* (Turgor refers to the elasticity of the skin.) Skin heals very slowly when an individual has suffered prolonged nutrient deficiency.

Exercise Exercise improves circulation, helping to bring a nourishing supply of blood to the surface tissues. It also aids in the elimination of waste products, both through the skin and other excretory routes.

Environment Weather affects the skin. In cold temperatures, the skin often becomes dry and chapped. Not only is the cold outside a factor, but the indoor environment, which is very dry in many homes with central heating, can also cause problems. Very warm weather can also be hard on the skin. We perspire more in the heat creating potentially harmful waste buildup on the skin. Frequent bathing will rid the skin surface of bodily wastes excreted via this route. Sunshine was once considered an important factor in healthy skin, but the thinning of the ozone layer now necessitates caution. Exposure to the sun's ultraviolet light has been linked to skin damage, premature aging and skin cancer.

Personal habits The health of the skin, hair and nails is affected by hygiene habits. Bathing and grooming rituals vary depending on factors such as culture, access to sanitation facilities, knowledge and personal preference. For example, in some cultures menstruating women believe they should not bathe or wash their hair. In rural Cambodia, salt or lemon is often used for dental care (Richardson, 1990).

Socioeconomic Maintaining hygiene is more difficult when facilities are not readily available. People who live in poor, crowded or unsanitary conditions often do not have the opportunity to practise good personal hygiene.

The person who has to cut a hole in the ice to obtain water in the wintertime or share a bathroom with several other people may not bathe frequently. Teeth may be neglected because an individual cannot afford visits to the dentist.

Health status General health status is very important, both in relation to the ability to maintain hygiene and with respect to the effect of health problems on the skin. Poor health, for whatever reason, is usually reflected by the condition of the skin. The ill person is more susceptible to infection, malnourishment, gastrointestinal problems and other disturbances of body functioning that can affect the condition of the skin. Many types of disorders also specifically affect the skin.

Physical and mental status affects the ability to carry out personal hygiene. Motor abilities, mental capacity and the severity and nature of an illness may impact greatly on the level of independence. If a patient is unable to bathe, the nurse's role is to assist as necessary.

Excessive moisture causes the skin to be more susceptible to damage. Fever causes increased perspiration and excretion of wastes through the skin. Irritating drainage seeping onto the skin from wounds can cause problems. Incontinence of urine or feces is a major factor in skin breakdown. Prolonged pressure on any area decreases blood supply and can lead to injury. Friction from rubbing on the bed linen causes additional trauma. Wrinkled sheets or crumbs in the bed increase the irregularity of the sheet surface and hence increase the friction. A smooth, firm foundation on the bed helps to lessen this friction and aids in preventing tissue breakdown.

Drugs and therapy Drugs and other forms of therapy may cause reactions in the skin. Many drugs may cause an allergic skin reaction. Radiation therapy, used to treat cancer, must penetrate the skin to reach and destroy malignant cells. The skin and its underlying tissues may also suffer some damage. Mucous membranes, which contain rapidly dividing cells, are frequently affected, leading to sores in the mouth.

HYGIENE NEEDS THROUGHOUT THE LIFE CYCLE

PREGNANCY

One of the first changes that a pregnant woman notices is increased pigmentation (colouring) of the nipples and areola of her breasts. *Striae* (stretch marks) and accentuated venous patterns appear over the breasts as they enlarge and prepare to nourish the infant. The tendinous middle line of the abdomen also shows increased pigmentation (*linea nigra*) and stretch marks usually appear on the abdomen. Darkened brown areas may also appear on the face; these are known as chloasma or the "mask of pregnancy." The changes in skin pigmentation are due to the melanocyte-stimulating hormone secreted by the pituitary gland. As the pregnancy progresses, there is often an increase of vascular spider-like spots, particularly on the legs, and *palmar erythema* (reddened areas on the palms of the hands) is common. These changes are thought to be due to the increased estrogen levels that accompany pregnancy. Sweat gland activity increases during pregnancy, causing increased perspiration. Thus, a daily bath or shower is usually recommended for pregnant women. The gums often become soft and edematous because of increased vascularity. They are sensitive and tend to bleed easily, even with the mild trauma of brushing or flossing.

INFANCY

The newborn's skin is usually red, wrinkled and covered with *vernix*, a white waxy coating that has protected the skin in utero. Some newborns are also covered with a downy hair called *lanugo*; premature babies almost always have this additional protective coating. Newborns have many skin variations such as *milia* (white pinpoint papules found on the nose) or *erythema toxicum* (newborn rash) which appear at birth or in the first few days after birth. These require no special care and disappear as the infant's structures mature. Infants need to be handled carefully as their skin is less resistant to injury and infection than an adult's. Mild soaps which are non-irritating to the skin may be used in the infant's bath. Soap should not be used on an infant's face. Daily bathing is not recommended since frequent washing removes natural oils and may dry the skin, increasing the risk of infection.

The infant's skin is very sensitive to heat and cold. A warm room for bathing and body temperature bath water provide comfort. After bathing, immediately wrapping the infant in a towel reduces heat loss. The hair and the head of an infant should be washed and dried separately, before the rest of the body because most heat is lost through the head. The nails of infants must be kept short to prevent scratching.

Diaper rash is a common skin problem with infants. "Diapering places a unique set of stressors on the skin. Factors affecting the diaper area include the type of diaper, skin vulnerability, consistency of the stool and diapering practices such as frequency of changing diapers and application of topical preparations and medications" (Wong et al, 1992, 41). Cleansing the skin before applying a clean diaper is important for removing urine and feces which are irritating to the skin. Often, getting the infant to take more water will help the problem, because it dilutes the urine and makes it less irritating.

Cradle cap is an oily yellowish crust that develops on the scalp of some infants, particularly in those who are breastfed. It is caused by an excessive amount of secretion from the sebaceous glands of the scalp. Applications of a mild oil (such as mineral oil) or a bland ointment, and frequent shampoos will usually remove the crust within a few

Children can find creative ways to meet their hygiene needs.

days. *Thrush* is a mild fungal infection of the mouth. Having the baby drink approximately a half ounce of sterile water after a milk feeding helps to prevent this problem.

CHILDHOOD

Usually, school age children have learned basic hygienic practices at home. Teachers and the school nurse may need to reinforce the early home teaching.

Due to vigorous play and still-developing motor skills, children suffer cuts, bruises and scrapes during the preschool and primary school period. The school nurse — and parents — should keep a good supply of mild disinfectant and simple bandage materials on hand to protect childhood wounds from infection. Another common childhood skin problem is allergic eczema, which can be very distressing for both the child and parents. Medical guidance is important in caring for the child with this problem. Children who have a problem with enuresis should have a morning shower or bath, so that they are not sent off to school or to play with the odour of urine on the body, an unpleasant reminder of the problem.

ADOLESCENCE

The adolescent's skin may be problematic. Acne is a common problem in many teenagers. Hormonal changes occurring at this stage of the life cycle, blockage of the excretions of the sebaceous glands onto the skin surface and bacterial infection are thought to be factors that contribute to teenage acne. Cleanliness, diet and exercise are important factors that help prevent secondary infections. Severe acne requires medical attention.

Adolescents usually demonstrate increased concern over personal appearance and hygiene. This is the time when sweating from the axilla commences, and the teenager is usually very self-conscious about the odour of perspiration.

ADULTHOOD

As a person advances in age, two kinds of skin change take place. First, wrinkling, sagging, and increased pigmentation occur due to exposure to sunlight. Secondly, there is a general thinning of the skin accompanied by increased dryness and inelasticity. This aging takes place in the epidermis, dermis and in the subcutaneous fat. The epidermis is generally thinned and flattened, and sometimes there is an increased growth of the outer layer of the epidermis. A decrease in oil secretions leads to increased dryness and scaliness, and as a result, older people tolerate soap less well than younger adults. If older adults bathe too frequently, the skin will become very dry. Oily liquids and skin creams are often better for the older patient than too much soap and water or alcohol rubs.

The aging process also takes its toll on the hair, the nails, the teeth and other structures in the mouth. Hair often becomes thin and loses its texture. Fingernails and toenails become tougher and more difficult to cut. The mucous membranes lining the mouth become thinner and more fragile with age. After age 20, the teeth are less susceptible to cavities and more susceptible to gum diseases. Half of all Canadians are completely toothless by age 60 (Canadian Dental Association, undated).

COMMON PROBLEMS

Problems resulting from an inability to maintain hygiene are numerous. The skin, the hair and the teeth may become dirty, and offensive odours from the body may cause discomfort, both physical and mental. Ingrown nails frequently result from uncut toenails, and may interfere with the ability to walk. If skin care is neglected or carried out inadequately, pressure areas may develop and the skin may break down, causing considerable discomfort and pain and rendering the patient more vulnerable to infection.

ORAL PROBLEMS

If the patient has been unable to look after oral hygiene and has not been assisted with it, the teeth and the mucous membranes lining the mouth soon show evidence of this. **Gingivitis,** or inflammation of the gums, is one problem. When oral hygiene is inadequate, a film of mucus and

bacteria (*plaque*) and *calculus* (tartar) accumulate on the surface of the teeth and particles of food gather around the teeth and in the crevices of the gums. These substances are removed by brushing the teeth, flossing and regular professional cleaning. Without proper cleaning, the substances accumulate and become a source of mechanical irritation. The tissues of the gums become swollen and inflamed and may separate from the teeth.

Gingivitis not only is uncomfortable for the patient, it also leads to poor nutrition and is a potential source of infection, in the parotid glands or the gastrointestinal or respiratory tracts. When oral hygiene is neglected, the teeth and the tongue also suffer. Decay of the teeth (**dental caries)** may result, which requires the assistance of dental health professionals to correct. Lack of oral hygiene also causes the tongue to become coated with a thick, furry substance that is often referred to as **sordes**. This adds to the patient's discomfort and diminishes the ability of the taste buds to receive stimuli, which in turn contributes to nutritional problems such as anorexia and malnourishment.

HAIR PROBLEMS

One common problem affecting the hair and scalp is excessive dandruff. Normally, dandruff is removed by combing, brushing and washing the hair. These procedures also help to remove the accumulation of excess sebum, the oily secretion of the sebaceous glands that keeps the hair supple and pliable. People whose hair is oily owing to the excessive secretions of sebum need to shampoo frequently to remove the oil. People with an irritation of the scalp should be referred to a physician.

The nurse may encounter patients whose hair and body are infested with lice or other vermin. Head lice is a frequent problem in schools, where the infestation is quickly spread from one child to another.

PRESSURE ULCERS

Pressure ulcers, also known as decubitus ulcers, bedsores or pressure sores, are areas from which the skin has sloughed. *Decubitus*, which is a Latin word meaning "lying down," is the traditional term for this type of ulcer, because it occurred originally in people who were bedridden. However, pressure ulcers do not only occur in people who are lying down. While decubitus ulcers often develop in people who are ill in bed for a long period of time, especially immobile people, they also occur in people who sit in wheelchairs for several hours at a time. Since the primary cause of these ulcers is prolonged pressure on a body part, the term *pressure ulcer* is considered more appropriate, because it "describes both the cause and the condition" (Colburn, 1990, 63).

Pressure ulcers are the result of prolonged pressure on one part of the body with resultant loss of circulation to the area and subsequent tissue destruction. Although pressure ulcers may occur in any patient if there is sufficient pressure on one area to cause *ischemia* (a decreased supply of oxygenated blood to a body part or organ, often accompanied by pain and dysfunction), they are seen most frequently in individuals with poor nutritional status, especially if there is a negative nitrogen balance. Pressure ulcers are most often seen on the bony prominences of the body such as sacrum, coccyx, hips, heels, ankles and elbows. Secondary infection may complicate the problem.

The conditions that predispose to pressure ulcers include continuous pressure on one area, dampness, a break in the skin surface, poor nutrition, dehydration, poor blood circulation and thinness (bony prominences unprotected by adipose tissue). Pressure ulcers develop in stages as illustrated in Figure 30.1. Early signs of a pressure ulcer include redness and tenderness of an area. Erythema (redness) lasting more than 30 seconds after pressure is removed is considered a Stage One ulcer (Colburn, 1990). Unless special measures are taken at this time to relieve pressure and increase local tissue nourishment, a break in the patient's skin usually follows. The sore then increases in depth and the skin tissue gradually sloughs off. Pressure ulcers are difficult to cure; some require surgical intervention. Consequently, preventive measures are crucial.

STAGE OF PRESSURE ULCER	WHAT YOU SEE

A. Stage One:

Nonblanchable erythema of intact skin; the heralding lesion of skin ulceration.

B. Stage Two:

Partial-thickness skin loss involving epidermis and/or dermis. The ulcer is superficial and presents clinically as an abrasion, blister or shallow crater.

C. Stage Three:

Full-thickness skin loss involving damage or necrosis of subcutaneous tissue that may extend down to, but not through, underlying fascia. The ulcer presents clinically as a deep crater with or without undermining of adjacent tissue.

D. Stage Four:

Full-thickness skin loss with extensive destruction, tissue necrosis, or damage to muscle, bone or supporting structures (e.g., tendon, joint capsule).

FIGURE 30.1   Stages of pressure ulcers

SOURCE: ConvaTec, (1992). *DuoDERM® "S.O.S" wound care: Clinical applications guide.* Pamphlet 581-1136. Princeton, NJ: E.R. Squibb & Sons.

HEALTH HISTORY GUIDE

Hygiene

Health and Illness Patterns

USUAL HYGIENE PATTERN AND PRACTICES

- Describe your usual hygiene routine and your usual practices for maintaining hygiene.
- How and when do you bathe? How often?
- How do you care for your teeth? What products do you routinely use?
- Do you take any special measures to care for your hair?
- How and when do you clean your ears?
- Do you wash your hands at specific times?
- Do you use any special products for hygiene such as soaps, lotions, creams, deodorants, perfumes?

For women:

- What type of sanitary protection do you use during menstruation?
- Do you have any special hygienic practices during menses?

RECENT CHANGES IN HYGIENE PATTERN AND PRACTICES

- Have you had a recent illness or health problem that has affected your hygiene practices?
- Is there anything else that is affecting your ability to keep yourself clean?
- What assistance will you need to meet your hygiene needs?

PRESENTING HEALTH PROBLEM

- Do you have any problems with your skin? Any dry-

ness, oiliness, rashes, open areas, changes in pigmentation or moles?
- Where on your body did the skin problem begin?
- When did you first notice the problem?
- How does your skin feel?
- Have you noticed skin changes in other areas?
- Does anything make the problem worse? better?
- Have you used any home remedies or over-the-counter preparations to try to resolve your problem? What were the results?
- Have you recently had any other illnesses?
- Have you noticed any unusual or patchy hair loss?
- Have you noticed any changes in your nails?
- Have you had any allergic reactions?
- Has anyone in your family had a skin problem?
- What medications or treatments have you been taking recently?
- Do you have any problems with your mouth or teeth?
- Do you experience any unpleasant odours?

Health Promotion and Protection Patterns

- How do you try to keep your skin healthy? What things would you like to do for your skin but feel unable to?
- Do you visit the dentist? How often?

ASSESSING HYGIENE NEEDS

The nurse begins an assessment of hygiene by exploring the patient's usual cleansing and grooming practices. The importance and meaning of these rituals should be identified. At the same time, the nurse can assess the patient's knowledge of hygiene. This information is obtained from the nursing history. Following the history, the nurse conducts a physical exam which uses observation and palpation techniques to add information to the data base.

The nurse also takes into consideration factors that affect the patient's ability to carry out hygienic practices. For example, do motor abilities allow the patient to provide

for hygiene? Does the physical environment provide the basic necessities for hygiene, such as fresh water? Other health problems may also affect the condition of the skin and need to be considered.

NURSING HEALTH HISTORY

The nurse may begin the hygiene health history by asking a broad, open-ended question such as "What are your usual routines and practices for maintaining hygiene?" More specific questions can be used to elicit more detail, if necessary. For women, the nurse may explore hygienic practices during menstruation. "Feminine hygiene" is a topic infrequently discussed and many misconceptions exist. Especially with adolescent girls, the nurse may use this opportunity for teaching hygiene practices during menses.

In taking a hygiene health history, the nurse ascertains if the patient has had any changes in usual hygiene practices and determines any assistance that may be required to meet hygiene needs. When the patient's presenting health problem relates to the skin or oral cavity, the nurse will then ask specific questions to gather information about it. Finally, as with all needs, the nurse examines the patient's health-promoting behaviours to determine learning needs and opportunities for health teaching. Above is a health history guide to facilitate the gathering of subjective data about hygiene needs.

PHYSICAL ASSESSMENT

The physical assessment for hygiene can be divided into two parts. In the first part, the nurse examines the hair, eyes, ears, mouth, teeth and skin that can be seen without the patient undressing. The second part involves examining areas under clothing. Depending upon the circumstances, this part of the exam may be postponed to a later time such as during the patient's bath. In any case, a thorough assessment includes an examination of all skin surfaces.

VISIBLE SKIN EXAMINATION

During the first encounter with the patient and during the history-taking, the nurse gains an overall impression of the patient's state of hygiene. Factors which might affect this impression include general cleanliness, tidiness and any unusual odour. The visible skin is assessed for colour, lesions, moisture (flaking or oiliness) and dirt.

The hair is examined for texture, dryness or oiliness, dandruff or lice. The scalp is carefully checked for any lesions. Is the hair short or long, combed, tied, or tangled and matted? The eyes are assessed for redness, swelling, tearing or discharge. The ears are checked for any discharge or wax buildup in the auditory canals. It is important to note any obvious hearing impairment as it may be related to accumulated cerumen (Ney, 1993). It is helpful to examine hearing aids, if the patient wears them, as they may be plugged with wax. The nurse checks the skin of the external ear and behind the ear.

Touching the skin provides information about temperature, texture and moisture. The skin of the hand or arm is gently "pinched" to assess turgor. The hands are examined for lesions and the nails are checked for shape, texture and cleanliness.

EXAMINATION OF ALL SKIN SURFACES

When the patient disrobes, the skin is examined for the same things — colour, temperature, moisture and lesions.

It is important for the patient's comfort that only one part of the body is exposed and examined at a time. Special attention is needed for any skin folds such as those under breasts or in the groin region and the buttock crease. The accumulation of moisture and lack of air circulation makes these areas especially susceptible to skin breakdown. The perineal area is examined for any unusual odour and/or discharge. Any evidence of incontinence is noted because hygiene is of added importance when bladder or bowel control is lost. The feet are examined for odour and lesions. The toenails are checked, with special attention to any signs of redness or inflammation due to ingrown nails. The feet may have red or blistered areas due to poor-fitting footwear.

DIAGNOSING HYGIENE PROBLEMS

When patients have difficulty performing any aspect of hygiene care by themselves, the diagnosis *Bathing/hygiene self-care deficit* is used. This may include problems in washing, combing the hair, shaving, brushing the teeth, manicuring the nails and applying lotions, creams, deodorants or makeup. The defining characteristics of this diagnosis include situations in which the person is unwilling or unable to wash or to obtain water or regulate the water flow. A hygiene self-care deficit is also indicated by the inability to perceive the need to keep clean (Carpenito, 1993). A multitude of factors, such as severe pain, extreme weakness or paralysis, immobility due to trauma or surgery and activity intolerance secondary to heart and respiratory problems, can contribute to a bathing/hygiene self-care deficit.

Impaired skin integrity identifies a state in which the patient experiences or is at risk for experiencing damage to the epidermal or dermal tissue (Carpenito, 1993). Patients who are immobilized necessarily have a high risk for skin breakdown due to the effects of pressure on body parts and the forces of shearing and friction if the skin sticks to or rubs against bed linen. Moisture, poor nutrition and dehydration also contribute to the problem. Redness and tenderness of an area, particularly over a bony prominence, is the first sign of impaired tissue integrity. A break in the epidermal or dermal tissue is the major defining characteristic of this nursing diagnosis. For example, the nurse in an extended care facility identifies a resident at risk for skin breakdown. The diagnosis might be stated as *High risk for impaired skin integrity related to incontinence and partial immobility*. This nurse has identified a problem for which health protecting strategies (preventive measures) need to be implemented.

Like the skin, the oral mucous membrane is prone to breakdown if oral hygiene is inadequate or not performed at all. In patients whose oral hygiene is inadequate, the diagnosis *High risk for altered oral mucous membrane* is used (Carpenito, 1993). Disruptions in the mucous membrane, such as lesions, coated tongue, gingivitis or dry mouth, indicate actual problems.

For patients who engage in poor hygiene practices because of an unhealthy lifestyle or lack of knowledge of how to handle a condition, the diagnosis *Altered health maintenance* may be used. Because people are responsible for their own health, this diagnosis indicates a problem that the patient must be motivated to treat, but for which the nurse has a responsibility to raise the patient's awareness that better health is possible (Carpenito, 1993). For example, for a patient with dental caries due to poor oral hygiene practices and a lack of dental care, the nurse can provide information about oral hygiene and dental services and encourage the patient to consider changing dental health practices.

The diagnostic label *Knowledge deficit* may also be used in cases where individuals have a need to learn hygiene self-care. For example, the school nurse may discover an adolescent girl who has just started menstruating and has questions about sanitary products and hygiene practices. A suitable nursing diagnosis might be *Knowledge deficit of menstrual practices related to change in physical functioning and lack of family discussion of sexuality issues*. This diagnosis illustrates an opportunity for the nurse to practise health promotion.

A bathing or hygiene self-care deficit may become the etiology of other problems for a patient. For example, patients unable to maintain their preferred pattern of hygiene may experience negative feelings about their body and express embarrassment about how they look. In such cases, the diagnosis *Body image disturbance* may be used. Patients may also experience feelings of powerlessness or lack of personal control if they are dependent on others to perform hygiene measures for them. Further, when a break in the integrity of the skin or mucous membranes occurs, the risk of infection increases because the first line of defense against harmful agents is interrupted. These diagnoses may be stated as *Powerlessness* and *High risk for infection*, respectively.

PLANNING HYGIENE INTERVENTIONS

Planning follows naturally from the identification of a problem or nursing diagnosis and involves establishing patient goals or expected outcomes. Hygiene is very personal and goals need to be set individually, taking into account special circumstances and preferences. Goals need to be clearly written, measurable and achievable.

The resident of an extended care facility who is at risk for skin breakdown would have a long-term goal, such as "The resident will show intact skin as evidenced by a lack of redness or open areas." For the adolescent newly experi-

KEY PRINCIPLES

Principles Relevant to Hygiene

1. Intact skin and mucous membranes are the body's first line of defence against infection and injury.

2. Individual differences exist in the nature of the skin, hair and nails.

3. Changes occur throughout the lifespan in the skin, the mucous membranes, the hair, the nails and the teeth.

4. The health of the skin and mucous membranes is highly dependent on adequate nourishment, fluid intake and exercise.

5. General health affects both the status of the skin, the teeth and the mouth, and the ability to maintain proper hygiene.

6. Hygiene practices are learned.

7. Hygiene practices vary with cultural norms, personal idiosyncrasies and values and the ability to maintain good habits of cleanliness and grooming.

8. The ability to maintain proper hygiene is an important independent function in older children and adults.

9. The skin, hair and nails may be affected by drugs and other forms of therapeutic intervention.

encing menstruation, one goal might be "The young woman will list four methods for managing menstrual flow." If she has identified that she would like to try using tampons, goals might include "The young woman will list three necessary precautions when using tampons which decrease risk of toxic shock syndrome." This goal deals with the prevention of illness as opposed to health promotion.

Assisting patients who need help in carrying out hygiene measures is among the nurse's most important priorities. Serious problems can develop if basic skin care and oral hygiene are not attended to on a regular, planned schedule. As with problems in mobility, *prevention* is the key. Deterioration of a patient's skin or mouth can develop very rapidly, sometimes with little forewarning. Repair of the damage is a slow process that entails much discomfort and suffering on the patient's part and much work on the nurse's part — work that can be avoided if simple precautionary measures are taken.

IMPLEMENTING HYGIENE INTERVENTIONS

HEALTH PROMOTING STRATEGIES

Hygiene is a basic requirement for health and well-being. Cleanliness promotes comfort, maintains skin and mucous membrane integrity and reduces the risk of infection from contaminants on the skin. While most people value cleanliness, not everyone engages in healthy hygiene practices; some do not because they lack knowledge of healthy hygiene measures; others do not because they lack the necessary means. For instance, people living in impoverished or crowded conditions may not be able to perform adequate hygiene care. Strategies for promoting healthy hygiene care involve education and referrals to appropriate resources or to other health care professionals. For example, community health and home care nurses may give advice to parents of young children regarding dental health and the need for regular dental visits in this age group. School nurses often teach hygiene care such as washing hands before eating and after using the toilet, brushing the teeth and using dental floss, as well as bathing and shampooing regularly. Hygiene practices for healthy living are given in the box below.

For patients who need help to acquire good hygiene habits, a teaching plan is incorporated into the nursing care plan. Much of the teaching may be done while carrying out specific nursing interventions such as the bed bath. Because hygiene is a very personal matter, tact is needed in this teaching, and care should be taken to protect the patient's self-esteem in the process. Putting the teaching in terms of promoting optimal health and including an explanation of the reasons for the development and maintenance of good hygiene practices help to put the teaching on a more objective and less personal basis.

HEALTH PROTECTING STRATEGIES

A very common function of nurses in acute care hospitals, long-term care facilities and in the home is assisting patients who are unable to maintain their own hygiene independently. These individuals may be experiencing an acute illness following traumatic injury or surgery that necessitates temporary assistance. Others may have a chronic or permanent condition such as paralysis following a stroke. This section focusses on procedures nurses employ when helping others with hygiene.

Most inpatient health care agencies have established routines for providing hygiene care. These include morning care, a daily bath and evening care. The routines are in place to ensure that every patient's need for hygiene is met on a consistent basis. Because these routines take into account staffing patterns, daily baths are usually scheduled in the morning, since there are generally more staff members on the day-shift.

GENERAL MORNING CARE

Before breakfast is served, patients are usually awakened. They are offered a bedpan or urinal, or assisted to the bathroom if they can get up. Patients who must remain in bed are provided with the necessary materials for washing hands and face and for mouth care, and are assisted with these activities if they require help. Patients are then prepared for the meal — the bed is straightened, they are assisted to the most comfortable position for eating and a place is prepared for the tray.

GENERAL EVENING CARE

The evening care routine is somewhat similar in that the patient is offered a bedpan or urinal (or assisted to the bathroom), and is given the opportunity to wash the hands and face and clean the teeth. In many agencies, the bed patient's back is washed and a back massage is given as part of the evening routine. The bottom sheet and drawsheet (if one is used) are tightened, and top bedclothes straightened and tucked in. If the patient needs an extra blanket, this is provided. The patient is assisted to a comfortable position and side rails, if needed, are put up on *both* sides of the bed. The call signal is put within easy reach, and any other items the patient wants near at hand, such as a clock or a jug of water and a glass, are placed within easy reach on the bedside table.

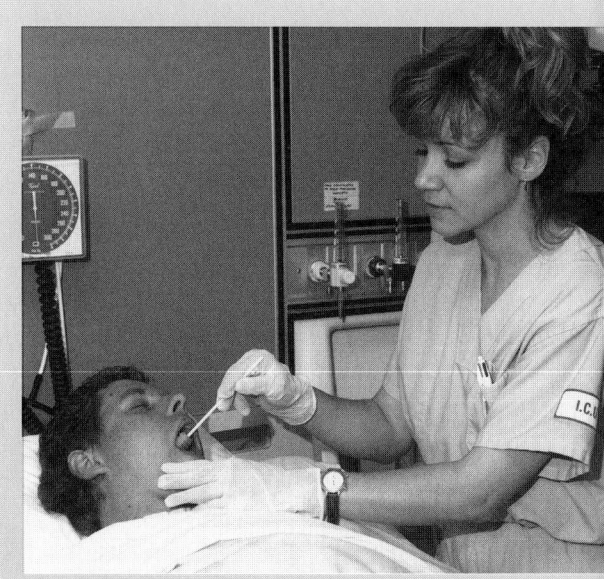

Good oral hygiene is essential for the patient's comfort.

HEALTH PROMOTING STRATEGY

Promoting Healthy Hygiene Practices

HAND WASHING

- Always wash your hands before starting the day, when visibly dirty, after using the toilet, after blowing your nose, after handling garbage, before eating or drinking, after finishing work and before going to bed at night.
- Use running water to wash your hands. Bacteria can multiply rapidly in standing water even when a germicidal agent is used.
- Use plain or antimicrobial soap depending on the purpose.
- Always dry your hands thoroughly. Individual or paper towels are best. Wet dirty towels can spread germs.

ORAL HYGIENE AND DENTAL CARE

- Brush your teeth regularly at least twice a day.
- Use a gentle, circular massaging action to work bristles into the sulcus (the shallow crevice where the tooth and gum meet).
- Brush all other tooth areas — fronts, backs and chewing surfaces.
- Use a soft brush with rounded bristles. A worn brush won't get your teeth clean; if it is worn, replace it.
- Floss your teeth at least once a day. Tartar builds up in 36 hours if plaque (invisible bacterial film) is not removed.
- Work the floss gently between the teeth and then below the gum line. Wrap the floss in "C" shape around each tooth and wipe away from the gum several times.
- If the floss catches and shreds, try waxed floss.

- Visit your dentist and have your teeth professionally cleaned regularly.

BATHING

- Bathe regularly. If you perspire a lot or have oily skin, daily bathing may be necessary.
- If you are elderly, avoid daily bathing. Frequent washing dries the skin and removes the natural protective oils.
- Showers are best for cleansing because running water washes away contaminants.

FOOT CARE

- Keep the feet clean and the toenails cut.
- Cut toenails after the bath or shower; otherwise soak the feet in a basin of water to soften the nails.
- Cut or file the nail straight across; avoid trimming the lateral corners as this can cause ingrown toenails.
- Use lotions and moisturizing creams to keep the skin soft and prevent callouses.
- Consult a podiatrist for treatment of corns and callouses.

HAND CARE

- Use lotions and moisturizing creams to keep the skin soft and prevent drying and cracking.
- Regularly trim the nails and push back the cuticles. Keep the cuticle softened with lotion.
- Cut the nails straight across and round the ends with a file.

SOURCES: WHO, 1988; Canadian Dental Association.

MOUTH CARE

Oral care includes daily cleansing of the teeth as well as regular care by dental professionals. Brushing the teeth removes food particles that provide a likely medium for bacterial growth. Brushing also massages the gums and stimulates circulation. It helps to keep the tongue, the mucous membranes lining the mouth and the lips moist as well as clean. A clean, fresh taste in the mouth is important to the desire for and the enjoyment of food. Thus, good oral hygiene helps to promote good nutritional status.

The Canadian Dental Association recommends brushing the teeth regularly at least twice a day, although many people brush more often. Some people prefer to brush first thing in the morning while others wait until after eating breakfast. Flossing is equally important in order to clean the spaces between the teeth which cannot be reached by brushing. Daily flossing is recommended as tartar forms in a minimum of 36 hours.

The nurse helps those patients who cannot brush their teeth unassisted. Patients whose food and fluid intake is restricted or who are unable to eat and drink sufficiently (for example, very weak patients and those who are unconscious), require mouth care at frequent intervals (*q.4h* and as indicated is usually recommended) to keep the tongue, teeth, gums and mucous membranes lining the oral cavity clean, moist and in good condition, and to keep the lips from drying out and cracking. The technique for providing mouth care is outlined in Procedure 30.1.

Preparing the Patient

Assess the patient's needs and preferences for oral hygiene. Explain the procedure and tell the patient how to be of assistance. If patients know what to do, they are better able to participate in the procedure.

Assembling Equipment

Patients usually supply their own toothbrush, dentifrice (toothpaste) or denture cleaner and dental floss. A mouthwash provided by the agency may be used if necessary and depending on the patient's preference. Water or normal saline solution is recommended for oral care. Commercially prepared normal saline swabs are available. Swabsticks can also be made by wrapping soft gauze around one end of a tongue depressor. Nurses traditionally used lemon-glycerine swabs for routine mouth care; however, the use of these kinds of swabs is no longer recommended. Research has shown that lemon-glycerine products may actually harm the patient. Warner (1986) reviewed a number of studies which found that lemon-glycerine dries mucosal membranes, irritates broken tissues and decalcifies the teeth. Petroleum jelly may be used on the lips to prevent drying and cracking. An emesis basin and a towel will also be needed. The nurse should always wear gloves when performing mouth care to prevent exposure to blood and bloodborne pathogens such as HIV and Hepatitis B.

When performing mouth care on unconscious patients, a large syringe may be used to rinse the mouth. A catheter connected to a suction unit may be necessary to remove liquid and loosened debris from the patient's mouth to avoid aspiration.

Dentures require special care. Most institutions provide plastic containers for storing dentures that are removed at night or taken out for special procedures such as surgery. Lost dentures is not an uncommon occurrence in hospitals. It is important that denture containers are safely stored and clearly labelled with the patient's name.

PROCEDURE 30.1

Performing Mouth Care

ACTION	RATIONALE
1. Assess the patient's needs and preferences for mouth care.	Provides individualized care.
2. Gather equipment: • Gloves • Toothbrush • Toothpaste • Warm water or normal saline *Optional:* • Mouthwash • Dental floss • Petroleum jelly • Denture cup • Large swabsticks • Large syringe • Catheter and suction unit	Ensures efficiency and economy of time.
3. Wash hands.	Reduces risk of transmitting infection to the patient.

ACTION	RATIONALE
4. Explain the procedure to the patient.	Promotes well-being and enables patient participation in care.
5. Assist the patient into an upright or side-lying position. Position the unconscious patient in a side-lying position. Put towel and basin next to the mouth.	Prevents aspiration of fluid.
6. Apply gloves.	Protects both patient and nurse from infection.
7. Clean the teeth:	
For dentures:	
• Remove the upper plate first, using a wiggling motion.	Helps to break suction.
• Hold the dentures over a plastic basin or towel placed in the sink.	Prevents breakage if inadvertently dropped.
• Clean dentures with a toothbrush.	
• Rinse with warm water.	Hot water may damage the dentures.
• Return dentures to the patient.	
For teeth:	
• Place the toothbrush with toothpaste at gum line.	
• Gently vibrate the toothbrush using a circular, massaging action.	Loosens food particles. Minimizes gum irritation.
• Brush front, back and chewing surfaces.	
• If it is the patient's usual routine, wrap dental floss around each tooth and pull away from gum, repeating this several times for each tooth.	Cleans the area between the teeth where the brush cannot reach.
• Have the patient rinse with warm water as needed.	Removes food particles and toothpaste.
8. Clean the mouth.	
• *If able*, have the patient rinse with warm water or half-strength mouth wash.	Removes food particles and debris from the mouth.
• *If unable*, use the large syringe to gently rinse the patient's mouth.	Gentle force reduces the risk of aspiration.
• If necessary, suction out any fluid remaining in the mouth.	Prevents aspiration of remaining fluid.
• Gently wipe the patient's gums and inside of the mouth and tongue with the swab.	Removes any debris. Moistens mucous membranes.
9. Apply petroleum jelly to lips.	Maintains moisture.
10. Examine the mouth for any open areas, redness, secretions or odour.	Provides data for ongoing evaluation of care.
11. Clean and/or dispose of equipment. Wash hands.	Maintains cleanliness and safety in the workplace.
12. Document care given and any pertinent observations.	Facilitates continuity of care.

BATHING

Bathing has several purposes: it cleanses, promotes comfort, stimulates blood circulation and affords an opportunity to exercise. When assisting a patient to bathe, nurses have an excellent opportunity for assessment and health teaching. For example, during the bath the nurse can observe the condition of the patient's skin, note such factors as the presence of edema, the quality of respirations and any difficulty or pain the patient experiences when moving. The nurse can provide teaching such as emphasizing the importance of avoiding pressure over areas of skin breakdown.

Due to the very personal nature of bathing, many patients find it much easier to talk to the nurse during the bath than at other times. It has been suggested that the reason for this is that the act of giving physical attention is perceived by many patients as a sign of caring (Davis, 1970). Thus, the bath provides an excellent opportunity for the nurse to establish rapport with the patient and to facilitate communication.

The type of bath depends on several factors including the patient's medical condition and restrictions, mobility and mental capacity. (A patient with advanced Alzheimer's disease might be physically capable of bathing alone but for safety reasons should not be left unsupervised.)

The three types of baths are the tub bath, the shower and the bed bath. Special aids are available such as pneumatic lifts for raising immobile patients in and out of large bathtubs and shower chairs for patients who cannot stand. Regular bathtubs are often equipped with railings, non-slip surfaces and special seats to reduce the risk of falls.

Not all patients require a bath every day, nor is it necessary for all patients to receive a bath in the morning. For the patient who tires very easily or who is very ill, the bath may be contraindicated. Because older people's skin will often become overly dry if they bathe too frequently, a partial bath may be indicated. This includes washing the patient's hands, back, axillae and perineal area, as well as providing for oral hygiene and massaging bony prominences. The nurse makes these judgements based on the needs of the patient and the assessment of the situation. In many long-term care facilities, residents receive a tub bath or shower on scheduled days of the week and partial baths on the other days.

THE BED BATH

The steps for giving a complete bed bath are detailed in Procedure 30.2. This basic procedure, however, can be adapted according to patients' abilities to perform some parts of the bath themselves. For instance, some patients may be able to wash the face and hands only, while others may be able to wash most of the body, with the nurse cleansing the back and feet.

Preparing the Patient

Before gathering the equipment, determine the patient's requirements and any personal preferences for bathing. Establish how much of the bath the patient will be able to perform and how much assistance will be needed.

Assembling Equipment

The equipment required for the bed bath includes bath towels, washcloths, a water basin and soap. A bath blanket is also required to cover the patient to avoid embarrassing exposure and to keep the patient warm. The kind of soap used will depend largely on the individual needs of the patient and on the policy of the health agency. In many agencies, patients are permitted, and sometimes even required, to supply their own soap. A moisturizing lotion is supplied by the agency, although many patients may wish to use their own products.

The skin is sometimes irritated by the chemical composition of certain soaps. Soap can be irritating to a patient's skin and particularly to the eyes. Therefore, patients are often advised not to use soap on the face.

THE TUB BATH

Tub baths are taken for hygienic and therapeutic reasons. The physician may order a therapeutic bath for some patients — Sitz baths, for example, may be ordered for the patient who has had rectal surgery. Patients with skin diseases often have oatmeal or medicated baths. A tub bath is often a pleasurable experience, but it is important to remember that it can also be very frightening for someone who is weak, unwell or confused.

Bathtubs in hospitals frequently have rails; if they do not, the adjacent wall is often equipped with handles to help the patient climb in and out of the tub. Most tubs also now have safety strips on the bottom which help to prevent slipping. No sick person should lock the bathroom door while unattended; help may be required. The nurse or attendant should know when a patient is bathing, and often it is wise to check on the patient every so often. If a patient is out of bed for the first time after even a few days of bedrest, it is generally unwise to leave the patient unattended in the bath. An attendant can stay just outside the curtains if the patient prefers privacy.

The bathtub is filled one-third full of water. Unless otherwise ordered, the water is drawn at 40.5° C, a comfortable and safe temperature for most people. The length of time that a patient bathes depends upon endurance and strength. A lengthy bath may cause unnecessary fatigue. A very hot bath will cause the blood to be diverted away from the vital centres of the brain to the surface areas of the body. As a result, the patient may feel faint and may even lose consciousness.

Giving a Complete Bed Bath

ACTION	RATIONALE
1. Assess the patient's needs and personal preferences for bathing.	Provides individualized care.

2. Gather equipment:
  • Bath blanket
  • Towels
  • Washcloths
  • Wash basin
  • Soap
  • Gloves
  • Skin lotion
	Ensures efficiency and economy of time.

3. Wash hands.	Reduces the risk of transmitting microorganisms to the patient.
4. Explain procedure to the patient.	Enables patient participation in care.
5. Partially fill the basin with water slightly hotter than desired.	Water cools quickly.
6. Draw the bed curtains, cover the patient with the bath blanket and remove the top bed linen. If a bath blanket is not available, use the top sheet as a cover.	Provides privacy and keeps patient warm during the bath. Prevents the bed linen from getting wet and allows reuse if clean.
7. If the patient or the nurse has any open areas on the skin, wear gloves.	Prevents the spread of infection either to or from the patient.
8. Encourage the patient to do as much as possible.	Promotes independence and provides active ROM.
9. If the patient is unable to do so unassisted, begin by washing the face using clear water. Cleanse each eye from the inner canthus, using a clean area of washcloth for each stroke. Then wash the face, ears and neck.	Prevents soap irritation in the eyes and on sensitive facial skin. Prevents transmission of infection from one eye to the other.

10. Suggested order for bath:
  • face, ears, neck
  • arms, hands, axilla
  • chest, breasts
  • abdomen
  • legs, feet
  • groin and front of perineum
  • **Change the water**
  • **Turn the patient to the side**
  • back, buttocks
  • perineal area, rectal area
	Proceeds generally from clean to dirty areas while minimizing position changes for the patient.

Continued on the next page

ACTION	RATIONALE
11. Exposing one area at a time, wash, rinse and dry each part well, then cover with the bath blanket or sheet. Place a towel under the extremity or next to the part being washed.	Keeps patient warm and comfortable. Prevents embarrassment from excessive exposure. Protects the bottom sheet(s) from water and facilitates drying.

ACTION	RATIONALE
12. Use long strokes on the arms and legs directed from the distal to the proximal areas.	Promotes venous return.
13. Change the water as it becomes dirty or cool and as above.	Maintains hygiene and comfort.
14. Apply gloves before perineal and rectal care, if gloves were not used up to this point.	Prevents the spread of infection either to or from patient.
15. Apply lotion to the back, feet, and legs as needed.	Promotes comfort and lubricates dry skin.
16. Help the patient put on a clean gown, pajamas or clothing as appropriate. Replace sheets, remove the bath blanket, and assist the patient to a comfortable position. Ensure that the call bell is in reach and side rails are up.	
17. Clean and/or dispose of equipment. Wash hands.	Maintains cleanliness and safety in the workplace.
18. Document care given and any pertinent observations.	Facilitates continuity of care.

Getting into and out of the bathtub is often a difficult manoeuvre, and the patient may need assistance from the nurse. Usually it is easiest if the patient first sits on the edge of the tub with feet inside the tub, then reaches over to grasp the rail on the other side and gradually eases down. In helping the patient out of the tub, it is a good practice to let the water out before the patient attempts to stand up. There are many mechanical devices available today for assisting with the tub bath procedures. A mechanical lift, for exam-

ple, can be used in either hospital or home situations. Shower stools, on which patients can sit while showering, are also available.

PERINEAL CARE

Perineal care involves washing the external genitalia with soap and water or with water alone. It may be carried out as part of the patient's bath or as a separate procedure. Patients

A mechanical lift facilitates transfer into the bathtub.

FROM RESEARCH TO PRACTICE

Lindell, M.E. and Olsson, H.M. (1990).Personal hygiene in external genitalia of healthy and hospitalized elderly women. *Health Care for Women International, 11,* 151-158.

This study, undertaken in Orebro, Sweden, compared the hygiene practices of two groups of elderly women: an investigation group consisting of 28 women hospitalized for long-term care and a comparison group of 35 healthy elderly women living in the community. All of the investigation group had identified symptoms of vaginal discomfort including erythematous (redness as a result of dilatation of superficial capillaries) mucous membranes and other vulvovaginal symptoms. In the comparison group, 20 percent of the women had experienced mild discomfort from pruritis (itching) in the extra-vaginal area.

The information was gathered from case records, documentation of customary care routines and observations, interviews of hospitalized patients and a questionnaire distributed to the comparison group. Most women in the investigation group were bedridden; all but two were incontinent and wore protective padding, as well as thick cotton briefs and often nylon pantyhose during the daytime. All received help with personal hygiene with soap and water used for morning and, in some cases, evening care and for showers (usually given once a week). Women in the comparison group had three to four showers a week and more than half used soap and water for personal hygiene five to eight times a week.

The study suggests that caregivers need to be more aware that low estrogen levels contribute to the fragility of the urogenital mucous membranes of older women and that these tissues are easily damaged in chronically ill elderly women. The protective padding and tight underclothes worn by patients in long-term care produce pressure. With the acidity of urine from incontinence, the pressure provides a perfect environment for bacteria growth and skin breakdown. The authors suggest that caregivers should be educated about the physiological function of the vaginal mucous membranes and the changes occurring during aging. They should also be aware that the remains of soap in the genital area may cause damage to the tissues and discomfort for the woman. Thus, it is important to rinse out the area thoroughly or, if this is not possible, to use water alone.

who are unable to take care of their own hygiene needs, who are incontinent or who have indwelling or condom catheters require specific perineal care two or three times a day. Perineal hygiene for incontinent patients removes irritating urine and feces which can cause skin breakdown and infection. Patients with condom catheters should have the condom removed, the skin washed and dried and the condom replaced twice daily. The perineal area is inspected regularly for signs of redness or skin breakdown.

Regular and antibacterial soaps are commonly used for perineal hygiene. Soap remaining in the genital area can cause damage to the genital tissues and discomfort for the patient (Lindell and Olsson, 1990; Ravnskov, 1984). In fact, Ravnskov has shown that soap is a major cause of dysuria (1984). It is therefore essential that soap be rinsed off thoroughly. If soap cannot be rinsed out completely, warm water alone should be used for perineal cleansing.

Perineal care varies for male and female patients owing to anatomical differences. Procedures 30.3 and 30.4 outline the steps for performing perineal care on female and male patients respectively.

Preparing the Patient

Providing perineal care can be an embarrassing matter for both the nurse and the patient. When at all possible, patients should do their own perineal care with assistance from the nurse. The nurse will find that if the genital organs are regarded as ordinary body structures and the sexual function (which is often at the root of the nurse's anxiety) is mentally deemphasized, tasks involving these areas will become less strained (Berger and Williams, 1992). Using a confident, matter-of-fact approach when explaining and performing the procedure will help the nurse and the patient feel more comfortable.

PROCEDURE 30.3

Performing Female Perineal Care

ACTION	RATIONALE
1. Gather equipment: • Towel • Washcloth(s) • Soap • Wash basin • Gloves	Ensures efficiency and economy of time.
2. Prepare the patient.	Enhances the patient's comfort.
3. Prepare a basin of warm water.	
4. Draw bed curtains and assist the patient to a supine or side-lying position. Expose only the perineum.	Promotes privacy, comfort and warmth.
5. Apply gloves.	Prevents transmission of infection.
6. Wash, rinse, and dry the groin area and the external labia.	
7. Using the nondominant hand, separate the labia and assess for redness, open areas, swelling, odour or unusual secretions.	Provides data for ongoing evaluation of care.
8. Using a washcloth, cleanse down the centre (over the urethral and vaginal openings), from the mons pubis to the base of the labia.	Prevents bacteria from the rectal area from coming into contact with the vagina and urethra.
9. If an **indwelling catheter** is present, stabilize it with one hand and wash approximately 5 cm of catheter proximal to the patient.	Prevents pulling on the balloon inside of the bladder and thus prevents injury to the bladder. Removes mucus that collects on the tube which can become a medium for bacterial growth and lead to urinary tract infection.
10. Using a clean part of the cloth for each stroke, cleanse each side of the labia minora from front to back.	Prevents transmission of infection from dirtiest to cleanest areas.
11. Gently pat dry.	Prevents injury to the fragile mucosa and prevents patient discomfort.
12. Leave the patient in a comfortable position.	
13. Clean and/or dispose of supplies. Wash hands.	Maintains cleanliness and safety in the workplace.
14. Document care given and any pertinent observations.	Facilitates continuity of care.

HAIR CARE

Care of the patient's hair is important both to grooming and to the sense of well-being. As a part of daily care, each patient's hair needs to be brushed and combed. Thorough brushing stimulates circulation to the scalp and improves the nourishment of the epithelium. Most patients can attend to this themselves, but the nurse may have to assume this responsibility for the aged or very ill patient.

The nurse, by seeing to daily hair care, can ensure that the patient's hair does not become matted. Long hair may

PROCEDURE 30.4

Performing Male Perineal Care

ACTION	RATIONALE
1. Gather equipment: • Towel • Washcloth(s) • Soap • Wash basin • Gloves	Ensures efficiency and economy of time.
2. Prepare the patient.	
3. Prepare a basin of warm water.	
4. Draw the bed curtains, and assist the patient into a supine or semi-Fowler's position. Expose only the perineal area.	Promotes privacy, comfort and warmth.
5. Apply gloves.	Prevents transmission of infection.
6. Wash, rinse and gently pat dry the groin area and scrotum.	Proceed from cleanest to dirtiest areas.
7. Remove condom catheter, if present.	
8. Wash, rinse and dry the shaft of the penis.	
9. Using a circular motion, wash around the urinary meatus, rinse and dry well.	The urinary meatus is usually considered to be the dirtiest area due to the presence of secretions.
10. If an **indwelling catheter** is present, reverse the order of cleansing, beginning with meatus; also wash and rinse approximately 5 cm of catheter proximal to the patient. Stabilize the catheter with one hand while washing meatal area and catheter.	When a catheter is present, the meatus is washed first to prevent the introduction of contaminants via the tube thereby reducing the risk of urinary tract infection. Prevents pulling on the balloon inside the bladder.
11. Reapply a condom catheter.	
12. Leave the patient comfortable.	
13. Clean and/or dispose of supplies. Wash hands.	Maintains cleanliness and safety in the workplace.
14. Document care given and any pertinent observations.	Facilitates continuity of care.

be braided so that it will stay neatly in place. Patients who are in the hospital for long periods will require a shampoo. Permission for a shampoo may have to be obtained from the physician depending on the patient's medical condition. For example, hair shampooing may be contraindicated for someone with a neck or spinal injury. Baby powder or corn starch, which absorb oily secretions, may be used as "dry" shampoo.

Patients on bedrest may have the hair shampooed while in bed or they may be transferred to a stretcher. When a stretcher is used, it is best to move the patient to a sink and support the head on the edge of the sink. If transferring the patient to a stretcher is not possible, the nurse can use a folded plastic sheet or a specially constructed hair washing trough to direct the water from the patient's hair into a pail (see Figure 30.2). The nurse uses pitchers of water to wet

FIGURE 30.2 Shampooing hair while a patient is in bed

SOURCE: Berger, K.J. and Williams, M.B. (1992). *Fundamentals of nursing: Collaborating for optimal health.* Norwalk, CT: Appleton & Lange, 1015.

and rinse the hair, taking precautions to keep the patient's bed dry. The patient's hair needs to be dried quickly after the shampoo in order to avoid chilling. Today, many large hospitals have hairdressing and barber services for patients.

Shaving

The nurse may sometimes have to shave the male patient who cannot shave himself. If the patient has an electric razor this is often not a problem, but a safety razor requires more skill. Very warm water is needed to give an adequate shave. After the skin has been lathered with shaving soap, the skin is held taut and the razor is drawn over the skin in short strokes. The nurse will find that the safest way to shave the patient is to stretch the skin over the bone in a particular area and then to shave in the direction in which the hair is growing. Areas around the mouth and nose are particularly sensitive; in these areas the nurse's motions need to be firm but gentle.

NAIL CARE

Care of the nails is another area of grooming that most patients can attend to themselves. For the very ill patient or the patient who has difficulty moving, however, nail care may be the nurse's responsibility. Often nail polish is not advised for a patient, because oxygenation can be assessed by checking the colour and capillary return of the nailbeds. For this reason, many hospitals required the removal of nail polish prior to surgery.

Toenails are cut straight across. Fingernails are also cut straight across; the edges are rounded with a file. For patients who are particularly prone to infection — for example, patients with diabetes mellitus or circulatory problems — it is advisable that the patient be referred to a podiatrist (foot specialist) for care.

To prevent hangnails, it is best to keep the cuticle of the nail pushed well back and lubricated with oil. Some patients have very hard fingernails and toenails. If the patient soaks the feet for 10 to 15 minutes in warm water, the nails will soften sufficiently to be cut with nail cutters. Special nail clippers are available for thick toenails.

EYE CARE

Special eye care may be required when the eyes have become irritated or infected. The physician usually orders a special solution to cleanse the eyes. Tap water or normal saline may also be used. With absorbent cotton dipped in the solution, the eye is wiped from the inner canthus to the outer canthus. The nurse uses a clean piece of cotton for each stroke. Water or normal saline will soften crusts so they can be easily removed. The motion from the inner to the outer canthus washes the discharge away from the nasal lacrimal duct, which is located on the inner aspect of the orbit of the eye.

Unconscious patients require special attention to protect the eyes from damage. The upper and lower lids should be kept clean and free from discharge. The lids should be closed when the patient is being turned to prevent scratching of the cornea. Special eye lubricants and "artificial tears" are available to prevent dryness and possible scratches.

Patients' glasses, contact lenses, and other prostheses should be looked after carefully and patients should be assisted with care of these articles if necessary.

EAR CARE

Hygiene for the ear consists of gentle washing of the external ear. The use of cotton-tipped applicators or other objects to remove ear wax (cerumen) is discouraged because the wax may be pushed further into the ear canal or the ear canal or tympanic membrane may be damaged (Ney, 1993). Special protocols are used to remove impacted cerumen which involve irrigation of the ear. A physician's order is usually needed to perform this procedure.

PREVENTIVE CARE FOR PRESSURE ULCERS

There are many preventive measures for pressure ulcers. Frequent changes in position rotate the weight-bearing areas and relieve pressure on any single group of bony prominences. The normal healthy individual shifts body position every few minutes. For the patient who is unable to do this unassisted, it is the nurse's responsibility to ensure that the position is changed. A regular schedule should be set up for turning the patient to keep the skin in good condition. Usual recommendations are to turn the patient every two hours and as needed.

Massage and exercise stimulate circulation and thus improve the nourishment to the skin cells. Keeping the skin dry and clean inhibits the growth of disease-producing bacteria and prevents skin from becoming excoriated; body secretions and excreta are particularly irritating to the skin. The nurse should take particular care that a patient's linen and dressings are dry and clean. In areas where secretions cannot be prevented, protective ointments, such as zinc oxide or petroleum jelly, can be used to prevent excessive irritation.

Another preventive measure for pressure ulcers is the use of devices to relieve pressure on specific areas of the patient's body. An overbed cradle will keep bedclothes off the patient, and other aids such as alternating pressure mattresses, oscillating beds and fluidized air or water mattresses may also be used. The use of sheepskin under pressure areas may be helpful.

Attention to the patient's nutritional status is essential. Since pressure ulcers occur most frequently in patients with a negative nitrogen balance, the protein intake should be increased. Foods that contain complete proteins, such as eggs, milk and meat, are recommended. Proteins are needed for the regeneration of body tissue. Usually, supplementary amounts of vitamin C are also prescribed because of this vitamin's role in the healing process. Care must also be taken to ensure an adequate fluid intake, since dehydration and poor tissue turgor predispose patients to the development of ulcers.

HEALTH RESTORING STRATEGIES

Helping patients to restore their hygiene status involves implementing activities related to specific problems of the

skin, hair, nails and oral cavity. Therapeutic care for many of these conditions — for example, skin disorders (such as psoriasis), skin and oral infections or tumours of the skin and mouth — is dealt with in more advanced nursing courses. Problems with a person's gums and teeth, such as gingivitis and dental caries, are referred to a dentist for care.

Care of Patients with Pediculosis

Occasionally a patient will have **pediculosis** (infestation with lice). Therapy involves killing and removing all the pediculi (lice) and their eggs (nits) that have infested the skin, hair and clothing. There are three main types of pediculosis: *pediculosis capitis* or infestation of the scalp with lice, *pediculosis corporis* or infestation with body lice, and *pediculosis pubis* or infestation of the pubic hair with lice. There are several methods of ridding patients of pediculi. For body lice, the patient's clothing is removed for washing or cleaning and the patient is usually given a cleansing bath, and then drugs are applied. In the case of head lice, or if body lice have infected the scalp, medicated shampoo is used. A number of drugs are available that are effective with only one application.

Pediculi are spread by direct contact and through vehicles such as clothing, eating utensils and combs. Pediculi are usually found in environments where poor hygienic measures are practised. However, infestation is not necessarily an indication of poor hygiene. For example, in schools pediculi may be acquired even by children who practise daily bathing.

Care of Patients with Pressure Ulcers

When a pressure ulcer develops, the nurse faces a challenge in restorative care. The amount of tissue breakdown is often less extensive on the outside area than the inside area of the ulcer. Healing of the ulcer may sometimes be difficult. The preventive measures just mentioned are also employed therapeutically. Specific measures may also be ordered to promote the healing of the ulcer. These may include wound irrigations, wet-to-dry dressings, topical enzymes which dissolve **necrotic** (dead) **tissue** and dressings which promote autolytic debridement, maintain a moist wound environment, absorb exudate and promote wound healing. **Autolytic debridement** refers to the removal of dead tissue from a wound by using dressings that allow enzymes in the wound fluid to dissolve the dead tissue (Maklebust, 1991). Pressure ulcers are prone to infection by bacteria; the moist, poorly nourished tissue provides a good medium for the growth of pathogenic bacteria. The use of aseptic technique in the care of an infected ulcer prevents secondary infection and the transfer of bacteria to other areas of the body and to other patients.

EVALUATING HYGIENE INTERVENTIONS

Evidence of successful nursing interventions is found in the healthy state of the patient's skin, hair, nails and mouth. Continuous reassessment of all of these is required.

More and more criticism is being directed at the ritualistic nature of nursing's hygienic practices. Financial constraints in the health care system also challenge nurses to provide the most efficient and effective care possible. Not only do nurses need to continually evaluate the effectiveness of their care for individual patients, but more evaluation in the form of research studies is also needed. In no area of nursing is the lack of research more evident than in the area of hygiene. Fortunately, this situation is slowly beginning to change

KEY TERMS

epidermis p. 966

dermis p. 966

dandruff p. 966

sebaceous glands p. 966

sweat glands p. 966

ceruminous glands p. 966

gingivae p. 967

gingivitis p. 969

plaque p. 969

dental caries p. 969

sordes p. 969

pressure ulcers p. 969

pediculosis p. 985

necrotic tissue p. 985

autolytic debridement p. 985

IN REVIEW

Hygiene is the science of health. On a personal basis, the term refers to those measures people take to keep their skin, teeth and mouth clean and in good condition. The body's first line of defence against infection is the skin. Composed of two layers, the epidermis or thin outer layer and the dermis or thick inner layer, the skin overlies the subcutaneous and adipose tissues.

Skin and oral integrity are influenced by a number of factors including the individual's general state of physical and mental health, nutritional and hydration status, fitness level and personal hygiene practices as well as drugs and other therapies the person may be having. Environmental conditions, such as the weather, and socioeconomic factors that determine the availability of facilities necessary for good hygiene also affect an individual's ability to maintain skin and oral cavity integrity.

Hygiene needs vary during the life cycle. More bathing is needed during pregnancy because of perspiration. Since frequent washing removes natural oils and may dry the sensitive skin of infants, daily bathing is not recommended. However, the skin must be cleansed before applying a clean diaper to prevent skin irritation. Children are particularly prone to minor cuts and scrapes which must be treated. Adolescents often have skin and perspiration problems due to hormonal changes taking place in their bodies so that cleanliness, diet and exercise are important. Older adults have special needs because of a lack of skin oils and a thinning of the skin layers as well as thinning hair, thickening nails and problems with gum disease. Inadequate hygiene measures at any age result in dirty skin, hair and teeth, often with offensive odours.

In assessing hygiene needs, the nurse uses information from the health history to determine the patient's hygiene practices and health promotion behaviours. The nurse's assessment includes visual inspection of the mouth, ears, eyes, scalp and all skin surfaces and assessment of the individual's ability for self-care. Deficits are noted for preventive measures and knowledge needs.

Common nursing diagnoses include *Bathing/hygiene self-care deficit, Impaired skin integrity* or *High risk for impaired skin integrity* (related to incontinence or other factors), and *Altered mucous membranes* (e.g. in oral cavity), or high risk for this condition. *Altered health maintenance* is the diagnosis used when hygiene practices are poor, e.g. related to unhealthy lifestyle or lack of knowledge. *Knowledge deficit* may also be used.

The main focus of nursing interventions is the promotion of healthy and intact skin, mucous membranes and oral cavity and the prevention of problems. In promoting healthy hygiene practices, hand washing and skin care are stressed as well as good oral and dental care, adequate bathing and hand and foot care.

Many inpatient agencies caring for the sick include health protection measures on a routine basis, such as morning and evening care, oral hygiene and bathing. Bathing usually includes perineal care, hair care, nail care and measures for the prevention of pressure ulcers. Special care for eyes and ears may be necessary.

Restorative care is needed if there are breaks in the skin, loss of integrity of the mucous membranes or problems in the oral cavity. Interventions to promote healing of pressure ulcers include changing the patient's position, exercise, massage, special mattresses and other devices to relieve pressure as well as ensuring cleanliness and dryness of the area. Topical enzymes and dressings to promote wound debridement, maintain a moist wound environment and absorb exudate may also be used. Continual reassessment and reevaluation of the patient's hygiene condition is essential for updating nursing planning and interventions.

LEARNING ACTIVITIES

1. **Case Study**: Mr. Charles Rose was admitted to hospital yesterday for investigative procedures. He is a 32-year-old bachelor and has been working on a trapline in the north woods for the past 2 years. He lives alone in a remote cabin, coming into town occasionally to replenish his supplies, which consist mainly of canned and dried foods. The cabin does not have electricity or running water; it is heated by a wood stove and Mr. Rose has to fetch his water from a stream 500 metres away.

   He spends several days at a time out in the woods inspecting his lines with only his dog for company. He hit his head 2 or 3 weeks ago on a fallen tree trunk when he was straightening up after looking at a trap and he hasn't been feeling too well since. He had headaches of increasing severity, so he went to the doctor in town, who admitted him to the hospital. Mr. Rose is thin, his skin is dry, and he has some lesions on his arms and legs; his long hair is matted, his nails are dirty and chipped, and his teeth and fingers are stained with nicotine. The physician has ordered bedrest.

   a. What problems can you identify relative to Mr. Rose's hygiene? to the status of his skin, hair, nails and teeth?

   b. What factors do you think contributed to these problems?

   c. What are the expected outcomes for these problems?

   d. What principles can assist you in planning hygiene measures for Mr. Rose?

   e. What specific nursing interventions would you implement?

   Mr. Rose's condition deteriorates over the next few days; he appears to be very weak and drowsy. The physician and a neurosurgeon who has been called in are contemplating surgery.

   f. What additional nursing interventions would you plan for Mr. Rose with regard to hygiene?

   g. How would you evaluate the effectiveness of your interventions?

REFERENCES AND READINGS

ASHTON, B., GELBIER, S. and PLAMPING, D. (1983). Improving dental health education. *Health Visitor, 56*, 362–363.

BERGER, K.J. and WILLIAMS, M.B. (1992). *Fundamentals of nursing: Collaborating for optimal health.* Norwalk, CT: Appleton & Lange.

BRADBY, M. (1990). Status passage into nursing: Undertaking nursing care. *Journal of Advanced Nursing, 15*, 1363–1369.

BUSH, T. (1984). Double handicap: The sense of well-being. *Nursing Times, 80*(1), 31–32.

CANADIAN DENTAL ASSOCIATION (circa 1994). *Gum disease.* (Pamphlet). Ottawa: Author.

COLBURN, L. (1990). Preventing pressure sores. *Nursing 90, 20*(12), 60–63.

CONVATEC. (1992). *DuoDERM® "S.O.S" wound care: Clinical applications guide.* Pamphlet 581-1136. Princeton, NJ: E.R. Squibb & Sons.

DASCHNER, F.D. (1985). Useful and useless hygienic techniques in intensive care units. *Intensive Care Medicine, 11*, 280–283.

DAVIS, E.D. (1970). Giving a bath? *American Journal of Nursing, 70*, 2366–2367.

GREIFZU, S., RADJESKI, D. and WINNICK, B. (1990). Oral care is part of cancer care. *RN, 53*(6), 42–46.

LINDELL, M.E. and OLSSON, H.M. (1989). Lack of caregivers knowledge causes unnecessary suffering in elderly patients. *Journal of Advanced Nursing, 14*, 976–979.

LINDELL, M.E. and OLSSON, H.M. (1990). Personal hygiene in external genitalia of healthy and hospitalized elderly women. *Health Care for Women International, 11*, 151–158.

MAKLEBUST, J. (1991). Pressure ulcer update. *RN, 54*(12), 56-62.

McGOVERN, M. and KUHN, J. K. (1992). Skin assessment of the elderly patient. *Journal of Gerontological Nursing, 18*(4), 39–43.

THE NEW LEXICON WEBSTER'S DICTIONARY OF THE ENGLISH LANGUAGE (1988). New York: Lexicon Publications.

NEWMAN, G.R. (1987). An oral-hygiene program for long-term care facilities. *The Journal of Long-Term Care Administration, 15*(2), 11–14.

NEY, D.F. (1993). Cerumen impaction, ear hygiene practices, and hearing acuity. *Geriatric Nursing, 14*(2), 70–73.

PILLITTERI, A. (1992). *Maternal and child health nursing: Care of the childbearing and childrearing family.* Philadelphia: Lippincott.

RAVNSKOV, U. (1984, May). Soap is the major cause of dysuria. *Lancet*, 1027–1028.

RICHARDSON, A. (1987). A process standard for oral care. *Nursing Times, 83*(32), 42–46.

RICHARDSON, E. (1990). The Cambodians and Laotians. In N. Waxler-Morrison, J. Anderson and E. Richardson (Eds.). *Cross-cul-*

tural caring: A handbook for health professionals in western Canada. Vancouver, BC: University of British Columbia Press.

SIMONS, W. (1989). Feminine hygiene. *Nursing, 3*(35), 31–34.

SMITH, S. and DUELL, D. (1992). *Clinical nursing skills: Nursing process model (Basic to advanced skills).* (3rd ed.). Norwalk, CT: Appleton & Lange.

WAGNILD, G. (1986). Personal-care complaints: A descriptive study. *Journal of Long-Term Care Administration, 14*(3), 27–29.

WARNER, L.A. (1986). Lemon-glycerine swabs should be used for routine oral care. *Critical Care Nurse, 6*(6), 82–83.

WOLF, Z.R. (1986). Nurses' work: The sacred and the profane. *Holistic Nursing Practice, 1*(1), 29–35.

WONG, D.L., BRANTLY, D., CLUTTER, L., DE SIMONE, D., LAMMERT, D., NIX, K., PERRY, K., SMITH, D. and WHITE, K. (1992). Diapering choices: A critical review of the issues. *Pediatric Nursing, 18*(1), 41–54.

WOOD, M., and BRIDGES, S. (1987). Resident grooming program draws praise as prototype. *Provider, 13*(1), 45–46.

WORLD HEALTH ORGANIZATION (WHO). (1988). *Manual for infection control in health facilities.* New Delhi: WHO Regional Office for South East Asia. (Catalogue SEARO – Regional Health Papers No. 18)

WRIGHT, L. (1990). Bathing by towel. *Nursing Times, 86*(4), 36–39.

The Prevention and Control of Infection

CENTRAL QUESTIONS

1. Why is the prevention and control of infection important to health?

2. What is the chain of infection and how does it relate to the infectious process?

3. What are some of the common pathogens that infect people and how are pathogens spread?

4. What are the major responses of the body to infection?

5. What factors determine the body's response to infectious agents?

6. How do infection prevention and control needs vary throughout the life cycle?

7. What age groups are the most susceptible to infection and why?

8. What are five of the most common infections?

9. What basic principles does the nurse apply in assisting individuals with the control and prevention of infection?

10. How does the nurse assess infection prevention and control needs?

11. What are the common nursing diagnostic statements for patients with infection-related problems?

12. How does the nurse develop a plan of care for patients with infection-related problems?

13. What strategies does the nurse implement in helping individuals, families or groups promote healthy infection control practices?

14. What health protecting measures does the nurse implement to maintain infection control and to prevent the spread of infection from one person to another?

15. What health restoring and supportive strategies does the nurse implement in the care of patients with infection-related problems?

16. How does the nurse evaluate the patient's response to nursing interventions?

INTRODUCTION

Infectious diseases have plagued humans throughout the centuries. It is only in the past one hundred and fifty years that successful measures to control infection have been developed. One of the principal reasons for the dramatic reduction in infant and child mortality, and the consequent lengthening of the life span in developed countries (and increasingly in developing countries), has been the implementation of infection control programs. The following factors have contributed to this achievement:

- the development and widespread use of specific immunizations against many of the common communicable diseases
- the discovery and widespread use of antimicrobial agents (antibiotics)
- the application of basic sanitary measures to protect the safety of water, milk, and food supplies and to ensure the safe disposal of garbage and sewage
- the overall increases in standards of living, with the resulting improvement in the general health of people (from factors such as better nutrition and better housing).

While significant gains have been made in controlling infectious diseases, we have by no means eliminated all illnesses caused by infections. Respiratory infections continue to be a leading cause of death and of acute illness throughout the life span. Gastrointestinal infections are one of the most common causes of short-term illness. Sexually transmitted diseases (STDs) have attained epidemic proportions in the past few years, and such diseases as chickenpox and viral hepatitis remain prevalent. AIDS (acquired immunodeficiency syndrome), which is caused by the human-immunodeficiency virus (HIV), appeared in the late 1970s and early 1980s. AIDS is a life-threatening disease which suppresses the body's immune system and renders it unable to fight infections. Infection is found world wide but sociodemographic factors determine the prevalence of disease in a given population. Institution-acquired infections (called *nosocomial infections*) continue to plague hospitals throughout the world and represent significant concerns regarding morbidity, mortality, and cost. Personnel in health care services also have concerns about the risk of disease, particularly from the blood-borne pathogens associated with hepatitis and AIDS.

The prevention and control of infection is a primary goal of all health personnel, whether in ambulatory care settings, in the community or in inpatient facilities. Infections are caused by microorganisms. Wherever there are sick people, microorganisms that are capable of producing infection pose a constant and serious threat to well-being. Many patients are highly susceptible to infection owing to a number of risk factors, such as underlying disease, altered immune status, the extremes of age, poor nutrition, invasive procedures, drug therapy and irradiation. This is especially true in tertiary care hospitals. It is in fact ironic that medical science is increasingly able to support patients through life-threatening illness or injury which would have been fatal only a few years ago, and yet the risks of infectious complications are rising markedly. The close proximity of patients to one another further serves to increase the risk of transferring infection as does the intimate contact required when giving care.

Microorganisms are everywhere around us. They are found on our bodies, inside our bodies, in the air, on horizontal surfaces, such as floors, table tops and counters, and on equipment and furniture and to a lesser extent on walls and ceilings. Although we cannot generally see microorganisms, their impact on our lives is profound and our interaction with them both constant and variable. It is safe to say that life as we know it on this planet would not exist without their presence. Being human, we constantly touch both the animate (persons) and the inanimate (things) environment, thus continually exchanging one lot of microorganism (those on our hands) for another (those on whatever we touch). Fortunately, for the most part our relationship with microorganisms is a symbiotic (mutually beneficial) one and in fact constitutes part of the balance in nature. It is when that balance is upset that people are at risk. This is especially true for patients in hospitals and to a much lesser extent for health care providers who must care for those harbouring potentially pathogenic (disease producing) microorganisms. Most microorganisms do not constitute a great threat to a healthy person, but there are a few pathogens which always have the potential to cause infectious disease.

Microorganisms are spread mainly by contact, through the air, by ingesting contaminated food and water and by carriers such as mosquitoes, flies and birds. Health personnel sometimes unknowingly act as carriers of pathogens, creating a potential risk to themselves or to coworkers and an even greater risk to patients. When hand washing techniques break down, for example, microorganisms are passed on to others. In spite of careful cleaning practices, microorganisms cannot be totally eliminated from the environment. Sometimes an organism highly capable of producing disease may be present and a worker with an open cut or lowered body resistance becomes infected. Workers primarily face the risk of blood-borne diseases such as hepatitis B or C and HIV, while patients may be at greater risk for acquiring infections from their own endogenous flora which gain entrance through an invasive procedure such as the insertion of a urinary catheter, a vascular catheter or surgery. People are increasingly vulnerable to common microorganisms that have developed resistance to previously reliable and usually tolerable antibiotics. The issue of multiple-resistant microorganisms is a growing threat to patients and a sometimes frustrating challenge for infection control. Multiple-drug resistant microorganisms will be one of the more significant infection control issues as we enter the twenty-first century.

In order to understand the rationale behind nursing measures taken to protect patients and staff from infections, it is important to keep in mind the sources, methods of transfer and modes of spread of microorganisms. Knowledge about the infectious process and the body's responses to it, as well as about specific communicable diseases, will be gained in microbiology and anatomy and physiology courses. Nursing interventions for specific infectious health problems such as care for persons with AIDS or pneumonia will be learned in more advanced nursing courses. In this chapter, we will review the history of infectious diseases, briefly describe the infectious process and the body's response to it, and outline common infectious problems in order to provide a framework for understanding the nursing care of individuals with existing or potential problems of infections. Measures to prevent and control the spread of infection, namely immunization, medical and surgical asepsis, as well as the use of universal and body substance precautions are also outlined.

HISTORICAL PERSPECTIVE

Infectious disease has been cited as the leading cause of morbidity and mortality throughout the world (Hoeprich, 1972). Hospital-acquired infections account for half of all infectious diseases seen in the Western world (Barrett-Connor, 1978). That figure, which is still largely undefined, is even higher in developing countries (Wenzel, 1987). With a moment's thought, it is easy to see that the people of the Western world were in a similar, perhaps even worse, situation just over a century ago. From earliest times, an aura of mysticism and helplessness pervaded communities when their members were stricken with illness. Faced with what was thought to have been divine anger, witchcraft or the work of demons, early peoples resorted to ritual, incantation and noxious potions as cures. Eventually a rudimentary awareness of the need to isolate infected people developed, but the real causes of disease continued to be elusive. Lepers in biblical times were considered "unclean" and were required to announce their presence when approaching a city or a group of people. Some travellers were kept in huts outside cities for 40 days under observation for evidence of contagion, while sailors entering port were required to remain on board for 40 days. If no one became ill, they could all go ashore. (Quarantine comes from the Italian "quaranta giorni" meaning 40 days).

The Black Death, or plague (due to the bacterium *Yersinia pestis*), decimated the population of medieval Europe. The plague doctor who went from door to door looking for victims of the dreaded disease wore an outfit that has interesting parallels today. A long hooded gown covered his entire body. On top of the hood he wore a large brimmed hat. A mask which covered his face was equipped

with round glass lenses which allowed him to peer out. Attached to the mask was a beak-like projection about seven inches long. The beak contained pungent herbs and strong-smelling spices. In the fourteenth century the population of Europe was 105 million. In the four years between 1346 and 1350, 25 million persons died of plague (LaForce, 1991). Remote though it seems now, the Black Death remains the most virulent epidemic in human history.

The Christian church in Europe has a history of caring for the sick and the poor. However, as they believed care of the soul to be of much greater importance than care of the body, washing and general care thereof was opposed. Nevertheless, a sixteenth century Italian by the name of Girolamo Fracastora suggested that disease spread from person to person via clothes or other possessions (fomites) or through the air. The scientific knowledge was not available at the time to prove this assumption. However, in 1678, Anton Van Leeuwenhoek, a Dutch merchant, whose hobby was microscopy, took scrapings from his teeth and observed them under the glass lenses he had ground himself by hand. There he observed small creatures believed to be various bacteria and protozoa, which he referred to as his little animalcules. It was Louis Pasteur who in 1855 established the relationship between microorganisms and the occurrence of disease. Robert Koch in 1876 outlined the steps, known as Koch's postulates (shown in the box below), which lead to the production of disease.

Koch's Postulates

1. The microorganism is found in a high proportion of hosts (human or animal) with disease, but not normally in healthy hosts.

2. The microorganism is isolated and propagated serially in pure culture in the laboratory.

3. The microorganism in pure culture induces a comparable disease in susceptible hosts and can be isolated from these hosts.

(McLean and Smith, 1991)

The Hungarian physician, Ignasz Semmelweis, promoted hand washing as a result of his observations when working at the Allgemeines Krankenhaus (lying-in hospital) in Vienna in 1847. While his findings were recognized far afield, his colleagues in Vienna ridiculed him. Ironically, he died of septicemia in a mental institution in 1865 without the recognition he deserved.

Fairly recently, in 1965, Professor Sydney Selwyn in England uncovered the virtually unknown work of Sir John Pringle who, in the 1740s, was a professor at Edinburgh University and a physician to the British Army. He insisted that uncrowded wards and adequate ventilation helped stop the spread of disease. He seems to have been ignored (Selwyn, 1991). Not quite a century later, Florence Nightingale, after observing appalling conditions in the Crimea, returned home to England. Working with William Farr, a noted British health statistician, she prevailed against a hostile military bureaucracy and an indifferent government to show that the mortality rate in British Army hospitals could be significantly reduced by improving hygienic practice, avoiding overcrowding and developing a standardized reporting system for army deaths. It has often been pointed out that Nightingale eschewed the germ theory of disease and did not believe the findings of Koch and Pasteur. However, she did appreciate the importance of a clean environment. In her book, *Notes on Hospitals*, she clearly stated that there was a direct relationship between the sanitary conditions of a hospital and postoperative complications due to infectious disease. The type of wards she advocated had high ceilings, had adequate space between beds, were well ventilated and were kept clean (Nightingale, 1861).

There were at least three cholera outbreaks in England in the first half of the nineteenth century. Dr. John Snow observed that all those who became ill obtained drinking water from the same pump. He persuaded authorities to remove the handle, preventing use. It was later discovered that the well was contaminated with raw sewage.

In Glasgow in the 1860s, Joseph Lister (later Lord Lister), who had studied Pasteur's work, decided to try using an antiseptic to dress and pack wounds. He went on to soak the instruments, ligatures and even his fingers in a carbolic acid solution prior to surgery. With this approach he demonstrated a dramatic drop in surgical wound infections and became known as the father of antiseptic surgery. Eventually, Halstead, a U.S. surgeon, introduced the concept of rubber gloves, first to protect the nurse and then to protect the patient. Also around the turn of the century in U.S. hospitals, gowns and masks began to be used for surgery, and the concept of asepsis through sterilization of supplies and equipment was well established by 1910.

However, highly communicable diseases continued to be a source of fear and concern. During the Middle Ages, leprosaria (hospitals for lepers) were common. (We know today, however, that leprosy is *not* a highly contagious disease and requires close prolonged contact for transmission of the pathogen to occur.) Lazarettos were built to confine plague victims and in the nineteenth century a large number of infectious disease hospitals were established. Sometimes called fever hospitals, they were used to house those with smallpox and a variety of other communicable diseases. Smallpox had been a dreaded disease for centuries. It decimated populations, sometimes all but wiping out whole communities. Because military personnel became infected very readily due to crowded living conditions, it influenced the outcomes of wars. About 30 percent of children born in eighteenth century England died of smallpox before they reached maturity (Parker, 1990). When introduced by Europeans to the native populations of North America who had never encountered the disease before, smallpox had a devastating effect and was largely responsible for reducing the population to one-tenth of what it had been before contact.

In 1796, Sir Edward Jenner discovered that a person who had had cowpox developed lifelong immunity to smallpox. He observed that the virus causing cowpox was immunologically related to smallpox and that the body could be fooled into producing effective antibodies to smallpox. These observations led Jenner to develop the first vaccine (vacca is Latin for cow). He subsequently published his findings and vaccination was gradually made available to all. Gradually other vaccines were developed including pertussis, diphtheria and polio. Today we also have routine immunization for measles, mumps, rubella and hemophilus influenzae, with others being given according to the requirements of the individual. The antibiotic era dawned with the discovery of penicillin in 1928 and the introduction of sulfonamides in 1935. The antibiotic armamentarium is now quite impressive but not without its drawbacks due to unfortunate side effects, expense and bacterial resistance.

Despite these advances, infectious disease hospitals, leprosaria and tuberculosis (TB) sanatoria continued to be used past the middle of the twentieth century. The last surviving Canadian leper who had lived and worked much of his life with his fellows in a leper colony on Bentinck Island off Vancouver Island died in 1956. It was only then that the colony was formally shut down by the Federal Government. Similar colonies existed across Canada, as did TB sanatoria in places such as Tranquille near Kamloops, British Columbia and Fort San near Fort Qu'Appelle in Saskatchewan. At Vancouver General Hospital, the infectious disease hospital was closed as recently as 1983. By this time, those who practised in the field of infection control had long been advocating the use of decentralized isolation that is done today.

Slowly, over the centuries we have seen the gradual understanding of the role of microorganisms in our environment, how they can cause disease and how disease can be prevented. We now know that certain basic hygienic measures can help ensure a safe community. These include a clean supply of drinking water, clean food and sanitary disposal of sewage. We also know that there are basic measures of hygiene that anyone can practise to help control the spread of infection, such as hand washing and safe disposal of body secretions and excretions.

Today, we also know enough about our relationship with microorganisms to make informed decisions about our own health and how to care for others so as to prevent the spread of disease. New diseases may arise to challenge us, such as HIV, while old diseases such as tuberculosis or *Staphylococcus aureus* may renew their imperative to survive and multiply by developing resistance to antibiotics that were previously effective. Whatever challenges we meet, it is important to remember the lessons we have learned and to apply that knowledge, understanding and wisdom.

THE INFECTIOUS PROCESS

Infection is the deposition or invasion and multiplication of microorganisms on surfaces of the body or in body tissues causing adverse or ill effects. Such adverse effects are always assumed in the definition. The disease-producing agent is referred to as a *pathogen*. In certain circumstances, any microorganism may cause disease, even those with which we usually enjoy a *symbiotic* (mutually beneficial) *relationship*. This is especially true of people who are *immunocompromised,* that is, people whose immune system is impaired. Fortunately, only two to three percent of all microorganisms are considered to be true human pathogens. In other circumstances, people may acquire a pathogen, for example, Hepatitis B, but never experience any adverse or ill effects. These people become *carriers* of that pathogen and, while they remain symptom free, they are capable of passing the disease to someone else who can get sick from it. Microorganisms with which we enjoy a symbiotic relationship — which are the vast majority of microorganisms on and in our bodies — are called *commensals*.

THE CHAIN OF INFECTION

An infection does not necessarily begin because a pathogen is present in the environment. Infection is the result of a number of interrelated factors that follow sequentially one after another in a cycle, commonly referred to as the chain of infection. The chain of infection is best visualized as a chain with its various links (see Figure 31.1). There must first of all be an infectious or *causative agent*. The agent must have a place *(reservoir)* in which it grows and multiplies. It leaves the reservoir, now referred to as a *source*, by an exit route *(portal of exit)*, and uses a means of travel (vehicle), or a *mode of transmission*. By using this vehicle, it gains entrance through a *portal of entry* to the body of a susceptible human being, who then becomes its *host* and constitutes a potential reservoir to start the cycle again. It is important to understand the various features of all the links in the chain as well as other terms used to define infection.

CAUSATIVE AGENTS

The chain of infection begins with an infectious agent capable of causing disease in humans. Causative agents may be bacteria, viruses, fungi, protozoa or helminths that normally inhabit or have recently entered the body or attached to the skin. **Pathogenic bacteria** are microorganisms capa-

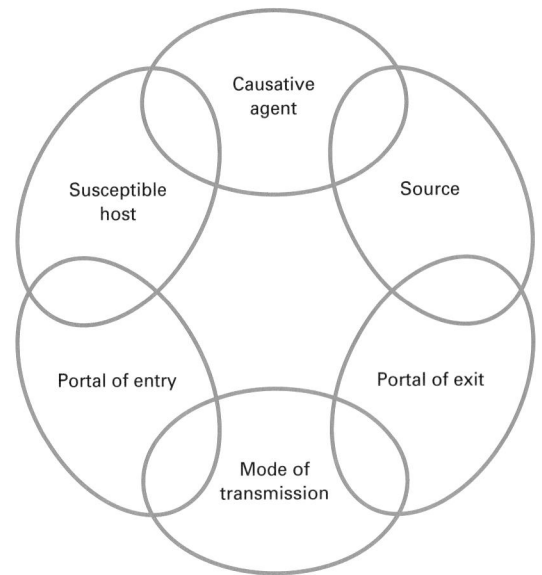

FIGURE 31.1   Chain of infection

ble of invading healthy tissue and causing injury to the body or body part. An example is *Salmonella* which invades the mucosal surface of the bowel, causing an acute form of gastroenteritis. Other bacteria may invade body tissue when given the opportunity and when present in sufficient numbers. These include, for example, some of the streptococci and staphylococci, which can cause wound and other soft tissue infections. Some bacteria do not invade body tissue but produce toxins which produce disease; *Clostridium (C.) tetani*, for example, is the causative agent of tetanus, which may cause paralysis and muscle spasm. Some microorganisms, such as *Salmonella*, can cause disease in more than one way, for instance, by inducing local inflammation and producing toxins. Another example is *Staphylococcus (S.) aureus* which may invade tissue, spread systematically, or produce a toxin in the gastrointestinal tract which in turn acts on the vomiting centre in the brain to cause vomiting and eventually dehydration and possibly even cardiac failure.

Many of the common communicable diseases are *viral* infections (measles, mumps, chickenpox) which usually occur in children. Diseases in the viral hepatitides group, HIV, influenza and the common cold are all viral infections. *Fungal* infections include those caused by yeasts and moulds, such as ring worm and athlete's foot. In hospitals, fungal infections most frequently include thrush in newborns (caused by *Candida*), or candidiasis of the esophagus which is sometimes seen in the immunocompromised patient and may develop into a potentially fatal systemic disease. Another disease seen in the immunocompromised patient is aspergillosis, usually in the form of pneumonia.

Protozoa are single-celled animals which can behave pathogenically. An example is *Entamoeba histolytica*, which causes the intestinal infection of amoebiasis, characterized by colicky abdominal pain, frequent bloody stools and possibly liver tenderness. Hemorrhage may occur in rare cases of amoebiasis. Another example is the protozoan *Giardia lamblia* which causes an enteric disease called giardiasis, popularly known as beaver fever since the parasite spends part of its life cycle in water-loving animals such as beavers. Infected people may be asymptomatic, have only mild diarrhea or have watery diarrhea with epigastric tenderness, flatulence, malaise or nausea.

The helminths are worms. Some are common parasites in humans, as, for example, the pinworms often found in children. In Canada, patients admitted to hospital who have worm infestations most frequently have acquired them from other parts of the world and since these particular parasites generally do not survive in our temperate climate, there is little risk to others. There is, however, the very rare exception of acquiring *Strongyloides* from skin contact with an infected person who has acquired it in the tropics. Wild meat (game) should always be well cooked to ensure that one does not ingest parasites which the animal has acquired.

Infection may be endogenous or exogenous in origin. In **endogenous infection,** the infection has been acquired from a person's own microbial flora. **Microbial flora** refers to microorganisms that live on or within the body and provide a natural immunity against certain infections. A primary endogenous infection occurs when normal flora becomes the causative agent of disease and a secondary endogenous infection when normal flora has been altered by therapeutic intervention. An example of a secondary endogenous infection would be diarrhea caused by antibiotic usage. **Exogenous infection** is infection acquired from the local animate or inanimate environment. Nosocomial infections are most commonly caused by bacteria and viruses.

RESERVOIR OR SOURCE

A reservoir is the agent's natural habitat for growth and multiplication. The most common reservoir for human infectious pathogens is the human body itself. Other reservoirs may include animals, birds, plants, soil and arthropods, such as mosquitoes, fleas, ticks and lice.

PORTAL OF EXIT

The portal of exit is the primary route by which organisms leave their source. Common exit routes in humans include the body systems such as the respiratory tract, the urinary tract, the gastrointestinal tract and reproductive tract, as well as breaks in skin and mucous membranes, discharges from wounds and especially blood.

MODES OF TRANSMISSION

An infectious agent may be transmitted from its reservoir to a host by a number of routes. Some agents can be transmitted by more than one route or mode.

Contact Transmission

An organism may be transmitted by direct or indirect contact. Direct contact involves direct physical transfer from the source of infection to the susceptible host. Touching wound drainage from a patient or kissing or engaging in sexual activity with an infected individual are examples of direct contact. Indirect contact involves contact with an intermediate object that has become contaminated from either an animate or inanimate source. For example, infection can be transferred by touching a contaminated bed rail or using a diagnostic instrument that was not properly disinfected after use on a patient. Inanimate objects which carry infectious agents are referred to as **fomites.** Another form of indirect contact is by droplet spread in which infectious agents are propelled through the air in droplets by coughing, sneezing or even speaking, travelling only a few feet before landing on an inanimate surface or on a susceptible host. For example, droplet spread occurs when someone's mucous membrane comes in contact with measles virus or a *Streptococcus* that can cause pharyngitis. Contact spread is by far the most common cause of nosocomial disease transmission and potentially is the easiest to interrupt.

Common Vehicle Transmission

Common vehicle spread is a mode of transmission in which a contaminated inanimate vehicle serves as a source of infection to multiple people. Examples of transmission include *Salmonellae* in foods that have become contaminated by an infected food handler or Hepatitis A in sewage-contaminated seafood. Another type of common vehicle is contaminated blood. A blood donation from someone with Hepatitis C or HIV may be fractionated, resulting in a number of people becoming infected from one person's blood. Due to blood screening, this is now a rare but not impossible event.

Airborne Transmission

Airborne transmission refers to the spread of microbes through the air. Organisms may be contained within droplet nuclei, dust particles or on skin squames. Droplet nuclei occur as a result of moisture evaporating from droplets. These droplet nuclei, which are 5 μm or less in size, may then become suspended in air, remain there for a long time and travel long distances. Thus, true airborne spread by droplet nuclei is distinguished from spread by indirect contact through droplets which are large and travel only a few feet through the air. Two of the most common examples of diseases transmitted by droplet nuclei are tuberculosis and chicken pox.

While dust particles will gravitate to horizontal surfaces, they can be readily resuspended by physical activity and serve as a means of transfer for many microorganisms, although this does not necessarily mean that infection will ensue. All of us shed skin squames on an ongoing basis. These dead epithelial cells carry with them the microbial flora associated with the parts of the body from which they were shed. Outbreaks most commonly associated with shedding skin squames include staphylococcal and streptococcal infections. However, spread of these microorganisms by airborne transmission must be kept in perspective, as contact spread is much more likely to occur as is endogenous acquisition of infection from one's own staphylococci or streptococci. Infectious aerosols are not created easily, and people with rapidly desquamating skin conditions are not admitted to hospital as frequently as in the past.

Vector-Borne Transmission

Vectors include animals, insects and birds which carry infection from a source to a host. For example, flies carry *Salmonella*, the anopheles mosquito carries protozoa which cause malaria and ticks carry *Rickettsia rickettsii*, the organisms responsible for Rocky Mountain spotted fever (tick-borne typhus fever).

PORTALS OF ENTRY

Portals of entry are generally the same as portals of exit. Infectious agents gain access to the body via the respiratory tract, the urinary tract, the gastrointestinal tract, mucous membranes, non-intact skin and percutaneously, for example by needlestick or blood transfusion.

HOST

The host is the final link in the chain, and becomes in turn a new reservoir and a potential source of infection. **Susceptibility** refers to the degree of resistance of a host to a pathogen. If people are susceptible to the pathogen, that is, if their resistance is weakened, they are more likely to develop an infection. Susceptibility may also be stated as the degree of vulnerability to a microorganism.

For disease transmission to occur, a potential pathogen must be present in sufficient quantities and with sufficient virulence. **Virulence** refers to an organism's ability to cause disease. The pathogen must be able to leave its source, acquire a mode of transmission and gain entry into the tissues of a susceptible host. All of these factors must be present simultaneously for disease transmission to occur. The acquisition and multiplication of a microorganism (pathogen or commensal) is referred to as **colonization**. The period leading up to disease manifestation is **incubation** and infection is the destructive pathological process that ensues.

THE BODY'S RESPONSE TO INFECTIOUS AGENTS

Humans are equipped with various mechanisms that help to prevent the invasion of body tissues by infectious agents and to control their growth and multiplication in the body if they get past the first lines of defence. However, it should be noted that the quality and quantity of these various defence mechanisms may vary greatly from one person to another. These defences may be divided into two major categories, non-specific defence mechanisms and specific defence mechanisms.

NON-SPECIFIC DEFENCE MECHANISMS

Non-specific defence mechanisms include the skin, the mucous membranes and some body secretions. Intact skin and mucous membranes form a barrier that cannot (with a very few exceptions) be penetrated by microorganisms. The skin and mucous membranes are considered to be the body's first line of defence. Skin and mucous membrane secretions also have antibacterial activity, sometimes combined with mechanical action. Tears, for example, contain an antibacterial enzyme and at the same time mechanically wash away bacteria and other debris. In the nose and upper respiratory tract, mucous serves to entrap infectious agents while cilia sweep out debris and microorganisms. In the lower respiratory tract, which should remain sterile, tissue macrophages (large phagocytic cells) mobilize to engulf and destroy unwanted invaders. Acid in the gastrointestinal tract acts against enteric organisms and peristalsis moves ingested products through the gastrointestinal tract reducing the time that organisms have to multiply and (or invade mucosa). Additionally, acid secretions of the genitourinary tract help to ward off pathogens.

Should a microorganism, through injury or deliberate therapeutic intervention, bypass these outer defences by transecting skin or mucous membrane, a local inflammatory response provides another non-specific host defence mechanism. The **local inflammatory response** is a readily observable phenomenon which nurses must become familiar with in their day-to-day care of patients. The four classic symptoms of inflammation are dolour (pain), rubor (redness), tumour (swelling) and calor (heat). Loss of function may also occur. In all but neutropenic patients the white blood cell (**leucocytes**) count will be elevated. The presence of pus (purulence) confirms the presence of infection. It should be noted that, as neutropenic patients do not have sufficient white blood cells to respond to the microbial invaders, the classic signs and symptoms of infection may be muted or absent.

In **acute inflammation** (which is not *always* due to infection) the initial response is vasodilation, which causes the redness. Fluid is lost from cells into tissue causing edema (swelling). Leucocytes, mostly neutrophils, collect in the tissues. Acute inflammation then will be manifested by a cellulitis that diffuses through adjacent tissues. The suffix "itis" is added to a word to indicate inflammation, for example, cellulitis, appendicitis, pharyngitis. The cellulitis may spread via the lymphatic system (lymphangitis) and is seen as red lines extending from the infected area towards the lymph nodes which become tender and enlarged, causing lymphadenitis.

When pus is evident, the wound is *suppurating*. Pus is the debris that accumulates as a result of the encounter between microbe and neutrophil (granular leucocyte). Tissue necrosis may be present. Should the area become walled off with fibrous connective tissue, an abscess will form. If the abscess consists of pockets or subdivisions, it is referred to as a loculated abscess.

Our environment, both animate and inanimate, is colonized by microbial flora. Organisms can always be found colonizing various parts of the body without causing visible signs of tissue damage. When they cause no problems and are part of our normal flora, microorganisms are called commensals. Whether commensal or pathogen, colonization always precedes infection.

Once someone has been exposed to a significant amount of the infecting agent and the host response does not overpower the invader, the period of *incubation* ensues. This period of time varies from one situation to another. During this interval of time the host enters the *symptomatic period* when signs and symptoms of infection are present.

However, in some situations, the infection may be described as inapparent or *asymptomatic*. This happens in the absence of signs or symptoms of infection. In these cases, infection may be demonstrated by laboratory test results, for example, a rise in antibody titre. Inapparent infection also occurs during the carrier state, in which an infectious agent may be present without signs and symptoms of infection. It may be part of the incubation period or it may follow a recovery from infection. Inapparent infection represents a potential source of infection to others.

SPECIFIC DEFENCE MECHANISMS

Specific defence mechanisms refers to an immunity that may be either naturally acquired or artificially induced. **Natural immunity** occurs from having had certain diseases such as measles or chicken pox. This contact evokes an antigen-antibody response in which antibodies specific to the disease are formed. These antibodies circulate in the blood and have the ability to recognize the same agent on subsequent encounters. Such immunity generally endures for the life of the host. Natural immunity also can develop after an inapparent infection. Some diseases, most notably those in the herpes group of viruses, may manifest themselves again when natural immunity against the retained

and now resident virus falters. One of the most frequently seen examples of this phenomenon is the appearance of shingles in a patient who previously has had chicken pox or the recurrence of herpes virus infections.

Artificial immunity can be active or passive. **Active artificial immunity** is conferred by vaccines. Vaccines may be attenuated during the manufacturing process during which the causative agent is weakened to the point of still being able to provoke an antibody response, yet unable to cause disease. "Killed vaccines" (vaccines prepared from dead microorganisms) are also produced. These vaccines are still able to evoke a satisfactory antigen-antibody response. In some instances when the infectious agent produces a toxin which is responsible for disease, a toxoid or antitoxin must be given to ameliorate the effects of the toxin. While active artificial immunity often is life-long, there are a few diseases for which a booster may be recommended. Pertinent information is readily available through public health agencies.

Passive artificial immunity results from antibodies that are passed from the mother to the fetus through the placenta or to the newborn in the first few weeks of life through ingestion of breast milk. Passive artificial immunity also results from giving immune serum globulin (serum which contains antibodies) to those thought to have been exposed to a specific disease. However, while protection from disease may be conferred with passive artificial immunity, the protection is short-lived, usually no longer than a few weeks to a few months at most.

OTHER RESPONSES OF THE BODY TO INFECTION

The body has both a generalized reaction to stress and a localized reaction that occurs at the site of stress. The early general reaction of the body to the stress of invasion by infectious agents is the same as the "just feeling sick" phenomenon described by Selye (see Chapter 8). This usually includes headache, malaise, a feeling of tiredness, slight elevation in temperature and loss of appetite (sometimes followed by nausea and vomiting). In response to infectious agents, there is usually a swelling of the lymph nodes as well.

DETERMINANTS OF THE BODY'S RESPONSE TO INFECTIOUS AGENTS

The response of the body (host) to a microbial invader may range from inapparent infection where there are no observable signs and symptoms, to clinical signs and symptoms of varying degree, to acute fulminating disease and death. The degree of response is influenced by a number of factors including agent characteristics and host susceptibility. The inoculum or dose of the infecting organism, its predilection for a particular body site (for instance, hepatitis in the liver or meningococcus in the meninges), its pathogenicity (ability to cause disease) and its virulence (strength), invasiveness and portal of entry, all influence the host response. In the host itself, the quality and quantity of both non-specific and specific defence mechanisms and the degree of resistance to infection also help determine the onset, spectrum and course of disease. Thus, the same microbial agent may produce a varying degree of illness in different people, in different body sites and at different times of life.

The state of physical, mental and emotional health affects the susceptibility to infection. Proper nutrition, regular exercise, sufficient rest and sleep, emotional well-being, absence of stress and good hygiene practices all contribute to increasing the body's ability to fight off infections. To supplement this general type of resistance, immunization provides acquired immunity against many communicable diseases such as whooping cough, smallpox, measles, tetanus, typhoid fever and poliomyelitis.

Infants and small children are particularly vulnerable to infections, as are older adults. People who are acutely ill and those with chronic conditions are more susceptible to infection because of general debility and often altered nutrition patterns. A well-balanced diet with an adequate intake of protein and vitamins is necessary for the production of antibodies and the maintenance and repair of body tissues. When these nutrients are lacking in the diet, healing is impaired and the body's defence mechanisms against infection are lessened.

Poor hygiene practices, unsafe sex and the sharing of intravenous needles increase vulnerability to infection by providing a portal of entry for microbes. People with lesions or cuts in the skin or wounds of any kind (for example, the surgical patient) have an obvious entry route. Patients who have experienced trauma with excessive blood loss are particularly susceptible due to inadequate cellular oxygenation and insufficient white blood cells with which to resist infection. Conditions in which the blood supply to a part is lessened, such as peripheral vascular disease, also increase susceptibility.

Any condition which weakens the body's natural defence mechanisms decreases resistance to microbes. Diseases of the immune system, such as leukemia and AIDS, impair the production of white bloods cells and compromise the body's defences. Radiation therapy and medications, like anticancer drugs, suppress bone marrow function and consequently the production of white blood cells (lymphocytes) needed to fight infection. The use of anti-inflammatory drugs like adrenal corticosteroids increases infection risk by suppressing the immune system and inhibiting inflammatory response.

Stress and poor coping ability can also impair the immune system and increase susceptibility to infectious disease. As part of the body's general response to a stressor, the adrenal cortex secretes cortisone which increases blood sugar levels and suppresses immune and inflammatory responses. If stress is prolonged, the body's natural immune system is jeopardized, glucose stores are depleted, and exhaustion ensues, all of which compromise defences against infection. Additionally, when a person is fatigued or in poor physical condition from lack of exercise, susceptibility to infection is necessarily increased because the efficiency of all bodily processes, including the immune system, is reduced.

INFECTION CONTROL NEEDS THROUGHOUT THE LIFE CYCLE

PREGNANCY

Certain infections can be transmitted from the mother to the fetus in utero and can seriously affect the health of the fetus and newborn. The most potentially harmful infections are TORCH, HIV and genitourinary infections (Kenner and MacLaren, 1993). TORCH stands for Toxoplasmosis, Other infections (chlamydia, group B beta-hemolytic streptococcal, syphilis and varicella zoster), Rubella (German measles), Cytomegalovirus and Herpesvirus type 2 infection. This group of infections can cause congenital abnormalities in the newborn, neonatal infection and death. The human immunodeficiency virus (HIV) readily crosses the placenta and may cause AIDS in the baby. Genitourinary infections include sexually transmitted diseases and urinary tract infections. Some of these, chlamydia, gonorrhea and herpes for instance, can be transmitted to the fetus as it passes through the birth canal during birth. Women are vulnerable to urinary tract infection during pregnancy owing to urinary stasis and asymptomatic bacteriuria. If infection travels up the urinary tract to the kidneys, high fever and a severe systemic reaction may occur. Pyelonephritis has been associated with premature labour, premature rupture of the membranes and fetal loss (Fihn, 1988).

Protecting the fetus from infection during pregnancy is complicated because the disease may be asymptomatic in the mother, and yet it may injure the fetus. Pregnant women are usually tested for syphilis and immunity to rubella. An HIV-screening test is also offered to women who are at high risk for contracting AIDS. Cervical cultures are taken to identify the presence of specific infections such as gonorrhea and chlamydia, common vaginal infections like candidiasis (yeast infection), as well as group B beta-hemolytic streptococcus. Throughout pregnancy the woman must take precautions to avoid infection. If infection should occur, prompt evaluation and treatment may prevent fetal complications.

INFANCY

The first year of life is the period of greatest susceptibility to infection. All newborn infants are to some degree immunologically deficient, their passive immunity being limited to IgG (immunoglobulin G) antibodies received from the mother.(Immunoglobulin G is synthesized in the body in response to bacteria, fungi and viruses that have invaded the body.) Some protection may also be afforded the breast-fed infant by specific immunoglobulin in breast milk and colostrum. Specific IgA (immunoglobulin A) antibodies may be present and become active in the infant's gastrointestinal tract. (Immunoglobulin A is found in body secretions such as saliva, mucus, tears, sweat and bile and provides defence against pathogens on exposed sufaces, especially the intestines and bronchi.) Other protective substances include lysozyme, an enzyme that breaks down bacterial walls, lactoferrin which can be bacteriostatic for some organisms and macrophages which can engulf and destroy bacteria. By about two months of age, many of the maternally acquired antibodies are depleted and the infant's body begins to produce its own immunoglobulins. At this point immunization is begun in order to confer artificial immunity against dangerous infections including diphtheria, pertussis, tetanus and poliomyelitis. Mumps, measles and rubella vaccine is administered at 12 months of age, since maternal antibodies for these agents have a longer life span.

Infants are particularly susceptible to infections caused by gram-negative bacteria such as *Hemophilus (H.) influenzae*, gram-positive bacteria such as group B beta-hemolytic streptococci and *S. aureus* and viruses such as varicella (chickenpox) and cytomegalovirus (Kenner and MacLaren, 1993). They are vulnerable to infections that may be present in health agencies, such as the nosocomial infections caused by *S. aureus* and to infections that may be harboured by staff, as in the case of a person with a herpes simplex eruption (cold sore). Personnel working in newborn nurseries and pediatric units must be meticulous in their technique and make sure that they are free from infection themselves in order to protect the infants entrusted to their care.

CHILDHOOD

There has been a marked decline in the death rate from infections in children since the 1920s. Infection is now the fourth leading cause of death in children aged one to four years (King, Gartrell and Trovato, 1991). Young children succumb very easily to colds, intestinal infections and the common contagious diseases. Smaller children, of course, suffer more quickly from dehydration when they have a fever, are not eating well or are losing fluids from the gastrointestinal tract with vomiting and diarrhea. Children build up their immunity to the common pathogens in their environment upon exposure. Regular immunization boosters are usually given at age 18 months and 4 to 6 years.

ADOLESCENTS

Adolescents are susceptible to all types of viral and bacterial infections. Effective immunization has reduced the number of cases of the childhood diseases, so that it is rare for a teenager to come down with measles, mumps or other contagious diseases. One disease that seems to attack adolescents particularly is infectious mononucleosis, a viral infection that has a low communicability and is transmitted by droplet infection. A polio booster and an adult type of tetanus and diphtheria toxoid is given at 14 to 16 years of age.

ADULTHOOD

The occurrence of viral hepatitis reaches its peak in the 30- to 39-year-old group, predominantly among males. Among young women, urinary tract and genital chlamydial infections are common (Health and Welfare Canada, 1991). Many young adults develop immunological disorders such as allergic rhinitis (hay fever) and sinusitis, which reach their peak incidence in this age group. Eczema and asthma are also common, and arthritis begins to show up as a major problem.

During the middle years, viral infections are common, especially those affecting the respiratory tract. Most people have built up sufficient immunity by this stage of life, however, to ward off the more serious complications of these infections. Bacterial infections are not usually a severe problem, unless the defence mechanisms have been weakened by other stressors. Alcoholics and those who have disorders such as cancer, for example, seem to be much more vulnerable to infections than most middle-aged adults. Allergies causing hay fever or bronchial asthma as well as drug allergies may emerge or become more severe during middle age.

Among older adults, the respiratory tract is the principal site of serious viral infections. Pneumonia is common, and influenza is often fatal, particularly if there are existing cardiopulmonary problems such as heart disease or chronic bronchitis. Older people are also prone to urinary tract infections, which is often related to two factors: most do not drink enough fluids and there is a general slowing down of all bodily processes, with more of a tendency towards stasis of urine in the bladder. Diminishing skin integrity increases the risk of infection for the older person. With aging, there is also a decline in the efficiency of immune response to infectious agents. Neoplastic disorders (such as cancer) tend to reduce it further. Treatment of disorders by drugs that suppress the immune reaction, as for example chemotherapy, which is often used in treating cancer, may further impair resistance to infection.

COMMON PROBLEMS

People can develop an infection in almost any tissue of the body. Five of the most common infections will be outlined here. These are urinary tract infections, lower respiratory tract infections, wound infections, gastroenteritis and bacteremia.

URINARY TRACT INFECTION

Urinary tract infection (UTI) involving only the mucosal surface of the bladder is called cystitis. When the interstitial tissue of the kidney is involved, it is referred to as pyelonephritis. While urine is normally sterile, occasionally an asymptomatic bacteriuria may occur, which is the persistence of bacteria in urine without any symptoms.

Common Causes and Risk Factors

The bacteria most commonly associated with UTI are for the most part those that colonize the lower gastrointestinal tract such as *Escherichia coli* (E. coli), *Klebsiella*, *Proteus*, enterococci, *Enterobacter*, *Serratia* and *Pseudomonas*. In the immunocompromised, *Candida albicans* is occasionally the causative agent.

About 40 percent of all nosocomial infections are due to UTI (Stamm, 1991). While 10 percent of hospitalized patients require a catheter, up to 25 percent of these patients may acquire an infection during their stay, usually as a result of the catheter (APIC, 1983). After 14 days of indwelling catheterization, fully 50 percent of patients become infected (Stamm, 1991; APIC, 1983). After one month, few escape acquiring an infection. Major risk factors include not only catheterization, especially lengthy catheterization, but also other instrumentation of the urinary tract. Females are at greater risk for infection because of a shorter urethra. Improper catheter care techniques and periurethral colonization with bowel flora further add to the risk. Certain diseases such as diabetes or multiple sclerosis may predispose patients to UTI.

Bacteria gain entry to the bladder either by ascending the thin mucous layer between the outer catheter surface and the urethra (periurethrally), or intraluminally within the column of urine inside the catheter. The infecting organism may have colonized the meatus and lower urethra. Bacteria may have originated not only from bowel flora but possibly from the hands of hospital staff manipulating the catheter or touching the perineal area. This can happen whether gloves are worn or not. Good technique is mandatory whether or not gloves are worn. Hand washing must always be done immediately before and after any catheter manipulation or procedure.

Pathogenesis

The microorganism that enters the urinary tract intraluminally most likely enters the catheter collecting system at some point where it can be opened, either the junction between the catheter and tubing or from the emptying spigot when the bag is drained. Organisms ascend the column of urine in the drainage tube. They also may enter the bladder by reflux should the drainage bag be inadvertently lifted above bladder level.

Signs and Symptoms

Signs and symptoms specific to UTI include suprapubic pain and urethral burning. If a catheter is not present, the typical symptoms include urgency, frequency and dysuria. Fever is usually absent. Should a catheter be in situ, those symptoms are obscured. However, at least half of all patients with UTI will not have any of the above symptoms, but only a bacteriuria.

About one to two percent of patients with UTI will develop bacteremia (presence of bacteria in the blood), which is manifested by fever, chills, sweats and possible even septic shock. Mortality is less than 10 percent if appropriately treated (APIC, 1983). Rare complications include epididymides and prostatitis with localized and systemic signs and symptoms of infection.

Prevention and Control Measures

The risk of acquiring a UTI is much greater in the catheterized patient. Many hospitals follow guidelines published by the Centers for Disease Control (CDC) in the United States and by the Laboratory Centre for Disease Control (LCDC) in Ottawa. If at all possible, catheterization should be avoided altogether. If catheters are necessary, the duration of catheterization should be kept as short as possible or the use of intermittent catheters may be considered, and a condom catheter may be considered for male patients. Insertion of catheters must be done aseptically following hospital procedure. The closed drainage system must be considered sterile and aseptic precautions must be maintained when entering the system. However, the system must not be entered unless absolutely necessary. Because drainage bags may become colonized (from repeated emptyings) it is important to avoid causing reflux of urine, which can occur if the bag is lifted above bladder level or if the bag is compressed. The perineum is an area that is heavily colonized with microbial flora. Therefore, it is important to ensure that patients are kept clean and at the same time to inspect the catheter site and collecting system for signs of crusting or soreness.

The perineum should be washed with soap and water, rinsed well and dried once a shift. The meatus should be inspected, ensuring that the catheter can rotate freely. Any crusting or other problems must be reported. There is no set time for changing urinary catheters; however, problems such as bypassing or blocking may indicate a need for change.

Very often then it is the nurse member of the health care team who can exercise the greatest influence and have the greatest impact on catheter-related infection. In summary, this is done by recommending alternatives or reducing the duration of catheterization, maintaining asepsis in all catheter-related procedures, maintaining gravity drain and maintaining good hygiene when caring for the patient.

LOWER RESPIRATORY TRACT INFECTIONS

Pneumonia, the most common expression of lower respiratory infection, may be described as infection of the pulmonary parenchyma (the functional elements of the lung) with consolidation (solidification) and exudation (the escape of fluid from blood cells with deposition in tissues). Once regarded as the "old man's friend" because it eased the elderly and debilitated to a reasonably quick death, pneumonia remains the most significant cause of death due to infection acquired in inpatient facilities.

Common Causes and Risk Factors

The bacteria most commonly associated with nosocomial pneumonia include *Klebsiella*, *Enterobacter*, *Proteus*, *Pseudomonas* and *Serratia* among gram-negative microorganisms, while *Streptococcus pneumoniae* and *S. aureus* predominate among gram-positive organisms. In immunocompromised patients, pathogens may include *Aspergillus* (a yeast), cytomegalovirus (CMV) or *Pneumocystis carinii* (PCP, which is a protozoan). Opportunist bacteria such as *Actineobacter* may pose a risk to ventilated patients. Occasionally during a community epidemic of influenza, a viral pneumonia may spread among hospitalized patients generally while pneumonia due to respiratory syncytial virus (RSV) may be seen in children.

Nosocomial pneumonia develops in about one to two percent of hospital patients, occurring with greater frequency in high-risk patients (APIC, 1983). High-risk patients include those in Intensive Care Units and those who are postoperative, intubated or immunocompromised. The major risk factors for individuals include intubation, intermittent positive pressure breathing apparatus, recent abdominal or thoracic surgery, immunosuppression and decreased level of consciousness, which may lead either to aspiration or impaired cough reflex. Other risk factors include pre-existing pulmonary disease or injury and exposure to smoke. In healthy individuals, the respiratory tract is lined with cilia which continuously sweep foreign bodies including microorganisms outward and away from the lower respiratory tract. This defence mechanism is bypassed when patients are intubated. Prolonged exposure to smoke will destroy cilia.

Pathogenesis

All people are colonized with bacteria particularly in the oropharynx. Normally mostly gram-positive cocci reside in the mouth and oropharynx, although a few species of gram-negative rods may be found there also. The stomach, due to its acidity, contains relatively few microorganisms. In sick hospitalized patients, however, this all changes. The oropharynx becomes colonized heavily with gram-negative bacteria. This predisposition to upper airway colonization increases with the severity of illness, prolonged antibiotic treatment and length of hospitalization. Patients may aspirate these microorganisms into the lower tracheobronchial tree and, if clearance mechanisms cannot get rid of these intruders, then nosocomial pneumonia may ensue. Should an endotracheal tube be in situ, contaminated aerosols may be delivered directly into the tracheobronchial tree. These aerosols may contain gram-negative rods as these organisms require moisture. The presence of an endotracheal tube or a tracheostomy or suctioning will facilitate the entry of these organisms to the lower respiratory tract. When patients are intubated and expected to be hospitalized for some time, antacids or histamine-2 receptor antagonists are administered to prevent possible erosion and ulcer formation in the stomach lining. Decreasing the natural acidity provides a more hospitable environment for gram-negative organisms adding to the risk of nosocomial pneumonia through the aspiration of stomach contents.

Signs and Symptoms

Patients with pneumonia usually have fever, cough, chest pain and produce purulent sputum. On examination, the patient may exhibit signs of pulmonary consolidation indicated by abnormal breath sounds such as crackles or bronchial breathing. Fever and tachypnea may be noted and may be the only signs present in an immunocompromised patient. When patients are on a ventilator, have just had surgery or have a reduced level of consciousness, it may be difficult to elicit these signs. As well, other clinical syndromes may confuse the picture when presentations are similar to those of nosocomial pneumonia. Such diseases might include congestive heart failure, pulmonary embolus, adult respiratory distress syndrome, atelectasis and aspiration. Radiological findings may help confirm the diagnosis of pneumonia. Findings include a new infiltrate (usually segmental, patchy or lobar) occasionally accompanied by a pleural effusion. A previously present infiltrate may enlarge, suggesting a new super-imposed infection, while cavitation of the lung is very suggestive of infection.

Prevention and Control Measures

The CDC and LCDC have issued guidelines for the prevention and control of nosocomial pneumonia to which many hospitals look for guidance. Briefly, it is important that the hospital have policies and procedures in place to ensure that respiratory therapy equipment is properly managed and reprocessed. Certain patients will require particular attention. For example, those undergoing anesthesia, especially those having abdominal or thoracic surgery, and patients with chronic pulmonary dysfunction or musculoskeletal chest abnormalities are at increased risk. Patients should be brought to an optimum state of health whenever possible before surgery, for example, they should stop smoking, lose weight and infections should be resolved. Preoperative teaching is essential to prepare the patient for coughing, deep breathing and whenever feasible, early ambulation. To achieve these ends postoperatively it will be necessary to control pain. Incisional support may be needed to help the patient cough effectively.

Hand washing remains the keystone of infection control practice. Hands must be washed after any contact with respiratory secretions, even after removing gloves, and hands must also be washed after contact with patients who have a tracheostomy or those who are intubated. Emphasis must be placed on good hand washing after suctioning and any manipulation of respiratory therapy equipment, including care of a tracheostomy.

Fluids being used in nebulizers or humidifiers must be sterile and must be dispensed aseptically. Any unused fluid in dated supply bottles should be discarded after 24 hours and a new bottle used when needed. Multi-dose vials for respiratory therapy must be stored according to manufacturer's instruction and discarded on expiry. Fluid reservoirs on equipment should be filled immediately before use only and not set up "just-in-case." Fluid in reservoirs should be discarded first before refilling rather than just "topping up." Water in tubing should be discarded. Newer types of tubing may make opening the system for this purpose unnecessary. Hospital policy regarding the frequency of change for particular pieces of equipment must be observed. All tubing and breathing circuits must be changed between patients and properly reprocessed. Adequate cleaning of all equipment must be done first whether equipment is to receive high-level disinfection or sterilization. Suctioning should be done only as indicated by the patient's condition using clean gloves on both hands. Sterile fluid only must be used to rinse the catheter. Suction bottles and tubing must be changed between patients except bottles which may be used for more than one patient in short stay areas such as the recovery room. However, these must be changed at the end of the day. In all instances, this equipment must receive high-level disinfection or sterilization. Room air humidifiers (the sort bought in hardware stores) are not to be used as they become contaminated readily and are difficult to clean and all but impossible to disinfect.

SURGICAL WOUND INFECTIONS

Postoperative surgical wound infection accounts for approximately 25 percent of all nosocomial infections (Haley et al., 1985). The likelihood of any surgical wound becoming infected varies according to its site, the general condition of the patient and the degree and type of contamination to which a wound is exposed. Surgical wound infections may be deep or superficial and they may involve implants such as artificial joint replacements, cardiac valves or synthetic vascular patches, for example.

Common Causes

Surgical wound infections are almost always bacterial in origin. The specific bacteria likely to cause infection at a given site usually are predictable according to the likely source of contamination. When contamination occurs from an exogenous source, the most likely agents are S. aureus and Group A beta-haemolytic streptococci. Contaminating bacteria from endogenous sources can usually be linked to the flora at the operative site. For example, in bowel surgery, the most common causative organisms include the enteric gram-negative rods found in the gut (E. coli, Klebsiella, Group D Streptococci, Bacteroides fragilis, Clostridum, to name a few). In very clean procedures where only sterile tissue is entered, such as in cardiac bypass surgery, the infecting microorganisms are likely to be skin flora such as S. epidermidis or S. aureus. Many of these endogenous infections are polymicrobial in nature.

Risk Factors and Pathogenesis

Risk factors for increased likelihood of infection associated with the host include advanced age, extreme obesity, malnutrition, anemia, chronic obstructive lung disease and diabetes mellitus. Some of these factors may indicate a reduced blood supply to the operative site, thus decreased oxygenation and lessened phagocytic activity. Other factors include a decreased antibody-antigen response and hypoalbuminemia.

Infection remote from the operative site, for instance, a pressure ulcer, is likely to contain a large amount of bacteria. Similarly, certain skin conditions may contribute to heavier colonization of the operative site. Alternatively, bacteria may travel via the lymphatic system from its source to the operative field. Areas of the body better supplied with blood, such as the head and upper trunk, generally have a lower rate of infection due to better perfusion and greater phagocytic activity. Another important factor in surgical wound infection is trauma, in particular when trauma results in heavy contamination of the area, as happens in some motor vehicle or industrial accidents.

The events in the intraoperative period are of prime importance in determining whether or not wound infection will ensue. Much depends on the skill of the surgeon and the particular techniques used. Influencing the situation at the same time are the two other factors already discussed: host susceptibility and the degree of contamination present.

Good operative technique includes expeditious surgery, gentle handling of tissue, controlling bleeding and hematoma formation, eradication of dead space, minimizing the presence of devitalized tissue, removal of foreign materials, choice of suture material and avoiding drains, especially penrose drains, where possible. There are however specific indications for closed drains which are preferable to penrose drains. Drains should not exit through the operative wound, but through an adjacent small incision. Depending on the degree of wound contamination that has occurred, the surgeon may choose to delay closure of the wound until the amount of contamination has been reduced, which is usually about five days.

It has been shown that the more people present in an operating theatre, the higher the bacterial air count. Few personnel who are carriers of pathogenic bacteria actually transmit bacteria to patients during surgery. Nevertheless, it seems prudent to restrict the number of people in a theatre during surgery, to reduce the flow of traffic in and out of the room and to ensure that operating theatres are constructed so that air changes occur about 25 times per hour. All of these considerations will reduce the bacterial air count during the course of an operation.

Signs and Symptoms

The classical signs and symptoms of surgical wound infection are pain, redness, induration (hardening), poor healing, dehiscence (separation of all the layers of a surgical wound) and purulent drainage. Systemic manifestations, such as fever, anorexia and malaise, may also be present.

Prevention and Control Measures

The prevention of surgical wound infections relies largely on the skill of the surgeon. However, there are some host factors and occasionally environmental factors in which the nurse can play a role. Whenever elective surgery is planned, the patient should be brought to a state of optimum health. For example, he or she should lose weight and stop smoking, nutrition should be improved, and chronic diseases such as diabetes should be brought under control and remote infections should be treated. Preoperatively, patients must understand the importance of frequent deep breathing and coughing when secretions are present so that nosocomial pneumonia does not develop and interfere with

oxygen perfusion. The importance of early ambulation must be stressed. The duration of hospital stay preoperatively must be as short as possible. A preoperative wash with a hospital-approved antiseptic may be desirable, and hair removal must be done by clippers or depilation only as close to the time of surgery as possible and only as much as needed to facilitate surgery. Should prophylactic antibiotics be ordered, timing of the first and subsequent doses is important to ensure that antibiotic levels are highest when surgery is actually taking place. The dose and timing will vary from one antibiotic to another. Personnel must adhere to hospital policy in regards to preoperative scrubbing and operating room attire. Personnel with infections or draining wounds *must not* work in an operating room suite. Intraoperatively, the charge nurse in the operating room may be responsible for seeing that traffic is controlled, that the air system has a maintenance schedule, that necessary supplies and equipment are at hand and that the operation proceeds expeditiously.

Postoperatively, the nurse may be responsible for ensuring that prophylactic antibiotics are administered until finished, that patients ambulate as soon as they are able, that deep breathing and coughing is done and that the wound is inspected regularly and any signs and symptoms of infection are noted and reported. In addition to the previously described signs and symptoms, nurses should also be alert to the presence of fluid collections, such as seromas or hematomas which may lead to infection. As always, meticulous hand washing and careful disposal of secretions and excretions are mandatory. Hands must be washed before dressing changes and after the disposal of used dressings. "No-touch" technique using sterile instruments must be used to maintain asepsis. Alternatively, sterile gloves may be used where direct contact is required.

GASTROENTERITIS

Gastroenteritis may be defined as increased bowel activity or impaired bowel function caused by an infectious agent. Diarrhea or vomiting may be present with or without associated systemic symptoms. The identity of the infectious agent may or may not be established.

Common Causes

The most common bacterial agents that cause gastroenteritis seen in patients admitted to hospital in Canada include *Salmonella, Shigella, Yersinnia, Campylobacter* and *Aeromonas*. Some bacteria produce toxins in food (for example, *S. aureus, C. botulinum*, and *E. coli*). Also, pathogenic *E. coli* is a significant cause of diarrhea in newborn nurseries. Viral agents most commonly seen in pediatric facilities include rotavirus, parvovirus, enterovirus and adenovirus, although laboratories in Canada do not always test for these agents. The two parasitic infestations most commonly seen in Canada are *Entamoeba histolytica* and *Giardia lamblia* (beaver fever). Occasionally patients may return from tropical countries with parasitic infestation, for example, *Strongyloides*. However, tropical parasites do not survive in our northern climate once excreted from the host.

For hospitalized patients, *C. difficile* becomes a significant pathogen, causing pseudomembranous colitis. This particular disease can be attributed to antibiotic usage. With certain antibiotics, normal bowel bacteria may be suppressed allowing the very small numbers of *C. difficile* present in some people to grow out of proportion in comparison to the usual ratio. When *C. difficile* exists in large quantities, it is capable of behaving pathogenically, causing toxin production during severe diarrhea and the formation of a false membrane along the walls of the lower bowel. There have been a number of *C. difficile* diarrhea outbreaks in hospitals involving person-to-person transmission via fecal–oral transmission. This happens easily when due care is not taken, as this organism is very hardy and can survive in the environment for long periods of time.

Risk Factors

For the most part, enteric pathogens are either food- and water-borne or are transmitted by the fecal–oral route. Some also are transmitted by direct contact such as in oral–anal intercourse. In food- or water-borne illness, the spread of disease may be attributed to fecal contamination through lack of adequate sewage facilities or, in some countries, the use of night soil. Food handlers who lack good hygiene and carriers of enteric disease may spread it readily to others. In crowded living conditions, the spread of infection is facilitated by the very real difficulties of maintaining both safe sewage disposal and a clean food supply. These conditions are exacerbated in times of war or natural disaster and the subsequent displacement of large numbers of people. In developed countries, contamination of well water or of shellfish can occur quite readily if proper precautions or adequate community planning are not undertaken.

Occasionally, food-borne illness or food poisoning can result from a single source. This may typically arise when a number of people become ill who have shared a single meal at a restaurant or social gathering. It is possible to make a relatively accurate assumption about the etiologic agent based on clinical signs and symptoms, the time frame and the likely food vehicle. In some daycare centres the parasite *Giardia lamblia* has been found in over 90 percent of the attendees who are not toilet trained, suggesting person-to-person spread (Plorde, 1990). Hepatitis A virus has also been spread under similar circumstances. Several enteric diseases are spread by receptive anal intercourse or oral–anal intercourse. Disease that can be spread in these ways include Hepatitis A, *Salmonella*, *Shigella*, *Campylobacter*, *Entamoeba histolytica* and some venereal diseases.

Impaired host defences may predispose a person to acquiring a gastrointestinal infectious disease. Gastric acid in the stomach usually provides protection by reducing or eliminating ingested organisms. A lowering of gastric acidity occurs most often in premature infants or in older adults. Medications designed to reduce stomach acidity may actually provide a favourable environment for potential pathogens, and those with partial gastrectomy or vagotomy are at higher risk. In hospitals, overcrowding and lack of proper hand washing facilities may contribute to the risk. Another contributing factor in some outbreaks is the ability of some bacteria such as *C. difficile* to survive in the environment or on equipment that is improperly processed after use.

Pathogenesis

Microorganisms responsible for enteric illness characterized by frequent fluid intestinal evacuations attack the host in several different ways. Some organisms, for example, *Vibrio parahaemolyticus*, will act directly on the wall of the intestine, stimulating secreting action and producing a watery diarrhea. Others, such as *Shigella*, invade the mucosa, producing dysentery (inflammation of the intestine), possibly bloody stools, and tenesmus (ineffectual straining at stool), while others, for example *Salmonella typhi* (typhoid fever), may penetrate to local lymphatic tissue and enter the blood stream, possibly producing a bacteremia. Some bacteria produce a toxin which, in the case of *S. aureus*, acts on the vomiting centre of the brain. This can quickly create problems with dehydration and cardiac disease in an older adult host. Some microorganisms can cause disease in several ways.

Signs and Symptoms

The frequent fluid intestinal evacuations that occur with gastroenteritis can be characterized in three different ways. The most common form is watery diarrhea. The loss of fluid occurs from the proximal small intestine. The diarrhea may be accompanied by nausea, vomiting, fever and abdominal pain. In most instances, the course is intense but brief, generally lasting from one to three days.

Dysentery begins rapidly, but stool may be of smaller volume and contain blood or pus. Fever, abdominal pain, cramps and tenesmus frequently accompany dysentery but vomiting is not as frequent. The colon is affected by direct invasion or by production of cell toxins. While blood and pus may be present, fluid loss is relatively small as the colon does not absorb or secrete fluid at the same rate as the small bowel. Most cases of dysentery are resolved in two to seven days.

Enteric fever is a systemic infection which originates in the intestinal tract. Diarrhea is usually mild and develops *after* fever and abdominal pain. The causative microorganism spreads through the mucosa of the small bowel to adjacent organs such as the liver and biliary tree. Bacteremia occurs frequently. The most common disease associated with this infection is *Salmonella typhi*, otherwise known as typhoid fever.

Prevention and Control Measures

A sanitary sewage disposal system and a safe water supply are fundamental to building a safe community. Additionally, the food supply must be delivered to the end-user free of harmful pathogens. People handling food and water for other's consumption must understand and practise good hygiene.

The most important and most common mode of transmission for enteric pathogens is the fecal–oral route via the hands of personnel. Therefore, hand washing remains the most important activity in preventing the spread of disease. Hands must be washed as necessary, before, during and after patient care, before eating or handling food, after using the toilet and after touching equipment in the patient care environment. Some enteric pathogens can survive for long periods of time in the environment. Not only is hand washing important, then, but a regular maintenance cleaning schedule and provision for spot cleaning and adequate reprocessing of items such as bed pans are important as well. Yet staff should be aware that spores of some microorganisms, notably C. *difficile*, survive exposure to hospital disinfectants. This reemphasizes the importance of good hygiene and good hand washing. Protective attire must be used when there is likely to be direct contact with stool. Gloves and water-impermeable gowns or aprons should be used. Gloves must be changed on completion of each task and hands must be washed. They must not be worn from one patient to another nor used for subsequent tasks on the same patient. Gowns must be changed between patients and whenever they become soiled. In some instances (in pediatric units, for example), patients must be isolated. Those with the same pathogen may be placed together in the same room (sometimes referred to as "cohorting" patients).

Hand washing and excretory disposal facilities (bedpan decontaminators) must be adequate, overcrowding must be avoided and the staff-patient ratio must be balanced so as to mitigate risks of cross-infection. These factors are crucial to good infection control in any care setting. Finally, staff should be aware that some people are asymptomatic excreters of certain pathogens, and so care with all secretions and excretions (including hand washing) is mandatory to all aspects of patient care.

Therapy for gastrointestinal infections is generally supportive, using fluid replacement and maintaining electrolyte balance. In cases of viral diarrhea, it is the only therapy available and may be necessary also for patients with bacterial diarrhea.

BACTEREMIA

Bacteremia is the presence of microorganisms (bacteria) in the blood. Terms also used specifically are viraemia, fungemia and parisitemia. These organisms are present either as part of an infectious disease (Hepatitis B, for example) or reflect a serious and uncontrolled disease process such as the seeding of microbes into the blood stream from pneumonia or pyelonephritis or direct introduction through a vascular device. Bacteremias may therefore be defined as primary or secondary. Primary bacteremias occur in patients who have no recognized site of infection. However, the two major sources for primary bacteremia are related to intravascular catheters and infusion systems or the gut flora of immunocompromised hosts. Two-thirds of bacteremias are considered secondary as there is a recognizable source of infection such as pneumonia, UTI or a surgical wound (APIC, 1983). Patients are described as septic or having septicemia when the bacteremia is accompanied by oliguria, hypotension, dulling of consciousness and acidosis progressing to septic shock. Occasionally a transient bacteremia will manifest itself after manipulation of, or trauma to, a body site that has a population of normal flora. This usually is of no lasting importance, except that it may be a significant factor in the development of infective endocarditis.

Common Causes and Risk Factors

The most common causes of primary nosocomial bacteremias are *Klebsiella, Enterobacter, Serratia* and *Pseudomonas*. In secondary bacteremia, the causative organism will be found both in blood and at the site from which the infection spread. Thus, in bacteremias associated with UTI, the agent is likely to be a gram-negative organism such as E. *coli*, while staphylococci would more likely be found in a surgical wound.

In primary bacteremia, the use of an intravascular catheter provides a ready pathway into the bloodstream. The organism may come from the patient's own microbial flora or from the hands of hospital personnel inserting or manipulating the catheter or its dressing. Infusion fluids are rarely contaminated at the time of manufacture, but can become contaminated in use by injection of medications, accidental disconnection, monitoring procedures or careless handling of the tubing or ports. Catheter-related sepsis occurs about ten times as often as infusion-related sepsis (APIC, 1983). In secondary bacteremia, the risk factors are as those for the underlying disease.

Pathogenesis

Patients with bacteremia are seriously ill, and require careful observation and immediate treatment. With septicemia, there is increased cardiac output and decreased total peripheral venous resistance. As shock progresses, decreased urinary output occurs as does acidosis, lactate accumulation, hyponatremia and elevation of serum creatinine. This may be followed by disseminated intravascular coagulation (DIC) resulting in a low platelet count, prolonged prothrombin time, low fibrinogen concentration and the presence of fibrin degradation products in the blood.

Signs and Symptoms

The signs and symptoms include fever, chills, perspiration, weakness and myalgia. The signs and symptoms pertinent to disease in the underlying site also will be evidenced in secondary bacteremia. Septic shock which leads to death in over fifty percent of cases proceeds to hypotension, oliguria and DIC (APIC, 1983).

Prevention and Control Measures

Primary bacteremia can be prevented by taking care when inserting and maintaining vascular lines. First, the use of intravascular lines should be done only as necessary or in anticipation of the need for access. A higher rate of infection is associated with lower extremity use, as in the development of phlebitis. Due to this, lines should be inserted in upper extremities. Hands must be washed before insertion or manipulation, and gloves may be needed according to hospital policy for some procedures. The area of insertion should be cleaned with a hospital-approved skin antiseptic first. The catheter should be kept as secure as possible using a sterile dressing. The intravenous site must be inspected daily and any problems, such as redness or purulence, should be reported immediately. Lines and catheters must be changed according to hospital policy for each particular type of catheter and line as well as after blood products or lipid emulsion. The system must not be entered unnecessarily. Irrigation and blood sampling must also be avoided. Should primary bacteremia occur, it is quite likely that the vascular catheter will be removed if it is considered the source of the microorganism circulating and being seeded into the blood. Removal of a foreign body also will facilitate antimicrobial therapy.

Secondary bacteremias occur less frequently. Then prevention is aimed at dealing with the source of infection and eradicating it, for example, by treatment of pneumonia, UTI, surgical wound or abscess by antibiotics and/or drainage. When the source of infection is not known or patients are very ill or immunocompromised, the physician likely will order broad-spectrum antimicrobial coverage empirically.

ASSESSING INFECTION PREVENTION AND CONTROL NEEDS

Every patient in a health agency has the potential for developing infection, as does every health care worker. The nurse must always be observant for infections in patients. In the nursing history and physical assessment, information is collected about factors that may influence the development of infection, the general health status of the patient (for example, the current state of functional abilities and state of health at the time of admission to the agency), and any existing infectious process. This information is supplemented by data about the patient's past and current health problems, and the physician's diagnostic and therapeutic plans of care as found in the patient's record. Laboratory tests and x-ray reports also provide valuable information.

NURSING HEALTH HISTORY

Much of the health history pertaining to infection prevention and control is incorporated into the data collection for each individual need. For instance, information about the usual patterns of hygiene and nutrition, recent changes in these patterns or problems that might suggest infection or place the patient at risk for infection are gathered during the specific need assessment. In addition, information is obtained about general susceptibility to infections, recent exposure to infectious agents, any factors that may place the patient at risk of infection and immunization status.

PHYSICAL ASSESSMENT

Ultimately, the nurse's observations of the patient are of primary importance in identifying infections. The nurse watches for signs and symptoms of the body's systemic and local responses to invasion. The vital signs — temperature, pulse and respirations — are particularly helpful in early detection of infection. Statements of tiredness, loss of energy, headache, loss of appetite or generally not feeling well are also among the early warning signs of a systemic reaction to infection. If a patient makes any of these statements, it is always wise to check the temperature, pulse and respirations to see if they are elevated. Lymph nodes draining the infected area may also be enlarged. Both subjective and objective findings should be reported promptly.

As we discussed earlier, tissue invasion may be manifested by localized signs and symptoms, namely pain or tenderness, redness, swelling, warmth and some loss of function of the affected body part. A foul odour may also be present due either to the by-products of bacterial metabolism or to the death of cells and tissue. These signs and symptoms vary according to the system or body site involved.

Infection Prevention and Control

Health and Illness Patterns

- Do you frequently experience infections? If so, how often? What type? Do you know what usually causes these infections? How were they treated?
- When did you last have an infection? How was it treated?
- Have you recently been exposed to any infectious diseases that you know of? If yes, where? How?
- Do you have a history of any acute or chronic illnesses (for example, asthma, diabetes, multiple sclerosis or leukemia) that may place you at risk for infection? Have you had surgery recently?
- Are you taking any medications or treatments (for example, radiation therapy, anti-cancer drugs or anti-inflammatory drugs) that might increase the risk of infection?

Health Promotion and Health Protection Patterns

- What do you ordinarily do to prevent infection?
- Have you been immunized against communicable diseases? If so, what immunizations have you had? When were they done?
- Are you on any precautionary measures for infection? If so, why? What precautions are being taken?

Other signs of infection the nurse should observe for include secretions from the nose and throat, coughing, sneezing or the expectoration of sputum by a patient. Exudates from wounds or other breaks in the skin, or from any of the body orifices, should also warn the nurse of the possibility of infection, as should any vomiting or diarrhea.

DIAGNOSTIC TESTS

Blood tests are usually ordered to determine the presence of infection in the body. These include a white blood cell (leucocyte) count, differential white blood count (different types of white blood cells) and erythrocyte sedimentation rate. Generally, increases in the total white blood count, neutrophils, lymphocytes and erythrocyte sedimentation rate are associated with acute and chronic bacterial and viral infections. Specimens of body fluids and wound drainage are also taken to identify the pathogen(s) causing the infection. When collecting specimens for microbiological examination, care must be taken to ensure that the specimens are not contaminated with organisms in the environment.

Urine specimens   In order that patients with urinary tract infections receive the best possible treatment, great care must be taken in the procuring and subsequent handling of urine specimens. Voided specimens must be obtained by the clean catch (midstream) method while catheter specimens must be obtained aseptically, either on insertion, before the drainage tube is connected, or after-

wards by aspirating through the puncture port or the catheter tubing itself. Foley catheter tips are not acceptable for culturing. The techniques for obtaining these specimens are detailed in Chapter 20.

Sputum specimens   Obtaining a good sputum sample is a challenge because expectorated sputum will become contaminated with whatever microorganisms are present as it passes through the oropharynx. However, there are a few steps the caregiver can take to help achieve a more accurate result. Because secretions tend to accumulate when one is asleep, an early morning specimen is best. The patient should be instructed to cough deeply since the *lower* respiratory tract is affected. It is advisable to have patients remove dentures first if necessary and to rinse the mouth out with plain water. This will help decrease the amount of contamination from the oropharynx. Once a proper specimen has been obtained, it should be sent to the laboratory as quickly as possible. The tests most frequently ordered are for culture and sensitivity and gram stain. However, if a search for tuberculosis, pertussis or legionella is ordered, this must be noted on the requisition. Otherwise, laboratories will not routinely do these tests, nor will they process specimens which appear to be saliva.

Wound specimens   It is important when obtaining a specimen from surgical wounds that the specimen reflect as accurately as possible the agents that are responsible for the infection. The wound should be cleansed first with normal saline. Fresh pus should be expressed from what appears to be the most affected part of the wound. This is important as fresh pus is most likely to contain live bacteria. Care must be taken to avoid contaminating the specimen with surrounding skin bacteria. The specimen should be sent for processing as soon as possible. The same procedures generally apply to taking a sample from any wound including pressure or vascular ulcers or traumatic wounds that appear to be infected.

Stool specimens   Stool specimens ("walnut-sized" or the liquid equivalent) are placed in clean, non-sterile containers for culture and sensitivity and for toxin detection. If other than culture and sensitivity is ordered, it must be specified on the requisition so that laboratory personnel can select the appropriate testing method. With some tests, the specimen must reach the laboratory minutes after it has been obtained, so one should ascertain the proper procedure for each test.

Blood specimens   Bacteremia is a serious disease with a thirty percent mortality rate overall and a fifty percent rate in the event of septic shock (APIC, 1983). Expeditious treatment aimed at eradicating the causative organism(s) is imperative. To this end, a sample of the patient's blood is obtained by aseptic venipuncture and sent to the laboratory for culture and sensitivity. Meticulous technique is critical if an accurate result is to be obtained. The skin over the venipuncture site must be cleansed thoroughly with a hospital-approved antiseptic and left to dry. Blood is drawn aseptically through a needle into a syringe or tube. The operator must avoid palpating the site once it has been prepared. The only time that blood can be drawn through a vascular catheter is if it cannot be obtained by venipuncture. Whenever possible at least ten millilitres should be collected from adults with a correspondingly smaller amount from children. Two to three samples of adequate volume are collected. Timing of samples will be dependent on the nature of the bacteremic episodes or underlying disease.

DIAGNOSING INFECTION-RELATED PROBLEMS

When patients are at risk for developing an infection, the diagnosis *High risk for infection* is used. This diagnosis describes people whose host defences are compromised, rendering them susceptible to pathogenic agents from endogenous or exogenous sources. Any number of health problems and conditions may contribute to the risk of infection including pathophysiological factors such as chronic diseases (such as respiratory diseases, cancer or diabetes), immunodeficiency, impaired skin and mucous membrane integrity or impaired circulation; treatment related factors, such as medications (steroids, insulin or immunosuppressants), intravenous therapy or enteral feedings; situational factors, such

as a history of recurrent infections, malnutrition, stress or lack of immunizations; and maturational factors, such as age. Treatment measures the nurse may implement focus on minimizing the patient's exposure to microorganisms and increasing the resistance to infection, for example, by improving nutritional status and infection control self-care practices in a person with diabetes. If infection is present in the patient, the diagnosis may be stated as a collaborative problem, for example, *Potential Complication: Septicemia* (Carpenito, 1993). This indicates the nurse's dependent functions in providing care — to implement medical treatments and monitor the patient for related complications.

A known or suspected infection brings additional problems such as controlling the spread of infection to others. In cases where the patient is at risk for transferring opportunistic or pathogenic agents to others, the diagnosis, *High risk for infection transmission*, may be used to direct protective measures towards preventing the spread of infection (Carpenito, 1993). People who are separated or isolated because of airborne communicable disease such as meningitis may experience associated problems. Some may worry and feel anxious about the cause of infection, about spreading it to others and about the seriousness of infection and what it means. These people may experience feelings of hopelessness or powerlessness if they think they have lost control over the situation. They may also feel socially isolated because of limited contact with others or they may experience sensory deprivation because they are unable to engage in customary leisure and recreational activities. Some common examples of diagnoses for infection-related problems are listed below.

- *High risk for infection related to malnutrition, skin lesions, and poor hygiene practices.*
- *High risk for infection related to suppressed immune response secondary to corticosteroid therapy.*
- *High risk for infection related to the presence of a Foley catheter.*
- *Social isolation related to airborne isolation precautions.*
- *High risk for diversional activity deficit related to isolation for airborne infection.*

PLANNING INFECTION PREVENTION AND CONTROL INTERVENTIONS

The prevention and control of infection is inherent in the planning and implementation of all nursing activities. The basic goals of nursing action in regard to infection are: to prevent infection, to control infection, to promote comfort and lessen or prevent problems associated with infection and to promote infection control self-care practices. The specific plan of care for a patient is based on the nursing diagnoses and must take into account the nature of the infection, the portal of entry of the opportunist or pathogen, its exit routes from the body and its mode of transfer.

Some examples of goals or expected outcomes for patients who are at risk for infectious processes are listed below.

- Patient will describe factors that may cause infection and the precautions that must be taken to prevent infection.
- Patient will demonstrate effective hand washing technique.
- Patient will remain free of nosocomial infection while in hospital.
- Patient will remain free of surgical wound infection.

IMPLEMENTING INFECTION PREVENTION AND CONTROL INTERVENTIONS

During the late eighteenth and throughout the nineteenth and twentieth centuries, discoveries about the role of microorganisms were made that enabled scientists and other leaders to develop strategies that controlled and prevented the spread of infection. Try to imagine what a hospital or a long-term care facility would be like if concern with the microbial world were unnecessary. There would be no need for protective attire such as gloves, gowns or masks. There would be no need for sterile equipment. Industries devoted to providing hospitals with sterile goods simply would not exist. However, that is not the way the world is. We do have to deal with the unseen microbial world around us and its profound impact on our day-to-day lives.

HEALTH PROMOTING STRATEGIES

Not only is the prevention and control of infection important, the promotion of healthy attitudes and practices can enhance the quality of our lives. It is important that the health care provider promote good health in individuals. It is also important to practise what you preach. To practise, teach and exemplify good health, it is necessary to keep informed and up to date on the health care issues of the day. Taking the time to discuss these issues with colleagues will better enable the nurse to deal with patient concerns later. Physical activity in the form of daily exercise and an adequate amount of rest and sleep helps the body to maintain its defences against infection. Ensuring good nutrition by eating a balanced diet and also maintaining good dental health will help to maintain defences. Recent research suggests that a positive attitude towards life is beneficial and humour may boost the immune system (Hall, 1988).

HEALTH PROTECTING STRATEGIES

The best strategies for dealing with infectious diseases are always preventative. Immunization against infectious diseases, hygiene and aseptic practices are primary forms of health protection.

An understanding of basic asepsis lays the foundation for good infection control practices. While traditionally aseptic technique was developed to protect the patient, it also protects the health care provider. *Asepsis* can be defined as an absence of contamination. What that really means in practice

HEALTH PROMOTING STRATEGY

Promoting Healthy Infection Control Practices

- Perform meticulous hand washing:
  - After using the toilet
  - Before eating or handling food
  - Whenever the hands are soiled
  - After sneezing or coughing.
- Cover the nose or mouth with tissues when coughing or sneezing.
- Keep physically fit and in good condition.
- Obtain adequate rest and avoid fatigue.
- Eat a well-balanced diet and make sure your teeth and gums are in good repair.
- Avoid stress and keep a positive attitude towards life. Humour is said to help maintain resistance against infection.

- If you suffer from a chronic disease, are over 65 years of age or work in an institution such as a daycare centre or extended care, check with your doctor about getting an annual *"flu shot."* This vaccine can help prevent many cases of influenza.
- Keep other immunizations (for example, polio, diphtheria and tetanus) up to date (about every ten years).
- Keep informed about health care issues. Infection control programs are found throughout local community health agencies or hospitals.

SOURCE: Walker, 1991.

according to Sue Crow, a noted American infection control practitioner, is the purposeful prevention of the transfer of infection from one person to another by keeping the microbial count to an irreducible minimum (1989). A hospital environment, both animate and inanimate, including supplies and equipment, must always be kept as clean as is reasonably possible. In some instances, this means that some items must be entirely devoid of microbial life (sterile), and every effort must be made to keep them that way. While it is inevitable in the course of patient care that some items will become soiled, it is essential to know what is dirty, what is clean, what is sterile and how to keep them separate. *Medical asepsis* refers to practices which maintain cleanliness and limit the spread of microorganisms. In this method, also known as "clean technique," objects are described as clean or dirty. Using clean towels for a bed bath, cleaning a bedpan and washing hands before preparing oral medications are examples of medical asepsis. *Surgical asepsis* refers to practices which eliminate microorganisms from objects or areas. This method is known as "sterile technique"; objects are described as sterile or unsterile. Surgical asepsis is the basis of operating room procedure. Nurses practise surgical asepsis at the bedside when they perform such activities as administering injectable medications, inserting urinary catheters or changing sterile dressings.

IMMUNIZATION

The first organized efforts to immunize a segment of the population occurred as a result of Sir Edward Jenner's publication in 1798 citing evidence to support his observations that milk maids infected by cowpox acquired immunity to the dreaded smallpox (White and Shackelford, 1983). Today in Canada and other countries, federally supported immunization programs ensure that everyone can receive protection from diseases that once were leading causes of morbidity and mortality. Tables 31.1 and 31.2 outline immunization schedules for infants, children and adults as recommended by Health Canada (1993).

The widespread immunization of infants and children has drastically reduced the incidence of diseases such as measles, mumps, rubella, diphtheria and whooping cough (pertussis), and even tetanus and polio, over the past few decades. Many parents today have not experienced the tragic epidemics that used to sweep the country and ended in the deaths of so many infants and children not too many years ago. Many people have, as a result, become unconcerned about the need for immunization. Yet children are just as vulnerable to these diseases today as they were before the vaccines were developed. The nurse who is counselling young mothers is in an excellent position to give advice on the needed immunizations for children at different ages.

Those who have concerns about immune status or the need for immunization should be encouraged to talk it over with a physician or a knowledgeable person at the local public health office. Those who work in hospitals must be able to provide, whenever possible, a written record of immunization and may be required to demonstrate immunity to certain specified diseases.

TABLE 31.1   Routine Immunization Schedule for Infants and Children

AGE OF VACCINATION	DPT	POLIO	HIB[1]	MMR	TD[2]
2 months	X	X	X		
4 months	X	X	X		
6 months	X	X[3]	X		
12 months				X	
18 months	X	X	X		
4-6 years	X	X			
14-16 years		X[3]			X

DPT: Diphtheria, pertussis and tetanus vaccine
Hib: Hemophilus b conjugate vaccine
MMR: Measles, mumps and rubella vaccine
Td: Tetanus and diphtheria toxoid, "adult type"

[1] Hib schedule shown is for HbCC or PRP-T vaccine. If PRP-OMP is used, give at 2, 4 and 12 months of age.

[2] Td (tetanus and diphtheria toxoid), a combined adsorbed "adult type" preparation for use in persons greater than or equal to seven years of age, contains less diphtheria toxoid than preparations given to younger children and is less likely to cause reactions in older persons. Repeat every ten years throughout life.

[3] Omit this dose if OPV (oral polio vaccine) is used exclusively.

SOURCE: Health Canada. (1993). *Canadian immunization guide* (4th ed.). Ottawa: Minister of Supply and Services, 21, 22. (Catalogue H49–8/1993E) Reproduced with permission.

TABLE 31.2 Summary of Selected Immunization for Adults

VACCINE	INDICATION	FURTHER DOSES IF RISK CONTINUES
BCG	High-risk exposure	None
Hepatitis B	Occupational, lifestyle or environmental exposure	None
Japanese Encephalitis	Travel to endemic area or other exposure risk	See page 66*
Meningococcal	High-risk exposure	See page 79
Pertussis	Not indicated	
Plague	High-risk exposure	See page 90
Poliomyelitis	Travel to endemic area or other exposure risk	See pages 97 and 98
Rabies Pre-Exposure Use	Occupational or other risk	Every 2 years See page 106
Typhoid	High-risk exposure	Every 3-4 years See page 120
Yellow Fever	Travel to endemic area or if required for foreign travel	Every 10 years

*These page numbers refer to pages in the source

SOURCE: Health Canada. (1993). *Canadian immunization guide* (4th ed.). Ottawa: Minister of Supply and Services, 26. (Catalogue H49–8/1993E) Reproduced with permission.

CLEANING, DISINFECTION AND STERILIZATION

Cleaning

Cleaning is the removal of any foreign material (soilage or organic matter) from an object. A clean environment provides the background against which all patient care activities are carried out to the required standards of hygiene and asepsis. A clean environment inspires confidence in the hospital's ability to meet these standards. Hospital administrators are responsible for ensuring an adequate routine maintenance cleaning schedule. Those who are involved in direct patient care must ensure that any spillage is cleaned up immediately to remove the potential for microbial contamination as well as to prevent accidents. A good neutral detergent properly diluted is acceptable for basic cleaning. It is essential that nurses and other caregivers develop good work habits that aid in the process of maintaining a clean environment.

On nursing units, there are areas referred to as *clean* or *dirty utility rooms*. The clean area is used for storage of sterile and clean supplies and for set-up of treatment trays. The dirty area is used for dismantling reusable trays and preparing supplies for reprocessing. It also holds garbage containers for disposal of materials and is usually equipped with a "hopper" or clinical sink for the disposal of fluids and excretions (see Figure 31.2).

A clean utility room contains clean and sterile supplies.

Supplies to be discarded should be placed securely in appropriate garbage containers according to agency policy.

FIGURE 31.2   Hopper or clinical sink

Equipment to be reprocessed should have gross soilage removed prior to the return to the appropriate department. Containers should be rinsed carefully (to avoid splashing) with cold water first, to remove any proteinaceous matter that may coagulate, then with copious amounts of hot water. This will achieve a degree of disinfection as long as gross soilage is removed. These procedures will vary somewhat from one facility to another depending on which supplies and equipment are reusable and which are disposable. On no account should items such as full urine bags be placed in garbage containers destined for landfill. All fluids must be discarded down a hopper or toilet before placing the container in the garbage. An alternative method of disposal such as incineration must be used when it is not possible to open containers safely.

Sanitization

Sanitization is generally used in public health terminology and usually refers to what in hospitals is considered low-level disinfection — the removal of vegetative bacteria, fungi and some viruses. Sanitization is used, for example,

in the reprocessing of bedpans. For many years, bedpan decontaminators functioned by flushing the contents followed by a steam cycle of one minute or more. In the last few years an improved technology has been introduced. The bedpan and contents (stool, urine, blood, toilet paper) are placed in the decontaminator which automatically flushes, then washes the utensil with warm water and detergent inside and out, rinses, steams, and then allows a cool down. Most stainless steel or plastic utensils can be reprocessed in these machines, and returned to circulation once they are dry. In some institutions, hoses have been attached to patient toilets for cleaning of soiled bedpans. This is *not* acceptable because of the difficulty involved in proper cleaning with them and because there is a strong likelihood for aerosolization of stool particles onto the caregiver's clothing or into the environment.

Disinfection

Disinfection is a process wherein all pathogenic microorganisms are removed from an inanimate object with the exception of bacterial spores. Various levels of disinfection (low, intermediate and high) may be used for different items in the hospital depending on usage. The degree of asepsis required will determine the choice of chemical disinfectant, but proper cleaning *must* be done first. An example of low-level disinfection was described in the sanitization of bedpans. An example of intermediate-level disinfection would be using an approved disinfectant on a hydrotherapy tank. High-level disinfection is applied to respiratory therapy equipment by pasteurization or reprocessing endoscopes with glutaraldehyde.

Many health agencies have separate departments in which supplies and equipment are cleaned and sterilized for use.

Sterilization

Sterilization is the complete destruction or elimination of all forms of microbial life. Any item that penetrates skin and mucous membrane must be sterile. This is achieved principally with steam under pressure, dry heat, ethylene oxide gas or chemicals. New technologies are emerging constantly.

MEDICAL ASEPSIS

Medical asepsis is practised to prevent the spread of infection. At a very basic level, medical asepsis is clean technique based on thorough hand washing and the careful disposal of supplies and equipment. Proper hand washing before and after giving care to each patient is *the* most important means of preventing the spread of infection from one patient to another. Medical asepsis also involves the use of techniques to protect health care providers, patients and others from known or potential pathogens through what is called universal or body substance precautions and isolation practices.

Body Substance Precautions

Throughout this century, but especially since the 1950s, a lot of emphasis has been placed on preventing the spread of disease from patient to patient in hospitals and long-term care facilities. To this end, agencies established infection control committees to review the problem. The first Infection Control Nurse position was established in England in 1960 because of concerns regarding how infection was transmitted from one end of a big open ward to another. The findings of these infection control pioneers led to a renewed emphasis on the importance of simple activities such as hand washing and the careful handling and disposal of all body secretions and excretions.

Concerns about safety for the health care worker had focussed on immunization and ways to protect staff from tuberculosis and polio in the first half of the twentieth century. Eventually in the 1970s, risks to health care workers from hepatitis B were recognized and changes in specimen handling in particular were implemented. It was, however, the advent of HIV (responsible for AIDS) that once again forced another look at safety for the health care provider. Following the report in May 1987 of three health care workers who became infected with HIV in work-related incidents, the Centers for Disease Control (CDC) in Atlanta, Georgia, published their first guideline on **Universal Precautions** (CDC, 1987). This guideline stated that all

Body substance precautions by all health care providers and agency personnel are necessary to safeguard against infectious disease.

blood from all people, as well as cerebrospinal fluid, pericardial fluid, pleural fluid, peritoneal fluid-amniotic fluid, and synovial fluid, should be treated as though potentially infectious. This guideline was supported by the Laboratory Centre for Disease Control (LCDC), Health and Welfare Canada.

At the same time that this guideline was published (August 1987), infection control practitioners in Seattle and San Diego published their approach to the issue of patient protection and worker safety which was referred to as Body Substance Isolation (BSI). Many hospitals in Canada were quick to recognize the simplicity and practicality of this generic system but chose to call it instead **Body Substance Precautions** or **BSP**. Policies and procedures in Infection Control manuals and other resources were developed to describe the activities in the system. The guidelines for Body Substance Precautions in the box below are consistent with good infection control practice in any hospital situation. The associated techniques for implementing these guidelines are outlined in Procedure 31.1.

Body Substance Precautions

1. Hand Washing

Hand washing **MUST** be done:

- before, during and after patient contact as necessary
- before eating or handling food
- after using the toilet
- after removing gloves
- whenever the hands appear soiled
- whenever the health care worker's intact skin is penetrated

NB: Neither jewellery nor nail polish should be worn by caregivers as both jewellery and chipped nail polish may harbour microorganisms and hand washing may not be as effective with jewellery in the way.

2. Hand Disinfection

Hands may be disinfected using an antiseptic hand rub made of chlorhexidine, isopropyl alcohol and an emollient. This combination is very effective in reducing the numbers of bacteria on the skin and may be less drying than actual hand washing. It may be used when circumstances require hand washing yet the hands appear superficially clean.

Procedure:

i. Apply 3–5 ml of antiseptic hand rub.

ii. Massage vigorously all skin surfaces of hand and lower wrist until dry.

3. Gloves

a) Sterile gloves are worn to protect patients from contamination during an aseptic procedure. They also provide protection for the wearer.

b) Clean gloves are worn to protect the wearer from sources of contamination.

c) Gloves **MUST** be worn:

- when touching body secretions and excretions
- when touching mucous membrane
- when touching non-intact skin
- if the nurse's hands are chapped, cracked or have open lesions

d) Hands must be washed and wedding band (if allowed by hospital policy) must be removed before donning gloves.

e) If a puncture occurs, remove gloves and wash hands before continuing.

f) Glove use must be task-specific.

g) Gloves must be removed and discarded and hands must be washed after every task is completed.

4. Gowns

a) Hand hygiene must be done before donning gown.

b) Gowns **MUST** be worn:

- when caring for patients with communicable disease
- when clothes are likely to be soiled from infective secretions or excretions
- to prevent visible soilage of clothing
- for certain procedures when the patient is highly compromised, for example, when changing dressings on severely burned patients (according to hospital policy)

c) Gowns are used only once in patient's room and then discarded in an appropriate receptacle.

d) Hand hygiene must be done when the gown is removed.

5. Masks (Also see 6. *Masks and Goggles*)

a) Masks are worn:

- by personnel to protect patient during aseptic procedures (Policies may vary from agency to agency and in some instances, they may not be worn.)
- by *susceptible individuals* when entering room of patient on isolation for airborne disease (Restrictive Isolation)
- by *personnel* to protect the patient who is immunocompromised (physician's order)
- by *patients* on isolation when leaving room as necessary

b) Masks must be handled by strings (ties) only and removed completely when not needed.

c) Hand hygiene must be done when mask is removed.

6. Masks and Goggles (or face shields)

a) Masks and goggles are worn to protect the mucous membrane and conjunctiva whenever aerosolization of blood or other body fluids is likely.

b) Goggles and face shields may be decontaminated by washing under running water with detergent. After drying, wipe with buffered bleach, alcohol swab or other approved hospital disinfectant and leave to dry.

7. Garbage Handling and Disposal

The principle behind garbage disposal in institutions is that all garbage should be packaged so that it does not:

a) pose a risk to the workers

b) contaminate the environment

It must remain safely packaged until it reaches its final destination whether incinerator, autoclave or landfill. Policies will vary from one hospital to another and from one jurisdiction to another.

8. Linen Disposal

The principle behind linen handling in institutions is that all linen must be safely packaged so that it does not:

a) pose a risk to the worker

b) contaminate the environment

Avoid overfilling bags so that they may be secured properly for transport and subsequent handling. Laundry workers must wear protective attire where needed and procedures must ensure adequate processing so that properly disinfected linen is returned to service in all situations.

9. Disinfection — The Environment and Equipment

Maintaining cleanliness is the most important part of the disinfecting process. This is always the first step to be taken. All floors, whether visibly contaminated or simply being routinely cleaned, need only to be cleaned with the hospital supplied neutral cleaner and left to dry. Areas above the floor and all equipment must be cleaned first with the neutral cleaner and where visibly contaminated, a hospital approved disinfectant must be applied. The following guidelines should be observed:

a) Don gloves and, using paper towels or other appropriate method, physically remove contaminating matter into garbage.

b) Ensure item or area appears clean, using neutral cleaner as necessary.

c) Apply disinfectant, leaving thin film.

d) Allow to dry.

e) Liquids may be poured down a hopper or toilet and the container then thoroughly rinsed before being

returned to the patient or for reprocessing, as appropriate.

A popular disinfectant for general use in all areas is sodium dichloroisocyanurate (NADCC). This is a buffered bleach solution prepared at approved strength for appropriate task. Isopropyl alcohol 70 % may be used alone in very small items, such as medication vials. Other disinfectants used in institutions may include:

a) Chlorhexidine gluconate 0.5 % with anti-rust

b) Phenolic germicidal 2 %

c) Glutaraldehyde 2 % or glutaraldehyde-phenate solution

d) Quaternary ammonia compounds

e) Hydrogen peroxide 3–6 %

f) Povidone-iodine

N.B: All equipment being passed on or returned to another department must do so with grossly contaminating matter removed.

Disinfectants (for inanimate objects) and antiseptics (for skin) are *not* interchangeable.

10. Disposable Food Trays

These are not required for any patient. Rather, the standard is that used cutlery, crockery and trays, etc., must be reprocessed so they may be used safely by anyone. Automatic dishwashers are preferred over hand washing.

11. Manual Ventilation Units

These may accompany any patient being transported throughout the hospital if there is thought to be a risk of cardiac or respiratory arrest.

12. Sharps Disposal Containers

Sharps containers that are puncture resistant must be readily available for disposal of used needles and sharps. Used needles MUST NOT be recapped, purposefully bent or broken.

PROCEDURE 31.1

Using Body Substance Precautions

ACTION

A. Hand Washing

1. Gather equipment:
   - Liquid or bar soap
   - Warm running water
   - Fingernail stick
   - Paper towel

RATIONALE

Soap and paper towel are usually provided in dispensers at each sink. Fingernail sticks (orangewood or plastic) should be found in the utility room.

ACTION

RATIONALE

2. Remove or push watch above the wrists. Long sleeves should be well above the wrists.

Cleanses the wrist area under the band and prevents the watch or the sleeves from becoming wet or contaminated.

3. Stand with clothing clear of sink.

Prevents transfer of microorganisms harboured in sink onto uniform.

4. Using paper towel, adjust water flow to a comfortable temperature. Avoid splashing, leave water running.

Prevents the spread of contaminants from hands to taps. Hot water depletes natural oils and causes drying of skin. Microorganisms in the sink are transferred onto the nurse's uniform through splashing. Running water washes away microorganisms.

5. Wet hands and wrists, keeping the hands pointing downward and lower than the elbows.

The hands and fingertips are more contaminated than the elbows. Allows water to flow from cleanest to dirtiest area.

6. Apply soap and massage all skin surfaces of hands and lower wrist vigorously for 10–15 seconds.

Dislodges and suspends contaminants in the lather.

If using bar soap, rinse it before and after use.

Bar soap harbours microorganisms.

7. Clean fingertips and fingernails thoroughly. Use a fingernail stick as necessary.

Removes microbes that lodge around and under the nails.

Continued on the next page

ACTION

RATIONALE

8. Rinse thoroughly and dry hands, holding hands downward. Take care not to abrade the skin. Discard towel.

Contaminants and microbes are washed away with flowing water. Drying the hands completely but gently prevents chapping and cracking.

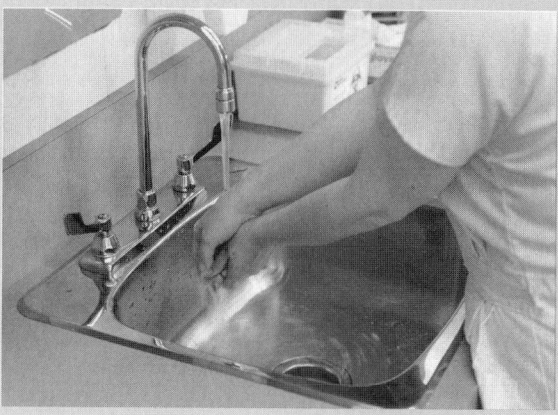

9. Use paper towel to turn off tap.

Prevents contamination of clean hands with microbes harboured on the taps.

10. When not at work, use hand lotion liberally if problems with dry skin develop.

Replaces moisture lost during handwashing and thereby maintains skin integrity.

B. Applying and Removing Clean Gloves

1. Obtain gloves.

Clean gloves are supplied in boxes which are kept in central areas such as clean and soiled utility rooms and, in some agencies, in patients' rooms.

2. Apply the gloves in a convenient manner, making sure the cuff covers the wrists and wrist watch.

Prevents contamination of hands, wrists and watch.

3. To remove the first glove, grasp the cuff area with the other gloved hand and pull the glove over the fingers turning it inside out. Hold the glove in the fingers of the gloved hand.

Prevents touching the outside of either glove.

Allows the first glove to be contained in the second glove when removed.

ACTION	RATIONALE

4. To remove the second glove, slide two fingers of the ungloved hand inside the cuff and roll the cuff downward onto the hand. With thumb and fingers grasp the inside of the glove and peel it off inside out over the first glove. Discard into appropriate container.

Avoids touching the outside of the gloves with bare hands.

5. Wash hands thoroughly.

Removes microorganisms that may have contaminated the hands during the procedure or that may have multiplied in the warm, moist environment of the glove.

C. Donning and Removing a Gown

1. Obtain gown.

Gowns may be made of reusable fabric or disposable paper. They open in the back and have ties at the neck and waist.

Continued on the next page

ACTION	RATIONALE

2. Put on a clean gown and fasten the neck ties. Overlap the gown at the back and tie it together at the waist.

Ensures the clothing is covered to avoid inadvertent contamination.

3. To remove the gown, untie the waist ties and wash hands.

Removes any microorganisms that may have transferred to back of gown.

4. Untie the neck ties and, without touching the outside of the gown, slide your hands into the sleeves, pull the gown off the shoulders, and slip out of the gown.

Prevents the transmission of microorganisms from the outside of the gown to the hands.

5. While still holding the gown on the inside, fold the outside surfaces inward and roll it into a ball. Discard into a laundry bag or garbage container.

As above.

ACTION

6. Wash hands thoroughly.

D. Applying and Removing a Mask

1. Obtain a mask.

2. To apply a mask, first bring the upper strings above the ears and then tie them at the back of the head. Adjust the mask to fit over the nose and under the chin. If wearing glasses, the top edge of the mask should fit under the glasses. Tie the lower strings at the back of the neck.

3. To remove the mask, handle only the ties. Unfasten the ties and discard the mask into a garbage container.

4. Wash hands thoroughly.

RATIONALE

Reduces spread of microorganisms.

Masks are supplied in boxes and kept in a central area such as the clean utility room or outside the patient's room.

Most masks have a metal strip that helps to secure the mask to the nose. Reduces fogging of the glasses.

The central part of the mask is dirty; the ties are clean.

Reduces spread of microorganisms.

Isolation Precautions

While the preceding activities are implemented to ensure proper practice of BSP, further precautions are taken to prevent transmission of infectious diseases. These include isolation for airborne and respiratory infection, protective isolation and multiple-drug resistance isolation.

Isolation for airborne and respiratory infections

Isolation precautions are implemented for patients with chicken pox, diphtheria, measles (rubeola, red), meningococcal disease, mumps, pertussis (whooping cough), including parapertussis, rabies and rubella (German measles). Children with respiratory symptoms or those suspected of having influenza, parainfluenza, respiratory syncytial virus (RSV), adenovirus or rhinovirus routinely may be isolated because it is sensible to contain respiratory secretions as much as possible despite the fact that in some instances (as with RSV), there is little evidence that masks offer any protection. Children with *Hemophilus influenzae* infection also should be isolated until appropriately treated.

The term for this type of isolation may vary from one institution to another. Originally, either *strict* or *respiratory isolation* were used. More recently, the preferred term has been *contact isolation* (a modification). Some hospitals have combined respiratory and strict isolation using a new term *restrictive isolation*. Others use the term *airborne precautions*. Occasionally, the term *AFB isolation* (acid-fast bacillus) has been used for patients with tuberculosis. The application of isolation precautions differs between adult and pediatric units. Nursing staff, including students, must become acquainted with the infection control and isolation protocols when receiving orientation to any new hospital or any new unit.

Protective isolation

Patients who are severely immunocompromised may be placed on *protective isolation* to decrease the numbers of contacts they have with others in order to reduce the chances of acquiring exogenous infection. However, the value of this practice is in some doubt and is not done in all hospitals.

Multiple-drug resistance isolation

Some bacteria have developed a high degree of resistance to antibiotics that at one time were effective against them. One of the most common of these bacteria is Methicillin-resistant *Staphylococcus aureus* (MRSA). Many hospitals now are adopting a modified form of Strict Isolation referred to as *Multiple-drug resistance isolation* to prevent these microorganisms from joining the resident microbial flora in the hospital. This likely will continue to be one of the major challenges of the twenty-first century.

Maintaining Psychosocial Well-Being on Isolation

Patients for whom isolation precautions are being maintained have special needs for emotional support. They are separated from other patients, are frequently in a private room and contact with people is limited. Some patients attach a moral significance to the disease; they feel unworthy and think they are creating extra work for the nurse. Feelings of unworthiness, social isolation and sensory deprivation can seriously affect well-being.

Providing education to patients on isolation precautions is crucial to care. Most people want to participate in their own therapy; moreover, the success of medical asepsis is largely dependent upon the patient's willingness to help. The nurse's explanations are based on the needs of the patient to understand the reason for the various precautionary measures, the possible causes of the infection, what it means in terms of the health problem and how to provide protection from further infection and help to prevent infection in others. The spread of pathogens from the respiratory tract of patients is thought to be best controlled by teaching safe hygiene practices, which include frequent hand washing under running water. A patient with a pulmonary infection is taught to use several thicknesses of paper handkerchief to cover the nose and mouth when sneezing or coughing. Also, covered waterproof containers are provided for sputum. Facilities are also made available for the adequate disposal of paper handkerchiefs and sputum containers after they have been used.

Diversional activities and sensory stimulation are very important in the care of patients on isolation precautions. Such activities should be designed so that they do not interfere with the barrier technique, yet still meet the patient's needs. A television set may help to relieve monotony, and items such as magazines, playing cards or hobby materials can be made safe after they are removed from the contaminated area. Keeping the room clean and providing space for personal items such as cards and pictures will help create a pleasant environment. Taking time to listen and talk to patients or providing comfort measures such as a back rub will help patients to feel less isolated and better about themselves.

Sterile technique is carried out in the operating room.

SURGICAL ASEPSIS

Surgical asepsis or sterile technique is the method of asepsis carried out to keep an object or area free of microorganisms. In the operating room, a birthing room or a specialized diagnostic area, it is basic infection control practice to ensure that all items transecting the patient's skin (scalpel), or entering a body cavity or tissue (instruments), are sterile. Not only must the "set-up" procedure ensure that supplies and equipment used for the procedure are kept sterile, but the actions of all personnel involved in the procedure must be such that the sterile field is maintained. The microbial count must be kept to an irreducible minimum during the entire procedure.

Surgical asepsis is also practised at the bedside in the performance of techniques that involve entry into a body part or cavity or penetration of skin and mucous membranes. Some of the more common procedures performed by nurses that require sterile technique are administration of injections, insertion of intravenous catheters, urinary catheterization, tracheobronchial suctioning and dressing changes. A sterile field is created with sterile equipment, towels and drapes. Sterile gloves or forceps are used to maintain asepsis. In the following section, we will focus only on the application of sterile technique in performing procedures at the bedside. The student wishing information on surgical asepsis in the operating room should refer to a text on operating room procedure. Basic guidelines for surgical asepsis are listed in the accompanying box. The techniques for putting on sterile gloves and setting up a sterile field are outlined in Procedures 31.2 and 31.3.

Preparing the Patient

In addition to preparing the patient for the specific procedure to be undertaken, the nurse should also explain sterile technique and enlist the patient's participation in ensuring sterility. The patient is asked to avoid touching sterile areas, to avoid sudden movement of body parts covered by the drapes and to refrain from talking, sneezing or coughing over the sterile field. If there is a chance that breathing or coughing may transmit airborne organisms, the patient should be given a mask to wear. If the procedure is anticipated to last a long time, the patient's comfort needs should be attended to first. For instance, the nurse may administer pain medication, assist the patient to the bathroom, or help them assume as comfortable a position as possible.

Assembling Equipment and Setting Up a Sterile Field

The nurse begins by gathering all of the equipment and supplies that will be needed for the procedure. In most hospitals today, commercially prepared trays or kits are provided which contain the basic supplies for a procedure. For

---

Basic Guidelines for Surgical Asepsis

1. A sterile field must be set up only immediately before use to help ensure sterility.

2. Hands and wrists must be washed thoroughly for one minute, preferably with an antiseptic agent such as chlorhexidine (CHG) or povidone-iodine.

3. The table on which the sterile field is set up must be clean and dry.

4. A sterile package is considered to be unsterile if it passes its expiration date, has been previously opened or if it is wet.

5. The only objects that can touch sterile objects or the sterile field are other sterile objects. If touched by a clean or contaminated object, or by an object of questionable sterility, the sterile object or field must be considered unsterile. If there is any doubt about an object's sterility, it must be considered contaminated.

6. Sterile objects that are out of the range of vision or below waist level are considered to be unsterile. A sterile field must never be left unattended. Edges of a sterile wrapper or towel that hang down over the edge of the table are considered contaminated. The top surface will remain sterile.

7. The outer, approximately 2.5 cm edge of a sterile field is considered unsterile. This area may be touched with clean hands.

8. Sterile objects are contaminated by transfer of airborne microorganisms. Avoid activities that create air currents such as talking, sneezing, reaching over the sterile field or shaking drapes vigorously.

9. Pour sterile solutions so that they do not splash on the field. When a sterile object or field lying on an unsterile surface becomes wet or damp, it is no longer sterile. Microbes can migrate from the unsterile surface to the sterile field through capillary action.

10. Meticulous aseptic technique must be practised when performing all sterile procedures. A break in technique can lead to infection.

---

example, a dressing tray contains a compartment for cleansing solution, two or three forceps, and some 5 x 5 cm and 10 x 10 cm gauze sponges. Equipment and supplies are added to the tray depending on the circumstances of each particular situation. The nurse will find it prudent to take a few extra supplies along in case of accidental contamination because once a tray is opened and a sterile field is established, it must not be left unattended.

Establishing the sterile field   A sterile field is set up on a clean, dry surface at about waist level. A bedside table is commonly used for this purpose. The table should be cleared of all items to provide ample surface area and avoid the risk of contamination from unsterile objects. The size of the sterile field depends on the procedure and the amount of equipment needed. In some cases, a sterile field is established by using the inside wrapper of a sterile package; in others it is created with sterile drapes. Supplies are added to the field either directly or with the use of sterile transfer forceps.

Opening sterile packages   Sterile items such as catheters, syringes or dressing materials are packaged in plastic or paper packages that are impenetrable by microorganisms as long as they remain dry and intact. Many of these items are wrapped in "peel packs" or "peelback" containers. Reusable equipment such as forceps, towels or drapes are wrapped in paper or cotton (or cotton blend) fabric. An "envelope" method of wrapping is used in which the four corners of the outer wrapper are folded around the object in a uniform manner. The box below shows illustrations of how to open the various types of sterile packages.

Using sterile forceps   A variety of forceps are used in sterile procedures (see Figure 31.3). For example, transfer forceps are used for transferring sterile supplies on a sterile field and thumb forceps are used for handling sponges and dressings or for anchoring a tube. Forceps are included in prepackaged and reusable trays but individually wrapped forceps may also be available in some agencies. As with all sterile objects, forceps must always be held above waist level and within full view. The handles are considered contaminated if held with ungloved hands. Dry, sterile forceps that are used with bare hands may be placed on the sterile area so that the tips rest within the sterile field and the handles outside it. Forceps must always be held with the tips downward, especially if they become wet. This prevents contamination from the backflow of moisture from contaminated handles to the sterile tips.

Guidelines for Opening Sterile Packages

Inspect all packages for dryness, intactness, indication of sterility and expiration date. Do not use any packages marked sterile that appear damp or whose wrappers are damaged.

Peel Packs

1. Grasp the tabs above the sealed edge as shown.

2. Peel edges apart to break seal.

3. Package may be placed on a flat surface and top wrapper removed to completely expose contents as shown, creating a small sterile field for contents of package.

4. Contents may be dropped on another sterile field.

Peelback Containers

1. Hold the bottom of the container with one hand.
2. Grasp corner tab of peelback top; pull to remove top.

3. Container may be used as self-contained sterile field for contents.
4. Sterile solution may be added if needed, or contents may be placed on another sterile field and container used to hold sterile solution.

Envelope Wrapped Package on a Surface

1. Centre the package on the work area so the outer flap of the wrapper faces away from you.

2. Reach around, not over, the package and open the flap, pulling it away from you. Touch only the outside of the wrap.

3. Open flaps in sequence, using right hand for right flap and left hand for left flap. Touch outside surface only, as shown. Avoid reaching over package.

4. Open inner flap by pulling turned-down corner towards you. If flap is large, step away from the table so wrapper does not contact your uniform. If inner corner is not turned down, touch outside of wrap only, as in step 3.

5. Wrapper may be used for sterile field. Additional items may be added as necessary.

Envelope Wrapped Package Held in Hand

1. Hold the package in one hand so the outer flap of the wrapper faces away from you.

2. Open the package as in steps 2 to 4 above, pulling the flaps back towards you as you open each one.

3. Gather the opened flaps with your free hand and hold them against the opposite arm, as shown. The sterile item can now be placed on a sterile field without risk of contacting the field with the parts of the wrapper that you have touched.

SOURCE: Berger, K.J. and Williams, M.B. (1992). *Fundamentals of nursing: Collaborating for optimal health.* Norwalk, CT: Appleton & Lange, 804–805. Reproduced with permission.

FIGURE 31.3   Forceps used in sterile procedures

Pouring sterile solutions   Sterile solutions are supplied in glass or plastic bottles. The inside of the bottle and cap are considered to be sterile; the outside surfaces clean. The cap must be removed carefully and held in the hand or placed on a flat surface inside up to prevent the inside from becoming contaminated. The bottle is held with the label facing upward to avoid wetting and possibly obliterating the label. The bottle should also be held outside the edge of the sterile field and about 10 cm above the receiving container to prevent contamination of the sterile field. The lip of the bottle should never touch the receiving container. Solution must be poured carefully to avoid splashing. Only the outside of the cap should be touched when replacing it on the bottle. As with all sterile supplies, check the expiration date on the solution container. Do not use solutions that have expired.

Donning sterile gloves   Sterile gloves are supplied in a variety of sizes. A proper glove size is necessary for comfort, dexterity and safety. Gloves that fit loosely will make the manipulation of objects difficult, whereas gloves that are too tight may tear and cause contamination.

PROCEDURE 31.2

Donning and Removing Sterile Gloves

ACTION	**RATIONALE**

A. Applying Gloves

1. Select correct glove size.

2. Wash and dry hands thoroughly.

   Removes transient microorganisms and reduces microbe growth in a dark moist environment.

3. Carefully open the outer package, remove the inner package, and place it on a clean, dry surface.

   Prevents the inner package from inadvertently opening and becoming contaminated.

4. Open the inner package, touching only the 2.5 cm border. Pull the wrapper gently but firmly to keep it flat. Gloves will be positioned so that the left-hand glove lies on the left and the right-hand glove on the right. Palms will face upward, with thumbs to the outside.

   Creates a sterile field for the gloves. If the wrapper falls back to its folded position after being touched, the gloves and inside of wrapper may become contaminated.

5. With the dominant hand* grasp the glove for the nondominant hand by the cuffed edge, lift it from the wrapper and hold it away from your body.

   Prevents contamination of the sterile glove by contact with unsterile objects.

* If right-handed, the left glove is put on first and vice versa if left-handed.

Continued on the next page

ACTION

RATIONALE

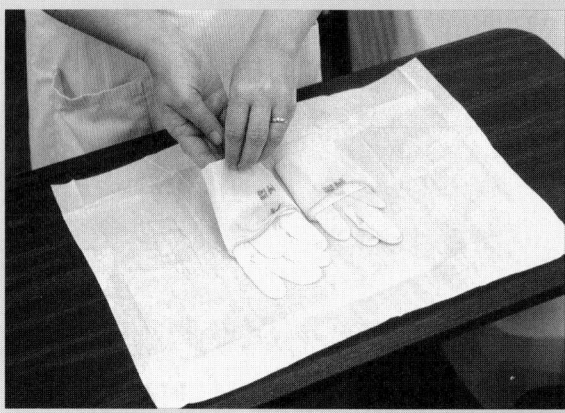

6. Slide the nondominant hand into the glove and pull it on. Do not adjust the cuff or placement of fingers inside the glove.

This is accomplished more easily when both gloves are on.

7. Slide the fingers of the gloved hand under the cuff of the remaining glove, and lift it up as above.

Maintains sterile to sterile contact. The cuff protects the gloved fingers.

ACTION	RATIONALE
8. Carefully slide the dominant hand into the glove, keeping the thumb abducted and pulling the cuff up over the wrist with the nondominant (gloved) hand, which is still under the cuff. The cuff of the nondominant glove may then be pulled up over the wrist by slipping the fingers of the now gloved dominant hand under the cuff of the remaining glove and carefully pulling it up over the wrist. Adjust both gloves, touching only sterile areas.	Avoids contact with exposed hand.

Maintains the technique of sterile surface to sterile surface.

Smooth fit is necessary for dexterity. |

ACTION	RATIONALE
9. Keep gloved hands in full view and above waist level at all times.	Prevents unintentional contamination.

B. Removing Gloves

ACTION	RATIONALE
1. Grasp the outside of one glove near the wrist and pull it over the hand. The glove will turn inside out.	Prevents transfer of organisms on the gloves (from contact with patient's skin or body substances) to the nurse's hands.
2. Hold onto the glove with the still gloved hand or discard it with other supplies.	If held, the first glove will be encased in the second glove when removed.
3. Slip the fingers of the ungloved hand inside the remaining glove and pull it off by turning it inside out.	Prevents contamination of the nurse's hands with organisms on the outside of the gloves.
4. Discard gloves and other equipment as per agency policy.	Promotes cleanliness and safety in the workplace by limiting the transmission of microorganisms.
5. Wash hands thoroughly.	Removes organisms on the skin.

PROCEDURE 31.3

Setting up a Sterile Field

ACTION	RATIONALE
1. Prepare the sterile field immediately before the procedure.	Prevents unnecessary exposure to air and contaminants.
2. Gather necessary supplies and equipment. Check packages for date of expiration, tears, punctures or wetness. Check the solution container for date of expiration.	Promotes efficiency and avoids having to leave the sterile field unattended. Checking packages ensures sterility.
3. Clear a surface area for the sterile field and make sure it is dry. If using an overbed table adjust the height to waist level.	Avoids contamination with unsterile objects. Sterile objects held below waist level are considered contaminated.
4. Don a mask if required by agency policy for the procedure.	Reduces the risk of spreading microbes from the nurse's mouth and respiratory tract to the sterile field.
5. Wash hands thoroughly.	Reduces the spread of microorganisms.
6. Create the sterile field.	

Using a sterile drape:

- Open the outer covering using proper guidelines.
- Pick up the corner that is folded back, touching only the outer 2.5 cm edge.
- Lift the drape from the wrapper, hold it away from your body, and let it open without touching any unsterile object. Discard the wrapper with your other hand.
- Grasp the adjacent corner of the drape with the other hand and lay it on the table. Position the drape on the table, without leaning or reaching over it.

The entire 2.5 cm border of a drape is considered unsterile and may be touched with bare hands.

Facilitates positioning the drape on the table. Avoids contamination by air transmission of organisms.

Using a commercially prepared tray:

- Centre the tray on the work area and open it using the guidelines for an envelope wrapped package.

Use of these techniques maintains sterility of the field.

ACTION

On top of the inner flap, there will be a transfer forceps which must be removed before opening the flap.

- Flatten the wrapper by gently pulling on the sides, touching only the 2.5 cm border.
- Position the wrapper on the table.

- Arrange items on the tray, placing the handles of the forceps on the 2.5 cm border of the sterile fields.

RATIONALE

Prevents it from falling on the floor.

Prevents corners of the wrapper from falling back on the sterile field and contaminating it.

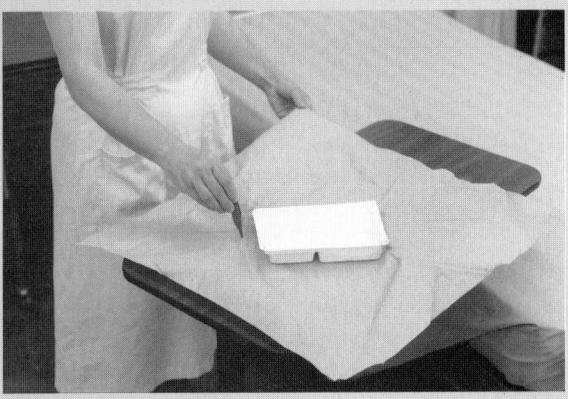

Prevents contamination of the sterile field when forceps are picked up with bare hands.

Continued on the next page

ACTION

RATIONALE

7. Add supplies to the sterile field as needed.
   - Open packages.
   - Drop small items onto the field from a distance of about 15 cm or use transfer forceps.

Prevents contamination of the sterile field with the outer wrapper.

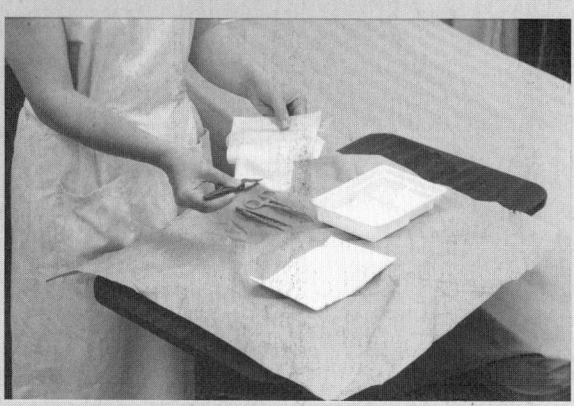

   - Add heavier items such as basins or scissors by holding one edge of the item in its wrapper and covering the hand and wrist with the corners of the wrapper.

The wrapper provides a barrier between the sterile item and the hand.

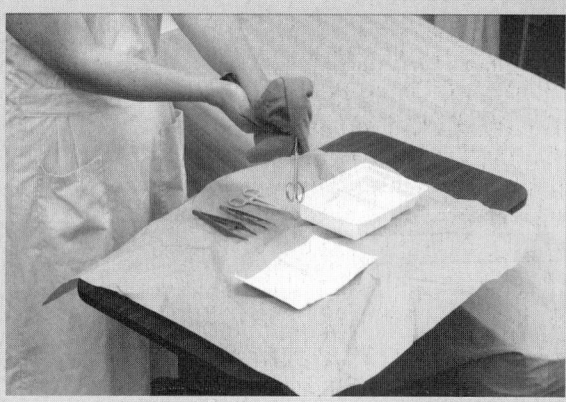

   - Be sure to place the items within the 2.5 cm border.

Ensures sterility by avoiding contact with an unsterile area.

8. Pour sterile solution.
   - Remove the cap and hold it in the hand or place it on a flat surface, inside up.
   - Hold the bottle with the label facing upward.
   - Hold the bottle outside the edge of the sterile field and about 10 cm above the receiving container.

Prevents the inside of the cap from becoming contaminated.

Avoids wetting and possibly obliterating the label.

Prevents contamination of the sterile field.

ACTION

- Pour the solution carefully. Avoid splashing.

- Grasp the outside of the cap and recap the bottle securely.

RATIONALE

Moisture facilitates the movement of microbes from the unsterile table to the sterile field through capillary action.

Maintains sterility of the solution.

HEALTH RESTORING STRATEGIES

Nosocomial infections have long been recognized as serious complications of disease or treatment with significant morbidity, mortality and cost. It would appear that even as we continue to find new and more sophisticated ways of supporting people through life-threatening injury or illness, we also expose them to greater risks of infection. Notwithstanding the fact that prevention of illness, coupled with health promotion, is the ideal in a healthy society, in developed countries approximately five to ten percent of people admitted to hospital develop infection as a result of their stay. This figure remains fairly constant despite best efforts to understand and prevent disease acquisition. It is inevitable that measures must be taken to tip the balance in favour of the infected person. This usually means prescribing antibiotics. The physician doing so will base his or her decision on clinical evidence for disease, possibly with microbiological and radiological support. The decision may be empirical, that is, it may be based on previous experience.

The nurse should have knowledge of the antibiotic agent being administered. The most important aspects include usual dosage and timing, route(s) of administration, potential adverse effects, contraindications and possible drug reactions. In the event of adverse effects or reactions, the nurse must know how to obtain help, especially in a sudden emergency, such as a severe anaphylactic reaction.

It also is useful to know the nursing measures that can be undertaken to relieve uncomfortable side effects that may not need medical intervention. Ideally, a specimen for culture and sensitivity should be obtained before initiation of antibiotic therapy. Once the specimen is obtained, therapy should be started immediately. The nurse must also monitor and assess whether or not the prescribed treatment appears to be effective. Sometimes a new infection (a *superinfection*) will superimpose itself on the original one, or sometimes the infecting microorganism may have developed resistance to the prescribed antibiotic.

Good nutrition is important to promote good health, and it is vital that someone fighting an infection have proper nutrients. Good nursing care means that the patient will be encouraged to eat and drink and that intake will be monitored. With some patients, especially older adults, it may be necessary to ensure that dentition is in good repair or that their dentures fit properly. The more conscientious the approach to good basic nursing care, the more likely a patient will return to a healthy life.

STAFF EXPOSURE TO INFECTIOUS AGENTS

Health care providers and personnel such as housekeeping staff are at risk for exposure to infectious agents. The greatest concerns expressed are exposure to blood-borne pathogens such as HIV and hepatitis B. The following measures are recommended for health care providers and hospital personnel should they sustain injury from a needle or other sharp instrument that has been used on a patient or should blood be splashed onto an open lesion or mucous membrane.

1. Wash area thoroughly with soap and water.
2. If stuck with a needle or sharp, squeeze blood from wound.
3. Soak affected area in buffered bleach 1400 ppm (or household bleach 1/2–1%) for 10 minutes.
4. Flush eyes and mucous membranes with normal saline at an eye wash station.

Report promptly to the employee health service (or Emergency, depending on hospital policy) and to the supervisor for follow up.

EVALUATING INFECTION PREVENTION AND CONTROL INTERVENTIONS

Evaluation of the effectiveness of nursing intervention is based on outcome criteria established in the patient's plan of care and by the absence of the infection in other patients, in visitors and in staff. Guidelines the nurse might use in evaluating the effectiveness of care are listed below.

1. Are aseptic practices keeping organisms within defined areas?
2. Are other people in the environment free of the infection?
3. Does the patient (and family) have the knowledge and skills required to prevent the spread of infection and to participate actively in care as much as possible?
4. Does the patient have misconceptions about the infection?
5. Does the patient indicate in any way feelings of isolation? For example, does the patient make verbal statements or show signs of depression?
6. Does the patient have the desired contact with family, hospital personnel and other patients without endangering health?
7. Does the patient get adequate exercise to meet needs?
8. Does the patient demonstrate an active interest in and is the patient encouraged to participate in care as much as possible?
9. Does the patient have diversionary materials of interest?

THE ROLE OF THE INFECTION CONTROL SERVICE

The vast majority of hospitals in Canada and the U.S. today have active infection control programs. The basic aim of these programs is to control and prevent the spread of nosocomial infection and to bring its incidence to an irreducible minimum. Three activities form the framework for an effective program. They are surveillance, education and consultation. Surveillance means the "systematic, active, ongoing observation of the occurrence and distribution of disease within a population and of the events or conditions that increase or decrease the risk of such disease occurrence" (Haley et al., 1991). This means that data are gathered according to pre-set criteria, are analyzed regularly and information is presented to those persons who can effect appropriate corrective action. Types of surveillance may vary from one hospital to another and may be refocussed or retargeted as changing circumstances indicate. Surveillance may also include outbreak investigation and communicable disease reporting to the appropriate authorities.

Educational programs include orientation for all new staff and ongoing service sessions as required. Educational needs are identified, programs implemented and evaluation done on a regular basis.

Consultation is an ongoing process both internally within the facility and externally from the community. Hospital staff at any level are encouraged to bring questions and concerns to the infection control department. Consultation is carried on externally through liaison with other hospitals, health care agencies and facilities, universities, community colleges and other organizations. This is especially true for infection control practitioners in teaching hospitals or in regional referral centres. Infection control practitioners may also sit on a variety of committees and policy-making bodies that deal with issues where infection control aspects must be addressed.

In Canada, the vast majority of people working on a daily basis in infection control are nurses. Usually these nurses have had broad clinical experience and have taken, or are expected to participate in, infection control educational programs. Goals and objectives for such programs have been developed by the Community and Hospital Infection Control Association — Canada (CHICA — Canada). These courses are available through several different educational institutions. Other disciplines active in infection control include laboratory technologists (or others with a science background), infectious disease physicians and medical microbiologists. It is absolutely essential that infection control practitioners have a close working relationship (preferably formalized) with the medical microbiology laboratory. In the larger institutions, a multidisciplinary approach is usual and is in fact desirable. It is contingent on all hospital staff that they support the hospitals' infection control program and there should be administrative recognition that infection control activities represent continuous quality improvement. In other words, *infection control is everybody's business!*

KEY TERMS

IN REVIEW

The prevention and control of infection is a primary goal of all health personnel. It is only in the past 150 years that successful measures to control infection have evolved. These include the development and widespread use of specific immunizations and antimicrobial agents, the implementation of basic sanitary measures as well as higher living standards. Important events in the history of infection control include Leeuwenhoek's discovery of the microscope (1678); Jenner's development of the first vaccine for smallpox (1796); Semmelweis' emphasis on hand-washing in lying-in hospitals (1847); Lister's introduction of antiseptics to cleanse the skin prior to surgery (1860s); Florence Nightingale's demonstration that improved hygiene, reduced overcrowding and standardized reporting of deaths could reduce mortality rates in army hospitals (1861); Koch's postulates on the relationship between microorganisms and disease (1876); and the discovery of penicillin (1928) and the sulfonamides (1935).

The infectious process starts with the invasion and multiplication of microorganisms on or in the body, causing ill or adverse effects. A causative agent (pathogen) grows in a reservoir which becomes its source, leaves through a portal of exit via a vehicle (mode of transmission) to a portal of entry in a susceptible host who becomes the new source. The portal of entry or of exit may be the respiratory, urinary, gastrointestinal or reproductive tracts, breaks in the skin or mucous membrane lining body cavities, wound discharges or blood. Modes of transmission include direct and indirect contact, inanimate objects (vehicle transmission), airborne transmission by droplet and vector (animal or insect) transmission. The host must be susceptible to the pathogen or have a low degree of resistance and the pathogen must be in sufficient quantity or of sufficient virulence to cause disease. A period of incubation precedes manifestation of symptoms or the appearance of infection.

The body has both non-specific and specific defences against infection. Non-specific mechanisms include the skin, mucous membranes, some body secretions and the local inflammatory response. There may also be a generalized stress reaction. Specific defence mechanisms include natural immunity and active or passive artificial immunity. The host's reaction to an infection may range from no symptoms to acute distress. Factors influencing the reaction include agent characteristics and host susceptibility. The host's state of physical, mental and emotional health affect susceptibility as well as the person's immunization history. The young and the old and the acutely or chronically ill are most vulnerable.

At different stages in the life cycle people are prone to different types of infections. During pregnancy infections in the mother can infect or injure the fetus. Genitourinary infections can be transmitted to the infant during birth. During infancy, deficiencies in the immune system make the danger of infection great, with dehydration a frequent concomitant. Respiratory infections affect all age groups with the young and the old being most susceptible.

The most common infections are those of the urinary tract, the lower respiratory tract, wound infections and gastroenteritis. Almost forty percent of nosocomial infections are in the urinary tract with fifty percent of patients with indwelling catheters developing an infection within two weeks and most within a month. The pathogens gain entry from outside or inside the catheter from either bowel flora or the hands of health care workers. Bacteremia develops in some cases. Of the lower respiratory tract infections, pneumonia is the most common and most frequent cause of death in the elderly and the debilitated. It may be viral or bacterial in origin. Wound infections after surgery account for 25% of nosocomial infections. These are almost always bacterial in origin and often polymicrobial. Gastroenteritis is a problem at all ages but particularly in children where it can quickly lead to dehydration. Its cause may be bacterial or viral agents or parasitic infestation. Enteric pathogens are usually either food- or water-borne or transmitted by the fecal-oral route. Bacteremia may be primary or secondary. Primary bacteremia is usually related to intravascular catheters, infusion systems or gut flora. Secondary bacteremias have a recognizable source such as pneumonia, urinary tract or surgical wound infections. Bacteremia can lead to septic shock and death. The best prevention strategy for all of these infections is good nursing techniques.

Assessing the infection prevention and control needs for each patient starts with the nursing history which includes the person's health practices and general susceptibility to infections and the physical examination. Temperature, pulse and respiration increases are often the first sign of infection with localized or systemic symptoms. Sputum, wound exudate, discharges or nausea and vomiting may also be present. Diagnostic tests include laboratory tests on blood, exudates, sputum, discharges, urine or stool as needed to identify the infecting agent(s).

Diagnosing infection problems includes identifying individuals at risk because of chronic disease, immunodeficiency, impaired skin or mucous membranes, impaired circulation, treatment-related factors, IV therapy, enteral feedings, malnutrition, lack of immunization or age.

Prevention and control of infection is inherent in the planning and implementing of all nursing activities. The basic goals are to prevent infection, control infection, prevent problems associated with infection and promote the patient's comfort. It is also important to promote infection control in self-care practices.

Health promoting strategies include the use of good handwashing techniques, maintaining good health through adequate exercise, nutrition and rest, reducing stress and maintaining immunization levels. Communities control infection through ensuring clean water and food supplies, proper sewage disposal and a clean environment.

Health protecting strategies include immunization, good hygiene and aseptic practices. Asepsis protects both the patient and the health worker. Cleaning, sanitization and disinfection are used to maintain a clean environment. The method and agent are chosen for the degree of asepsis required. Sterilization destroys all microbes and must be used for anything that will pierce the skin or mucous membranes. Medical asepsis is clean technique with thorough handwashing and careful disposal of supplies and equipment and is practised to prevent the spread of infection. Proper handwashing before and after the care of each patient is the most effective method of prevention.

Body substance precautions include handwashing and careful handling and disposal of all body substances and excretions, including laboratory specimens. Gloves must be worn when touching body excretions and secretions, touching mucous membranes or non-intact skin and when the caregiver's hands are cracked, chapped or cut. Punctured gloves are renewed and hands washed before continuing. Gloves are task specific, that is, they must be discarded and hands must be washed after completion of each task. Gowns are worn to protect patient and caregiver. Masks are worn to protect patients during aseptic procedures, when the patient is immunocompromised and when the patient is on restrictive isolation. Garbage and linen disposal consists of safe packaging to prevent contamination of workers and environment, and equipment is cleaned according to agency policy and procedures. Sharps disposal containers must be used.

Medical asepsis includes isolation procedures to protect others from a patient's infection or to protect the patient who is immunocompromised or has a multiple-drug resistant infection. Either way, the patient needs considerable emotional support as social contact is limited, feelings of unworthiness increase and sensory deprivation may occur. Teaching is essential and the patient's willingness to participate in his or her care is important to prevent spreading the infection through contamination.

Surgical asepsis is used to keep an object or area free of microorganisms. Anything entering the body or transecting the skin and all linen used in a procedure must be sterile. A sterile package is unsterile if wet, previously opened or past the expiry date. Only sterile objects can touch sterile fields or objects, otherwise they are contaminated. If in doubt, consider the field or object contaminated.

Health restoring strategies include the use of careful technique to prevent nosocomial infections, monitoring for the effects and side effects of antibiotic treatment, good nutrition and fluid intake and good basic nursing care.

LEARNING ACTIVITIES

1. **Case Study**: Mrs. Rose Jackson is admitted to a hospital for an operation to remove an ulcer on her left leg. Three days after her surgery, Mrs. Jackson's wound appears reddened and has a purulent discharge. A wound culture has been ordered to identify the infecting organism. Mrs. Jackson, who is 54 years old, is in a room that has four beds and a shared bathroom.

   a. What specific precautions should be taken?

   b. What factors would you consider prior to explaining these precautions to this patient?

   c. If feasible, what would be the advantages of moving Mrs. Jackson to a single room?

   d. The infecting organism is found to be *Staphylococcus aureus*. What do you need to know about this organism in order to establish a safe environment?

   e. Mrs. Jackson's wound is dressed at least twice a day. After this measure what should be done with the (i) old dressing, (ii) used dressing equipment and supplies, (iii) unused supplies and (iv) unused disinfectant?

2. "The safety of an environment is related to the number of pathogenic organisms in it." What measures in medical asepsis are based on this principle?

REFERENCES AND READINGS

ASSOCIATION FOR PRACTICE IN INFECTION CONTROL (APIC). (1983). *Curriculum for infection control practice.* Dubuque, IA: Kendall/Hunt.

BARRETT-CONNOR, E. (1978). Nosocomial infection: Definitions and magnitude. In E. Barrett-Connor, S. L. Brandt, H. J. Simon, and D. C. Dechairo. *Epidemiology for the infection control nurse.* St. Louis: Mosby.

BENENSON, A.S. (1990). *Control of communicable diseases in man* (15th ed.). Washington, D.C.: American Public Health Association.

BENNETT, J.V. and BRACHMAN, P.S. (Eds). (1991). *Hospital infections* (3rd ed.). Boston: Little Brown.

BERGER, K.J. and WILLIAMS, M.B. (1992). *Fundamentals of nursing: Collaborating for optimal health.* Norwalk, CT: Appleton & Lange.

CARPENITO, L.J. (1993). *Nursing diagnosis: Application to clinical practice* (5th ed.). Philadelphia: Lippincott.

CENTRES FOR DISEASE CONTROL (1987). Recommendations for prevention of HIV transmission in health care settings. *Morbidity and Mortality Weekly Report, 36* (Supplement 25), 15.

CENTRES FOR DISEASE CONTROL. (1988). Update, universal precautions for prevention of transmission of human immunodeficiency virus, hepatitis B virus and other blood borne pathogens in health care settings. *Morbidity and Mortality Weekly Report, 37*(24), 377.

CROW, S. (1989). *Asepsis, the right touch.* Bossier City, LA: Everett Companies Publishing Division.

DAVEY, F. (1991). Glove talk. *Canadian Nurse, 87*(4), 17–18.

DEDHAR, J. and ENQUIST, G. (1992). Practical guidelines for body substance precautions in long-term care. *Canadian Journal of Infection Control, 7*(3), 77–80.

EARNEST, V.V. (1993). *Clinical skills in nursing practice* (2nd ed.). Philadelphia: Lippincott.

FIHN, S.D. (1988). Urinary tract infection in primary care obstetrics and gynecology. *Clinical Obstetrics and Gynecology, 31*, 1003.

FLYNN, J.M. and HACKEL, R. (1990). *Technological foundations in nursing.* Norwalk, CT: Appleton & Lange.

HALEY, R.W., CULVER, D.H., WHITE, J.W., MORGAN, W.M., EMORI, T.G., MUNN, V.P. and HOOTON, T.M. (1985). Surveillance by objective: A new priority-directed approach to the control of nosocomial infection. *American Journal of Epidemiology, 121*, 182–205.

HALEY, R.W., GAYNES, R., ABER, R. and BENNETT, J. V. (1991). Surveillance of nosocomial infections. In J.V. Bennett and P.S. Brachman (Eds).*Hospital infections* (3rd ed.). Boston: Little Brown.

HALL, N. (1988). *Psychoneuroimmunology.* Paper presented at the 15th Annual Educational Conference of APIC, Dallas, TX.

HEALTH CANADA. (1993). *Canadian immunization guide* (4th ed.). Ottawa: Minister of Supply and Services. (Catalogue No. H49–8/1993E)

HEALTH AND WELFARE CANADA. (1991). *Notifiable diseases annual summary.* Ottawa: Minister of National Health and Welfare.

HEALTH AND WELFARE CANADA (Health Services and Promotion Branch). (1986). *Long-term care facilities.* Ottawa: Minister of National Health and Welfare.

HEALTH AND WELFARE CANADA (Health Services and Promotion Branch). (1988) *Infection control guidelines.* Ottawa: Minister of National Health and Welfare.

HEALTH AND WELFARE CANADA (Health Services and Promotion Branch). (1988). *Perinatal care.* Ottawa: Minister of National Health and Welfare.

HEALTH AND WELFARE CANADA (Health Services and Promotion Branch). (1990). *Isolation and precaution techniques.* Ottawa: Minister of National Health and Welfare.

HEDRICK, E.R. (1988). Infectious waste management — Will science prevail? *Infection Control and Hospital Epidemiology, 9*, 488–490.

HOEPRICH, P. D. (Ed.). (1972). *Infectious diseases.* Hagerstown, MD: Harper and Row.

JACKSON, M.M. and LYNCH, P. (1985). Isolation practices: A historical perspective. *American Journal of Infection Control, 13*(1), 21–51.

KENNER, C.A. and MACLAREN, A. (1993). *Essentials of maternal and neonatal nursing.* Springhouse, PA: Springhouse.

KING, M., GARTRELL, J. and TROVATO, F. (1991, Summer). Early childhood mortality 1926–1986. *Canadian Social Trends.* Ottawa: Minister of Supply and Services, 6–10. (Statistics Canada catalogue 11–008E)

LABORATORY CENTRE FOR DISEASE CONTROL. (1987). Recommendations for prevention of HIV transmission in health care settings. *Canada Diseases Weekly Report, 13* (Supplement 3).

LABORATORY CENTRE FOR DISEASE CONTROL. (1988). Update, universal precautions for prevention of human immunodeficiency virus, hepatitis B virus and other blood borne pathogens in health care settings. *Canada Diseases Weekly Report, 14*, 27.

LAFORCE, M.F. (1991). The control of infections in hospitals: 1750–1950. In R.P. Wenzel (Ed). *Prevention and control of nosocomial infections.* Baltimore, MD: Williams and Wilkins, 1–12.

LYNCH, P., JACKSON, M.M., CUMMINGS, M.J. and STAMM, W.E. (1987). Rethinking the role of isolation practices in the prevention of nosocomial infections. *Annals of Internal Medicine, 107*, 243–246.

MacDONALD, K.S., McLEOD, J. and NICOLLE, L. (1993). Clostridium difficile in a Canadian tertiary care hospital. *Canadian Journal of Infection Control, 8*(2), 37–40.

McLEAN, D.M. and SMITH, J.A. (1991). *Medical microbiology synopsis.* Philadelphia: Lea and Febiger.

NIGHTINGALE, F. (1861). *Notes on hospitals* (3rd ed.). London: Longmans.

PARKER, L. (1990). From pestilence to asepsis. *Nursing Times, 86*(49), 63–67.

PHILLIPS, C. (1989). Hand Hygiene. *Nursing Times Supplement — Journal of Infection Control Nursing, 85*(37), 76–79.

PILLITERI, A. (1992). *Maternal and child health nursing: Care of the child bearing and childrearing family.* Philadelphia: Lippincott.

PLORDE, J.J. (1990). Flagellates. In J. C. Sherris (Ed.). *Medical microbiology: Introduction to infectious disease* (2nd ed.). New York: Elsevier Science, 734.

SELWYN, S. (1991). Hospital infection: The first 2500 years. *Journal of Hospital Infection, 18* (Supplement A), 5–64.

SHOVEIN, J. and YOUNG, M.S. (1992, February). MRSA: Pandora's box for hospitals. *American Journal of Nursing.* 49–52.

SKIDMORE, A.G. (1993). Clostridium difficile — the only important nosocomial pathogen in developed countries. *Canadian Journal of Infection Control, 8*(2), 33.

STAMM, W.E. (1991). Urinary tract infection. In J.V. Bennett and P.S. Brachman (Eds). Hospital infections (3rd ed.). Boston: Little Brown, 597.

WALKER, M. (1991). What you should know about infection control today — A patient information booklet. *Canadian Journal of Infection Control, 6* (2), 43–45.

WENZEL, R.P. (Ed). (1987). *Prevention and control of nosocomial infections*. Baltimore, MD: Williams and Wilkins.

WHITE, P.J. and SHACKELFORD, P.G. (1983). Edward Jenner, MD, and the scourge that was. *American Journal of Diseases in Children, 137*, 846–869.

CHAPTER 32

Preoperative and Postoperative Care

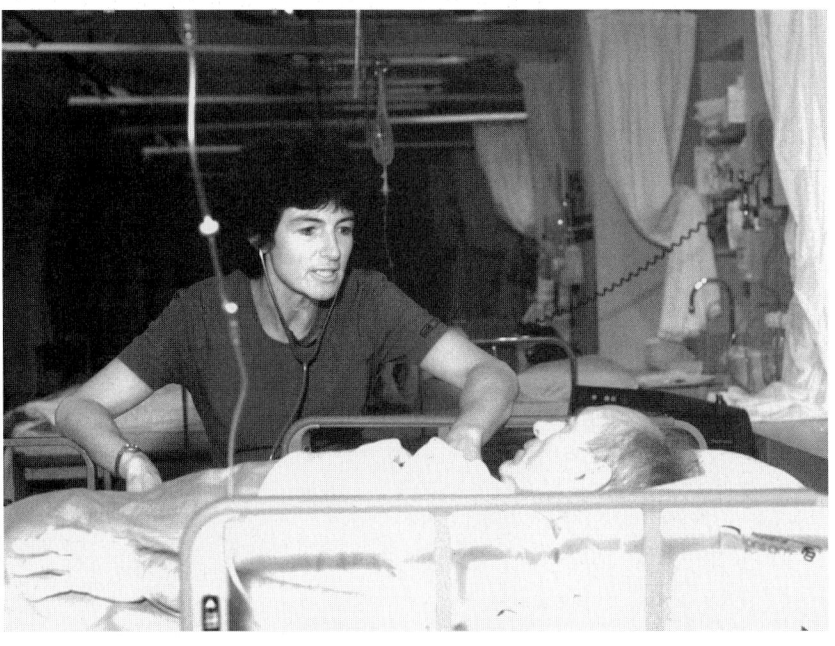

CENTRAL QUESTIONS

1. Why is surgery safer today than in previous times?

2. What are the major goals of nursing care for surgical patients?

3. What are the determinants of a patient's ability to cope with surgery?

4. What is involved in the nurse's preoperative assessment of the surgical patient?

5. What are the common nursing diagnostic statements for patients experiencing surgery?

6. What health promoting and health protecting strategies are indicated for preoperative and postoperative patients?

7. What is included in a preoperative teaching program?

8. What are the nursing responsibilities in the immediate and continuing postoperative periods?

9. How do surgical wounds heal and what determines healing?

10. What restorative strategies promote wound healing and facilitate recovery from surgery?

11. How does the nurse evaluate the effectiveness of nursing interventions?

INTRODUCTION

Surgery involves the deliberate and planned alteration of anatomical structures in order to arrest, alleviate or eradicate a pathological process, or to repair a traumatic injury. When surgery is recommended, a period of psychological and physiological stress begins and personal control of some aspects of life is surrendered in order to obtain relief from symptoms, restore normal bodily functions or to retain life itself. In some situations, such as after an accident, there may be no time for the patient to prepare for the surgical experience. In others, there may be ample time to think about and become prepared for surgery.

Nursing care of patients whose illness experience involves surgery is complex and varied. The major goals of nursing practice are to prepare the patient for surgery and to promote a healthy recovery. These goals can be fostered by the nurse who strives to maximize the patient's abilities to cope with the physiological and psychological stressors involved in a surgical experience. Assisting the patient to maintain self-care abilities, ensuring a sense of participation in care, protecting the patient from injury or harm and educating the patient and significant others to effectively manage recovery once home also help to foster these goals.

This chapter outlines the basic knowledge needed to care for patients whose illness experience involves surgery. The developments important to the care of the patient undergoing surgery and the determinants of the ability to cope with surgery are briefly described. Next, the events of the preoperative phase of the illness experience are discussed, along with the factors which increase physiological and psychological stress, and the nursing intervention of preoperative education. The impact of surgery on basic needs is identified and potential or actual problems which may be encountered in surgical illnesses are explored within a nursing process framework. The process of wound healing and basic wound procedures are also described.

SURGERY AND HEALTH CARE

Surgery has been used in the treatment of disease and injury from the beginning of humanity, but it was not until the middle of the nineteenth century that surgery began to evolve as a specific type of medical treatment. At that time, surgery was hazardous and it was limited either to measures that were essential to save a life, such as amputating a smashed limb, or to minor procedures such as removing a tooth, or draining an infected wound. Aseptic techniques were unknown, and surgery was performed by doctors who did not wear gloves or change instruments between successive operations. The rates of infection and mortality were so high that the treatment was not often beneficial.

Today, surgery has become a safe and humane method of treating disease. Advances in surgery have been made possible by the development of knowledge and techniques in the areas of hemostasis, asepsis, anesthesia and technology. The development of critical care units and the increase of research-based knowledge in nursing also have improved the outcomes of the patient undergoing surgery.

Hemostasis is the control of bleeding. Without adequate methods to control bleeding, the patient may die from hemorrhage. The methods used to control bleeding include pressure, cauterization (burning), tying the ends of the blood vessels with some type of material and tissue sealants which are sprayed on areas to retard or halt blood capillary oozing.

Prior to the development of the science of bacteriology, death from infection was common. The modern concept of asepsis is based on the knowledge that microorganisms are capable of causing disease. Factors that need to be controlled in order to prevent microorganisms from gaining access to wounds have been identified, and the application of this knowledge has decreased mortality and morbidity. The development of antibiotics has contributed to the decrease in infection rates after surgery. However, with heavy reliance on antibiotic therapy, the danger always exists that aseptic techniques will be relaxed or that antibiotic-resistant strains of microorganisms will develop causing massive problems of infection.

The development of anesthesia has made the prevention of pain during surgery possible. The physician can now take time to handle the tissues gently and perform the procedures with care. A variety of chemical anesthetic agents are used for inducing unconsciousness, controlling pain and removing the sensation in a region of the body or in a small area of the skin or mucous membrane. Chemical agents are delivered by gases which are inhaled and by liquids which are either injected into the skin, veins, sensory nerves or spinal cord or applied directly onto the skin.

Technological advances such as the use of video endoscopes, lasers and microsurgery have improved outcomes for the patient treated by surgery. In video endoscopy, a small telescope-type instrument with a camera is put into a body cavity through a small incision. Another small incision is made for the tiny tools which are used to perform the surgery. The reduction of tissue trauma decreases postoperative pain and diminishes the time of hospitalization and disability. The removal of a gallbladder by video endoscopy (laparoscopic cholecystectomy) is now a common procedure.

The manner of health care delivery is changing as the cost of prolonged hospital care has become a financial burden to society and many aspects of care are now delivered safely and effectively in the community. By the year 2000, the majority of patients will be admitted to the hospital on the morning of surgery, and 60 percent of them will return home the same evening (Connolly, 1991). At the same time as these advances are taking place, people are exercising their rights and assuming responsibility for health care. The patient undergoing surgery has the right to informed consent and the responsibility to assume a significant portion of presurgical and postsurgical care. The nurse is responsible for the patient education that will allow the patient to fulfil these responsibilities. Much of the education will occur at an outpatient clinic in the hospital or a community centre.

TYPES OF SURGICAL INTERVENTION

The classification of surgical procedures relates to the seriousness, urgency or purpose of surgery. A surgical procedure may fall into one or more categories. Surgical seriousness is designated as *major* or *minor* depending on the hazards involved and the physiological effects of the procedures on the body. For example, removal of an ingrown toenail or the incision and drainage of a boil are considered minor surgery, and may not even be done in an operating room. A hysterectomy (removal of the uterus), on the other hand, is considered a major surgical procedure and would be performed in an operating room.

Surgical interventions are also classified by urgency of the problem or time. Surgery for life-threatening problems such as bleeding is termed *immediate* or *emergency* surgery. When intervention is required within 24–48 hours, the surgery is classified as *urgent*, and when a procedure is needed but may be performed within a few weeks, such as seen in thyroid disorders, it is classified as *required* or *elective*. *Optional* surgery, such as cosmetic surgery, occurs when patient preference determines the time of the surgery.

The purpose of surgery varies. Surgery may be *diagnostic*, such as when a tissue sample is obtained **(biopsy)**, or it may be *curative*, such as when an inflamed appendix is removed. *Reparative* surgery is done, for example, when multiple wounds are repaired. *Palliative* surgery is done to lessen the distressing symptoms of a pathological process such as when a portion of the intestine is used to bypass an obstruction caused by a cancer growth. Surgery may also be constructive, reconstructive or cosmetic. *Constructive* surgery involves building or correcting a body part to improve its function or appearance, such as when the upper lip of a child with a congenital cleft is repaired. *Reconstructive* surgery is performed to repair damage to the appearance or functioning caused by trauma or disease in a previously intact anatomical structure. Reconstructive surgery is done, for example, when rebuilding a breast after the removal of a breast due to cancer. *Cosmetic* surgery may be done to improve physical appearance and, although it is not necessary for physical health, it is important for self-esteem.

The specific type of surgical procedure performed is described by the use of prefixes and suffixes. Prefixes identify the organ or body part and suffixes explain the procedure. For example, the prefix *gastro-* means stomach; the suffix *ectomy-* means the surgical removal of an organ or gland. Thus *gastrectomy* refers to the surgical removal of the stomach.

THE PREOPERATIVE PERIOD

During the preoperative period, the nature of the illness is determined and a plan of treatment is made. The time before diagnosis may be confusing to the patient who is undergoing a variety of procedures which are time-consuming, embarrassing, strenuous or even painful. Once the decision to have surgery is made, the patient will be asked to have more tests done. Frequently, an electrocardiogram is done, a chest x-ray is taken and blood and urine samples are tested again. The patient must make arrangements to be absent from school or work and to have someone assume

TABLE 32.1 Common Surgical Procedures

SUFFIX	DEFINITION	EXAMPLE OF PROCEDURE
-ectomy	Removal of organ or gland	Nephrectomy (removal of a kidney)
-ostomy	Forming an opening or stoma	Colostomy (an artificial opening from the colon to the surface of the abdomen)
-otomy	Making an incision or cutting into	Laparotomy (a surgical incision through the abdominal wall, often for diagnostic purposes)
-plasty	Repairing or restoring a body part	Mammoplasty (surgical reconstruction of a breast)
-rrhaphy	Suturing an organ or part in place	Osteorrhaphy (surgical fixation of bone fragments with sutures or wires)
-scopy	Visual examination by means of a fibreroptic instrument	Gastroscopy (visual examination of the stomach)

responsibilities that cannot be ignored. In addition, patients must cope with fears about the surgery. The illness experience causes changes in the interactions, roles and relationships between the patient and those involved with the illness experience. The result is a loss of a normal way of life (Morse and Johnson, 1991).

The overall goal of the preoperative period is to optimize the patient's psychological and physiological health. The patient who is in physiological hemostasis and is emotionally prepared for surgery has the best chance of tolerating surgery well. Preoperative assessment is done to determine the risk of surgery. Factors such as age, extent of planned surgery and the presence of other health problems may affect the ability to tolerate surgery. If possible, interventions are taken to minimize problems which exist. An essential nursing intervention in preparing for surgery is decreasing the patient's psychological stress and enhancing the patient's ability to participate in health care.

DETERMINANTS OF THE ABILITY TO COPE WITH SURGERY

Surgery involves an invasion of the body tissues. Some people are more vulnerable and at higher risk to develop complications than others. The principal factors affecting surgical risk are discussed below.

EXTENT OF SURGERY

The risk of shock, infection and other complications increases in proportion to the amount of tissue damage, manipulation or removal. The more that tissues are damaged, manipulated or removed, the higher the risk of complications. The patient who undergoes two or more surgical procedures close together in time is more at risk. The body requires time to recover from one surgery before another is imposed upon it.

AGE

The very young and the older patient are more at risk. Before the age of six months, the child's circulatory and renal functions are not fully developed and therefore they do not withstand the stress of surgery as well as older children and adults. Children have small amounts of subcutaneous tissue and fragile thermal regulating mechanisms and are sensitive to chilling and exposure. The child may have adequate heart muscle reserve but small alterations in fluid and electrolytes may impose significant problems. For example, a small volume of blood loss which would be easily compensated for in an adult may represent a large decrease in the total blood volume of a child.

KEY PRINCIPLES

Principles of Preoperative and Postoperative Care

1. Surgery evokes a major stress reaction in the body.
2. Surgery is a major assault on the body and lowers the ability to cope with other stressors.
3. Surgery affects the ability to meet basic needs.
4. The skin is the body's first line of defence against harmful agents, and penetration of the skin by surgical incision provides a portal of entry for invading pathogens.
5. The very young and the very old are vulnerable to the adverse effects of surgery, as are those with respiratory problems, cardiovascular disease, abnormal blood coagulation patterns, diabetes or disorders causing vascular insufficiency.
6. People who are extremely fearful are poor surgical risks.
7. Fear of the unknown is a potent factor in presurgical anxiety, and information may help to alleviate some of this fear.

The very young and the older patient are more vulnerable to the stress of surgery.

The physiological changes in older people increase vulnerability to the stresses of surgery. Some of the changes are decreased heart and lung reserves, disturbances in fluid and electrolyte regulation, decreased liver and renal function, decreased gastric and gastrointestinal tract motility, decreased immunological function, decreased sensory abilities, decreased amount of subcutaneous tissue and increased susceptibility to complications from bedrest (King, 1991; White, Thurston, Blackmore, Green and Hannah, 1987).

The decreased reserves of the heart and the lungs of older people make it difficult for the body to maintain hemostasis in the face of continued strain. The fluid and electrolyte changes include a decline in the ability of the kidney to conserve water and retain sodium which increases the risk of dehydration. Additionally, there is a decrease in thirst perception, which means that the older patient may not respond to dehydration by independently increasing fluid intake (Miller, 1987).

The decreased liver function in an older patient may alter or prolong the metabolization of drugs which, combined with the decline in the ability of the renal tissues to excrete end products, makes the administration of drug therapies difficult. The decrease in intestinal motility prolongs the time of drug absorption and decreases the ability to feel hungry, to take and absorb the nutrients essential for healing and to excrete waste products. A decreased amount of subcutaneous tissue increases the vulnerability to a loss of body heat and decreases the resistance to mechanical trauma of the integument. The decreased immunologic activities increases the susceptibility to infection.

Despite the increased risk, the older patient who has a good outlook, is well nourished and has reasonable cardiac, pulmonary and renal reserves will cope with the stress of a single surgical procedure well.

NUMBER OF OTHER HEALTH PROBLEMS

The patient who has a number of other health problems or is in general poor health is at greater surgical risk than one who is physically fit. Particularly vulnerable to postoperative problems are those with chronic respiratory tract disease such as chronic obstructive pulmonary disease (emphysema), those with respiratory tract infections or cardiovascular disease, those with blood coagulation problems and those with metabolic disorders such as diabetes.

OBESITY

The patient who is obese is at increased risk for impaired wound healing and wound infections owing to the decreased circulation to adipose tissue and the strain of the adipose tissue on the incision. The patient who is obese may have shallow breathing or may breathe poorly when lying on the side, causing an increased incidence of pulmonary complications. In addition, there is an increased incidence of abdominal distention and phlebitis (inflammation of the veins) with increased weight.

PSYCHOLOGICAL STRESS

The patient who is extremely anxious or has multiple life stressors is at increased risk for developing problems during or after surgery. The psychological stressors increase the level of the surgical stress response and may make it difficult for the patient to learn about activities such as deep breathing and coughing which can improve the outcome of the surgery.

MEDICATION THERAPY

Many prescribed and over-the-counter medications have the potential to affect the physiological functions of the body and may interact with anesthetic agents causing serious problems. Of particular concern are adrenal corticosteroids, which must be continued to avoid circulatory collapse; diuretics, which can cause electrolyte imbalance; antidepressants, which can increase the hypotensive effects of anesthetics; tranquilizers, which can cause seizures if withdrawn too quickly; insulin, which must be adjusted to account for the rise in blood sugar associated with the stress of surgery; some antibiotics which can interact with anesthetic agents; and, of course, anticoagulants, which alter the normal pattern of blood coagulation. The patient with an addiction to narcotic drugs or alcohol is also at increased risk for developing postoperative complications.

ASSESSING PREOPERATIVELY

A preoperative nursing assessment should begin with the first nurse who is in contact with the patient after surgery is planned. The nurse may work in an outpatient clinic, a preadmission testing centre or an inpatient unit of a health care facility. A nursing assessment of each need, as outlined in previous chapters, is done by the nurse who should have knowledge of the basic nature of the patient's health problem and the purpose of the surgery being planned. The health history is very important in order to establish a data base for future comparisons. Increased attention to oxygen, nutrition, elimination and immune needs is suggested. Each nurse who cares for the patient is responsible for adding to the data base. As the patient will move through several geographical locations in a surgical experience, it is essential to communicate specific information to other nurses and members of the health care team.

SPECIFIC ASSESSMENT OF NEEDS

Oxygen

The lungs are carefully assessed as pulmonary complications are the largest single cause of prolonged hospitalization and death after surgery. Assessment should include information about chronic lung conditions, medications taken for these conditions, smoking history, coughing, wheezing, shortness of breath, orthopnea, ankle edema, cyanosis, clubbing of the fingers, asthma, chest pain on exertion and barrel chest. Signs and symptoms of a cold or other respiratory infection, however minor, are reported and surgery in non-life threatening illnesses may be cancelled due to this information. A chest x-ray is done on patients over the age of 45 before surgery, and on younger patients if a respiratory problem is present or suspected. Preoperatively, an improvement in lung reserve may be fostered by encouraging those who are able to walk one mile per day. All patients who smoke are asked to stop six weeks prior to elective surgery.

Fluid and Electrolytes

A careful assessment of the circulatory system is essential. Existing problems such as chronic heart conditions, high blood pressure, varicose veins, circulatory disorders causing cold extremities and diabetes are noted. These problems increase the risk of surgery and may contribute to vulnerability to the formation of blood clots in the extremities. The patient should be asked about any medications taken for circulatory health problems. The circulatory system is assessed in relation to the reserve capacity of the heart and blood vessels. Poor exercise tolerance, presence of chest pain, irregularities of the pulse and in adults a blood pressure of below 90 systolic or above 120 diastolic may indicate a diminished or inadequate ability to tolerate the stress of surgery. Deviations from normal should be reported to the doctor. Surgery may be delayed until treatable problems are corrected. Extremities and the site of planned surgery should be examined for pallor and coldness which may indicate poor blood supply with a decreased ability to heal. An electrocardiogram is taken in all patients over the age of 45 and all patients who report heart problems.

An assessment of the quality and quantity of the blood components and volume is done preoperatively. The red blood cell count and hematocrit or hemoglobin are determined. A group and screen of the blood type is done in case a transfusion is needed. In situations involving major surgery, a cross-match is done the evening prior to or the morning of surgery. Patients undergoing elective surgery may be able to donate their own blood for use if needed. The availability of the patient's own (autologous) blood should be documented. Prothrombin time (a blood test to assess clotting) is done to identify potential or actual problems in the blood clotting mechanism. Tests are carried out to assess the electrolyte balance. Of particular importance are the levels of potassium, sodium, chloride and bicarbonate.

Nutrition

Important factors to consider in nutritional assessment are body weight, blood hemoglobin and recent weight loss. Correction of malnutrition before surgery decreases the risk of surgery. If body weight is ten percent below the ideal weight for height and if time permits, patients can be referred to a dietitian for dietary counselling, given nutritional supplements, referred to a community resource which delivers meals to the home or helped by family and friends to improve intake (Beckermann and Galloway, 1989). It is important to document information on the food and fluid preferences and any food allergies. Cultural or religious practices in relation to food and any special dietary needs such as a sodium-restricted or diabetic diet should be noted and the information given to the dietary department. If the patient is overweight and if preoperative time permits, a program of exercise and weight reduction may be advised to reduce the risk of surgery.

Elimination

Kidney function is carefully assessed because the kidneys are involved with the excretion of anesthetic drugs and their end products. Urinary elimination is assessed in relation to the patient's normal voiding pattern and any problems which are currently present. Recent problems in urinary functions, such as kidney infections, are noted as they may have to be investigated prior to surgery. A routine urinalysis is usually done. The nurse is responsible for instructing the patient how to collect the sample, or assisting with the collection if the patient is unable to do so. Results of the urinalysis should be examined for abnormalities. The presence of sugar in the urine is of particular importance and may be indicative of a diabetic condition. Normal bowel function is assessed and information about any longstanding or recent problems or aids used for bowel function is gathered.

Immunological Needs

It is important to determine the presence of a history of allergies, including a description of signs and symptoms experienced. Allergies to any medications, blood products or contrast media used in radiological procedures are of special significance. Some medications such as corticosteroids, radiotherapy and chemotherapy produce immunosuppression, and careful assessment of these factors is essential.

Body temperature is taken, and even the mildest deviation should be reported to the physician.

IMPACT OF SURGERY ON SECURITY AND SELF-ESTEEM

Surgery may be judged as a stressful event that threatens the patient's security and self-esteem. Anxiety is a common problem before surgery. Anxieties may arise if the patient fears death on the operating room table, mutilation or disfigurement, postoperative pain and separation from family and friends. Often the patient is afraid that the surgeon will find evidence of cancer, or worse still a cancer that is too large to remove. The patient may be anxious about how to cope after surgery both in the hospital and at home. The extent of the surgery, including the discomfort and changes that are anticipated, is often related to the amount of anxiety experienced. The patient who is having surgery for a small hernia may be less anxious than the one who is to have open-heart surgery. Young children may be very anxious prior to any surgery.

During the preoperative period, discharge planning is begun. The patient may be anxious and may express concerns about managing care after hospital discharge. Assistance may be required to plan for care once the patient returns home. The health care system may provide rehabilitative care or professional community nursing care such as that required for wound care. Convalescent care, however, is the responsibility of the patient and significant others. If the patient is unable to make arrangements for help at home, referral to a social worker or a community nurse to assist in this process is beneficial.

The patient may seek information to help control anxiety. The information may be used to formulate a picture of the events to be encountered, to increase the understanding and interpretation of specific elements in the surgical experience and to make plans to minimize the negative aspects of the illness (Johnson and Lauver, 1989). Research studies have shown that nursing interventions related to providing accurate relevant information, reassurance and attention to individual concerns produce positive outcomes in the postoperative period. These outcomes include improved satisfaction with care, reduced pain, decreased anxiety and minimized postoperative complications (Devine and Cook, 1986; Hathaway, 1986).

DIAGNOSING PREOPERATIVELY

Two major nursing diagnoses of the preoperative period are *Knowledge deficit regarding the preoperative procedures and protocols and the postoperative expectations* and *Anxiety related to the surgical experience and the outcome of surgery*.

PLANNING AND IMPLEMENTING PREOPERATIVELY

PREOPERATIVE EDUCATION PROGRAMS

The health promoting strategy which assists the patient and family to prepare for the psychological and physiological stress of surgery is preoperative education. Preoperative education programs are given prior to hospital admission in preadmission testing centres and outpatient clinics or after admission in the hospital. In situations where there is limited time for education, such as before emergency surgery, patients are given small amounts of situational information and psychosocial support. Information about skills training or role expectations are given during the postoperative period.

At times, preoperative teaching is done in groups, and at times it is done on a one-to-one basis. Whatever the method, it is important to determine the level of understanding of the surgical process and the type of surgery that is to be done. It is important to assess the ability to learn, and to identify any problems that might interfere with learning, such as poor eyesight, a hearing loss, extreme anxiety or limited mobility. Children and those with special learning needs require an alteration in the type and amount of preoperative education. The preoperative assessment and teaching should involve the family or significant others. The family is then able to provide the support and assistance the patient needs in order to review what the nurse has said and to help in the application of the information. Many facilities have excellent teaching aids, but they are not substitutes for education by the nurse who understands about the specific type of surgery, the sensations to expect and the role to be taken in recovery.

The types of information that are given preoperatively are situational information, sensation and discomfort information, patient role information, psychosocial support and skills training (Schoessler, 1989). Situational information includes descriptions of nursing care activities, equipment and explanation of the sequence and timing of events. Information about sensations and discomfort includes explanation about the sensations and discomforts that the patient may experience and how discomforts can be managed. Role information describes the ways in which the patient will be expected to participate in care so that the treatment goals are met. For example, information that the patient is to call a nurse for assistance the first time out of bed after surgery is role information. The information indicates to patients the action that is necessary to assist in protecting themselves from harm after surgery. Psychosocial support refers to the interactions between the nurse with the patient which are aimed at alleviating anxiety and/or enhancing coping. Skill training is the explanation and guided practice of skills, such as deep breathing and coughing, that aid the patient in protecting or restoring health.

An example of a preoperative education program is presented in the following pages. This includes the goals, expected outcomes, educational content and evaluation of a teaching program provided at the Scarborough Grace Hospital and Sunnybrook Health Sciences Centre, Toronto, Ontario (Desjardins, Noble, Bubela, McKibbon and Galloway, 1992. Reproduced with permission.).

Preoperative Education Program

GOALS

1. To provide information regarding the surgery and sensations to be expected.

2. To assist the patient to manage preoperative anxiety, and thus optimize coping abilities.

3. To assist patients in identifying roles and responsibilities in the preoperative, postoperative and recovery periods.

EXPECTED OUTCOMES

The patient will be able to

1. state the nature and purpose of the surgery, and the anticipated course of the surgical illness experience.

2. describe the sensations to be expected after surgery and identify strategies to manage the sensations. The patient will postoperatively report pain to the nurse and take analgesics as necessary.

3. perform deep breathing and coughing and leg exercises.

4. identify his or her role and responsibilities preoperatively and postoperatively.

5. adhere to the dietary and smoking restrictions and the other preoperative instructions.

To promote continuity of care, an education checklist is placed on the chart. An example of an education checklist is given in the box below, followed by a description of the information which is given in each category. The content is individualized to reflect the surgical procedure and the circumstances.

1. Information provided specific to the procedure Document the information provided that is specific to the surgical procedure such as the nature of the procedure, postoperative nursing care and expected course in hospital.

Preoperative Education Checklist

Content Given

1. Information Provided Specific to the Procedure

2. Type of Anesthetic: General, Neuroleptic or Local

3. Dietary Restrictions:
   Pre-OR_____ Post-OR_____

4. Medications:

5. IV Therapy:

6. Dressings and Drainage Tubes:

7. Oxygen Therapy:

8. Sensations Experienced: (Pain)

9. Smoking Restriction:

10. Deep Breathing and Coughing Exercises:

11. Leg Exercises:

12. Coping:

13. Hospital Policies: Visiting, Smoking, Discharge Time

---

2. Anesthetic Many patients are afraid of being awake or in pain during surgery. Some patients fear not waking up after surgery. Reassure the patient that modern anesthesia is effective and that the anesthetist will monitor the patient carefully. Give general information about how a local or general anesthetic works, and what sensations, such as a sore throat, may be experienced afterwards. Ask the patient to write down other questions for the anesthetist. The anesthetist will see the patient the evening before surgery or the morning of surgery. Ask if the patient has had any experience or problems with anesthetics before. Notify the Anesthesia Department or the on-call anesthetist of the patient's name and unique hospital number if any concerns exist.

3. Dietary restrictions All patients are to be NPO (nothing by mouth) from midnight of the night prior to surgery, unless ordered differently by the physician. Postoperatively, a diet as tolerated is usual. After abdominal surgery, the patient will usually be NPO until they have passed gas through the rectum.

4. Medications People on cardiac medications such as digoxin, antiarrhythmics or antihypertensives (but not diuretics) may be asked by the anesthetist to take medications with a sip of water the morning of surgery. No other medications are to be taken.

5. Intravenous therapy An intravenous (IV) may be inserted preoperatively. The IV is needed to give fluids and medications. It will be removed when the patient is drinking well. Instruct the patient to report pain, swelling or redness at the IV insertion site.

6. Dressings and drainage tubes Ascertain what the surgeon has described to the patient about dressings and drainage tubes and correct any misconceptions.

7. Oxygen therapy The patient may have oxygen given in the Post Anesthetic Care Unit (PACU or Recovery Room) only. Instruct people who are smokers and those with respiratory disease that they may be required to wear an oxygen mask or nasal prongs for longer.

8. Sensations experienced Pain is a major sensation experienced after surgery. Describe the type and severity of pain that the patient can expect. The type of questions asked by patients before surgery (Pogue, 1993) are outlined in a following box. Explain other sensations that the patient can expect preoperatively or postoperatively such as nausea, plugged nose or sore throat.

9. Smoking Patients who smoke must stop prior to surgery as smoking causes an increase in mucous production causing more coughing, and increases risk for respiratory complications postoperatively. Identify methods that will help stop smoking such as relaxation exercises and discontinuing activities associated with smoking such as drinking alcohol or coffee.

10. Deep breathing and coughing Review the method for deep breathing and coughing and have the patient give a repeat demonstration. Explain the rationale for the exercises and, if available, give the patient a copy of the instructions.

11. Leg exercises Review leg exercises to be done postoperatively. Instruct the patient to call for assistance the first time of ambulation and at any time if feeling unsteady or dizzy.

12. Coping Ask if the patient anticipates any problems coping with the surgery, hospitalization and after hospital discharge. Ascertain if the patient has any recent emotional problems or major losses (for example, loss of a spouse, very ill family member or depression) which may increase the stress response to surgery.

13. Hospital policies Explain the visiting hours, the no smoking policy, and the discharge time.

The evaluation of the effectiveness of the preoperative teaching is done after surgery. A nurse evaluates the effectiveness on a questionnaire similar to the one depicted in the box on page 1051.

IMMEDIATE PREOPERATIVE CARE IN THE HOSPITAL

No matter how well prepared, people are often anxious at the time of hospitalization and feel dehumanized. They are labelled with an arm band, most of their possessions are taken away and they are given a hospital gown to wear. They may be told when and where they can come and go, they are stabbed with needles and have numerous personal questions asked of them by a variety of health care providers. These events happen at a time when they are anxious about the surgery which is planned.

The nurse is responsible for taking or completing the nursing assessment, and reviewing or giving information in the preoperative period to ease the patient's anxiety. In addition, the nurse is responsible for ensuring that the patient is safely prepared for surgery. Vital signs are taken to obtain baseline data and to observe for deviations that indicate the patient is not in good general health. An elevated temperature, irregular heart beat or abnormal blood pressure are vitally important to document and to report. The safe preparation includes nutritional, fluid and integumentary considerations.

Nutrition and Bowel Elimination

A normal diet may be allowed until eight to ten hours prior to the administration of an anesthetic. Food and fluids are then withheld so that the stomach will be empty while the patient is under anesthetic. Ensuring that the patient understands and complies with the food and fluid restrictions is vital to prevent the aspiration of regurgitated stomach contents. Such material in the lungs causes irritation, an inflammatory reaction and decreases adequate air exchange. If the surgery being planned involves the gastrointestinal tract or surrounding area, the intestinal tract is cleared of stool the night prior to surgery. A variety of bowel preparations are used to accomplish the cleaning. These will be ordered by the surgeon or administered according to agency policy.

Skin Preparation

The first line of defence of the body against injury or invading agents is a healthy and intact skin. The objective of preoperative skin preparation is to decrease bacterial sources without injuring the skin. The patient may have a bath or shower using a detergent-germicide to cleanse the skin. The patient is asked to wash the hair and to clean under the fingernails. The nurse may be responsible for performing certain scrubs or instructing the patient in these procedures.

Questions Patients Ask About Pain After Surgery

Being comfortable after surgery is important. You can work with your nurses and doctors to manage your pain after surgery.

What is pain?

People call pain many things. They may say pain is a soreness, a hurt, a pang, an ache, a sting or a cramp. Only the person who has pain knows when it is there, and can describe what it is.

Why is it important to decrease pain after surgery?

With less pain, moving is easier. By moving, you may avoid problems that can delay your recovery. Getting out of bed and walking after surgery keeps your muscles strong and prevents blood clotting. Deep breathing after surgery helps prevent lung problems.

Why will I have pain after surgery?

Pain after surgery may be due to the cutting of skin and tissues, drainage tubes and muscle soreness from the position in which your body was during surgery.

Where will I have pain?

Pain is often in the area of the surgery. Ask your doctor or nurse where you may expect to have pain.

How much pain will I have?

This is a hard question to answer. Two people having the same type of surgery may have different amounts of pain. Medications are available to help decrease your pain.

How will the nurse know how much pain I have?

Tell your nurse how much pain you have. The nurse may ask you how much pain you have on a scale of 0 to 10. No pain is 0. The worst pain you can think of is 10.

When should I tell the nurse about my pain?

Tell your nurse when you start to have pain, if your pain medication does not help or if you have a different type of pain.

When will I get pain medication?

Pain medication will be ordered by your doctor. Ask your nurse for pain medication when you start to have pain. Do not wait until you have severe pain. Ask for pain medication half an hour to an hour before activity.

What medication will I get for my pain?

Medication containing a narcotic is usually given for pain after surgery. This medication may be given by a needle at first. When you can drink, a pain pill is often given. Other ways are used to give pain medication for some patients. If this applies to you, your doctor or nurse will discuss this with you.

Can I become addicted to pain medication?

People seldom become addicted to medication taken for pain after surgery. Unless you have had a problem with drug addiction, this should not worry you. If you have or had a problem with drug addiction, let your doctor know.

Do pain medications have any side effects?

Possible side effects include constipation, nausea or drowsiness. Please ask your nurse or doctor how to manage these symptoms in the hospital and at home.

What can I do to decrease pain?

- Do not wait until you have severe pain before you ask for pain medication.

- Change your position in bed. Ask your nurse if you need help to change your position.

- If you had surgery in the area of your stomach or chest, hold a pillow against your incision while you do breathing and coughing exercises.

- If you have gas pain, walk at least three times per day.

- If you have worries about being in hospital, talk to your nurse.

- Try reading, watching television, listening to music, talking on the telephone, visiting or other quiet activities. These things can help your pain at any time or when you are waiting for pain medication to work.

SOURCE: Pogue, P. (1993). *Questions patients ask about pain after surgery.* Sunnybrook Health Science Centre: Toronto, Ontario. Reproduced with permission.

The skin and the area around the site of the incision are *not* shaved (Cruse and Foord, 1980; Seropian and Reynolds, 1971) as research has shown that shaving destroys the natural skin defence and can create superficial bacterial growth (Alexander, Fischer, Boyaijian, Palmquist and Morris, 1983). If removal of hair at the operative site is necessary, the area is cleaned with a depilatory cream or by electric clippers.

Depilatory creams have a che...ical base to remove the hair. They result in a clean, smooth and intact skin. The electric clipper with a disposable head is also a safe effective method for hair removal and leaves an intact skin (Alexander et al., 1983). If removal of hair by shaving is necessary, it is done 30 minutes or less prior to surgery (AORN, 1992) to minimize the risk of infection.

Evaluation of Effectiveness of Preoperative Education Questionnaire

Circle the appropriate response

Rate this patient in relation to	Poor		Good		Excellent
1. knowledge of the surgical procedure	1	2	3	4	5
2. knowledge of sensations to expect	1	2	3	4	5
3. knowledge of expected hospital course	1	2	3	4	5
4. knowledge of post-op exercises	1	2	3	4	5
5. compliance with post-op exercises	1	2	3	4	5
6. reporting of post-op pain	1	2	3	4	5
7. appropriate taking of analgesics	1	2	3	4	5
8. adherence to NPO and dietary restrictions	1	2	3	4	5

NURSING INTERVENTIONS ON THE DAY OF SURGERY

There are a number of nursing interventions aimed at safety and at protecting the patient from injury that are performed on the day of surgery. These provisions are instituted prior to the administration of the preoperative medication. Most facilities have a checklist which guides the nurse in completing all of the activities (see Figure 32.1). The nurse checks the list to ensure that everything has been done before the patient goes to the operating room.

Informed consent   Determine whether the patient or a legal representative of the patient has given written Informed Consent. The word "consent" literally means to feel together that something should be done. Physicians have a nontransferable legal duty to obtain a patient's informed consent for any medical or surgical treatment (Curtin, 1993). If the patient has signed a consent form, but the nurse finds that the patient has withdrawn consent, or expresses confusion or uncertainty about the planned surgery, the nurse informs the physician who is then obligated to explain the matter again to the patient.

The patient's record   Physician orders are reviewed to ensure that all recommended preparations have been instituted. All pertinent laboratory and preoperative test results are to be present on the chart.

Identification label   Ensure that the patient's identification label is correct. The correct spelling of the name and the unique hospital number are carefully checked. The unique hospital number will be used to identify the unconscious patient and to label tissue specimens sent to the laboratory. The patient who has a medic alert bracelet is either to wear it or to have it taped securely to the hospital record.

Hygiene and dress   After bathing, the patient is given a hospital gown to wear. All nail polish is removed from fingers and toes to facilitate observation of tissue perfusion in the extremities. All jewellery and hair pins are removed. If the patient does not wish to remove a wedding ring, it is secured with a piece of tape placed around the finger.

Dentures   Check for, remove and store dentures or partial dental appliances. These appliances are removed to decrease the risk of inadvertent aspiration and obstruction of the airway during the surgery. Research has shown that many patients who wear dentures are distressed at having to remove them (Cobley, Dunne and Sanders, 1991). The nurse should not ask the patient to remove dentures until necessary, and if the patient's distress is high, explore the possibility of the patient keeping them in place until in the operating room.

Health aids and prosthetic devices   Other health aids and prosthetic devices are identified. Contact lenses are removed, as are glasses. If a patient is unable to hear without a hearing aid, the hearing aid is often left in place. The nurse in the operating room will need to be informed of the hearing aid. Other prosthetic devices such as artificial limbs are removed and placed in a secure location on the nursing unit.

Family and support people   The family or support persons are identified by the patient. The patient's wishes about who is to be notified by the physician after the surgery are determined. Family and support people are given guidance about where to wait during surgery, the anticipated length of the surgery and when the physician will speak to them after surgery.

Vital signs   The patient's pulse, blood pressure, respiratory rate and temperature are taken and documented before administration of preoperative medications or within several hours of the planned surgery if no preoperative medication is ordered. Deviations from the patient's baseline vital signs are reported to the doctor.

Urinary bladder   The patient is to void so that the bladder is emptied. A distended bladder can obscure the operative area in pelvic and abdominal surgery, increase the risk for inadvertent penetration of the bladder and increase the chance of reflex bladder emptying as muscles relax during anesthesia.

Preoperative medication   If ordered, the preoperative medication is given. The medication may be ordered to decrease anxiety, make the induction of anesthesia less stressful or decrease secretions in the mouth and throat. Once the medication is given, the patient is asked to remain in bed and, as a safety precaution, the side rails are raised.

Final check   The nurse makes a final check to make sure that everything has been done for the patient's safety.

When the operating room notifies the nursing unit, the patient is taken to the operating room area on a stretcher. Patients may be transported on a bed if the bed has special attachments, such as traction. The patient's chart is sent to the operating room. A porter may take the patient from the nursing unit to the operating room. The nurse should accompany those individuals who are unable to communicate easily, who are not hemodynamically stable or who are unduly anxious.

Patient awaiting transfer to the operating room.

Preparing the postoperative unit   The postoperative unit is set up directly after the patient goes to surgery. It involves making a postoperative bed and assembling necessary equipment for postoperative care. The postoperative bed, also called an *anesthetic bed* or *recovery bed*, is a variation of the basic hospital bed. Its purpose is to provide a safe, clean area into which a patient can be easily moved. It is set up so that bed linen can be changed with a minimum of disturbance to the patient.

Making a postoperative bed is similar to making an unoccupied bed (Procedure 25.1). Usually the foundation for an unoccupied bed is completed, and then a cotton drawsheet or flannelette sheet is placed over it to protect the bottom sheet. This is done because a short sheet can be changed more easily than an entire bottom sheet and therefore causes the least disturbance to the patient. Flannelette sheets are preferred by some because they provide additional warmth. A disposable incontinence or reusable drainage pad may also be placed over these sheets. The top covers are applied and then fan-folded to the bottom of the bed in preparation for the patient's transfer into bed upon return to the unit.

Once the bed is made, it is raised to the high position so that it will be the same level as the stretcher and a check is made to ensure that the wheels are locked. This will facilitate a safe transfer of the patient from the stretcher to the bed. The other furniture and equipment in the room are arranged to make room for the stretcher.

Supplies and equipment needed for postoperative care are gathered and placed for convenient access. The patient's personal belongings are put safely away, and the overbed table is left clear. Tissues and a kidney basin should be immediately available. Side rails should be attached to the bed. An intravenous pole should be either attached to the bed or available in the patient's room.

THE POSTOPERATIVE PERIOD

A patient's postoperative response to surgical intervention can be varied and complex. Any one of the patient's basic needs can be affected, depending on the nature of each situation. The nurse assesses the patient, diagnoses problems and plans, implements and evaluates care by applying knowledge of the impact of the surgery on basic human needs. In this section, we will discuss the immediate postoperative care of the patient and the initial assessment of the patient upon return to the nursing unit. The impact of surgery on the patient's basic needs and an outline of care organized according to the nursing process will follow. This includes examples of nursing diagnoses and expected outcomes, as well as nursing strategies to achieve patient goals. Evaluation of the effectiveness of care is based on the goal being achieved.

LIONS GATE HOSPITAL — PRE-OPERATIVE CHECKLIST

Date of Surgery: _____

Surgical Procedure: _____

Date & Time Of Last Food Or Drink

Preparation of Chart:	Yes	No	N/A	Preparation For Surgery:	Yes	No	N/A
Consent for Surgery				Skin / Shave Prep			
F3100d Refusal Form				Bowel Prep			
History				NG Tube Inserted			
Old Chart				Foley Catheter Inserted			
Addressograph (in Jacket)				IV Started			
M AR				Pre-Op IV Meds			
Clipboard Sheets				**Specimens & Tests:**			
Preparation For Transport:				Urinalysis			
Identiband				HGB - (Results on Chart)			
Allergy Band				Blood X-Match			
Wt/ VS Charted				Chest X-Ray			
Voided				ECG - (Results on Chart)			
Pre-Op Med. Given				Other: ____ Results On Chart			
Cosmetics Removed							
Jewelry Removed							
Contact Lenses Removed							
Dentures Removed							
Teeth: Loose, Caps,							
Bridgework							

Special Messages:

e g. Blind, Deaf, Physical Limitations, Preferred Language, Implants & Prostheses, Respiratory Precautions

Signatures:

1. Ward

   Time: _____ Signature: _____

2. Holding Area:

   Time: _____ Signature: _____

FIGURE 32.1 Preoperative Checklist Form

IMMEDIATE POSTOPERATIVE CARE

Most patients go to a Post Anesthesia Care Unit (PACU) directly from the operating room. In the PACU, nurses are responsible for the patient's recovery from anesthesia. The nursing care includes assessing the patient's level of consciousness, vital signs and presence or absence of reflexes, as well as drainage from dressings, tubes and collecting bags on arrival and at frequent intervals. Immediate postoperative orders for medications, x-rays, oxygen, intravenous and blood infusions or laboratory work are instituted. Pain control strategies are implemented. This may include setting up and initiating patient-controlled analgesia (PCA) (Maxwell, 1992). The nurse is responsible for coaching patients who are ordered PCA for pain control and providing emotional support and comfort.

The patient is assessed as ready for transfer from the PACU to the nursing unit when vital signs are stable; orientation to person, place and time or the preanesthetic level of consciousness has returned; airway is satisfactory; no significant bleeding is present; and, if regional anesthesia was used, movement of extremities has returned (Fraulein, 1987). Patients with acute problems and those who are predicted to need constant monitoring or nursing care are taken to another critical care unit.

IMMEDIATE POSTOPERATIVE ASSESSMENT ON THE NURSING UNIT

When the patient is ready for transfer to the nursing unit, the PACU nurse telephones the nurse on the floor and describes any special equipment that is required. The PACU nurse verbally communicates information about the operative procedure, the patient's response during and after the surgery and the nursing management during recovery from anesthesia. The physician's written orders are reviewed. The patient is transferred to the nursing unit on a stretcher and is assisted to transfer to the bed. The nurse who is assuming responsibility for care makes the patient comfortable and assesses the position of the dressing and any tubes, contents of collecting bags and equipment. The assessment is done to ensure that there have been no alterations in the patient's condition during transportation. Safety precautions, such as putting the bed in a low position and positioning the patient so that the airway is patent and secretions can drain easily from the mouth, are implemented.

The nurse immediately assesses the blood pressure, pulse and respirations, and continues to monitor the vital signs every 4 hours for 24 hours, or more frequently if ordered or if needed. Level of consciousness, colour, temperature and condition of the skin are assessed, as well as the location of any wound or drainage tube. The dressings,

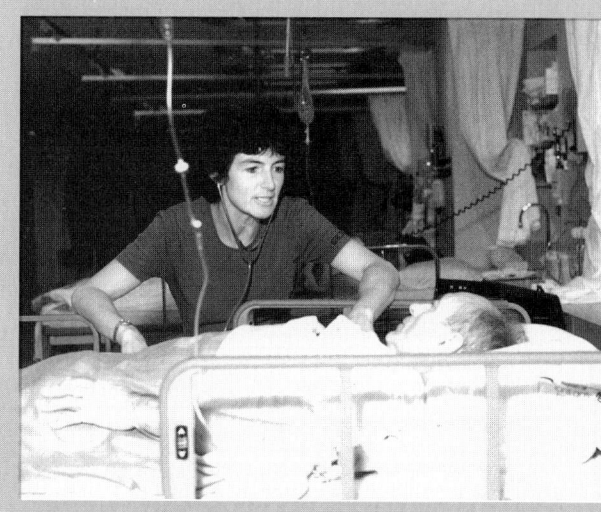

Immediate postoperative care in the PACU.

drainage and functioning of the equipment is reassessed every 4 hours for the first 24 hours, and then as needed.

ONGOING POSTOPERATIVE ASSESSMENT AND INTERVENTION

OXYGEN: BREATHING AND AIRWAY

Oxygen needs during and after surgery are of major concern. During general anesthesia, the central nervous system is depressed, and the body's muscles are relaxed. Both the anesthetic and the artificial airway inserted to assist in breathing are irritating, and they cause an increase in the secretion of mucous in the throat. The lack of muscle tone means that the patient is unable to keep the tongue from falling back and occluding the airway and is unable to expel the mucous and any other debris that collects. When a patient is recovering from the anesthetic, the nurse must protect the patient's airway by ensuring that it is clear and by assisting the patient to clear the throat and lungs of excess mucous. The patient's body movements may be restricted, and the lack of movement increases the tendency for secretions and other debris to collect in the respiratory tract. The patient is encouraged and assisted to deep breathe, cough and, if necessary, change positions to prevent the stasis of fluids in the lungs.

Diagnosing: Sample Diagnosis

• *High risk for ineffective breathing and airway clearance related to poor cough effort associated with depressant effects of anesthesia and some medications (for example, narcotic* analgesics, muscle relaxants), *pain, fatigue, tenacious secretions associated with fluid loss and decreased fluid intake*.

Planning: Sample Expected Outcome

- The patient will maintain a clear airway and an effective breathing pattern as evidenced by quiet, easy breathing and normal rate, rhythm and depth of respiration.

Implementing: Health Promoting Activities

- Promote effective airway clearance by performing actions to decrease pain so that deep breathing and coughing are done with ease. Assist and encourage mobilization as allowed and as tolerated.
- Implement measures to liquefy tenacious secretions by maintaining a fluid intake of at least 2500 ml per day unless contraindicated, and humidify inspired air.
- Instruct and assist with effective deep breathing techniques every one to two hours unless contraindicated. Monitor the performance of deep breathing exercises. Assist the patient to cough effectively if secretions are present in the lungs. Encourage the patient to take pain medication if pain is interfering with deep breathing and coughing. Use a small pillow to splint abdominal incisions. Encourage the patient to use an incentive spirometer if available.

Implementing: Health Protecting Activities

- Monitor for rapid, shallow respiration, dyspnea and use of accessory respiratory muscles, restlessness, irritability and confusion.
- Monitor for signs of respiratory distress such as the sounds of rasping heard when an airway is partially blocked, wet or noisy breathing and changes in skin colour.
- Monitor for and report signs and symptoms of pneumonia such as cough productive of purulent, green or rust-coloured sputum, chills and fever.

Splinting the incision with a pillow helps the patient cough more effectively.

- Position the patient on the side so that the tongue does not occlude the airway and any secretions and vomitus can drain from the mouth rather than being aspirated.
- Encourage and assist the patient to change position every two to four hours to prevent the accumulation of secretions and debris in the respiratory tract.
- Perform actions to reduce risk of aspiration such as withholding food and fluids if gag reflex is absent or if the patient experiences severe nausea and/or vomiting. Place the patient in a semi- to high Fowler's position during eating or drinking and 30 minutes after unless contraindicated.
- Administer narcotic analgesics, sedatives and tranquilizers judiciously. Withhold medication and consult physician if respiratory rate is less than 12 per minute.

OXYGEN: CIRCULATION AND BLOOD VOLUME

Shock and hemorrhage are always potential problems after surgery. Bleeding may result from the rupture of small surface blood vessels or from trauma to larger, deeper-lying ones. It may be caused by spontaneous rupture of a vessel that is weakened in the process of trauma, by the giving way of sutures that are used to repair damaged vessels, or by problems in the clotting mechanism resulting from a lack of certain clotting factors in the blood.

The presence of bright red blood on dressings from a wound is always a sign of actual or potential hemorrhage, and should be reported promptly. A registered nurse must check a wound when fresh red blood is observed and report to the physician immediately. A bleeding wound is monitored frequently (every 15 to 20 minutes) to see if the bleeding is increasing. If bleeding becomes excessive, the patient may show signs of shock. Evidence of shock is observed through changes in the vital signs (such as falling blood pressure), a rapid weak pulse, pallor, cold and clammy skin, weakness and restlessness. If any of these signs are detected, a registered nurse is alerted immediately and interventions, such as increasing intravenous fluids, are initiated.

Diagnosing: Sample Diagnosis

- PC: *Hypovolemic shock associated with hemorrhage and dehydration*.

Planning: Sample Nursing Goal

- The nurse will manage and minimize postoperative bleeding (Carpenito, 1993).

Implementing: Health Protecting Activities

- Monitor and report bleeding, gastrointestinal and wound drainage, persistent vomiting and/or difficulty taking oral fluid intake.

- Monitor for and report signs of hypovolemic shock such as
  - restlessness
  - agitation
  - confusion
  - decrease in BP below 90 systolic in a normotensive patient and 30 systolic below baseline in a hypertensive patient
  - decline in BP of 15 with concurrent rise in pulse when patient changes from lying to standing or sitting position
  - resting pulse rate greater than 100 beats per minute
  - rapid or laboured respirations
  - cool, pale or cyanotic skin
  - diminished or absent peripheral pulses
  - urine output less than 30 ml per hour
- Implement measures to prevent hypovolemic shock such as administering fluid volume replacement as ordered. Perform actions to prevent nausea and vomiting. When oral intake is allowed, maintain a fluid intake of at least 2500 ml per day unless contraindicated.
- If bleeding occurs, apply firm, prolonged pressure to area if possible.
- If signs and symptoms of hypovolemic shock occur, notify the physician, continue above measures to control bleeding. Place patient flat in bed with legs elevated 20 degrees unless contraindicated. Monitor vital signs frequently (every 10–15 minutes). Provide emotional support to the patient and significant others.

OXYGEN: OTHER CIRCULATORY DISTURBANCES

One potential problem is the development of an embolus. Emboli are clots in the blood that have broken off and travel through the circulatory system until they reach a point where the vessel is too small for them to pass through. They then lodge in the vessel, blocking the passage and cutting off blood flow to or from the tissues supplied by the artery or drained by the vein. Pulmonary embolism, when the clot travels to the lungs, is a potential hazard for all patients after surgery.

The nurse needs to observe for signs of phlebitis (inflammation of the veins), which predisposes clot formation. A common site for phlebitis is the thigh. Characteristic signs are redness, edema, pain and warmth in the area. Postoperatively, one of the best measures to prevent clot formation is to get the patient mobile as quickly as possible.

Diagnosing: Sample Diagnosis
- PC: *Thromboembolism associated with venous stasis resulting from decreased activity and/or trauma to vein walls during surgery.*

Planning: Sample Nursing Goal
- The nurse will manage and minimize complications of phlebitis and pulmonary embolism (Carpenito, 1993).

Implementing: Health Promoting Activities
- Implement actions to prevent peripheral pooling of blood such as teaching and supervising active leg exercises five minutes every hour when awake, and mobilization at a minimum of three times a day. Maintain a minimum fluid intake of 2500 ml per day unless contraindicated to prevent dehydration and increased blood viscosity, which leads to hypercoagulability.
- Discourage positions that compromise blood flow (for example, pillows under knees, crossing legs, sitting for long periods).
- If ordered, put on antiembolic stockings to decrease pooling of blood in the legs. Remove once a shift and provide skin care (see Figure 32.2).

Implementing: Health Protecting Activities
- Monitor for and report signs and symptoms of venous thrombus such as tenderness and pain in extremity, increase in circumference of calf or thigh (measure at the same place(s) on leg once a shift), unusual warmth and redness in extremity.
- If signs and symptoms of a venous thrombus occur, maintain bedrest until activity orders are received. Prepare the patient for diagnostic studies such as Impedance Plethysmography (IPG). Do not rub the affected area, as it may dislodge a formed clot.
- Provide emotional support to the patient and significant others if thromboembolism occurs.

WATER, SODIUM, POTASSIUM AND ACID–BASE BALANCE

Surgery always results in a loss of fluids from the body, from the blood vessels, from the interstitial spaces and from cells as tissues are cut during the surgical procedure. The body's protective mechanisms are activated and there is an increased production of antidiuretic hormone (ADH) and aldosterone. The antidiuretic hormone increases the reabsorption of water by the kidney, protecting the volume of circulating fluid. The aldosterone increases sodium and water retention, enhancing plasma volume and blood pressure. With surgery, there is also a loss of potassium, as large amounts are released from damaged cells and excreted in the urine.

There is usually a disturbance of the body's acid–base balance, with a tendency towards alkalosis. This may be caused by a number of factors. There is a decrease in the ability of the kidneys to excrete sodium bicarbonate, which results in a more acid urine. The retention of sodium and increased loss of potassium appear to reinforce this tendency.

FIGURE 32.2 Antiembolism stockings. Antiembolism stockings force blood out of smaller vessels into the deep veins and also prevent pooling of blood in the legs. The stockings are removed several times a day to check the colour of skin. To assure that the stockings are not exerting too much pressure and reducing circulation to the legs, toenail colour can be checked more frequently through the opening in the stocking at the toes.

Hyperventilation in the early postoperative period also contributes to the acid loss, as carbonic acid (in the form of carbon dioxide and water) is expired from the lungs. If the patient is on nasogastric suctioning following surgery, there is further depletion of acid from the gastric secretions, and this aggravates the tendency towards alkalosis. The nurse should also be watchful for disturbances in the acid–base balance as evidenced by physical signs and symptoms and by laboratory findings.

Dehydration and edema are among the common potential postoperative problems. In order to maintain fluid volume and offset the anticipated loss of fluid during surgery, intravenous infusions are given. The intravenous infusions are maintained following surgery if the patient is receiving no oral intake. An important set of signs to watch for are those indicating a potassium deficit. The patient may experience general malaise, anorexia and gas in the intestinal tract. Muscles become soft and the patient may have tremors and may become disoriented. It is necessary to be alert for signs of agitation, such as the patient's plucking at the bedclothes, and for signs of disorientation or confusion. If the potassium deficit is severe, muscles in the arms and legs may become flaccid, and there may be paraesthesia. A heart block, and/or cardiac arrest, can occur with severe potassium depletion.

Diagnosing: Sample Diagnoses

- *High risk for fluid volume deficit related to vomiting, nasogastric tube drainage and profuse wound drainage.*
- *High risk for fluid volume excess related to vigorous preoperative fluid therapy and increased production of antidiuretic hormone (ADH) and aldosterone (output of these hormones is stimulated by trauma, pain, anesthetic agents and narcotic analgesics).*
- *PC: Hypokalemia*

Planning: Sample Expected Outcome

- The patient will maintain fluid balance as evidenced by normal skin turgor, moist mucous membranes, stable weight, BP and pulse both within the patient's normal range and with position change, urine output greater than 30 ml per hour, balanced intake and output within 48 hours following surgery, mental status, quiet, easy breathing and absence of edema.

Planning: Sample Nursing Goal

- The nurse will manage and minimize episodes of potassium deficits (Carpenito, 1993).

Implementing: Health Protecting Activities

- Monitor for and report signs and symptoms of fluid volume deficit such as
  - poor skin turgor
  - dry mucous membranes
  - thirst
  - weight loss greater than 0.5 kg/day
  - low BP and/or decline in BP of 15 mm Hg with concurrent rise in pulse when patient sits up
  - weak, rapid pulse
  - urine output less than 30 ml/hour.
- Implement measures to prevent and treat fluid and electrolyte imbalance such as performing actions to prevent vomiting and maintaining a fluid intake of at least 2500 ml per day unless contraindicated. When oral intake is ordered and tolerated, assist the patient to select foods/fluids high in potassium (bananas, oranges, tomatoes, fruit juices) and sodium (for example, soups, bouillon).
- Weigh patient daily, if possible.

- Provide mouth care if tongue, lips and oral mucous membranes are dry.
- Monitor for and report signs and symptoms of fluid volume excess such as significant weight gain (greater than 0.5 kg/day), elevated BP and pulse, intake that continues to be greater than output 48 hours postoperatively, change in mental status, dyspnea, peripheral edema.
- Implement measures to prevent and treat fluid volume excess such as administering fluid replacement therapy judiciously especially within first 48 hours after surgery.
- Maintain fluid restriction as ordered, restrict sodium intake as ordered.
- Consult physician if signs and symptoms of fluid volume excess persist or worsen.

NUTRITION

All types of injury to the body, including surgery, result in an increased metabolic rate. The body mobilizes its forces to repair the damaged tissue and tissue protein, especially in the skeletal muscles, is metabolized as an energy source. The excess nitrogen is excreted in the urine. There is a breakdown of fat, which becomes a major source of energy in the immediate postoperative period.

At the same time that nutritional needs are increased to keep up with the increased metabolic rate, there is a decrease in food and fluid intake. Most patients having surgery are not allowed any food or fluids for eight to ten hours prior to surgery. Some are unable to tolerate food and fluids for varying lengths of time postoperatively. Some anesthetic agents may cause nausea and vomiting. The patient's nutritional needs must be met, and intravenous fluids are usually given until the patient is able to tolerate a sufficient amount of nourishment by mouth to meet nutritional needs.

When oral intake is allowed, the patient is started on clear fluids, with the diet modified as tolerance for food and fluids increases. Some patients are on nasogastric feedings postoperatively. Some are maintained on nothing by mouth for a lengthy period of time, in which case total parenteral nutrition may be required.

Diagnosing: Sample Diagnosis

- *Nutrition, altered: Deficit due to food and fluid restrictions preanesthetic, postoperative nausea, vomiting or paralytic ileus.*

Planning: Sample Expected Outcome

- The patient will maintain adequate nutrition as evidenced by tolerance of fluids and nutrients, and will maintain weight.

Implementing: Health Promoting Activities

- The nurse should observe food and fluid intake and encourage the patient to increase intake gradually as tolerance improves.

Implementing: Health Protecting Activities

- Monitor signs of nausea and vomiting particularly in a patient who is recovering from anesthetic, is under sedation, or has limited mobility.
- Assess patient to determine factors that contribute to nausea and vomiting (for example, abdominal distention, pain, anxiety, certain foods, medications, constipation).
- Implement measures to prevent nausea and vomiting such as eliminating noxious sights and smells from the environment. Instruct the patient to change positions slowly.
- Provide oral hygiene every two hours or before meals if oral intake is allowed, and after each emesis.
- Keep a careful record of the patient's intake and output.
- When oral intake is allowed, advance the diet slowly (usually beginning with clear liquids and progressing to solid food). Instruct the patient to ingest foods and fluids slowly. Foods/fluids that irritate the gastric mucosa such as spicy, acidic and/or caffeine-containing items should be avoided. Encourage dry foods (toast, crackers) and avoid drinking liquids with meals if nauseated. Rest after eating with head of bed elevated will facilitate gastric emptying.
- Consult a clinical nutritionist for help in providing the patient's preferred foods or fluids.
- Monitor for therapeutic and non-therapeutic effects of antiemetic if administered.
- Consult the physician if the above measures fail to control nausea and vomiting.

ELIMINATION NEEDS

The loss of body fluids during surgery stimulates secretion of the antidiuretic hormone which directly reduces urinary output lessening the loss of water from the body. The retention of sodium also helps to hold fluid in body tissues, further contributing to a decreased output of urine. A relative oliguria is seen in the postoperative period for the first two to three days. The central nervous system depressant effect of anesthesia and analgesics depress neuromuscular functioning causing muscle spasm of the sphincter in the bladder and may result in an inability to void — a not uncommon occurrence.

Elimination from the gastrointestinal tract is also disturbed by surgery. There is a lack of solid food intake in preparation for surgery and usually for a few days postoperatively, so that there is insufficient bulk to stimulate the bowel. The restrictions imposed on activity following surgery also contribute to a sluggish bowel. A paralytic or adynamic ileus (obstruction of the intestines resulting from an inhibition of motility of the gastrointestinal tract) is also a fairly common occurrence following major surgery, especially if the peritoneum has been entered.

Diagnosing: Sample Diagnoses

- *Urinary elimination, altered pattern due to the decrease in the amount of urine produced (caused by increase in ADH and aldosterone), the decrease in the amount of fluid intake, the effect of anesthetic and analgesics in increasing vasoconstriction of bladder sphincter, and in some cases by having to void in a prone position.*

- *Constipation related to decreased physical mobility, decreased motility of gastrointestinal tract, and decreased intake of solid food.*

Planning: Sample Expected Outcomes

- The patient will have adequate urinary output as evidenced by voiding eight hours after surgery, by voiding every three to four hours with output of at least 30 ml per hour and by emptying bladder when voiding.

- The patient will have adequate bowel elimination as evidenced by a bowel movement at least every three days with easy passage of stool.

Implementing: Health Promoting Activities

- Establish a regular pattern of urinary elimination by assisting the patient to the bathroom to void every three hours.

- Encourage adequate fluid intake, if permitted, to 2500 ml per day.

- Encourage ambulation as soon as possible

- Provide privacy in bathroom at time the patient usually evacuates bowel.

Implementing: Health Protecting Activities

- Monitor the amount and time of first postoperative urination. If the patient has not voided by eight hours after surgery notify the doctor.

- Monitor the amount, frequency, colour and odour of urine.

- Monitor for and report signs and symptoms of urinary tract infection (for instance, cloudy, foul-smelling urine; complaints of frequency, urgency and/or burning on urination; elevated temperature; chills).

- Implement measures to prevent urinary tract infection by acting to prevent urinary retention. Such actions include helping the patient assume a normal position to void (for females, sitting; for males, standing). Instruct females to wipe from front to back after urinating or defecating. Increase activity as tolerated to decrease urinary stasis.

- Request that a stool softener be considered if the patient is taking analgesic medications which contribute to constipation.

- Monitor for frequency of bowel movements.

COMFORT, REST AND SLEEP

Pain is usually experienced following surgery because of the tissue damage from mechanical disruption, inflammation and stretching. The pain disturbs comfort and may interfere with rest and sleep. If there has been tissue damage in part of the body that is involved in mobility, movement is likely to induce and/or increase pain. The intensity of the pain may vary with the extent of surgery, the location of the incision, the degree of intraoperative trauma and the meaning of the surgery to the patient. The intensity of postoperative pain does vary, but it is more severe after intrathoracic, intraabdominal and renal surgery, and after extensive surgery of the spine, major joints and large bones of the hand and foot (Wasylak, 1992).

The assessment of pain includes the location, the intensity and the quality of pain. The intensity of pain may be assessed by asking the patient how much pain is present on a scale of 0 to 10. The 0 means no pain, and 10 means the worst pain that can be imagined. Pain intensity scales are available for children and adults. Descriptions of the quality of pain, such as "sharp," "shooting" or "dull," are determined. The assessment includes the impact of pain on usual activities and the patient's satisfaction with interventions which are used to control pain.

Diagnosing: Sample Diagnosis

- *Pain related to tissue trauma and reflex muscle spasm associated with surgery.*

Planning: Sample Expected Outcome

- The patient reports satisfaction with pain control, has a relaxed facial expression. Body positioning and activities are not limited by pain.

Implementing: Health Promoting Activities

- Provide instruction and coaching if the patient is receiving patient-controlled analgesia.

- Provide or assist with non-pharmacological measures for pain management (for example, back rubs, position changes, relaxation techniques, a restful environment).

Implementing: Health Protecting Activities

- Monitor for nonverbal signs of pain such as facial grimaces, restlessness.

- Monitor the location, intensity and quality of pain every four hours and following any event that might be expected to cause pain, such as treatments.

- Implement measures to reduce pain such as administering analgesics as ordered and monitoring for therapeutic and non-therapeutic effects.

- Instruct and assist the patient to support abdominal or chest incisions with a pillow or hands when turning, coughing and deep breathing.

- Consult physician if above measures fail to provide adequate pain relief.

MOVEMENT AND EXERCISE

During the Second World War, it was observed that the patient who got up and walked around in the early postoperative period recovered sooner and had fewer complications than the patient who remained in bed. Since then, early ambulation has become an important concern for nurses. The patient often needs a great deal of physical and psychological support in order to ambulate. Surgery limits mobility in several ways. If a general anesthetic is given, the patient will be unconscious and unable to move. During surgery, the patient is often maintained in one position for a prolonged period of time. Anesthesia causes muscle paralysis. When the anesthetized patient is positioned, the muscles cannot contract against the stretching effects of certain positions. The patient may later complain of soreness in the muscles. With a spinal anesthetic, the patient is unable to move parts of the body below the site of the injection of the anesthetic. Even a local anesthetic causes immobility in and around the area being manipulated.

After surgery, pain, the extent and type of tissue damage, weakness and equipment may interfere with mobility. Pain is a major factor limiting mobility. The strain on tissues in the operative area may induce pain when turning in bed or trying to sit up, get out of bed or walk. The patient who has an abdominal incision may not realize the extent to which the abdominal muscles are involved in respiration until asked to breath deeply or cough after surgery.

With some types of surgery, it may be important to immobilize a limb or other part of the body to allow time for the tissues to heal. The immobility may be achieved by enclosing the part in a cast, or attaching it to various pieces of equipment which severely hamper movement. Often, the patient's freedom of movement is restricted due to intravenous infusion, various tubes or drains that must accompany the patient during ambulation.

Immobility can cause many problems, such as congestion in the lungs and a peripheral pooling of blood, as well as a loss of muscle tone through disuse. Peripheral pooling of blood makes the patient more vulnerable to clot formation in the blood vessels, with the potential risk of emboli to the lungs and heart. There is also a depletion of protein from the muscles and calcium from the bones of immobilized patients, which further interferes with mobility.

The nurse should be observant of the patient's difficulty in carrying out the necessary activities to maintain bodily functions because of limited mobility. Problems with hygiene (for example, because one arm has an intravenous infusion running into it), with feeding, in using a bedpan or in turning over in bed may arise. It is a nursing responsibility to provide the assistance the patient needs.

Diagnosing: Sample Diagnosis

- *High risk for impaired physical mobility related to pain, weakness and fatigue, orthostatic hypotension associated with peripheral pooling of blood and blood loss during surgery, central nervous system depressant effects of some medications, presence of drainage tubing or equipment that must accompany the patient, and anxiety at hurting the operative area.*

Planning: Sample Expected Outcome

- The patient will ambulate unless contraindicated three times per day, will perform hygiene in a bathroom and will sit up for all meals.

Implementing: Health Promoting Activities

- Explain the importance of movement and exercise in promoting healthy recovery from surgery.
- Explain the importance of requesting medication for pain, so that exercises can be done comfortably.
- Keep the bed in low position. Encourage the patient to request assistance whenever needed.
- Assist to a chair for all meals.
- Assist back to bed for frequent rest periods.
- Alternate frequent (every three hours) short walks (for example, one hall length) with periods of rest. Increase length, then frequency as tolerance improves.
- Give positive acknowledgement of the patient's efforts during and after movement and/or exercise.

Implementing: Health Protecting Activities

- Determine the existence of conditions predisposing the patient to immobility (weakness, pain, preoperative problems in movement, narcotic analgesics, presence of long tubing and equipment, fear of hurting incision).
- Instruct the patient to wear shoes with nonskid soles and low heels when ambulating. Position tubing and equipment carefully so that they will not interfere with ambulation.
- Accompany the patient during ambulation. Ambulate in well-lit areas and use handrails if needed. Do not rush and allow adequate time for trips to the bathroom and for ambulation. Increase level of activity as tolerated. Assist in changes of position slowly to reduce dizziness associated with orthostatic drop in BP.
- Consult a physiotherapist if the patient is immobilized or is having difficulty walking.

TEMPERATURE REGULATION

Many general anesthetics cause vasodilation which results in a loss of body heat during the intraoperative period. The effect of the vasodilation is compounded by surgical exposure. As a result, the immediate postoperative body reaction is shivering. The shivering requires an increased metabolism. Increased metabolism is also required for tissue repair, and body temperature is usually slightly elevated in the early postoperative period. This is generally considered to be a good sign that the body's recuperative mechanisms are functioning. An elevation of temperature should alert the nurse to the possibility of infection, which causes the body's metabolism to be greatly speeded up in efforts to combat the invading pathogens.

INFECTION CONTROL

One of the most important needs for all patients undergoing surgery is protection from infection. Cutting through the skin penetrates the body's first line of defence, and provides a ready access to deeper tissues for infectious agents. The trauma of surgery, the stress of the illness which necessitated the surgery, the pain and decreased nutrients all are stressors which increase vulnerability to infection. The nurse should also be alert to the possibility of generalized infection following surgery. Observations the nurse should make in regard to both generalized and localized infectious processes were discussed in Chapter 31. They include signs of redness, pain, swelling, unusual discharge, elevated temperature and increased white blood cell count.

Diagnosing: Sample Diagnoses

- *Impaired tissue integrity related to surgical trauma.*
- *High risk for infection related to surgical incision.*

Planning: Sample Expected Outcome

- The patient will show normal healing of the surgical wound as evidenced by the gradual reduction of redness and swelling at wound site and the presence of granulation tissue or intact, approximated wound edges.

Implementing: Health Promoting Activities

- Perform actions to maintain optimal nutritional status and adequate circulation to the wound area (for instance, do not apply dressings tightly unless ordered as excessive pressure impairs circulation to the area).

Implementing: Health Protecting Activities

- Monitor and report signs and symptoms of impaired wound healing (such as increasing redness and swelling at wound site and separation of wound edges).
- Inspect dressings, wounds, and skin areas in contact with wound drainage (drains or puncture sites) and tape for signs of irritation and breakdown.
- Use aseptic techniques in all wound contacts.
- Decrease stress on wound by instructing and assisting the patient to support the involved area when moving and to splint abdominal and chest wounds when coughing.
- To protect the wound from mechanical injury, ensure that dressings are secure enough to keep them from rubbing and irritating the wound.
- Cleanse the skin and change dressings if appropriate.
- To prevent skin irritation due to drainage, maintain the patency of drainage tubes to decrease the risk of leakage around the tubes. Apply a collection pouch over drains or paste to skin areas likely to be in contact with drainage. Caution the patient against lying on drainage tubes. Secure all tubing to prevent excessive movement which can irritate mucous membranes or skin.
- To minimize skin irritation resulting from tape, use necessary amounts of tape only, and use hypoallergenic tape whenever possible to secure tubing and dressings. Use elastic netting or montgomery ties to avoid repeated tape application and removal. Apply skin sealants or barriers such as stomadhesive before application of tape if necessary. Remove tape by pulling in the direction of hair growth and using adhesive solvents if necessary.
- If skin irritation or breakdown occurs, notify the physician. To prevent further irritation and breakdown monitor closely and report signs and symptoms of infection (such as elevated temperature; redness, warmth and edema around incision or area of breakdown; unusual drainage from site).

SENSORY FUNCTIONING

General anesthetics depress all sensation, and the patient is maintained in an unconscious state for the length of time the surgery takes. After surgery sensory perception may be dulled by the administration of sedatives and analgesics. These drugs may result in confusion, poor defence responses and postural imbalance. If surgery was done on the nose or mouth, vision, smell or taste may be affected. Neural pathways may have been disturbed, by accident or by design, during the course of surgery and any deviations from the initial baseline data in regard to sensory functioning must be observed. If deviations occur, adequate precautions are taken to assure safety and the doctor is notified.

PROTECTION AND SAFETY

After surgery, mental function may be affected by a number of factors, including medication, anesthesia and disturbances in physiological processes. The patient will have experienced varying levels of consciousness during induction and recovery from anesthesia. Some people have untoward reactions to sedation and to anesthetic agents. Older people are particularly sensitive to drug reactions. All of these factors may interfere with the patient's capacity for self-protection. Protective strategies for the confused and disoriented patients and those with altered levels of consciousness were discussed in Chapter 29.

SELF-ESTEEM, SECURITY AND HEALTH MAINTENANCE

After surgery, anxiety may arise concerning pain, the dependency on health care providers, equipment and about the outcome of surgery itself. The nurse assists in decreasing anxiety by attending to the need for comfort, by providing competent technical care, by providing clear explanations about what is expected in the patient role and by encouraging the expression of emotions related to the surgical illness experience.

The patient may express many emotions after surgery. There may be uncertainty related to the future outcome of illness or relief that the surgery has been successful. If the surgery has altered a body part, the patient may express grief over the alteration in body image. The predischarge and early postdischarge periods may be times which are particularly distressful for the patient. The distress may be associated with the recognition that recovery will now be a personal responsibility and the patient may be concerned about how to manage at home. Nursing research has shown that at hospital discharge, people feel it is important to know what complications may occur and if a complication occurs, what actions to take, how to manage symptoms such as pain and fatigue, what diet and activity guidelines to follow and how to take medications (Bubela, McKibbon, McCoy and Ross, 1990; Galloway et al., 1993).

Diagnosing: Sample Diagnosis

- *Knowledge deficit related to safe management at home after hospital discharge.*

Planning: Sample Expected Outcome

- The patient will be able to manage recovery at home, as evidenced by verbalizing what complications to monitor for, what activity and dietary guidelines to follow, how to care for the incision and how to take medications as directed.

Implementing: Health Promoting Activities

- Refer to community support groups specific to the health problem if the patient is agreeable.
- Encourage to remain a non-smoker if the patient smoked preoperatively.
- Provide information about adequate nutritional intake to promote wound healing.
- Explain that frequent rest periods during the day may be needed, but that energy level will begin to return in several weeks.
- Encourage exercise. Unless contraindicated, the best exercise is walking.

Implementing: Health Protecting Activities

- Provide teaching about complications specific to surgical procedure. For example, after bowel surgery, instruct about what action to take if diarrhea or constipation occurs.
- Provide teaching about wound care. Instruct the patient to keep the wound clean and to notify doctor if signs of infection develop (for example, if the wound becomes red, swollen or warm to the touch or discharge becomes green or yellow).
- Explain that a shower may be taken, but that perfumes, creams or powder should not be put on wounds.
- Provide information about prescribed medications to take and how to take them.

WOUND HEALING AND RESTORATIVE CARE

A physical wound is an injury caused by anything that disrupts the normal continuity of the body's structure. Wounds are classified as open or closed. An **open wound** refers to tissue injury with a break in the skin or mucous membrane. A surgical incision is one example of an open wound. Injury to the skin and underlying tissues without a break in the skin is called a **closed wound**. A contusion is a closed wound. The names of wounds correspond to the manner in which they are acquired and to the extent of injury to the skin. Table 32.2 presents a description of the common types of wounds. The major goals of restorative wound care are to promote wound healing, prevent damage to surrounding tissues and to prevent infection.

THE PROCESS OF HEALING

Normal healing is a series of complex events that leads to the restoration of tissue continuity. The localized response of the body to tissue injury begins at the time of injury and occurs in three major phases: the inflammatory phase, the proliferative phase and the remodelling phase (Stotts, 1986).

Inflammatory Phase

The inflammatory phase lasts for three or four days. The small vessels initially contract and the body activates the coagulation mechanisms which allow clots to form. The initial vasoconstriction lasts for only five to ten minutes and if effective, it will cause the cessation of bleeding. Then, there is vasodilation with increased capillary permeability and blood flow. Lymph channels swell as they become plugged with fibrin. Increased capillary permeability allows plasma to leak into the interstitial spaces adding to the edema at the wound site. The wound will appear slightly red, feel warmer than the tissue away from the injury, look swollen and be tender or painful. During this phase, the

TABLE 32.2	Types of Wounds	

TYPE	CAUSE	CHARACTERISTICS
Open:		
Incision	Surgical or traumatic cut with a sharp instrument (scalpel or knife).	A clean cut; straight, smooth edges. A surgical incision is more likely to heal well, with less chance of infection, because it is made under controlled, aseptic conditions.
Abrasion	Surgical or traumatic scraping off of the outer layer of the skin.	Superficial wound of the skin only. Often painful because nerve endings are exposed. Prone to infection.
Puncture	Surgical or traumatic stab with a penetrating object or instrument.	Well-defined penetration of skin and underlying tissues. May damage nerves and arteries. Traumatic wounds may have concealed blood loss and foreign objects.
Laceration	Traumatic tearing apart of skin and underlying tissues.	Opening of the skin with ragged, irregular edges. Not likely to heal well.
Closed:		
Contusion	Direct blow from a blunt object.	Damage to tissues and blood vessels under the skin; a bruise. Edema and tenderness are often present.

SOURCES: Flynn and Hackel, 1990; Earnest, 1993.

epithelial cells start to migrate (travel) from the margins of the wound. These cells are able to proliferate by mitosis and differentiate into mature cells.

Proliferation Phase

The proliferation phase of healing begins on the fourth or fifth day after tissue injury and lasts for 17 or more days. During this time, granulation and collagen tissue formation occur. The granulation tissue provides the foundation for scar tissue and the formation of new blood vessels which come from capillary buds arising from existing vessels. During this time, the tensile strength of the tissue begins to build slowly but is only three to five percent of the original skin strength at 14 days, and only 40 percent of the original strength at 28 days.

Remodelling Phase

The remodelling phase begins at about 21 days and can take six to 24 months to complete. During this period, the organization and the tensile strength of the collagen fibres increase and the bulk of the scar decreases. The colour of the scar changes from bright pink to white.

DETERMINANTS OF WOUND HEALING

The factors which affect the speed and character of the healing process may be either systemic or local (Harding, 1990; Neuberger and Reckling, 1990). Systemic factors refer to conditions within the body, while local factors are conditions in the area near the wound which may impair wound healing. Some of the systemic and local factors are described below.

SYSTEMIC FACTORS

Extent of the injury   The process of repair and regeneration depends upon the extent of the tissue damage. Wounds with minimal tissue damage or loss, for example, clean surgical incisions or simple lacerations, heal very quickly by what is termed *primary intention*. On the other hand, wounds in which tissue loss is extensive, for example, burns or ulcerated areas, heal by *secondary intention*.

   Primary intention healing occurs when there is little or no tissue loss. The wound edges are approximated (brought together) and secured with sutures, staples or tapes. This enhances the migration of epithelial cells from the wound edges. Because epithelialization is rapid, the risk of infection is decreased. Some inflammation may occur. Granulation tissue is not noticeable and scar formation is minimal.

Secondary intention healing occurs when damage and loss of tissue is extensive. In secondary intention healing, wounds cannot be approximated and secured with sutures or staples. The wound edges remain open until scar tissue fills the wound site. The phases of healing are prolonged because drainage, necrotic tissue and debris in the wound space must be removed. Granulation tissue replaces the tissue that has been destroyed, providing a connective tissue base for the growth of epithelial (skin) cells. Inflammation persists and infection is a high risk. Scar formation is sometimes excessive and may result in a permanent loss of function.

Age Healing is more rapid in children than in adults. It is slowed in older patients due to the lessened efficiency of circulation which can result in inadequate nutrients, blood cells and oxygen being delivered to the wound.

Nutrition Nutrients are essential for normal healing as they provide the ingredients for cellular repair and regeneration. Specific nutrients needed for healing include protein, carbohydrates, fats, vitamins, minerals and oxygen. Protein is needed for revascularization, lymphatic formation, fibroplastic proliferation, collagen synthesis and wound remodelling. Carbohydrates and fats are needed for cellular energy. Vitamin C is needed for the formation of new capillaries and is involved in the maturation of collagen fibres during the later stages of healing. Vitamin K deficiencies may cause bleeding and result in anemias or hematomas which may interfere with wound healing. Although injury increases the use of specific B vitamins, the mechanism by which they influence protein, fat and carbohydrate metabolism is not well understood.

Obesity Patients who are obese may have poorer wound healing. Adipose tissue has poor vascularization and, combined with the increased tension of the excess tissue, increases the incidence of incisional hernias, infections and dehiscence (the breaking open of a wound).

Diabetes Diabetes is one of the most common metabolic disorders. It causes disturbances in carbohydrate, protein and fat metabolism, and makes the patient more vulnerable to impaired or prolonged wound healing. Wound infections are more common in patients with diabetes as the leucocytes malfunction with hyperglycemia. It is also possible that there is poor oxygenation to the healing tissue due to the thickened capillaries which are related to diabetes.

Immunosuppression The immune system of the body is important for the regeneration and repair of wounds and for other functions such as promoting phagocytosis dur-

ing the inflammatory phase. The normal immune response may be artificially prevented or diminished by radiotherapy or by the administration of steroids, antimetabolites, antilymphocyte serum or specific antibodies. The nurse must be aware of the effects of immunosuppression, and protect the surgical wound from pathogenic organisms. The normal signs and symptoms of infection may not all be present although a fever is often seen.

Radiation Healing is slowed after radiotherapy due to the systemic effects of immunosuppression and the local effects of decreased blood supply and increased fibrotic (scar) tissue. If an area is to be radiated before surgery, the best operative time is considered to be four to six weeks after the therapy is completed. This is because the tissues are in the proliferative stage of healing before fibrosis and vascular narrowing occur. Complications which are common with patients who have received radiotherapy are delayed healing, dehiscence and fistula formation. The tissues of the irradiated area are more friable than normal and require very gentle handling.

LOCAL FACTORS

Chemical, mechanical or thermal The disinfectants and medications used to cleanse and treat a wound and the surrounding tissue should be strong enough to be effective but should not irritate healthy tissue. Protective ointments such as sterile petrolatum can be used to protect the skin when it is necessary to use irritating disinfectants on open wounds. Mechanical stress such as friction over a new wound may strip the new epithelial cells and delay healing of a wound. To avoid mechanical injury all wounds should be handled gently. Adhesive tape near the wound must be removed carefully. Special solvents may be used to loosen the adhesive. Thermal injury can be avoided by the use of solutions at a temperature which is not dangerous to tissue. Room temperature is generally considered to be safe for most tissues.

Suture material Some people have an allergic response to the sutures, staples or wound care supplies. Each patient is asked about prior allergies, and in patients with no known allergies, the wound should be observed for localized reactions.

Infection The major complication in surgical wounds is infection. Infectious processes result in tissue destruction, delay the healing process and contribute to increasing the size of surgical scars. All solutions, dressings and equipment that come into contact with an open wound should be sterile. There are several organisms that are commonly found in wound infections. Of the gram-positive group, *Staphylococcus (S.) aureus* and *S. epidermidis* are found most commonly. These spherical asymmetric bacteria are normally found in the nose, skin and feces. The alpha- and beta-hemolytic streptococci also cause many infectious processes. An estimated eight percent of all people carry these bacteria in the nasopharynx.

Of the gram-negative bacteria, *E. coli* and species of *Aerobacter* and *Alcaligenes* are frequently found in wounds. These, together with *Proteus* and *Pseudomonas*, are the principal inhabitants of the intestine. They can also often be isolated in the anogenital area, and are frequent causes of urinary tract infections.

Blood supply   Blood supply is necessary for healing as it brings the nutrients, blood cells and oxygen to the wound. Factors which impede circulation such as damaged arteries, restrictive bandages or casts, restraints and gross edema will interfere with wound healing and render the area more vulnerable to infection. Healing is also slowed in patients with anemia or blood disorders that cause vascular insufficiency, such as atherosclerosis, in which there is a buildup of fatty deposits in the walls of large and medium-sized arteries.

ASSESSING WOUNDS

A wound is assessed every eight hours for signs of healing, infection and discharge. Approximation of skin edges is observed. The skin edges may be held together by metal skin clips (staples) or sutures. After three to seven days the clips or sutures are removed. The incision and surrounding area are assessed. Normally, there is slight redness along an incision for 48 hours. Redness extending 2 cm or more away from incision, edema and tissue heat are signs of infection which are reported to the doctor. Surgical wound infections are not uncommon. The incidence is markedly reduced by shortening preoperative stays (Cavanillas et al., 1991), avoiding preoperative shaving of hair, flawless aseptic technique and elimination of drains in clean wounds. If infection is suspected, the patient's temperature is taken, and an assessment is done for pain in the area, headache and malaise. The latter are indicators of systemic infection.

The colour, type and amount of discharge is observed. **Serous discharge**, from the clear portion of blood, is amber in colour. **Sanguineous discharge** is blood, which may be bright red, indicative of fresh blood, or dark red which is old blood. A combination of blood and serum is called **serosanguineous drainage**. **Purulent drainage** contains pus and may be white, yellow, green or pink. The colour is associated with the type of organism which is growing. The drainage is thick and may have an unpleasant odour.

The amount of discharge from a wound is monitored. The nurse first determines what amount of discharge is usual. For example, an abdominal incision is not expected to have more than a few drops of drainage after 24 hours. An

KEY PRINCIPLES

Principles Relevant to Wound Care

1. Skin and mucous membranes normally harbour microorganisms.

2. Microorganisms are present in the air.

3. Moisture facilitates the growth of microorganisms. Dressings that are wet with drainage are more likely to foster the growth of organisms than are dry dressings. Dressings should be changed when they become wet.

4. Moisture facilitates the movement of microorganisms. When a dressing becomes soaked, movement of microorganisms towards the wound is facilitated as the moisture provides a vehicle for their transport. Because the outside of a dressing is generally highly contaminated, the movement of organisms from the outside inward must be prevented. Maintaining dry dressings inhibits the multiplication and the transfer of organisms.

5. Fluids move through materials by capillary action. Loosely woven fabrics such as gauze provide a good surface for capillary action. The fluid is absorbed through the material as each thread in the material conducts the fluid away from the wound by the action of the surface tension of the fluid and the forces of adhesion and cohesion. Adhesion and cohesion are forces that draw two things together.

6. Fluids flow downward as a result of gravitational pull. In a draining wound, the area of greatest contamination is likely the lowest part, where the drainage collects.

7. The respiratory tract often harbours microorganisms.

8. Blood transports the materials that nourish and repair body tissues. When dressing and bandaging a wound, exercise care to ensure that circulation to the area is not restricted. Dressings are never made restrictively tight, and they are applied starting at the distal portion of the body and proceeding to the proximal portion as a means of promoting venous flow.

incision in the perineum, however, may have 20 to 30 ml of drainage every 12 hours for several days. The amount of drainage is given in millilitres (ml) whenever possible.

Wounds are assessed for the presence of complications such as hematoma, dehiscence or evisceration. A *hematoma* occurs when there has been bleeding and a clot forms beneath the skin. The old clot (hematoma) may be absorbed, or may have to be removed. Removal is accomplished by a doctor who opens a small area of incision allowing the hematoma to drain out. *Dehiscence* occurs when there is a disruption of a surgical wound, whereas *evisceration* is the protrusion of body organs through the wound.

IMPLEMENTING RESTORATIVE STRATEGIES

Operative wounds may be sutured with a wide variety of nonabsorbable sutures, including those made of polyester, polypropylene or silk, or with absorbable sutures made from surgical gut or a synthetic fibre or metal clips (staples). A wound is covered with a sterile dressing to provide a proper environment for healing, to absorb drainage, to protect the new epithelial tissue from mechanical injury, to promote hemostasis in a pressure dressing and at times to reduce anxiety in patients who are distressed by an incision in their body. Some wounds are clean, dry wounds; others are draining wounds.

CLEAN, DRY WOUNDS

The initial dressing that is applied to a clean dry incision is left in place until the wound edges are sealed. Wound edge sealing usually occurs in 24 hours. Then, the dressing is removed and the area is gently cleaned and left uncovered. The absence of a dressing is beneficial as it allows easy observation of the area, eliminates conditions of warmth, moisture and darkness that promote microorganism growth, and avoids reactions from tape. Occlusive dressings allow insulation of a wound and have been shown to reduce the rate of wound infection when compared to nonocclusive dressings such as gauze (Hutchinson and McGuckin, 1990). Occlusive dressings that are impermeable to bacteria, that are transparent and that are gas and vapour permeable are preferred for some wounds such as intravenous insertion sites. The occlusive dressings are changed when dirty or damaged, or according to the guidelines of the specific product.

DRAINING WOUNDS

Wounds heal more quickly if accumulated blood clots and if body fluids, pus or debris are adequately drained. The accumulated materials provide a rich medium for microorganism growth; thus, soiled dressings need to be changed several times a day. If a wound is draining, the skin is not completely closed and a pathway exists for the entry of microorganisms. The placing of a dressing is done by sterile technique so that microorganisms are not introduced into the area. If a wound is expected to drain excessively, a drain or packing is inserted by the physician to facilitate this process. Soft and firm rubber drains as well as plastic drains are used for this purpose. Packing is usually made of a long strip of gauze, often impregnated with an antiseptic or antibiotic. Drains and packing are sometimes withdrawn a little each day to encourage healing from the depth of the wound towards the surface. Drainage can be anticipated from wounds of this nature. Some drains are sutured in place, others are freely movable. Soft rubber drains (Penrose drains) have a sterile safety pin attached to the distal portion of the drain to prevent it from slipping completely inside the wound. When dressings on draining wounds are wet they need to be changed. The drainage is irritating to the skin and increases the risk of infection. The dressing procedure is called a dry dressing change because the wound is cleansed and dry dressings are then applied to the wound.

CHANGING A DRY DRESSING

Dry dressings are usually applied to wounds that heal by primary intention. A dressing is changed to cleanse the wound, to remove excessive drainage and to apply a clean covering. It also provides an opportunity for careful assessment of wound healing. The technique for changing a dry dressing is detailed in Procedure 32.1.

Preparing the Patient

Prior to the dressing of a wound, the patient is given information about the procedure to be done. If the patient will be seeing the wound for the first time, information about its appearance and what will happen during the dressing change is given. Often a wound has meaning for the patient, and concerns may be discussed. The nurse should be careful that words such as "contaminated" and "dirty" are not used since they may make a patient feel uncomfortable and not acceptable. A wound infection is, however, a legitimate cause for concern, and the patient needs to know if it is present. The patient may ask whether changing a dressing is painful and may worry about coping with the pain. Most dressing procedures have some discomfort but the pain is usually mild. If the procedure is going to be uncomfortable, the patient should be offered a pain medication before the procedure. Dressings that stick to the skin because of dried discharges can be removed with little discomfort by soaking them with sterile normal saline or sterile water. Another possible source of discomfort is the use of a cleansing solution with an alcohol base. These agents may feel cold and may sting when in contact with an open wound. The use of a cleansing solution without an alcohol base is often advisable. The patient can participate in the procedure by lying still and keeping hands away from the wound area so that the wound and the equipment do not accidentally become contaminated.

Before assembling equipment for the dressing change, the nurse inspects the patient's dressing to determine the supplies and equipment that will be needed. Once a dressing tray is opened and set up, the nurse cannot leave the sterile field to obtain additional supplies, since doing so would constitute a break in sterile technique. Because of this, the nurse needs to make a quick check to determine the type of dressings, the presence of drainage tubes and the type of tape used to anchor the dressing. At the same time, the nurse should clear space on the patient's bedside or overbed table for the dressing equipment and supplies.

Assembling Equipment

Changing a dry dressing is a sterile procedure. Supplies and equipment are needed for removing the old dressing, for cleansing the wound and for redressing the wound. The specific cleansing solution and the dressings that will be needed depend upon the kind of wound, the physician's order and the agency policy.

The safest aseptic technique in wound care is carried out by using individual trays containing only materials and equipment which can be discarded or sterilized after the wound is dressed. In most agencies, it is standard practice to use a disposable tray, referred to as a "dressing set." While variations may exist from one manufacturer to another, the dressing set consists of a tray with a compartment for the cleansing solution, some 5 cm × 5 cm gauze sponges, some 10 cm × 10 cm gauze sponges, a metal thumb forceps, a

plastic thumb forceps, a plastic locking forceps and a drape (see Figure 32.3). Separately packaged dressing materials are added to the set according to the specific needs of the patient. Sterile scissors may also be needed to shape the dressings and tape. Many agencies no longer require masks to be worn for sterile dressing changes, but the nurse should consult agency policy.

Supplies for removing old dressing   A large moisture-proof bag is needed to contain the old dressing materials. Clean gloves are required for removing the outer dressing. The inner dressings may be removed using a transfer forceps (from the dressing set) or sterile gloves. Because sterile gloves are costly, their use should be reserved for special circumstances only. In some cases, the adhesive surface of the tape anchoring the dressing adheres to the patient's skin after the tape is removed. When this happens, an adhesive remover such as acetone may be used to loosen the adhesive. It is applied with clean 10 cm × 10 cm gauze sponges and the area is then washed with soap and water.

Cleansing solutions and supplies   Normal saline is commonly used to cleanse wounds; however, other topical solutions may be ordered by the physician. These are outlined in Table 32.3. Incisions are cleansed with sterile 5 cm × 5 cm gauze pads or cotton balls. Sterile supplies are handled with sterile forceps.

Dressings   The most commonly used dressings are fine mesh gauze pads made of cotton or rayon fabric or synthetic materials, such as viscose polyester. Gauze is beneficial in wound care because it is highly absorbent and draws drainage away from the wound. In addition, the inert nature of gauze minimizes wound irritation. Gauze dressings come in a variety of sizes and textures, including 5 cm × 5 cm

FIGURE 32.3   Dressing set. A. Unopened set. B. Set-up tray.

TABLE 32.3   Solutions Used in Wound Care

AGENT	EFFECT	USES
Normal Saline	Removes debris from wound without injury to cells.	Cleansing, debriding and maintaining moist wound surface.
Povidone-iodine (Betadine)	Kills bacteria, fungi, viruses, protozoa and some spores.	Cleansing minor wounds, infected wounds, abrasions; topical applications.
Sodium hypochlorite (Dakin's Solution)	Kills some bacteria, fungi; dissolves necrotic tissue.	Wound irrigations.
Hydrogen peroxide	Retards bacterial growth; liquefies organic matter.	Cleansing and debriding wounds.

SOURCES: McKenry and Salerno, 1992; Spencer, Nichols, Lipkin, Henderson and West, 1993.

FIGURE 32.4   Montgomery straps

and 10 cm × 10 cm squares, 10 cm × 20 cm rectangles and gauze bandage rolls. The gauze dressings are placed directly over the wound to form the inner dressing. In some cases, a dressing with a nonadherent surface is first applied to the wound. This is done to prevent further injury to the delicate healing surface when the dressing is removed. There are many nonadherent dressings on the market. These include dressings made of silicone and silk, gauze pads with a non-adherent surface (for example, Telfa) and gauze rolls permeated with petroleum jelly. The external or outer dressing is usually a large, thick cotton pad, commonly called an abdominal or combination pad. Its purpose is to absorb drainage and protect the wound from external contaminants. An abdominal pad is more absorbent on one side than on the other. The more absorbent side is placed against the inner gauze dressings; the less absorbent side faces outward. Some manufacturers mark the outward side with a blue line running through the centre.

Dressings are secured by adhesive tape, elasticized tape, waterproof tape, adhesive ties, binders, bandages or plastic tape. The type of tape used and the method by which it is applied depend upon the site of the wound and the specific needs of the patient. For the patient who is allergic to adhesive tape, some other type of commercially prepared bandage can be used. Adhesive ties or Montgomery straps, illustrated in Figure 32.4, are selected when frequent dressing changes are necessary, since only the ties are undone when the dressing is changed. The adhesive portion is not removed from the skin unless the tape becomes soiled. Use of Montgomery straps prevents skin irritation and breakdown caused by frequent removal and application of tape.

PROCEDURE 32.1

Changing the Dry Dressing

ACTION	RATIONALE
1. Check the physician's order for specific instructions.	Promotes accuracy and avoids error.
2. Prepare the patient and check the existing dressing.	Promotes the patient's well-being and participation in care. Indicates the supplies and equipment that will be needed.
3. Wash hands thoroughly.	Maintains aseptic technique.
4. Gather equipment:	Facilitates efficiency and economy of time.

4. Gather equipment:
   * Dressing set
   * Cleansing solution
   * Moisture-proof bag
   * Clean gloves
   * Cotton balls or gauze squares
   * Gauze dressings and abdominal pad(s) as necessary
   * Tape, bandage or binder
   * Sterile scissors (optional)
   * Sterile gloves (optional)
   * Mask (optional)
   * Acetone and clean 10 cm × 10 cm gauze squares (optional)

ACTION	RATIONALE
5. Help the patient into a comfortable position. Expose the wound area; drape the patient with a sheet or bath blanket.	Provides privacy and avoids unnecessary exposure of the patient.
6. Fold down the top of the moisture-proof bag to make a cuff. Place the bag within easy reach and in an area away from the sterile field such that soiled dressings and sponges are not passed over the wound and sterile field.	Prevents contamination of the outside of the bag, protecting the nurse from contact with contaminants. Placing the bag within reach and away from the sterile field facilitates the nurse's work and reduces the risk of contaminating sterile areas.
7. Apply a mask if required.	Some agencies require masks to be worn to prevent droplet contamination of the wound from the nurse's respiratory tract.
8. Apply clean gloves and remove tape, ties, or bandages. To loosen tape, apply gentle pressure to the skin and pull the tape in the direction of hair growth and towards the wound.	Protects the nurse from contaminants on the outer dressing. Prevents stress on the wound and lessens patient discomfort.

Continued on the next page

ACTION	RATIONALE
9. Remove the external dressing. Note the amount and character of drainage. Fold the dressing inward and discard it into the moisture-proof bag. Avoid touching the outside of the bag. Remove and discard gloves.	Provides data for ongoing evaluation of wound healing. Prevents the transmission of microorganisms.
10. Open the sterile dressing tray on the overbed table. Add solution. Open packages and add supplies ensuring aseptic technique.	Readies the equipment for the dressing change.
11. Using a sterile forceps, remove the inner dressings, taking care not to dislodge any drains. If the gauze sticks to the drain, use another forceps to anchor the drain while taking off the dressings.	Prevents contamination of the nurse's hands from wound drainage.
12. Observe the dressings for amount and character of drainage and discard. Place the forceps aside (on the sterile area but away from the supplies).	Provides data for ongoing evaluation of wound healing. Reserves the forceps if needed for anchoring a drain during the cleansing procedure.
13. Using a forceps and sponges moistened with solution, cleanse the wound: • Use one gauze pad for each stroke. • Work from clean to dirty (see Figure 32.5). Discard the gauze sponge. • After cleaning the wound itself, work away from the wound to a distance of about 5 cm. • If a drain is present, clean it after the incision is cleaned. • Keep the tips of the forceps lower than the handle. • Do not carry contaminated sponges over sterile areas. • Do not reach over a sterile field.	Prevents the spread of microorganisms from dirty to clean areas. The drain is dirtier than the incision since moisture harbours microorganisms. Prevents contamination of the tips with backflow of solution. Prevents contamination from solution dropping on sterile equipment. Prevents contamination from the nurse's arms or uniform.
14. Dry the wound with gauze as necessary, using the same sequence as for cleansing.	
15. Inspect the wound for appearance, integrity, and drainage.	Provides data for ongoing evaluation of healing and effectiveness of care.
16. Using sterile forceps, place the new dressing over the wound. It should be dropped in place rather than moved over the skin. The outer dressing should extend at least 5 cm beyond an open wound.	Avoids transfer of microorganisms from the skin to the centre of the wound and prevents mechanical injury to the wound.
17. Secure the dressing as appropriate with tape, ties, bandages or binders.	Prevents contamination of the wound should the edges be accidentally turned back.
18. Using acetone, remove tape surfaces that have adhered to the skin and are outside the dressing. Wash the area with soap and water.	Prevents skin irritation.

ACTION	RATIONALE
19. Assist the patient into a comfortable position.	Promotes patient well-being.
20. Discard supplies and wash hands.	Maintains cleanliness and safety in the workplace.
21. Document the procedure, the condition of the wound, the cleansing solution, and the type of dressing applied.	Fulfils requirement for nurse accountability. Promotes continuity of care.

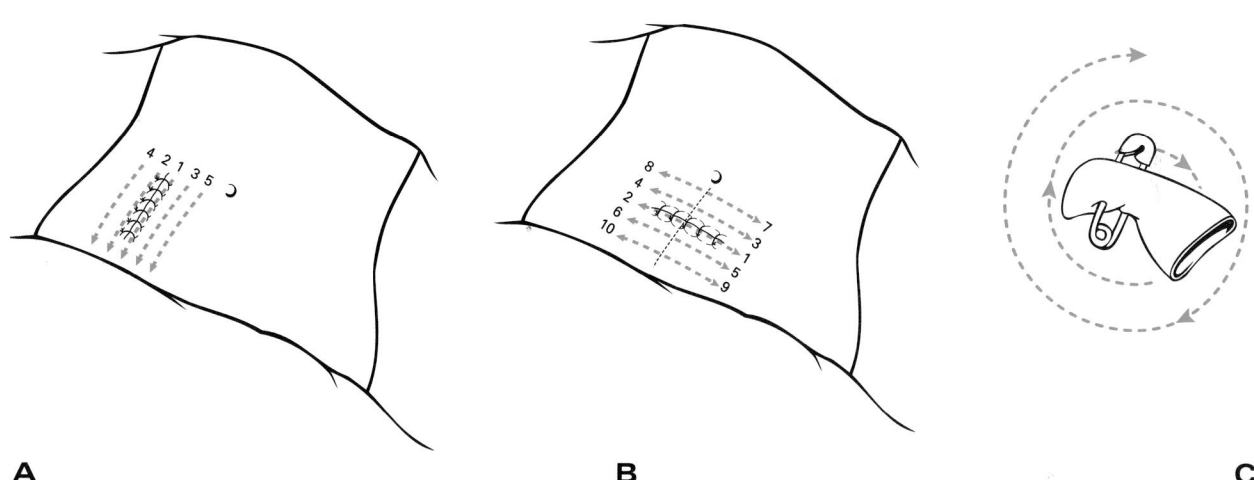

A **B** **C**

FIGURE 32.5   Cleansing wounds. A. A vertical wound is cleaned from the top, where there is the least amount of drainage, to the bottom, where drainage is the greatest. B. A horizontal wound is cleaned from the centre of the incision outward. C. A drain or stab wound is cleaned in a circular fashion, working from the centre outward.

CHANGING A WET-TO-DRY DRESSING

Wet-to-dry dressings are ordered as a means of removing drainage and debriding (removing necrotic tissue and debris) wounds that heal by secondary intention. Moistened dressings are placed over the wound and then covered with a dry dressing. The moist dressing traps drainage and necrotic tissue as it slowly dries. Wound debris is removed with the dressing when it is changed. Dressings are changed every six to eight hours. Wet dressings must not be excessively wet or else skin maceration and bacterial growth may occur in the dark, moist environment. A method for applying a wet-to-dry dressing is given in Procedure 32.2.

Preparing the Patient

The wet-to-dry dressing can be painful. Therefore, the nurse should discuss the need for analgesia with the patient prior to the procedure. If needed, pain medication is given about 30 minutes before the dressing change.

Assembling Equipment

The equipment for a wet-to-dry dressing change is similar to that for a dry dressing. Additional 10 cm × 10 cm gauze squares will be needed. If the wound is large, sterile gloves are recommended to expedite the wound packing procedure. Sterile forceps are sufficient if wounds are small. Normal saline is commonly used to cleanse and debride wounds; however, other solutions may be ordered.

Changing the Wet-to-Dry Dressing

ACTION	RATIONALE
1. Follow steps 1 to 10 of Procedure 32.1. In addition to equipment necessary for changing a dry dressing, gather: • Extra 10 cm × 10 cm sterile gauze pads • Normal saline or solution as ordered	
2. Apply clean gloves.	Protects the nurse's hands from wound contaminants.
3. Using a sterile forceps, remove the contact dressing. If it adheres, warn the patient of discomfort. Do not moisten it to ease removal. Discard dressings and gloves into the moisture-proof bag.	Moistening the dressing would counteract the effectiveness of debridement.
4. Observe the dressings for amount and character of drainage and discard. Inspect the wound for appearance, necrotic tissue and drainage.	Provides data for ongoing evaluation of healing.
5. Put on sterile gloves.	Maintains sterile technique.
6. Saturate 10 cm × 10 cm gauze pads with solution. Wring out excess solution so that they are damp but not dripping.	Creates an optimal environment for absorbing and trapping exudate.
7. Pack the wound with the moistened gauze pads, making sure that all surfaces are covered. Forceps may be used to tuck the gauze into deep areas.	Effective debridement requires complete contact between the wound surface and the dressing.
8. Place dry, sterile 10 cm × 10 cm gauze pads over the moist dressings and cover the wound with an abdominal pad.	
9. Complete the procedure as for a dry dressing change (Steps 17 – 21, Procedure 32.1).	

CHANGING AN OCCLUSIVE DRESSING

Occlusive dressings are used on ulcerated areas, pressure sores, minor burns, abrasions, lacerations and postoperative wounds. They might also be used to protect skin areas from irritation and breakdown, for example, around a stoma. The transparent occlusive dressing is commonly used to anchor venipuncture devices in intravenous therapy. Occlusive dressings are self-adhesive. They adhere to the skin around the wound, not the wound itself. The advantage of these dressings is that they keep wounds moist, thereby speeding the healing process. Moreover, the dressings are left in place until healing has occurred or until they have loosened away from the skin (up to a week or more). This protects the healing basin (the migration of epithelial cells across the open area) from damage caused by the shearing effect of frequent removal and reapplication of dressings. The technique for changing an occlusive dressing is outlined in Procedure 32.3.

Assembling Equipment

There are two types of occlusive dressings: transparent and hydrocolloid (see Figure 32.6). These dressings come in a variety of sizes. The nurse should choose a size that will extend about 5 cm beyond the wound edge.

Transparent dressing   The *transparent dressing,* such as OpSite™ or Tegaderm™, is a thin selectively permeable membrane that is applied to a wound. It permits moisture vapour and oxygen to move towards the wound while providing a barrier against bacteria and fluids. Because it is pliable, this dressing conforms easily to irregular skin surfaces and can be placed over joints without disrupting the patient's mobility. The dressings are commercially prepared to facilitate ease of application. Wounds are assessed through the dressing since it is transparent. In addition, some dressings (as OpSite™) have a grid incorporated into the film which permits accurate measurement of the healing process. Transparent dressings, however, are not absorbable. Wound drainage can accumulate and cause the dressing to separate from the skin. A transparent pouch dressing is now available for containing wound drainage. With a pouch dressing, some of the drainage is eliminated through evaporation, extending the integrity of the dressing.

Hydrocolloid dressings   *Hydrocolloid dressings* (for example, DuoDERM®) are used for covering wounds that yield a lot of drainage and for wounds that heal by secondary intention. The underside of the dressing contains a preparation which absorbs moisture and wound secretions to form a gelatinous substance, hence the label "hydrocolloid." The moist environment promotes healing and protects the newly formed epithelial tissue from damage and contamination. The dressing may remain in place for up to a week unless it becomes loosened.

MANAGING WOUND DRAINS AND DRAINAGE SYSTEMS

Wound healing is hastened if accumulated blood clots, and if body fluids, pus and debris are adequately drained. This process is facilitated by the insertion of a drain or packing at the time of wound closure in the operating room. Soft and firm rubber drains as well as plastic drains are used for this purpose. They may be inserted through the incision line or, more commonly, through a stab wound situated a few centimetres away from the incision. This allows the fluid to drain from the wound without excessive moisture accumulating on the incision line. Some drains are sutured in place, whereas others are freely movable.

Soft rubber drains (Penrose drains) have a sterile safety pin attached to the distal portion of the drain to prevent them from slipping completely inside the wound (see Figure 32.7). These drains are open drains because liquid secretions flow by gravity from the wound into the dressings. Similarly, microorganisms can migrate upward to the wound through contaminated dressings. A closed drain, on the other hand, is a perforated plastic tube connected to a drainage receptacle which draws secretions from the wound by vacuum action. The Hemovac or Davol units are examples of portable wound suction devices (see Figure 32.8). A closed drain may also be connected to a wall suction unit or a suction machine set at low pressure. Because the system is closed, the possibility of microorganisms entering the

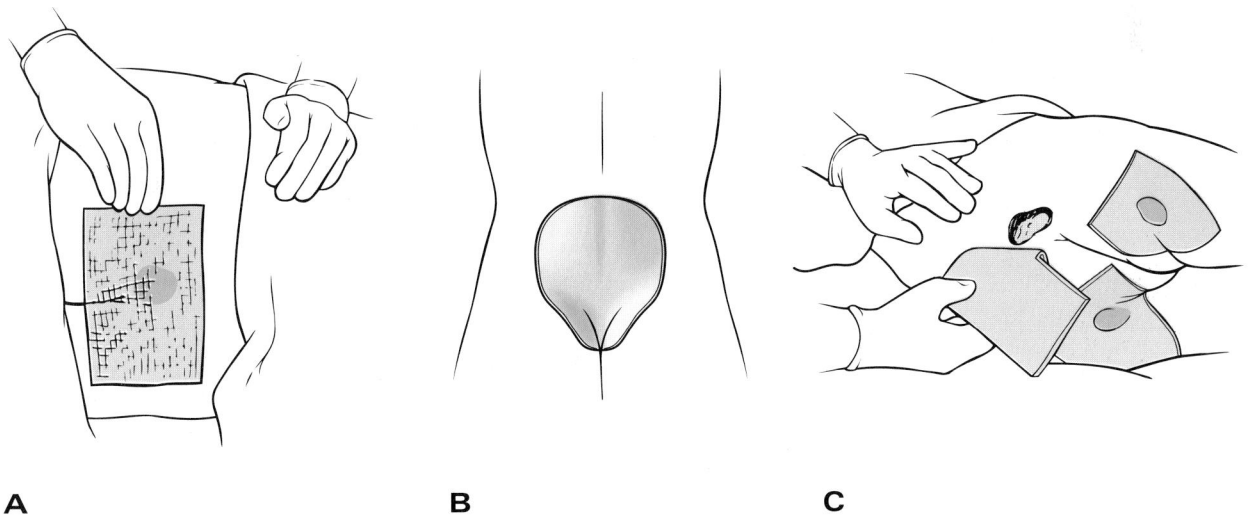

A   **B**   **C**

FIGURE 32.6   Occlusive dressings. A. Transparent dressing. OpSite™ Flexigrid. B. Hydrocolloid dressings. DuoDERM® CGF® Border TRI-ANGLE dressing C. DuoDERM® CGF® Control Gel Formula dressing.

SOURCES: A. Smith & Nephew Inc., Lachine, QC. B. ConVatec. (1992). 581-1136. Princeton, NJ: E.R. Squibb & Sons, Inc. Reproduced with permission.

Changing an Occlusive Dressing

ACTION	RATIONALE
1. Follow steps 1 to 7 of Procedure 32.1, but gather the following only: • Dressing set • Cleansing solution and supplies • Occlusive dressing • Clean gloves • Moisture-proof bag • Mask (optional) • Soap and water	
2. Don clean gloves.	Protects the nurse from contact with contaminants and secretions.
3. Gently press down on the skin at the edge of the dressing with one hand and, with the other, peel the dressing away from the wound. Work from the edges towards the centre of the dressing.	Avoids tearing the newly healed surface that could be pulled away with the dressing.
4. Discard dressing and gloves into the moisture-proof bag.	Reduces spread of contaminants.
5. Cleanse the wound in an appropriate manner, making sure to remove loose necrotic tissue and debris. If a solution other than normal saline is used to clean the wound, rinse with normal saline.	The wound must be clean and free of necrotic tissue and debris for effective healing to occur.
6. Wash the skin around the wound with soap and water. Dry it well.	Removes secretions and dried exudates.
7. Inspect the wound for appearance, integrity and drainage.	Provides data for ongoing evaluation of healing and effectiveness of care.
8. Remove the paper backing from the dressing. Centre the dressing over the wound and gently press it in place. Working from the centre outward, smooth out wrinkles and mould the dressing to the contour of the skin surface.	Avoids air bubbles being trapped beneath the dressing.
9. If necessary, secure the dressing edges with tape.	
10. Assist the patient into a comfortable position.	Promotes patient well-being.
11. Discard supplies and wash hands.	Maintains cleanliness and safety in the workplace.
12. Document the procedure, the condition of the wound, and the type of dressing applied.	Fulfils requirement for nurse accountability. Promotes continuity of care.

wound through the drain is reduced. Packing is usually made of a long strip of gauze, often impregnated with an antiseptic or antibiotic. Open drains and packing are some- times withdrawn a little each day to encourage healing from the base or depth of the wound. Closed drainage systems are left in place until the wound is free of drainage (three to seven days). When the drainage receptacle fills to a designated level, it is emptied and the amount of drainage is measured. Procedures 32.4 and 32.5 outline how to shorten a drain and how to empty a closed drainage receptacle.

Preparing the Patient

Drain shortening should be a relatively comfortable procedure. The patient may experience a pulling sensation when the drain is withdrawn.

Assembling Equipment

A sterile safety pin, sterile scissors and sterile gloves are needed in addition to the equipment for a dry dressing change. Suture scissors are added for the first drain shortening if the drain is anchored with a suture. Clean gloves and a calibrated pitcher are required for emptying a closed wound drainage receptacle.

FIGURE 32.7 Penrose drain exiting from a stab wound

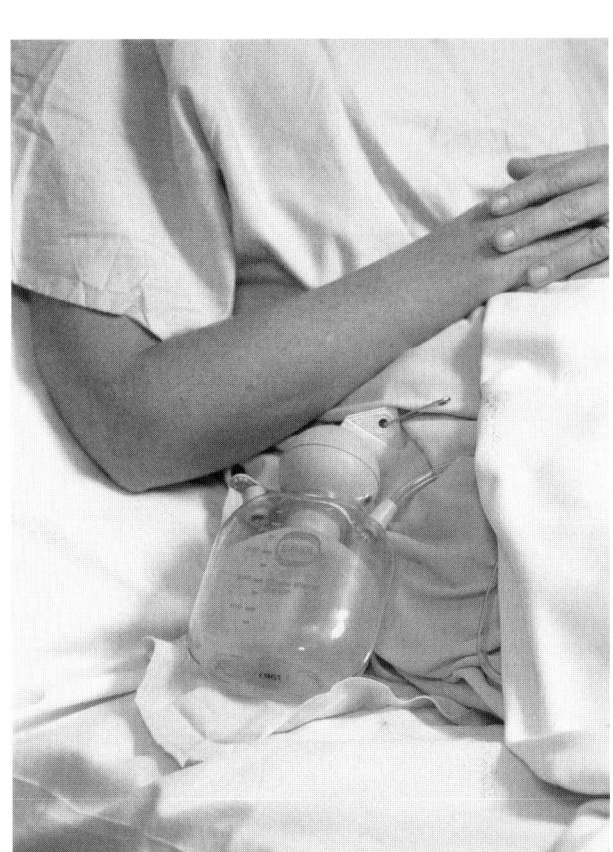

FIGURE 32.8 Closed drainage system

PROCEDURE 32.4

Shortening a Wound Drain

ACTION	RATIONALE
1. Follow steps 1 to 12 of Procedure 32.1. In addition to the equipment necessary for changing a dry dressing, gather: • Sterile safety pin • Sterile scissors • Sterile gloves • Sterile suture scissors (for first drain shortening)	

Continued on the next page

PROCEDURE 32.4
continued

ACTION	RATIONALE
2. Cleanse and dress the incision as in Procedure 32.1.	
3. Cleanse the drain wound.	
4. Put on sterile gloves.	Maintains sterile technique and expedites the procedure.
5. If necessary, clip and remove the suture securing the drain, as in Step 6, Procedure 32.7.	Provides a measurement marker for shortening the drain.
6. Open a 5 cm × 5 cm gauze and wrap it around the drain adjacent to the skin. Place another piece of gauze on the skin beside the drain site.	Facilitates application of countertraction needed for drain withdrawal.
7. With the nondominant hand, withdraw the drain as required. Then, with the dominant hand, insert the sterile pin about 1.5 cm away from the skin.	Allows space for placing dressings between the drain and the skin. The pin prevents the drain from slipping back into the incision.
8. Using sterile scissors, cut the drain between the pins. Discard the piece of drain and the gloves.	Reduces the spread of microorganisms.
9. Using forceps, cleanse the wound again.	Removes secretions that may have accumulated when the drain was withdrawn.
10. Dress the drain site. Cut several 10 cm × 10 cm gauze pads on one side across to the centre or use precut gauze. Layer the gauze snugly under the drain. Encircle the drain with the dressings and make sure the edges overlap. Apply gauze dressings (uncut) over the drain.	Provides a surface for absorption of drainage and protects the skin.

11. Cover the incision and the drain area with an abdominal pad.

12. Complete steps 17 to 20 of Procedure 32.1.

Emptying a Closed Wound Drainage Receptacle

ACTION	RATIONALE
1. Gather equipment: • Measuring pitcher • Clean gloves • Water-proof protective pad	
2. Lay a protective pad on a flat surface and place the measuring pitcher on it.	Catches spills that might occur when the receptacle is emptied.
3. Apply gloves and maintain aseptic technique when emptying the receptacle.	Prevents the introduction of contaminants into the system.
4. Open the receptacle cap, invert the receptacle, and empty the contents into the measuring pitcher.	
5. Reestablish suction mechanism according to the manufacturer's directions.	Suction mechanisms vary according to the manufacturer.
6. Measure the amount of drainage and note the colour, odour, and consistency.	Provides data for ongoing evaluation of care.
7. Record the procedure and the characteristics of drainage in the patient's record. Enter the amount of drainage on the intake and output record.	Fulfils requirements for nurse accountability and communicates assessment information to members of the health care team.

IRRIGATING WOUNDS

"A *wound irrigation* is the introduction of a solution called an irrigant into the wound to wash out exudate, drainage and debris so that the wound can heal" (Earnest, 1993, 920). Wound irrigations are often done to cleanse deep wound cavities or to debride large open wounds. A wound may also be irrigated to apply warmth to an area or to administer medication. Because wounds constitute a break in skin integrity, wound irrigations are performed using sterile technique. Procedure 32.6 outlines the steps for executing a wound irrigation.

Preparing the Patient

Wound irrigations are painful. Therefore, the nurse should ascertain the patient's need for pain medication. If necessary, the analgesic agent should be administered at least 30 minutes before performing the procedure.

Assembling Equipment

A wound irrigation is usually done in conjunction with a dressing change. The irrigation procedure itself will require a syringe, an irrigant, and a collecting basin. A large catheter tip syringe is used for flushing out large wound cavities. Sometimes, deep wound cavities have small surface openings. In such cases, a soft, straight catheter is necessary to reach the base of the wound. Normal saline is a common irrigant; however, other solutions, such as Dakin's solution or hydrogen peroxide, may also be prescribed. Approximately 200 ml of solution may be required to cleanse the wound; a large sterile basin is needed to hold the irrigant. The irrigant should be warmed to 32.2° to 35°C. This can be done by placing the solution container in a basin of warm water. The collecting basin for irrigant return does not have to be sterile since it will not come in direct contact with the wound. A clean large kidney basin is sufficient for this purpose. If an irritating irrigant, such as Dakin's solution, will be used, a skin protectant, such as zinc oxide or petroleum jelly, will also be necessary.

Irrigating a Wound

ACTION	RATIONALE
1. Check the physician's order for type of irrigant and specific instructions.	Promotes accuracy and avoids error.
2. Prepare the patient and check the existing dressing. If necessary, administer pain medication 30 minutes prior to the procedure.	Promotes the patient's well-being and participation in care. Indicates the supplies and equipment that will be needed.
3. Wash hands thoroughly.	Maintains aseptic technique.
4. Gather equipment:	Facilitates efficiency and economy of time.

- Dressing set and dressing materials as necessary
- Catheter-tip syringe
- Soft, straight catheter (optional)
- Irrigant as ordered
- Sterile basin
- Clean kidney basin
- Sterile gloves
- Clean gloves
- Moisture-proof bag
- Water-proof protective pad
- Skin protectant (for example, petroleum jelly)
- Sterile tongue blade
- Mask (optional)

ACTION	RATIONALE
5. Help the patient into a position in which the wound is accessible and drains downward. Make sure the patient is comfortable. Expose the wound and drape the patient with a sheet or bath blanket.	The force of gravity is used to flush and drain the wound.
Put a protective pad under the wound area. Position the clean kidney basin below the wound.	Protects the bed linen from drainage.

ACTION	RATIONALE
6. Prepare the sterile equipment for the irrigation and subsequent dressing application.	Promotes efficiency and ease of performing procedure.
7. Remove the dressing and discard it as in Procedure 32.1.	
8. If necessary, apply a skin protectant to healthy skin around the wound and especially between the wound and the collecting basin.	Provides a barrier against the irritating solution.
9. Don sterile gloves and fill the syringe with irrigant. If using a catheter, attach it to the syringe.	
10. **Syringe:** Gently flush the entire wound surface, beginning at the top and working downward, using slow, continuous pressure.	Flow of solution with gentle force loosens debris and washes it downward, without damaging the fragile healing surface of the wound.
Catheter: Insert the catheter into the wound until resistance is felt and then pull back about one to two centimetres. Gently flush the wound using slow, continuous pressure.	Ensures that catheter tip is off the fragile surface of the wound.
11. Continue irrigation until all of the irrigant is used up or the returning solution is clear.	
12. Using sterile forceps or gloves, dry the wound edges with gauze.	
13. Inspect the wound for appearance, integrity and drainage.	Provides data for ongoing evaluation of healing and effectiveness of care.
14. Dress the wound as required.	
15. Assist the patient into a comfortable position.	Promotes patient well-being.
16. Discard supplies and wash hands.	Maintains cleanliness and safety in the workplace.
17. Document the procedure, the irrigant used, the appearance of the returning fluid and the condition of the wound.	Fulfils requirement for nurse accountability. Promotes continuity of care.

REMOVING SUTURES AND STAPLES

Sutures and staples hold the skin and underlying tissues together in wounds that heal by primary intention. Some sutures are made of absorbable materials which slowly dissolve as the wound heals. These require no care. Nonabsorbable sutures are made of natural fibres, such as silk, or synthetic materials, such as polyester or polypropylene. Some are made of wire. Staples are wide metal clips made of wire or silver. They resemble ordinary paper staples. Staples do not fully encircle the wound edges. They simply form a trough which keeps the wound edges together (see Figure 32.9).

Sutures and staples remain in place until the wound has healed sufficiently. This can be as soon as three days or as long as 14 days postoperatively. A physician's order is required for removal of both sutures and staples.

There are many different types of suturing methods the surgeon may use for skin closure. You will learn more about these as you advance through your course of study. Here, we will discuss two methods of suturing skin: intermittent and continuous suturing. With intermittent suturing, separate sutures are placed in the skin and tied in a knot (see Figure 32.9). In continuous suturing, one suture is woven through the tissues just below the surface of the

FIGURE 32.9 Examples of suturing methods and staples. A. Intermittent sutures. B. Plain continuous sutures. C. Staples.

FIGURE 32.10 A. Staple remover. B. Suture scissors.

skin. A knot is tied at either end. Often, a piece of tubing is placed between the skin surface and the knot to prevent the knot from entering the incision. Sometimes, if incisions are long, the surgeon brings one or more loops of suture over the surface of the skin to facilitate removal. Sutures are removed by clipping the side next to the skin surface and then pulling them out with forceps. The most important principle to remember in removing sutures is to **never** pull loops of suture from the surface of the skin through underlying tissue. Doing so can cause infection. The techniques for removing sutures and staples are detailed in Procedure 32.7.

Preparing the Patient

The removal of sutures and staples may be uncomfortable for some people. As with all procedures, knowing what to expect eases some of the discomfort. A stinging sensation and a feeling of pressure is commonly experienced as a continuous suture is being pulled out. Patients often express the most discomfort when an intermittent suture is being lifted away from the skin so that it can be cut with the suture scissors. Removal of intermittent sutures and staples cause a pinching or "mosquito bite" sensation. Tension can worsen the discomfort. The patient will find that use of relaxation and distraction techniques described in Chapter 26 will significantly help cope with the discomfort accompanying suture and staple removal. The nurse should also assess the patient's pain level and administer analgesia prior to the procedure, if necessary.

Assembling Equipment

Suture and staple removal are sterile techniques. The incision is cleansed first; a dressing set and cleansing solution are required. Sutures are clipped with special suture scissors that have a short, curved cutting tip which slides easily under the suture. Staples are taken out with a special surgical staple remover (see Figure 32.10). In some cases, a bit of wound dehiscence may occur when the sutures and staples are removed. When this happens, the separated edges are brought and held together with tape strips, such as butterfly tape or Steri-Strips. The wound may be left exposed, or covered with a light dressing such as a 10 cm × 20 cm gauze rectangle or an adhesive wound dressing (such as Hypafix® or Mepore plaster®) may be applied following the procedure.

PROCEDURE 32.7

Removing Skin Sutures or Staples

ACTION	RATIONALE
1. Validate the physician's order.	Promotes safety; avoids error.
2. Prepare the patient. Determine the need for analgesia and administer medication if necessary.	Promotes the patient's well-being and participation in care.
3. Wash hands thoroughly.	Maintains aseptic technique.
4. Gather equipment: • Dressing set • Cleansing solution • Sterile suture scissors or staple remover • Steri-Strips or butterfly tape • Light wound dressing (optional) • Moisture-proof bag • Clean gloves	Facilitates efficiency and economy of time.
5. Remove the dressing and cleanse the incision as outlined in Procedure 32.1.	Removes surface microorganisms and moistens sutures which may ease removal.
6. **Removing Intermittent Sutures** • Using forceps, grasp and lift the knot. Slide the scissors under the suture, away from the knot.	Facilitates insertion of the scissors underneath the suture.
• Cut the suture as close to the skin as possible.	Prevents surface suture material from being pulled through underlying tissue.
• Gently pull the freed stitch up and out.	
• Remove alternate sutures. If there is no evidence of dehiscence remove the remaining sutures. Should a large dehiscence occur, cover the wound with sterile gauze and notify the physician immediately.	Provides support to the incision should dehiscence occur.

Continued on the next page

ACTION	RATIONALE
Removing Plain Continuous Sutures	
• Grasp the first loop of suture with a forceps. Lift it gently and cut it at the end opposite to the knot. Then cut the same end of the adjacent suture.	As above.
• Grasp the knot of the freed suture and pull the suture out, pulling parallel to the body.	Reduces patient's discomfort.
• Next, grasp the freed end of the suture and cut it off close to the skin.	
• Grasp the next loop, pull out the underlying suture and cut it off. Repeat this sequence until all loops have been removed.	
• Grasp the remaining knot and pull out the suture.	
Removing Staples	
• Slide the lower tips of the staple remover under the middle of the staple. Squeeze the handle and when both edges of the staple are visible, lift it from the skin. Remove staples in the same alternate fashion as for intermittent sutures.	Bends the centre of the staple and straightens the embedded ends.

ACTION	RATIONALE
7. If necessary, clean the incision again.	Sometimes, bleeding may occur.
8. If small areas of wound separation are present, bring the wound edges together with butterfly tape or Steri-Strips. These tapes may be placed intermittently along the entire length of the wound.	Holds the wound edges together and provides support to the wound.
9. Cover the incision with a light dressing, if necessary.	Protects the wound from external contaminants.
10. Assist the patient into a comfortable position.	Promotes patient well-being.
11. Discard supplies and wash hands.	Maintains cleanliness and safety in the workplace.
12. Document the procedure, the condition of the incision, any wound separation, whether tape strips or a dry dressing was applied.	Fulfils requirement for nurse accountability.

APPLYING BANDAGES

A bandage is a piece of material that is used to wrap a part of the body. The purposes of applying a bandage are:

1. to limit movement
2. to apply warmth (for example, to a rheumatoid joint)
3. to secure a dressing
4. to keep splints in position
5. to provide support (for example, to the legs to aid venous blood flow)
6. to apply pressure in order to control bleeding, promote the absorption of tissue fluids or prevent the loss of tissue fluids

Materials Used in Bandaging

Gauze   Gauze is one of the most frequently used materials for bandaging. It is a soft, woven cotton that is porous but not bulky, light in weight and readily moulded to any contour. Gauze is sometimes impregnated with various ointments such as petrolatum. Cotton gauze is not commonly used anymore because of its cost. It is the safest bandage material, however, when there is concern about pressure on the wound.

Kling gauze or Kerlix gauze   Kling gauze and Kerlix gauze are woven to allow the gauze to stretch, moulding to body contours. The gauze has a crepe-like texture and tends to cling to itself, an attribute that helps keep it in place after it has been applied.

Stockinet   Stockinet is a stretchable material in the shape of a tube. It comes in various widths and can be applied to many parts of the body, such as the head, chest, arms, legs or fingers. It is easy to use, moulds well to the body and provides uniform pressure.

Flannel   Flannel makes a soft and pliable bandage. It is heavy and keeps in the heat of the body; it can be used to apply warmth to body joints.

Muslin   Muslin (factory cotton) is a strong heavy cotton that is not pliable. It is used to provide support, as for splints, or to limit movement.

Elasticized bandages   Elasticized bandages made of cotton with an elastic webbing (Ace bandages) are often used as tensor bandages to apply pressure. They are expensive but can be washed and reused.

Elastic adhesive   Elastic adhesive (Elastoplast) is a woven bandage with an adhesive side. It is applied to give support, for example, when dressings are being secured.

Plastic adhesive   Plastic adhesive is a waterproof bandage with an adhesive side. It is somewhat elastic and

KEY PRINCIPLES

Principles Relevant to Bandaging

1. *Microorganisms flourish in warm, damp and soiled areas.* A bandage is applied only over a clean area; if it is to be placed over an open wound, the wound is dressed aseptically beforehand. Skin surfaces are dry and clean and are not pressed together when bandaging. Adjacent skin surfaces may be kept separated by inserting a 5 cm × 5 cm piece of gauze between them. Bandages are removed at regular intervals and the skin surfaces are washed and dried. Soiled bandages are never reused.

2. *Pressure exerted upon the body tissues can affect the circulation of blood.* A bandage is applied from the distal to the proximal part of the body to aid the return of the venous blood to the heart. Bandages are always applied evenly so that they do not restrict circulation. They should be checked frequently to make certain that there is no interference with blood supply to the part.

3. *Friction can cause mechanical trauma to the epithelium.* A bony prominence of the body is padded before it is bandaged, so that the bandage does not rub the area and cause an abraded wound. Skin surfaces are separated to prevent friction and maceration.

4. *The body is maintained in the natural anatomical position with slight flexion of the joints to avoid muscle strain.* Bandages are applied with the body in good alignment to avoid muscle extension, which is fatiguing and produces strain. In particular, adduction of the shoulder and hip joint is avoided.

5. *Excessive or uneven pressure upon body surfaces can interfere with blood circulation and therefore with the nourishment of the cells in the area.* Bandage evenly and, if possible, leave the distal portion of the bandaged limb exposed so that any restriction in circulation can be detected. Signs and symptoms of restricted circulation are pallor, erythema, cyanosis, tingling sensations, numbness or pain, swelling and cold.

   When a bandage is applied over a wet dressing, allowances are made for shrinkage as the bandage becomes wet and subsequently dries.

can be used to apply pressure and at the same time keep an area dry.

FIGURE 32.11 Types of bandages. A. A spiral reverse bandage on the calf. B. A figure-eight turn on the elbow. C. A recurrent turn on the hand. D. A finger bandage with the tip covered. E. A thumb spica.

Fundamental Turns in Bandaging

There are five fundamental turns in bandaging, and it is these turns that are used to make up the variety of bandages applied to the various parts of the body.

The **circular turn** is used to bandage a cylindrical part of the body or to secure a bandage at its initial and terminal ends. In a circular turn, the bandage is wrapped about the part in such a way that each turn exactly covers the previous one. Two circular turns are usually used to initiate and to terminate a bandage. For comfort, the initial and terminal ends are not situated directly over the wound.

The **spiral turn** is used to bandage a part of the body that is of uniform circumference. The bandage is carried upward at a slight angle so that it spirals around the part. Each turn is parallel to the preceding one and overlaps it by two-thirds of the width of the bandage. A spiral turn is used on parts of the body such as the fingers, arms and legs.

The **spiral reverse turn** is used to bandage cylindrical parts of the body that are of varying circumference, such as the lower leg. To make a spiral reverse turn, the thumb of the free hand is placed on the upper edge of the initial turn; the bandage is held firmly. The roll is unwound about 15 cm and then the hand is pronated so that the bandage is directed downward and parallel to the lower edge of the previous turn, overlapping it by two-thirds of the width. The roll is then carried around the limb and another reverse is made at the same place so that the turns are in line and uniform.

The **figure-eight turn** is usually used on joints but may also be used for the entire length of an arm or leg bandage. It consists of repeated oblique turns that are made alternately above and below a joint in the form of a figure eight. After the initial circular turns are made over the centre of the joint, the next turn is superior to the joint and the next is inferior to the joint. Thus the turns are worked upward and downward, with each turn overlapping the previous turn by two-thirds of the width of the bandage.

The **recurrent turn** is used to cover distal portions of the body, such as the tip of a finger or the toes. After the bandage is anchored with a circular turn, the roll is turned and brought directly over the centre of the tip to be covered.

It is then anchored inferiorly, and alternate turns are made, first to the right and then to the left, over the original turn covering the tip so that each turn is held above and below. Each turn overlaps the preceding one by two-thirds of its width. The bandage is secured by circular turns that gather in the ends.

Generally speaking, bandages for the hands, arms and feet are made with circular, spiral and spiral reverse turns. Bandages for the joints are made with figure eights, and bandages for the distal portions of the body are done with recurrent turns. In addition, there are many special bandages, such as the thumb spica, ear and eye bandages and skull bandages. It is suggested that the nurse consult a bandaging text for more detailed information.

APPLYING BINDERS

Binders can be used to retain dressings, to apply pressure, to support an area of the body and to provide comfort. Binders are generally made of a heavy cotton material that is strong and durable. Scultetus binders are occasionally lined with flannel, which absorbs moisture and provides additional comfort. When the purpose of the binder is to provide support to abdominal muscles, a two-way stretch type of binder, similar to a girdle, is sometimes used.

Guides to Bandaging

1 Face the patient being bandaged.

2. Start a roller bandage by holding the roll of the bandage upward in one hand, the initial end in the other hand.

3. Bandage from the distal to the proximal and from the medial to the lateral.

4. Do not initiate or terminate a bandage directly over a wound or an area where the patient is likely to exert pressure.

5. Bandage evenly and firmly, overlapping the preceding turn by two-thirds of the width of the bandage.

6. Use the bandage material that best serves the purpose of the bandage.

7. Cover a dressing with a bandage that extends past each side of the dressing.

8. Separate the skin surfaces and pad bony prominences and hollows to prevent friction and to apply even pressure.

9. Check the bandage and look for any signs of restricted circulation.

10. A bandage should be safe, durable, neat, therapeutically effective and economical.

Guides for the Applying of Binders

1. Binders are applied in such a manner as to provide even pressure over an area of the body.

2. Binders should support body parts in their normal anatomical position, with slight joint flexion.

3. Binders are secured firmly so that they do not cause friction and irritate the skin or mucous membrane.

Types of Binders

There are five basic types of binders: T-binder, straight abdominal binder, scultetus (many-tailed) binder, breast binder and triangular binder.

The *T-binder* is made of two strips of cotton attached in the shape of a *T*. The top of the *T* serves as a band which is then placed around the patient's waist. The stem of the *T* is passed between the patient's legs and is then attached to the waistband in front. In some T-binders, the cotton strip that goes between the patient's legs is split into two tails about 22.5 cm from the end. These tails provide wider support to the perineal area and add to the comfort of the male patient particularly. T-binders are used chiefly to retain perineal dressings. Because of the profuse drainage that often occurs from this area, they are usually changed frequently.

The *straight abdominal binder* is a rectangular piece of cotton from 15 cm to 30 cm wide, and long enough to encircle the patient's abdomen and overlap at least 5 cm in front. This type of binder is used to retain abdominal dressings or to apply pressure and support to the abdomen.

The *scultetus binder,* which is also known as the many-tailed binder, is a rectangular piece of cotton, usually 22.5 cm to 30 cm wide and 37.5 cm long, with 6 to 12 tails attached to each side. It is usually used to provide support to the abdomen, but it can also be used to retain dressings. It can be applied to the chest as well. The advantage of the scultetus binder is that it fits the contours of the body closely.

The *breast binder* is a rectangular piece of cotton shaped roughly to the contours of the female chest. It usually has straps that fit over the shoulders and pin to the binder in front.

Various forms of the *triangular binder* (sling) are used to support a limb, to secure a splint (as a first aid measure) and to secure dressings. The triangular binder is made of heavy cotton, is triangular in shape, and has two sides approximately 1 m in length. It can be applied as a full triangle or folded for a variety of applications.

As a full triangle, the binder is used frequently to make a *large arm sling.* Folded into a broad bandage, it can be used as

FIGURE 32.12 A. Types of binders. B. A large arm sling. C. A small arm sling. D. A triangular sling.

a *small sling* to support the patient's wrist and hand. A triangular binder can also support a patient's arm in such a manner as to elevate the hand. This is called a *triangular sling*.

Problems Related to the Use of Binders

Binders are most often used for large areas of the body, and since they are not secured to skin surfaces, they have a tendency to slip out of position. A binder should be changed or reapplied as often as necessary to maintain its intended function of support, comfort or application of pressure.

Soiling is also a problem with binders. Because a dirty binder can be a source of both irritation and infection, it is essential to see that soiled binders are changed promptly.

When a binder is applied, it should be secured firmly, but the nurse should be careful that there is no interference with normal body functioning. An abdominal or breast binder that is too tight, for example, can restrict movements of the chest wall and interfere with respiration. In postoperative patients this could lead to serious complications. The nurse should be alert for signs of impaired respiration, such as shallow breathing, which could indicate that a binder is too tight and should be loosened.

KEY TERMS

biopsy p. 1043
open wound p. 1062
closed wound p. 1062
primary intention healing p. 1063
secondary intention healing p. 1064
serous discharge p. 1065
sanguineous discharge p. 1065
serosanguineous drainage p. 1065

purulent drainage p. 1065
hematoma p. 1066
dehiscence p. 1066
evisceration p. 1066
occlusive dressings p. 1072
wound irrigation p. 1077
circular turn p. 1084
spiral turn p. 1084

spiral reverse turn p. 1084
figure-eight turn p. 1084
recurrent turn p. 1084
T-binder p. 1085
straight abdominal binder p. 1085
scultetus (many-tailed) binder p. 1085
breast binder p. 1085
triangular binder p. 1085

IN REVIEW

Surgery involves the deliberate and planned alteration of anatomical structures to arrest, alleviate or eradicate a pathological process or to repair a traumatic injury. The major nursing goals for people experiencing surgery are to prepare them for and promote healthy recovery from surgery. Due to the development of knowledge and techniques in the areas of hemostasis, asepsis, anesthesia and technology, surgery today is a safe and humane procedure.

Surgery may be major or minor depending on its extent; it is classified as immediate, urgent, elective or optional depending on the severity of existing pathology. The purpose of surgery may be diagnostic, curative, constructive, reparative or palliative.

The determinants of a person's ability to cope with surgery include not only the extent of the surgery but also the person's age, physiological and psychological health, overall coping capabilities, ability to assist in postoperative planning and the support received from family and significant others.

The nurse's preoperative assessment of the patient includes a health history and assessment of basic needs. Particular attention is paid to oxygen, nutrition, fluid and electrolyte and elimination needs as well as immunological status and security and self-esteem needs.

Two major preoperative nursing diagnoses are *Knowledge deficit regarding preoperative procedures and*

protocols and postoperative expectations and *Anxiety related to the surgical experience and the outcome of surgery.*

Preoperative teaching is an important health promoting and protecting strategy. This teaching, which may be done singly or in groups, can be given before admission in either testing centres or outpatient clinics or it may be given after admission in the hospital. Teaching includes situational, sensational/discomfort and patient role information, psychological support and skills training.

In the immediate preoperative period, the nurse is responsible for completing the nursing assessment, reviewing or giving information to ease patient anxiety and ensuring the patient is safely prepared for surgery. Most agencies have specific protocols for pre- and postoperative care that are essential for the health and safety of the patient on the nursing unit, in the post-anesthesia care unit and after transfer back to the nursing unit.

Following surgery, the patient goes to a post-anesthesia care unit where vital signs, reflexes, dressing drainage, tubes and collecting bags are immediately assessed and checked as often as necessary. When conscious and in a stable condition, the patient is returned to the nursing unit where all basic needs are monitored on a regular basis and as necessary for the patient's comfort and safety and to avoid or identify complications. Particular problems to watch for are ineffective breathing and airway clearance; shock and hemorrhage; the development of phlebitis and embolism; water, sodium, potassium and acid-base balance; altered nutritional status; altered urinary elimination; constipation; pain and anxiety. Because of impaired tissue integrity, the risk of infection is high.

A surgical incision is a type of physical wound. Drains and packing may be inserted at the time of surgery to facilitate drainage from the wound. Healing is a restoration of tissue continuity after any injury, including surgery. Healing occurs by primary intention when there is little or no tissue loss or by secondary intention when damage and tissue loss are extensive. The healing response of a surgical wound has three phases: inflammatory, proliferatory and remodelling. Both systemic and local factors may impede healing of the wound. Systemic factors include the extent of the injury, the patient's nutritional status, obesity, diabetes, immunosuppression and use of radiation in treatment. Local impediments may be chemical, mechanical or thermal in origin; they may be caused by the suture material, by infection or by the blood supply to the area. A wound is assessed for signs of healing, infection or discharge and for approximation of skin edges.

Restorative strategies include the use of aseptic technique for cleansing and changing dressings and in the management of wound drains and drainage systems. Clean dry dressings and asepsis are essential. Specific techniques are used for changing dressings, shortening drains, irrigating wounds and removing sutures and staples. Bandages may be used to secure a dressing, apply warmth, keep splints in place, provide support, apply pressure or limit movement. The purpose determines the type of bandage, type of material used and method of application. Binders are used to retain dressings, apply pressure or provide comfort. Common binders are T-binders, straight and scultetus binders, breast binders and various forms of triangular binders. The type of binder used depends on its purpose.

LEARNING ACTIVITIES

Case Study: Mr. John Smith is a 30-year-old law enforcement officer who is married, has four children, and is in excellent physical condition. He was admitted to hospital 3 days ago with a bullet wound to his right shoulder. The bullet has been removed, but since there may still be particles of foreign matter present, the physician has not sutured the wound. The physician's orders for Mr. Smith include: Change dressings b.i.d. and as necessary; Flush wound with normal saline; Fluids to diet as tolerated.

When you arrive to change his dressing, Mr. Smith complains of headache and a burning sensation in the region of his wound. You notice a yellow discharge seeping through the previous dressing. Mr. Smith also remarks that he feels hot, although a fresh breeze is blowing through the open window beside his bed.

Mr. Smith has been worried that he may not regain full use of his right arm, and since he is right-handed, he fears he may have to resign from active duty.

1. What would you do first when faced with this situation?
2. What might be causing the yellowish discharge from the wound?
3. What other observations might you expect to note in the area of Mr. Smith's wound?
4. What other observations might you note about his general condition?
5. How would you record your observations concerning Mr. Smith?
6. What could you do to assist in relieving his anxiety?

REFERENCES AND READINGS

ALEXANDER, J.W., FISCHER, J.E., BOYAIJIAN, M., PALMQUIST, J. and MORRIS, M.J. (1983). The influence of hair-removal methods on wound infections. *Archives of Surgery, 118,* 347–352.

AORN RECOMMENDED PRACTICES (1992). Proposed recommended practices skin preparation of patients. *AORN Journal, 55*(2), 555–562.

BECKERMANN, S. and GALLOWAY, S. (1989). Elective resection of the liver: Nursing care. *Critical Care Nurse, 9*(10), 40–48.

BUBELA, N., GALLOWAY, S., MCCAY, E., MCKIBBON, A., NAGLE, L., PRINGLE, D., ROSS, E. and SHAMIAN, J. (1990). Factors influencing patients' informational needs at time of hospital discharge. *Patient Education and Counselling, 16,* 21–28.

CARPENITO, L.J. (1993). *Nursing diagnosis: Application to clinical practice.* Philadelphia: Lippincott.

CAVANILLAS, A.B., RODRIGUEZ-CONTRERAS, R., RODRIGUEZ, M.D., ABRIL, O.M., GIGOSOS, R.L., SOLVAS, J.G. and VARGAS, R.G. (1991). Preoperative stay as a risk factor for nosocomial infection. *European Journal of Epidemiology, 7*(6), 670–676.

COBLEY, M., DUNNE, J.A. and SANDERS, L.D. (1991). Stressful preoperative preparation procedures. *Anaesthesia, 46,* 1019-1022.

CONNOLLY, M.L. (1991). Ambulatory surgery and prepared discharge. *Nursing Clinics of North America, 26*(1), 105-112.

CRUSE, P. and FOORD, R. (1980). The epidemiology of wound infection: A 10 year prospective study of 62,939 wounds. *Surgical Clinics of North America, 60,* 27–40.

CURTIN, L.L. (1993). Informed consent: Cautious, calculated candor. *Nursing Management, 24*(4), 18-20.

DESJARDINS, L., NOBLE, J., BUBELA, N., MCKIBBON, A. and GALLOWAY, S.C. (1992). *Preoperative Education Program, Scarborough Grace Hospital/Sunnybrook Health Science Centre.* Toronto, Ontario.

DEVINE, C. and COOK, T. (1986). Clinical and cost-savings effects of psycho-educational intervention with surgical patients. A meta-analysis. *Research in Nursing and Health, 9*(2), 89–105.

EARNEST, V.V. (1993). *Clinical skills in nursing practice* (2nd ed.). Philadelphia: Lippincott.

FLYNN, J.M., and HACKEL, R. (1990). *Technological foundations in nursing.* Norwalk, CT: Appleton & Lange.

FRAULEIN, K.E. (1987). After anesthesia: *A guide for PACU, ICU, and medical-surgical nurses.* Norwalk, CT: Appleton & Lange.

GALLOWAY, S.C., BUBELA, N., MCKIBBON, A., MCCAY, E. and ROSS, E. (1993). Perceived information needs and effect of symptoms on activities after surgery for lung cancer. *Canadian Oncology Nursing Journal, 3*(3), 116–119.

HARDING, K.G. (1990). Wound care: Putting theory into clinical practice. *Wounds: A compendium of clinical research and practice, 2* (1), 21–32.

HATHAWAY, D. (1986). Effect of pre-operative instruction on postoperative outcomes: A meta-analysis. *Nursing Research, 35*(5), 269–275.

HUTCHINSON, J.J. and McGUCKIN, M. (1990). Occlusive dressings: A microbiologic and clinical review. *American Journal of Infection Control, 18*(4), 257–268.

JOHNSON, J.E. and LAUVER, D.R. (1989). Alternative explanations of coping with stressful experiences associated with physical illness. *Advances in Nursing Science, 11*(2), 39–52.

KING, M.S. (1991). Preoperative evaluation of the elderly. *Journal of the American Board of Family Practice, 4*, 251–258.

MAXWELL, L. (1992). Acute pain management: IV patient controlled analgesia places the patient in control. *Canadian Operating Room Nursing Journal, 10*(3), 12–15.

McKENRY, L.M. and SALERNO, E. (1992). *Mosby's pharmacology in nursing.* St. Louis: Mosby.

MILLER, M. (1987). Fluid and electrolyte balance in the elderly. *Geriatrics, 42*(11), 65–76.

MORSE, J.M. and JOHNSON, J.L. (Eds.). (1991). *The illness experience: Dimensions of suffering.* Newbury Park, CA: Sage.

NEUBERGER, G.B. and RECKLING, J.B. (1990). Preventing wound complications in an age of DRGs. *Chronic Wound Care, 49*.

POGUE, P. (1993). *Questions patients ask about pain after surgery.* Sunnybrook Health Science Centre: Toronto, Ontario.

POTTER, P. A. and PERRY, A. G. (1993). *Fundamentals of nursing: Concepts, process and practice* (3rd ed.). St. Louis: Mosby.

SCHOESSLER, M. (1989). Perceptions of pre-operative education in patients admitted the morning of surgery. *Patient Education and Counselling, 14*, 127–136.

SEROPIAN, R. and REYNOLDS, B.M. (1971). Wound infections after preoperative depilatory versus razor preparation. *American Surgeon, 121*, 251–254.

SPENCER, R.T., NICHOLS, L.W., LIPKIN, G.B., HENDERSON, H.S. and WEST, F.M. (1993) *Clinical pharmacology and nursing management* (4th ed.). Philadelphia: Lippincott.

STOTTS, N.A. (1986). Impaired wound healing. In V.K. Carrieri, A.M. Lindsey and C.M. West (Eds.). *Pathophysiological phenomena in nursing: Human responses to illness.* Philadelphia: Saunders.

TIMBY, B.K. and LEWIS, L.W. (1992). *Fundamental skills and concepts in patient care* (5th ed.). Philadelphia: Lippincott.

WASYLAK, T.J. (1992). Surgical pain management. In J. Watt-Watson and M. Donovan (Eds.). *Pain management: A nursing perspective.* St. Louis: Mosby.

WHITE, H., THURSTON, N.E., BLACKMORE, K.A., GREEN, S.E. and HANNAH, J. (1987). Body temperature in elderly surgical patients. *Research in Nursing and Health, 10*, 317–321.

CHAPTER 33

Administering Medications Safely

CENTRAL QUESTIONS

1. *Why do some drugs have several different names?*

2. *How do drugs produce their effects in the body? What is pharmacokinetics?*

3. *What determines the action and effects of drugs on different people?*

4. *What controls exist on drugs in Canada?*

5. *How are standards for drugs determined?*

6. *What information is required for medication orders to be valid?*

7. *What are the nurse's responsibilities in administering drugs safely?*

8. *How does the nurse assess the medication needs of patients?*

9. *What are some problems associated with drug therapy?*

10. *In order to promote healthy medication use, what advice should nurses give patients?*

11. *What is involved in teaching the self-administration of drugs?*

12. *What are the five rights of drug administration?*

13. *What methods are used for administering drugs? How are these carried out?*

14. *How does the nurse record the administration of medications?*

15. *How does the nurse evaluate the effectiveness of medications?*

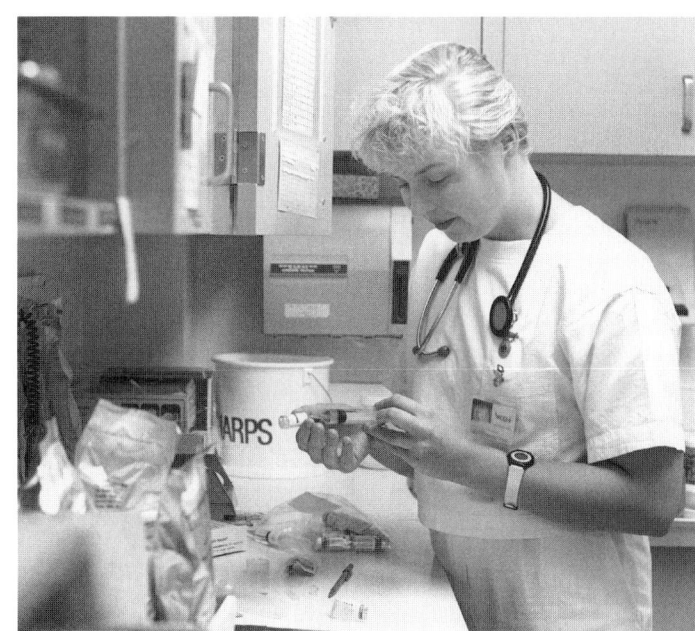

INTRODUCTION

By definition, a *medication* is a substance taken to treat a disease or condition. This may include pharmaceutical agents (also referred to as drugs) and other "medicines" such as laughter, therapeutic touch or hugging. In this chapter we will deal only with the administration of pharmaceutical agents.

Medications have been used throughout history to promote, maintain and restore health. In recent years, however, the number of different medicines manufactured commercially for distribution has increased exponentially. We take drugs to go to sleep, to reduce pain, to settle our nerves, to reduce ulcers, to provide vitamins and minerals — the list goes on. We are at the point in North American society when we almost expect to take a drug of one type or another. Health care professionals have the enormous task of keeping up-to-date with the new drug products that are introduced each year, so that they may safely prepare and administer the drugs and provide the patient with adequate information for self-administration. Medications can offer huge benefits for our health, but they are not without potential hazards. We must always be aware of these.

The administration of medications is a therapeutic nursing function that is chiefly dependent upon the orders of the physician. Some medication orders state the exact time of administration, others leave this to the nurse's judgement. For example, ferrous sulphate is usually prescribed three times a day after meals; morphine sulphate, on the other hand, is often ordered so that it can be given when the patient *requires* medication for pain. While the administration of medications is a delegated task, the responsibility for safe and effective administration rests with the nurse. Legally, nurses are responsible for any medications they administer. Safe, effective administration of medications begins with a basic understanding of pharmacology and the legal implications of drug administration. It requires knowledge and skill in preparing, administering and recording the administering of medications. It also requires knowledge and skill in assessing the patient's health status, in identifying problems and in implementing nursing interventions to enhance the effectiveness of drug therapy, minimize adverse reactions and promote patient safety and well-being.

BASIC PHARMACOLOGY

The term *pharmacology* comes from the Greek *pharmakon*, which means "drugs," and *logos*, which stands for "science." By definition, pharmacology means the study of drugs, their actions and their effects on living organisms. An understanding of the basic concepts of pharmacology is fundamental to the safe administration of drugs.

NAMES OF DRUGS

A drug usually has at least three names: its trade name, a chemical name and a generic name. The beginning nurse often finds it difficult to decipher these names when first learning to administer drugs, because the same drug may be referred to with three or more names.

The *trade* name, also called *brand* name or *proprietary* name, is the name of a drug chosen and copyrighted by the manufacturer. An example of a trade name is Valium. Manufacturers market drugs under the trade name. One drug may therefore have several trade names, since the same drug may be manufactured by several drug companies, each one giving it a different trade name. The *chemical* name of the drug is a description of its chemical constituents. For instance, the chemical name for Valium is 7-chloro-1,3-dihydro-1-methyl-5-phenyl-2H-1,4-benzodiazepin-2-one. A *generic* name is the original name assigned by the individual or company that develops the drug. It is usually a simpler representation of the drug's chemical name. The generic name for Valium is diazepam.

An increasing number of health agencies are promoting the use of generic names of drugs for writing prescriptions. This practice eliminates confusion about the nature of the drug prescribed. It also means that products from different drug companies can be used alternatively, except in cases where the physician requests a specific product. In addition, if the drug is ordered in its generic form, the patient can often save money, since brand name products are frequently more expensive.

MECHANISMS OF DRUG ACTION

Drugs act on the body in a number of different ways. The study of the mechanisms of drug action and the effects on cellular function is called *pharmacodynamics*. Drugs act by replacing missing or deficient substances, by altering the environment of the cell or by affecting the rate of cellular functions. Replacement therapy consists of administering an essential component of the body such as insulin in diabetes mellitus or iron in iron-deficiency anemia. Drugs may alter the environment of cells through physical and chemical processes. For example, some drugs act by the mechanism of lubrication. Mineral oil given orally acts as a lubricant on the surface of the bowel which facilitates the passage of feces. Other drugs act by altering the chemistry of body fluids. Administering intravenous fluids and electrolytes will change the serum levels of the individual ions and may influence the pH level of body fluids as well. Drugs that affect the rate of cell functions do so by acting on *receptors* found on cell membranes to stimulate (activate) or depress (block) a tissue response. Mechanisms of stimulation "increase the rate of cellular activity or increase the secretion from a gland" (Kee and Hayes, 1993, 14). Mechanisms of depression decrease or block cellular activity and reduce organ function. Drugs that stimulate or produce a response are called **agonists**. For example, epinephrine, which acts on alpha and beta adrenergic receptors to stimulate an adrenergic response, is an agonist. Drugs that block a cellular response are called **antagonists**. For example, cimetidine is an antagonist because it blocks the histamine$_2$ (H$_2$) receptors of the parietal cells of the stomach, thereby reducing gastric acid secretion.

A drug's action in the body is related to the amount of drug that reaches its target sites, or sites of action. Drug action is influenced by the dose of the medication (the quantity or concentration of the drug in a unit of volume or weight) and four basic processes: absorption, distribution, metabolism and excretion. The study of these four processes is called **pharmacokinetics**. *Absorption* is the process by which a drug moves from its site of entry to circulating body fluids, the bloodstream and the lymphatic system. Absorption occurs in the mouth when medication is placed under the tongue (sublingual), in the gastrointestinal tract, in subcutaneous tissue, in muscle tissue and in the skin. Drugs given intravenously are injected directly into the bloodstream and thus do not have to be absorbed. Once the drug molecules are absorbed, they are transported throughout the body and to their sites of action. Drug molecules are also delivered to sites in the body where they are chemically changed into active or inactive compounds. This process is called biotransformation or *metabolism* and it takes place primarily in the liver. Most drugs are deactivated by this process and converted into water-soluble compounds for excretion from the body. However, some drugs are modified into active forms which can produce new pharmacological effects. *Excretion* is the process which eliminates drugs from the body. Excretion occurs primarily through the kidneys. Other routes of excretion include bile, feces, lungs, saliva, sweat and breast milk.

There is an ever-changing balance between the processes that increase active drug levels in the blood (absorption and distribution) and those that reduce active drug levels (metabolism and excretion). This balance "determines how soon the drug's actions will appear, how intense and widespread they will be, and how long they will last" (Shlafer, 1993, 46). The **onset of action** is the time it takes for a drug to enter the bloodstream and begin its action on the body (or reach its minimum effective concentration). The point at which a drug reaches its highest blood level (concentration) and maximum effect is called **peak action** or **peak effect**. Once the peak effect and concentration are reached, levels begin to fall as a result of metabolism and excretion.

The term **half-life** is generally used to indicate the time it takes for 50 percent of the plasma concentration of a drug to be eliminated from the body. For instance, if a person takes 325 mg of acetaminophen and the half-life is 3 hours,

the plasma concentration would drop to 162 mg in 3 hours, 81 mg in 6 hours, 40 mg in 9 hours, and so on. **Duration of action** refers to the length of time a drug produces a pharmacological effect. This may be hours, days or months depending on the half-life of the drug. Most drugs have a half-life of only a few hours. Therefore, dosages must be repeated regularly to maintain the concentration of the drug in the blood at a relatively constant level (the **plateau**). The object of drug therapy is to keep the plateau in a safe therapeutic range. This is accomplished by spacing repeated doses according to known influences on the absorption, distribution, metabolism and excretion, as well as the half-life of drugs. Drugs with a short half-life, such as aspirin or penicillin, are given several time a day. Those with a long half-life, for instance digoxin, are given every one or two days.

DRUG ACTION AND EFFECTS

Drugs are administered to produce desired or intended effects on the body. The desired response of drug action is called the **therapeutic effect.** Generally, drugs are administered for one of two therapeutic effects: systemic or local. A **systemic effect** refers to the action of a drug on the whole body after it is absorbed and distributed to the tissues. In a **local effect,** drug action is confined to the specific area of application. Eyedrops, eardrops or ointments are examples of preparations administered for their local effects. Drugs that are administered locally, however, can produce systemic effects if they are absorbed into the bloodstream. For example, an anticholinergic agent instilled into the eyes may cause systemic effects such as flushing of the skin, a dry mouth or a rapid pulse rate.

No drug exerts a single effect on the body. All drugs have the potential to affect more than one body system and to produce physiological responses that are unrelated to the therapeutic effect. These responses are called **adverse reactions** or **side effects.** Side effects are often predictable and occur with normal doses. Most side effects are undesirable; however, some may be desirable. For example, diphenhydramine (Benadryl), which may be used as an antihistamine to counteract allergic itching, also causes drowsiness. This sedative effect may be helpful to patients who are feeling distressed by the itchiness and cannot relax. Side effects may be harmless or they may cause mild to severe injury. Some side effects may even be lethal; for example, a severe allergic reaction can cause death.

An **allergic reaction** is a hypersensitive (antigen–antibody) reaction to a drug in a person who was previously exposed to the drug or a related chemical and has developed antibodies to it. The reactions may vary from mild to severe itching, skin rashes and urticaria (hives) to exfoliative dermatitis and fever, rhinitis or bronchospasm to life-threatening respiratory distress and cardiovascular collapse known as *anaphylactic reaction*. Although patients with a history of allergies are more likely to develop hypersensitive drug reactions, all patients must be carefully monitored for allergic responses to medications. A mild allergic reaction should be regarded as a warning that if the drug is continued, a more serious reaction will likely occur. The drug should not be administered again and the physician should be notified.

A *toxic effect* "may be thought of as a poisoning" (Shlafer, 1993, 115). **Drug toxicity** refers to the effects produced by an overdosage, an accumulation of a drug in the body or an abnormal sensitivity. Drug accumulation is a common cause of toxicity, which often results when a drug is metabolized or excreted more slowly than it is being administered. Older adults or people with hepatic and renal impairment are prone to drug accumulation. However, toxicity is not always the result of drug overdosage or accumulation. It can also occur as an abnormal reaction to a drug taken in therapeutic doses (Shlafer, 1993). Toxic effects may appear as exaggerated therapeutic or side effects. For example, a drug used for sedation may cause coma. Careful monitoring of the serum levels of drugs can avoid toxicity.

Drug tolerance describes the circumstance in which a therapeutic response to a dosage lessens after days or weeks of continued administration. A larger dose of the drug is often required to maintain the desired effect. Patients commonly develop tolerance to opiate analgesics and sedative drugs.

Effects resulting from the combined actions of two or more drugs are called **drug interactions**. The interaction of two or more drugs can modify the mechanisms of action and alter the way in which any of the drugs are absorbed, distributed, metabolized and excreted from the body, all of which ultimately influence the therapeutic effects. Two drugs that are administered simultaneously may have an additive, potentiating or antagonistic effect. An **additive effect** is the result of administering two drugs with similar actions. For example, if nitroglycerin (for angina) is taken with an alpha-adrenergic blocker such as prazosin, the blood pressure will drop significantly causing syncope or faintness. A **potentiating** or **synergistic effect** is one in which the combined effect of two drugs is greater than the intended effect of the single drug. For example, promethazine (Phenergan), an antihistamine, is often given with meperidine hydrochloride (Demerol) to enhance the analgesic effect of meperidine. In fact, when combined with promethazine, less meperidine is necessary to produce a therapeutic effect. An **antagonistic effect** occurs when two drugs in opposing categories cancel out the effects of both drugs. For instance, if an adrenergic beta stimulant such as isoproterenol (Isuprel) were given with an adrenergic beta blocker such as popranolol (Inderal), the actions of each drug would nullify the other. There would be no therapeutic effect in this case (Kee and Hayes, 1993).

DETERMINANTS OF DRUG ACTION AND EFFECTS

A number of factors determine the action and effects of any medication and the nurse must be aware of them all. These factors can alter the effects of medication to varying degrees within and among patients. One patient may respond differently to repeated doses of a medication after a period of time. Similarly, the same dose of a drug may cause different effects in different patients.

Age The age groups at opposite ends of the life cycle are the most greatly predisposed to alterations in the effectiveness of medications. Very young people and older adults are particularly affected, children because of the immaturity of the entire system and older adults because of changes associated with aging. Both of these age groups are discussed more fully later in this chapter.

Body size, weight and sex The actions, and therefore the effectiveness of a medication, are greatly influenced by body size, weight and sex. Generally, the greater the body weight, the higher the dosage required to produce a therapeutic effect. Children, for example, usually require smaller dosages of a medication, as do severely emaciated patients. Conversely, obese people may require larger doses in order to obtain an effective action from a medication.

Males and females respond differently to certain drugs because of differences in body size and weight, as well as differences in the distribution of fat and water and hormones. Typically, males have more body water than women and women have more body fat than men. Drugs that are soluble in water are more readily adsorbed in men, whereas those soluble in fat are better adsorbed in women.

Environment The physical, mental and spiritual environment has an impact on the effectiveness of a medication. Environments that are disruptive may provoke anxiety in some patients which will reduce the maximum effect of an analgesic. Similarly, a patient who is completely isolated and feels shut out and uncared for, in spite of the nurse's intentions to protect the patient, often experiences less pain relief from analgesics. Finally, environmental temperature affects the action of medications. For example, topical medications are absorbed more quickly in a warm environment because warm temperatures cause peripheral vasodilation. Conversely, topical preparations absorb more slowly in cold temperatures because the peripheral blood vessels constrict. For the most part, the patient's environment is an aspect of preference and the nurse should attempt to create an environment in which the patient can feel comfortable.

Genetic makeup   Genetic variations cause some individuals to react differently to certain medications. Frequently, these differences are hereditary and family members experience similar drug sensitivities or reactions. When taking a medication history, the nurse should ask the patient if other family members have particular sensitivities.

Disease and illness   The actions and effects of many medications depend on the proper functioning of body organs and processes within the individual, particularly gastrointestinal absorption and circulatory, hepatic and renal function. Thus, in addition to the problem being treated, the nurse must explore other health problems the patient may have, such as chronic illnesses or secondary problems.

Patients' experiences with medications
Many patients have had past experience with medications and carry beliefs about the effectiveness of these drugs. Often, the medication that the patient believes will work has a much greater effect than if the patient does not believe in the medication. On the other hand, if a patient has been using a medication, such as an analgesic, for a long period of time, the dosage may need to be altered since the degree of tolerance developed will decrease its effectiveness.

Psychological factors   Lack of trust in health care professionals and negative emotions such as anger, sadness and high anxiety will inhibit the action of medications; on the other hand, positive emotions and beliefs will enhance the effects. It is therefore crucial that the nurse develop a trusting relationship with the patient and acknowledge and assist the patient to cope with negative emotions.

Time of administration   The time that oral medications are administered can affect the action of drugs and cause unpleasant side effects. The existence of food in the stomach generally slows the absorption of medications; thus, oral medications should be given on an empty stomach. Notwithstanding, some medication must be administered with food or milk to prevent gastric irritation.

DRUG ACTION AND EFFECTS THROUGHOUT THE LIFE CYCLE

While the nurse must be prudent about administering medications to any age group, there are certain stages of the life cycle that have special needs and warrant further attention. These include pregnant women, infants, children and older adults.

PREGNANT WOMEN

As a general rule, pregnant women are advised to avoid all medications except acetaminophen, since most drugs will cross the placental barrier and affect the fetus. The fetus is most susceptible to the effects of drugs during early pregnancy (the first three months) when the brain and other organs are developing. Drugs administered during this time may cause *teratogenesis*, the creation of physical defects in the fetus during development. Some drugs (such as alcohol, nicotine to a lesser degree and opiates) may cause mental deficiencies and growth retardation in the developing fetus. If fetal growth has been retarded by medications, there is usually no major "catch up" growth after birth.

Smoking has been linked to both low-birth-weight babies and prematurity (Naeye, 1981; Shiono, Klebanoff and Rhoads, 1986). Alcohol, in any amount, affects fetal development and birth weight. Excessive alcohol taken in early pregnancy can affect the development of the fetal facial features and central nervous system (CNS) or cause a full-blown fetal alcohol syndrome. Fetal alcohol syndrome is characterized by craniofacial abnormalities, growth retardation, CNS dysfunction (hypotonia, irritability), mental retardation, hyperactivity, poor coordination and fine motor dysfunction. It is also associated with congenital defects of the cardiovascular, genitourinary and musculoskeletal systems. There is some evidence, although not conclusive, to suggest that caffeine in ordinary tea, coffee and cola, if consumed in large quantities, may harm the fetus (Aaronson and MacNee, 1989). The narcotic addiction of a pregnant woman can cause neonatal dependency and withdrawal trauma (neonatal abstinence syndrome) during the first few days or weeks of life. Drugs that are given to a woman during labour also cross the placenta and affect the newborn. Women who have been given opiate analgesics and sedatives during labour usually find that their babies are drowsy for the first two to three days after birth.

INFANTS

Infants require a smaller amount of medication than adults do. The dosage of medications for infants is usually ordered according to body weight. Infants are often more sensitive to the pharmacologic effects of drugs because of smaller body size and rapidly developing tissues. They are more prone to drug accumulation and side effects due to immature functioning of the liver and kidneys. Infants are unable to swallow tablets or pills; oral medications are given in liquid form. They may be administered by dropper, on a spoon or with a medicine dispenser that is specially designed for children.

CHILDREN

With older children, drug dosage is usually calculated in relation to height and weight, with weight being considered the more important factor. When an exact dosage for size is necessary, surface area may be used. Surface area is estimated from both height and weight measurements.

ADOLESCENTS AND YOUNG AND MIDDLE-AGED ADULTS

Allergies to drugs often begin to develop in adolescence and young and middle adulthood. The nurse should be particularly alert for allergic reactions in patients in these age groups. The problem of drug abuse, which is discussed at the end of this chapter, is also most prevalent among people of these ages.

OLDER ADULTS

Drug overdoses in older patients have become fairly common. They may result from a number of factors related to dosages, multiple prescriptions, drug interactions, the aging process and intentional overdose.

Kidney and liver function declines with age, and often older people simply cannot process and excrete the drugs as efficiently as before. Drug concentrations increase, which result in cumulative effects and the potential for toxicity (Matteson and McConnell, 1988). The nurse must be aware that a dosage may be too large for the older patient to process.

With the increase in life expectancy and the concomitant increase in the incidence of chronic illness, older adults often take many medications. Some of these medications may be taken once a day, two or three times a day or every other day; the frequency of dosages can vary tremendously. All this can be very confusing for the older person, who may have difficulty reading the label on the prescription bottle because of failing vision. The patient may not understand what medications to take or when to take them. The nurse often has to help the older adult set up a simple orderly system for ensuring that the right dosage of the right drug is taken at the right time. Dispensing a week's supply of pills into small envelopes for daily consumption or distributing them in egg cartons are two potential methods.

Drug interactions are a potential problem for older adults on multiple drug regimens. This frequently happens when a patient is being treated by more than one physician for different conditions. The patient's general practitioner may prescribe medications for a heart problem and other long-standing maladies, but the urologist who is treating a urinary tract obstruction may order other drugs. The two sets of drugs are not always compatible. The nurse should encourage the patient to keep a current list of medications readily available for different members of the health care team to consult. It is also wise to give a copy of this list to a family member in case of emergency.

Idiosyncratic reactions to drugs because of the age factor are also possible. Older people often react poorly to certain drugs. Barbiturates and tranquilizers are two groups of drugs that many older people do not tolerate well. Barbiturates often cause excitement in older patients instead of putting them to sleep, while tranquilizers may cause mental disturbances such as delusions.

Malnourishment is a factor which contributes to adverse drug reactions in older adults. Malnourished patients have less plasma protein to bind with highly protein-bound drugs. Consequently, plasma concentration of the drug is greater and there is more free drug to enter cells. Dehydration also contributes to altered drug distribution, since it leads to increased plasma concentrations of drugs. The results are more intense drug effects. Factors influencing nutrition and hydration in the older patient include finances, physical ability, disease, condition of teeth or dentures, mental status, decreased thirst drive and a decreased ability to concentrate urine.

Intentional overdose is the final factor that must be considered. Suicide rates are high among older people. Because sedatives and tranquilizers are so commonly prescribed, they are readily available, and drug overdose is a common method of committing suicide among older people. The nurse must be aware of older patients who appear depressed, lonely or despondent, as they are at a greater risk for intentional overdose.

Nurses are often in the best position to assist older adults with safe medication administration. The nurse can frequently both identify and intervene in problems that the older person is experiencing in taking medications. The nurse's responsibilities include explaining the actions of various medications, reviewing the administration schedule and helping the patient to set up a simple medication regimen that is physically manageable. The nurse is also frequently the first person to observe untoward reactions to drugs in patients. Therefore, the nurse must be alert to side effects and possible interactions with other drugs the patient is taking. Often the nurse is in the position of patient advocate, who can discuss the patient's difficulties with taking certain medications with the physician.

LEGAL ASPECTS OF MEDICATION ADMINISTRATION

Nurses are not only responsible for knowing the pharmacological aspects of drug therapy. They must also be knowledgeable of the legal implications of drug administration and abide by established laws and regulations.

DRUG LEGISLATION

All aspects of drug production, distribution, advertising and sale are governed by laws. In Canada, the drug laws include the *Food and Drugs Act* of 1953 (with yearly amendments) and the *Narcotics Control Act* of 1961 (with periodic amendments). Table 33.1 outlines the provisions of these laws. Both laws are administered under the Health Protection Branch of Health Canada. Enforcement of the *Narcotics Control Act* is delegated to the Royal Canadian Mounted Police. In the United States, the *Food, Drug and Cosmetics Act* (1938), and the *Controlled Substances Act* (1970), both with amendments, provide the governing laws.

Drug laws regulate the availability and use of drugs in a country, the purpose being to ensure that all drugs available for use are safe, effective and wisely administered. Under the law, the term "drugs" covers a diverse group of substances including nonprescription preparations that may be purchased in any retail outlet or in a pharmacy (drug store); prescription preparations that are available for medical management by a physician or dentist; and restricted preparations, obtainable only by a research institution that has received authorization from Health Canada. Many of the regulations pertaining to the availability of drugs are based on federal law, but provincial laws may further restrict the distribution of a drug. For example, ephedrine is a nonprescription drug at the federal level, but in British Columbia, ephedrine, as the single active ingredient for internal use, is ruled to be a prescription drug. Provincial laws may be more, but not less, restrictive than federal law. Drugs placed on the list of prescription drugs by federal law may not be removed by provincial regulation (*Health Protection and Drug Laws*, 1991). Table 33.2 outlines the categories of drug control and availability of drugs for public use in Canada.

DRUG STANDARDS AND CONTROL

Drugs are derived from natural sources (plants, animals or inorganic substances such as minerals) or they are produced from synthetic chemicals. For example, digitalis is extracted from a plant called the purple foxglove; some insulins are obtained from the pancreases of cattle and pigs; and biosynthetic insulin is synthesized in the laboratory. Natural sources of drugs are not uniform in their pharmacological quality or strength, and synthetic processes may not always be consistent. Therefore, drugs can vary in strength and purity and thereby produce unpredictable effects. Drug standards ensure that drugs meet requirements for purity, that dosages are uniform and that effects are predictable. Many countries have official or recognized formularies or pharmacopeiae that prescribe standards for drugs and drug use.

TABLE 33.1   Canadian Drug Legislation

LEGISLATION	PROVISIONS
Canada Food and Drugs Act (1953)	• Provides for regulation of the manufacture, distribution, advertising and sale of drugs.
	• Prohibits the sale of drugs that are contaminated, adulterated or unsafe.
	• Prohibits the sale of drugs whose labels are false, misleading or deceptive.
	• Drugs must comply with the professed standards of the manufacturer or the standards set out in recognized pharmacopeiae or formularies.
	• Prohibits the advertising and sale of food, drugs, cosmetics or devices for diseases listed in Schedule A of the Act (such as alcoholism, arteriosclerosis and cancer).
	• Classifies drugs into groups with varying degrees of control over distribution and sale.
Canadian Narcotics Control Act (1961)	• Restricts the manufacture, sale, possession and distribution of narcotics.
	• Allows authorized professionals to prescribe and dispense narcotics to those patients for whom the drug is prescribed.
	• Requires the maintenance of complete records of the disposition of the narcotic drugs.

TABLE 33.2 Categories of Drug Control and Availability

CATEGORY	DESCRIPTION	AVAILABILITY AND IDENTIFICATION
Nonprescription Drugs		
• *Proprietary medicines*	For treatment of minor self-limiting illness that does not require advice of a health professional; for example, cough drops, medicated shampoos, fluoride toothpastes.	Any retail outlet. Have letters **GP** (General Public) on labels.
• *Over-the-counter drugs*	For treatment of minor self-limiting illness but may require the advice of a health professional for proper use; for example, decongestants, laxatives, many vitamins, mild analgesics.	Any pharmacy. Have letters **DIN** (Drug Identification Number) followed by an eight-digit number.
• *Limited public access*	For use only after consultation with and upon recommendation of physician; for example, muscle relaxants, insulin, nitroglycerine, analgesic preparations containing low doses of codeine (not more than 8 mg per tablet or 20 mg per 30 ml oral solution).	Dispensed by pharmacist. Not on open shelves.
Prescription Drugs		
• *Vitamins A, D, K, and folic acid*	When recommended daily dose of vitamin A and D exceeds 10000 IU and 1000 IU respectively; when recommended daily dose for folic acid is greater than 1 mg; and all vitamin K preparations.	By prescription.
• Schedule *F Drugs*	Diversity of drug classes ordered by a physician or dentist to treat diagnosed conditions; for example, antibiotics, diuretics.	By prescription. Have the symbol **Pr** on the label.
• *Controlled Drugs (Schedule G)*	Stimulants and sedatives that have mood-modifying effects, are habit-forming and may be abused; for example, amphetamines and barbiturates.	By prescription. Have the symbol ◇**C**◇ on the label.
• *Narcotic Drugs*	Drugs that are controlled by the *Narcotics Control Act* and Regulations; for example, cocaine, opium derivatives (codeine, morphine), phencyclidine, and *cannabis* (marijuana).	By prescription. Have the letter **N** on the label.
• Restricted *Drugs (Schedule H)*	Drugs that have no recognized medicinal use but cause dangerous physiological and psychological effects; for example, LSD (lysergic acid diethylamide).	Available only to authorized institutions involved in highly specialized research.

SOURCE: Health and Welfare Canada. (1991).

In Canada, drugs are evaluated according to the manufacturer's own standards and those of *The United States Pharmacopeia* and *The British Pharmacopeia*. The manufacturer's standards for a drug must be equal to or more stringent than the standards of the recognized pharmacopeiae. Once drugs are approved they are entered into the *Compendium of Pharmaceuticals and Specialties* (CPS). The CPS is a drug reference book compiled and revised annually by the Canadian Pharmaceutical Association for the use of all health care professionals. The World Health Organization (WHO) also publishes a guide entitled *Specifications for the Quality Control of Pharmaceutical Preparations*. This is an international pharmacopoeia listing important drugs used in many countries. The World Health Organization publication has been a major step towards establishing international standards for drugs.

THE NURSE'S LEGAL RESPONSIBILITY

As members of a profession and as individuals who administer medications to patients, nurses must be accountable under the laws regulating drug administration. The Nursing Act in every province further outlines the nurse's legal responsibility for conduct. It is illegal for a nurse to practise in a manner that is beyond or does not adhere to the defined limits of the law. The nurse must know the legal specifications in his or her region, because practices can vary between provinces. For example, nurses employed in the Yukon and Northwest Territories prescribe a range of drugs according to standard protocols; in other provinces this practice would be illegal.

As professionals, nurses are responsible and accountable for all of their actions, including the administration of medications. It is important for nurses to maintain an adequate knowledge base, clarify orders when necessary and refuse to administer a prescribed medication if a potential problem is indicated. For example, a nurse may refuse to administer a dosage that is beyond the recommended safe limits or if the patient's condition is in jeopardy.

Unfortunately, even the most careful nurse may make a medication error at some point. When this happens, it is important for the nurse to confront the error in an honest and professional manner so that patient safety can be maintained and the occurrence can be documented swiftly and accurately. A medication error is reported immediately to the physician and the nurse in charge so that immediate steps can be taken to protect the patient from injury. The error is also analyzed to determine the exact cause as a safeguard against making the same mistake again. Most agencies also have unusual occurrence forms that the nurse fills out, describing the details of the error. Mistakes do happen, and it is important for the nurse to acknowledge them, learn from them and seek appropriate support. Finally, no nurse ever *plans* to make a medication error and so must forgive him- or herself once the incident is over.

BASIC FOUNDATIONS FOR ADMINISTERING MEDICATIONS

The safe administration of medications is based on knowledge and skill, and requires collaboration with other health care professionals. The physician, the pharmacy department and the agency administrators are also responsible for safe drug therapy. To this end, health care agencies have established policies and systems for ordering, processing, communicating, storing and dispensing medications. Medications are not always supplied in the exact dosages ordered. Therefore, mathematical skills are needed for the computation of individual drug dosages.

KNOWLEDGE ABOUT MEDICATIONS

It is never acceptable to administer a medication without having an adequate knowledge base. Knowledge of the drug and its effects helps to safeguard against the administration of a medication that could harm a patient. For example, if a patient has very slow respirations (for example, 10 per minute), morphine may be contraindicated, because it can depress the respirations even further. This knowledge helps the nurse to make intelligent observations that assist in the assessment of the effectiveness of both the medication and the nursing care.

In an ideal world, the nurse would be able to take the time to review the overall classification of the drug and follow through with research on information about the specific drug to be given. The information the nurse should gather includes indications for use (the diagnoses and conditions that are treated with the drug); actions, therapeutic effects and adverse reactions; food and drug interactions; dosage; contraindications (problems or conditions in the patient in which giving the drug may be harmful); and nursing implications (specific concerns related to administration of a drug).

On the other hand, the realities of the situation must also be recognized. Nurses are at times faced with the situation of administering an unfamiliar medication with little time to research it. However, the nurse can still gain a safe level of knowledge and administer the medication within minutes. While shortcuts are possible, it is never acceptable to administer a medication without knowing the following basics: classification and main action, key adverse effects, safe dosage and nursing considerations. A quick search will often only take one to two minutes and the nurse can pursue a more complete review later.

There are a number of sources of drug information available in the agency for the nurse's use. These may include the CPS, the agency pharmacy department, physicians, professional nursing and medical journals and information supplied by commercial drug firms. In many health agencies, the pharmacy department maintains an up-to-date *formulary* which lists and describes drugs currently used in the agency. Copies of the formulary are usually distributed to all nursing units, where they are readily available for reference. In addition, many head nurses like to keep a drug file on the units containing information about new drugs. The pharmacist is, of course, an excellent reference source, and the nurse should not hesitate to request information from this health professional. Physicians, too, are usually very willing to explain the nature and purpose of new drugs they have prescribed for patients.

MEDICATION ORDERS

Medications are, in most instances, ordered or prescribed by a physician. In an ambulatory care setting, the physician usually writes the prescription on a form the patient later gives to the pharmacist. The prescription should tell the pharmacist what medication(s) the patient is to have, the dosage required, the amount to be supplied, how to prepare it and the instructions the patient is to be given. In many places, the name of the drug and the unit dosage must be included on the label of the medication the patient receives.

In an inpatient facility, the prescription is usually in the form of a written order that is dated and signed by the physician, although in some health agencies, physicians are permitted to issue orders to the nursing staff by telephone. In such cases, the physician is usually required to countersign the order within a defined period of time. In an emergency situation, medications are often prescribed via verbal orders that are later written and countersigned. Generally speaking, *written* orders are considered to be the safest practice.

TYPES OF MEDICATION ORDERS

There are two types of written orders: the self-terminating order and the standing order.

Self-Terminating Orders

Self-terminating orders have a time limit on them. A *stat order* is a type of self-terminating order that is to be carried out immediately and only once; for example, meperidine hydrochloride (Demerol) 100 mg IM stat (IM means intramuscularly). The order is not repeated unless there are specific instructions to do so. Another type of self-terminating

order is an order in which the time limit is actually specified; for example, the physician orders acetaminophen (Tylenol) 0.65 g for six doses, or digitalis 0.1 g June 12th and 14th. Sometimes a self-terminating order is dependent upon the condition of the patient, such as when an order is written, acetylsalicylic acid 0.65 g q.4h. until temperature remains below 37.8°C for 24 hours. Some agencies have policies that place a time limit on orders regardless of how they are worded. For example, a narcotic order often remains in effect for 72 hours, after which time it is automatically discontinued unless the physician writes another order.

Standing Orders

Orders that are carried out indefinitely are called *standing orders* (for example, vitamin C 25 mg p.o. b.i.d.). Some standing orders contain the direction "prn" which means the medication is to be given "as necessary." The administration of a drug under a **prn order** is left to the nurse's judgement and the patient's need. These orders, however, often specify minimum time intervals between doses, for example, lorazepam, 1–2 mg q.h.s. prn.

COMPONENTS OF A MEDICATION ORDER

There are a number of essential components to a medication order. An order should *always* include the patient's name, the date of the order, the name of the drug, the dosage, the route of administration, the time and frequency of administration and the prescriber's signature.

Patient's name   The patient's full name should appear on the drug order form to avoid confusion among patients of the same surname. Most agencies require an imprint of the patient's name and identification number on the physician's order form.

Date of the order   The date of the order must include the day, month and year. Many agencies also require that the prescriber specify the time the order is written. Specifying the time is essential for orders that are automatically terminated because it indicates precisely when the order should end.

Name of the drug   The name of the drug should be clearly written and correctly spelled. Many agencies require the use of generic names in the drug order; however, a large number of agencies still use common trade names.

Dosage   The order must specify the exact strength and amount of drug to be administered. Sometimes a range of amount may also be given. For example: "acetaminophen 325 mg (**strength**) 1 or 2 tabs (**range of amount**)."

Route of administration   A medication may be administered by a number of different routes. Thus, it is necessary to specify the route in the drug order. The route of administration is often indicated through the use of common abbreviations, such as p.o. (oral route) or IV (intravenous route).

Time and frequency of administration   The time and frequency of giving medications must be indicated. Again, common abbreviations may be used, for example, "ferrous gluconate 300 mg b.i.d." Many inpatient facilities have standard times for administering medications. For example, b.i.d. or twice a day medications may have standard times of 1000 hours and 2200 hours. If the physician wishes a medication to be given at a time other than the standard time, this should also be specified. Thus, the order "ferrous gluconate 300 mg b.i.d. with meals" would be written.

Signature   The signature of the prescriber is a legal requirement on all medication orders. An order that is not signed is not valid in a court of law. When a medication order is obtained over the telephone, the nurse must indicate that it is a telephone order, identify from whom the order was taken and sign the order. In most agencies, the physician who gave the telephone order will then countersign the order at a later date.

If any one of the components is omitted in a medication order, it is appropriate for the nurse to contact the physician and seek clarification. The nurse has an obligation to question any order that is ambiguous or seems to be unsafe for a patient. It is not acceptable to administer a medication merely because it was ordered by the doctor. It never hurts to clarify orders and if the dosage exceeds the limits defined by the medication manuals, it is unwise to administer it. In health agencies, it is a customary practice for all of a patient's orders to be written on a doctor's order sheet, which may be kept in the patient's chart or in a central book. Hospitals use a variety of methods of flagging charts to indicate that a patient has new orders.

PROCESSING AND COMMUNICATING MEDICATION ORDERS

Once an order has been written, it is then *processed*. A nurse or a unit clerk may process the order. When an order is processed, it is transcribed onto appropriate forms and the pharmacy department is notified. In some agencies, the order is copied onto the medication record in the patient's chart and the nursing unit Kardex or nursing care plan. In addition, a medication card is filled out. In other agencies, the new order is entered on the patient's medication administration record, called the MAR.

Medication cards are still used in some agencies, although the use of this system is not as widespread as it was in the past. With this system, each medication is recorded on a separate card which includes the patient's name, the medication, dosage, route and times to be administered (see Figure 33.1-A). Often these cards are filed on a central shelving system that is divided into each hour of the day. The nurse then searches through all the medication cards at the specific time, pulls the cards and prepares those medications. Once the medication has been administered, the card is advanced to the next time slot when the medication is to be given. The nurse must be especially careful when using the card system because cards may get lost or put into the wrong time slot or they may go home in the nurse's pocket.

The MAR set-up is a computerized system that is being used with increasing frequency in hospitals. Once a day, the pharmacy department prints out the medications that have been ordered for a patient and sends the computer printouts to the nursing units (see Figure 33.1-B). These printouts are often stored in binders so the nurse has easy access to them. When new orders are written or when medications are terminated, notations are made on the existing MAR. The changes are then displayed on the next day's computer printouts. The MAR printout often groups medications according to solutions, oral medications and prn and/or stat dosages of medications. The time of administration is printed beneath each regular medication, to cue the nurse. The nurse simply looks through the patients' MARs and notes the times that the medications are to be prepared and administered. The MAR system has several advantages over the card system. It offers a more complete picture of the medications that each patient is taking and it avoids the problem of losing medication cards.

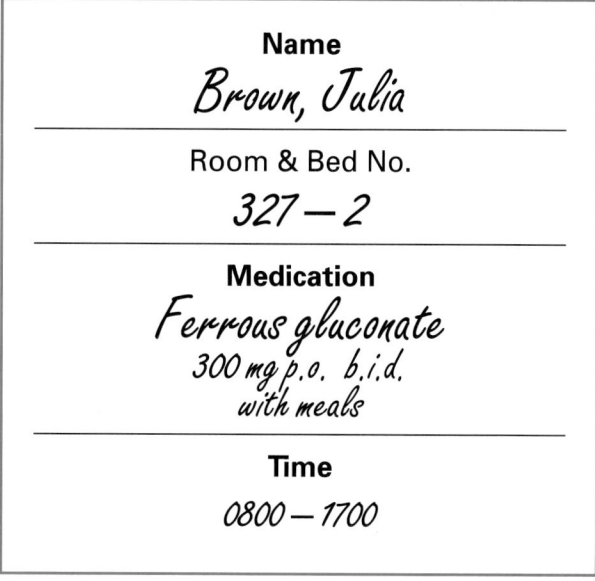

Name

Brown, Julia

Room & Bed No.

327 – 2

Medication

Ferrous gluconate 300 mg p.o. b.i.d. with meals

Time

0800 – 1700

FIGURE 33.1 A   Medication card

```
M E D I C A T I O N   A D M I N I S T R A T I O N   R E C O R D

24 HOURS FROM 0100 09DEC94 THRU 2400 09DEC94          PAGE 1
```

NAME:	SMITH JOHN	UNIT: 6 WEST	BED NO. 627-2
BIRTHDATE:	12JAN49	PATIENT ID: 92-1234567	
SEX:	MALE	DR.: WELLS	
DIAGNOSIS:	ASTHMA, CONGESTIVE HEART FAILURE	ADMITTED: 0800 08DEC94	
ALLERGIES:	PENICILLIN, CODEINE		

COMMENTS:_____

```
01 02 03 04 05 06 07 08 09 10 11 12 13 14 15 16 17 18 19 20 21 22 23 24
```

—— M E D I C A T I O N ——

ORDER #   1   DIGOXIN TAB 0.25MG

0.25MG (1 TAB) PO DAILY

10

ORDER #   2   HYDROCORTISONE CRM 1%

APPLY TID TO AFFECTED AREA

10   14   22

ORDER #   4   AMINOPHYLLINE VIAL 500MG/10ML

500MG (10ML)/500ML D5W. INFUSE AT

50MG (50ML)/HOUR

```
01 02 03 04 05 06 07 08 09 10 11 12 13 14 15 16 17 18 19 20 21 22 23 24
```

P R N   M E D I C A T I O N S

ORDER #   1   ACETAMINOPHEN TAB 325MG   PO

325-650MG (1-2 TABS)   PO Q3-4H PRN

FIGURE 33.1 B   Medication Administration Record (MAR)

Although different methods of posting medication orders are used in various agencies, the nurse should remember that the original written order is the primary source of information. Whenever orders are copied, whether onto a Kardex file, a nursing care plan, a medicine card or an MAR, the possibility of error is always present. The nurse who administers the medication should always check the original order to make certain that communication has been accurate.

Agencies have different methods of indicating that a medication has been discontinued. In hospitals, it is common practice for "discontinued" to be imprinted across the physician's order once it is no longer valid. In agencies that use the MAR system, the discontinued medication is often highlighted in yellow. If the card system is used, the medication card is destroyed and an appropriate notation is made on the medication record. In a public health agency, the notation "discontinued" and the date are entered on the nursing care record.

MEDICATION DISTRIBUTION AND STORAGE

Every agency has a system for the distribution and storage of medications. Some medications are considered stock, while others are specifically obtained for the individual patient (private drugs). Additionally, some agencies use a unit dose system. Each of these systems is designed to minimize error and maximize efficiency.

Stock Drugs

Stock drugs are the more commonly used medicines and a supply is kept on the unit at all times. Stock drugs are sometimes grouped according to action; for example, all vitamin preparations are kept together. Another method of grouping stock drugs is to arrange them alphabetically according to generic or trade names. Either method facilitates finding a specific preparation quickly.

Private Drugs

Private or personal drugs are specially prepared for a patient, and a small supply is obtained from the pharmacy department with the patient's name on it. The drug is then stored in either a common drawer with all the other personal drugs, or in the individual's medication drawer if the medication cart system is used.

Unit Dose System

The unit dose system is the safest method of distributing medications. In this system, each dose of the patient's prescribed medication is individually packaged. The nurse simply double checks the order and takes the entire packet supplied by pharmacy. Normally, the pharmacy department sends enough doses for a 24-hour period. This method is advantageous to the nurse because it saves nursing time and decreases the opportunity for error.

STORAGE OF CONTROLLED DRUGS

Narcotics, barbiturates and other controlled drugs are under strict governmental control. In hospitals, narcotics and other controlled drugs are kept in locked containers and distribution is closely managed. The administration of these drugs is recorded not only on the patient's chart but also in a special book commonly referred to as the narcotics book. The information recorded in the narcotics book includes the name of the patient to whom the narcotic will be administered, the name of the physician who ordered the drug, the drug, dosage, date and time and the signature of the nurse administering the drug. Any narcotics that are wasted are also recorded along with the quantity of drug wasted. In addition, wastages must be co-signed by another nurse, who validates the wastage.

The narcotics book is usually kept in close proximity to the narcotics cupboard. Narcotics, barbiturates and other controlled drugs are counted at specific times and totals are recorded in the narcotics book. For example, narcotics and controlled substances are often counted at the end of each shift, and the number distributed plus the number remaining on hand must equal the number assigned to the nursing unit or agency. The count is usually done by two nurses, a nurse going off duty and a nurse coming on duty. This practice helps to protect the nurses on both shifts. Any discrepancies in the count must be reported immediately and the appropriate paperwork filed.

CALCULATIONS OF DRUG DOSAGES

In order to prepare and administer medications safely, the nurse must be adept at converting measurements from one system to another and calculating dosages.

Systems of Measurement

There are three systems of measurement used to prescribe drugs: the apothecary, the household and the metric systems.

Apothecary system The apothecary system is based on the "troy pound" with 5760 grains as a standard pound. The pound is divided into 12 ounces, ounces divided into 8 drachms (also spelled drams), drachms into 3 scruples, and scruples into 20 grains. Fluid measures use the quart of 32 oz, which is subdivided into 2 pints, pints to 16 ounces, fluid ounces to 8 fluid drams, and fluid drams into 60 minims. Roman numerals are used to express numbers (grains X) and quantities less than one are written as fractions. This system is seldom used anymore, as it is inconvenient and not as accurate as the metric system.

Household measurements The household system is widely used in the home environment. Most people are likely to be familiar with the basis of the household system, as it is frequently used in cookbooks. The teaspoon, tablespoon, teacup and glass are commonly used household measures. As this system is the least accurate of the three, it is rarely used in professional health care settings.

Metric system The metric system is the most accurate and convenient system of measurement. It is based on multiples of 10 with the basic units being the metre (linear), the litre (volume) and the gram (weight). The

TABLE 33.3 Conversion of Metric Calculations

LINEAR		VOLUME		GRAM	
10 millimetres	= 1 centimetre	1000 millilitres	= 1 litre	1000 micrograms	= 1 milligram
100 centimetres	= 1 metre			1000 milligrams	= 1 gram
1000 metres	= 1 kilometre			1000 grams	= 1 kilogram

nurse should become familiar with the metric units outlined in Table 33.3.

Computing Drug Dosages

It is not uncommon for the nurse to have to calculate drug dosages. While calculations may be done in the pharmacy department, it is not always possible nor do all nurses work directly with a pharmacy. Further, it is prudent for the nurse to double check all calculations. Given all of this, the nurse must be familiar with formulas for computing drug dosages. Several methods can be used, but the dosages to be calculated must always be in the same unit of measurement. One common method uses a formula based on simple algebra:

$$\frac{\text{Dose available}}{\text{Quantity available}} = \frac{\text{Dose desired}}{X \text{ (Quantity desired)}}$$

Example 1

Order: Morphine sulphate 100 mg p.o. q.4h. is ordered for a patient with cancer pain. The morphine is supplied as a solution 5mg/1ml.

1. Set up proportions: $\dfrac{5 \text{ mg}}{1 \text{ ml}} = \dfrac{100 \text{ mg}}{X \text{ ml}}$

2. Cross multiply: $5X = 100$

3. Compute X: $100 \div 5 = 20$ ml to be administered

Example 2

Order: Digoxin 0.125 mg p.o. once a day. Supplied: Digoxin 0.25 mg pills.

1. Set up proportions: $\dfrac{0.25 \text{ mg}}{1 \text{ tablet}} = \dfrac{0.125 \text{ mg}}{X \text{ tablet}}$

2. Cross multiply: $0.25X = 0.125$

3. Compute X: $0.125 \div 0.25 = 1/2$ tablet to be administered

Calculating Pediatric Dosages

The administration of medications to infants and children requires extra caution. Due to the smaller size of children, the administration of adult doses could be lethal. Special methods have been developed to convert adult dosages to safe dosages for children. The method most often used is based on Body Surface Area (BSA) and uses a nomogram to estimate the BSA according to the child's height and weight. As shown in Figure 33.2, a child's BSA is obtained by drawing a straight line on the nomogram from the child's height on the left side to his or her weight on the right side. The point on the surface area (S.A.) column indicates the body surface area (m²). The BSA is then used in a formula for calculating the safe dosage for the child. This formula is a ratio of the child's BSA to the body surface area of an average adult (which is 1.7) times the normal adult dose. Thus:

$$\text{Child's dose} = \frac{\text{surface area of child (m}^2)}{1.7} \times \text{adult dose}$$

ASSESSING MEDICATION-RELATED NEEDS

Nothing in the human body happens in a completely isolated fashion; the nurse must consider the entire person when assessing medication-related needs of patients. This involves an appraisal of factors in the patient's health history pertaining to the use of medications that would contribute to health or place the patient at risk for complications. The nurse should be aware of disease or illness states, such as chronic conditions or secondary problems, that may impact on the effectiveness of medications or cause adverse effects. Physical and psychological assessments may indicate actual and potential problems that may influence if, when or how a drug is given and provide a baseline for evaluating the patient's response to medication. In addition, an understanding of the patient's medical plan of care and the desired therapeutic effect of the prescribed medications is essential. The nurse cannot evaluate the effectiveness of medications unless the indications or reasons for their use are known. Personal concerns, cultural values and religious beliefs that may cause the patient difficulty in accepting drug therapy or maintaining a medication regimen must also be examined.

FIGURE 33.2 Nomogram of body surface area for infants and children. To find the BSA, draw a straight line from the child's height (on the left column) to the child's weight (on the right column). The point at which the line intersects the S.A. column is the estimated BSA.

SOURCE: Modified by West, C.D. from data of Boyd, E. In Behrman, R.E. and Nelson, V.C. (1987). *Nelson textbook of pediatrics.* Philadelphia: Saunders. Reproduced with permission.

Throughout all aspects of assessment, the nurse must be aware of the special needs of patients throughout the life cycle and those with specific health challenges.

The patient's medical history should provide the nurse with information about physical and emotional conditions that may affect the overall response to a new drug or contraindicate its administration. For example, patients with congestive heart failure may be at risk for altered drug responses owing to the generalized slowing of drug distribution throughout the body. Similarly, the potential for cumulative effects is common in patients with renal and hepatic diseases because of impaired biotransformation and excretory functions. The medical history may also provide information about a patient's physical capabilities to self-administer medications at home, for example, physical deficits such as poor eyesight, impaired mobility or inability to remember dosages and times for medications.

NURSING HEALTH HISTORY

The patient's medication history is one facet of the nursing health history. In the medication history, the nurse focusses on the patient's patterns of drug use, both current and in the recent past, responses to the medications and any related problems. Health promotion and protection patterns pertaining to medication use are also explored. This includes the patient's understanding about the drug action, purpose, administration and adverse effects, as well as any associated expectations and concerns. The patient's ability to self-administer and adhere to a medication regimen must also be determined. This information is necessary in order to identify actual and potential problems with the use of drugs and find opportunities for assisting and teaching people how to use, or not to use, medications that will promote optimum health for themselves or their family members.

In the event the patient is admitted in an unconscious state, the nurse should attempt to contact a member of the family or close friend for a medication history. Many drugs interact with one another; therefore, it is necessary to know about all types of drugs the patient uses including prescription and nonprescription drugs, recreational drugs (for example, marijuana, tobacco) and alcoholic beverages. It is important to note that patients may not openly admit to using illegal drugs or alcohol. Nevertheless, the nurse should attempt to explore the patient's use of these substances. This information might also be found in the physician's history. Knowledge of medications used in the past few months is important because such medications can have an effect on newly prescribed preparations. It is wise to encourage patients to carry with them a current list of medications they take. The patient's food and eating pattern is reviewed because the adsorption of drugs can vary with the kinds of foods ingested. In addition, some foods are incompatible with certain drugs, for example, foods high in active amines (aged cheese, beer, yeast or chocolate, for example) can provoke a dangerously high blood pressure if consumed by a person taking monoamine oxidase (MAO) inhibitors, such as procarbazine (Matulane). The patient's age, weight and any allergies are also noted.

MEASUREMENTS AND DIAGNOSTIC TESTS

Vital signs and laboratory tests necessary for assessing medications and for monitoring the effectiveness. For example, blood pressure readings are

Medication
Health and Illness Patterns

CURRENT MEDICATION PATTERN

- What medications are you presently taking that have been prescribed by your doctor? What are the medications for? What dosage are you taking? How frequently? By what route are you taking them?
- Describe the response to these medications. What are the therapeutic effects? adverse effects? Do you have problems taking these medications?
- What nonprescription medications do you use, for example, vitamins, laxatives, sleep aides, aspirin or acetaminophen, decongestants or antihistamines? What for? How often do you take them? How much do you take? By what route do you take them? What is your response to these medications?
- Do you smoke or use recreational or street drugs? If so, what kind? How often do you take them? How much do you take? By what route do you take them? What is the response when habitual use of these substances is interrupted?

PAST MEDICATION PATTERNS

- What medications have you taken during the past few months? What for? How frequently? What dosage? What route?
- Describe your response to these medications. What are the therapeutic effects? adverse effects? allergic reactions? What problems occurred taking these medications?
- Do you have medications saved from past use? How are they stored? What is the expiration date?

Health Promotion and Protection Patterns

- What do you know about the medications you are currently taking? How much do you want to know?

- Do you want to know the reasons for the medications? the expected therapeutic effects? side effects? what to do if side effects occur? when medications should be taken? any special precautions? whether there is a need for follow-up?
- What do you expect from the current drug therapy as prescribed by the doctor? as self-prescribed? For example, a patient may be taking self-prescribed garlic pills in conjunction with a prescribed antihypertensive drug to control blood pressure problems.
- What are your personal views about the use of medications?
- Do you have any concerns about taking the medications? any fear of medications? fear of side effects? any religious or cultural influences?
- What things help or prevent you from taking your medications as prescribed?
- How do you usually take oral medications at home? With water? milk? juice? food?
- Do you usually take your medications with meals? before meals? at bedtime?
- If taking multiple medications, how do you keep track of the medications you take?
- Do you have any problems self-administering medications? reading and understanding labels? knowing or remembering when to take the medication? with using special techniques, for example, eyedrops, injecting insulin? If so, do you have a relative or a friend who can help you take your medications as prescribed?
- Where do you store your medications? Are they kept out of reach of small children?
- Do you have any concerns about the cost of the medications? Would you require help with financing the medication?

taken to assess the therapeutic effectiveness of antihypertensive medications. Serum potassium levels are monitored for the development of hyperkalemia, a potentially dangerous side effect when patients are given a daily potassium supplement in conjunction with a potassium-sparing diuretic such as triamterene (Dyrenith). Dosages of some medications are based on serum levels of certain substances. For instance, insulin dosage is ordered according to blood glucose

and prothrombin times determine dosage adjustments for the anticoagulant, Coumadin. The plasma levels of drugs that have a very narrow therapeutic index (margin of safety), such as digoxin or anticonvulsants, must be monitored frequently because they pose a high risk for the development of toxic effects. In collecting data for determining medication-related problems and needs, the nurse must examine vital signs and review laboratory results as required.

PHYSICAL ASSESSMENT

During physical assessment, the nurse examines the patient for indications of therapeutic and adverse effects of the specific medications the patient is on. For instance, if a patient is prescribed a heart pill and a diuretic for congestive heart failure, the physical examination would focus on such things as colour, shortness of breath, ease of breathing, coughing, activity tolerance and edema to determine therapeutic effectiveness. When the prescribed diuretic is a potassium-wasting agent, the physical assessment would include observations for signs of hypokalemia and digitalis toxicity, since the most common cause of digitalis toxicity is hypokalemia secondary to associated use of potassium-wasting diuretics.

The physical assessment also includes an appraisal of the patient's ability to take medications and any indicators that may contraindicate the administration of a particular medication. For example, nausea and vomiting may contraindicate the use of an oral medication. The nurse observes the patient for wakefulness, alertness, ability to swallow and ability to participate in the administration procedure. For example, can the patient assume the necessary position for administering eardrops? If the patient is going home while still on the medication, the nurse must also observe the patient's self-administering capabilities. This includes the patient's visual acuity, mobility, mental processes and manual dexterity. For instance, someone with arthritis may have difficulty opening and closing containers or self-administering insulin.

DIAGNOSING MEDICATION-RELATED PROBLEMS

Problems pertaining to safe medication administration may relate to the drug therapy itself or to the distinctive circumstances of patients taking the drugs. Potential problems caused by the side effects of drugs that may be prevented independently by the nurse are labelled *High risk for injury*. For instance, if the side effect of a drug is dizziness and orthostatic hypotension, the nursing diagnosis would be *High risk for injury related to dizziness and fainting secondary to medication*. However, adverse effects of drugs may cause potentially serious reactions that require medical intervention for treatment or prevention. These are collaborative problems and, in drug therapy, they are identified as *Potential complications: medication therapy adverse effects*. For example, for a patient taking anticancer drugs, the diagnosis would be *PC: antineoplastic adverse effects* (Carpenito, 1993).

A wide range of problems may apply to the distinctive circumstances of patients on medication therapy. When a new drug is prescribed to a patient there is always the need to learn about the drug's actions, its therapeutic and side-

effects and self-administration. Lack of knowledge about the use of nonprescription and recreational drugs may lead to unhealthy lifestyles and problems with health maintenance. In addition, personal concerns, cultural values and religious beliefs may cause difficulties for patients in accepting drug therapy or maintaining a medication regimen. Sensory/perceptual impairments, such as poor vision, inability to read, forgetfulness or drowsiness, may interfere with the ability to self-administer and maintain a medication schedule. Likewise, physical problems such as difficulty swallowing or difficulty handling medication supplies and equipment may affect the ability to take medications. Examples of nursing diagnoses are listed below.

- *Knowledge deficit about drug action, therapeutic and adverse effects, and administration.*
- *Altered health maintenance related to unhealthy lifestyle and lack of knowledge about over-the-counter drugs and substance abuse.*
- *Altered health maintenance related to personal concerns, cultural values and religious beliefs about the prescribed medication.*
- *Ineffective management of therapeutic regimen related to sensory/perceptual or physical impairments affecting correct self-administration of medication.*
- *High risk for injury related to lack of knowledge or sensory/perceptual or physical impairments affecting correct self-administration of medication.*

PLANNING MEDICATION ADMINISTRATION

As with all needs, a plan for the safe administration of medications is based on goals or expected outcomes which are derived from the nursing diagnoses. Planning must be done jointly with the patient and/or family and must consider individual beliefs and values, lifestyle practices, preferences and socioeconomic factors. Emphasis is placed on strategies to enable the optimal use of medications for therapeutic interventions and health maintenance. This includes health teaching about drug actions, effects and safe use, as well as safe self-administration. The patient may need help developing a dosage schedule and arranging for follow-up evaluation and care.

Some examples of goals or expected outcomes pertaining to safe medication administration are listed below.

- Patient will explain the reasons for and expected effects of the medication, describe the route and method of administration, state the times for self-administration and describe interventions for common side effects.
- Patient will correctly and independently administer the prescribed dose of insulin.prepare written medication schedule.

IMPLEMENTING MEDICATION ADMINISTRATION

HEALTH PROMOTING STRATEGIES

We are in an age of empowerment, where people want to actively participate in health care and have some control over the situation. In medication therapy, this means having the right to make an informed consent, having the right to refuse medication and taking responsibility for self-administration. Patient education, teaching and supportive care are key nursing strategies for helping patients to promote optimal health through the use of medications.

INFORMED CONSENT

Patients have the right and want to make informed decisions about care and the prescribed medications. Informed consent requires adequate knowledge on which to make a decision. The patient needs to know the reasons for drug therapy, the effects and the resulting alterations in habits and lifestyle. Simple explanations given in terms the patient can understand are not only reassuring but also help to provide conditions of acceptance that can enhance the effectiveness of the drug. In the rare occurrence when a physician does not want the patient to receive information about a medicine from the nurse, it can be suggested that the patient confer with the physician.

RIGHT TO REFUSE MEDICATION

Sometimes a patient may refuse to take a medication. With rare exceptions, it is *not* the nurse's duty to administer the medication no matter what. The patient has the right to refuse treatment. It is the nurse's responsibility to determine, if possible, why the patient is refusing the medication and to take reasonable action to gain the patient's consent. There are a myriad of reasons why patients refuse medications and it is imperative that the nurse explore these. Often, the problem can be remedied and the medication administered. Some of the common reasons for refusal along with suggested interventions are outlined in Table 33.4. If the patient refuses to take a medication, the nurse must inform the physician and document the event immediately.

PATIENT EDUCATION AND TEACHING

All people taking medication should be aware of the nature of the drugs they are taking, the reasons

for the drug, the dosage, possible side effects, the route and method of administration and any specific things that should or should not be done when taking the medication. They should also be alerted to adverse signs and symptoms to watch for and the dangers of altering the dosage or neglecting to take medications. Unfortunately, some people mistakenly believe, "If one tablet is good for me, two tablets are twice as good." Some people also need help to understand why they should take a prescribed dose and require realistic explanations of the action and anticipated effects of the drug. Not only is this a need for hospitalized patients, it is also crucial for people who take medicines in the home. People experience various reactions to specific drugs. The patient's reaction to any single drug is important and should be recorded. Thus, patients require information about what reactions to report to the nurse or the physician. This is particularly true for the person who is taking medicine at home and does not have constant contact with health personnel.

A checklist for patient teaching in drug therapy is given in the box below. Many agencies provide written information about medications for patient use; some agencies print this information in a variety of languages so that non-

---

Checklist of Teaching in Drug Therapy

- Comprehensive health and medication history
- Reason for medication therapy
- Expected results
- Side effects and other adverse reactions
- When to notify physician, pharmacist, or health care provider
- Drug–drug and drug–food interactions
- Required changes in activities of daily living (ADL)
- Demonstration of learning; may take several forms, such as listening, discussing or return demonstration of psychomotor skills (for example, insulin injection)
- Medication schedule, associated with ADL as appropriate
- Recording system
- Discussion and monitoring of access to financial resources, medication and associated equipment
- Community resources

SOURCE: Kee, J.L. and Hayes, E.R. (1993). *Pharmacology: A nursing process approach.* Philadelphia: Saunders, 22. Adapted with permission.

TABLE 33.4   Refusal to Take Medications

REASON FOR REFUSAL	NURSING INTERVENTION
• Finds the medication to be nauseating and causes vomiting.	• Administer antiemetic as ordered 30–60 minutes prior or administer with food.
• Is allergic to the medication. A record of the patient's allergies should be noted on admission; however this is not always possible. For example, the patient may have been unconscious upon admission.	• Notify the pharmacy department and initiate appropriate references on the patient's chart, Kardex and wristband and at the bedside.
• Believes the medication does not help.	• Explain medication effects to the patient in terms that he or she can understand.
• Thinks it is the wrong medication.	• When this occurs, always double check the order and the medication. If it is the correct medication, spend time discussing the issue with the patient. It may be a different brand than the patient is used to taking and will appear different.
• Believes the physician has changed the order.	• Check the physician's orders. The doctor may have changed the order and it may not be processed yet or the physician may have intended to change the order, but has not written it yet.
• Finds injections painful.	• Use techniques to minimize the pain of injections. Give the patient as much choice as possible.
• Finds the medication has an unpleasant taste.	• Administer the medication with a pleasant tasting juice or food. Give with a cold fluid. This helps to decrease the sensitivity of the taste buds.
• Does not want medication because of religious or cultural beliefs. A Hindu patient may refuse a hormonal preparation that contains extracts from cattle. A patient who belongs to the Jehovah's Witness sect may refuse a blood transfusion. Many people who believe in naturopathic remedies will refuse any medicine prepared from inorganic chemicals.	• Respect the patient's beliefs and collaborate with the physician and the patient to determine alternatives.
• Does not understand the purpose of the medication and is afraid it will be harmful.	• Provide information and pamphlets in terms the patient can understand.
• Thinks the medication is given at an inconvenient time, such as when visitors are present.	• If possible, collaborate with the patient to find a more convenient time. If this is not possible, minimize time spent in the room.
• Is afraid of becoming addicted to the medication.	• Explain that addiction is a remote possibility when medications are used for short periods of time.

English-speaking people can benefit as well. If a patient is unable to self-administer medications, a family member or friend should be given the necessary instruction. Patient teaching is an ongoing process. It is wise to review medications periodically, even if the patient has been taking the same drugs for some time. The nurse will often be surprised at the gaps in knowledge. In addition to teaching about specific medications, there are a number of general things people can do to facilitate the effectiveness of medication use and promote optimum health.

HEALTH PROTECTING STRATEGIES

Safe administration of medications is imperative, as mistakes can lead to dangerous effects. Because the possibility of error is always present, special precautions are taken to avoid mistakes. Nursing has adopted the practice of checking medications using the "five rights" when preparing and administering medications as a means of avoiding error. The five rights include the right drug, the right dose, the right time, the right route and the right patient. If the nurse

HEALTH PROMOTING STRATEGY

Promoting Healthy Medication Use

- Take all of the medication as prescribed by your physician. Do not stop taking the medication just because you feel better.
- Consult your physician if you are experiencing undesirable side effects.
- Keep the medication in its original container. Make sure the label remains clear.
- Keep all medications in a cupboard *well out of reach of children*. Remind visitors to keep any medications they bring with them safely out of children's reach.
- When taking prescribed medications, check with your physician or the pharmacist about using over-the-counter drugs such as cold remedies, deconges-

tants, aspirin, acetaminophen, antihistamines, or laxatives.
- Take all medications with you when you visit your physician.
- Know why you are taking each medication and the reactions you should immediately report to your physician or health care provider.
- Avoid using alcoholic beverages because these alter the action of medications. Abstain from alcohol when it is absolutely contraindicated.
- Nicotine affects the actions of some drugs. If you are a smoker, check with your physician or the pharmacist for specific information.

SOURCE: Kee and Hayes, 1993, 21.

consistently practises the five rights for each medication, the potential for error is reduced dramatically.

RIGHT DRUG

The nurse uses the MAR or medication card to chose the appropriate medication. When using the MAR, if a number of medication orders are present on the same page, it is wise to cover up the other orders while pouring a particular medication. This practice will help to prevent errors. To ensure the right drug is obtained, the nurse uses a three-check system when pouring the medication. The first check occurs when the nurse obtains the medication from the drawer or cupboard. He or she then compares the MAR or medication card with the label on the medication container, making sure the drug name is the same on both. The second check is done when the nurse plans to pour the medication into the cup or container. The third check is made when the nurse replaces the remaining medication in the drawer or cupboard. If the unit dose is used, the package will be empty, but the nurse will compare the information on the package.

RIGHT DOSE

The dose of a drug is ordered by the physician in consideration of the weight, age, sex, physical condition and level of drug tolerance. Therefore a medicine must be administered in the exact dose that is ordered by the physician. When calculating the right dose, the nurse will check the

MAR or medication card and compare the information to the supplied medication. It is important to calculate the dosage considering what the pharmacy supplies and what is ordered, since there may be a difference. Again, it is prudent to use the three-check system described above. Frequently, the pharmacy department calculates the ordered dose, particularly when small doses are required (for example, for children) and includes the information on the MAR or personal medication package. It is still important for the nurse to calculate the dosage as well since errors can occur anywhere, and the nurse administering the medication is ultimately responsible. In situations requiring dose calculation, the safest practice is for a second nurse to check the calculations made by the first nurse.

The nurse should *never* "guestimate" a dosage. It is not safe practice to break an unscored tablet to obtain a dosage, since the amount of drug in an unscored tablet is not evenly distributed. When pouring liquid medications, the receptacle should be placed on a flat surface and kept at eye level in order to obtain an accurate dosage.

RIGHT TIME

Many agencies have standard times for administering medications and the nurse should become familiar with these. Many oral medications that are ordered for more than once per day are given during waking hours, while intravenous medications are given around the clock. Thus, if an intravenous antibiotic is ordered three times per day, the nurse would administer it at regular eight-hour intervals such as

0600, 1400, 2200. Also, if patients have been taking medications at home, their usual schedule should be considered. Wherever possible, medication times should be similar to the patient's usual schedule.

Finally, the realities of nursing are such that it is rarely possible to give every medication at the exact moment of the exact hour that it is ordered. Thus, the rule of 30 minutes is used. This gives the nurse 30 minutes on either side of the time the medication is due in which to administer it. Having said that, the nurse must consider the medications to be administered and consider certain medications as higher priorities than others. Insulin, for example, must be administered before meals and not 30 minutes after the meal has been consumed.

RIGHT ROUTE

It is important to verify that the medication supplied coincides with the prescribed route. The nurse can only administer the medication by the ordered route; the route cannot be arbitrarily changed. If the nurse believes the ordered route is not appropriate, he or she must contact the physician. Sometimes, the physician will provide some variance with the route order. For example, the physician may order dimenhydrinate 25–50 mg p.o., IM, or IV q.6h. and the route can be decided by the nurse and patient together.

RIGHT PATIENT

One of the most important factors in the administration of a medication is the identification of the patient. Any method that accurately identifies a patient is satisfactory. Some agencies provide each patient with an identification band. Many protocols suggest asking the patient his or her name before administering a medication. If this is the case, the nurse should not say, "Are you Mr. Smith?" nor should the nurse rely on the patient to answer to the name he or she uses. In both situations, the patient may give an automatic affirmative answer. It is better to say, "What is your name?" or "Please state your full name." The habit of relying on bed numbers and even room numbers in order to identify patients is also dangerous. Patients' rooms often change and patients also move to other units. Situations in which patients are continually reassigned to new rooms make identification especially difficult. Further, it is not entirely unheard of for patients to lie down in the wrong bed. Therefore, it is prudent to check the patient's identification band prior to the administration of *every* group of medications.

The beginning nurse often feels foolish pursuing this suggestion, since this person often only administers medications to one or two patients. The nurse who administers a number of medications to a multitude of patients knows only too well that lack of time, not knowing what

The safest method of ensuring the "right patient" is to check the patient's identification band.

each patient looks like and being constantly distracted carries with it a huge potential for error. The measure of checking wristbands is the final stopgap to prevent the wrong medication from being given to the wrong patient. Good habits formed early in a career save errors later.

OTHER STRATEGIES FOR PREVENTING MEDICATION ERRORS

If a nurse is ever in doubt about whether or not to give a medication, he or she should consult a reliable source before going ahead. As mentioned earlier, most agencies have literature to which the nurse can refer. If the agency possesses no resources and the nurse is routinely unable to contact a pharmacist or physician, it is imperative that the nurse carry a current drug book.

The pharmacist should be the only one to label a container of drugs. Therefore, when the nurse finds an unlabelled container or a label that has been partially obscured, the entire container is returned to the pharmacy for clarification. It is also considered safe practice not to return medications to a container once they have been removed; instead, they should be disposed of by flushing down a toilet or hopper. Most agencies require a witness to be present when narcotics and controlled substances are discarded. Finally, medications should not be transferred from one container to another even when two containers with the same medication are in use.

In order to avoid error, the nurse who prepares a medication should administer it immediately after it has been prepared. If prepared medicines are left unattended, the chances of the drug being misplaced or taken by another patient are increased. Moreover, the nurse is legally responsible for the medications to be administered and only if the nurse has prepared a medication can he or she testify to the actual drugs in the medication container. The identification of medication by its appearance alone is dangerous practice, since many drugs have similar appearances. If it happens that medications are distributed when a patient is unavailable to take the medication (for example, if the patient is having a test done in another department), that medication can be returned to the nursing unit and locked in the cupboard with the identifying medication card.

HEALTH RESTORING STRATEGIES

The administration of medications is a therapeutic nursing function, often implemented on the order of the physician to treat a specific illness and disease. The nurse requires not only knowledge but also psychomotor skills in preparing and giving the medications. In this section we will focus on the skills required to administer medications by the various methods and routes.

METHODS OF ADMINISTERING MEDICATIONS

Medications can be administered using a variety of methods and routes. These will be described here.

Oral The most common method of administering medications is by mouth (*orally*). Not only is it simple, it is also the most economical way. Capsules, liquids, lozenges, tablets and powders are all administered by mouth. A *capsule* contains a powder, oil or liquid within a gelatinous covering. A *lozenge* or *troche* contains a drug in a flavoured base and releases the drug as it dissolves in the mouth. *Tablets* are solid dosages of medication that are often coloured. Some tablets are *enteric coated*. These tablets are coated with a substance that is insoluble in gastric acids, thereby reducing gastric irritation. Finally, *powders* may be a single dose or a mixture of finely ground drugs.

Sublingual *Sublingual administration* involves placing the drug (for example, nitroglycerin) under the patient's tongue, where it is dissolved and absorbed.

Parenteral *Parenteral* refers to the administration of drugs by a needle. Intramuscular, intradermal, subcutaneous and intravenous injections are common methods of parenteral therapy. Intracardiac, intrapericardial, intrathecal (intraspinal) and intraosseous (into bone) injections are less common methods that may be used by physicians. All parenteral therapy involves the use of sterile equipment and sterile, readily soluble solutions.

Inhalation *Inhalation* is the administration of a drug into the respiratory tract where it is almost immediately absorbed. Volatile and nonvolatile drugs can be inhaled, the latter by means of a vehicle such as oxygen.

Instillation *Instillation* is a method of putting a drug in liquid form into a body cavity or orifice, for example, the ears, the eyes, the urinary bladder or the rectum. Liquid medications can be instilled with a dropper (into the ear) or with a syringe (into the urinary bladder).

Topical Medications are also applied to the skin and mucous membranes; this process is called *topical application*. Antiseptics, astringents and emollients can be applied as liquids or ointments. An ointment is a semisolid mixture that is applied topically to mucous membranes or skin.

Suppository A *suppository* is moulded into a firm base and is most commonly used for insertion into a body cavity or orifice, such as the rectum or vagina. As the suppository gradually dissolves at body temperature, the drug is released and is absorbed through the mucous membrane. Although a suppository is sometimes used to administer drugs when a systemic action is desired, as for example, an antipyretic, it is not considered as efficient as a medication administered by other routes. Suppositories are therefore used principally for local action. They may be used, for instance, to administer an analgesic to the rectal area, or to stimulate peristalsis and bring about a bowel movement.

PREPARING MEDICATIONS

There are two common places for preparing medications: a medication room and a medication cart. A medication room is usually in or near the nursing unit office, yet separate from it so that medications can be prepared with minimal disturbance. If the nurse prepares the medication in a medication room, the medication is placed on a tray for transport to the patient's room. The trays often have special slots so that the medicine card stands upright and can be read easily.

Medication carts are similar to medication rooms, except that they are portable. They are designed to save the nurse time by allowing preparation and administration of the medication directly from the cart. Trays for medications are not needed. The cart can be positioned close to the area where the medications will actually be administered. Nurses should take time to familiarize themselves with the cart, as it is often possible to prepare all medications without leaving the cart.

A hospital medication cupboard is sometimes locked, the key being kept by the head nurse or the nurse responsible for administering medications (if this system is used).

Adjacent to the medication cupboard are usually a locked narcotic cupboard and a refrigerator. Drugs that lose their potency unless kept cold are stored in the refrigerator.

The first step in preparing medications is to obtain the medication card or MAR and verify the order. This is done by checking the MAR or medication card against the original doctor's order. Errors in transcription occur, especially with medication cards and less often with MAR. In some agencies, all medication orders are checked with the doctor's orders during the night shift. Any discrepancies are communicated to the pharmacy department, who contact the physician.

The second step in the preparation of any medication is to get the complete order and make sure it is understood. Sometimes agency policy or the medication order governs the administration of a specific drug or the special nursing measures that accompany its administration. For example, an order might read "withhold drug if apex is below 60 beats per minute." Specific directives in the order may influence how the medication is poured, as we will discuss later. Occasionally medications are inadvertently ordered to which the patient has an allergy. Because allergies can cause severe and sometimes life-threatening reactions, the nurse must always check for allergies. The presence of allergies is noted at the top of the physician's order form. Additionally, in many agencies, patients with allergies are given a red identification band and the label on the chart is also red.

The medication is obtained from the patient's personal medication package, from the stock drug section in cart or medication room or from the refrigerator. Often the MAR will distinguish whether the medication is a personal or a stock drug. The techniques for preparing medications vary according to the route of administration. These are outlined in the specific procedures that follow.

Medications may be prepared at the bedside table from the medication cart.

When a nurse is preparing a variety of medications for a group of patients, the medicines for one patient are separated from those for another. Generally, all medicines that are administered by the same route for one patient can be placed in the same container, except for specific drugs when the administration is dependent upon some specified criterion. For example, if digitalis 0.125 mg is to be withheld when the patient's pulse is below 60 beats per minute, this drug is put in a separate container from the other oral medications for that particular patient.

A

B

FIGURE 33.3 A. Medication cart B. Medication tray

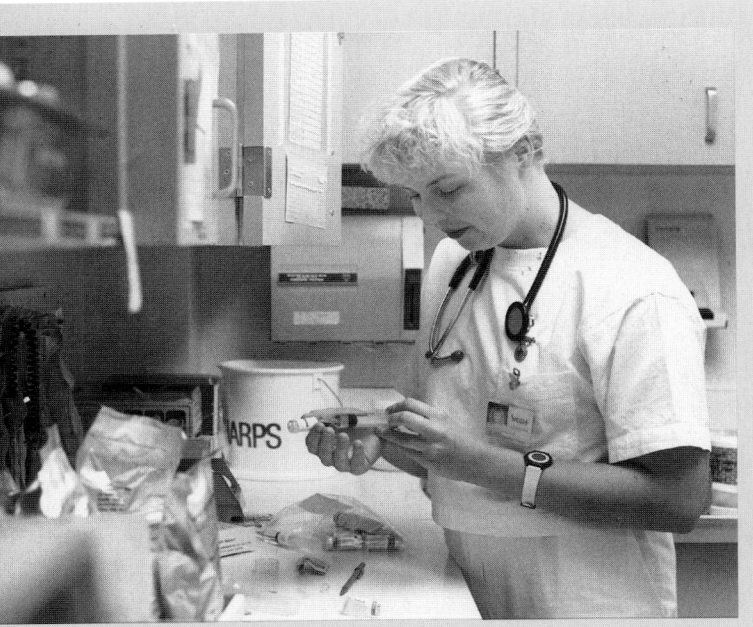

This nurse prepares medications in a medication room.

ADMINISTERING MEDICATIONS

Preparing the Patient

Medications are given to individuals, and the nurse will find that each individual is different. Some people want to know about medications; others prefer not to know. The amount of knowledge that a patient desires is highly dependent upon individual circumstances. The seriously ill patient in a hospital may be too ill to learn about the drug. The information that each patient should have depends on intelligence, age, education, illness and emotional needs. The nurse is guided by the patient and the physician as to the amount of information provided. When a patient does express a desire to learn about the medication, the patient should be informed, in an understandable manner, of the basic action of a medication, the main adverse effects, dosage and how to take the medication. It is always wise to ask the patient about allergies, even if these are not indicated in the chart. Sometimes, people don't recall allergies when first asked. It is also possible that the physician unintentionally orders a medication the patient has known allergies to.

Giving the Medication

Any technician can safely administer medications, but the nurse who views the patient in a holistic way will be better able to assist. Complementary to the administration of many medications is the provision of nursing care measures that serve to supplement the action of a drug. For example, giving the patient a back rub and straightening the bed might increase the effectiveness of a sedative and teaching a patient

to drink fluids properly can help prevent the crystallization of sulfonamides in the kidneys. Similarly, spending a few extra moments to ensure the patient has the preferred type of juice, or gets the pills in the preferred order, lets patients know they matter as individuals. It is *how* the medications are administered that makes the difference.

Sometimes the administration of a drug is contingent upon some factor, such as the patient's apical rate or blood pressure, and this is assessed first. With few exceptions the nurse stays with a patient until the medication has been taken. The exceptions are drugs that have been ordered to be left with a patient; for example, a drug that the patient has for immediate use (such as nitroglycerin for cardiac pain) or a drug that is contained in an intravenous infusion for gradual administration. If medications are left at the patient's bedside, it is the nurse's responsibility to check at frequent intervals to ascertain the dosage that has been consumed. Such intervals vary depending upon the drug; the nurse is referred to the agency policy manual for these.

Some circumstances call for a number of different forms of oral medications to be administered at the same time. In these cases, tablets and capsules should be administered before liquid forms, particularly syrups and antacids. This will ensure that the benefits of syrups and antacids on the oropharynx, esophagus and stomach are not washed away with the water consumed with the tablets or capsules.

When administering medications to children, the nurse should attempt to make it fun and incorporate play into the session. Generally, it takes longer to administer medications to children than to adults. At all times, be honest, and negotiate with the child. Give medications in as small amounts of food or fluid as possible, since large quantities often cause difficulties. Abstain from bribing the child with a favourite food as a mixing agent — this may turn the child against the favourite food.

Assessing for Adverse Effects

An important part of administering a medication is assessing the patient afterward for drug effectiveness, side effects or allergic reactions. The patient should be observed within an hour of taking the medication for adverse reactions. If the reaction is severe (such as difficulty breathing), notify the doctor immediately and prepare to administer interventions as ordered.

RECORDING MEDICATION ADMINISTRATION

As for all nursing procedures, medications must be recorded to provide legal documentation that they have been administered. The record also keeps other members of the health care team informed. It is important to note the exact time and dosage (if a range is provided) with prn or stat medications. Medications are recorded immediately after they have been administered. The recording should include the name of the drug, the time it was administered, the exact dosage, the method of administration and the signature of the nurse. Some agencies also require that the status of the person administering the drug also be designated, for example R.N. or S.N.

When the card system is used, the nurse enters the time of administration and his or her name on the medication record in the patient's chart. The MAR system often requires the nurse to take the MAR to the bedside to provide a final check for the correct patient. Once the medication has been administered, the nurse then signs the MAR. In some agencies, prn and stat medications are recorded in the nurses' notes, along with the assessment of the patient's condition and the reason the medication was given. In other agencies, these are recorded on the MAR. In both systems, a notation should be made later in the nurses' notes or on the MAR describing the patient's re-

sponse to a prn or a stat medication. Additionally, many agencies require that the nurse also indicate on the doctor's order sheet that stat dosages have been administered.

ORAL MEDICATIONS

Oral medications are taken by mouth. They are chiefly absorbed in the small intestine, although they can also be absorbed in the mouth and the stomach. Drugs in liquid form, either upon administration or upon dissolution within the stomach, are absorbed through the gastric mucosa. Absorption of a drug is slowed by the presence of food in the stomach as well as by its administration in concentrated form. Dilution, an alcoholic base and an empty stomach facilitate absorption. Table 33.5 gives an outline of the advantages and disadvantages of oral medications.

PROCEDURE 33.1

General Steps in Preparing a Medication

ACTION	RATIONALE
1. Obtain MAR or medication card and verify order.	Protects the patient from injury and promotes accuracy.
2. Check for allergies.	Ensures safety and economizes time.
3. Clear working surface on medication cart or in medication room.	Allows nurse to focus and prevents errors.
4. Wash hands.	Prevents spread of microorganisms.
5. Gather equipment.	Facilitates efficiency and economy of time.
6. Maintain cleanliness and aseptic technique as necessary.	Prevents contamination and the spread of microorganisms.
7. Prepare medications using the "five rights."	Ensures safety and accuracy.

TABLE 33.5　Advantages and Disadvantages of Oral Medications

ADVANTAGES	DISADVANTAGES
• convenient: simple method of administration	• taste: can stimulate nausea and vomiting
• economic: cost less to manufacture	• gastric irritation
• safe: do not invade body defences	• destroyed by gastric secretions
	• harmful to the teeth: can damage enamel and discolour teeth
	• inaccurate measure of absorption: some drugs are destroyed to a variable extent by gastrointestinal secretions
	• limited use: patient must be able to swallow or have a feeding tube
	• patient must be able to retain medication

Nursing measures can often minimize the disadvantages of oral medications. For example, drugs that are administered in a liquid or partially dissolved form tend to activate taste buds more than drugs in tablet or capsule form. These often unpleasant tasting fluids can be given with cold fluids or with ice, since cold is less stimulating than warmth and helps to desensitize taste buds.

Irritation of the gastric mucosa, caused by some drugs, can be minimized by administering the drug after a meal, while food is still in the stomach. Also, the more diluted the medicine is, the less irritating it will be to the mucosa. A medicine that is particularly irritating can sometimes be given with another drug or with food, such as bread, in order to modify its undesirable effect.

Medications that are *destroyed by the gastric secretions* can still be administered by the oral route if they are manufactured with an enteric coating so that they do not dissolve in the stomach. Otherwise, these drugs may be ordered to be given via parenteral administration.

Medications such as hydrochloric acid and liquid iron preparations are *harmful to the teeth.* These undesirable effects can be avoided by giving highly diluted forms and by using a straw in order that the teeth do not come in contact with the liquid. It is also wise to have the patient rinse the mouth with water or a mouthwash after taking these medicines.

Another disadvantage of the oral administration of medications is the relative inability to *measure absorption accurately* in the gastrointestinal tract. Certain disorders affect absorption; for example, accelerated peristalsis will decrease absorption because of the drug's speedy propulsion through the gastrointestinal tract. Moreover, some medications are destroyed to a variable extent by gastrointestinal secretions. In addition, the adequacy of the circulation of the blood to the tract affects the rate of absorption. If a patient vomits after ingesting a medicine, the amount of drug retained in the body is questionable. Generally the physician is consulted in order to assess the patient's need for a repeated dose of the medicine when this happens.

Considering the list of disadvantages, it quickly becomes evident that the use of oral medications is *limited* to patients who are able to swallow and retain them. The unconscious patient, the patient who is unable to swallow and the vomiting patient cannot take oral medications. Patients who are restricted to taking nothing by mouth are occasionally allowed oral medications. Some patients cannot take oral medications because of gastric suction and some find swallowing difficult because of surgery or paralysis. Frequently, it is the nurse who first becomes aware that a patient has difficulty swallowing a medicine. The nurse needs to inform the physician so that a change to a more easily consumed drug can be made. Tablets can be crushed and a scored tablet can be broken for easier administration, but the protective coverings of capsules or enteric-coated pills should not be removed to facilitate administration. The techniques for preparing and administering oral medications are outlined in Procedure 33.2

Assembling Equipment and Supplies

Dry medications are generally distributed in disposable paper cups. Liquid medications are given in plastic or waxed paper containers. The advantages of using disposable containers are obvious: cleanliness is assured and washing and sterilizing are eliminated. It is difficult to pour the exact amount of tablets into a medication cup. This poses a problem when a number of tablets are being poured into the same container. Therefore, pills should first be dropped onto the bottle cap or into an empty medicine container and then transferred to the medication cup. Medications should not be handled indiscriminately. Pouring pills into the hands increases the transmission of microorganisms. If there is any doubt about administering a specific drug, the drug is kept separately from the other tablets for a specific patient. For example, Digoxin is poured into a separate container, since the nurse cannot administer the medication until the patient's apical beat has been determined to be above the specified rate.

In order to obtain an accurate measurement when pouring liquids, the dose is measured from the bottom of the concave meniscus. It is important to visualize the container at eye level with the container on a flat surface (see Figure 33.4). Excess amounts are sometimes poured into the cup. These should not be returned to the medication container but should be discarded instead. Some liquids separate after standing in a bottle and need to be shaken before they are used. The medication container should be held so that the medication flows from the side opposite to the label. This prevents medication from staining and obstructing the label. Drips from the lip of the bottle can be wiped with a clean damp paper towel before the lid is replaced. Minims (0.06 ml) and drops are not interchangeable measures. Special droppers or glasses and, in some agencies, syringes, are used for measuring small amounts of liquid medications.

FIGURE 33.4   When pouring liquid solution, the dose is measured from the bottom of the meniscus. A meniscus is the result of the surface tension of the solution against the wall of the container, which causes a concave curvature on the surface of the solution.

PROCEDURE 33.2

Administering Oral Medications

ACTION	RATIONALE
1. Follow steps in Procedure 33.1.	
2. Gather equipment: • MAR or medication card • Medication container • Prescribed medication • Food or fluid • Drinking straw (optional) • Mortar and pestle (optional)	Facilitates efficiency and economy of time.
3. Pour medications: **Tablets or capsules:** Pour into lid of container and then transfer to medication cup. **Liquids:** Set plastic container on flat surface and bend (using correct body mechanics) so that eyes are at the level of the cup. Place lid of medication container top down on table. Pour medication into container until meniscus reaches desired level. **Separate** drugs that require special consideration.	Ensures safety and accuracy. Prevents contamination of lid. Ensures accuracy of measurement.
4. Place medication cup in medication tray with appropriate medication cards or notation on MAR.	Allows correct identification of medications.
5. Return medication to appropriate storage place (such as a drawer or refrigerator) and tidy area.	Promotes cleanliness and safety.
6. Take medication, medication card or MAR and selected fluid (water, juice) to patient's room. Identify the patient.	Ensures the correct patient is receiving the medication.
7. Explain the medication(s) to the patient and encourage questions.	Facilitates the patient's well-being and participation in care.
8. Ask the patient to sit upright, if possible, or roll the head of bed (HOB) up unless contraindicated.	Assists patient to swallow and prevents choking.
9. Give the medication cup to the patient and offer selected fluids.	Gives patient control and individualizes care.
10. Ensure the patient has swallowed oral medications.	Ensures effective administration. Some people may require more fluids. Patients with paralysis may not feel whether medications have been swallowed. Rarely, patients will collect medications inside mouth and remove later.
11. Position the patient for comfort and offer any further explanation regarding medications.	Promotes patient well-being.
12. Record administration of medication on appropriate form.	Provides legal record of medication administration.
13. Assess the patient for therapeutic effects, side effects, or allergic reactions.	Provides evaluation of care and promotes patient safety.

Occasionally, patients require tablets to be crushed. In this instance, it is more palatable to administer crushed medications with food such as jam, pudding or ice cream to enhance the taste. The choice will depend upon the type of medication and the patient's preference. It is not wise to try to "hide" the medication in these foods and administer them without the patient knowing. This may threaten the patient's trust in the nurse and it may turn the individual against that particular food. A mortar (small ceramic bowl) and pestle (little hammer with a rounded end) is used to crush tablets. Fluid, such as water, juice or milk, will also be required for swallowing tablets and capsules and following liquid medications. A drinking straw will be needed for any liquid medication that stains the teeth.

ADMINISTERING ORAL MEDICATIONS THROUGH A TUBE

Some patients cannot tolerate oral medications because of the presence of a nasogastric (NG) tube. Fortunately, it is still possible to administer some oral medications. Ideally, it is best if the medication is in a liquid form, but some tablets and capsules can be administered as well. For example, some tablets can be crushed and administered with water, and some capsules can be punctured or opened and the contents removed. Table 33.6 outlines the tablets and capsules that should not be given via nasogastric tube.

The administration of medications by nasogastric tube is a relatively simple procedure, but because clogging of the tube is a common problem, care must be taken to flush the tube properly. Procedure 33.3 outlines the steps for administering oral medications via a tube.

SUBLINGUAL MEDICATIONS

Sublingual medications are basically prepared and administered like oral medications. The difference is that the patient places the medication under the tongue rather than swallowing it. Absorption occurs swiftly through the epithelial layer under the tongue. Sublingual medications bypass the liver and do not come into contact with contents of the gastrointestinal tract, resulting in a higher concentration of the drug in the blood.

PARENTERAL MEDICATIONS

It is becoming more common to administer medications by the parenteral route. In fact, next to oral administration, parenteral administration is the most common route. Parenteral medications are delivered through a needle into the dermal layer of the skin (intradermal injection), into subcutaneous tissue (subcutaneous injection), into designated muscle tissue (intramuscular injection) and into veins (intravenous injection). Drugs administered by parenteral routes are absorbed more quickly than by oral routes, and because of this, have a more rapid effect. Additionally, once administered, parenteral medications are not retrievable. Therefore, caution and precision are essential when preparing and administering parenteral medications. Considerable skill and dexterity are needed to perform the procedures safely and accurately. Furthermore, because parenteral injections penetrate the skin barrier, the risk of infection is always present. Solutions and equipment must be sterile and aseptic technique must be used throughout the procedure. The techniques for administering medications by each of the parenteral routes will be outlined separately. All parenteral medications are prepared in the same basic way.

Assembling Equipment

The basic equipment for administering parenteral medications consists of syringes, needles and medication containers, namely vials and ampoules.

Syringes A syringe consists of the barrel, the plunger and the tip which attaches to a needle. The parts of a syringe

---

TABLE 33.6 Oral Medications that Cannot be Given by Tube

MEDICATION	RATIONALE
Buccal or sublingual tablets	These medications are intended to be absorbed by veins under the tongue, or in the cheek.
Enteric-coated tablets	The enteric coating prevents release of active drug until the drug passes through the stomach. Administration without coating would cause premature release of medication.
Uncoated gastric irritants	May cause adverse gastrointestinal reactions.
Sustained-release tablets and capsules	Since they are designed to release medication slowly and contain two to three doses, crushing them could cause overdose.

PROCEDURE 33.3

Administering Oral Medication by Nasogastric Tube

ACTION	RATIONALE
1. Follow steps in Procedure 33.1.	
2. Gather equipment: • MAR or medication card • Prescribed medication • 2 paper medication cups (if pills to be crushed) or plastic medication cup (if liquid suspension) • Mortar and pestle • 50 ml syringe • Water	Facilitates efficiency and economy of time.
3. Pour medications using the "five rights." Prepare medication according to type: **Tablets:** crush between 2 paper cups. **Capsules:** open and pour into plastic medication cup. Some capsules may need to be pierced with a needle.	Ensures safety and accuracy.
4. Continue as in steps 4 to 7 of Procedure 33.2	
5. Aspirate fluid from the NG tube and test for acidity with a pH test strip (see Procedure 19.1).	Checks placement of the tube.
6. Flush NG tube with 15–30 ml water.	Ensures patency of the tube.
7. Administer each medication separately with at least 5 ml of water.	Dilutes medication in order to prevent clogging of the tube.
8. Repeat step 7 for each medication.	
9. When all medications have been administered, flush the NG tube with 15–30 ml water.	Maintains patency and prevents clogging of the tube.
10. If the NG tube is attached to suction keep the suction off for 30 minutes.	Allows absorption of medications.
11. Rinse large syringe with water and keep at patient's bedside.	Economizes use of supplies.
12. Follow steps 11 to 13 of Procedure 33.2.	

are shown in Figure 33.5-A. Syringes are made of glass or plastic material. Plastic syringes are usually disposable and are commonly used in hospitals, offices and clinics. Syringes are supplied in sizes ranging from 0.5 cc to 50 cc capacities. The *standard* 3 cc ("cc" stands for cubic centimetre) syringe is commonly used for subcutaneous and intramuscular injections. The standard syringe is calibrated in millilitres (1 ml equals 1 cc) and minims (M), as shown in Figure 33.5-B. A larger syringe may be needed for preparing intravenous medications. An *insulin* syringe is used specifically for administering insulin. The units of measurement on the syringe are equated to the concentration of insulin in units per ml. Since most insulins are manufactured in concentrations of 100 units per ml, the most common insulin syringe

FIGURE 33.5   A. Parts of a syringe B. Calibrations of a 3 cc syringe

FIGURE 33.6   A. U-100 insulin syringe
B. Low-dose insulin syringe

FIGURE 33.7   Calibrations of a tuberculin
syringe

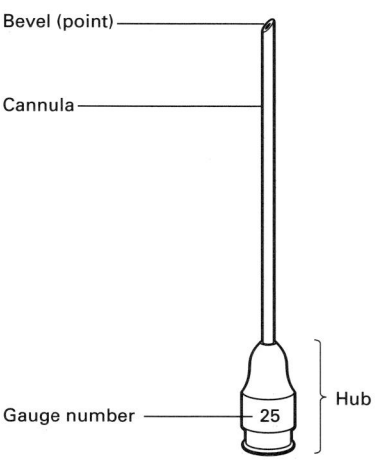

FIGURE 33.8   Parts of the needle

FIGURE 33.9   Needle length and gauge

is the U-100, which is calibrated in 100 units per cc (Figure 33.6). A low-dose insulin syringe is also available for patients requiring 50 units or less of U-100 insulin. The *tuberculin* syringe, originally designed to administer tuberculin, is now used to enable accurate measurement of small volumes of solution. A tuberculin syringe is calibrated in tenths and hundredths of a cubic centimetre and in 0.5 and 1 minim scales (16 minims equals 1 cc), as shown in Figure 33.7.

Needles   A needle consists of the hub, the shaft or cannula and the bevel (see Figure 33.8). The hub is the larger section that connects to the barrel of the syringe; the shaft is the long narrow part. The weakest point in a needle is where the cannula joins the hub. The bevel is the sharp slanted tip at the end of the cannula. Bevels vary in slant or length. A longer bevel means a sharper needle which minimizes discomfort when the needle penetrates the tissues. It is used for subcutaneous and intramuscular injections. A short or small bevel is used when the risk of occlusion in a larger bevel is high, as in intravenous injections in which the bevel could rest against the side of the vein.

Needles vary in the length and diameter of the shaft. The length may range from about one to five centimetres. The diameter of the needle shaft is expressed as the *gauge*. The higher the gauge, the smaller the needle diameter. For example, an 18 gauge needle is larger than a 26 gauge needle. Needles used for parenteral administration range from 18 to 26 gauge. Figure 33.9 is a representation of the various needle lengths and sizes.

A needle used for any injection should be straight and sharp. Since the use of disposable needles is increasing, the problem of the bent or dull needle is disappearing. Reusable needles are checked for sharpness and the presence of barbs before they are sterilized. A needle may be checked for the presence of barbs by passing the tip lightly over a piece of absorbent cotton. If the needle catches on the cotton, it may have a barb and will be uncomfortable for a patient. Needles that have barbs should not be used. A needle that is bent should not be used either, because it could possibly break off in a patient.

Medication containers   Parenteral medications are usually prepared from vials and ampoules containing sterile powdered or liquid medication. A *vial* is a glass container with a self-sealing rubber stopper that may contain one or more doses of medication. An *ampoule* is a sealed glass container that contains a single dose of medication (see Figure 33.10). Vials contain liquid or dry, powdered medication. Medications that are unstable in solution are packaged as powders which have to be reconstituted before use. A vial is a closed system and, as such, requires the creation of positive pressure inside the container in order to withdraw medication from it. This is accomplished by injecting air equal to the amount of medication to be removed. The neck of an ampoule must be broken in order to withdraw the medication. Many ampoules are prescored to facilitate opening; scoring is depicted with a coloured ring around the neck. Those that are not prescored should be scored with a file to facilitate opening.

A **B** **C**

FIGURE 33.10   A. Vial B. Prescored ampoule C. Unscored ampoule

Preparing Injections

Parenteral medications are supplied in liquid or powder form. Both of these forms must be kept sterile during preparation and administration. The techniques for preparing injections depends on the form of the drug and on the container (ampule, single-dose vial, multidose vial or a two-compartment vial). Sometimes two drugs are ordered by the same route. Providing the drugs are compatible, they can be mixed together in one syringe, saving the patient the unnecessary discomfort of another injection. Medications may be mixed from two ampules, from two vials or from a vial and an ampule. The various techniques for preparing drugs for parenteral administration are outlined in the following Procedures 33.4–33.8.

Body Substance Precautions

The disposal of syringes and needles requires a special word of caution. Nurses must be meticulous in discarding needles and syringes. This is an area where short cuts are not acceptable as carelessness can lead to disastrous results. One of the problems that can occur relates to people who may be looking for needles and syringes to assist their habit of illicit drug use. Nurses can prevent these opportunities from occurring by swiftly disposing of needles and syringes into sharps containers. In many hospitals and clinics sharps containers are placed in every room. Needles and syringes should *never* be put in the garbage can after use. Uncapped needles can easily prick an unsuspecting housekeeping person and cause injury. Furthermore, the nurse should *never* recap syringes once an injection has been administered. Current literature indicates that most needlestick injuries occur when the nurse recaps the needle following an injection (Ford, 1990). Needlestick injuries carry the risk of transmitting Hepatitis B and HIV. Therefore, the safest method is to deposit the syringe into a sharps container directly after giving the injection.

It is permissible to recap a needle before it is used on a patient. Once the medication has been prepared the needle is covered to keep it sterile and to protect others from needlestick injury. The needle may be recapped by sliding it into the protective cover (cap). *Do not* use the other hand. This prevents needle stick injury and fosters safe habits.

PROCEDURE 33.4

Preparing a Medication from an Ampoule

ACTION	RATIONALE
1. Follow the steps in Procedure 33.1.	
2. Gather equipment: • Medication card or MAR • Prescribed medication • Syringe and needle • Cotton ball or alcohol swab	Facilitates efficiency and economy of time.
3. Hold the top of the ampoule upright and rotate it in a swift motion or using a windmill movement.	Transfers solution from the top of the ampoule into the bottom from which it is withdrawn.

PROCEDURE 33.4
continued

ACTION

RATIONALE

4. Wrap the neck of the ampoule with a cotton ball or alcohol swab.

Prevents cuts when opening.

5. Grasp the ampoule with one hand and with the thumb of the other hand on the neck, apply pressure to the neck while bending it backward away from the face.

Prevents injury from splinters.

6. Deposit the top with alcohol swab directly into the sharps container.

Swift disposal prevents injury and keeps working area clean.

7. Twist the needle onto the syringe, and remove the needle cap. Leave the cap on a flat, accessible surface.

Prepackaged syringes and needles are not always tightly fastened.

8. Insert the needle into the ampoule without touching the neck of the ampoule.

Maintains sterility of needle.

Continued on the next page

ACTION	RATIONALE

9. Withdraw the desired amount of solution:

A. Hold the inverted ampoule and syringe in one hand and gently pull on the plunger with the other hand until the desired amount of solution is withdrawn. Ensure that the ampoule is directly upright and that the tip of the needle is below the level of solution.

Pulling on the plunger creates a negative pressure in the syringe, drawing fluid from the ampoule into the syringe. Air will also be drawn into the syringe if the needle tip is not in solution. Solution will not drip out of ampoule because of surface tension. *DO NOT push solution or air into an ampoule while it is inverted or it will drip out.*

B. Place the ampoule on a flat surface and gently pull on the plunger until the desired amount of solution is withdrawn. Make sure the tip of the needle is below the level of solution.

10. Place the ampoule on a flat surface and remove the syringe.

Facilitates manual dexterity.

11. Hold the syringe upright and tap the barrel using a pen or the heel of a hand (*Hint: flicking with finger-tips tends to be ineffective and causes sore fingers*).

Causes air bubbles to rise to the hub of the syringe.

PROCEDURE 33.4
continued

ACTION	RATIONALE

12. Aspirate approximately 0.25 ml.

Any time the syringe is tapped, small amounts of solution escape into the needle. Aspirating draws this solution back into the syringe and prevents spurting when dosage adjustments are made.

13. With the syringe in a vertical position, eject any air remaining in the syringe.

Syringe must be exactly vertical as even a slight tilt causes air bubbles to sequester in the syringe.

14. Check the dosage in the syringe against the MAR. Expel excess solution into a paper towel or container.

Ensures accuracy of dosage.

15. Recap the needle.

Ensures safety for nurse and others.

16. Discard the ampoule into a sharps container.

Correct disposal ensures workplace safety.

PROCEDURE 33.5

Preparing a Medication from a Vial

ACTION	RATIONALE

1. Follow the steps in Procedure 33.1.

2. Gather equipment:
- Medication card or MAR
- Prescribed medication
- Syringe and needle
- Alcohol swab

Facilitates efficiency and economy of time.

3. Remove the metal or plastic cap from the top of an unopened vial.

Continued on the next page

ACTION

RATIONALE

4. Cleanse the rubber top of a previously opened multidose vial with an alcohol swab. If the surface of a newly opened vial has not been touched, this step is unnecessary.

Removes surface microorganisms.

5. Twist the needle onto the syringe and remove the needle cap. Leave the cap on a flat accessible surface.

Prepackaged syringes and needles are not always tightly attached.

6. Draw back on the plunger to fill the syringe with an amount of air equal to the amount of solution to be withdrawn.

Because a vial is a closed container, the amount of fluid withdrawn must be replaced with air to keep the pressure inside the vial equalized. This prevents the formation of a vacuum which would make the withdrawal of medication difficult.

7. With the vial placed firmly on a flat surface, insert the needle into the vial and inject the air into the space above the solution.

Prevents the formation of air bubbles which could cause difficulty in withdrawing the correct amount of medication.

ACTION	**RATIONALE**
8. Invert the vial and syringe unit, ensuring that the needle tip is below the level of fluid in the vial.	Prevents air from being drawn into the syringe.

9. Holding the syringe at eye level, pull down on the plunger to withdraw the required amount of solution.

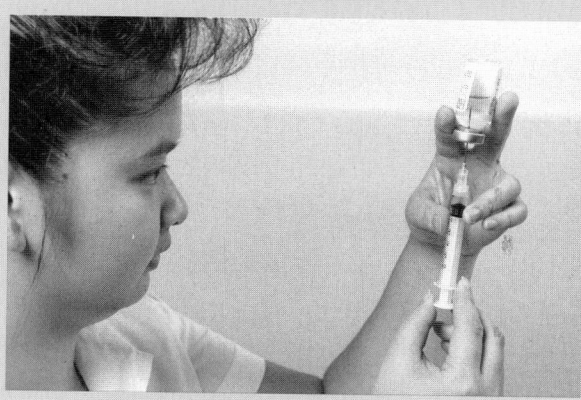

| 10. With the needle still in the vial, and holding the syringe upright, tap on the barrel. | Dislodges air bubbles and displaces any air to the top of the syringe. |

Continued on the next page

PROCEDURE 33.5
continued

ACTION	RATIONALE
11. Inject air at the top of the syringe into the vial.	
12. Check the amount of solution in the syringe. Return excess or withdraw more solution as necessary.	Ensures accuracy of measurement.
13. Place the vial in an upright position on a flat surface. Remove the needle.	Removing the syringe with the vial inverted may cause spraying of medication.
14. Recap the needle.	Ensures safety for nurse and others.
15. Return a multidose vial to storage. Discard empty vial and used supplies.	Promotes cleanliness and safety in the workplace.

PROCEDURE 33.6

Preparing a Medication from a Powder

ACTION	RATIONALE
1. Follow the steps in Procedure 33.1.	
2. Gather equipment: • Medication card or MAR • Prescribed medication • Diluent (as specified on label) • Syringe and needle • Alcohol swab	Facilitates efficiency and economy of time.
3. Read the instructions on the package insert.	Provides specific instructions regarding reconstitution.
4. Withdraw air from the vial equal to the amount of diluent to be added.	Prepares the vial for the diluent, to balance the pressure in the vial.
5. Draw the required amount of diluent into the syringe and inject it into the upright medication vial.	Mixes with powder to reconstitute the medication.
6. Remove the syringe and without using a second hand, replace the needle by sliding it into the needle cap. Set it aside.	Promotes safe habits and prevents needlestick injuries.
7. Roll the medication vial between the palms of the hands. *Do not shake!*	Rolling promotes mixing, whereas shaking often causes multiple bubbles or foaming to occur. This wastes time and can impede accuracy of measurement.
8. Withdraw the desired amount of medication as in Procedure 33.5.	
9. Label the vial indicating the date, time, type, amount of diluent and amount of drug per ml if it is to be reused. Store the vial as directed.	Ensures safe reuse. Many reconstituted drugs are effective for a limited period of time.

Common Problems in Preparing Medications From a Vial

There are several problems commonly associated with drawing fluid from a vial into a syringe. One problem occurs when the nurse begins to draw the fluid into the syringe only to find that large air bubbles form in the syringe. There are two basic reasons for this. First, if the needle has not been tightly secured to the syringe, air from the outside is drawn into the syringe. Second, the needle may be above the level of the fluid inside the vial, in which case air will be drawn into the syringe instead of fluid. Another problem occurs when the nurse forgets to put air into the vial prior to withdrawing solution. When this step has been forgotten, the solution will flow sluggishly into the syringe because of the resulting negative air pressure inside the vial. The air pressure inside the vial must be positive (greater than atmospheric) for fluid to flow freely.

Using Two-Compartment Vials

Some drugs are commercially prepared in two-compartment vials. One compartment contains the powdered medication and the second contains the sterile liquid for dissolving the drug. The insertion of a sterile needle or pressure exerted upon a rubber diaphragm releases the liquid to mix with the powder, which is then ready for injection. Some drugs are packaged this way because they are more stable in a dry state and can be kept for a longer period of time in this form.

PROCEDURE 33.7

Mixing Medications in One Syringe Using Two Vials

ACTION	RATIONALE
1. Follow the steps in Procedure 33.1.	
2. Gather equipment: • Medication card or MAR • Prescribed medications • Syringe and needle • Alcohol swab	Facilitates efficiency and economy of time.
3. Check a compatibility chart.	Protects the patient by ensuring that two medications can be mixed in the same syringe.
4. Determine which drug will be withdrawn first (Vial 1) and which will be withdrawn last (Vial 2).	
5. Prepare vials as in Procedure 33.5.	
6. Inject an amount of air equal to the volume to be withdrawn into Vial 2 and remove the syringe.	Creates a positive pressure in the vial.
7. Repeat Step 6 for Vial 1 but do not remove the needle. Invert the vial and withdraw the correct dose. Ensure that this amount is accurate and that no air bubbles are present.	Since two medications are being mixed in the same syringe, accuracy is essential for correct dosage.
8. Insert the needle into Vial 2, taking care not to depress the plunger. Withdraw the exact dose. Check the dosage.	Prevents contamination of medication in Vial 2 and ensures accurate dosage. Excess medication cannot be returned to the vial because the syringe now contains a mixture of the two medications.
9. With one hand, recap the needle.	Ensures safety for nurse and others.

Preparing Medication from an Ampoule and a Vial

ACTION	RATIONALE
1. Follow the steps in Procedure 33.1.	
2. Gather equipment:	Facilitates efficiency and economy of time.
• Medication card or MAR	
• Prescribed medications	
• Medication ampoule	
• Syringe and needle	
• Alcohol swab	
3. Check a compatibility chart.	Protects the patient by ensuring that two medications can be mixed in the same syringe.
4. Prepare the ampoule as outlined in Procedure 33.4.	
5. Withdraw the correct dose from the vial as outlined in Procedure 33.5.	Prevents contaminating a multidose vial with medication from the ampoule.
6. Ensure that the dosage from the vial is accurate and no air bubbles are present.	Since two medications are to be mixed, accuracy is essential for correct dosage.
7. Withdraw the exact dose from the ampoule as in Procedure 33.4.	
8. Recap the needle.	Ensures safety for nurse and others.

TABLE 33.7   Recommended Quantity of Solution for Route

ROUTE	AMOUNT OF SOLUTION
Subcutaneous	0.1–1.0 ml
Intramuscular	
Adults:	
deltoid	0.1–2.0 ml
ventrogluteal	0.1–5.0 ml
dorsogluteal	0.1–5.0 ml
vastus lateralis	0.1–5.0 ml
Children:	
vastus lateralis	0.1–1.0 ml
Intravenous	
Adults and Children	0.1–1000 ml/hr (children are at the lower end)
Infants	0.1–10 ml/hr

SUBCUTANEOUS INJECTIONS

Injections into subcutaneous tissues entail the delivery of medication into the loose connective tissues between the dermis and muscle layer. This route has been used since the 1860s and has been traditionally called the hypodermic injection. It has a relatively slow rate of absorption — about one to two millilitres per hour per injection site. The result is a lower concentration of drug in the body but with longer lasting effects. The onset of action begins within minutes but, depending upon the drug, this may also be hours. The duration of action is from hours to weeks. As outlined in Table 33.7, the maximum volume of solution that can be given comfortably by this route is thought to be less than 1.0 ml. Certainly anything greater than 1.5 ml will cause pressure on surrounding tissues and will therefore be painful. The advantages and disadvantages of subcutaneous injections are presented in Table 33.8.

TABLE 33.8 Advantages and Disadvantages of Subcutaneous Injections

ADVANTAGES	DISADVANTAGES
• virtually complete absorption, as long as patient's circulation is adequate • accurate measure of the amount of drug absorption as a result of complete absorption and no disruption in absorption from gastric secretions • not dependent upon consciousness or rationality of the patient	• invasive; breaks natural barrier (skin) against infection • skin changes with repeated injections can lead to development of lipomas or leathery skin • absorption rate varies with the patient's exercise, temperature and position following injection

The nurse can minimize the risk of infection by using strict aseptic technique for all injections. Unfortunately, it is not possible to entirely prevent the development of lipomas or leathery skin in patients who require repeated injections over a long period of time, such as with insulin dependent diabetics. However, it is possible to minimize the potential by rotating sites appropriately and allowing sites to rest for at least a month between injections. The variability in the rate of absorption can be reduced with consistent exercise and by remaining in the same position following injection for about fifteen minutes. In addition, if the patient's temperature is elevated, every effort should be made by the nurse to reduce it to a normal range. The technique for administering a subcutaneous injection is outlined in Procedure 33.9.

Preparing the Patient

As with many procedures, patients are concerned about the impending discomfort an injection may cause. The nurse should explain to the patient that the subcutaneous tissue is just below the cutaneous tissue or skin. It has fewer sensory receptors than the skin itself; therefore, once a needle is through the skin, an injection is relatively painless. Some drugs sting upon injection, but an isotonic solution can usually be administered painlessly. The term isotonic refers to a concentration that is the same as the saline composition of body fluids.

Assembling Equipment

The MAR or medication card, a syringe, a needle, the medication and an alcohol swab are collected. The standard 3 ml or the 1 ml tuberculin syringe with a 24, 25 or 26 gauge needle is commonly used for subcutaneous injections. An insulin syringe is required for administering insulin. The length of the needle may vary from 1 cm to 2.5 cm depending on the amount of subcutaneous fat and the degree

of hydration of the patient. A longer needle is needed for the obese patient, a shorter needle for the dehydrated or emaciated person. Generally a 25 gauge, 1.6 cm needle is used for the average adult.

There are two variations to the traditional method of administering subcutaneous injections. These are the injector syringe and the jet injection. The injection syringe is equipped with a spring which releases the needle for rapid insertion. The jet injector introduces the medication into the subcutaneous tissue by means of high pressure rather than through a needle. Although these methods are preferred in some instances, they have not replaced the usual subcutaneous injection by hypodermic syringe.

Choosing Subcutaneous Injection Sites

The exact site for a subcutaneous injection depends on the need of the specific patient, on the medication and to some extent, on the policy of the institution. There are, however, exceptions to this rule, such as with insulin and heparin, and these will be discussed separately. Generally, areas of the anterior and lateral aspects of the thigh, lower ventral abdominal wall, and the fat pads on the lower back and posterior aspect of the arms are recommended as usable sites (see Figure 33.11). In the past, the anterior aspect of the upper arms and the back of the thighs have been portrayed as potential injection sites, but these are no longer advocated (Drass, 1992). The skin and subcutaneous tissue should be free of irritation, such as itching, and any signs of inflammation, such as redness, heat, edema, tenderness or pain. Areas in which scar tissue is present should be avoided.

Rotating injection sites   If a patient is receiving a series of repeated injections, the sites are rotated to minimize trauma and to allow unused areas the chance to heal completely between use. An anatomic region is selected, for example, the lower ventral abdominal wall, and injections

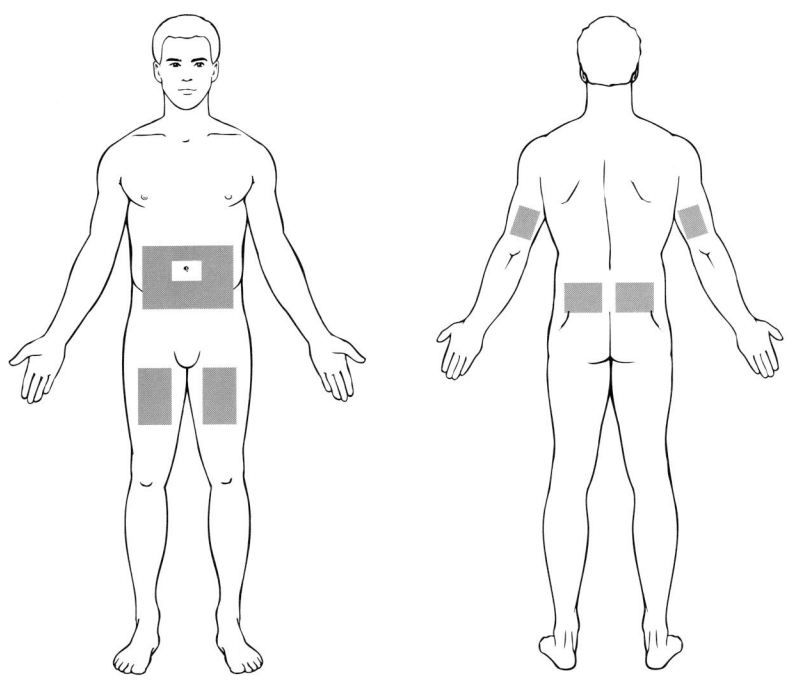

Intrasite Rotation
1. Mark the injection site with a spot bandage.
2. Regard the circle formed by the bandage as a clock.
3. Administer subsequent injections at the 1200, 1500, 1800 and 2100 points.
4. Start a new circle 2.5 cm away from previous intrasites.

Injection Sites

FIGURE 33.11 Subcutaneous injection sites and intrasite rotation

SOURCE: Drass, J. (1992). What you need to know about insulin injection. *Nursing 92, 22*(11), 40-43.

are made into that region until all of the sites have been used. This is called intrasite rotation. The sites progress in clockwise direction and each injection should be 2.5 cm away from the previous one. A region should not be reused for a month (Drass, 1992). It is important to chart the site every time it is used so that two consecutive doses are not given in the exact same area. Sometimes a map is made indicating the sites to be used for rotating injections, or a chart may be attached to the nursing care plan for the patient. Another method for keeping track of used sites is to put a spot bandage on the first site used in a region. The nurse can then rotate the sites as described above.

Subcutaneous Injection of Insulin

The subcutaneous injection of insulin is virtually the same as other subcutaneous injections, but with a few variations. The nurse must be especially aware of the types of insulins that can be mixed in the same syringe. Only insulins of the same brand should be mixed together. Similarly, there should never be cross-mixing of insulins with different bases, such as pork-based insulins and humulin insulins.

Regular insulin can be mixed with most other types, that is, Lente and NPH (Neutral protamine hagedorn) insulin. However, care must be taken to ensure that the vial containing the Regular (short-acting) insulin is not contaminated with longer-acting insulins. The accidental instillation, on repeated occasions, of a drop of longer-acting insulin into a vial of short-acting insulin can appreciably decrease the insulin's onset, peak and duration of action. Short-acting insulin should always be drawn up first, followed by the longer-acting insulin (Drass, 1992; Drury, 1986).

When administering insulin, the nurse does not need to pull back on the plunger before injecting the solution. The potential for entering a blood vessel is minimal and tissue disruption is at risk. However, Drass recommends that the nurse should consider aspiration "for children, thin adults, or any patient who has many superficial blood vessels at the injection site or well-developed underlying muscle (common among diabetic athletes)" (1992, 42). The insulin is slowly injected into tissues. The syringe is then withdrawn and firm pressure is applied with an alcohol swab. The area must not be massaged because this will cause inconsistent absorption.

PROCEDURE 33.9

Administering Subcutaneous Injections

ACTION	RATIONALE
1. Explain the procedure and the medication(s) to the patient. Encourage questions.	Facilitates patient well-being and participation in care.
2. Follow the steps in Procedure 33.1.	
3. Gather equipment: • MAR or medication card • Prepared medication with appropriate needle attached • Alcohol swab	Facilitates efficiency and economy of time.
4. Identify the patient.	Ensures the right patient.
5. Select the appropriate injection site. Assess the area for redness, birthmarks, scars, swelling and lesions. Ask the patient if the area is tender, itchy or burning. If any of these conditions are present, choose another site.	Facilitates consistent absorption of medication. Ensures a clean site which promotes absorption and prevents discomfort and inflammation.
6. Open the alcohol swab, loosen the needle cap from the syringe and move to within close proximity of the selected area.	Readies supplies for injection. Maintains safe body mechanics.
7. Cleanse the injection site with the alcohol swab using a circular motion, starting at the site and moving outward. Allow the area to dry completely.	Removes surface contaminants and bacteria. A circular motion pushes microorganisms away from the selected site.
8. **Patients with ample subcutaneous tissue:** With the thumb and forefinger of the nondominant hand, spread a fold of skin surrounding the site.	Assists in penetration of needle and causes less discomfort.
Patients with minimal subcutaneous tissue: With the nondominant hand, pinch a fold of skin around the site.	Pinching the skin elevates it from muscle tissue.

Continued on the next page

ACTION

RATIONALE

9. Hold the syringe, bevel upward, between the thumb and four fingers or the thumb and forefinger of the dominant hand and swiftly insert the needle using a 45–90° angle to the skin.

Most patients have enough subcutaneous tissue to warrant a 90° angle; very thin patients may require a 45° angle to prevent injection into the muscle.

10. Release the nondominant hand and move it to the plunger end of the syringe.

Once the syringe is in the patient, it is no longer necessary to stretch or pinch the skin. *Never leave a syringe unattended while in a patient's body!*

11. Aspirate by pulling back slightly on the plunger and inspect the syringe for the presence of blood. If this happens, prepare a new syringe.

Blood in the syringe indicates the needle is in a vessel and should be removed.

12. If no blood is present, slowly inject the solution.

Prevents rapid tissue distention and discomfort.

13. Swiftly remove the needle and massage the site with an alcohol swab unless contraindicated for the specific drug. If blood appears on site, cover the alcohol swab with the swab package.

Swift removal decreases discomfort. Massaging the site decreases bleeding and facilitates distribution of the medication. If bleeding does occur, the package from the swab will act as a barrier between the nurse and the patient and prevent the need for gloves.

14. Do not recap the needle. Discard directly into the nearest sharps container.

Prevents the potential for needlestick injury.

15. Ensure patient comfort, wash hands and record medication.

Promotes patient well-being, prevents the spread of microorganisms and fulfills requirements for nurse accountability.

TABLE 33.9 Advantages and Disadvantages of Intramuscular Injections

ADVANTAGES	DISADVANTAGES
• provides a less painful route for medications • muscles can absorb larger amounts of fluid than subcutaneous tissue • absorption is more rapid than the subcutaneous route. • can be used for potent drugs that are not cytotoxic • can be used for aqueous suspensions and solutions in vegetable oil that may cause emboli if give intravenously	• greater danger of damaging nerves and blood vessels • invasive; breaks skin thus potentiates infection • many patients fear intramuscular injections

Subcutaneous Injection of Heparin

Heparin is frequently administered via the subcutaneous route and has several variations from the routine procedure. Heparin is prepared and administered using an *air-lock technique*. The air-lock technique makes use of a minimal amount of air which is injected into the tissues after the medication has been administered. The purpose of this technique is to deliver all of the drug into the tissues, including the amount ordinarily left in the needle. This prevents trauma to tissues caused by leakage of solution from the needle when it is removed. After the correct dose of heparin has been drawn up, 0.1 ml of air is drawn into the syringe. The needle is changed and the syringe is inverted. The air is flicked to the plunger end of the syringe, so that it follows the injection of medication. A clean needle will be free of any heparin that may cause tissue damage.

Another variation in administering heparin subcutaneously pertains to site selection. The arms should not be used as sites. Arms are moved frequently, and are at greater risk for tissue disruption and bruising. As with insulin administration, the plunger is not aspirated prior to injection. The medication is injected slowly including the 0.1 ml air.

The syringe is swiftly removed and firm pressure is applied with an alcohol swab. Massaging is not recommended as it can cause greater tissue disruption.

INTRAMUSCULAR INJECTION

Intramuscular injections are administered under the muscle fascia below the subcutaneous layer. This route is often the choice for administering some medications, particularly those that are viscous and irritating, since the scarcity of sensitive nerve endings in deep muscle tissue results in less pain. Because muscles have a good vascular supply, medications are absorbed more quickly than when they are ad-

ministered subcutaneously. However, there is the danger of damaging nerves and injecting drugs into blood vessels. Medications administered by this route begin to work in less than an hour and the duration may last from hours to weeks, depending on the medication. Table 33.9 outlines some advantages and disadvantages of intramuscular injections.

While there are disadvantages to the intramuscular route, it is possible to minimize them. Nurses who consistently use proper techniques in locating injection sites (landmarking) will minimize damage to blood vessels and nerves. In addition, as with any injection, it is important to maintain aseptic technique in order to decrease the chance of infection. Many people fear and shy away from intramuscular injections because they are uncomfortable. Although injections are not as easy to take as an oral medication, the nurse can often minimize the discomfort. A number of suggestions are given in the box below. The technique for administering intramuscular injections is detailed in Procedure 33.10.

Assembling Equipment

The MAR or medication card and the prescribed medication are gathered. If the medication is in a powdered form a diluent will also be necessary. Most intramuscular injections require a 3 ml or 5 ml syringe. The standard prepackaged 3 ml syringe with a 21 or 22 gauge, 3.8 cm needle is commonly used for adults. If more than 5 ml of solution is ordered, the amount is given in two injections. Viscous fluids require a larger needle, 19 gauge for example. The length of the needle depends on the injection site, the size of the patient's muscle and the amount of adipose tissue that is present. A person with a large amount of adipose tissue will need a longer needle in order to reach the muscle tissue; a thin person will need a shorter needle. Smaller, shorter needles are required for infants and small children.

Reducing the Pain of Intramuscular Injections

1. Involve the patient in the choice of site. Any patient who has had more than a few injections may have a preference.

2. Choose the smallest gauge of needle possible giving consideration to the site and solution to be administered.

3. Assist the patient to relax the muscle to be used. If the gluteal muscle is to be used, have the patient lie prone, or stand with toes pointed inward, or lie on the side with knees flexed. If the vastus lateralis muscle is to be used, ask the patient to point the toes inward so the hips rotate internally. If the deltoid muscle is to be used, flex the elbow and support the lower arm.

4. Avoid sensitive areas. Roll the selected muscle mass with thumb and forefinger to assess for twitching.

5. Numb the site with ice if the patient is very apprehensive.

6. Make sure that the antiseptic used to wipe site is dry. Wet antiseptic can cling to needle and cause discomfort during insertion.

7. Change the needle if it was used to puncture a rubber stopper during preparation. This will also obliterate any medication on the needle which can be another cause for discomfort.

8. Insert and remove the needle quickly and smoothly. If possible, distract patient by asking them to wiggle the toes, take a deep breath and exhale or participate in discussion.

9. Inject the medication slowly to minimize the creation of high pressure in the muscle.

10. Never leave the needle unattended while it is in the patient. Instead, hold it steady.

11. Use all possible sites.

12. Massage muscle following injection, unless contraindicated.

13. Administer only recommended amount of fluid into muscle.

Locating Intramuscular Injection Sites

Regardless of the site chosen, the area must be exposed adequately so that the nurse can clearly see it. The selection of an area for an intramuscular injection depends on a number of factors: the size of the patient and the amount of muscle tissue available for injection; the proximity of nerves and blood vessels; the condition of the skin around the area; the nature of the drug to be administered; and the patient's preference. There are four recommended sites for administering intramuscular injections all of which are anatomically safe. Each area has little potential of hitting a nerve or large blood vessel. When choosing a particular site, the nurse must inspect the tissue in the area to make sure it is free from bruises or soreness. There should be no abrasions on the skin, and areas with hardened tissue (such as scar tissue) should be avoided.

It can sometimes be difficult to locate a suitable site on a patient who has had repeated injections. The patient should be involved in picking the general area of safe sites where he or she would feel comfortable getting the injection. If a patient has been receiving intramuscular injections over a long period of time, the nurse should collaborate with the physician to evaluate the effectiveness of this route and to consider alternatives.

Three areas of the body are commonly used for intramuscular injections: the gluteus muscles in two areas of the buttocks, the quadriceps muscles of the thigh and the deltoid muscles of the upper arm. Generally, it is best to rotate the areas when a series of injections are given. The gluteal muscles are thick and permit the injection of larger quantities of fluid. The use of these muscles in many normal daily activities also aids in the absorption of drugs.

The dorsogluteal muscle   The *dorsogluteal site* uses the gluteus maximus muscle. The site may be located by dividing the buttock into quadrants. The crest of the ilium and the inferior gluteal fold act as landmarks for describing the buttock. The injection is given in the upper outer quadrant of the buttock, 5 to 7.5 cm below the crest of the ilium (see Figure 33.12). By using this area, large blood vessels and the sciatic nerve are avoided. Another method for locating a safe gluteal site is to draw an imaginary line from the posterior superior iliac spine to the greater trochanter of the femur. This line runs lateral and parallel to the sciatic nerve, and consequently an injection lateral and superior to it is in a safe area.

To position a patient for an intramuscular injection in the gluteal muscle, ask the patient to lie in a prone position with his or her toes internally rotated in plantar flexion. In this position the gluteal muscles are relaxed and there is good visualization of the injection site. If the patient is unable to lie prone, ask the patient to lie on the side with knees flexed.

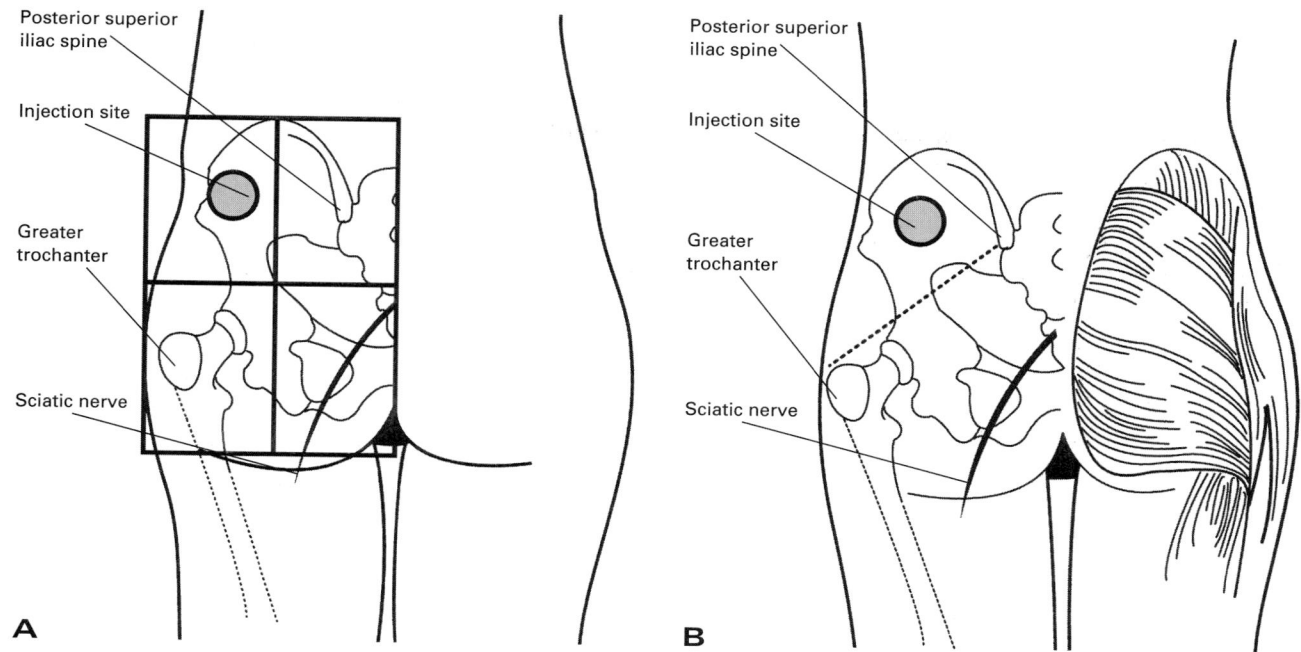

FIGURE 33.12 Locating the dorsogluteal injection site

SOURCE: Nursing Department, Langara College, Vancouver, BC. Reproduced with permission.

The ventrogluteal muscle The use of the *ventrogluteal site* is increasing because there are no large nerves or blood vessels in the area. In addition, the ventrogluteal area is usually less fatty than the buttocks, meaning that more medication is administered directly to the muscle.

When the ventrogluteal site is used, the injection is made into the gluteus minimus and the gluteus medius muscles. The site is situated in a triangle within three palpable bony landmarks: the iliac crest, the anterior superior iliac crest and the greater trocanter of the femur (Figure 33.13-A). The site may be located by placing the palm of the hand on the lateral part of the greater trocanter with the index finger on the anterior superior iliac spine. Then the middle fingers are stretched dorsally as far along the iliac crest as possible (Figure 33.13-B). An alternate method of locating the ventrogluteal site has been developed by Rhoda Brooke through her nursing experiences with adults and children. With this method it is not necessary to lay the nurse's hands on the body. Rather, the individual's anatomy is relied on more specifically. In this method, an imaginary line is drawn from the top of the iliac crest down to the trocanter. Then another line, parallel to the waistline, is drawn from the anterior superior iliac spine (hip bone) to join the first line. The point of intersection is the ventrogluteal site (Figure 33.13-C). It is important to palpate the injection site; it should feel soft and fleshy. If it feels hard, the site is likely too close to the bone and it will have to be adjusted accordingly.

An injection may be given into the ventrogluteal site with the patient in a prone, supine or side-lying position. The beginning student may find it easier to locate the site when the patient is side-lying. If the patient's gluteal muscles are tense, flexing the knees will help to relax them for the injection.

The vastus lateralis The *vastus lateralis* muscle on the lateral aspect of the thigh is also being used more frequently for intramuscular injections. The area is free of major blood vessels and nerve trunks. By virtue of its length, the vastus lateralis muscle provides a long area which is useful when numerous injections have to be given. The muscle extends the full length of the thigh from mid-anterior to mid-lateral and is approximately 7.5 cm wide. The injection may be given anywhere from approximately 10 cm above the knee to approximately 10 cm below the hip joint (see Figure 33.14). While this muscle is excellent to use because it lacks major nerves or vessels, the injection can be painful for individuals with large musculature on the upper leg.

The deltoid muscle The *deltoid muscle* of the arm is also used for intramuscular injections. This site is two to three finger-breadths down from the acromion process on the outer aspect of the arm (see Figure 33.15). In most people this is a smaller muscle than the gluteal muscle and therefore is not capable of absorbing a large volume of medicine comfortably. The danger of administering an injection in this area is that harming the radial nerve is a possibility.

With careful technique, complications from intramuscular injections can be avoided. Abscesses, nerve injuries, cysts and necrosis of tissue do occur as a result of intramuscular injections. Aseptic technique, the correct use of landmarks in determining injection sites and the alternate use of sites help to avoid these complications.

A   **B**   **C**

FIGURE 33.13   Locating the ventrogluteal injection site A. Ventrogluteal site B. Standard method C. Brooke method

Greater trochanter

Vastus lateralis (middle third)

Lateral femoral condyle

Deep femoral artery

Sciatic nerve

Femoral artery and vein

FIGURE 33.14   Locating the vastus lateralis injection site

SOURCE: Nursing Department, Langara College, Vancouver, BC. Reproduced with permission.

Acromian process

Clavicle

Deltoid muscle

Axilla

Humerus

Deep brachial artery

Scapula

Radial nerve

FIGURE 33.15   Locating the deltoid muscle injection site

SOURCE: Nursing Department, Langara College, Vancouver, BC. Reproduced with permission.

PROCEDURE 33.10

Administering Intramuscular Injections

ACTION	RATIONALE
1. Explain the procedure and the medication(s) to the patient. Encourage questions.	Facilitates patient well-being and participation in care.
2. Follow the steps in Procedure 33.1.	
3. Gather equipment: • MAR or medication card • Prepared medication with appropriate needle attached • Alcohol swab	Facilitates efficiency and economy of time.
4. If agency policy requires, draw 0.1 or 0.2 ml of air into syringe and flick it to plunger end (air-lock technique).	Clears the needle and locks medication in the muscle which helps to prevent reflux leakage of solution into subcutaneous tissues.
5. Follow steps 4 and 5 of Procedure 33.9.	
6. Once the general site has been selected position patient and provide privacy.	Promotes physical comfort and emotional well-being.
7. Place the syringe and alcohol swab in close proximity to selected site.	Maintains safe body mechanics.
8. Locate the injection site by identifying the correct landmarks. Cleanse it as in Procedure 33.9. It is often possible to mark the site with the corner of the alcohol swab.	Essential for a safe injection. Positioning the alcohol swab pointing towards the selected area allows the nurse to obtain the syringe without losing the site.
9. With the dominant hand, take the syringe and slide the needle cap off of the needle.	
10. Using the thumb and forefinger of the nondominant hand, pull the skin taut within 5 cm of the selected site. If the patient is emaciated, it may be necessary to pinch the skin.	Facilitates needle insertion and lessens pain when the injection is given.

Continued on the next page

ACTION

11. Ask a question or instruct the patient to take a big breath, or wiggle the toes.

12. Hold the syringe between the thumb and forefinger of the dominant hand and with a swift, smooth motion, insert the needle at a 90° angle to the skin, completely into the muscle.

RATIONALE

Distracts the patient and decreases the discomfort of the injection.

A quick motion decreases the patient's discomfort.

13. Follow steps 10 to 15 of Procedure 33.9.

Z-TRACK INJECTIONS

Some medications are best given by the Z-track method. The Z-track method permits the injection of highly irritating medications or those which discolour tissues. It is also used for people who have had multiple intramuscular injections and reflux leaking becomes a problem. The Z-track injection is prepared and administered in the same way as a routine intramuscular injection, with the following exceptions. The needle is always changed after the medication has been drawn up. This ensures that there is no medication on the needle that could cause irritation to the tissues. In the Z-track method the skin and subcutaneous tissues are laterally displaced and traction is maintained while the medication is injected. Release of the tissues after injection seals the medication in the muscle and creates a leak-proof zigzag path (see Figure 33.16). With the nondominant hand, the skin and subcutaneous tissue are displaced about 2 cm over the target muscle. The needle is inserted at a 90° angle and the medication is injected while lateral traction is being maintained. Once the medication has been administered, the needle is quickly removed and then the traction is released. An alcohol swab is held firmly over the site but the site is not massaged. Massage may cause seepage of medication into delicate tissue resulting in discomfort or staining.

INTRADERMAL INJECTION

An intradermal injection is the administration of a small amount of fluid (0.1 or 0.2 ml) into the dermal layer of the skin. It is frequently done as a diagnostic measure, as in tuberculin and allergy testing. Since the blood supply to the dermis is decreased, medications absorb very slowly and the effects are generally localized. It is important to reassess the area for the next few days, as this is generally when reactions appear.

Assembling Equipment

A tuberculin syringe with a very fine 26 or 27 gauge, 1 cm to 1.25 cm needle is used for intradermal injections.

Choosing Intradermal Sites

The areas of the body commonly used for intradermal injections are the fat pads over the medial aspect of the forearms, the upper arms, the scapula and the upper chest (see Figure 33.17). The area should be free of hair, veins and discolouration.

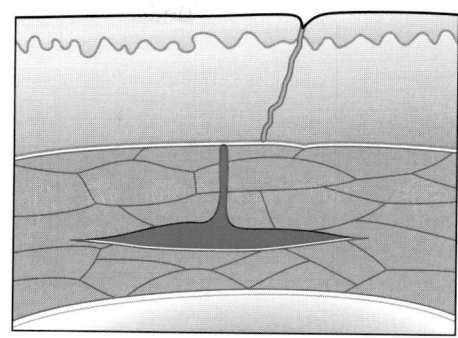

FIGURE 33.16 Z-Track method. This technique converts the needle track into a zigzag, which prevents leakage of solution into tissues.

FIGURE 33.17 Intradermal injection sites

PROCEDURE 33.11

Administering an Intradermal Injection

ACTION	RATIONALE
1. Explain the procedure and the medication(s) to the patient. Encourage questions.	Facilitates patient well-being and participation in care.
2. Follow the steps in Procedure 33.1.	
3. Gather equipment: • MAR or medication card • Prepared medication with appropriate needle attached • Alcohol swab	Facilitates efficiency and economy of time.
4. Follow steps 4 to 7 of Procedure 33.9.	
5. With the nondominant hand, pull the skin taut between thumb and forefinger with selected site in the centre.	Taut skin is easier to pierce and less painful for the patient.
6. Using the dominant hand, allow loosened needle cap to slide off. Position the needle with bevel facing up and fingers below the syringe, almost parallel to the skin.	Hand position provides stability.
7. Using a 15° angle to the skin, insert the needle gently but firmly through the epidermis into dermis.	Using a greater angle will ultimately inject solution into the subcutaneous tissue, instead of the dermal tissue.
8. Without aspirating, slowly inject the fluid into the dermis to produce a small bleb (blister) under the skin.	Intradermal tissue contains no large blood vessels, thus aspiration is not necessary. Slow injection causes gradual distention and is less painful for the patient.

9. Remove the needle swiftly and at the same angle as insertion.	Maintains patient comfort.
10. Do not recap needle. Discard directly into the nearest sharps container.	Prevents the potential for needlestick injury.
11. Ensure patient comfort, wash hands and record medication.	Promotes patient well-being, prevents the spread of microorganisms and fulfills requirements for nurse accountability.

TABLE 33.10 Advantages and Disadvantages of Intravenous Medications

ADVANTAGES	DISADVANTAGES
• No absorption problems. The medication is administered directly into the patient's circulation, thus rapidly achieves therapeutic levels.	• Potential incompatibility when any two drugs are mixed in a syringe or solution.
• Accurate titration due to accurate absorption.	• Poor vascular access. In emergencies with venipunctures, or with infusions of extended irritating drugs, normally accessible veins may collapse or develop scarring.
• Less discomfort. The pain associated with IM and sc routes is generally avoided since the veins have a much higher pain threshold.	• Severe adverse reactions may occur quickly due to high blood levels.
• Alternative to the oral route when the patient is unconscious, uncooperative or NPO.	
• Immediate discontinuation. If an adverse drug reaction does occur, the infusion can be stopped.	

INTRAVENOUS ADMINISTRATION

The use of the intravenous route to administer medications is also increasing. Intravenous medications begin to work immediately and that can be both an advantage and a disadvantage. They are very beneficial when a rapid effect is needed but adverse reactions or errors can cause serious, life-threatening complications. Intravenous medications can be delivered through a variety of methods: by adding a medication to a primary IV container (continuous infusion); by using a separate container connected to the primary line with secondary tubing (secondary line or piggyback set-up); or by the direct push method (small amount of solution is injected directly into an existing IV line). These same methods can also be used for the patient who has an intermittent infusion device, commonly referred to as a saline or heparin lock. The duration of action of a medication administered intravenously varies from a few seconds to hours. Table 33.10 outlines some of the advantages and disadvantages of using the intravenous route for administering medications.

The most effective way to deal with the noted disadvantages of intravenous medications is to prevent their occurrence. Drug incompatibilities can largely be prevented by scrupulous checking of the compatibility of the solution, the medication and the diluent. Most agencies have current compatibility charts available, and the nurse can always contact the pharmacist to double check. Effective vascular access is sometimes beyond the nurses control; however, the insertion of intravenous needles can be performed with excellent technique, thus avoiding repeated attempts which serve only to cause discomfort and injure the patient. When irritating drugs are to be infused, the nurse must follow recommendations for solution quantities and times. Adverse reactions can occur either immediately or following an infusion and the nurse must be alert to this pos-

sibility. While the nurse can not necessarily prevent adverse reactions, he or she can check carefully for known allergies or drug sensitivities prior to the administration of the medication.

ADDING MEDICATION TO A PRIMARY IV CONTAINER

Some drugs are best administered by continuous infusion in a large volume (500 ml or 1000 ml) of compatible solution. Multiple vitamins and potassium chloride are two examples of medications administered in this way. Procedure 33.12 outlines the steps for adding medication to a primary IV container.

A nurse adds medication to an IV container.

Assembling Equipment

The procedures for establishing and maintaining a primary IV line are described in Chapter 22. It is generally recommended that medication be added to a new solution container rather than an existing one. In some agencies the medication is prepared in the pharmacy department, while in others this is done by the nurse in the unit. The supplies and equipment the nurse will need include the IV solution (as ordered by the physician), the prescribed medication, a diluent if the medication is to be first reconstituted, a syringe with a 3.8 cm needle, alcohol swabs and a medication label. The IV container must be clearly labelled with the name of the medication, the dose, the duration of infusion and the infusion rate of flow in order to avoid inadvertent error in administration.

PROCEDURE 33.12

Adding Medication to a Primary IV Container

ACTION	RATIONALE
1. Explain the procedure and the medication(s) to the patient. Encourage questions.	Facilitates patient well-being and participation in care.
2. Follow the steps in Procedure 33.1.	
3. Check compatibility of diluent, medication and IV solution.	Prevents adverse reactions.
4. Gather equipment: • MAR or medication card • IV solution as ordered • Prescribed medication • Diluent • Syringe with 3.8 cm needle • Alcohol swabs • Medication label	Facilitates efficiency and economy of time.
5. Prepare the medication as in Procedure 33.4 or 33.5.	
6. Lay the solution container on a flat surface.	Facilitates ease of injecting medication.
7. Clean the resealable injection port.	Removes surface microorganisms.
8. Hold the injection port with thumb and forefinger of nondominant hand, keeping the container horizontal on the flat surface.	Acts as a guide to insert the needle. If the bag is kept in a vertical position, the needle can easily travel through the side and poke the nurse. The nondominant hand will feel if the needle is coming through the side and it can easily be repositioned.
9. With the syringe in the dominant hand, slowly insert the needle into the centre of the port up to the hub. Inject the medication.	The needle must be inserted to the hub to ensure that the medication is injected into the container, not the port.

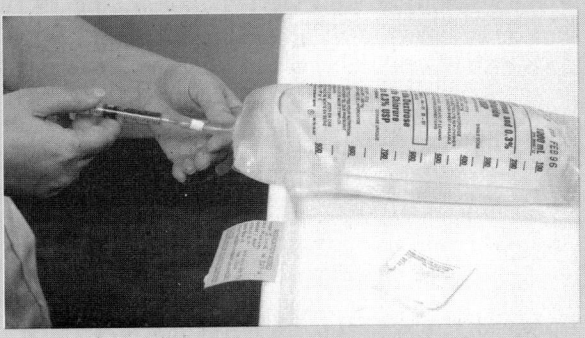

ACTION

10. Remove the needle and dispose of syringe in the nearest sharps container.

11. Prepare the medication label with the patient's name, medication, dosage, date and time and infusion rate of flow. Apply the label right side up on the solution container.

12. Gently agitate the solution container 4–5 times.

13. Identify the patient.

14. Change the solution container using principles of IV therapy outlined in Chapter 22.

15. Ensure patient comfort, wash hands. Record medication and enter the solution in the fluid balance record according to agency policy.

16. Carefully monitor the IV infusion and the patient for therapeutic and adverse effects of the medication.

RATIONALE

Prevents needlestick injury.

Provides identification. When preparing numerous medications, an added safety measure is to put the label half way on during preparation and remove the backing completely once the medication is in the bag.

Distributes medication evenly and prevents a bolus of medication from forming.

Ensures the right patient.

Promotes patient well-being, prevents the spread of microorganisms. Fulfills requirements for nurse accountability and promotes continuity of care.

Promotes safety and establishes need for care.

ADMINISTERING MEDICATION THROUGH A SECONDARY IV LINE

Many intravenous medications are administered intermittently through the use of a separate, small-volume container that is connected to the patient's primary IV line. The medication is delivered over a short period of time, usually 30 to 60 minutes. This method permits the infusion of medications that are not compatible with the solution in the primary line or those that are stable in solution for only short periods of time (for example, antibiotics). Diluting the drug in a small amount of solution also decreases the risk of immediate drug reactions or local vein irritation. The steps in administering medication via a secondary IV line are outlined in Procedure 33.13.

Assembling Equipment

A secondary IV line is made up of a small solution bag, usually of 50 or 100 ml capacity (but may be more), that is connected to the highest injection port of the primary IV line by a short section of tubing, called a secondary medication set. This system is often called a *piggyback* set-up because the secondary unit "borrows the use of the primary line and equipment" (Earnest, 1993, 885). The secondary line is connected to the primary infusion by an 18 gauge needle, equipped with a protective needle lock which protects the nurse from needlestick injury. The highest injection port is used because it has a backcheck valve that stops the infusion from the primary container when solution flows from the secondary container. Since IV flow is assisted by gravity, the secondary container is held higher by

The use of an infusion pump facilitates accurate infusion of medications administered by continuous infusion.

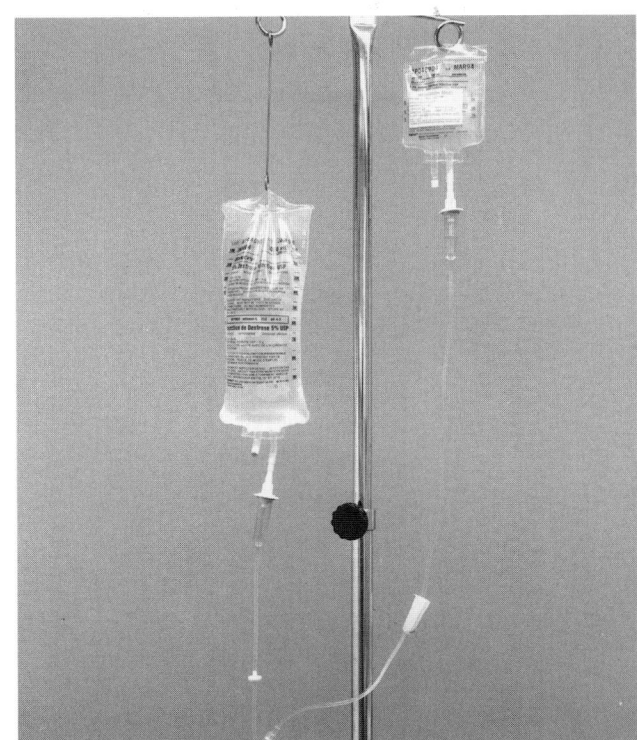

FIGURE 33.18 Secondary IV line (piggyback set-up)

lowering the primary container on an extension hook. When the secondary infusion is finished and the level of fluid in the secondary tubing is lower than the fluid in the drip chamber of the primary line, the backcheck valve opens and the primary infusion begins to flow again. An extension hook is included in each secondary medication set. Figure 33.18 illustrates a secondary IV (piggyback) line.

When patients receive intermittent IV medications, for example q.6h., the secondary tubing is not changed every time a dose is given. Only a new solution container is put up each time. The container is left hanging after the medication has infused to maintain a closed system and reduce the risk of contamination. The secondary IV line is changed every 24 hours or as per agency policy.

PROCEDURE 33.13

Administering Medication Through a Secondary IV Line

ACTION	RATIONALE
1. Explain the procedure and the medication(s) to the patient. Encourage questions.	Facilitates patient well-being and participation in care.
2. Follow the steps in Procedure 33.1.	
3. Check compatibility of diluent, medication and IV solution.	Prevents adverse reactions.
4. Gather equipment: • MAR or medication card • 50 or 100 ml solution bag	Facilitates efficiency and economy of time.

ACTION

- Prescribed medication
- Diluent
- Syringe with 3.8 cm needle
- Alcohol swabs
- Medication label
- Secondary medication set

5. Add the medication to the solution bag and label it as in Procedure 33.12.

6. Calculate the infusion rate of flow based on the amount of solution, the time in which it is to be administered and the drop factor of the tubing.

7. Assemble the secondary medication set. Close the roller clamp.

8. Remove the protective cover from the tubing port on the secondary bag. Uncap the spike and, while holding the port with one hand, insert the spike with the other hand using a firm, twisting motion.

9. Prime the tubing by slowly opening the roller clamp. Close the roller clamp when the tubing is primed.

10. At the bedside, hang the secondary bag on the IV pole.

11. Identify the patient.

    NOTE: If a secondary line is already set up, the medication container is changed using principles of IV therapy outlined in Chapter 22, and then steps 14 to 21 are implemented.

12. Clean the highest injection port on the primary tubing with alcohol.

13. Remove the protective cap from the needle on the secondary tubing and insert it into the injection port of primary line.

14. Lower the primary bag using the extension hook.

15. Completely open the clamp on the secondary set.

16. Regulate the rate of flow by adjusting the roller clamp in the primary tubing.

17. Monitor the patient and the infusion.

18. When the secondary infusion is finished, clamp the secondary tubing, raise the primary bag to its original position, and regulate the flow rate.

RATIONALE

Promotes efficiency and economy of time at the bedside.

Prevents solution from leaking out while tubing is being primed.

Pulling downward quickly removes the cover and maintains sterility of the port. A twisting motion is needed to puncture the seal on the bag.

The tubing is short and will prime quickly.

Facilitates manual dexterity.

Ensures the right patient.

Removes contaminants from port.

Connects the secondary set to the primary line.

Force of gravity assists the flow of solution from the secondary bag.

Establishes flow of the secondary infusion.

Solution ultimately flows into primary tubing thus it will regulate rate of flow.

Ensures safety.

Reestablishes primary infusion at the required flow rate.

Continued on the next page

ACTION	RATIONALE
19. If the secondary line is to be reused, leave the empty bag attached to the system.	Decreases risk of contamination by minimizing disruption of the closed system.
20. If the secondary line is not to be reused, remove it and discard. Make sure the needle is disposed of into a sharps container.	Promotes safety of nurse and others.
21. Record the medication and enter the solution and amount absorbed into the fluid balance record as per agency policy.	Fulfills requirements for nurse accountability and promotes continuity of care.

ADMINISTERING MEDICATION BY IV PUSH

Some medications are administered into the systemic circulation by direct injection (push) through an existing intravenous line. This route is selected when a rapid response is necessary and therefore is used frequently in emergency situations. It is also used to deliver drugs that cannot be diluted, such as digoxin. Extreme caution must be used since the complete dose of a medication is delivered in a short period of time and the drug is irretrievable. Many agencies have policies which specify the nurses permitted to administer drugs by this route, as well as the drugs they can administer. Some IV push drugs may only be given by the physician. All nurses, including students and graduates, must check agency policies before giving a medication by di-

rect push. The steps in delivering medications by push through an existing IV line are outlined in Procedure 33.14.

Assembling Equipment

The size of the syringe will depend upon the amount of solution to be delivered. A larger needle is needed to draw up the medication and a smaller one to administer it. Usually a 22 gauge, 2.5 cm needle is used for giving the medication in order to minimize the puncture holes created in the injection port with repeated instillations. In agencies employing a needleless IV administration (access) system, a blunt syringe cannula will be used instead of the needle. A watch with a second hand is also needed because the medication must be administered carefully over a specified period of time.

PROCEDURE 33.14

Administering a Medication by IV Push Through a Primary Line

ACTION	RATIONALE
1. Explain the procedure and the medication(s) to the patient. Encourage questions.	Facilitates patient well-being and participation in care.
2. Follow the steps in Procedure 33.1.	
3. Check the type and amount of diluent and the recommended administration time.	Ensures safety. The length of time required for injection varies with each medication. It is usually between one and five minutes.
4. Gather equipment: • MAR or medication card • Prescribed medication	Facilitates efficiency and economy of time.

ACTION	RATIONALE
• Syringe	
• 22 gauge, 2.5 cm needle or syringe cannula if using a needleless IV access system	
• Diluent	
• Alcohol swabs	
• Watch with second hand	
5. Prepare the medication as in Procedure 33.4 and 33.5.	
6. Identify the patient.	Ensures the right patient.
7. Inspect the IV site for redness, swelling, discharge, and ask if the patient feels discomfort.	Ensures a patent site.
8. Sit on a chair or on the patient's bed and bring the tubing in close proximity.	IV push medications take several minutes and sitting will allow the nurse to use proper body mechanics and talk to the patient.
9. Cleanse the port closest to IV insertion site with an alcohol swab.	Removes surface particles.
10. Turn off the primary IV if indicated.	
11. Insert the needle or syringe cannula completely into the port.	Inserting the needle part way into the port will sequester the medication in the port and it will not be delivered to the patient.
12. Administer the medication over the recommended period of time while monitoring the injection rate with a watch.	Permits the medication to disperse, and thus decreases irritation to the vein wall and promotes patient comfort. A bolus of medication delivered too fast may cause shock or embolism.
13. Reopen the primary IV and infuse slowly for 2–5 minutes.	Some of the medication will remain in the primary tubing. Resuming the original primary rate will permit ample dispersion and prevent the problems mentioned above.
14. Reestablish the prescribed rate.	
15. Observe the patient closely for reactions.	IV medications begin to work immediately.
16. Do not recap needle. Discard directly into nearest sharps container.	Prevents the potential for needlestick injury.
17. Ensure patient comfort, wash hands and record medication.	Promotes patient well-being, prevents the spread of microorganisms and fulfills requirements for nurse accountability.

ADMINISTERING MEDICATION THROUGH AN INTERMITTENT INFUSION DEVICE

An intermittent infusion device is a reusable membrane or injection site connected to either a winged-tip needle with tubing or an angiocatheter placed in the patient's vein and maintained for regular, intermittent use (see Figure 33.19). Medications are administered either through a secondary IV line piggybacked to a primary IV line that is attached to the infusion device or by the direct push method. Between use, the infusion device is kept patent with normal saline or

FIGURE 33.19   Intermittent infusion device connected to an angiocatheter

a dilute solution of heparin, thus the name saline or heparin lock. The advantage of a saline or heparin lock is that it allows intermittent access for intravenous medications while affording the patient freedom of movement when it is not being used.

An intermittent infusion device may be inserted specifically for administering medications or an existing IV line may be converted to a heparin or saline lock when the patient no longer requires continuous infusion of fluids. The technique for inserting an intermittent infusion device is the same as for inserting a peripheral venipuncture device (see Procedure 22.2). However, instead of attaching a primary IV administration set to the venipuncture device, a male adapter plug is inserted into the needle or cannula hub. The infusion device is flushed after each use and according to agency policy with normal saline or dilute heparin solution to keep it patent. The care for the venipuncture device and site is the same as for peripheral intravenous infusion, outlined in Chapter 22. In this section we will describe the technique for converting an existing IV line to a saline or heparin lock (see Procedure 33.15). We will also detail how to administer medications through an intermittent infusion device using an IV line (see Procedure 33.16) and by IV push (see Procedure 33.17).

Assembling Equipment

An intermittent infusion device consists of an injection site or cap at one end and one of two basic types of adapter plugs at the other. The two types are the long male adapter plug (slip lock) which slides into the needle or cannula hub by friction and the short male adapter plug (luer lock) which twists into place. The injection site is a membrane made of the same resealable rubber material similar to the injection ports on IV administration sets. The sites are usually accessed with a 22 gauge, 2.5 cm needle. In agencies using the needleless IV access system, a needleless blunt syringe cannula is used for piercing the injection site.

As we mentioned in the previous section, intermittent infusion devices must be flushed regularly to maintain patency. Agencies vary with regard to the type and amounts of solution used for flushing these devices. Heparin lock flush procedures call for 0.5 ml to 1 ml of dilute heparin solution, either 100 units per ml or 10 units per ml. Saline lock flushes require from 1 ml to 2 ml of normal saline.

When a medication is administered via an intermittent infusion device using an IV line, the procedure is similar to that for administering medication through a secondary line (see Procedure 33.13). A primary line is set up and a secondary administration set is usually piggybacked to it. A solution of 5 % Dextrose in water (D_5W) is usually used in the primary line because it is the solution with which most medications are compatible. The exception to this rule is the diabetic patient for whom sugar is contraindicated; normal saline is used for these patients instead.

PROCEDURE 33.15

Converting an IV Line to an Intermittent Infusion Device

ACTION	RATIONALE
1. Check physician's order.	Ensures safety and avoids error.
2. Gather equipment: • Intermittent infusion device as per agency policy • Dilute heparin or normal saline in a syringe with a 22 gauge, 2.5 cm needle or a syringe cannula if using needleless IV access system • Sterile gauze sponges • Sterile protective cover • Alcohol swab • Gloves	Facilitates efficiency and economy of time.
3. Identify the patient and explain the procedure.	Avoids error and promotes patient well-being.
4. Wash hands and maintain sterile technique throughout the procedure.	Prevents the spread of microorganisms.
5. Ready the equipment. Remove the tape anchoring the IV tubing and place a gauze sponge under the connector site. Open the sterile packages containing the intermittent infusion device and the protective cover. Place them within easy reach.	Facilitates efficiency. The gauze sponge absorbs moisture.
6. Turn off the IV.	
7. Apply gloves.	Protects the nurse from backflow of blood during the conversion.
8. Grasp the hub of the venipuncture device firmly with the nondominant hand and, at the same time, apply pressure to the distal end of the catheter tip with the little finger. With the dominant hand, disconnect the IV tubing from the venipuncture device and quickly insert the male adapter plug, keeping all ends sterile.	Stabilizes the venipuncture device and prevents it from becoming displaced during the procedure. Prevents backflow from the venipuncture device.
9. Apply the sterile protective cover over the connecter end of the tubing.	Maintains sterility of the connector end between uses.
10. Clean the injection cap with alcohol.	Avoids possible contamination.
11. Slowly inject the normal saline or heparin flush solution.	Prevents trauma to the vein wall and avoids a burning sensation.
12. Do not recap needle. Discard directly into the nearest sharps container.	Prevents the potential for needlestick injury.
13. Ensure patient comfort, discard supplies, wash hands.	Promotes patient well-being and ensures cleanliness and a safe work environment.
14. Document the procedure, noting the time, the type of intermittent infusion device inserted, and the amount and type of flush solution.	Fulfills requirements for nurse accountability and promotes continuity of care.

Administering Medication Through an Intermittent Infusion Device Using an IV Line

ACTION	RATIONALE
1. If one has not been established, prepare a primary IV line as outlined in Procedure 22.1, Chapter 22. Place a protective covering over the connector end of the tubing.	Provides the IV line for the secondary medication set. Prepares for connection to the intermittent infusion device.
2. Prepare medication and secondary medication set as in Procedure 33.13. In addition gather, as per agency protocol: • 1 ml or 2 ml of normal saline solution in a syringe with a 22 gauge, 2.5 cm needle or needleless blunt syringe cannula • Alcohol swabs	Promotes efficiency and economy of time.
3. Connect the secondary medication set to the primary IV line as in Procedure 33.13. (This is done at the bedside if there is an existing primary IV line.)	
4. At the bedside, identify the patient.	Avoids error.
5. Cleanse the injection cap with alcohol and flush the device with normal saline.	Determines patency and placement of the venipuncture device. Checks patient comfort of the site.
6. Cleanse the injection cap with alcohol and connect the primary IV line. NOTE: If using an existing primary line, first attach a sterile 22 gauge, 2.5 cm needle or a needleless locking cannula to the connector end of the tubing.	Prevents entry of surface contaminants into the system. Ensures sterility of connector.
7. Establish the infusion from the primary line, then lower the primary container and open the roller clamp on the secondary tubing. Regulate the rate of flow.	Establishes flow of medication.
8. Monitor the patient and the infusion.	Ensures patient safety.
9. When the medication infusion is finished, prepare dilute heparin or normal saline solution as per agency policy.	Prepares for disconnection of primary IV line and flush procedure.
10. Close the roller clamp and disconnect the primary line. Remove and discard the needle into a sharps container. Place a sterile protective cover over the connector end of the tubing.	Maintains sterility of connector end between use.
11. Cleanse the injection cap with alcohol and slowly inject heparin or normal saline solution.	Maintains patency of the venipuncture device and vein.
12. Do not recap needles. Discard directly into the nearest sharps container.	Prevents the potential for needlestick injury.
13. Ensure patient comfort, discard supplies, wash hands and record medication.	Promotes patient well-being, prevents the spread of microorganisms and fulfills requirements for nurse accountability.

PROCEDURE 33.17

Administering an IV Push Medication Through an Intermittent Infusion Device

ACTION	RATIONALE
1. Prepare medication as in Procedure 33.14. In addition gather, as per agency policy: • Syringe with 1 ml to 2 ml normal saline • Syringe with 2 ml to 3 ml normal saline • Syringe with dilute heparin or normal saline solution • 3 22 gauge, 2.5 cm needles or needleless blunt syringe cannulas (one for each syringe) • Alcohol swabs	
2. At the bedside, identify the patient.	Ensures the right patient.
3. Inspect the IV site for redness, swelling, discharge, and ask if the patient is experiencing discomfort.	Assesses for inflammation and patency of site.
4. Sit on a chair or on the patient's bed and bring the extremity with the infusion device in close proximity.	IV push medications take several minutes and sitting will allow the nurse to use proper body mechanics and talk to patient.
5. Cleanse the injection cap with an alcohol swab each time a needle or needleless cannula is inserted.	Removes surface particles and prevents entry of contaminants into system.
6. Attach the syringe with 1 ml or 2 ml normal saline and flush the intermittent infusion device.	Determines patency and placement of the venipuncture device. Checks patient comfort of the site.
7. Administer the medication over the recommended period of time while monitoring the injection rate with a watch.	Permits the medication to disperse, decreasing irritation to the vein wall and promoting patient comfort. A bolus of medication delivered too fast may cause shock or embolism.
8. Attach the syringe with 2 ml to 3 ml normal saline and slowly instill the solution into the infusion device.	Flushes medication out of the venipuncture device, ensures medication is dispersed into the system and prevents a bolus effect.
9. Attach the syringe with dilute heparin or normal saline and slowly instill the solution.	Maintains patency of the venipuncture device and vein.
10. Do not recap needles. Discard directly into the nearest sharps container.	Prevents the potential for needlestick injury.
11. Ensure patient comfort, discard supplies, wash hands and record medication.	Promotes patient well-being, prevents the spread of microorganisms and fulfills requirements for nurse accountability.

TOPICAL APPLICATIONS

Medications may be applied to the skin or mucous membranes in the form of aerosol sprays and foams, creams, gels and jellies, liniments, lotions, ointments, pastes and powders.

Aerosol sprays provide a thin layer of medication onto a designated area. They are generally used when large areas of the skin are to be treated or when manual application would be uncomfortable for the patient.

Aerosol foams provide a layer of medicated foam and are generally used in hairy areas such as the rectum or vagina.

Application of Topical Medication

ACTION	RATIONALE
1. Follow the steps in Procedure 33.1.	
2. Gather equipment: • MAR or medication card • Container of prescribed medication • Sterile 5 cm × 5 cm gauze or cotton balls • Tongue depressor • Nonsterile gloves • Possibly sterile gloves and dressing tray if the area is covered	Facilitates efficiency and economy of time.
3. At the bedside, identify the patient.	Ensures the right patient.
4. Explain the procedure and purpose of medication.	Promotes patient well-being and enables participation in care.
5. Ensure the area to be treated is clean.	Removes drainage, reduces microorganisms and enhances effectiveness of application.
6. Observe the area for discharge, redness, swelling, bleeding or odour and ask if the patient is experiencing discomfort itchiness, burning.	Provides information that is necessary for ongoing evaluation of treatment.
7. Apply gloves, if necessary.	Gloves reduce transmission of microorganisms and adhere to body substance precautions. It is also often easier to apply some medications with gloves than with tongue depressors.
8. Place a small amount of medication on a sterile gauze or a tongue depressor. If a tongue depressor is used, do not return it to the container.	Prevents the transmission of microorganisms.
9. Apply the medication to the desired area according to package directions (for example, liniments should be rubbed in long smooth strokes).	Each preparation if different. Some require massage, others should be put on skin with minimal disruption of tissue.
10. Remove gloves: peel from the wrist downward, and collect one glove inside the other.	Prevents transmission of microorganisms.
11. Wash hands and apply a sterile dressing, if necessary.	Keeps medication from soiling bed linen and patient's gown.
12. Wash hands and record procedure.	Prevents the spread of microorganisms and meets requirements for nurse accountability.

Creams are semisolid, nongreasy, water-soluble preparations that are usually applied on an area where esthetics is a consideration or on moist areas.

Gels and *jellies* are semisolid preparations that are often clear or translucent. These preparations contain water or alcohol. They liquefy when applied to the skin and are especially useful for lubrication.

Liniments are liquids that are applied to the skin by rubbing. They are frequently used to warm an affected area through the superficial dilation of blood vessels. This also helps to relax tight muscles. The application of lotions or liniments is often a clean rather than a sterile procedure in a home situation. In a hospital or other inpatient facility, however, it is advisable to use sterile cotton balls or gauze to apply the liquid. More commonly, clean disposable gloves are worn on the hand being used for the application, unless the skin is broken, which would require the use of sterile gloves.

Lotions are liquid preparations that are usually applied to protect, soothe or soften surface areas; to relieve itching; or to prevent the growth of microorganisms.

Ointments are preparations with a fatty base, such as lard, petroleum jelly or oils. They may be applied to the skin or mucous membranes where they are melted by the heat of the body and absorbed. Ointments are frequently used for antiseptic or antimicrobial purposes. As with lotions and liniments, it is advisable in an institutional setting to use sterile equipment for the application of an ointment. Sterile gloves are not needed since the ointment is applied with a sterile tongue depressor.

Pastes are similar to ointments, but they do not penetrate the skin, they contain more powder and they are stiff in consistency. They may absorb secretions and provide protection from secretions such as urine and feces.

Powders are nonabsorbable, finely ground preparations that are applied as protection to reduce friction on dry areas. However, they cause clumping on wet areas and must be used selectively.

INSTILLATIONS INTO THE EAR

Instillation means to introduce small amounts (drops) of a medication into a body opening. Common sites for instillations are the ear, eye, nose, throat, vagina and rectum.

Liquid medications are instilled into the ear cavity usually for one of two purposes: to insert a softening agent so that earwax can be removed easily or to introduce an antibiotic suspension in cases where the ear canal or the eardrum is infected. The technique of instilling medication into the ear is presented in Procedure 33.19.

Assembling Equipment

A medicine tray, a sterile medicine dropper, the bottle of medication and some sterile cotton balls will be needed. Many preparations are packaged for individual use and come with an attached dropper.

The medication should always be warmed before being inserted into the ear. A temperature of 40.6° C is recommended. Cool solutions are not comfortable and may cause dizziness or nausea because the equilibrium sense receptors in the semicircular canals are stimulated. The bottle of ear drops may be placed in a small open container of warm water for a few minutes before it is to be used. The temperature of the solution may be tested by dropping a small amount on the inner aspect of the wrist. If it feels comfortable (neither hot nor cool), the solution should be comfortable for the patient.

PROCEDURE 33.19

Instilling Medication Into the Ear

ACTION	RATIONALE
1. Follow the steps in Procedure 33.1.	
2. Gather equipment: • MAR or medication card • Container of prescribed medication • Medicine tray • Sterile medicine dropper • Sterile cotton balls • Cotton tipped applicators	Facilitates efficiency and economy of time.
3. At the bedside, identify the patient.	Ensures the right patient.
4. Explain the procedure and the purpose of the medication to the patient.	Promotes patient well-being and enables participation in care.
5. Ask the patient to lie on the side with the ear to be treated facing upward.	Facilitates instillation and absorption of medication.

Continued on the next page

ACTION

6. Observe the auditory meatus for discharge, redness, swelling, bleeding or odour and ask if patient experiences discomfort, itchiness or burning.

7. Clean the auditory meatus with a cotton tipped applicator.

8. Draw medication into applicator.

9. With nondominant hand, straighten the auditory canal.
   Adult: *gently pull the pinna upward and back.*

Children under 3 years: *gently pull the pinna down and back.*

10. With dominant hand, instill the medication along the side of the ear canal, counting the correct number of drops.

11. Gently massage tragus (cartilaginous protrusion at the entrance to the ear canal).

12. Loosely place a cotton ball at the meatus of the auditory canal and leave there for 20 minutes. Encourage the patient to remain on the side for 5 minutes following treatment.

13. Wash hands and record the procedure.

RATIONALE

Provides information that is necessary for ongoing evaluation of treatment.

Removes any drainage.

Facilitates instillation and absorption.

The anatomy of the ear canal of adults and children is quite different and must be taken into account.

Facilitates distribution of medication into the ear canal.

Prevents medication from escaping out of the ear canal.

Prevents the transfer of microorganisms and meets requirements for nurse accountability.

INSTILLATIONS INTO THE EYE

Liquid medications in the form of eye drops or ointments are instilled into the eye for several reasons: to soothe the irritated eye, to dilate the pupil for an eye examination, to apply an anesthetic or to combat infection. It is best to use aseptic technique since the eye is vulnerable to infection. Eye medications should *never* be shared between patients. The technique for instilling medications into the eye is outlined in Procedure 33.20.

Assembling Equipment

Most eye medications come in bottles with their own dropper or in tubes of ointment. A soft cloth or cotton balls and warm water may be necessary to remove secretions and crusting on the eyelids.

PROCEDURE 33.20

Instilling Medications into the Eye

ACTION	RATIONALE
1. Follow the steps in Procedure 33.1.	
2. Gather equipment: • MAR or medication card • Prescribed eye drops or ointment • Medicine tray • Soft cloth or cotton balls • Warm water • Sterile eye pad if needed	Facilitates efficiency and economy of time.
3. At the bedside, identify the patient.	Ensures the right patient.
4. Explain the procedure and the purpose of the medication to the patient.	Promotes patient well-being and enables participation in care.
5. Cleanse secretions or crusts on the eyelid and lashes with a soft cloth or with cotton balls dipped in warm water.	Cleaning the eye will give the medication the opportunity to work, and it is more esthetically pleasing for the patient.
6. Give the patient a cotton ball or tissue to use after the instillation.	With some medications, it is necessary to block the nasolacrimal duct after liquid applications to prevent systemic effects. The cotton ball or tissue can also be used to catch excess medication and prevent it from running down the cheek.
7. If possible, have the patient sit or lie supine with the head tilted back.	Permits absorption of the medication into the canthus or cornea.
8. Observe the eye for redness, discharge, swelling. Ask if the patient experiences burning, itching, blurring diplopia or photophobia.	Provides information that is necessary for ongoing evaluation of treatment.
9. Open the medication container and, if there is a dropper, fill it with the prescribed amount of medication.	
10. Ask the patient to look towards the ceiling.	Lessens the urge to blink by partially protecting the cornea.

Continued on the next page

ACTION	RATIONALE
11. While resting the nondominant hand on the cheek and using the thumb and forefinger, gently pull downward on skin below the eye.	Exposes the conjunctiva and provides stability. Prevents fingers from poking cornea, does not put pressure on eyeball, and prevents the patient from blinking.

ACTION	RATIONALE
12. Hold the medication in the dominant hand and rest the hand on patient's forehead.	Provides stability and prevents the potential for poking the cornea.
13. **Eye drops:** Squeeze the bulb of the dropper gently being careful to dispense only the required amount of drops. **Ointment:** Gently squeeze the tube to fill the length of lower canthus moving from inner to outer canthus.	
14. Ask the patient to close the eye for 2–3 minutes, but avoid tightly squeezing the eye shut.	Allows medication to absorb and disperse. Squeezing the eye will force the medication out of the eye.
15. Instruct the patient to block the nasolacrimal duct for 30 seconds.	Prevents medication from running out of eye and into duct.
16. Gently wipe the eyes from inner to outer canthus.	Collects excess medication.
17. If necessary, apply a sterile eye pad.	
18. Wash hands and record procedure.	Prevents transmission of microorganisms and meets requirements for nurse accountability.

INSTILLATIONS INTO THE NOSE

The usual purpose of instilling medication into the nose is either to heal infection or to shrink swollen membranes. The instillation of medication into the nose is not usually a sterile procedure. The technique is presented in Procedure 33.21.

Assembling Equipment

Nasal instillations may be in the form of drops, administered with a dropper that is attached to the medication bottle. They may also come in the form of an inhaler or an atomizer.

PROCEDURE 33.21

Instilling Medications into the Nose

ACTION	RATIONALE
1. Follow the steps in Procedure 33.1	
2. Gather equipment:	Facilitates efficiency and economy of time.
• MAR or medication card	
• Prescribed medication with dropper	
• Medicine tray	
• Towel or tissues	
3. At the bedside, identify the patient.	Ensures the right patient.
4. Explain the procedure and the purpose of the medication to the patient.	Promotes patient well-being and enables participation in care.
5. Ask the patient to blow the nose and assess the discharge noting colour, consistency and odour.	Provides information that is necessary for ongoing evaluation of treatment.
Ask the patient to describe any congestion or difficulty breathing, and note facial discomfort and any discharge from the nares.	
6. Position the patient according to the area to be used.	
Eustachian tube: back-lying position. The drops will flow into the nasopharynx.	Eustachian tube opens into the nasopharynx.
Ethmoid and sphenoid sinuses: Proetz position. That is, back-lying with the head over the edge of the bed or place a pillow under the shoulders to tip the head backwards.	Allows drainage into ethmoid and sphenoid sinuses.

Maxillary and frontal sinuses: Parkinson position. That is, the same as Proetz position except that the head is turned to the side to be treated. Assure patient comfort by supporting the head.

Allows drainage into maxillary and frontal sinuses.

Continued on the next page

PROCEDURE 33.21
continued

ACTION

7. Draw up prescribed amount of solution into dropper.

8. With the dropper slightly above the nostril, instill the medication towards the midline. Do not touch the mucous membranes of the nares with dropper.

9. Ask the patient to remain in the position for 5–10 minutes.

10. Reassess the patient immediately and when medication is expected to be effective.

11. Leave the patient comfortable.

12. Wash hands and record procedure.

RATIONALE

Allows maximum solution to be absorbed. Touching mucous membranes with dropper would contaminate it and cause potential cross-contamination of the medication.

Allows the solution to disperse into the entire area.

Provides information for evaluation of care.

Prevents transmission of microorganisms and meets requirements for nurse accountability.

INSTILLATIONS INTO THE THROAT

The throat may be either sprayed or painted as means of applying an antiseptic or an anesthetic. The steps in administering medications into the throat are outlined in Procedure 33.22.

Assembling Equipment

Cotton tipped applicators are used to paint medications onto tissues of the throat. A tongue depressor is needed to keep the tongue out of the way. A flashlight will help to visualize the area.

PROCEDURE 33.22

Administering a Medication into the Throat

ACTION	RATIONALE
1. Follow the steps in Procedure 33.1	
2. Gather equipment: • MAR or medication card • Prescribed medication • Medicine tray • Cotton tipped applicators • Tongue depressor • Flashlight	Facilitates efficiency and economy of time.
3. At the bedside, identify the patient.	Ensures the right patient.
4. Explain the procedure and the purpose of the medication to the patient.	Promotes patient well-being and enables participation in care.
5. Ask the patient to sit upright. Stand directly in front of the patient and look down into the throat. A good light is essential for this procedure.	Provides the best position to visualize and instill the medication.
6. Ask the patient to tilt the head backward (or help him or her to do this) and to open his or her mouth. Using the nondominant hand, hold down the tongue with a tongue depressor.	Permits the nurse to visualize the throat.
7. Apply the spray or medication, using either an atomizer for spraying or cotton tipped applicators for painting the tissues.	Ensures the prescribed dose has been delivered.
8. Inspect the area and ensure the entire area has been covered.	Promotes patient well-being.
9. Leave the patient comfortable.	
10. Wash hands and record procedure.	Prevents transmission of microorganisms and meets requirements for nurse accountability.

INSTILLATIONS INTO THE VAGINA

Medications are usually instilled into the vagina to combat infection or to relieve discomfort. They may be applied in the form of a suppository or an ointment. Suppositories are inserted with the index finger of the nurse's gloved hand. Ointments for use in the vagina usually come in a narrow tube with an attached plunger. Procedure 33.23 outlines the steps for administering vaginal instillations.

Assembling Equipment

In addition to the medications, the nurse will need clean gloves. A water-soluble lubricant will be necessary for suppositories that do not come prelubricated. A perineal pad may be used to absorb any leakage.

PROCEDURE 33.23

Administering a Medication into the Vagina

ACTION	RATIONALE
1. Follow the steps in Procedure 33.1	
2. Gather equipment: • MAR or medication card • Prescribed vaginal cream or suppository • Lubricant, if necessary • Clean gloves • Perineal pad, if necessary	Facilitates efficiency and economy of time.
3. At the bedside, identify the patient.	Ensures the right patient.
4. Explain the procedure and the purpose of the medication to the patient.	Promotes patient well-being and enables participation in care.
5. Ask the patient to void prior to the procedure and, if possible, to wash the perineum.	An empty bladder will promote patient comfort. A clean perineum facilitates accurate assessment. A clean surface promotes absorption.
6. Ensure privacy.	Promotes patient well-being and decreases embarrassment.
7. Apply gloves.	Prevents the spread of microorganisms and adheres to body substance precautions.
8. Ask the patient to lie on her back with knees flexed and hips rotated laterally. If the patient can tolerate it, place a pillow under the hips. Drape the patient so that only the perineum is exposed.	A pillow will help to prevent the medication from leaking out. Ensures comfort and warmth and decreases embarrassment.
9. Observe the vagina and perineum for redness, lesions, discharge or odours. Ask if patient experiences discomfort, itchiness, burning or other symptoms.	Provides information that is necessary for ongoing evaluation of treatment.
10. **Vaginal suppository:** Remove the suppository from the package, lubricate it if necessary.	Facilitates insertion and decreases discomfort.
Using the nondominant hand, separate the labia majora and minora. With the middle and forefinger of the dominant hand, insert the suppository approximately 8–10 cm along the posterior wall of the vagina.	Exposes the vaginal orifice. The posterior aspect of the vagina is longer than the anterior wall, because of the protrusion of the cervix into the anterior wall.
Vaginal cream, jelly, foam: Using manufacturer's directions, instill the required amount of medication into the applicator. Insert the applicator approximately 5 cm and slowly inject the plunger until medication has been distributed. Remove the applicator and place it on a paper towel or directly into garbage.	
11. Remove gloves: peel from the wrist down and collect one glove inside the other.	Turning the gloves inside out will minimize spread of the vaginal discharge and microorganisms.
12. Assist the patient to straighten her legs, and instruct her to remain supine for 10 minutes following treatment.	Returns the patient to a position of comfort and ensures the medication will be absorbed into the posterior fornix once it has melted.
13. Apply a clean perennial pad.	
14. Wash hands and record procedure.	Prevents the spread of microorganisms and meets requirements for nurse accountability.

INSTILLATIONS INTO THE RECTUM

Medications are inserted into the rectum to provide local or systemic effects. Rectal suppositories are commonly used to stimulate bowel function. The steps in administering a rectal instillation are given in Procedure 33.24.

Assembling Equipment

The medication, clean gloves, water-soluble lubricant and a disposable incontinent pad will be needed. If the suppository is used to stimulate defecation in a patient, a commode or toilet should be in close proximity.

PROCEDURE 33.24

Administering a Medication into the Rectum

ACTION	RATIONALE
1. Follow the steps in Procedure 33.1.	
2. Gather equipment: • MAR or medication card • Prescribed suppository • Lubricant, if necessary • Clean gloves • Incontinent pad	Facilitates efficiency and economy of time.
3. At the bedside, identify the patient.	Ensures the right patient.
4. Explain the procedure and the purpose of the medication to the patient.	Promotes patient well-being and enables participation in care.
5. Provide privacy and ask the patient to lie on the left side with knees flexed.	In this position, the sigmoid is in the lowest position and decreases the potential for feces to be expelled.
6. Drape the patient so that only the buttocks are exposed.	Ensures comfort and warmth and decreases embarrassment.
7. Apply gloves	Prevents the spread of microorganisms.
8. Assess the anal area for redness, swelling, lesions, hemorrhoids, discharge and odour and ask if patient experiences any burning, itchiness or discomfort.	Provides information that is necessary for ongoing evaluation of treatment.
9. Remove the suppository from the wrapper and, if necessary, lubricate it. Lubricate the middle finger of the dominant hand.	Facilitates insertion.
10. Ask the patient to breathe through the mouth. Touch the anal sphincter with middle finger.	Facilitates relaxation of anal sphincter.
11. Using the middle finger, insert the suppository into the anal sphincter (small pointed end first) as far as possible along the wall of the rectum. This will be approximately 10 cm for an adult and 5 cm for a child.	The middle finger is the longest and will be able to insert the farthest. The pointed end will facilitate insertion and decrease discomfort. The suppository will be absorbed by the mucosa of the wall of the rectum.
12. Remove the finger and peel off the glove by pulling down from the wrist and turning it inside out.	Reduces possibility for transmission of microorganisms.
13. Cover the patient and advise him or her to lie in this position for up to 30 minutes (if possible).	Facilitates absorption of the medication.

SPECIAL CHALLENGES IN ADMINISTERING MEDICATIONS

Alterations in Consciousness or Orientation

It is important for the nurse to assess for and report *any* difficulties that are encountered when administering a medication, as they could lead to further problems for the patient. For example, a patient with a decreased level of consciousness may not have a gag reflex and is at risk for aspirating an oral medication. The nurse may request that another route be ordered or that a feeding tube be inserted. Similarly, the disoriented patient may simply refuse to swallow an oral medication. The nurse must consider other routes, and also whenever possible give medications when the patient is most alert and oriented.

Illness

Some illnesses do not affect the patients ability to take and retain medications, others do. The nauseated patient may not be able to retain oral medications. In this instance, an antiemetic may be administered one hour prior to the administration of other oral medications, or another route may be considered. On the other hand, some patients are so fatigued that it is overwhelming to attempt to swallow numerous oral medications. The nurse can often work around this by offering medications at spaced intervals throughout the day, giving the medications when the patient has the most energy or considering another route.

Other Potential Challenges

Another area of nursing practice is concerned with idiosyncratic reactions to medications, overdoses of drugs and the ingestion of poisonous materials. Many medical centres provide immediate information to people about the antidotes and emergency measures for common poisons. Poison control centres are located in many large cities. A list of poison control centres in Canada is contained in the *Compendium of Pharmaceuticals and Specialties of Canada* (CPS).

EVALUATING MEDICATION ADMINISTRATION

After the administration of any therapeutic agent, the nurse should observe the patient for effectiveness and reaction. The criteria by which the nurse judges the effectiveness of a medication are dependent upon the purpose for which it

Quick Guide to Evaluating the Effectiveness of Medications

1. Is the patient taking the medicines that have been prescribed?
2. Have the medications been administered safely?
3. Does the patient show signs or symptoms which indicate that the medications are effective (or ineffective)?
4. Has the administration of the medications been accurately reported on the patient's record? Have pertinent observations been recorded and reported to appropriate personnel?

Quick Guide to Safe Medication Administration

1. Does the patient have any allergies?
2. How old is the patient?
3. What medications have been prescribed for the patient?
4. Why is the patient receiving these medications?
5. What observations should the nurse make relative to the effect of these medications on the patient?
6. Are specific nursing measures indicated because of the action of drugs contained in these medications?
7. How are the patient's medications to be administered?
8. What precautions should be taken in administering these medications? Are there special precautions that should be taken because of the patient's age, physical condition or mental state?
9. Do any of the medications require special precautionary measures for administration?
10. Does the patient have learning needs relative to medicinal therapy?
11. Does the patient or family require specific skills or knowledge in order to continue medicinal therapy at home?

was administered. It can be the alleviation of pain, the reduction of fever, a decrease in swelling or even the appearance of orange-coloured urine. These are anticipated results and they reflect the effectiveness of the particular medication. The observations are recorded in detail on the patient's chart. Adverse reactions to the medication are always reported to the charge nurse and the physician. If a reaction is severe, that is, if the patient is acutely uncomfortable or essential body functions are impaired, the physician is notified immediately so that measures to stop the reaction can begin. In severe allergic reactions, the tissues of the throat may become so edematous that breathing is difficult. Prompt intervention at the earliest sign of an allergic reaction is required. These reactions are also recorded in detail on the patient's chart.

ILLEGAL USE OF DRUGS

While drug abuse can result from the use of drugs for therapeutic purposes, it is a more widespread problem among those who use drugs illegally. Experimentation with drugs such as marijuana, hashish, cocaine and alcohol is common among young people under the influence of peer groups. It may constitute both a new experience and an "escape from reality" for the user.

There is a considerable lack of public understanding about the effects of drug abuse. Professional controversy exists regarding the consequences of the use of "soft" drugs such as marijuana, both in regard to the direct effects of these drugs and in regard to the question of whether use of these drugs leads to use of "hard" drugs. Attempts are under way by several groups to decriminalize the possession and use of marijuana. However, it is clear that marijuana, like alcohol, can severely impair the user's ability to drive and can lead to automobile accidents.

Health professionals are in contact with drug users in all types of settings. However, the effects of "hard" drugs such as cocaine, heroin and LSD (lysergic acid diethylamide) are seen and dealt with more and more in overdose or emergency units. These drugs are mind-altering and mood-changing. The sense of being "high" on these drugs is usually followed by a "low" or hangover of some type, which may be difficult for the patient to cope with alone. Someone may be needed to "guide" or "talk down" the person on an LSD "trip" who is hallucinating badly and experiencing a distorted sense of reality.

As we mentioned earlier in the book, drug overdose has become a leading cause of death among teenagers. Drug overdoses often seen in emergency units include both accidental overdoses of illegal drugs and deliberate attempts at suicide, which may involve the use of either illegal drugs or prescribed sedatives. The combination of sedatives with alcohol is particularly dangerous.

On the other hand, several drugs that are widely used illegally may also have uses in medical therapy. Cocaine and morphine are used as anesthetics, and it has been proposed by some people that heroin, which like morphine is derived from opium, should be used to alleviate pain in terminally ill patients. Marijuana is currently administered to some cancer patients to lessen the nausea and vomiting that often accompany radiation therapy and chemical therapy. Marijuana has also been proposed as a treatment for the eye disease glaucoma.

KEY TERMS

medication p. 1092
pharmacology p. 1092
trade (brand/proprietary) name p. 1092
chemical name p. 1092
generic name p. 1092
pharmacodynamics p. 1092
agonists p. 1093
antagonists p. 1093
pharmacokinetics p. 1093
onset of action p. 1093

peak action (peak effect) p. 1093
half-life p. 1093
duration of action p. 1093
plateau p. 1093
therapeutic effect p. 1093
systemic effect p. 1093
local effect p. 1093
adverse reactions (side effects) p. 1093
allergic reaction p. 1093
anaphylactic reaction p. 1094

drug toxicity p. 1094
drug tolerance p. 1094
drug interactions p. 1094
additive effect p. 1094
synergistic (potentiating) effect p. 1094
antagonistic effect p. 1094
stat order p. 1100
prn order p. 1100

IN REVIEW

Throughout history, medications prepared from pharmaceutical agents have been used to promote, maintain and restore health. Often referred to as "drugs" or "medicines," they are ordered in most instances by a physician. The administration of medications is, however, a therapeutic nursing function and the nurse has a legal responsibility to do so safely. This means the nurse must have knowledge and understanding of pharmacology; knowledge and skill in assessing the patients' health status; skill in preparing, administering and recording medications; and skill in monitoring the effectiveness of their action. It also means implementing nursing interventions to enhance the therapy, minimize adverse reactions and promote patient safety and well-being.

Each drug usually has at least three names: its trade name, a chemical name and a generic name. Drugs manufactured by different companies may be marketed under several different trade names.

Drugs act by replacing missing or deficient substances, altering the cell environment or affecting the rate of cellular function. The drug reaction in the body is influenced by the dose of the drug reaching its target site and by pharmacokinetics — the absorption, distribution, metabolism and excretion of the drug. In order to maintain the drug at a therapeutic level in the blood, dosages must be repeated at regular intervals. The length of time between intervals depends on the half-life of the drug.

The determinants of drug action and effects include age, sex, body weight and size, genetic makeup, presence of disease or illness, medication history, psychological factors and time of administration as well as environmental conditions. Because drugs can cause adverse effects or allergic reactions, all patients should be monitored. Special monitoring is necessary for pregnant women, infants, children and older adults, all of whom may react unpredictably to a medication. Older adults are particularly prone to problems with medications because of failing vision, lessened efficiency of excretion of drugs and the possibility of malnourishment and dehydration. They may have multiple conditions with different physicians' orders resulting in possible drug interactions exacerbated by the widespread use of over-the-counter drugs. Older adults may become confused about dosages and administration times, they may have idiosyncratic reactions and they may even take an intentional overdose.

In Canada, all aspects of drug production, distribution, advertising and sale are governed by the Federal Food and Drug Act and the Federal Narcotics Control Act, with some provinces having additional drug legislation. Provincial Nursing Acts outline the nurse's legal responsibility regarding medications. Each nurse must understand the requirements in her or his jurisdiction.

Drugs are derived either from natural substances (plants, animals or inorganic substances) or from synthetic chemicals. They must be standardized by the manufacturers to recognized pharmacopeiae. Once approved for use in Canada, they are entered into the Compendium of Pharmaceuticals and Specialities, a drug reference book compiled and revised annually by the Canadian Pharmetical Association. An international pharmacopoeia of important drugs used in many countries is published by the World Health Organization.

All health care agencies have their own policies and procedures for the ordering, processing, communicating, storing and dispensing of medications so that standard procedures are followed throughout the agency. Before administering a new drug, the nurse should know its classification and main action, key adverse effects, safe dosage limits and nursing considerations. These can be obtained from the CPS, the drug formulary, the pharmacy department, physicians, commercial drug information and professional journals. Medication orders may be self-terminating or standing orders, either of which is invalid without the required information about patient, drug, dosage, frequency, route of administration and prescriber's signature.

The nurse is obligated to question any drug or dosage order that is ambiguous or felt to be unsafe. The nurse is also responsible for checking the original order for the medications of her or his patients to be sure of the validity of the order and to verify that no mistakes have been made in the transfer of information. Agencies use many different methods to minimize errors and maximize efficiency. The nurse should always follow the "five rights" in giving medications — the right drug, the right dose, the right time, the right route, and the right patient. A medication error must be reported to the charge nurse and physician immediately it is detected so that patient safety can be protected. Unusual occurrence forms are usually required for reporting the error.

Controlled drugs are stored in locked containers, and distribution is closely managed because of the strict government regulations. Controlled drugs are recorded on the patients' record and also in the "narcotics book." At designated times during every 24 hours, the dosages administered and wasted plus the remaining stored drugs are counted to ensure that the total equals the amount assigned to the nursing unit. The narcotic count is usually checked by two nurses and any discrepancy reported immediately.

When the dosage ordered of a drug is different from the dosage supplied, the nurse needs mathematical skills to compute the exact dosage. Calculating drug dosages can be done by the apothecary, household or metric systems and the nurse must be able to convert from one to another as well as calculate the dosages. This is particularly so with pediatric drug orders which are usually calculated by body surface areas (BSA).

A nursing history includes assessment of the medication-related needs of the patient (including medication and medical history) and actual or potential problems that might influence the effectiveness of a drug, as, for example, visual problems or mental confusion could limit a patient's ability for self-administration of drugs at home after discharge from hospital. In order to assess the effectiveness or adverse effects of many drugs it is necessary to monitor the patient's vital signs and/or laboratory tests, particularly with drugs that have a narrow therapeutic index since dosages are calculated according to laboratory results.

Many problems associated with drug therapy are collaborative problems which require accurate observation of the patient to assess the effectiveness of the therapy as well as adverse effects. Potential problems that may be prevented independently by nurses are labelled *High risk for injury related to .....* Nurses must also be aware of personal concerns, cultural values and religious beliefs which may cause difficulties for patients to accept the therapy or maintain it at home. Common nursing diagnoses include *Knowledge deficit, Altered health maintenance, Ineffective management of therapeutic regime, High risk for injury related to patient problems such as inability to read, difficulty in swallowing, or inability to handle medication supplies or equipment, a history of substance abuse or unhealthy lifestyles.*

Patient education and supportive care are key nursing strategies to promote optimal health. The goals or expected outcomes of teaching self-administration of medications are that the patient can repeat information on the drug and its intended results, on any adverse effects, on the exact dosage and reasons for it, and that the patient is able to safely and correctly carry out the procedure. If the patient is unable to administer the drug, a family member or a friend may be taught to do so.

Medications are administered orally, sublingually, parenterally or topically, and by inhalation, instillation or suppository. Sterile equipment and supplies and aseptic technique must be used for all parenteral administration because the skin barrier is broken and the danger of infection is always present. After parenteral injections, needles are NOT recapped but deposited immediately in a sharps container and NEVER in the garbage. Patients having multiple injections should have the sites rotated in an orderly fashion.

Intramuscular injections are given into anatomically safe sites which avoid large blood vessels and nerves. With irritating medications, the needle is changed after the solution is drawn into the syringe and the Z-track method is usually used.

Intravenous medications may be delivered by adding a medication to a primary solution, by means of secondary tubing (piggyback set-up), or by injection directly into the existing intravenous line (push method). An intermittent infusion device may be used for patients who require frequent but not continuous intravenous infusions or medications. Because of their immediate effect, adverse reactions occur quickly; careful prechecking and careful monitoring are essential.

After the administration of any medication, the nurse observes the patient for effectiveness and reactions, and documents any changes. When there is an untoward reaction, the symptoms are reported to the charge nurse and the physician promptly so necessary intervention can be started.

LEARNING ACTIVITIES

1. **Case Study:** You are a home care nurse assigned to an 86-year-old lady whose memory is failing and who has difficulty reading because of poor eyesight. She tells you she has to take medications for a heart ailment, for high blood pressure, for joint pain and for indigestion. How can you help this lady effectively manage her medication regimen?

2. In the health agency in which you are having clinical practice, find out the following information:

    a. The method of ordering medications for patients.

    b. The methods of processing and communicating medication orders.

    c. The location of medications on a nursing unit, storage facilities and system for arranging medications.

    d. The equipment used for preparing and administering medications.

    e. Safety precautions taken in the preparation and administration of medications.

    f. The approved method of recording medications by various administration routes, including narcotic and controlled drugs.

    g. The location of resources and reference material on drugs.

    h. Pertinent agency policies regarding the administration of medications.

REFERENCES AND READINGS

AARONSON, L.S. and MACNEE, C.L. (1989). Tobacco, alcohol, and caffeine use during pregnancy. *JOGNN, 18*(4), 279–287.

ANDERS, J. and MOELLER, P. (1982). Topicals: What to use, how to apply. *RN, 44*(9), 32.

BEHRMAN, R.E. and NELSON, V.C. (1987). *Nelson textbook of pediatrics*. Philadelphia: Saunders.

CARPENITO, L.J. (1993). *Nursing diagnosis: Application to clinical practice*. Philadelphia: Lippincott.

CLAYTON, B.D., STOCK, Y.N. and SQUIRE, J.E. (1985). *Basic pharmacology for nurses* (8th ed.). St. Louis: Mosby.

DICKERSON, R. (1992). 10 tips for easing the pain of intramuscular injections. *Nursing 92, 22*(8), 55.

DRASS, J. (1992) What you need to know about insulin injections. *Nursing 92, 22*(11), 40–43.

DRURY, M. (1985). *Diabetes mellitus.* (2nd ed.) Oxford: Blackwell Scientific.

EARNEST, V.V. (1993). *Clinical skills in nursing practice* (2nd ed.). Philadelphia: Lippincott.

EDMOND, M., KHAKOO, R., McTAGGART, B. and SOLOMON, R. (1990). Effect of bedside needle disposal unit on needle recapping frequency and needlestick injury. *Canadian Intravenous Nurses Association, 6*(1), 10–11.

FLYNN, J.B.M. and HACKEL, R. (1990). *Technological foundations in nursing.* Norwalk, CT: Appleton & Lange.

FORD, C. (1990). Disposal of sharps. *Journal of Intravenous Nursing*, 13(1), 42–47.

HART, S.J. (1993). Drug administration. In Springhouse. *Nursing procedures: Student version.* Springhouse, PA: Springhouse.

HEALTH AND WELFARE CANADA. (1991). *Health protection and drug laws.* Ottawa: Minister Supply and Services Canada. (Health and Welfare Canada Catalogue No. H49–5/1991E)

HUSSAR, D. (1993). Reviewing drug interactions. *Nursing 93, 23*(9), 50–57.

IV THERAPY (1990): CLINICAL SKILLBUILDERS. Springhouse, PA: Springhouse.

JOHNSON, G.E., HANNAH, K.J. and ZERR, S.R. (1992). *Pharmacology and the nursing process* (3rd ed.). Philadelphia: Saunders.

KEE, J.L. and HAYES, E.R. (1993). *Pharmacology: A nursing process approach.* Philadelphia: Saunders.

KEEN, M. (1986). Comparison of intramuscular injection techniques to reduce site discomfort and lesions. *Nursing Research*, 35(4), 207–210.

KNOR, E. R. (1987). Substance abuse. In E. R. Knor (Ed.). *Decision making in obstetrical nursing.* Toronto: B.C. Decker, 56–59.

LEHMANN, S. and BARBER, J. (1991). Giving medications by feeding tube. *Nursing 91,* 21(11), 58–61.

MACISAAC, A., RIVERS, R. and ADAMSON, C. (1989). Multiple medications – is your elderly patient caught in the storm? *Nursing 89, 19*(7), 60–64.

MAILHOT, R. (1986). The Canadian drug regulatory process. *Journal of Clinical Pharmacology, 26,* 232–239.

MATTESON, M. and McCONNELL, E. (1988).*Gerontological nursing – concepts and practice.* Philadelphia: Saunders.

McGOVERN, K. (1992) 10 golden rules for administering drugs safely. *Nursing 92, 22*(3), 49–56.

McKENRY, L. and SALERNO, E. (1989). *Mosby's pharmacology in nursing.* (17th ed.). St. Louis: Mosby.

MORRISON, R. (1993). Medication non-compliance. *The Canadian Nurse, 89*(4),15–18.

NAEYE, R. (1981). Influence of maternal cigarette smoking during pregnancy on fetal and childhood growth. *Obstetrics and Gynecology, 57*(1), 18–21.

NEWTON, M., NEWTON, D. and FUDIN, J. (1992). Reviewing the "big three" injection routes. *Nursing 92, 22*(2), 34–42.

O'DONNELL, J. (1992). Understanding adverse drug reactions. *Nursing 92, 22*(8), 34–40.

PETROSINO, B.M., CHRISTIAN, B.J., WOLF, J. and BECKER, H. (1989). Implications of selected problems with nasoenteral tube feedings. *Critical Care Nursing Quarterly, 12*(3), 1-18.

SHIONO, P., KLEBANOFF, M. and RHOADS, G. (1986). Smoking and drinking during pregnancy: Their effects on preterm birth. *JAMA, 255*(1), 82–84.

SHLAFER, M. (1993). *The nurse, pharmacology, and drug therapy: A prototype approach* (2nd ed.). Redwood City, CA: Addison-Wesley.

WEBBER-JONES, J. (1992, April). How to declog a feeding tube. *Nursing 92, 22*(4), 62–64.

WHALEY, L. and WONG, D. (1991). *Nursing care of infants and children* (4th ed.). St. Louis: Mosby.

Psychosocial Needs

Sexuality Needs

OUTLINE

CENTRAL QUESTIONS

1. What is sexuality?

2. Is there a difference between sex and sexuality?

3. What are the structures and functions of the male and the female reproductive systems?

4. What are the four phases of the human sexual response cycle?

5. What are the major determinants of sexual functioning?

6. How do sexuality needs vary throughout the life cycle?

7. What are some sexual behaviours, orientations and variations?

8. What are some common sexual concerns and problems?

9. What basic principles does the nurse apply in assisting individuals to meet sexuality needs?

10. How does the nurse assess an individual's sexuality needs?

11. What are the common nursing diagnostic statements for patients with sexuality problems?

12. How does the nurse develop a plan of care for individuals with sexuality problems?

13. What strategies might the nurse implement in helping individuals, families or groups promote and protect sexual health?

14. How does the nurse assist in providing restorative and supportive care for individuals with sexuality problems?

15. How does the nurse evaluate the patient's response to nursing interventions?

INTRODUCTION

The recognition and acceptance of sexuality as an important aspect of health and well-being is a relatively recent development. Prior to the twentieth century, sexual intercourse was thought to be for procreation and not pleasure, at least as far as women were concerned. Sexual mores were dictated by religious and cultural doctrines alone and it was considered inappropriate for a woman to initiate or enjoy sexual activity. As the disciplines of psychiatry and psychology developed, and beginning with the work of Freud and others, an interest in sexuality as a separate concept emerged and evolved into the science of sexology. The Kinsey Reports (1948 and 1953) and the works of researchers such as Masters, Johnson and Kolodny in the 1960s did much to provide a clearer understanding of sexual attitudes and practices and to encourage open discussion of sexuality. This stage in the development of sexology was dominated by a biomedical model which did not deal with the psychosocial aspects of sexuality. Furthermore, it was a common belief that female sexuality should be a "mirror image" of male sexuality, without consideration of the vast differences in male and female sexual needs. For example, from a male perspective, "normal" sexual behaviour was believed to be coital activity which resulted in orgasm. In developed countries today, however, the sexual needs of women are beginning to be viewed as distinctly different from those of men. Safety, trust, intimacy and sensuality are considered to be more important to women than the physical aspects of sex alone. Unfortunately, in some areas of the world, women are not yet allowed sexual rights and are still legally considered the property of their husbands.

In 1975, the World Health Organization recognized sexuality as a health entity. It defined sexual health as "the integration of the somatic, emotional, intellectual, and social aspects in ways that are positively enriching and that will enhance personality, communication, and love" (WHO, 1975, 2). Furthermore, WHO recommended that health care professionals become involved in the education, counselling and treatment of sexual health problems (WHO, 1975).

Social developments in the latter half of the twentieth century have increased public awareness of sexuality and the sexual needs of people. Television, music videos and movies provide a source of education about sexuality for many people, particularly children and adolescents. Whether these sources are positive or negative depends upon the content and the context in which they are viewed. Political and social pressures from factions in society opposed to sexuality education and reproductive choice have resulted in limited access to safe, effective birth control measures and to safe, legal abortion in many areas of the world. HIV infection (which leads to AIDS) and Hepatitis B viral infections, the results of which may be fatal, have emerged as major health and social problems, along with other health-damaging sexually transmitted infections. There is an increasing incidence of child sexual abuse and sexual assault — crimes which have devastating effects on the emotional and physical health of victims unless effective intervention is available.

All of these developments present a strong challenge to providers of sexual health education and services. There is a need to counteract negative influences and inaccurate information, while empowering people to care for their own sexual and reproductive health. The challenge for nurses in promoting sexual and reproductive health or in providing restorative care when sexual problems occur is to be a helpful, accurate and culturally sensitive resource. Comfort, competence, confidence and a nonjudgemental attitude will enable nurses to address issues related to sexual needs of individuals in an appropriate and professional manner. Talking to someone about sex and sexuality is not easy. In order to deal competently with the sexuality needs of patients, nurses must first of all feel comfortable discussing sexuality with others. A solid base of knowledge and understanding of sexuality and sexual health problems will help to reduce a nurse's discomfort in this area. Nurses must also examine their own values and beliefs around sexuality and be able to recognize situations where personal biases could interfere with meeting the needs of patients. An awareness of the changing sexual needs throughout the life cycle and a sensitivity to variations in values, beliefs and behaviours will enhance the nurse's effectiveness in providing care.

HUMAN SEXUALITY

"Where do babies come from?"

"I'm 13 and my period hasn't started yet. All my friends have theirs. What's wrong with me?"

"Is it harmful for a man to get all excited and then nothing happens?"

"I'm a virgin. Is intercourse always painful at first for the woman?"

"I'm 70 now and I guess sex shouldn't even be on my mind anymore."

"I feel inadequate, less than a woman, because I can't conceive a baby."

"I look like a man, but inside I feel like a woman."

Questions and statements such as these reflect concerns of individuals with regard to sexuality. Human sexuality is a multifaceted phenomenon which "encompasses the biological, psychological, social, cultural, and ethical aspects of sexual behaviour" (Knowlton, 1988, 420). It involves two related concepts — sex and sexuality. **Sex** refers to the

KEY PRINCIPLES

Principles of Human Sexuality

1. Sexuality is an integral aspect of the human personality.
2. Sexuality is a life-long component of the personality.
3. The components of sexuality include physical, biological, psychological, social and cultural aspects.
4. Everyone has the right to be recognized as a sexual being, regardless of age, physical, emotional or cognitive status, or sexual orientation.
5. Sexuality may be expressed in many physical and emotional ways, only one of which is sexual intercourse.
6, Everyone has the right to consent to activity related to sexuality or reproduction.
7. Everyone has the right to possess personal values.
8. No one has the right to impose sexual values on another person.

biological distinctions that identify a person as male or female based on the characteristics of the sex organs. This is called **biological sexual identity**. Sex also refers to the sexual functions for reproduction and pleasure, namely sexual intercourse. **Sexuality** is a broad concept which brings together the expression of self and the totality of feelings, attitudes, beliefs and behaviours related to being male or female. Sexuality is expressed in how people relate to others, how they dress and look, how they behave and how they express feelings of intimacy, tenderness and love. It includes the need for emotional attachment with another human being, for tenderness, intimacy and affection, for sensuality and for procreation (Knowlton, 1988).

The concept of sexuality includes a number of components. **Gender definition** or **identity** is the perception of self as a male or female. This definition may or may not coincide with one's biological sexual identity as in the case of the man who said, "I have a man's body but inside I feel like a woman." **Gender role identity** refers to behaviours identified by one's culture as appropriate to that gender, in other words, how a person behaves as a male or female. It includes all of the learned behaviours pertaining to masculinity or femininity, sexual behaviours and orientations (how sexuality is expressed) and sexual relationships (how sexuality is shared). Sexuality also includes attitudes and values, feelings and judgements that people have about sex-

ual behaviour. And it includes choices people make about reproduction (whether or not to become a parent) and about sexual pleasure (whether or not to engage in a physical relationship with a sexual partner).

Human sexuality exists in two dimensions: private and public. The private dimension includes feelings, values and beliefs that are very personal. The public dimension manifests itself through behaviours that are influenced by values and beliefs and may disclose how the person is feeling. Illness, chronic disease or disability can have an impact on both dimensions. For example, someone who holds the belief that sexuality is limited to the domain of healthy, able-bodied, young people may be devastated by the onset of a debilitating disease or disability. In the public dimension, this same person may also develop poor personal hygiene and grooming as well as a "what's the use?" attitude.

Sexuality pervades virtually every aspect of life, from birth to death. It is an integral part of the human personality and a significant factor in a person's self-identity. Successful gender identification in early childhood is important for health and well-being throughout life. Sexual fulfillment is a very basic need. Actual or potential damage to the integrity of an individual's sex organs poses a considerable threat to self-esteem and self-identity.

SEXUAL ANATOMY AND PHYSIOLOGY

EMBRYOLOGY

All human body cells, with the exception of the *gametes* (germ cells), contain 23 pairs of *chromosomes*. Twenty-two of these are homologous pairs; they are like each other and bear genes for the same traits. The twenty-third pair are the sex chromosomes. Females have two similar sex chromosomes, designated as X *chromosomes*. Males have two dissimilar sex chromosomes; one is an X *chromosome*, and the other, a Y *chromosome*.

During the process of maturation, the gametes (the male sperm and the female ovum) divide, and the number of chromosomes each carries is reduced by half to 23. The mature ovum always contains an X chromosome, while the sperm cell may contain either an X or a Y chromosome. If the ovum is fertilized by a sperm carrying an X chromosome, the resultant embryo will be a (XX) female who will develop a female reproductive system. If the sperm carries a Y chromosome, a (XY) male embryo will result and the *gonads* (sex organs) will develop into testes. Under the influence of the Y chromosome, further testicular development occurs. This is a major function of the Y chromosome since the embryonic testes secrete the hormone *testosterone* which stimulates the formation of the male external genitalia, duct system and accessory sex organs. In the absence of the influence of testosterone, female reproductive organs develop. Testosterone is also responsible for sex differentiation in the brain.

HORMONAL CONTROL OF THE REPRODUCTIVE SYSTEM

The master gland controlling the sex hormones in both sexes is the *hypothalamus*. This gland, located in the brain, secretes *gonadotropin-releasing hormone* (GnRH) which stimulates the pituitary gland to secrete the gonadotropic hormones, *follicle-stimulating hormone* (FSH) and *luteinizing hormone* (LH). FSH stimulates maturation of germ cells in the ovary and testes, while LH stimulates production of estrogen (female) and testosterone (male).

The hypothalamus is sensitive to external stimuli such as physical or emotional stress. Altered hypothalamic function can affect the pituitary gland, with resulting changes in ovarian or testicular function. For example, a woman who is undergoing extreme training for a competitive sport may cease menstruating because of stress or a lowered body fat content. Men who have a severe systemic illness will likely have a temporary lowering of the sperm count.

The male hormones are collectively known as *androgens*. The principal male hormone is *testosterone*, the functions of which are listed below.

1. To induce sexual differentiation during embryonic development.
2. To stimulate growth and development of the genitalia and secondary sex characteristics.
3. To initiate and maintain the process of spermatogenesis.
4. To promote body growth through protein anabolism.
5. To stimulate the sex drive.

Hormone production in the male is not cyclic as it is in women, although minor fluctuations of testosterone levels do appear to occur within a 24-hour period. Recent research has indicated that men's testosterone levels and sperm counts are up to 17 % higher in the winter (Levine, 1993). This may account for the higher birth rates in summer and early fall. The production of male hormones declines with aging, but since this is a gradual change, it should not necessarily cause concern.

The principal female hormones are the *estrogens* and *progesterone*. The estrogens are secreted by the ovarian follicle, by the corpus luteum and, during pregnancy, by the placenta. The functions of these hormones are listed below.

1. To stimulate growth of the reproductive organs and development of secondary sex characteristics at puberty.
2. To induce regeneration of the endometrium following menstruation.
3. To promote growth of the duct system of the mammary glands.
4. To maintain matrix formation in bone.
5. During labour and delivery, to increase the motility of the uterus and its sensitivity to oxytocin.

Progesterone is secreted by the corpus luteum and during pregnancy by the placenta. Its primary functions are listed below.

1. To cause the vascular and glandular structure of the endometrium to assume its mature form during the luteal (post-ovulatory) phase of the cycle, ready to supply glucose to the blastocyst (embryonic stage) and to create an environment hospitable to implantation. If pregnancy does not occur, corpus luteum function declines, estrogen and progesterone levels fall and endometrial shedding (menstruation) occurs.
2. To promote growth of the mammary gland alveoli.
3. To decrease motility of the uterine muscle.

Female hormone levels vary in a cyclic fashion from the onset of puberty until menopause occurs. During childhood and after menopause, the levels of estrogen and progesterone are consistently lower than during the reproductive years.

THE MALE REPRODUCTIVE SYSTEM

The male reproductive system includes the organs which produce both the male hormone and germ cells, a duct system to transport the germ cells to the exterior of the body, various internal structures which aid in the process and the penis which, during sexual intercourse, allows the deposit of the germ cells into the reproductive tract of the female. A successful outcome — achieving a pregnancy — depends upon a complex interplay of physical and emotional factors.

Testes

The testes are a pair of ovoid organs which produce testosterone and spermatozoa (germ cells) in the mature male. They develop within the abdominal cavity and descend into the scrotal sac during fetal development. As is the case with many mammals, human sperm production and viability require a narrow range of temperatures just below normal body temperature. The *scrotum* acts as a thermostat, relaxing with warmth to keep the testes away from the body, and contracting when cold to bring the testes up towards the perineum.

Each testicle consists of about 250 wedge-shaped lobes, each of which contains a few narrow coiled tubes, known as the *seminiferous tubules*, which produce the spermatozoa. Also located in the testes are *Sertoli's cells*, which supply

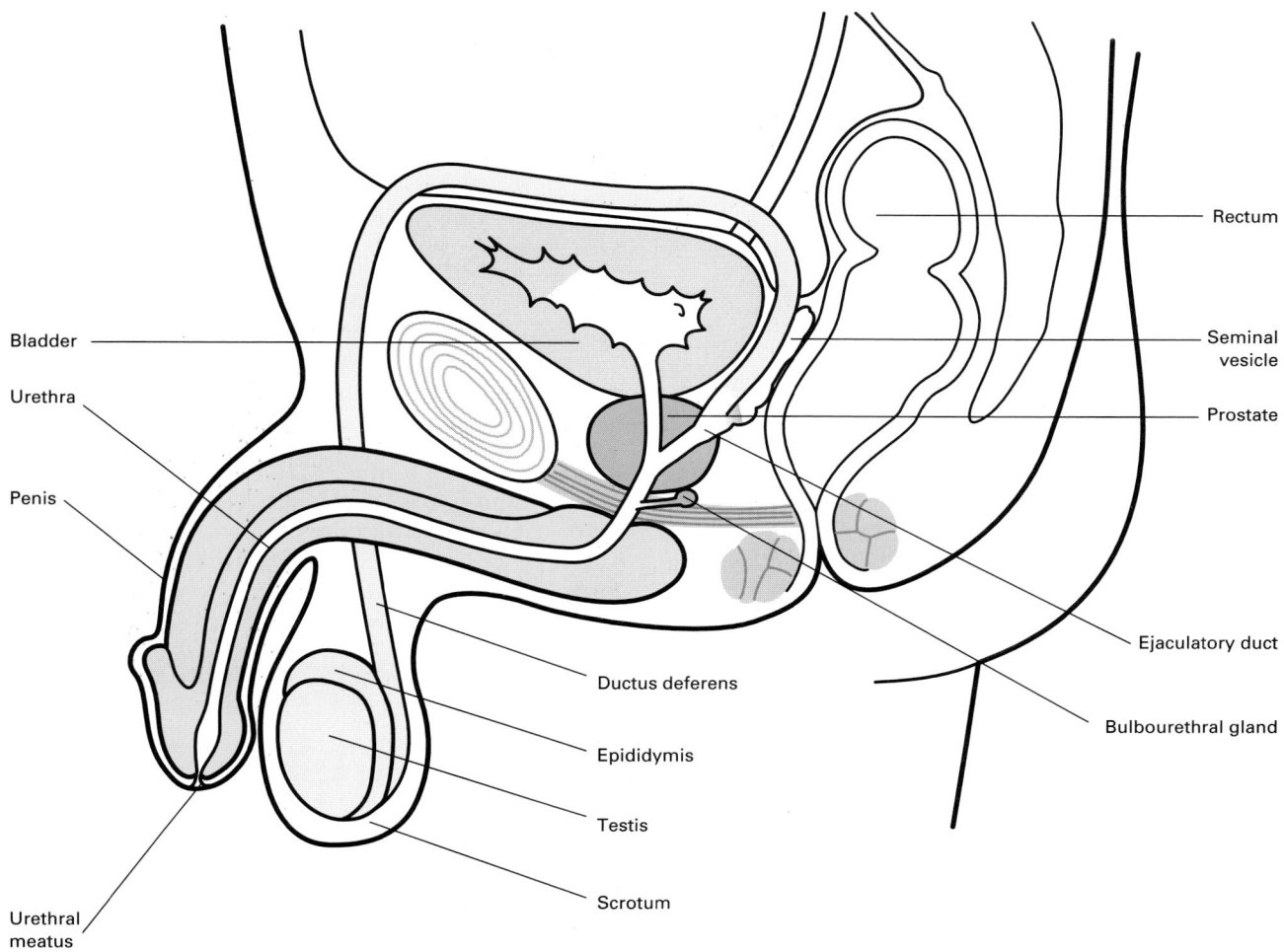

FIGURE 34.1   Male reproductive organs

nutrients to the sperm, and *Leydig's cells*, which produce testosterone.

Duct System

The process of spermatogenesis takes about 60 days in the seminiferous tubules. After another 14 days in the *epididymis*, the sperm are usually motile (able to move) and capable of fertilizing an ovum.

The sperm then move through the *vas deferens* towards the *urethra*. Several glands in this area contribute secretions which ensure the survival of the sperm. The first of these are the *seminal vesicles*, which lie behind the bladder and secrete a thick nutrient-containing fluid which mixes with the sperm. The *prostate gland* surrounds the urethra at the neck of the bladder. It secretes a thin, milky alkaline fluid essential for

maintaining viability of the sperm. The *bulbourethral (Cowper's) glands* are a pair of pea-shaped structures that lie along the lower portion of the urethra. They secrete a mucus substance during sexual stimulation, referred to as pre-ejaculatory fluid. This fluid is slightly alkaline and is thought to protect the sperm from residual acidity of urine in the urethra. It may also contain significant numbers of sperm.

The combination of spermatozoa and fluids from the various glands is known as *semen* or *seminal fluid*. During the process of ejaculation, about 2 ml to 6 ml of seminal fluid containing several hundred million sperm are discharged by a healthy male. The average normal sperm count is about 120 million per ml, of which an average of 60 % to 80 % will be motile. Semen is thick and milky when first ejaculated, but rapidly becomes watery due to the action of hydrolytic enzymes from the prostate gland.

Penis

The penis is the male organ of copulation. In the flaccid or non-erect state there is some degree of difference in size in different individuals. In the erect state, however, size variations are less marked (average is about 15 cm by 2.5 cm). The penis consists of three cylindrical structures (cavernous bodies) of erectile tissue bound together by fibrous bands. They extend into the pelvis where they are attached to the anterior and lateral walls of the pubic arch by muscle fibres. Two of these structures located in the dorsal portion of the penis are called the *corpus cavernosa*. The third structure, located more ventrally, is called the *corpus spongiosum*. The corpus spongiosum also forms the *glans penis*, the enlarged conical structure at the end of the penis. The urethra is contained within the corpus spongiosum and the opening in the glans penis is called the *urethral meatus*. The glans is covered by a fold of retractable skin, the *foreskin* or *prepuce*, which may be removed by circumcision for cultural, religious or health reasons.

During sexual arousal or in situations where nerve reflexes are activated, blood flow increases to the pelvic area and the cavernous bodies, causing the penis to become erect. Vascular pressure increases, thereby slowing blood flow out of the penis and allowing the erection to be maintained. Erection of the penis is essential in order for vaginal intercourse to take place.

THE FEMALE REPRODUCTIVE SYSTEM

The female reproductive system forms the other half of the equation in terms of human reproduction. Its functions are to produce and transport the female germ cells, receive the sperm, support conception and furnish an environment which promotes growth and development of the fetus. The system includes a birth canal for the passage of the mature fetus and a mechanism for suckling the infant after it is born.

Ovaries

The ovaries are small ovoid organs located in the pelvic region of the abdominal cavity. They are suspended from the lateral pelvic wall by a section of the broad ligament. At birth, the ovaries contain approximately 10 million *primordial follicles* (primitive ova), of which about 350 to 500

FIGURE 34.2 Female reproductive organs

will mature to become graafian follicles during the woman's reproductive years.

A few years before puberty, the ovaries begin to secrete increased amounts of the hormones estrogen, progesterone and some androgens (male hormones). Puberty starts when the production of female hormones becomes cyclic and continues in a regular pattern. Approximately every 28 days, the pituitary hormone FSH stimulates the maturation of a small number of oocytes within their follicles. The follicles secrete ever-increasing amounts of estrogen. One or two mature ova are extruded from the surface of the ovary in a process called *ovulation*. An ovum is capable of being fertilized for about 24 to 36 hours, after which it disintegrates. The cyst-like structure left on the surface of the ovary then begins to secrete progesterone.

Fallopian Tubes (Oviducts)

The fallopian tubes or oviducts are two small tube-like structures of approximately 10 cm in length, which extend from the uterus to the ovaries. They are attached to the broad ligaments and open into the lateral aspects of the uterus about one-third of the way down. The distal end of each tube has a fringe of finger-like projections, called *fimbria*, which lie in close proximity to the ovaries. They help to direct the ovum into the outer (distal) portion of the fallopian tube, where fertilization usually takes place. Over the three or four days following conception, the fertilized ovum is transported to the uterus for implantation. The ovum is propelled through the tubes by a series of peristaltic waves and the wave-like motion of *cilia*, which line the fallopian tubes.

Uterus (Womb)

The uterus is a hollow muscular organ, about the size of a fist, located in the pelvic portion of the abdominal cavity between the rectum and the bladder. The lining of the uterus consists of a specialized layer of tissue, the *endometrium*, which is the primary site for implantation of the fertilized ovum. If conception does not occur, the hormone levels decrease, and about 14 days following ovulation the endometrium is shed in a process called *menstruation*.

Cervix

The cervix is the muscular, conical neck of the uterus. It is firm to the touch and protrudes into the posterior vault of the vagina. It has a narrow opening in its centre, the cervical os. The cervical os leads to the cervical canal, which forms the passageway from the vagina to the uterine cavity. During pregnancy, the muscle in the cervix helps to keep the developing pregnancy within the uterus by keeping the cervix tightly closed. A mucus plug, present in the cervical canal during pregnancy, helps to prevent entry of substances from the vagina.

Vagina

The vagina is an elastic tube lying, with its walls against each other, between the bladder and the rectum. It is approximately 10 cm long and 4 cm wide in its resting state, but expands during sexual arousal. The vagina functions as the birth canal and is capable of expanding to allow passage of a full-term fetus. During coitus (sexual intercourse), the erect penis is inserted into the vagina. When ejaculation occurs, sperm are deposited at the cervical os to make their way through the uterus to the fallopian tubes.

Vulva

The external female genitals are collectively known as the vulva (Figure 34.3). The *mons pubis* is a soft pad of adipose tissue located over the symphysis pubis and is covered with pubic hair. The *labia majora*, which are somewhat similar to the scrotum in the male, are longitudinal folds of skin which cover and protect the opening of the vagina, the urethral meatus and the labia minora. The *labia minora* are small folds of erectile tissue which extend from the *clitoris* to the *fourchette*.

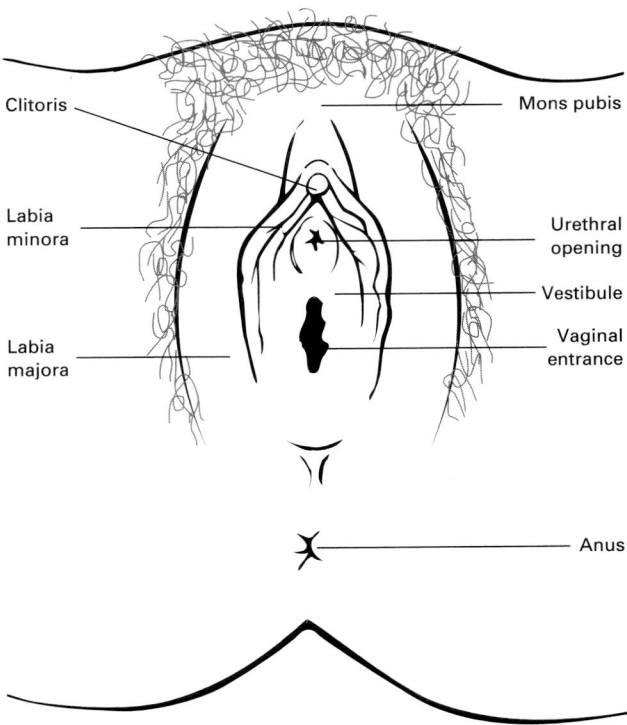

FIGURE 34.3 External female genitalia (vulva)

The clitoris is a short, erectile organ located just below the mons pubis and just above the urinary meatus. It is the female organ corresponding to the glans penis of the male, but contains a relatively greater concentration of sensory nerve endings. It is highly sensitive to tactile stimuli.

The vestibule is the ovoid area between the labia minora which contains the vaginal introitus (opening), the urethral meatus, the hymen and the openings of several glandular ducts. The *hymen* is an elastic fibrous membrane that may or may not be visible at the introitus. The presence or absence of the hymen is not an accurate indicator of whether or not a woman has had sexual intercourse, although the presence of a very thick membrane (imperforate hymen) would likely be an impediment to vaginal intercourse.

Mammary Glands (Breasts)

The mammary glands are accessory sexual structures in the female. Their purpose is to excrete milk to nourish an infant. Each breast contains lobes separated by adipose tissue and made up of lobules. The lobules contain grape-like clusters of milk-secreting cells called *alveoli*. The milk is conveyed to storage areas (ampullae), and thence to the lactiferous ducts which lead to the nipple. During pregnancy, increased levels of estrogens and progesterone begin to prepare the breasts for milk production and after childbirth, the hormone prolactin stimulates this function.

THE MENSTRUAL CYCLE

The average length of the menstrual cycle is 28 days, counting the first day of menstrual flow as Day 1 of that cycle. Ovulation consistently occurs an average of 14 days before the onset of menstrual flow. The length of cycles may vary from woman to woman, and also in the same woman from cycle to cycle, reflecting variations in the follicular phase. The duration of menstrual flow can also vary, ranging from two to seven days on average, with about 40 ml to 50 ml of blood loss. The menstrual cycle consists of three phases: the menstrual phase, the proliferative or follicular phase and the secretory phase.

The Menstrual Phase

The menstrual phase occurs about 14 days after ovulation when the hormone secretion of the corpus luteum decreases

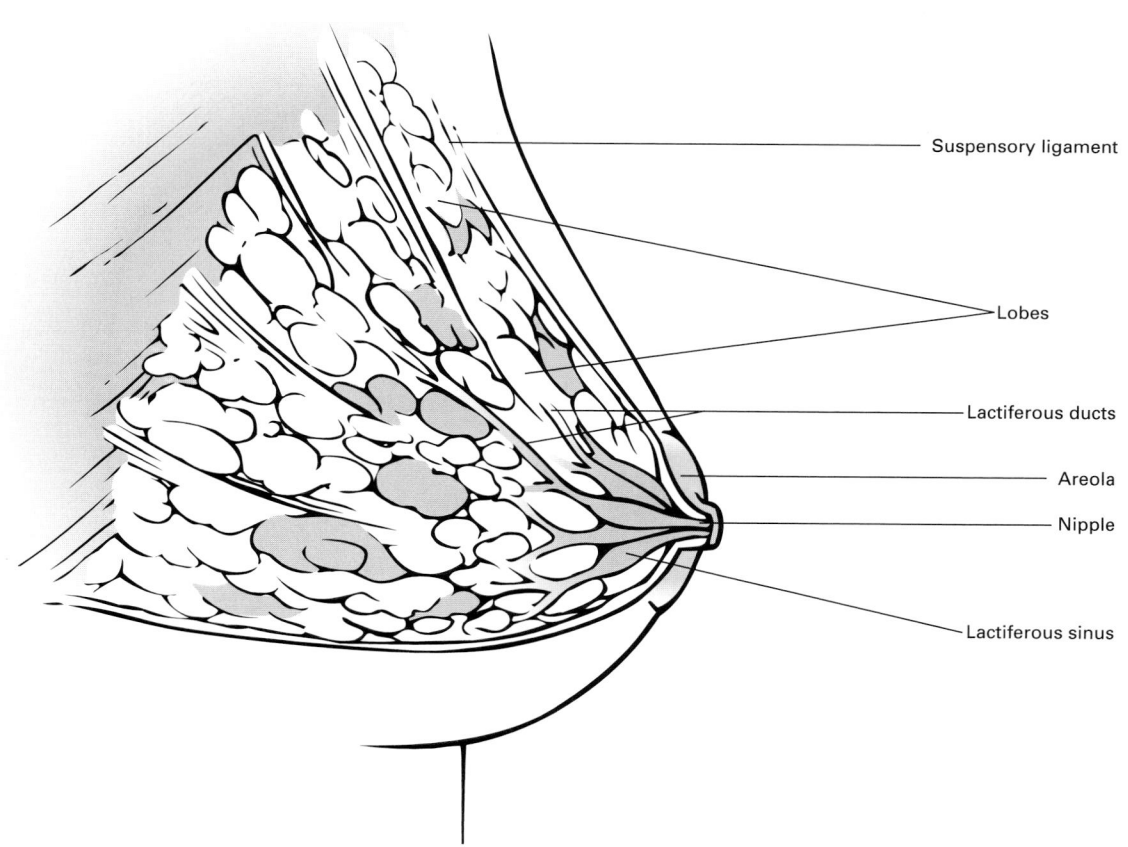

Suspensory ligament

Lobes

Lactiferous ducts

Areola

Nipple

Lactiferous sinus

FIGURE 34.4   Lateral view of the breast

and the endometrium disintegrates. Separation between the innermost basal layer of the endometrium takes place, with shedding of the two outer layers lining the uterus.

The Proliferative (Follicular) Phase

Under the influence of FSH, the ovarian follicle begins to develop and secrete increasing levels of estrogen. This initiates regeneration of the endometrium and glycogen storage.

The Secretory (Luteal) Phase

As the ovum matures, the hypothalamus and pituitary glands respond to increased estrogen levels by lowering production of FSH and sharply increasing production of LH (luteinizing hormone). The mature ovum ruptures the surface of the ovarian follicle and is released into the pelvic cavity. This process is called *ovulation*. Ovulation occurs 10 to 12 hours after the peak level of LH. The ruptured follicle forms the *corpus luteum*, which secretes progesterone. Under the influence of progesterone, the vascular and glandular structure of the endometrium assumes its mature form as a hospitable environment for implantation. If conception occurs, *Human Chorionic Gonadotropin* (HCG) is produced by the developing pregnancy and supports the continued function of the corpus luteum until the placenta is able to provide these hormones at six to eight weeks gestation. If conception does not occur, the corpus luteum degenerates, estrogen and progesterone levels fall, and a new menstrual cycle begins.

Menarche and Menopause

The onset of the first menstrual period is called **menarche**. In North America, the average age of menarche is 12 years with the "normal" range extending from age 9 to age 16.

Menopause is considered to have occurred when a woman has not experienced menstrual flow for one to one and a half years. The average age of menopause is 51 years, and ranges from age 45 to 55 (Droegemuller, Herbst, Mishell and Stenchever, 1987).

Menopause is a normal physiological event which results from the lowered response of the ovaries to hormone stimulation. "Surgical menopause" can occur at any age if the ovaries are removed or rendered non-functional in the treatment of life-threatening diseases such as cancer within the reproductive system.

In addition to marking the end of a woman's reproductive years, lowered estrogen levels can produce a variety of effects on the body as outlined in Table 34.1. These effects are more acute in women who have had a surgical menopause. Some women experience few if any problems with menopause. Others have a difficult time with physical symptoms and/or emotional reactions to this significant life event and may require support and counselling from a health care professional. These women may also benefit from hormone replacement therapy.

THE SEXUAL RESPONSE CYCLE

The human sexual response can be triggered by a variety of stimuli. These may be mental, as in sexual fantasies or thoughts; or sensory, involving vision, smell, taste, hearing, or touch. Responsiveness to any particular stimulus is highly individual and can vary in the same person from time to time. Sexual responsiveness and function also depend upon the emotional status of the individual. Some "turn-offs" are anxiety, pain, lack of privacy or lack of trust in one's partner.

Physiologists divide the human sexual response cycle into four phases: excitement, plateau, orgasm and resolution.

TABLE 34.1   Menopausal Effects of Lowered Estrogen Levels

EFFECT	SYMPTOMS EXPERIENCED
Vasomotor disturbance	Hot flashes Flushing Dizzy spells Headaches
Atrophy of the vaginal walls	Dyspareunia (painful intercourse)
Decrease in perineal muscle tone	Urinary stress incontinence
Loss of calcium from the bone matrix	Osteoporosis

This commonly used definition of the human sexual response cycle evolved from laboratory situations in which the researchers Masters and Johnson (1966) used male and female volunteers who were chosen because of a history of sexual responsiveness. The conclusions were reached after measuring physiological changes in a laboratory setting and so probably do not reflect the great variation in sexual responses of people in general. Because of this same fact, it is not likely to reflect those variations that happen within each person on different occasions either. Any person may experience varying degrees of the sexual response cycle. Therefore, the human sexual response cycle definition might best be used as a guideline, but not as a standard against which all sexual experiences should be evaluated.

In general, two main physiological changes take place during sexual response: vasocongestion and myotonia. Vasocongestion occurs when the sexual response is triggered. There is a rise in heart rate and blood pressure. The blood vessels (chiefly the venous system) in the lower pelvic area and the genitals become engorged with blood. Myotonia is the increase in muscle tension, which in turn enhances the response to sensory stimuli. The awareness of these physical changes also contributes to the arousal process.

EXCITEMENT PHASE

If a woman is receptive to sexual activity, touching and caressing of various body parts can promote arousal. These are called the "erogenous zones," after Eros, the Greek god of love. The most sensitive areas in many women are the breasts and the genitals, particularly the clitoris. As the woman becomes sexually aroused, vaginal lubrication begins, the inner two-thirds of the vagina expands, the outer lips of the vulva open and the clitoris enlarges. The vaginal walls become a dark purplish colour due to vasocongestion. As the excitement phase continues, the breasts increase in size, the nipples become erect and the areolae become engorged. A redness or maculopapular rash appears on the skin of the epigastric region and breasts, known as a "sex flush."

In men, the response to sexual stimuli may appear to be more rapid than that of females, although the physiological changes are the same. The most obvious sign of male sexual arousal is erection of the penis. At the same time, the scrotal sac is pulled up towards the body and the scrotal skin becomes thick and rigid.

As the stimulation continues, the blood pressure and heart rate in both sexes continue to increase. Rising sexual tension causes involuntary tensing of the intercostal and abdominal muscles.

PLATEAU PHASE

During the plateau phase in women, the uterus is elevated within the pelvis and the vaginal barrel elongates.

Vasocongestion causes swelling of the labia minora and the outer third of the vagina. The colour of the labia minora changes from bright red to dark purple. The Bartholin's glands secrete a small amount of mucoid material and the clitoris retracts against the symphysis pubis. The muscles of the pelvic floor retract, allowing for comfortable insertion of the penis.

In the male, the plateau phase includes a further increase in size of the head of the penis and the testicles. The glans may also darken in colour and clear fluid (pre-ejaculatory fluid from Cowper's glands) may appear at the urethral meatus. As muscle tension increases, the blood pressure becomes markedly elevated. Just prior to ejaculation, a valve located in the urethra at the bladder neck closes, in order to prevent discharge of urine and to create a path through the penile urethra for the semen.

ORGASM

In both men and women, orgasm is characterized by a series of involuntary muscle contractions. In the female, there may be 5 to 12 contractions at 0.8 second intervals. They involve the uterus, the muscles of the lower abdomen and the pelvic floor. Contractions of the anal sphincter also occur.

In the male, clonic contractions along the length of the urethra transport the semen and expel it from the urethral meatus. The epididymis, vas deferens, seminal vesicles and prostate gland also contract at 0.8 second intervals. The contractions become less frequent as the ejaculatory process is completed (within a few seconds). Separate but closely related reflex centres in the spinal cord govern erection, ejaculation and orgasm. These three events are thus interrelated, but can occur independently.

Sexual response can occur regardless of the type of sexual activity that is taking place. It may occur during a fantasy or a dream, during sexual activity with a partner or during self-stimulation. The experience of orgasms is highly individual and subjective. It can be different each time, depending on how it is achieved (for instance, fantasy, vaginal intercourse, anal intercourse, partner or self-masturbation or use of sexual aids). Following orgasm, a woman may be able to become sexually aroused again almost immediately and experience a second, third or further orgasm. In males, however, a period of 10 to 45 minutes (or more depending upon the age and health status of the man) is required before the arousal cycle can recur. This is called the *refractory period*.

RESOLUTION

The resolution phase involves the relaxation of muscles and a decline in vasocongestion, called detumescence. This process begins within seconds after orgasm occurs.

Factors Influencing Sexual Function

Psychosocial Factors	Biological Factors
Cognitive	Age
Emotional	Genetics
Educational	Health related:
Personal and Societal	Acute illness
Situational	Chronic illness
	Disability
	Treatment related:
	Medications
	Other treatments
	Recreational substance use

DETERMINANTS OF SEXUAL FUNCTIONING

Probably there is no other area of human functioning that is affected by so many factors as sexuality. Successful sexual functioning combines a range of sensory and motor responses that are mediated by cognitive, emotional, social and biological influences. These determinants are listed in the box above. A disturbance in any one area can interfere with sexual functioning. In a way, the experience of healthy sexuality depends upon the absence of negative factors almost as much as it depends on the presence of positive ones.

PSYCHOSOCIAL FACTORS

Cognitive

As a child grows towards maturity, the development of cognitive skills provides the ability to seek out and maintain relationships, to understand the concept of consent, to evaluate possible risks and benefits and to recognize and adopt rewarding behaviours. With regard to sexual functioning, the stage of cognitive development is as important as chronological age. For example, someone who has well-developed cognitive skills may prefer to seek sexual gratification through masturbation rather than through more risky involvement with a partner.

Emotional

Mental health professionals have long been aware that depressive illnesses have a dampening effect on sexual function. The primary effect is a decrease of desire and subsequent loss of sexual interest. Emotional well-being is integral to a positive self-image, which in turn contributes to a healthy interest in all aspects of life, including sexuality.

Educational

Myths and misinformation about human sexuality abound, often causing individuals to make decisions which have unfortunate results. For example, a young woman who thinks that pregnancy cannot occur the first time she has intercourse may not even consider using a condom for birth control nor for protection from sexually transmitted diseases. Studies have shown that access to accurate, relevant information, such as that provided through comprehensive health education programs in the schools, promotes healthy sexual decision making (Orton and Rosenblatt, 1986).

Personal and Societal

Every society in history has attempted to control sexual behaviour to some degree through societal norms. Children learn very early about what constitutes acceptable sexual behaviour within their culture. These early lessons are very powerful and can have a life-long influence on personal values. For example, a person raised in an atmosphere of strict sexual repression may have difficulty learning to be sexually responsive even in a marital situation where sexual behaviour is sanctioned.

Although there may be some variation from one culture to another, certain sexual taboos seem to be nearly universal. One of these is prohibition of incest, which is sexual intercourse between members of the same family (father with daughter, mother with son, or between siblings). Sexual taboos are frequently enforced by legal controls. Sexual assault (the violent sexual assault on one person by another); sexual activity by an adult with a child; and indecent exposure (inappropriate exposure of the body) are all illegal acts described in the Canadian Criminal Code. In addition to major impacts on emotional health in general, sexual abuse or assault during or after childhood can have a damaging influence on subsequent sexual function. Although many survivors of childhood sexual abuse and trauma are able to develop into sexually healthy adults, therapists note that a high percentage of people who seek help for sexual problems have a history of sexual abuse (Maltz, 1991; Beitchman, Zucker, Hood, DaCosta, Akman and and Cassavia, 1990).

The various religions exert important influences on the sexual behaviour of followers and in a general way on society at large. For example, the Judeo–Christian and Islamic faiths have strict codes allowing sexual contact only within marriage and teach that the principal objective of marriage is to form a family unit for the production of children. Although not strictly adhered to, these codes of behaviour influence general attitudes in subtle ways.

Personal factors also have a significant bearing on sexual functioning. Restrictive attitudes, ignorance and fear have tended to shroud with feelings of guilt, repression and anxiety what is in fact a normal biological function. During the latter part of this century, societal attitudes have changed, with more general acceptance of consensual sexual activity regardless of marital status, with a recognition of the right of women to sexual satisfaction in relationships and with a tolerance of pregnancy and parenthood in unmarried women. The availability and widespread use of contraception has provided women with reproductive choices that were not possible even 50 years ago. With the ability to postpone childbearing, women have been able to exercise other life choices in the areas of career, relationships and lifestyle.

Other issues related to sexuality remain controversial. One such area is homosexuality, which is still considered abnormal and deviant by many religious and cultural groups. The scientific community, however, now recognizes that sexual preference is inherent. Homosexuality is not a perversion but a reflection of one facet of the large spectrum of human sexual preference.

Situational

A number of situational factors may influence sexual functioning. These include the availability of a compatible partner, the capacity to sustain an intimate relationship with a sexual partner and opportunities for sexual expression. For instance, a young couple, both trying to pursue successful careers while at the same time raise a family, may find little time or energy for intimacy and sexual expression. Freedom from anxiety about sexual performance, pregnancy and sexually transmitted diseases are other factors which affect sexual functioning.

BIOLOGICAL FACTORS

Age

Age and physical development are very important factors in determining sexual function. Neurological pathways for sensory input and for certain reflex responses are intact and functioning even prior to birth. For example, erection of the penis may be observed on ultrasound scans of the fetus, and small children are known to be capable of experiencing orgasm. The anatomical structures required for reproduction are present at birth but do not become capable of this function until puberty.

The sexual response cycle, from arousal to orgasm, can occur, if conditions allow it, in either sex throughout the lifetime. Women are capable of childbearing from the onset of puberty until menopause and can fulfill this function even if the sexual response cycle is absent. After puberty, the male produces sperm on a more or less continuous basis and is capable of biological fatherhood, even in old age. For reproductive purposes, an erection response is necessary in order to insert the penis into the vagina. The only other requirement is for ejaculation to occur within the vagina. For most males, orgasm and ejaculation occur simultaneously or within seconds of each other. Although increasing age can have a negative effect on general health, which in turn can affect sexual function, sexual response patterns change with age, but do not disappear.

Genetics

The primary biological agents controlling reproductive and sexual function are the genes and the hormones. Initial differentiation of the sexual organs in utero is determined by the XX or XY chromosome combination in the newly-formed embryo. Further development of the sexual organs is controlled by hormones produced under the influence of these chromosomes. Defects in the sex chromosomes or disturbance of hormone balance can give rise to problems in growth, development, future sexual function and fertility. One example is *Klinefelter's syndrome*, which occurs in males. It is caused by the presence of an extra X chromosome and can result in low testosterone levels, small testicles, a nonmasculine stature and no sperm production. *Turner's syndrome* is an example of a genetic defect which affects females. This syndrome results from the absence of one of the X chromosomes. The ovaries fail to develop adequately, breast development and menarche do not appear and stature may remain short. Women with Turner's syndrome are no less feminine than other women, and if treated with female hormones, can develop an adult female body type. However, pregnancy is not possible.

Health-Related Factors

Sexual function can be altered by a disease or disability if sensory loss, motor disability, loss of reflexes or muscle weakness occur as part of the disease process. Some of the effects of illnesses, such as pain, fatigue, depression, anxiety, grief reaction, altered self-image or changed sex roles, can also impact on sexual function, as can some medications and other treatments. Therapeutic medications and recreational drugs can affect sexual function by causing a decrease in the sex drive or by interfering with the vascular or neuromuscular systems. Examples of acute and chronic illnesses which affect sexual function may be found in the box below. Table 34.2 outlines the effects of treatments and recreational drugs on sexual functioning.

Acute or Chronic Illness Which Can Affect Sexual Function

ENDOCRINE DISORDERS:

Diabetes mellitus	Addison's disease
Pituitary dysfunction	Gonadal disease
Thyroid disease	Acromegaly

GENITOURINARY DISORDERS:

Chronic renal failure	Vaginismus
Retrograde ejaculation	Priapism
Altered structures	Infections

NEUROMUSCULAR AND SKELETAL DISORDERS:

Spinal cord injury	Arthritis
Multiple sclerosis	Brain injury
Amyotrophic lateral sclerosis	Cerebral vascular accident

CARDIORESPIRATORY DISORDERS:

Peripheral vascular disorders	Chronic obstructive pulmonary disease
Myocardial infarction	Congestive heart failure

GASTROINTESTINAL DISORDERS:

Ulcerative colitis	Crohn's disease
Liver disease	Colostomy/ileostomy
Cancer	

SEXUALLY TRANSMITTED DISEASES:

HIV/AIDS	Hepatitis B
Herpes	Chlamydia
Syphilis	Gonorrhea
Human papilloma virus (HPV)	Parasites and fungal infections

OTHER DISORDERS:

History of sexual abuse or assault

Major psychiatric illnesses, such as schizophrenia, unipolar and bipolar major affective disorders

Infertility

SOURCE: Carpenito, 1993; Shrover and Jensen, 1988

SEXUALITY NEEDS THROUGHOUT THE LIFE CYCLE

The biological purpose of the sex drive is to ensure continuation of a species. In most other species, coital activity is mostly limited to episodes when the female is fertile and biologically programmed to be receptive. In human beings, however, sexual needs include more than the physical need to propagate the race. The cognitive abilities of human beings allow recognition that sexual activity is inherently rewarding. The pleasure obtained from physical contact with another person and from positive sensory stimulation is reinforced by the pleasurable experience of orgasm. The "reward" of orgasm is probably a factor in the desire for sexual contact whether or not procreation is intended. Human sexuality involves a complex set of interrelationships between people. These include the need to develop and express the self as a male or female within society, the need to engage in close, reciprocal relationships with others and the need to mate and reproduce children.

INFANCY

As has been mentioned, sex differentiation begins in utero, and sexual and reproductive organs are intact but immature at the time of birth. The first "sexual" experiences of an infant are related to gratification of basic needs for nourishment, warmth and touch. If these early experiences are positive, the infant's feelings of love, trust and self-worth are engendered. These form a solid basis for a personality which allows people to take risks and extend themselves to others in future relationships.

CHILDHOOD

One of the most important developmental tasks of childhood is the establishment of gender identity and gender (sex) role identity. The child learns his or her gender, that he is a "boy" or she is a "girl," and incorporates the appropriate sex role at the same time. Gender role behaviours include mannerisms, deportment, demeanour, preferences for play or recreational activities, daydreams and fantasies, life goals and performance on projective tests. Over-emphasizing the importance of gender roles can have the unfortunate consequence of sex role stereotyping. In the absence of rigid sex role behaviour guidelines, children are able to learn more complete life skills and enjoy the expression of creativity.

It is thought that gender identity and role are imprinted during the first three years of life, by which time the child's self-concept includes the gender-appropriate label. Some children may briefly experiment with the opposite gender identity by role playing behaviours specific to that gender.

TABLE 34.2   Effect of Medications and Recreational Drugs on Sexual Function

DRUG	EFFECT ON SEXUAL FUNCTION
Alcohol	Small amounts: decreased inhibitions, increased libido Chronic use: lowered testosterone, erectile and ejaculatory dysfunction, infertility

Tobacco	Long-term use:
	    Men: erectile dysfunction, infertility
	    Women: infertility

Cocaine	Short-term use: said to enhance sexual pleasure. Long-term use: decreased libido, impaired erectile, ejaculatory and orgasmic responses
Marijuana	Long-term use: Same as cocaine, infertility
Anabolic steroids	*Women:* menstrual disturbances, infertility *Men:* testicular atrophy, lowered testosterone, low sperm production, possibly permanent sterility
Tricyclic antidepressants *Monoamine oxidase inhibitors* *Anticholinergic drugs* *Antihypertensives* *Antihistamines* *Antispasmodics* *Beta blockers* *Radiation therapy*	All of these commonly used medications can affect sexual function, depending on dosage and individual response. The most common effects in men are problems with erection, orgasm or ejaculation. In women, libido and orgasmic response may be affected. May have a negative effect on general health as well as on the reproductive glands and organs.
Surgery	Includes structural and functional changes in the body, altered body image and grief in reaction to perceived loss

Although a same-sex role model is helpful in early childhood, children need role models of both sexes in order to develop a sexual identity and later to be able to establish comfortable relationships with others. A safe, loving and nurturing environment is now considered to be a much more important factor than the gender of a parent. In addition, during the preschool years, children need clear, honest answers to questions about sexuality. They need to know the correct names for reproductive anatomy and should have a basic understanding of the male and female roles in reproduction.

Sex roles are firmly entrenched during the early school years. By age nine or ten, segregation of the sexes is reflected in different interests and play activities. Boys may prefer sports such as soccer, baseball and football, while girls seem to enjoy such activities as skipping rope, dancing and skating. As barriers based on gender are lowered, the differences in activity preferences are becoming less marked.

Children explore and derive pleasure from their own bodies, including the genital area. *Masturbation*, the stroking and stimulation of one's own genital area, is quite common throughout childhood. School-aged children are usually very curious about sexual matters as they develop the ability to understand abstract concepts, such as relationships and consequences of behaviours. They need to know about the physical and emotional changes that occur during puberty before they are experienced, about sexuality and reproductive function, about sexual assault and about sexually transmitted diseases. Decision making and communication skills are also important for a healthy sexuality to develop.

PUBERTY

Puberty is defined as the process by which the body gains the physical ability to reproduce. In girls, estrogen levels

In developing gender role identity, a girl often imitates her mother.

begin to rise at about age eight or nine. There may be a marked increase in height, and breast development begins with growth of the "breast buds." Axillary and pubic hair appears, hips broaden and further breast development is followed by menarche.

The first few menstrual cycles may be anovulatory; that is, the ovaries do not release an ovum. However, ovulation obviously does take place in some early cycles as pregnancies have occurred in young women who have not yet had a menstrual period. Adolescent women may experience difficulties with menstruation, including irregular cycles, amenorrhea (absence of menstruation) or dysmenorrhoea (painful menstruation). The fluctuations of hormones can produce uncomfortable premenstrual symptoms and strong emotional reactions. Dysmenorrhoea can be treated successfully in most cases by medications such as non-steroidal anti-inflammatory drugs which have an anti-prostaglandin (antispasmodic) effect on smooth muscle.

Societal or cultural attitudes tend to be very negative towards menstruation, as reflected by commercial advertising of sanitary products where the need for deodorants and for internal (unseen) protection (tampons) is emphasized. Positive attitudes towards the natural phenomenon of menstruation can be fostered in young women by female relatives, by peer groups and by health professionals, particularly nurses and health educators.

In boys, the levels of testosterone are low until about eight. The early physical changes of puberty are not as obvious as they are in girls. Nonetheless, they include enlargement and an increase in pressure sensitivity of the testes, reddening and stippling of the scrotal skin, an in-

crease in penis size, the appearance of axillary, pubic and facial hair, activation of axillary sweat glands, voice change, nocturnal emissions ("wet dreams") and an increase in height and broadening of the shoulders. These changes can begin as early as age eight or nine but may not be completed for several years. The age range for puberty in boys is about age nine to age seventeen, with the average age of first ejaculation of semen at about age twelve.

ADOLESCENCE

The period of adolescence encompasses the physical changes of puberty, and includes the psychological, cognitive and social transition from childhood into adulthood. Adolescence is a process which involves coming to terms with a new physical appearance as well as with an emerging self-identity.

Up until the early part of the twentieth century, puberty was generally followed closely by marriage, with childbearing occurring as a natural consequence. Adolescents now seem to reach puberty about three years earlier than is thought to have been the average one hundred years ago. The need to attain greater levels of education and to "grow up" before seeking a spouse causes a delay between the onset of biological maturity and the time when sexual behaviours are officially sanctioned.

Adolescents frequently find themselves caught between their own biological urges and desires, the need to conform to peer pressure and the "pro-sex" messages in advertising, and the equally powerful messages about the dangers of sex from parents, religious groups and well-meaning health educators. In the book *The Dynamics of Psychological Development*, Thomas and Chess outline the developmental tasks involved in attaining sexual adulthood, expressed in terms of *cultural norms*. There is no end-point to these tasks, some of which require lifelong effort. These developmental tasks are listed below.

1. Establishment of basic identity as a male or female (usually by age three or four).
2. Adopt appropriate sex role behaviours as dictated by the particular cultural milieu (an ongoing process).
3. Develop sexual attraction to the opposite sex.
4. Know how to give and receive sexual pleasure.
5. Have ability to establish intimacy in a relationship.
6. Establish sufficient self-control over pleasure-seeking to control reproduction (and to practise safer sex).*

Achievement of these developmental tasks requires that the adolescent learn behaviours involved in giving and receiving sexual pleasure. Skills required for establishing intimate relationships must also be gained. The challenge for our society is to allow adolescents sufficient

* Thomas and Chess (1980).

opportunities to learn these behaviours and skills while ensuring that there will be few if any undesired consequences. Society must also learn to tolerate and accept the fact that a percentage of people are unable to conform to the expectation that they will develop heterosexual attraction. When one considers the strong need for social and peer group conformity and the desire to be "normal," any uncertainty about sexual preference could be devastating to an adolescent. Mental health professionals have observed a higher suicide rate among homosexual youth (*Suicide among gay and lesbian youth*, 1993). Other problems associated with adolescence are high rates of unplanned pregnancy, sexual assault and abuse and very high rates of sexually transmitted infections. For example, 33.7 % of all chlamydia genital infections reported in Canada in 1991 were in people aged 15 to 19 (Health and Welfare Canada, 1991).

In order to become sexually healthy adults, adolescents need comprehensive health education with curricula that include all topics relevant to sexuality. Whether they are gay or straight, adolescents need access to health care and other resources which will allow them to make responsible decisions about managing sexuality safely. And when they make mistakes, special support services are needed to help diminish any negative effects which may occur.

YOUNG ADULTHOOD

Young adulthood marks the period of life when pair-bonding takes place and families begin to be established. Although the traditional concept of family as a basis for bearing and raising children is still strongly in evidence, the definition of family could be expanded to include any group of two or more people who share interests and mutual support. Families may also be "blended"; with higher rates of divorce and remarriage, new families may be formed with children from two or more previous relationships.

In addition to reproductive functions, sexual behaviour during young adulthood may also foster closeness and intimacy, give pleasure and bolster self-esteem. Although there is a widespread belief that young adults are at their "sexual peak," the demands involved in raising and supporting a family and establishing an acceptable standard of living can be detrimental to relationships and sexual function. Fatigue, stress and unrealistic expectations about sexual performance can lead to dissatisfaction and distress. Approximately 15 % to 20 % of the population will experience infertility which contributes to stress and sexual problems (Canadian Research Institute for the Advancement of Women, 1989). The incidence of both cancer of the cervix and infertility is associated with increased rates of sexually transmitted diseases within the general population. The rates of unplanned pregnancy and sexually transmitted diseases are also very high in the group between the ages of 20 to 30. Taking the example of chlamydia genital infections, 52.2 % of reported cases occurred in this age group (Health and Welfare Canada,

1991). The incidence of testicular cancer is also highest in this age group, affecting, for example, about 4 of every 100,000 white males per year (Reinisch, 1990).

Young adults need ongoing access to reliable information about sexual function, contraception and safe sex practices. Some of the sexual difficulties in this age group can be addressed through health promoting education and lifestyle changes.

MIDDLE ADULTHOOD

During the years commonly referred to as "middle age," ongoing changes in sexual and reproductive anatomy and function become more noticeable. Some women experience an increase in sexual drive while others note a decline in sexual interest and activity. The lowering of female hormone levels with menopause can cause vasomotor disturbances such as hot flushes, dizziness or headaches, and disturbed sleep patterns. Lowered estrogen levels can also cause atrophy of the vaginal mucosa, leading to dryness, painful intercourse and increased susceptibility to vaginal infections. Prior to menopause, pregnancy is possible, unless reliable contraception is used. The risk of sexually transmitted diseases does not disappear with menopause. Because the risks of cancer in the reproductive system increase with age, women in the middle years need information on how to promote sexual health and access to regular health screening including mammography and gynecological examinations.

Although there is no such phenomenon as "male menopause," many men are distressed with changes which affect sexual function and may become concerned about sexual performance. These changes may include a slower erectile response, a decrease in the degree of erection or a decrease in the intensity of orgasm and/or force of ejaculation (or occasionally no ejaculation). Many men require more direct manual stimulation in order to become aroused and have a longer refractory period following orgasm. In some men, the interval between arousal and orgasm is prolonged, which could have the beneficial effect of allowing more time for a partner to achieve orgasm. Male fertility declines gradually with the lowering of testosterone levels, but healthy men have been known to father children even in old age.

Men in their middle years are at increased risk for either benign or malignant overgrowth of the prostate gland. In addition to reassuring information about the normal and gradual changes in sexual function, they need regular health examinations which include a rectal examination of the prostate gland.

OLDER ADULTHOOD

During the later years, the changes which occurred in the middle years may become more pronounced. The myth that older adults are not interested in sex was shattered by a Canadian study on sexuality by Judith Stryckman. She

---

Respecting the Sexuality of Older Adults

- Support and encourage interest in appearance and individuality.
- Encourage children to accept their parents' sexuality and their need for intimate contact.
- Recognize that sexuality may be expressed in many physical and emotional ways, only one of which is sexual intercourse.
- Ensure that older adults have the opportunity to meet members of the opposite sex.
- Do not deprive older adults the privacy they need in order to develop an intimate relationship.
- Encourage older adults to speak up for themselves and make others aware of their right to make decisions about their own sexuality.

SOURCE: DuGas, 1993, 152.

---

found that "seven out of ten couples who do not have major health problems were sexually active, sometimes into their late eighties" (Government of Canada, 1990). "Age, it seems, has less of an effect on interest in sexual activity than previous patterns of sexual activity. Those with a strong interest in sex in their younger days continue to have it as they grow older" (DuGas, 1993, 148).

An older adult who has access to a willing and capable partner can enjoy a full range of sexual activities. A loving sexual relationship, even one that does not include sexual intercourse, contributes significantly to the health and well-being of an older person. Because women in general have a longer life span than men, older women are more likely to lack a partner and may suffer from loneliness or even touch deprivation. Some suggestions for respecting the sexuality of older people are higlighted in the box above.

The incidence of cancer and degenerative diseases is higher in older people and these diseases can have a negative impact on sexual function. If sexuality is recognized and validated, older people are more likely to seek assistance with sexual difficulties, especially if these are associated with a health concern.

SEXUAL BEHAVIOURS, ORIENTATIONS AND VARIATIONS

There are many possible sexual behaviours known to most sexually active adults. Some other behaviours are not so familiar, or may be viewed as strange, risky or not even interesting. Generally, an activity can be considered within the range of "normal" if it is mutually desired and enjoyed

when shared, if it provides sensual pleasure and if it causes no mental or physical harm.

Some sexual behaviours such as fantasies and dreams require little or no physical effort. These could be called ***autosexual activities***, referring to self-involvement only. Masturbation is also an autosexual behaviour, and often takes the form of rhythmic stroking of the genital area. As recently as 50 years ago, masturbation was considered to be unhealthy and a probable cause of mental illness and other ailments which commonly afflicted young people. It is now being accepted more and more as a natural and healthy manner of sexual expression for people of all ages and as a safe way for young women and men to learn about their own sexual responses.

Heterosexual behaviours include activities that are often called *foreplay*, or a prelude to sexual intercourse. Many people who are unable for one reason or another to have intercourse discover, to their delight, that the activities usually called foreplay can be just as satisfying as intercourse. Stimulation of a woman's genitals by a partner's mouth or tongue is called *cunnilingus*, and the same activity performed on a man's genitals is called *fellatio*. Both activities are called "oral sex" and may or may not be a prelude to intercourse. Couples may also engage in *outercourse*, or the rubbing of the penis between the thighs or breasts. This is often done as a form of contraception.

Although anal intercourse has been generally considered a homosexual form of activity, in two recent surveys, between nine and thirteen percent of women reported that they engaged in anal intercourse regularly. Another survey indicates that up to forty-three percent of heterosexual couples engage in anal intercourse at least occasionally (Reinisch, 1990).

Homosexual behaviours can include any possible combinations of the previously mentioned activities, but take place between partners of the same gender. **Homosexuality** is a sexual orientation, defined as the romantic and sexual attraction to a same-sex partner. There is no clear explanation for homosexuality, but it is known to have existed in ancient cultures, and is considered, as is heterosexual preference, to be an inherent aspect of a person's identity. **Bisexuality** refers to the preference and attraction to either sex.

There are a number of other variations in human sexual identity and sexual behaviour. Gender dysphoria, commonly known as ***transsexualism***, occurs when an individual's gender identity does not match the biological gender. In this situation, a man may feel like a woman trapped in a male body or a woman may view herself as a man encased in a woman's body. ***Transvestism***, or cross-dressing, refers to individuals who enjoy dressing like the opposite sex for sexual pleasure or psychological comfort. Another variation in sexual behaviour is ***paraphilia***. In Greek, "para" means beyond or outside of the usual and "philia" means love. Paraphilias range from sexual preferences generally not considered unusual as, for example, a desire to see one's partner dressed in seductive underwear to more extreme or possibly dangerous activities such as bondage or asphyxiation. A more thorough discussion of these variant sexual preferences and behaviours is beyond the scope of this book.

COMMON SEXUAL CONCERNS

A large number of factors can influence sexual function. Problems may arise when people feel that patterns of sexual interest or response which are normal for them have been impaired. For instance, fear of the effect of sexual activity on the heart following a heart attack may inhibit sexual desire for both partners. Sometimes sexual problems are not so much problems as they are culturally based differences in expectations. For example, a male partner may view his female partner's sexual arousal and orgasm as a direct reflection of his masculinity. His partner, however, may not be easily aroused or may not need frequent orgasm. The pressure of his expectations can generate feelings of inadequacy and stress which can further suppress sexual desire. Table 34.3 presents an outline of some common sexual concerns that people may have.

Treatment of Sexual Concerns

Treatment of sexual problems may involve both psychological and physical treatment and will depend upon the cause of the dysfunction and the context in which it occurs. Sexual therapy begins with a detailed assessment which includes the time of onset of the problem (whether it has existed since the onset of sexual experiences or whether it began after a period of satisfactory sexual experiences); the extent of the problem (whether it is present in all situations or only in particular situations or with certain partners); and an exploration of the effects of the problem on the person and his or her partner. An educational component is often required. If problems are evident within the relationship in general, couple therapy may be required before sexual issues can be addressed. In most cases, and especially those in which the sexual problem has had an impact on both partners and the relationship, therapy is most effective if both partners participate.

SEXUALLY TRANSMITTED DISEASES

There are a number of diseases caused by bacterial or bacteria-related organisms which are spread by infected people through intimate or sexual contact. These diseases are called sexually transmitted diseases or STDs. The Human Immunodeficiency Virus (HIV) and the Hepatitis B Virus are STDs that may be contracted through sexual or other contact with body fluids such as blood, semen, urine or feces.

STDs may also be found in areas of the body other than the sexual organs. For example, gonorrhea and chlamydia can infect other warm, moist areas such as the throat, the nasopharynx or the eyes. A person may be infected by more than one STD at a time. In addition, many STDs have similar or overlapping symptoms. Therefore, in Table 34.4, the more common and serious STDs are listed as *syndromes*, or groups of symptoms which result from one or more infective agents.

Treatment of Sexually Transmitted Diseases

STDs are usually treated successfully with antibiotics. Unfortunately, reinfection can occur, and bacteria (such as the gonococcus) may form resistance to antibiotics, which necessitates the development of ever more potent medications.

The virus which causes Herpes Simplex usually can only be treated symptomatically until the infection subsides. The virus may then be harboured within the nerve pathways and becomes symptomatic and infectious when the body's natural defences are weakened through stress or illness.

Viruses such as Hepatitis B (HBV) and HIV are capable of surviving within the body for many years often without symptoms, but they may be transmitted through unprotected sexual contact or by sharing needles used for injecting street drugs. Treatment for both HBV and HIV/AIDS is aimed at treating opportunistic infections and diseases and supporting the body's natural defences as much as possible. A vaccine is available for the prevention of Hepatitis B, but as yet a vaccine preventing HIV infection has not been developed. Neither disease is as yet curable, which leads to an emphasis on prevention.

ASSESSING SEXUALITY NEEDS

An assessment of a patient's sexual health status is an essential part of the general health assessment. This includes an appraisal of physical or functional status and an exploration of the psychosocial aspects of sexual health. Reproductive health issues will be briefly discussed here because the reproductive system is involved in both sexual function and childbearing.

NURSING HEALTH HISTORY

When taking a health history, a thorough exploration of the patient's sexual practices and patterns of sexual functioning is neither appropriate nor necessary in the majority of cases. For instance, when a patient comes into the hospital for the

TABLE 34.3   Common Sexual Concerns

PROBLEM	WOMEN	MEN
Impaired sexual desire	Also called *low libido*. Most frequent problem in women. May be associated with relationship problems, depression or organic causes.	In both primary and secondary cases, organic causes (for example, hypogonadism) may be a factor. In secondary cases, relationship with partner or depression may be a factor.
Impaired sexual arousal	Lack of sensations associated with sexual excitement. Absence of vaginal lubrication and engorgement. May occur secondary to impaired sexual interest following childbirth or menopause, and in women with strong sexual inhibitions.	Manifested as erectile dysfunction. Most common problem in men who seek help.
Orgasmic problems	Absent or very infrequent orgasm in both men and women. If orgasm can occur with masturbation but not with the partner, this may be associated with relationship problems.	
Ejaculatory problems		*Premature ejaculation*: Ejaculations occur consistently before or very soon after vaginal penetration. Common in first sexual encounters and in stressful situations. *Retarded (delayed) ejaculation*: Relatively uncommon. Can affect both ejaculation and orgasm. *Retrograde ejaculation*: Usually due to physical causes (surgery to bladder neck, spinal cord injury). Orgasm may be experienced but ejaculation is directed into the bladder.
Other problems	*Dyspareunia* (Pain during intercourse): May be localized at introitus or deeper. Causes include lack of arousal or lubrication, vaginal or pelvic infection, endometriosis or constipation. *Vaginismus*: Involuntary muscle spasm at introitus, which occurs with attempted penetration. May be a primary problem or secondary to vaginal trauma or infection. Most women with vaginismus are otherwise sexually responsive.	

removal of a gallbladder, it is not necessary to inquire about sexual practices but when admitted for an investigation of genitourinary symptoms, a sexual health history becomes necessary. It is important in the nursing history to discover any effects the current illness or treatment measures may have on sexual functioning and on sexual self-image. For example, how has gallbladder disease and the need for surgery affected a woman's ability to function as a mother and as a wife?

When taking a sexual health history, the nurse begins with questions about the effects of the current illness on sexual functioning. If it is known that sexuality is likely to be affected by a specific illness, treatment regimen or surgery, more specific information about sexual functioning may be gathered. Furthermore, should significant sexual needs and concerns become evident, a more thorough examination may then ensue. A guide for obtaining a brief sexual health

TABLE 34.4   Common Sexually Transmitted Diseases

SYNDROME AND CAUSATIVE AGENT	SYMPTOMS
Urethritis • Gonococcus • Chlamydia and others	Penile pain or itching Dysuria Urethral discharge (30 % to 50 % asymptomatic)

Vaginitis
• Candida albicans
• Bacterial vaginosis:
   Gardnerella
   Trichomonas
	Vulval, vaginal itching
	Abnormal vaginal discharge
	Redness, edema of vulva
	Dyspareunia
	Dysuria
	Unpleasant odour

Cervicitis • Chlamydia • Gonorrhea • Herpes simplex 2	Often asymptomatic Abnormal vaginal discharge Systemic symptoms (herpes) Dyspareunia Menstrual spotting Post-coital bleeding
Pelvic Inflammatory Disease • Chlamydia • Gonorrhea • Other non-STDs • HIV in women	Lower abdominal or back pain Menstrual spotting Abnormal vaginal discharge Fever, general malaise Dyspareunia

Ulcerative Skin Lesions
• Syphilis
  (Treponema Pallidum)
	Painless ulcer at area of contact
	Skin rash, fevers, general malaise
	Late stage: deterioration of neurological
	  and cardiovascular systems, death

• Herpes simplex virus	**Primary infection**: malaise, fever itching, pain
	  in genital area, blister-like genital lesions lasting
	  for three to six weeks
	Recurrences: same as primary but without malaise

Non-Ulcerative Skin Lesions
• Condyloma acuminata
  (Human Papilloma Virus)
• Certain sub-types of HPV
  are implicated in some types of genital cancers,
  for example, cervix, vulva, penis, rectum
	Cauliflower-like growths on genitals,
	  in oral cavity, vagina or rectum, may
	  be difficult to see

Other Viral Infections
• HIV: causative agent of
  Acquired Immunodeficiency
  Syndrome (AIDS)
	Early infection: usually no symptoms
	Later stages: symptoms are related to loss of immune
	  defences. Opportunistic infections and cancers develop in
	  the majority of cases so far, leading to death.
	AIDS-related symptoms vary widely from person to
	  person and for men and women.
	Tests for antibodies, indicating infection with HIV, may be
	  negative for up to six months following exposure, but the
	  person may infect others during that time.

• Hepatitis B Virus	**Symptoms of acute hepatitis:** • malaise • fever • jaundice **Late complications:** • cirrhosis of the liver • cancer of the liver

history is given in the box below. The beginning student who does not feel ready to pursue this level of examination should seek the help of an instructor or experienced nurse.

Many people view sexuality as very private and are often reticent to discuss sexual health with others. As a result, they may be reluctant to talk openly about sexual matters. In some cultures, discussing female and male physiologic functions and problems is taboo. It is therefore necessary to first obtain the patient's permission before asking sex-related questions. Patients may be more willing to discuss sexual functioning if they know why the information is needed and that the information will be kept strictly confidential. If the patient chooses not to discuss sexual functioning, nurses should accept this decision. At the same time, nurses should stress that they will be available to talk about any concerns the patient may have in the future.

In order to generate a level of trust which will allow for open discussion of personal issues, nurses must arrange for privacy and they must be sensitive to the patient's concerns in this regard. Because confidentiality is a critical point when information about sexual matters is being shared, nurses must emphasize that what is said in the interview will remain confidential. Taking the history when the patient is dressed and using terms they understand will enhance comfort. Terminology and anatomical language may pose barriers to obtaining accurate data about body functions. The use of slang terms may be necessary to impart meaning. Only those areas that are pertinent to the needs of the patient should be discussed.

PHYSICAL ASSESSMENT

Physical assessment begins with a general inspection of appearance. This includes body shape and stature (Is it appropriate for gender?), hair distribution, skin texture and growth patterns. These aspects vary according to the age and developmental stage of the individual. The nurse must apply knowledge of growth and development patterns throughout the life cycle to determine whether findings are normal or abnormal. Inspection and palpation techniques are used to assess the genital structures of both men and women. Just as many people do not like talking about sexual matters, they also do not like others looking at their genitals. Nurses must therefore exercise the same consideration and sensitivity to patient privacy during physical assessment as they do during the history-taking. A confident, thoughtful and reassuring approach along with proper draping will do much to enhance patient ease and reduce embarrassment. In addition, unless the patient is admitted with a sexual health problem, conducting the physical assessment while performing routine measures may alleviate embarrassment. For instance, the nurse might wait to carry out an external genital appraisal on an older adult until administering perineal hygiene care.

FEMALE PATIENTS

Female physical appraisal involves examination of the breasts, the external genitalia and an internal (pelvic) examination. Breast examination provides a good opportunity

---

HEALTH HISTORY GUIDE

Sexuality

Health and Illness Patterns

- Are you sexually active?

- Has your illness or anything else affected your sexual function? If so, how?

- How has your illness or anything else affected your ability to function in your role as a spouse/ sexual partner/parent?

- How has your illness or anything else affected the way you feel about yourself? As a man/woman?

- Do you have any concerns about your sexuality and sexual function?

- What do you expect from health care professionals in promoting your sexual health?

Health Promotion and Protection Patterns

For Females:

- Do you have regular health checkups? Pap smear? Mammography?

- Do you examine your breasts on a monthly basis?

For Males:

- Do you examine your testes regularly?

For Both Sexes:

- Do you practise safe sex?

- Would you like some information on sexual self-care and on safe sex practices?

SOURCES: Carpenito, 1993; Woods, 1984.

for teaching breast self-examination. The breasts are examined for contour appropriate for age, symmetry of structures, areas of skin pigmentation, the presence of redness, rashes, lesions and edema, as well as discharge from the nipple. It is not unusual for breasts to be slightly asymmetrical and unequal in size, particularly in growing women. The breasts, nipples and axillary and clavicular nodes are palpated for consistency of tissues, masses and tenderness.

The external genitalia are examined for the size, shape and colour of structures and the presence of lesions, inflammation and discharge. A mirror can be used to teach women about their own anatomy, showing them the mons pubis, the clitoris, the labia majora and minora, the urethral and vaginal openings and the openings of the ducts of Bartholin's and Skene's glands. Normally, the vulva is darker in colour than other skin areas, and the mucous membranes are dark, pink and moist. Abnormalities that should be noted include tenderness, irritations or lesions of the skin, discolouration, lumps or swelling in any area, abnormal size or adhesions of the clitoris and unusual discharges from the vagina. A small amount of clear or whitish discharge is normal.

The vaginal and internal pelvic examinations are ordinarily performed by physicians, midwives and nurses specializing in sexual health care. However, nurses may be called upon to assist with the procedure and certainly to prepare the patient and answer questions. The vaginal examination involves the use of a speculum and light source to examine the vagina and the cervix. The examiner looks for lesions, discolouration or unusual discharges from either the vaginal walls or the cervix, abnormalities in size or position of the cervix and signs of infection, damage or growths in either area. If the speculum is metal, it should be warmed prior to use. The speculum should also be lubricated with a water-base jelly or warm water. While the speculum is in place, specimens may be obtained for laboratory examination, which will be discussed later. During the internal pelvic examination, the examiner inserts two gloved fingers into the vagina and exerts pressure to move the uterus and other organs towards the front of the abdominal wall, allowing palpation with the other hand. Any pain or abnormality in the size or consistency of the internal organs are noted.

In preparation for a vaginal or internal pelvic examination, the woman is asked to void immediately prior to the procedure. This facilitates ease of examination, since a full bladder distorts the position of the pelvic organs. A full bladder also makes the procedure more uncomfortable for the patient. The patient is usually placed in a lithotomy position to permit full visualization of the genital area. A lateral Sim's position may be used for patients who are unable to assume a lithotomy position, for example, women with arthritis or musculoskeletal deformity.

MALE PATIENTS

The genital examination includes visual inspection of the size and shape of the organs, the condition of the skin and the presence of lesions, edema, inflammation or discharge. The inguinal region is observed for hernias. Using a gloved hand, the penis is palpated for masses or tenderness. The tip of the glans is compressed to determine the presence of penile discharge (an abnormal finding). The scrotal contents are examined by holding the scrotum in the palm of one hand and gently palpating the structures with the thumb and first two fingers of the other hand. The testes are examined for size, shape, consistency and mobility; the epididymis and spermatic cord for masses, tenderness and swelling. Normally, the testes are asymmetrical, the left usually being slightly lower than the right. Their size varies; approximately two centimetres in diameter at the larger end is average. The testes feel firm on palpation and move around easily. Because testicular cancer is common in young adult men, men should learn how to perform testicular self-examinations on a periodic basis. Again, a good time for patient teaching is during the physical assessment.

DIAGNOSTIC TESTS

A number of laboratory tests are performed on a regular basis on any woman who is sexually active, regardless of age, and on every woman beyond the age of twenty. The *Papanicalou (Pap) test* is done to screen for cervical cell dysplasia (abnormal changes which can lead to cancer). The Pap test may also indicate chronic inflammation or the presence of trichomonas, herpes simplex and/or human papilloma virus. A small amount of tissue for laboratory examination is scraped from the cervix during a pelvic examination. Culture samples are taken to identify infectious diseases, caused mainly by *Candida albicans* (yeast), *Gardnerella vaginalis* (bacterial vaginosis), *Trichomonas vaginalis*, *Chlamydia trachomatis* and N. *Gonorrhoeae*. At the same time, the vaginal walls and cervix are carefully scrutinized for herpes or HPV lesions. Reproductive hormone level assays are also done. Abnormal hormone levels may be a factor in disrupted sexual function or reproductive (fertility) problems. Reproductive hormone level changes can also confirm that menopause has occurred. The levels of male reproductive hormones may also be tested to confirm or rule out hormonal factors in sexual or fertility problems. Males who have ever had sexual intercourse should have routine cultures taken for chlamydia and gonorrhea. Cultures should also be obtained if any suspicious skin lesions are present.

DIAGNOSING SEXUALITY PROBLEMS

Sexuality problems that fall under the domain of nursing therapy are labelled *Altered sexuality patterns*. This diagnostic statement represents problems in which the patient is experiencing or is at risk for experiencing a change in sexual health (Carpenito, 1993). It is used primarily when patients express concern about sexuality. For example, a diagnosis of *Altered sexuality pattern* applies to the problem experienced by a woman who worries about her femininity and ability as a sexual partner following a radical mastectomy; or the problem of a middle-aged male who expresses concern about altered sexual function as a result of antihypertensive medications. Patients may experience a range of responses to conditions affecting sexuality. In these cases, nursing diagnoses reflecting these responses should be used. For instance, in an adolescent who is sexually active but lacks knowledge of contraception and safe sex practices, the more appropriate diagnosis would be *Knowledge deficit*. Similarly, the diagnosis for a patient who is anxious about the effects of treatment on body image would be stated as *Anxiety related to altered body image*.

PLANNING SEXUALITY INTERVENTIONS

As with all nursing needs, the nurse formulates a plan of care based on the established nursing diagnoses. In many cases, patients' problems fall outside the domain of independent nursing intervention. A nursing plan of care might centre on examining feelings, providing information and making referrals to appropriate health care professionals. For instance, impaired sexual function due to physical problems may be referred to gynecologists or urologists or, if available, physicians or mental health professionals with training in sexual therapy. Marital difficulties and relationship problems might be referred to mental health professionals or to sex therapists. Collaboration with the patient and, if appropriate, the sex partner is essential in identifying patient goals and in formulating the plan of care. Effective achievement of goals or expected outcomes is more likely if the patient is involved in setting goals and has a desire to achieve them. Some examples of expected outcomes are listed below.

- Patient will identify limitations on sexual activity caused by health problem.
- Patient will express positive statements about body image and desirability as a sexual partner.
- Patient will report increase in sexual desire and arousal.
- Patient will verbalize proper use of contraceptive methods.
- Patient will verbalize safe sex practices.

IMPLEMENTING SEXUALITY INTERVENTIONS

There are three principal goals of nursing action with regard to human sexual health and sexuality.

1. To provide the knowledge and skills that will enable people to promote and protect their sexual health.
2. To assist in the detection of illness, abnormality or other disorders which can have a damaging impact on sexual health.
3. To assist with or carry out therapeutic measures and to provide support which may improve or restore sexual health.

THE PLISSIT MODEL

Many nurses and health care providers are reluctant to address sexual issues, often because of their own discomfort or lack of special training. They may also be concerned about invading the privacy of patients. One model that is used frequently in sexual counselling is the PLISSIT Model, developed by Annon in 1978. Annon's PLISSIT model identifies four levels of intervention and provides a guideline based on the skills and training of the health care provider. The first level, "Permission," would always be included in any intervention because it is important to promote questions and communication about concerns at every level. The PLISSIT model clearly defines the roles of health care providers at each level.

PERMISSION

The primary element of the *Permission* level of intervention is the encouragement of discussion about sexual matters. The message is given that "sex is spoken here." The role of the nurse at this level is to be sensitive to verbal or behavioural cues about sexual concerns (questions, inappropriate comments or sexual acting out). The nurse then

---

> ### The PLISSIT Model
>
> P
> (PERMISSION)
> LI
> (LIMITED INFORMATION)
> SS
> (SPECIFIC SUGGESTIONS)
> IT
> (INTENSIVE THERAPY)

acknowledges that any changes in a patient's sexual life can be of great concern, that many people have questions but are reluctant or unable to ask them. The other aspect of *Permission* is listening respectfully to patients' concerns, and, if knowledge and training are appropriate, providing the next level of intervention. If not, the nurse may assist in locating an appropriate other resource.

Mr. G. is a 68-year-old man who is in a rehabilitation facility starting his recovery from a cerebral vascular accident (stroke). Whenever a female staff member enters his room, he greets her flirtatiously, invites her into his bed "for a good time," and requests back rubs for his "lower back pain."

The *Permission* level of intervention in this situation could involve a gentle but firm setting of behavioural limits for Mr. G., pointing out that his behaviour causes the staff discomfort, making them feel reluctant to enter his room and provide the care that he needs. The nurse could then state that many people who have had Mr. G.'s type of illness also have concerns about what changes may have occurred sexually and that arrangements could be made for him to talk to someone who is knowledgeable in that area.

Many people will not express questions or concerns unless directly encouraged to do so. The nurse can anticipate this and, once rapport is established with the patient, the topic of sexuality may be introduced. One method which promotes comfort is the making of a "ubiquity" statement — a statement that validates the "normality" of such concerns. For example, the nurse might say, "Many people who have had a spinal cord injury have concerns about what their sexual function might be like when they go home from hospital. Is this something you have thought about?"

LIMITED INFORMATION

The next level of the PLISSIT model is *Limited Information*. The patient is provided with information that pertains to the specific situation. For example, myths or misinformation may be clarified, the basic sexual response cycle may be explained, contraception or safer sex practices may be discussed or the possible effects of certain medications on sexual function may be outlined.

Sally is a 16-year-old secondary school student who has been visiting the health office at school frequently, with a number of minor concerns. The nurse's time in the school is limited, with only one session per year in each classroom. The session in Sally's class dealt with making healthy decisions. It was enthusiastically received because of the nurse's creative approaches to the topic and non-judgemental manner. Later, Sally comes to the nurse's office complaining of a sore throat. While the nurse is checking Sally's throat, she asks, "You can't get pregnant the first time you have sex, can you?"

The nurse, who has had training in counselling and adolescent health, encourages Sally to talk about her concerns. The *Permission* level is applied here (and was im-

plicitly applied in the classroom). The nurse could provide information about the possibility of pregnancy in that situation (*Limited Information*) and then assist Sally in finding appropriate resources.

SPECIFIC SUGGESTIONS

The use of the *Specific Suggestions* level usually requires a level of specialized expertise which is achieved through training and experience. This may be viewed as the "problem-solving" level, where the health care provider's knowledge and skills can assist the patient in improving the quality of sexual experiences.

Mrs. H. is a 31-year-old woman whose first baby is now six weeks old. During a visit to the well-baby clinic, the nurse inquires about how things are going at home, sleeping habits, breast feeding and concerns about contraception. Mrs. H. states, "Sex is pretty well a non-event at our house these days. Not only am I too tired most of the time, but it also hurts when we try to have intercourse."

The nurse is aware that in the postpartum period and during the time the mother is breast feeding her baby, there can be a decline in sexual desire. In addition, hormonal changes involved in lactation can decrease the amount of vaginal lubrication which in turn can cause dyspareunia. The nurse could discuss some strategies (*Specific Suggestions*) with Mrs. H. to promote positive sexual functioning, for example, finding some time to herself and getting some extra rest by having her partner bottle-feed the baby once during the night with breast milk that has been collected and stored by freezing. The use of water-soluble vaginal lubricants for intercourse can relieve the discomfort when Mrs. H.'s interest in sex returns. In the meantime, Mrs. H. and her partner might explore some mutually acceptable alternate approaches.

INTENSIVE THERAPY

Intensive Therapy is the final level of intervention and is usually provided by specialized health care professionals. It includes such approaches as medications, surgery, counselling, sexual therapy or other specialized techniques. The use of intensive therapy requires very careful assessment of all aspects of sexual function and consideration of the impact that such treatment may have on the person and, if appropriate, on the partner.

Mrs. T. is a 24-year-old woman whose marriage was arranged by her family. Shortly after the wedding, the couple moved to Canada and Mrs. T. began to learn to speak English. She was referred for sexual therapy because all attempts to have sexual intercourse had been extremely painful and unsuccessful.

In this situation, the sexual therapist, who could be a nurse with special training, would conduct a sexual health assessment from a physical perspective and within a psychosocial and cultural context. The diagnosis of vaginismus, confirmed by a careful examination, would provide a basis for a comprehensive therapeutic approach. This includes sexual and relationship counselling and sexuality education for both partners, the use of vaginal introducers to relieve spasm of the vaginal muscles and referral to community agencies which provide social contact for women from other cultures who are also isolated from customary support systems. The nurse is aware that the use of vaginal introducers alone, without the other interventions, would likely be unsuccessful.

NURSE–PATIENT RELATIONSHIPS

One of the most difficult challenges for nursing practice is the setting of boundaries between professional and personal relationships. Situations involved in nurse–patient interactions, particularly where personal care or sexuality issues are involved, can engender a form of intimacy which could then "spill over" into other interactions between the nurse and patient. A patient may become sexually attracted to or infatuated with a nurse. This attraction could become mutual.

Many institutions have developed guidelines or regulations regarding relationships between patients and staff, but some have not. In any case, the onus is on the nurse to behave in a responsible manner which also recognizes and respects the patient's needs. Below are some approaches the nurse may find helpful in such situations.

1. Recognize and accept that sexual attraction can and does occur between people. Also recognize that there is no need to act on this attraction just because it is there.

2. Recognize that the physical closeness and dependency inherent in a health care setting is different from the usual mutuality and independence found in healthy relationships.

3. Whether or not the feelings of attraction are mutual the nurse has to address this in a calm, professional manner which recognizes and affirms the patient's sexuality and needs, while clarifying the need for the relationship to remain asexual and professional.

4. Recognize that many people are embarrassed and sensitive about sexual matters and have a strong need for privacy. Nurses may become so accustomed to nudity or exposed genitalia that the patient's discomfort may not be acknowledged or dealt with. Providing suitable coverings during a complete physical examination can help preserve a sense of dignity.

5. Before asking about sexual matters, it often helps to alleviate patient discomfort by asking permission. For example, "Would it be all right if I asked you a few questions about what your sex life has been like since your illness?" Respect the right of the person to decline this discussion and respond with a statement such as, "I understand that this is a very private matter for you. If you have any questions later on, I would be happy to try to find you some answers."

6. Avoid making assumptions and avoid expressing them in your terminology. For instance, ask, "Are you currently in a relationship?" rather than, "Are you married?" And refer to a "partner" rather than "wife" or "husband." Use phrases such as "people who have a spinal cord injury" or "people with disabilities" rather than "the spinal cord injured" or "the disabled." A balance between a professional manner and the warmth of genuine caring is most beneficial in the nurse–patient relationship.

HEALTH PROMOTING STRATEGIES

Sexuality is a fundamental aspect of life that is influenced by a complex system of physiological, psychological, developmental and social factors. In order to assist patients to achieve an optimum level of sexual health, the nurse must understand these influences and recognize differences in sexual orientation and experience. Nurses can help patients and if appropriate their partners to maintain optimum sexual health in two basic ways. First, nurses can encourage people to explore lifestyle factors, cultural and personal values and health practices that might have an impact on sexual health. Second, nurses can provide information which will enable patients to make informed decisions and take responsibility for sexual health. Sexuality education and supportive care are the chief nursing strategies in helping to promote optimal sexual health.

SEXUAL DECISION MAKING

An underlying element in the promotion of healthy and responsible sexual decision making is the concept of empowerment and ownership of the sexual self. People who lack a sense of control over situations may have difficulty making decisions about sexual health. For example, someone whose low self-esteem is the result of sexual or other forms of abuse may be unable to make decisions about the use or care of his or her own body and may continue to be victimized. Many people who have not been victimized also lack this ability. With proper support, a sense of self-ownership and an ability to exercise control over one's sexual life can be gained.

In addition to a sense of control, people need sufficient information to allow informed decision making. Very often, health promoting measures are not followed because of a lack of information or because the information is incorrect. An example might be a woman who not only believes

HEALTH PROMOTING STRATEGY

Promoting Healthy Sexuality

- Develop a sense of control over your sexual life. Learn about sexual health and sexual functioning so that you can make the best decisions for your needs. Information may be obtained from school health nurses, occupational health nurses or community clinics.

- Develop a Reproductive Life Plan so that you can make choices about your sexual health.

- If appropriate, learn about contraception or birth control to enable you to make an informed decision. Information and counselling may be obtained from community clinics, such as Planned Parenthood, community health agencies and women's health clinics.

- If single, become involved in activities where you can meet people of the opposite sex (or of the same sex if you are homosexual) such as church groups, sports and health clubs, special interest groups.

- Maintain physical fitness. This helps you feel good about yourself and enhances relationships with others.

- Remember that sexuality is expressed in many physical and emotional ways, not only in sexual intercourse. Enjoy close relationships with others you care about and who love you; share feelings, give hugs; and accept touch as an expression of warmth, caring and love.

---

that oral contraceptives cause heart attacks and cancer, but also rejects condoms "because men don't like to use them." Access to appropriate health screening services and safe, effective contraceptive methods also facilitates decisions that need to be made about sexual health. People who know where to go and how to find the available services are much more likely to act responsibly in regard to sexuality needs.

from a long-term perspective offers the opportunity to make choices. In so doing, it provides a sense of control over life. People who choose to use safe sex practices and protection from unwanted pregnancy will be much more likely to have a positive attitude towards these practices instead of considering them bothersome intrusions with negative potential consequences.

SEXUALITY EDUCATION

Just as sexuality is a life-long issue, the need for education and counselling exists throughout the life span. Three common areas of sexuality education in which nurses play a key role include reproductive health, contraceptive education and the prevention of sexually transmitted diseases (STDs). Teaching about preventive measures for STDs is a health protecting strategy. The role of the nurse in providing sexuality education or counselling depends on the nurse's level of training and expertise and on the policies of the health care agency.

Reproductive Health

One way of assisting people to promote optimal sexual health is the concept of a *Reproductive Life Plan*. A Reproductive Life Plan allows individuals to consider sexuality from a long-term perspective. This would include an exploration of hopes and dreams for future relationships, career plans and whether or not to have children. The impact of sexually transmitted diseases on health and fertility would be discussed as would possible options if an unplanned pregnancy were to occur. The management of sexuality

Contraceptive methods permit couples to regulate the number and timing of children.

Contraceptive Education

The use of contraception or birth control is a personal choice. The nurse's primary role in contraceptive teaching and counselling is to provide accurate, unbiased information to enable the patient to make an informed decision. The selection of a contraceptive method is a collaborative endeavour between the health care provider and the patient. There are several factors that must be considered when selecting a contraceptive method:

1. The effectiveness of the method in preventing pregnancy.
2. The safety and possible side effects.
3. The cost.
4. The long-term effects on future fertility.
5. The effectiveness of the method in protection from STDs.

Table 34.5 gives a description of common birth control methods along with typical failure rates and contraindications for use. The typical failure rates are expressed as a percentage of typical couples who initiate use of a method and experience accidental pregnancy during the first year, and do not stop use of the method for any other reason.

TABLE 34.5   Birth Control Methods

METHOD AND DESCRIPTION	FAILURE RATE	CONTRAINDICATIONS
Coitus Interruptus Removal of the penis from the vagina prior to ejaculation.	16 % – 23 %	Any situation in which pregnancy is absolutely contraindicated.
Fertility Awareness Methods Methods of determining probable fertile period during a menstrual cycle (Calendar Method, Sympto-Thermal or Billings).	2 % – 25 %	Women who have irregular menstrual cycles or where pregnancy is absolutely contraindicated.
Vaginal Spermicides Foams, suppositories, tablets or jellies inserted intravaginally prior to intercourse.	10 % – 21 %	Sensitivity to chemicals or perfumes in the product; physical or mental disability.
Vaginal Contraceptive Sponge Small, pillow-shaped polyurethane sponge, containing 1 gm nonoxynol 9, inserted intravaginally prior to intercourse, effective for 24 hours.	18 % – 28 %	History of Toxic Shock Syndrome, vaginal infection, including *S. Aureus*; allergy to polyurethane or nonoxynol 9; anatomic abnormalities of the pelvis or vagina; physical or mental disability.
Female Condom A polyurethane pouch which is held in the vagina by an inner flexible ring. An outer ring holds the condom in place, covering the entire area of the labia. Provides better protection from STDs for the female than does the male condom.	Not yet available	Allergy to condom material; physical or mental disability.
Male Condom Latex sheaths worn over the penis during genital contact; the latex forms a barrier to transmission of semen and/or organisms that cause sexually transmitted diseases.	12 %	Allergy to latex or spermicidal agent; mental or physical disability; some men cannot maintain erections if condoms are used.

continued on next page

TABLE 34.5

continued

METHOD AND DESCRIPTION	FAILURE RATE	CONTRAINDICATIONS
Diaphragm, Cervical Cap Vaginal barrier methods used in combination with spermicidal creams or jellies.	18 % – 23 %	History of Toxic Shock Syndrome, vaginal infections, including *S. Aureus*; repeated urinary tract infections, pelvic inflammatory disease; allergies to rubber or spermicides; anatomic abnormalities; cervical biopsy or cryosurgery within past six weeks (cervical cap); full-term delivery within past six to twelve weeks.
Intrauterine Device Plastic device usually wrapped with copper, or may have hormone added; inserted into the cavity of the uterus where it prevents passage of sperm to fallopian tubes, may also prevent implantation if fertilization occurs.	1.5 % – 5 %	Risk factors present for sexually transmitted diseases, acute pelvic infection, history of ectopic pregnancy, known or suspected pregnancy; anatomic abnormalities or malignancy of the reproductive system; valvular heart disease, bleeding disorders, anemia; concern for future fertility.
Oral Contraceptives **a. Combined**: tablets containing estrogen and progesterone taken in a series; suppress ovulation, diminish growth of endometrium, increase viscosity of cervical mucus.	0.5 % – 3 %	Personal or family history of cardiovascular disorders, risk factors for thrombosis, known or suspected estrogen-dependent neoplasms; pregnancy; liver disease; age over 40 combined with any other risk factor; smoking, (15 or more cigarettes per day), headaches, hypertension, inability to take pills consistently or correctly.
b. Progestin-Only: The "mini-pill" has fewer estrogen-related health risks than combined pill. 40 % to 60 % of women on mini-pill have ovulatory cycles. Possible method once lactation is well established in breast-feeding mothers.	1 % – 3 %	A history of functional ovarian cysts or ectopic pregnancy, unexplained abnormal or irregular vaginal bleeding during previous three months; inability to take pills consistently and correctly.
Long-Acting Progestin Provides long-term contraception. Most common side effects are irregular bleeding and some weight gain. May be a delay of six to twelve months in return of fertility following use.		
a. Norplant (levonorgestrel): Progestin is contained in small silastic capsules that are inserted subcutaneously. Provides contraception for up to five years.	0.04 %	Acute liver disease, jaundice, unexplained vaginal bleeding, history of blood clots in legs (thrombophlebitis), lungs (pulmonary embolism) or eyes; pregnancy, within six weeks postpartum in lactating women, smoking. The presence of other medical conditions such as diabetes, epilepsy, hypertension; elevated cholesterol or triglycerides should be carefully reviewed prior to administering Norplant.

TABLE 34.5

continued

METHOD AND DESCRIPTION	FAILURE RATE	CONTRAINDICATIONS
b. DepoProvera (medroxyproges-terone acetate): Progestin is given by injection every three months.	0.3 %	Same absolute contraindications as in combined oral contraceptives, (except DepoProvera does not appear to increase the risk of thromboembolic disease), unexplained irregular vaginal bleeding, and where a rapid return to fertility will be desired.
Post-Coital Methods		
a. Hormonal: Can prevent pregnancy if taken within 72 hours of unprotected intercourse, must be only episode of unprotected intercourse in that cycle. Consists of 2 tablets of 50 μg ethinyl estradiol, 0.5 mg D1-norgestrel (Ovral-Wyeth), and 2 tablets 12 hours later.	less than 1 %	Same as for combined oral contraceptives but because post-coital use is short-term, the advantages of using may outweigh possible risks.
b. Intrauterine Device: A copper-bearing IUD can be inserted within five days of unprotected intercourse. Left in place, it can then provide ongoing contraception.	1 % – 3 %	Same as for IUD.
c. Menstrual Extraction: Insertion of a sterile cannula into the uterine cavity and removal of uterine contents by suction, if menstrual period more than two weeks late.	Not well documented	Any situation where risks of hemorrhage or infection outweigh other considerations.
Sterilization A permanent method which involves surgical procedures.		Where informed consent cannot be obtained, where future pregnancy might be desired, or where surgical risks outweigh other considerations.
Female: Tubal ligation, in which the fallopian tubes are ligated or sealed by cautery.	0.4 %	
Male: Vasectomy, in which the vas deferens is cut and either ligated or cauterized through an incision made into the scrotal skin.	0.15 %	

Unreliable Methods

A. Attempting to calculate ovulation by using a calendar alone.
B. Douching or washing out the vagina following intercourse. This cannot prevent sperm from entering the uterus immediately after ejaculation. Douching should only be used if a special solution is prescribed for treatment of vaginal infection. The use of strongly acidic solutions can cause severe damage to the vaginal mucosa.
C. Coitus interruptus or withdrawal is not effective because of the difficulty of interrupting sexual intercourse at the peak of sexual feelings and because the pre-ejaculatory fluid may contain a significant number of sperm.
D. The insertion of spermicidal products into the vagina following intercourse is unlikely to be effective (see item B).
E. Lactation decreases fertility in some women particularly if the breast feeding is constant and the infant has no other source for suckling. However, lactating women may ovulate without warning as their menstrual cycles resume. Conception can occur at this first post-partum ovulation.

SOURCES: Hatcher, et al., 1992; International Planned Parenthood Federation, Family Planning Policy Statements.

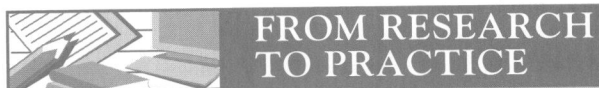

FROM RESEARCH TO PRACTICE

Menstrual Hygiene and Toxic Shock Syndrome

Hatcher et al. (1992). *Contraceptive technology, 1990–1992.* New York: Irvington.

Toxic Shock Syndrome (TSS) is a rare but serious disease which can occur when a toxin produced by the S. Aureus bacteria enters the bloodstream and causes a systemic illness. This can occur when the bacteria are present in a wound or in the vagina during menstruation. TSS was first noted in 1980 and at that time was associated with the use of a particular brand of super-absorbent tampon. The tampon has since been removed from the market. TSS occurs in males with infected wounds and in females who use tampons, contraceptive sponges and diaphragms.

The rates of TSS are low, estimated at 3 to 14 cases per 100,000 menstruating women. The risk of TSS in tampon, sponge, cap and diaphragm users can be minimized by ensuring that tampons are changed frequently during menstruation and that birth control methods are left in place for no longer than the recommended length of time.

The symptoms of TSS are fever, rash with desquamation of the skin, conjunctivitis, pharyngitis, vomiting, myalgia, weakness, hypotension, fatigue and severe diarrhea. In severe cases, TSS can rapidly lead to shock, coma and death. Immediate medical intervention is mandatory.

HEALTH PROTECTING STRATEGIES

Many aspects of reproductive health screening, such as breast and testicular examinations and the teaching of breast and testicular self-examination, are performed by nurses. In some agencies Pap tests and tests for STDs may also be performed by nurses. This offers a unique opportunity to discuss sexual anatomy and sexual function in a non-threatening setting. Another major element of health protection is the teaching of safe sex practices and prevention of sexually transmitted diseases. Guidelines for safe sex practices and the prevention of STDs are presented in the box below. Figures 34.5 and 34.6 outline methods for breast self-examination and testicular self-examination. Nurses can also assist individuals to maintain safe sexual health by promoting public education and access to resources that encourage healthy sexual behaviours and awareness of possible risks.

In addition, there are a number of strategies that health care providers can implement to prevent the transmission of STDs. Because many STDs, including HIV/AIDS and Hepatitis B, are infectious even when asymptomatic, body substance precautions must *always* be exercised by health care providers when in contact with any body fluids just as safer sex practices must always be used by all sexually active people. Blood, tissues, organs and sperm that will be used for transplant or donation must be carefully screened as blood is screened for transfusion.

HEALTH PROTECTING STRATEGY

Protecting Strategies

Promoting Safe Sex Practices

- Take some time to get to know your sex partner. Share your sexual health histories with one another.
- Avoid anal intercourse.
- Use latex condoms for vaginal intercourse.
- Use latex condoms or dental dams for oral sex.
- Minimize the number of sexual partners.
- Avoid sharing sex toys or devices.

Prevention of Sexually Transmitted Diseases

- Do not share needles used for injecting drugs.
- Practice safe sex and, in addition:
  - Avoid any sexual behaviour that involves exchange of or contact with body fluids.
  - Limit sexual activity to one partner who is guaranteed not to be infected.

BEFORE MIRROR   **LYING DOWN**

1. With your arms relaxed at your sides, inspect your breasts carefully for any changes in size or shape. Look for any rashes, puckered or dimpled skin, and for any discharge or change in the nipples.

Turn and inspect each side view of the breast. Observe for any flattening in side view. When turned, inspect back and bra line areas for moles and skin irritations.

2. Raise your arms over your head and bend forward from your waist, inspecting both breasts for any changes.

3. Standing straight, raise your arms over your head and move them *slowly* up and down (3 times), observing that the breasts move freely over the chest wall. Turn left and right, observing sides of breasts in same manner.

4. Press hands together at chin level and push firmly (3 times) to flex your chest muscles. Turn left and right, observing sides of breasts and underarm breast tissue in the same manner.

5. Regular inspection shows what is normal for you and will give you confidence in your examination.

1. To examine your left breast, place the back of your left hand on your forehead. This distributes breast tissue more evenly on the chest. With the fingers of your right hand held together flat, press gently but firmly with small circular motions around an imaginary clock face, feeling the breast tissue between your fingers and your chest wall.

2. Begin at the outermost top of your left breast for 12 o'clock, and without lifting your fingers from your breast, feel slowly and carefully with small circular motions all the way around the rim of your breast back to 12. A ridge of firm tissue in the lower curve of each breast is normal. Now move your fingers in towards the nipple about 2 cms and feel all the way around again. Repeat this action as many times as necessary to be sure you have covered the entire breast, finishing over the nipple.

3. Bring your left arm down to your side and, still using the flat part of your fingers, feel under your armpit, since breast tissue is found there as well.

4. Now slowly repeat the entire procedure using your left hand on your right breast.

Examine your breasts *regularly* once a month, seven to ten days after each menstrual cycle begins, when breasts are usually not tender or swollen. If you are not menstruating, pick a special day, the first day of the month or your birthdate, to practise BSE. Doing BSE will protect your health.

When you practise BSE you quickly learn what is usual for you, so if anything unusual develops you'll discover it at a very early stage. If a lump, thickening or *any change* is discovered during BSE, it is important to see your doctor right away. Don't be frightened. Most breast lumps or changes are *not* cancer, but only your doctor can make that diagnosis.

FIGURE 34.5   Breast self-examination

SOURCE: Canadian Cancer Society. (1989). *BSE: Breast self-examination*. (Pamphlet). Vancouver: Author. Reproduced with permission.

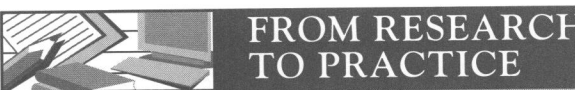

FROM RESEARCH TO PRACTICE

Lierman, L.M., Young, H.M., Cope, G.P., Georgiadou, F. and Benoliel, J.Q. (1994). Effects of education and support on breast self-examination in older women. *Nursing Research, 43,* 158–163.

The purpose of this study was to determine how an educational program and structural support affects the frequency of breast self-examination (BSE) by middle-aged and older women, their proficiency in doing the examination and their perceptions of their skill in BSE. The study population consisted of 175 women 50 years of age or older from a prescreened group of health maintenance organization (HMO) subscribers who volunteered to participate. The women were divided into three groups. One received only the basic teaching program with no support. The second group were paired with peer partners assigned by the researcher. The third group brought their partners of choice to the instructional sessions. Women in both partner groups contracted to work together for six months after instruction, using self-determined strategies of support.

The educational program consisted of a sound/slide presentation about BSE and a discussion of risk factors for breast cancer and factors influencing the performance of BSE. This was followed by individualized one-on-one instruction and supervised practice with a registered nurse. An initial interview was held with each participant and data was gathered in two subsequent interviews (six and twelve months after the educational program).

Data analysis based on the differences between initial interviews and the follow-up interviews indicated that the educational program was very successful in increasing the frequency of breast self-examination, the women's proficiency in carrying it out and their perceived skill in doing it. There was no significant difference in the scores of women in the three groups which the authors feel may have been due to the high level of motivation of all participants. The study shows that older women are willing and able to change their behaviour, given the needed instruction, skills and support.

HEALTH RESTORING STRATEGIES

Sex therapy is a specialized area for nurses as well as for other health care providers such as social workers, psychologists and mental health counsellors. A discussion of restorative care for sexual health challenges is beyond the scope of this book. However, this topic will be covered in more advanced courses.

1. The best time to examine your testicles is right after a hot bath or shower because the scrotal skin is more relaxed and the contents can be felt more easily.
2. Place your index and middle fingers on the underside of the testicle and your thumbs on the top. Gently roll your testicle between your thumb and fingers. The normal testicle feels slightly soft with an even consistency and a smooth surface. The epididymis can be felt at the back of the testicle and feels slightly different in consistency. Examine both testicles.
3. Any thickening or lump, however small (even pea size), should be reported to your physician.

FIGURE 34.6 Testicular self-examination

SOURCE: Canadian Cancer Society. (1989). *TSE: The most important minute in a man's life.* (Pamphlet). Vancouver: Author. Reproduced with permission.

EVALUATING SEXUALITY INTERVENTIONS

Evaluation of the effectiveness of sexual health care follows implementation and is based on the patient goals and the plan for care. The criteria listed below represent the range of nursing interventions that a general staff nurse or student may implement in meeting patients' sexuality needs.

1. Has the patient gained the knowledge and skills which will enable the promotion of sexual health in the course of living? to be able to exercise informed consent in areas of sexual behaviour? to prevent unwanted pregnancy? to protect against sexually transmitted diseases? to identify the presence of disorders of sexual or reproductive function and be able to seek and obtain appropriate treatment?

2. Are you, the nurse, aware of your personal values and beliefs, and sufficiently comfortable with them to be able to deal with patients' sexuality issues in a matter-of-fact manner? Does your patient show embarrassment or distress when sexual issues are discussed? If so, what steps have you taken to alleviate the distress?

What could you have done differently or in addition that might have been more effective?

3. Have female patients learned and demonstrated skills in breast self-examination? Are they aware of the importance of Pap testing and infection screening? Are male patients able to practise regular testicular self-examination? Are they able to discuss and use condoms appropriately?

KEY TERMS

sex p. 1174

biological sexual identity p. 1175

sexuality p. 1175

gender definition
  (gender identity) p. 1175

gender role identity p. 1175

menarche p. 1181

menopause p. 1181

puberty p. 1186

autosexual activities p. 1189

homosexuality p. 1189

bisexuality p. 1189

transsexualism p. 1189

transvestism p. 1189

paraphilia p. 1189

IN REVIEW

Sexuality is a broad concept which brings together not only the functions for reproduction and sexual pleasure but also the needs for love, personal fulfillment and self-expression and the totality of feelings, attitudes, beliefs and behaviours related to being male or female. Sex refers to the biological distinctions that identify a person as male or female and to the sexual functions for reproduction and pleasure.

Sexual functioning combines a range of sensory and motor responses that are mediated by cognitive, emotional, social, and biological influences. The experience of healthy sexuality depends on the presence of positive factors and the absence of negative ones.

Sexual needs change throughout the life cycle. Through gratification of basic needs for nourishment, warmth and touch, the infant develops feelings of trust and self-worth. These form a solid basis for a personality which allows people to form satisfying relationships with others. In childhood, gender identity and gender (sex) role identity develop. Puberty is the age of hormonal changes affecting growth and secondary sex characteristics. The period of adolescence encompasses the physical changes of puberty and includes the psychological, cognitive and social transition from childhood to adulthood. It is a process which involves coming to terms with a new physical appearance along with an emerging self-identity. Marriage and families are often established during young adulthood. In addition to reproductive functions, sexual behaviour during young adulthood may foster closeness and intimacy, give pleasure and strengthen self-esteem. The middle years of adulthood produce changes in sexual and reproductive anatomy and function. Some women experience an increase in sexual interest while others note a decline. Changes in sexual function may cause distress and concern for many men. The sexual function is still active in older adults provided a capable partner is available.

Throughout the teen and adult years there may be problems with sexually transmitted diseases, pregnancy into the menopausal years and cancer of the reproductive organs (breast and cervix in women and prostate in men). In older adults degenerative diseases can have a negative effect on sexual function. Common sexual concerns may need physical and psychological treatment of both partners. Sexually transmitted diseases (STDs) are spread through intimate or sexual contact and through contact with any body fluid.

A nursing health history should include sexual health questions that are relevant to the patient's condition or expressed concern. Many people view sexuality as a private matter. The patient's permission is necessary before asking sex-related questions. Privacy, trust and the assurance of confidentiality will facilitate expression of sexual issues and concerns.

Altered sexuality patterns is a nursing diagnostic label which may be used for problems in which patients are experiencing changes in sexual health or expressing concern about their sexuality. In many cases, patients' problems fall outside the domain of independent nursing intervention. Referrals to other professionals are made with the patient's participation.

The PLISSIT model, often used in sexual counselling, provides a guideline based on the skills and training of the health care provider. The letters stand for Permission, Limited Information, Specific Suggestions and Intensive Therapy.

Optimal sexual health can be promoted by giving patients and their partners sexuality education and supportive care, especially in the areas of self-empowerment and the ability to exercise control over one's sexual life. Correct information is usually needed in reproductive health, safe sex practices, contraceptives and the prevention of STDs. Reproductive health screening includes the nurse's examination of the breasts and testicles and the teaching of self-examination.

LEARNING ACTIVITIES

1. **Case Study**: Mr. Ivanovitch is a divorced 70-year-old patient in extended care with a leg injury. He likes to play cribbage, and he frequently tells you that he is lonely. According to Sarah, another nurse on the unit, he requests her attention often. Over the past week, he has started to make overtures and then direct passes at her, saying ``I just want a woman.'' Apparently, it is fairly typical of his cultural background to be direct.

    a. How should Sarah deal with his behaviour?

    b. What are some of the ways to redirect his attention?

    c. What community resource groups can be called upon to help this gentleman?

2. **Case Study**: Candy Lane, 18, is a very unkempt girl who shows up repeatedly in the women's health clinic for treatment of STD. Her records indicate she is slightly retarded and has a ninth-grade education. She lives with her family. Her five brothers and sisters have various learning disabilities. Her father is an occasional labourer; her mother stays at home. Both parents are alcoholics. Apparently she engages in prostitution.

    a. How can you assist Candy in improving her situation?

    b. Which resource people can be contacted?

    c. What are some of the factors affecting her situation?

    d. Should Candy be sterilized?

    e. Should prostitution be legalized? Why or why not?

REFERENCES AND READINGS

ANNON, J.S. (1976). The PLISSIT model: A proposed conceptual scheme for the behavioural treatment of sexual problems. *Journal of Sex Education and Therapy, 2*, 211–215.

BANCROFT, J. (1989). *Human sexuality and its problems*. New York: Churchill Livingstone.

BARBACH, L. (1975). *For yourself: The fulfillment of female sexuality*. Garden City, NY: Doubleday.

BARBACH, L. (1982). *For each other: Sharing sexual intimacy*. New York: Doubleday.

BEITCHMAN, J., ZUCKER, K., HOOD, J., DACOSTA, G., AKMAN, D. and CASSAVIA, E. (1990). *A review of the long-term effects of child sexual abuse*. (Revised version of a final report submitted to Health and Welfare Canada.)

BOSTON WOMEN'S HEALTH BOOK COLLECTIVE. (1992). *The new our bodies ourselves*. New York: Simon and Schuster.

BRICK, P. (1989). Toward a positive approach to adolescent sexuality. *SIECUS Report, 17*(5).

BUTLER, R.N. and LEWIS M. (1988). *Love and sex after 60*. New York: Harper and Row.

CAMPION, M.J. (1992). *The baby challenge: A handbook on pregnancy for women with a physical disability*. New York: Tavistok Rutledge.

CANADIAN CANCER SOCIETY. (1989). *BSE: Breast self-examination*. (Pamphlet). Vancouver: Author.

CANADIAN CANCER SOCIETY. (1989). *TSE: The most important minute in a man's life*. (Pamphlet). Vancouver: Author.

THE CANADIAN RESEARCH INSTITUTE FOR THE ADVANCEMENT OF WOMEN. (1989). *What you should know about infertility and sterility*. Ottawa: Author.

CARPENITO, J.B. (1993). *Nursing diagnosis: Application to clinical practice*. Philadelphia: Lippincott.

COLLEGE OF FAMILY PHYSICIANS OF CANADA. (1993). *A Report on the Task Force on Adolescent Health*. Mississauga: Author.

DIVISION OF VITAL STATISTICS, B.C. Ministry of Health and Ministry Responsible for Seniors. (1993, May). *Adolescent childbearing rates: Live births and stillbirths*. Victoria: Queen's Printer.

DROEGEMULLER, W., HERBST, A., MISHELL, D. and STENCHEVER, M. (1987). *Comprehensive gynaecology*. St. Louis: Mosby.

DUGAS B. W. (1993). Healthy life-styles. In A. C. Beckingham and B. W. DuGas (Eds.). *Promoting healthy aging*. St. Louis: Mosby.

FISHER, W. (1990). All together now: An integrated approach to preventing adolescent pregnancy and STD/HIV infection. *SIECUS Report, 18*(4).

FOGEL, C.I. and LAUVER, D. (1990). *Sexual health promotion*. Philadelphia: Saunders.

GENDER, A.R. (1992). An overview of the nurse's role in dealing with sexuality. *Sexuality and Disability, 10*(2), 71–78.

GLASS, J.C. and DALTON, J.A. (1988). Sexuality in older adults: A continuing education concern. *The Journal of Continuing Education in Nursing, 19*(2), 61–64.

GOVERNMENT OF CANADA. (1990-91). Sexuality: A lifelong issue. *Seniors' Info Exchange*, Winter, 1990, 2, 3.

HATCHER, R.A., STEWART, F., TRUSSELL, J., LOWAL. D., GUEST, F., STEWART, G. and CATES, W. (1992). *Contraceptive technology, 1990–1992*. New York: Irvington Publishers.

HEALTH AND WELFARE CANADA. (1991). *Notifiable diseases annual summary*. Ottawa: Minister of National Health and Welfare.

INTERNATIONAL PLANNED PARENTHOOD FEDERATION. *Family planning policy statements*. London: Author.

KATCHADOURIAN, H.A. (1985). *Fundamentals of human sexuality* (4th ed.). New York: Holt, Reinhart and Winston.

KING, A., BEAZLEY, R., WARREN, W., HANKINS, C. ROBERTSON, A. and RADFORD, J. (1988). *Canadian youth and AIDS study*. Ottawa: Health and Welfare Canada.

KINSEY, A.C., POMEROY, W.B. and MARTIN C.E. (1948). *Sexual behaviour in the human male*. Philadelphia: Saunders.

KINSEY, A. C. et al. (1953). *Sexual behaviour in the human female*. Philadelphia: Saunders.

KNOWLTON, C. N. (1988). Human sexuality. In J.M. Flynn and P.B. Heffron (Eds.). *Nursing: From concept to practice* (2nd ed.). Norwalk, CT: Appleton & Lange.

KOZIER, B., ERB, G. and OLIVIERI, R. (1991). *Fundamentals of nursing: Concepts, process and practice* (4th ed.). Redwood City, CA: Addison-Wesley.

KROLL, K. and KLEIN, E. L. (1992). *Enabling romance: A guide to love, sex and relationships for the disabled*. New York: Harmony Books.

LERNER, H.G. (1989). *The dance of intimacy*. New York: Harper and Row.

LEVINE, R. (1993). Unpublished Report. U.S. National Institute of Child Health and Human Development.

LIERMAN, L.M., YOUNG, H.M., COPE, G.P., GEORGIADOU, F. and BENOLIEL, J.Q. (1994). Effects of education and support on breast self-examination in older women. *Nursing Research, 43*, 158-163.

MALTZ, W. (1992). *The sexual healing journey*. New York: Harper Perennial.

MARTINI, F. (1989). *Fundamentals of anatomy and physiology*. Englewood Cliffs: Prentice Hall.

MASTERS, W.H. and JOHNSON, V.E. (1966). *Human sexual response*. Boston: Little, Brown.

MASTERS, W.H., JOHNSON, V.E. and KOLODNY, R.C. (1986). *Masters and Johnson on sex and human loving*. Boston: Little, Brown.

McNAUGHT, B. (1988). *On being gay: Thoughts on family, faith and love*. New York: St. Martin's.

MONTREAL HEALTH PRESS. (1990). *Menopause: A well woman book*. Toronto: Second Story Press.

NEISTADT, M. and FREDA, M. (1987). *Choices: A guide to sex counselling with physically disabled adults*. Florida: Kreiger.

ORTON, M. J. and ROSENBLATT, E. (1986). *Adolescent pregnancy in Ontario: Progress in prevention*. Toronto: Planned Parenthood Association of Ontario.

PILLITTERI, A. (1992). *Maternal and child health: Care of the childbearing and childrearing family*. Philadelphia: Lippincott.

REINISCH, J. (1990). *The Kinsey Institute new report on sex: What you must know to be sexually literate*. New York: St. Martin's.

SCHROVER, L. and JENSEN, S.B. (1988). *Sexuality and chronic illness: A comprehensive approach*. New York: Guilford Press.

SUICIDE AMONG GAY AND LESBIAN YOUTH. (1993). Anecdotal Report. Annual AIDS Conference, Vancouver.

THOMAS, A. and CHESS, S. (1980). *The dynamics of psychological development*. New York: Brunner/Mazel.

WOODS, N. (1984). *Human sexuality in health and illness* (3rd ed.). St. Louis: Mosby.

WORLD HEALTH ORGANIZATION. (1975). *Education and treatment in human sexuality: The training of health professionals*. (Technical Report Series No. 572.) Geneva: Author.

ZILBERGELD, B. (1992). *The new male sexuality*. New York: Bantam Books.

CHAPTER 35

Self-Esteem Needs

CENTRAL QUESTIONS

1. Why is self-esteem important to well-being?

2. What are the main determinants of self-esteem?

3. How is the sense of self-esteem developed and nurtured throughout the life span?

4. What sort of problems stem from a lack of fulfilment of the need for self-esteem?

5. How does the nurse assess self-concept?

6. What are some problems related to low self-esteem?

7. What specific nursing diagnoses might apply to patients with problems related to low self-esteem?

8. What basic principles are applicable in planning care to promote, protect and restore self-esteem?

9. What strategies might be used for promoting self-esteem? for protecting self-esteem? for helping to restore self-esteem?

10. How does the nurse evaluate the individual's or the group's response to nursing interventions?

INTRODUCTION

Self-esteem is to the mind as food is to the body; and all human beings need self-esteem for both physical and psychological well-being.

— Simmermacher, 1989

Self-esteem, it has been said, is the key to a person's behaviour. It influences thinking processes, emotions, desires, values and goals. It affects virtually all aspects of our lives, how we function in school, at work, in love and as parents and how successful we will be in life (Simmermacher, 1989). Maslow (1970) contended that attainment of self-esteem is only possible when lower level needs have been fulfilled. Healthy self-esteem can only develop when we feel secure. Our sense of security depends on having basic physiological needs met, feeling safe from harmful elements in the environment and feeling safe and secure in our relationships with other people.

Self-esteem is the way we judge ourselves; it has an evaluative component, as opposed to self-concept which is the "sum total of perceptions, feelings and beliefs about oneself" (Haber, Leach, McMahon, Price-Hoskins and Sideleau, 1992, 806). Self-esteem has three interrelated aspects. The first aspect is **body image** — the mental image we have of our physical being and our attitudes towards our body and its various parts and functions (the perceptual aspect). The second aspect is **self-respect** — the feeling that we are worthwhile and that what we are doing, or have done, is "right" according to our values (the emotional aspect). The third aspect is **self-confidence** — believing that we are and have the ability to do things or the power to make things happen (the cognitive aspect) (Haber et al., 1992).

Self-esteem involves a critical self-evaluation. How do I measure up physically, socially, psychologically and in my behaviour to the standards and values I have chosen for myself? People are constantly judging themselves in relation to the standards they themselves have established. Although they may not be aware of their self-evaluation on a conscious, verbalized level, they experience it as a feeling about themselves. People feel "good" about themselves if, in their opinion, they have done something well, or they feel small and miserable because they never seem to be able to do things right.

The way we see ourselves, and the way we feel and think about ourselves, is learned through our interaction with others and through their responses to us. It is not something we are endowed with at birth (Chartow, 1983). If the way we see ourselves is learned, it follows that positive self-esteem can be promoted or negative self-esteem can be transformed into a positive one through successful learning experiences.

Poor self-esteem has been linked as a causative factor to illnesses such as anxiety, depression and other psychosomatic disorders and to numerous social problems, such as delinquency, child abuse, prejudice, alcoholism and drug addiction (Chartow, 1983). Poor self-esteem is a common factor among the groups of people in Canadian society who are most vulnerable to poor health — those in poor socioeconomic situations, the unemployed, older adults, single mothers, new immigrants and people of the First Nations (Epp, 1986).

Today we are hearing a lot about the need to "empower" people so that they can assert control over factors that affect their health. **Empowerment** is a key concept in the socioeconomic model of health. Empowerment has been defined as a "social process of recognizing, promoting and enhancing people's abilities to meet their own needs, solve their own problems, and mobilize necessary resources to take control of their own lives" (Gibson, 1991. Cited in Jones and Meleis, 1993). If health is viewed as "the ability (of people) to realize their aspirations and satisfy needs and, on the other hand, to change or cope with the environment" as defined by the World Health Organization (1980), then empowerment is a vital component in helping people realize their health potential (Epp, 1986).

In this chapter, we will look at the determinants of self-esteem, its development throughout the life cycle, and some of the common problems experienced by people when these needs are unfulfilled. We will also discuss the nurse's role in helping to promote people's self-esteem, in protecting feelings of self-worth and in helping people to overcome feelings of low self-esteem.

DETERMINANTS OF SELF-ESTEEM

Basic Needs

Self-esteem is derived from a number of different elements, including the fulfilment of basic physiological and security needs. Physiological needs must be met first. People need food, clothing and protection from the elements for themselves and their families. They do not feel very secure if their stomachs are empty and they do not know where the next meal is coming from; or if they are constantly worrying about paying the rent; or, if they are among the growing number of homeless in this country, where they are going to sleep at night. People also need freedom from pain. In addition to having physiological needs met, people also have to feel that they can go about their daily activities without fear, that they are safe in their home at night, and that their children are safe. These are very basic components of feeling safe that are essential for a sense of security.

Money is important to provide the basic essentials of security — food for the table, adequate housing, clothing and the other necessities of life. An economic recession puts strains on individuals and families, especially when there is not enough money to pay all the bills and still buy necessary items. The uncertainty of not knowing whether there will be a job tomorrow is devastating to anyone's security and self-esteem.

Money is also the way our society rewards people for the work they do. The higher the income, the more valuable the position is considered to be. Although we would like to think otherwise, in this materialistic world of ours, success is to a large extent judged by the amount of income earned.

Love and a Sense of Belonging

Meeting basic physical needs is not enough. People also need a sense of belonging and a feeling that they are part of a particular segment of the population. They also need love and companionship of other people, although sometimes a pet will provide its owner with the needed affection. People also need attention and recognition from others — an acknowledgement that they are accepted members of society.

Social Support

Of primary importance in both the development and nurturing of self-esteem are the significant people who inhabit our social world. These include family members, peers and teachers at school, colleagues and supervisors in the workplace and friends and neighbours in the social networks of the community.

Home   The importance of the family in helping people grow up comfortable and secure with themselves and their environment cannot be stressed too much. It is the family or significant others who provide people with the support they need to make their way in the outside world.

School   People also need attention and recognition from others outside the family — acknowledgement that they are accepted members of society. The school is usually the first place where the outside world is confronted. The way children are accepted and the way that their development is nourished in classrooms and on the playing field is crucial to formation of feelings of security and self-esteem that are carried throughout life (Government of Ontario, 1993). Level of education is probably more important now than ever before in helping people to meet security needs and in contributing to self-esteem. Today, a minimum of a high school education is required to even begin to compete in the job market. To enter most professions and occupations requires post-secondary education in a community college, technical institute or a university. A high school diploma provides a sense of achievement and a certain amount of security when obtaining employment; a

certificate or diploma from a college program or a university degree gives both more security and increased feelings of self-worth (Oderkirk, 1993; Gilbert and Orok, 1993).

Workplace   Work, how people feel about it, the pleasure they receive from it, and the companionship and respect they obtain from co-workers and supervisors all contribute to feeling comfortable and secure in daily living. A warm, supportive atmosphere at home can often nullify the damaging effects of a work environment filled with stress. More and more, however, employers are finding it advantageous to make the workplace more conducive to developing employees' self-esteem. Employers are fostering a cooperative team spirit that gives people the feeling of being an important part of the organization, and not just a cog in the machinery.

Community   Social networks in the community are also important in contributing to feelings of self-worth. These social networks include the friends we have, the people we know in our neighourhood, the clubs and other organizations we belong to and the community of worship we attend. These networks provide emotional, material and companionship support. People who lack this support are much more likely to experience feelings of low self-esteem, anxiety, depression, self-blame and helplessness than those with strong social support systems (RNABC, 1992; Government of Ontario, 1993). The supportive (nurturing) community fosters social contacts by providing places where people can meet and interact such as the library, the school, the churches, the parks and playgrounds and the community centre. A supportive community also provides services that people need to feel secure such as health and social services and law enforcement services.

Cultural Customs and Mores

The traditional customs and mores of a community also play a part in self-esteem. They help maintain a sense of the continuity of life and to give people a sense of identity. There is an order that is reassuring, for example, in the fact that Thanksgiving comes in fall every year. The ceremonies that mark life events — starting, for example, with the circumcision of the male Jewish child a few days after birth and the baptism of the Roman Catholic infant, and continuing through the marriage ceremony and the death service — are all important in that they help family members to develop a sense of continuity. The ceremonies also contribute to meeting self-esteem needs for participants and their families, since the event is being marked in the approved manner. It has been government policy in Canada to help ethnic groups to maintain their own cultural identity, and many of the traditional customs have been passed down from generation to generation. Vancouver is noted for its Chinese New Year celebrations, for example,

Edmonton for its celebrations of the Ukrainian Christmas, Toronto for Caribana and Kitchener-Waterloo for Oktoberfest. These events all help people whose roots are outside Canada to feel more at home.

Religion

Many ceremonies and traditional events are religious in nature. Religion has always provided many people with a refuge from the uncertainties of life. It can be reassuring for people to feel that there is an order to the universe and that a Supreme Being is in charge to whom they can go for comfort, support and guidance. The stress of living in today's fast-paced world, with all the uncertainties brought about by rapid change, has no doubt contributed to the growth of many churches in recent years. People seem to be looking for a semblance of order and a meaning to life to renew their faith and security in the world.

A Purpose in Life

Rapid changes in institutions and in the economic situation have an effect on human roles and on our sense of security and the way in which we view ourselves. According to Toffler, we derive our sense of purpose, our feeling that our lives "count," from our relationships with family, our place of work, our community of worship or our political involvement. We also need to be able to see ourselves as part of a cosmic scheme of things (1981).

Health-Related Factors

Self-esteem is threatened by illness — sometimes very much so — particularly in the case of sudden illness or accident that requires hospitalization. Sometimes in health agencies, personnel are so busy taking care of the technical aspects of health care that they may forget that people are attached to all the tubes and wires. An important responsibility of the nurse is to look after the people — to help them to feel secure and to support both self-confidence and self-respect. This responsibility is part of the *caring* aspect of the nurse's role which is the core of nursing.

The loss, or potential loss, of independence, for example, poses a very real threat to people with health problems. It can cause them to lose self-esteem and to think that other people will not respect them. It is important therefore to make sure that nothing the nurse does or says causes patients to think that they are any less themselves because of the health problem.

Illness can interfere with people's careers, or with the fulfilment of the need to make the best of their potential in any sphere. The loss or threatened loss of the ability to use the hands, for instance, would be a major blow to a pianist or people who use the hands in pursuing one of their prin-

---

> ## Determinants of Self-Esteem
>
> * Fulfilment of basic physiological needs
> * A safe physical environment
> * An adequate income to purchase the necessities of life
> * Supportive, nurturing family, school and work environments
> * A strong support network of family and friends
> * A nurturing community
> * Cultural customs and mores
> * A sense of purpose in life
> * Good health
> * Successful transitions through developmental stages in the life cycle

cipal interests. Similarly, someone whose hobbies are mainly outdoor ones that require motor skills, such as skiing or riding, would be very anxious about being able to continue with these activities if a health problem, actual, potential or imagined, threatens the loss of motor functioning abilities.

Developmental Crises

At certain times in the life span, major changes, often referred to as *developmental crises,* take place as transitions from one developmental stage to another are made. These transitions were discussed extensively in Chapter 8. These crises cause a considerable threat to self-esteem as people wonder if they can cope with the demands that will be made upon them in the next stage of development.

SELF-ESTEEM NEEDS THROUGHOUT THE LIFE CYCLE

PREGNANCY

Building self-esteem is probably our most important developmental task (Simmermacher, 1989). It begins in infancy — some say even before, when the fetus is still in the womb.

During pregnancy, many women say that they have never looked or felt better, and they feel a sense of satisfaction and completion that they have not known before. The woman's needs now may become secondary to those of the fetus. She is planning more and more for the coming birth. During this period some men feel excluded. Both

Prospective fathers need to feel they are an important part of the birthing process.

men and women need reassurance at this time. Women have to deal with clumsiness and ungainly proportions and a sense that their earlier self-image has been distorted and their equilibrium disturbed. Pregnant women need to know that they are still attractive and that the changes in appearance are normal. They should be encouraged to see the beauty of the body during pregnancy, exemplified by the many paintings and sculptures focussing on the subject of motherhood. A woman can invest her emotions in the care of the fetus better when she feels secure. There is a desire for deeper intimacy during this period of life, and a new sense of family develops.

Some single women have children on their own. Single pregnant women need a supportive environment such as a nuclear family, a cooperative housing arrangement or an extended family environment.

Prenatal classes are invaluable for both the mother and her partner; the latter also needs to be an important part of this process and needs reassurance and peer support. The birth of a child causes a major change in the lives of a man and woman. After birth, the family must be reorganized to accommodate the new member. Feelings of security and a sense of self-esteem develop from the moment of birth. Considerable emphasis is now put on the importance of parental bonding during the first few hours after birth and throughout the first week to give the infant a sense of security. At one time, the mother's partner was barred from the delivery room in most Canadian hospitals. If there is no "birthing room," a separate room is usually set aside where the mother, her partner and baby can get to know

each other immediately after birth. The quality of the contact — with an emphasis on touching and caressing — is considered more important than the quantity of interaction. The voice of the mother is very important, as it gives positive reassurance of her presence to the infant.

INFANCY

Erikson (1963) felt that one of the major developmental tasks of infancy is the development of trust — in oneself, in the environment and in other people. At first, infants do not distinguish between themselves and the environment. They can, however, sense and respond to feelings of approval or disapproval on the part of a mother or a nurse. Approval leads to a sense of well-being, and disapproval causes discomfort. At three months, children begin to explore their sense of self. They watch their hands and their feet with great interest and examine other areas of their body. At four months, children are aware of themselves as distinct from the rest of the world. They begin to explore this world, using the mother as a security base. Infants who have developed security in their attachment to mother are more likely to actively explore the world around them, although they will cry if she leaves them showing happiness only when she returns.

Anxious infants may be more passive, showing less curiosity and less interest in exploring their environment than secure ones. "Stranger anxiety" is a common trait at six to ten months, the time when infants distinguish between mother and others.

An infant's emotional security rests to a considerable extent on the relationship that develops between the mother and the baby. If the relationship is a positive one, a rapport is established that permits interaction on a nonverbal basis, with the mother responding empathetically to her infant's needs. If the mother–infant relationship is cold, inconsistent or rejecting, mistrust and insecurity are built into the personality of the infant. Parents who respond promptly to their infant's cries have happier, calmer and more outgoing children as a general rule. Inconsistency or lack of response to the infant's needs can lead to infant anxiety, which is manifested by crying and clinging behaviour.

Body-image — the way we perceive our physical being — begins to develop in infancy from sensory input. Infants begin to notice the parts of their body that they can see, and to explore both their own body and that of their mother, using touch, smell, taste, sight and hearing. As children become a little older, they begin to associate the reflections they see in the mirror with themselves and they hear other people complimenting them on their appearance. Because the bony prominences of the body (such as the knees and the elbows) and the body openings are what come into contact most often with other objects, they serve as the most immediate points of reference in orienting children to their environment and are particularly important in developing body image. People's attitudes towards their body and its parts and functions are largely a product of their early socialization. Children absorb without question the attitudes of their parents regarding "clean" and "unclean" parts of their body, the appropriate state of cleanliness of the body generally, and whether it is good to be fat or lean.

CHILDHOOD

During the toddler stage, children gain new motor skills, learn to walk, and extend their range of activities to investigate different aspects of their surroundings. Verbal and intellectual abilities develop at a rapid rate. They begin to comprehend and test out the meaning of the word "no." For the first time, children learn that there are restrictions and limitations on behaviour. This is a time when the house needs to be childproofed, so that the restrictions and limitations can be kept to the minimum needed for the child's safety. During the toddler stage and until about age four, the principal developmental task is to gain a sense of autonomy without developing doubt or a sense of shame. Thus, the child needs to learn to negotiate the stairs (under watchful eyes) when they are ready to do so, without too many admonishments about being careful. Positive reinforcement will greatly enhance the situation. Toddlers' burgeoning communication skills enhance the development of self. Their first and most deeply learned perception of themselves is a composite reflection of how significant persons around them — their parents (or others taking a parental role), siblings and grandparents — perceive them.

The preschooler needs to learn initiative and to develop skills that build self-confidence. It is important for preschoolers to be given the opportunity to try new things and to receive the support of their parents while doing so. The self-confidence that is gained is reflected in the children's sense of eagerness, their spontaneity and the "bounce" in their steps. The development of routine times for meals, bedtime and outings helps to provide security for the child because it develops a sense of expectation with reinforcement. During the preschool stage, the child is beginning to develop a conscience. Until approximately age seven, however, children are still very egocentric in thought. As they mature, they begin to think more about other people's needs and wishes.

When children enter school, they are suddenly confronted with an expanding circle of people and new activities. They must learn how to interact and cooperate with others. In school, children also have a wider range of roles to emulate as teachers and older students provide models to choose from. They learn how others (teachers, students and principal) evaluate their strengths and how others care for them as people. They learn the difference between work and play and they learn to enjoy work for the rewards it brings. If children feel a sense of inferiority or mediocrity,

Through sports, school-age children learn to interact and cooperate with others their same age.

they may tend to withdraw and be discouraged. The school may provide reinforcement for a child's self-esteem through recognition of achievements, which can often offset an adverse atmosphere at home. On the other hand, problems at school may counteract the benefits of a supportive home environment. The chief task of this age group is to develop a sense of industry rather than inferiority to others.

ADOLESCENCE

The adolescent stage begins at approximately 12 years and lasts until about 18. During puberty, when adolescents tend to be very self-conscious, a sense of identity and belonging is gradually achieved, usually through the stabilizing influence of peer groups. Adolescence is a period of great ambivalence, with the desire to be free of authority forms, most importantly parents and school, conflicting with the need to be dependent upon them for emotional and financial support. Adolescents are dealing with who they are, what they want to work at and what they want to do with their lives. The major task at this stage is to gain a sense of identity. Failure to resolve this may lead to confusion, depression or an identification with a group or cult that supplies an identity. It may also lead people to seize the first job or the first mate that offers a sense of identity, or else to "opt out" through the use of alcohol and drugs to ease the difficult transition from adolescence to adulthood.

Positive reinforcement is vital during this period. One goal of education is to reinforce adolescents' identity through teamwork and the development of skills that can support them throughout their lifetime. In order to achieve a secure identity, adolescents need a sense of community in which they can exchange learning skills and support each

Adolescents need their own space to help them develop a sense of their own identity.

MIDDLE ADULTHOOD

Erikson (1963) felt that during middle age, there is a need to focus on a sense of "generativity" as opposed to stagnation in one's life, socially, at work and in the community. He felt that emphasis should be placed on the ability to impart wisdom to the young and on innovation, rather than simply going through life in a mechanical routine. Many men often tend to become more concerned with feelings and less aggressive in the middle years. Parents feel more free as their children become less dependent. A person's sense of security comes from the home one has created and the abilities one has developed. Somatic disorders frequently develop in response to psychic stress and anxiety. Diarrhea, colitis, bronchial asthma, hyperventilation and diabetes insipidus are among the health problems that are thought to have a strong psychosomatic component. Essentially, middle age is a time for stock-taking and reevaluation. A sense of order in this world and a sense of how one's life is an aspect of history has been developed.

OLDER ADULTHOOD

During the older years, there is increased attention to the maintenance of dignity to preserve the sense of self-esteem. Older people value their independence above all else. Home care services are now making it possible for them to stay in their own homes when they become ill. An increasing number of people are choosing to die at home, surrounded by friends, relatives and belongings until they die. Although sometimes this is not possible, home care and palliative care are increasing the feasibility of this option.

During the older adult years, security is ensured partially through financial means such as pensions, savings and retirement plans and partially through the ability to adapt, often to the situation of being dependent upon others. The main task during this period of the life cycle, according to Erikson (1963), is the maintenance of integrity as opposed to despair: accepting what has been, feeling useful and receiving respect. The older years are a time period for looking back; the self-concept is related to past experience.

The problem of dependency upon others for support and assistance may weigh heavily on older adults' sense of integrity. Depression may follow the loss of spouse, friends, home and income coupled with a feeling of rejection by society. Help in dealing with daily situations is usually welcome, along with visits from friends and relatives. The problem of decreased mobility may deepen the sense of isolation, although many communities have transportation systems geared to serving older adults. A large number of older people live alone and many are lonely. The alienation of the elderly is reflected in the high percentage of suicides among the older population. Older people need a social support network within their own communities, such as seniors clubs that are located in many community centres that help

other, especially since a vast number of adolescents are now being raised in single-parent homes. Parents today tend not to put high expectations on young people to achieve material success, recognizing that life is much more complicated than it used to be and that other values are important, such as a sense of purpose in life.

YOUNG ADULTHOOD

The young adult is mainly concerned with developing more intimate relationships with others. Without these relationships they experience a feeling of isolation. Intimacy has traditionally centred on marriage, although an increasing number of people are postponing marriage and devoting the early part of the adult years to establishing careers. It is necessary for the young adult to have a firm sense of identity at this point, although in today's society, people often experience a sense of isolation and insecurity. Young women in particular appear to have a difficult time at this stage because of conflicting societal expectations to marry and have children on the one hand, and to have a career on the other.

There is a tendency to view oneself during young adulthood as being "indestructible" and able to "burn the candle at both ends." This attitude often leads to accidents and to the physical and mental state known as "burn out." This in turn may alter the self-image and adversely affect self-esteem. Damaged self-esteem and feelings of helplessness contribute to many of the suicides and homicides committed by people in this age group. Stable young adults, however, who are married or in an intimate relationship with another and have careers underway tend to see their lives as more secure, productive and self-actualized.

FROM RESEARCH TO PRACTICE

Mitchell, G.J. (1993). Time and a Waning Moon: Seniors describe the meaning to later life. *The Canadian Journal of Nursing Research.* 25(1), 51 – 66.

Personal meaning plays a crucial role in relation to health and quality of life. This study was undertaken to learn more about the meaning of aging to older adults. The researchers used a phenomenological approach, gathering data from narratives written by six hundred voluntary participants over the age of 65 years. Two analyses of the data were made. The first identified three recurring phenomena in the narratives: simile, paradox and humour. The second identified and synthesized descriptions of these phenomena.

Among the similes, a number of common themes compared life to a journey or a wearing down or diminishing and likened old age to freedom or sudden release. Old age was also likened to various colours, to works of art or to aspects of nature (such as wrinkles being marks of a long and meaningful life). The most common paradox was that people felt no differences in themselves but, at the same time, they saw change and differences. Humour, the third recurring phenomenon, was described as essential to survival: one laughs at oneself and one's personal frailties and also enjoys sharing humour and laughter with others.

The authors suggest that nurses wanting to understand the meaning of aging to older patients might ask them what their life is like. The general question could be followed with an exploration of the meaning of similes if these are used or a request for more detail if the "same yet different" paradox appears. Nurses should also be alert to older people's need for humour and help them create it.

to provide older adults with a sense of belonging. A network of friends helps to fulfill the need for love and affection that is vitally important to security and self-esteem.

COMMON PROBLEMS

People whose self-esteem needs are unfulfilled are anxious people, unsure of themselves, usually unhappy and afraid to take the chance of doing something for fear of failing. People with low self-esteem often blame themselves for their problems: they believe that it is their fault that they are inadequate, that they didn't try hard enough or that they did something wrong. Often there is an associated feeling of guilt and a need for punishment. People with low self-esteem may punish themselves with self-destructive behaviour to atone for wrongdoing. Alternatively, they may blame others for their problems and become hostile and angry. People with low self-esteem are often prone to illnesses that originate in the body's reaction to real or imagined threats. People in low income brackets such as some single mothers living in low rental housing complexes, older adults who have insufficient income to live comfortably, many people of the First Nations and some unemployed people often experience a pervasive feeling of powerlessness — they feel that there is nothing they can do to make their situation better (Epp, 1986).

Disturbances of self-concept and many of the problems related to negative self-esteem, such as anxiety, depression, negative body image, ineffective individual and family coping and powerlessness are addressed in depth in psychiatric/mental health nursing. The effects of low self-esteem are so pervasive, however, affecting so many aspects of a person's well-being that it is important to develop early in your course of study some beginning skills in assessing self-concept and identifying some of the common problems. It is also essential that nurses incorporate measures to promote positive feelings of self-worth and to protect this aspect of the patient's self into the nursing care of all patients from the beginning of their career.

In this chapter, we will focus on three of the most common problems related to lack of fulfilment of the need for self-esteem: feelings of powerlessness (hopelessness/helplessness), anxiety and depression. These problems often tend to cluster together with other problems such as negative body image, social isolation and ineffective individual or family coping; one problem is often related to another so that a patient may have several problems in one. For example, a patient may develop a poor body image because of the loss of a leg in an accident; the patient may become depressed and may tend to withdraw from contact with friends.

POWERLESSNESS

Powerlessness has been defined as "The state in which an individual or group perceives a loss of personal control over certain events or situations which impacts outlook, goals and lifestyle " (Carpenito, 1993, 561). It is probably the most devastating problem related to self-esteem — the feeling that nothing you can do is going to make any difference. It is an unpleasant feeling when people believe that it is impossible to obtain the things they want or need in order to protect themselves or their family and it leaves people feeling very vulnerable and insecure. The future looks bleak and people become anxious and uneasy and constantly worried.

People often react to feelings of powerlessness with anger and hostility towards the government, employers, the school system — whatever is seen as the power that is controlling their lives. Violent behaviour, such as the vandalism and destruction that sometimes occurs during labour strikes, is often the result of feelings of powerlessness. We mentioned in Chapter 3 that the social unrest, the strikes and the riots during the 1930s were due to feelings of powerlessness on the part of unemployed workers who were unable to do anything themselves to remedy the situation. If a patient is ill and the prognosis is poor, there is often anger towards the physician, the hospital and the nurses (Staples, Baruth, Jefferies and Warder, 1994). Sometimes friends and family bear the brunt of this anger as the patient fights against his or her fate. The anger may fade into apathy or turn into depression as the patient becomes resigned to the situation.

ANXIETY

Anxiety is defined as "…an unpleasant feeling of tension and apprehension, accompanied by physiological, psychological and behavioural symptoms, that serves as an early warning signal that alerts people to impending real or symbolic threat to self, significant others or a way of life" (Haber et al., 1992, 794). There are varying degrees of anxiety, ranging from mild apprehension to overwhelming panic. Unresolved anxiety, or anxiety in more than mild degree, can be incapacitating. In Chapter 8, in the section on stress, we discussed the individual's reaction to perceived threats. The material in Chapter 8 provides a theoretical background for our discussions in this chapter about anxiety.

Threats to the individual cause certain physiological reactions to take place within the body. These reactions vary to a certain extent depending on physical makeup; however, there are many reactions that are common to most anxious people. Anxiety also brings about changes in a person's behaviour. Again, these changes vary, depending on the basic personality structure and the ways in which people have coped with anxieties in the past. There are also changes in *feeling tone (affect)* and in the person's *mental functioning (cognitive ability)*. Physical condition affects the ability to tolerate anxiety. Something that may constitute only a minor worry when healthy may create an overwhelming anxiety when the body's defences are lowered.

Physiological Manifestations

The principal physiological mechanism operating in anxiety is the fundamental stress reaction as the body attempts to protect itself from harm. The most easily observable physical signs of anxiety in an individual are the circulatory changes that take place. The action of the heart is strengthened and accelerated. Blood pressure may be elevated by 10 mm of mercury or more above normal. Pulse rate may be as much as 30 percent above normal, and respiratory pattern is often disturbed as well — there may be increases in rate and depth, or there may be irregularities. There may be a marked pallor of the skin or sometimes a flushing of the face, and often the skin surfaces are cold.

Muscular tension is almost invariably present with anxiety. In some people this tension may be observed in a taut expression of the face or in a clenching of the fists. Some people assume a very rigid posture. At times, muscular tension is revealed by a tremor of the hands, in a facial, arm or shoulder tic, or in a generalized shivering or trembling of the body. The tightening of the abdominal muscles and the "butterflies" in the stomach that are commonly experienced with anxiety are the result of muscular tension. The tension headache is another common symptom of anxiety.

Many people perspire excessively in anxiety-provoking situations. The palms of the hands or the soles of the feet may be the most affected. This increased perspiration combined with a coldness and pallor of the skin (due to lessened peripheral circulation) results in the typical cold and damp hands of very anxious people.

Gastrointestinal symptoms often accompany anxiety. The "knot" or "butterflies" in the stomach may progress to nausea and vomiting. Often people say they cannot face the thought of food when they are going to take an exam or have an important interview. Some people vomit before every exam they take. Diarrhea is also a common symptom of anxiety, and people often have urinary frequency as well.

Feeling Tone (Affect)

People react to threatening situations in a variety of ways. Behaviour usually reflects the ways in which people have learned to cope with life's dangers. While some people can talk easily about their fears, and openly express them to the nurse, others may be expressing fear in less easily recognizable forms. Some people attempt to deny the existence of anxiety. These people ask no questions and frequently make a point of keeping conversation off the subject of themselves. In our culture, many men still feel that it is "unmanly" to express fear, particularly to a woman. Men (and sometimes women) frequently cover up feelings of anxiety with loud assurances that they are not frightened, and may joke and laugh in an attempt to minimize the seriousness of the condition.

Some people react to the threat of danger with anger and hostility. They may criticize the care they are receiving and be loud and insistent in demanding special treatment. People who react in this way often engender hostility on the part of nurses and other staff, who label them consciously or unconsciously as "difficult" patients. If nurses can accept this type of behaviour as being indicative of the patient's anxiety and not take it as a personal attack they will be in a better position to take positive measures to help the patient.

Severe anxiety may become *panic,* in which the patient is unable to say or do anything meaningful. Behaviour may be completely out of context — people may laugh when they should be crying — and thoughts and speech become incoherent. People who have "panicked" need someone calm to stay with them, to take charge of the situation and to tell them what to do. People cannot think for themselves at this point.

We said in Chapter 9 that a little anxiety is a good thing because it stimulates us to put forth the effort needed to accomplish things. However, when the anxiety persists too long, or is too overpowering, the body defences break down and illness results.

Mental Functioning (Cognitive Functioning)

In patients experiencing anxiety, mental activity is usually increased. When anxiety is mild, increased mental activity may mean that the individual is simply more alert and better able to think clearly. As anxiety mounts, however, perceptual awareness decreases. People become unaware of their immediate surroundings, except possibly one thing upon which their attention is focussed. Anxious people often have difficulty concentrating on anything other than that one thing. Attention span is usually short and people may be unable to answer even simple questions. Worried parents bringing a sick child into the emergency unit are sometimes so distraught that they cannot remember their own address.

With increasing anxiety, heightened mental activity may hinder rest, and insomnia frequently results. If anxious people do manage to get to sleep, they are often troubled by nightmares. They may awaken early in the morning and be unable to get back to sleep.

Behavioural Manifestations

People seek relief from muscular tension in a number of ways: by biting nails, drumming fingers on the table or pacing, for example. Restlessness and overactivity are usually fairly reliable indications of anxiety.

Changes in the patient's voice and speech patterns are also possible indications of anxiety. Some people talk very rapidly or constantly when anxious and sometimes the voice becomes very loud or high-pitched; sometimes it may quaver. In others, there may be a hesitancy of speech; people may appear to be having difficulty finding the right words. Stammering and stuttering are not uncommon in people with anxiety.

Some people react to anxiety with crying. Many nurses are embarrassed to find a patient in tears and find it difficult to know what to say or do. Attempts to reassure patients

---

Common Manifestations of Anxiety

Physiological

- increased pulse and blood pressure rates
- altered respirations; increased or irregular
- skin pale (sometimes flushed)
- increased perspiration
- muscular tension (clenched fists, rigid posture, nervous tics, trembling or shivering, headache)
- lack of interest in food
- diarrhea
- frequency of urination

Affective

- feelings of tension
- uneasiness
- a sense of dread; a feeling that something bad is about to happen
- anger and hostility

Cognitive

- heightened mental activity
- insomnia, nightmares, early morning wakening
- inability to focus on any topic other than the one that is the centre of attention
- short attention span

Behavioural

- rapid speech in a loud, high pitched or quavery voice; sometimes hesitancy of speech with stammering and stuttering
- restlessness, may become agitated as tension mounts
- rapid movements, hurried gait
- verbal or physical hostility towards others
- inappropriate behaviour (for example, laughing when should be crying)
- crying
- use of defence mechanisms

---

that "everything is going to be all right" are not usually effective in helping them to cope with their feelings. Crying often denotes a feeling of helplessness and an inability to handle certain problems. Tears serve to relieve tension, and the nurse can perhaps be most helpful by staying with the patient and being ready to listen when the crying episode is over.

DEPRESSION

Depression has been defined as "a feeling of profound sadness, low self-esteem and hopelessness about one's life" (Haber et al., 1992, 797). It may range from being minor and transitory (the "blues" that everyone has once in awhile) to a severe feeling of sadness that is pervasive and persistent. Someone whose security is threatened and who feels helpless in a situation may react with depression rather than anxiety. Often the same stressors that cause anxiety in some people give rise to sadness and melancholy in others. Depression may also be caused by a situation or an event that would normally cause a person to be sad, such as the death of a spouse or a good friend; this is called *reactive* or *situational depression.*

Depression is said to be the single most common problem that nurses and other health professionals encounter (Haber et al., 1992). Social surveys undertaken in recent decades in Canada indicate that people in lower socioeconomic groups are "on the average, more unhappy, more worried, and [tend to be] less hopeful about the future" (Stolzman, 1988). We noted in Chapter 12 the high rate of suicide among people of the First Nations and the high incidence of depression among recent immigrants, especially refugees.

Depression is a common problem among people of all age groups. Although it was once more common among adults in the 25–44 age bracket, it appears to be becoming more prevalent among 18–24 year olds; the age when depression is prevalent is decreasing with each generation (Haber et al., 1992). In Canada, suicide and motor vehicle accidents are the leading causes of death in young adults from age 15 upward. Generally speaking, depression affects women more than it does men except in the older age group when more men than women suffer from depression (Branckner, 1992; Ross and Casey, 1993).

Depression is so prevalent among the population that it is said to be the "common cold" of mental illness. It is often hidden by people who may wear a mask of joviality to cover sadness, or it may masquerade as physical illness. Nurses encounter depression among people living in the community and in patients on all units of an inpatient facility. Nurses should be particularly watchful for depression in teens and young adults who are having difficulty "finding themselves," in people who are going through middle-age turmoil and in older people, particularly those living alone in the community.

Depression and anxiety both cause certain physiological reactions to occur within the body. They also both give rise to specific behavioural manifestations, although the two sets of responses are quite different. The observant nurse should be able to distinguish between these two problems in most cases. Sometimes, however, a person will show manifestations of both anxiety and depression, a state which is called *agitated depression.*

Physiological Manifestations

Gastrointestinal functioning slows down, and depressed patients tend to become constipated. They usually have no appetite and will say that they no longer enjoy food. As a result, depressed people will probably lose weight. A loss of anywhere from five to twenty pounds is not unusual. On the other hand, some people overeat when they are depressed. Men tend to lose their sex drive when they are depressed, and women may have a cessation of menses.

Feeling Tone (Affect)

Three basic feelings are experienced as part of depression and these feelings are evident in the behaviour of depressed people. They often do not want to socialize, and in fact they often do not want to do anything at all. They have feelings of worthlessness and experience a loss of self-esteem. They also may want to hurt or even destroy themselves because they feel they are not worthy to live.

Even if people have accomplished a great deal in life, when depressed they often speak of their achievements as meaningless. Sometimes people turn to alcohol or drugs to find temporary relief from depression.

Depressed people may describe their feelings in terms such as "blue," "down," "low," "sad" or even "depressed." Others may complain of being irritable. Often, people say they feel "hopeless," "worthless" or "no good."

Mental Functioning (Cognitive Functioning)

Depressed people usually find it difficult to concentrate and hard to remember things. They may forget appointments or they may feel that it is too much effort to go. Often, activities are started but not completed. People either lose interest or just do not have the energy to finish.

Behavioural Manifestations

In most types of depression, people claim to feel as if everything is happening in slow motion. They feel less active, their movements are slow and their reaction time is longer. They are less responsive to any form of stimulation and they talk less; their speech is slower than normal. Severely depressed people may be totally unresponsive.

Depressed people usually walk with a stooped, slouching gait, the head down near the chest, often shuffling along. They seem to want to make themselves as small as possible. They are also not much concerned about what they wear. It is such an effort just to get out of bed in the morning. Depressed people begin to neglect their appearance, and not bother to take a bath or shave. Most depressed people find that the worst time of the day is when they are waking up (Haber et al., 1992; Morales-Mann, 1990).

Many different theories, such as cognitive, social and family role theories as well as a "learned helplessness" theory, have been proposed to account for the phenomenon of depression. There is no single theory, however, that accounts for all types of depression. Rather, it is important to look at all the factors in an individual's life in order to understand the reasons for depression (Haber et al., 1992).

OTHER PROBLEMS
NEGATIVE BODY IMAGE

Body image is the mental picture we have of our body (Haber et al., 1992). It reflects the perceptual image we have of our physical being and our attitudes towards our body and its various parts and functions. This mental picture of our bodies is derived from sensory input over the years, from our social interactions with other people and from our responses to them. How we see our bodies is very much a cultural matter. Children whose appearance is different from those of other children in the prevailing culture, for instance, soon become aware of the fact that they are different. If they are teased by the other children, they begin to feel that they are not as good as the others.

Whether a child develops a positive or a negative body image is a product of the early social environment. Children's body image reflects the image parents project of them and it is subsequently modified by others in the home, school and playground. Our body image changes over the years as our bodies change. People are always disturbed by changes in their body — adolescents wonder how to cope with the physical signs and inward changes in their maturing body. Pregnant women may be disturbed by changing body shape. With the emphasis in our society on a lean and physically fit body, people who do not fit this image tend to think poorly of themselves. People in their middle years often regret the loss of physical prowess and view the sight of the first grey hairs with dismay. Older adults often perceive themselves as having lost their physical attractiveness and will make depreciating remarks about themselves.

Any alteration in body image can seriously upset a person's equilibrium. Alterations may be caused by illness or accident as well as by developmental changes in body structure and functioning. A scar on the face may result from a motor vehicle accident; a person with diabetes may lose a limb from complications of the disease; a loss of hair commonly happens with radiation therapy for cancer. The loss of hair with chemotherapy is usually temporary — ending when the treatment does — but it is nonetheless traumatic. Almost all illnesses cause temporary or permanent changes in the body — even the common cold makes the eyes water, the nose run and the body function less ef-

---

Common Manifestations of Depression

Physiological
- loss of appetite leading to loss of weight
- constipation, may have retention of urine in severe cases
- slow movements
- lessened response to stimulation
- lessened sex drive
- amenorrhea

Affective
- feeling of sadness, melancholy; loss of enjoyment of usual activities
- feelings of worthlessness and low self-esteem
- anger towards self
- feelings of hopelessness

Cognitive
- poor concentration
- difficulty remembering things
- may become obsessed with one topic
- difficulty making decisions
- disturbed sleep patterns, often waken in the night, may sleep excessively

Behavioural
- stooped posture, slouching gait
- lack of interest in clothes, grooming
- withdraw from social contacts
- reluctant to talk, speech slow
- may use drugs or alcohol in seeking temporary relief
- difficulty finishing tasks

---

ficiently. People can be disturbed by even the slightest change in the body's appearance or its functioning. Major changes can be devastating.

People who are worried about body image may feel ashamed, or embarrassed about the defect they see in their body. They may also feel guilty if they think the perceived defect is the result of some wrongdoing on their part. It is not uncommon for people who have had a mastectomy or a colostomy to show revulsion towards their body. Some people are able to express their feelings openly. For others, the disturbance in self-image may be inferred from a reluctance to look at or touch the offending part. These people may try to hide the disturbance in self-image although some over-expose it with a "Let the world see me for what I am" show of bravado. Often, people with self-image problems are preoccupied with the change or loss; they may express feelings of depression and they may engage in self-destructive behaviour. They will often limit contact with other people and some may use denial, refusing to believe what has happened or trying to convince themselves that the affected part of their body does not belong to them (Carpenito, 1993).

SOCIAL ISOLATION

People who have low opinions of themselves are usually hesitant about making social contacts. Social support is one of the most important factors in the development and maintenance of self-esteem, but people with low self-esteem are often unable to make the contact with others that is necessary to gain this support. Being alone should not be confused with loneliness, however. Some people are "loners" and quite content with solitary pursuits; these people make the choice to be alone. It is important to validate that the reason for not having many social contacts is a matter of personal choice, not because of difficulty in making friends, or fear of reaching out to other people. We all need the company of other human beings; some more than others. People who have difficulty in meeting and interacting with other people are lonely.

INEFFECTIVE INDIVIDUAL OR FAMILY COPING

People with low self-esteem have many problems coping with life's stresses. They may have difficulty making decisions, solving problems and resolving conflicts. Often angry at themselves as the cause of their failures, they may become self-destructive or hostile and aggressive in their behaviour towards others. Playground bullies, for example, are frequently the children who receive more punishment than love and affection at home and consequently grow up with strong negative feelings about themselves. People who have been abused as children are likely to abuse their own children in a vicious cycle that may persist for generations. People often turn to alcohol or drugs which give them temporary respite from feelings of inadequacy. Some join cults which provide them with the security of a supportive group and give them a sense of identity (Morales-Mann, 1990; Haber et al., 1992).

We have mentioned the links between poverty and self-esteem, poverty and educational attainment, educational attainment and self-esteem and self-esteem and family violence. A recent Ontario study found that more people with a low income, and more people with a low level of education (the two frequently go hand in hand), reported living in dysfunctional families than those with higher incomes and higher educational attainment. According to the report, "...people with lower incomes and less education report poorer personal and social well-being..." (Government of Ontario, 1992, 13).

ASSESSING SELF-ESTEEM NEEDS

Low self-esteem may be the result of a number of causes and it may be manifested in many ways. It is therefore sometimes difficult to identify. The assessment process is ongoing. It begins with the nursing health history and continues as the nurse and the patient interact during the process of nursing care.

NURSING HEALTH HISTORY

The amount of information disclosed during the health history depends on the relationship that is established between interviewer and interviewee. Trust is essential in this relationship and as patients develop security in the relationship with the nurse, they are more open in talking about feelings, thoughts and perceptions. Most people will talk quite freely if the nurse has established a climate in which the patient feels free to communicate, and if the nurse takes the time to be an attentive listener.

In order to assess self-concept and identify actual or potential problems related to negative self-esteem, the nurse needs to know something about the patient as a person, the present stage of physical and psychosocial development, and about lifestyle, health status and immediate concerns.

The nurse needs to know the patient's personality characteristics and value systems. What are the most important things in the patient's life? The patient's interests, especially those that can be enjoyed in spite of the health problem(s), should also be determined.

The nurse considers age and the current stage of physical and psychosocial development. Is there a possibility that the patient is going through a developmental crisis? The nurse should also be aware of marital and family status, and how the patient fits into the family structure. The patient's friends and significant others may also influence self-esteem.

The patient's occupation and socioeconomic status may be sources of insecurity leading to self-esteem problems. Where does the patient stand in relation to the fulfilment of basic needs? Is self-actualization important at this point in life, or is the patient struggling to make enough money to provide the basic essentials of food, shelter, and security?

Another matter to consider is whether there have been any major changes in the patient's life recently. If so, what sort of changes were they? Did they necessitate major readjustments in the patient's life?

HEALTH HISTORY GUIDE

Assessing Self-Concept

1. How old are you?

2. What is your marital and family status?

3. Do you live with someone other than a family member?

4. Do you have many friends? Do you feel lonely?

5. What is your occupation?

6. Have you experienced major changes in your life recently? If so, what were they? What kind of adjustments to your life did they require?

7. What are some of your immediate concerns? Do you have any fears or worries?

8. What is your health problem? Are you worried about pain, surgery, disfigurement or death related to this problem? Are you afraid that this problem will prevent you from pursuing your normal lifestyle?

9. What are some sources of stress in your life?

10. How do you usually handle stress?

11. Briefly describe your personality. Are you happy? sad? optimistic? pessimistic? outgoing? self-sufficient? an idealist? a realist? a perfectionist?

12. Do you usually feel better in the morning or at night?

13. What things are important to you?

14. Do you have any hobbies? What leisure activities do you enjoy?

15. Are you a member of any religious or cultural groups? If so, would you like to meet with representatives of these groups?

16. Can you think of any resource people on our staff whom you would like to see?

In regard to health status, the nurse considers the patient's main concerns at present about recognized or perceived health problems. What brought the patient to the health agency? Verbalizations of feelings, and statements made in regard to physical or mental symptoms being experienced, also help the nurse to identify low self-esteem or problems associated with it. The patient's attitude towards the illness and the hospital staff — lightheartedness, joking, hostility or crying — may also reflect self-esteem needs. Even the patient's willingness or reluctance to talk about their social, emotional or health problems may indicate self-esteem needs.

Some questions that have been found helpful in assessing the self-concept of individuals to identify problems related to low self-esteem are listed in the Health History Guide above.

PHYSICAL ASSESSMENT

During both the nursing health history and the physical assessment of the patient, the nurse looks for behavioural manifestations of negative self-esteem. For example, does the patient avoid eye contact? In Chapter 16, we discussed non-verbal behaviour as a means of communicating attitudes and feelings.

During the physical assessment, the nurse notes general appearance. Is the patient well-groomed or untidy in appearance? Does it appear that the patient has taken care of his or her appearance? With the exception of the very ill, most people like to put on a good appearance when they come to the health centre or when the nurse or physician is visiting them.

The nurse also looks for physical signs of anxiety or depression, such as altered heart rate, constipation or diarrhea, change in appetite, poor posture or altered rates of speech and movements. Does the patient speak in monotone or in a high-pitched voice? Does the patient show signs of muscular tension?

DIAGNOSING SELF-ESTEEM PROBLEMS

The effects of low self-esteem are pervasive and related to numerous problems that are in the domain of nursing practice. Carpenito (1993) lists body image disturbance, personal identity disturbance, self-esteem disturbance, chronic low self-esteem and situational low self-esteem in one broad category that she calls self-concept disturbance. The person who has had a debilitating health problem may have a *disturbance of the self-concept related to* [the health problem]. For the woman who has had a mastectomy the diagnosis would be written as *body image disturbance related to surgery*. For a young man who has never done well in school and drops out in Grade 10 the nursing diagnosis might be written as *self-esteem disturbance due to repeated failures*. In other problems where low self-esteem is a major factor, the nursing diagnosis would be written as PROBLEM *related to* CAUSE, for example, *anxiety related to low self-esteem* or *anxiety related to actual or perceived threat to self-concept*. "Depression" is not on the NANDA list of nursing diagnoses. Any of the following nursing diagnoses may be related to depression:

powerlessness, any of the *self-care deficit* family of diagnoses, such as *self-care deficit in dressing and grooming*, also, *high risk for self-harm, self-mutilation or suicide* and *social isolation* (Carpenito, 1993).

PLANNING SELF-ESTEEM INTERVENTIONS

Nursing care is based on planning to meet the nursing needs of individuals and groups. As we noted in discussing the determinants of security and self-esteem, self-esteem is the product of many factors including home life, the school environment, the workplace and the social networks people have. To nurture self-esteem, then, requires a multisectoral approach involving collaboration with people in numerous fields. In planning nursing care to promote, protect, support and restore self-esteem, the nurse works in collaboration with the members of many disciplines.

Basic principles regarding self-esteem that are relevant to planning nursing measures to nurture self-esteem are shown in the box below.

The nurse's responsibilities are:
- to work with parents and families to foster the development of self-esteem in children
- to work with others at the community level and in the public forum to promote conditions that will nurture feelings of self-worth
- to protect the self-esteem of individuals, families and groups
- to plan and implement nursing care for individuals and

KEY PRINCIPLES

Principles of Self-Esteem

- Self-esteem is an internal evaluation of the sum total of people's perceptions, feelings and beliefs about themselves
- Self-esteem exists in relation to the individual's total psychological environment
- Fulfilment of the basic physiological, security and love and belonging needs is necessary for the development of a positive self-esteem
- Self-esteem is acquired through the process of growth and development
- Negative (or low) self-esteem has been linked to numerous physical and social ills
- Negative self-esteem can be transformed into a positive one through successful learning experiences

groups to meet the needs of people with specific nursing diagnoses

It is essential that the individual or group participate in identifying goals and in planning strategies to meet these goals. It is important that the goals become the patient's own, with the nurse acting as a facilitator, instead of as an authority.

Some examples of outcome criteria for nursing diagnoses related to low self-esteem and to specific problems are given in Table 35.1.

TABLE 35.1 Examples of Outcome Criteria for Nursing Diagnoses Related to Low Self-Esteem

NURSING DIAGNOSES RELATED TO LOW SELF-ESTEEM	SAMPLE OUTCOME CRITERIA
Low self-esteem	• The person will identify ways of exerting control influencing outcomes (Carpenito, 1993). • The person will verbalize and demonstrate acceptance of appearance (grooming, dress, posture, eating patterns, presentation of self) (Carpenito, 1993). • The person will describe strategies to promote effective socialization (Carpenito, 1993).
Powerlessness	• The person identifies and explores how she (he) can update employable skills (Haber et al., 1992). • The person will make decisions regarding his (her) care, treatment, and future when possible (Carpenito, 1993).
Anxiety	• The person will describe his (her) own anxiety and coping patterns (Carpenito, 1993).
Depression	• The person will state the desire to live (Carpenito, 1993).

IMPLEMENTING SELF-ESTEEM INTERVENTIONS

The specific goals of nursing care related to the need for self-esteem are:

- to promote the fostering of self-esteem in individuals, families and other groups and communities
- to protect the individual's or group's feelings of self-worth
- to enhance the individual's power to improve the life situation
- to facilitate the acquisition of knowledge and the development of skills that will enable people to take control of their lives, make decisions about choices and improve their life situation

HEALTH PROMOTION STRATEGIES

Nursing interventions to promote self-esteem include individual counselling, teaching, working with groups and working with people in other sectors, such as school teachers and employers, to foster environments in which self-esteem is nurtured. Nursing interventions to promote self-esteem also involve political action at times, such as forming coalitions and lobbying.

The Epp Framework for Health Promotion suggested three mechanisms for health promotion: self-care, mutual aid and healthy environments. Nurses use all three in fostering self-esteem.

SELF-CARE

"Simply put, encouraging self-care means encouraging healthy choices" (Epp, 1986, 6). In this context, **self-care** refers to the decisions people make and the practices they adopt to promote and protect their own health. In order to make healthy choices, people need access to information and they need motivation and a supportive environment to adopt healthy practices. Nurturing self-esteem is a lifelong process that begins before a child is born. To nurture self-esteem, the nurse works with:

- prospective parents to provide them with access to the information they need to become nurturing parents
- the mother and partner during labour and delivery to foster "bonding" between parents and child
- the new mother to encourage breastfeeding and with both parents to help them gain the knowledge and skills needed to care for their infant and develop a good relationship with the child
- the parents of young and school-age children to help them learn how to help their children grow up with positive feelings of self-worth

Children need friends to help them develop a sense of belonging.

Children reflect the image their parents have of them. If parents communicate to their children that each one is loved, wanted and an important being, children are much more likely to grow up with a positive concept of themselves than children who are constantly criticized. Parents communicate their feelings to daughters and sons in basically the same ways as they communicate other feelings. The different ways we have of communicating are summarized in the box below.

Different Ways of Communicating

- verbally — through spoken or written words
- non-verbally — non-verbal sounds (for example, groans, laughter, facial expressions, body positions and movements)
- behaviourally — our actions communicate our thoughts, feelings and desires very clearly. For example, if someone says "I really want to lose weight" but continues to overeat, it looks as if eating is more important than losing weight.
- silently — silence can mean "I do not want to communicate with you" or "I am afraid to communicate with you" or "I am too angry to communicate with you."

SOURCE: Holloway, S. (1991). *Critical skills for communicating in conflict*. Vancouver: Justice Institute of B.C. Reproduced with permission.

Some of the ways parents can help children grow up with positive feelings of self-worth are shown in the box below.

Some Ways Parents Can Help Children to Grow Up with Positive Self-Esteem

Verbally

- telling the child "I love you" on a daily basis
- praising children with honest praise for each accomplishment
- telling children "I like what you did (or said)" often
- demonstrating unqualified love by saying, for example, "I love you, but I don't like what you are doing," rather than "I won't love you if you aren't a good boy (or girl)."

Non-Verbally

- hugging and kissing children often
- smiling at children more often than frowning at them
- being approachable

Behaviourally

- spending time with children, for instance by reading to them at bedtime
- giving autonomy consistent with the child's age and developmental level
- setting limits and being consistent in their application
- helping children to make friends with other children outside the family circle
- taking pride in your family's ethnic background and heritage and encouraging children to do the same
- celebrating birthdays and other family events
- keeping photo albums and other reminders of family events and family history around the home

Silently

- being there when the child wakes up at night
- being there (or having a parent substitute there) when the child comes home from school
- being there when the children are ill

SOURCE: Canadian Mental Health Association (1993). *Children and Self-Esteem.* (Pamphlet). Toronto: Author. Adapted with permission.

MUTUAL AID

Mutual aid refers to the concept of people helping other people. Much of the nurse's work with parents is done with groups of people such as "Prospective Parents" classes or with young mothers, helping them to learn to foster self-esteem in their children. It is reassuring for a young mother to learn that their child's behaviour is not so different from that of other children the same age, and to share with other mothers ways to help their children grow up confident and sure of their worth in this world. We talked in Chapter 4 about self-help groups, and in Chapter 16, the Enterostomal Therapist talked about working with the "Ostomy Association," a self-help group for people with colostomies or ileostomies. Associations such as these help people and their families to feel comfortable with their illness by sharing experiences, feelings and ways of coping with the stresses of their everyday lives. In so doing, feelings of self-worth are nurtured; people are part of a group with similar problems.

In working with all of these groups, it is important for nurses to remember that their role is that of *resource* for the group — a source of information and professional expertise when it is needed, a teacher of skills and sometimes an advocate for the group with official governmental and other agencies. The nurse's task is to *facilitate* the work of the group.

HEALTHY ENVIRONMENTS

Self-esteem requires fostering in the home, school, workplace and community. The nurse works with parents and other family members, with teachers and school principals, with employers and with other people in the community to foster environments that will nurture people's self-esteem. Nurses are also involved in promoting the fostering of self-esteem as citizens and through professional associations with the development of healthy public policies to provide a supportive environment for everyone.

Characteristics of a healthy school environment and a healthy workplace taken from the Ontario document *Nurturing Health* (1993) are shown in the boxes on the next page. The information in these boxes emphasizes the importance of nurturing self-concept in the promotion of health and suggests strategies for doing this.

HEALTH PROTECTING STRATEGIES

In Chapter 5 we discussed the writings of some of the "human care" theorists in nursing, including Leininger, Watson, Orem and Roach. That material is particularly pertinent to our discussion here on protecting self-esteem. Watson, for example, has stated that "the end [goal of

A Healthy School Environment

- Involves students, staff and parents in decisions affecting the school and community

- Ensures that students and teachers have safe working conditions and access to support services

- Builds students' and teachers' self-esteem and fosters values such as mutual responsibility, caring and personal power

- Provides instruction in health matters and gives opportunities to practise decision-making skills

- Prepares students for productive employment, positive social relationships and full participation in the community

SOURCE: Government of Ontario. (1993). *Nurturing Health.* Report of the Premier's Council on Health. Toronto: Queen's Printer. (Catalogue No. 01–93–20m.) Reprinted with permission.

A Healthy Workplace Environment

- Provides a healthy and safe physical environment

- Invests in employees by offering ongoing training and by rewarding good work

- Recognizes that fairness, job security, recognition, good management, teamwork and personal wellness are important to employees

- Involves employees in making decisions, and in defining and responding to workplace needs

- Offers flexible work hours that alleviate the stress of balancing home and workplace responsibilities

- Offers workplace health promotion programs and opportunities for positive interactions with co-workers

SOURCE: Government of Ontario. (1993). *Nurturing Health.* Report of the Premier's Council on Health. Toronto: Queen's Printer. (Catalogue No. 01–93–20m.) Reprinted with permission.

nursing] is protection, enhancement and preservation of human dignity" (Watson, 1988, 35). The treatment of people in health care agencies has become increasingly impersonal as our predominantly "cure-oriented" care has become more technological and the institutions more bureaucratized (Watson, 1988). The reforms that are taking place in health care across the country are attempting to make the system more humane by deemphasizing institutional care and bringing health care closer to the homes of people and by encouraging people to be partners in the health care process rather than simply the recipients of services.

Still, there are many agencies where the patient feels like a cog in a machine. To cite one example, an individual phoned to make an appointment with her physician who is in a busy family practice clinic. The office nurse who answered the phone told the woman she did not need her name, just her clinic number. One cannot blame the woman for changing her family physician to one in a smaller practice where she would be treated as a person instead of a number.

Hospitals have been especially criticized for the impersonal manner in which admission procedures have been carried out, and the depersonalization that results from the routines many hospitals have considered necessary. First, patients are asked a lot of personal questions, to which they are expected to give answers to a stranger. They are then given a number and "tagged" with an armband. They are taken to a nursing unit that is usually also designated with a number, not a name, and assigned to a room or bed, likewise numbered. Once there, patients are stripped of all their clothes and most of the valuables that help to identify them as people. A procession of strangers then begin to arrive at their bedside, to ask more personal questions and perform various examinations. Sometimes, these strangers do not even introduce themselves, and the patient is left to guess who they are by the uniform they are wearing. If patients are assigned to a room where there are other patients, they often have to make introductions themselves.

Many agencies have changed admission procedures to make them less impersonal. Preadmission clinics make the procedure of admission more "people-oriented." The introduction of primary nursing on nursing units has also been helpful because it gives patients one person to whom they can relate throughout their stay in hospital, one person they feel really cares about them. Regardless of whether primary nursing is in operation or not, nurses can do a great deal to dispel the impression of agency impersonality and to minimize patients' feelings of depersonalization.

Nurses protect the self-esteem of the people they care for by conveying feelings of respect for the personhood of the individual. This is done in the same ways as other feelings are communicated. Some of the ways the nurse conveys to the individual or group respect for their personhood are listed in the box on the next page.

Ways of Conveying Respect for Personhood

Verbally

- addressing patients by the name they wish to be called

- using "active listening" skills

- telling patients what the nurse or others are going to do to them, or for them, and asking permission

- giving praise for each accomplishment

Non-Verbally

- using non-verbal sounds like "Mmmm" to convey interest in what is being said

- being conscious of facial expressions and careful not to show negative feelings such as hostility, anger, disinterest or disgust

- looking at the patient's face when talking and using frequent eye contact (in some cultures, eye contact is considered disrespectful)

- avoiding quick movements that give the impression of being in a hurry

Behaviourally

- carrying out requests that have been made, such as phoning a patient's child and reporting back on the conversation

- seeing that members of the patient's family feel welcome

- ensuring the patient's (family or group's) privacy when discussing personal matters

- getting an interpreter to help patients to communicate if they do not speak English

- adapting care so that the individual can maintain traditional religious and ethnic customs

- respecting the patient's modesty

Silently

- being there when the patient needs support, for example, during a painful procedure

- holding patient's hands, touching the arm or putting an arm around the shoulder

HEALTH RESTORATION AND SUPPORTIVE STRATEGIES

STRATEGIES FOR POWERLESSNESS

The most pervasive problem related to low self-esteem is the feeling of powerlessness (helplessness/ hopelessness) it engenders. Strategies used to restore self-esteem so that people are able to meet their own needs, solve their own problems and mobilize resources so that they can take control of their lives are referred to as "empowering" strategies.

The overall goals of empowering strategies are twofold: (1) "…to transform internal feelings of powerlessness (hopelessness/helplessness); and (2) to initiate changes in the physical and social living conditions that create or reinforce inequalities in power" (Rappaport, 1987; Labonte, 1990. Both cited in RNABC, 1992, 9).

These goals imply that there needs to be a continuum of empowering strategies that begin with the individual through personal empowerment, and include small group development, community organization, coalition advocacy and political action. This continuum of empowering strategies is shown in Figure 35.1.

Nurses work at the individual and group development level and, increasingly, in community development; they work through their professional organizations, in coalition advocacy and in political action to improve physical and social conditions. You will learn more about working with groups and community development in more senior courses on community nursing and more about coalition advocacy and political action in courses on issues in nursing. We will focus here on personal empowerment strategies. The following assumptions suggested by Gibson (1991) and summarized here are pertinent to our discussion of nursing strategies for personal empowerment.

- Individuals are primarily responsible for their own health
- The individual has the right and the capacity for self-determination
- Individuals empower themselves but nurses provide the resources that foster empowerment
- Individuals' input into decisions must be valued, and their opinions must be the bottom line
- Mutual respect must exist between the individual and the nurse
- Trust is a necessary part of empowerment

Some *personal empowerment strategies* are listed below.

- Provide people with the information they need to change their behaviour or their environment, for example, information about courses in assertiveness training; courses to upgrade skills; services that are available such as a rent

X **Personal Empowerment**	X **Small Group Development**	X **Community Organization**	X **Coalition Advocacy**	X **Political Action**

PERSONAL EMPOWERMENT:
- Developmental case-work
- Enhancing personal perceptions of control and power

SMALL GROUP DEVELOPMENT:
- Improving social support
- Promoting personal behaviour change
- Providing support for lifestyle choices

COMMUNITY ORGANIZATION:
- Developing local actions on community-defined health issues
- Critical community/professional dialogue
- Raising conflict to the conscious level

COALITION ADVOCACY:
- Lobbying for healthier public policies
- Achieving strategic consensus
- Collaboration and conflict resolution

POLITICAL ACTION:
- Support for broad-based social movements
- Creating vision of sustainable, preferred future
- Enhancing participatory democracy

FIGURE 35.1   A continuum of empowering strategies

SOURCE: Registered Nurses Association of British Columbia (RNABC). (1992). *Determinants of health: Strategies for nursing practice — A background paper.* (Publication No. 24) Vancouver: Author, 10.

ombudsman, health services, shelters for battered wives; government grant programs such as New Horizons, which provides funds for senior citizen projects.

- Encourage participation in decisions regarding the person's own actions — to take a course, to go to the Family Services Bureau, and to make decisions regarding the small things in everyday life. For people in an inpatient facility, it means giving them the opportunity to make as many decisions on their own as possible, such as when they are going to take their bath, what they want to eat for breakfast, lunch and dinner, what they are going to wear for the day, what services they want to have.
- Help people to develop positive coping skills.
- Help people to derive power from other sources, such as prayer, or stress-reduction techniques; help people to maintain religious or cultural rituals; offer to call the patient's religious leader or leader in their ethnic community (Carpenito, 1993).

- Encourage the patient to participate in groups, such as self-help and support groups (Carpenito, 1993).
- Help people to form a group with other people in similar situations. Quarrington (1992) discusses starting a patient self-help group on a psychiatric unit and helping the patients to overcome feelings of powerlessness and low self-esteem by letting them have a say in their care and the services they receive and by encouraging them to share successful coping strategies with each other.

We discussed in Chapter 11 numerous other examples of ways to help people form groups to tackle problems which they feel powerless to do anything about on their own. Forming these groups is part of the nurse's role in community development, and is a role which is shared with other workers in the field, such as social workers and health educators.

STRATEGIES FOR ANXIETY

In the course of daily practice, nurses meet many people who are anxious. Most people are at least a little nervous when they visit a health agency for the first time. Even if they are going for a routine checkup, there is always the nagging worry that something may be wrong. Anxiety almost invariably accompanies the person who is being admitted to a hospital or coming into the emergency department. When dealing with people who are anxious, the nurse must take into account the fact that the plan of care has to be individualized to suit each individual. No two people are alike in regard to the nature of anxieties, reactions to these, or the type of help needed to overcome them. The nurse also considers whether this patient needs the help of another member of the health team. There is therefore no easy set of rules for the nurse to follow. The assumptions about anxiety listed below can be used to guide your selection of strategies that may be helpful with a particular individual.

- It is easier to allay a known fear than to ease anxiety from an unknown source
- People generally feel less anxious when they know what is going to happen to them
- Anxiety is lessened when people feel they have some control over their situation
- Loneliness aggravates anxiety
- A feeling of depersonalization contributes to anxiety
- Physical activity helps to relieve muscular tension
- Anxiety can often be relieved by diversional activity

The following nursing interventions are based on the assumptions listed above and might be considered in the care of specific individuals.

Identify the cause of the anxiety, if possible. We have already discussed some of the ways the nurse can gather information to help identify the sources of a patient's potential or actual problem of anxiety. The nurse always verifies with the patient that the interpretation of the source of the anxieties is consistent with the patient's perceptions. The nurse may think that the patient is very worried about the treatment, for example, when in actual fact the patient may be anxious about a family member who has not come in to visit.

Help the patient to explore the problem. It is important to remember, too, that talking with the patient can also be therapeutic. It gives the patient an opportunity to explore the causes of anxieties, to discuss them with someone and to work out solutions to some of the things that are worrisome.

Refer the individual to specialized counselling services. Beginning nurses should not feel that they can be skilled counsellors at this stage in their career. If you do not feel comfortable dealing with a patient's anxieties, or feel the patient needs more highly skilled counselling than you are able to provide, you should not hesitate to call in someone else. Nor should you feel guilty in doing so. The clinical instructor, or the charge nurse on the unit (case manager in

home care), may be able to help the patient. If a clinical nurse specialist in psychiatric/mental health nursing is available, this person is often able to help patients with their anxieties more effectively than someone else. A psychiatric/mental health nurse may also be able to provide the beginning nurse with help in the approach to caring for the patient. Some patients need the counselling services of a psychologist or psychiatrist, and they should be referred for these services.

Provide the individual with the information they need. Providing information is important both in preventing and in allaying anxiety. If patients know what is going to be done during a laboratory test, they are usually less apprehensive about it. Similarly, the patient who has been told that a certain procedure may hurt a little is better able to face the pain. Teaching plans that identify patient information needs should form a part of every nursing care plan.

Encourage the person to take some control of the situation. Enlisting patient cooperation and having the patient participate in care whenever possible helps to give a feeling of control over the situation. The use of self-administration techniques for pain-relieving medications has been helpful in this regard. Giving patients a voice in the scheduling of their activities or in the way some intervention is carried out is one way of helping them to feel they still have some control over events.

Promote social contacts. People need the company of other people and a group with whom they can identify. We have mentioned the importance of social support in nurturing self-esteem. Family, friends and a group identity help to provide individuals with the security and support needed to overcome threats to self-concept. Many groups, such as fraternal organizations, churches and alumni associations, have visitors committees to visit the sick, people who are confined to their homes and lonely elderly people in the community. Senior citizens centres in connection with community centres help to fill the need for socialization and the provision of a group identity. For inpatients, the nurse needs to be alert to patients who have no visitors, to encourage family to visit, or if the patient has no family close by, to arrange for visits from the patient's church, lodge or other organization.

Show respect for the patient as an individual. When patients feel that they have lost their identity, that they are just a health agency number or an interesting "case," their confidence in the care they are receiving is diminished. It is important to help patients to retain the feeling that they are respected.

Provide opportunities for exercise and/or relaxation techniques. Exercise to a patient's limits of tolerance is a good way of relieving the muscular tension that accompanies anxiety. Relaxation exercises and techniques can also help. The assistance of the physical therapist is often helpful for teaching people relaxing exercises or for suggesting other measures to reduce muscular tension.

STRATEGIES FOR DEPRESSION

The subject of depression will be treated in more detail in psychiatric nursing courses. The beginning student, however, should be alert to the possibility that depressed people may try to injure themselves, and they may attempt to commit suicide. Most of the time, someone who is contemplating suicide will signal their intentions. They may say, "I wish I could do away with myself" or "I'd like to kill myself," and may even discuss ways of doing so. The nurse should always be watchful of any patient who seems to be getting more depressed. The nurse may notice that the physiological and behavioural manifestations are becoming more pronounced. It is important to remember that depressed patients are not always on a psychiatric unit in a hospital; they may be on a surgical or a medical ward or at home in the community. The patient's physician should be alerted if the nurse suspects that the patient is becoming more depressed, so that psychiatric counselling and appropriate therapy can be instituted promptly. Often, mood-elevating drugs are administered.

In selecting specific strategies to help depressed people, the nurse may find the following assumptions helpful.

- A person who is depressed will show changes in physiological functioning, in feeling state, in cognitive functioning and in behaviour.
- Prolonged or deep depression may cause general metabolic retardation, mental confusion and/or dullness.
- Emotions tend to be contagious.
- Emotions are influenced by physiological state.
- Depressed people usually have very low self-esteem.
- Depressed people may not want to live because they feel unworthy.

Nursing interventions for the depressed patient are directed towards three principal goals: preventing patients from injuring themselves or taking their own lives; supporting and maintaining the patient's basic physiological processes, such as nutrition and elimination; and helping the patient to overcome the depression.

Protect the patient from self-injury. Constant vigilance is needed to protect severely depressed patients from injuring themselves or committing suicide. Patients who are seriously depressed are usually placed on a psychiatric nursing unit so that the specialized care they require is available. If they are on a general ward, often a private duty nurse or one staff nurse may be assigned to care for the patient. The nurse who has a depressed individual among the regular patient load should be particularly careful to make sure that the depressed patient takes all medications. There should be no opportunity for the person to collect a large number of sleeping pills or other drugs. When visiting a patient in the home, the nurse should make sure the patient who shows signs of depression is not collecting too many tranquilizers or other drugs. In tidying up the drawer of the bedside table of patients in hospital each day, it is important to make sure that medications are not being collected there. Sharp instruments and glass items that could be broken to provide depressed patients an instrument with which to hurt themselves should not be accessible. The medication cupboard on the ward should be kept locked at all times, unless a nurse is actually in the process of dispensing medicines. This is a good general rule, in any case. Nurses should not go off to answer a patient's signal light and leave the medication cupboard keys dangling from the door or leave the door open.

If the patient is known to be suicidal, all potential sources of self-injury, such as belts and shoe laces, are removed. There should also be a check on the patient at irregular but frequent intervals. Depressed patients who wake up in the early morning hours (when a person's body processes are at their lowest ebb) often need someone to talk to, and the nurse should take time to stop and chat for a few minutes. Occasionally, patients will need to be physically restrained to keep them from injuring themselves. This is most likely to be seen in the Emergency Unit, where a person may be coming out of the effects of a drug; LSD, for example, is noted for causing suicidal tendencies in people as they are recovering from its effects.

Maintain physiological processes. Because depressed people are inactive, nutritional status may suffer. Depressed people often have no appetite and must be encouraged to eat. Appetite often improves in mildly depressed people if they have company during meals. Some community organizations have "pot-luck" suppers on a regular basis so that people who live by themselves do not have to eat dinner alone.

The nurse should be alert to the problem of constipation in depressed people because of the slowing down of gastrointestinal functioning and the inactivity. These people need to be encouraged to take a sufficient amount of fluids. The slowing down of physiological functioning also causes a tendency for urine to be retained in the bladder for too long, and bladder infections could result from a combination of inadequate intake of fluids and stasis of urine. Because depressed people tend to sit a lot, they may develop edema in the dependent limbs, or in the sacral area.

Help with hygiene and grooming. Depressed people often need help with hygiene and grooming, since it requires too much effort for them to do it themselves. Often, assisting a person to improve their personal appearance will help to lift a mild depression. A new article of clothing may also stimulate an individual, helping with mild depression.

Promote socialization. People who are lonely often get depressed. Everyone needs the stimulation of other people (or a pet) to stay alert and responsive. One of the things the nurse can do for lonely people is to encourage them to participate in group activities. Loneliness is a common companion to old age. Community centres have a wide variety of activities for seniors and have become the "drop-in centres" for older people in many places. Many long-term care facilities employ activity aides who help to get residents interested in doing things with other people. Often, there are also transportation aides, so that people who are not mobile can be taken by wheelchair to activities or special programs.

In long-term care agencies, a resident's depression will often lift when a companion with shared interests can be found. It is good to discover patients' interests, and to try to match them with someone else who is interested in the same things.

Use non-verbal communication. Unlike the anxious patient, the person who is depressed may not like to talk with the nurse — or with anyone — because talking really does not help. Still, the presence of the nurse, with a touch on the arm or an arm around the shoulder, often goes a long way towards making a depressed person feel that someone still cares.

Try music therapy. Music is being used quite extensively now to assist in overcoming depression. Happy lively music will most times lift spirits. Some people may not like lively music, however; for them, something light but not too strident may be more effective. Many people come out of depressed moods when they start to play a tune on a musical instrument.

However, it is important not to try to force severely depressed patients into activities to "cheer them up." Sitting beside the person and giving quiet companionship is often helpful in gradually drawing a response. Very often the patient needs to work through a problem, as in the case of a woman who has had a mastectomy and must adjust to her altered figure. Many people need the help of a psychiatric nursing specialist or a psychiatrist to help them to overcome depression.

Encourage good nutrition and regular exercise. One should not forget the vital role of good nutrition and regular exercise both in helping to prevent depression and in helping people overcome it. Some of the most enthusiastic marathon runners took up the sport to overcome the effects of depression. All report that they feel a "high" when they are reaching their maximum potential in running. Vigorous exercise also helps to promote sleep and better quality rest. It encourages good nutrition and promotes a more regular daily schedule. There is much truth in the old adage, "healthy mind, healthy body."

EVALUATING SELF-ESTEEM INTERVENTIONS

In evaluating the effectiveness of interventions for self-esteem, the nurse observes the patient for changes in affect, behavioural patterns, cognitive functioning and physiological status indicating progress towards resolution of the specific problem(s) the individual had. The nurse observes whether the outcome criteria established in planning care for patients have been met.

Examples of Evaluative Observations
For low self-esteem:
- Does the person (or group) identify factors that he or she can control?
- Has the person verbalized acceptance of his or her appearance?
- Has the person demonstrated acceptance of his or her appearance, for example, by taking more care with grooming and dress, standing tall and presenting themselves better and eating better?
- Does the person describe strategies to promote effective socialization? Does the person demonstrate use of these strategies?
- Has the person identified and explored ways to update employable skills, e.g. obtained calendars or brochures about educational programs or sought the advice of an employment counsellor?

For powerlessness:
- Does the person have the information needed to make decisions about his or her care or situation?
- Does the person appear more confident in making decisions about his or her care, treatment and future?
- Does the person verbalize feelings of greater control of situations?

For anxiety:
- Is the person able to express his or her own anxiety and coping patterns?
- Have the physical and behavioural manifestations of anxiety lessened or disappeared? For example, is the patient's facial expression more calm and relaxed? Is muscle tension reduced? Are speech and voice patterns more normal? Have distressing symptoms such as diarrhea, urinary frequency, or headache disappeared?
- Can the patient describe techniques for stress reduction? Does the patient use these techniques?
- Does the patient state that he or she is feeling better?

For depression:
- Does the person state that he or she wants to live?
- Have the physical and behavioural manifestations of depression been lessened? For example, are movements faster? Is posture improved? Is the person more animated? Does the patient sleep well at night? less in the daytime?
- Does the patient socialize more with other people?
- Is the patient eating well? Gaining weight?

KEY TERMS

self-esteem p. 1210

body image p. 1210

self-respect p. 1210

self-confidence p. 1210

empowerment p. 1210

developmental crises p. 1212

powerlessness p. 1216

anxiety p. 1217

panic p. 1218

depression p. 1219

reactive (situational) depression p. 1219

agitated depression p. 1219

self-care p. 1224

mutual aid p. 1225

IN REVIEW

Self-esteem includes self-image, the perceptual aspect of ourselves; self-respect, the emotional aspect; and self-confidence, the cognitive aspect. It is said to be the key to our behaviour, affecting virtually all aspects of our lives — our thinking, emotions, desires, values and goals. Low self-esteem has been linked to numerous illnesses and social problems.

The determinants of self-esteem include the fulfilment of basic physiological needs, freedom from pain and fear, a sense of belonging and the love and companionship of others. Social support in home, school, workplace and community, cultural customs and mores, religion and the feeling of having a purpose in life also contribute to self-esteem. Health-related factors and developmental crises can threaten it.

The building of self-esteem is probably our most important developmental task. The successful accomplishment of other developmental tasks at each stage of the life cycle builds self-confidence and is important in fostering self-esteem. The lack of accomplishment of these tasks establishes feelings of worthlessness, inferiority and low self-esteem, which are often lifelong feelings. People with low self-esteem feel anxious and unsure of themselves; they are often unhappy and afraid of failing. Frequently, they feel responsible for their own problems and guilty because of this; sometimes, they blame others for their failures.

Three of the most common problems related to lack of fulfilment of self-esteem needs are feelings of powerlessness (hopelessness/helplessness), anxiety and depression. People experiencing powerlessness feel unable to control their own destiny. They often react with anger and hostility to whatever is seen as the power controlling their lives. As they become resigned to the situation, the anger and hostility may fade into apathy and depression.

The unpleasant feeling of anxiety alerts people to real or symbolic threats to themselves, their significant others or their way of life. Ranging from mild anxiety to overwhelming panic, it is manifested in changes in feeling tone (affect), physiological reactions, behavioural changes and changes in cognitive ability. Feelings include tension, uneasiness, a sense of dread or anger and hostility. Physiological changes may include increased blood pressure, pulse and respirations, pallor or flushing, cold skin, loss of appetite, increased frequency of voiding, muscular tension, tension headaches, perspiration, nausea and vom-

iting or diarrhea. Behavioural changes include biting nails, drumming fingers, pacing, restlessness and overactivity, talking rapidly or constantly, difficulty in finding words, stammering or crying. Movements are usually rapid and behaviour may be inappropriate. Increased mental activity usually accompanies anxiety and may range from simply being more alert to inability to rest.

Depression is a common problem among all segments of the population but is particularly prevalent in young and older adults, immigrants (especially refugees) and people in low socioeconomic groups. Feelings expressed include sadness, lack of enjoyment, low self-esteem, self anger and feelings of hopelessness. Physiological changes include lack of appetite with resultant loss of weight, slow movements, constipation, amenorrhea, lessened response to stimulation and lessened sex drive. Behavioural changes include stooped posture and slouching gait, a lack of interest in clothes and grooming, a withdrawal from social contacts, a reluctance to talk, slow speech and difficulty in finishing tasks. Cognitive changes include poor concentration, obsession with one topic, disturbed sleep patterns and an inability to make decisions. Depressed people may use drugs or alcohol for temporary relief.

Other problems resulting from unfulfilled self-esteem needs include negative body image, social isolation and ineffective individual or family coping.

The assessment of self-esteem is an ongoing process which starts with the nursing health history. At this point, the nurse learns about the patient's personality, present stage of physical and psychosocial development, lifestyle, health status and immediate concerns. During both the health history and the physical examination, the nurse looks for affective and behavioural manifestations of negative self-esteem and during the physical examination for physiological changes that might indicate anxiety, depression or other problems related to low self-esteem.

Nursing diagnoses related to low self-esteem are usually written as specific problem related to cause as, for example, anxiety related to pending surgery. For depression, common diagnoses include powerlessness, self-care deficits, high risk for self-harm, self-mutilation or suicide and social isolation.

The nurturance of self-esteem requires a multisectoral approach and the nurse works in collaboration with people in many different disciplines in planning nursing care. Nursing interventions for health promotion include counselling, teaching, working with groups and with people in other sectors such as school teachers and employers to promote an environment that fosters self-esteem. Nurses protect the self-esteem of people by conveying respect for the personhood of the individual.

A continuum of empowering strategies is needed to restore self-esteem when people feel powerless. Nurses work at the individual and group level of the continuum, increasingly, in community development and, through their professional organizations, in coalition advocacy and in political action. Personal empowering strategies nurses can use include providing people with information, encouraging them to participate in making decisions about their own actions, helping them develop positive coping skills, teaching them to derive power from sources such as prayer or stress-reduction techniques and helping them form and participate in groups with people in similar situations.

Nursing interventions for anxiety include identifying the cause of the anxiety where possible, helping the individual explore the problem, providing needed information, encouraging the individual to take some control of the situation, showing respect for the person as an individual, promoting social contacts, providing opportunities for exercise and relaxation techniques and referring to specialized counselling services as needed.

Nursing interventions for people who are depressed include protecting the patient from self-injury, maintaining physiological processes, helping with hygiene and grooming, encouraging good nutrition and regular exercise, promoting socialization, music therapy and using non-verbal communication to convey care.

In evaluating self-esteem interventions, the nurse looks for changes in the patient's feeling tone, behaviour, cognitive ability and physiological status that would indicate progress is being made towards resolution of the problem(s); for example, the patient may be better able to take control of his or her situation, may have lessened anxiety or may be less depressed.

LEARNING ACTIVITIES

Delcina Arias is a thirty-eight-year-old single mother of two boys, aged nine and twelve. Recently divorced, she returned to teaching after a refresher course and is now in her first full-time position at a local elementary school as a Grade 4 teacher. During the Easter vacation period, she noticed a small lump in her right breast. Her family doctor referred her to the Cancer Clinic where she underwent a number of diagnostic tests and examinations before being admitted to hospital for a mastectomy.

1. What threats does the impending surgery pose for Delcina's self-esteem?

2. How would you assess Delcina's self-esteem?

3. What emotional, physiological, behavioural or cognitive manifestations might you observe in Delcina that would indicate that she:

a. was anxious about the surgery?

b. depressed when told she had to have radiation therapy after the surgery?

c. felt that she no longer had any control over her life?

4. What nursing diagnoses might be applicable in Delcina's care?

5. What nursing interventions might you use to promote and protect Delcina's self-esteem? to relieve her anxiety? to help her overcome depression if this occurs? to regain feelings of control over her situation?

6. How would you evaluate the effectiveness of your interventions?

REFERENCES AND READINGS

BERGER, K.S. (1993). *The developing person through the life span.* (3rd ed.). New York: Worth Publishers.

BERGER, K.S. (1991). *The developing person through childhood and adolescence.* (3rd ed) New York: Worth Publishers.

BRANCKER, E. (1992). Highlights: causes of death 1990. *Health Reports, 4.* Ottawa: Minister of Supply and Services, 185-189. (Statistics Canada Catalogue No. 82–003)

CANADIAN MENTAL HEALTH ASSOCIATION. (1993). *Children and self-esteem.* (Pamphlet) Toronto: Author.

CARPENITO, L.J. (1993). *Nursing diagnosis: Application to clinical practice.* Philadelphia: Lipincott.

CHARTOW, L. (1983). *The stress protection plan.* London: Thorson's.

DU GAS, B.W. (1993). Healthy Lifestyles. In A. Beckingham and B.W. Du Gas (1993). *Promoting healthy aging. A nursing and community perspective.* St. Louis: Mosby.

DWORETSKY, J.P. and DAVIS, N.J. (1989) *Human development — A lifespan approach.* New York: West Publishing.

EBERSOLE, P. and HESS, P. (1990). *Toward healthy aging: Human needs and nursing response.* St. Louis: Mosby.

EPP, J. (1986). *Achieving health for all: A framework for health promotion.* Ottawa: Minister of Supply and Services.

ERIKSON, E. (1963). *Childhood and society.* New York: Norton.

FOSTER, R.L.R., HUNSBERGER, M.M. and ANDERSON, J.J.T. (1989). *Family-centred nursing care of children.* Philadelphia: Saunders.

GIBSON, C.H. (1991). A concept analysis of empowerment. *Journal of Advanced Nursing, 16,* 354–361.

GILBERT, S. and OROK, B, (1993, Autumn). School leavers. *Canadian social trends, 30,* 2–7.

GOVERNMENT OF BRITISH COLUMBIA. (1992). *Health indicator workbook*. (1st ed.). Victoria, B.C.: Office of Health Promotion, B.C. Minister of Health and Minister Responsible for Senior Citizens.

GOVERNMENT OF ONTARIO. (1992). *Ontario health survey 1990 highlights*. Toronto: Ontario Minister of Health.

GOVERNMENT OF ONTARIO. (1993). *Nurturing health*. Report of the Premier's Council on Health, Well-being and Social Justice (1987–1991). Toronto: Ontario Minister of Health.

GRAINGER, R.D. (1990). Self-confidence: A feeling you can create. *American Journal of Nursing, 90*(10), 12.

HABER, J., LEACH, McMAHON, A., PRICE-HOSKINS, P., and SIDELEAU, B.F. (1992). *Psychiatric nursing*. (4th ed.). St. Louis: Mosby.

HOLLOWAY, S. (1991). *Critical skills for communicating in conflict*. Vancouver: Justice Institute of British Columbia.

JONES, P.S. and MELEIS, A.I. (1993). Health is empowerment. *Advances in Nursing Science, 15*(3), 1–14.

MASLOW, A. (1970). *Motivation and personality*. (2nd ed.). New York: Harper and Row.

MORALES-MANN, E.T. (1990). Child with depression. In A. Baumann, N.E. Johnston and Antai-Otong, D. (1990). *Decision in psychiatric and psychosocial nursing*. Toronto: B.C. Decker Inc., 58–59.

ODERKIRK, J. (1993, Autumn). Educational achievement. An international comparison. *Canadian Social Trends*, 30, 8–12.

PAPALIA, D.E. and OLDS, S.W. (1986). *Human development*. (3rd ed). Toronto: McGraw-Hill.

QUARRINGTON, D. (1992). The power of self help. *The Canadian Nurse, 88*(2), 26–28.

REGISTERED NURSES ASSOCIATION OF BRITISH COLUMBIA (RNABC). (1992). *Determinants of health: Strategies for nursing practice. A background paper*. (Publication No. 24). Vancouver: Author, 10.

ROSS, M. and CASEY, A. (1993). Health concerns associated with aging. In A. Beckingham and B.W. Du Gas. *Promoting healthy aging*. St. Louis: Mosby.

SIMMERMACHER, D. (1989). *Self-image modification*. (Revised ed.). Dunfield Beach, Florida: Health Communications Inc.

STAPLES, P., BARUTH, P., JEFFERIES, M., and WARDER, L. (1994). Empowering the angry patient. *The Canadian Nurse, 90*(4), 28–30.

STOLZMAN, J.D. (1988). The distribution and treatment of mental disorders by social class: A review of the research and theoretical implications. In B.S. Bolaria and H.D. Dickinson. (1988). *Sociology of health care in Canada*. Toronto: Harcourt Brace Jovanovich.

TOFFLER, A. (1981). *The third wave*. New York: Bantam.

WATSON, J. (1988) *Nursing: Human science and human care*. New York: National League for Nursing.

WORLD HEALTH ORGANIZATION. (1980). *Health for all by the year 2000*. (Pan-American Health Organization). Washington, DC.: Regional Office for the Pan American Sanitary Bureau.

36

Death, Loss and Grief

CENTRAL QUESTIONS

1. What are the meanings of loss, death, bereavement, grief and mourning?

2. What are some different types of loss?

3. What are some common manifestations of the grief response?

4. What are the most common causes of death?

5. What physical changes occur in the body as death approaches?

6. How do the frameworks of Kubler-Ross and Weisman explain the psychological responses to death and dying?

7. How does a bereaved person work through the process of grieving?

8. What are the determinants of bereavement and grief?

9. How do the concept and understanding of death and grief vary throughout the life cycle?

10. How does the nurse assess the needs of dying patients and their families?

11. What are some common nursing diagnoses related to death, dying and grieving?

12. How does the nurse plan and implement appropriate interventions to assist dying patients and their families meet their needs?

13. How does the nurse evaluate the effectiveness of care?

INTRODUCTION

Inextricably involved in nursing is the preservation of life, the alleviation of suffering and the restoration of health. Our society celebrates health, life and youth. Death is a subject that generally is avoided; even when death is imminent, it is frequently denied. Yet death is not an uncommon occurrence on hospital wards, in nursing homes or among the sick in the community. By the very nature of their work, nurses and physicians encounter death more often than most people.

Encountering death as part of their job does not make it easy for nurses to deal with. Regardless of whether death is sudden or follows a lengthy illness, the care of the terminally ill patient and the comforting and consoling of the patient's family presents one of the most demanding and stressful situations in nursing practice. Yet, caring for the dying can also be one of the more satisfying nursing responsibilities.

The difficulty that nurses and other health care professionals have in caring for the dying stems in part from membership in the larger North American society which does not openly deal with death very well. As members of a society focussed on youth, productivity and activity, we are not prepared to accommodate into our lives what is seen as a deteriorating process, nor are we prepared to allow for the expression of the intense responses that accompany death. When a person becomes terminally ill, others are reminded of their own mortality. Death is an unfamiliar experience which provokes many feelings — fear, futility, uncertainty, joy, grief, loneliness, hope, anger, a longing for death and a longing to avoid it. These feelings are as much present in nurses as they are in patients and families. To provide comprehensive and compassionate care to dying people and their families, however, is to learn to cope with the strong emotions and to learn that death really is a part of life.

Coping with the prospect of one's own death and with the loss of loved ones through death is perhaps the greatest challenge human beings must face in the course of living. Death brings about disruptive changes in individuals and families which threaten the ability to satisfy needs and to change and cope with the environment. How people are able to resolve these challenges — to die peacefully and with dignity or to restore emotional, social and spiritual health and harmony after the death of a loved one — depends on a number of influences. These influences may include the coping strategies that individuals and families have learned in dealing with past loss experiences, as well as support systems, cultural, religious and spiritual beliefs and age. We will discuss these determinants in a later section. However, to cope with death in a healthy way, people need sensitive, caring support from health care professionals. In this chapter we will provide basic knowledge of loss, death, grief and grieving. This knowledge will enable nurses to

- assess the needs of dying patients and their families
- provide comprehensive and compassionate care for dying patients
- promote healthy grieving in individuals and families.

LOSS AND DEATH

All of us have experienced loss at some time in our lives. Perhaps our first encounter with loss came when we were weaned from our mother's breast or from the bottle and taught how to drink milk from a cup. As we grew and moved through the developmental stages of life, we weathered certain losses — our first day at kindergarten, taking the school bus by ourselves, graduating from high school or moving away from home to attend college or university. All of these experiences meant leaving behind both a degree of dependence on our parents and the security of a familiar environment. Some of us may also have lost something very significant to us, such as a husband, wife or partner through separation or divorce, a playmate whose family moved away, a coveted part in a school play or a valuable piece of jewellery. And some of us may have lost a part of our body functioning from illness or trauma or experienced the death of someone close to us. All of these losses have one thing in common: the individual who loses something is separated from and deprived of the lost person, object, status or relationship (Corr, Nabe and Corr, 1994).

Loss refers to any life event in which one is deprived of something that is valued. This may include loss of external objects, developmental loss, loss of a part of the self, secondary losses, symbolic losses, loss of a significant other or impending loss of self through death (Shapiro, 1993). The experience of loss through death is called ***bereavement*** (Corr, Nabe and Corr, 1994). The term "bereaved" is used as an adjective (the "bereaved" family) or as a noun (the "bereaved") to refer to those who have experienced the loss of a loved one through death. The different types of losses are defined in Table 36.1.

Loss brings about a variety of feelings, from shock and disbelief, to resentment, sadness, despair and even relief. For example, we may feel very saddened when a close friend dies from cancer, but at the same time we may feel relief that this friend is no longer suffering. The degree of loss one feels depends on the magnitude of attachment to what has been lost and on the availability of its replacement. For instance, the loss that might be felt when a perfect new car sustains its first scratch or dent may cause minor distress requiring minimal emotional adjustment and a trip to the automotive repair shop to reestablish a sense of well-being. On the other hand, the loss of something or someone very important and irreplaceable will cause profound distress and place heavy demands on adaptive resources and on the capacity for coping with adversity and change. Such losses might include the loss of a body part or function, a highly esteemed occupation or role in society or a significant other through separation or death. In addition, one's own impending death is a major loss that must be resolved (Kubler-Ross, 1969).

Although death is a biological process, it is accompanied by a multitude of social, emotional and spiritual experiences both for dying people and for their survivors. Death can have many meanings for the dying person. Some may view death as a punishment for past wrong-doings; others may see it as a loss of self and self-identity and missed future goals, opportunities, pleasures and relationships. For others, death may mean relief of prolonged suffering from a terminal illness or a reunion with loved ones in an afterlife. What death means for the survivors will depend upon the value of the lost person and on the ways in which they interpret that loss (Corr, Nabe and Corr, 1994). For instance, the death of a spouse may mean the end of sharing life experiences with a partner, loneliness and perhaps a loss of economic and domestic security. For parents, the death of a child may mean never seeing the child grow to be an adult or enjoying the gratification of watching their child's accomplishments in life. Bereavement is typically painful because death is final (Corr, Nabe and Corr, 1994). No two individuals will cope with death in the same way because people are different. Each person will approach the loss experience using available resources and coping strategies learned in dealing with other stressful events in life. Our goal as health care professionals is to try to understand other's ways of coping with death and to support his or her coping abilities. We will discuss this aspect further on in the chapter.

TABLE 36.1 Types of Losses

TYPE	DEFINITION	EXAMPLE
Loss of external objects	Loss of valued material things	A family loses financial security when the parent loses a job. Family residences and possessions are lost in a hurricane. A child's teddy bear wears to shreds.
Developmental loss	Maturational loss resulting from normal life transitions	Adolescents lose their childhood identity as they assume their own self-image. Elderly people lose their physical endurance as a result of aging.
Loss of a part of self	Loss of one's sense of identity, body image or physical functioning	Disfigurement due to trauma such as burns. Loss of a limb due to injury or illness. People with spinal cord injuries lose their independence in carrying out daily functions.
Secondary losses	Losses associated with other losses	Patients in hospital lose the comforts of home, their sense of autonomy and control. A person recuperating from a prolonged illness experiences financial loss.
Symbolic losses	Perceived losses associated with the psychological aspects of a physical loss	Women who lose a breast to cancer perceive a loss of sexual attractiveness and femininity. Men who develop sexual impotence feel "less than a man."
Loss of a significant other	Loss of significant other through death, separation or divorce	A family loses a loved one through death. Children lose a parent through divorce. An important friend moves to another country.
Impending loss of self	Personal losses experienced as one approaches death	Loss of ending relationships, status or roles. Missed experiences and opportunities in life.

SOURCE: Shapiro, 1993.

GRIEF AND GRIEVING

Grief refers to the total response to loss. When individuals suffer an irreversible loss, they grieve. Grief is a profound and painful state that involves strong emotions and affects how one thinks, feels, behaves and continues the functions of daily living. People who grieve exhibit a number of manifestations, which may be categorized as physical, psychological, behavioural, social and spiritual (Corr, Nabe and Corr, 1994). Examples of these manifestations are given in the accompanying box.

Mourning is associated with grief and grieving. "*Mourning* refers to the process of incorporating the experience of loss into our everyday lives" (DeSpelder and Strickland, 1992, 234). Also referred to as *grieving* or *grief work* (Lindeman, 1944, cited in Corr, Nabe and Corr, 1994), mourning denotes the long-term process of moving forward and working through the grief towards the resumption of a satisfying life. It involves an internal process in which individuals struggle with the grief response and an outward process in which they acknowledge the loss to others (Corr, Nabe and Corr, 1994). The outward display of loss is influenced by culture. Culture defines certain behaviours as socially appropriate for disclosing the fact that a person or family is mourning. For example, in some cultures, families who are in mourning often wear dark colours and abstain from social functions for a period of time after the death of a loved one. In others, such as the Hindu or Sikh religions, the mourning dress is traditionally white.

DEATH AND DYING

CAUSES OF DEATH

When considering death, a question often asked is, "What did the patient actually die from?" When death is not sudden (as from a myocardial infarction), its actual cause is most often cancer-related, since cancer is the second leading cause of death, next to cardiovascular problems. The most common causes of death in advanced cancer are infection, organ failure, infarction and hemorrhage.

Infection results in death in almost half of terminal cancer patients. There are various types and locations of infections.

- Septicemia and/or septic shock
- Major visceral infection including pneumonia, peritonitis and pyelonephritis
- Gram-negative bacteria, including *Escherichia coli*, *Klebsiella* and *Pseudomonas aeruginosa*

Organ failure is due to the consequence of tumour invasion, except for the heart. Failure leading to death occurs more often in some organs. In decreasing frequency, organ failure occurs in the lungs, heart, liver, central nervous system and kidneys.

Death attributable to infarction in cancer patients is uncommon. Pulmonary infarctions are more frequent than

---

Manifestations of the Grief Response

FEELINGS

- Profound sadness, emptiness, loneliness, sorrow, helplessness, anger, numbness or relief.

PHYSICAL SENSATIONS

- Hollowness in the stomach, dry mouth, tightness in the throat or chest, a frequent need for sighing, fatigue or muscle weakness.

COGNITIONS (THOUGHTS)

- Distress, confusion, events perceived as unreal, absentmindedness, difficulty concentrating, preoccupation with thoughts of the lost person or object, a sense of presence or hallucinations of the deceased person or object.

BEHAVIOURS

- Sleep pattern disturbances, loss of appetite, general restlessness or hyperactivity, searching for the deceased, talking incessantly about the deceased or visiting places and cherishing objects or pictures reminiscent of the deceased person.

SOCIAL

- Difficulties in interpersonal relationships, problems in functioning at home and at work.

SPIRITUAL

- Search for a sense of meaning or recognition that one's value framework is inadequate to cope with this particular loss.

SOURCES: Worden, 1991; DeSpelder and Strickland, 1992; Corr, Nabe and Corr, 1994.

---

myocardial infarction. Pulmonary emboli are derived in equal frequency from distal venous thrombosis and tumour cell emboli.

Death directly related to persistent or massive bleeding is rare. In descending order, hemorrhage is more common in the gastrointestinal system, the brain, the cardiovascular system and the lungs. The bleeding may be related to direct tumour invasion and erosion, thrombocytopenia or a coagulopathy.

PHYSICAL CHANGES AT THE END OF LIFE

Unless death occurs suddenly, there is usually a progressive failure of the body's homeostatic mechanisms as the individual becomes weaker. Changes are noted in every major body system. Table 36.2 gives a summary of the changes in body systems approaching death.

THE PSYCHOLOGICAL RESPONSE TO DYING

No two people react to dying or death in exactly the same way. Yet, most people experience characteristic responses as they face significant losses, such as the loss of physical ability, the loss of a loved one or the loss of one's own life from a terminal illness. Both the patient and the family experience grief. The concept and theories of grief are tools for the nurse to use in anticipating the needs of patients and families and in planning interventions to help them understand and cope with the grief.

STAGES OF COPING WITH DYING AND GRIEF

After considerable experience in counselling patients on death and dying, Kubler-Ross (1969) developed a theoretical model consisting of five stages in the process of death and dying. The stages include denial, anger, bargaining, depression and acceptance. According to Kubler-Ross these stages are "defense mechanisms" that "will last for different periods of time and will replace each other or exist at times side by side" (1969, 138). These stages do not necessarily proceed in an orderly fashion. They may occur in varying order and any one may recur a number of times during the course of a terminal illness. In addition, any one of the stages may be totally absent in some individuals.

The framework provided by Kubler-Ross is behaviour-oriented. The first stage is characterized by *denial* and *isolation*. The person may act as if nothing has happened. "No, that can't be so," "This cannot be happening to me!" and "There must be some mistake" are common reactions. This denial may be so pronounced that patients or family members may not even recall important relevant statements that have been made. Often the patient seeks reassurance

TABLE 36.2 Physical Changes Approaching Death

SYSTEM	AREAS TO DISCUSS	OUTCOME
Respiratory	Breathing patterns	Will decrease to death
	Respiratory congestion	Will be relieved if occurs
	Haemoptysis	Very rare
Neurological	Conscious level	Will decrease to death
	Pre-death restlessness	Treat if a problem
	Twitching	Treat if moderate
	Convulsions	Rare unless prior
Cardiovascular	Blood pressure	Will fall
	Heart rate	Often rapid and weak
	Heart failure	Part of dying process
	Pulmonary edema	Uncommon; treat if occurs
	Arrhythmias	Part of dying process
Skin	Temperature	Often cool; may be febrile
	Colour	Often pale, blue, blotchy
	Breakdown	Minor at end is OK
Excretory	Rectal incontinence	May occur
	Bladder incontinence	Common
Gastrointestinal	Food	Intake will become zero
	Fluid	Intake will become zero
	Medications	
	• Which to keep	Analgesics, antiemetics
	• Which to stop	
	• Which routes	
	Mouth care	Important
Prognosis	How long	
	When to call family	

SOURCE: Victoria Hospice Society. (1990). *Hospice resource manual. Volume 1: Medical care of the dying.* Victoria, B.C.: Author, Section 16, 17. Reproduced with permission.

from nurses and questions them regarding what the doctor has said. Further, there is often a sense of being totally alone, separate from all the others who are not dying.

Anger depicts Kubler-Ross's second stage of dying and grief. "Why me? What did I do to deserve this punishment?" patients may wonder. "Anger is almost constantly present on some level in both the dying and their loved ones, and may show itself in many contexts and in unexpected ways" (Gonda and Ruark, 1984, 33). Patients often lash out at those closest to them — family members, the physician, the nurses, the hospital, the health care system. They may be highly critical of the care they are receiving.

The distinctive reaction in the third stage is *bargaining*. In this phase the reality of the loss is postponed. The individual attempts to cope by making deals with a higher being to avert the loss. From early childhood, good behaviour is rewarded and bad actions are punished. Therefore, many people reason that promising to be very good may bring about a reversal of impending death.

Depression characterizes Kubler-Ross's fourth stage. When patients realize that their bargaining efforts are of no avail and they sense the full impact of the loss, they usually enter into depression. During this time people think about all that they value in life and mourn its loss. They may feel overpowering loneliness and withdraw from others, but during this stage they begin working through the challenges of death and dying.

The fifth stage of the dying process comes when patients have accepted that they are going to die soon and are prepared for it. Kubler-Ross stresses that acceptance is coming to terms with the situation rather than submitting to resignation or hopelessness. Acceptance of death may be one goal for terminal care. However, it must not be an expectation that patients, families and caregivers must meet in order to feel that their roles have been performed properly.

PHASES OF COPING WITH DYING

Weisman (1980, cited in Gonda and Ruark, 1984) describes the common reactions during the process of dying as phases that are connected to the course of terminal illness. The phases are existential plight, mitigation and accommodation, decline and deterioration and preterminality and terminality. The phases tend to occur in a particular order; however, they may persist or recur throughout illness and dying.

The first phase, *existential plight,* refers to the initial shock people experience when faced with the irrefutable evidence of their own vulnerability and mortality. During this phase patients and families may exhibit numbness, shock and bewilderment. Weisman's second phase, *mitigation and accommodation,* often follows initial treatment of the disease. During this time patients and families focus their attention on achieving a balance between new roles as potentially dying patients and old identities with their related

coping capacities. In this process, the acute threat of death is allayed or mitigated. An accommodation is made between the reality of the prognosis and the customary requirements for daily living. For example, a patient with ovarian cancer stated, "I know I have cancer. I will get sicker in time. But at the present time, I will carry on with life as usual."

The third phase of coping with dying is *decline and deterioration*. This phase occurs when the patient's disease advances, when they have minimal energy for daily functions, and when treatment brings shorter periods of freedom from symptoms. This period of a terminal illness may be the most difficult for patients and families. The signs of advancing illness are unavoidable and the prospect of death becomes real. While patients may continue the struggle to maintain their functioning, the ability to maintain hope and a positive attitude may begin to fade. The support of health care professionals which facilitates patients' autonomy and control of their life is vital during this time.

The fourth of Weisman's phases is *preterminality and terminality*. In this phase, the response to treatment is minimal and the focus shifts to palliative care of symptoms and management of discomfort. Both the patient and family may come to the realization that they have limited time together. Thus they may alter their goals to much narrower outcomes. For example, the goal might be living to see the birth of a grandchild, the graduation of a son or daughter, or the marriage of a favourite niece (Gonda and Ruark, 1984).

BEREAVEMENT AND GRIEVING

Bereaved people grieve the loss of a loved one in much the same manner as those anticipating their own death. The process includes periods of shock, disbelief and somatic distress, feelings of guilt, anger and hostility, disruption in the daily functions of living, preoccupation with thoughts of the deceased and finally, working through to a healthy resolution and an integration of the loss into life. The desired outcomes of grieving are to remember the loved one without major emotional pain and to preserve the capacity to love. Successful achievement of these outcomes requires that bereaved individuals face the pain by recognizing that what is happening is a normal part of life and by acknowledging and expressing the full range of feelings associated with grief (Martocchio, 1985).

Martocchio (1985) identified four elements in grieving:

1. breaking the emotional bond to the deceased;
2. readjusting to an altered environment;
3. developing new or renewed relationships; and
4. learning to live comfortably with memories of the deceased.

In breaking the emotional bond to the deceased, the survivor must work through unfinished business. "The content of unfinished business, how it is handled, and how the survivor is affected by it all have an impact on the experience of grief" (DeSpelder and Strickland, 1992, 255). An unresolved conflict, words that were unspoken or deathbed promises, for example, constitute unfinished business that must be resolved before normal grieving can continue. Suffering is heightened when survivors feel unable to resolve conflicts left by unfinished business. Such individuals may need the help of health care professionals to work through these aspects. "Perhaps the key to unfinished business is forgiveness; accepting the situation as it is" (DeSpelder and Strickland, 1992, 256). Breaking bonds with the deceased also includes establishing a new or renewed identity. This includes learning new skills and reestablishing roles. For example, a young widow who had been staying at home with children may have to reenter the workforce, take on the role of single parent and manage the household and family on her own. Readjustment to an altered environment means learning to live without the presence of the loved one and becoming comfortable with symbols of the deceased in everyday life. For example, an elderly widow now eats and sleeps alone and finds ways to replace the time and activities shared with her loved one. She may take a trip with a friend and develop new interests to fill the void in her life.

In developing new or renewed relationships, the survivor reenters social life and invests emotional energy in other people. Sometimes this takes the form of joining support groups and helping others who are experiencing crises or losses in life. This element of grieving may also include the renewal of the spiritual dimension in the survivor's life and the integration of the loss into his or her religious beliefs.

The last element, learning to live comfortably with memories of the deceased, requires that the survivor say good-bye to his or her loved one. The survivor achieves a level of resolution in which he or she can treasure memories of the deceased with a sense of peace and personal equilibrium. The process of grief is highly variable among individuals. Each person will progress and regress as he or she works to integrate the loss and reestablish a "normal" life. Time is also variable. It often takes two to five years for most people to work through grief and feel fully integrated into a new and satisfying life.

Grief work may not always be successful. Sometimes grief is complicated with unfinished business, personality variables or ineffective coping abilities. Grief may become prolonged or chronic, in which case the survivors experience a sense of hopelessness and a resistance to moving forward. Anger, self-blame and depression may be intensified. Grief can also be delayed. In delayed grief, survivors refuse to acknowledge grief and carry on with life as though nothing has happened. While people may appear to be doing well on the surface, they do so at great cost to themselves. Some people may never begin the normal process of grieving and may eventually require professional intervention (Martocchio, 1985).

DETERMINANTS OF BEREAVEMENT AND GRIEF

Several factors can influence how people experience loss and determine the ability to grieve and the capacity to cope. Principal among these are

1. the degree of prior attachment to the deceased;
2. the type of death;
3. the age of the deceased;
4. the personality and coping strategies of the bereaved individual; and
5. the social support the bereaved individual is able to draw upon.

Knowledge of these factors will help the nurse understand the nature of grief and facilitate the assessment of needs, strengths and coping abilities of bereaved persons and families.

Prior Attachment to the Dead Person

Bereavement and grief are greatly influenced by the prior attachment to (or the perceived value of the relationship with) the deceased person. How important was the deceased person in the survivor's life? How will the survivor's life change because of the loss? Generally speaking, the feelings of loss and grief are more intense when the deceased and the survivor shared a strong relationship and when the death causes significant changes in the survivor's life. Thus, the loss of a spouse, partner, parent, child or a close friend or relative has a far greater impact on the survivor than the loss of an acquaintance or co-worker. The quality of the relationship may also affect bereavement and grief. For example, a woman who was ambivalent about her relationship with an abusive husband may not find his death to be so devastating and she may even inwardly feel glad that he is gone. However, this very ambivalence may bring about feelings of guilt which will affect her grieving and coping capacity.

Type of Death

The way in which death takes place, whether expected or unexpected, affects one's bereavement and grief. Sudden, unexpected, traumatic deaths, for example, accidental death, homicide or suicide are overwhelming and very difficult to cope with. Furthermore, suicide is accompanied by guilt, self-reproach and blame on the part of the survivor. "Why didn't I see it coming?" "If I had done something better, this would not have happened!" As well, survivors may see suicide as a personal affront or "final insult" and consequently "direct strong feelings of anger and blame toward the person who committed suicide" (DeSpelder and Strickland, 1992, 252). Such feelings compound grief and grieving.

Knowledge of an impending death as a result of a terminal illness is believed to alter bereavement and the experience of grief. The "response to prior knowledge of an impending death, with the result that the survivor has time to contemplate its effect before it actually occurs" is called *anticipatory grief* (DeSpelder and Strickland, 1992, 251). Some believe that anticipatory grief facilitates mourning by lessening the intensity of feelings following the actual loss. However, anticipatory grief does not significantly diminish the grief experienced when the loss becomes an objective fact (DeSpelder and Strickland, 1992). Nevertheless, knowledge of an impending death does temper the element of shock that accompanies the news that a loved one has died.

Age of the Deceased

Human beings hold an intrinsic belief that people should live to an old age and enjoy a multitude of successes and opportunities in life before they die. Therefore, premature death, whether sudden or expected, is among the most difficult to cope with. The death of a child causes the most profound and intense grief in survivors (Rando, 1986). Corr, Nabe and Corr (1994) cite Sanders (1979), saying that research has shown that "adult bereavement is usually impacted most significantly by the death of a child, a spouse, and a parent — in that order" (302). In addition, they quote a familiar saying that, "the death of my parent is the death of my past; the death of my spouse is the death of my present; the death of my child is the death of my future" (Corr, Nabe and Corr, 1994, 302).

Personality and Coping Strategies

We noted earlier that people will cope with bereavement using skills they have acquired in dealing with past losses or crises in their lives. "Developing new and more effective coping skills requires more time and energy than are usually available in the immediate aftermath of a death or other significant loss" (Corr, Nabe and Corr, 1994, 174). Bereaved people draw upon known strengths for coping and grieve in much the same manner as they ordinarily function in life (Rando, 1988). Personality influences how a person relates to life events in general. A person with a healthy personality and a positive self-concept is likely to grieve in a more effective manner than someone with a dependent and emotionally immature personality (DeSpelder and Strickland, 1992).

Social Support

Social support is a crucial determinant in the ability to grieve and cope with death. In the period immediately after the death of a loved one, survivors experience profound feelings of grief and isolation. All energy is devoted to the loss and little is left to reach out to others or even feed and care for themselves. People cannot cope successfully with the challenges of mourning if they do not obtain adequate nutrition, hydration, rest and exercise (Corr, Nabe and Corr, 1994). The presence of caring people is paramount during this time. Having someone present who can give emotional support and ensure the bereaved person eats, drinks and gets some rest and exercise is essential for effective coping. In many communities and societies, relatives, friends and neighbours function in this capacity. Similarly, social support is necessary as bereaved individuals progress through the grieving process. This may be in the form of continued support from a close friend or relative, a health care professional or a community support group.

DEATH AND GRIEF THROUGHOUT THE LIFE CYCLE

A person's concept and understanding of death develops maturationally in accordance with cognitive and emotional readiness and past experiences with death. As with other developmental processes, children who have had "firsthand encounters with death may arrive at an understanding of death beyond that which is characteristic of children of the same age group" (DeSpelder and Strickland, 1992, 90). Regardless of this, there are certain characteristic responses to and levels of understanding of death at different ages and developmental stages.

Children Below the Age of Five

Generally, children below the age of five see death as a reversible state or a temporary departure; the deceased is still somewhere eating, sleeping and doing the things they usually do. This is evident in questions and statements such as: "Will Grandpa come back for Christmas?" "Who will cook for Grandpa in heaven?" "Can we take some birthday cake to Grandpa in his grave?" Although children under the age of five may use the word "death," they do not fully understand its meaning and have difficulty understanding abstract explanations of death. Because children at this age think in concrete terms, telling a four-year-old that his mother is in heaven and at the same time buried in her grave will cause confusion. "How can Mom be up in heaven when she is in a grave?" "Can we go to heaven to see Mom?" Because young children lack understanding of the finality of death, they may not show severe emotional response when told of someone's death. For example, they may want to go out and play shortly after hearing of a loved one's death and then come back later and ask when that person is coming back (Dyregrov, 1991).

Children Aged Five to Nine

Children between the ages of five and nine develop the understanding of death as a finality. They accept death as irreversible; however, they resist thinking that death is a possibility for themselves. They personify death as an external force — a "death man" or "bogey man" who takes people away. In this way, children view death as avoidable and not inevitable. They believe that "those whom the external force catches, do die; those who escape or get away from the clutches of that force do not die" (Corr, Nabe and Corr, 1994, 244). Children in this age group are still concrete in their thinking. Therefore, they need concrete expressions such as rituals, pictures and tombstones to support them in their grief work. In addition, because children in this age-span are less self-focussed, they are able to comprehend the perspective of others' loss and thereby are able to show empathic feelings and compassion towards others who are grieving a loss (Dyregrov, 1991).

Children Aged Ten Through Adolescence

After the age of nine, children recognize death as universal, inevitable and no longer avoidable. It is seen as something that "can happen to me" even though this thought is kept at a distance. Adolescents fear lingering death and view death in philosophical or religious terms (Murray and Zentner, 1993). Like all human beings, adolescents respond to death by grieving. However, their mourning processes may not correspond to those of adults; rather the processes may reflect characteristics of their developmental stage (Corr, Nabe and Corr, 1994). Adolescents may not outwardly display grief for a loved one because they may fear a loss of emotional control and worry how others will perceive them. Instead, adolescents will often occupy themselves with usual activities, for example, playing games, listening to music, studying or playing a musical instrument. At the same time, they will manifest distress in behaviours such as withdrawal, disturbances in eating and sleeping, fatigue or ambivalence in other relationships (Murray and Zentner, 1993; Corr, Nabe and Corr, 1994).

Adults

Adult attitudes, understandings and expressions of death and grief are influenced by personal, cultural and religious beliefs. These aspects differ among individuals and, furthermore, change within individuals over the course of a lifetime. In a study on death attitudes across the life span, Gesser, Wong and Reker (1987–1988) found that the fear of death and dying was relatively high among young adults; it peaked during the middle years, and fell to the lowest level among the elderly. Corr, Nabe and Corr (1994) maintain that the worries or concerns of young adults about

death are likely in relation to the deaths of others, perhaps grandparents or even parents. As they encounter the illness and deaths of others (peers, spouses or parents, for example) and learn from life's experiences, people in the middle years develop a new sense of mortality and the realization that they, too, will die someday. The developmental tasks of older adults (Erikson's *integrity versus despair*) relate directly to death and dying because they denote the end of our given course of life. As a developmental task, death "can be viewed as a goal and as fulfillment" (Murray and Zentner, 1993, 605). People who have lived happy, rich and productive lives and have achieved the developmental task of ego identity are able to accept the realization that life is limited and that the self will cease to be. They begin preparing for this eventuality, physically, emotionally, philosophically and spiritually, long before death actually takes place (Murray and Zentner, 1993).

ASSESSING THE NEEDS OF DYING PATIENTS AND THEIR FAMILIES

Assessment of loss, death and grief involves the patient who is dying and the family or significant others who are responding to the death. Effective care for dying patients and their families is based on an assessment of everyone's needs — physical, psychological, social and spiritual. The methods of data collection are the same as for standard assessments. The nurse uses communication and interviewing techniques, observation and physical assessment skills as well as interaction with other health care providers. However, data collection is an ongoing process rather than a one-time health history or physical examination, and is oriented towards understanding the strengths as well as the vulnerabilities of the dying patient and members of the family (Benoliel, 1985).

NURSING HEALTH HISTORY

The initial interview is an important tool for obtaining information about the patient and family, the understanding of the terminal illness, problems being encountered and coping capacities. During this time, the nurse will focus on patient and family goals and expectations; concerns about the challenges being faced; knowledge and understanding of the disease and medical treatment; knowledge about the patient's health status and prognosis; perceptions of relationships with physician and health care providers; how illness and treatment affect the patient's activities of daily living; environmental supports and barriers in the home; and the availability of support systems (Benoliel, 1985).

As we discussed in a previous section, the needs and coping capacities of dying patients and their families are complex and very personal. The nurse has to take into account social, cultural and religious factors as well as personal experiences and family beliefs and practices that are influencing individual and family responses at the time. This requires open communication with and active listening to those who are coping with dying and loss in order to identify, with them, their own needs.

The ability to cope with challenges in life is quite personal. People will cope with terminal illness, impending death and the resulting changes in daily living in ways of coping that they have learned from other losses and crises in life. Similarly, families will cope with death and grief in the same way. Thus, asking patients and families how they usually cope with loss and crises will give a good indication of how they will cope with this terminal illness and the eventual death and bereavement.

AWARENESS OF IMPENDING DEATH

In order to talk openly and freely with patients and families, the nurse must first identify the state of awareness of the impending death. Glaser and Strauss (1965) described four states of awareness of impending death: closed awareness, suspected awareness, mutual pretence and open awareness.

Closed Awareness

Closed awareness is the state in which the dying person does not realize the impending death. The family may or may not be aware. The physician, and perhaps the family, determine it may not be in the patient's best interest to disclose the diagnosis or prognosis. While the intention is to protect the patient, difficulties result for the family and the nurse. Families and patients are cheated of the opportunity to communicate openly, to express feelings, to share the burden of grief, to plan realistically for the family's future and to close life with the proper rituals. Likewise, nurses caring for the patient find it difficult because they are unable to communicate openly and freely (Murray and Zentner, 1993).

Suspected Awareness

However, dying patients do not remain unaware for too long. The deteriorating state of health, changes in physical appearance and altered behaviours of family members and health care professionals lead to *suspected awareness*. The patient begins to suspect that things are not as they are said to be. Because patients may feel that trust has been undermined, they may not voice suspicion to others, which further complicates communication.

Mutual Pretence

In *mutual pretence* the patient, family and health care provider all know that death is pending but continue to pretend otherwise. Patients may avoid talking about their death to protect the family from distress and nurses may not bring up the subject because they think they are preserving the patient's privacy. Mutual pretence is very demanding for everyone involved and interferes with a healthy response to death.

Open Awareness

In *open awareness*, the dying person, the family and the health care professional realize and are willing to discuss the impending death. While it is not easy, open awareness allows the patient and family to share grief, to support one another, to finish important business and to make appropriate future plans. "The anguish is not reduced but can be faced together" (Murray and Zentner, 1993, 619).

PHYSICAL ASSESSMENT

The physical assessment of a dying patient follows the format for assessing all needs. The patient will exhibit signs and symptoms related to the disease process and responses to it. In addition, certain signs are indicative of the imminence of death. These are outlined later in the chapter in the section dealing with care for the dying patient.

DIAGNOSING PROBLEMS RELATED TO DEATH, DYING AND GRIEVING

Patients who are in the terminal phase of illness and are facing the ending of life can experience the total range of nursing diagnoses, depending on individual circumstances. Dying people will have concerns about challenges being encountered and usual coping abilities may not always be effective. In a study on the concerns (fears and anxieties) about death among those coping with dying, Davidson (1979) found that the majority of terminally ill patients were concerned firstly about abandonment and rejection by significant others; secondly about losing control or ability to manage their lives; and thirdly about intractable pain (cited in Corr, Nabe and Corr, 1994). This study revealed that people who are dying have a mixture of physical, psychological, social and spiritual concerns and suggested that coping with dying "may be closely linked to what is involved in coping with living" (Corr, Nabe and Corr, 1994, 106). Thus, three diagnoses that may apply specifically to dying patients are *Fear*, *Anxiety*, and *Ineffective individual coping*. The diagnoses of *Fear* and *Anxiety* can take many forms since they are related to a number of different attitudes and beliefs individuals and societies hold about death and dying. The same is true for *Ineffective individual coping*, since people cope in ways that are vastly different.

People who are coping with the impending death of a loved one may also experience a range of problems including physical responses to the stresses being experienced. They may also have concerns related to the suffering of a loved one, as well as fears and anxieties related to the consequences of the death. For example, there may be fear of loneliness and of the anticipated changes the loss will bring. In fact, people may already be experiencing losses—for example, the loss experienced by a husband whose wife becomes too weak to participate in the activities of daily living. How effectively people will be able to cope with the impending death will depend on personality and on coping abilities.

Grieving is the diagnosis used for individuals and families who have experienced a loss, including bereavement (Carpenito, 1993). As we discussed earlier, people experience and manifest grief in many different ways. Normal grief and mourning may cause a variety of problems for individuals or families that nurses may independently treat. For example, a widow may experience *Sleep pattern disturbance*, *Social isolation* or *Altered role performance*; a family may experience *Decisional conflict* or *Ineffective family coping*. When grief is unresolved or when it is unusually long, the diagnosis of *Dysfunctional grieving* is used (Carpenito, 1993). *Dysfunctional grieving* constitutes an abnormality in the normal process of grief and mourning which is beyond the realm of this introductory work. You will learn about dysfunctional grieving in more advanced courses.

PLANNING INTERVENTIONS FOR DEATH, DYING AND GRIEVING

The goals for care of patients in the terminal phase of life and facing impending death are highly individual, reflecting patients' fears, anxieties, concerns and desires, as well as the physical needs brought about by the illness and the process of death. In general, expected outcomes of dying patients that may be used to guide interventions for care include the following.

- Patient will achieve a peaceful, dignified death.
- Patient will maintain physical comfort, primarily control of pain.
- Patient will verbalize fears, anxieties, concerns.
- Patient will maintain control over aspects of care.
- Patient will express positive feelings, optimism and hope about the present and future.
- Patient will share reflections of his or her life in a positive manner.

- Patient will share reflections of his or her values and the personal meanings of life and death.
- Patient will die with the support of loving family members and individuals who care.

As we discussed earlier, the general goals or expected outcomes of grieving for a bereaved person are "to remember the loved one without major emotional pain and to reinvest emotional energy in life so that the capacity to love is not lost" (Martocchio, 1985, 331). Understandably, these are long-term goals, the achievement of which will be determined by the multiplicity of factors that affect grief and mourning. The care for bereaved persons and families may be better guided by setting short-term goals based on their individual responses and perceived needs. Some examples of short-term expected outcomes are listed below.

- Survivor will verbalize the reality of the loss.
- Survivor will express the pain of the loss.
- Survivor will express feeling more hopeful about the future.
- Survivor will express regained interest in life.
- Survivor will establish new roles.

IMPLEMENTING INTERVENTIONS FOR DEATH, DYING AND GRIEVING

PRINCIPLES OF PALLIATIVE CARE

In recent years, the development of the hospice movement has fostered special programs to care for the dying. Hospices or programs of care for the dying began in Britain in the 1960s. In the 1970s, the first program in Canada was started in Montreal. The term "palliative care" was adopted to describe this program, and has become the term used more frequently than "hospice" in Canada. **Palliative care** is active, compassionate care of the terminally ill at a time when goals of cure or prolongation of life are no longer paramount and when the emphasis of care is on the comfort and quality of life until death. Care encompasses the terminal phase, death and period of grieving after death.

Palliative care programs may be located within special units of hospitals or as free-standing places, or they may operate through a variety of home care programs. Palliative care programs are increasing in numbers rapidly and exist in every province. Not every patient who dies, however, does so within the context of a palliative care program. Many deaths occur in critical care units and in nursing homes. Regardless of location of care at the time of death, the philosophy and principles of palliative care should guide the care of the terminally ill.

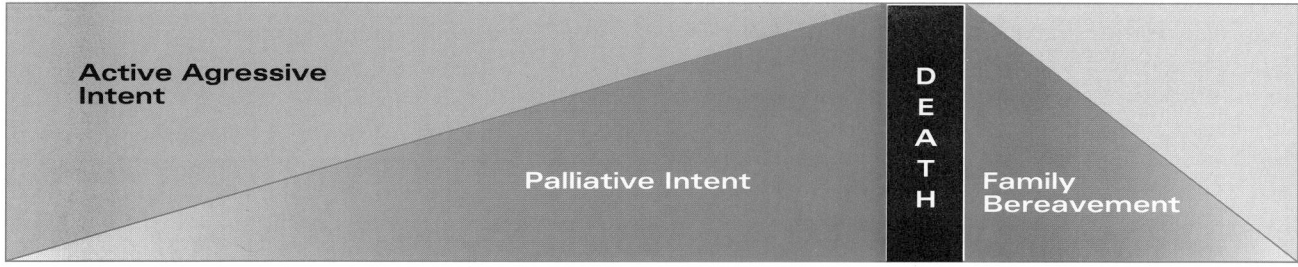

FIGURE 36.1   Hospice view of medical treatment

SOURCE: Health and Welfare Canada. (1989). *Guidelines for establishing palliative care services.* Ottawa: Department of National Health and Welfare, 2. Reproduced with permission.

THE HEALTH CARE TEAM

Roles and relationships among health care professionals also affect the care of the terminally ill and dying patients. Clearly, they greatly determine the emotional climate of any care setting. Traditional authoritarian relationships, which have in the past characterized physician–nurse relationships in particular, have no place in the care of the terminally ill. As professionals interested in providing optimal care to the dying, collaboration and cooperation are essential.

NEEDS OF DYING PATIENTS

Dying patients have many needs involving physical, psychological, social and spiritual dimensions. A summary of these needs appears in Table 36.3.

Perhaps the need that can best guide the nurse is the patient's need to die gracefully, or with dignity. What does it mean to assist another to die with dignity? To treat another with dignity is to acknowledge that each dying person is to be seen as a unique individual, one whose life history is solely his or her own. Further, this person is just as important as anyone else in the health care system and is entitled to the same rights and privileges. The dying person's bill of rights (illustrated in the following box) assures comprehensive and compassionate care.

CARE FOR THE DYING PATIENT

Nursing interventions for death and dying involve strategies that support the needs and goals of dying patients. Care focusses on maintaining physiological functioning as well as psychological, social and spiritual well-being. Ethical dilemmas may arise when serious decisions have to be made concerning death and dying. Throughout all aspects of care, the nurse implements activities that enable patient participation, foster a sense of control and promote a peaceful death with grace and dignity.

TABLE 36.3   Needs of Dying Patients

DIMENSION	NEED
Physiological	Good symptom control
Safety	A feeling of security
Belonging	The need to be needed
	The need not to be a burden
Love	Expressions of affection, human contact (touch)
Understanding	Explanation about the disease and its symptoms
	Opportunity to discuss process of dying
Acceptance	Regardless of mood and sociability
Self-esteem	Involvement in decision making, especially as physical dependency on others increases
	Opportunity to give as well as receive

SOURCE: Victoria Hospice Society. (1990). *Hospice resource manual. Volume 1: Medical care of the dying.* Victoria, B.C.: Author. Reproduced with permission.

Listening to patients warmly and affectionately is important in palliative care.

MAINTAINING PHYSIOLOGICAL FUNCTIONING

The physical needs of people who are dying are similar to the needs of all seriously ill patients. In addition, one of the most crucial needs is to control pain. Assisting patients and families through this period requires art and compassion. Knowledge of the process of dying is basic to supporting patients and families.

Sensory-Perceptual Needs

Changes in the level of consciousness may be the first symptom, occurring over a period of weeks or days in patients with cancer. In other diseases, such as with stroke or cardiac arrest, change in the level of consciousness may be an event, not a process.

Consciousness is an integral component of being human, of relating to the environment and to others and an indication of the extent of influence or control an individual has. Although patients may have intellectually accepted that they are dying and will lose consciousness, most have great difficulty in letting go of the conscious awareness of life. Some will be so fatigued from the disease and its limitations that "just going to sleep" becomes the wish and such patients often die very quickly once they "let go." For other patients, however, the inner drive to survive continues. Any impairment of consciousness creates a turbulent, restless phase during which they continually attempt to "climb up out of." The box on the next page summarizes the states of consciousness in dying patients, and is taken

---

The Dying Person's Bill of Rights

I have the right to be treated as a living human being until I die.

I have the right to maintain a sense of hopefulness, however changing its focus may be.

I have the right to be cared for by those who can maintain a sense of hopefulness, however changing this might be.

I have the right to express my feelings and emotions about my approaching death in my own way.

I have the right not be deceived.

I have the right to have help from and for my family in accepting my death.

I have the right to die in peace and dignity.

I have the right to retain my individuality and not be judged for my decisions which may be contrary to beliefs of others.

I have the right to participate in decisions concerning my care.

I have the right to expect continuing medical and nursing attention even though "cure'" goals must be changed to "comfort" goals.

I have the right not to die alone.

I have the right to be free from pain.

I have the right to have my questions answered honestly.

I have the right to discuss and enlarge my religious and/or spiritual experiences, whatever these may mean to others.

I have the right to expect that the sanctity of the human body will be respected after death.

I have the right to be cared for by caring, sensitive, knowledgeable people who will attempt to understand my needs and will be able to gain some satisfaction in helping me face my death.

SOURCE: Barbus, A.J. (1975). The dying person's bill of rights. *The American Journal of Nursing*, *75*(January), 99. Reprinted with permission. All rights reserved.

---

from the Victoria Hospice Society, *Hospice resource manual*, which was adapted from the classical states of altered consciousness described by Plum and Posner (1980).

Breathing Needs

Respiratory difficulty is one of the most distressing symptoms for patients, and it is agonizing for families to witness. As the patient's condition deteriorates, he or she may experience Cheyne-Stokes Respirations (CSR). Cheyne-Stokes Respirations are characterized by the following:

• regular alternation of hyperpnea and apnea
• smooth crescendo and smooth decrescendo
• hyperpnea usually greater than apnea period.

States of Consciousness in Dying Patients

A. Consciousness: To be fully conscious is to be aware of one's self and the surrounding environment. There are two aspects:

1. *Content.* The sum of mental processes including the ability to discriminate among both the sensory inputs and the internal cognitive aspects.

2. *Arousal.* A state of wakefulness or alertness to external and internal processes.

B. Clouding of Consciousness: Defined as a reducing state of wakefulness or through any or all of these as death approaches.

1. *Mild clouding.* For the terminal patient, fatigue and periods of drowsiness are common. After a period of rest, the patient remains fully conscious. Several other features may occur intermittently, and may be attributed to anxiety. They may not be observed or appreciated by caregivers in the early part of this phase. These are:

   - Excitability and irritability which alternate with drowsiness
   - Tendency to be startled by minor stimuli
   - Distractibility
   - Misjudging sensory perceptions, especially visual
   - Inability to think clearly or quickly.

2. *Advanced or subacute confusional state.* In this phase, the intensity and persistence of the symptoms is increased. The patient is "confused." Symptoms include:

   - Consistent misinterpretation of stimuli
   - Shortened attention span
   - Bewilderment including difficulty following commands
   - Disorientation to time and sometimes to place and person

   - Faulty memory
   - Drowsiness (which may alternate with nighttime agitation).

3. *Semi-consciousness.* This phase is frequently seen in toxic and metabolic states including poisoning, alcohol withdrawal, uremia, acute hepatic failure and severe systemic infections. Symptoms at this level include:

   - Intensified disorientation, fear or irritability
   - Misinterpretation of stimuli; often visual hallucinations
   - Lucid periods which often alternate with delirium (while lucid, the patient may be afraid of mental failure)
   - Delusions
   - Loud, talkative, offensive, suspicious or agitated behaviour.

4. *Stupor.* This state is reached when the patient is unresponsive but briefly arousable, only during vigorous and repeated stimuli and then immediately drifts back to unresponsiveness. In this phase, the patient may moan or be briefly restless when being turned or when given skin care. The nurse needs to ascertain whether this moaning is due to insufficient pain control or simply being partially aroused from a deeper level.

5. *Coma.* This is the true comatose state, defined as completely unarousable, unresponsive or the absence of any psychologically understandable response to external stimuli or inner need. The patient is breathing on his or her own, but is totally unarousable by any stimulus.

SOURCE: Victoria Hospice Society. (1990). *Hospice resource manual. Volume 1: Medical care of the dying.* Victoria, B.C.: Author, 10–12. Adapted with permission.

CSR appears to be due to a combination of abnormal increased response to carbon dioxide causing hyperpnea, an abnormal decreased forebrain ventricle stimulus, thereby allowing posthyperventilation apnea and bilateral cerebral dysfunction in the deep cerebrum or diencephalon. This breathing pattern may occur in conscious, frail patients, such as those in mild congestive heart failure or with chronic obstructive pulmonary disease, during sleep and may disappear upon awakening. CSR occurs very commonly in the terminally ill who are on moderate to high doses of narcotic agents and who are very weak. It must be pointed out that the narcotic dose should not be reduced if patients are on a stable dose and require this amount. If the dose is being titrated upward and the patient is now pain-free, the doses should be either continued at the present level or reduced slightly. However, it is exceedingly rare that CSR alone is a sign of drug toxicity. Finally, CSR also occurs in comatose patients who are imminently dying.

Tissue Perfusion (Cardiovascular)

Decreasing blood pressure, lessening heart rate and arrhythmias are part of the dying process. As blood circulation slows, the patient's extremities appear cyanosed or mottled and feel cool and clammy to touch, even though the patient may perceive warmth and even though the patient's body temperature is above normal. When circulation is considerably decreased, the effectiveness of analgesics administered intramuscularly or subcutaneously is decreased. As a consequence, the patient may require intravenous analgesia.

Elimination Needs

Dying patients experience inability to control urination and defecation. This is usually due to the loss of muscle tone. The sphincter muscles of the rectum and bladder relax and as a result there is involuntary micturition and defecation. A retention catheter may be required and absorbent pads can be used to help keep the patient dry and comfortable. Since patients are often embarrassed about the inability to control these functions, it is important that the nurse be discreet and understanding. Deodorants are frequently used to keep the air in the patient's room fresh and free from unpleasant odours.

Involuntary micturition and defecation predispose the patient to pressure ulcers. By helping patients to keep dry and clean and to change position regularly, the nurse can usually prevent these complications.

Movement and Activity Needs

Because of the progressive loss of muscle tone, dying patients find it increasingly difficult to maintain position in bed without support. If patients are conscious, Fowler's position is usually indicated in order to increase the depth of ventilation of the lungs. If they are unconscious, a semi-prone position promotes the drainage of mucus from the mouth. Family members may become anxious when they see the patient positioned in this manner, and it is wise to explain the reasons for it. Regardless of the position that the nurse judges to be most beneficial, the patient will need supportive measures, such as pillows, to maintain it. If possible, the various parts of the body should be kept out of dependent positions to prevent the pooling of blood.

Nutritional Needs

The inability to swallow (dysphagia) is also characteristic of the loss of muscle tone in the dying patient. Mucus tends to accumulate in the patient's throat and, as a result, the air passing through it causes a typical gurgling sound, the "death rattle." Throat suctioning usually helps to keep the airway patent.

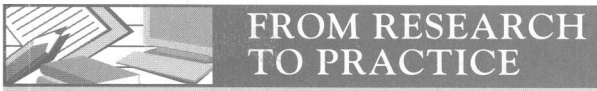

FROM RESEARCH TO PRACTICE

Waller, A., Hershkowitz, M. and Adunsky, A. (1994). The effect of intravenous fluid infusion on blood and urine parameters of hydration and on state of consciousness in terminal cancer patients. *The American Journal of Hospice & Palliative Care, 11*(4), 26-29. 1994.

Intravenous fluids are commonly administered in the treatment of terminal cancer patients. This study assessed the effect of IV fluids on the state of hydration of terminally ill cancer patients in the last 48 hours of their life. The population consisted of 68 patients consecutively admitted for palliative care. Fifty-five were hydrated orally; thirteen received IV fluids. Blood and urine specimens were collected and tested for parameters of hydration. The blood parameters were the values of Urea (mg%), Creatinine (mg%), Na+ (mEq/L), Uric acid (mg%) and Osmolality (mOsm/kg). Urine samples were tested for osmolality and electrolytes. At the same time as the blood samples were taken, patients were assessed for their state of consciousness, according to a local alertness scale.

The results indicated that the majority of patients (85%) were in a state of dehydration. Those treated with IV fluids did not show better biochemical parameters of hydration than those hydrated orally. In addition, although states of consciousness correlated significantly with serum sodium and urine osmolality, patients treated with IV fluids did not show a better state of consciousness than those not treated. The authors concluded that intravenous fluids should not be administered to advanced cancer patients. Recognizing that families may view IV infusion as a continuation of medical care and therefore may want to see it continued, they suggest that the preference of the dying patient and his or her family should prevail in the decision-making process regarding IV treatment.

There is a progressive diminution in peristalsis of the gastrointestinal tract of dying patients. The desire for food is usually minimal, but they may want frequent sips of water. The mouth may be dry, owing to dehydration and perhaps to a light fever, which sometimes precedes death. Good oral hygiene is essential. Because of the reduced peristalsis, flatus accumulates in the stomach and intestines, often distending the patient's abdomen and causing nausea. More than a few sips of water at a time, consequently, can cause vomiting. Dying patients are often given nourishment and fluids parenterally, but rarely are sips of fluid contraindicated.

Pain Management

One of the greatest fears of terminally ill patients is that they will have unbearable pain during their final days. However, research suggests that only 50% of cancer patients experience pain (Anderson, 1982; Fainsinger, Miller and Bruera, 1991). Pain control is important because pain alters sleep, appetite, mobility, energy levels and psychological functioning. The sooner that pain relief is provided, the more energy the patient has for maintaining activities which enhance quality of life. Analgesic drugs are more effective if administered regularly rather than on a prn basis. Medication for pain management can be supplemented by relaxation, guided imagery, distraction and peripheral nerve stimulators to provide relief for the patient.

MAINTAINING PSYCHOLOGICAL WELL-BEING

Denial and feelings of anger, fear, anxiety and sadness are common during the terminal illness and the period of dying. Throughout the denial state, the nurse must accept the fact that patients vary in the ability to acknowledge the seriousness of the illness. Most patients seem to experience these denial responses fairly often during the terminal illness. Some patients maintain denial up to the point of impending death, and continue to talk optimistically of future plans. Many patients, however, are aware of the prognosis, even though they have never been told in words; yet they may pretend not to know. Often, patients maintain a facade of cheerfulness for the benefit of families, in whom they sense a discomfort talking about death, or because they believe that they are expected to behave in this manner by the hospital staff. For these patients, it is frequently a relief to drop the facade in the presence of someone who understands what they are going through.

Expressions of anger, hostility, fear, anxiety or sadness are feelings nurses often have the most difficulty responding to because nurses innately want to find answers which will make the patient's pain and distress go away. Anger is especially hard to deal with, particularly because it is often projected onto the caregiver. The important element in providing psychological support is to realize that these feelings must be identified, acknowledged and expressed. Careful *listening* to the patient is the key. Giving patients "permission" to share feelings, to talk about what they feel and why they feel as they do may be the most helpful intervention (Corr, Nabe and Corr, 1994). The nurse can also use *touch* in some cases as a healing activity. However, not all people are comfortable with physical touching. Therefore, the nurse must pay attention to the patient's verbal and nonverbal responses when touch is used.

People lose their sense of dignity, self-esteem and self-worth when they become dependent on others for their care. This also happens when they lose control over their lives and their environment. Dying patients often feel this way. The nurse can do much to maintain a dying patient's psychological well-being by continually involving the patient in decisions, asking for preferences and offering choices in regards to care.

MAINTAINING SOCIAL WELL-BEING

Dying people need ongoing interaction with loved ones to maintain a sense of security and social well-being. Within the security of a loving relationship, one is able to talk about concerns, find meaning in experiences and work through problems. Sometimes all that is needed is the presence of a significant person. The nurse can best assist by providing support to family members and significant others in coping with their own grief so that they, in turn, are able to maintain meaningful relationships with the patient. When these individuals are not present, the nurse can facilitate the patient's well-being by showing an interest and encouraging the patient to talk about family members and significant others.

People who are coping with impending death also have concerns about changes in social roles and about family circumstances that will be left behind. For example, patients may worry about a work project not completed, the economic security of their family, and how their partner will cope as a single parent. Nurses can help by allowing patients to talk about such concerns and by enabling them to act for themselves. This is done by listening and helping patients explore problems, consider options and find resources to fulfill needs. Nurses may also become advocates for dying patients by finding needed resources, such as social workers, counsellors or lawyers.

MAINTAINING HOPE AND SPIRITUAL WELL-BEING

Hope is characterized by a confident yet uncertain expectation of achieving a future goal (Dufault and Martocchio, 1985). Hope is not a single entity, but rather a combination of thoughts, feelings and actions that change frequently. Even when there is not a shadow of a doubt in the nurse's mind that the present illness will result in death for the patient, it still proves possible to maintain hope in a realistic sense. The key is that the object of the hope is shifted to a shorter range. Patients shift from hoping for a cure to hoping for longer periods of remission. As things advance, the focus of hope changes to even more immediate objects, to hope for survival until a special occasion has passed, and then to hope for symptom-free days. Finally, patients may hope for a relatively peaceful and dignified death. If given the opportunity and the encouragement, patients will remain hopeful, often right until the moment of death.

As death approaches, patients will often seek comfort by analyzing values and beliefs related to life and death. If they have had questions about their life, those also come out when they are dying. A dying patient seeks to find purpose and meaning in life before surrendering to death (Conrad, 1985).

Providing a patient with spiritual comfort implies much more than arranging for clergy to visit. The nurse must support patients in the expression of a philosophy of life. The nurse or family can assist the patient with spiritual matters through careful listening, expressing empathy, reading scriptures and praying if that is in line with the patient's desires, or arranging for clergy to visit if the patient so wishes.

Attentive listening encourages patients to express feelings, clarify them and accept death. However, it is crucial that nurses are aware of and feel comfortable with their own spiritual beliefs and values before offering support to patients so that their own needs are not guiding the discussion.

ETHICAL ASPECTS OF CARE

There are many decisions to be made surrounding patients whose life is slipping away. Can the medical condition be reversed? Should present treatments be continued or stopped? If so, when?

Ethics and the decision-making process is a vast area which is rapidly increasing in importance in the health care system. Decisions concerning dying and death are at the very roots of medicine since one of its main goals is the reverse — to sustain and improve life. When the possibility of death enters, a host of reactions and decisions are necessary. The professional mandate of nurses is to promote health, to care for those who are ill, and in cases where cure is not possible, to provide comfort to those who are dying. Discrepant views about sustaining life and accepting an inevitable death are at the root of the ethical dilemmas that many nurses face.

Ethical issues arise in all facets of health care when serious decisions have to be made. Preferences are expressed or not expressed by patients about their care or future; differing futures are envisioned for the patient by others. When caring for the terminally ill, the goals of care must be revised. Patients, family members and health care professionals need to adjust to partial achievement of goals. What is possible and what is desirable must be considered in establishing goals. Several factors must be taken into account, including the nature of the disease, the patient's status and preference, the values of the patient, his or her family and health care providers and social, cultural, political and financial realities.

In recent years the concept of **advanced directives** has developed as a mechanism for dealing with some of the decisions which arise when caring for the terminally ill. Advanced directives apply when there is no hope of recovery. Their purpose is to speak for an incapacitated patient who cannot speak for himself or herself by outlining the patient's medical treatment wishes. Advanced directives incorporate the concepts of **living will**, the patient's right to refuse unwanted life support. Every state in the United States has passed some legislation authorizing the use of advanced directives, and the issue is being debated in many Canadian provinces. Figure 36.2 illustrates a living will form. A living will prepared by the organization Choice in Dying Inc. is presented in the box that follows.

Some patients will talk about and seriously consider euthanasia. They may feel their lives are without meaning, they have completed the life they enjoyed or they may feel a burden to themselves, their families or the community. **Euthanasia** means an easy or painless death, the word being derived from the Greek words meaning "good death." The term is often used synonymously with "mercy killing," a concept that has caused a considerable amount of controversy over the years. There are two forms of euthanasia. *Passive* or *negative euthanasia* means the withholding of life-preserving techniques. It involves an omission (or failure to do something). *Active* or *positive euthanasia* is the initiation of life-shortening measures and involves taking deliberate action to end life.

The issue is an ethical one which has not been fully resolved. It revolves around two fundamental beliefs, the right of individuals to decide their own time and means of dying and the equally strong argument that all measures must be tried before death is accepted as inevitable. Often, it becomes a matter of "to treat or not to treat." Passive euthanasia is much more widely accepted than active life-shortening measures and often, in hospitals and long-term facilities, directions will be left for care that prolongs life, particularly of an older person, only if the individual and/or family wish it.

Traditionally, hospice programs have acted as an alternative to the euthanasia movement by pointing out that patients often request euthanasia because they are in physical distress. As the symptoms are relieved, most patients regain a sense of life and wish to live until they die, but in comfort.

CARE WHEN DEATH IS IMMINENT

SIGNS OF IMMINENT DEATH

Patients' reflexes gradually disappear as they approach death and they are unable to move. Sensation and power of motion as well as reflexes are lost first in the legs and then gradually in the arms. Pressure on the legs is especially uncomfortable so sheets should not be snug, and special attention should be paid to the positioning of the legs. Respirations become increasingly difficult; Cheyne-Stokes Respirations may occur.

To My Family, My Physician, My Lawyer and All Others Whom It May Concern:

Death is as much a reality as birth, growth, maturity and old age — it is the one certainty of life. If the time comes when I can no longer take part in decisions for my own future, let this statement stand as an expression of my wishes and directions, while I am still of sound mind.

If at such a time the situation should arise in which there is no reasonable expectation of my recovery from extreme physical or mental disability, I direct that I be allowed to die and not be kept alive by medications, artificial means or "heroic measures." I do, however, ask that medication be mercifully administered to me to alleviate suffering even though this may shorten my remaining life.

This statement is made after careful consideration and is in accordance with my strong convictions and beliefs. I want the wishes and directions here expressed carried out to the extent permitted by law. Insofar as they are not legally enforceable, I hope that those to whom this Will is addressed will regard themselves as morally bound by these provisions.

Signed _____

Date _____

Witness _____

Witness _____

Copies of this request have been given to   _____

_____

_____

_____

FIGURE 36.2   Living will form

Typically a faint cyanotic pattern becomes discernible in the face. As peripheral circulation fails, there may be a "drenching sweat" and the body surface cools. The patient's skin feels cold and clammy. Most dying patients are not conscious of being cold, however, regardless of how cold the body surface becomes. Restlessness is often caused by the sensation of heat, and they tend to throw off the bedclothes. At that point, patients need lighter covering and fresh circulating air. The nurse may have to explain to family members that even though the patient feels cold to the touch, he or she is not aware of being cold, because the internal temperature is quite high.

The pulse accelerates and becomes weaker. With increasing anoxia, the pupils become dilated and fixed. Low blood pressure, an elevated temperature, and a rapid respiration rate are common.

For the comfort of the dying patients and their family, their room must be kept clean and tidy. Dying patients may be given a private room on the nursing unit in the hospital so that they may have privacy with their family. Staff must ensure frequent visits into the room so that the patient and family do not feel forgotten. As sight and hearing fail, the patient frequently sees only what is near and hears only what is spoken directly to him or her. Indirect lighting should be provided, and family members should be encouraged to sit near the patient's head. Nurses and family members should not draw the shades in the room, talk in whispers in a corner, or fail to answer honestly any of the patient's questions. There may be an interval of peace just before death occurs.

SIGNS OF DEATH

Death is considered to have occurred when the patient's respirations and heart have ceased to function for several minutes. Usually breathing stops first; the heart stops beating a few minutes later.

For the purpose of human transplants, it has become necessary to have a more precise definition than the cessation of breathing and heartbeat as the absolute signs of death. The absence of brain wave activity as measured by the electroencephalogram is usually used to confirm that death has occurred.

CARE AFTER DEATH

In caring for the body of the patient after death, whatever procedures are carried out are performed with dignity and respect. In some religious faiths, only family members are permitted to care for the body of the deceased. However, this is generally a nursing responsibility. Although each agency usually has its own specific procedures, there are some general guidelines for the care of the body after death which are fairly universal.

The body is generally placed in a supine position in bed with one pillow under the head. The head is slightly elevated to prevent post-mortem hypostasis of blood, which could discolour the face. The body is positioned immediately after death and before rigor mortis sets in.

Rigor mortis, a stiffening of the body after death, is a result of a chemical action within the muscles in which glycogen is coagulated and lactic acid is produced. It generally occurs shortly after death, progressing from the jaw down the trunk to the extremities. Once rigor mortis has set in, the body remains rigid for one to six days. When relatives wish to see the body, the nurse first tidies the room and removes extraneous equipment. The body should appear clean, comfortable and peaceful. A slightly shaded room affords a comforting effect.

In some hospitals, it is the policy to insert dentures immediately after death; other institutions send the dentures with the body to the morgue, where they are inserted later by the mortician. In most institutions, rings are removed; if a ring cannot be removed it is taped in place and a notation is made on the patient's chart and on the form that goes with the body to the morgue.

The preparation of the body by the nurse involves the application of pads to the perineal area or the insertion of packing into the rectum and vagina. Rarely is it necessary to bathe the body; this procedure is carried out by the mortician. It is, however, necessary to cleanse the body of any blood or drainage that may have accumulated after death.

After the family has left, the nurse places the identification tags on the body. At most hospitals, bodies are labelled twice: one label is attached to the ankles, the other to the shroud in which the body is wrapped. If a patient had a transmissible disease, this information also needs to be noted for the protection of others who will be handling the body. When agency protocol requires the ankles and wrists to be tied together, they should be well padded in order to prevent bruising. In some areas, it is the practice to treat the body as if the patient were still living, and no shroud is used. When the preparation of the body is complete, the body is taken to the hospital morgue. If the hospital does not have a morgue, the mortician should be notified to come for the body.

The patient's valuables and clothes should, whenever possible, be sent home with the relatives. If there is no one present who can assume responsibility for these, valuables should be placed in the hospital safe and the clothes labelled and stored until such time as the family collects them.

The laws of each province may vary with regard to the requirements of certifying death. This is usually the responsibility of a physician. For the medical record, nurses should note the time that respirations cease and the heart stops beating. In many agencies, it is the nurse's responsibility to inform families who are not present at the time of the death.

The physician often asks families about organ or tissue donation when the patient is a suitable donor. The nurse, however, may have to answer questions asked by the family and support them in their decision. In some provinces, it is common for individuals to indicate whether they want their eyes donated for corneal transplantation. Enucleation of the eyes for corneal transplant must follow a rigid procedure as developed by the CNIB and carried out by a physician. Nurses must be aware of the patient's choice and may assist with this procedure.

The decision to conduct an autopsy (post-mortem examination) usually rests with the family. The physician discusses with the family the need or the desire for an au-

topsy. The nurse should be aware of the nature of the discussion in order to provide appropriate follow-up should the family ask additional questions or express concerns about the procedure.

SUPPORT FOR THE GRIEVING FAMILY

Family members must be supported through the patient's dying and death and, at the same time, be encouraged to provide support to the patient. In the hospital setting, particularly outside of palliative care units, the family has greater difficulty in providing support. The nurse must recognize family members as potential resources in providing optimal care to the patient.

The family is more involved when the patient is being cared for at home. Most families prefer to have their loved one cared for at home, but to do so four factors must be present: a caregiver is able and available, support from health care providers is readily available, the patient's symptoms are under control and the physical environment of the home is conducive to patient's mobility (Brown, Davies, Reimer and Martens, 1990). Regardless of location of care, however, families sometimes have great difficulty coping with terminal illness. Benoliel (1985) describes circumstances that make it difficult to cope with demands of terminal illness. These include a lengthy period of dying, symptoms that are difficult to control, unpleasant sights and smells, limited coping resources, poor relationships with caregivers and a dying child.

It is important that the family feels the patient is receiving the best care possible. Helping the patient to die in a dignified and peaceful manner is perhaps one of the most valuable contributions the nurse can make to the comfort of both the patient and family.

The nurse must first determine the degree to which family members want to be involved in the patient's care. Giving family members an active role in the care of their loved one can help them feel useful and help preserve the relationship with the patient. Though relieved of some nursing chores, the nurse must still supervise the care given to the patient and support the family in the care they provide. Explanations of treatments, procedures and changes in the patient's condition in particular are crucial to helping the family cope with the impending death.

At times, it is up to the nurse to tell the family that a patient has died. Breaking such news requires a delicate and sensitive transaction. It is best to tell the family group in privacy. The nurse should anticipate that they will be upset and will look to him or her for supportive understanding. Care does not stop with the event of death. Dying with dignity means in part respect for the body and for those who remain. Suggestions for discussion with family members include the following:

1. Reassure family members about the normalcy of grief reactions. Allow them to sit with the body, if they so choose.

2. Reassure them that tears are very natural for some, and they are not abnormal or an indication that the person is "falling apart." For others, tears do not come easily, or the person may not feel any need to cry. This is also normal. It doesn't mean that the loss is any easier to bear.

3. Allow families to stay with the body and to decide for themselves when they wish to leave. Some families may want to stay with the body for a long time after death, others may want to leave immediately. Neither way is callous or morbid. On rare occasions, excess preoccupation or rejection of the dead may signal abnormality, but on the whole there is great variance in people within a normal range.

   Children require special attention. Allow them to touch the body. They may ask many questions which should be answered accurately at their level of understanding.

4. Provide families with an opportunity for prayer. Some families appreciate this opportunity, others do not feel it is necessary. The nurse can support a family's wishes to say their own prayer, offer to call the chaplain or the family's own minister, or in some cases, he or she might offer a Universal prayer which can be read:

   "Oh God, in whose presence we came into life, in whose care we live and die, we come at this moment of death to remember with one another the life of ——, who has lived with us. Our love goes with him/her as we now in silence commend him/her to your care."

5. Allow families to engage in other rituals that might be specific to their faith or cultural beliefs. Some ethnic groups expect that members of the immediate family will be very vocal in their outpouring of grief. With others, more stoical behaviour is expected.

Nurses should be prepared to provide support to the bereaved regardless of the mode in which their grief is expressed. Grief is the normal, natural response to loss and it is a very individualized process. Nurses, therefore, should avoid instructing the family on how to respond. Nurses need to listen and provide small acts of kindness that will make families feel cared for. Nurses can offer support even by making a cup of coffee, allowing adequate time to pack up the deceased's belongings (or helping with this painful task) or walking with the family to the front door of the agency. The gentle actions of the nurse at the time of death can greatly assist the family by starting them on a positive bereavement course.

EVALUATING INTERVENTIONS FOR DEATH, DYING AND GRIEVING

It is especially important to evaluate nursing interventions for effectiveness in the care of dying patients because their needs and goals change as death approaches. Outcome criteria should be evaluated and the plan of care revised on a regular basis to meet the changing needs of patients and their families.

KEY TERMS

loss p. 1238
bereavement p. 1238
grief p. 1240
mourning p. 1240

anticipatory grief p. 1244
palliative care p. 1247
advanced directives p. 1253
living will p. 1253

euthanasia p. 1253
rigor mortis p. 1255

IN REVIEW

People experience loss throughout their lifetime. When loss involves death it is called bereavement. Grief refers to the total response to loss. It is a profound and painful state, involving strong emotions and affecting how one thinks, feels, behaves and functions in daily living. People who grieve manifest a number of physical, psychological, behavioural, social and spiritual manifestations. Mourning refers to the process of incorporating the experience of loss into everyday life. It denotes the process of working through grief and resuming a satisfying life.

While each person reacts differently to death and dying, most people experience characteristic responses as they face a significant loss. Both dying patients and their families experience grief. The nurse can use theoretical models of dying and grief in anticipating the needs of patients and families and in planning interventions to help them understand and cope with their grief. Kubler-Ross's model consists of five stages: denial, anger, bargaining, depression and acceptance. These stages are regarded as defence mechanisms which may recur a number of times and in varying order during the course of illness. Weisman describes the common reactions during the process of dying as phases closely connected to the course of terminal illness. These are existential plight, mitigation and accommodation, decline and deterioration and preterminality and terminality. While the phases tend to occur in a particular order, they may persist or recur throughout illness and dying.

Bereaved people grieve the loss of a loved one in much the same way as those anticipating their own death. The bereaved need to express feelings associated with the loss and work through the steps of breaking the emotional bond with the deceased, adjusting to a new environment, developing new or renewed relationships and living comfortably with memories of the deceased.

Several factors influence how people experience loss and determine the ability to grieve and the capacity to cope. These include the degree of attachment to the deceased person, the type of death, the age of the deceased, the personality and usual coping strategies of the bereaved individual and the social support system.

Throughout the life cycle, responses to death and grief vary from the pre-schooler who believes death is temporary to the older adult who can usually directly relate to death.

Assessment of the dying patient and the grieving family is based on a holistic approach. The nurse uses communication and interviewing techniques, observation, physical examination and collaboration with other health care providers to determine all needs. Data collection is an ongoing process and is oriented towards understanding strengths and vulnerabilities of the dying patient and family members.

People who are in the terminal phase of illness and who are coping with impending death can experience the total range of nursing diagnoses. People who are dying have a mixture of physical, psychological, social and spiritual concerns. Three diagnoses that apply specifically to dying are *Anxiety*, *Fear* and *Ineffective individual coping*. The diagnosis *Grieving* is used for individuals and families who have experienced loss.

Palliative care is the active compassionate care of the terminally ill with emphasis on comfort and quality of life until death and the following care of the bereaved. Strategies for the dying patient include maintaining physiological, psychological, social and spiritual well-being. Ethical dilemmas often revolve around sustaining life or accepting inevitable death. The concept of advanced directives and the living will provide a mechanism for dealing with some of the decisions which arise when the patient is no longer capable of speaking for himself or herself. In a living will the patient can outline wishes for medical treatment including the refusal of unwanted life support.

Care after death is performed with dignity and respect. Specific agency policy and directives are followed. Some religions require that family members care for the body after death.

Nurses should be prepared to provide support to grieving families regardless of how grief is expressed. Supportive interventions include listening, providing warmth and kindness and making the family feel cared for.

LEARNING ACTIVITY

Case Study: Mr. John Edwards is in a hospital with a malignancy that the doctors consider terminal. He is 93 years old and has three sons and seven grandchildren. Mr. Edwards has been in a stuporous state and upon waking he experiences pain.

1. What are some of the nursing needs of this patient?

2. What is stupor?

3. What needs of the family could be met by the nurse?

4. Which other members of the health team might be able to assist Mr. Edwards and his family?

REFERENCES AND READINGS

ANDERSON, J. (1982). Nursing management of the cancer patient in pain: A review of the literature. *Cancer Nursing, 5,* 33.

ARCHER, D. and SMITH, A.C. (1988). Sorrow has many faces. *Nursing 88, 18,* 5.

BARBUS, A.J. (1975). The dying person's bill of rights. *The America Journal of Nursing, 75,* 99.

BENOLIEL, J. (1985). Loss and terminal illness. *Nursing Clinics of North America, 20,* 439.

BROWN, P., DAVIES, B. and MARTENS, N. (1990). Families in supportive care (Part II): Palliative care at home — A viable care setting. *Journal of Palliative Care, 6*(3), 21–27.

CARPENITO, L. J. (1993). *Nursing diagnosis: Application to clinical practice* (5th ed.). Philadelphia: Lippincott.

COLE, E. (1987). Guidelines for aiding the bereaved through death. *Thanatos, 12*(3), 2–3.

CONRAD, N. L. (1985). Spiritual support for the dying. *Nursing Clinics of North America, 20,* 415.

CORR, C. A., NABE, C. M. and CORR, D., M. (1994). *Death and dying, life and living.* Pacific Grove, CA: Brooks/Cole.

DAVIES, B., REIMER, J.C. and MARTENS, N. (1990). Families in supportive care (Part I): The transition of fading away — The nature of the transition. *Journal of Palliative Care, 6*(3), 12–20.

DESPELDER, L.A. and STRICKLAND, A.L. (1992). *The last dance* (3rd ed.). Mountain View, CA: Mayfield.

DUFAULT, K. and MARTOCCHIO, B.C. (1985). Hope: Its spheres and dimensions. *Nursing Clinics of North America, 20,* 379.

DYREGROV, A. (1991). *Grief in children: A handbook for adults.* London: Jessica Kingsley.

EVANS, M.A., ESBENSON, M. and JAFFE, C. (1981). Expect the unexpected when you care for a dying patient. *Nursing 81, 11,* 55.

FAINSINGER, R., MILLER, M. and BRUERA, E. (1991). *Journal of Palliative Care, 7*(1), 9–15.

FIELD, D. (1989). Nurse's accounts of nursing the terminally ill on a coronary care unit. *Intensive Care Nursing, 5*(3), 114–122.

GESSER, G., WONG, P.T.P. and REKER, G.T. (1988). Death attitudes across the life span: The development and validation of the death attitude profile (DAP). *Omega: Journal of Death and Dying, 18,* 113–128.

GLASER, B. and STRAUSS, A. (1965). *Awareness of dying.* Chicago: Aldine.

HEALTH AND WELFARE CANADA. (1989). *Guidelines for establishing palliative care services.* Ottawa: Department of National Health and Welfare.

JOHNSON, S.S. (1986). 10 ways to help the family of a critically ill patient. *Nursing 86, 16,* 50.

KUBLER-ROSS, E. (1969). *On death and dying.* New York: Macmillan.

LINDLEY-DAVIS, B. (1991). Process of dying: defining characteristics. *Cancer Nursing, 14*(6), 328–333.

MARTOCCHIO, C.B. (1985). Grief and bereavement. *Nursing Clinics of North America, 20,* 327–341.

McWHAN, K. (1991). Caring for dying patients in acute hospital wards: A review. *Nursing Practice, 5*(1), 25–8.

MOODY, R. (1976). *Life after Life.* Harrisburg, PA: Stackpole Books.

MULHERN, R.M. (1986) When there's no treatment left but the truth. *RN, 49,* 26.

MURRAY, R.B. and ZENTNER, J.P. (1993). *Nursing assessment and health promotion: Strategies through the life span* (5th ed.). Norwalk, CT: Appleton & Lange.

PLUM, F. and POSNER, J. (1980) *The diagnosis of stupor and coma.* (3rd ed.). Philadelphia: F. A. Davis.

RANDO, T.A. (1986). *Loss and anticipatory grief.* Lexington, MA: Lexington Books.

RANDO, T.A. (1988). *Grieving.* Lexington, MA: Lexington Books.

REIMER, J.C., DAVIES, B. and MARTENS, N. (1991). Palliative care: The nurse's role in helping families through the transition of "fading away." *Cancer Nursing, 14*(6), 321–327.

SAUNDERS, C. (1965). The last stages of life. *American Journal of Nursing, 65*(3), 70.

SHAPIRO, C. H. (1993). *When part of the self is lost.* San Francisco: Jossey-Bass.

STIKNEY, S.D. and GARDNER, E.R. (1984). Companions in suffering. *AJN, 84,* 1491.

STOCKDALE, L. and HUTZENBILER, T. (1986). How you can comfort a grieving family. *Nurs Life,* 23.

TYNER, R. (1985). Elements of empathetic care for dying patients and their families. *Nursing Clinics of North America, 20,* 393.

VICTORIA HOSPICE SOCIETY. (1990). *Hospice resource manual. Volume 1: Medical care of the dying.* Victoria, BC: Author.

WALBORN, K.A. (1980, March). A nursing model for the hospice: Primary and self-care nursing. *Nursing Clinics of North America, 15*(1), 205–217.

WALLER, A., HERSHKOWITZ, M. and ADUNSKY, A. (1994). The effect of intravenous fluid infusion on blood and urine parameters of hydration and state of consciousness in terminal cancer patients. *The American Journal of Hospice and Palliative Care, 11*(4), 26–29.

WORDEN, J.W. (1991). *Grief counselling and grief therapy: A handbook for the mental health practitioner.* New York: Springer.

CNA NURSE REGISTRATION/LICENSURE EXAMINATIONS[1]

• The Nature and Purpose of the Exam

The Criterion-Referenced (C-R) Nurse Registration/Licensure Examination (subsequently referred to as the Nurse Examination), like registration/licensure examinations in general, has a well-defined purpose: to protect the public by ensuring that those who are licensed possess sufficient knowledge and skills to perform important occupational activities safely and effectively (Canadian Psychological Association, 1987).[2] In the case of the Nurse Examination, the purpose is to determine whether or not examinees are prepared to practice nursing, without risk to their clients.

The examination content is based on nursing competencies—that is, the knowledge, abilities, skills, attitudes, and judgment expected of a beginning practitioner are expressed within the examination, according to explicit guidelines and specifications, such that accurate decisions can be made on the ability of examinees to practice safely and effectively.

• Use by All Provinces

Since August 1980, passing the Canadian Nurses Association Registration/Licensure Examination has been one of the requirements for registration/licensure in all provinces. (From 1970 to this date, candidates from Québec who wrote in French took an examination developed by the Order of Nurses of Québec.)

The registering/licensing authorities (see attached list) impose eligibility criteria (e.g., completion of an approved program of nursing education) which provide additional information required to decide on an individual's readiness to practice nursing.

• English and French Versions

Both English and French examinations are developed from a common document, entitled *The Blueprint for the Criterion-Referenced Nurse Registration/Licensure Examination (1993)*. Therefore, the content domain (i.e., the list of competen-

cies) is common, as are the specifications for structural and contextual variables. The examinations are developed in each official language; that is, items are written by nurses in French and English for the respective examinations. To facilitate equivalency between different versions of the examination (i.e., English/French, or from one year to the next), a psychometrically sound test equating method is employed.

• Minimum Passing Grade

The pass mark (standard) to be met on the Nurse Examination is established prior to the administration of the exam. The procedure used involves extensive input from a panel of content experts who are familiar with the roles and responsibilities, scope of practice and expectations of a beginning practitioner. In addition to the expert input, a variety of other relevant data is carefully considered to ensure that the standard that examinees are required to achieve is fair and valid.

• Who Is Eligible to Write

All graduates of diploma and baccalaureate nursing programs from Canadian schools are eligible to write the Nurse Examination. Nurses trained outside of Canada must apply through one of the provincial registering/licensing authorities to determine if they are eligible to write the examination.

• Where the Exams Are Written

The Nurse Examination is offered in all provinces and territories. The registering/licensing authorities are responsible for administering the examination in their province or territory. They determine the number and location of the examination writing centres in their jurisdiction. Writing centres are usually established in proximity to the nursing schools in each province.

• How Long the Exams Are

There are 240-260 operational items on the Nurse Examination, presented in two books. As well as the "operational" items (i.e., those on which the examinees are scored), there are a number of "experimental" items which are included in exam books, to study their suitability for use on future examinations. Examinees are not scored on these experimental items.

---

[1] The information in this section was provided by the Canadian Nurses Association Testing division.

[2] Canadian Psychological Association. (1987) *Guidelines for educational and psychological testing.* Old Chelsea, QC: Author

• *How Often They Are Written*

With a change to a criterion-referenced format (introduced in August 1995), the Nurse Examination will be offered in a one-day administration. The Nurse Examination is administered four times a year: in January, June, August, and October. However, the number of times the Nurse Examination is offered in a particular jurisdiction is at the discretion of each registering/licensing authority.

• *Explanation of Content*

The content domain for the Nurse Examination is a list of 238 competencies required for the safe and effective practice of beginning nurses in Canada. The content domain was developed from a nursing focus. This means that the metaparadigm of nursing—namely, the concepts of person (client), health, environment, and nursing—was accepted as a basic tenet.

In developing the list of competencies for nurses beginning to practice, a number of assumptions were made. Specifically, the competencies are assumed to:

- include knowledge, abilities, skills, attitudes, and judgement;
- focus on the individual client, who is a member of a family, a group, or a community;
- focus on the client's responses to common and predictable health situations throughout the life cycle;
- include health promotion, illness prevention, restoration and maintenance of health, and care of the dying;
- recognize that nurses beginning to practice are generalists prepared to practice collaboratively, in structured, supervised environments; and,
- be directed toward the practice of the beginning nurse, on entry into practice, regardless of education preparation.

The list of competencies is classified into seven categories, the first five representing the nursing process and the last two representing more general and ongoing aspects of nursing:

> Data Collection; Analysis and Interpretation of Data; Planning Care; Implementation; Evaluation; Collaboration and Coordination; and Professional Practice.

• *Criterion-Referenced Based*

Criterion-referenced means that the test (in this case the Nurse Examination) measures an individual's command of a specified content/skills domain. As well, scores on a criterion-referenced examination are interpreted in comparison to a predetermined performance standard, independent of the results obtained by other examinees.

• *Type of Questions and One or Two Examples*

Questions on the Nurse Examination are objective-type items presented in one of two formats: case-based (i.e., a brief introductory text accompanied by approximately five related items) or independent items (i.e., stand-alone items which are not specifically connected with any other text or items).

Sample Items: Case-Based

Case 1

Mr. Robert Lowry, an 82-year-old married man, collapses at home. Mr. Lowry is rushed to the community hospital where it is determined that he has suffered a cerebrovascular accident (CVA). Mrs. Lowry tells the nurse that, prior to this incident, her husband had been taking hydrochlorothiazide (Hydrodiuril) to control his hypertension.

ITEMS 1 to 5 refer to this case. (* indicates correct answer)

1. Which one of the following initial nursing assessments would determine Mr. Lowry's level of consciousness?
   1. Visual fields
   2. Auditory acuity
   3. Reaction to cold
   *4. Responses to painful stimuli

2. Mr. Lowry regains consciousness and is found to have loss of movement on his left side and hemianopsia. Which one of the following responses by the nurse would be appropriate to give Mrs. Lowry when she asks questions regarding her husband's potential for recovery?
   1. "It sounds as though you may be somewhat anxious to resume your former lifestyle."
   2. "It's difficult to know, but most people take at least a year to recover completely."
   *3. "Concern about recovery is common. Rehabilitation takes time and progress is often slow."
   4. "To be anxious is normal. Unfortunately, there is no way of estimating your husband's recovery potential."

3. Mr. Lowry is receiving a thiazide diuretic. Which one of the following manifestations would indicate mild hypokalemia?
   *1. Anorexia; irregular and weak pulse
   2. Agitation; redness and dryness of skin
   3. Hyperreflexia; numbness and tingling of fingers
   4. Abdominal cramps; anxiety and changes in personality

4. Which one of the following interventions should the nurse implement to encourage Mr. Lowry to feed himself?

1. Assist him to position the cutlery in his hands.

2. Suggest that Mrs. Lowry take him to the cafeteria.

3. Allow sufficient time for him to cut up his own food.

*4. Arrange food items on his tray so that he can see them.

5. Which one of the following nursing observations of Mrs. Lowry's behavior would best indicate her readiness to participate in her husband's care at home?

    1. She selects his daily menus.

    2. She visits her husband every day.

    3. She brings his shaving kit and pajamas from home.

  *4. She asks if she is correctly positioned to help him walk.

Sample Items: Independent

1. Which of the following nursing measures would most likely facilitate a client's acceptance of an altered body image following a total laryngectomy and tracheostomy?

    1. Emphasize what the client can do within the limitations resulting from the treatment.

2. Encourage the client's family to refrain from discussing the tracheostomy while visiting.

3. Demonstrate a sympathetic approach when providing the client's tracheostomy care.

*4. Reassure the client that following discharge there can be a complete return to prehospitalization activities.

2. What should the nurse do if, in the nurse's opinion, the physician's order for a postoperative analgesic seems excessive?

    1. Assess the client closely for side effects after giving the drug.

  *2. Seek clarification from the physician before giving the medication.

    3. Give the medication and document the concern in the nursing notes.

    4. Withhold the medication and document the reason in the nursing notes.

To obtain information on writing the Nurse Registration/Licensure Examination, contact any of the provincial registering/licensing authorities.

Alberta Association of Registered Nurses
11620-168th Street
Edmonton, Alberta T5M 4A6
(403) 451-0043
Fax: (403) 452-3276

Association of Nurses of Prince Edward Island
17 Pownal Street, Box 1838
Charlottetown, Prince
Edward Island C1A 7N5
(902) 368-3764
Fax: (902) 628-1430

Association of Registered Nurses of Newfoundland
55 Military Road
P.O. Box 6116
St. John's, Newfoundland A1C 5X8
(709) 753-6040
Fax: (709) 753-4940

College of Nurses of Ontario
101 Davenport Road
Toronto, Ontario M5R 3P1
(416) 928-0900
Fax: (416) 928-6507
Toll Free: 1-800-387-5526

Manitoba Association of Registered Nurses
647 Broadway Avenue
Winnipeg, Manitoba R3C 0X2
(204) 774-3477
Fax: (204) 775-6052

Northwest Territories Registered Nurses Association
P.O. Box 2757
Yellowknife, Northwest Territories X1A 2R1
(403) 873-2745
Fax: (403) 873-2336

Nurses Association of New Brunswick
165 Regent Street
Fredericton, New Brunswick E3B 3W5
(506) 458-8731
Fax: (506) 459-2857

Ordre des infirmières et infirmiers du Québec
4200 ouest, boulevard Dorchester
Montréal, (Québec) H3Z 1V4
(514) 935-2501
Fax: (514) 935-1799
Toll Free: 1-800-363-6048

Registered Nurses Association of British Columbia
2855 Arbutus Street
Vancouver, British Columbia V6J 3Y8
(604) 736-7331
Fax: (604) 738-2272

Registered Nurses Association of Nova Scotia
Suite 104, 120 Eileen Stubbs Ave.
Darmouth, Nova Scotia B3B 1Y1
(902) 468-9744
Fax: (902) 468-9510

Saskatchewan Registered Nurses Association
2066 Retallack Street
Regina, Saskatchewan S4T 2K2
(306) 757-4643
Fax: (306) 525-0849

Yukon Nurses Society
P.O. Box 5371
Whitehorse, Yukon Y1A 4Z2
(403) 667-4062
Fax: (403) 668-5123

GLOSSARY

abduction movement away from the central axis (midline) of the body.

abstract a brief summary of a study.

accessibility one of the five principles on which the Canadian health insurance plan is based; health services are available to all insured persons on uniform terms and conditions with no impediments to services, by charges or other means.

accessible population a population that is a feasible source of sample members.

accountability a person is answerable (or accepts responsibility) for his or her own actions.

accreditation/approval (of basic nursing education programs) (1) a process to ensure that schools of nursing meet certain minimum standards established by the registering body in a province (2) the process of certifying that an educational program has not only met minimum standards, but is considered "good" by national standards.

acculturation process whereby individuals learn the beliefs, values and lifeways of a culture other than the one into which they were born and accept these as their own.

acid a compound that releases hydrogen ions when dissociated in solution.

acidosis a condition in which there is an excessive proportion of acid (H^+ concentration) in the blood or a depletion of base (bicarbonate) reserves.

active artificial immunity immunity conferred by vaccines.

active ROM range of motion exercises carried out by the individual.

active transport the movement of solute particles from an area of lower concentration to an area of higher concentration with the use of a carrier molecule.

actual diagnosis represents a problem that has been validated by the presence of major defining characteristics.

actual problem situation in which data in the cluster are similar to the defining characteristics for a hypothesized problem.

acupressure massage technique which uses manual pressure to stimulate energy points on the body.

acute pertaining to a condition with a sudden, severe onset and a relatively short course.

adaptation a condition in which the brain no longer perceives the available stimuli because the receptors are not picking up enough stimuli or are picking up too much of the same stimulus.

additive effect the result of administering two drugs with similar actions.

adduction movement toward the central axis (midline) of the body.

advanced directives statements by people specifying the type of care they wish to receive when they are terminally ill in the event that they are incapable of expressing their wishes at that time.

adverse (side) effects physiological responses to a drug other than the therapeutic effect.

aerobic exercise sustained physical activity that uses the oxygen system to strengthen cardio-respiratory function and endurance.

affective domain the domain of learning tasks involving the changing of attitudes.

agonists drugs that stimulate or produce cellular response.

alkalosis a condition in which there is a reduced proportion of acid (H^+) in the blood or an excess of base (bicarbonate) reserves.

allergic reaction a hypersensitive reaction to a drug in a person who was previously exposed to the drug or a related chemical and has developed antibodies to it.

allophone a Canadian whose mother tongue is neither English or French.

amino acid the structural unit of protein.

amniotic sac the protective membrane filled with fluid that surrounds the developing embryo, providing warmth, moisture and relative freedom of movement.

anabolism the building process of metabolism in which simple substances are converted to more complex compounds; synthesis of enzymes and proteins needed by the body cells.

analgesic relieving pain; a pain relieving agent.

analogic usual nonverbal communication such as body posture, facial expression and tone, as well as creative expression such as music, poetry and painting.

anaphylactic reaction life-threatening respiratory distress and cardiovascular collapse as a result of an allergic reaction to a drug.

anion ion that carries a negative charge.

anointing of the sick a sacrament in the Roman Catholic Church interpreted as an aid to healing and a source of strength.

anorexia loss of appetite or lack of desire for food; it involves the subjective perception of a distaste for food.

antagonistic effect two drugs whose effects cancel each other out.

antagonists drugs that block cellular response.

anthropometric measurement measurements of the size and proportions of the body: height, weight and skinfold (fatfold) thickness.

anticipatory grief the response to prior knowledge of an impending death.

antidiarrheal agents agents which counteract diarrhea.

aphasia the state of being unable to speak at all.

apical pulse the beat of the heart auscultated at its apex.

apnea the absence of breathing.

appetite the desire for food.

aquathermia pad a type of heating pad, consisting of channels through which heated water circulates and transmits dry heat of a constant temperature.

aromatherapy makes use of aromatic essences extracted from wild or cultivated plants for beauty treatments and for therapies similar to those used in herbal medicine.

artificial airway a tube inserted into a person's airway by way of the mouth or nose, or through a tracheostomy.

asepsis the absence of contamination.

assault a threat to do physical harm to another and an apparent ability to carry out that threat.

assessment the first step in the nursing process; the collection and interpretation of clinical information.

assumptions provisional suppositions.

asymptomatic a condition without signs or symptoms.

auscultation listening to body sounds produced by the heart, lungs and abdomen.

authenticity genuineness; often manifested by spontaneity, self-disclosure and a lack of defensiveness.

authority the status attributed to individuals or groups giving them the power and right to command and be obeyed.

autocratic a teaching style in which the teacher makes all decisions about learning.

autolytic debridement the removal of dead tissue from a wound by using dressings that allow enzymes in the wound fluid to dissolve the dead tissues.

autonomy the right to self-determination.

autosexual activities sexual behaviours which involve the self only.

ayurvedic medicine based on natural phenomena as the cause of illness, rather than spirits, with treatment based on a belief in the body's innate ability to heal itself.

Baha'i a religion based on the belief that mankind is one human race; it teaches the unity of religions and the unity of mankind.

Balkan frame a metal frame that extends lengthwise above the bed supported at either end by a pole attached to the bed frame.

baptism a Christian ritual in which the individual is immersed in or sprinkled with water as a sign of purification and admission to the church.

basal metabolic rate (BMR) the minimum energy requirements of the body when the individual is awake and at digestive, physical and emotional rest.

base a compound that combines with acids to form salts; neutralizes the effects of acids.

base of support foundation that gives an object stability.

battery touching without consent.

bed cradle a device used to keep the weight of the top bed covers off the patient.

behaviour modification substituting desired behaviour for undesired behaviour using reinforcement.

behavioural model an approach to health based on the premise that there are four principal factors affecting both individual and group health; namely, heredity, environment, lifestyle, and health care organization. (Also known as the *health fields approach* or *lifestyles model*).

behaviourist school a theory that believes learning is observable and can be controlled by manipulating the environment.

beneficence an ethical principle that requires that we do good and prevent harm.

bereavement the experience of loss through death.

binuclear family families in which children are members of two households as a result of joint-custody arrangements following divorce.

biological sexual identity the biological distinctions that identify a person as male or female based on the characteristics of the sex organs.

biomedical model an empirical approach to health, based on scientific research and training, that focusses on the physiological determinants of health and disease.

biopsy surgery to obtain a tissue sample from the body.

bisexuality romantic and sexual attraction to partners of either sex.

blended or reconstituted family a husband and wife, at least one of whom has been married before. The blended family can include one or more children from a former marriage as well as offspring from the new union.

blood pressure   the pressure of the blood within arteries.

body alignment   relationship of body parts to the midline of the body.

body temperature   the balance between heat production and heat loss.

bonding   attachment that occurs between parent and newborn.

boundaries   filters which permit varying degrees of exchange between the system and the environment; in family systems theory, physical demarcations such as the family's property line or a member's bedroom, or abstract entities like rules, norms, attitudes and values which separate families and subsystems from their environments, and which require human interaction inside and outside the family.

brachial pulse   the pulse located on the anterior surface of the arm just below the elbow where the brachial artery passes over the ulna.

bradycardia   a very low pulse rate (less than 60 beats per minute).

bradypnea   an abnormal decrease in respiratory rate.

breast binder   a rectangular piece of cotton shaped roughly to the contours of the female chest with straps that pin to the binder in front.

bronchoscopy   an examination of the larynx, trachea and bronchi with the use of a fiberoptic bronchoscope, a tubular instrument with an attached light source.

Buddhism   a world-wide religion with no gods but encompassing various philosophical beliefs and ethical systems. A central belief is that the ultimate state is one of self-enlightenment.

calorie   a unit of heat; the amount of heat required to raise the temperature of one gram of water by one degree Celsius.

Canada Pension Plan (CPP)   a pension plan that is compulsory for all employed persons in Canada, except in the Province of Quebec which has its own Quebec Pension Plan (QPP).

carbohydrate   an organic compound composed of carbon, hydrogen and oxygen found in most plants, fruit sugars and natural starches; the primary source of energy for the body.

carcinogenic   pertaining to influences causing cancer.

cardiac output   the amount of blood ejected from the heart with the force of each ventricular contraction.

carotid pulse   the pulse found in the carotid artery.

carriers   individuals who acquire a pathogen but do not experience any adverse effects; however, these individuals may transmit the pathogen to others.

case mix groups (CMGs)   diagnosis-related groups of patients.

case study   a teaching strategy that uses an imaginary situation as the basis for questions and discussion.

catabolism   a complex metabolic process in which compounds are broken down or oxidized for energy.

cathartic   a substance that promotes the passage of watery soft stool accompanied by some cramping.

cation   an ion that carries a positive charge.

causality   relating of causes to the effect they produce; determination that one variable causes another.

certification   a legal document from an official body attesting that an individual or an institution has met certain standards or an individual has successfully completed a course of training.

ceruminous glands   skin glands located in the external ear canal that secrete cerumen (wax).

change agent   outside consultant who is called in to assist with the dissemination of information about new ideas and/or practices in an organization (or in a social system) and their adoption in practice.

channel   the means of conveying a message.

charting by exception (CBE)   documents only significant findings or exceptions to the norm.

chemical name   the description of a drug's chemical components.

Chi   the finite amount of energy we are endowed with at birth.

chill   involuntary contractions of the voluntary muscles with shivering and shaking.

Chinese/Oriental medicine   a doctrine revolving around theories of energy and elements, with 3 basic types of intervention: (1) herbal remedies, (2) acupuncture, and (3) exercise.

chiropractic medicine   a branch of medicine primarily concerned with the examination and treatment of the spine.

cholesterol   a fat-like substance (an alcohol) found in all animal fats and oils; an essential component of some body tissues and compounds.

Christianity   the doctrine of Christ and his apostles, based on the belief that Jesus is the Christ and the Son of God.

chronic   pertaining to a condition which develops slowly and persists for a long duration, often throughout the remainder of a person's lifetime.

circadian (diurnal) rhythm a regular pattern which recurrs in cycles of about twenty-four hours; the biological clock which regulates many body processes including the daily sleep-wake cycle.

circumduction circular movement, as of a limb or eye.

cleaning the removal of any foreign material from an object.

climate of trust a situation in which the patient feels able to trust the nurse as a person concerned first and foremost with the patient's welfare.

clinical laboratory technologist a member of the health team who collects specimens for laboratory tests, treats and analyzes these specimens and advises physicians and nurses on the results of these tests.

clinical nurse specialist a registered nurse who holds a master's degree in nursing and has expertise in a clinical nursing specialty.

clinical significance the usefulness of the findings of a study in clinical practice.

closed systems systems that limit interaction with their environment.

closed wound injury to the skin and underlying tissue without a break in the skin.

cluster categories or groups of data.

cluster sampling taking progressively larger random samples from different units within a population.

coenzyme an essential element needed for the activation or control of enzyme activity in the body.

cognitive appraisal a person's perception of a situation as harmful and an assessment of his or her ability to cope with it.

cognitive coping skills the mental processes used to regulate the emotional and physiological responses to stress by attempting to see at least some part of a stressful situation in a positive way.

cognitive domain the domain of learning tasks involving the acquisition of knowledge.

cognitive school a theory that believes learning is an intellectual process similar to information processing.

cohabiting family a man and a woman living together without the sanctity of marriage. Also known as a common-law relationship.

collaborative problem complications that occur or may occur in association with specific pathology and treatment.

collaborative research studies done in collaborative teams with colleagues, people in other agencies, people in other provinces or countries, or with members of other disciplines.

colonization the acquisition and multiplication of a microorganism.

colostomy a surgically created opening from the large intestine to the abdominal wall.

combustible material a substance capable of burning.

comfort a subjective experience indicating a sense of physical, psychological, social, spiritual and environmental ease.

commensals microorganisms with which people enjoy a symbiotic relationship.

commitment a complex, affective response characterized by convergence between one's desires and one's obligations and by a deliberate choice to act in accordance with them.

communal family an intimate network of unrelated adults and their children who make a commitment to live together as one large family unit.

communication the process by which people transmit information to one another through verbal and nonverbal messages or cues.

communion (or eucharist) a Christian sacrament in which the person partakes of bread and wine. The bread represents the body of Christ; the wine his blood.

community (1) a group of people living in a given geographical area (which may not necessarily be defined by legislation) who interact with one another and work collectively on matters of common concern. (2) Any group of people with a common bond.

community health centre a health agency that provides primary health care services in an ambulatory setting.

compassion a sensitivity to the pain and brokenness of another; a quality of presence which allows one to share with and make room for another.

compensation over-achieving in the same sphere or one different from that in which we feel inferior.

competence having the knowledge, judgement, skills, energy, experience and motivation required to respond adequately to the demands of one's professional responsibilities.

complete protein food that contains all of the essential amino acids in amounts and proportions for proper use in the body.

compliance the ease with which the lungs and the chest wall can expand to fill with air and contract to empty the air.

comportment bearing, demeanour, dress and language.

comprehensiveness one of the five principles on which the Canadian health insurance program is based. The term is used to mean the provision of all insured services provided by hospitals, medical practitioners, or dentist, and, where permitted, by other health care practitioners.

concept a complex mental formulation of an object, a property (characteristic) or an event that is derived from an individual's perceptual experience.

conceptual model (conceptual framework) the diagrammatic representation of a theory.

confidence the quality which fosters trusting relationships.

confirmatory data analysis involves the use of various techniques in order to (1) test proposed relationships between variables, (2) ascertain (infer) that the findings from a sample are representative of the total population, (3) examine causality (that a specific change in 'a' caused reaction 'b'), (4) predict that under similar circumstances, 'a' will probably cause 'b' again, and (5) infer from the sample to a theoretical model.

congenital problems encountered by the unborn infant *in utero*.

conscience a state of moral awareness which grows with experience.

constipation infrequent, hard, dry bowel movements.

consumers' bills of rights statements developed in both the United States and Canada that have sought to clarify an individual's basic rights as these are applicable to health care.

continent urostomy a urinary diversion procedure consisting of an internal pouch, a stoma and two nipple valves which prevent urine from draining out of the stoma; urine is stored in the pouch until it is emptied with a catheter passed through the stoma.

contracture a shortening or distortion of muscle tissue.

control group one that can be compared with the experimental group.

controlled drugs drugs whose use is controlled by federal legislation (in Canada, the Narcotic Control Act and Regulations). Included are the narcotics and certain other drugs such as barbiturates.

convenience sampling (accidental sampling) allows the entry of any available (convenient) subject into the study until the desired sample size is reached.

core temperature temperature of the internal, deep structures of the body as compared to temperature of peripheral tissues.

correlation the extent to which values of one variable are related to values of another variable.

crackles abnormal breath sounds described as discontinuous crackling sounds produced by air passing through fluid in the small airways.

crime a wrong committed against the public and punishable by the crown.

critical path an outline of care for an individual patient.

critique a critical assessment of a piece of research involving a systematic appraisal according to specified criteria.

cue a piece of information that one perceives from the environment.

cultural mosaic ethically plural society in which people retain a distinct sense of cultural identity.

cultural sensitivity (cross-cultural competence/intercultural effectiveness/ethnic competence) the ability to work effectively with people of different cultures in a way that people of these cultures find acceptable.

culture the basic beliefs, values and lifeways of groups of people.

cumulative trauma disorders a group of disorders caused by sustained, unnatural body postures and repetitive, forceful movements.

cyanosis bluish tinge in the skin and mucous membranes frequently associated with respiratory distress.

cybernetics the science of systems of control and communications in animals and machines.

cystitis inflammation of the urinary bladder.

cystoscopy an examination of a patient's bladder with a lighted instrument inserted up the urethra.

daily hassles the irritating, distressing and frustrating demands of everyday life.

daily uplifts things in a person's daily life that help to balance stressors such as relating well to one's spouse or lover, relating well to friends, completing a task or feeling healthy.

dandruff dry, scaly material shed from the scalp.

data information the researcher (investigator) collects from subjects or participants in the research study, or about objects in a non-human study.

data base a component of the POMR including the physician history and physical exam and the nursing history and functional health assessment.

data base assessment an evaluation of the patient, conducted on admission to a health care agency or upon initial contact with the patient.

deductive working from existing theory to hypothesize relationships that can then be tested.

defamation of character damage to a person's reputation by written or spoken words that tend to lower his or her esteem in the eyes of other people.

defecation the evacuation of feces.

defence mechanisms strategies that people commonly use in day-to-day life to buffer the emotional component of a stressful situation.

defining characteristic lists or categories of signs and symptoms or risk factors that depict hypothesized problems.

dehiscence the disruption of a surgical wound.

dehydration loss of water from body tissues.

delayed gratification the ability to put off immediate rewards in order to achieve long-term goals.

democratic a teaching style advocated by the humanists where the students participate in decisions about learning but are not the sole decision makers.

demonstration method of teaching by exhibition and explanation of a procedure.

demonstration project involves studying a new method of delivering health care in the community.

denial refusal to acknowledge a threat.

dental caries decay of the teeth.

dependent variable (outcome variable) the characteristic that is being measured to show results in a research study.

dermis the inner, thicker layer of skin.

diagnosis a deliberate, systematic process of data analysis and synthesis that ends with a clinical judgement, the nursing diagnosis.

diagnostic cue one that gives strong, valid information for making inferences.

diagnostic reasoning the process of critical thinking in which the nurse uses his or her clinical knowledge and experience to collect information, interpret the information collected, and form a conclusion about the patient's health or illness status (the nursing diagnosis).

diaphoresis sweating or perspiration.

diarrhea the frequent discharge of loose, watery stools.

diastolic pressure the force exerted against the arterial wall during ventricular relaxation.

dietitian a member of the health team usually responsible for planning meal service for patients and staff, supervising other workers in the preparation of food and counselling patients about their nutritional problems.

diffusion the process whereby dissolved particles (ions and molecules) distribute themselves equally within a given space; the particles move from an area of higher concentration to an area of lower concentration until equilibrium is reached.

digestion the process by which complex food forms are changed into simpler, soluble chemical parts so that they can be absorbed into the circulation for use by the body.

digital verbal communication.

disciplinary bodies monitor the practice of nurses to whom they have granted registration/licensure.

disease an interruption in the continuous process of health, manifested by abnormalities or disturbances in the structure and function of body parts, organs or systems.

displacement type of behaviour in which one transfers anger at one person to another person or object.

distal farther from a point of reference or point of attachment.

distress detrimental, harmful, unpleasant or damaging stress.

diuresis excretion of an increased amount of urine.

diuretic a drug given to increase the secretion of urine in the kidneys.

documentation the communication in writing of essential facts in order to maintain a continuous history of events over a period of time.

dorsal recumbent position lying on the back with the head and shoulders slightly elevated on a pillow.

dorsalis pedis pulse the pulse located on the dorsum of the foot in a line between the first and second toes, just above the longitudinal arch.

dorsiflexion flexion of a body part toward the back, such as upward bending of the fingers, hand, foot or toes.

drug addiction the psychological need to use drugs for other than medical reasons, such as pain relief.

drug dependence symptoms of withdrawal which occur when a drug is abruptly discontinued.

drug interactions the effects of two or more drugs on the body.

drug tolerance the circumstance in which a therapeutic response to a drug dosage lessens after continuous exposure to it.

drug toxicity the effects of a drug produced by an overdose, accumulation of the drug in the body or an abnormal sensitivity to the drug.

dual-career family a family in which both heads of the household pursue careers and at the same time maintain a family life together.

duration of action the length of time a drug produces a pharmacological effect.

dyspnea difficult or laboured breathing.

dyssomnias conditions characterized by difficulties with the quantity and quality of sleep; insomnia, hypersomnia and narcolepsy.

dysuria difficulty or pain on voiding.

ecological (environmental) equilibrium the balance maintained by human organisms in their interactions with the physical environment.

ecology the study of organisms and how they relate to their environment.

ecomap depiction of the family members' contact with their outside world.

ectoderm outer layer of the uterine wall.

edema the accumulation of excessive amounts of fluid in the tissues.

electrolyte a substance which, when dissolved in solution, splits into electrically charged ions of individual atoms or molecules that conduct an electrical current.

emancipated minor a teenager who no longer lives at home and is self-supporting.

emergency medical technician a member of the health team who has had training in advanced life support skills, can do basic and advanced first aid and CPR and can start intravenous infusions.

emesis stomach contents expelled during vomiting.

empathy the ability to recognize and understand another person's feelings.

empirical concrete, based on observation, experiment or experience, not on theory.

empirical abstract meaning inferred from examples of direct or indirect evidence in the real world.

empowerment the social process of recognizing, promoting and enhancing people's abilities to meet their own needs, solve their own problems, and mobilize necessary resources to take control of their own lives.

endoderm inner layer of the uterine wall.

endogenous infection infection originating from a person's own microbial flora.

endorphins large polypeptides with an opioid-like pharmacological action.

enema the instillation of fluid into the rectum to stimulate peristalsis and remove feces or flatus from the colon.

entrepreneurial health care model one in which health care services are provided by private agencies and paid for by the consumer of these services.

enuresis bedwetting.

environment both the social environment (the patient's family, friends and significant others) and the physical environment, that is, the surroundings.

enzyme a compound, almost always a protein, that speeds the rate of a chemical process but is not altered by the process.

epidemiological model basic components are (1) the systematic collection of health data through epidemiological surveys and (2) the search for causes of various states of health.

epidemiology the study of the distribution and determinants of various health-related states or events in specified populations and the application of this study in the control of health problems.

epidermis the outer, thinner layer of skin.

epidural analgesia a method of pain relief by injecting analgesic medication into the epidural space of the spinal column.

esteem needs need to feel that you are worthwhile as a human being.

ethical dilemma a problem with two or more moral claims.

ethnicity the ethnic or cultural group(s) to which an individual's ancestors belonged; it pertains to the ancestral roots or origins of the population and not to place of birth, citizenship, nationality or language.

ethnography the scientific description of human races (ethnic groups).

ethnomethodological a descriptive analysis of a culture or sub-culture which can be used as a basis to develop theories about that culture.

etiology the search for the causes of disease and other health states.

eupnea normal breathing (effortless, regular and noiseless).

eustress "good" stress.

euthanasia easy or painless death; often synonymous with "mercy killing."

evaluation a comparison against accepted standards.

eversion turning outward away from the body.

evisceration the protrusion of body organs through a wound.

examination an objective, systematic assessment of the patient's physical status.

excretion a substance discharged by the body.

exhalation the phase of breathing when air is passed out of the lungs; expiration.

exogenous infection an infection acquired from the local animate or inanimate environment.

expected outcome the behaviour the patient is expected to achieve.

experimental studies the researcher intervenes and changes one variable, then observes what happens.

expiration   breathing out.

exploratory or descriptive data analysis   involves tabulating, depicting and describing collections of data.

extended care   health services required by persons with long-term illness or disability and provided in nursing homes, intermediate care facilities, adult residential care, home care and ambulatory care.

extended family   network of two or more related nuclear families, known in everyday language as relatives or kinsfolk. This family unit consists of grandparents, aunts, uncles and cousins, who may live near by or far away from one another.

extension   the act of straightening.

external respiration   breathing.

extracellular fluid   fluids situated outside the cells of the body.

exudate   an inflammatory fluid discharged from an infected area of the body.

faith healing   based on the belief a person has in the healing power of an object or the healing ability of an individual.

false imprisonment   individuals who are unjustifiably detained, or confined against their will and without a legal warrant for detention.

family   two or more people, who may or may not be related by blood, marriage, or adoption, bound by strong emotional ties, a sense of belonging, and a commitment to live with and care for one another over time.

Family Allowance   a universal social program in Canada through which every family with children receives an allowance, based on a certain amount per child.

family crisis   state of disorganization in the family unit.

family dynamics   interrelationships among members of a family, namely their roles, relationships and communication patterns.

family functions   those activities a family performs in order to meet the needs of both individual family members and society as a whole.

family stress   a state of imbalance in the family.

family stressors   life events or demands that impact on the family, producing stress or having the potential of producing stress, and ultimately require change.

family structure   the way a family is organized.

family systems theory   views the whole family as a unit of care, such that the family is the patient or client.

family therapy   a branch of psychotherapy concerned with the use of family process to treat psychopathological conditions or other dysfunctions in families.

fantasy   day-dreaming.

fat   an organic water-insoluble compound found naturally in animals and plant seeds; also called lipid.

fatty acid   a unit of fat consisting of a chain of carbon atoms linked to hydrogen ions and an acid group attached; may be saturated, monounsaturated and polyunsaturated.

fecal impaction   a large, hardened mass of stool that cannot be expelled.

fecal incontinence   a lack of control over bowel evacuation.

feces   waste products excreted from the intestines.

feedback   a process created by the output of a system which permits the system to maintain stability of its internal function; in family systems theory, a continuous process

of input and output exchanges between families and the community that surrounds them.

femoral pulse   the pulse located in the middle of the groin where the femoral artery passes over the pelvic bone.

filtration   the process whereby water and dissolved substances are forced across a membrane from an area of high pressure to an area of low pressure by hydrostatic or fluid pressure.

First Nations   the earliest settlers in Canada; the term includes native North American Indians and the Inuit.

flexion   the act of bending.

flowsheet   graphic recording of interventions or observations that occur within a designated period of time.

focus assessment   information collected on an ongoing basis to determine changes in the patient's health status and the need for change in the nursing plan for care.

focus charting   a type of charting in which the nurse identifies client concerns rather than problems and focusses on a behaviour, change, event or a nursing diagnosis.

fomites   inanimate objects that carry infectious agents.

footboard   a device made of plastic or wood that is placed at the foot of the patient's bed to serve as a support for the feet.

Fowler's position   a sitting position in which the person's head and trunk are raised 45° to 90°.

fracture board   a board made of wood or plexiglass that is placed under the patient's mattress to increase support.

frail elderly   people who require nursing care or supervision.

fremitus   a vibration that can be felt on the exterior chest wall when a person speaks.

frequency distribution analysis method that involves determining how often scores or values appear in a data set.

function the dynamic interaction among component parts of a system.

gay or lesbian family form of cohabitation in which individuals of the same sex live together, with or without children, and share a sexual relationship.

gender definition (gender identity) the perception of self as male or female.

gender role identity the behaviour identified by one's culture as appropriate to that gender; how a person behaves as male or female.

general adaptation syndrome (GAS) the response of the body to physiological stress.

generic name a drug's original name assigned by the individual or company that originally marketed the drug.

genogram diagram of the family constellation. It shows the structure of the intergenerational relationships of a family.

gestation term used to describe the development of new life that takes place in the womb between conception and birth.

gingivae the gums.

gingivitis inflammation of the gums.

gliding movement in one plane, as in sliding.

gluconeogenesis the formation of glucose from proteins and fatty acids when carbohydrate stores are depleted.

glycogen a polysaccharide stored in the cells after the breakdown of carbohydrate.

glycogenolysis the conversion of glycogen to glucose in the liver.

good samaritan laws legislation designed to protect the professional practitioner from malpractice suits arising from care given to the injured at the scene of an accident or other emergency.

grand theory/mega theory a global statement that identifies phenomena (concepts or ideas) that are of interest to the discipline.

graph shows how many times each score has occurred, displaying the frequency of each score and illustrating the distribution of scores.

grief the total response to loss.

grounded theory a theory that has been grounded in reality derived from data systematically obtained from social research.

gurgles abnormal breath sounds described as a coarse, continuous sound produced by air flowing through large passages narrowed by secretions, mucosal swelling or obstruction.

gustatory pertaining to the sense of taste.

half-life (of a drug) the time it takes for 50 percent of the plasma concentration of a drug to be eliminated from the body.

hardiness a particular constellation of personality characteristics that helps people stay healthy despite facing stressful life events. It includes (1) commitment, (2) the ability to view change as a challenge, (3) a sense of personal control over life.

hazardous substance substance capable of causing injury upon exposure.

health (1) a positive state of being that includes physical fitness, mental (or emotional) stability, and social and spiritual ease. (2) the extent to which an individual or group is able, on the one hand, to realize aspirations and satisfy needs; and, on the other hand, to change or cope with the environment.

health educator a member of the health team who is responsible for the development of health education programs in a community.

health maintenance organization a form of prepaid group practice. They provide a comprehensive range of services on a fixed contract basis, which is paid for in advance by people enrolling in the organization.

healthy public policy public policy that is concerned with health and equity and with accountability for the health impact of the legislation.

hematoma a clot formed beneath the skin as a result of bleeding.

hemiplegic a person with loss of function on one side of the body.

hemodialysis a procedure in which waste products and excess water are removed from the body by circulating blood from an artery through an external dialyser (sometimes referred to as the artificial kidney).

hemoptysis the coughing up of sputum containing varying amounts of blood.

hemorrhoids swollen veins of the anus or rectum.

herbalist a person who treats people with potions, salves and brews made from various plants.

high-risk diagnosis describes a potential problem.

Hinduism a religion, a social system and a way of life for most of population of India with a belief in numerous gods and in reincarnation.

histogram a graphic display of a frequency table using rectangular bars with heights equal to the frequency in a particular class.

holistic focussing on the total person, the reaction to stress and the factors influencing the person's ability to cope with stress and restore equilibrium.

holistic health an approach to wellness that recognizes the interaction between the whole person and his or her environment, and emphasizes harmony within oneself, with nature and the world.

homeostasis the process by which the body brings into play certain mechanisms to maintain stability in its internal environment.

homeothermic warm-blooded.

homosexuality the romantic and sexual attraction to the same-sex partner; a sexual orientation.

hospice/palliative care refers to both a philosophy of care and an agency for inpatient and outpatient services for the dying person.

hospital postgraduate course an educational program in a clinical nursing specialty given in a hospital.

hot compress applications of either sterile or unsterile gauze sponges moistened with heated normal saline or antiseptic solution.

humanist school a theory that believes learning must involve the whole person (intellect and emotions).

humidifier a device that adds moisture to inspired air.

hunger an uncomfortable sensation that indicates a physiological need for nourishment.

hydrolysis a process of chemical digestion whereby nutrients are split into simpler elements by the addition of water to molecules.

hydrotherapy water treatments which include tubs, tanks and whirlpool baths.

hypercalcemia an excessive amount of calcium in the blood.

hyperextension straightening beyond the normal range of motion.

hyperkalemia an excessive amount of potassium in the blood.

hypernatremia an excessive amount of sodium in the blood.

hypersomnia excessive sleeping, especially during the day.

hyperthermia an abnormally high body temperature; fever.

hypertonic having more solute concentration than another solution, thus exerting greater osmotic pressure than the other solution.

hyperventilation increase in rate and depth of respirations; a condition in which the amount of air in the alveoli exceeds metabolic demands.

hypervolemia an abnormal increase in blood volume.

hypnotic a drug that acts to induce sleep.

hypocalcemia a decrease in the amount of serum calcium.

hypochloremia a reduced concentration of chlorides in the blood.

hypokalemia a reduction in the amount of potassium in the blood.

hyponatremia a decrease in the amount of sodium in the blood.

hypothermia excessively low body temperature.

hypothesis suggests solutions or answers by translating the problem into a precise prediction of expected outcomes.

hypotonic having less solute concentration than another solution, thus exerting less osmotic pressure than the other solution.

hypoventilation an irregular slow, shallow pattern of alveolar ventilation which does not meet metabolic demands.

hypoxemia a decrease in the oxygen content of the blood.

hypoxia an insufficient supply of oxygen to the tissues.

identification modelling oneself on a successful person.

ileal conduit a urinary diversion procedure consisting of a reservoir constructed from a portion of the ileum and a stoma.

ileostomy a surgically created opening from the ileum of the small intestine to the abdominal wall.

illness the personal experience of feeling unhealthy.

immunocompromised having an immune system that is impaired.

incidence the number of instances of illness commencing, or of people falling ill, during a given period in a specific population.

incubation the period leading up to a disease.

independent variable (experimental/intervention variable) a variable that the researcher establishes independently, e.g. treating Group A differently from Group B, or variations in population under study, e.g. age, sex.

inductive working from data collected to identify variables in order to generate theory.

industrial hygienist a member of the health team whose main concern is the detection and control of hazards in the work environment.

infection the deposition or invasion and multiplication of microorganisms on surfaces of the body or in body tissues causing adverse or ill effects.

inference the subjective interpretations of cues.

inflammation the protective response of body tissues to injury.

informed consent the consent must be consensual, freely given, informed, and specific to both the treatment and the caregiver.

inhalation the phase of breathing when air is taken into the lungs; inspiration.

input energy, information and resources that the system receives from the environment and then processes.

insomnia difficulty falling asleep or staying asleep, or excessive wakefulness.

inspection using the senses to assist in making judgements, comparisons and decisions.

inspiration breathing in.

instrument device used to record the data obtained from subjects.

intermittent pain exacerbations and remissions of acute episodes of pain.

interstitial fluid the fluid in the spaces between the cells.

intracellular fluid fluids situated within the cells of the body.

intrathecal analgesia a method of pain relief by injecting analgesic medication into the subarachnoid space for dispersion throughout the spinal fluid.

intravascular fluid the fluid in the blood and lymph vessels; plasma.

Inuit a separate group of the First Nations occupying small communities north of the treeline in Canada's Far North stretching from the Mackenzie River Delta, through the Arctic Islands and Baffin Island, along the coast of Hudson Bay and Ungava Bay in Quebec, to the east coast of Labrador.

inversion turning inward towards the body.

Islam the religion of the Muslims, based on the revelations of the god Allah through his prophet Mohammed.

isokinetic exercise exercise in which the speed of muscle short-ening is controlled by a machine or electronic device.

isometric exercise exercise in which muscle tension is increased with little movement of the joint or change in muscle length.

isotonic having the same solute concentration as another solution, thus exerting the same osmotic pressure as the other solution.

isotonic exercise exercise in which the tension of a muscle remains constant while its length changes to move the resistance (weight) through a range of motion.

jargon technical terms common to a particular field but not common outside of that field.

Judaism a religion of the Jewish people with a belief in one God and based on mosaic and rabbinical teaching.

kaccha in Sikhism, special undershorts worn by members of both sexes, as a reminder of modesty and sexual morality for women.

kanga a comb worn in the hair by Sikhs.

kara a steel bangle, worn on the right wrist by Sikhs.

kegel exercises pelvic floor strengthening exercises.

kilocalorie a thousand calories; the amount of heat needed to raise the temperature of one kilogram of water by one degree Celsius.

kinesiologist a member of the health team who specializes in human movement and human performance.

kinesthesia the sense that tells the person where body parts are in relation to one another.

Kirpan a symbolic dagger, worn under the clothes by Sikhs as a symbol of readiness to fight.

knowledge deficit not a nursing diagnosis; refers to the lack of knowledge a patient has about his or her condition or about aspects of his or her care.

Koran the Holy Scriptures of the Islamic religion.

Kosh uncut hair maintained by Sikhs.

labour the process by which the baby is expelled from the uterus.

laissez-faire a teaching style in which the students make all decisions about learning.

lanugo fine downy hair covering the body of the fetus.

lateral position lying on the side.

laxative a substance that promotes the passage of a soft stool.

laying on of hands the use of touch to promote healing, for example, the anointing of the sick.

learned resourcefulness learned repertoire of skills that people use to regulate their lives and overcome the stresses of life.

lecture uninterrupted talk that presents information.

leucocytes white blood cells.

libel term used for defamation of character through written words, as in a letter to a third party, or depicted in a cartoon that causes the person to be the subject of ridicule or contempt.

licence a permit granted by a government agency to an individual to engage in the practice of a profession and to use a particular title.

licensed practical nurse (LPN) (Registered Nursing Assistant (RNA) in Ontario and Certified Nursing Assistant (CNA) in Alberta). A person trained in basic nursing techniques and direct patient care who practises under the supervision of a registered nurse or a physician in hospitals and other health care settings.

lithotomy position   a position in which the patient lies on the back with the hips flexed and slightly abducted and the knees flexed.

living will   an advance directive in which an individual writes down preferences for treatment in the event that he/she cannot decide for him/herself.

local adaptation syndrome (LAS) localized reactions which occur when a specific part or organ of the body is affected by a stress.

local effect   drug action which is confined to a specific area of application.

long-term goals   goals that will be achieved over a long period of time, sometimes weeks or months.

loss   any life event in which one is deprived of something that is valued.

love and belonging need   the need for love and affection and for a supportive network of friends, family and/or significant others.

macrosystems   the whole individual is viewed as a part of larger systems.

malnutrition   a state of poor health resulting from a long-standing dietary intake that either fails to meet or greatly exceeds nutritional needs.

malpractice   negligent or incorrect treatment of a patient by a health professional; may include other claims such as breach of contract.

material justice   equal share according to need, effort or merit.

mature minor   one who has demonstrated that he/she has the intelligence, understanding, and independence to make his/her own decisions in regard to the acceptance or rejection of medical treatment.

mean (average)   a measure of central tendency derived by dividing the sum of the values in a data set by the total number of values, scores, or subjects in it; represented by the symbol $\bar{x}$, read as x bar.

measures of central tendency   a statistic that summarizes the data into one representative value.

meatus   an opening.

meconium   the first bowel movement of the newborn infant; a greenish black, tarry substance.

median   measure of central tendency that corresponds to the middle score.

Medicaid   a federal government program in the US that provides personal health care services for the poor.

Medicare   in Canada, a national medical insurance program that covers the total population. In the United States, a national government program that provides personal health care services for older people.

medication   a substance taken to treat a disease or condition.

melting pot   the blending of various nationalities who have come as immigrants into a homogenous identity.

menarche   the onset of the first menstrual period.

menopause   the cessation of the menstrual cycle, occurring when a woman has not experienced menstrual flow for one to one-and-a-half years.

meridian   the path of energy channels in the body.

mesoderm   middle layer of the uterine wall.

message   the thought, feeling or idea being conveyed in communication.

metabolism   the physical and chemical changes that nutrients undergo after their absorption from the gastrointestinal tract; the use of simple sugars, amino acids, and glycerol by the body cells.

microbial flora   microorganisms that live on or within the body and provide a natural immunity against certain infections.

micturition   the act of emptying the bladder; urination, voiding.

midwifery   the care of women and their families throughout the maternity cycle. Its mandate is to provide care for normal versus high-risk pregnancies and for normal newborns.

minimal justice   equals must be treated equally.

minimal responders   small reactions, such as a nod or single word, that signify a person is listening to a speaker.

mode   category or class that has the highest frequency. It is the simplest measure of central tendency.

modular nursing   in this method, the nurse is assigned a group of patients, usually eight to twelve, whose beds or rooms are close together in one geographic area of the nursing unit.

moral distress   term used when a person knows the right thing to do but is unable to do so because of agency constraints.

morbidity   the incidence of illness.

mortality rate   the number of deaths relative to the population.

motivation   the stimulus of interest in carrying out a task.

mourning   the process of incorporating the experience of loss into our everyday lives.

Muezzin   a crier in the Muslim religion who calls the faithful to prayer five times a day.

multi-service agency   the single entry point for people needing long-term care services at home or in the community, or who require care in a nursing home, or a charitable or municipal residential facility for older people. The range of services to be delivered includes visiting nurses, supporting housing, homemaking, friendly visiting, security programs, physiotherapy, nutrition counselling, meal programs and transportation as well as palliative care either at home or in the community.

multisectoral involving collaboration between different sectors, as, for example, actions that involve collaboration between the health care sector and the business, education, justice and law enforcement sectors, such as the passage of mandatory seatbelt legislation.

Muslim one who practises Islam.

mutagenic pertaining to influences causing permanent alterations in the genes.

narcolepsy sudden, irresistible sleep attacks.

narcotics drugs that depress the central nervous system, relieving pain and producing sleep when taken in moderate doses, producing unconsciousness, stupor, coma and possibly death in excessive doses.

narrative charting progress notes are written in simple paragraph form and in chronological order as patient issues are presented; also known as source-oriented medical recording.

national health insurance model (public insurance model) one in which the government is the insuring agency. People pay a predictable sum to government, or a quasi-governmental agency, either through a premium or through taxes, to cover their health care costs.

national health services model model in which health services are provided and organized by the national government of a country.

natural immunity immunity acquired from having had certain diseases.

naturopath practitioner of natural medicine.

naturopathy a health doctrine based on drugless therapy and natural therapeutic and healing techniques.

nausea gastric distress accompanied by an urge to vomit.

nebulizer a device that generates a fine spray (aerosol) that is inhaled deeply into the respiratory tract.

necrotic tissue dead tissue.

negative copers ineffective coping strategies.

negligence the omission to do something which a reasonable person, guided by those considerations which ordinarily regulate the conduct of human affairs, would do, or doing something which a prudent and reasonable person would not do.

nephron the functional unit of the kidney.

neutral thermal environment the relatively narrow range of environmental temperature in which an infant can maintain normal body temperature with the least amount of oxygen consumption.

neutropenia abnormal decrease in neutrophils in the blood.

neutrophil granular leucocyte necessary for phagocytosis and the removal of bacteria and cellular debris.

nightmare frightening dream causing the individual to wake up; occurs during REM sleep.

nociceptor free sensory nerve ending responsible for pain reception.

nocturia the need to get up during the night to void.

nonmaleficence an ethical principle that requires that we do no harm.

nosocomial infections institution-acquired infections.

noxious causing harm or injury.

nuclear family a husband and wife with their own or adopted children, who share a residence, divide their labour, and cooperate economically.

nuclear-dyad family comprised of a couple without children.

nuisances factors in the environment that may endanger health (such as excessive noise, offensive odours, and the like).

null hypothesis a hypothesis which, if rejected, indicates that the reverse is true and the relationship is considered to exist.

nurse manager charge nurse of a nursing unit.

nurse's aides also called nursing attendants, personal care attendants or health care aides, workers in this category are frequently trained on the job, or in a formal course of a few weeks' duration. The nature of the tasks varies from one agency to another.

nursing the actions taken by the nurse on behalf of, or in conjunction with the patient.

nursing audit method of evaluating nursing care through a review of patient records which document the care given.

nursing diagnosis a clinical judgement about individual, family, or community responses to actual or potential health problems/life processes.

nursing health history a primary tool for collecting baseline data which relies on skilful interviewing techniques.

nursing problems patients' problems, which can be helped by nursing action.

nursing process a systematic and logical approach to practice which embodies a series of interrelated steps the nurse takes in planning and giving nursing care.

nutrient a chemical substance found in foods that provides energy for human metabolism and is needed for growth and repair of tissues, synthesis of enzymes and hormones and regulation of body processes.

nutritionist a member of the health team who advises people about good dietary habits, counsels them about nutrition problems and undertakes nutrition education programs for people in the community.

objective data information that can be observed, perceived, or measured through the use of the sense organs or through the use of instruments.

observation the collection of information through the use of the physical senses (sight, sound, touch, smell, and taste).

occlusive dressings self-adhesive dressings used on ulcerated areas, pressure sores, minor burns, abrasions, lacerations and post-operative wounds.

occupational health a field of health concerned with the physical, mental and social well-being of people in relation to work and working environment and people's adjustment to work and the adjustment of work to people.

occupational therapist a member of the health team who is primarily concerned with the restoration of bodily functions through specific tasks or skills, rather than exercises and treatments.

Old Age Security a universal pension program in Canada that provides income security for older people.

olfactory pertaining to the sense of smell.

oliguria decreased production of urine; less than 30 ml per hour.

onset of action the time it takes for a drug to enter the bloodstream and begin its action on the body.

open system a system that exchanges energy, resources and information with its environment.

open wound tissue injury with a break in the skin or mucous membrane.

operational definition definition of a concept such that someone else will measure it in the same way.

ophthalmoscope an instrument used to examine the eyes.

oral airway a curved, plastic device which slides over the tongue to hold it down and forward.

orderlies nursing attendants who assist with the care of patients in hospitals, extended-care facilities, nursing homes and similar establishments.

orientation phase the time it takes for a nurse and patient to get to know each other and begin to trust each other.

orthopnea the inability to breathe except when in a sitting or standing position.

osmolality a measure of the number of osmotically active particles per kilogram of water (mmol/kg).

osmolarity the quantity (concentration) of dissolved substances in a solution.

osmosis the movement of a solvent, such as water, across a selectively permeable membrane from a solution that has a lower solute concentration to one that has a higher solute concentration.

osmotic pressure the force exerted by the nondiffusible particles in a solution which tends to draw water toward it; the amount of pressure required to prevent osmotic movement across a membrane.

otoscope an instrument used to examine the ears.

output energy, information and resources that are released back to the environment.

oxygenation the supply of oxygen to body cells.

pain a subjective experience; an unpleasant sensation resulting from the noxious stimulation of sensory nerve endings.

pain threshold the point at which a stimulus has reached sufficient intensity to activate pain receptors and produce a sensation of pain; the point at which the pain is first felt.

pain tolerance the amount of pain an individual is willing to endure.

palliative care active, compassionate care of the terminally ill at a time when goals of cure or prolongation of life are no longer paramount and when the emphasis of care is on the comfort and quality of life until death.

palpation using touch to detect characteristics of the body.

paralysis loss or impairment of motor or sensory function due to neural or muscular disease.

paraphilia sexual preferences beyond or outside the usual.

paraplegic a person who is paralysed from the waist down.

parasomnias conditions characterized by disruptions of the sleep cycle; somnambulism, enuresis and night terrors.

partial pressure the pressure exerted by a single gas in a mixture, with the pressure directly related to its relative amount to the total pressure of the mixture.

participant observation researcher involvement in the activities of the group.

passive artificial immunity immunity conferred by antibodies passed from the mother to the fetus through the placenta and/or breast milk.

passive ROM range of motion exercise performed by someone else.

pathogen the disease-producing agent of an infection.

pathogenic bacteria microorganisms capable of invading healthy tissue and causing injury to the body.

patient contract a systematic agreement between the patient and the nurse that grants reinforcement to the patient for performing a specific desirable behaviour.

patient record an account of the patient's history, present health status, treatment and response to treatment; a means of communication among health care providers.

patient-controlled analgesia a drug delivery system that permits patients to self-administer small amounts of predetermined doses of narcotic analgesics as they need them.

PCIS (Patient Care Information System) a computerized system that documents patient care; in hospitals known as HIS (Hospital Information System).

peak action (peak effect) the point at which a drug reaches its highest blood level and maximum effect.

pediculosis an infestation of lice.

peer review a method of assessing the quality of care provided by a practitioner through a review of his/her work by a group of peers.

perception the conscious recognition and interpretation of a sensory stimulus.

percussion striking or tapping the body surface to produce sounds that correlate with the type of underlying tissue density.

peripheral vascular resistance the resistance to blood flow primarily caused by friction within the vascular walls.

peristalsis the rhythmic wave-like muscular contractions that move food down the gastrointestinal tract.

peritoneal dialysis a procedure in which waste products and excess water are removed from the body by instilling and later removing a dialyzing fluid into the peritoneal cavity.

person the individual, family, group or community that is the recipient of nursing care.

personal space the amount of room a person prefers to keep between him- or herself and others.

pH the abbreviation for potential hydrogen, a measure of the hydrogen ion concentration in solution.

phagocytosis a process by which certain body cells engulf and destroy microorganisms and cellular debris.

phantom pain pain experienced after the cause of the pain has been removed, as pain in amputated limbs.

pharmacist a member of the health team whose primary area of responsibility is the preparation and dispensing of drugs and other chemical substances used in the detection, prevention and treatment of illness.

pharmacodynamics the study of the mechanisms of drug action and the effects on cellular function.

pharmacokinetics the study of a drug's four basic processes (absorption, distribution, metabolism and excretion).

pharmacology the study of drugs, their actions and their effects on living organisms.

phenomenological research concerned with how people perceive experiences.

physician's assistant (US) member of the health team usually employed by a physician who performs, under the supervision of the physician, many tasks traditionally considered a part of medical practice.

physiological needs include the need for water, for food, for air, for elimination, for rest and sleep, for temperature maintenance, and for the avoidance of pain.

physiotherapist a member of the health team who assists in assessing the patient's functional ability, strength and mobility; carries out therapeutic treatments, particularly those dealing with the musculoskeletal system; and teaches families and individuals exercises and other measures that can contribute to the patient's recovery and rehabilitation.

PIE charting acronym for Problem, Intervention and Evaluation (of nursing care); a problem-oriented approach to charting that eliminates the Care Plan and incorporates it into the daily documentation.

placenta organ that attaches itself to the uterine wall and to the fetus by means of the umbilical cord.

plan of care the written plan of nursing action (interventions) for a patient.

plantar flexion extension of the foot away from the body.

plaque a film of mucous and bacteria on the teeth.

plateau a relatively constant level of a drug in the blood.

policy a decision or an action taken in an organization by which other specific proposals are judged for their acceptability.

polyuria excretion of an excessive amount of urine.

popliteal pulse the pulse located on the inner aspect of the back of the knee.

population participants in a study.

populations at risk a group of people who, because of certain factors, are more likely to develop a disease or condition.

portability one of the five principles on which the Canadian health insurance plan is based. The term is used to mean that residents moving to another province continue to be covered by their home province until eligible for insured services in their new province (maximum 3 months), and that people absent from their home province temporarily will have insured services paid for (a) in another province at the rate set in the province of temporary residence (b) out-of-country at the rate normally paid in the home province.

post-basic education formal educational programs offered by educational institutions for graduate nurses.

posterior tibialis pulse the pulse located on the inner aspect of the ankle.

postural drainage a form of chest physiotherapy that uses positioning to aid in drainage of secretions by the flow of gravity and deep breathing.

potential problem presence of risk factors in a data base without the accompanying defining characteristics of a hypothesized problem.

power hierarchy the actual or potential ability of individual family members to control, influence or change the behaviour of other family members.

pressure ulcers areas from which the skin has sloughed; also known as decubitus ulcers, bedsores or pressure sores.

prevalence the number of instances of a given disease or other condition in a given population at a designated time.

primary intention healing the process of repair to a wound where there is little or no tissue loss.

primary nursing a system of delivering nursing services where the nurse is responsible for planning complete 24-hour care for each patient.

Priory Model a philosophy of restorative care for older people.

prn order a type of standing order that is to be carried out as necessary, as determined by the nurse's judgement and the patient's need.

probability sampling/random sampling measure to ensure that each element in the study population has an equal and independent chance of being selected.

Problem-Oriented Medical Record (POMR) a patient record organized by the patient's problems in which members of the health care team document issues relevant to their discipline.

problem statement/research question outlines the stated purpose and identifies the general problem under study.

problem-solving teaching strategy using problems the student might encounter in practice.

progress notes documentation of patient issues as these are presented.

projection ascribing one's own unacceptable feelings to others.

pronation turning down toward the ground.

prone position lying on the abdomen with the head turned to one side.

proprietary hospital a small hospital, providing specialized mental health or addiction-related services.

proprioceptors sensory nerve endings that provide information about movement and the position of the body in space.

protein a complex organic compound containing carbon, hydrogen, oxygen and nitrogen found in animals and plants.

proximal closer to the point of reference or the point of attachment.

psychomotor domain the domain of learning tasks involving the development of skills.

psychosocial equilibrium a balance in a person's relationships with other people.

puberty the period of sexual maturation in humans when they become functionally capable of reproduction; marked by menarche in females and the production of sperm in males.

public general hospital a non-profit general hospital.

public health inspector (US: "sanitarian") a member of the health team concerned with the elimination or control of "nuisances," ensuring the safety of water, milk, and food supplies, ensuring that garbage and sewage disposal is properly carried out, enforcing public health laws with regard to sanitation, and assisting in control of communicable diseases.

public policy a policy that has been established and legislated by a public body, duly constituted to make policy in the area of concern.

pulmonary function tests a number of tests performed to assess lung function and identify the presence and severity of respiratory disease.

pulse a wave of blood caused by the contracting of the left ventricle of the heart.

pulse pressure the difference between the systolic and diastolic pressure.

pulse rate the number of ventricle contractions per minute.

pulse rhythm the pattern of heart beats.

pulse tension the compressibility of the arterial wall.

pulse volume the size of the pulse wave.

purposive sampling selection of subjects based on the investigator's knowledge of the population under study and the elements of the study.

purulent drainage thick discharge which contains pus; white, yellow, green or pink in colour.

pyelogram a radiological procedure which outlines the renal pelvis, calices, ureters, and urinary bladder by means of a contrast medium.

pyrexia (fever) condition in which the body temperature is above normal.

quadraplegic a person who is paralysed from the neck down.

qualitative studies, usually descriptive in nature, in which knowledge is developed inductively from the data.

quality assurance a program designed to try to ensure that health care provided to patients is consistently of good quality.

quantitative includes experimental and non-experimental studies in which knowledge is derived deductively.

quasi-governmental agency one that is closely related to government and is responsible to it, although it operates autonomously, as, for example in Canada, a Crown Corporation.

Qui Gong the healing art of building up a person's energy.

quota sampling selecting participants by proportional representation of different groups or strata within the total population.

rabbi the spiritual leader in Judaism (a teacher—not a priest).

radial pulse the pulse located in the inner aspect of the wrist on the thumb side where the radial artery passes over the radius.

radiology technologist a member of the health team who carries out diagnostic and therapeutic measures involving the use of radiant energy.

range of motion exercises exercises in which a body part is moved through a range of motion.

rationalization giving socially acceptable reasons to defend one's actions.

reaction formation protesting too much against something for which someone secretly yearns.

reasonable prudence an individual acting with the care that any reasonable person with his or her knowledge, education and experience would take.

receiver the recipient of a message.

recreation specialist a member of the health team concerned with promoting health and physical fitness. Responsibilities include the development of recreation, sports, and physical fitness programs in the community.

refereed journal journal in which articles have been reviewed, assessed for accuracy, scholarliness and scientific merit and accepted for publication by an editorial board of experts.

referred pain pain that may be felt in one region of the body from a stimulus in another.

reflexes automatic responses to stimuli.

reflexology also known as "zone therapy," the study of the reflexes of the foot, which are believed to correspond to specific parts of the body.

registration the listing of an individual's name on the official roster of a governmental or nongovernmental agency.

regression reverting to a form of behaviour that was acceptable at one stage of our development but is no longer considered appropriate.

rehabilitation the restoration of an individual who has been ill to the most complete level of social, physical and mental functioning possible.

reliability the extent to which a measuring device yields the same results wherever the same quantity is measured.

remedial gymnast a member of the health team who specializes in rehabilitation through exercise.

renal anuria the cessation of urine production; urine output of less than 100 ml per day.

repetitive strain injuries a group of disorders caused by sustained, unnatural body postures and repetitive, forceful movements.

reporting the communication of information to another individual or a group of individuals; may be written or oral.

repression unconsciously forgetting that which we do not want to remember.

research concepts elements that are abstract and only measurable indirectly.

research design structure of an investigation, through which answers to research questions are sought.

research-based practice practice which includes three components: (1) the conduct of studies, (2) the dissemination of research findings, and (3) the utilization of research in practice.

respect the recognition of a person's worth and dignity.

respiration the exchange of oxygen and carbon dioxide between the atmosphere and the cells of the body.

respiratory character digressions from normal, effortless breathing.

respiratory depth the amount of air inhaled and exhaled with each breath movement.

respiratory rate the number of breath cycles per minute.

respiratory rhythm the regularity of the inhalation and exhalation cycles.

respiratory technologist a member of the health team who is an expert in diagnostic procedures and therapeutic measures used in the care of patients with respiratory problems.

rest repose or relaxation; implies freedom from emotional tension and physical discomfort.

return demonstration a demonstration performed by the patient in order to learn a skill previously demonstrated by the nurse.

rigor mortis a stiffening of the body after death.

risk the probability that an event will occur, e.g., that an individual will become ill within a stated period of time, or age.

role structure behaviours expected of members in designated positions.

role-play a teaching strategy in which students participate in a situation (real or imaginary) to learn appropriate actions or responses.

rotation turning in a circular motion around a fixed axis.

safety and security needs such fundamental components as adequate shelter from the elements and protection from harmful factors in the environment; includes feeling secure and protected from both real and imagined dangers.

safety to practise confirmation that beginning practitioners have the knowledge and skills necessary to practise their profession competently and without harming the people to whom they render care.

salwar kameze a traditional garment worn by Hindu and Sikh women consisting of a blouse or long tunic over loose trousers.

sample a small portion of a total population which serves to give information about the characteristics of the population sampled.

sanguineous discharge discharge of blood from a wound.

sari a traditional garment worn by Hindu and Sikh women consisting of a length of cotton or silk draped around the body as a skirt.

saturated fatty acid a form of fatty acid in which all carbon atoms are linked to hydrogen ions; it cannot take up any more hydrogen atoms.

scapegoating hostility directed at one particular person or group of people.

screening a preliminary examination or testing to determine whether or not a person might have a particular condition and whether further diagnostic testing is indicated.

scultetus (many-tailed) binder a rectangular piece of cotton with 6 to 12 tails attached to each side; used to provide support to the abdomen or to retain dressings.

seasonal affective disorder (SAD) a depression that affects people at certain seasons of the year, particularly in winter.

sebaceous glands skin glands that secrete oil; located with hair.

secondary intention healing the process of repair to a wound where there is extensive tissue loss.

secretion a product produced by a gland.

selectively permeable membrane a type of membrane that allows some substances to pass through it but not others.

self-actualization the need to attain one's highest potential and achieve one's ambitions in life.

self-efficacy a belief in personal responsibility for one's own behaviour and in one's ability to influence events.

sensorium the part of the consciousness that includes the special sensory-perceptive abilities and the mental awareness of time, place and person.

sensory deficit a lack of or a deficiency in one of the senses.

sensory deprivation a prolonged reduction in exposure to sensory stimuli that may result result from inadequate or monotonous stimuli, poorly functioning sense receptors, an inability to perceive environmental data, physical or social isolation, immobilization or restricted movement or sensory overload.

sensory overload an overabundance of sensory stimulation.

serosanguineous drainage discharge of a combination of serous and sanguineous matter from a wound.

serous discharge discharge of the clear portion of blood, amber in colour, from a wound.

sex biological sexual identity or sexual intercourse.

sexuality the expression of self and the totality of feeling, attitudes, beliefs and behaviours related to being male or female.

shaman medicine man who deals with the spirit world.

shared governance the organization of hospital patient services in which staff nurses have more autonomy and decision-making authority than in the traditional structure. Also called "participatory management."

shiatsu Japanese form of acupressure in which pressure is applied to the body along the meridians (energy lines).

short-term goal expected outcomes that can be met in a relatively short period of time (a week or less).

sickness a status defined by the social actions or roles that an individual assumes when he or she experiences illness or is diagnosed with a disease.

Sikhism an offshoot of Hinduism with a belief in one God and in reincarnation.

simple random sampling selecting a sample using a table of random numbers.

Sims' position a lateral position in which the patient is semi-prone (sometimes called 3/4-prone).

single-parent family a mother or father living with one or more dependent children.

sitz bath a special bath used to cleanse and to provide comfort and warmth to the perineal area.

slander defamation of character through spoken words.

sleep a period of decreased mental alertness and physical activity which is part of the normal daily pattern of living and is necessary for life.

sleep apnea a sleep disorder characterized by repetitive pauses in breathing lasting from 10 seconds to 2 minutes.

sleep deprivation a decrease in the amount, quality, or consistency of sleep.

SOAPIE format method of charting information in which information is organized on a POMR; SOAPIE is an acronym for Subjective data, Objective data,

Assessment, Plan, Interventions and Evaluation.

social climate atmosphere created by interpersonal relationships between people in a group.

social safety net a network of programs to protect people from the crippling effects of unexpected financial, social or health problems as, for example, by ensuring income security for those in need and universal health care.

social worker a member of the health (and social services) team who assists in evaluating the psychosocial situation of the patient and helps people with social problems.

socialization the process by which people learn the beliefs, values and lifeways of a culture.

socioeconomic model an approach to health that recognizes the importance of the relationship between health and the economic and social dimensions of a community.

solo research study conducted by a researcher working independently.

solute a substance that dissolves in a solution.

solvent the fluid (water) in which substances are either dissolved or suspended.

somatic pain pain which originates from the skin, muscles, or joints; it may be superficial or deep.

somatization expression of emotional and psychosocial discomfort through physical symptoms or body language.

somnambulism sleepwalking.

sordes a thick, furry substance which coats the tongue; caused by lack of oral hygiene.

source the sender of a message.

speciality a specifically defined area of clinical and functional nursing

with a narrowed, in-depth focus, necessary for the safe delivery of the full range of services required in that area of nursing.

specificity clarification of the nature of a patient's problems.

sphygmomanometer an instrument used to measure blood pressure consisting of an inflatable cuff, an inflation bulb with a release valve and a mercury manometer or an aneroid pressure gauge.

sputum mucous secretion from the lungs, bronchi and trachea; not saliva.

standard deviation the average distance of the deviations from the mean.

stat order a type of self-terminating order that is to be carried out immediately and only once.

statistics the systematic collection, organization, analysis and interpretation of numerical data.

stertor a snoring sound made when secretions are present in the trachea or large bronchi.

stoma an opening.

storytelling method of teaching using stories that present information, usually to children.

straight abdominal binder a rectangular piece of cotton long enough to encircle the abdomen and overlap at least 5 cm; used to retain abdominal dressings or to apply pressure and support the abdomen.

stratified sampling a random selection made from different subgroups within the population.

street clinics storefront or free clinics developed in the 1960s and 1970s in both Canada and the United States. Set up in poor neighbourhoods, they provide services for people who are reluctant to use the traditional agencies. The clinics offer readily accessible care, usually on a 24-hour free basis in a setting that is as devoid of 'red tape' as possible.

strengths physical and psychosocial capabilities, the cultural and religious values and beliefs, and the spiritual dimensions of persons or families which enable them to cope with the challenges of daily living.

stress the body's response to any demand made upon it.

stress incontinence the excretion of small amounts of urine involuntarily with exertions such as coughing or laughing.

stress response physiological response to stress which is modulated by the emotion a person attaches to the stressor.

stressor any factor that disturbs the organism's equilibrium.

stridor a harsh high-pitched "crowing" sound heard on inspiration caused by a narrowing of the larynx or trachea.

structure the arrangement of the specific parts of a system.

structured interview an interview controlled and directed by the interviewer for the purpose of gathering specific information.

subject in research, a participant in a study.

subjective data in nursing, information reported primarily by the patient or the patient's family or significant other.

sublimation channelling socially unacceptable motives into acceptable forms of behaviour.

subsystems hierarchies in family systems theory; two or more interrelating family members can form subsystems, such as the spousal subsystem, the parent-child subsystem, or the sibling subsystem.

superinfection a new infection superimposed upon a previous infection.

supination turning upward (the opposite of pronation).

supine position lying on the back without a pillow under the head and shoulders.

supporting cue information used to assure the certainty of the patient state when combined with other cues.

suppression deliberately putting something unpleasant out of one's mind.

suppuration the production and exudation of purulent matter or pus.

suprasystem in family systems theory, the physical, social and cultural environment with which the family interacts in order to sustain its life, continuity and growth.

susceptibility the degree of resistance of a host to a pathogen.

sweat glands skin glands that produce sweat.

symbiotic relationship a mutually beneficial relationship.

symptomatic period the stage of infection when signs and symptoms of the infection are present.

synagogue the Hebrew place of worship.

syndrome diagnosis cluster of actual or high-risk nursing diagnoses that are predicted to be present because of a certain event or situation.

synergistic (potentiating) effect the combined action of two drugs which is greater than the intended effect of a single drug.

system two or more connected elements or parts which mutually interact to form an organized whole.

systematic sampling taking every nth member of the population, e.g. every 10th name on a list.

systemic effect the action of a drug on the whole body after it is absorbed and distributed to the tissues.

systolic pressure the force exerted against the arterial wall as the left ventricle contracts.

tachycardia a very high pulse rate (over 100 beats per minute).

tachypnea an abnormal increase in respiratory rate; also called polypnea.

tactile pertaining to the sense of touch.

Tai Chi a form of medication in motion, used both as part of a spiritual quest and as a lifestyle health practice.

T-binder two strips of cotton attached in the shape of a T; used to retain perineal dressings.

temporal pulse the pulse located anterior to the ear at the mandibular joint, where the temporal artery passes over the temporal bone.

tenesmus painful straining in unproductive attempts at defecation.

teratogenic pertaining to influences during pregnancy that result in physical defects to the fetus.

termination phase the stage when the nurse ceases to care for the patient.

testator the individual making a will.

theoretical pluralism in the case of an educational program, the teaching of several nursing models.

theory a supposition, or system of ideas that has been proposed to explain a given happening in the world.

therapeutic effect the desired response of drug action.

therapeutic relationship the relationship between the nurse and a patient that enables the nurse to administer care.

therapeutic touch a non-invasive type of therapy involving the laying on of hands.

thermal injury tissue injury caused by exposure to extreme heat.

thermoregulation the physiological control of body temperature (heat production and heat loss).

thoracentesis the insertion of a needle through the chest wall and into the pleural space for the aspiration of fluid or air.

tort legal wrong committed by one person against the person or property of another.

trade (brand/proprietary) name the manufacturer's copyrighted name for a drug.

transformation the changing of input into meaningful forms that can be used for an organism's survival.

transsexualism also known as gender dysphoria; occurs when gender identity does not match biological gender.

transvestism cross-dressing; dressing like the opposite sex for sexual pleasure or psychological comfort.

triangular binder a triangular piece of cotton with two sides approximately one metre in length; used as a full triangle or folded for a variety of applications; often called a sling.

triglyceride a lipid compound made up of three fatty acids to one glycerol base.

type A personalities (workaholics) people who tend to drive themselves to the brink of exhaustion while ignoring the need for rest and relaxation.

ulnar pulse the pulse located on the opposite side of the wrist to the radial.

umbilical cord cord through which the fetus receives nourishment and oxygenated blood and disposes of wastes.

universality one of the five principles on which the Canadian health insurance plan is based—all insured persons of a province must be entitled to the services provided for by the plan on uniform terms and conditions.

unsaturated fatty acid a form of fatty acid which is capable of absorbing more hydrogen ions.

uremia an excessive amount of urea and other nonprotein waste products of metabolism in the blood.

ureter the tube that carries urine from the kidney to the urinary bladder.

urethra a short, muscular tube which carries the urine from the bladder to its exit point from the body.

urgency the need to void in a hurry.

urinalysis an examination of urine.

urinary bladder a distensible muscular sac which serves as a reservoir for urine.

urinary frequency voiding more often than usual.

urinary incontinence the inability to control urination.

urinary retention the inability to pass urine despite bladder distention.

urostomy an artificial opening or stoma made to divert urine from the kidneys to the abdominal wall.

vaccine a preparation of attenuated or dead microorganisms administered to induce active immunity against infectious diseases.

validate the knowledge base explore how a study relates to and builds on previous research and theory in the field.

validity the extent to which tests measure what they are intended to measure.

values the ideas, attitudes and beliefs about the worth of any entity that bind together the members of a common culture.

variable in research, a quality, characteristic or property of an object, a person, or a situation that can and does change in different circumstances.

vernix a creamy white substance which protects the baby's skin in the womb and eases its passage through the birth canal.

vestibular system a proprioceptive sense, located in the inner ear that conveys information about the position of the body in space; the sense of balance.

villi tiny finger-like projections within the folds of the mucosal surface of the small intestine which serve as sites of absorption of fluids and nutrients.

virulence an organism's ability to cause disease.

visceral pain pain which arises from sources in the abdominal cavity.

visual acuity the ability to see objects or persons clearly.

visual field the entire area an eye sees when it is fixed on a central point.

vital signs temperature, pulse and respirations; also known as cardinal signs.

vomiting the forceful ejection of the stomach's contents.

welfare society a society characterized by a multisectoral approach to the promotion of health, consumer participation in the formulation of health and social policies and partnerships in research and training between business, government, educational institutions and health agencies.

welfare state one which provides a wide range of health and support services for its people, as, for example, unemployment insurance, universal old age pensions, national health insurance.

well-being the personal experience of a feeling of ability, harmony and vitality.

wellness a state of optimal health or optimal functioning.

wellness diagnosis clinical judgement about an individual, family, or community in transition from a specific level of wellness to a higher level of wellness.

wheeze a high pitched "whistling" sound often made on inspiration when the airway is partially obstructed.

will a declaration of an individual's wishes regarding what is to be done with his/her property after death.

working phase the time when the nurse and patient determine and implement a plan of care.

wound irrigation the introduction of a solution called an irrigant into the wound to wash out exudate, drainage and debris so the wound can heal.

Yin Yang flow two opposing but complementary forces which Chinese philosophers believe balance everything in the universe.

Zoroastrianism the oldest monotheistic religion practised today with a highly moral belief system that salvation is the reward for those who follow "good thoughts, good words and good deeds."

zygote fertilized ovum.

Butterfly needle, 657, 658, *658*, 661
Buzzell, Mary, 75–76
Caffeine
    effect on fetus, 1095
    and urinary functioning, 535
Calcium, 470
    carbonate, 627
    deficit, 626–627, 630(t)
        interventions for, 631
    excess, 627
    and osteoporosis, 482
    role in body, 616
    sources of, 615(t)
Calculus, 969
Calgary Family Assessment Model
    (CFAM), 240–244
    branching diagram, 241(f)
Calorie, 470
Campbell, Margaret, 315, 321, 323
Canada
    community orientation of health care
        system, 256
    culture of, 280
    distribution of health care resources,
        296
    drug legislation, 1097
    education of aboriginal people, 300(f)
    health care reform in, 53–57
    immigrants, 281–285
        countries of origin, 283(f), 283(t)
        ethnic origin, 284(t)
        health care workers, 296
        refugees, 282
        20th century, 282
        in urban areas, 285(f)
    language statistics, 286(t), 287(t)
    languages, 286–287
    leprosy in, 984
    national health insurance, 256
    northern nursing, 104, 291, 299
    population statistics, 27, 282(f),
        282–287(t)
    religion, 287
    tuberculosis sanitoria, 984
Canada Evidence Act, 131
Canada Pension Plan (CPP), 45
Canada's Food Guide to Healthy Eating
    (Health and Welfare Canada), 498,
    499–500(f)
    key nutrients, 502(f)
Canada's Health Promotion Survey, 208
Canadian Association of Practical Nurses
    and Nursing Assistants (CAPNA),
    115
Canadian Association of University
    Schools of Nursing (CAUSN), 123
Canadian government
    Indian and Northern Affairs, 299
    Indian and Northern Health Services,
        300
    Medical Services Branch, 300
Canadian Healthy Communities project,
    260
Canadian Heart Association, 20
*Canadian Journal of Nursing Research
    (Nursing Papers),* 141

Canadian Journal of Public Health, 141
Canadian legislation
    Canada Health Act (1984), 46–47, 48,
        49, 107
        criteria for funding, 48
    Constitution Act (1982), 301
    Health Resources Act (1966), 40
    Multiculturalism Act (1988), 281
    Narcotics Control Act (1961), 1097
    Tobacco Control Act (1987), 41
Canadian Motor Vehicle Safety
    Standards, 946
*Canadian Nurse, The/L'infirmière
    Canadienne,* 115, 141
Canadian Nurses Association, 7, 188,
    195, 269, 299
    charting standards, 456
    Jeanne Mance Award, 225, 269
    and Metropolitan School of Nursing, 91
    origins of, 114–115
    and political action, 107
    and research, 144–147
    Standards for Nursing Practice, 324
Canadian Nurses Foundation, Ross
    Award for Leadership, 269
Canadian Pharmaceutical Association
    *Compendium of Pharmaceuticals and
    Specialties* (CPS), 1099
Canadian Public Health Association, 205
Canadian Red Cross, 693
Canadian Registered Psychiatric Nurses
    Association (CRPNA), 115
Canadian Safety Standards, 946
Canadian Student Nurses
    Association/L'Association des
    Étudiant(e)s Infirmiers et Infirmières
    du Canada (CSNA/AEIC), 115
Canadian Translators and Interpreters
    Council, 426
Cancer, cause of death, 31, 1240
Canes, 924–925
Cannon, Walter, 196
CAPNA. *See* Canadian Association of
    Practical Nurses and Nursing
    Assistants
Carbohydrate metabolism, 496
Carbohydrates, 466–467
    chemical digestion of, 465
    digestion and metabolism, 468(f)
Carbolic acid, 984
Carbon arc lamp, 788
Carbon dioxide, transport in
    oxygenation, 707, 708
Carbonic acid, 640
Carcinogenic, 934
Cardiac output, 385
Cardiopulmonary laboratory tests, 394
Cardiovascular disease
    cause of death, 31, 1240
Cardiovascular system, 704
    and aging, 710
    diseases, 708–709
Care paradigm, 88, 97–98
Care patient system, 318
Care priorities, 347
    for patients with limited mobility, 894

Carminative enema, 590
Carotid pulse, 380
Carpenito, L.J., 729
Carrier (of infection), 995
Case manager, 213
    in community health care, 212
    role of, 216
Case Mix Groups (CMGs), 455
Case study, 432
CAT (computerized axial tomography)
    scan, 393
Catabolism, 466
    and illness, 485
    indication for TPN therapy, 524
Cataplexy, 799
Cathartics, 589
Catheter. *See also* Urinary drainage
    for central venous therapy, 682–683,
        682–683(t)
    condom, 562–564
        procedure for applying, 563
    double-lumen, 546, 547(f)
    epidural, *852*
    Foley tips, 1008
    indwelling, 546, 547(f)
        bladder irrigation, 558
        care of, 554–555
        fluid intake, 554
        procedure for obtaining urine
            sample, 556
        removal, 556, 558
        removal procedure, 557
    insertion procedure
        for female patient, 548–552
        for male patient, 552–554
    over-the-needle, 657, 658, *658*, 661
    and perineal care, 981
    replacement of, 555
    retention, 546
    single-lumen, 546, 547(f)
    straight, 547(f)
    triple-lumen, 546, 547(f)
        closed system bladder irrigation,
            558(f)
    types of, 546–547
Catheterization, 546
    catheter-related sepsis, 1006
    kits, 546
    LCDC and CDC guidelines for, 1001
    risk of urinary tract infection (UTI),
        1001–1002
Catheter-tip syringe, 520
Catholic University of America
    (Washington, D.C.), 195, 225
Cations, 610, 614
Causality, 148
CAUSN. *See* Canadian Association of
    University Schools of Nursing
CBE. *See* Charting by Exception
CDC. *See* Center for Disease Control
    (CDC) (Atlanta, Georgia)
Cecum, *574, 574–575*
Center for Disease Control (CDC)
    (Atlanta, Georgia)
    guidelines
        catheterization, 1001